Sabiston & Spencer Surgery of the Chest

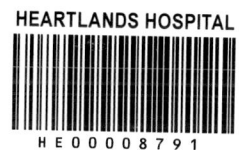

Sabiston & Spencer Surgery of the Chest, Volume II

Seventh Edition

Editor-in-Chief
Frank W. Sellke, M.D.
Johnson and Johnson Professor of Surgery
Harvard Medical School
Chief, Division of Cardiothoracic Surgery
Beth Israel Deaconess Medical Center
Boston, Massachusetts

Editors:
Pedro J. del Nido, M.D.
Professor of Surgery
Harvard Medical School
Chairman, Department of Cardiac Surgery
Children's Hospital Boston
Boston, Massachusetts

Scott J. Swanson, M.D.
Chief, Division of Thoracic Surgery
The Eugene W. Friedman Professor of Surgical Oncology
Mount Sinai School of Medicine
New York, New York

ELSEVIER
SAUNDERS

ELSEVIER
SAUNDERS
An Affiliate of Elsevier

The Curtis Center
Independence Square West
Philadelphia, Pennsylvania 19106-3399

Notice

Surgery is an ever-changing field. Standard safety precautions must be followed, but as new research and clinical experience broaden our knowledge, changes in treatment and drug therapy may become necessary or appropriate. Readers are advised to check the most current product information provided by the manufacturer of each drug to be administered to verify the recommended dose, the method and duration of administration, and contraindications. It is the responsibility of the treating physician, relying on experience and knowledge of the patient, to determine dosages and the best treatment for each individual patient. Neither the Publisher nor the author assumes any liability for any injury and/or damage to persons or property arising from this publication.

The Publisher

Library of Congress Cataloging-in-Publication Data

Sabiston & Spencer surgery of the chest.–7th ed./editor-in-chief, Frank W. Sellke;
editors, Pedro J. Del Nido, Scott J. Swanson.
p. ; cm.
Rev ed. of: Surgery of the chest/[edited by] David C. Sabiston, Jr., Frank C. Spencer.
6th ed. c1995.
Includes bibliographical references and index.
ISBN 0-7216-0092-1 (set)
1. Chest–Surgery. 2. Heart–Surgery. I. Title: Sabiston and Spencer surgery of the chest. II. Title: Surgery of the chest. III. Sellke, Frank W. IV. Del Nido, Pedro J. V. Swanson, Scott J. VI. Sabiston, David C., VII. Spencer, Frank Cole. VIII. Surgery of the chest.
[DNLM: 1. Thoracic Surgical Procedures–methods. WF 980 S116 2005]
RD536.S236 2005
617.5′4059–dc22

2004059212

£175.33

Publisher: Anne Lenehan
Editorial Assistant: Vera Ginsbergs

Printed in the United States of America.

Last digit is the print number: 9 8 7 6 5 4 3 2

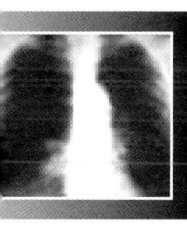

Dedication

This book is dedicated to my loving wife, Amy, who gives me unwavering support, inspiration, and love in all of my endeavors, and our children, Michelle, Eric, Nick, and Amanda. They provide us with limitless pleasure and humor and give us our purpose in life.

Frank W. Sellke

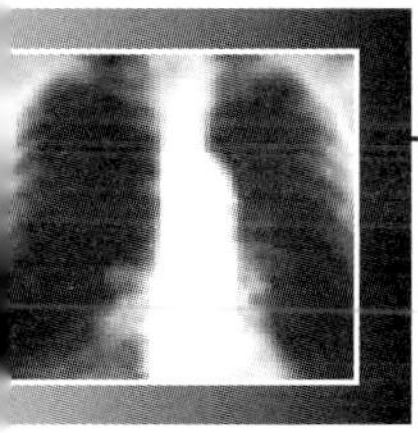

Contributors

Brian G. Abbott, M.D.
Assistant Professor of Medicine (Cardiology); Associate Director, Cardiology Fellowship Training Program, Yale University School of Medicine, Section of Cardiovascular Medicine; Chief, Cardiology Clinics, Veterans Administration Connecticut Healthcare System, West Haven, Connecticut
Nuclear Cardiology and Positron Emission Tomography in the Assessment of Patients with Cardiovascular Disease

David H. Adams, M.D.
Marie-Josée and Henry R. Kravis Professor, Department of Cardiothoracic Surgery, Mount Sinai School of Medicine; Chairman, Department of Cardiothoracic Surgery, Mount Sinai Medical Center, New York, New York
Acquired Disease of the Mitral Valve; Ischemic Mitral Regurgitation

Arvind K. Agnihotri, M.D.
Assistant Professor of Surgery, Department of Cardiac Surgery, Harvard Medical School; Attending Surgeon, Department of Cardiac Surgery, Massachusetts General Hospital, Boston, Massachusetts
Postinfarction Ventricular Septal Defect

Lishan Aklog, M.D.
Associate Chief, Cardiac Surgery, Department of Cardiothoracic Surgery, Mount Sinai Medical Center, New York, New York
Acquired Disease of the Mitral Valve; Ischemic Mitral Regurgitation

Mark S. Allen, M.D.
Professor of Surgery; Chair, Division of General Thoracic Surgery, Mayo School of Medicine, Rochester, Minnesota
Chest Wall Reconstruction

Nikki Allmendinger, M.D.
Surgical Research Fellow, Department of Surgery, Harvard University; Surgical Research Fellow, Department of Surgery, Children's Hospital Boston, Boston, Massachusetts
Congenital Diaphragmatic Hernia

Nasser Altorki, M.D.
Professor of Cardiothoracic Surgery, Department of Cardiothoracic Surgery, Weill Medical College of Cornell University, New York, New York
Screening for Lung Cancer

Robert H. Anderson, B.Sc., M.D., F.R.C.Path.
Joseph Levy Professor of Paediatric Cardiac Morphology, Cardiac Unit, Institute of Child Health, University College; Great Ormond Street Hospital for Children National Health Service Trust, Cardiac Services, London, United Kingdom
Surgical Anatomy of the Heart

David A. Ashburn, M.D.
Research Fellow, Congenital Heart Surgeons Society Data Center and Division of Cardiovascular Surgery, Hospital for Sick Children, Toronto, Ontario, Canada; Senior Administrative Resident in Surgery, Department of Surgery, Wake Forest University School of Medicine, Winston-Salem, North Carolina
Adult Congenital Cardiac Surgery

Simon K. Ashiku, M.D.
Instructor in Surgery, Department of Surgery, Harvard Medical School; Division of Cardiothoracic Surgery, Beth Israel Deaconess Medical Center, Boston, Massachusetts
Tracheal Lesions

Louis I. Astra, M.D.
Fellow, Department of Cardiothoracic Surgery, Ohio State University Medical Center, Columbus, Ohio
Surgical Treatment of Cardiac Arrhythmias

Erle H. Austin, III, M.D.
Professor of Surgery, Department of Surgery, University of Louisville; Chief, Department of Pediatric Cardiac Surgery, Kosair Children's Hospital, Louisville, Kentucky
Pulmonary Atresia with Intact Ventricular Septum

Eric H. Awtry, M.D., F.A.C.C.
Assistant Professor of Medicine, Boston University School of Medicine; Director, Education, Division of Cardiology, Boston Medical Center, Boston, Massachusetts
The Pharmacological Management of Heart Failure

Leon Axel, Ph.D., M.D.
Professor of Cardiac Imaging; Director, Cardiac Imaging, Department of Radiology, New York University School of Medicine, New York, New York
Ventricular Mechanics

Emile A. Bacha, M.D.
Assistant Professor of Surgery and Pediatrics; Director, Pediatric Cardiac Surgery, Department of Cardiothoracic Surgery, The University of Chicago Children's Hospital, Chicago, Illinois
Ventricular Septal Defect and Double-Outlet Right Ventricle

Carl Lewis Backer, M.D.
Professor of Surgery, Department of Surgery, Northwestern University Feinberg School of Medicine; A.C. Buehler Professor of Surgery, Division of Cardiovascular–Thoracic Surgery, Children's Memorial Hospital, Chicago, Illinois
Congenital Tracheal Disease; Surgery for Arrhythmias and Pacemakers in Children

Donald S. Baim, M.D.
Professor of Medicine, Harvard Medical School; Director, Center for Integration of Medicine and Innovative Technology, Brigham and Women's Hospital, Boston, Massachusetts
Nonatherosclerotic Coronary Heart Disease

Leora B. Balsam, M.D.
Research Fellow and Resident in Surgery, Department of Cardiothoracic Surgery, Stanford University School of Medicine; Stanford, California
Heart Transplantation

Michael K. Banbury, M.D.
Cardiothoracic Surgeon, Department of Cardiothoracic Surgery, The Cleveland Clinic Foundation Cleveland, Ohio
Acquired Aortic Valve Disease

Hendrick B. Barner, M.D.
Clinical Professor of Surgery, Department of Surgery, Washington University School of Medicine; Staff Surgeon, Department of Surgery, Forest Part Hospital, St. Louis, Missouri
Bypass Conduit Options

David J. Barron, M.D., M.R.C.P. (U.K.), F.R.C.S.(C.T.)
Consultant Cardiac Surgeon, Birmingham Children's Hospital, Birmingham, United Kingdom
Surgery for Congenitally Corrected Transposition of the Great Arteries

Céline Liu Bauwens, M.A.Sc.
Postdoctoral Student, Institute of Biomaterials and Biomedical Engineering, Department of Chemical Engineering and Applied Chemistry, University of Toronto, Toronto, Ontario, Canada
Tissue Regeneration

David P. Bichell, M.D.
Director, Department of Cardiovascular Surgery; Director, Children's Heart Institute; Children's Hospital and Health Center, San Diego, California
Atrial Septal Defect and Cor Triatriatum

Edward L. Bove, M.D.
Professor of Cardiac Surgery; Head, Section of Cardiac Surgery, Department of Surgery, University of Michigan, Ann Arbor, Michigan
Truncus Arteriosus and Aortopulmonary Window

William J. Brawn, F.R.C.S., F.R.C.T.
Cardiac Surgeon, Birmingham Children's Hospital, Birmingham, United Kingdom
Surgery for Congenitally Corrected Transposition of the Great Arteries

Christian P. Brizard, M.D.
Director, Cardiac Surgery Unit, Royal Children's Hospital, Melbourne, Victoria, Australia
Congenital Anomalies of the Mitral Valve

Malcolm V. Brock, M.D.
Assistant Professor of Surgery, Department of Surgery, Johns Hopkins University School of Medicine; Johns Hopkins Hospital, Baltimore, Maryland
Thoracic Trauma

Kelli R. Brooks, M.D.
Resident, Department of Surgery, Duke University Medical Center, Durham, North Carolina
Combined Modality Therapy for Esophageal Cancer

Redmond P. Burke, M.D.
Chief Cardiac Surgeon, Department of Cardiac Surgery, Miami Children's Hospital, Miami, Florida
Patent Ductus Arteriosus and Vascular Rings

Harold M. Burkhart, M.D.
Assistant Professor of Cardiothoracic Surgery, Department of Cardiothoracic Surgery, University of Iowa Hospitals and Clinics, Iowa City, Iowa
Congenital Lung Diseases

Whitney M. Burrows, M.D.
Assistant Professor of Surgery, Division of Thoracic Surgery, Department of Surgery, University of Maryland, Baltimore, Maryland
Staging Techniques for Carcinoma of the Esophagus

Christopher A. Caldarone, M.D.
Associate Professor of Cardiovascular Surgery, Department of Cardiovascular Surgery, The University of Toronto; Staff Surgeon, Department of Cardiovascular Surgery, The Hospital for Sick Children; Associate Scientist, Reseach Institute, The Hospital for Sick Children, Toronto, Ontario, Canada
Surgical Considerations in Pulmonary Vein Anomalies

Robert M. Califf, M.D.
Associate Vice Chancellor for Clinical Research, Director, Duke Clinical Research Institute; Professor of Medicine, Department of Medicine, Division of Cardiology, Duke University Medical Center, Durham, North Carolina
Medical Management of Acute Coronary Syndromes

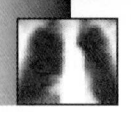

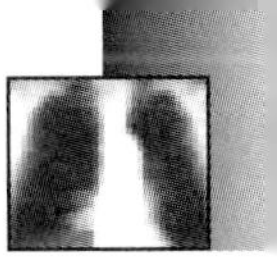

David N. Campbell, M.D.
Professor of Surgery, Department of Surgery, Section of Cardiovascular Surgery, University of Colorado Health Sciences Center; Surgical Director, Pediatric Cardiac Transplantation, The Children's Hospital, Denver, Colorado
Thrombosis and Thromboembolism of Prosthetic Cardiac Valves and Extracardiac Prostheses

Justine M. Carr, M.D.
Assistant Professor of Surgery, Department of Surgery, Harvard Medical School; Director, Clinical Resource Management, Department of Health Care Quality, Beth Israel Deaconess Medical Center, Boston, Massachusetts
Clinical Quality and Cardiac Surgery

Joseph P. Carrozza, Jr., M.D.
Associate Professor of Medicine, Harvard Medical School; Chief, Section of Interventional Cardiology, Beth Israel Deaconess Medical Center, Boston, Massachusetts
Interventional Cardiology

Robert J. Cerfolio, M.D.
Chief, Thoracic Surgery; Associate Professor of Surgery, Department of Surgery, University of Alabama at Birmingham; Chief, Thoracic Surgery, Birmingham Veterans Administration Hospital, Birmingham, Alabama
Benign Lesions of the Lung

A. Alfred Chahine, M.D.
Assistant Professor of Surgery and Pediatrics, Department of Surgery and Pediatrics, The George Washington University School of Medicine; Chief, Department of Pediatric Surgery, Georgetown University Medical Center; Attending Surgeon, Department of Pediatric Surgery, Children's National Medical Center, Washington, D.C.
Surgery for Congenital Lesions of the Esophagus

Dharmender Chandhok, M.B.B.S.
Assistant Professor of Anesthesia and Critical Care; Director, Cardiac Anesthesia and Perioperative Echocardiography; Director, Ancillary Service; Assistant Clinical Director, Department of Anesthesia and Critical Care, St. Louis University Hospital, St. Louis, Missouri
Adult Cardiac Anesthesia

W. Randolph Chitwood, Jr., M.D.
Professor of Surgery; Chairman, Department of Surgery, East Carolina University, Brody School of Medicine, Greenville, North Carolina
Robotic and Novel Visualization Systems

Neil A. Christie, M.D., F.R.C.S.(C.)
Assistant Professor of Surgery, University of Pittsburgh; Attending Surgeon, Division of Thoracic and Foregut Surgery, University of Pittsburgh Medical Center, Pittsburgh, Pennsylvania
Innovative Therapy and Technology

Andrew D. Cochrane, M.B.B.S., F.R.A.C.S., F.R.C.S.(C.Th.), M.P.H.
Consultant Cardiac Surgeon, Department of Pediatric Cardiac Surgery, Royal Children's Hospital; Consultant Cardiac Surgeon, Department of Cardiothoracic Surgery, Monash Medical Centre; Cardiothoracic Surgeon, Heart and Lung Transplant Service, Alfred Hospital, Melbourne, Victoria, Australia
Surgery for Congenital Anomalies of the Coronary Arteries

Herbert E. Cohn, M.D.
Anthony E. Narducci Professor of Surgery; Interim Chairman, Department of Surgery, Thomas Jefferson University, Philadelphia, Pennsylvania
Secondary Lung Tumors

William E. Cohn, M.D.
Associate Professor of Surgery, Department of Surgery, Transplant and Assist Devices, Baylor College of Medicine; Direct, Minimally Invasive Surgical Technology, Department of Transplant, Texas Heart Institute at St. Luke's Episcopal Hospital, Houston, Texas
Alternative Approaches to Surgical Coronary Artery Bypass Grafting

Yolonda L. Colson, M.D., Ph.D.
Assistant Professor of Surgery; Assistant Professor of Medicine; Thoracic Surgeon, Department of Surgery, Brigham and Women's Hospital; Thoracic Surgeon, Department of Thoracic Oncology, Dana-Farber Cancer Institute, Boston, Massachusetts
Interstitial Lung Diseases

Wilson S. Colucci, M.D., F.A.C.C., F.A.H.A.
Thomas J. Ryan Professor of Medicine; Director, Myocardial Biology Unit, Boston University School of Medicine; Chief, Cardiovascular Medicine Section, Boston University Medical Center, Boston, Massachusetts
The Pharmacological Management of Heart Failure

Andrew C. Cook, B.Sc., Ph.D.
British Heart Foundation Lecturer, Cardiac Unit, Institute of Child Health, London, United Kingdom
Surgical Anatomy of the Heart

Joel D. Cooper, M.D.
Evarts A. Graham Professor of Surgery; Chief, Division of Cardiothoracic Surgery, Washington University School of Medicine; Barnes-Jewish Hospital, St. Louis, Missouri
Surgery for Emphysema

Robert M. Cortina, M.D.
Attending Thoracic Surgeon, Department of Surgery, New Hanover Regional Medical Center, Wilmington, North Carolina
Chylothorax

Sabine H. Daebritz, M.D.
Professor of Surgery, Department of Cardiac Surgery, Ludwig Maximilians University; Ludwig Maximilians University Hospital Grosshadern, Munich, Germany
Atrioventricular Canal Defects

Thomas A. D'Amico, M.D.
Associate Professor of Surgery, Division of Thoracic Surgery, Department of Surgery; Director, Clinical Oncology, Duke Comprehensive Cancer Center, Duke University Medical Center, Durham, North Carolina
Lung Cancer: Minimally Invasive Approaches

Thomas M. Daniel, M.D.
Professor of Surgery; Section Chief, Department of Thoracic and Cardiovascular Surgery, University of Virginia Health System, Charlottesville, Virginia
Mediastinal Anatomy and Mediastinoscopy

Gordon K. Danielson, M.D.
Professor of Surgery, Division of Thoracic and Cardiovascular Surgery, Mayo Clinic School of Medicine, Rochester, Minnesota
Ebstein's Anomaly

Philippe G. Dartevelle, M.D.
Professor of Thoracic and Vascular Surgery and Heart–Lung Transplantation, Paris Sud University, Paris; Chairman, Department of Thoracic and Vascular Surgery and Heart–Lung Transplantation, Marie Lannelongue Hospital, Le Plessis Robinson, France
Anterior Approach to Pancoast Tumors

Tirone E. David, M.D.
Professor of Surgery, University of Toronto; Chief, Cardiac Surgery, Toronto General Hospital, Toronto, Ontario, Canada
Surgery of the Aortic Root and Ascending Aorta

Jonathan D'Cunha, M.D., Ph.D.
Cardiovascular and Thoracic Surgery Fellow, Department of Surgery, University of Minnesota; Fairview–University Medical Center, Minneapolis, Minnesota
The Use of Genetic Science in Thoracic Disease

Barbara J. Deal, M.D.
M. E. Wodika Professor of Pediatrics, Northwestern University Feinberg School of Medicine; Director, Electrophysiology Services, Department of Cardiology, Children's Memorial Hospital, Chicago, Illinois
Surgery for Arrhythmias and Pacemakers in Children

Joseph A. Dearani, M.D.
Associate Professor of Surgery, Division of Cardiovascular Surgery, Mayo Clinic, Rochester, Minnesota
Ebstein's Anomaly

Daniel T. DeArmond, M.D.
Thoracic Surgery Resident, Department of Cardiothoracic Surgery, University of Iowa Hospitals and Clinics, Iowa City, Iowa
Congenital Lung Diseases

Malcolm M. DeCamp, M.D.
Chief, Section of Thoracic Surgery, Beth Israel Deaconess Medical Center; Associate Professor of Surgery, Harvard Medical School, Boston, Massachusetts
Lung Cancer: Multimodal Therapy

Ralph De La Torre, M.D.
Chief, Section of Cardiac Surgery, Beth Israel Deaconess Medical Center; Instructor in Surgery, Harvard Medical School, Boston, Massachusetts
Occlusive Disease of the Supraaortic Trunk and Management of Simultaneous Surgical Carotid/Coronary Disease; Valve Replacement Therapy: History, Options, and Valve Types

Marc R. de Leval, M.D., F.R.C.S.
Professor of Cardiothoracic Surgery, Cardiothoracic Unit, University of London; Professor of Cardiothoracic Surgery, Cardiothoracic Unit, Great Ormond Street Hospital for Children National Health Service Trust, London, United Kingdom
Management of Single Ventricle and Cavopulmonary Connections

Pedro J. del Nido, M.D.
Professor of Surgery, Harvard Medical School; Chairman, Department of Cardiac Surgery, Children's Hospital Boston, Boston, Massachusetts
Surgical Approaches and Cardiopulmonary Bypass in Pediatric Cardiac Surgery; Atrioventricular Canal Defects; Transposition of the Great Arteries (Complex Forms)

Tom R. DeMeester, M.D.
Chairman, Department of Surgery, Keck School of Medicine, University of Southern California; Chief, Department of Surgery, University of Southern California University Hospital; University of Southern California Los Angeles County Hospital; Norris Cancer Center, Los Angeles, California
Esophageal Anatomy and Function

Philippe Demers, M.D., M.Sc.
Postdoctoral Research Fellow, Department of Cardiovascular Surgery, Stanford University School of Medicine, Stanford, California
Postpneumonectomy Empyema and Bronchopleural Fistula; Type A Aortic Dissection; Type B Aortic Dissection

Todd L. Demmy, M.D.
Associate Professor of Surgery, Department of Surgery, University of Buffalo; Chair, Department of Thoracic Surgery, Department of Surgery, Roswell Park Cancer Institute, Buffalo, New York
Malignant Pleural and Pericardial Effusions

Jean Deslauriers, M.D., F.R.C.S.(C.)
Professor of Surgery, Division of Thoracic Surgery, Laval University, Centre de Pneumologie de l'Hôpital Laval, Sante-Foy, Quebec, Canada
Postpneumonectomy Empyema and Bronchopleural Fistula

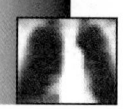

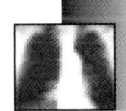

Eric J. Devaney, M.D.
Assistant Professor of Surgery, Department of Cardiac Surgery, University of Michigan, Ann Arbor, Michigan
Truncus Arteriosus and Aortopulmonary Window

Elisabeth U. Dexter, M.D.
Assistant Professor of Thoracic Surgery, Department of Surgery, State University of New York, Upstate Medical University; Chief, Thoracic Surgery, Syracuse Veterans Administration Medical Center, Syracuse, New York
Perioperative Care of Patients Undergoing Thoracic Surgery

Paul L. DiGiorgi, M.D.
Cardiothoracic Surgery Research Fellow, Division of Cardiothoracic Surgery, Columbia University, New York, New York
Left Ventricular Assist Devices

Abdul R. Doughan, M.D.
Internal Medicine Resident, Department of Internal Medicine, Emory University School of Medicine; Emory University Hospital, Atlanta, Georgia
Physiology of the Coronary Circulation

Robert D. Dowling, M.D.
Professor of Surgery, Department of Surgery, University of Louisville; Attending Surgeon, Department of Surgery, Jewish Hospital; Attending Surgeon, Department of Surgery, Norton's Hospital; Attending Surgeon, Department of Surgery, University Hospital, Louisville, Kentucky
Total Artificial Heart

Brian W. Duncan, M.D.
Associate Staff, Department of Pediatric and Congenital Heart Surgery, The Children's Hospital at The Cleveland Clinic, Cleveland, Ohio
Tetralogy of Fallot with Pulmonary Stenosis

Carlos M. G. Duran, M.D., Ph.D.
Professor and Chair, Department of Cardiovascular Sciences, The University of Montana; Cardiovascular and Thoracic Surgeon; President and CEO, The International Heart Institute of Montana, St. Patrick Hospital, Missoula, Montana
Acquired Disease of the Tricuspid Valve

Jeremy J. Erasmus, M.D.
Associate Professor of Radiology, Department of Radiology, University of Texas–Houston; University of Texas M. D. Anderson Cancer Center, Houston, Texas
Imaging the Thorax

Dario O. Fauza, M.D.
Assistant Professor of Surgery, Department of Surgery, Harvard Medical School; Associate, Department of Surgery, Children's Hospital Boston, Boston, Massachusetts
Congenital Diaphragmatic Hernia

Paul W. M. Fedak, M.D., Ph.D.
Clinical and Research Assistant; Professor of Surgery; Toronto General Hospital, University of Toronto, Toronto, Ontario, Canada
Cell Transplantation for Cardiovascular Disease

Hiran C. Fernando, F.R.C.S., F.R.C.S.Ed., F.A.C.S.
Assistant Professor of Surgery; Attending Surgeon, Division of Thoracic and Foregut Surgery, University of Pittsburgh Medical Center; Attending Surgeon, Department of Surgery, Veterans Administration Medical Center, Pittsburgh, Pennsylvania
Endoscopic Therapies for the Airway and the Esophagus; Innovative Therapy and Technology

Farzan Filsoufi, M.D.
Assistant Professor of Surgery; Director, Cardiac Valve Center, Department of Cardiothoracic Surgery, Mount Sinai Medical Center, New York, New York
Acquired Disease of the Mitral Valve; Ischemic Mitral Regurgitation

Mitchell P. Fink, M.D.
Professor and Chair, Department of Critical Care Medicine, University of Pittsburgh School of Medicine; Chairman, Department of Critical Care Medicine, University of Pittsburgh Medical Center Presbyterian Hospital, Pittsburgh, Pennsylvania
Shock and Sepsis

Rosario Freeman, M.D., M.S.
Assistant Professor of Internal Medicine, Division of Cardiology, University of Washington, Seattle, Washington
Diagnostic Echocardiography

Joseph S. Friedberg, M.D., FACS
Chief, Division of Thoracic Surgery, Department of Surgery, University of Pennsylvania Medical Center, Presbyterian, Philadelphia, Pennsylvania
Secondary Lung Tumors

Willard A. Fry, M.D.
Professor Emeritus of Clinical Surgery, Northwestern University Feinberg School of Medicine; Former Chief, Section of Thoracic Surgery, Evanston Northwestern Healthcare, Evanston, Illinois
Spontaneous Pneumothorax

David A. Fullerton, M.D.
Professor of Surgery, University of Colorado Health Sciences Center; Chief, Division of Cardiothoracic Surgery, Denver, Colorado
Prosthetic Valve Endocarditis

Lawrence A. Garcia, M.D., F.A.C.C., F.A.H.A.
Assistant Professor of Medicine, Harvard Medical School; Director, Peripheral Cardiovascular Program and Peripheral Interventions; Director, Interventional Cardiology Fellowship Program, Beth Israel Deaconess Medical Center, Boston, Massachusetts
Coronary Angiography, Valve and Hemodynamic Assessment; Peripheral Angiography and Percutaneous Intervention

J. William Gaynor, M.D.
Associate Professor of Surgery, Department of Surgery, University of Pennsylvania; Associate Professor of Surgery, Department of Cardiac Surgery, The Children's Hospital of Philadelphia, Philadelphia, Pennsylvania
Coarctation of the Aorta, Aortopulmonary Shunts, and Aortopulmonary Collaterals

Tal Geva, M.D.
Associate Professor of Pediatrics, Department of Pediatrics, Harvard Medical School; Senior Associate; Director, Cardiovascular Magnetic Resonance Imaging Program, Department of Cardiology, Children's Hospital Boston, Boston, Massachusetts
Diagnostic Imaging: Echocardiography and Magnetic Resonance Imaging

Sébastien Gilbert, M.D., F.R.C.S.C.
Clinical Instructor, Division of Cardiothoracic Surgery, University of Pittsburgh; Chief Resident, Division of Cardiothoracic Surgery, University of Pittsburgh Medical Center, Pittsburgh, Pennsylvania
Endoscopic Therapies for the Airway and the Esophagus

A. Marc Gillinov, M.D.
Staff Surgeon, Department of Thoracic and Cardiovascular Surgery; Surgical Director, Center for Atrial Fibrillation, The Cleveland Clinic Foundation, Cleveland, Ohio
Tumors of the Heart

Robert J. Ginsberg, M.D., F.R.C.S.C.†
Professor of Surgery, Department of Surgery, University of Toronto, Toronto, Ontario, Canada
Lung Cancer: Surgical Treatment

Donald D. Glower, M.D.
Professor of Surgery; Associate Professor of Biomedical Engineering, Duke University Medical Center, Durham, North Carolina
Pericardium and Constrictive Pericarditis

Sean C. Grondin, M.D., M.P.H., F.R.C.S.C.
Associate Professor of Surgery, Department of Surgery, University of Calgary; Attending Thoracic Surgeon, Department of Thoracic Surgery, Foothills Medical Centre, Calgary, Alberta, Canada
Spontaneous Pneumothorax

Frederick L. Grover, M.D.
Professor and Chairman, Department of Surgery, University of Colorado Health Sciences Center; Surgeon-in-Chief, Department of Surgery, University of Colorado Hospital, Denver, Colorado
Prosthetic Valve Endocarditis; Thrombosis and Thromboembolism of Prosthetic Cardiac Valves and Extracardiac Prostheses

†Deceased.

Kyle J. Gunnerson, M.D.
Chief Fellow, Critical Care Medicine, University of Pittsburgh School of Medicine, Pittsburgh, Pennsylvania
Shock and Sepsis

Constanza J. Gutierrez, M.D.
Associate, Capital Imaging Association, Austin, Texas
Imaging the Thorax

John R. Guyton, M.D.
Associate Professor of Medicine, Department of Medicine; Assistant Professor of Pathology, Duke University Medical Center, Durham, North Carolina
The Coronary Circulation: Dietary and Pharmacological Management of Atherosclerosis

Zane T. Hammoud, M.D.
Assistant Professor of Surgery, Division of Thoracic Surgery, Northwestern University Feinberg School of Medicine; Evanston Northwestern Healthcare, Department of Thoracic Surgery, Evanston, Illinois
Middle Mediastinum

David H. Harpole, Jr., M.D.
Professor of Surgery, Division of Thoracic Surgery; Thoracic Surgeon; Director, Cardiothoracic Surgical Intensive Care Unit, Duke University Medical Center; Chief, Cardiothoracic Surgery, Department of Surgery, Durham Veterans Affairs Medical Center, Durham, North Carolina
Combined Modality Therapy for Esophageal Cancer

David G. Harrison, M.D.
Director, Division of Cardiology, Department of Medicine, Emory University; Professor of Medicine, Department of Cardiology, Emory Hospital and The Emory Clinic; Professor of Medicine, Department of Cardiology, Atlanta Veterans Administration Medical Center, Atlanta, Georgia
Physiology of the Coronary Circulation

Chuong D. Hoang, M.D.
General Surgery Resident, Department of Surgery, University of Minnesota; General Surgery Resident, Department of Surgery, Fairview–University Medical Center, Minneapolis, Minnesota
The Use of Genetic Science in Thoracic Disease

Katherine J. Hoercher, R.N.
Director of Research, Kaufman Center for Heart Failure, The Cleveland Clinic Foundation, Cleveland, Ohio
Left Ventricular Reconstruction and the Surgical Treatment of the Failing Heart

Lauren D. Holinger, M.D.
Head, Division of Otolaryngology and Department of Communicative Disorders; Paul H. Holinger Professor; Professor of Otolaryngology, Head, and Neck Surgery, Northwestern University Feinberg School of Medicine; Head, Division of Pediatric Otolaryngology; Medical Director, Department of Communicative Disorders, Children's Memorial Hospital and Medical Center, Chicago, Illinois
Congenital Tracheal Diseases

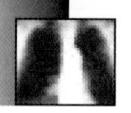

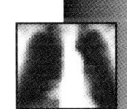

Keith A. Horvath, M.D.
Chief, Cardiothoracic Surgery Branch, National Institutes of Health, Bethesda, Maryland
Transmyocardial Laser Revascularization

Michael T. Jaklitsch, M.D.
Assistant Professor of Surgery, Department of Surgery, Harvard Medical School; Thoracic Surgeon, Division of Thoracic Surgery; Surgical Director, Lung Transplant Program, Brigham and Women's Hospital, Boston, Massachusetts
Surgery of the Diaphragm: A Deductive Approach

Stuart W. Jamieson, M.B., F.R.C.S., F.A.C.S.
Professor of Cardiothoracic Surgery; Head, Department of Cardiothoracic Surgery, University of California, San Diego School of Medicine, San Diego, California
Surgery for Pulmonary Embolism

Doraid Jarrar, M.D.
Chief Resident, Department of Surgery, University of Alabama at Birmingham, Birmingham, Alabama
Benign Lesions of the Lung

David W. Johnstone, M.D.
Associate Professor of Surgery and Oncology, Division of Cardiothoracic Surgery, University of Rochester Medical Center, Rochester, New York
Chylothorax

Mark E. Josephson, M.D.
Professor of Medicine; Chairman, Cardiovascular Division, Beth Israel Deaconess Medical Center, Boston, Massachusetts
Catheter Ablation of Arrhythmias

Lilian P. Joventino, M.D.
Cardiologist; Electrophysiologist, New England Heart Institute, Catholic Medical Center, Manchester, New Hampshire
Cardiac Devices for the Treatment of Bradyarrhythmias and Tachyarrhythmias

Amy L. Juraszek, M.D.
Instructor in Pathology, Department of Pathology, Harvard Medical School; Medical Director, Cardiac Registry, Department of Pathology; Assistant in Cardiology, Department of Cardiology, Children's Hospital Boston, Boston, Massachusetts
Cardiac Embryology and Genetics

Larry R. Kaiser, M.D.
The John Rhea Barton Professor and Chairman, Department of Surgery, University of Pennsylvania; Chief of Surgery, Hospital of the University of Pennsylvania, Philadelphia, Pennsylvania
The Posterior Mediastinum

Steven M. Keller, M.D.
Professor of Cardiothoracic Surgery, Albert Einstein College of Medicine; Chief, Thoracic Surgery, Department of Cardiothoracic Surgery, Montefiore Medical Center, Bronx, New York
Surgical Treatment of Hyperhidrosis

Kemp H. Kernstine, M.D., Ph.D.
Professor and Director, Department of Thoracic Surgery; Director, Lung Cancer Program, City of Hope National Medical Center, Duarte, California
Congenital Lung Diseases

Shaf Keshavjee, M.D., M.Sc., F.R.S.C.S., F.A.C.S.
Professor of Surgery, Department of Surgery, University of Toronto; Head, Division of Thoracic Surgery; Director, Thoracic Surgery Research, Toronto General Hospital, University of Toronto, Toronto, Ontario, Canada
Lung Cancer: Surgical Treatment

Leslie J. Kohman, M.D.
Professor of Surgery, Department of Surgery, State University of New York Upstate Medical University; University Hospital, Syracuse, New York
Perioperative Care of Patients Undergoing Thoracic Surgery

Robert J. Korst, M.D.
Associate Professor of Cardiothoracic Surgery, Department of Cardiothoracic Surgery, Weill Medical College of Cornell University; Attending Cardiothoracic Surgeon, Department of Cardiothoracic Surgery, New York Presbyterian Hospital—Cornell Campus, New York, New York
Screening for Lung Cancer

Peter C. Kouretas, M.D., Ph.D.
Cardiopulmonary Transplant Fellow, Department of Cardiothoracic Surgery, Stanford University, Stanford, California
Heart–Lung Transplantation

Mark J. Krasna, M.D.
Professor of Surgery; Chief, Thoracic Surgery, University of Maryland Medical School; Associate Director, Echocardiography Laboratory, Greenebaum Cancer Center, Baltimore, Maryland
Staging Techniques for Carcinoma of the Esophagus

Judy Krempin, M.S.
Clinical Data Manager, Department of Cardiac Surgery, Beth Israel Deaconess Medical Center, Boston, Massachusetts
Clinical Quality and Cardiac Surgery

John C. Kucharczuk, M.D.
Assistant Professor of Surgery, Section of General Thoracic Surgery, University of Pennsylvania School of Medicine; Chief, Thoracic Surgical Section, Philadelphia Veterans Affairs Administration Medical Center, Philadelphia, Pennsylvania
Anterior Mediastinal Masses

Eugene L. Kukuy, M.D.
Cardiothoracic Surgery Resident, Department of Cardiothoracic Surgery, Weill Medical College of Cornell University; New York Presbyterian Hospital—Cornell Campus, New York, New York
Left Ventricular Assist Devices

Alan P. Kypson, M.D.
Assistant Professor of Surgery, Division of Cardiothoracic Surgery, East Carolina University, Brody School of Medicine, Greenville, North Carolina
Robotic and Novel Visualization Systems

Roger J. Laham, M.D.
Associate Professor of Medicine, Department of Medicine; Director, Angiogenesis Research Center and Basic Angioplasty Research, Department of Cardiology, Beth Israel Deaconess Medical Center, Harvard Medical School, Boston, Massachusetts
Nonatherosclerotic Coronary Heart Disease

Peter Lang, M.D.
Cardioc Catheterization

Christine L. Lau, M.D.
Fellow, Lung Transplantation, Division of Cardiothoracic Surgery, Washington University School of Medicine, St. Louis, Missouri
Lung Transplantation

Peter C. Laussen, M.B.B.S.
Associate Professor of Anaesthesia, Department of Anaesthesia, Harvard Medical School; Director, Cardiac Intensive Care Unit, Department of Cardiology, Children's Hospital Boston, Boston, Massachusetts
Mechanical Circulatory Support; Pediatric Anesthesia and Critical Care

Richard Lee, M.D., M.B.A.
Assistant Professor of Surgery, Department of Surgery, St. Louis University; Active Staff, Department of Cardiothoracic Surgery, St. Louis University Hospital, St. Louis, Missouri
Left Ventricular Reconstruction and the Surgical Treatment of the Failing Heart

Robert B. Lee, M.D., F.A.C.S.
Associate Clinical Professor of Cardiac and Thoracic Surgery, Department of General Surgery, University of Mississippi Medical Center; Chief, Surgery, Central Mississippi Medical Center, Jackson, Mississippi
Empyema Thoracis

Sidney Levitsky, M.D.
David W. and David Cheever Professor of Surgery, Department of Surgery, Division of Cardiothoracic Surgery, Harvard Medical School; Director, Cardiothoracic Surgery, CareGroup; Senior Vice Chairman, Department of Surgery, Beth Israel Deaconess Medical Center, Boston, Massachusetts
Myocardial Protection

Ren-Ke Li, M.D., Ph.D.
Professor of Surgery, Division of Cardiac Surgery, Department of Surgery, University of Toronto; Senior Scientist, Toronto General Research Institute, Toronto General Hospital, Toronto, Ontario, Canada
Cell Transplantation for Cardiovascular Disease

John Liddicoat, M.D., M.B.A.
Assistant Professor of Surgery, Department of Surgery, Harvard Medical School; Division of Cardiothoracic Surgery, Beth Israel Deaconess Medical Center, Boston, Massachusetts
Tumors of the Heart

Chien-Chih Lin, M.D.
Assistant Professor of Surgery, Department of Thoracic Surgery, KaoHsiung Medical University; Assistant Professor of Surgery, Department of Thoracic Surgery, KaoHsiung Medical University Attached Chung-Ho Memorial Teaching Hospital, KaoHsiung, Taiwan
Surgical Treatment of Hyperhidrosis

Philip A. Linden, M.D.
Instructor in Surgery, Harvard Medical School; Staff Surgeon, Division of Thoracic Surgery, Brigham and Women's Hospital, Boston, Massachusetts
Pleural Tumors; Esophageal Resection and Replacement

John C. Lipham, M.D.
Assistant Professor of Surgery, Department of Surgery, Keck School of Medicine; University of Southern California University Hospital; University of Southern California Los Angeles County Hospital; Norris Cancer Center, Los Angeles, California
Esophageal Anatomy and Function

Michael J. Liptay, M.D., F.A.C.S.
Assistant Professor of Surgery, Northwestern University Feinstein School of Medicine; Chief, Division of Cardiothoracic Surgery, Department of Surgery, Evanston Northwestern Healthcare, Evanston, Illinois
Middle Mediastinum

Andrew J. Lodge, M.D.
Assistant Professor of Surgery, Department of Surgery, Duke University Medical Center, Durham, North Carolina
Transposition of the Great Arteries

Gary K. Lofland, M.D.
Professor of Surgery, University of Missouri–Kansas City School of Medicine; Joseph Boon Gregg Chair, Section of Cardiac Surgery, Children's Mercy Hospital, Kansas City, Missouri
Interrupted Aortic Arch

James D. Luketich, M.D.
Associate Professor of Surgery, Department of Thoracic Surgery, University of Pittsburgh; Chief, Division of Thoracic and Foregut Surgery; Department of Thoracic Surgery, University of Pittsburgh Medical Center Health System, Presbyterian University Hospital; Shadyside Hospital; St. Margaret Hospital; Pittsburgh, Pennsylvania
Endoscopic Therapies for the Airway and the Esophagus; Innovative Therapy and Technology

Bruce W. Lytle, M.D.
Staff Surgeon, Department of Cardiovascular Surgery, The Cleveland Clinic Foundation, Cleveland, Ohio
Redo Coronary Artery Bypass Surgery

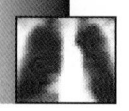

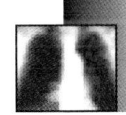

Michael A. Maddaus, M.D.
Professor of Surgery, Department of Surgery, University of Minnesota; Fairview–University Medical Center, Minneapolis, Minnesota
The Use of Genetic Science in Thoracic Disease

Feroze Mahmood, M.D.
Instructor in Anesthesia, Department of Anesthesia and Critical Care, Harvard Medical School; Director, Division of Thoracic Anesthesia, Department of Anesthesia and Critical Care, Beth Israel Deaconess Medical Center, Boston, Massachusetts
Adult Cardiac Anesthesia

Abeel A. Mangi, M.D.
Fellow, Department of Cardiac Surgery, Columbia Presbyterian Medical Center, New York, New York
Postinfarction Ventricular Septal Defect

Warren J. Manning, M.D.
Professor of Medicine and Radiology, Harvard Medical School; Section Chief, Noninvasive Cardiac Imaging, Cardiovascular Division, Beth Israel Deaconess Medical Center, Boston, Massachusetts
Cardiovascular Magnetic Resonance in Cardiovascular Diagnosis

Edith M. Marom, M.D.
Associate Professor of Radiology, Department of Radiology, University of Texas–Houston; University of Texas M. D. Anderson Cancer Center, Houston, Texas
Imaging the Thorax

Audrey C. Marshall, M.D.
Instructor of Pediatrics, Harvard Medical School; Assistant in Cardiology, Department of Cardiology, Children's Hospital Boston, Boston, Massachusetts
Cardiac Catheterization; Catheter-Based Interventions

David P. Mason, M.D.
Assistant Professor of Surgery, Division of Thoracic Surgery, Johns Hopkins University School of Medicine, Baltimore, Maryland
Thoracic Trauma

Douglas J. Mathisen, M.D.
Hermes C. Grillo Professor of Surgery, Harvard Medical School; Chief Emeritus, General Thoracic Surgery Unit, Department of Thoracic Surgery, Massachusetts General Hospital, Boston, Massachusetts
Tracheal Lesions

Constantine Mavroudis, M.D.
Professor of Surgery, Department of Surgery, Northwestern University Feinberg School of Medicine; Willis J. Potts Professor of Surgery, Division of Cardiovascular–Thoracic Surgery, Children's Memorial Hospital, Chicago, Illinois
Congenital Tracheal Disease; Surgery for Arrhythmias and Pacemakers in Children

Patrick M. McCarthy, M.D.
Professor of Surgery, Department of Surgery, Northwestern University Feinberg School of Medicine; Chief, Cardiothoracic Surgery; Co-Director, Northwestern Cardiovascular Institute, Northwestern Medical Faculty Foundation, Inc., Chicago, Illinois
Left Ventricular Reconstruction and the Surgical Treatment of the Failing Heart

James D. McCully, Ph.D.
Associate Professor of Surgery, Department of Surgery, Harvard Medical School, Division of Cardiothoracic Surgery, Beth Israel Deaconess Medical Center, Boston, Massachusetts
Myocardial Protection

Edwin C. McGee, Jr., M.D.
Assistant Professor of Surgery, Department of Surgery, Northwestern University Feinberg School of Medicine; Northwestern Memorial Hospital, Chicago, Illinois
Valve Replacement Therapy: History, Options, and Valve Types

Francis X. McGowan, Jr., M.D.
Professor of Anesthesia, Department of Anesthesia (Pediatrics), Harvard Medical School; Chief, Division of Cardiac Anesthesia, Department of Anesthesiology, Children's Hospital Boston; Director, Anesthesia/Critical Care Medicine Research Laboratory, Children's Hospital Boston, Harvard Medical School, Boston, Massachusetts
Surgical Approaches and Cardiopulmonary Bypass in Pediatric Cardiac Surgery

Roger B.B. Mee, M.B., Ch.B., F.R.A.C.S.
Chairman, Department of Pediatric and Congenital Heart Surgery, The Children's Hospital at The Cleveland Clinic, Cleveland, Ohio
Tetralogy of Fallot with Pulmonary Stenosis

Bryan F. Meyers, M.D.
Associate Professor of Surgery, Department of Surgery, Washington University School of Medicine; Attending Physician, Barnes-Jewish Hospital, St. Louis, Missouri
Surgery for Emphysema

Robert E. Michler, M.D.
John G. and Jeanne B. McCoy Chair, Department of Cardiothoracic Surgery; Associate Director, Davis Heart and Lung Institute, The Ohio State University; Chief, Cardiothoracic Surgery and Transplantation, The Ohio State University Medical Center, Columbus, Ohio
Surgical Treatment of Cardiac Arrhythmias

Carmelo A. Milano, M.D.
Assistant Professor of Surgery, Department of Surgery, Duke University; Director of Surgical Cardiac Transplantation, Department of Surgery, Duke University Medical Center, Durham, North Carolina
Critical Care for the Adult Cardiac Patient

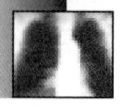

D. Craig Miller, M.D.
Thelma and Henry Doelger Professor of Cardiovascular Surgery, Department of Cardiothoracic Surgery, Stanford University School of Medicine; Medical Staff of Cardiovascular Surgery, Department of Cardiothoracic Surgery, Stanford University Hospitals and Clinics, Stanford, California
Type A Aortic Dissection; Type B Aortic Dissection

John D. Mitchell, M.D.
Chief, Section of General Thoracic Surgery, Division of Cardiothoracic Surgery, University of Colorado Health Sciences Center; University of Colorado Hospital; Consulting Surgeon, National Jewish Medical and Research Center, Denver, Colorado
Infectious Lung Diseases

R. Scott Mitchell, M.D.
Professor, Department of Cardiovascular Surgery, Stanford University School of Medicine, Stanford, California
Endovascular Therapy for the Treatment of Thoracic Aortic Aneurysms and Dissections

Susan D. Moffatt-Bruce, M.D., Ph.D.
Assistant Professor of Surgery, Department of Cardiovascular Surgery, University of British Columbia, Vancouver, British Columbia, Canada
Endovascular Therapy for the Treatment of Thoracic Aortic Aneurysms and Dissections

Bassem N. Mora, M.D.
Instructor in Surgery, Harvard Medical School; Assistant in Cardiac Surgery, Department of Cardiac Surgery, Children's Hospital Boston, Boston, Massachusetts
Atrioventricular Canal Defects

Ivan P. Moskowitz M.D., Ph.D.
Instructor in Pathology, Department of Pathology, Harvard Medical School; Scientific Director, Cardiac Registry, Department of Pathology, Children's Hospital Boston, Boston, Massachusetts
Cardiac Embryology and Genetics

Nabil A. Munfakh, M.D.
Associate Professor of Surgery, Department of Cardiothoracic Surgery, Washington University School of Medicine; Chief, Cardiothoracic Surgery, Christian Hospital, St. Louis, Missouri
Bypass Conduit Options

Sudish C. Murthy, M.D., Ph.D.
Staff Surgeon, Department of Thoracic and Cardiovascular Surgery, The Cleveland Clinic Foundation, Cleveland, Ohio
Lung Cancer: Multimodal Therapy; Surgical Treatment of Benign Esophageal Diseases

Sacha Mussot, M.D.
Fellow, Department of Thoracic and Vascular Surgery and Heart–Lung Transplantation, Paris-Sud University, Paris; Thoracic Surgery Fellow, Department of Thoracic and Vascular Surgery and Heart–Lung Transplantation, Marie-Lannelongue Hospital, Le Plessis Robinson, France
Anterior Approach to Pancoast Tumors

Yoshifumi Naka, M.D., Ph.D.
Herbert Irving Assistant Professor of Surgery, Department of Cardiothoracic Surgery, Columbia University, College of Physicians and Surgeons, New York, New York
Left Ventricular Assist Devices

Siyamek Neragi-Miandoab, M.D.
Division of Thoracic Surgery, Brigham and Women's Hospital, Boston, Massachusetts
Pleural Tumors

Kurt D. Newman, M.D.
Professor of Surgery, Department of Surgery and Pediatrics, George Washington University School of Medicine; Executive Director, Center for Surgical Care, Children's National Medical Center, Washington, D.C.
Surgery for Congenital Lesions of the Esophagus

L. Wiley Nifong, M.D.
Assistant Professor of Cardiothoracic Surgery, Department of Surgery, East Carolina University, Brody School of Medicine; University Health Systems of Eastern Carolina, Greenville, North Carolina
Robotic and Novel Visualization Systems

Chukwumere Nwogu, M.D.
Assistant Professor of Surgery, Department of Surgery, University at Buffalo; Attending, Department of Thoracic Surgery, Roswell Park Cancer Center, Buffalo, New York
Malignant Pleural and Pericardial Effusions

James E. O'Brien, Jr., M.D.
Assistant Professor of Surgery, University of Missouri–Kansas City School of Medicine; Attending Surgeon, Section of Cardiac Surgery, Children's Mercy Hospital, Kansas City, Missouri
Interrupted Aortic Arch

Kirsten C. Odegard, M.D.
Assistant Professor of Medicine, Harvard Medical School; Senior Associate in Anesthesia, Department of Anesthesia, Children's Hospital Boston, Boston, Massachusetts
Pediatric Anesthesia and Critical Care

Richard G. Ohye, M.D.
Assistant Professor of Surgery, Department of Surgery, University of Michigan, Ann Arbor, Michigan
Truncus Arteriosus and Aortopulmonary Window

William C. Oliver, Jr., M.D.
Associate Professor of Anesthesiology, Department of Anesthesiology, Mayo Clinic College of Medicine, Rochester, Minnesota
Blood Coagulation, Transfusion, and Conservation

Mark Onaitis, M.D.
Resident, Thoracic Surgery, Department of Surgery, Duke University Medical Center, Durham, North Carolina
Lung Cancer: Minimally Invasive Approaches

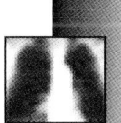

Catherine M. Otto, M.D.
Professor of Medicine; Director, Cardiology Fellowship Programs, Division of Cardiology, Department of Medicine, University of Washington; Associate Director, Echocardiography Laboratory; Co-Director, Adult Congenital Heart Disease Clinic, University of Washington Medical Center, Seattle, Washington
Diagnostic Echocardiography

Mehmet C. Oz, M.D., F.A.C.S.
Professor of Surgery, Department of Cardiothoracic Surgery, Columbia University; Director, Cardiovascular Institute; Vice Chairman, Cardiovascular Services, Department of Cardiovascular Surgery, New York Presbyterian Hospital—Columbia University, New York, New York
Left Ventricular Assist Devices

Peter C. Pairolero, M.D.
Chair, Department of Surgery, Mayo Clinic College of Medicine, Rochester, Minnesota
Chest Wall Tumors

Bernard J. Park, M.D.
Clinical Assistant Surgeon, Thoracic Service, Department of Surgery, Memorial Sloan-Kettering Cancer Center; Cornell University Medical College, New York, New York
Lung Cancer Workup and Staging

Kyung W. Park, M.D.
Associate Professor of Anesthesia, Department of Anesthesia, Harvard Medical School; Department of Anesthesia, Critical Care, and Pain Medicine, Beth Israel Deaconess Medical Center, Boston, Massachusetts
Adult Cardiac Anesthesia

Amit N. Patel
Department of Surgery, University of Texas Southwestern Medical School, Dallas, Texas
Thoracic Outlet Syndrome and Dorsal Sympathectomy

G. Alexander Patterson, M.D.
Joseph C. Bancroft Professor of Surgery; Chief, General Thoracic Surgery, Division of Cardiothoracic Surgery, Washington University School of Medicine, St. Louis, Missouri
Lung Transplantation

Edward F. Patz, Jr., M.D.
James and Alice Chen Professor of Radiology; Professor of Pharmacology and Cancer Biology; Professor of Pathology, Department of Radiology, Duke University Medical Center, Durham, North Carolina
Imaging the Thorax

Subroto Paul, M.D.
Chief Resident, General Surgery, Department of Surgery, Brigham and Women's Hospital, Boston, Massachusetts
Interstitial Lung Diseases

Glenn Pelletier, M.D.
Assistant Professor, Department of Cardiovascular Surgery, Drexel University College of Medicine; Department of Cardiothoracic Surgery, St. Christopher's Hospital for Children, Philadelphia, Pennsylvania
Atrial Septal Defect and Cor Triatriatum

Frank A. Pigula, M.D.
Assistant Professor of Surgery, Department of Surgery, University of Pittsburgh School of Medicine; Director, Department of Pediatric Cardiothoracic Surgery, Children's Hospital of Pittsburgh, Pittsburgh, Pennsylvania
Surgery for Congenital Anomalies of the Aortic Valve and Root; Hypoplastic Left Heart Syndrome

Duane S. Pinto, M.D.
Instructor in Medicine, Harvard Medical School; Co-Director, Cardiology Fellowship Training Program, Division of Cardiology, Interventional Section, Beth Israel Deaconess Medical Center, Boston, Massachusetts
Interventional Cardiology

Marvin Pomerantz, M.D.
Professor of Surgery, Division of Cardiothoracic Surgery, University of Colorado Health Sciences Center; University of Colorado Hospital; Consulting Surgeon, National Jewish Medical and Research Center, Denver, Colorado
Infectious Lung Diseases

Jeffrey L. Port, M.D.
Assistant Professor of Cardiothoracic Surgery, Department of Cardiothoracic Surgery, Weill Medical College of Cornell University; Assistant Attending Cardiothoracic Surgeon, Department of Cardiothoracic Surgery, New York Presbyterian Hospital—Cornell Campus, New York, New York
Screening for Lung Cancer

D. Dean Potter, Jr., M.D.
Research Fellow, Division of Cardiovascular Surgery, Mayo Clinic, Rochester, Minnesota
Blood Coagulation, Transfusion, and Conservation

Harry Rakowski, M.D., F.R.C.P.C., F.A.S.E.
Professor of Medicine, Department of Medicine, University of Toronto; Director, Hypertrophic Cardiomyopathy Clinic, Department of Medicine, Toronto General Hospital, University Health Network, Toronto, Ontario, Canada
Surgical Management of Hypertrophic Cardiomyopathy

Anthony C. Ralph-Edwards, B.Sc., M.D.
Lecturer, Department of Surgery, University of Toronto; Staff Surgeon, Department of Cardiovascular Surgery, Toronto General Hospital, Toronto, Ontario, Canada
Surgical Management of Hypertrophic Cardiomyopathy

Daniel P. Raymond, M.D.
Surgical Resident, Department of Surgery, University of Virginia Health System, Charlottesville, Virginia
Mediastinal Anatomy and Mediastinoscopy

Brian L. Reemtsen, M.D.
Resident, Department of Cardiothoracic Surgery, University of Washington, Seattle, Washington
Endoscopic Diagnosis of Thoracic Disease

John J. Reilly, Jr., M.D.
Associate Professor of Medicine, Department of Medicine, Harvard Medical School; Clinical Director, Pulmonary and Critical Care Medicine, Department of Medicine, Brigham and Women's Hospital, Boston, Massachusetts
Preoperative Assessment of Patients Undergoing Thoracic Surgery

Bruce A. Reitz, M.D.
The Norman E. Shumway Professor, Department of Cardiothoracic Surgery, Stanford University School of Medicine, Stanford, California
Heart–Lung Transplantation

Thomas W. Rice, M.D.
Head, Section of General Thoracic Surgery, The Cleveland Clinic Foundation, Cleveland, Ohio
Lung Cancer: Multimodal Therapy; Surgical Treatment of Benign Esophageal Diseases

John R. Roberts, M.D., M.B.A.
Co-Director, Thoracic Oncology, Department of Thoracic Surgery, Sarah Cannon Cancer Center; Oncology Thoracic Surgeon, Centennial Medical Center, Baptist Hospital, Nashville, Tennessee
Other Primary Tumors of the Lung

Robert C. Robbins, M.D.
Associate Professor of Cardiothoracic Surgery, Department of Cardiothoracic Surgery, Stanford University; Stanford University School of Medicine, Stanford, California
Heart Transplantation

Evelio Rodriguez, M.D.
Cardiothoracic Surgery Fellow, Department of Surgery, Division of Cardiothoracic Surgery, Thomas Jefferson University, Philadelphia, Pennsylvania
Secondary Lung Tumors

Audrey Rosinberg, M.D.
Postdoctoral Fellow, Department of Surgery, Columbia University Medical Center; New York Presbyterian Hospital, New York, New York
Nonatherosclerotic Coronary Heart Disease; Alternative Approaches to Surgical Coronary Artery Bypass Grafting

Stephen J. Roth, M.D., M.P.H.
Associate Professor of Pediatrics, Department of Pediatrics, Stanford University School of Medicine; Director, Cardiovascular Intensive Care Unit, Division of Pediatric Cardiology, Lucile Packard Children's Hospital, Palo Alto, California
Mechanical Circulatory Support in Children

Fraser D. Rubens, M.D., M.Sc., F.R.C.S.(C.)
Associate Professor of Surgery, Department of Cardiac Surgery, University of Ottawa Heart Institute, Ottawa, Ontario, Canada
Cardiopulmonary Bypass: Technique and Pathophysiology

Marc Ruel, M.D., M.P.H.
Cardiac Surgeon; Assistant Professor of Surgery; Director, Cardiac Surgery Laboratory Research, Division of Cardiac Surgery, Cross-Appointed to the Department of Epidemiology, University of Ottawa Heart Institute, Ottawa, Ontario, Canada
Coronary Artery Bypass Grafting; Therapeutic Angiogenesis

Valerie W. Rusch, M.D.
Chief, Thoracic Service, Department of Surgery; William G. Cahan Chair of Surgery, Memorial Sloan-Kettering Cancer Center; Professor of Surgery, Cornell University Medical College, New York, New York
Lung Cancer Workup and Staging

Sacha P. Salzberg, M.D.
Research Fellow, Department of Cardiothoracic Surgery, Mount Sinai Medical Center, New York, New York
Acquired Disease of the Mitral Valve

Hartzell V. Schaff, M.D.
Stuart W. Harrington Professor of Surgery; Chair, Division of Cardiovascular Surgery, Mayo Clinic, Rochester, Minnesota
Blood Coagulation, Transfusion, and Conservation

Jess M. Schultz, M.D.
Senior Resident, Department of Surgery, Oregon Health and Science University, Portland, Oregon
Right Ventricle-to-Pulmonary Artery Conduits

Frank W. Sellke, M.D.
Johnson and Johnson Professor of Surgery, Harvard Medical School; Chief, Division of Cardiothoracic Surgery, Beth Israel Deaconess Medical Center, Boston, Massachusetts
Physiology of the Coronary Circulation; Coronary Artery Bypass Grafting; Therapeutic Angiogenesis

Michael V. Sefton, Sc.D.
University Professor and Director, Institute of Biomaterials and Biomedical Engineering, University of Toronto, Toronto, Ontario, Canada
Tissue Regeneration

Rohit Shahani, M.D.
Chief Resident, Department of Cardiothoracic Surgery, Mount Sinai Medical Center, New York, New York
Anatomy of the Thorax

Robert C. Shamberger, M.D.
Robert E. Gross Professor of Surgery, Department of Surgery, Harvard Medical School; Chief, Department of Surgery, Children's Hospital Boston, Boston, Massachusetts
Congenital Chest Wall Deformities

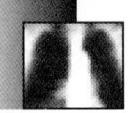

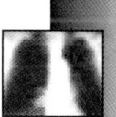

Irving Shen, M.D.
Associate Professor of Surgery, Division of Pediatric Cardiac Surgery, Doernbecher Children's Hospital, Oregon Health and Science University, Portland, Oregon
Right Ventricle-to-Pulmonary Artery Conduits

Joseph B. Shrager, M.D.
Assistant Professor of Surgery, Department of Surgery, University of Pennsylvania School of Medicine; Chief, Section of General Thoracic Surgery, Hospital of the University of Pennsylvania; Director, Department of General Thoracic Surgery, Pennsylvania Hospital, Philadelphia, Pennsylvania
Anterior Mediastinal Masses

Dhruv Singhal, M.D.
Surgery Resident, Department of Surgery, Brigham and Women's Hospital, Boston, Massachusetts
The Posterior Mediastinum

Peter K. Smith, M.D.
Professor and Chief, Department of General Thoracic Surgery, Duke University Medical Center, Durham, North Carolina
Critical Care for the Adult Cardiac Patient

R. John Solaro, Ph.D.
University Professor and Head, Department of Physiology and Biophysics, University of Illinois at Chicago, Chicago, Illinois
Physiology of the Myocardium

Thomas L. Spray, M.D.
Professor of Surgery, Department of Surgery, University of Pennsylvania; Alice Langdon Warner Endowed Chair in Pediatric Cardiothoracic Surgery, Department of Surgery, Children's Hospital of Philadelphia, Philadelphia, Pennsylvania
Transposition of the Great Arteries

William Stanford, M.D.
Professor of Radiology, Department of Radiology, University of Iowa Hospitals and Clinics, Iowa City, Iowa
Applications of Computed Tomography in Cardiovascular Disease

William L. Stanford, Ph.D.
Assistant Professor, Institute of Biomaterials and Biomedical Engineering, University of Toronto; Associate Scientist, Samuel Lunenfeld Research Institute, Mount Sinai Hospital, Toronto, Ontario, Canada
Tissue Regeneration

Michael Straznicka, M.D.
Instructor in Surgery, Department of Thoracic and Cardiovascular Surgery, University of Texas M. D. Anderson Cancer Center, Houston, Texas; Surgeon, Department of Thoracic Surgery, John Muir Medical Center, Walnut Creek, California; Surgeon, Department of Thoracic Surgery, Mount Diablo Medical Center, Concord, California
Lung Cancer: Surgical Strategies for Tumors Invading the Chest Wall

David J. Sugarbaker, M.D.
Richard E. Wilson Professor of Surgical Oncology, Department of Surgery, Harvard Medical School; Chief, Division of Thoracic Surgery, Department of Surgery, Brigham and Women's Hospital, Boston, Massachusetts
Pleural Tumors

Lars G. Svensson, M.D., Ph.D.
Director, Center for Aortic Surgery, Marfan Syndrome, and Connective Tissue Disorder Clinic, The Cleveland Clinic Foundation, Cleveland, Ohio
Surgery of the Aortic Arch; Descending Thoracic and Thoracoabdominal Aortic Surgery

Scott J. Swanson, M.D.
Chief, Division of Cardiothoracic Surgery, Mount Sinai School of Medicine; Eugene W. Friedman Professor of Surgical Oncology, Mount Sinai Hospital, New York, New York
Esophageal Resection and Replacement

Patricia A. Thistlethwaite, M.D., Ph.D.
Associate Professor of Surgery, Division of Cardiothoracic Surgery; Professor and Head, Division of Cardiothoracic Surgery, University of California, San Diego, San Diego, California
Surgery for Pulmonary Embolization

David F. Torchiana, M.D.
Associate Professor of Surgery, Department of Surgery, Harvard Medical School; CEO and Chairman, Massachusetts General Physical Organization, Boston, Massachusetts
Postinfarction Ventricular Septal Defect

Ross M. Ungerleider, M.D.
Professor of Surgery; Chief, Pediatric Cardiac Surgery, Doernbecher Children's Hospital, Oregon Health and Science University, Portland, Oregon
Right Ventricle-to-Pulmonary Artery Conduits

Harold C. Urschel, Jr., M.D., L.L.D.(Hon.), D.S.(Hon.)
Clinical Professor of Cardiovascular and Thoracic Surgery, University of Texas Southwestern Medical School; Chair, Cardiovascular and Thoracic Surgical Research, Education, and Clinical Excellence, Baylor University Medical Center, Dallas, Texas
Thoracic Outlet Syndrome and Dorsal Sympathectomy

Glen S. Van Arsdell, M.D.
Associate Professor of Surgery, Department of Surgery, University of Toronto; Head, Division of Cardiac Surgery, CIT Chair, Cardiovascular Surgery, Department of Surgery, Hospital for Sick Children, Toronto, Ontario, Canada
Pulmonary Atresia and Ventricular Septal Defect; Adult Congenital Cardiac Surgery

Carin van Doorn, M.D. F.R.C.S.(C./Th.)
Senior Lecturer in Cardiothoracic Surgery, Cardiothoracic Unit, Institute of Child Health; Honorary Consultant Cardiothoracic Surgeon, Cardiothoracic Unit, Great Ormond Street Hospital for Children National Health Service Trust, London, United Kingdom
Management of Single Ventricle and Cavopulmonary Connections

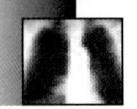

Timothy L. Van Natta, M.D.
Assistant Professor of Surgery, Department of Surgery, University of Iowa Hospitals and Clinics, Iowa City, Iowa
Congenital Lung Diseases

Richard Van Praagh, M.D.
Professor Emeritus of Pathology, Department of Pathology, Harvard Medical School; Director Emeritus, Cardiac Registry, Departments of Pathology, Cardiology, and Cardiac Surgery, Children's Hospital Boston, Boston, Massachusetts
Segmental Anatomy

Jeffrey S. Veluz, M.D.
Chief Resident, Division of Cardiothoracic Surgery, Beth Israel Deaconess Hospital; Harvard Medical School, Boston, Massachusetts
Occlusive Disease of the Supraaortic Trunk and Management of Simultaneous Surgical Carotid/Coronary Disease

Gus J. Vlahakes, M.D.
Professor of Surgery, Department of Surgery, Harvard Medical School; Chief, Division of Cardiac Surgery, Massachusetts General Hospital, Boston, Massachusetts
Valve Replacement Therapy: History, Options, and Valve Types

Garrett L. Walsh, M.D.
Professor of Surgery, Department of Thoracic and Cardiovascular Surgery, University of Texas M. D. Anderson Cancer Center, Houston, Texas
Lung Cancer: Surgical Strategies for Tumors Invading the Chest Wall

Thomas J. Watson, M.D.
Associate Professor of Surgery, Division of Thoracic and Foregut Surgery, University of Rochester School of Medicine and Dentistry; Attending Physician, Strong Memorial Hospital, Rochester, Minnesota
Fibrothorax and Decortication of the Lung

Ronald M. Weintraub, M.D.
David S. Ginsburg Associate Professor of Surgery, Harvard Medical School; Chief Emeritus, Division of Cardiothoracic Surgery, Beth Israel Deaconess Medical Center; Chief, Surgery, Department of Surgery, Cambridge Health Alliance, Boston, Massachusetts
Clinical Quality and Cardiac Surgery

Richard D. Weisel, M.D., F.R.C.S.C.
Professor and Chairman, Division of Cardiac Surgery, University of Toronto; Surgeon, Division of Cardiovascular Surgery, Toronto General Hospital, Toronto, Ontario, Canada
Cell Transplantation for Cardiovascular Disease

Margaret V. Westfall, Ph.D.
Assistant Professor of Surgery, Department of Surgery, University of Michigan, Ann Arbor, Michigan
Physiology of the Myocardium

Daniel C. Wiener, M.D.
Resident, Department of General Surgery, Dartmouth Hitchcock Medical Center, Lebanon, New Hampshire; Research Fellow, Department of Adult Oncology, Dana-Farber Cancer Institute, Boston, Massachusetts
Surgery of the Diaphragm: A Deductive Approach

Dennis A. Wigle M.D., Ph.D.
Resident in Thoracic Surgery, Department of Surgery, University of Toronto, Toronto, Ontario, Canada
Lung Cancer: Surgical Treatment

Ernest D. Wigle, M.D.
Professor Emeritus of Medicine, Department of Medicine, University of Toronto; Staff Physician, Department of Medicine (Cardiology), Toronto General Hospital, Toronto, Ontario, Canada
Surgical Management of Hypertrophic Cardiomyopathy

Benson R. Wilcox, M.D.
Professor of Surgery, Department of Cardiothoracic Surgery, University of North Carolina, Chapel Hill, North Carolina
Surgical Anatomy of the Heart

William G. Williams, M.D., F.R.S.C.(C.)
Cardiac Surgeon, Department of Cardiac Surgery, Toronto General Hospital, Toronto, Ontario, Canada
Surgical Management of Hypertrophic Cardiomyopathy; Adult Congenital Cardiac Surgery

Jay M. Wilson, M.D.
Associate Professor of Surgery, Department of Surgery, Harvard Medical School; Senior Associate in Surgery, Department of Surgery, Children's Hospital Boston, Boston, Massachusetts
Congenital Diaphragmatic Hernia

Douglas E. Wood, M.D.
Professor and Chief, Section of General Thoracic Surgery, University of Washington, Seattle, Washington
Endoscopic Diagnosis of Thoracic Disease

David Wrobleski, M.D.
Staff Electrophysiologist, Department of Cardiology, St. Vincent Hospital, Indianapolis, Indiana
Catheter Ablation of Arrhythmias

Stephen C. Yang, M.D., F.A.C.S., F.C.C.P.
Chief, Thoracic Surgery; Associate Professor of Surgery and Oncology, Department of Surgery, The Johns Hopkins Medical Institutions; Chief, Thoracic Surgery, Department of Surgery, The Johns Hopkins Bayview Medical Center, Baltimore, Maryland
Thoracic Trauma

Susan B. Yeon, M.D., J.D.
Instructor in Medicine, Harvard Medical School; Department of Medicine, Cardiovascular Division, Cardiac Magnetic Resonance Center, Beth Israel Deaconess Medical Center, Boston, Massachusetts
Cardiovascular Magnetic Resonance in Cardiovascular Diagnosis

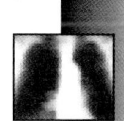

Peter Zandstra, Ph.D.
Associate Professor, Institute of Biomaterials and Biomedical Engineering, University of Toronto; Canada Research Chair in Stem Cell Bioengineering, Toronto, Ontario, Canada
Tissue Regeneration

Barry L. Zaret, M.D.
Robert W. Berliner Professor of Medicine; Chief, Section of Cardiovascular Medicine, Department of Internal Medicine, Yale University School of Medicine, New Haven, Connecticut
Nuclear Cardiology and Positron Emission Tomography in the Assessment of Patients with Cardiovascular Disease

Peter J. Zimetbaum, M.D.
Assistant Professor of Medicine, Harvard Medical School; Director, Clinical Arrhythmia Service, Department of Medicine, Division of Cardiology, Beth Israel Deaconess Medical Center, Boston, Massachusetts
Cardiac Devices for the Treatment of Bradyarrhythmias and Tachyarrhythmias

Preface

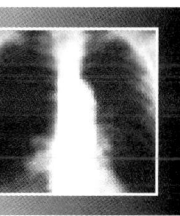

When first asked to be editor of the 7th Edition of *Sabiston and Spencer Surgery of the Chest*, I considered it a great honor and privilege, since this textbook is widely regarded as one of the premier resources in cardiothoracic surgery. Drs. David Sabiston and Frank Spencer have been regarded as leaders in the field of surgery for nearly the past half century. When asking some of my esteemed colleagues if they would be willing to contribute a chapter to this new edition, they almost universally said yes, but in a few cases their initial reply was, "In these days of electronic publishing and web based information gathering, why do we need another printed textbook?" While much information can be obtained from the web, including the contents of most peer-reviewed journals, I believe that the most efficient, authoritative method to obtain clinical information remains reading the textbook. This can be in the traditional hard copy, printed form, or an electronic version. Considering that the sales of cardiothoracic surgery textbooks has not diminished recently, I can say that most of my surgical colleagues would agree with this assertion.

Despite being one of the best regarded textbooks in the field, the other editors and I felt that the next edition should be totally rewritten. This is, in fact, what we did. The format has been reorganized to better reflect the modern practice of cardiothoracic surgery. Virtually all authors contributing chapters in the 7th Edition are new. In fact, none of the authors were given the related chapter from the previous book. The content was changed to reflect recent major changes in adult and pediatric cardiac surgery and general thoracic surgery. Even when a chapter was thought to be acceptable in the previous edition, it was usually reassigned to a new author to revitalize and modernize the book. The content of several previous chapters was eliminated, and many new chapters were added, again reflecting these recent changes in the field. Chapters were included covering most areas of basic science that the editors believed should be in the knowledge base of practicing cardiac and thoracic surgeons. These chapters include those covering coronary physiology, myocardial contractile function, congenital and adult cardiac anatomy, and pulmonary and esophageal physiology. In addition, new chapters that overlap with the surgical treatment of cardiothoracic diseases were added. These chapters include catheter-based treatment of cardiac disease, electrophysiology, cell-based treatment of cardiac disease, and multimodality treatment of thoracic malignancies. Not to lessen the impact or importance of these chapters dealing with "peripheral or supporting information," the chapters dealing with the "heart" of cardiothoracic surgery are certainly the major thrust of the current edition. We are very pleased to have recruited those who we believe to be internationally recognized experts in their respective subspecialties. One of the strengths of this book is that all areas of cardiothoracic surgery are covered in one edition: adult and pediatric cardiac surgery and general thoracic surgery. Almost everything that needs to be known for practice, with the exception of basic operative techniques and clinical judgment, is included. This ranges from basic science to medically-based approaches to cardiac and thoracic disease. As the boundary between the classical medical and surgical treatments of many disorders seems to be disappearing, we feel that it is critical that surgeons are aware of a broad range of treatment options.

As with most textbooks, one of the main jobs of the editors was to hound delinquent authors for their contributions. We hope that these authors will not hold a grudge and apologize if we were too abrupt at times. We hope most will consider contributing to the next edition.

I wish to express my sincere thanks and gratitude to my co-editors, Drs. Pedro del Nido and Scott Swanson. Their knowledge of the field and perseverance made this book the success that it is. Finally, I would like to thank the staff at Elsevier for their unwavering support of this book. Despite some of the not unexpected initial inconveniences, they were always available for the duration of the project and especially when problems occurred, and I cannot thank them enough for all of their hard work. My assistant, Mrs. Susan Lerman, was a tremendous asset with organization and loyalty and provided comic relief, not just in regard to this book.

Frank W. Sellke
Pedro J. del Nido
Scott J. Swanson

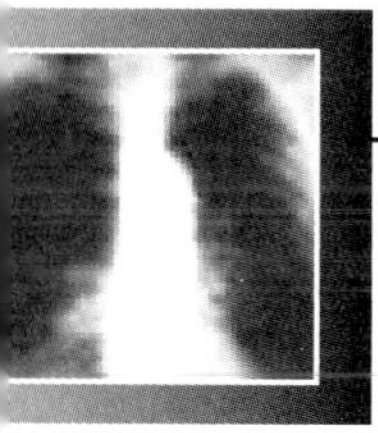

Table of Contents

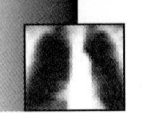

SECTION III

Congenital Heart Surgery

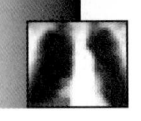

Sabiston & Spencer Surgery of the Chest

Color Plates

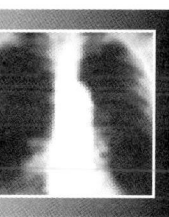

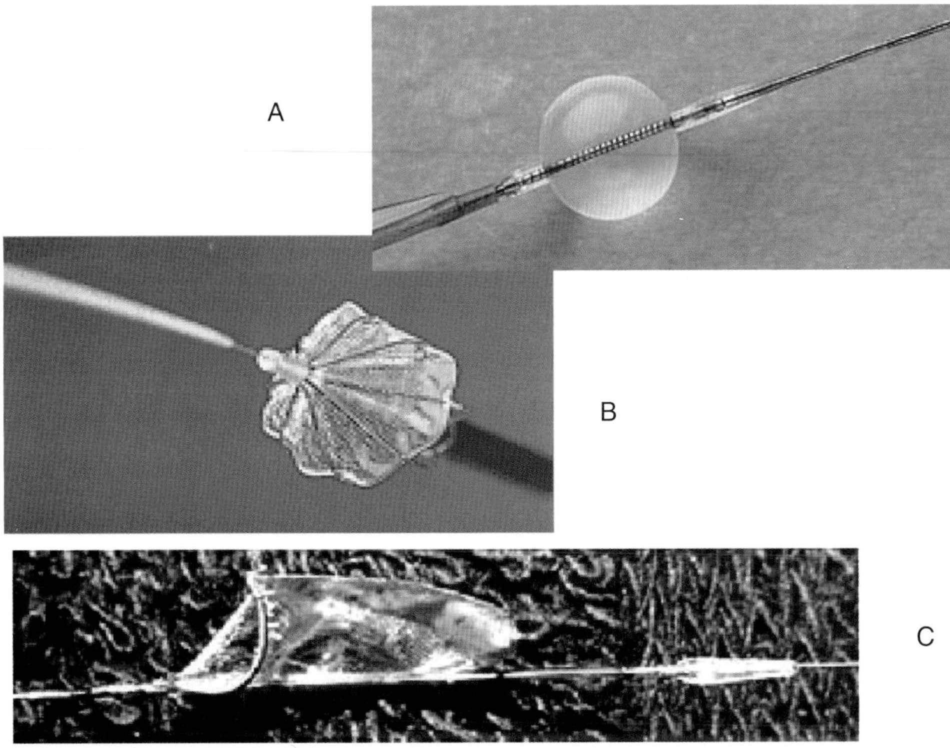

Figure 71B-12 Distal protection devices: GuardWire (PercuSurge, Inc., Sunnyvale, CA) **(A),** Angioguard (Cordis, Warren, NJ) **(B),** and EPI filter **(C)** (EPI, Inc., Boston, MA).

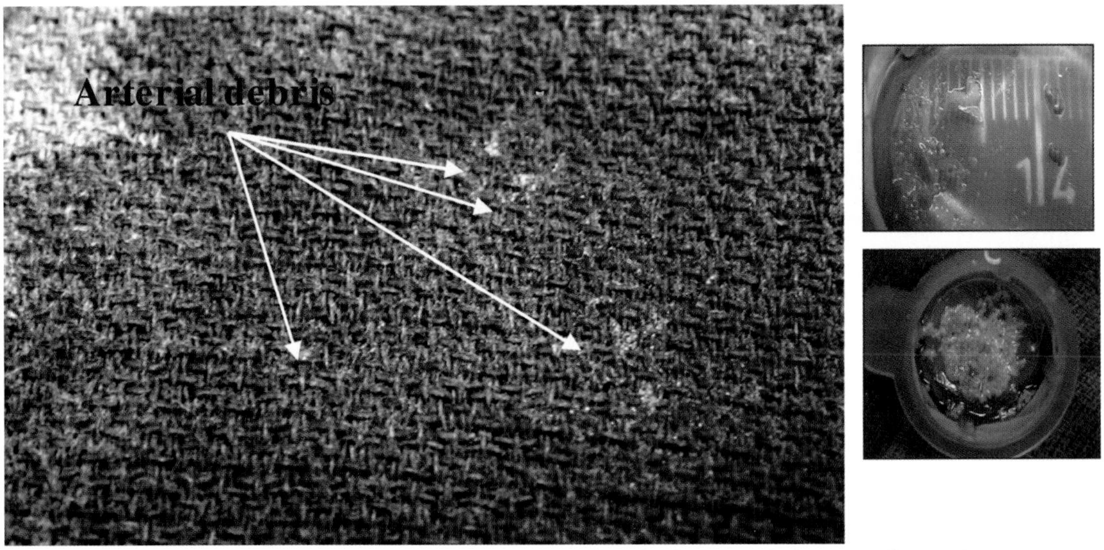

Figure 71B-13 Distal macroscopic emboli captured with the use of the GuardWire (PercuSurge, Inc., Sunnyvale, CA) in an ulcerated left internal carotid lesion following predilatation with angioplasty prior to stenting.

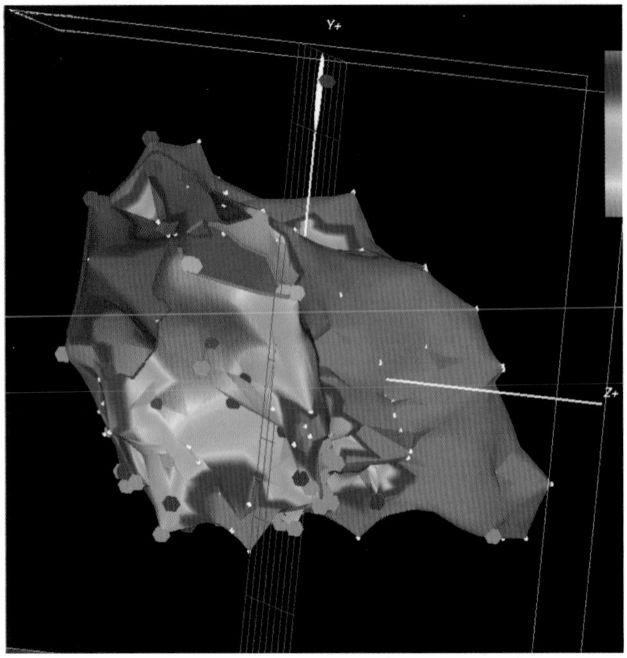

Figure 80-7 Substrate mapping guided ablation of untolerated VT. A voltage map demonstrates low voltage *(scar)* in the center of an old, inferior infarction. Induced unstable VT had morphology that was replicated by pacing the exit site at the border zone. RF lesions from exit site to center of scar abolished VT. (See text.) SP, split potential.
(Reproduced with permission from Josephson, ME: Clinical Cardiac Electrophysiology. Philadelphia: Lippincott Williams & Wilkins, 2002.)

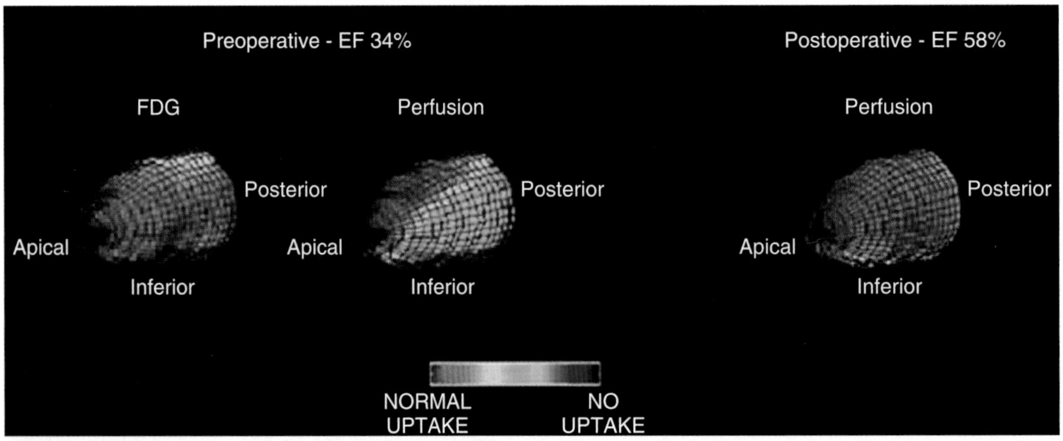

Figure 82-2 Preoperative myocardial viability assessment. This patient with CHF symptoms and inferior wall akinesis was evaluated prior to CABG with ^{18}F–2–deoxyglucose (FDG) positron emission tomography (PET) and perfusion scintigraphy. Depressed ejection fraction (EF), viable myocytes (indicated by the normal FDG uptake), and the presence of a large posteroinferior perfusion defect were identified preoperatively. After CABG the perfusion defect disappeared and the ejection fraction normalized.
(Images courtesy of Robert S. Beanlands, MD, Division of Nuclear Cardiology, University of Ottawa Heart Institute.)

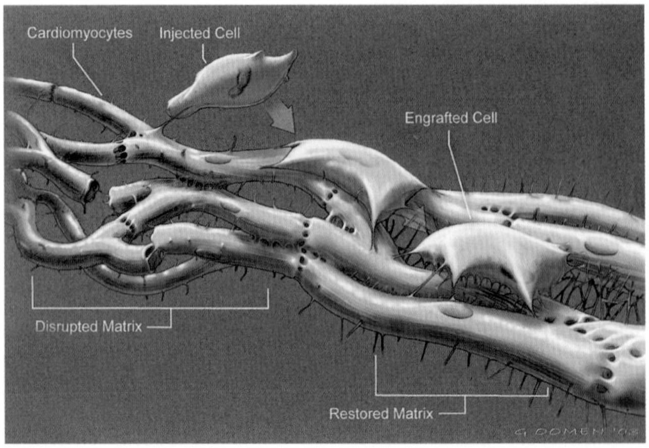

Figure 97-3 Cell engraftment in the failing heart. The interstitial matrix provides the structural support for cardiomyocytes, maintaining ventricular shape and function. The myocardial matrix is disrupted and degraded in the failing heart. The process of cell engraftment may replace and reorganize damaged structural elements after cell transplantation, preventing cardiac dilatation and restoring myocardial function in the failing heart.

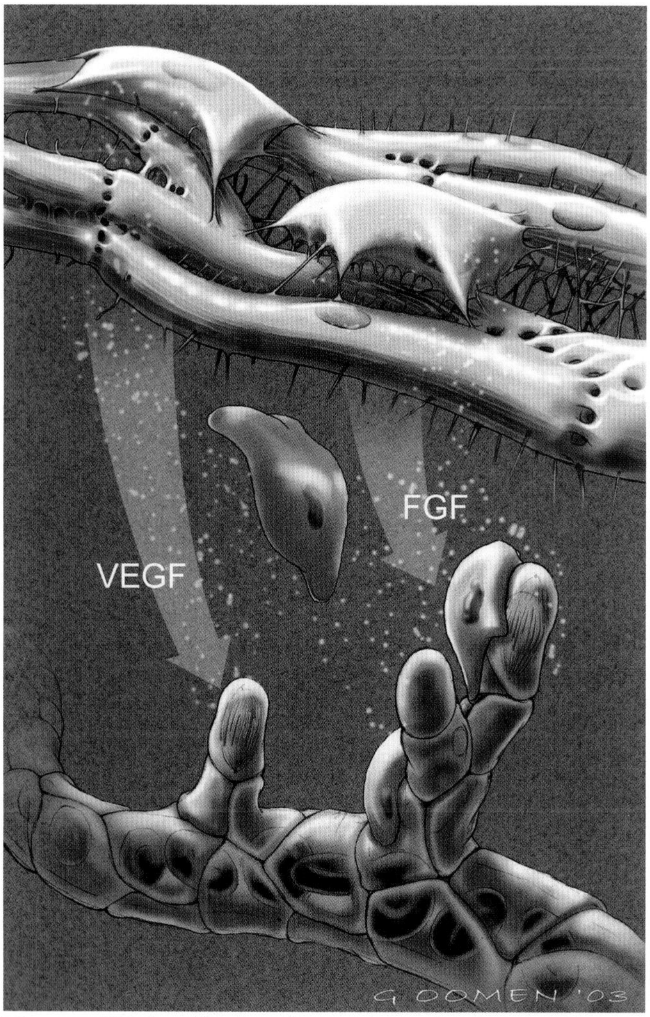

Figure 97-4 Cell transplantation and angiogenesis. Engrafted cells stimulate angiogenesis after transplantation by releasing growth factors and by directly participating in the formation of new vessels.

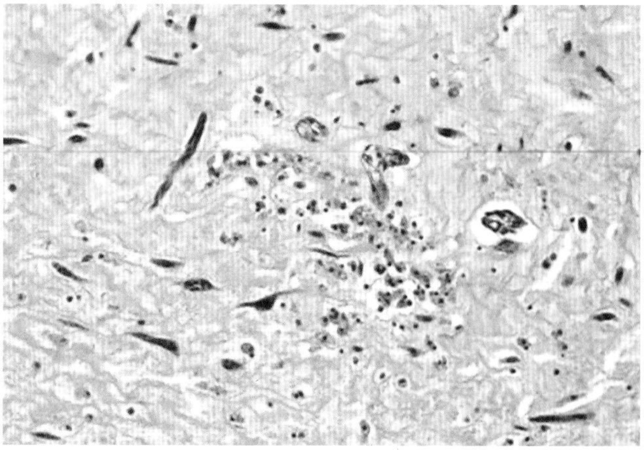

Figure 99-2 Hematoxylin and eosin (H & E) stain of myxoma.

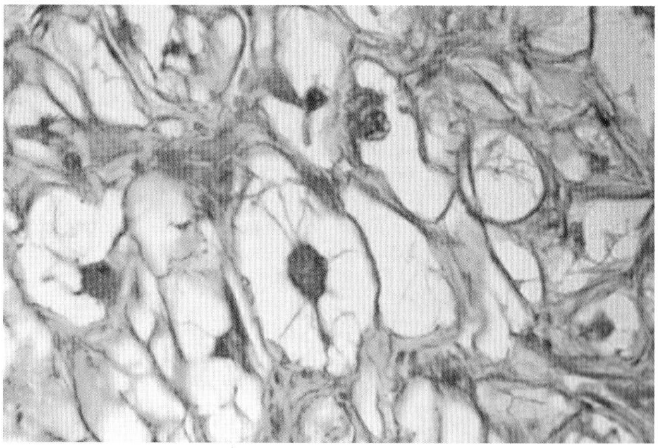

Figure 99-3 Rhabdomyoma spider cell.

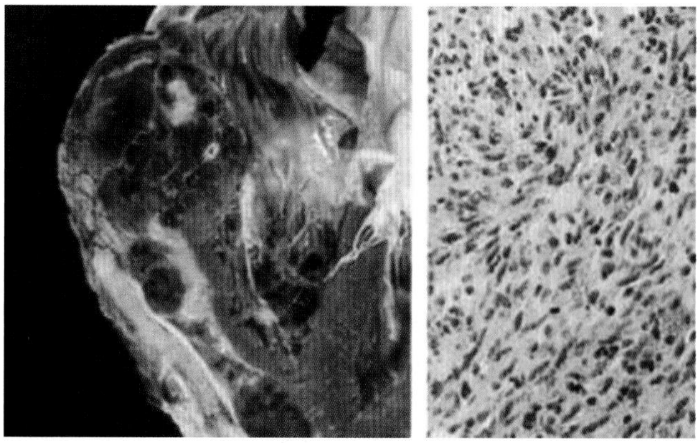

Figure 99-4 Angiosarcoma.

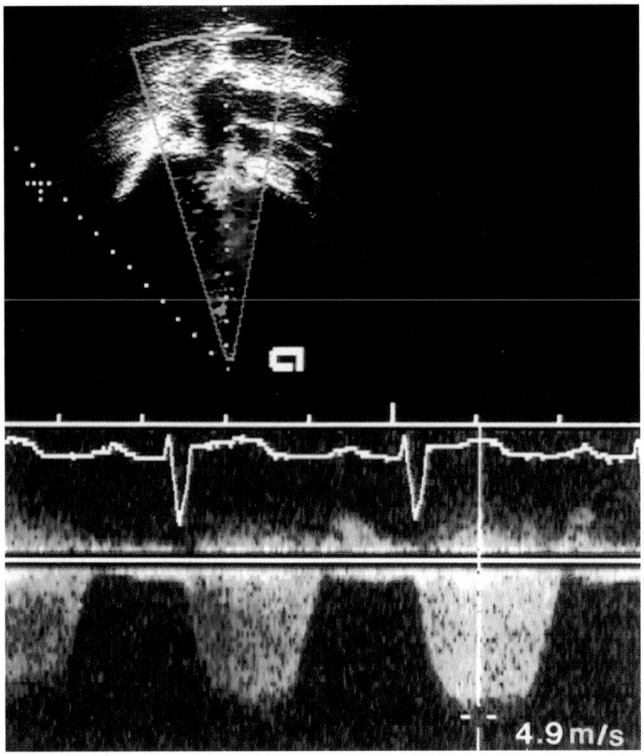

Figure 102-4 Doppler echocardiography. Visualization of a high-velocity jet by color Doppler aids in aligning the continuous wave Doppler cursor in a patient with {S,L,L} transposition of the great arteries with severe subpulmonary stenosis (predicted maximal instantaneous gradient ~96 mm Hg).

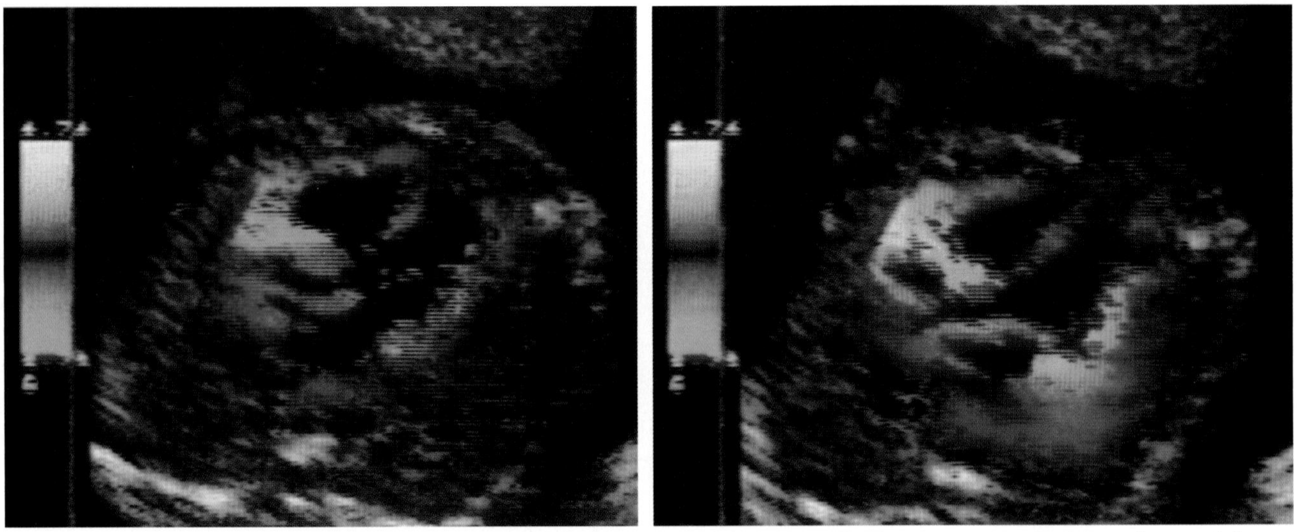

A B

Figure 102-8 Use of tissue Doppler imaging to determine heart rhythm in the fetus. A, Diastolic frame showing left ventricular relaxation. **B,** Systolic frame showing ventricular contraction.

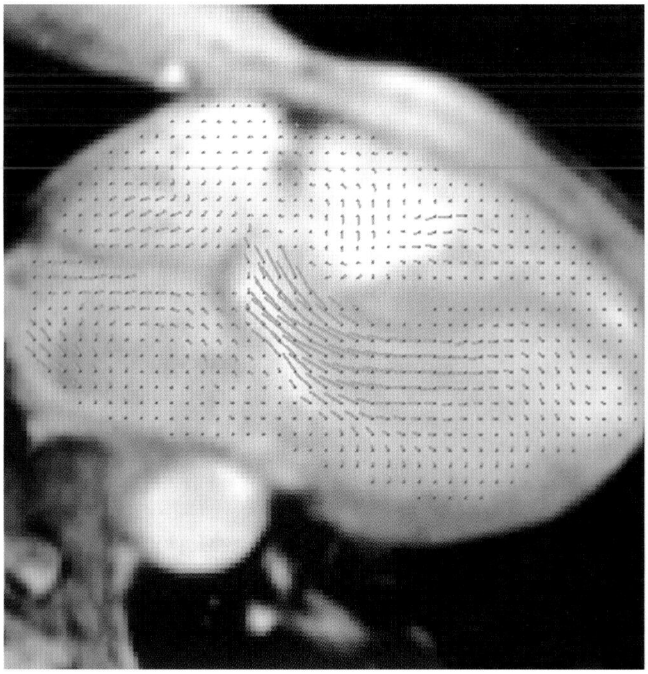

Figure 102-16 **Three-dimensional (3D) flow vector map showing intracardiac diastolic (A) flow pattern.** The orientation of the vector corresponds to the instantaneous in-plane direction of blood flow, whereas the vector's length is proportional to instantaneous velocity.

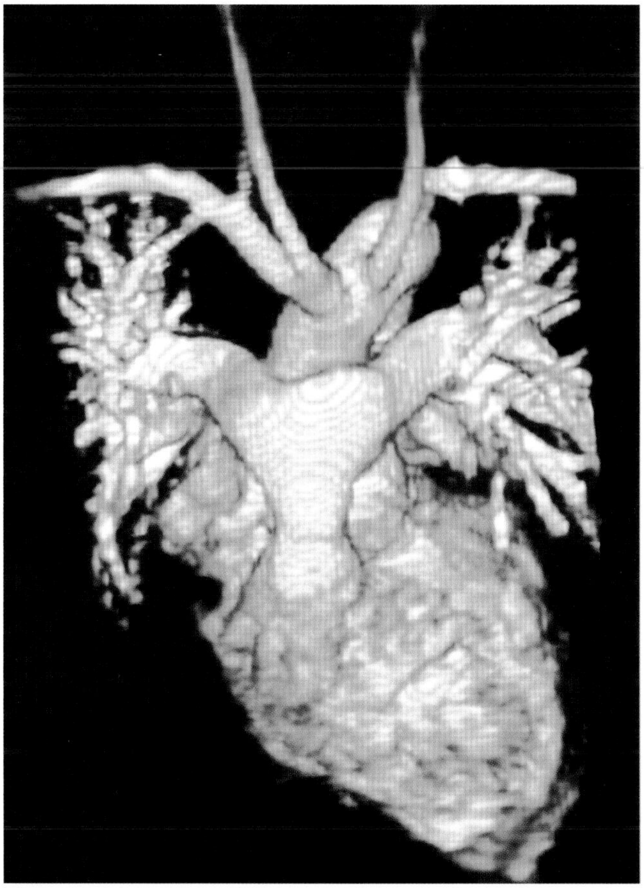

Figure 102-17 **Gadolinium-enhanced three-dimensional (3D) magnetic resonance angiography (MRA) in a patient with D-loop transposition of the great arteries after an arterial switch operation. D,** 3D volume reconstruction provides enhanced perception of the relationships between the great vessels.

A 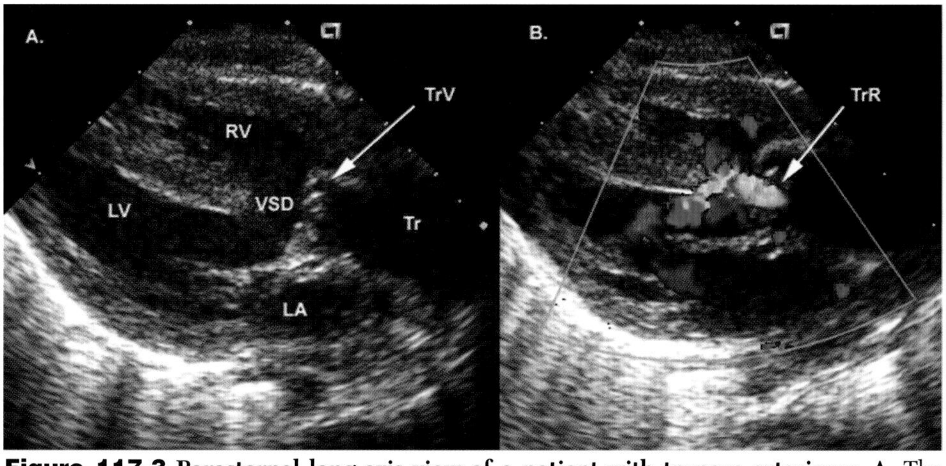 B

Figure 117-3 **Parasternal long-axis view of a patient with truncus arteriosus. A,** The large truncus (Tr) overriding the ventricular septal defect (VSD) is demonstrated. **B,** The addition of Doppler reveals a jet of truncal regurgitation (TrR). LA, left atrium; LV, left ventricle; RV, right ventricle; TrV, truncal valve.

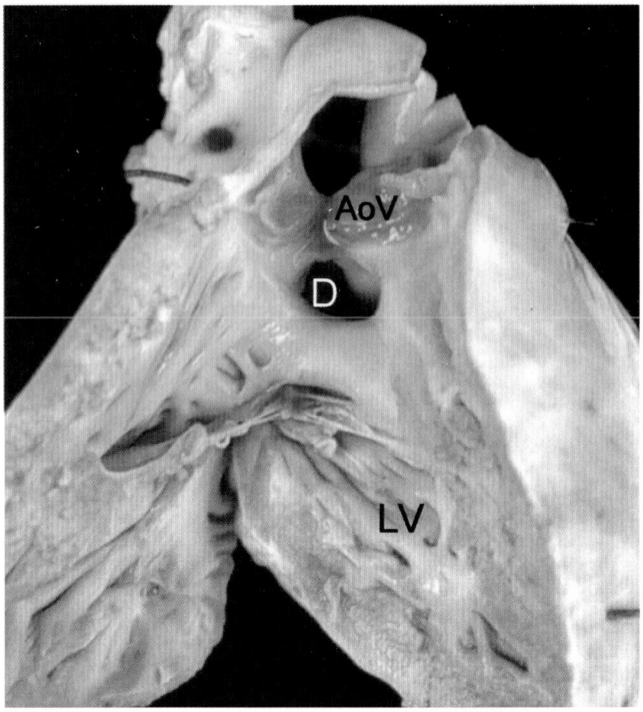

Figure 128-3 **Aortic valve insufficiency in subarterial doubly committed ventricular septal defect (VSD). A,** The anatomy specimen viewed through the right ventricle (RV) demonstrates the position of a doubly committed subarterial defect (D). There is fibrous continuity between the aortic (AoV) and pulmonary valve, and the VSD is adjacent to both great arteries. **B,** The echo illustrates the position of the VSD (D) relative to the pulmonary and aortic valves (PV and AV). The arrow marks the fibrous continuity between the valves. The close proximity of the aortic valve to the VSD usually results in aortic valve prolapse that progresses to aortic regurgitation.

Surgical Management of Aortic Disease

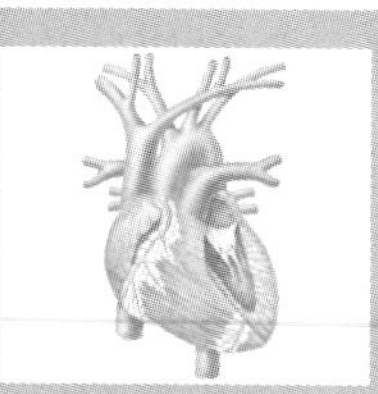

CHAPTER 68

Surgery of the Aortic Root and Ascending Aorta

Tirone E. David

FUNCTIONAL ANATOMY OF THE AORTIC ROOT

The aortic root is the anatomical segment between the left ventricle and the ascending aorta. It contains the aortic valve and other anatomical elements, which function as a unit. The aortic root has four anatomical components: the aortic annulus, the aortic cusps, the aortic sinuses or sinuses of Valsalva, and the sinotubular junction.

The aortic annulus is a fibrous structure that attaches the aortic root to the left ventricle. It is attached directly to the myocardium in approximately 45% of its circumference and to fibrous structures in the remaining 55%, as shown in Figure 68-1. The aortic annulus has a scalloped shape. Histological examination of the aortic annulus reveals that the aortic root has a fibrous continuity with the anterior leaflet of the mitral valve and membranous septum, and it is attached to the muscular interventricular septum through fibrous strands (Figure 68-2). The fibrous tissue that separates the mitral valve from the aortic valve is called the intervalvular fibrous body. An important structure immediately below the membranous septum is the bundle of His. The atrioventricular node lies in the floor of the right atrium between the tricuspid annulus and the coronary sinus orifice. This node gives origin to the bundle of His, which travels through the right fibrous trigone along the posterior edge of the membranous septum to the muscular interventricular septum. At this point the bundle of His divides into left and right bundle branches, which run subendocardially along both sides of the interventricular septum.

The normal aortic valve has three cusps. Each cusp has a semilunar shape and has a base and a free margin. The base is attached to the aortic annulus in a crescent fashion. The point at which the free margin of a cusp joins its base is the commissure, and the ridge in the aortic wall that lies immediately above the commissures is the sinotubular junction. The spaces contained between the aortic annulus and the sinotubular junction are the aortic sinuses or sinuses of Valsalva. There are three cusps and three sinuses: left cusp and sinus, right cusp and sinus, and noncoronary cusp and sinus. The left main coronary artery arises from the left aortic sinus and the right coronary artery from the right aortic sinus.

The triangular spaces underneath two aortic cusps are part of the left ventricular outflow tract but they are important for aortic valve function. The subcommissural triangle beneath the right and left aortic cusps is muscular, whereas the other two subcommissural triangles are fibrous (Figure 68-1).

The normal aortic root has a fairly consistent shape, and the sizes of the cusps, the aortic annulus, the aortic sinuses, and the sinotubular junction are somewhat interdependent.[8,57,81,90] Thus, large cusps have proportionally large

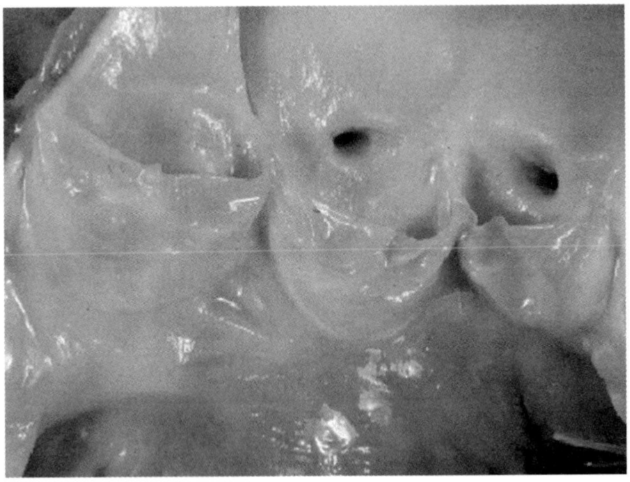

Figure 68–1 **A photograph of the inside of the aortic root.**

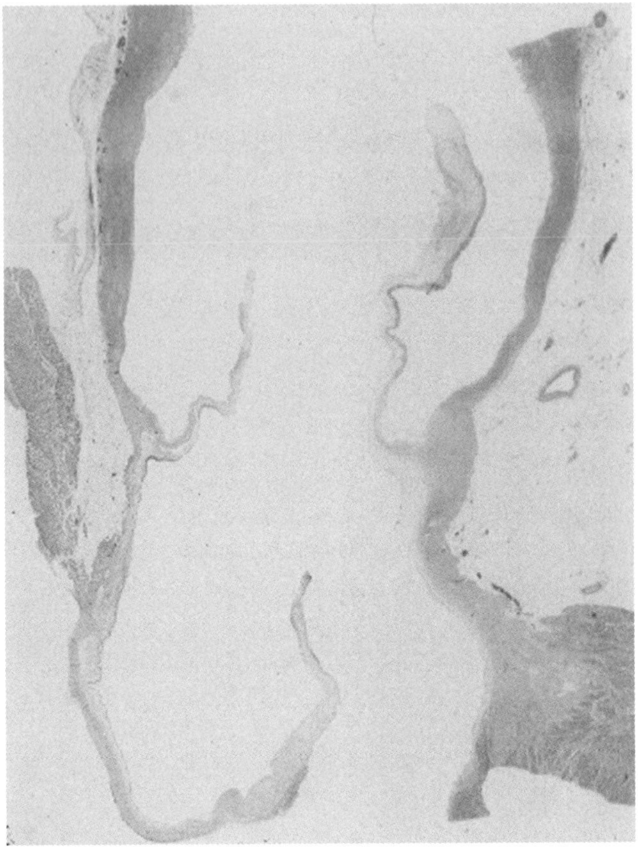

Figure 68–2 **Microphotographs of the aortic annulus, cusps, and sinuses.**

annulus, sinus, and sinotubular junction. The three aortic cusps often have different sizes in a person, and the right and noncoronary cusps are usually larger than the left cusp.[81] The same cusp may have different sizes in individuals with the same body surface area.[81,90] There are, however, certain geometric parameters that are fairly constant among the various components of the aortic root, and this knowledge is indispensable to understand the principles of aortic valve repair or replacement with stentless biological valves.

The free margin of an aortic cusp extends from one of its commissures to the other. The length of the free margin of an aortic cusp is approximately 1.5 times the length of its base (Figure 68-3). During diastole, the free margins and part of the body of the three cusps touch each other approximately in the center of the aortic root to seal the aortic orifice. Thus, the average length of the free margins of three aortic cusps must exceed the diameter of the sinotubular junction to allow the cusps to coapt centrally and render the aortic valve competent. If a pathological process causes shortening of the length of the free margin of a cusp or if the sinotubular junction dilates, the cusps cannot coapt centrally resulting in aortic insufficiency (Figure 68-4). If the length of a free margin is elongated, the cusp prolapses, and depending of the degree of prolapse, aortic insufficiency ensues (Figure 68-5).

The diameter of the aortic annulus is 10–20% larger than the diameter of the sinotubular junction of the aortic root in young patients (Figure 68-3). As the number of elastic fibers in the arterial wall decreases with age, the sinotubular junction dilates, and its diameter tends to become equal to that of the aortic annulus in older patients.

Dilation of the aortic annulus pulls the belly of the aortic cusps apart decreasing the coaptation area and eventually causes aortic insufficiency (Figure 68-6). With dilation of the aortic annulus, the subcommissural triangles of the noncoronary cusp tend to become more obtuse as the crescent shape of the aortic annulus along its fibrous insertion flattens (Figure 68-6). The subcommisural triangle beneath the

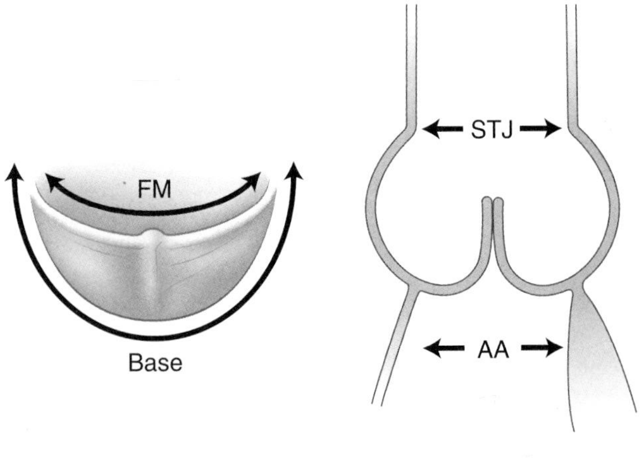

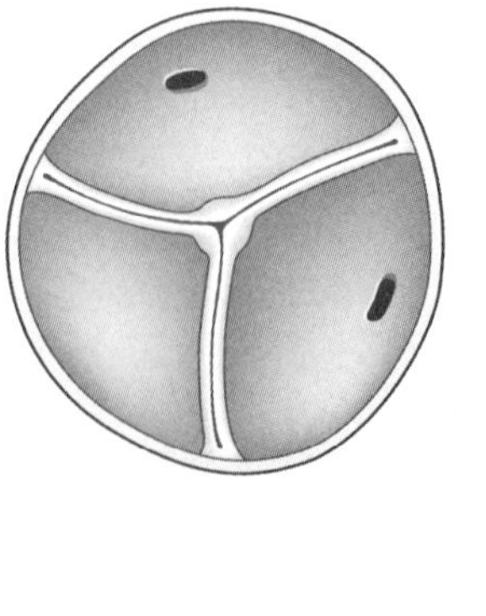

Figure 68–3 **Geometric relationship between the free margin (FM) and base of the aortic cusps, sinotubular junction (STJ), and aortic annulus (AA).**

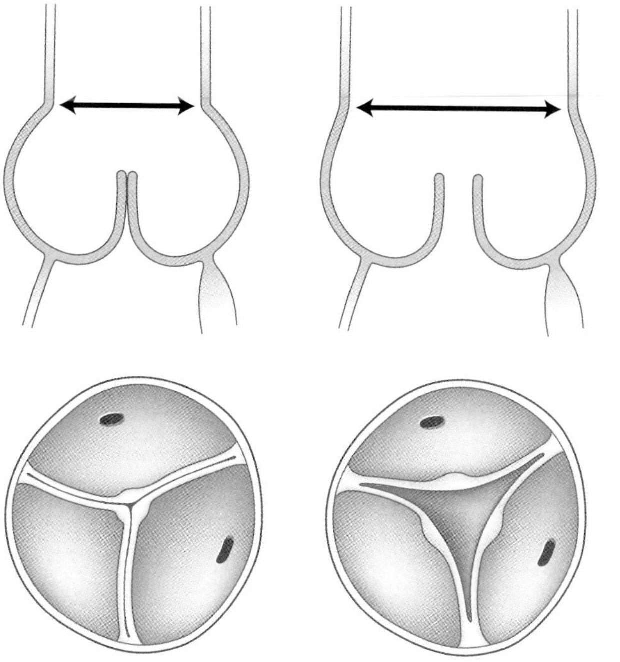

Figure 68–4 Dilation of the sinotubular junction causes aortic insufficiency.

right and left cusps does not change much in patients with annuloaortic ectasia because it is part of the muscular interventricular septum and it is not affected by the connective tissue disorder that causes dilation of the fibrous skeleton of the heart.

The aortic sinuses facilitate closure of the aortic valve by creating eddies currents between the cusps and arterial wall (Figure 68-7). They also prevent the cusps from occluding the coronary artery orifices during systole, thus guaranteeing myocardial perfusion during the entire cardiac cycle. Isolated dilation of the aortic sinuses does not cause aortic insufficiency.[40] That is why patients with congenital aortic sinus aneurysm can have a competent aortic valve.

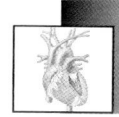

The aortic root of young individuals is elastic and very compliant. It expands and contracts during the cardiac cycle. Expansion and contraction of the aortic annulus are heterogeneous probably because of its attachments to contractile myocardium and to fibrous structures such as the membranous septum and intervalvular fibrous body. On the other hand, the expansion and contraction of the sinotubular junction are more uniform. The aortic root also displays some degree of torsion during isovolumic contraction and ejection of the left ventricle.[18] Compliance decreases with aging because of loss of elastic fibers, and the movements of the aortic annulus, cusps, sinuses, and sinotubular junction also change.

PATHOLOGY OF THE AORTIC ROOT AND ASCENDING AORTA

The wall of the aorta is composed of three layers: intima, media, and adventitia. The intima is a thin layer of ground substance lined by endothelium, and it is easily traumatized. The media is the thickest of the three layers, and it is made of elastic fibers, which are arranged in spiral fashion to increase the tensile strength. The adventitia is a thin fibrous layer and contains the vasa vasorum, which carry the nutrients to the media. The aorta is very compliant and expands and contracts during the cardiac cycle because of the elastic fibers in the media. Compliance decreases with aging because of fragmentation of the elastic fibers and an increase in the amount of fibrous tissue in the media. Hypertension, hypercholesterolemia, and coronary artery disease cause premature aging of the aorta.[19,66,85] Exercise seems to protect the elasticity of the aorta.[66]

Degenerative diseases of the media with aneurysm formation are the most common disorders of the aortic root and ascending aorta. A broad spectrum of pathological and clinical entities is grouped under degenerative disorders, and it ranges from severe degeneration of the media, which can become clinically important early in life in cases such as Marfan syndrome in children, to cases of the not so important mild dilation of the ascending aorta in elderly patients. Bicuspid and unicusp aortic valve disease are often associated with dilation of the aorta. Atherosclerosis, infectious and noninfectious aortitis, and trauma are other pathological entities with which the cardiac surgeons must be familiar. Primary tumors of the aortic root and ascending aorta

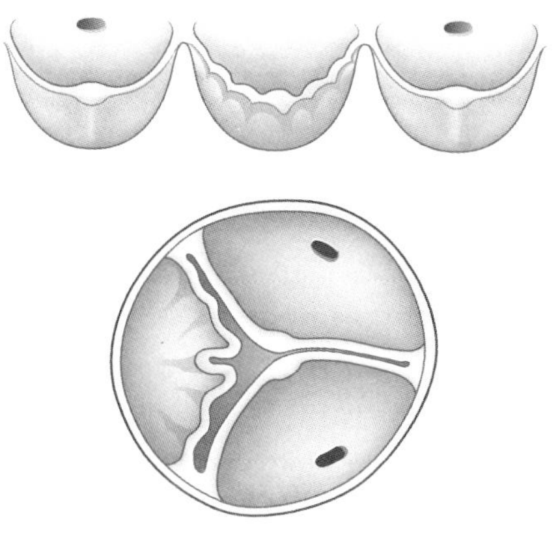

Figure 68–5 Elongation of the free margin of an aortic cusp causes prolapse with resulting aortic insufficiency.

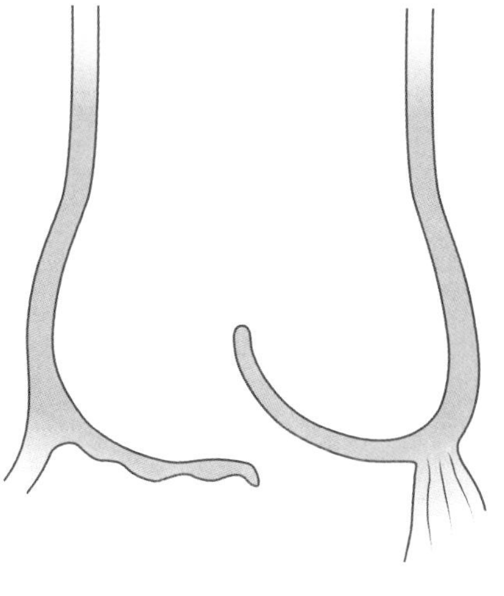

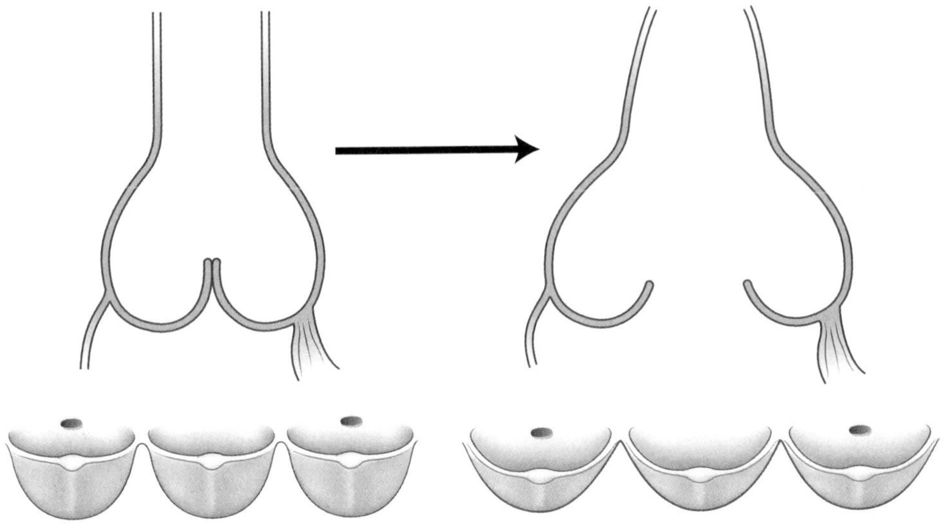

Figure 68–6 Dilation of the aortic annulus. The subcommissural triangles of the noncoronary cusp become more obtuse.

are very rare. False aneurysms and aortic root abscess are problems commonly encountered in clinical practice.

Degenerative Aneurysm of the Ascending Aorta

Aneurysms of the ascending aorta are often caused by cystic medial degeneration (cystic medial necrosis). Histologically, necrosis and disappearance of muscle cells in the elastic lamina, and cystic spaces filled with mucoid material are often observed. Although these changes occur more often in the ascending aorta, it may affect any portion or the entire aorta. These changes weaken the arterial wall, which dilates and forms a fusiform aneurysm. The aortic root may be involved in this pathological process, and in patients with Marfan syndrome, the aneurysm usually begins in the aortic sinuses. A large proportion of patients with aortic root aneurysms do not fulfill the criteria of diagnosis of Marfan syndrome but the gross appearance of the aneurysm and the histology of the arterial wall may be indistinguishable from that of Marfan syndrome. These cases are referred to as forma frusta of Marfan syndrome. Patients with aortic root aneurysms are usually in their second or third decade of life when the diagnosis is made. Other patients have relatively normal aortic roots but develop ascending aortic aneurysms. These patients are usually in their fifth or sixth decade of life. Finally, certain patients have extensive degenerative disease of the entire aorta and develop the so-called megaaorta syndrome with dilation of the thoracic and abdominal aorta.

Ascending aortic aneurysms tend to increase in size and eventually rupture or cause aortic dissection. The transverse diameter of the aneurysm is the most important predictor of rupture or dissection. In a study by Coady and associates[15] of 370 patients with thoracic aneurysms (201 ascending aortic aneurysms), during a mean follow-up of 29.4 months, the incidence of acute dissection or rupture was 8.8% for aneurysms <4 cm, 9.5% for aneurysms of 4–4.9 cm, 17.8% for 5–5.9 cm, and 27.9% for those >6 cm. The median size of the ascending aortic aneurysm at the time of rupture or dissection was 5.9 cm.

The growth rates of thoracic aneurysms are exponential.[15] In Coady's study, the growth rate ranged from 0.08 cm/year for small (<4 cm) aneurysms to 0.16 cm/year for large (8 cm) aneurysms.[15] The growth rates for chronic dissecting aneurysms were much higher than for chronic nondissecting aneurysms. Other studies found greater annual growth rates than Coady's.[48,86] In addition, the growth rates for aortic root aneurysms may be different of ascending aortic aneurysms.

Most patients with aortic root or ascending aortic aneurysms are asymptomatic, and the aneurysm is usually found during routine chest X-rays, which shows widened mediastinum.[72] Tracheal and esophageal displacement may be observed in the posterolateral view of the chest X-rays. Approximately one-third of the patients complain of vague chest pain.[72] In patients with a massive ascending aortic aneurysm, signs of superior vena cava obstruction may be present. If aortic insufficiency is present, there may be cardiac enlargement and the physical findings associated with

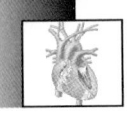

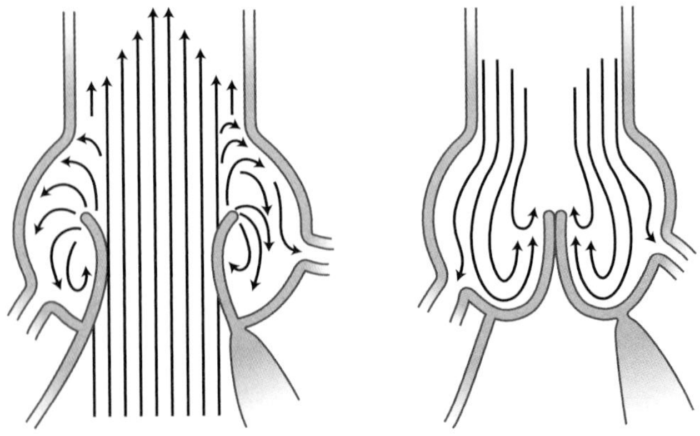

Figure 68–7 The aortic sinuses create eddies and currents and facilitate aortic valve closure.

it. The diagnosis of aortic root and/or ascending aortic aneurysm can be confirmed by echocardiography.

Transesophageal echocardiography is the best diagnostic tool to study aortic root aneurysm and the mechanism of aortic insufficiency. The echocardiographer should obtain information on each component of the aortic root and particularly the aortic cusps. The number of cusps, their thickness, the appearance of free margins, and the excursion of each cusp during the cardiac cycle must be carefully observed. The coaptation areas of the cusps should also be investigated in multiple views and Doppler imaging recorded. Information regarding the morphological features of the aortic sinuses, sinotubular junction, and ascending aorta is also important. The diameters of the aortic annulus, aortic sinuses, sinotubular junction, and ascending aorta should be obtained in multiple views. The lengths of the free margins of the cusps should be estimated if possible. The mechanism of aortic insufficiency can often be determined by transesophageal echocardiography. Dilation of the sinotubular junction is a common cause of aortic insufficiency in patients with ascending aortic aneurysm and normal aortic cusps. Dilation of the aortic annulus and of the sinotubular junction is usually the cause of aortic insufficiency in patients with aortic root aneurysm. Although fenestrations in the cusps are not easily seen by echocardiography, a regurgitant jet in a commissural area is suggestive of fenestration.

Computed tomography (CT) with intravenous contrast enhancement permits accurate evaluation of the extent and size of the aneurysm. Three-dimensional imaging techniques can provide additional information on the extensiveness and type of aneurysm (fusiform or saccular).

Magnetic resonance imaging (MRI) provides even more information than CT scan because it visualizes the arterial wall and surrounding structures with greater contrast. In addition, it has been increasingly used in the diagnosis and management of patients with heart diseases.[39,71] Magnetic resonance angiography (MRA) is replacing contrast angiography, and eventually it may even replace coronary angiography.[6]

Marfan Syndrome

Marfan syndrome is an autosomal dominant variably penetrant inherited disorder of the connective tissue in which cardiovascular, skeletal, ocular, and other abnormalities may be present to a variable degree. The prevalence is estimated to be around 1 in 3000–5000 individuals. It is caused by mutations in the gene that encodes fibrillin-1 (FBN1) on chromosome 15. This is a large gene (approximately 10,000 nucleotides in the mRNA), and identification of the mutation is a complex task. More than 300 mutations in FBN1 have been described. The phenotype presents to a highly variable degree because of varying genotype expression.

The clinical features are the result of weaker connective tissues due to defects in fibrillin-1, a glycoprotein and principal component of the extracellular matrix microfibril. The diagnosis of Marfan syndrome is made on clinical grounds, and it is not always simple because of the variability in clinical expression. A multidisciplinary approach is needed to diagnose and manage patients afflicted with this syndrome. Table 68-1 shows the criteria for the diagnosis of Marfan syndrome. The presence of major criteria in two separate systems and involvement of a third (minor or major) are needed to establish the diagnosis.[28]

The most common cardiovascular features are aortic root aneurysm and mitral valve prolapse. These anatomical abnormalities may cause aortic rupture, aortic dissection, aortic insufficiency, and mitral insufficiency.

Mitral valve prolapse is age dependent and is more common in women. It is caused by myxomatous degeneration of the mitral valve apparatus, which is present in up to 80% of patients with Marfan syndrome, but only 25% of them develop mitral insufficiency. The posterior mitral annulus is grossly dilated in patients with mitral insufficiency and it is often displaced posteriorly.[50] The mitral annulus may also become heavily calcified and display a "horseshoe" appearance on X-rays.

The dilation of the aortic root is often progressive, and the rate of expansion, which varies somewhat, is usually less than 1 or 2 mm/year. Shores and colleagues[86] randomized 70 patients with Marfan syndrome into propanolol-treated and placebo groups. The growth rates of the aortic root aneurysms in untreated patients were slightly more than three times that of patients who received β-adrenergic blockage. This study has been the scientific basis to treat these patients with a β-blocker agent.

Aortic dissection is rare in patients with aortic root aneurysm of less than 50 mm, unless they have family history of aortic dissection. The dissection in most patients starts at the level of the sinotubular junction (Stanford type A aortic dissection). In approximately 10% of the patients it starts just beyond the left subclavian artery (Stanford type B aortic dissection). Without surgery most patients with Marfan syndrome die in the third decade of their lives from complications of aortic root aneurysm such as rupture, aortic dissection, or aortic insufficiency.[67,87]

Patients with Marfan syndrome should be followed up at regular time intervals. Doppler echocardiography is the best diagnostic tool for monitoring changes in the mitral valve and aortic root. Patients with an aortic root >40 mm should be followed with echocardiographic measurements twice yearly. Magnetic resonance images of the remaining thoracic and abdominal aorta should also be obtained when indicated.

Pregnancy in women with Marfan syndrome has two potential problems: the risk of having a child who will inherit the disorder and the risk of acute aortic dissection during the third trimester, parturition, or the first month postpartum. The offspring has a 50% risk of inheriting the syndrome. The risk of aortic dissection is less known, but it appears to be low in patients with normal aortic root and cardiac function.[79]

Ehlers–Danlos Syndrome

This syndrome encompasses a group of heterogeneous connective tissue disorders that involves the skin and joints causing hyperelasticity and fragility of the former and hypermobility of the latter. It may also involve the cardiovascular system. Vascular Ehlers–Danlos syndrome is a rare autosomal dominant inherited disorder of the connective tissue resulting from mutation of the COL3A1 gene encoding type III collagen.[42] Affected individuals are prone to serious vascular, intestinal, and obstetrical complications.

Table 68–1

Diagnosis Criteria for Marfan Syndrome

Criteria	*Major*	*Minor*
Family history	Independent diagnosis in parent, child, sibling	None
Genetics	Mutation FBN1	None
Cardiovascular	Aortic root dilation Dissection of ascending aorta	Mitral valve prolapse Calcification of the mitral valve (<40 years) Dilation of the pulmonary artery Dilation/dissection of the descending aorta
Ocular	Ectopia lentis	Two needed Flat cornea Myopia Elongated globe
Skeletal	Four needed Pectus excavatum needing surgery Pectus carinatum Pes planus Wrist *and* thumb sign Scoliosis >20° or spondylolisthesis arm span–height ratio >1.05 Protrusio acetabulae (X-ray, MRI) Diminished extension elbows (<170°)	Two major or one major and two minor signs Moderate pectus excavatum High narrowly arched palate Typical facies Joint hypermobility
Pulmonary		Spontaneous pneumothorax Apical bulla
Skin		Unexplained stretch marks (striae) Recurrent or incisional herniae
Central nervous system	Lumbosacral dural ectasia (CT or MRI)	

These problems are rare during infancy but occur in up to 25% of affected persons before the age of 20 years and in 80% before the age of 40. Median survival is 48 years. Spontaneous rupture without dissection of large and medium-caliber arteries such as the abdominal aorta and its branches, the branches of the aortic arch, and the large arteries of the limbs accounts for most deaths. Intestinal perforation, usually involving the colon, is less fatal. Pregnancy is a high risk for women with this syndrome. Aortic root dilation was present in 28% in a series of 71 patients with Ehlers–Danlos syndrome.[94] Aortic dissection is uncommon.

As with many rare diseases, delayed or incorrect diagnosis can lead to inadequate or inappropriate management. Diagnosis is based on clinical findings including specific facial features, thin translucent skin, propensity to bleeding, and rupture of vessels and/or viscera. Diagnosis can be confirmed either by biochemical assays showing qualitative or quantitative abnormalities in type III collagen secretion or by molecular biology studies demonstrating mutation of the COL3A1 gene. Varied molecular mechanisms have been observed with different mutations in each family. No correlation has been established between genotype and phenotype. Diagnosis should be suspected in any young person presenting with arterial or visceral rupture or colonic perforation. There is currently no specific treatment for this syndrome.

Bicuspid Aortic Valve Disease

Congenital aortic valve malformations may reflect a phenotypic continuum of unicuspid valves (severe form), the various types of bicuspid aortic valves (moderate form), tricuspid valves (normal), and the rare quadricuspid valves.[38]

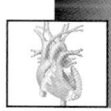

Bicuspid aortic valve is the most common of these malformations and occurs in 1–2% of the population. Males are affected more than females at a ratio of 4:1. There is a relatively high incidence of familial clustering, which suggests an autosomal dominant inheritance with reduced penetrance.[14,49] However, it remains unproven that bicuspid aortic valve is an inherited disorder. Patients with bicuspid aortic valve usually have three aortic sinuses and two cusps of different sizes. The larger cusp, usually the one attached to the interventricular septum, contains a raphe, which probably represents an incomplete commissure. Bicuspid aortic valves with two cusps and two sinuses are far less common than bicuspid aortic valves with two cusps and three sinuses. Most patients with bicuspid aortic valves have a dominant circumflex artery and a small right coronary artery. Normally functioning bicuspid aortic valve may last the patient's lifetime. Others become stenotic by the fourth or fifth decades of life. Aortic insufficiency may also occur, and it is often associated with dilated aortic annulus.[80] It is more common in younger patients and it is due to prolapse of one cusp, usually the one that contains the raphe.

Both bicuspid and unicuspid aortic valves are often associated with premature degenerative changes in the media of the wall of the aortic root and ascending aorta.[29,69] These patients are at risk of developing chronic degenerative aneurysms of the ascending aorta and type A aortic dissection.[32]

Atherosclerosis

Atherosclerosis of the ascending aorta and transverse arch is a common cause of stroke.[2,64] Sometimes atherosclerosis can cause extensive calcification of the aortic root, ascending aorta, and transverse arch, which is often associated with coronary artery disease, stenosis of one or both coronary arteries orifices, and aortic valve stenosis. Extensive calcification of the ascending aorta is clinically described as "porcelain aorta."[9,53,84,97]

Atherosclerotic aneurysms of the ascending aorta are uncommon. They are more common in the abdominal aorta and to a lesser degree in the descending thoracic aorta. Atherosclerosis often causes irregular and saccular aneurysms of the ascending aorta rather than a more fusiform shape as those caused by degenerative disease of the media.

Infectious Aneurysms

Syphilis was a common cause of aneurysm of the ascending aorta but it is now rare. The spirochetal infection destroys the muscular and elastic fibers of the media, which are replaced by fibrous and other inflammatory tissues. The ascending aorta is the most common site of involvement and the aneurysm is usually saccular.[47] The wall of the ascending aorta is frequently calcified. Syphilitic aortitis also causes coronary ostial stenosis and aortic valve insufficiency.[1] Although rare, other bacteria can also cause aneurysm of the ascending aorta.

Aortitis

Various types of aortitis may involve the ascending aorta.* Giant cell arteritis is among the more common and it involves medium-sized arteries, but the aorta and its branches are involved in approximately 15% of the cases.[77] The etiology is unknown. The characteristic lesion is a granulomatous inflammation of the media of large and medium-caliber arteries such as the temporal artery. This disease is also referred to as "temporal arteritis." Narrowing of the aorta is rare. Occasionally the inflammatory process weakens the aorta leading to aneurysm formation, aortoannular ectasia, and aortic insufficiency.[68] Patients are usually older than 50 years with a mean age of 67 years and mostly are women. Diagnosis is established by biopsy of the involved artery, usually the temporal artery.

Takayasu's arteritis is a chronic inflammatory disease that often involves the aortic arch and its major branches. The pulmonary artery may also be involved. The lesions are purely stenotic in 85% of patients, aneurysmal in 2%, and mixed in 13%.[61,73] Aortic insufficiency occurs in approximately 25% of the cases. It has been classified in type I when the aortic arch is involved, type II when the arch is free of disease but the thoracoabdominal aorta and its branches are affected, type III when both areas are affected, and type IV when the pulmonary artery is involved.[61,91] The etiology is unknown but it is probably an autoimmune disorder. It occurs worldwide but most cases are seen in Asia and Africa. The disease affects women more than men at a ratio of 8:1.[61,73] The mean age at the time of the diagnosis is 29 years.

Ankylosinsg spondylitis, Reiter's syndrome, psoriatic arthritis, and polyarteritis nodosa can cause aortic insufficiency because of annuloaortic ectasia. Behçet's disease can cause aneurysm of the ascending aorta.

Aortic Dissection

Aortic dissections are discussed in Chapter 70.

Ascending Aorta Tumors

Primary tumors of the ascending aorta are extremely rare. Most aortic tumors are located in the descending thoracic or abdominal aorta and are usually sarcomas.[41,95]

Ascending Aorta Trauma

Nonpenetrating traumatic injuries of the ascending aorta are often fatal and diagnosed at autopsy.[37] Penetrating trauma is usually secondary to bullet or stab wounds and causes cardiac tamponade when the intrapericardial portion of the aorta is involved. These injuries are frequently fatal.

SURGICAL TREATMENT OF ASCENDING AORTIC ANEURYSMS

Although ascending aortic aneurysms may present themselves as isolated lesions, more often they are associated with aortic valve disease. Both bicuspid and tricuspid aortic valve disease may be associated with degenerative aneurysms of the ascending aorta, but bicuspid aortic valve disease appears to be associated with premature degeneration of the media of the aorta.

*References 52, 54, 61, 68, 73, 77, 91.

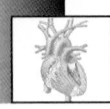

Ascending aortic aneurysm may cause aortic insufficiency in patients with anatomically normal aortic valve cusps if the sinotubular junction becomes dilated as illustrated in Figure 68-4. These patients may develop symptoms related to the aortic insufficiency, but more often the aneurysm is asymptomatic and it is discovered during routine chest X-rays or echocardiogram, which is done as part of the workup for an unrelated problem. Surgery is recommended when the transverse diameter of the ascending aorta exceeds 55 mm.[15] If there is moderate or severe aortic insufficiency and the aortic valve cusps are normal by echocardiography and the valve is judged to be repairable, operation is justifiable when the ascending aorta reaches 50 mm in diameter.[20,21,23]

Operative Techniques

Surgery for ascending aortic aneurysm is performed under cardiopulmonary bypass, which is established by cannulating the transverse aortic arch, right axillary artery or femoral artery, and the right atrium. Because the aneurysm frequently extends up to the origin of the innominate artery, a brief period of circulatory arrest is necessary to resect the arch aneurysm and perform the distal anastomosis (see Chapter

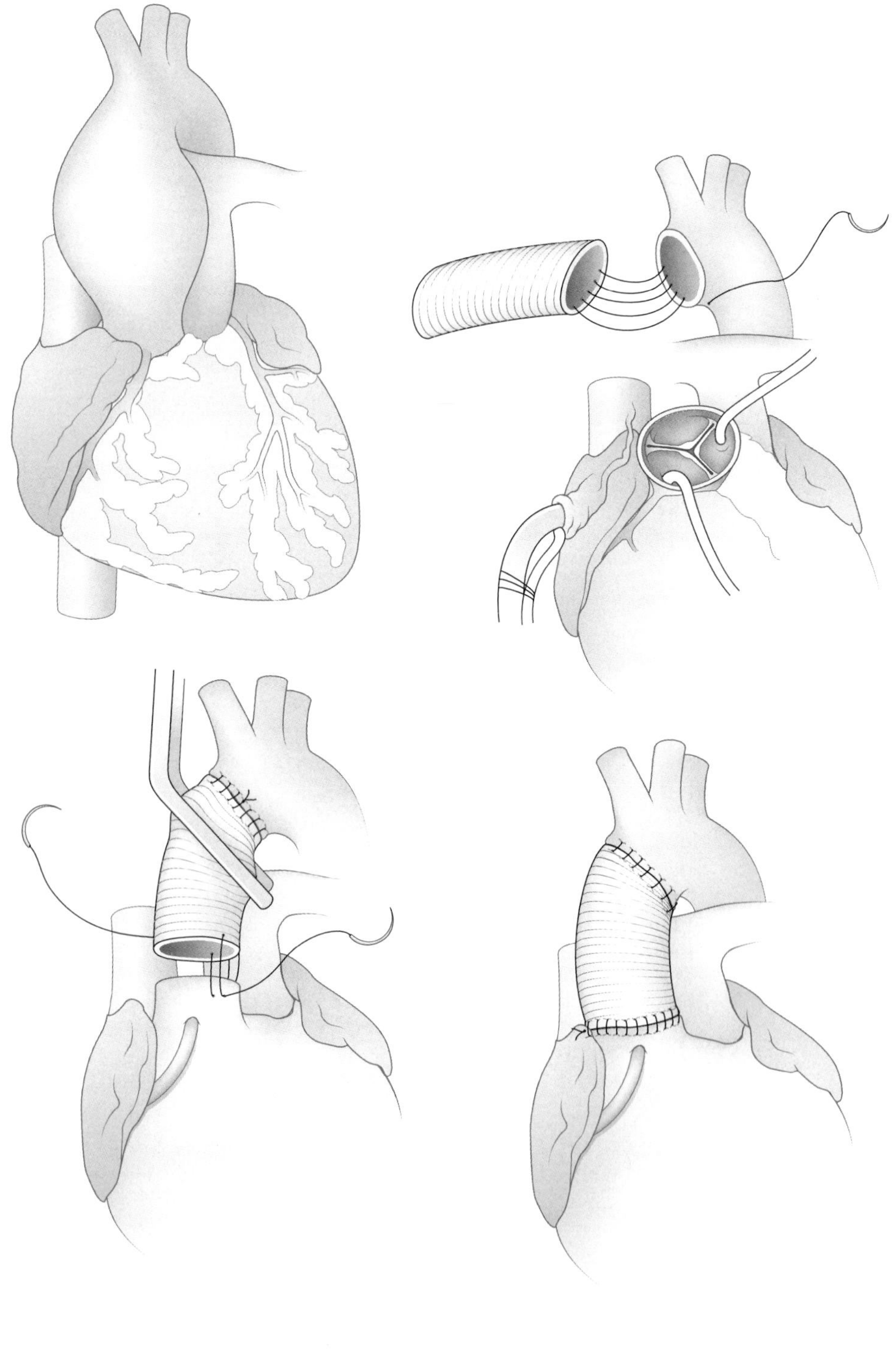

Figure 68–8 Replacement of the ascending aorta for aneurysm.

70 for techniques of cerebral protection). The proximal anastomosis should be performed at the level of the sinotubular junction. The Dacron graft used to replace the ascending aorta should not be too long or too large. It is important to remember that when the ascending aorta expands to develop an aneurysm it also becomes elongated. Thus, during its replacement, the graft should be much shorter than the aneurysm. Actually, a graft of 5 or 6 cm in length is all that is needed to replace the entire ascending aorta from sinotubular junction to the level of the innominate artery. Longer grafts may kink and cause partial obstruction and even hemolysis. A single graft can be used but it should be beveled at the distal anastomosis, and its shorter side should be aligned with the medial part of the arch as illustrated in Figure 68-8. The diameter of the graft should be between 24 and 30 mm, depending on the patient's body surface area. When the diameter of the graft used is larger than the diameter of the sinotubular junction by more than a couple of millimeters, its caliber should be reduced to that of the sinotubular junction at the level of the anastomosis. This is easily done by plication of that end of the graft. Matching the diameter of the graft to that of the sinotubular junction is important to prevent late development of aortic insufficiency.

If the aortic valve is incompetent but the aortic cusps are normal and the sinotubular junction is dilated, all that is needed to reestablish valve competence is to reduce the diameter of the sinotubular junction to allow the cusps to coapt again. The ascending aorta is transected 5 mm above the sinotubular junction. All three commissures are pulled upward and approximate to each other until the cusps coapt centrally. The diameter of an imaginary circle that contains all three commissures is the correct diameter of the sinotubular junction. A graft of that diameter is then sutured to the remnants of ascending aorta wall at the level of the sinotubular junction. Because the aortic cusps are frequently of different sizes, the spaces between the commissures should reflect that during performance of the proximal anastomosis. Aortic valve competence can be assessed by injecting cardioplegia solution under pressure in the graft and observing the left ventricle for distention. We prefer to use two separate segments of grafts when aortic valve repair is necessary and the entire ascending aorta and/or transverse arch needs replacement. We usually do the distal anastomosis first (under hypothermic circulatory arrest) and work on the aortic valve during rewarming of the patient. The distal and proximal grafts are trimmed and sutured to each other (Figure 68-9).

If the noncoronary aortic sinus is aneurysmal, it should be replaced along with the ascending aorta. This is accomplished by selecting a graft of an appropriate diameter as described above and then creating a neoaortic sinus in one of its ends. The width of the neoaortic sinus is equal to the distance between the commissure of the cusp and the height is approximately equal to the diameter of the graft. This neoaortic sinus is sutured directly to the remnant of arterial wall and aortic annulus, as illustrated in Figure 68-10.

Sometimes one aortic cusp may be slightly elongated and its free margin coapts at a level lower than the other two cusps. The free margin can be shortened by plication of the central portion as illustrated in Figure 68-11. If the free margin is elongated and thinned or has a fenestration near a commissure, it can be reinforced with a double layer of a 6-0 expanded polytetrafluoroethylene suture as shown in Figure 68-12.

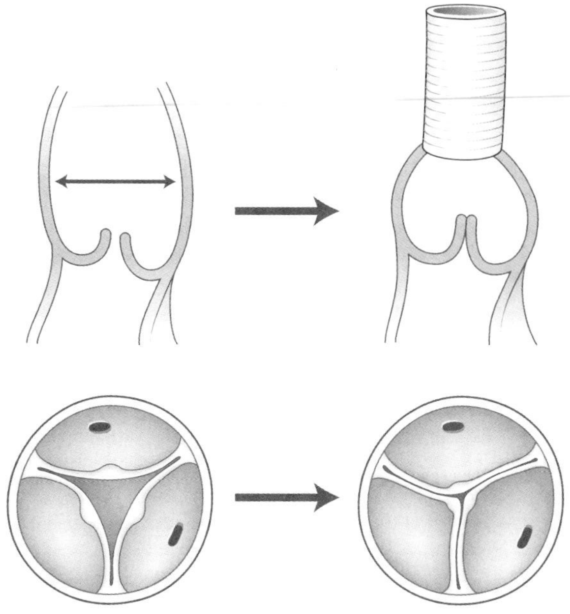

Figure 68–9 Replacement of the ascending aorta with adjustment of the diameter of the sinotubular junction.

Patients with a normally functioning bicuspid aortic valve, normal aortic root, and ascending aortic aneurysm can be treated by simple replacement of the ascending aorta.

Patients with aortic valve disease not amenable to repair and ascending aortic aneurysm are treated by aortic valve replacement and supracoronary replacement of the ascending aorta. If only the noncoronary aortic sinus is dilated, aortic valve replacement of the ascending aorta with a graft extension into the noncoronary sinus as illustrated in Figure 68-10 are preferable to composite replacement of the aortic valve and ascending aorta with reimplantation of the coronary arteries. If two aortic sinuses are dilated, composite replacement of the aortic valve and ascending aorta with reimplantation of the coronary arteries should be performed as described for aortic root aneurysm.

Clinical Outcomes

Isolated replacement of the ascending aorta for chronic aneurysm is uncommon.[22,24] Patients with ascending aortic aneurysm often have aortic insufficiency or aortic valve disease that may also need surgical attention. Whether the operation is done in isolation or combined with other procedures the operative mortality for elective surgery is low.[16,22,24] In our experience with 79 patients who had aortic valve-sparing operations for ascending aortic aneurysm and aortic insufficiency only one patient died perioperatively.[24] We reviewed our experience with aortic valve replacement and supracoronary replacement of the ascending aorta at Toronto General Hospital during the past 12 years and identified 132 patients. There were six operative deaths, and the series included acute aortic dissections, acute infective endocarditis, and reoperations. Cohn et al[16] also reported low operative mortality for replacement of the ascending

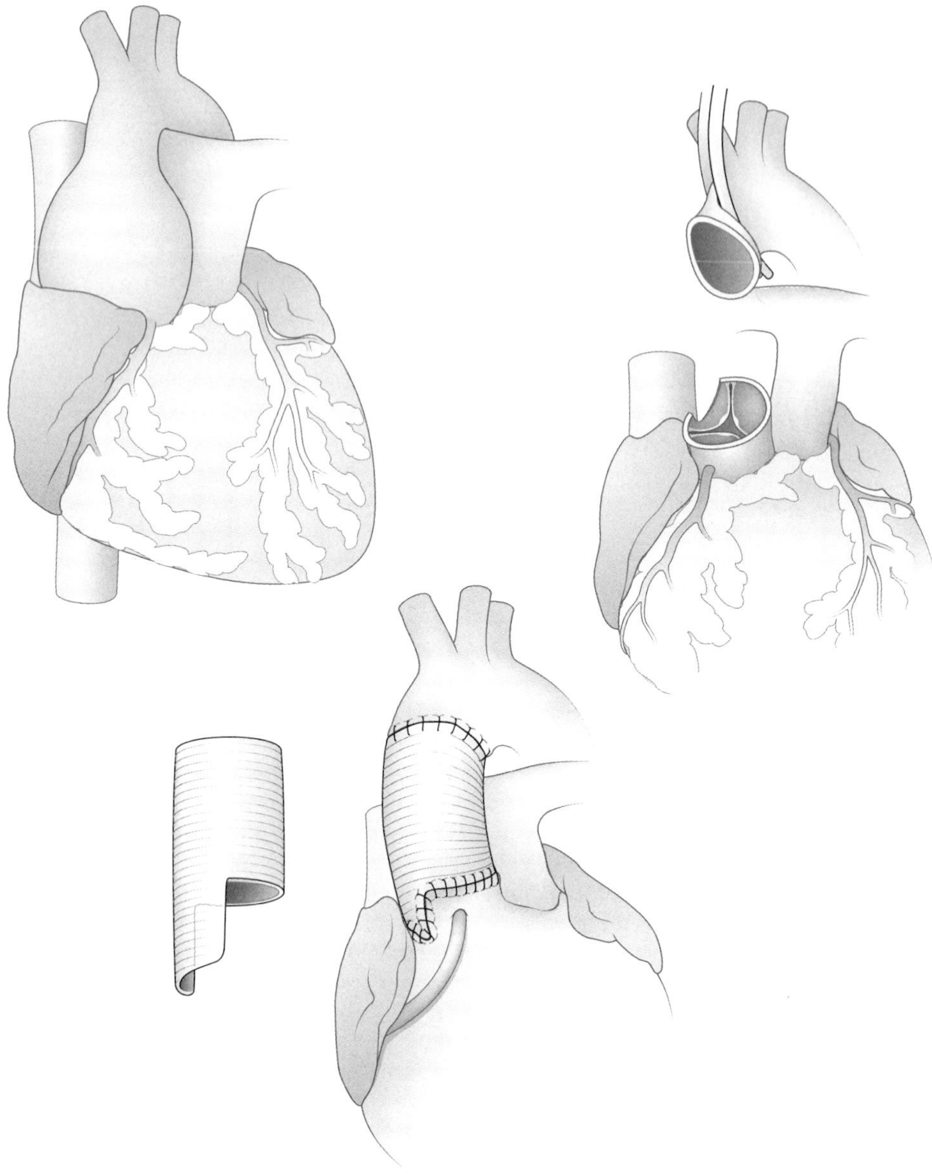

Figure 68–10 Replacement of the ascending aorta and noncoronary aortic sinus.

aorta. The operative mortality for ascending aortic surgery has decreased over the past four decades.[58] Age, functional class, and associated diseases play an important role in the operative risk.

The long-term survival of our 79 patients who had aortic valve-sparing operations for ascending aortic aneurysm and aortic insufficiency was only 36% at 8 years, but most of them had extensive vascular disease including transverse aortic arch disease or megaaorta syndrome.[24] Our patients who had aortic valve replacement and supracoronary replacement of the ascending aorta had a 10-year survival of 70% but they were younger than those who had aortic valve repair and had less extensive vascular disease.

Patients who had replacement of the ascending aorta with or without aortic valve surgery must be evaluated annually with echocardiography to assess the size of the retained aortic root and function of the aortic valve; they should also have CT scans or MRI of the remaining thoracic and abdominal aorta. Aneurysms of the aortic root, false aneurysms, valve dysfunction, and infections in the graft or aortic valve are problems that may develop and need surgical treatment.[58]

Patients who had aortic valve repair or replacement with bioprosthetic valves do not need anticoagulation if they are in sinus rhythm. Obviously those with mechanical valves should be anticoagulated with warfarin sodium. Other systemic disorders are common among these patients, particularly hypertension and coronary artery disease, which should also be treated.

SURGICAL TREATMENT OF AORTIC ROOT ANEURYSMS

Aortic root aneurysm may or may not be associated with Marfan syndrome. Composite replacement of the aortic valve and ascending aorta with reimplantation of the coronary arteries was the standard operation for patients with aortic root aneurysm with or without aortic insufficiency.[44,45,55]

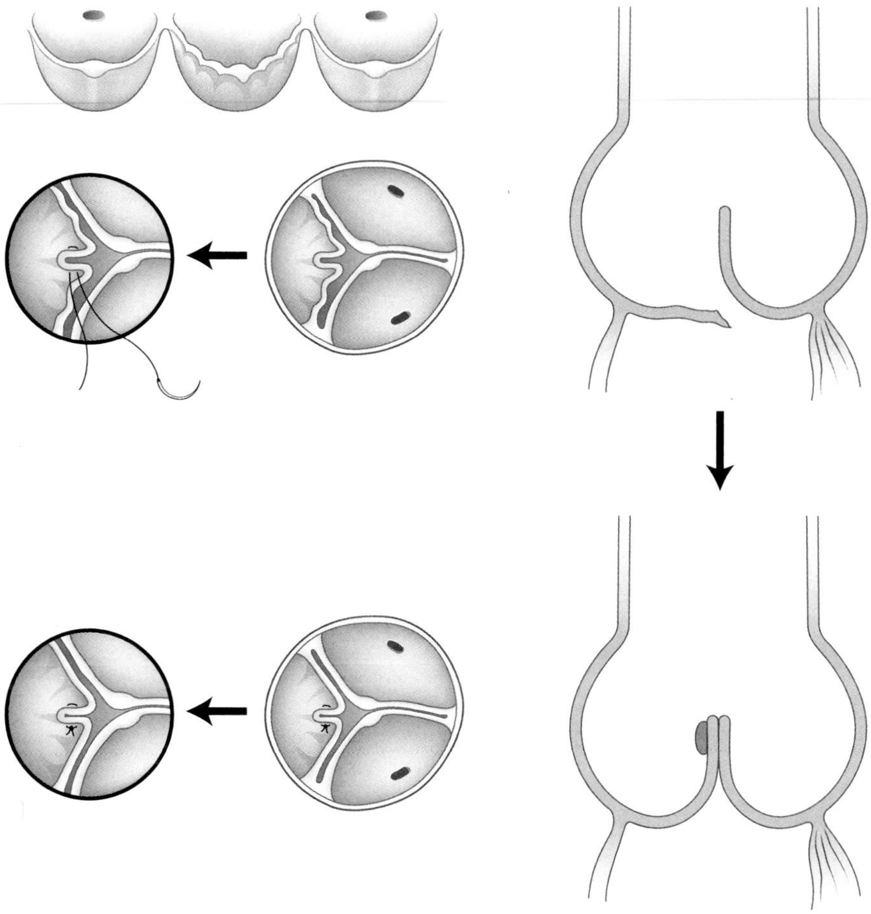

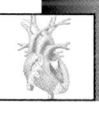

Figure 68–11 Repair of aortic cusp prolapse by shortening of its free margin.

During the past decade, an increasing number of these patients have undergone aortic valve-sparing operations.* Consequently, surgery is now being recommended when the diameter of the aortic root reaches 50 mm in patients with Marfan syndrome or 55 mm in those without this syndrome if an aortic valve-sparing operation is feasible.[27] If a patient has a family history of aortic dissection, surgery should probably be done when the aortic root reaches 45 mm in diameter.

Operative Techniques

There are basically two types of aortic valve-sparing operations for patients with aortic root aneurysms: remodeling of the aortic root and reimplantation of the aortic valve.[20,21,23]

Remodeling of the Aortic Root

The aortic root is dissected circumferentially down to the level of the aortic annulus, and the three aortic sinuses are excised, leaving approximately 5 mm of tissue attached to the aortic annulus and around the coronary artery orifices. The three commissures are gently suspended upward and approximated until the three cusps coapt. The diameter of an imaginary circle that includes all three commissure is approximately the diameter of the tubular Dacron graft to be used for reconstruction of the aortic sinuses as illustrated in Figure 68-13. One of the ends of this graft is tailored to create neoaortic sinuses. The widths of the

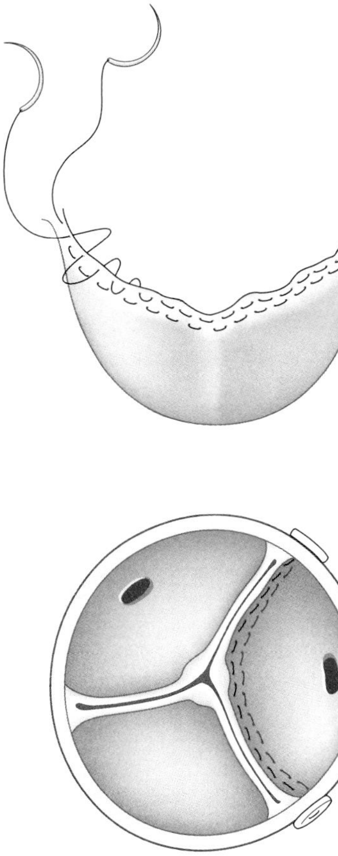

Figure 68–12 Reinforcement of the free margin of the aortic cusp with a double layer of a 6-0 expanded polytetrafluoroethylene suture.

*References 5, 20–24, 27, 51, 82, 96.

neoaortic sinuses are based on the distance between commissures of each cusp when they are pulled upward to determine the diameter of the graft. The heights of the neoaortic sinuses should be approximately equal to their width. The three commissures are secured on the outside of the graft immediately above the neoaortic sinuses, and the remnants of aortic wall and aortic annulus are sutured to the neoaortic sinuses with a continuous 4-0 polypropylene as illustrated in Figure 68-13. The coronary arteries are reimplanted into their respective sinuses. If an aortic cusp coapts at a level lower than the other two, shortening of the free margin corrects the problem (Figures 68-11 and 68-12).

Reimplantation of the Aortic Valve

The aortic root is dissected circumferentially and prepared as described above. Next, multiple 3-0 or 4-0 polyester sutures are passed from the inside to the outside of the left ventricular outflow tract through a single horizontal plane corresponding to the lowest portion of the aortic annulus along its fibrous components and following the scalloped shape of the annulus along its muscular component as illustrated in Figure 68-14. If the fibrous portion of the left ventricular outflow tract is thin, Teflon felt pledgets should be used in those sutures. The diameter of the sinotubular junction is estimated by pulling the three commissures upward until the cusps coapt. A tubular Dacron graft 4–6 mm larger

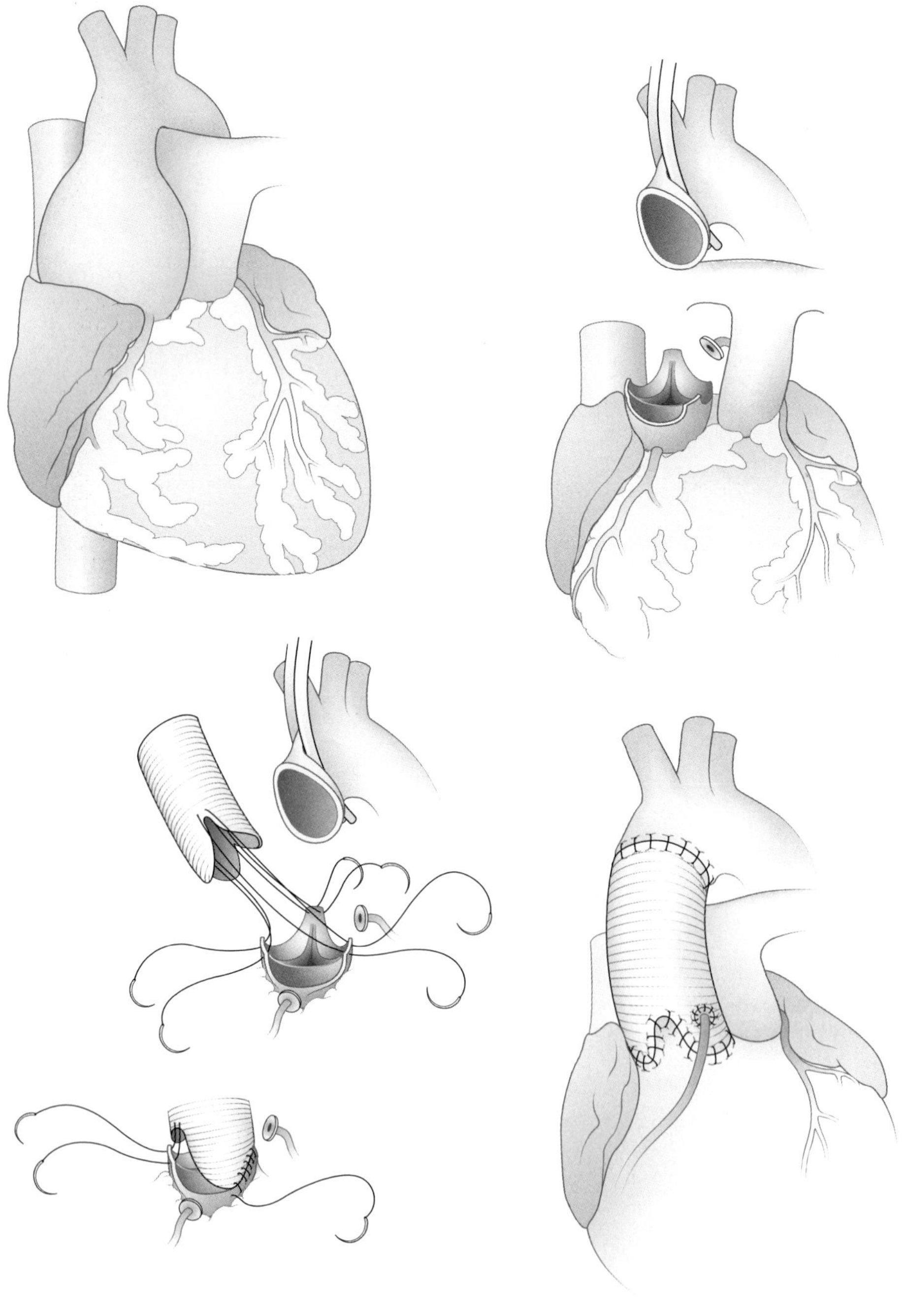

Figure 68–13 Aortic valve-sparing operation: Remodeling of the aortic root.

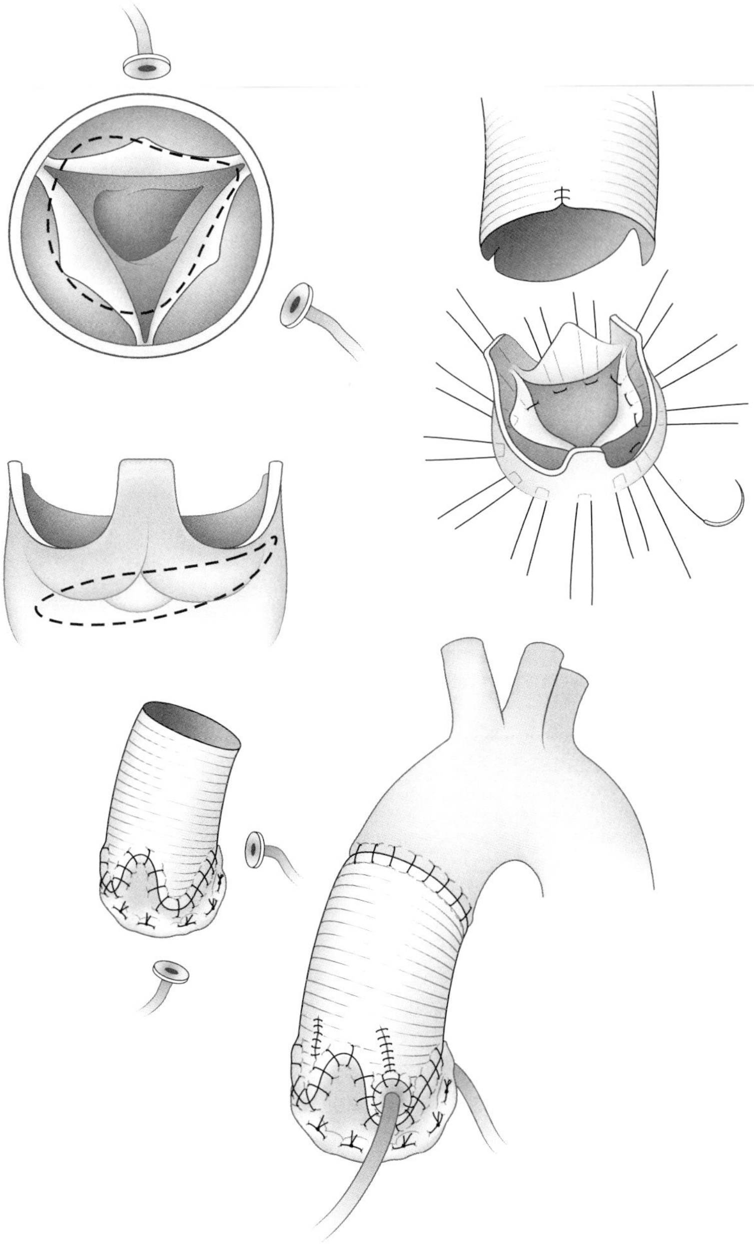

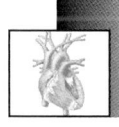

Figure 68–14 Aortic valve-sparing operation: Reimplantation of the aortic valve.

than the diameter of the sinotubular junction is selected and a small triangular excision if made in one of its ends and the remaining portion is plicated in two or three places to reduce its diameter by 3–4 mm. Most grafts we currently use are 30–34 mm in diameter, depending on the size of the patient and aortic cusps. The sutures passed through the left ventricular outflow tract are then passed from the inside to the outside of the tailored end of the graft. If reduction in diameter of the aortic annulus is desirable, it is done beneath the commissures of the noncoronary cusp. This is accomplished by placing the sutures closer in the graft than they are beneath the commissures of the noncoronary cusp. The aortic valve is placed inside the graft and all sutures are tied on the outside. The three commissures are suspended inside the graft and secured to it with 4-0 polypropylene sutures. These sutures are then used to secure the aortic annulus and remnants of aortic sinuses to the graft. The coronary arteries are reimplanted into their respective sinuses. The spaces between commissures are plicated to create a slight bulge in the neoaortic sinuses and to reduce the diameter of the graft to that of the desirable sinotubular junction. Cusp prolapse or reinforcement can be done if needed as illustrated in Figures 68-11 and 68-12.

Patients with a normally functioning bicuspid aortic valve and aortic root aneurysm are also candidates for aortic valve-sparing operations.

Aortic Root Replacement

Replacement of the aortic root is performed when the aortic cusps are abnormal and cannot be safely repaired.[21,82] The aortic cusps are excised and the coronary arteries detached from their sinuses with 5 or 6 mm of aortic sinus wall around them. A valved conduit is then used to replace the aortic root. This conduit can be a commercially available Dacron tube with a mechanical valve already attached to one of its ends or a glutaraldehyde-fixed porcine aortic root such as the Medtronic Freestyle (Medtronic, Minneapolis, MN) or the Toronto Root (St. Jude Medical, St. Paul, MN). The valved conduit is sutured to the aortic annulus and the coronary arteries are reimplanted into the graft as illustrated in Figure 68-15.

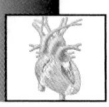

An aortic homograft can also be used for aortic root replacement. It is not wise to use a pulmonary autograft for replacement of the aortic root in patients with aortic root aneurysms because the pulmonary autograft may become aneurismal when subjected to systemic pressures. Finally, aortic root replacement also can be performed with a conduit prepared in the operating room. When the use of a stented bioprosthetic valve is desirable, the bioprosthesis and the Dacron tube can be secured to the aortic annulus using the same sutures. Another method is to secure the bioprosthetic valve inside a tubular Dacron graft 1 cm from one of its ends and secure the Dacron graft alone to the annulus as illustrated in Figure 68-16. This approach allows for aortic valve rereplacement without taking down the original graft or the coronary arteries when the bioprosthetic valve fails. The technique of securing a tubular Dacron graft in the left ventricular outflow tract before implanting a prosthetic valve into it is very useful in situations such as a narrow or destroyed aortic annulus by multiple previous operations, calcification, or endocarditis. The Dacron graft can be tailored to conform to the anatomy of the left ventricular outflow tract before it is sutured to it.

In the original description of aortic root replacement by Bentall and DeBono in 1968, the aneurysm was opened and a tubular Teflon graft containing a mechanical valve was sutured to the aortic annulus, to the coronary arteries by suturing the graft to the aortic sinus wall around their orifices, and to the distal aorta.[4] The aneurysm wall was wrapped around the graft and closed tightly for hemostasis. Pseudoaneurysm formation at the coronary artery and the aortic anastomoses was a complication of this technique.[55] To decompress the space between the graft and aneurysm wall, Cabrol and colleagues described the creation of a shunt between that space and the right atrium.[10] Kouchoukos et al[55] stressed the importance of not wrapping the graft with the aneurysm wall to avoid tension on the anastomoses when accumulation of blood occurs between the aneurysmal wall and the graft. They recommended an open technique in which the coronary arteries are detached from the aortic sinuses and sutured to the tubular Dacron graft.[55] Cabrol et al described a technique whereby the two coronary arteries were connected to each other with a smaller graft and anastomosed side to side to the valved conduit.[11] This technique, however, has not provided as good long-term results as direct coronary artery reimplantation.[3]

Clinical Outcomes

Surgery for aortic root aneurysm is associated with low operative mortality and morbidity, particularly when performed electively. In a recent report of our experience with aortic valve sparing operations, there were only 2 operative deaths among 151 patients operated for aortic root aneurysms, including 15 with acute type A aortic dissection.[24] Other investigators reported similarly low operative mortality with aortic valve-sparing operations.[5,51,82,96] The long-term survival of these patients is excellent. In our experience the survival at 8 years was 83% for all patients and 96% for those with Marfan syndrome.[24,27] Yacoub and colleagues[96] reported an 80% 10-year survival for all patients. Birks et al[5] from the same group reported an 84% 10-year survival for those with Marfan syndrome. Most late deaths are due to dissection or complications of aortic dissection. Aortic valve insufficiency is also a potential problem after aortic valve-sparing operations. Although 99% of our patients were free from reoperations for aortic insufficiency at 8 years, one third of them developed moderate aortic insufficiency.[24] Increased experience, better operative techniques, and perfect aortic cusps coaptation by shortening of the free margins of the cusps when needed are expected to improve the long-term results of these operations. We believe that aortic valve function is more stable in patients with annuloaortic ectasia who had reimplantation of the aortic valve than the remodeling of the aortic root. We found that the aortic annulus and sinotubular junction do not change with time after reimplantation as they do with remodeling.[24,27] The principal advantages of aortic valve-sparing operations over aortic valve replacement are the low risk of thromboembolism, hemorrhage, and infective endocarditis.[27]

In a report by Gott et al[45] on the outcomes of aortic root surgery in patients with Marfan syndrome operated on at 10 experienced surgical centers the operative mortality was 1.5% among 455 patients who had elective surgery, 2.6% among 117 who had urgent surgery, and 11.7% among 103 who had emergency surgery, mostly for acute aortic dissection. However, in the experience of Gott and colleagues at the Johns Hopkins Hospital,[44] there was no operative death among 235 patients who had elective surgery and only 2 deaths among 36 who had urgent or emergent surgery. In our personal experience with 105 patients with Marfan syndrome in whom 44 had root replacement and 61 had aortic valve sparing, there was only one operative death in a patient in preoperative cardiogenic shock because of end-stage aortic insufficiency.[27] Patients with Marfan syndrome are usually young when they require aortic root surgery and that is one of the reasons the operative mortality is low. Surgery in older patients is associated with higher risk.[3,65] Not only age but also the clinical presentation is an important determinant of outcome.[3,30,56,65] Surgery in patients with acute type A aortic dissection is associated with higher operative and late mortality (see Chapter 70). Overall the operative mortality for aortic root replacement is around 5–10%.[3,30,56,65]

The long-term survival after aortic root replacement in patients with Marfan syndrome is very good. Gott et al[45] reported from multiple institutions that the 10-year survival after aortic root surgery ranged from 60 to 80%, depending on the clinical presentation, but in their experience at Johns Hopkins the 10-year survival was 81%.[44] Dissection or rupture of the residual aorta and dysrhythmias were the leading causes of late death.

Thromboembolism, hemorrhage, and endocarditis remain problematic for patients who had aortic root replacement with mechanical valves,* and tissue degeneration and reop-

*References 3, 27, 30, 44, 45, 56, 65.

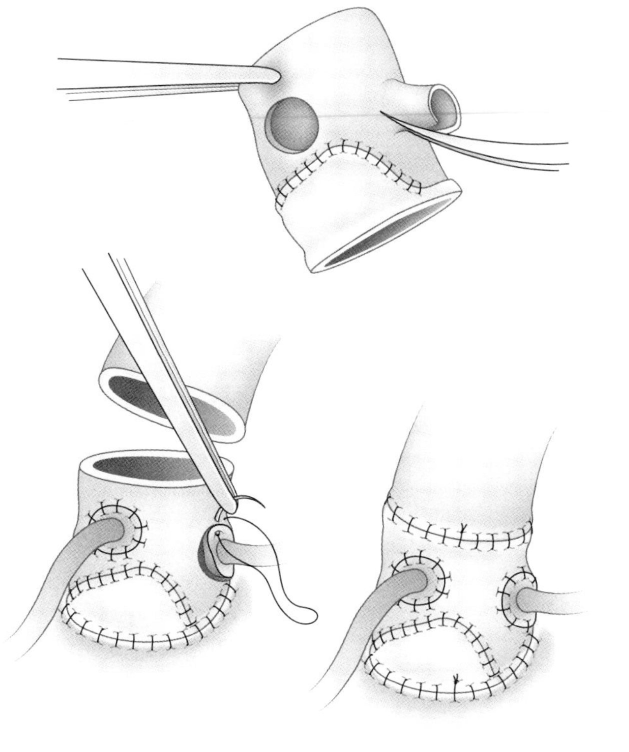

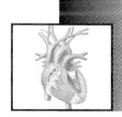

Figure 68–15 **Composite replacement of the ascending aorta and aortic valve with a stentless porcine aortic root.**

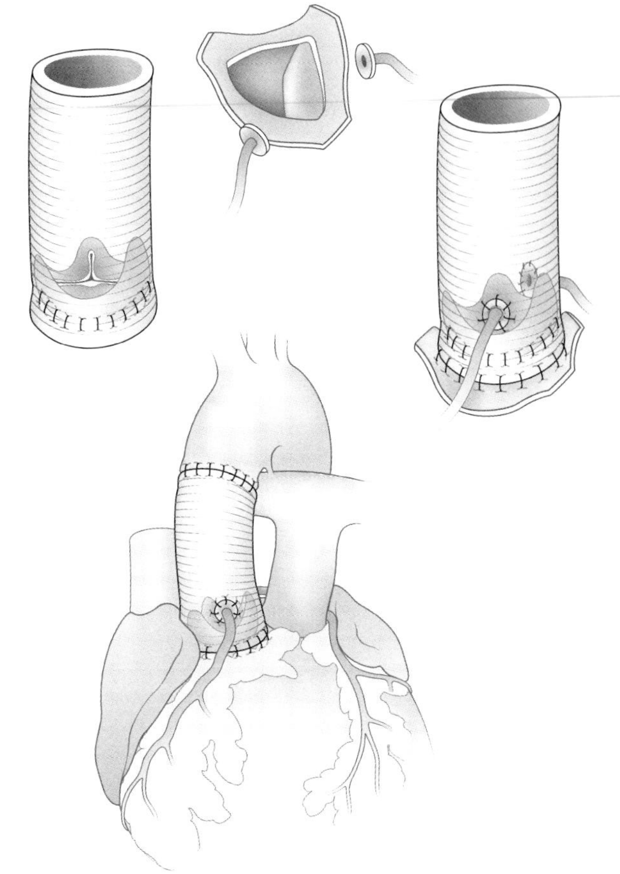

Figure 68–16 **Composite replacement of the ascending aorta and aortic valve with a bioprosthetic valve.**

eration are problems for those who had biological aortic valve.[27]

Patients who had aortic root replacement require periodical check-ups including a transthoracic echocardiogram and CT scans or MRI of the residual aorta. Patients with Marfan syndrome should take a β-blocker permanently if tolerated.

Reoperations in the aortic root after replacement with valved conduits can be difficult, but in the hands of experts can be done with relatively low operative mortality.[59,74] When the problem is graft infection, the use of an aortic homograft is believed to offer the patient the best chance of cure.[62,93] Others and we have obtained similar results by using an approach of radical resection of infected tissues and reconstruction with synthetic grafts.[31,46,76]

ROSS PROCEDURE

The Ross procedure is a type of aortic valve replacement. It is a complex operation whereby the diseased aortic valve is replaced with the patient's own normal pulmonary valve, and a biological valve, usually a pulmonary homograft, is used to replace the pulmonary valve. This operation was first described in the experimental laboratory by Lower et al in 1960[60] and clinically performed by Ross in 1967.[78] The original technique consisted in implanting the pulmonary autograft into the aortic root in a subcoronary position. For the next two decades Ross was, practically, the only surgeon performing this procedure.[63] Interest in this operation increased after the initial report by Stelzer and colleagues in late 1980s, who performed it using the technique of aortic root replacement, a more reproducible method.[88]

The Ross procedure is ideal for children because the pulmonary autograft grows with the child.[34,43] Although the Ross procedure can be used in patients of any age,[7,13] most surgeons prefer to use it in children and young adults.[12,33] Some surgeons consider it ideal to treat patients with active infective endocarditis.[70] The Ross procedure also has been performed in patients with dilated ascending aorta or even aneurysms.[36] It should not be used in patients with Marfan syndrome or in others with connective tissue disorders.

Operative Techniques

There are basically three methods to transfer the pulmonary autograft into the aortic position: subcoronary implantation, aortic root replacement, and aortic root inclusion.

Subcoronary Implantation

The aortic valve should be exposed through a transverse aortotomy 1 cm above the sinotubular junction. The diseased aortic valve is excised and all calcified tissues are completely debrided from the aortic annulus, membranous septum, and anterior leaflet of the mitral valve. The diameters of the aortic annulus and sinotubular junction are measured with a

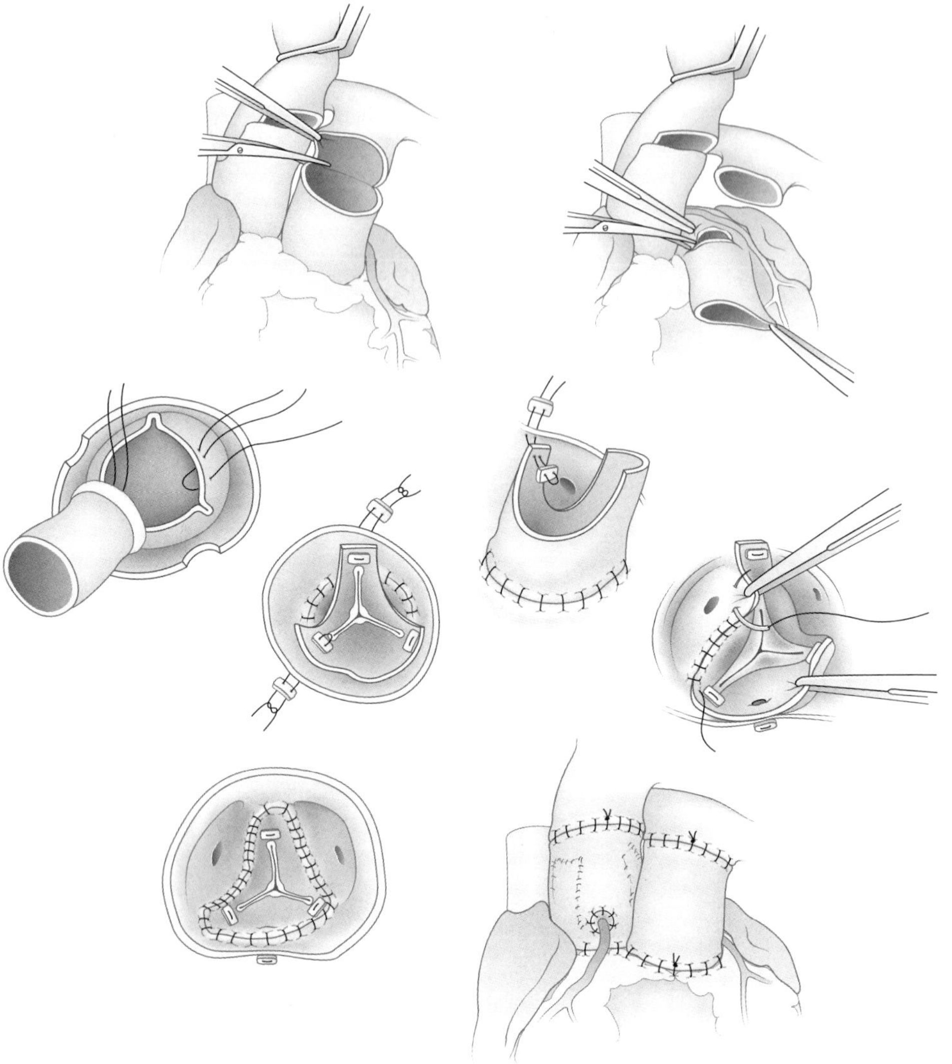

Figure 68–17 The Ross procedure: Subcoronary implantation.

metric sizer. The pulmonary artery is opened just before its bifurcation and the valve cusps are inspected. If they are normal, the pulmonary root is excised. The incision in the right ventricular outflow tract is made along a single horizontal plane approximately 3 mm below the lowest level of the pulmonary annulus. Care must be exercised to prevent damage to the left anterior descending artery and the first septal perforator branch. It is difficult to measure the diameter of the pulmonary annulus because it is entirely attached to distensible muscle, but it can be estimated by measuring the diameter of the sinotubular junction of the pulmonary root. The diameter of the pulmonary annulus is 15–20% larger than the diameter of the sinotubular junction. If the diameters of the aortic annulus and sinotubular junction of the two roots are similar, the technique of subcoronary implantion will work well. If there is mismatch in size, an alternate technique should be used and the difference in diameters corrected.[26] When the pulmonary annulus is slightly larger than the aortic annulus, it can be reduced by placing the sutures beneath the subcommissural triangles close together in the left ventricular outflow tract rather than in the pulmonary autograft. The smallest pulmonary sinus (usually the posterior sinus) should be oriented toward the left aortic sinus. The pulmonary autograft is secured to the left ventricular outflow tract and aortic annulus with multiple interrupted 4-0 polyester sutures. It is very important that all sutures be precisely distributed along a single horizontal plane at a level where the pulmonary annulus coincides with the level of the aortic annulus. The three commissures are precisely suspended in the aortic root and stay sutures through both arterial walls are placed immediately above the commissures. The sinuses of the pulmonary autograft that face the left and right aortic sinuses are partially excised and sutured to the aortic sinuses around the coronary arteries with a continuous 5-0 polypropylene suture. The sinus of the pulmonary autograft that faces the noncoronary aortic sinus need not to be excised and it is sutured to the aortic root. It is important not to alter the diameter of the sinotubular junction of the pulmonary autograft when it is being sutured to the aortic root or when the aortotomy is closed. The right side of the heart is reconstructed with a pulmonary homograft. This homograft should be larger than the pulmonary autograft. Figure 68-17 illustrates the technique of subcoronary implantation.

Aortic Root Replacement

Aortic root replacement with a pulmonary autograft is done as described above for aortic root aneurysm. The aortic valve is excised and so are the sinuses, leaving 5 mm of arterial wall around the coronary artery orifices. The same steps described above are used to harvest the pulmonary autograft and measure it. If the aortic annulus is larger than the pulmonary annulus, a reduction annuloplasty is necessary. This can be accomplished by closing the subcommissural triangles of the noncoronary sinus of the aortic root as illustrated in Figure 68-18. The pulmonary autograft is secured to the left ventricular outflow tract with simple multiple interrupted 4-0 polyester sutures along a single horizontal plane. A strip of Teflon felt in this suture line improves hemostasis and may prevent annular dilation.[25] The coronary arteries are reimplanted into the respective sinuses. The pulmonary autograft is sutured to the ascending aorta. If the ascending aorta is dilated, it may need replacement or plication as illustrated in Figure 68-19. A strip of Dacron fabric or Teflon felt along this anastomosis prevents late dilation of the sinotubular junction.[25] Figure 68-18 illustrates a Ross procedure using the technique of aortic root replacement.

Aortic Root Inclusion

Another method of implanting the pulmonary autograft is the aortic root inclusion technique. The noncoronary aortic sinus should be incised vertically toward the aortic annulus to enhance exposure of the aortic root. The pulmonary autograft is secured to the aortic annulus using the same technique as described above. After suturing the pulmonary autograft in the left ventricular outflow tract, the three commissures are pulled gently upward to determine the positions of the right and left coronary artery orifices in the pulmonary autograft. Small openings (5 or 6 mm in diameter) are made in the sinuses of the pulmonary autograft sinuses that correspond to the coronary artery orifices. The arterial wall of the pulmonary sinus is then sutured to the aortic sinus around the coronary artery orifices with a continuous 6-0 polypropylene. The three commissures of the pulmonary autograft are also sutured to the aortic wall, and the aortotomy is closed including the aortic and pulmonary arterial walls. The incision made in the noncoronary sinus of the aortic root should be closed only if there is no bleeding between the two roots and if closure causes no distortion of the pulmonary autograft after unclamping the aorta. Figure 68-19 illustrates the technique of aortic root inclusion.

We believe that the techniques of aortic root inclusion and aortic root replacement are ideally suited for patients with mild or moderate dilation of the aortic root whereas subcoronary implantation should be reserved for patients with aortic and pulmonary roots of similar dimensions. Most surgeons, however, prefer the technique of aortic root replacement even in patients with normal aortic root because it is easier to perform and it is more reproducible than the other techniques.[7,13,33,70]

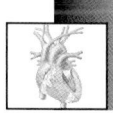

Clinical Outcomes

In spite of its technical complexity, the operative mortality associated with the Ross procedure is reportedly low. It ranges from 0 to 5%, and this variation is largely due to

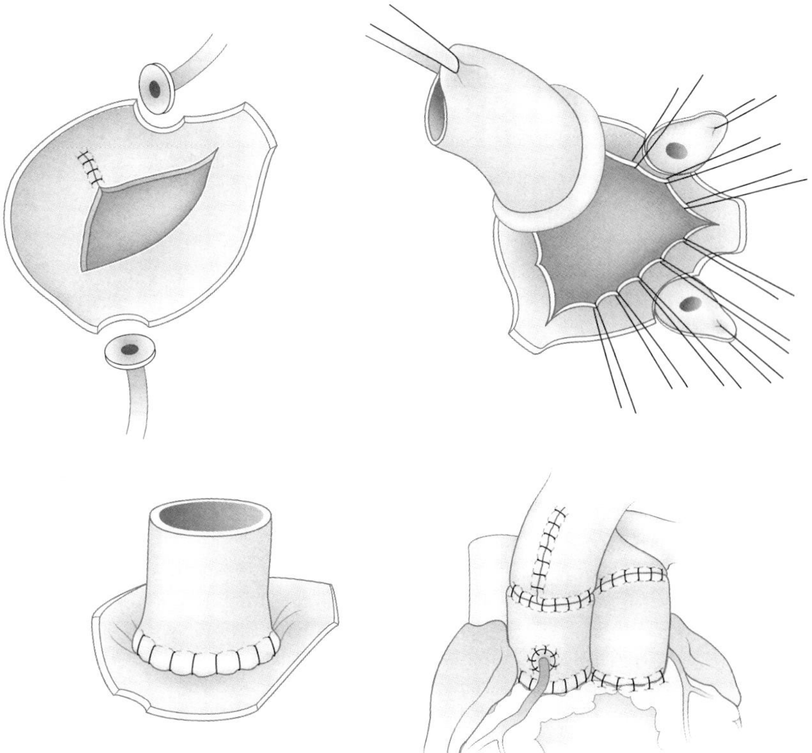

Figure 68–18 The Ross procedure: Aortic root replacement.

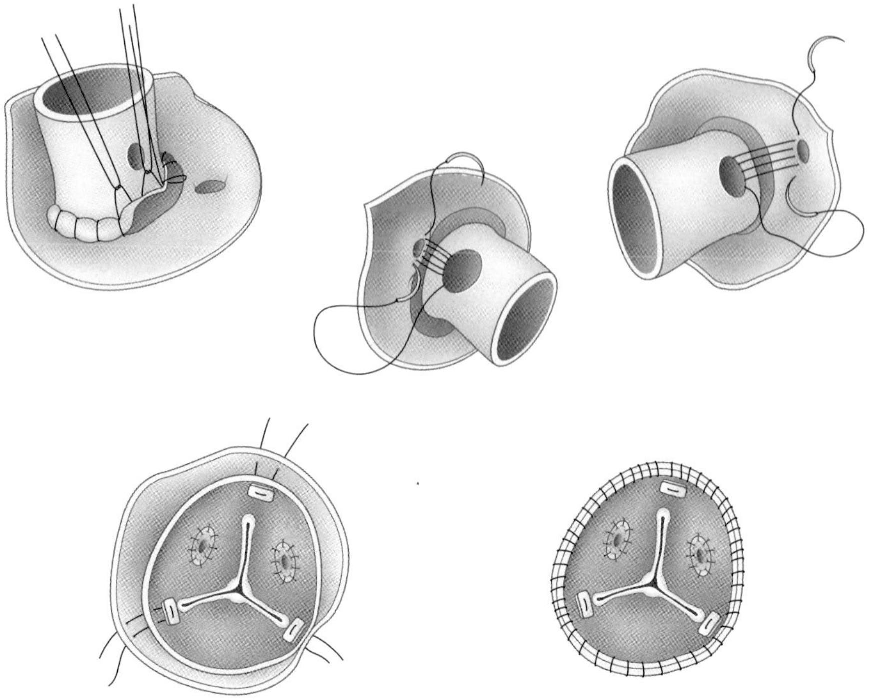

Figure 68–19 The Ross procedure: Aortic root inclusion.

associated procedures.* Postoperative bleeding may be a problem because of extensive dissection and suturing during the Ross procedure.[88] Another serious problem is early aortic insufficiency due to technical errors.[26] Thromboembolic complications are rare because of the nature of the valves used and the patients' age. Once the autograft is healed within the aortic root it should not be thrombogenic. We have documented a few episodes of transient ischemic attacks during the first few weeks after surgery but never after the first couple of months. The risk of infective endocarditis is also very low but patients who had the Ross procedure should have antibiotic prophylaxis as should any patient with heart valve disease.

Patients who had the Ross procedure should have annual Doppler echocardiography to assess the function of the aortic and pulmonary valves and measure the size of the aortic root. Dilation of the aortic annulus and/or sinotubular junction may occur after the Ross procedure and cause aortic insufficiency.[25,34] Dilation of the sinuses of the pulmonary autograft may occur, particularly after the technique of aortic root replacement.[25] We have shown that this problem is less likely to occur among patients who had the aortic root inclusion technique.[25] Aneurysms of the sinuses of the pulmonary autograft have been described.[25,83,89] If the pulmonary cusps remain normal, an aortic root reconstruction with preservation of the pulmonary valve is feasible; otherwise the patient needs replacement of the entire pulmonary autograft.[22,83,89] In the original experience of Ross, the freedom from autograft failure that needed reoperation was 75% at 20 years.[12] In the series by Elkins and colleagues, which is the largest in North America, freedom from reoperation or dysfunction of the pulmonary autograft (aortic insufficiency of 3+ or greater) was 83% at 9 years.[33] Many surgeons believe patients who had aortic root replacement with pulmonary autograft should be treated with a β-blocker and/or angiotensin-converting enzyme inhibitor during the first postoperative year to prevent dilation during the adaptation of the graft to systemic pressures but there are no scientific data to support this treatment.

Another problem with the Ross procedure is dysfunction of the biological valve used to reconstruct the right ventricular outflow tract.[12,33,34,75] A pulmonary homograft is probably the best conduit to use but it is not free from complications, and a number of patients develop stenosis of the graft.[75] Stenosis of the pulmonary artery rather than the valve is usually the case. When the peak gradient reaches 50 mm Hg or the patient develops symptoms, percutaneous balloon dilation with stenting or pulmonary valve rereplacement is indicated. In the series by Elkins and colleagues freedom from reoperation on the pulmonary homograft was 94% at 8 years.[33]

*References 7, 13, 25, 26, 33, 34, 36, 43, 70.

REFERENCES

1. Aizawa H, Hasegawa A, Arai M, et al: Bilateral coronary ostial stenosis and aortic regurgitation due to syphilitic aortitis. Intern Med 37:56–59, 1998.
2. Amarenco P, Cohen A, Tzourio C, et al: Atherosclerotic disease of the aortic arch and the risk of ischemic stroke. N Engl J Med 331:1474–1479, 1994.
3. Bachet K, Termignon JL, Goudot B, et al: Aortic root replacement with a composite graft. Factors influencing immediate and long-term results. Eur J Cardiothorac Surg 10:207–213, 1996.
4. Bentall HH, DeBono A: A technique of complete replacement of the ascending aorta. Thorax 23:338–339, 1968.
5. Birks EJ, Webb C, Child A, et al: Early and long-term results of a valve-sparing operation for Marfan syndrome. Circulation 100(Suppl. II):II29–35, 1999.
6. Blankenship J, Iliadis L: Coronary magnetic resonance angiography. N Engl J Med 346:1413–1414, 2002.

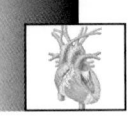

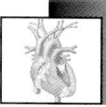

7. Böhm JO, Botha CA, Hemmer WB, et al: Older patients fare better with the Ross operation. Ann Thorac Surg 75:769–801, 2003.
8. Brewer R, Deck JD, Capati B, Nolan SP: The dynamic aortic root: Its role in aortic valve function. J Thorac Cardiovasc Surg 72:413–417, 1976.
9. Byrne JG, Aranki SF, Cohn LH: Aortic valve operations under deep hypothermic circulatory arrest for the porcelain aorta: "no touch" technique. Ann Thorac Surg 65:1313–1315, 1998.
10. Cabrol C, Pavie A, Gandjbakhch I, et al: Complete replacement of the ascending aorta with reimplantation of the coronary arteries: new surgical approach. J Thorac Cardiovasc Surg 81:309–315, 1981.
11. Cabrol C, Pavie A, Gandjbakhch I, et al: Complete replacement of the ascending aorta with reimplantation of the coronary arteries. New surgical approach. J Thorac Cardiovasc Surg 91:17–25, 1986.
12. Chambers CC, Sommerville J, Stone S, et al: Pumonary autograft procedure for aortic valve disease. Long term results of the pioneer series. Circulation 96:2206–2214, 1997.
13. Chemidtke C, Bechtel MF, Noetzold A, et al: Up to seven years experience with the Ross procedure in patients >60 years of age. J Am Coll Cardiol 36:1173–1177, 2000.
14. Clementi M, Notari L, Gorghi A. et al: Familial congenital bicuspid aortic valve: a disorder of uncertain inheritance. Am J Med Genet 62:336–338, 1996.
15. Coady MA, Rizzo JA, Hammond GL, et al: Surgical intervention criteria for thoracic aortic aneurysms: a study of growth rates and complications. Ann Thorac Surg 67:1922–1926, 1999.
16. Cohn LH, Rizzo RJ, Adams DH, et al: Reduced mortality and morbidity for ascending aortic aneurysm resection regardless of cause. Ann Thorac Surg 62:463–468, 1996.
17. Crawford ES, Svensson LG, Cosseli JS, et al: Surgical treatment of aneurysm and/or dissection of the ascending aorta, transverse aortic arch, and ascending aorta and transverse aortic arch. Factors influencing survival in 717 patients. J Thorac Cardiovasc Surg 98:659–674, 1989.
18. Dagum P, Green GR, Nistal FJ, et al: Deformational dynamics of the aortic root. Modes and physiologic determinants. Circulation 100(Suppl. II):II-54–II-62.
19. Dart AM, Lacombe F, Yeoh JK, et al: Aortic distensibility in patients with isolated hypercholesterolemia, coronary artery disease, or cardiac transplant. Lancet 338:270–273, 1991.
20. David TE: Remodeling of the aortic root and preservation of the native aortic valve. Oper Tech Card Thorac Surg 1:44–56, 1996.
21. David TE: Surgery of the aortic valve. Curr Probl Surg 36:421–504, 1999.
22. David TE, Armstrong S, Ivanov J, et al: Results of aortic valve-sparing operations. J Thorac Cardiovasc Surg 122:39–46, 2001.
23. David TE, Feindel CM, Bos J: Repair of the aortic valve in patients with aortic insufficiency and aortic root aneurysm. J Thorac Cardiovasc Surg 109:345–352, 1995.
24. David TE, Ivanov J, Armstrong S, et al: Aortic valve-sparing operations in patients with aneurysms of the aortic root or ascending aorta. Ann Thorac Surg 74:S1758–1761, 2002.
25. David TE, Omran A, Ivanov J, et al: Dilation of the pulmonary autograft after the Ross procedure. J Thorac Cardiovasc Surg 119:210–220, 2000.
26. David TE, Omran A, Webb G, et al: Geometric mismatch of the aortic and pulmonary roots causes aortic insufficiency after the Ross procedure. J Thorac Cardiovasc Surg 112:1231–1239, 1996.
27. de Oliveira, NC, David TE, Ivanov J, et al: Results of surgery for aortic root aneurysm in patients with the Marfan syndrome. J Thorac Cardiovasc Surg 125:1143–1152, 2003.
28. De Paepe A, Devereux RB, Dietz HC, et al: Revised diagnostic criteria for the Marfan syndrome. Am J Med Genet 62:417–426, 1996.
29. de Sa M, Moshkovitz Y, Butany J, et al: Histologic abnormalities of the ascending aorta and pulmonary trunk in patient with bicuspid aortic valve disease: clinical relevance to the Ross procedure. J Thorac Cardiovasc Surg 118:588–594, 1999.
30. Dossche KM, Schepens MA, Morshuis WJ, et al: A 23-year experience with composite valve graft replacement of the aortic root. Ann Thorac Surg 67:1070–1077, 1999.
31. d'Udekem Y, David TE, Feindel CM, et al: Long-term results of operation for paravalvular abscess. Ann Thorac Surg 62:48–53, 1996.
32. Edwards WD, Leaf DS, Edwards JE: Dissecting aortic aneurysm associated with congenital bicuspid aortic valve. Circulation 57:1022–1025, 1978.
33. Elkins RC: The Ross operation: a 12-year experience. Ann Thorac Surg 68:S14–18, 1999.
34. Elkins RC, Knott-Craig CJ, Ward KE, et al: Pulmonary autograft in children: realized growth potential. Ann Thorac Surg 57:1387–1394, 1994.
35. Elkins RC, Lane MM, McCue C: Pulmonary autograft reoperation: incidence and management. Ann Thorac Surg 62:450–455, 1996.
36. Elkins RC, Lane MM, McCue C: Ross procedure for ascending aortic replacement. Ann Thorac Surg 67:1843–1845, 1999.
37. Feczko JD, Lynch L, Pless JE, et al: An autopsy case review of 142 nonpenetrating (blunt) injuries to the aorta. J Trauma 33:846–849, 1992.
38. Fernandez MC, Duran AC, Real R, et al: Coronary artery anomalies and aortic valve morphology in the Syrian hamster. Lab Anim 34:145–154, 2000.
39. Friedrich MG, Shculz-Mdgnder J, Poetsch T, et al: Quantification of valvular aortic stenosis by magnetic resonance imaging. Am Heart J 144:329–334, 2002.
40. Furukawa K, Ohteki H, Cao ZL, et al: Does dilatation of the sinotubular junction cause aortic insufficiency? Ann Thorac Surg 68:949–953, 1999.
41. Fyfe BS, Quintana CS, Kaneka M, Griepp RB: Aortic sarcoma four years after Dacron graft insertion. Ann Thorac Surg 58:1752–1754, 1994.
42. Germain DP: Clinical and genetic features of vascular Ehlers-Danlos syndrome. Ann Vasc Surg 16(3):391–397, 2002.
43. Gerosa G, McKay R, Ross DN: Replacement of the aortic valve or root with a pulmonary autograft in children. Ann Thorac Surg 51:424–429, 1991.
44. Gott VL, Cameron DE, Alejo DE, et al: Aortic root replacement in 271 Marfan patients: a 24-year experience. Ann Thorac Surg 73:438–443, 2002.
45. Gott VL, Greene PS, Alejo DE, et al: Replacement of the aortic root in patients with Marfan's syndrome. N Engl J Med 340:1307–1313, 1999.
46. Hagl C, Galla JD, Lansman SL, et al: Replacing the ascending aorta and aortic valve for acute prosthetic valve endocarditis: is using prosthetic material contraindicated? Ann Thorac Surg 74:S1781–1785, 2002.
47. Heggtveit HA: Syphilitic aortitis: a clinicopathologic autopsy study of 100 cases, 1950 to 1960. Circulation 29:346–352, 1964.
48. Hirose Y, Hamada S, Takamiya M. et al: Aortic aneurysms: growth rates measured with CT. Radiology 185:249–252, 1992.
49. Huntington K, Hunter AG, Char KL: A prospective study to assess the frequency of familial clustering of congenital bicuspid aortic valve. J Am Coll Cardiol 30:1809–1812, 1997.
50. Hutchins GM, Moore GW, Skoog DK: The association of floppy mitral valve with disjunction of the mitral annulus fibrosus. N Engl J Med 314:535–540, 1986.

51. Kallenback K, Karck M, Leyh RG, et al: Valve-sparing aortic root reconstruction in patients with significant aortic insufficiency. Ann Thorac Surg 74:S1765–1768, 2002.
52. Kerr LD, Chang YJ, Spiera H, Fallon JT: Occult active giant cell aortitis necessitating surgical repair. J Thorac Cardiovasc Surg 120:813–815, 2000.
53. Kerut EK, Hanwalt C, Everson CT, et al: Left ventricular apex to descending aorta valved conduit: description of transthoracic and transesophageal echocardiographic findings in four cases. Echocardiography 18:463–468, 2001.
54. Klein RG, Hunder GG, Stanson AW, Sheps SG: Larger artery involvement in giant cell (temporal) arteritis. Ann Intern Med 83:806–812, 1975.
55. Kouchoukos NT, Marshall WG Jr, Wedige-Stecher TA: Eleven-year experience with composite graft replacement of the ascending aorta and aortic valve. J Thorac Cardiovasc Surg 92:691–705, 1986.
56. Kouchoukos NT, Wareing TH, Murphy SF, Perrillo JB: Sixteen-year experience with aortic root replacement. Ann Surg 214(3):308–320, 1991.
57. Kunzelman KS, Grande J, David TE, et al: Aortic root and valve relationships: impact on surgical repair. J Thorac Cardiovasc Surg 107:162–170, 1994.
58. Lawrie GM, Earle N, DeBakey ME: Long-term fate of the aortic root and aortic valve after ascending aneurysm surgery. Ann Surg 217:711–720, 1993.
59. LeMaire SA, DiBardino DJ, Koksoy C, Coselli JS: Proximal aortic reoperations in patients with composite valve grafts. Ann Thorac Surg 74:S1777–1780, 2002.
60. Lower RR, Stoffer RC, Shumway NE: Autotransplantation of the pulmonic valve into the aorta. J Thorac Cardiovasc Surg 39:680–687, 1960.
61. Lupi-Herrera E, Sanches-Torres G, Marcushamer J, et al: Takayasu's arteritis. Clinical study of 107 cases. Am Heart J 93:94–103, 1977.
62. Lytle BW, Sabik JF, Blackstone EH, et al: Reoperative cryopreserved root and ascending aorta replacement for acute aortic prosthetic valve endocarditis. Ann Thorac Surg 74:S1754–1757, 2002.
63. Matsuki O, Okita Y, Almeida RS, et al: Two decades' experience with aortic valve replacement with pulmonary autograft. J Thorac Cardiovasc Surg 95:705–711, 1988.
64. Matsumura Y, Osaki Y, Fukui T, et al: Protruding atherosclerotic aortic plaques and dyslipidaemia: correlation to subtypes of ischaemic stroke. Eur J Echocardiogr 3:1–2, 2002.
65. Mingke D, Dresler C, Stone CD, Borst HG: Composite graft replacement of the aortic root in 335 patients with aneurysm or dissection. Thorac Cardiovasc Surg 46:12–19, 1998.
66. Mohiaddin RH, Underwood SR, Bogren HG, et al: Regional aortic compliance studied by magnetic resonance imaging: the effects of age, training, and coronary artery disease. Br Heart J 62:90–96, 1989.
67. Murdoch JL, Walker BA, Halpern BL: Life expectancy and causes of death in the Marfan syndrome. N Engl J Med 286:804–808, 1972.
68. Nesi G, Anichini C, Pedemonte E, et al: Giant cell arteritis presenting with annuloaortic ectasia. Chest 121:1365–1367, 2002.
69. Niwa K, Perloff JK, Bhuta SM, et al: Structural abnormalities of great arterial walls in congenital heart disease: light and electron microscopic analyses. Circulation 103:393–400, 2001.
70. Oswalt JD, Dewan SJ, Mueller MC, Nelson S: Highlights of a ten-year experience with the Ross procedure. Ann Thorac Surg 71:S332–335, 2001.
71. Paelinck BP, Lasbm HJ, Bax JJ, et al: Assessment of diastolic function by cardiovascular magnetic resonance. Am Heart J 144:198–205, 2002.
72. Pressler V, McNamara JJ: Aneurysm of the thoracic aorta. Review of 260 cases. J Thorac Cardiovasc Surg 89:50–54, 1985.
73. Procter CD, Hollier LH: Takayasu's arteritis and temporal arteritis. Ann Vasc Surg 6:195–198, 1992.
74. Raanani E, David TE, Dellgren G, et al: Redo aortic root replacement: experience with 31 patients. Ann Thorac Surg 71(5):1460–1463, 2001.
75. Raanani E, Yau TM, David TE, et al: Risk factors for late pulmonary homograft stenosis after the Ross procedure. Ann Thorac Surg 70:1953–1957, 2000.
76. Ralph-Edwards A, David TE, Bos J: Infective endocarditis in patients who had replacement of the aortic root. Ann Thorac Surg 35:429–433, 1994.
77. Rojo-Leyva F, Ratliff NB, Cosgrove DM 3rd, Hoffman GS: Study of 52 patients with idiopathic aortitis from a cohort of 1,204 surgical cases. Arthritis Rheum 43:901–907, 2000.
78. Ross DN: Replacement of aortic and mitral valves with a pulmonary autograft. Lancet 2:956–958, 1967.
79. Rossiter JP, Morales AJ, Repke JT, et al: A prospective longitudinal evaluation of pregnancy in the Marfan syndrome. Am J Obstet Gynecol 173:1599–1604, 1995.
80. Sadee A, Becker AE, Verheul HA, et al: Aortic valve regurgitation and the congenitally bicuspid aortic valve: a clinico-pathological correlation. Br Heart J 67:439–441, 1992.
81. Sands MP, Rittenhouse EA, Mohri H, Merendino K: An anatomical comparison of human, pig, calf and sheep aortic valves. Ann Thorac Surg 8:407–414, 1969.
82. Schäfers HJ, Aicher D, Langer F: Correction of leaflet prolapse in valve-preserving aortic replacement: pushing the limits? Ann Thorac Surg 74:S1762–1764, 2002.
83. Schmidtke C, Stierle U, Sievers HH: Valve-sparing aortic root remodeling for pulmonary autograft aneurysm. J Heart Valve Dis 123:437–441, 2002.
84. Shapira OM, Cruz HA, Shemin RJ: Endarterectomy of the ascending aorta: an alternative method in patients with extensively calcified (porcelain) aorta requiring aortic valve replacement. J Card Surg 12:160–164, 1997.
85. Shimojo M, Tsuda N, Iwasaka T, Inuda M: Age-related changes in aortic elasticity determined by gated radionuclide angiography in patients with systemic hypertension or healed myocardial infarcts and in normal subjects. Am J Cardiol 68:950–953, 1991.
86. Shores J, Berger KR, Murphy EA, et al: Progression of aortic dilatation and the benefit of long-term β-adrenergic blockage in Marfan's syndrome. N Engl J Med 330:1335–1341, 1994.
87. Silverman DI, Burton KJ, Gray J: Life expectancy in the Marfan syndrome. Am J Cardiol 75:157–160, 1995.
88. Stelzer P, Jones DJ, Elkins RC: Aortic root replacement with pulmonary autograft. Circulation 80(Suppl. III):III209–213, 1988.
89. Sundt TM, Moon MR, Xu R: Reoperation for dilatation of the pulmonary autograft after the Ross procedure. J Thorac Cardiovasc Surg 122:1249–1252, 2001.
90. Swanson WM, Clark RE: Dimensions and geometric relationships of the human aortic valve as a function of pressure. Circ Res 35:871–882, 1974.
91. Ueno A, Awane G, Wakabayachi A: Successfully operated obliterative brachiocephalic arteritis (Takayasu) associated with elongated coarctation. Jpn Heart 8:538–544, 1967.
92. Veinot JP: Congenitally bicuspid aortic valve and associated medial disease. Ann Thorac Surg 71:1067–1068, 2001.
93. Vogt PR, Brunner-LaRocca HP, Carrel T, et al: Cryopreserved arterial allografts in the treatment of major vascular infection:

a comparison with conventional surgical techniques. J Thorac Cardiovasc Surg 116:965–972, 1998.
94. Wenstrup RJ, Meyer RA, Lyle JS, et al: Prevalence of aortic root dilation in the Ehlers-Danlos syndrome. Genet Med 4:112–117, 2002.
95. Wright EP, Glick AD, Virmani R, Page DL: Aortic intimal sarcoma with embolic metastases. Am J Surg Pathol 9:950–957, 1985.
96. Yacoub MH, Gehle P, Chandrasekaran V, et al: Late results of a valve-preserving operation in patients with aneurysms of the aorta and root. J Thorac Cardiovasc Surg 115:1080–1090, 1998.
97. Yasuda T, Kawasuji M, Sakakibara N, Watanabe Y: Aortic valve replacement for calcified ascending aorta in homozygous familial hypercholesterolemia. Eur J Cardiothorac Surg 18:249–250, 2000.

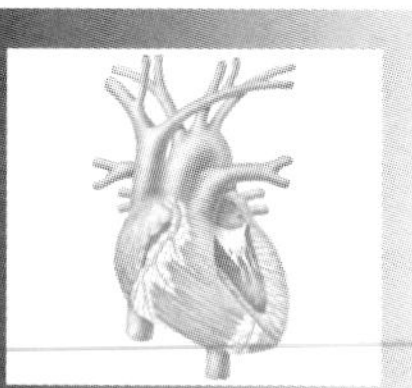

CHAPTER 69A

Surgery of the Aortic Arch, Descending Thoracic and Thoracoabdominal Surgery, and Aortic Dissection

Surgery of the Aortic Arch

Lars G. Svensson

HISTORICAL NOTE

The history of cardioaortic surgery is replete with new techniques being developed for ascending or aortic arch repairs starting with the operation on August 18, 1956, when Denton Cooley and Michael DeBakey replaced the ascending aorta with a homograft using cardiac bypass.[1–41,43–63] In 1957, DeBakey and colleagues[12] first described aortic arch replacement using antegrade brain perfusion. Prior to this, one of the few successful ascending aortic repairs was reported in 1932 by Blalock, who repaired a stab wound of the ascending aorta caused by an ice pick.[47] By removing the occluding clot, Blalock noted "bright red blood that shot over the screen at the head of the table on the anesthetist's clothes." Using only nitrous oxide and oxygen during the anesthetic in a patient with cardiac tamponade most likely contributed to the hypertension and description of the procedure.

With the advent of cardiopulmonary bypass, technical problems in doing aortic arch surgery became considerably simpler. In 1950, Bigelow[47] first published the results of his experiments in dogs using deep hypothermia for cardiovascular operations without cardiopulmonary bypass. Nonetheless, it was not until 1963 that Barnard[2] combined deep hypothermia with circulatory arrest and cardiopulmonary bypass for aortic arch operations and dissection. In 1964 Borst[47] reported using deep hypothermia and circulatory arrest to repair an arteriovenous fistula between the innominate vein and the aorta caused by shrapnel. The routine use of deep hypothermia and circulatory arrest did not, however, become popular until 1975 when Griepp[47] reported a series of aortic arch replacements using deep hypothermia and circulatory arrest. In 1983 Borst et al[3,4,22] reported replacing the aortic arch and leaving a tube graft lying free in the descending aorta, which they called the "elephant trunk" technique. In 1990, Crawford, Svensson, and colleagues[47,57] reported replacement of the entire aorta as a planned stage procedure using a modified elephant trunk technique. The modification of inverting the graft into the descending aorta while sewing the distal anastomosis resulted in a more secure anastomosis with less risk of bleeding or rupture.[57] Subsequently, in 1993, Svensson and colleagues[47] successfully replaced the entire aorta from the aortic valve to the aortic bifurcation during a single operation using a combined mediastinal and thoracoabdominal incision with deep hypothermia and circulatory arrest.[12]

Currently, aortic arch surgery has become relatively common and safe with a mortality risk of 2% and a stroke risk of 2%.[55] In 2002, we performed 999 aorta operations, 423 on the ascending aorta and aortic arch. Our approach is discussed later.

This chapter will discuss the potential etiologies of aortic arch aneurysms, the association with some pathological entities, diagnostic workup, brain protection, perfusion methods, different operative approaches, and outcomes after aortic arch surgery.

DEFINITIONS AND CLASSIFICATION

Anatomically, the aortic arch is defined as the segment of aorta between a line at a right angle proximal to the innominate artery origin and extending to a line drawn at a right angle distal to the origin of the left subclavian artery.[47] Aneurysms are irreversible dilatations of the aorta exceeding the normal diameter for the age and height of the patient.[47] The exact size at which the aorta is labeled "aneurysmal" varies. Definitions vary from 1.5 times to twice the normal aorta. In patients with Marfan syndrome, we suggest that when the cross-sectional area (in square centimeters) divided by the patient's height (in meters) exceeds a ratio of 10, this should then be considered significant and an indication that the patient requires surgical repair.[50] Thus, in some respect, the definition of an aneurysm is not absolute, but rather refers to the significant dilatation of the aorta.

Aneurysms can be divided further into aortic aneurysms without penetration through the aortic adventitia (true aneurysms) and those that penetrate through the adventitia and are contained by the surrounding tissue that prevents exsanguination of the patient (false aneurysms).[47] In addition, aneurysms are classified according to their likely etiology: medial degenerative aneurysms (typically showing loss of elastic tissue); those related to aortic dissection; other disorders of connective tissue, particularly loss of collagen as in Ehler–Danlos syndrome or loss of elastic tissue as in Marfan syndrome; those associated with blunt trauma; aortitis; primary aortic infections or following previous cardiovascular surgery, especially graft infection in the ascending aorta; and congenital abnormalities.[47]

We prefer the term medial-degenerative aneurysms to atherosclerotic aneurysms simply because not all medial-degenerative aneurysms have atherosclerosis within them.[47] Furthermore, atherosclerosis does not appear to be necessarily the sole etiological factor in the development of medial-degenerative aneurysms. It appears that atheroma formation, fibrosis, and calcification are results of degeneration that follow the primary injurious event that caused the aneurysm.

Aneurysms can be either fusiform, showing uniform dilatation, or saccular in appearance.[47] The three most common sites for saccular aneurysms are on the lesser curve of the aortic arch, the descending aorta, and opposite the visceral vessels.[47] The saccular aneurysms in the aortic arch are usually related to penetrating ulcers, often with localized dissection or mycotic aneurysm formation.[47] Fusiform aneurysms of the aortic arch are typically associated with dilatation of the ascending aorta, particularly when associated with inflammatory aortitis. Medial-degenerative aneurysms of the root are known as annuloaortic ectasia, a term coined by Cooley.[47] This results in a flask-like or hourglass appearance of the aortic root (Erdheim deformity), which is also associated in particular with Marfan syndrome. For example, in Marfan syndrome, initiation of aortic root dilatation results early in the annuloaortic ectasia stage and, if not treated, there is subsequent development of aortic root, ascending aorta, and aortic arch aneurysm formation. In fact, at this late stage, aortic dissection will often precede aortic arch aneurysm formation.

The human artery consists of five distinct layers. The first or innermost layer (the endothelial layer, which lies on a basement membrane) is known as tunica intima. Between the tunica intima and the tunica media is a fenestrated sheath of elastic fibers known as the internal elastic lamina. The tunica media has several layers of elastic tissue lamellae arranged concentrically along the length of the aorta and forms the bulk of the aortic wall. The amount of elastic tissue decreases in an amount from the sinotubular ridge as the aorta progresses down to the aortic bifurcation. Within the tunica media lies smooth muscle cells and the ground substance of the aorta. The latter consists of proteoglycans. The outer third of the tunica media receives its nutrition from the vasovasorum, lymphatics, and nerves. On the outside of the tunica media is the external elastic lamina, which separates the media from the adventitia. The tunica adventitia consists of strong, tough layers of collagen and elastic fibers. Because of its strength, this is the critical layer wherein the surgeon must sew the sutures for graft placement.[47]

To date, there has been no clear, systematic classification of aortic pathology in the literature with different pathologists coining a variety of terms. In our experience, we favor a definition of aortic pathology based on hematoxylin and eosin (H&E) findings and elastic tissue stains. Thus, medial-degenerative disease is defined as a loss of elastic fibers and medial necrosis as a loss of smooth muscle cells. The presence of atherosclerosis superimposed on degenerative disease is described as atherosclerotic with or without calcification. Atheroma is also frequently superimposed. Inflammatory disease is diagnosed when there is evidence of chronic inflammatory cell infiltrates. The intima and adventitia may also show various degrees of hyperplasia.[47]

ETIOLOGICAL AND PREDISPOSING FACTORS

Congenital Aneurysms

Congenital aneurysms of the aortic arch are extremely rare, although they may be associated with aberrant right subclavian arteries from a Kommerell's diverticulum situated in either the distal aortic arch or proximal descending aorta (Figure 69A-1A and B).[47] Similarly, aneurysms can be associated with one of two types of right-sided congenital arches (Figure 69A-1C and D). For the Felson and Palayew type I right-sided arches, there is a vascular ring that encircles and compresses the esophagus and trachea (Figure 69A-1C).[36] The distal arch and descending aorta may be aneurysmal. In patients with type II right-sided arches (Figure 69A-1D), the anatomy is basically a mirror image of an aberrant right subclavian artery with a Kommerell's diverticulum. Thus, an aberrant left subclavian artery comes off the right-sided descending aorta.[36] More frequently, however, the aortic arch, in association with these two varieties, is hypoplastic unless the hypoplasia is severe enough to cause aortic stenosis and prestenosis or poststenosis aneurysm formation occurs. Coarctation of the aorta is often associated with a bicuspid valve and ascending aortic aneurysm but, if left untreated, may sometimes be associated with aortic arch aneurysm formation. A history of patent ductus arteriosus or ventricular septal defect may also be noted.

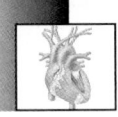

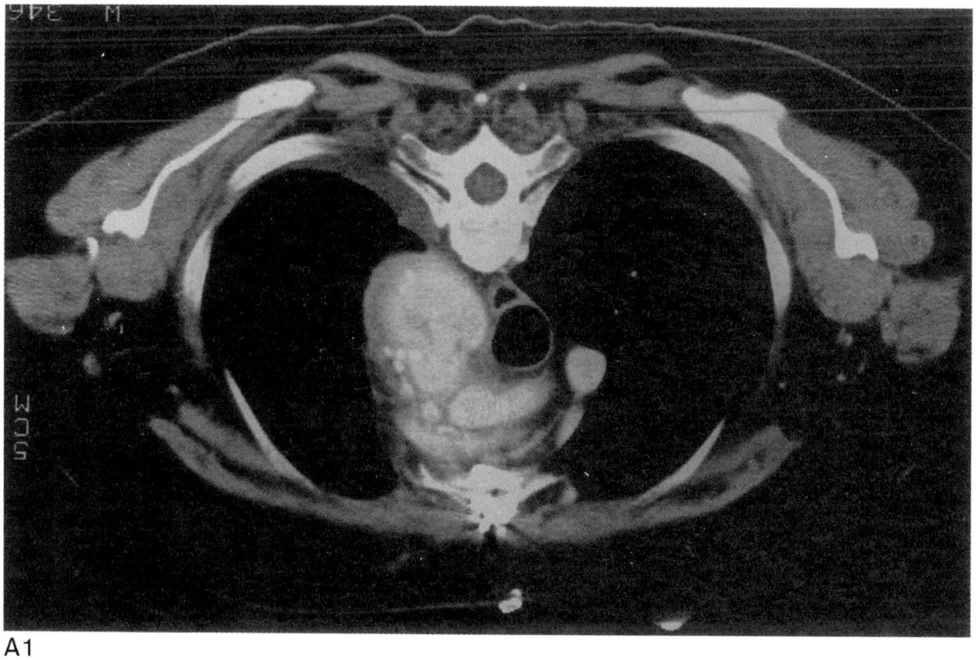

A1

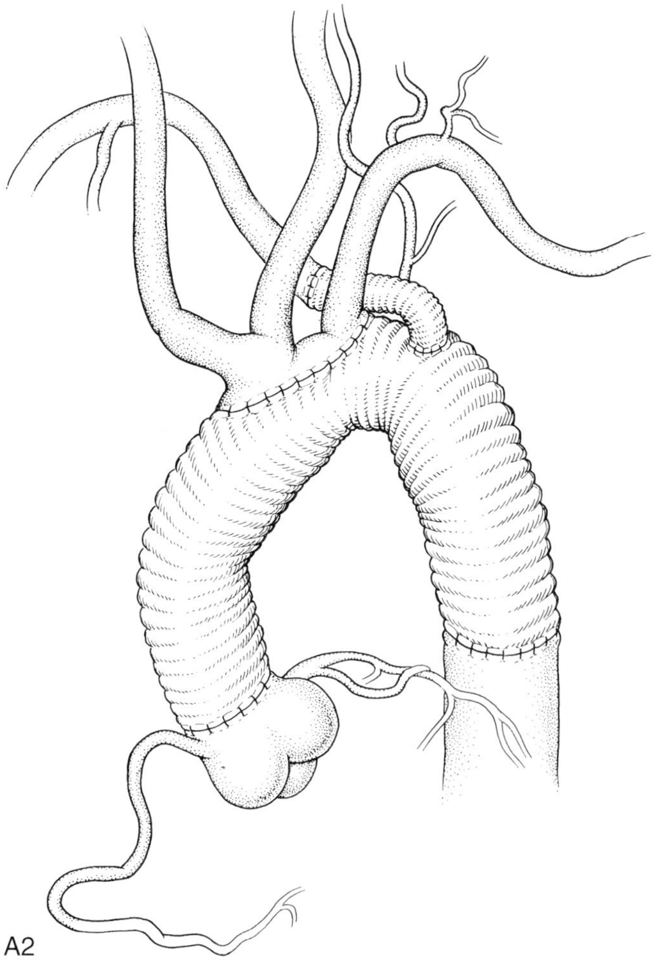

A2

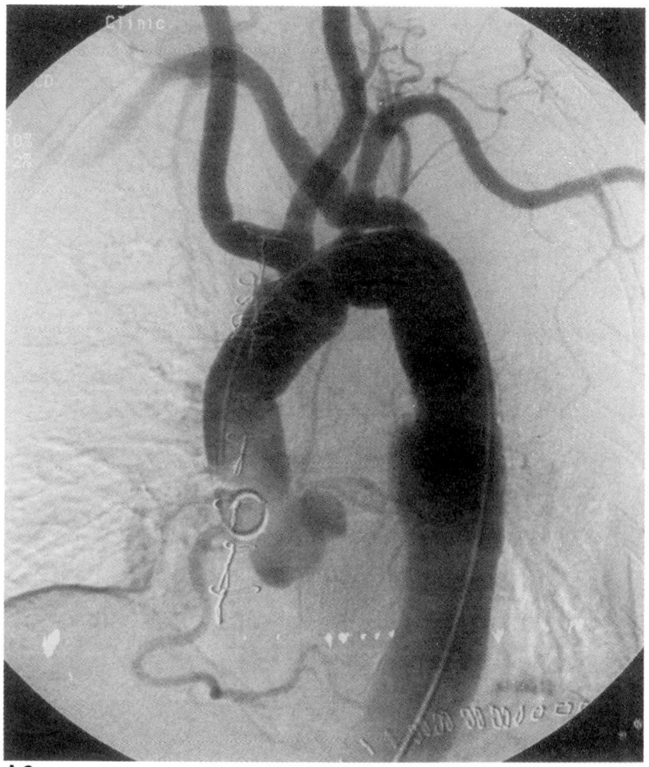

A3

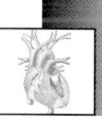

Figure 69A–1 A, Example of an aortic arch aneurysm associated with an aberrant right subclavian artery that was treated by a modified elephant trunk technique. (1) The first stage elephant trunk procedure was done with an anastomosis between the left subclavian artery and the aberrant right subclavian artery. (2) The second stage elephant trunk procedure was performed with an interposition graft to the right subclavian artery. (3) The completed repair and angiogram. Note the tube graft to the right subclavian artery arising from the more distal part of the aortic arch.

(Continued)

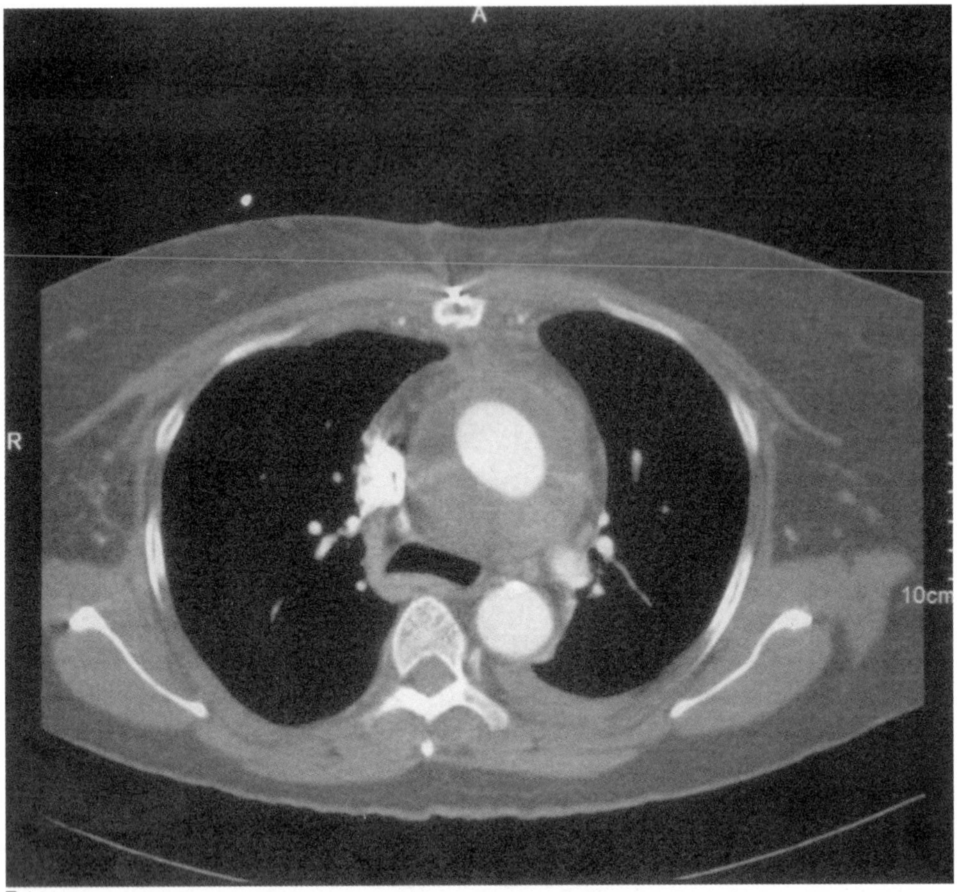

B1

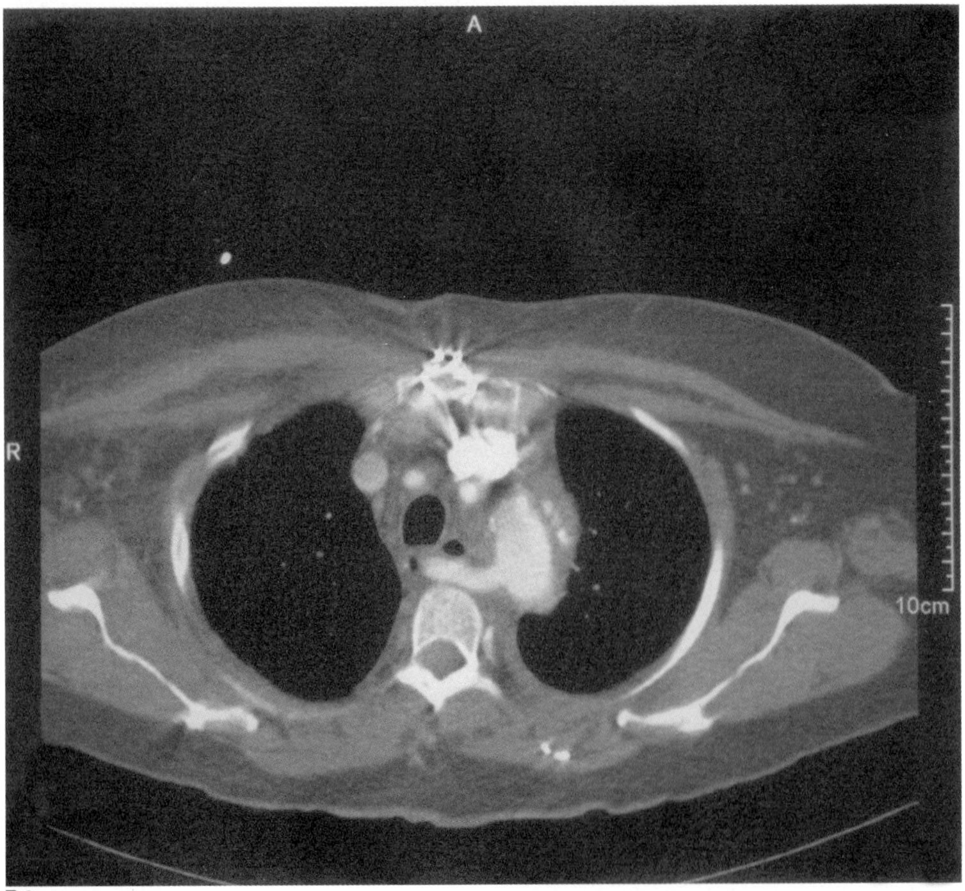

B2

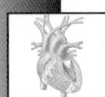

Figure 69A–1 cont'd B, (1) Example of a patient with an ascending and arch aneurysm with extensive clot formation within the aneurysm associated with a right aberrant subclavian artery. (2) The CT scan after the repair. The repair was done from the aberrant right subclavian artery ostium, through the aortic arch, using a long "tongue" extension into the descending aorta. The ascending aorta was replaced with a composite valve graft. Note the aberrant right subclavian artery coming off the distal aorta and running posterior to the esophagus and trachea.

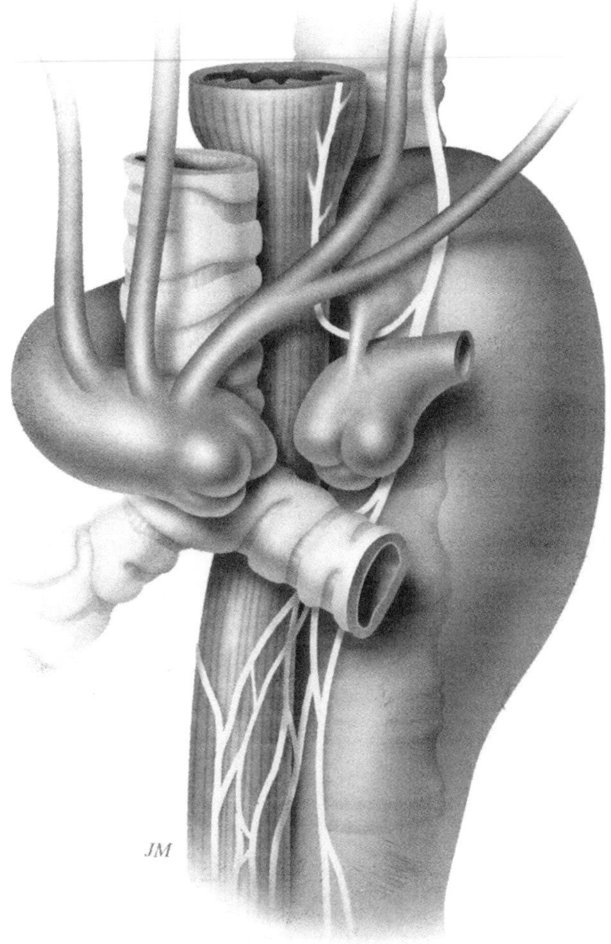

C1

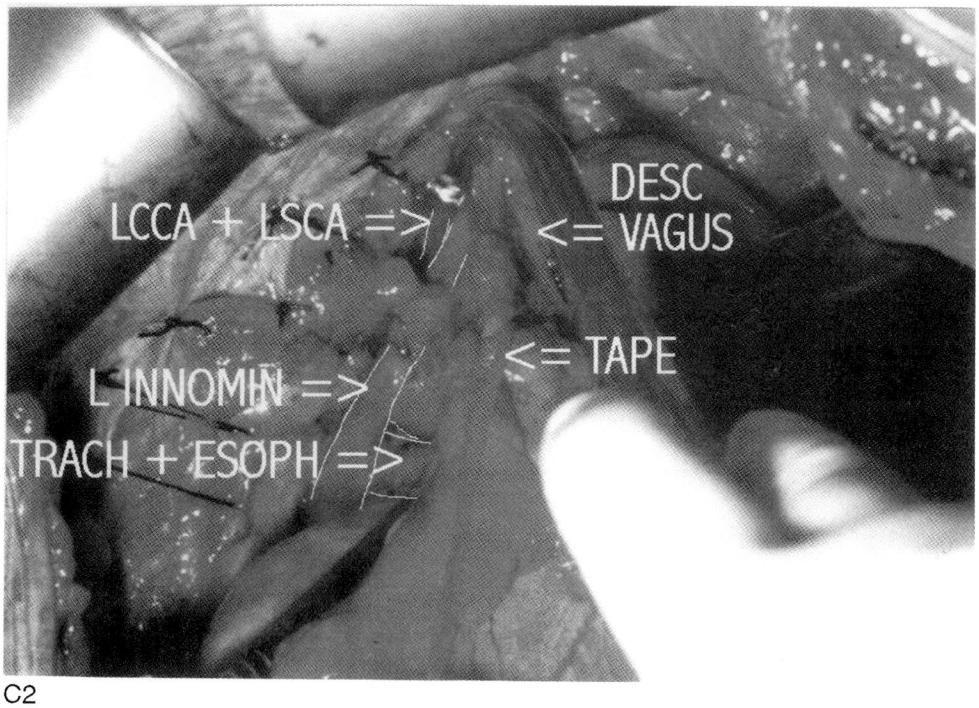

C2

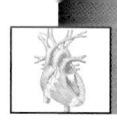

Figure 69A–1 cont'd C, (1) Illustration of right-sided aortic arch with vascular ring and (2) intraoperative findings. DESC, descending aorta; LCAA + LSCA, left common carotid artery and left subclavian artery; L INNOMIN, left innominate artery; TRACH + ESOPH, trachea and esophagus.

(Continued)

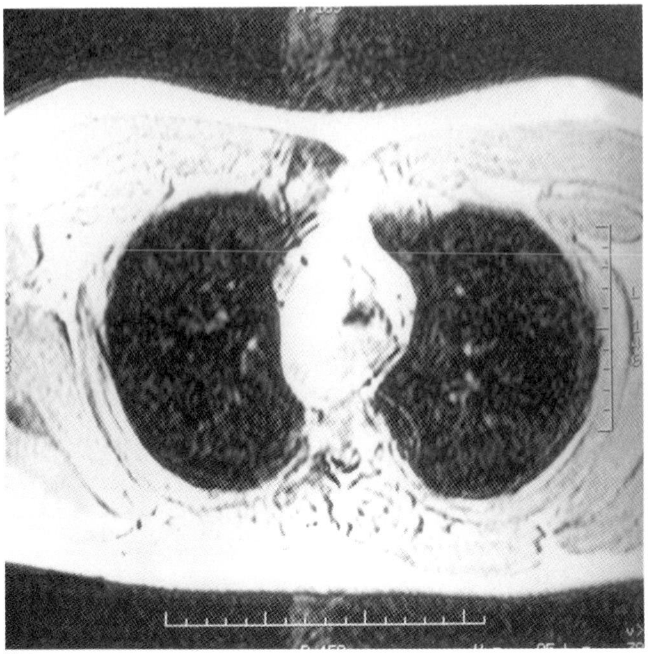

D1

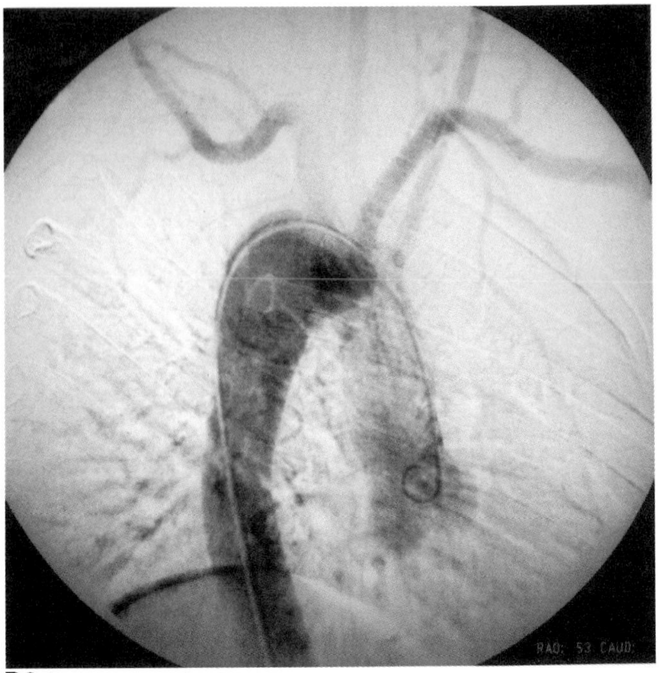

D2

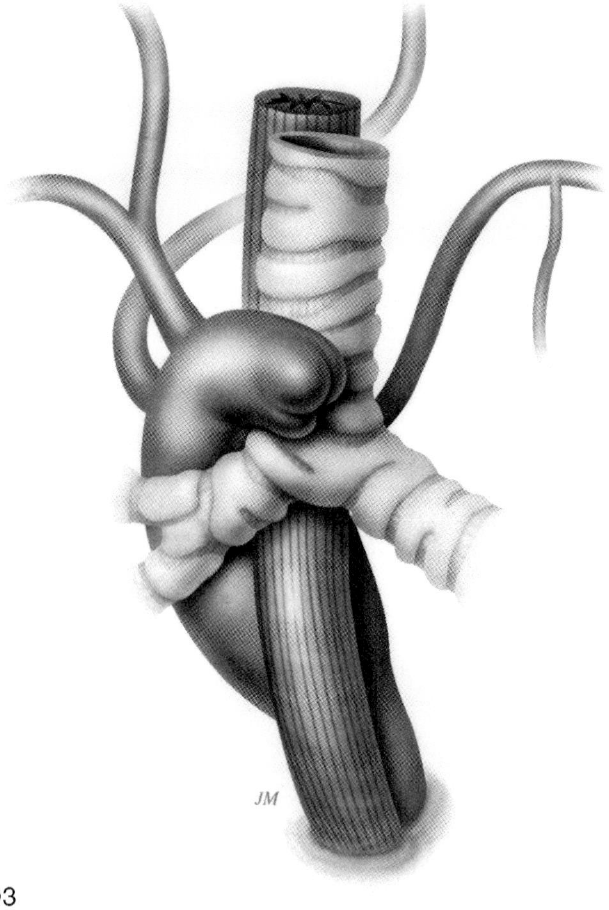

D3

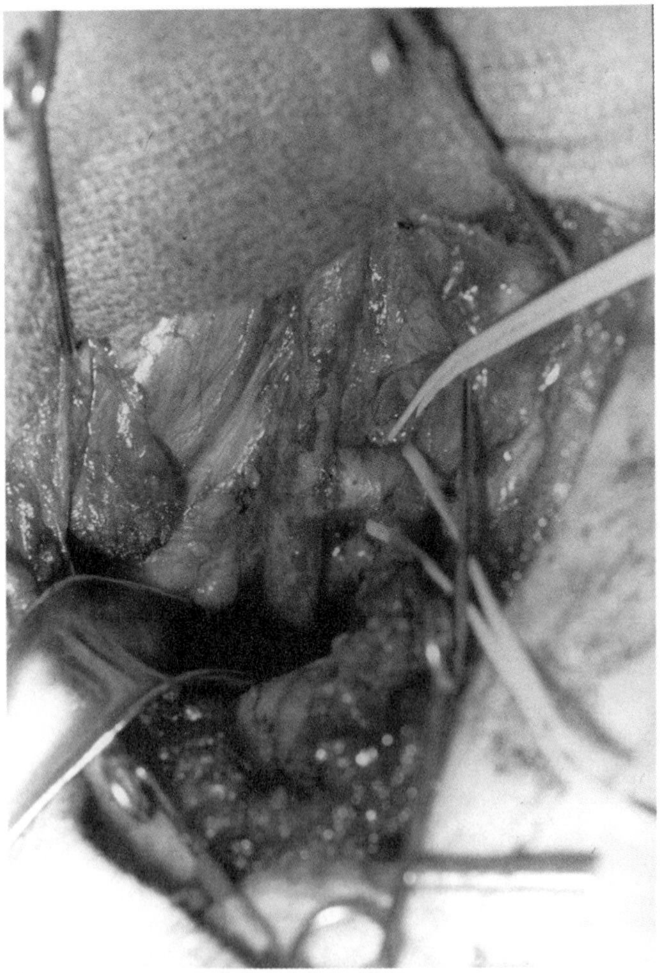

D4

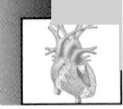

Figure 69A–1 cont'd **D,** (1) MRI of right-sided arch compressing the trachea, bronchus, and esophagus. (2) Angiogram. (3) Anatomy illustration. (4) Left subclavian to carotid anastomosis.

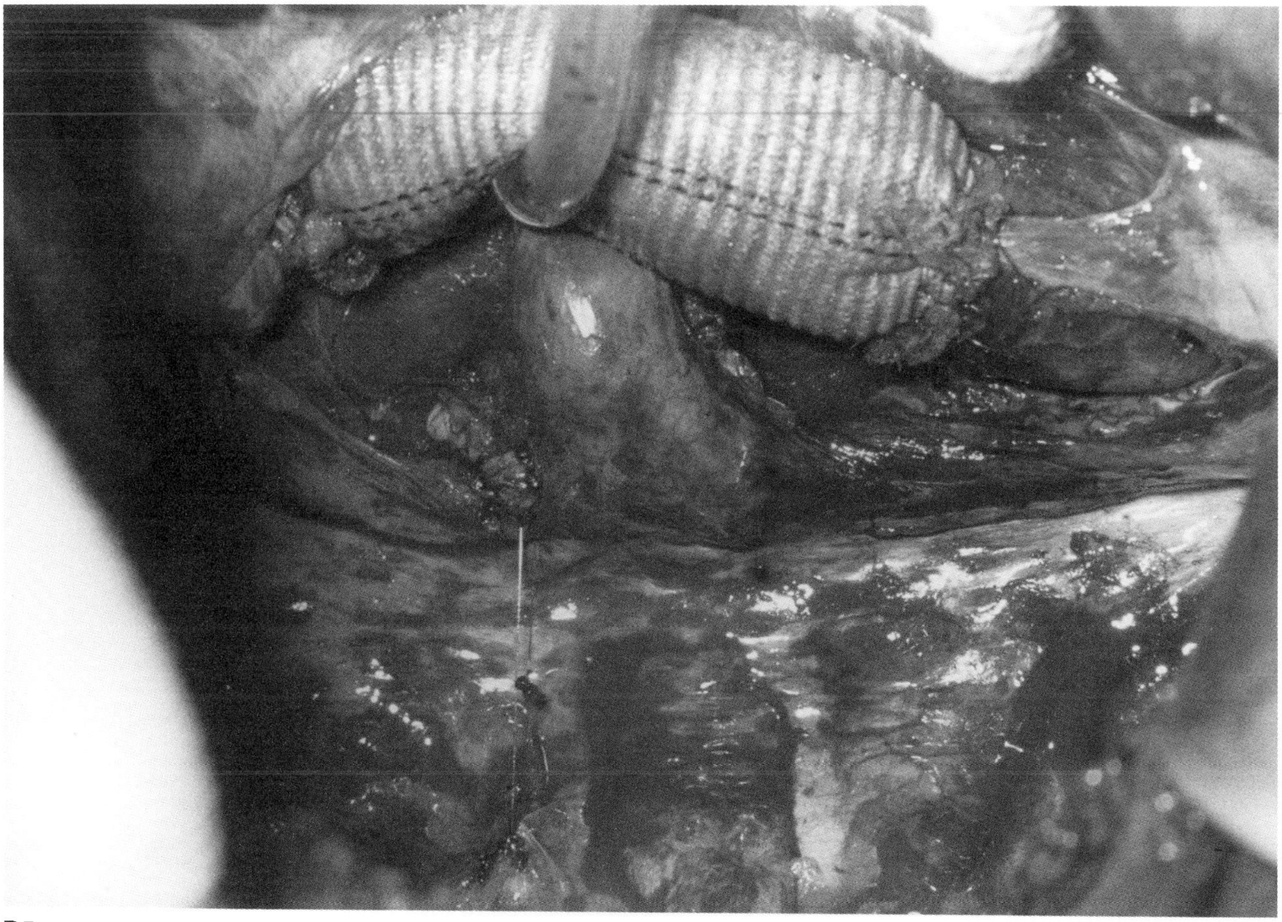

D5

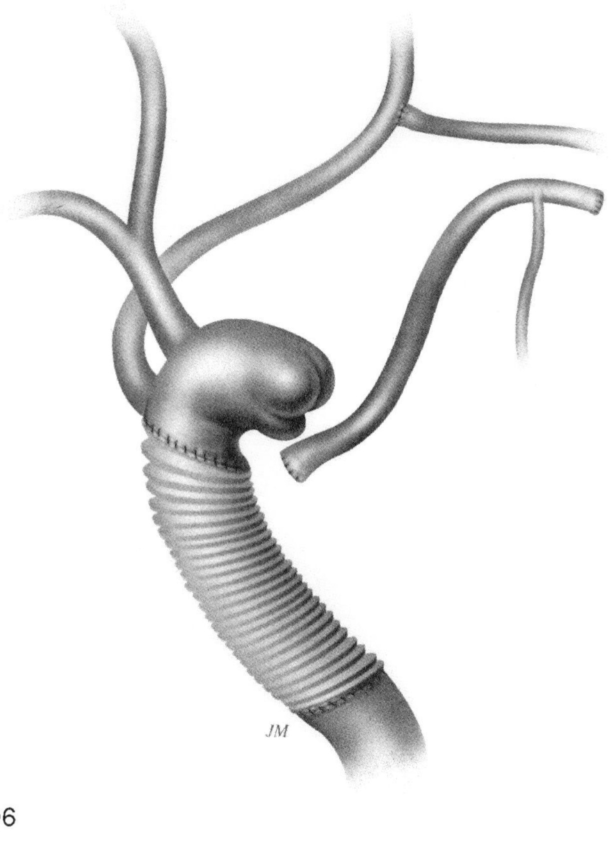

D6

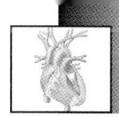

Figure 69A–1 cont'd (5) Distal arch and descending aorta replacement with Kommerell's diverticulum oversewn (a stay suture is attached to the stump). (6) Illustration of repair.

(Continued)

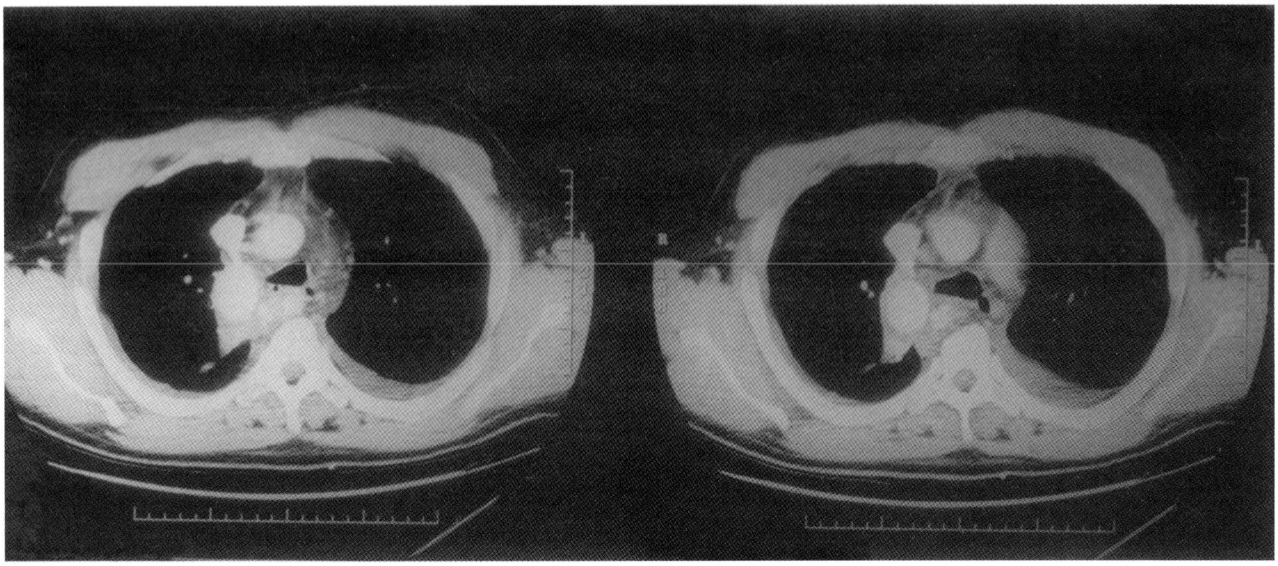

D7

Figure 69A–1 cont'd (7) Postoperative CT with tracheal compression relieved.

More rarely, adult patients with ascending and aortic arch aneurysms, who have been previously operated upon for an interrupted aortic arch, may present.[47]

Medial-Degenerative Aneurysms

Medial degenerative aneurysms typically occur in elderly patients who have been long-term smokers or who have had a long history of hypertension. If the smoking history is severe and there is presence of chronic obstructive pulmonary disease (COPD), then extensive atheroma formation may also be found within the aneurysms. These types of aneurysms, with extensive atheroma and atherosclerosis formation, typically will involve not only the ascending aorta and the aortic arch but also the descending and thoracoabdominal aorta. Coronary artery disease and carotid artery disease are also common associations. At the time of inspection of the aorta, small ulcers are often observed and these can later form penetrating ulcers that result in dissection in the media adventitial plane or false aneurysm formation if the adventitia is penetrated.[47] Less typically, medial degenerative aneurysms are associated with systemic inflammatory disease and various types of arthritis or vasculitis (see later).

Aortic Dissection

Aortic dissection is discussed later in this chapter. It is important to keep in mind the difference between the DeBakey and Stanford classifications and also the different classes of dissection[51] (Figure 69A-2) when replacing the aortic arch. The class of intimal tear will also influence the aortic arch repair technique.[51]

Mycotic Aneurysms

For reasons not entirely clear, true primary mycotic aneurysms of the aorta, as described by Svensson and Crawford,[47] have a tendency to occur either on the lesser curve of the aortic arch with a variable extent of involvement or opposite the visceral vessels in the abdomen. Whether this is related to the structure of the aorta or because of flow patterns resulting in turbulence in these areas opposite branches of the aorta is unclear. The typical infective organisms are *Escherichia coli*, staphylococcal species, *Salmonella*, and streptococcal species including strep pneumococcus. Other strains, however, may sometimes be detected. Some of these may be related to atherosclerotic ulcers that initially act as a nidus for subsequent infection to occur. Mycotic aneurysms frequently penetrate through the aortic arch wall resulting in false aneurysms or free rupture. The reason Osler labeled these aneurysms as mycotic was because the gray slimy lining often seen in these aneurysms reminded him of fungal growth. Human fungal infections are, on the whole, very rare, with the exception of patients who have had previous graft infections.[47]

Vasculitis and Aortitis

Inflammatory infiltrates of the aorta are not infrequent. In a prospective examination of histological specimens by both H&E and elastic tissue stains, inflammatory infiltrates were found in over 2570 of the specimens.[53] Although these inflammatory infiltrates consist of various types of leukocytes, often associated with the diseases listed below, an associated systemic illness may be absent. This would suggest that the etiological factor had gone unrecognized, causing aortic injury, which subsequently presents as a medial-degenerative aneurysm, including formation of atherosclerosis and calcification. Previous chest radiation for Hodgkin's disease or breast malignancies may also be noted in the history. Radiation-induced vasculitis is associated with severe calcification and a porcelain aorta. A stiff left ventricle, scarred right ventricle, and fixed cardiac output increase the risk of surgery.

Inflammatory systemic diseases may result in aneurysms. For example, the development of aortitis is commonly associated with Takayasu's disease (nonspecific aortoarteritis) (Figure 69A-3); giant cell arteritis (Horton's disease); temporal arteritis; polymyalgia rheumatica; Behçet's, Buerger's, Logan's, Sjögren's, Reiter's, or Kawasaki's disease; relapsing

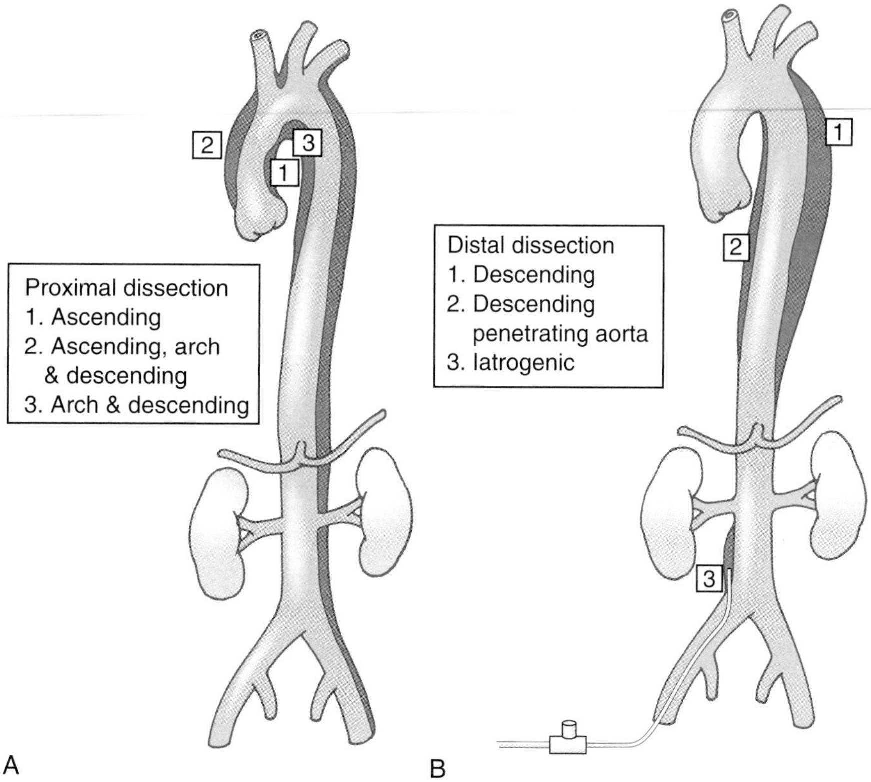

Figure 69A–2 **A,** Aortic dissection classification. A proximal dissection indicates: (1) ascending only involvement; (2) ascending, aortic arch and descending aorta involvement; and (3) arch and descending involvement. **B,** Distal dissection: (1) involvement of the descending aorta with or without the abdominal aorta; (2) penetrating aortic ulcer with descending dissection; and (3) abdominal dissection, most iatrogenic.

polychondritis; systemic lupus erythematosus (often mycotic); rheumatoid arthritis; sarcoid and ankylosing spondylitis; osteoarthritis of unknown origin; ulcerative colitis; and potentially autoimmune disease of the thyroid such as Hashimoto's.

Histologically, Takayasu's disease has panaortitis, severe intimal hyperplasia, severe adventitial fibrosis with perivascular inflammation. In contradistinction, giant cell aortitis has inflammatory margins around areas of medial necrosis and inflammation of the media. Fibrosis and intimal hyperplasia are minimal.

Trauma

Ten percent of traumatic lesions of the aorta occur in the aortic arch. The remaining 90% occur in other segments that will be discussed in Chapter 69B. The aneurysms are most often related to tears at the hinge point of the aorta during acceleration or deceleration injuries. Thus, the usual sites of primary tears occur at either the origin of the innominate artery or the subclavian artery (70–80%), although the origin of the common carotid artery may also be involved.[47] Although blunt trauma is the most common etiology in the United States, for traumatic arch injuries, penetrating injuries from shrapnel or bullets or knife injuries are more frequently observed in the third world. With penetrating lesions, involvement of the trachea, esophagus, venous system, nerves, and vertebral column significantly complicates the management of the injuries.

Tumors of the Arch

Tumors of the aortic arch are extremely rare and when they do occur are usually found distal to the subclavian artery. Very rarely have tumors been related to prosthetic grafts.[47]

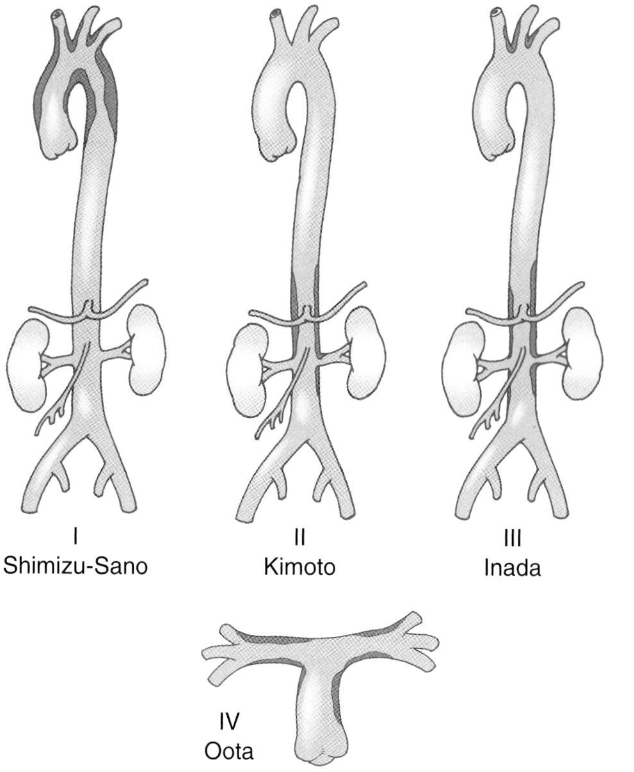

Figure 69A–3 **Classification of Takayasu aortitis with the extent and subtypes depicted in the illustration.** PA, pulmonary artery.[47]

Reoperations

Patients who have undergone previous cardiovascular surgery may require reoperation either for new aneurysm formation or for false aneurysm formation. Approximately half of all patients undergoing arch operations have had previous cardiovascular surgery. Two typical scenarios are presented below.

The first case is the patient who earlier underwent acute dissection repair and subsequently presents with an aortic arch aneurysm because the weakened aorta from the dissection dilates over time. This situation occurs commonly in patients with Marfan syndrome. We have previously argued that it is better to repair only the ascending aorta at the time of acute dissection repair.[46,47] The two main reasons are that first, the first priority is to save the patient's life and second, trying to repair the aortic arch simultaneously carries a much higher mortality risk.[46,47] Furthermore, the risk of a patient requiring another operation after acute dissection repair is, in most cases, small.[46,47] It is, however, important that the initial acute dissection repair should be performed with circulatory arrest unless the dissection is a DeBakey Type II. This is so that the inside of the aortic arch can be inspected and a more complete hemiarch repair can be performed at the initial operation. If the tear is in the aortic arch, this can often be repaired with pledgeted 4-0 Prolene running sutures.[46,47]

The second scenario for reoperation will usually involve the patient in whom either there was progression of the aneurysm formation in the aortic arch after initial ascending aorta repairs or, at the time of the ascending aorta repair, not enough of a hemiarch was repaired, particularly when circulatory arrest was not performed.

An uncommon group of patients who require reoperations are those who form aneurysms at either the origin of the greater vessels, most typically the innominate artery, or the site where a Carrel patch of the aorta was used for reattachment of the greater vessels becomes aneurysmal and enlarges. This latter scenario should particularly be watched for in patients with Marfan syndrome, especially if they have suffered aortic dissection and the aorta is fragile.[43,46,47]

Fortunately, aortic graft infections are rare in our own experience, although we are often referred such cases. These cases require extensive debridement and repair, usually with homografts (allografts). If prosthetic material is present, omental or muscle flaps are used. Patients are kept on lifelong antibiotics or, for fungal infections, fungal antimicrobials, particularly the newer, less toxic form of amphotericin B (Figure 69A-4).

Syndromes Associated with Aortic Arch Pathology

Aneurysms may form in association with genetically based diseases such as Marfan syndrome, Ehlers–Danlos syndrome, Erdheim's syndrome (annuloaortic ectasia), Noonan's syndrome, hereditary polycystic kidney disease, osteogenesis imperfecta, and Turner's syndrome.[47]

HISTORY AND PHYSICAL EXAMINATION

Questioning patients about symptoms and physical examination in patients with aortic arch aneurysms usually are not particularly informative about the aneurysm. During the questioning, however, any history of aortic valvular disease associated with aortic root aneurysms needs to be sought along with any history of neurological or neurocognitive events. Based on computed tomography (CT) scans or magnetic resonance image (MRI) studies prior to aortic arch surgery, between 40 and 60% of patients have evidence of brain injury. In a prospective randomized study (see below), 38% of our patients, excluding those who had strokes with residual deficits and those >75 years of age, had a neurocognitive deficit prior to undergoing aortic arch surgery.[48,54]

If the aortic arch aneurysms are particularly large, hoarseness may develop, particularly if the distal aortic arch is enlarged. The reason is that the left recurrent nerve wraps around the distal aortic arch at the ligamentum arteriosis and can get stretched by the aneurysm.

Dysphagia may also occur but is more frequent with congenital lesions (Figure 69A-1). In 1794, Bayford called this "lusoria," referring to the Latin term *lusus naturae* meaning "a freak of nature." This is often described as dysphagia lusoria or *arteria lusoria*. Dyspnea can also be a symptom when the pulmonary artery or left bronchus is constricted.[47]

Patients may complain of occasional mid-scapular pain if the aneurysms are large, although this is associated more with enlarged descending or thoracoabdominal aorta aneurysms. With aortic dissection or a false aneurysm related to a penetrating ulcer or mycotic aneurysm, severe chest pain may be present. This may be anterior or posterior chest pain with extension into the neck (see Chapters 69C and 69D).

On examination, most patients do not have any physical findings specifically related to the aortic arch aneurysm, although, when the aneurysm is large, the anterior chest wall may be pulsatile and, in the worst of circumstances, may have eroded through the sternum or manubrium, particularly if infected. An associated pulsatile mass or a fullness of the neck with a pulsatile mass in the lower neck may be present. Displacement of the arch cranially may result in tortuosity of the carotid arteries. Palpation above the clavicle on the left side, at the thoracic outlet, may reveal a pulsatile mass.

During examination, the patient's arm, neck, and head pulses should be checked since there may be discrepancies or absent pulses related to aortic dissection or aortitis, particularly giant cell arteritis or Takayasu's disease.

Preoperative Studies

In addition to routine laboratory work, preoperative investigations include pulmonary function tests because many patients may have predisposing factors such as a smoking history, Marfan syndrome with bullae formation, obstructive lesions related to the arch aneurysms (particularly with a congenital aberrant right subclavian artery lesions), and right-sided aortic arches (see Figure 69A-1). We have seen patients treated for a number of years for asthma because of expiratory wheezes caused by compression of the trachea or bronchi by aneurysms.[47]

Routine brain MRIs or CTs should be obtained prior to surgery to detect any asymptomatic infarcts or brain lesions that may have occurred.[62] Most patients undergo carotid ultrasound studies if a history of coronary artery disease, peripheral vascular disease, or left main coronary artery stenosis is present. All patients undergo echocardiography prior to surgery[5,15,32] and, if possible, good views of the ascending aorta and descending aorta are obtained by transesophageal echocardiography to check for atheromatous disease since this will affect the method of cannulation for arterial inflow. All patients should also undergo cardiac catheterization to identify any presence of coronary artery disease or valvular heart disease. Routine 24-h Holter monitor examinations are also included in the preoperative workup because many of these patients have cardiac arrhythmias. This is most likely related to valvular heart disease, chronic hypertension, coronary artery disease, or displacement of the left ventricle and the heart downward and to the left by the aneurysm. Indeed, it should be noted that aneurysms have not only enlarged in diameter but also in length. Arrhythmias may also be related to abnormal vagal and sympathetic innovation stimulation.

At the time of cardiac catheterization, cardiologists are requested to obtain left anterior-oblique views of the aortic arch with injection of contrast immediately proximal to the innominate artery. This is one of the best methods for obtaining good views of the aortic arch and determining the extent of the aortic arch repair that is required, including the need for an elephant trunk procedure. In the preoperative workup, prior to referral, patients have normally undergone CT scans with contrast of the chest or MRI studies. Neither of these two studies, however, is the best technique for deciding the extent of aortic arch repair that will be required. We recommend magnetic resonance angiography (MRA) studies be obtained to provide the most accurate information.

In addition, we used to obtain aortography in all patients, but this is no longer done because of the time period needed for scheduling, the invasive nature, and the dye load, often used on the day prior to the patient undergoing surgery, potentially compromising renal function.

The operative procedure planned is then discussed with the patient. Based on preoperative studies, it can usually be predetermined with accuracy whether a hemiarch, a total

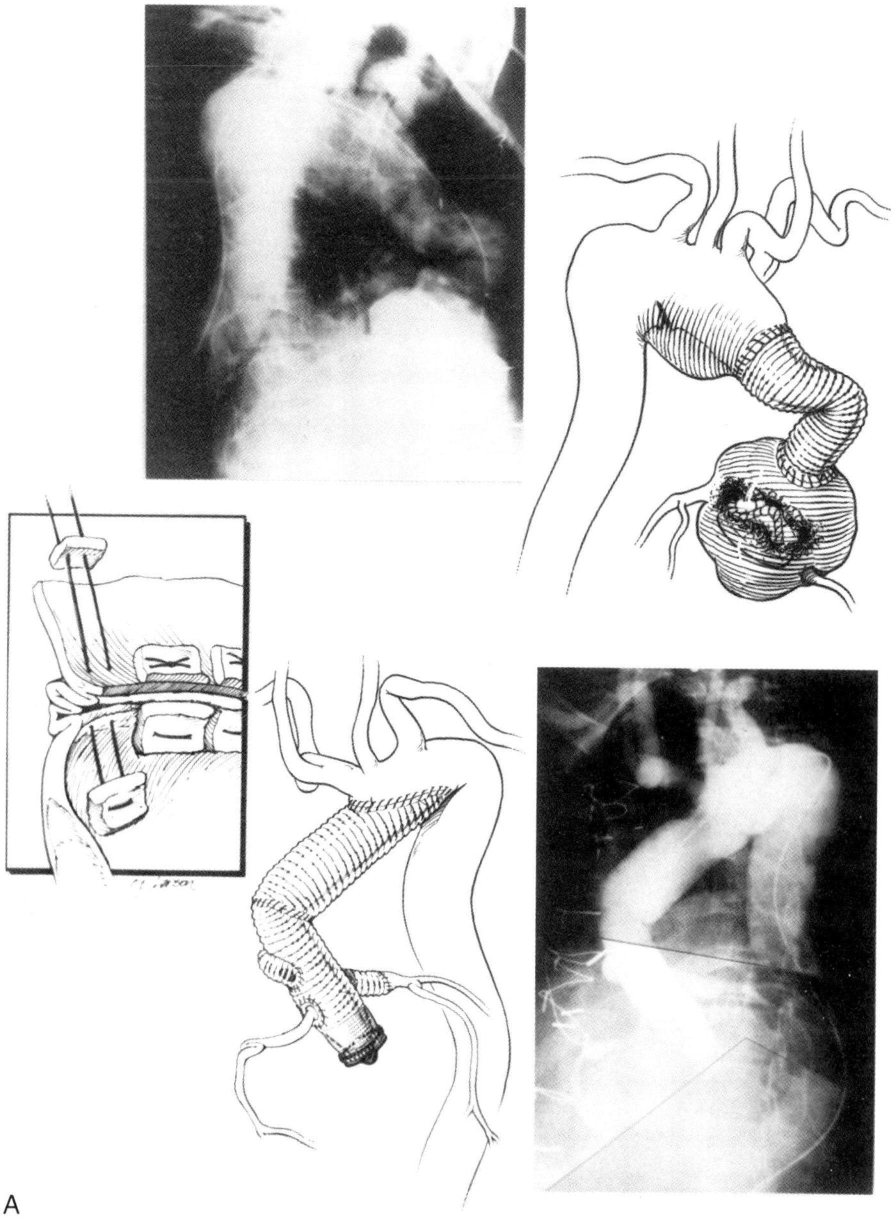

A

Figure 69A–4 **A,** Illustration of an infected ascending aorta graft after initial aortic valve replacement followed by reoperation with graft insertion done elsewhere and then the third procedure shown with a new composite valve graft with a tube graft to the left main and the right coronary artery reattached as a button and the hemiarch replaced by a separate graft. The annulus had to be reconstructed because of extensive annular abscess. Although the organism was *Staphylococcus aureus*, the patient, on suppressive antibiotics, has continued to be free of further infection. An omentum flap was swung into the chest to fill dead space.

(*Continued*)

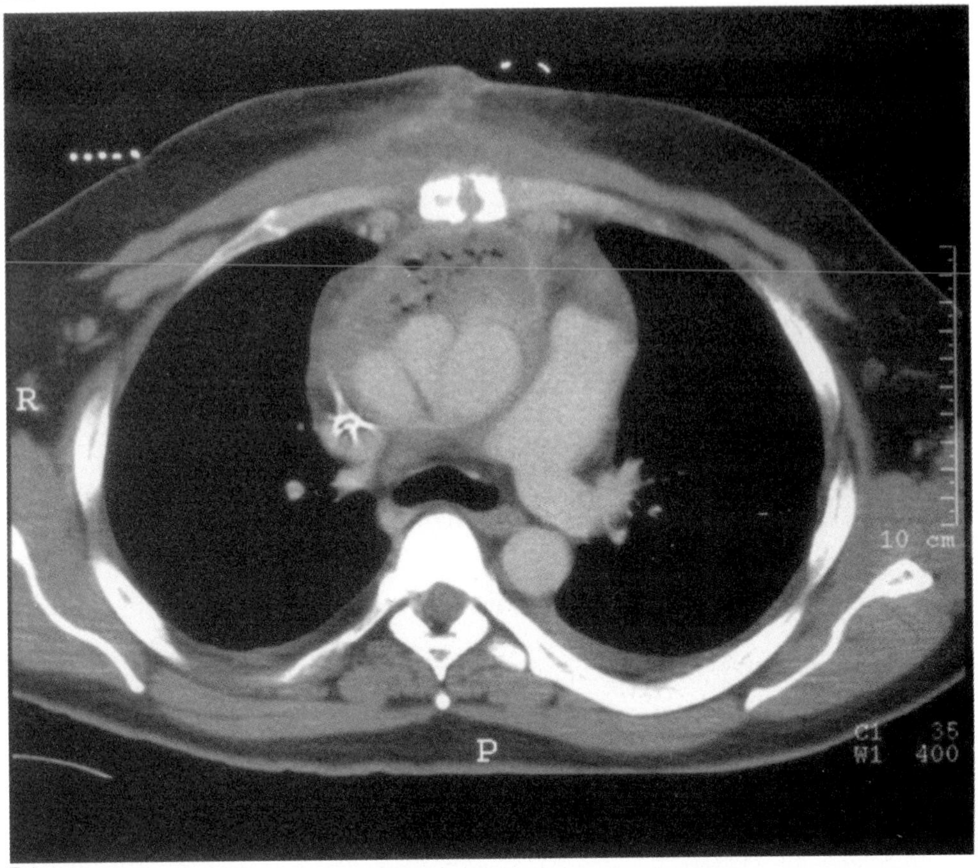

B1

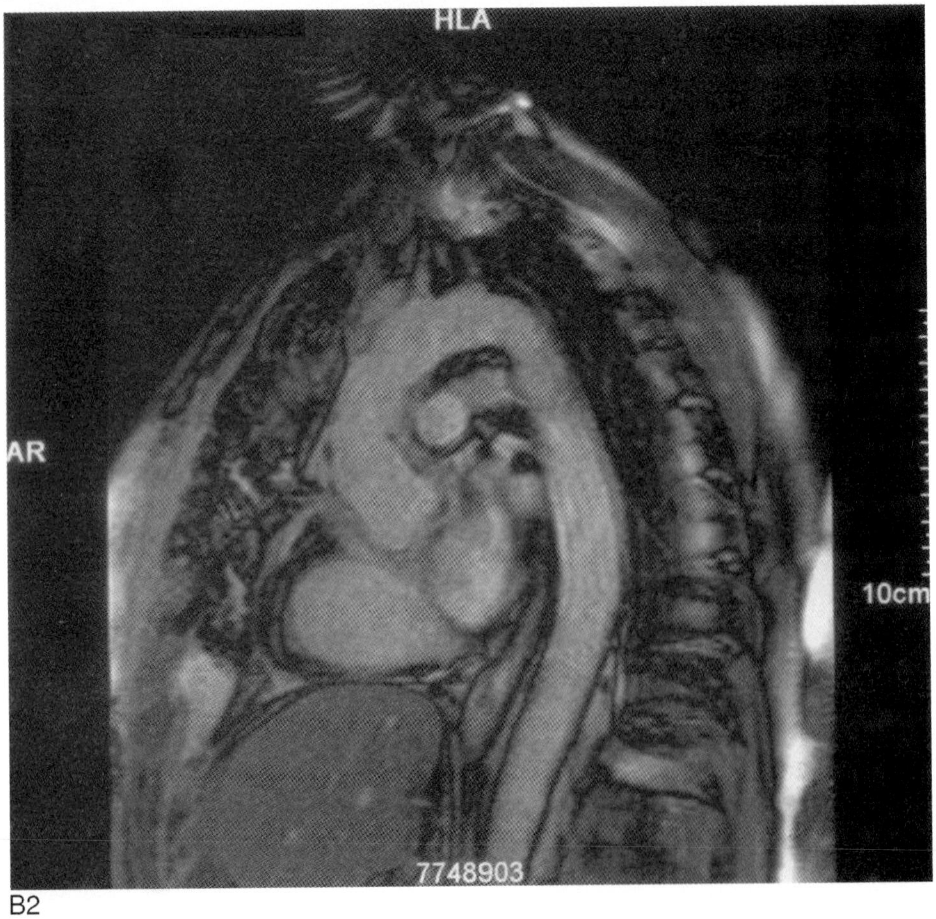

B2

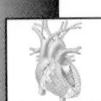

Figure 69A–4 cont'd B, (1) Patient who had undergone two previous heart operations, including a composite valve graft insertion that became infected. The patient also underwent a limited sternal debridement elsewhere but later presented to us with an abscess under the skin and associated air in the mediastinum. (2) The postoperative MRA after the repair. The patient had two allografts (homografts) inserted to replace the aortic root and the aortic arch. In addition, an omentum flap was swung into the chest to fill the dead space.

arch, or a total arch plus elephant trunk procedure is necessary. Additionally, it can be ascertained whether the greater vessels require bypasses because of stenotic lesions or aneurysmal disease, particularly in association with aortic dissection.

Next, again determined from preoperative studies, a decision must be made as to the site of the arterial inflow for the operation. For most patients undergoing aortic arch surgery, the right subclavian artery for arterial inflow is preferentially used. In young patients, however, who need only a hemiarch procedure, particularly for Marfan syndrome, the right femoral artery is most often used. Usually, the left femoral artery is not used in patients with aortic dissection because the dissection typically extends into the left iliac artery and, thus, the femoral artery perfusion cannula may perfuse the false lumen resulting in a flutter-valve effect and inadequate perfusion. Similarly, the aortic arch is not used because first, it limits the extent of the repair; second, the cannula gets in the way of the operation; third, aortic dissection may be precipitated; and fourth, if a graft is inserted, the cannula must be repositioned, either through a side graft or directly into the new aortic graft. Occasionally, the right subclavian artery is dissected and the femoral artery or aorta is used.

CARDIOPULMONARY PERFUSION ASPECTS

When the right subclavian artery is used, the technique is similar to that previously reported by Sabik and Lytle and colleagues.[26,47,48,54] These authors describe the method for complex cardiovascular surgery. In a prospective randomized study, it was thought this would be a useful means for antegrade brain perfusion.[48,54] To do this, the innominate artery was occluded with a balloon catheter in addition to the common carotid artery. The balloon catheter in the common carotid artery allowed perfusion of the left side of the brain (Figure 69A-5). This has proven to be a safe and effective technique (see later discussion).

Our preference is to attach a side graft to the subclavian artery, defined as the part of the artery proximal to the lateral edge of the first rib. The reason for this is that there are fewer branches in this area and the nerve that swings across the artery to the pectoral muscles more distally does not obstruct the view. It does, however, require that the subclavius muscle be divided with electrocautery under the clavicle. Caution should be taken that the vein is not injured during this procedure. To dissect the axillary artery more laterally, care should be taken to retract the nerves out of the way and also not injure the arterial branches. We have found the safest and best method for obtaining perfusion of the subclavian artery is to attach an 8-mm side graft, end to side. This is sewn into position with a 5-0 Prolene suture and any leaks are oversewn with 6-0 Prolene. This allows for perfusion of the vessel both proximally and distally and for greater flow rates. Thus, by avoiding direct cannulation of the subclavian artery, there are fewer tears and less difficulty in repairing the artery at the end and one circumvents the problem that if the cannula was inserted too far into the subclavian artery, occlusion of the common carotid artery could occur or result in inadequate flows if pressing up against the innominate artery wall. In a recent report by us on 1336

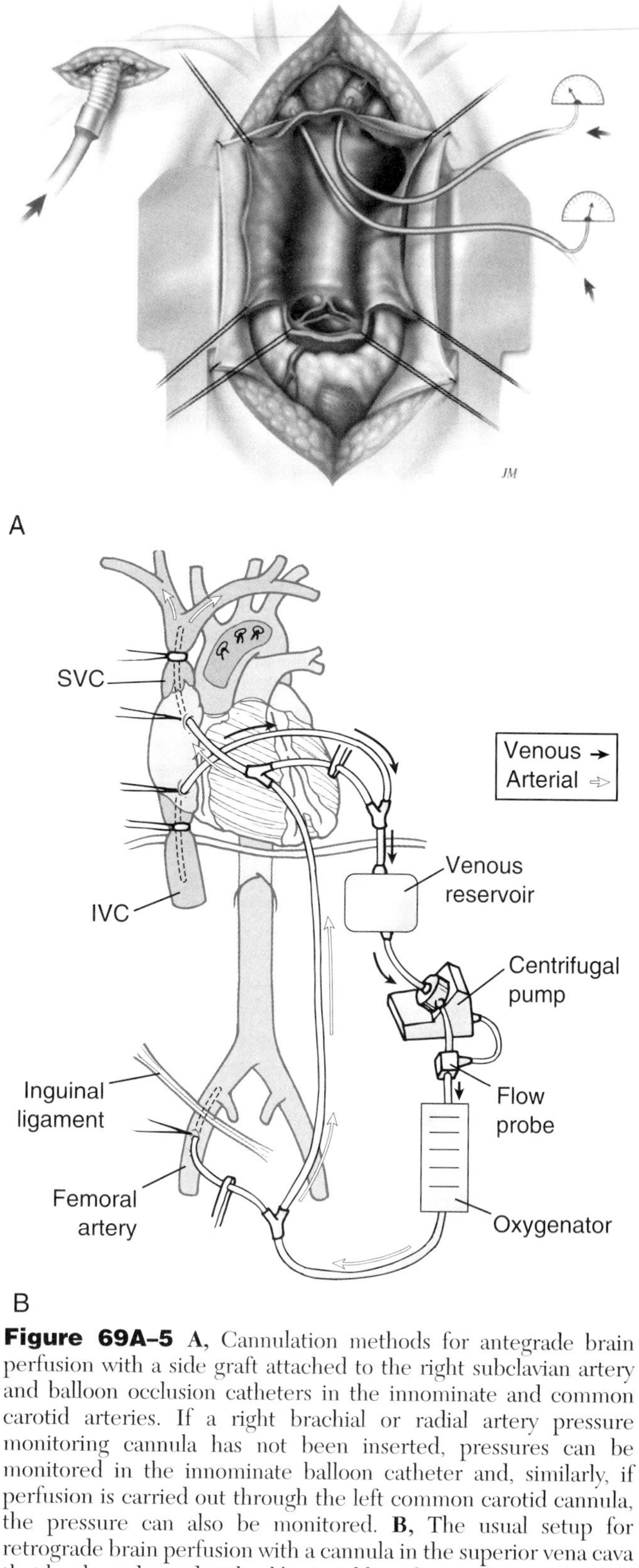

Figure 69A–5 **A,** Cannulation methods for antegrade brain perfusion with a side graft attached to the right subclavian artery and balloon occlusion catheters in the innominate and common carotid arteries. If a right brachial or radial artery pressure monitoring cannula has not been inserted, pressures can be monitored in the innominate balloon catheter and, similarly, if perfusion is carried out through the left common carotid cannula, the pressure can also be monitored. **B,** The usual setup for retrograde brain perfusion with a cannula in the superior vena cava that has been looped with a Y arterial line that can be run through the superior vena cava.

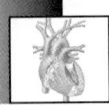

circulatory arrest patients, use of a side graft in the subclavian artery reduced the risk of stroke by 40%.[58]

An exception to the use of the subclavian artery, however, is that it should be avoided in those patients who have had aortic dissection and when the extension of the aortic dissection is noted in the vessel (Figure 69A-5A). In three patients in whom we used the subclavian artery, when dissection was present in the artery, two suffered postoperative strokes, probably from malperfusion related to the dissection. In patients exceeding 250 pounds, a larger 10-mm side-graft is usually used.

The graft is attached after the patient is heparinized and to collect any blood that accumulates within the subclavian incision pocket, a basket or coil sucker is placed in the wound to collect any leaking blood. The graft is carefully deaired and connected to a three-eighths inch to quarter-inch perfusion connector that is then connected to the arterial line of the cardiopulmonary bypass machine.

As indicated previously, when the femoral artery is used, the right femoral artery is preferable. In patients in whom the femoral artery is used, care must be taken, as much as possible, to ascertain that there is no atheroma present in the arterial system that may potentially embolize with retrograde pumping through the femoral artery up to the brain. Thus, the femoral artery is avoided in patients who are elderly, with evidence of atherosclerotic disease, aneurysms of the descending thoracoabdominal and abdominal aorta, reoperations, DeBakey Type I and Type III aortic dissections, and extensive aortitis. Similarly, in patients on whom we are planning to use antegrade brain perfusion or elephant trunk procedure (see later discussion) or acute dissection, the subclavian artery is the vessel of choice.[48,54,55]

BRAIN PROTECTION

Discussions of brain protection could be very extensive since multiple viewpoints are held by authors on how to best protect the brain during aortic arch surgery. The reasoning and some of the research that we have performed resulting in the techniques we recommend will be discussed later. A summary of our findings include the subclavian artery is the preferred cannulation site (see earlier discussion) whereas the femoral artery is less so, deep hypothermia to 20° C is preferable,[7] EEG silence is desirable,[7] retrograde brain protection may not be as effective as originally thought and may have some side effects, antegrade brain perfusion should be considered for longer circulatory arrest times exceeding 30 min, long cardiopulmonary bypass times are harmful (particularly with inadequate filtration), and excessive rewarming may be harmful.[11,14,53]

Brain protection will be discussed from three aspects: (1) avoidance of doing harm during aortic arch surgery, (2) prevention of stroke, and (3) prevention of neurocognitive deficits.

Primum Non Nocere, First Do No Harm

Prior to the safe use of cardiopulmonary bypass, aortic arch operations were designed to use bypass shunts from the ascending aorta to the greater vessels to avoid using a heart–lung machine. These operations were generally limited to patients who had a normal aortic root and not extensive aneurysms, but these techniques were associated with a high incidence of stroke and death. With the advent of cardiopulmonary bypass, the operations became considerably safer. Nevertheless, attempts by Crawford and others[9] to directly cannulate aortic arch greater vessels for perfusion of the brain during aortic arch operations were associated with a high incidence of stroke, up to one third of the patients. The view of Crawford was that this was related to injury of the greater vessels by balloon catheters and occluding clamps or by atheroma resulting in stroke. Barnard and Schrire[2] and Borst et al[3,4] independently pioneered deep hypothermia for arch surgery; however, the technique was popularized by Griepp in 1975. Deep hypothermia and circulatory arrest, without perfusion of the greater vessels, thus became popular.[16,19,47,55] Cooley and Livesay[6] emphasized the usefulness of doing an "open" distal anastomosis.

In a series of 656 patients with deep hypothermia and circulatory arrest alone for aortic arch operations,[44] we reported 10% mortality and 7% stroke rate (Figure 69A-6). In this paper, however, we describe retrograde brain perfusion in 50 patients with initial encouraging results (Figure 69A-5B). Our subsequent study in animals also showed promising findings.[37,47] At that time, the consensus was that strokes were related to embolic events or ongoing brain metabolism during deep hypothermia with circulatory arrest. As reports showed increasing success with retrograde perfusion of the heart during cardiac arrest, it was felt retrograde brain perfusion may have a potential protective role. Mills and Ochsner[28] reported using retrograde brain perfusion in a patient in whom air embolization occurred to the brain from the arterial inflow cannula.[47,62,63] They placed the patient on cardiopulmonary bypass with arterial blood flow into the superior vena cava to try to "retrograde flush-out" air from the arterial system. Subsequently, Lemole reported using retrograde brain perfusion for aortic arch operations.[47] This was later popularized by Ueda.[47,62,63] More recent studies by Griepp's group, Okita and colleagues, and others, however, have indicated that retrograde brain perfusion may also be associated with harmful side effects, including a higher incidence of stroke or neurocognitive deficits and depression.[20,25,55] It has been speculated that brain edema may be a factor. In our initial use of retrograde brain perfusion, we were careful not to exceed a perfusion pressure between 25 and 30 cm H_2O because we knew patients with congestive heart failure with a central venous pressure to these levels could tolerate this. Subsequently, studies by Griepp's group showed a higher perfusion pressure is needed to obtain any retrograde perfusion of the brain. Furthermore, this group demonstrated that perfusion pressures that exceed 60 cm H_2O resulted in brain edema. Retrospective studies, however, show that in comparison with historical controls, results are improved.[26] There is no doubt this method is effective in removing embolic material from the aortic arch, including atheromatous emboli. Nevertheless, the technique may be associated with harmful side effects. In our prospective, randomized study, depression appeared more common in this group of patients and there appeared to be no neurocognitive benefit over deep hypothermia and circulatory arrest alone. Thus, retrograde brain perfusion is used less frequently.* Currently, we are performing a randomized study for total arch replacements to evaluate this further.

*References 11, 14, 16, 17, 19, 20, 25, 26, 28, 34, 37, 44, 48, 53–55, 59, 60, 62, 63.

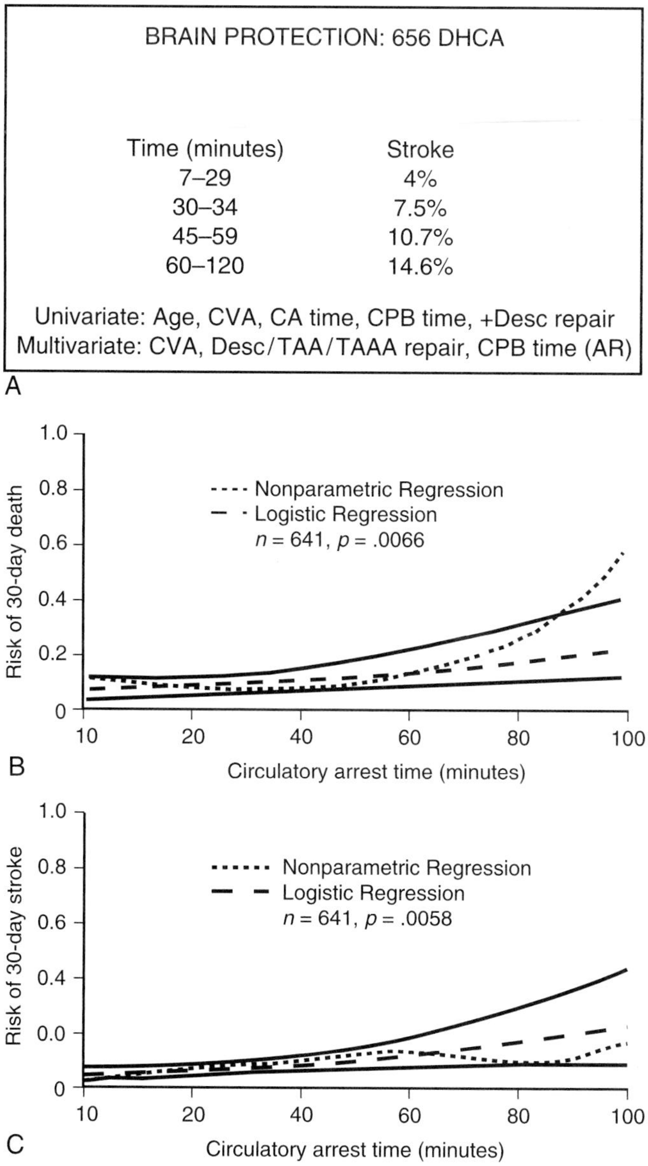

Figure 69A–6 **A,** Incidence of stroke in 656 patients undergoing deep hypothermia with circulatory arrest according to the time of circulatory arrest shown in the left column. DHCA, deep hypothermia and circulatory arrest; CA, circulatory arrest; CVA, cerebrovascular accident history; CPB, cardiopulmonary bypass time, plus DESC, including descending aorta repair at the same time; TAA, thoracoabdominal aneurysm repair; AAA, abdominal aneurysm repair; AR, aortic valve regurgitation, shown in parentheses because aortic valve regurgitation was significantly associated with lower risk. (The univariate and multivariate predictors are also shown.) **B,** Relationship between circulatory arrest time and the risk of 30-day death. Note that after 65 min, there is an exponential increase in the risk of death. **C,** Relationship between circulatory arrest time and the risk of 30-day stroke. Note that after 40 min, there is an increase in the risk of stroke; however, at 60 min, it appears to decline. This is a statistical aberration because, after 60 min of circulatory arrest, there is a rapid increase in the risk of death and, therefore, patients could not be necessarily assessed for neurological function.

Prevention of Strokes

As our knowledge of cardiopulmonary pathophysiology improved, it became clear that most strokes after cardiac surgery are related to microemboli. Most of these emboli seem to be the result of atheromatous or calcific debris from the aorta. For most patients undergoing aortic arch surgery, other sources, such as from the left atrium in patients with chronic atrial fibrillation or transiting through an atrial septal defect, is less of a problem. Another potential source of emboli is from the descending aorta or abdominal aorta or iliac and femoral arteries during femoral artery perfusion. With modern cardiopulmonary bypass techniques, massive air embolism or pump failure that can result in strokes has been greatly lessened.[21,47]

Various techniques, methods, and procedures have been used in attempts to reduce the risk of embolic-related strokes. We have not tested every method, although, early on, we established a protocol based on the current level of knowledge at the time that we considered of value (Table 69A-1). With reference to cardiopulmonary bypass, it appears that the following are beneficial: a centrifugal pump, arterial line filtration (at least 25 μm), leukocyte filtration, closed-bag venous reservoir, cell saver, avoiding pump suction, and reducing cardiopulmonary bypass time. If a leukocyte filter is used, it is important to use immediate preoperative plasmapheresis to remove platelets and clotting factors from the patient because

Table 69A–1

Brain Protection Protocol

All patients	Electroencephalogram silence Temperatures less than 20° C Head packed in ice Mannitol prime and after arrest Alpha-stat pH control Leukoguard filter CO_2 flooding of field Thiopental 5 mg/kg 5 min before arrest Lidocaine 200 mg before arrest Magnesium sulfate 2 g Centrifugal pump Membrane oxygenator Closed circuit bag venous reservoir Prebypass plasmapheresis Routine cell saver
Antegrade brain perfusion	Right subclavian and side graft Innominate and carotid balloon occlusion (retrograde cardioplegia balloon occlusion catheter) Pressure maintained at 40–60 mm Hg Sequential removal of catheters as arch anastomosis completed
Retrograde brain perfusion	Superior vena cava cannula Snared below azygous vein 300–500 ml/min but less than 25–35 mm Hg

leukocyte filters tend to remove platelets from the circulation. The platelet-rich plasma is reinfused at the end of the operation. For pH management during cardiopulmonary bypass and circulatory arrest, we favor using the alpha-stat method. In the pediatric age group, there is more convincing evidence that the pH-stat method works better. In adults, however, the alpha-stat method is generally preferred, although there are no prospective or randomized studies that have definitely answered the question of which is best in adults. An advantage with the alpha-stat method is that lactic acid that accumulates in the brain during circulatory arrest can, to some extent, be buffered by histamine molecules on hemoglobin.[47,53,55]

We advise flooding the field with carbon dioxide at 10 l/min so any air accumulating in the heart or the field will be displaced.[30] This includes the aortic arch so that when circulation to the brain is restarted, any potentially gaseous material is carbon dioxide rather than air. Carbon dioxide is reabsorbed approximately 25 times faster than air, reducing the risk of microcirculation obstruction related to gaseous material.

In addition to perfusion aspects and the site of cannulation, we recommend packing the patient's head in ice because it reduces the risk of the ambient operating room temperature raising the temperature of the patient's head during circulatory arrest. Patients are also given 5 mg/kg of thiopental prior to circulatory arrest. It is impressive to see on EEG monitoring that EEG activity is frequently abolished by giving the thiopental when patients are cold. Of note, controversy exists regarding the merits of using thiopental. We have found, however, that at 20 mg/kg, patients developed myocardial depression from the thiopental and some patients had to be placed on left ventricular assist devices from 24 to 48 h to recover from the myocardial depression. The use of this protocol in patients undergoing ascending and aortic arch procedures in combination with the perfusion techniques discussed below resulted in approximately a 2% incidence of stroke as outlined in our report of a series of 403 ascending and aortic arch operations.[53]

Prevention of Neurocognitive Deficits

With improved results for aortic arch surgery and fewer complications such as strokes, interest has focused on prevention of postoperative neurocognitive deficits. As stated previously, 38% of patients in our prospective randomized study were found to have, prior to surgery, neurocognitive deficits.[48,54] The reason for this is not entirely clear although, as indicated, it may be related to silent brain injury prior to surgery. There is also a correlation between neurocognitive deficits and other preoperative factors such as heart failure and New York Heart Association degree of dyspnea.[53] This would be in keeping with patients exhibiting a greater degree of systemic cardiovascular disease experiencing more neurocognitive deficits. The reasons may be due to inadequate brain perfusion, brain edema, similar etiological factors affecting the brain vasculature, and general overall poor health. Indeed, it is our impression that patients with preoperative neurocognitive deficits do not tolerate deep hypothermia and circulatory arrest as well. In a previous study of 656 patients undergoing deep hypothermia and circulatory arrest,[44] older patients did not tolerate circulatory arrest as well as younger patients, putting them more at risk for stroke. The same probably holds true for the risk of neurocognitive deficits, but this has not been formally studied.

The incidence of neurocognitive deficits after cardiac surgery remains controversial.[14,48,54] So much depends on the method of defining when neurocognitive deficits occur. There are multiple reasons why deficits could occur, (e.g., preoperative neurocognitive dysfunction or atherosclerosis of the microvasculature of the brain, similar to that affecting coronary arteries). Some of the large studies that have been undertaken to examine neurocognitive dysfunction after coronary bypass surgery have used cardiopulmonary bypass pump setups that were out of date. It is also instructive that some studies have shown no differences between off-pump and on-pump incidences of neurocognitive deficits, suggesting other factors, such as anesthesia management, are important. Studies have also shown no differences between coronary artery bypass surgery and major abdominal aortic surgery. It is well known that any patient who undergoes an anesthetic often has neurocognitive dysfunction after surgery despite no obvious risk factors causing neurological dysfunction. In our prospective, randomized study, although over 90% of patients had neurocognitive dysfunction 3–6 days after surgery, by 2–3 weeks only 9% had a new neurocognitive deficit and by 6 months, all had recovered.[48,54] The entire field of neurocognitive dysfunction requires further study to determine when a deficit occurs in an individual patient and what the change in global scores for an entire group of patients means. In our prospective randomized study (Figure 69A-7A), we found the patient's IQ improved after circulatory arrest over time. Although desirable, clearly, this would not be the case! The reason for this was the patients underwent repeated IQ tests (four) and learned to do the tests over time. Nevertheless, it was gratifying to note that the patient's IQs did not deteriorate after deep hypothermia and circulatory arrest. Indeed, the practice effect on reported neurocognitive scores is difficult to compensate for. Figure 69A-7B shows the S-100 changes by group studied.

The reason for potential neurocognitive dysfunction after surgery is multiple. Anesthetic gases and pharmacological agents, including barbiturates, are factors. Other potential

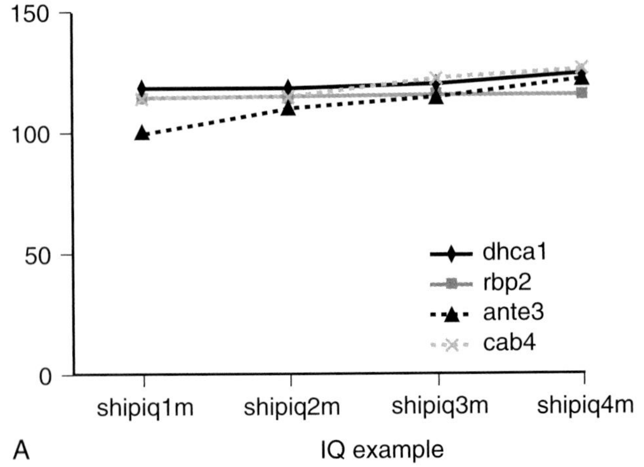

Figure 69A–7 A, Illustration of Shipley (Shipiq) IQ scores over time in patients who underwent deep hypothermia with circulatory arrest (DHCA), retrograde brain perfusion (RBP), antegrade brain perfusion (ANTE), and coronary artery bypass (CAB). The first tests were done preoperatively (1M), then 3–6 days after surgery (2-M), 2–3 weeks after surgery (3M), and 6 months after surgery (4M).

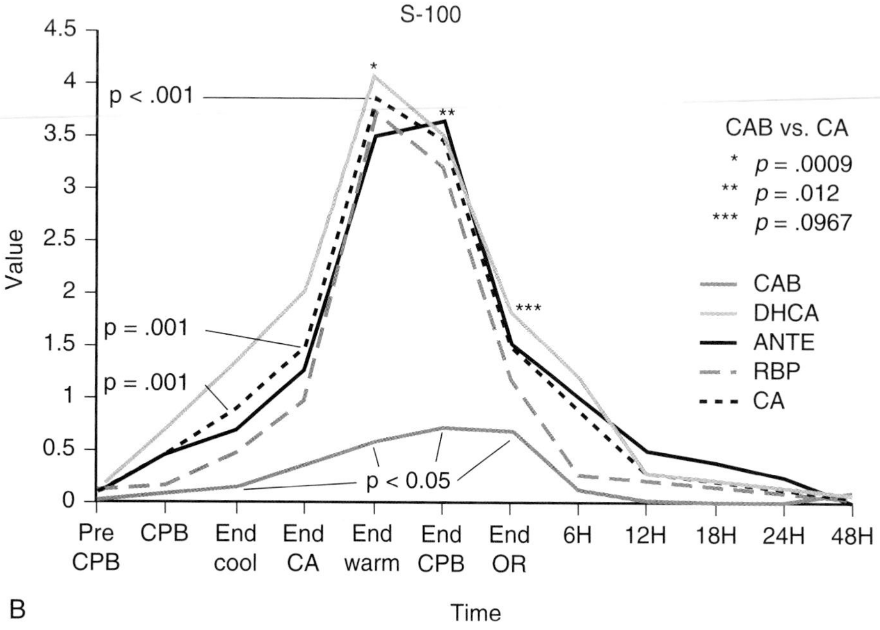

Figure 69A–7 cont'd B, Relationship of time to S-100 value. CAB, coronary artery bypass; DHCA, deep hypothermia and circulatory arrest alone; ANTE, antegrade brain perfusion; RBP, retrograde brain perfusion; CA, all circulatory arrest patients; CPB, cardiopulmonary bypass; CA, circulatory arrest; OR, operating room; H, time after surgery in the intensive care.

reasons are brain edema and swelling from third space fluid accumulation. Undoubtedly, chemical and metabolite accumulation also play a role. Microemboli may also be a factor and these may be in the form of small fat globules or air or carbon dioxide gaseous emboli.

It was once thought that emboli to the frontal lobes were largely silent and that there was selective streaming of emboli, including platelet aggregates, to the middle cerebral artery resulting in middle cerebral artery territory infarcts. Because of this, a study was done using radioactive platelet aggregates in a baboon model to test this theory.[41] We found injection of the platelet aggregates into the left atrium resulted in equal distribution across the brain including occipital lobes and distribution to the eye, as expected from an anatomical point of view. Injection into the common carotid arteries had a similar effect, although the occipital lobes were spared. Injection into the internal carotid artery did not reveal any preferential streaming into the middle cerebral artery. From this we infer that the emboli to the frontal lobes do cause infarcts of equal frequency, although these may be more silent in the sense that critical motor and sensory functions are not affected. We do, however, ascertain these so-called silent infarcts do affect neurocognitive function as expected from a more recent understanding of brain pathophysiology. Some of the neurocognitive decline after cardiopulmonary bypass may thus be related to microemboli to the frontal lobes and infarction. This is an evolving field and the correlation with microembolic and postoperative neurocognitive function will need to be further defined. For example, it is unclear how high-intensity transient Doppler signals (HITS), produced by aortic valve prostheses, affect neurocognitive function both early and long term. Studies in patients with various types of aortic valve prostheses suggest many of these are microgaseous emboli but are usually transient and rapidly return into solution without causing any permanent brain dysfunction.[42,55]

In our prospective randomized study, we failed to show any benefit from antegrade brain perfusion or retrograde brain perfusion regarding neurocognitive function when compared with deep hypothermia with circulatory arrest alone. There are several caveats: first, the circulatory arrest was relatively short and for hemiarch repairs, antegrade brain perfusion resulted in significantly longer circulatory arrest time. This was due to the time required to insert the common carotid artery catheter and the innominate artery catheter. For total arch replacement, there were no differences in circulatory arrest times. Retrograde brain perfusion was associated with slightly longer circulatory arrest times compared with circulatory arrest alone, probably because retrograde brain perfusion results in blood accumulating in the operative field, which obscures the field when suturing. Based on these findings and our current level of knowledge, we do not use antegrade or retrograde brain perfusion for brief circulatory arrest periods (e.g., a hemiarch repair that may take 5–15 min of deep hypothermia and circulatory arrest). If, however, we expect atheroma in the aorta at the time of surgery and the patient may require endarterectomy, we will use antegrade perfusion via the right subclavian artery as discussed above or retrograde brain perfusion to flush out embolic material. Whether a balloon perfusion catheter is required in the left common carotid artery during antegrade brain perfusion via the subclavian artery and deep hypothermic arrest is unclear. Certainly, if the aortic arch is being repaired at moderate hypothermia, this would be advisable.*

In patients undergoing total arch replacement, in which the circulatory arrest time may exceed 30–40 min, antegrade or retrograde brain perfusion is used for the repair. Data in the pediatric cardiac surgical literature show, as with pulmonary embolectomy in adults for thrombotic material, circulatory arrest with intermittent periods of brain perfusion followed by circulatory arrest is better than one long period of circulatory arrest. In one patient undergoing a fourth complex cardiac reoperation at deep hypothermia, we were able to successfully protect his brain for more than 90 min by running antegrade brain perfusion for 5-min periods every 30 min. He was extubated the day after surgery

*References 1, 47, 48, 54, 55, 59, 62.

without a neurological deficit. We, therefore, usually run antegrade brain perfusion, if not throughout the period of circulatory arrest for total arches, at least at intermittent intervals when convenient from the point of view of visualizing the field and suturing. The balloon occlusion catheter can easily be led out of the field so it does not obstruct the view. Because the right subclavian artery is perfused in these patients, once the balloon catheter is withdrawn from the arch, the arch is flushed of any embolic material prior to completing the anastomosis. If an elephant trunk procedure is being used, a side graft to the elephant trunk is not required for antegrade perfusion since the right subclavian artery is being perfused. Similarly, in patients undergoing acute dissection repairs, a side graft to the aortic arch is not required because the subclavian artery is being perfused.[1,47,48,54,55]

Future research is needed to determine the best perfusion method for brain protection during total arch replacements, including the best temperature.

OPERATIVE TECHNIQUES

The operative procedures for aortic arch replacement are most commonly hemiarch repairs or entire arch repairs, with or without a distal descending elephant trunk procedure.[47] Other unusual types of operations are options in specific situations. To a large extent, the choice of aortic arch procedure is influenced by the proximal aortic root or the ascending aorta operative technique whether composite graft, root remodeling, separate valve and graft, valve reimplantation, Ross procedure, or no valve procedure. Also, in choosing a valve type, it is important to consider durability, particularly for biological valves, since a third or fourth operation will be complicated.[42]

Hemiarch Replacement

Hemiarch replacement of the aortic arch is the simplest and quickest operative technique. The anastomosis can be achieved in 5–15 min depending on the aortic arch pathology. Once the patient has been cooled down, the method of brain protection and perfusion techniques decided upon and pentothal administered, the patient's circulation is stopped with the patient in the head down position. In patients undergoing reoperations, we use one of two approaches: either full median sternotomy or a minimally invasive approach (see below). The ascending aorta is then opened between stay sutures. A decision is made as to whether the aortic arch should be transected for the anastomosis. Briefly, transection of the aorta is indicated for acute aortic dissections in those patients who have had an aortic root procedure where the aorta has already been transected proximally and for most patients who need hemiarch replacements. The reason is that it is easier to obtain hemostasis at the distal anastomosis if the aorta was transected and, thus, the risk of false aneurysm formation is also less. The transection line usually runs from the proximal base of the innominate artery to the mid-point of the lesser curve of the aortic arch. In patients with acute dissections, it is important to be certain that all layers are transected, the adventitia freed of the posterior lying pulmonary artery and a bit further cranial to the pulmonary artery to ensure adequate tissue is present for effective suturing. The anastomosis is performed with a running 4-0 or 3-0 Prolene suture, dependent on the pathology. For patients with acute dissections, it is best to use 4-0 or even 5-0 Prolene. When the anastomosis is near completion, the graft and arch are filled with blood by restarting the arterial flow from the pump. Any potential embolic material is sucked away and gaseous pockets are evacuated. To further reduce risk of gaseous embolism, carbon dioxide is run into the operative field during the procedure. The anastomosis is completed and the suture is tied down. The patient is rewarmed and the proximal ascending aorta anastomosis or aortic root procedure is completed.

In patients who have either had aortic root remodeling using techniques described by David and Feindel,[10] Sarsam and Yacoub,[39] or us[52] or who have a modified valve reimplantation procedure, an interposition graft is usually required between the aortic root procedure graft and the aortic arch.[61] If, however, the valve remodeling was done while cooling, an interposition graft may not be necessary. In patients, however, who have undergone aortic valve replacement only, the hemiarch graft is used to suture the proximal anastomosis immediately above the aortic valve and coronary arteries. In patients in whom a composite valve graft will be inserted, the proximal anastomosis of the composite valve graft to the aortic valve annulus and the left main coronary artery anastomosis can first be performed while cooling the patient and the hemiarch anastomosis done directly to the composite graft without using an interposition graft, but always being careful to deair the graft. Alternatively, if the patient cools quickly, a separate hemiarch graft is placed and later anastomosed to the proximal composite valve graft with a graft-to-graft anastomosis while the patient is rewarmed. In patients who have had a homograft inserted with an aortic root repair, a decision needs to be made as to whether prosthetic polyester graft material should be used for the hemiarch or whether a homograft (without an aortic valve) (see Figure 69A-4) should be used to bridge the gap between the aortic valve and the homograft. In patients with extensive infection of a previous inserted graft (e.g., a composite graft), we replace the aortic root with a new homograft and use another homograft to bridge the gap between the root homograft and aortic arch so that there is no prosthetic material other than Prolene suture material (see Figure 69A-4B). In most cases, these grafts are wrapped with omentum to further obliterate any dead space. For those patients undergoing reoperations with extensive scar tissue formation that restricts the ability to transect the proximal and distal aorta, the hemiarch anastomosis may be done inside the aortic arch without transecting the aorta. Rarely, if bleeding cannot be controlled, a Cabrol fistula can be performed from the aneurysm sac to the right atrium or the superior vena cava.

A variation on the hemiarch replacement is a long tongue of the graft used to replace the entire aortic arch, potentially down onto the descending aorta to approximately the middle third of the descending aorta, depending on the aortic arch aneurysm size (Figure 69A-1B). When using a long tongue for the total aortic arch replacement and down the descending aorta, there are some points worth noting. First, if the anastomosis is quite far down the descending aorta, parachuting the distal anastomosis makes it easier. Second, the patient should be warned prior to surgery that hoarseness may occur because the recurrent laryngeal nerve often cannot be preserved where it wraps around the distal aortic arch. Third, hemostasis at the distal anastomosis must be secure prior to continuing the operation after doing the arch repair since obtaining hemostasis is much more difficult once the graft is pressurized and connected proximally. Fourth, the extent distally to which the anastomosis can be performed may be judged, to some extent, by examining the CT scan or the left anterior oblique view of the arch on MRA or cardiac catheterization. As a rule, an anastomosis can be easily performed no more than a few centimeters beyond the lowest level of the lesser curve of the aortic arch: the larger the size of the aortic arch aneurysm, the further down the descending aorta within the descending aorta the anastomosis can be performed. If the anastomosis cannot be performed through the aortic arch, an alternative method needs to be considered (see below).

It is important when doing a hemiarch with these long "tongues" that great care be taken that the aortic graft does not become stenosed or badly kinked. This may obstruct blood flow through the repaired aortic arch resulting in excessive cardiac afterload. This may progress to either early acute heart failure or later ventricular hypertrophy and congestive heart failure if the gradients are too large.

Replacement of the Entire Aortic Arch

Replacement of the entire aortic arch can be done with or without a distal elephant trunk procedure. This latter variation of the operation will be discussed first (Figure 69A-8).

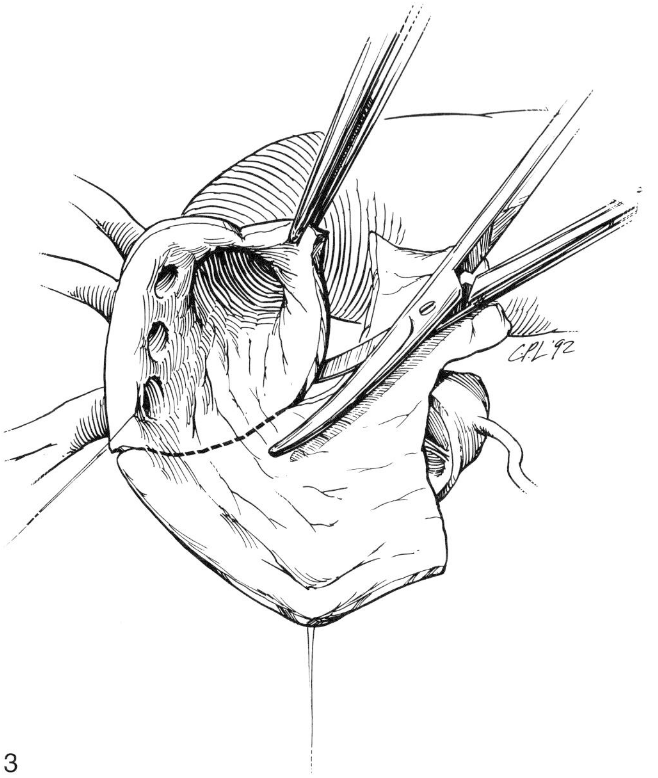

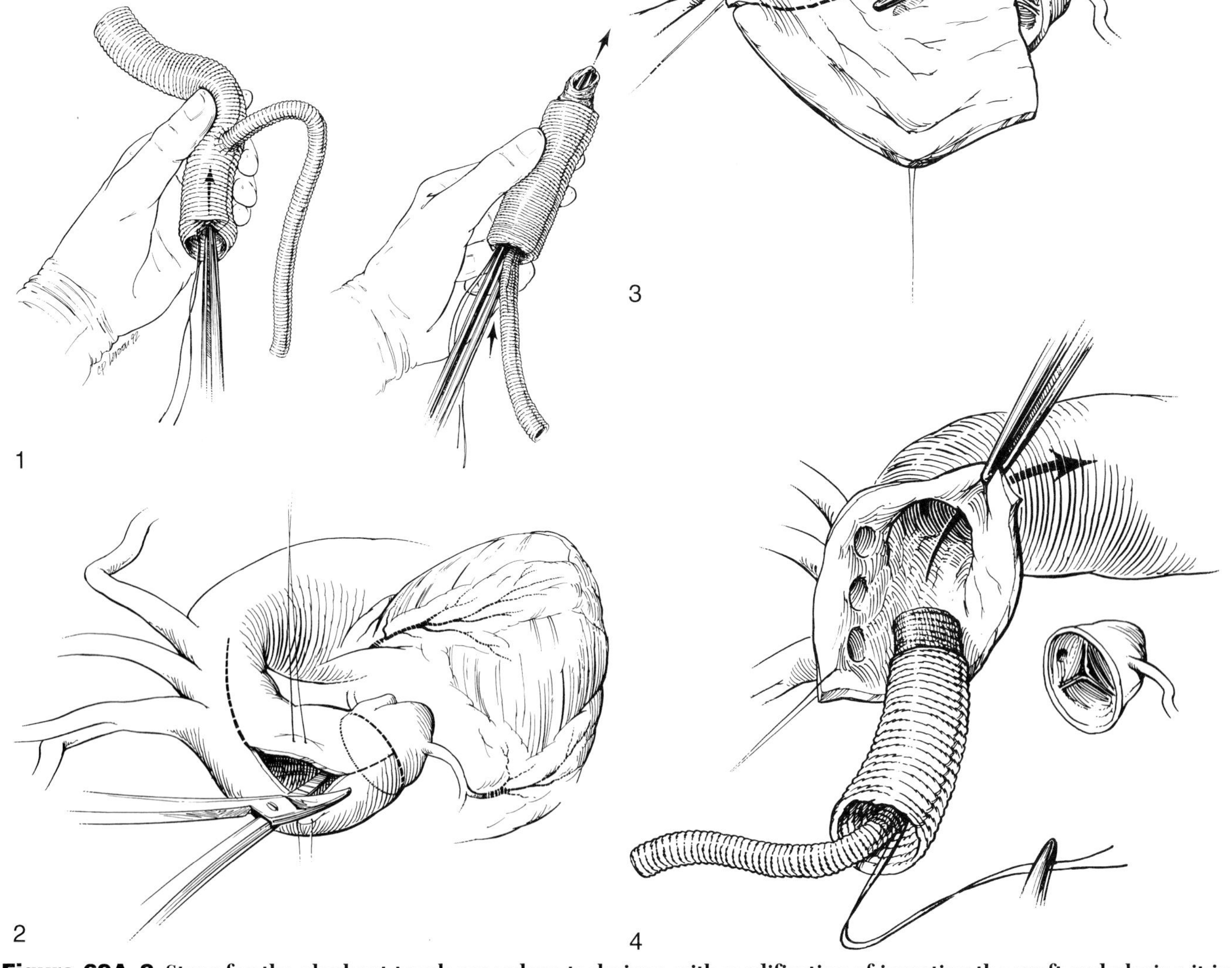

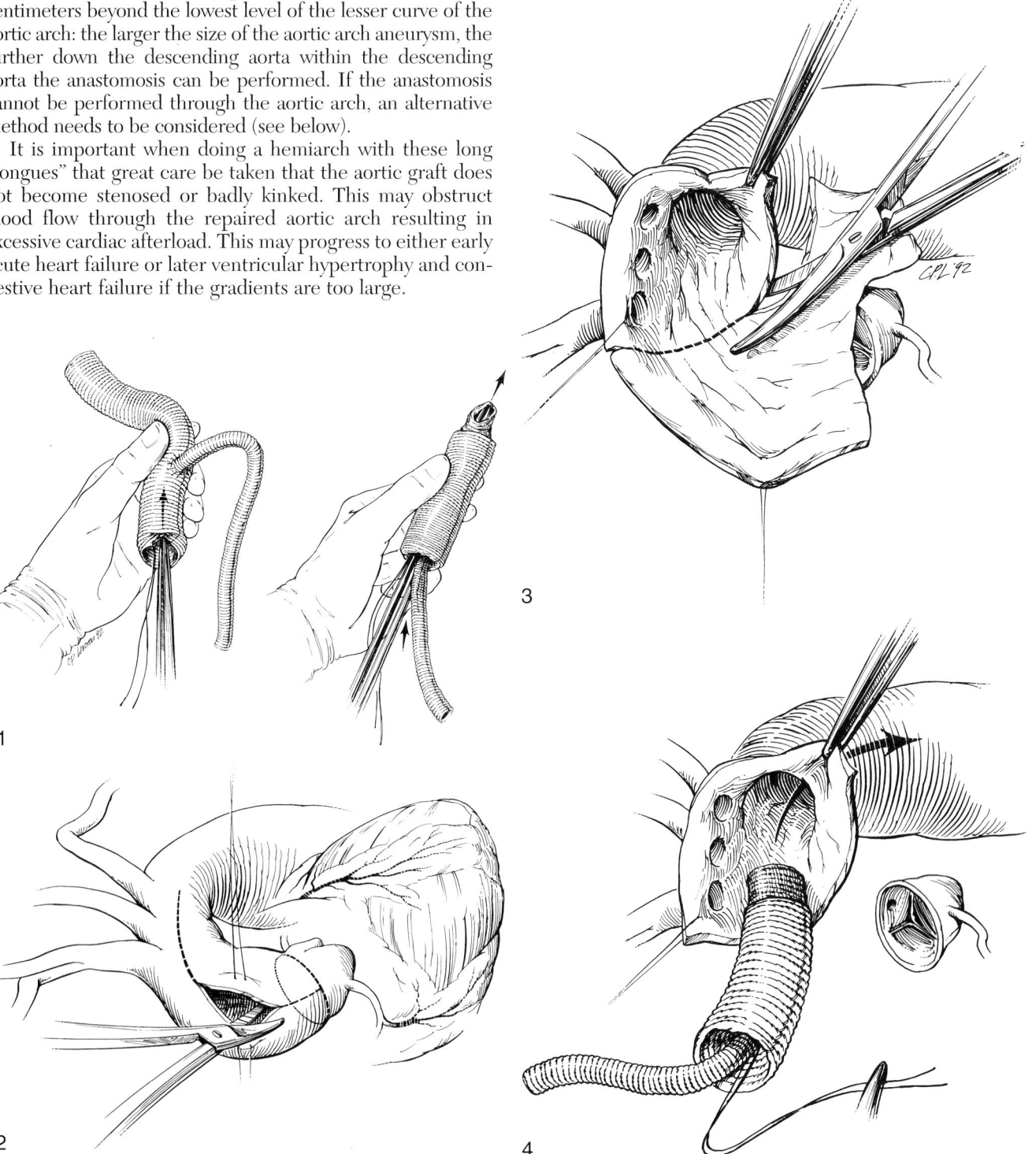

Figure 69A–8 Steps for the elephant trunk procedure technique with modification of inverting the graft and placing it in the descending aorta. (1) A side graft is sewn to the graft that will be used for the aortic replacement and then the graft is inverted on itself, including the side graft. The distal extent of the elephant trunk should be 10–15 cm in length and an approximately 1–2 cm rim is left between the side graft and the inverted edge turned down for sewing. If the right subclavian artery is used for arterial inflow, then the side graft is not necessary. (2) Once the patient is cold enough, circulation is arrested and the aorta is opened. (3) The aorta can be transected to improve exposure, if needed. (4) The previously prepared graft is then placed in the descending aorta.

(Continued)

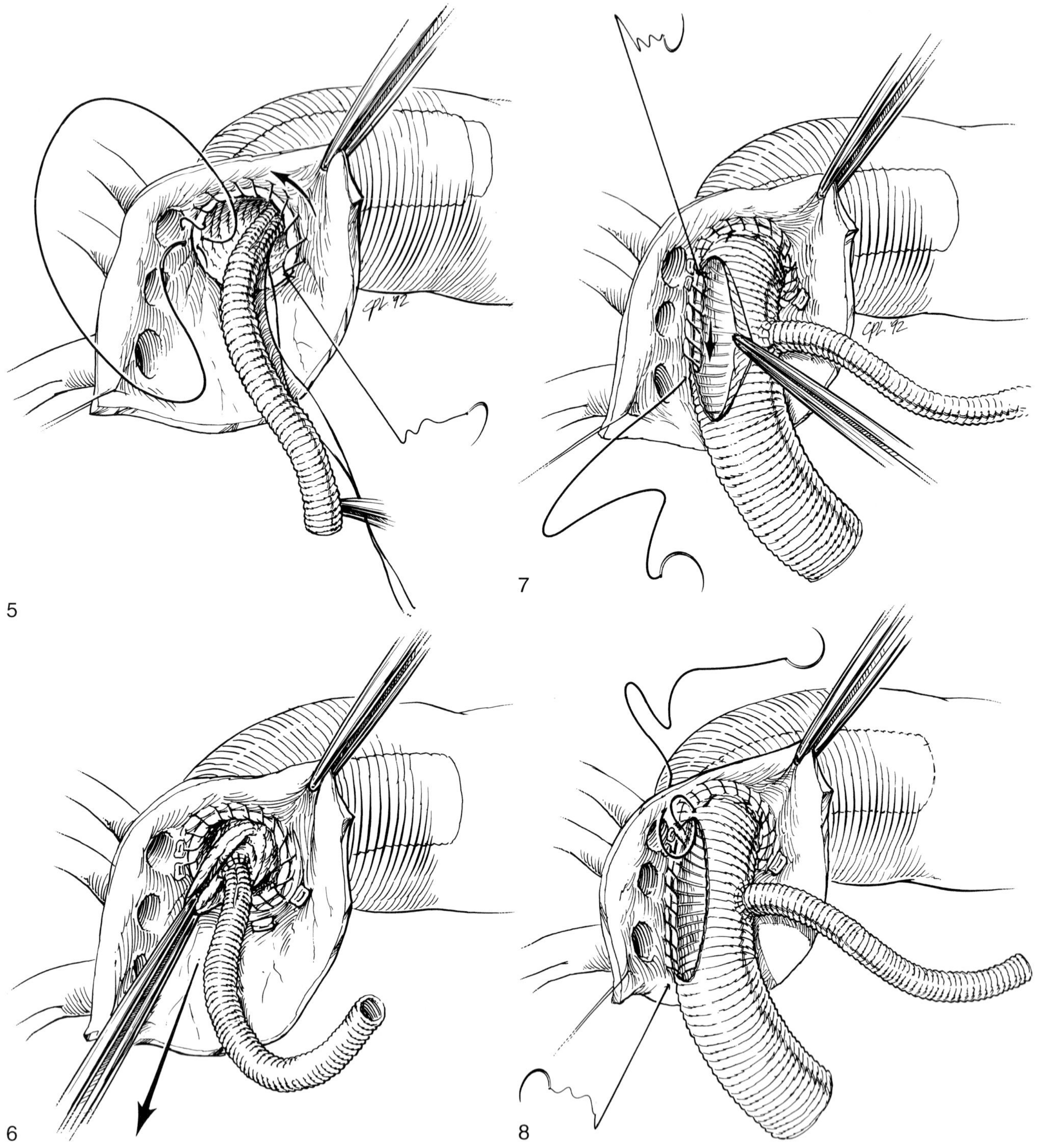

Figure 69A–8 cont'd (5) The distal anastomosis is performed starting at the three o'clock position as the surgeon looks at the anastomosis. (6) The inner inverted tube is then pulled back into the operative field. (7) The posterior suture line is then performed for the aortic arch. (8) The anterior suture line is then performed. Once the anastomosis is completed, arterial inflow is started through the side graft again to perfuse the brain if the right subclavian artery has not been used.

To shorten the period of circulatory arrest, the elephant trunk and inverted graft should be prepared while the patient is cooled. This is done by first suturing and tying a silk stitch to the end of the graft that will be used for the proximal repair of the ascending aorta. The distal elephant trunk should be approximately 10–15 cm in length. If the second stage will be done with stent grafts because of comorbid disease (e.g., chronic pulmonary disease), then metal clips and a loop of wire (pacing) are attached to the distal end. The proximal part with the stitch attached to it is then inverted into the distal elephant trunk. It is important to ensure that the edge of the inversion is at the same level and smooth. If retrograde brain perfusion or circulatory arrest alone is used and the subclavian artery has not been

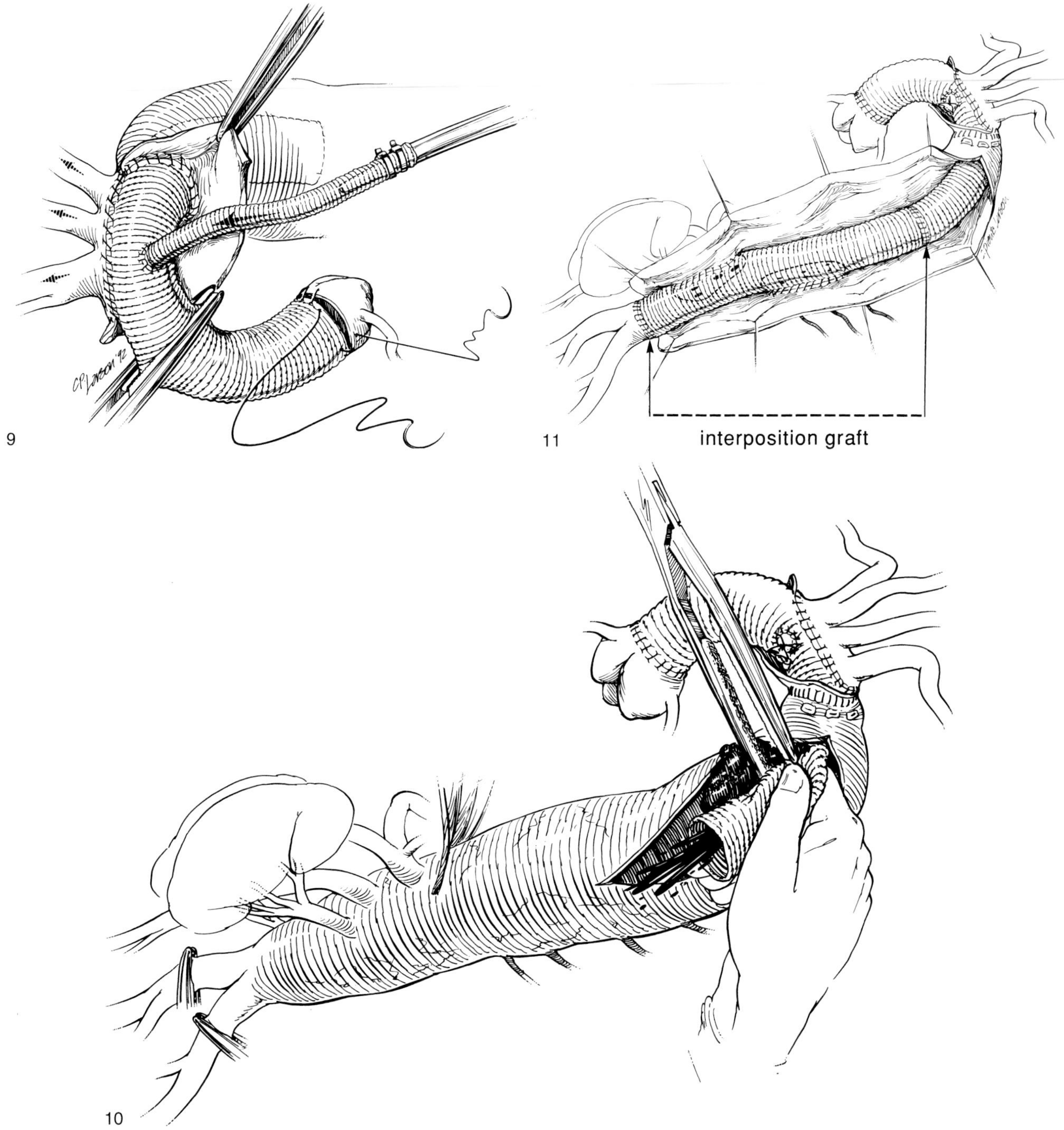

Figure 69A–8 cont'd (9) At the second stage operation, the graft is exposed within the aneurysm and clamped. It is not necessary to encircle the aorta to perform this since the graft is surrounded by clot and can be exposed without much bleeding and then digitally clamped it before applying a mechanical clamp. (10) The remainder of the aorta is then repaired. (11) For thoracoabdominal aneurysms, an interposition graft is necessary to complete the repair.

used for arterial inflow, a side graft needs to be attached to the aortic arch and inverted into the distal elephant trunk. This side graft should be attached approximately 2–4 cm proximal to the edge of the inverted graft. If the right subclavian artery is used for arterial inflow, there is no need to attach a side graft to the elephant trunk graft.

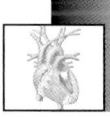

Once circulatory arrest is established and the patient is in a head-down position, the graft is fed into the descending aorta, ensuring it is neither kinked nor twisted into a spiral. In patients with chronic dissection, the septum or flap should be excised as much as possible so that the graft perfuses *both* the true and false lumens. Perfusion of either the true or false lumen alone may result in paraplegia or renal failure. It is also important that the elephant trunk is not excessively long. In a previous review of 84 elephant trunk procedures,[57] three patients developed paralysis postoperatively, one with dense paraplegia and the other two with paraparesis from excessively long elephant trunks. Subsequent to shortening the length of the elephant trunk, this has not been a problem. The reason for this appears to be either that the elephant trunk is too long and perfusion of the intercostal arteries is inadequate or that, as noted at the second-stage procedure, extensive clot formation occurs around the elephant trunk, which can occlude critical intercostals. Because of this clot formation, when using the elephant trunk, patients often require multiple platelet transfusions as the clot builds up around the elephant trunk in the descending aorta.

The elephant trunk graft material should be one of the collagen-coated woven grafts and not a gel-coated graft. In the gel-coated grafts, the gel is absorbed quickly. At the time of the second stage operation, bleeding from a proximal elephant trunk can be excessive and potentially uncontrollable since the graft is porous after the gel has been absorbed.

The anastomosis between the inverted edge of the elephant trunk graft and the distal aortic arch beyond the left subclavian artery is then performed. The patient should be warned that hoarseness may occur postoperatively since this procedure is in the region of the recurrent laryngeal nerve.

Reasons for inverting the graft on itself and placing it in the descending aorta are several, as previously explained.[57] First, the anastomosis is easier to perform, even though it can be difficult to drive the needle through a double layer of graft material. However, with collagen-coated grafts, this is not much of a problem. Second, when the inverted graft is withdrawn from inside the elephant trunk, it has the effect of tightening the anastomosis, improving hemostasis at the distal anastomosis. Third, the larger contact surface area between the graft and aortic wall is increased so that there is less bleeding past the anastomosis. Fourth, if the graft is not inverted, suturing in a tight space between a graft and the aorta in a deep "V" results more often in the aorta tearing with a potential for disastrous rupture in the postoperative period. This problem of rupture was experienced in the early period of using the elephant trunk technique and not inverting it.[57]

One of the problems with elephant trunk procedures is the risk of rupture during the interval between the first operation and second stage operation. Rupture of the descending aorta continues to be a potential risk of the elephant trunk procedure during the postoperative period because the systemic inflammatory response results in release of collagenase and elastinase, which can result in rupture of the aneurysm. Furthermore, the aneurysm may grow in the interim while the patient is recovering from the first operation.

A second stage operation is usually planned after the patient's recovery from respiratory problems related to the first operation, usually 6 weeks to 4 months after the first stage. Alternatively, if the patient is in poor condition after the first operation, including respiratory problems, we will electively proceed to stent grafting the elephant trunk as part of the second stage procedure, provided that the descending aorta down to the celiac artery can be stented. On occasion, a limited thoracoabdominal incision has been used to place bypasses from the iliac artery to the visceral vessels and, thereafter, a stent graft has been inserted to replace the remaining aorta from the elephant trunk down to the aortic bifurcation or iliac arteries (see Chapter 69B). Surprisingly, these few patients have tolerated this procedure well without development of leg weakness or paralysis.

In patients with acute dissection, total arch replacement is avoided as much as possible. If total arch replacement must be done, an elephant trunk can be placed in the true lumen in the descending aorta after transecting the aorta beyond the left subclavian artery. Transecting the aorta ensures that all layers are cut and a completely hemostatic suture line achieved with a rim of Teflon felt around the aorta. The recurrent nerve usually ends up being transected.

An alternative for a dilated distal arch is to sew the anastomosis between the common carotid and left subclavian artery (Figure 69A-9).[49] If the distal aortic arch beyond the left subclavian artery is enlarged and there is no "landing site" for doing the distal anastomosis, then the aortic arch is often more narrow between the left common carotid and left subclavian artery. Thus, doing the anastomosis at this site results in a shorter circulatory arrest period because the suture line is shorter and also because exposure is better. The downside of doing the anastomosis between the left common carotid and left subclavian arteries is that the left subclavian artery needs to be anastomosed to the elephant trunk during the second stage operation. This is typically done with an interposition graft. The results using this technique have been satisfactory in our experience with over 20 patients. An alternative method described by Kieffer is to attach the left subclavian artery to the left carotid artery at the first stage operation.

Once the distal anastomosis is performed, the inner inverted graft is withdrawn and an opening is made opposite the greater vessels. The posterior suture line is performed followed by the anterior suture line. The graft is flushed and any potential embolic material removed and then the graft clamped. The graft is checked for hemostasis at both the distal anastomosis and the aortic arch. The proximal anastomosis is performed to the ascending aorta, depending on the root technique used.

Increasingly, patients are referred for descending thoracic or thoracoabdominal operations but have severe cardiac disease, either valvular or coronary.[60] If the proximal descending aorta or distal arch is also enlarged, we will place a descending thoracic elephant graft with the proximal anastomosis sewn just beyond the left subclavian artery in preparation for the second stage operation or stent grafting. One reason for this is that the left subclavian artery can also be used. If not, the distal arch could not be clamped at the second operation with a patent left internal mammary artery.

In our recent review of 142 elephant trunk procedures, the survival rate for the first operation was 98%. In our previous review of 84 elephant trunk procedures, the survival rate was 92%. Safi and colleagues[38] recently reported their experience with the elephant trunk procedure with a survival rate of 95%.

If the entire thoracic aorta or the entire aorta is going to be replaced through both a mediastinal and left thoracoabdominal incision, the distal anastomosis in the aortic arch does not need to be done, only the anastomosis to the greater vessels. This operative technique will be discussed in Chapter 69B. Also, if the descending aorta, arch, and ascending aorta are replaced through a "clam-shell" incision, a distal arch anastomosis is not needed.

If the elephant trunk procedure is not used for the distal anastomosis, the distal anastomosis is performed in the descending aorta with a simple running suture (Figure 69A-10). Usually, the aorta is not transected because of the risk of cutting the recurrent laryngeal nerve. The transition

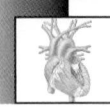

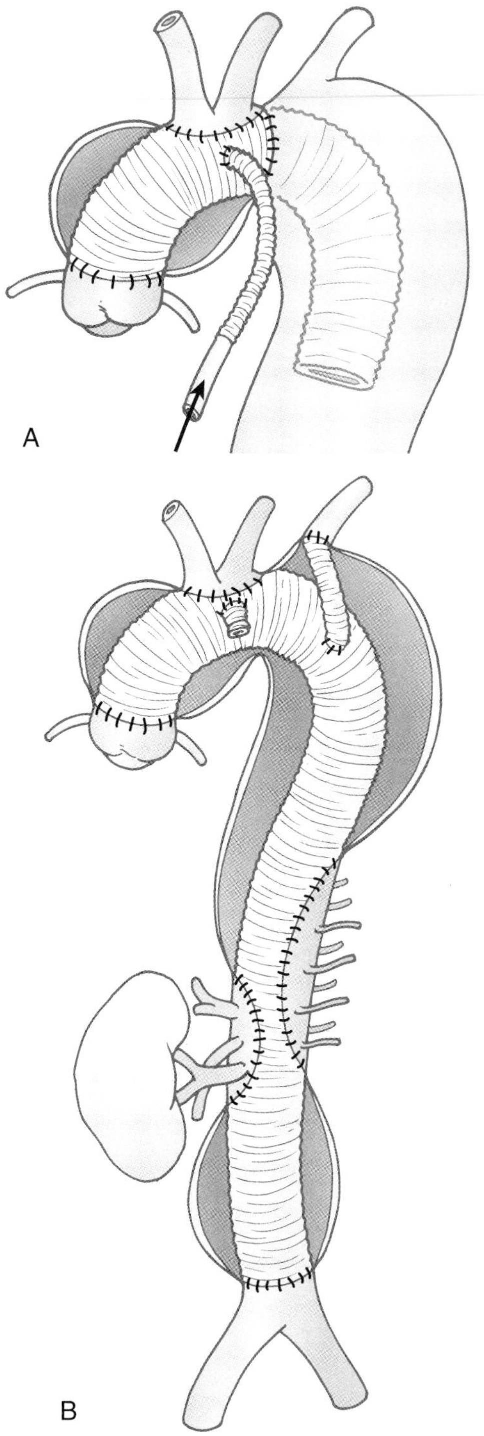

Figure 69A–9 Example of modified elephant trunk technique with an anastomosis performed between the left common carotid and left subclavian arteries (A and B). Completion of the second stage elephant trunk procedure with a tube graft to the left subclavian artery.

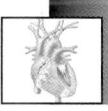

between the aneurysm to the normal aorta usually has fairly tough tissue to suture. As indicated previously, if this is within the proximal third of the descending aorta, the anastomosis can be performed without a problem, particularly if the parachuting technique is used. If there is an aberrant right subclavian artery without a Kommerell's diverticulum aneurysm, it can be included within the repair (see Figure 69A-1B). An alternative is a technique described by Griepp in which the graft is placed in the descending aorta while the anastomosis is performed and then the inverted graft in the descending aorta is withdrawn for the aortic arch repair.[47]

Less Commonly Used Techniques

In patients with saccular aneurysms with a fairly narrow neck, a patch of graft material can be sewn to the neck in the aortic arch, usually on the lesser curve. One needs to ensure that the edge of the aorta is strong and will hold sutures. This technique is also useful for saccular aneurysms of the proximal descending aorta. A decision, however, has to be made as to whether a mediastinal approach or left thoracotomy is better. When a patch technique is used, because there is usually extensive atheroma, it is advisable to use the right subclavian artery for arterial inflow to ensure that any potential embolic material is not flushed back up into the brain but rather washed into the descending aorta.

Griepp and the Mt. Sinai group have described a technique of suturing a large graft to the greater vessels island and then perfusing this graft from the pump while another graft is used for doing both the distal and proximal anastomoses in the aorta.[16,17,19] Finally, an anastomosis between the graft to the greater vessels and the separate aortic arch graft is performed. This technique allows for shorter circulatory arrest to the brain but does require additional anastomoses be performed.

Japanese surgeons, when doing aortic arch replacements, like to use branch grafts to the greater vessels. Branch grafts have a neoaortic larger graft with four-sided grafts attached end to side, typically 8 or 10 mm in size. The distal anastomosis is first performed between the neoaortic graft and the descending aorta, followed by the greater vessel anastomoses. The left subclavian artery and the left common carotid and innominate artery are anastomosed to the branch grafts in sequential order. Cannulas within the transected greater vessels are used to maintain antegrade perfusion while these anastomoses are performed. The fourth side graft is used for perfusing the aortic arch and reestablishing blood flow to the greater vessels as they become attached to the branch graft. This approach is not generally favored by most European and United States surgeons, although there is some virtue to this technique in patients with extensive calcification and atheroma of the aortic arch when suturing beyond the atheroma and calcification in the greater vessels is required. Disadvantages of this technique are a very long pump time, prolonged total body systemic circulatory arrest, and the longer period of nonpulsatile flow to the brain. Indeed, for aortic arch surgery, the pump time is the best predictor of mortality and risk of stroke.[44,47] A method we have used in conjunction with subclavian arterial perfusion is to sew a bifurcated graft to the innominate artery and carotid artery first and then do an elephant trunk procedure and left carotid bypass. These are then connected to the neoaortic graft. The advantage is that the brain arrest time is 5–15 minutes.

A technique that can occasionally be used is to place a bifurcated graft on the ascending aorta, suturing the other ends of the bifurcated graft to the greater vessels so that the native greater vessel stump in the aortic arch can be oversewn. Later, the aortic arch and descending aorta are

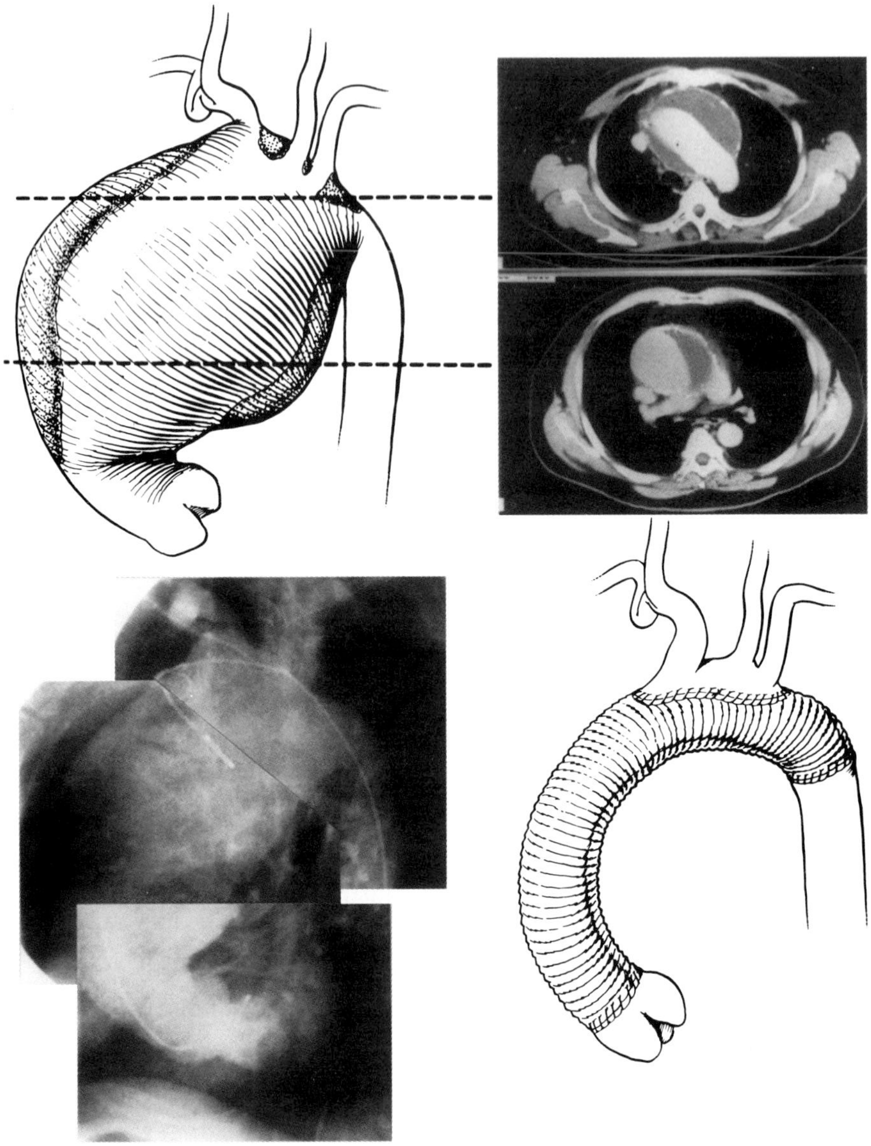

Figure 69A–10 Example of an aneurysm involving only the ascending and aortic arch and proximal descending aorta for which the elephant trunk procedure was not necessary. Note the extensive clot formation within the aneurysm shown on the CT scan. The arch was repaired by sewing the graft into the proximal descending aorta and then reattaching the greater vessels as a Carrel patch.

stented as needed. This technique may be useful in patients who cannot be placed on cardiopulmonary bypass or who have significant comorbid disease that prevents more definitive operations from being used.

In patients with extensive atheroma and calcification, endarterectomy of the aortic arch may also be required. In our experience with 45 patients, the results have been surprisingly good when doing endarterectomies at the same time as aneurysm repairs of the aortic arch.[53] When performing endarterectomies of the aortic arch and greater vessels, a meticulous technique must be used to ensure that no embolic material gets into the ostia of the greater vessels. For this reason, we use antegrade brain perfusion and often combine this with retrograde brain perfusion to ensure maximum flushing of the greater vessels while doing these types of repairs.[53]

Increasingly, we have favored using a minimum invasive approach for redo aortic arch surgery and have found that this does not limit our exposure. The advantage of using this method at reoperations is that the rest of the heart and the right atrium do not need to be dissected out. Because the patient has typically undergone a previous aortic root procedure, an elephant trunk procedure can be done distally and the proximal anastomosis performed to the ascending aorta. We have used this method now in 125 patients with a 95% survival and a 2.6% stroke incidence.[21,31,56]

We do not use the new biological glues extensively for aortic arch repairs. In our experience, patients who return for reoperations who have had repairs with these glues often have tissue that is extremely thick, hard, and often calcified, making it difficult to work with. There is also the potential risk in using glue in aortic arch surgery in that some of the glue may embolize distally, especially with the GRF glues that are made with formaldehyde. Infection and false aneurysms may also be a problem.

In patients with aneurysms or stenosis of the greater vessels, various operative techniques can be used at the time of aortic arch surgery. Most of these involve placing bypasses from the neoaortic graft to a more distal normal segment of the greater vessel. Sometimes, if only the origin of the greater vessels of the aortic arch is involved, these procedures can be performed without placing the patient on cardiopulmonary bypass (Figure 69A-11). For example,

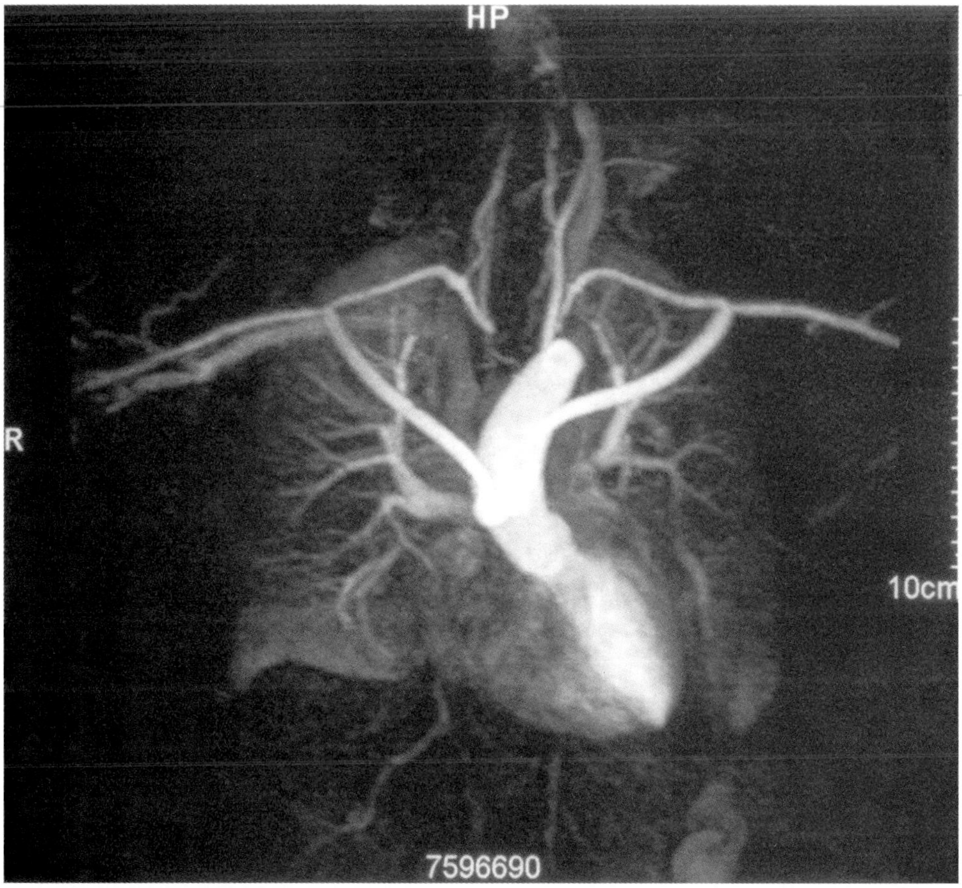

1

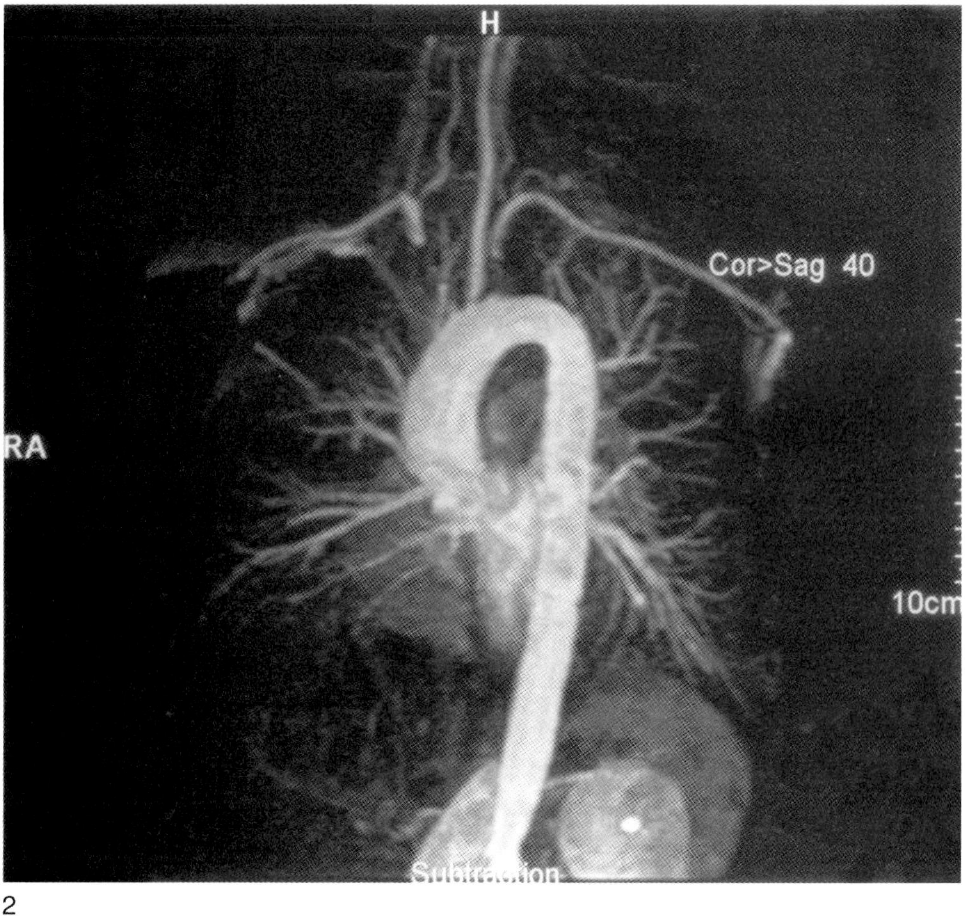

2

Figure 69A–11 (1) MRA of a patient with occluded innominate and left subclavian arteries and 50% narrowing of the left common carotid artery. (2 and 3) Postoperative MRA after off-pump insertion of a bifurcated graft from the ascending aorta to both axillary arteries with a transpleural approach.

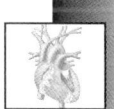

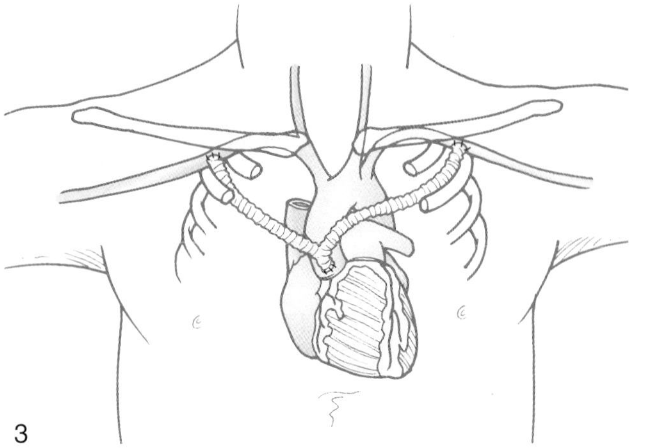
3

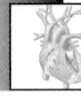

Figure 69A–11 cont'd

a side-biting clamp can be placed on the ascending aorta and a bifurcated graft sewn to the ascending aorta. The distal grafts can then be used to bypass the innominate, the common carotid, or the subclavian arteries. Figure 69A-11 demonstrates a patient in whom this technique was used to attach the bifurcated graft to the ascending aorta using a side biting clamp: the two distal grafts were routed through the chest pleural spaces and through the first intercostal space to the bilateral axillary arteries where anastomoses were performed.

Occasionally, the aortic arch cannot be replaced or operated upon. A left ventricular apex to descending aorta valved conduit is one option (Figure 69A-12).

OUTCOMES

In a previous analyses of 656 patients who underwent deep hypothermia and circulatory arrest, mostly for aortic arch replacements, the mortality rate was 10% and the stroke rate was 7%.[44] This large study noted that the longer the circulatory arrest the greater the risk of stroke. It is of interest that some patients tolerated circulatory arrest periods of up to 120 min without developing frank strokes. In this series of patients, the predictors of stroke by multivariate analyses were ($p < .05$) history of cerebrovascular disease, previous aortic surgery beyond the left subclavian artery, and cardiopulmonary bypass time.[44]

Results with aortic arch surgery continue to improve. In a recent prospective randomized study, we reported a survival rate of 100% and no patient suffered stroke after aortic arch repairs. Although 91% of patients had a neurocognitive deficit when tested between 3 and 6 days after undergoing aortic arch repairs, by 2–3 weeks after surgery with repeat testing using 51 neurocognitive tests, 9% had a deficit and by 6 months, all the patients with new neurocognitive deficits had recovered. As noted previously, 38% of patients had a preoperative deficit. In another analysis of 403 patients undergoing ascending and aortic arch operations using a protocol to protect the brain as much as possible from strokes and neurocognitive deficits, the survival rate was 98%, stroke rate 2%, and incidence of neurocognitive gross clinical deficits 2.5%. The predictors of death by

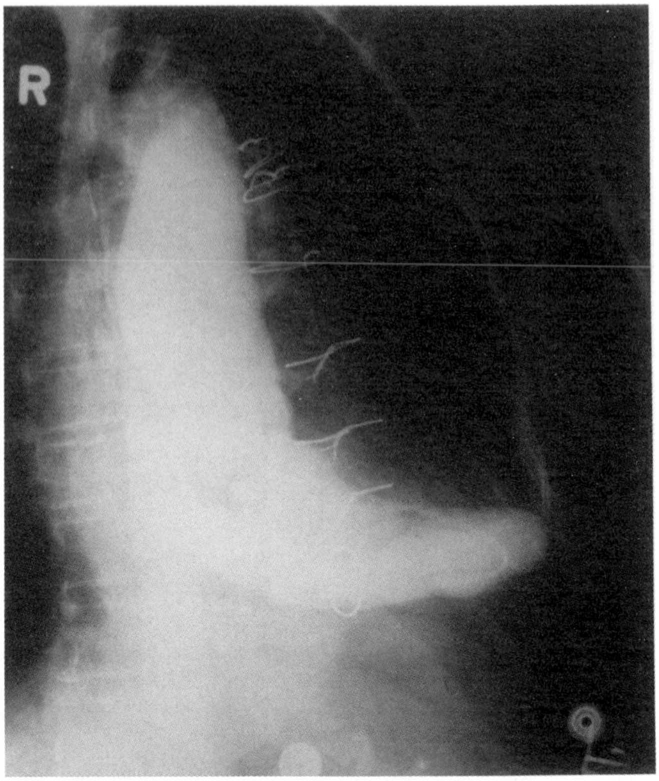

1

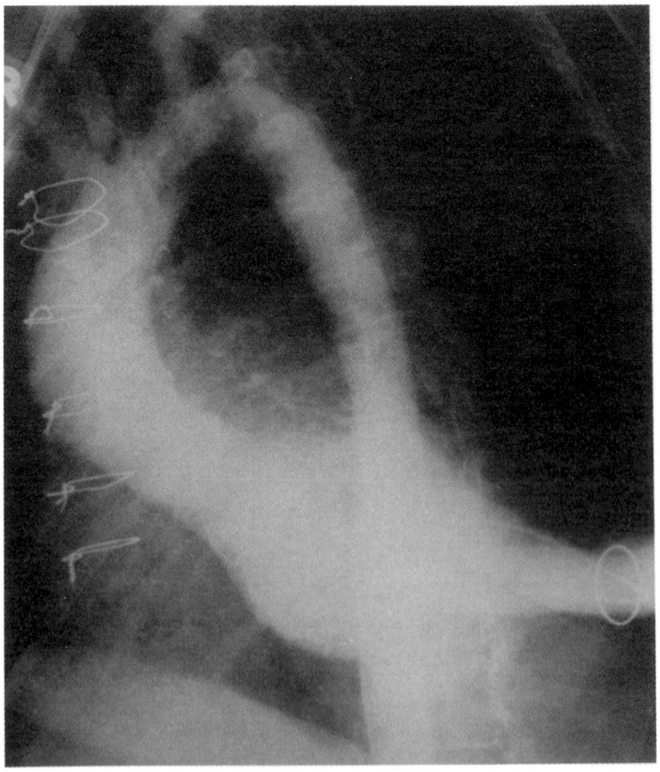
2

Figure 69A–12 (1 and 2) Example of a left ventricle apex to descending aorta valved tube graft for extensive calcification of the ascending aorta and aortic arch including modest stenoses of the greater vessels. The patient had undergone previous coronary artery bypass surgery, had systemic lupus and renal disease, was on high-dose steroids, and had heart failure from aortic valve stenosis. The operation was done without cardiopulmonary bypass.

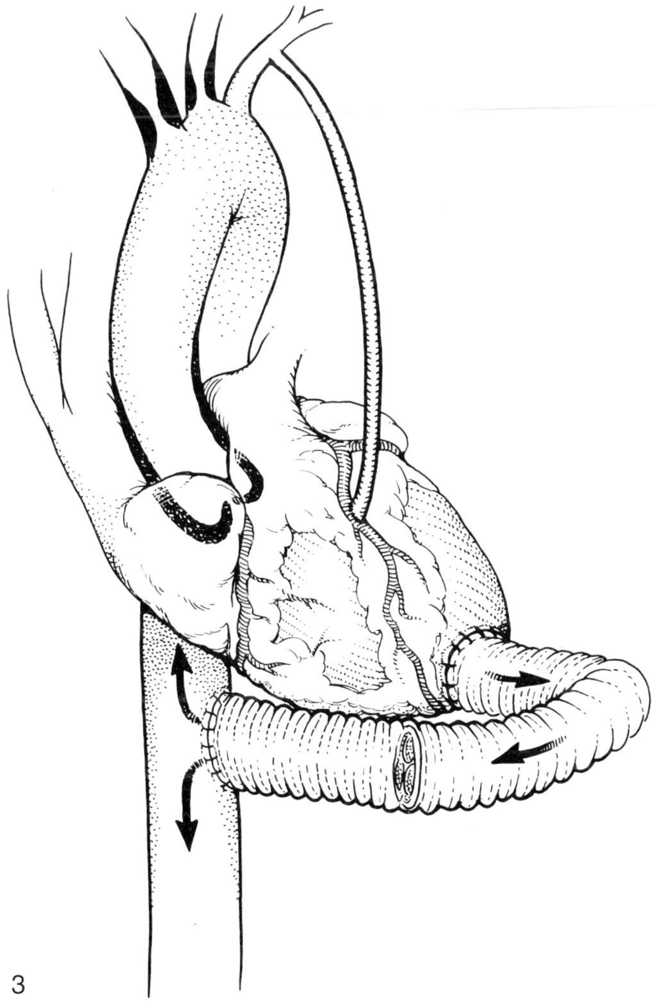

3

Figure 69A–12 cont'd (3) Illustration, diagrammatically, of the operative procedure.

multivariate analyses were pump time; for stroke, aorta symptom grade, peripheral vascular disease and pump time; and for neurocognitive dysfunction, New York Heart Association dyspnea class, pump time, arrest time, day extubated, and antegrade perfusion. These latter two studies emphasize the importance of awareness that patients may have suffered silent strokes and developed neurocognitive deficits prior to undergoing aortic arch surgery.[53,59]

SUMMARY

In the past aortic arch surgery was considered among the most formidable of cardiovascular operations. With modern techniques, surgery for the aortic arch is considerably safer and satisfactory results can be achieved in most patients.

REFERENCES

1. Bachet J, Guilmet D, Goudot B, et al: Antegrade cerebral perfusion with cold blood: a 13-year experience. Ann Thorac Surg 67:1874–1878, 1999.
2. Barnard CN, Schrire V: The surgical treatment of acquired aneurysms of the thoracic aorta. Thorax 18:101–105, 1963.
3. Borst HG, Frank G, Schaps D: Treatment of extensive aortic aneurysms by a new multiple-stage approach. J Thorac Cardiovasc Surg 95:11–13, 1988.
4. Borst HG, Walterbusch G, Schaps D: Extensive aortic replacement using "elephant trunk" prosthesis. Thorac Cardiovasc Surg 31:37–40, 1983.
5. Cigarroa JE, Isselbacher EM, DeSanctis RW, Eagle KA: Diagnostic imaging in the evaluation of suspected aortic dissection: old standards and new directions. N Engl J Med 328:35–43, 1993.
6. Cooley DA, Livesay JJ: Technique of "open" distal anastomosis for ascending and transverse arch resection. Bull Tex Heart Inst 8:421–426, 1981.
7. Coselli JS, Crawford ES, Beall AC Jr, et al: Determination of brain temperature for safe circulatory arrest during cardiovascular operation. Ann Thorac Surg 45:638–642, 1988.
8. Crawford ES, Saleh SA: Transverse aortic arch aneurysm: improved results of treatment employing new modifications of aortic reconstruction and hypothermic cerebral circulatory arrest. Ann Surg 194:180–188, 1981.
9. Crawford ES, Svensson LG, Coselli JS, et al: Surgical treatment of aneurysm and/or dissection of the ascending aorta, transverse aortic arch, and ascending aorta and transverse aortic arch: factors influencing survival in 717 patients. J Thorac Cardiovasc Surg 98:659–674, 1989.
10. David TE, Feindel CM: An aortic valve-sparing operation for patients with aortic incompetence and aneurysm of the ascending aorta. J Thorac Cardiovasc Surg 103:617–622, 1992.
11. Davis EA, Gillinov AM, Cameron DE, Reitz BA: Hypothermic circulatory arrest as a surgical adjunct: a 5-year experience with 60 adult patients. Ann Thorac Surg 53:402–406, 1992.
12. DeBakey ME, Cooley DA, Crawford ES, Morris GC Jr: Successful resection of fusiform aneurysm of aortic arch with replacement by homograft. Surg Gynecol Obstet 105:656–664, 1957.
13. Eichelberger JP: Aortic dissection without intimal tear: case report and findings on transesophageal echocardiography. J Am Soc Echocardiogr 7:82–86, 1994.
14. Engelman RM, Pleet AB, Rousou JA, et al: Does cardiopulmonary bypass temperature correlate with postoperative central nervous system dysfunction? J Card Surg 10:493–497, 1995.
15. Erbel R, Mohr-Kahaly S, Oelert H, et al: Diagnostic strategies in suspected aortic dissection: comparison of computed tomography, aortography, and transesophageal echocardiography. Am J Card Imaging 4:157–172, 1990.
16. Ergin MA, Galla JD, Lansman SL, et al: Hypothermic circulatory arrest in operations on the thoracic aorta. J Thorac Cardiovasc Surg 107:788–799, 1994.
17. Ergin MA, Uysal S, Reich DL, et al: Temporary neurological dysfunction after deep hypothermic circulatory arrest: a clinical marker of long-term functional deficit. Ann Thorac Surg 67:1887–1890, 1999.
18. Gott VL, Gillinov AM, Pyeritz RE, et al: Aortic root replacement: risk factor analysis of a seventeen-year experience with 270 patients. J Thorac Cardiovasc Surg 109:536–544, 1995.
19. Griepp RB, Ergin A, McCullough JN: Use of hypothermic circulatory arrest for cerebral protection during aortic surgery. J Card Surg 12:312–321, 1997.
20. Griepp RB, Juvonen T, Griepp EB, et al: Is retrograde cerebral perfusion an effective means of neural support during deep hypothermic circulatory arrest? Ann Thorac Surg 64:913–916, 1997.
21. Guiraudon GM, Ofiesh JG, Kaushik R: Extended vertical transatrial septal approach to the mitral valve. Ann Thorac Surg 52:1058–1062, 1991.

22. Heinemann MK, Buehner B, Jurmann MJ, et al: Use of the "elephant trunk technique" in aortic surgery. Ann Thorac Surg 60:2–7, 1995.
23. Hilgenberg AD, Akins CW, Logan DL, et al: Composite aortic root replacement with direct coronary artery implantation. Ann Thorac Surg 62:1090–1095, 1996.
24. Hirst AE Jr, Johns VJ Jr, Kime SW Jr: Dissecting aneurysm of the aorta: a review of 505 cases. Medicine (Baltimore) 37: 217–219, 1958.
25. Juvonen T, Weisz DJ, Wolfe D, et al: Can retrograde perfusion mitigate cerebral injury after particulate embolization? A study in a chronic porcine model. J Thorac Cardiovasc Surg 115: 1142–1159, 1998.
26. Lytle BW, McCarthy PM, Meaney KM, et al: Systemic hypothermia and circulatory arrest combined with arterial perfusion of the superior vena cava. Effective intraoperative cerebral protection. J Thorac Cardiovasc Surg 109:738–743, 1995.
27. Miller DC, Mitchell RS, Oyer PE, et al: Independent determinants of operative mortality for patients with aortic dissections. Circulation 70(Suppl. I):I-153–I-164, 1984.
28. Mills NL, Ochsner JL: Massive air embolism during cardiopulmonary bypass. J Thorac Cardiovasc Surg 80:708–717, 1980.
29. Mohr-Kahaly S, Erbel R, Kearney P, et al: Aortic intramural hemorrhage visualized by transesophageal echocardiography: findings and prognostic implications. J Am Coll Cardiol 23:658–664, 1994.
30. Nadolny EM, Svensson LG: Carbon dioxide field flooding techniques for open heart surgery: monitoring and minimizing potential adverse effects. Perfusion 15:151–153, 2000.
31. Navia JL, Cosgrove DM III: Minimally invasive mitral valve operations. Ann Thorac Surg 62:1542–1544, 1996.
32. Nienaber CA, von Kodolitsch Y, Nicolas V, et al: The diagnosis of thoracic aortic dissection by noninvasive imaging procedure. N Engl J Med 328:1–9, 1993.
33. Nienaber CA, von Kodolitsch Y, Petersen B, et al: Intramural hemorrhage of the thoracic aorta: diagnostic and therapeutical implications. Circulation 92:1465–1472, 1995.
34. Reich DL, Uysal S, Sliwinski M, et al: Neuropsychologic outcome after deep hypothermic circulatory arrest in adults. J Thorac Cardiovasc Surg 117:156–163, 1999.
35. Robbins RC, McManus RP, Mitchell RS, et al: Management of patients with intramural hematoma of the thoracic aorta. Circulation 88(Suppl. II):II-1–II-10, 19.
36. Robinson BLAC, Nadolny EM, Entrup MH, Svensson LG: Management of right-sided aortic arch aneurysms. Ann Thorac Surg 72:1764–1765, 2001.
37. Safi HJ, Brien HW, Winter JN, et al: Brain protection via cerebral retrograde perfusion during aortic arch aneurysm repair. Ann Thorac Surg 56:270–276, 1993.
38. Safi HJ, Miller CC III, Estrera AL, et al: Staged repair of extensive aortic aneurysms. Morbidity and mortality in the elephant trunk technique. Circulation 104:2938–2942, 2001.
39. Sarsam MAI, Yacoub M: Remodeling of the aortic valve annulus. J Thorac Cardiovasc Surg 105:435–438, 1993.
40. Sundt TM, Kouchoukos NT, Saffitz JE, et al: Renal dysfunction and intravascular coagulation with aprotinin and hypothermic circulatory arrest. Ann Thorac Surg 55: 1418–1424, 1993.
41. Svensson LG, Robinson MF, Esser J, et al: Influence of anatomic origin on intracranial distribution of micro-emboli in the baboon. Stroke 17:1198–1202, 1986.
42. Svensson LG, Blackstone E, Cosgrove DM: Valve selection in young adults. Curr Probl Cardiol 28(7):417–480, 2003.
43. Svensson LG, Crawford ES, Coselli JS, et al: Impact of cardiovascular operation on survival in the Marfan patient. Circulation 80(Suppl. I):I-233–I-242.
44. Svensson LG, Crawford ES, Hess ER, et al: Deep hypothermia with circulatory arrest: determinants of stroke and early mortality in 656 patients. J Thorac Cardiovasc Surg 106:19–31, 1993.
45. Svensson LG, Crawford ES, Hess KR, et al: Composite valve graft replacement of the proximal aorta: comparison of techniques in 348 patients. Ann Thorac Surg 54:427–439, 1992.
46. Svensson LG, Crawford ES: Aortic dissection and aortic aneurysm surgery, II: Clinical observations, experimental investigations, and statistical analyses. Curr Probl Surg 29:915–1057, 1992.
47. Svensson LG, Crawford ES: Cardiovascular and Vascular Diseases of the Aorta. Philadelphia: W. B. Saunders, 1997, pp. 42–83.
48. Svensson LG, Hussain A, Penney DL, et al: Brief communication. A prospective randomized study of neurocognitive function and S-100 protein after antegrade or retrograde brain perfusion with hypothermic arrest for aortic surgery. J Thorac Cardiovasc Surg 119:163–166, 2000.
49. Svensson LG, Kaushik SD, Marinko E: Elephant trunk anastomosis between left carotid and subclavian arteries for aneurysmal distal aortic arch. Ann Thorac Surg 71:1050–1052, 2001.
50. Svensson LG, Khitin L: Aortic cross-sectional area/height ratio timing of aortic surgery in asymptomatic patients with Marfan syndrome. J Thorac Cardiovasc Surg 123:360–361, 2002.
51. Svensson LG, Labib SB, Eisenhauer AC, Butterly JR: Intimal tear without hematoma: an important variant of aortic dissection that can elude current imaging techniques. Circulation 99:1331–1336, 1999.
52. Svensson LG, Longoria J, Kimmel WA, Nadolny E: Management of aortic valve disease during aortic surgery. Ann Thorac Surg 69:778–784, 2000.
53. Svensson LG, Nadolny EM, Kimmel WA: Multimodal protocol influence on stroke and neurocognitive deficit prevention after ascending/arch aortic operations. Ann Thorac Surg 74:2040–2046, 2002.
54. Svensson LG, Nadolny EM, Penney DL, et al: Prospective randomized neurocognitive and S-100 study of hypothermic circulatory arrest, retrograde brain perfusion, and antegrade brain perfusion for aortic arch operations. Ann Thorac Surg 71:1905–1912, 2001.
55. Svensson LG: Antegrade perfusion during suspended animation? J Thorac Cardiovasc Surg 124:1068–1070, 2002.
56. Svensson LG: Minimal-access "J" or "j" sternotomy for valvular, aortic, and coronary operations or reoperations. Ann Thorac Surg 64:1501–1503, 1997.
57. Svensson LG: Rationale and technique for replacement of the ascending aorta, arch, and distal aorta using a modified elephant trunk procedure. J Card Surg 7:301–312, 1992.
58. Svensson LG: Invited commentary. (In press.) Ann Thor Surg.
59. Svensson LG: Signing for modified David's reimplantation procedure. Ann Thor Surg 76: 1751–1753, 2003.
60. Svensson LG, Kim KH, Blackstone EH, et al: Elephant trunk procedure: Newer indications and uses. Ann Thorac Surg 78: 109–116, 2004.
61. Swain JA, McDonald TJ, Griffith PK, et al: Low-flow hypothermic cardiopulmonary bypass protects the brain. J Thorac Cardiovasc Surg 102:76–84, 1991.
62. Ueda T, Shimizu H, Ito T, et al: Cerebral complications associated with selective perfusion of the arch vessels in patients undergoing surgery of the thoracic aorta. Ann Thorac Surg 70:1472–1477, 2000.
63. Ueda Y, Miki S, Kusuhara K, et al: Deep hypothermic systemic circulatory arrest and continuous retrograde cerebral perfusion for surgery of the aortic arch aneurysm. Eur J Cardiothorac Surg 6:36–41, 1992.

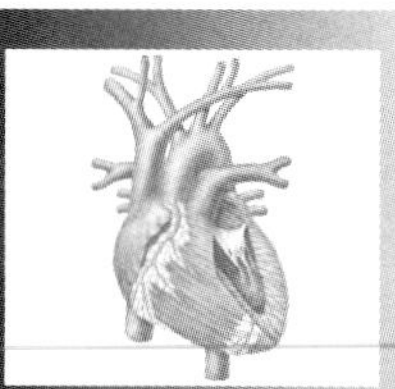

CHAPTER 69B

Surgery of the Aortic Arch, Descending Thoracic and Thoracoabdominal Aortic Surgery, and Aortic Dissection

Descending Thoracic and Thoracoabdominal Aortic Surgery

Lars G. Svensson

INTRODUCTION

Chapter 69A on aortic arch surgery dealt with definitions and the micropathology of aortic diseases. The discussion of brain protection during deep hypothermia and circulatory arrest is also relevant to descending and thoracoabdominal aortic surgery when deep hypothermia and circulatory arrest are used. The reader is referred to Chapter 69A for a more detailed review. In this chapter, the discussion on central nervous system protection will focus mainly on protection of the spinal cord against injury during descending and thoracoabdominal aortic surgery. The etiological and predisposing factors, preoperative workup, and operative procedures will also be reviewed.

In 2003, we performed 999 aorta operations at our Cleveland Clinic Aorta Center, 180 on the descending thoracic or thorocoabdominal aorta. Our approach is discussed below.

CLASSIFICATION OF DESCENDING THORACIC AND THORACOABDOMINAL ANEURYSMS

This chapter discusses the issues associated with nondissecting types of aneurysms of the descending thoracic aorta and thoracoabdominal aorta.[1–59] Aortic dissection and dissecting aneurysms will be dealt with in Chapters 69C, 69D, and 70.

Previously, descending thoracic aortic aneurysms were classified according to the extent of involvement and replacement at the time of surgery.[45] In a study of 832 descending thoracic aortic aneurysms,[45] this classification was used to evaluate the outcome after surgery: namely, the risk of developing a spinal cord neurological deficit resulting in either paraplegia or paraparesis. After data collection for the analyses, the descending aorta was divided into three equal extents: extent A was the proximal third, extent B was the middle third, and extent C was the distal extent. For the purposes of statistical analyses, these extents were used to determine the incidence of neurological deficit. The influence of replacing the entire descending aorta was also analyzed. The results of the analyses will be discussed under outcomes.

Thoracoabdominal aneurysms were classified by Crawford and colleagues[38,44,48] into four extents (Figure 69B-1). Type I thoracoabdominal aneurysms involved the

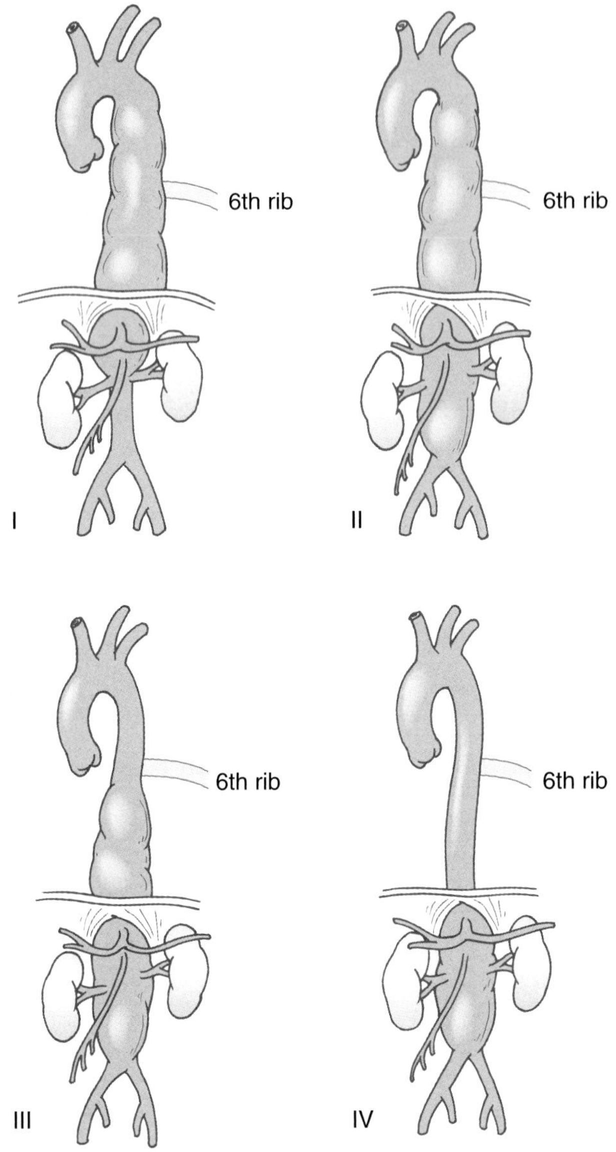

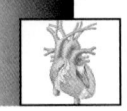

Figure 69B–1 Crawford classification of thoracoabdominal aneurysms. Type I aneurysms extend from the proximal descending aorta to the renal arteries. Type II extends from the proximal descending aorta above the level of T_6 to below the renal arteries. Type III extends from below the level of T_6 in the descending aorta and into the abdomen in varying extents. Type IV involves predominantly the abdominal aorta.

descending aorta proximal to the level of the sixth rib to above the renal arteries; type II thoracoabdominal aneurysms involved the descending aorta proximal to the level of the sixth rib but beyond the renal arteries; type III thoracoabdominal aneurysms involved the distal descending aorta beyond the sixth rib and a variable extent of the abdominal aorta; type IV thoracoabdominal aneurysms involved the abdominal aorta without involvement of the descending aorta. These classifications revealed marked differences between the groups of both the expected risk of neurological deficits involving the spinal cord and, to some extent, the risk of renal failure and mortality. Type II suffered the worst outcomes. Subsequent analyses showed the risk of developing paralysis in Crawford type I aneurysms varied, according to whether the aorta was replaced below the celiac artery.[48] Later, it was suggested that type III thoracoabdominal aneurysms should be further divided into a separate group according to the extent of abdominal involvement.[26] These aneurysms, however, are seldom seen and their influence on outcome was not strong enough to warrant a separate classification. Crawford type II thoracoabdominal aneurysms also have varying outcomes according to the involvement of the distal aortic arch and whether the entire abdominal aorta down to the iliacs needs to be replaced.

ETIOLOGICAL AND PREDISPOSING FACTORS

Congenital Lesions

Congenital lesions of the descending aorta are fairly frequent in contrast to the thoracoabdominal aorta where they are rarely observed.[38] The most common congenital lesions involve the distal aortic arch and the proximal third of the descending aorta. In this area, the most frequently occurring lesion is coarctation of the aorta,[38] either missed in childhood or seen in patients who have undergone previous surgery for coarctation of the aorta. Not infrequently, multiple operations have been done and patients present as adults with restenosis, an aortic replacement graft or repair that is of inadequate size for an adult, aneurysm formation proximally or distally to the previous repair, or rupture of an old previous repair including, for example, knitted grafts inserted in childhood. Sometimes, a lesion takes the form of an interrupted aortic arch associated with descending aorta pathology. Other congenital lesions include a large Kommerell's diverticulum associated with an aberrant right subclavian artery or a right-sided aortic arch (see Chapter 69A). Rarely is thoracoabdominal aortic congenital coarctation (sometimes referred to as the middle-aortic syndrome) seen. Some of these thoracoabdominal coarctation lesions may be related to other diseases such as Takayasu's disease or neurofibromatosis.[38] Occasionally, aneurysms may be observed in the descending or thoracoabdominal aorta and are most probably the result of chronic congenital infections, particularly from the use of intravenous or arterial cannulas that became infected. We observed this in one of our pediatric patients.[38]

Medial-Degenerative Aneurysms

Medial-degenerative aneurysms of the descending or thoracoabdominal aorta are associated with loss of elastic tissues in the aortic wall. Depending on whether cigarette smoking and chronic pulmonary disease are associated factors, there is a variable extent of atherosclerosis within the aortic wall. As aneurysms enlarge, there is an increasing amount of atheromatous material deposition and clot formation within the aneurysms. Areas of clot even appear on computed tomography (CT) scans or magnetic resonance imagings (MRIs) to resemble aortic dissections. Aneurysms are typically fusiform in nature, although there may be areas of weakness that have a bubble appearance on angiography or magnetic resonance angiography (MRA) studies. A variant usually seen in older women with long histories of pulmonary disease and cigarette smoking is a penetrating ulcer that can either lead to dissection or, if successfully healed, a saccular aneurysm.[38] These are most frequently seen in the distal part of the proximal-third or middle-third of the descending aorta.

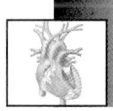

Because of extensive atheroma and clot formation in the aneurysms, patients may present with evidence of distal embolization such as "trash foot," pancreatitis, abdominal angina, bowel infarction, progressive intermittent claudication, and progressive renal failure. Very rarely, patients are seen with distal embolization from atheromatic and thrombotic lesions in the arch or descending aorta without aneurysms being present. In these patients, a hypercoagulable state is usually found.[38]

At the time of surgery, if there is extensive clot formation within the aorta in addition to the presence of atheroma, the intercostal vessels will often be obstructed, especially in patients with large aneurysms. In such patients, therefore, collateral sources of blood flow to the spinal cord become critical to maintain spinal cord function.

Furthermore, those patients who have large aneurysms and a long history of medial degenerative aneurysms with extensive atherosclerosis in the aortic wall will show evidence of visceral artery lesions such as renal artery, celiac artery, and superior mesenteric artery stenoses.[42,43] Over a period of time, total vessel occlusions will occur.[43] Of note, CT scans should be carefully examined for both formation of calcium and atheroma in the distal aortic arch to check if the aortic arch can be safely clamped for more proximal extending medially degenerative aneurysms. The reason for this is the obvious risk of stroke in these patients. If atheroma, clot, or calcium is found, alternative methods for doing the proximal anastomosis should be considered.

Mycotic Aneurysms and Infected Grafts

Mycotic aneurysms involving only the descending aorta are quite uncommon. More frequently these occur either in the lesser curve of the aortic arch or, for thoracoabdominal aneurysms, in the area opposite the visceral vessels. Nevertheless, saccular aneurysms of the descending aorta can become infected, resulting in mycotic aneurysms. (Figure 69B-2). Similarly, bacterial cultures done on clots removed from descending or thoracoabdominal aneurysms are often found to have bacteria growing within the aneurysms. Of interest, these bacteria appear to have little influence on the postoperative risk of graft or wound infections.

Infection in previously inserted descending or thoracoabdominal grafts can be a very complicated problem to manage. They may or may not be associated with a left-sided chest empyema, particularly if the patient has recently undergone an operation. Diagnosis can be difficult to obtain. CT-guided aspiration of any fluid around the graft is the most accurate method of determining graft infection.

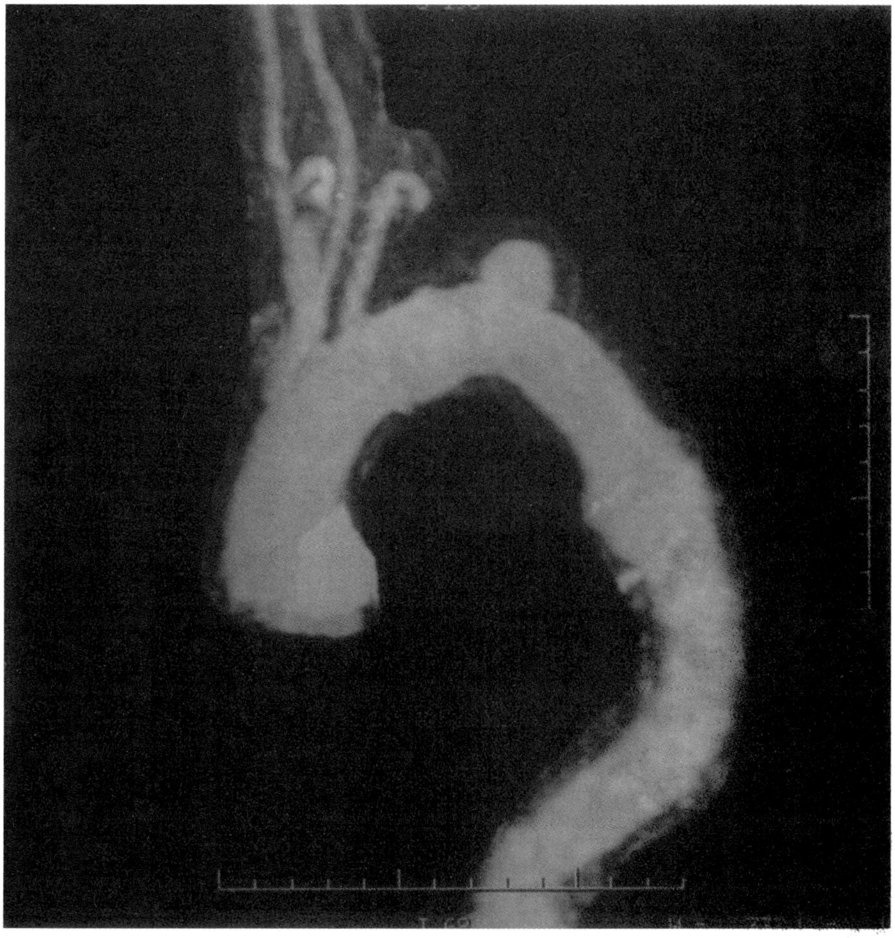

Figure 69B–2 Saccular aneurysm of the proximal descending aorta.

Treatment options include irrigating the cavity with antibiotics, resecting the infected graft material and placing a new tube prosthetic graft or an allograft, or resecting the segment of the aorta and oversewing the aortic stumps and doing extra anatomical bypasses, either aorto-to-abdominal aorta or bilateral axillary-femoral bypasses.[32,34,38,44]

Traumatic Injuries of the Aorta

Traumatic injuries of the aorta are either penetrating or blunt injuries.[38] Penetrating injuries require immediate attention since most patients are in shock and have lost large volumes of blood. Most injuries can be repaired by direct suture repair and usually do not require graft insertion. High-velocity missile injuries from either shrapnel or bullets are rarely survived; if the patient does survive long enough to reach the operating room, extensive destruction and secondary injury are usually found.

Blunt injuries of the aorta most commonly occur in the proximal descending aorta at the isthmus.[38] Parmley and associates[24] performed a study of 275 autopsies and noted 45% were at the isthmus, 23% in the ascending aorta, 13% in the descending aorta, 8% in the transverse aortic arch, 5% in the abdominal aorta, and 6% in multiple sites. It should be noted that clinically ascending aortic injuries rarely undergo operation since patients do not survive long enough to reach a hospital. In contrast, approximately 90% of patients undergo operation for descending aortic tears.[38] In approximately one fifth of autopsies in fatal motor vehicle accidents, victims show a ruptured aorta.

Multiplane angiography has been the gold standard for identification of tears; however, spiral CT with three-dimensional (3D) reconstruction or transesophageal echocardiography is being increasingly used for diagnosis.[38]

Patients with ruptured aortas are often hemodynamically unstable, because of either shock or hypertension. Prior to surgery, while the operating room is being prepared, the patient's blood pressure needs to be stabilized.

The method to use ("clamp and sew," or distal perfusion with pump, shunt, or cardiopulmonary bypass) to protect the spinal cord during aortic cross-clamping is still debated.

In a previous review of 596 patients,[40] there were no differences in spinal cord injuries; however, mortality rate was higher with cardiopulmonary bypass. In a more recent review of 1742 patients, Von Oppell et al found cardiopulmonary bypass and distal perfusion reduced the risk of paralysis.[38,58] A prospective multicenter trial reported "clamp and sew" ($p = .002$) and an aortic cross-clamp time exceeding 30 min ($p = .01$) were associated with postoperative paraplegia.[12]

Available results suggest both distal perfusion with centrifugal pump and "clamp and sew" can be equally safe for less than 30 min of aortic cross-clamping (Figure 69B-3). With increasing cross-clamp times, usually because of related, more complicated lesions and tears, the risks of paralysis and/or renal failure increases with both techniques, although less so with distal perfusion.[12,38,39,58]

Full cardiopulmonary bypass with circulatory arrest is usually reserved for complicated lesions involving the aortic arch. These lesions are best treated with circulatory arrest after the patient recovers from the initial injury and scar tissue forms so it will hold sutures. In a review of the literature[40] of 44 patients initially treated with medical management and subsequently treated with elective surgery, results were excellent. Initial management of patients with traumatic rupture of the aorta associated with complicated injuries of other organ systems or of the aorta is similar to the management of acute aortic dissections of the descending aorta. Patients must be carefully observed in the intensive care unit and treated with antihypertensive medications to ensure no leakage occurs. It is important to continue to monitor patients carefully for any evidence of leaks for the first week or two.

In patients with traumatic tears of the aorta, the classic site of tears is at the isthmus. These simple tears can often be repaired with a running suture and with the aid of pledgets. In more complicated lesions, a tube graft with a resection of the aorta with end-to-end anastomoses is required (Figure 69B-4). Occasionally, aortic dissection is precipi-

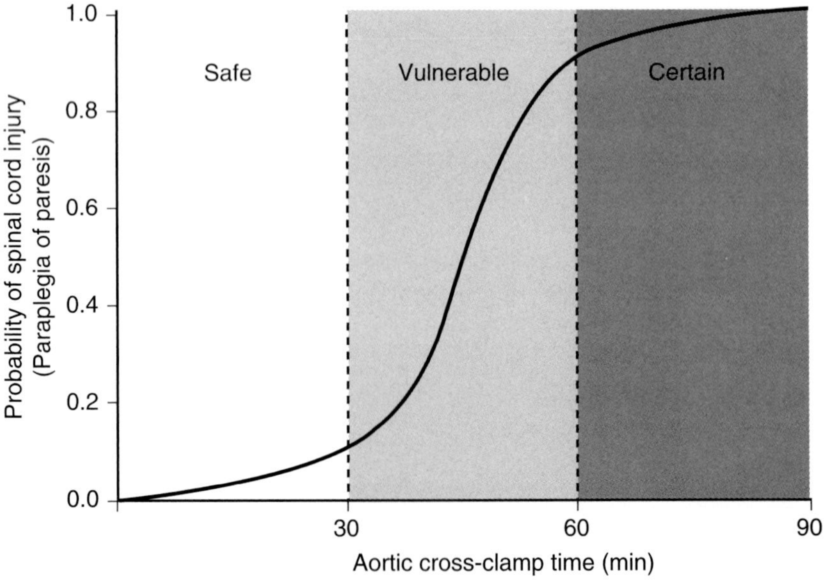

Figure 69B–3 Relationship between aortic cross-clamp time and the probability of spinal cord injury based on data from traumatic rupture of the aorta and repairs for descending acute dissections. Note: The clamp time for the first 30 min is safe; between 30 and 60 min, patients are vulnerable; more than 60 min, the risk of paralysis is almost certain in this group of patients who have no collateral blood flow and are often in shock. For patients with other types of chronic aneurysms, the curve is shifted further to the right.

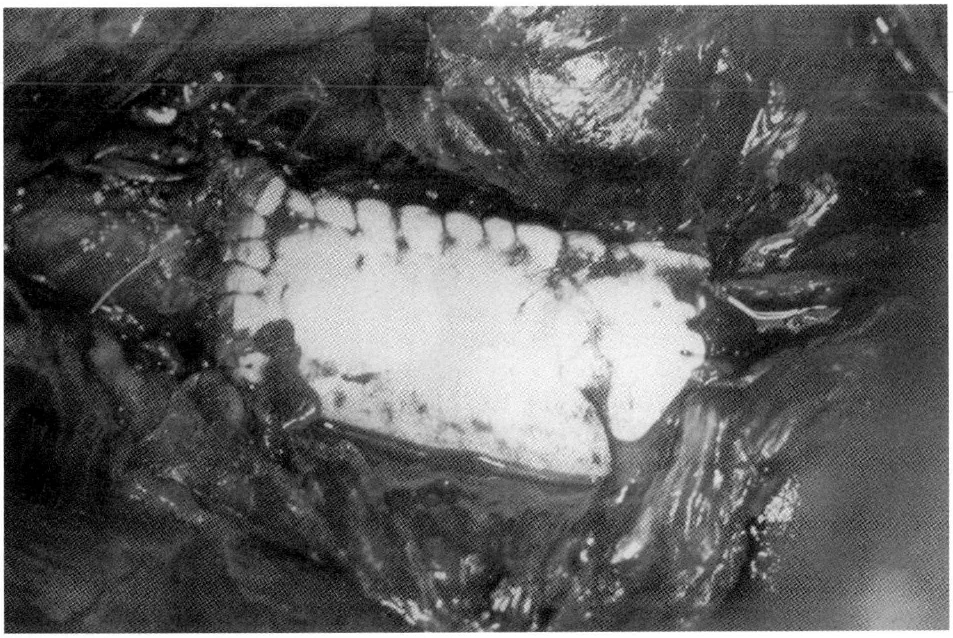

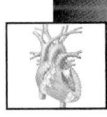

Figure 69B–4 Traumatic rupture of the aorta repair by insertion of a tube graft that is initially opened lengthwise and then resutured again.

tated by trauma, and in this situation, the site of the tear is repaired. The remaining aorta, however, is managed conservatively with careful blood pressure control and follow-up, as with classic types of DeBakey III or Stanford B dissections. Rarely, chronic traumatic saccular aneurysms may resolve spontaneously over time[28] (Figure 69B-5). Increasingly, we are now treating traumatic tears with stent grafts.

Aortitis

There is an increased frequency of aortitis associated with giant cell arteritis in the United States and in other countries such as Iceland.[38] The reason for this is unknown. In patients with giant cell arteritis of the aorta, it appears that about one third have a history of polymyalgia rheumatica. In addition, approximately 10% of patients with temporal arteritis will typically progress many years later to giant cell arteritis of the aorta.

In patients with giant cell arteritis, the ascending aorta and the aortic arch are enlarged pari passu with the descending aorta or thoracoabdominal aorta. The infrarenal aorta, however, is often spared. Whether this is related to increased collagen content in the infrarenal segment of the aorta or a high elastic content in other segments is not clear.

Tubercular aortitis frequently involves the descending aorta, particularly the mid-descending aorta. This is a rare complication of tuberculosis but appears to be related to common antigens found on both the tuberculous bacillus and aortic wall antigens. In contrast, syphilitic aortitis involves the ascending aorta more frequently then the descending or thoracoabdominal aorta.

In the United States Takayasu's disease is uncommon, although it is more frequent in patients with a Mediterranean family background. Takayasu's disease of the aorta has been classified into various categories as illustrated in Chapter 69A. Diagnosis is usually based on a symptom complex rather than aneurysm type. The disease may also transition from an acute phase to a subacute phase before progressing to a chronic phase. Most aneurysms are detected at the chronic stage. Should an aneurysm form at the acute phase, we recommend treatment with steroids, but there is an increased risk of aortic dissection or rupture. It should also be noted that in Takayasu's disease, segments of the aorta may be skipped and spared of inflammatory lesions (see Chapter 69A).[38] Erythrocyte sedimentation rate and C-reactive protein levels (>1 mg/dl) are useful for following long-term risk of reoperation and activity.

Tumors

Tumors of the aorta are rare, although when they are found, they tend to occur in the descending and thoracoabdominal aorta segments. In a collected series of these patients from the literature, the prognosis has generally been poor.[38] Treatment usually involves resection and graft replacement with or without chemotherapy and radiotherapy.[38]

Reoperations

Reoperations on the descending and thoracoabdominal aorta are increasing in frequency. For example, in a recent analyses of our patients undergoing surgery, one third had undergone previous descending or thoracoabdominal aneurysm operations, excluding patients who had had previous abdominal aneurysm repairs or ascending arch repairs.[50] The reason for this is the natural course of dilatation of the aorta in other unresected segments, particularly if dissected.

The main reasons for reoperation include progression of aneurysmal dilatation of unresected segments of the aorta and either false aneurysm or saccular aneurysm formation after previous repair. In patients who have had previous acute dissection repairs of the ascending aorta, aneurysm formation in the aortic arch and descending or thoracoab-

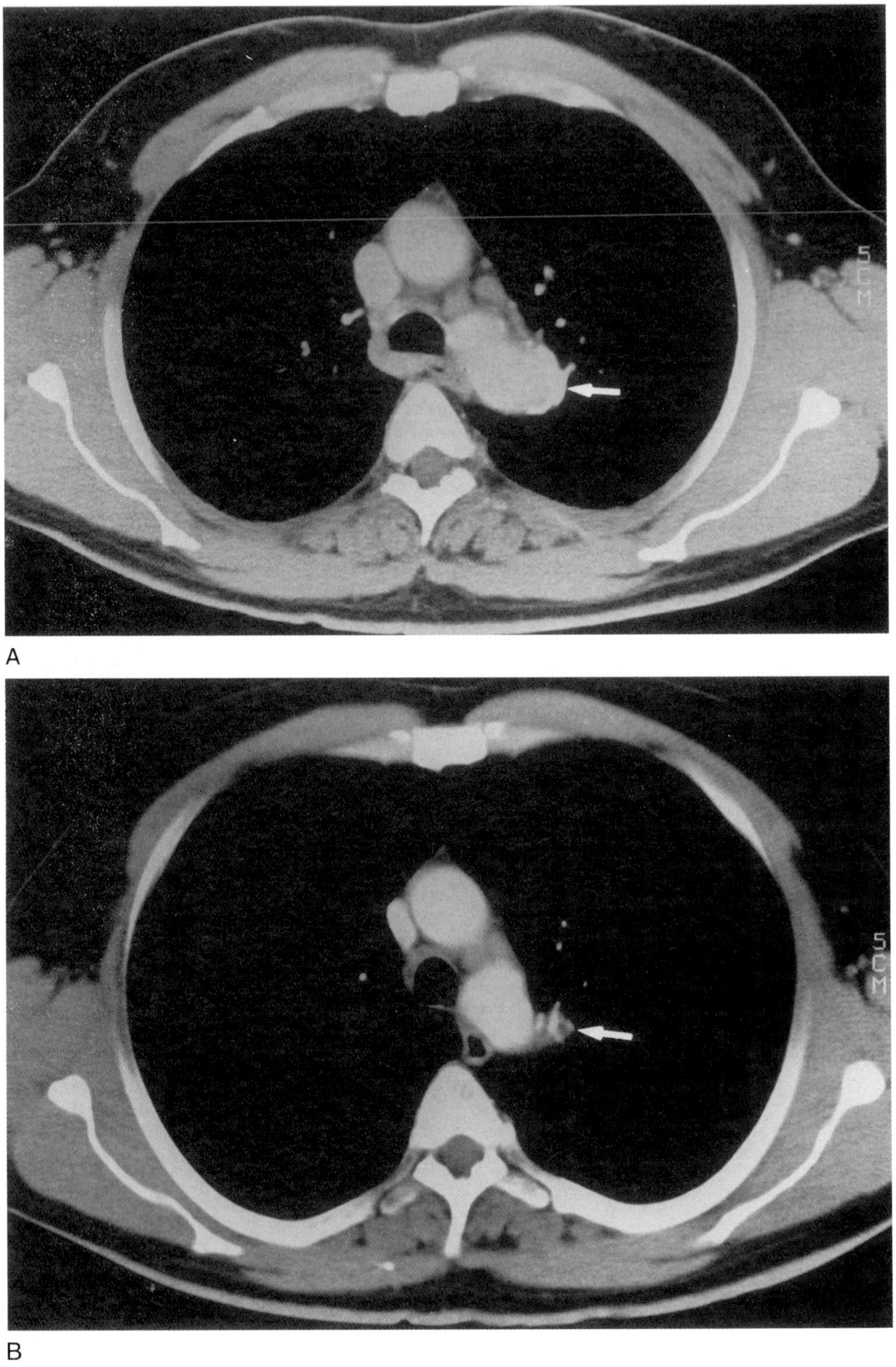

A

B

Figure 69B–5 **A,** CT of patient with a chronic partially calcified traumatic rupture of the aorta (*white arrow*). **B,** Repeat CT several years later with absorption of the aneurysm (*white arrow*).

dominal aorta is a common entity. Patients who have had previous descending aortic aneurysm replacements will quite often present with distal degenerative thoracoabdominal aneurysms below the previous descending repair. Less commonly seen are patients who either develop false aneurysms at the various anastomoses or who develop saccular aneurysms of the Carrel patches where intercostal lumbar or visceral vessels have been reattached to a new aortic graft. Albeit rare, this is a problem that should particularly be watched for in patients with Marfan syndrome. Another problem that is more frequently observed is in that subset of patients with previous stent grafts inserted in the descending aorta who present with complications related to the stent graft (e.g., migration, kinking, and/or leaks and broken stents) or because of aneurysm formation distal to the stent grafts. These latter problems are not surprising in that the formation of aneurysms in the aorta tends to be of a progressive nature. Because stent grafts do not limit expansion

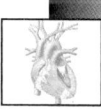

of the aorta, aneurysm formation at the anastomotic landing sites will often extend beyond the previous stent grafts.[38]

HISTORY AND PHYSICAL EXAMINATION

In questioning patients with descending or thoracoabdominal aneurysms, the most important symptom to elicit and to establish is the presence of back pain. The reason for this is that patients with ongoing pain related to the aneurysms are at greater risk of leaking or rupture and operative complications. Back pain, however, can be difficult to distinguish from chronic backaches related to arthritis of the spinal column. Thus, for diagnosis, it is important to search CT scans or MRI scans for any possible evidence of erosion of the vertebral bodies or the ribs by an aneurysm or if the aneurysm is indented by bony structures. Such a finding would indicate that the back pain is related to the aneurysm.

Arch aneurysms, particularly descending or thoracoabdominal aneurysms involving the distal aortic arch, may present with associated hoarseness or respiratory problems, particularly wheezing related to compression of the left bronchus. The esophagus may also be compressed by the aneurysm at the junction of the aortic arch and the descending aorta or if the descending aorta aneurysm swings into the right chest by being pinched between the vertebral bodies and the aorta. On CT scan, this may appear as a dilated proximal esophagus with fluid and results in dysphagia. Hoarseness is caused by the recurrent nerve being stretched by the aneurysm as the nerve wraps around the isthmus of the aorta and the ligamentum arteriosum.[38]

As mentioned above, evidence of distal embolism should be sought in patients with extensive and large aneurysms with contained clot and atheroma. A diagnosis of peripheral vascular disease is often made in these patients, although the reason for peripheral ischemia is related to chronic embolization of atheroma into distal vessels resulting in arterial occlusion. In patients with medial degenerative aneurysms, presentation of sudden leg weakness and paralysis is uncommon and is more frequently seen with acute dissections. This arises because of interference with spinal cord blood flow, either in the descending or thoracoabdominal segments. In both patients with medial degenerative aneurysms and congenital lesions, chronic hypertension is often a factor. Whether chronic hypertension will resolve after the repair of coarctations of the aorta is not certain but is variable. Historical studies have generally shown that approximately two thirds of patients who present as adults with coarctation of the aorta or previous coarctation repairs will continue to have hypertension but usually not as severe as prior to surgery. Some patients may be normotensive at rest, but during exercise hypertension is induced as a result of restricted flow to the descending aorta. Thus, a stress test with blood pressure measurement is of value in these patients, both preoperatively and postoperatively. It is also important to note that if patients experience exercise-induced hypertension after surgery, even if the surgery is apparently successful, it is often because of an inadequate size graft or the presence of aortic lumen after the repair. For this reason, we recommend that at least a 20-mm tube graft be used in females and, preferably, a 22-mm tube graft or greater in males (see below).

For reasons yet to be determined, smoking plays a much larger role in descending and thoracoabdominal aneurysm formation than ascending or arch aneurysms. Tobacco addiction with patients currently smoking is a common preoperative problem in patients presenting for descending or thoracoabdominal aneurysm repair. Thus, a history of respiratory problems and a determination of respiratory capacity are essential prior to descending or thoracoabdominal aneurysm surgery. In a previous prospective study[47] examining pulmonary function tests prior to thoracoabdominal surgery, there was no single cut-off point at which the risk of postoperative respiratory failure, defined as more than 5 days of postoperative ventilation, became significant. Nevertheless, at a forced expiratory volume in 1 s (FEV_1) of less than 1.2 liters/min, the risks increased considerably. Of course, the patient's body habitus, including the smaller size of a woman, must be factored into this. Furthermore, if the aneurysm is relatively large, occupying much space in the left chest, respiratory function may improve after resection of the aneurysm, although this is not always the case. Forced expiratory flow $FEF_{25-75\%}$ was found in our prospective study to be the most effective predictor of postoperative respiratory complications. The reason for this is that it gives some indication of the patient's strength of coughing and, thus, the ability to clear secretions postoperatively. Also, the presence of significant carbon dioxide retention on resting blood gases is a relative contraindication for surgery as is the case for patients on chronic supplemental oxygen therapy.[38,47]

During the history and physical examination, it is clearly important to establish any potential risk factors for and any history of cardiac disease. Thus, patients with atherosclerotic coronary artery disease have significantly greater risk of in-hospital mortality after these types of operations and a poorer long-term survival.[38,44] In a previous study, two thirds of the late deaths were related to coronary artery disease.[38,44] For this reason and the perioperative risk of myocardial infarction, the presence of coronary artery disease needs to be thoroughly examined. In addition to checking for coronary artery disease, any valvular disease, particularly aortic valve regurgitation, needs to be investigated because during aortic cross-clamping, even with atriofemoral bypass, there is a significant increase in cardiac afterload. If this is associated with aortic valve regurgitation, the patient may go into acute heart failure from myocardial distention. The patient's left ventricular muscle strength and ejection fractions are also strong determinants of early and late outcome after surgery. Part of the reason for this is that the increased afterload presented to the left ventricle results in a temporary left ventricular dysfunction after surgery and, if the patient has a poor ejection fraction, both the early and late mortality rates are increased. In a study of 132 patients undergoing descending or thoracoabdominal repairs, an interesting finding was that patients that had modest coronary artery disease and did not have coronary bypasses or stents had a higher risk of myocardial infarction and poorer long-term survival than those that did have bypass surgery. This could be in keeping with our current understanding of coronary disease.

A careful search for any presence of renal disease should also be done.[42] An increased preoperative creatinine level in the blood has a very strong correlation with both operative and late postoperative outcomes. Indeed, it is one of the most important risk factors for both early and late mortality by multivariable analyses.[38,42–44] Furthermore, if significantly elevated levels of creatinine are present, evidence for renal artery stenosis should also be investigated.

PREOPERATIVE TESTING

Our choice of preoperative testing prior to descending or thoracoabdominal repair is directed, first, by determining the extent of resection required and, second, by the prevention of postoperative complications. Most patients will have undergone CT scans, MRI scans, or both of the chest and abdomen, which will document the extent of the aneurysms. In patients with coarctation of the aorta, of particular importance is the need to determine the extent and any gradients. The extent and site of coarctation should be carefully examined by left anterior-oblique views of the aortic arch. Those patients who have had thoracic trauma from either acceleration or, especially, deceleration injuries should have extensive views performed of the distal aortic arch and proximal descending aorta. Of note, accelerating injuries may also cause traumatic rupture of the aorta. We have treated a patient who developed a traumatic rupture of the aorta after being kicked in the chest by a horse. Patients who have extensive aneurysms, especially with a lot of clot and atheroma and renal dysfunction, must have their visceral vessels examined for potential renal artery or celiac or superior mesenteric artery stenoses. This may require a separate MRA of the visceral vessels.

Cardiac Catheterization and Angiography

All our patients, prior to elective descending or thoracoabdominal aneurysm surgery, undergo cardiac catheterization and angiography. We ask the cardiologists to do a left anterior-oblique view of the aortic arch at the time of catheterization so that the proximal extent of the aneurysm can be determined, since this will influence the operative technique. If coronary artery disease is found at the time of cardiac catheterization, a decision must be made as to the best course of repair management. For example, if it is a single stenosed vessel or a large vessel with a critical area of muscle dependent upon it, angioplasty with or without stenting is performed. After this, patients are kept on Plavix for 30 days prior to scheduling elective descending or thoracoabdominal aneurysm surgery. Drug-eluting stents are avoided since they require about 3–4 months of treatment before open surgery. If extensive three-vessel coronary artery disease is present, the patient should undergo coronary artery bypass surgery prior to the repair. It is important to note that if the aneurysm involves the proximal descending aorta and the aortic arch, the left subclavian artery may need clamping and this can interfere with the left internal mammary artery blood supply to the heart. Thus, the options in this situation are either to use a right internal mammary artery bypass graft to bypass the left internal descending coronary artery or to insert an elephant trunk beyond the left subclavian artery at the time of the use of the left internal mammary artery for the coronary artery bypass surgery. We have successfully used these approaches in seven patients, including one patient in whom we elected to do a Dor ventricular aneurysm procedure at the time of the cardiac surgery prior to the thoracoabdominal aneurysm repair. Lastly, if the patient is found to have more than a 2+ aortic valve regurgitation, the aortic valve needs to be replaced or repaired before surgery. This is due to the potential for acute left ventricular distention leading to heart failure and intraoperative cardiac arrest.

Preoperative 24-h Holter ECG Examination

All patients undergo a 24-h Holter examination because of the high incidence of arrhythmias in this group of patients. This is particularly useful to know because, with arrhythmias, patients who have cooling during the operative procedure may be at greater risk for developing supraventricular arrhythmias, either atrial fibrillation or supraventricular tachycardia.

Pulmonary Function Tests

As indicated above, all patients undergo pulmonary function tests prior to surgery.[47] If the patients are actively smoking and are scheduled to undergo a pulmonary function test, an effort is made to wean the patients off their tobacco dependency and improve their pulmonary function prior to surgery. Patients who are actively smoking and undergo thoracoabdominal descending aortic surgery are more prone to prolonged intubation and bronchial secretions after the operation that will complicate their postoperative recovery.

Creatinine Levels

It is essential that all patients have their creatinine levels checked prior to surgery because this measure of kidney function will have a very strong influence on early and late outcomes after surgery. Curiously, for reasons that are not entirely clear, the creatinine level after surgery can be surprisingly variable. In most patients, in the first 5 days after surgery, the creatinine level increases. In most of these patients with quite high creatinine levels after repair of the aneurysm (2–3 mg/dl), there is a rapid return to a normal creatinine level as long as the renal arteries have not been treated for stenoses. In a few patients with high preoperative levels, there is a rapid decline to normal levels. This observation occurs in patients with relatively large aneurysms. An explanation could be that normal pulsatile flow to the renal arteries is interfered with because of the large aneurysms. In patients with significant renal dysfunction (>3 mg/dl) and small kidneys, it is difficult to determine whether their renal function will recover after surgery. One possibility is to stent the renal arteries stenoses prior to surgery to see if renal function improves. Although not formally studied, it is our impression that patients with high creatinine levels above 4–5 mg/dl prior to surgery may benefit from preoperative dialysis.

SPINAL CORD PROTECTION

Both the pathophysiology and etiological factors causing paralysis after descending and thoracoabdominal aneurysm surgery have been extensively reviewed elsewhere.[27,36,38,49,50] Briefly, based on both animal and human studies, there are three main mechanisms by which postoperative neurological deficits and paralysis can arise. First, duration and degree of ischemia during the period of aortic cross-clamping are important. In patients with coarctation of the aorta, there is an extensive collateral network of blood to the spinal cord so the degree of ischemia is not as severe as in a patient with traumatic rupture of the aorta or acute dissection where no collaterals have been established to the spinal cord.[38,39] In an extensive aneurysm (such as Crawford type II thoracoabdominal aneurysms), the degree of ischemia is more severe because of a greater amount of interference to the spinal cord blood supply. Multiple studies have shown the duration of ischemia is an important factor. The best way of showing this is by logistic regression analysis of the aortic cross-clamp time or the intercostal ischemia time versus the risk of neurological deficit (Figures 69B-3 and 69B-6). The relationship is an "S"-shaped sigmoid curve with a risk of paralysis rapidly increasing after 30 min of aortic cross-clamping in patients with acute dissection or traumatic rupture of the aorta.[38,39] Of interest, in patients with thoracoabdominal aneurysms, because of the extensive collateral blood supply that has been established, the curve is not quite as steep.[38,44] Similarly, for descending aortic aneurysms, when there is more direct blood supply below the repair or collateral blood supply, the risk of paralysis after 30 min is less. Thus, research shows the curve is moved to the right by interventions that successfully reduce the risk of spinal cord injury. Over the past two decades, interventions have successfully reduced the risk of this aspect of spinal cord injury.[8,26,27,49,50]

Second, failure to reestablish spinal cord blood flow after clamping the aorta increases the risk of spinal cord injury. Thus, both animal and human studies have shown intercostal and lumbar arteries supplying the spinal cord need to be reattached to reduce the risk of postoperative spinal cord and neurological deficits.*

Third, after the initial ischemic event to the spinal cord, secondary injury can result related to postoperative hemo-

*References 27, 33, 36, 38, 46, 48, 52.

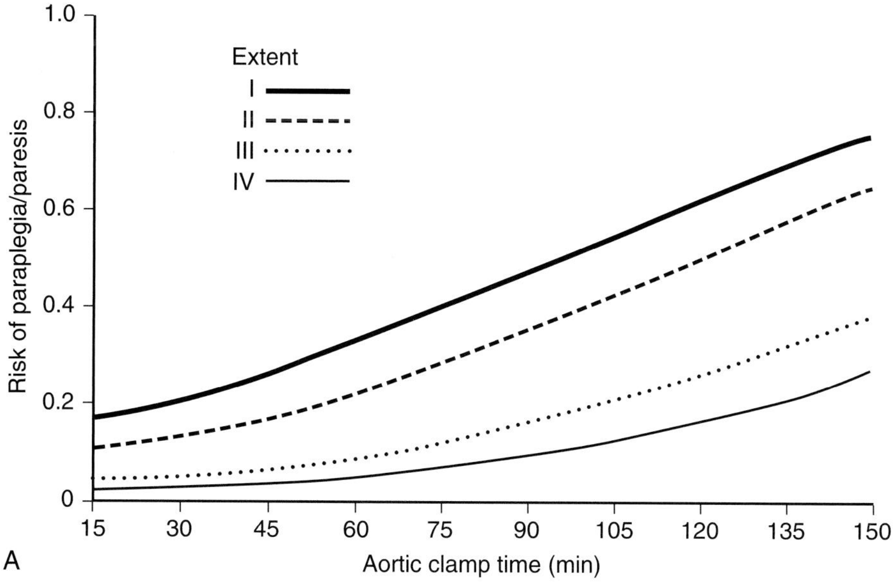

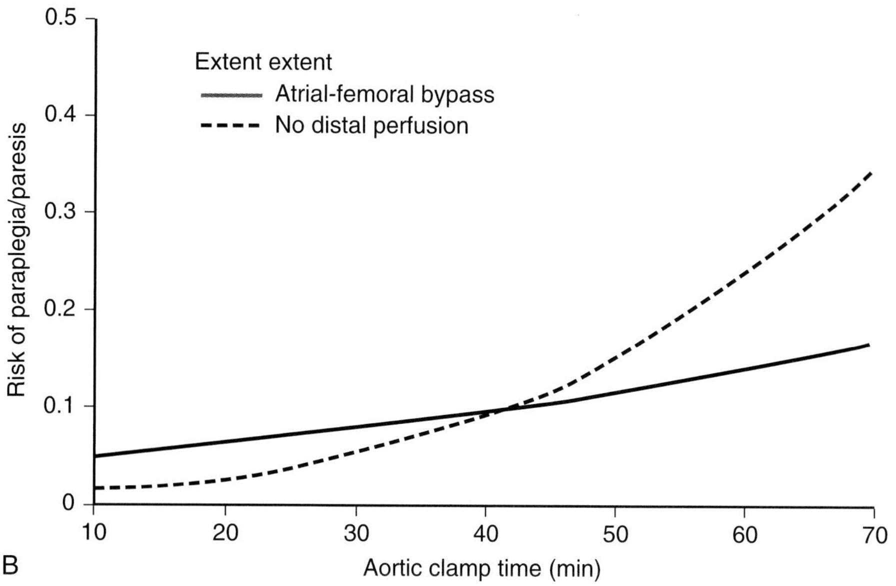

Figure 69B–6 **A,** The relationship between aortic cross-clamp time and the risk of paraplegia/paraparesis based on 1508 patients undergoing thoracoabdominal aneurysm repairs according to the Crawford classification of extent (see definitions for extent in the text). **B,** Influence of aortic cross-clamp time on the risk of paraplegia or paraparesis based on 832 patients with the entire descending aorta replaced. The solid line in black is for atriofemoral bypass and the dashed line is for no distal perfusion. Based on logistic regression analysis, after 40 min of aortic cross-clamping, atriofemoral bypass did show a protective effect. Atriofemoral bypass was only for the proximal anastomosis at normothermia.

(Continued)

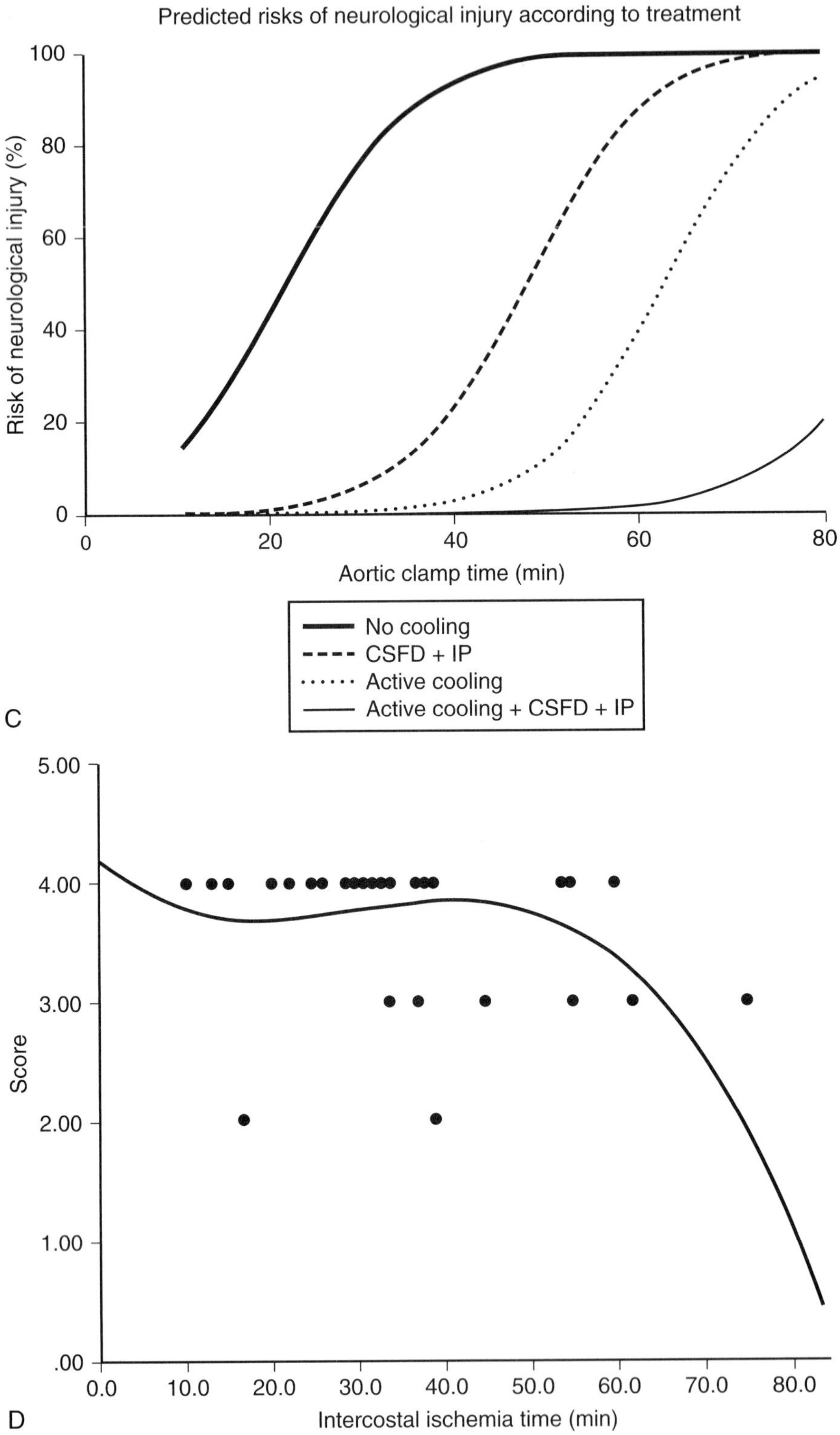

Figure 69B–6 cont'd **C,** The relationship between aortic cross-clamp time and the risk of neurological injury based on a prospective randomized study showing the risk according to no cooling nor CSF drainage nor intrathecal papaverine, then the greater protective effect with CSF drainage and intrathecal papaverine (CSFD + IP), the further greater protective effect of active cooling with atriofemoral bypass, and the greatest protective effect by combining active cooling plus CSFD + IP. Note that this allows for a safe aortic cross-clamp time out to approximately 60–70 min. **D,** Influence of intercostal ischemia time on motor function scores. Note the drop after approximately 50 min. Motor score 0 = no movement; 1 = flicker of movement, e.g., big toe; 2 = movement but not against gravity, e.g., sliding a leg while in bed; 3 = against gravity but weak, e.g., leg raising; 4 = normal.

dynamic instability in the intensive care unit after surgery or because of the complex biochemical cascade that is set in motion by the initial ischemic injury and results in secondary reperfusion injury including the development of apoptosis. This complex cascade of multiple pathways of events has been extensively reviewed previously in detail.[35,38,56]

Based on the pathophysiology involved in causing neurological deficits, operative techniques and both experimental and intraoperative maneuvers have been developed to reduce the risks of developing postoperative neurological incidents.[38,44,49,50] Indeed, to address the first etiological factor (i.e., degree of ischemia and duration of ischemia) certain intraoperative techniques are used. To reduce the risk of ischemia, every attempt is made to shorten both the aortic cross-clamp time and the intercostal ischemia time. Recently, we showed[50] the intercostal ischemia time to be a

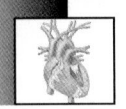

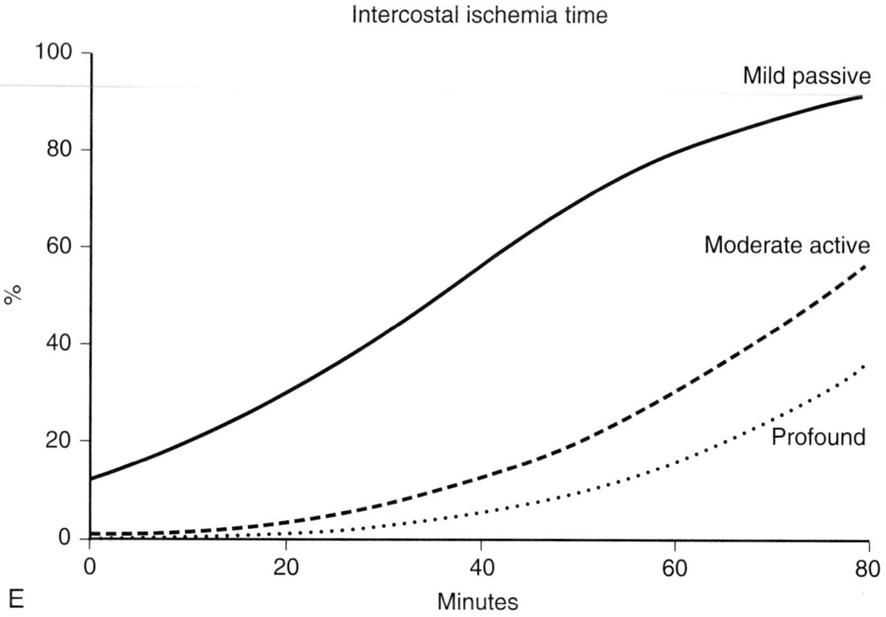

Figure 69B–6 cont'd E, Intercostal ischemia time influence on percentage risk of paraplegia/paraparesis based on logistic regression analysis. Note that profound hypothermia and moderate active hypothermia did not have a significantly different risk, however, mild passive hypothermia was associated with a significantly greater risk of paralysis than either moderate active or profound hypothermia ($p < .04$).

more important variable with respect to neurological injury than total aortic cross-clamp time. Therefore, quick and efficient anastomoses must be performed during the operation. We recommend the use of techniques that shorten the length of aortic cross-clamp time: for example, the use of second-stage elephant trunk procedures whenever indicated. A method we developed in 1992 based on animal experiments was a segmental sequential repair that reestablished spinal cord blood flow.[37,39,49,52] Once proximal anastomosis has been accomplished, the proximal descending aortic and subclavian clamps are removed to reperfuse the subclavian artery and to improve blood flow via vertebral arteries and the posterolateral spinal arteries. The mid-descending aorta is cross-clamped during the initial cross-clamping as frequently as possible so that the remaining portion of the aorta below is perfused by the atriofemoral bypass circuit. The intercostal vessels in this segment, down to T6, are oversewn with a 1-0 suture. This segmental level is conveniently in line with the sixth rib, which has been resected during the initial thoracotomy. Next, the aorta is opened down to the clamp placed immediately above the celiac artery and the intercostal arteries, between T6 and the celiac artery, including any upper lumbar arteries, are then reanastomosed to the graft. If possible the graft is then deaired and the intercostal Carrel patches reperfused reestablishing further blood flow to the spinal cord via the thoracic radicular arteries, so that these collateral vessels can perfuse the anterospinal artery both up and down the length of the spinal artery. Following the above, the visceral segment of the aorta is repaired including any lumbar arteries that need to be reattached. This segment is also reperfused to both increase spinal cord blood flow and reestablish visceral blood flow. In Crawford types II and III thoracoabdominal aneurysms, the lumbar arteries in the abdominal segment are reattached to reperfuse them as well as the median central artery if it is present. Hence, this sequential segmental technique minimizes the period of ischemia to the spinal cord. Both our studies and those by others[38,49,50,52] have confirmed that this approach reduces the risk of spinal cord injury. In addition, we have found that cooling the patients prior to aortic cross-clamping, either to moderate hypothermia levels, particularly between 30° C and 32° C with an atriofemoral bypass circuit,[49] or to profound hypothermia levels with cardiopulmonary bypass reduces the risk of spinal cord injury.[50] Both methods appear to be equally effective in protecting the spinal cord.

Other methods of locally cooling the spinal cord include injection of cold solution into the occluded aorta, intrathecal cooling, epidural cooling, and intrapleural cooling alongside the vertebral bodies. Most of these techniques have been shown to be protective in animal studies but human studies have shown variable degrees of success.[2,4,38,46,50]

To address the protection of the spinal cord and the influence of segmental intercostal or lumbar arteries, it is important to briefly review the anatomy of the spinal cord (Figure 69B-7).

The segmental intercostal and lumbar arteries arise from the aorta to perfuse the various vertebral segments. In neonates, the radicular arteries arise from the segmental arteries at each vertebral foramina, but with increasing age, many of these arteries at most vertebral levels involute. Typically, this results in two or three radicular arteries coming off the vertebral arteries supplying the cervical segment of the spinal cord, two or three supplying the thoracic segment of the spinal cord, and two or three to the lumbar segment of the spinal cord. Because these radicular arteries do not arise from the aorta, per se, examining the inside of the aorta to try to determine which vessels need to be reattached is of little value. Furthermore, the size of the vessel and the degree of backflow have no relationship to whether the segmental arteries arising from the aorta actually supply the spinal cord. The thoracic radicular arteries, once they reach the anterior spinal artery, bifurcate and can perfuse the spinal cord both upward and downward via the anterior

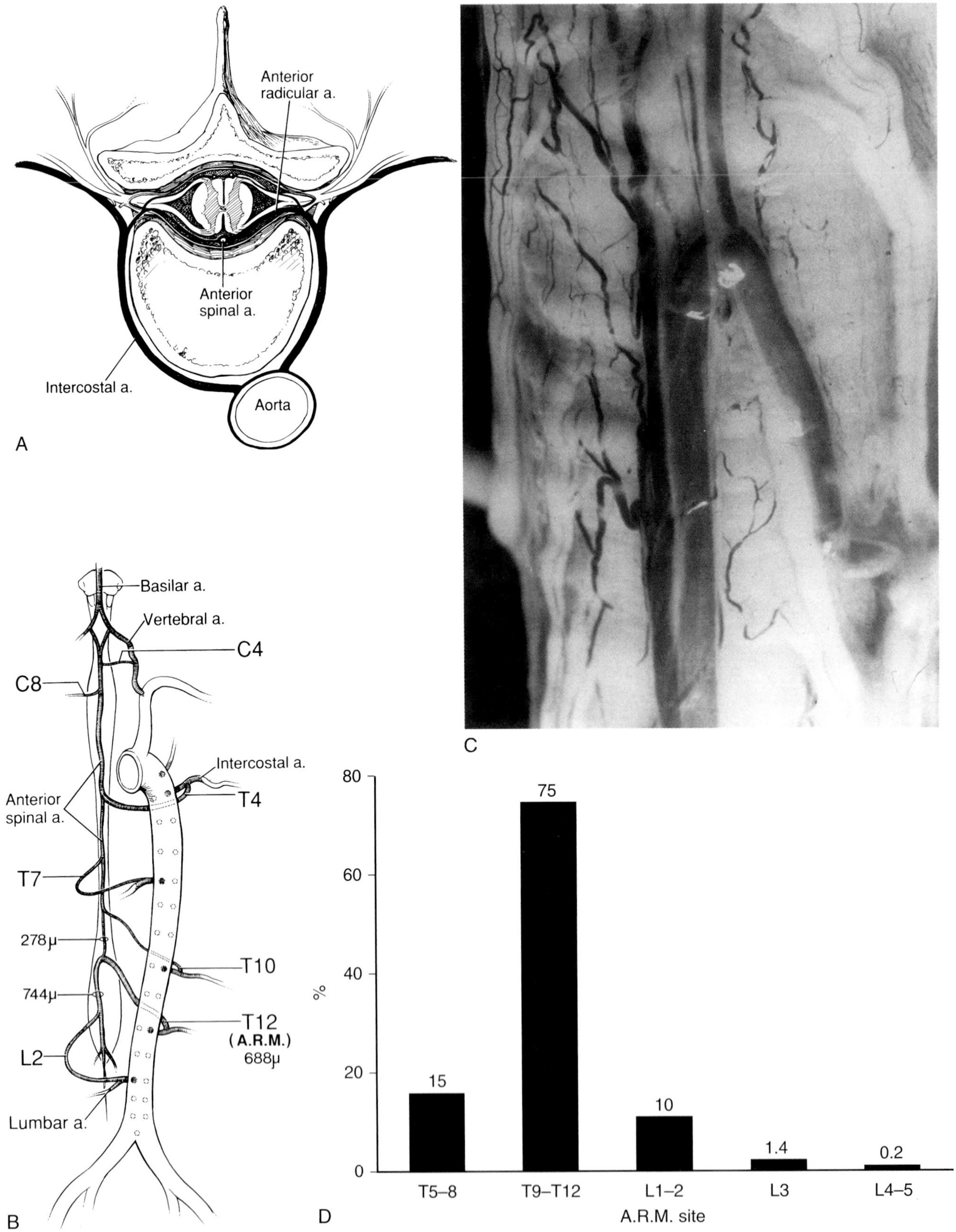

Figure 69B–7 **A,** The aorta gives off intercostal arteries that in turn give off small anterior or posterior radicular arteries that join the anterospinal or posterolateral arteries. **B,** The anterior radicular arteries join the anterospinal artery that runs the length of the spinal cord. The *arterio radicularis magna* (ARM) joins the anterospinal artery as a hairpin bend. The sizes are shown. **C,** Photograph of ARM and anterospinal artery from postmortem specimen. **D,** Distribution of ARM origin by vertebral level.

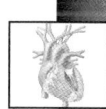

spinal artery. Small twigs also supply the two posterolateral networks of spinal arteries.[38,39,41,53]

Arising from the lower intercostal or the upper lumbar arteries, there is a larger radicular artery known as *arterio radicularis magna* (ARM), also known as the artery of Adamkiewicz (Figure 69B-7B). This vessel arises anywhere from T7 to L2 but most often arises from between the segments T8 and L1. Approximately 80% of these vessels arise from the left side of the pair of intercostal-lumbar arteries. This ARM joins the anterior spinal artery and forms a hairpin bend that preferentially perfuses the lumbar spinal cord below its level or junction of the anterior spinal artery.[53,56] Based on Poiseuille's equation that says resistance to flow is inversely proportional to the radius to the fourth power, very little blood flows up the anterior spinal artery to the lower thoracic spinal cord via this vessel. The reason for this is that where the anterior spinal artery is joined by the ARM, the anterior spinal artery is significantly smaller above than below the ARM. In contradistinction, the lower lumbar spinal cord at its expansion typically receives a lumbar vessel that is quite large and this artery allows both upward and downward blood flow in contrast to the ARM, which perfuses blood only down the length of the anterior spinal artery. At the end of the spinal cord, at the beginning of the cauda equina, there is a cruciate anastomosis that communicates between vessels on the cauda equina and also between the anterior spinal artery and the posterolateral spinal arteries. These lower vessels may arise from the median sacral artery, particularly in lower animals, or from the iliac and hypogastric vessels. The anterospinal artery is a continuous vessel that is formed by the union of two branches from the basilar artery with feeding branches from the vertebral arteries that then join at a variable level on the cervical spinal cord. The artery continues down the length of the spinal cord to the cruciate anastomosis. Multiple anatomical studies by Dommisse,[38] Svensson et al,[41,53,56] and Biglioli et al[3] have shown this to be a continuous vessel. This is important because in older literature on spinal cord anatomy it was suggested that the anterospinal artery was not a continuous vessel.[38] This was based on radiological examinations of the anterospinal cord in dogs. Clearly, the above technique was defective in establishing that the anterospinal artery was continuous. Furthermore, in other studies of baboon spinal cords and pig spinal cords, the anterospinal artery was found to be continuous in every specimen.[37,41,49,52,53] This has significant consequences regarding the method of operative technique. Thus, Biglioli et al,[3] based on the anterospinal artery being a continuous vessel, advocated a very rapid clamp-and-sew technique because of the collateral flow via this vessel. Furthermore, based on our experiments in baboons and a prospective randomized study in humans,[49,50,55,56] we have used intrathecal papaverine to dilate the anterospinal artery and the posterolateral spinal artery to improve blood flow to the spinal cord. In certain respects, the posterolateral vessels are more like a network of vessels that migrates along the posterolateral aspects of the spinal cord. In humans, based on anatomical dissections,[39,41] the vessels can vary in individual spinal cords as to how clearly defined the vessels are. Nevertheless, this network forms an important source of blood supply to the posterior one third of the spinal cord. The anterior two thirds, including the anterior horn cells and the muscle fibers, are more dependent on the anterospinal artery and the central perforating arterioles and capillaries.[38]

Based on these anatomical studies that we have performed, we carried out a study of intraoperatively identified segmental arteries.[36,48] This study showed the high risk of paralysis if lower thoracic patent segmental arteries are not reattached. Thus, in summary, for thoracoabdominal aneurysms we recommend reattachment of all patent vessels from T6 down to and including L2. Furthermore, in patients with aortic dissection, we also try to reattach all lumbar arteries in the lower abdominal aorta if the segment needs to be replaced. In the prospective study of reattaching intercostal vessels, we found that if in the segment of the aorta from T11 to L1 the vessels were patent but not reattached, then there was a significantly greater risk of neurological deficit compared to patients in whom patent vessels were reattached.[36,48] Also, there was a trend toward a lower risk of paralysis when patent vessels at each segment from T6 down to T11 were reattached.[36,48]

For descending aortic aneurysms, however, the decision to reattach intercostal arteries is not as clearly defined.[15,21,38,45] Based on our study of 832 descending aortic aneurysm repairs,[45] most patients who developed paraplegia and paraparesis had the entire descending aorta repaired (segments A, B, and C) or had the distal third of the descending aorta replaced. Similarly, Borst,[38] in a study of 132 patients, found that only patients who had intercostals oversewn below T_8 developed postoperative neurological deficits. Griepp et al[15] showed that the more intercostals that are sacrificed, the greater the risk of developing paraplegia and paraparesis, although multiple intercostal arteries can be sacrificed in the chest for descending aortic repairs. Safi and Kron also confirmed that sacrificing the vessels in the distal third of the descending aorta increased the risk for thoracoabdominal aneurysm repairs.[27]

It has been noted that the use of stent grafts placed in the distal descending aorta is associated with a greater risk of postoperative paraplegia and paraparesis[14]; this risk is particularly increased if a patient has had previous abdominal and aortic aneurysm repairs. The association between the development of paraplegia and paraparesis in patients who had previous infrarenal abdominal aneurysm repairs followed by descending aortic repairs was also found in our study of 832 aortic aneurysm repairs.[45] Thus, it appears that if descending aortic repairs extend below T8, then the lower intercostal vessels need to be reattached. This may be the observation because if the upper thoracic intercostals are sacrificed, then there is still adequate collateral blood flow from other thoracic and radicular arteries that are able to perfuse the anterospinal artery both up and down its length. If the lower thoracic intercostals are sacrificed, it may involve the artery of Adamkiewicz or the lower thoracic radicular arteries, which may, in turn, compromise spinal cord blood flow. We advocate the reattachment of intercostal arteries above the ARM because they could potentially supply thoracic radicular arteries and reattaching these vessels can perfuse the spinal cord both upward and downward at the time of thoracoabdominal aneurysm repairs. Clearly, the artery of Adamkiewicz is not the sole vessel that requires attachment, because the lower thoracic spinal cord would then still be at risk. How critical the artery of Adamkiewicz is to the spinal cord blood flow has been debated. In animal studies by Di Chiro, between 50% and 100% of animals have become paralyzed when the ARM has been identified and ligated.[38] Furthermore, ligating the anterospinal artery below the artery of Adamkiewicz has been associated with 100% risk of paralysis.[38] It is likely, however, in the human situation with associated aneurysms and occlusion of many segmental arteries that the ARM is not quite so vital to spinal cord blood flow since there is a more extensive collateral network of vessels supplying the spinal cord, particularly if the ARM has been occluded by clot. Clearly, in patients who have stent grafts inserted, the ARM may be occluded in the lower thoracic spinal cord and yet the patients tolerate this.[14] Nevertheless, if extensive intercostal segments are sacrificed, in addition to ARM, the risk of paralysis is increased. Based on both research in a porcine model and human studies, patients with increased dependence on collateral blood flow were at greater risk of developing delayed paraplegia and paraparesis during episodes of postoperative hypotension.[10,50,52]

In the animal laboratory, we tried to preoperatively identify vessels supplying the spinal cord.[38,51,52] In baboons we were able to successfully do this by highly selective angiography.[38] Other authors use this routinely for these repairs.[17,59] Of caveat, highly selective angiography, per se, may sometimes result in paraplegia/paraparesis, renal failure, or even death because this is an extensive and long procedure that may take, in our experience, 3–5 h to perform.[33] Apart from the risks involved, when a vessel has been identified as supplying the spinal cord, at the time of surgery it can be difficult to ascertain which exact intercostal vessel this is.[33] This is aided to some extent by counting the vertebral bodies from the level of T6 where the incision has been made but does not guarantee that the correct vessel is reattached. We have also used highly selective angiography in the postoperative period to establish how accurately we identified vessels supplying the spinal cord using a hydrogen and platinum electrode polargraphic technique.[33] In both animal and human studies,[33,38,51,52] we performed hydrogen mapping, placing a platinum electrode along the spinal cord and sensitized it by using the polargraphic technique. Hydrogen in solution was then injected into vessels potentially supplying the spinal cord and if these vessels gave off radicular arteries that supplied the spinal cord, hydrogen in contact with the platinum electrode produced a weak current that then could be measured. This indicated the vessel had been injected and needed to be preserved or reattached at the time of surgery to maintain spinal cord blood flow. Both in animal and human studies, this was found to be an accurate and highly significant influence on the development of postoperative paraplegia/paraparesis. Also, in the human studies, this tended to result in shorter cross-clamp times since not all intercostal and lumbar arteries needed to be reattached. This technique requires a lot of time and effort and is very sensitive to movement and other sources of interference with the measurement of a current. This technique will require further refinement before it can be used regularly in the clinical setting. In addition to measuring hydrogen, the polargraphic technique, by changing the polarity and a different voltage, can be used to detect oxygen. The studies we performed in both animals and humans measuring oxygen on the surface of the spinal cord were very sensitive in detecting when blood flow was reduced to the spinal cord. When blood flow was reestablished to the spinal cord with the delivery of oxygen, the instrumentation was very sensitive in detecting that oxygen was reaching the spinal cord. This method of monitoring spinal cord function has been further developed and may become a useful technique in selected situations.[29]

Spinal motor-evoked potentials have also been used to test spinal cord function.[53,56] Motor-evoked potentials are useful in measuring spinal cord function because the anterior horn cells contain motor cells that are more sensitive to ischemia than the posterior sensory conduction pathways of fibers. The anterior horn cells and the motor cells and the axons are predominantly in the anterior two thirds of the spinal cord, which tend to become initially ischemic, whereas the long sensory fibers are in the posterior aspect of the spinal cord. Thus, in many patients who develop paraplegia/paraparesis after surgery, the motor function has been lost but the sensory function remains intact. Studies have also shown the spinal somatosensory-evoked potentials are not as sensitive as motor-evoked potentials in detecting spinal cord ischemia.[38] Although we found motor-evoked potentials to be accurate in both animal models and in humans,[33,52,53,56] the problem was that for motor-evoked potentials to be monitored, the compound muscle potential had to be monitored. This was done by placing electrodes into the muscles of the lower limbs. However, to maintain these motor-evoked potentials, a muscle relaxant could not be used to paralyze the animal or in patients. Thus, while stimulating the motor cortex or spinal cord, the legs would jerk during stimulation. This did not appear to have harmful effects but was disconcerting. Subsequently, de Haan et al, Jacobs, Schepen's group, and others[11,35,38,57] have developed a technique of titrating the amount of muscle relaxant by using thenar or hypothenar muscle amplitudes as a comparative parameter. This has allowed the use of some muscle relaxant while not completely abolishing the compound action potentials from the muscles in the lower limbs. This has been found to be highly accurate and useful but it has not been widely adopted. Part of the problem has been that the use of motor-evoked potential monitoring devices in humans in the United States required both institutional review board (IRB) and Food and Drug Administration (FDA) approvals. Recently, the testing method was approved by the FDA and we are presently evaluating the newer devices. The degree to which these devices will help during operative procedures is debatable. In a previous commentary, we stated this would probably affect the method of protection in only approximately 15% of patients.[11] This is a useful technique, particularly from a research point of view, and considerable data have been gained from the technique. It remains to be seen what role it will play in the general management of patients.

As earlier stated, postoperative events may contribute to paraplegia and paraparesis. In the postoperative period, high blood pressure is maintained by inducing hypertension using inotropes and vasoconstrictors.[50] Because delayed paraplegia is related to episodes of hypotension, it is important to maintain blood pressures at a high level (greater than a mean of 85 mm Hg) in the intensive care unit for 2–3 days after surgery. Patients are also best kept intubated longer in contrast to other patients undergoing cardiovascular surgery because postoperative respiratory dysfunction leading to distress can result in delayed neurological deficits. It is also important to ensure that patients return to the intensive care unit hemodynamically stable, particularly from the point of view of bleeding, since patients who have postoperative bleeding are at increased risk of developing paraplegia or paraparesis.[38,44] Prevention and control of atrial and ventricular arrhythmias are also important.

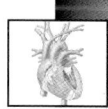

Whenever possible, patients undergo cerebrospinal fluid (CSF) drainage during descending and thoracoabdominal operations.[49,50] The exact reason why this is effective is not entirely clear and, indeed, there may be multiple reasons. CSF drainage was first tried in a dog model by Cooley and Blaisdel and was found to be advantageous.[38] Miyamoto also found this to confer a positive benefit.[38] He suggested this was possibly because the relative perfusion pressure of the spinal cord was improved, namely that the spinal cord perfusion pressure was directly dependent on the systemic pressure minus the CSF pressure. It should be noted that the perfusion pressure at the level of the spinal cord and the anterior spinal artery or posterolateral spinal arteries or in the spinal arterioles is unknown and may have very little correlation with the systemic mean arterial pressure in a patient whose aorta has been cross-clamped.[38] In both animal experiments and human studies, we noted the CSF pressure best correlated with the central venous pressure (Figure 69B-8).

There has also been some evidence that during ischemic events or injury to the spinal cord, removal of the CSF may remove negative neurotrophic factors such as one related to TPA. CSF drainage may also remove false neurotransmitters that may cause deficits or delayed recovery from the period of ischemia.[35,49]

Three prospective randomized studies have been performed to evaluate the benefits of CSF drainage in high-risk Crawford types I and II thoracoabdominal aneurysms.[7,10,49] In the first one we performed,[10] however, we were limited by the IRB to draining only 50 ml of CSF during the period of aortic cross-clamping. Thus, in the first study, we failed to show any benefit of CSF drainage. Furthermore, in that particular study, apart from limiting the amount of CSF drainage performed, the CSF pressure was only lowered to

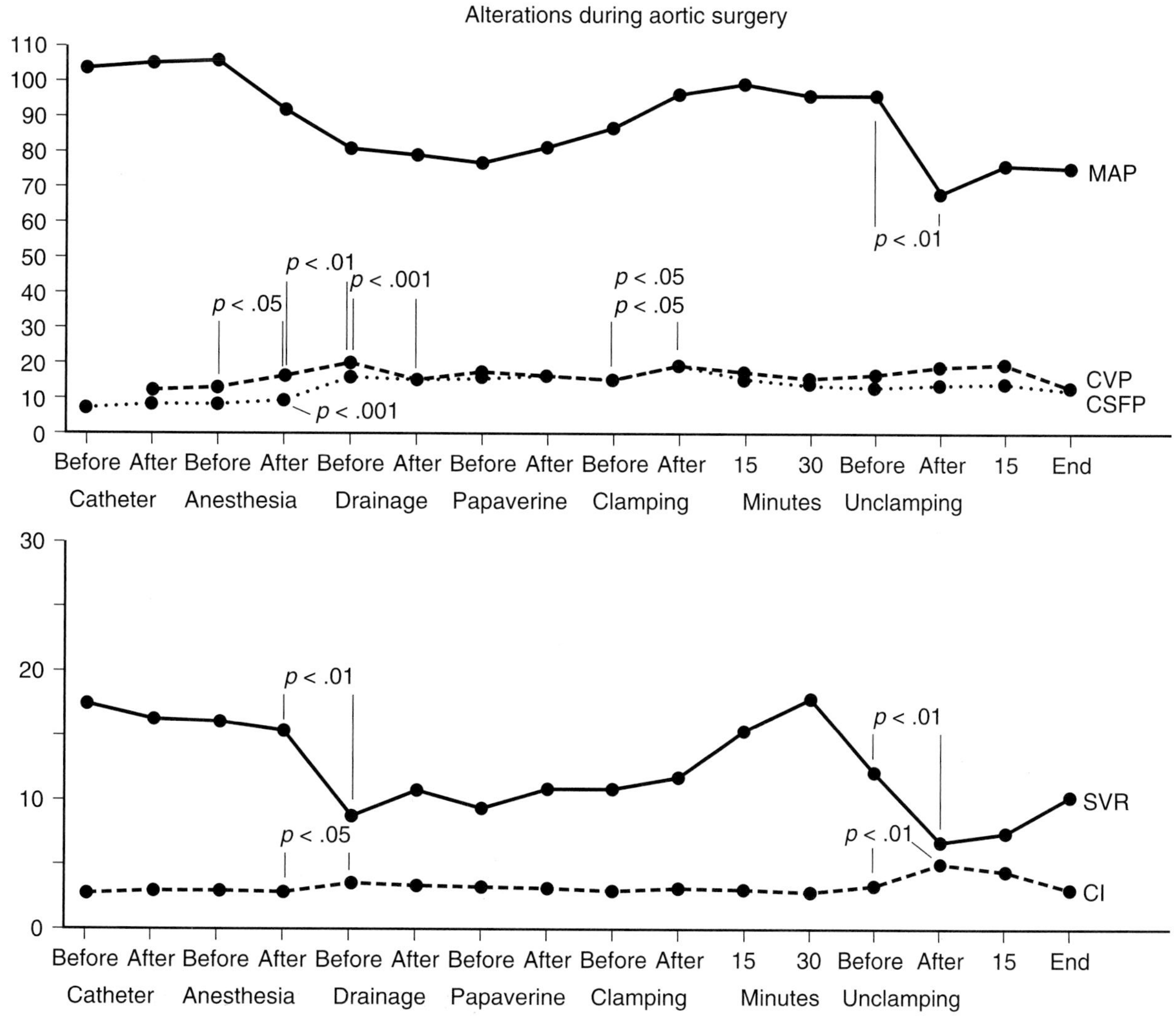

Figure 69B–8 Hemodynamic and cerebrospinal fluid pressure (CSFP) alterations during surgery. MAP, mean arterial pressure; CVP, central venous pressure; SVR, systemic vascular resistance; CI, cardiac index.

10 mm Hg. Also, postoperative CSF drainage in the intensive care unit was not performed. Although no significant benefit was demonstrated when we compared the two groups with or without CSF drainage, we observed that there was a trend toward a lower incidence of postoperative delayed neurological deficits in the group that had CSF drainage ($p = .08$). In a subsequent study,[49] we randomized patients with type I and type II thoracoabdominal aneurysms to a control group and a group who received preservative-free intrathecal papaverine prior to aortic cross-clamping. CSF was drained during a period of aortic cross-clamping by free-gravity drainage. This was continued in the intensive care unit for the first 2 days after surgery, keeping the pressure between 7 and 10 cm H_2O above the level of the spinal cord. This study showed a significantly beneficial effect from CSF drainage and intrathecal papaverine use (Figures 69B-3 and 69B-9), although the use with atriofemoral bypass with cooling also showed a protective effect.[49] Indeed, the combination of the two (i.e., CSF drainage and intrathecal papaverine) and combined cooling of the patient to 30–32° C with atriofemoral bypass had the most significant protective effect.[49] Subsequently, Coselli and colleagues[7] have also performed a prospective randomized study in which Crawford types I and II patients were randomized to CSF drainage to keep the pressure below 10 mm Hg. This study also showed that CSF drainage was associated with a protective effect.[7]

The reason for delayed postoperative deficits that occur in the intensive care unit after the initial arrival of patients with functioning and intact spinal cords remains to be fully elucidated. There are three main reasons to consider.[10,38,50,52] First, if extensive involvement of the intercostal and lumbar arteries has been sacrificed, the patient's collateral blood flow may be precarious and periods of hypotension, for whatever reason, may result in delayed deficits. Second, respiratory problems, particularly reintubation for respiratory failure, are associated with the occurrence of delayed deficits. Third, it is clear from animal experiments[52] and our understanding of the biochemistry of the spinal cord after ischemic events[38,56] that secondary injury can occur within the spinal cord resulting in delayed deficits. The most likely scenario appears to be RNA and DNA fragmentation that leads to programmed death (apoptosis) of anterior horn cells or fibers in the spinal cord. Although there are animal studies that show some agents may be effective in reducing this biochemical cascade of harmful events, none has been put to the test by prospective randomized studies in humans. Indeed, no pharmacological agent has yet been shown in humans to be protective by prospective randomized studies. In our first prospective randomized study of CSF drainage,[10] there was a trend for patients given lidocaine for ventricular arrhythmias to have a lower risk of postoperative spinal cord deficits ($p = .1$). We, therefore, routinely give patients 200 mg of lidocaine prior to aortic cross-clamping. In addition, this may reduce the risk of ventricular arrhythmias during the period of aortic cross-clamping.

Protection of the spinal cord for most patients undergoing thoracoabdominal aneurysm surgery without circulatory arrest is dependent upon the following[35,49,50]: establishing atriofemoral bypass including cooling the patients to approximately 31–32° C prior to aortic cross-clamping, giving the patients intrathecal papaverine prior to aortic cross-clamping, draining CSF by gravity during aortic cross-clamping, and performing quick and efficient aortic repair during the period of aortic cross-clamping with reestablishment of blood flow to all intercostal and lumbar arteries in the segments between T6 and L2. This is followed by drainage of CSF for the first 2 days of the postoperative period. Induced hypertension is also protective of the spinal cord based on retrospective studies and porcine animal model studies.[35,38,49,52] Nevertheless, as we observed in our first CSF drainage study, neurological deficits could occur up to 3 weeks after surgery. Indeed, we have seen deficits occur even later after the initial operation, related to periods of severe hypotension and shock.

OPERATIVE TECHNIQUE

The operative technique for descending and thoracoabdominal aneurysm surgery is aimed at making the repair as efficient

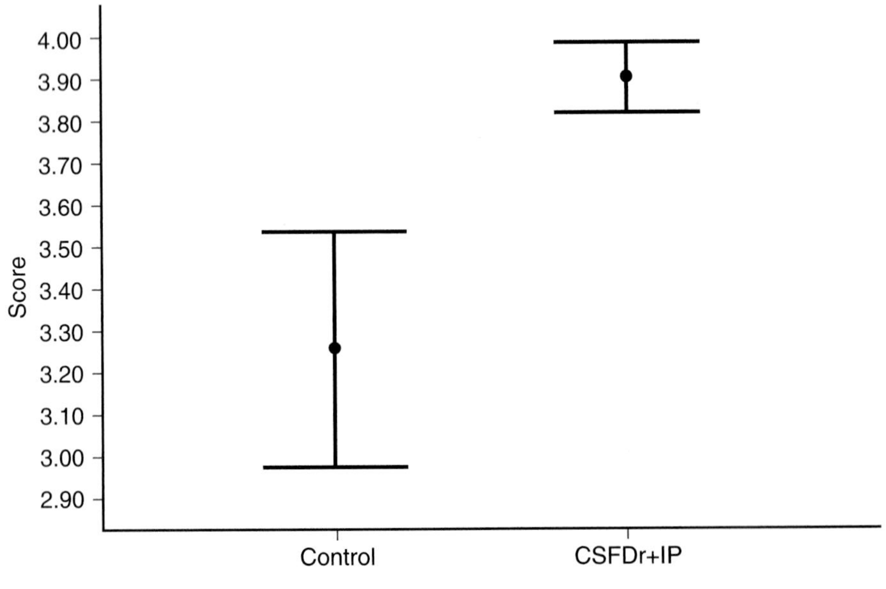

Figure 69B–9 Randomized study of CSF drainage with intrathecal papaverine. Mean motor scores of patients in the control group and cerebrospinal fluid drainage plus intrathecal papaverine (CSF Dr + IP) group ($p < .05$).

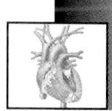

and expeditious as possible by ensuring that it is accurately performed so that the risk of spinal cord injury and renal failure is reduced.* Further techniques are also used to lower the risks of respiratory failure after these operations. With careful attention to preoperative factors, particularly atherosclerotic coronary artery disease and aortic valvular disease, the mortality risk is lessened if, in addition to preventing paralysis and renal failure, cardiac complications are prevented.[38,50]

OPERATIVE PROCEDURES

Descending Thoracic Aorta

Tubular graft replacement of the descending aorta is the most common and the easiest of the distal aortic operations to perform other than infrarenal aneurysm repairs.[45] A spinal catheter is inserted under local anesthetic at the level of L3/4, L4/5 with the plastic catheter fed up inside the intrathecal space approximately 20–25 cm from the skin. The reason for this is that the spinal cord ends at approximately the level of L1, L2 and to deliver preservative-free intrathecal papaverine to the vulnerable area beginning in the lower thoracic spinal cord, the catheter must be fed this distance into the intrathecal space. Chest X-rays done after placement of the catheter corroborate that this length of catheter is required. Because the patient is awake, any paresthesia or pain that does not subside is noted and the patient is asked to move his or her legs to ensure that spinal cord injury has not occurred. Next, the soft Silastic catheter is transected at the skin, the connectors attached to it, and the arterial pressure line connected to the Silastic catheter approximately 3–5 cm from the site of skin entry. The reason for this is that the Silastic catheter has a small lumen and since flow is inversely proportional to the fourth power of the radius, using a larger lumen arterial line reduces the resistance to drainage when CSF is being drained. It is also important to put 4 × 4 sponges under the Silastic catheter at the site of skin entry so that it does not kink-off and stops CSF drainage. A 4 × 4 sponge is also placed on top of this and covered with sterile dressings so that when the patient lies on his or her back in the intensive care unit, the connector does not press onto the skin.[38]

The patient is then given a general anesthetic and the double lumen endobronchial tube is inserted. Often if the left bronchus is compressed, the anesthesiologist will find it useful to put in a separate balloon bronchial occluder with fiberscopic assistance. The femoral arterial line is inserted on the right side while the patient is still flat on his or her back. This is to measure femoral arterial pressure generated by the atriofemoral bypass circuit. The patient is then turned onto his or her right side for a left thoracotomy. The angle of the shoulder to the table is dependent on the planned operative procedure. For patients having descending aortic aneurysm repair, the angle is typically 70 degrees so that the hips can be rotated more toward 45 degrees, which allows access to the femoral artery on the left side. The patient is cleaned and sterile drapes placed around the intended operative sites. The left femoral artery is first exposed and encircled with umbilical tape.

*References 35, 38, 44, 45, 49, 50.

A skin incision is made from behind the scapula and following the rib line to approximately the mid-axillary line, but then is angled toward the umbilicus and across the subcostal margin for approximately 1 or 2 inches (Figure 69B-10). The muscle layers are then divided with electrocautery and the ribs counted; the fifth rib is identified by both counting and identifying the interdigitations of the posterior superior serratus muscle attaching to the posterior aspect of the fifth rib just beyond the neck.

A decision needs to be made as to which rib will be removed. If the most complex part of the operation is proximally, particularly if the distal arch or subclavian artery is involved and the aorta needs to be clamped between the left common carotid and the left subclavian arteries and especially if the aneurysm extends up to the apex of the left pleural cavity, the fifth rib is removed and the subcostal margin is divided just beyond the attachment of the xiphoid to the rib cage. A segment of the subcostal margin (approximately 1.5 inches) is also removed. If this does not result in adequate exposure, the posterior aspect of the fourth rib is divided after placing heavy sutures both proximally and distally around the rib at the site of the intended division of the posterior fourth rib. In patients undergoing operations predominantly of the lower segments of the descending aorta, the sixth rib is removed and the subcostal margin is divided. The lateral chest wall below the incision is then freed from the diaphragm at the anterior costophrenic angle. Some of the fibers of the abdominal muscles are also divided.[38]

The inferior ligament of the lung is divided to expose the inferior pulmonary vein. The aorta is then dissected free circumferentially from surrounding tissues both proximal and distal to the aneurysmal segment or area of planned repair. If the distal arch is involved, the left subclavian artery is also dissected out. Tapes are not placed around the aorta since these may become sutured into the anastomoses and they tend to be in the way during suturing.[38]

The patient is heparinized with a low dose of heparin. A purse string suture is placed in the inferior left pulmonary vein. A drainage cannula is placed through an incision in the inferior pulmonary vein into the left atrium, carefully excluding all air from the system, and then connected to the drainage side of the atriofemoral bypass centrifugal pump circuit. The femoral artery is clamped and opened; the arterial cannula is inserted into the femoral artery and is secured into

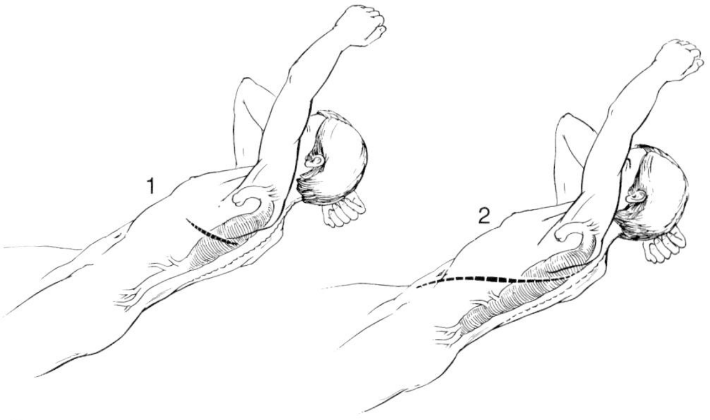

Figure 69B–10 (1) Positioning for descending thoracic aortic repair and (2) thoracoabdominal repair.

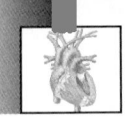

position. The patient is placed on atriofemoral bypass and cooled to approximately 32° C for descending aortic repair.[39]

While cooling, the patient is slowly given (over 5 min in duration) 30 mg of intrathecal preservative-free papaverine that has been kept at about 37° C. This precaution prevents the risk of a sympathetic response occurring, which may happen with any cold solution when it is injected into the intrathecal space, and results in a low blood pressure. The injected papaverine is followed with 3–5 ml of previously withdrawn CSF to flush the arterial and Silastic cannula of any papavarine.[38]

When the patient reaches the target temperature, based on Swan-Ganz temperature monitoring, the aorta is cross-clamped and CSF drainage is allowed to occur freely by gravity. The cross-clamped aorta is then opened and the graft sewn into position with a running suture. As this graft is being sewn into position in the aortic arch, it is important to try to preserve the recurrent laryngeal nerve, although this is not always possible. If the distal artery and subclavian artery have been clamped for the proximal anastomosis, a clamp is placed on the graft once the proximal anastomosis has been done and the graft allowed to flush and the proximal clamps are completely removed. Hemostasis is then ensured at the anastomosis.[38]

If the anastomosis is in the distal third of the descending aorta, it is often easier to do the distal anastomosis at the diaphragm, for example, parachuting it into position and placing a clamp on the graft and using atriofemoral bypass to retrograde fill the graft and check for hemostasis at the distal anastomosis. In this situation, the proximal anastomosis is then done.

More typically, once the proximal anastomosis has been performed, the distal anastomosis is done. If the graft does not go beyond the level of approximately T7 or T8, the intervening intercostal arteries are oversewn without any reimplantation. If the graft distally needs to go down to the diaphragm, for example, then, in most patients, a long beveled distal anastomosis is performed. Thus, for example, intercostals from T7 down to T11 or T12 will be preserved yet the cuff of beveled anterolateral graft is carried down to the diaphragm with a long running suture and anastomosis. The graft is then first flushed distally, then proximally, prior to tying the final suture knot down and the patient is placed in a head-down position.[39]

It is important that once the graft is unclamped, the perfusionist keeps the distal pressure below the proximal pressure during rewarming. The reason for this is that if any clot or air remains in the graft, or atheroma, this can be forced by the pump to embolize to the brain if the distal pressure exceeds the proximal arterial pressure. Hemostasis is then ensured and the graft wrapped with the old aneurysm sac as much as possible.[38]

In patients in whom repair needs to be carried down to the level of the celiac artery, the posterior diaphragm at the aortic hiatus can be divided to gain exposure without dividing the entire diaphragm. Next, a Parks retractor is placed in the hiatus and pulled downward to give exposure to the celiac artery. It is important that this retractor is carefully placed so the spleen is not injured. By doing this, exposure can be achieved without dividing the diaphragm circumferentially all the way down to the hiatus. This approach reduces the risk of postoperative respiratory problems.[38]

In performing descending aortic repairs, some special situations necessitate the use of different techniques. For example, in adults undergoing coarctation repairs or interrupted aortic arch repairs, a side-biting clamp is usually placed on the distal arch and left subclavian artery. A tube graft (at least a 20-mm graft for an average female and a 22-mm graft for an average male) is sewn to the distal arch and, if necessary, up onto the subclavian artery. Next, the distal end of this graft is sewn onto the descending aorta also with a side-biting clamp. The reason for using this technique is two-fold. First, the risk of a patient developing hoarseness is reduced; second, the risk of developing paraplegia or paraparesis is reduced. We believe this approach reduces this latter risk because the aortic blood flow through the aorta is not completely cut off during the repair and also because none of the collateral intercostal arteries and aberrant sources of blood flow to the spinal cord (Abbott's artery) needs to be divided. Another consideration is that in adults, the incidence of false aneurysm formation around patches is greater. Furthermore, doing an end-to-end anastomosis in adults carries a greater risk of developing paraplegia or paraparesis because the well-developed collateral source of blood flow to the spinal cord may be interfered with. As stressed earlier, it is very important to use a large sized graft, otherwise patients, during exercise, may develop gradients across the graft. In fact, we have seen patients who had grafts inserted that were too small and who were not relieved of their hypertension. These patients required second or third reoperations to fix the problem, including ascending to descending or ascending to abdominal extraanatomical grafts to relieve the gradients across previously placed grafts.[38]

Traumatic injuries were discussed previously, although it should be noted that many of these injuries can be repaired with a primary suture closure without insertion of a tube graft. If a tube graft is used, the anastomosis can often be done, because the gap is small, by opening the tube graft longitudinally and sewing the graft into position as a patch. After the proximal and distal anastomoses are performed, the tube is reformed by sewing together the cut longitudinal edge (Figure 69B-4). As indicated above, if the aortic arch is involved and there is no evidence of significant leak, attempts will be made to treat these traumatic injuries with hypotensives and later operating on the patients using deep hypothermia and circulatory arrest. We first used this technique in 1993 with satisfactory results.[40] Increasingly, this has become a popular approach for complex injuries, particularly if associated with multiple trauma (typically head injuries with hemorrhage).

In patients with saccular aneurysms of the distal aortic arch or the descending aorta, often related to penetrating ulcers, the saccular aneurysm can be repaired by using either total occlusion clamps or a side-biting clamp. The opening in the aorta is then cut back to good tissue and a patch is sewn into position.

In patients with an aberrant right subclavian artery and an enlarged Kommerell's diverticulum, a graft is usually inserted to replace the descending aorta and the stump of the aberrant right subclavian artery is oversewn where the size is of a normal diameter.[22,25,31] The patient is then turned onto his or her back at the end of the operation, redraped, and an interposition graft is placed between the right subclavian artery and the right common carotid artery (see Chapter 69A). Alternatively, this part of the operation can be done before doing the thoracotomy, although we issue a caveat that if this sequence is used, the graft may clot off either from competitive flow from the native aberrant right subclavian artery or because of kinking during the positioning of the patient.[23,25,38]

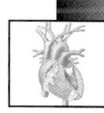

Patients in whom the descending aorta and the varying extents of aortic arch or ascending aorta need to be done through the left chest will be positioned at approximately a 30° angle with a large pillow behind the left shoulder so that a gap is present underneath the patient's back to beyond the scapula.[23] The patient's left arm is placed on an anesthesia screen support; the right arm is placed alongside the patient's side. The right subclavian artery is then included in the sterile field so that it can be dissected out for later suturing of the arterial inflow side graft to the right subclavian artery. This way, circulatory arrest can be established and if antegrade brain perfusion is needed, the innominate artery and common carotid balloon catheters can be placed in the origins of these vessels for antegrade flow.[23]

Occasionally, patients will present with "porcelain" aortas. Such patients have often had previous cardiac surgery. Endarterectomy and tube replacement of the ascending aorta and arch are usually performed at the time of aortic valve replacement, however, sometimes this is not feasible. In these patients, we recommend that a left ventricular to descending aorta valve tube conduit be used (see Chapter 69A). In most patients, we do not use partial cardiopulmonary bypass support but this is certainly an option to consider. The technique is somewhat similar to insertion of the left ventricular assist device. The apex of the left ventricle is first exposed. If the patient has had previous cardiac surgery and adhesions to the pericardium are quite dense, it is better to remove approximately a 4-cm-wide area of pericardium at the apex. Valve pledgeted sutures are then placed circumferentially around the site of the intended placement of the right angled ventricular connector. Next, a side-clamp is positioned in the descending aorta and a distal anastomosis performed for the tube graft. A "cork" or "cookie-cutter" of the desired size is then used to core out the apex of the left ventricle. Because this will clearly result in ejection of blood, the surgeon's thumb is used to plug the hole until the connector is sewn into the left ventricle. The previously placed valve sutures are placed through the cuff and tied into position. Additional running sutures are used to further strengthen this anastomosis. The connector and valve conduit are then connected to the distal graft. The sequence of these connections and insertions can be varied according to what is best suited to the individual patient. We particularly stress the importance of ensuring that the sections of the conduits are carefully deaired using large bore needles.

In some patients, reentry into the left chest for second or third reoperations may be considered too difficult, for example, in patients who have had multiple procedures for coarctation of the aorta.[31] In these patients, an extraanatomical graft from the ascending aorta to the distal aorta can be inserted. Also, the distal anastomosis can be performed at various sites. If a decision is made to place the anastomosis to the descending aorta, then it is best to put the patient on cardiopulmonary bypass, arrest the heart, reflect the heart up, and open the posterior pericardium to expose the descending aorta behind the pericardium. It is important to ensure the esophagus is not in the way when doing this. Next, a side-biting clamp is placed on the descending aorta and a tube graft sewn into the site of the descending aorta, typically using a parachuting technique. The graft is then clamped and the side-biting clamp removed. Hemostasis is ensured distally. The graft is brought up around the right side of the heart, past the inferior margin of the heart, and, keeping to the right, past the right atrium to the ascending aorta. Next, a side-biting clamp is placed in the ascending aorta and the graft proximal anastomosis is performed. The tube graft is carefully deaired and hemostasis is ensured. Alternatively, a distal anastomosis can be made above the celiac artery or to the infrarenal abdominal aorta. To do the anastomosis above the celiac artery, a hole is made in the central part of the diaphragm; the lesser sac opened superior to the stomach. The crura of the diaphragm are divided so that a side-biting clamp can be placed. This anastomosis is a bit more difficult to perform than a side-biting anastomosis in the posterior pericardium for the descending aorta, but has the advantage that the patient does not need to be placed on cardiopulmonary bypass. Another approach, for reasons of either sepsis or middle aortic coarctation syndrome, is for the graft to be taken through a hole in the diaphragm, brought posterior to the stomach and down to the infrarenal aorta. In this situation, we recommend wrapping the graft with omentum to reduce the risk that the graft will erode into surrounding gastrointestinal tissues.

Of note, in patients with coarctation of the aorta and ascending dissections, particularly if acute, the coarctation of the aorta may cause problems with cardiopulmonary bypass and perfusion of the distal aorta. In these patients, we prefer to suture a graft to the descending aorta or to the abdominal aorta and perfuse it with a side-graft from the pump at the same time as perfusing the ascending aorta or right subclavian artery during the establishment of deep hypothermia and circulatory arrest. In most of these patients, because bicuspid aortic valves are associated with the aortic pathology, we insert a composite valve graft, extend it into the aortic hemiarch to resect the dissection, and then reattach the distally placed tube graft to the ascending aorta. Indeed, the first person in whom we used this technique did not even require a blood transfusion for the operation.[31,38]

Graft infections in the descending aorta can be very difficult to successfully manage.[32,34] As indicated above, the aneurysm cavity can sometimes be cannulated by CT guidance and irrigated with antibiotics. This has occasionally resulted in the successful sterilization of an infected graft, but is, by no means, a foolproof approach. Alternatively, the graft has to be excised and then the course of management decided. There are studies by Kieffer et al[18] suggesting that insertion of a homograft (allograft) is useful in this situation. In most patients, however, we prefer to resect the graft, carefully debride the entire area, insert a new tube graft, and wrap it with an omentum flap. In addition, we position a percutaneous irrigation catheter into the area of infection and place surrounding drainage cannulas, either chest tubes or Jackson–Pratt type drainage catheters. It is important, when using chest tubes, to ensure that the omentum does not get caught in the holes and tears when the chest tubes are withdrawn. Antibiotic irrigation is then cycled to this area by running antibiotics, for a period of 15 min, through the percutaneous catheter and then aspirating the area through the drainage tubes for three-quarters of an hour. This cycle must be repeated every hour for 5–7 days. When doing this, specimens are sent daily for bacterial and fungal cultures. The antibiotic is selected on the basis of sensitivity. In most patients we have successfully used gentamicin, penicillin, vancomycin, or imipenem. In addition, if a gel-impregnated graft is used, the graft can be soaked in 600 mg of rifampicin or amphotericin B and then inserted. The rifampicin or amphotericin B remains active up to 4–5 days after insertion. Alternatively, the two stumps of the aorta can be oversewn and a bypass graft placed extraanatomically from the ascending aorta to the abdominal aorta or bilateral femoral arteries. These latter two alternatives, however, have not been reported in the literature as being optimal because of potential stump "blow-out" after oversewing the stumps. In addition, a Carpentier clamp that has been used on the aorta and the subclavian artery can result in a high mortality rate from the clamp eroding through the aorta.[32,34,38]

When the ascending aorta and aortic arch need to be replaced simultaneously through the left chest, the pulmonary artery limits exposure to the aorta proximal to the mid-ascending aorta. A technique Turina (personal communication) has used is to divide the pulmonary artery and retract it out of the way so that the aortic valve can be exposed. Thus, the tube graft can then be carried down to the sinotubular ridge and, if need be, the aortic valve can also be replaced. Next, the pulmonary artery is repaired in the usual manner as for a heart transplant. Another technique is to use modified incisions that gain exposure of the ascending aorta. These include the use of bilateral clam shell-type incisions and the use of two different levels of intercostal incisions such as the second or third interspace for the aortic arch section on the left side and a mediastinal incision and a sternal vertical incision and then extending the clam shell into the fourth or fifth intercostal space on the right side. Alternatively, the thoracotomy can be done in the fourth intercostal space and the incision carried across the sternum into the right chest with division of the internal mammary arteries.[20] Another technique (the "reversed elephant procedure") is to sew a graft inverted on itself into position just beyond the subclavian artery and then, at a later date, perform a mediastinal incision for the ascending and arch section. We recommend, in most patients, the technique, as described above, of using a right subclavian artery for arterial inflow and then replacing the ascending aorta through a left thoracotomy.[23]

In patients in whom complex aortic root procedures have also been required at the same time, we prefer to use a minimally invasive "J" incision or median sternotomy combined with a separate thoracoabdominal incision.[38,50,54]

In patients in whom an elephant trunk has been sutured into position between either the common carotid and left subclavian arteries or beyond the left subclavian artery and once the patient is placed on atriofemoral bypass, the distal aorta is clamped and the aorta incised beyond the proximal anastomosis (see Chapter 69A). In most patients, when this area is incised, there is a considerable amount of clot around the elephant trunk that prevents exsanguination when the aorta is incised. A finger should be inserted and wrapped around the elephant trunk, which is then removed through the aortic incision and clamped. This brief and quick maneuver results in minimal blood loss and is well-tolerated. An important caveat is that the amount of blood that can be lost during this maneuver is equal to the cardiac output times the length of time that is required to clamp the graft! Thus, the anesthesiologist and perfusionist should be prepared for rapid infusion of blood. Apart from the advantage of not needing to do the proximal anastomosis again, another advantage of the second-stage elephant trunk is that the densely thickened and inflamed aorta does not need to be dissected out to clamp it to do the proximal anastomosis. If, however, the anastomosis is done between the left common carotid and left subclavian arteries, then once the elephant trunk has been clamped, an end-to-end graft anastomosis should be performed to the left subclavian artery. Next, a distal anastomosis is performed with the elephant trunk and, finally, the subclavian graft is sutured to the descending aortic graft. Alternatively, a graft prosthesis with a side graft can be sewn to the elephant trunk and the side graft sewn to the left subclavian artery, taking care to judge the length of the side graft exactly (see Chapter 69A).

Occasionally, the aorta has to be clamped between the innominate artery and the left common carotid artery. It is surprising how well-tolerated this is by patients as long as atheroma is not present in the aortic arch. We have even clamped the ascending aorta and angled it up to the base of the innominate artery to replace the aortic arch. This had been done under emergency situations for a ruptured aortic arch and usually is not something that would be performed as an elective surgical procedure, particularly when a cardiopulmonary bypass pump is available and the patient can be cooled and circulatory arrest established.[6,30,50,57]

If cardiopulmonary bypass is used, the venous drainage is established usually for primary cases by placing a purse string suture around the right auricle and then placing a two-stage catheter into the right auricle through the left thoracotomy approach. Although this may appear to be a difficult procedure to do, this can be performed with comparative ease. If, however, the patient has had previous cardiac surgery, then it is preferable to dissect out the right femoral vein and place a long venous drainage catheter through the right femoral vein up into the right atrium, using transesophageal echo to make sure it is positioned correctly.[38]

Thoracoabdominal Aneurysm Repair

For thoracoabdominal aneurysm repairs the anesthesia and insertion of cerebrospinal catheters are the same as for descending aortic repairs. The positioning of the patient, however, is slightly different; the chest and shoulders should be positioned approximately 60 degrees to the table and when the patient is draped, it is essential that the umbilicus and the abdomen down to the public bone are within the operative field (Figure 69B-10). In addition, if an aortic bifurcated graft needs to be inserted down to the iliac or external iliac or even femoral arteries on the right side, the right groin must also be prepared and draped into the sterile field. Similarly, if a right iliac to renal artery bypass needs to be placed, then this part of the abdomen and groin must also be prepared within the sterile field. The femoral artery on the left side is dissected out as described above. Next, the incision is performed from behind the scapula across the subcostal margin aiming for the umbilicus. The incision is then carried down to the pubic bone for type II aneurysms. The muscle layers are divided and the subcostal margin exposed. The sixth rib is resected and the subcostal margin divided and the diaphragm is mobilized circumferentially. We now routinely use an extraperitoneal approach without opening the peritoneum and, thus, do not have to deal with the abdominal viscera and intestines when closing patients. Next, a retractor is inserted and the aorta encircled proximal and distal to the intended sites of repair. As indicated above, to reduce the period of intercostal ischemia, we try to perform a sequential segmental repair as much as possible. In the patient with extensive thoracoabdominal aneurysm, we mobilize the following: the aorta and aortic arch between the left common carotid and left subclavian arteries; the left subclavian artery; the aorta, approximately at the level of the sixth rib; immediately above the celiac artery where there is often a neck; below the renal arteries around the proximal infrarenal aorta; and the distal aorta and/or the left iliac artery. This allows us to perform a segmental sequential repair while maintaining perfusion of the spinal cord as much as possible during this period.[38,49,50]

Atriofemoral bypass is then established as described previously. In patients with type III or type IV thoracoabdominal aneurysms, we cannulate the descending aorta for inflow into the centrifugal pump bypass circuit. The reason for this is that we find hemodynamic stability is easier to control because cardiac output and blood pressure are not quite so dependent on left atrial volume and ventricular preload and it is then possible to establish a constant blood pressure.[38,49,50]

The operative sequence for Crawford type II thoracoabdominal aneurysms involves clamping the distal aortic arch, the left subclavian artery, and the aorta at T6 (Figure 69B-11). The aorta is opened and a proximal anastomosis performed at the distal aortic arch or at the left subclavian artery. The left subclavian artery is then unclamped to fill the graft and check for hemostasis. Once this is ensured, the aortic arch clamp is also removed to further test the anastomosis. Next, the intercostal vessels down to the level of T6 are oversewn. The aorta is clamped at the diaphragm above the celiac artery after the new aorta graft has also been clamped. The aorta down to the diaphragmatic clamp is then opened, flushed out of any debris, and the intercostal vessels carefully identified and reattached to the new graft as needed with Carrel patches. These are done from the level of T6 down to the clamp.[38]

A clamp is placed below the renal arteries on the proximal infrarenal aorta and the intercostal vessels reperfused and the visceral segment opened. Of note, whether inserting a cardioplegia-type cooling coil and using a separate roller pump to maintain higher pressures to perfuse the renal arteries with cold blood may be more protective than cold crystalloid remains to be established.[42] Once the kidneys have been cooled (Figure 69B-12A), a decision needs to be made as to how the visceral segment should be managed.[43] If there are further intercostal lumbar arteries that are patent, these are reattached, particularly because at this segment they are critical for spinal cord perfusion and preventing spinal cord injury. In most patients, especially if they do not have either dissection or Marfan syndrome, the visceral vessels can be reattached as a single patch or as a patch for the superior mesenteric, celiac, and right renal arteries with the left renal artery being reattached as a mobilized button to the graft directly or with an interposition graft. For those patients with either Marfan syndrome or young patients with aortic dissections, we usually place individ-

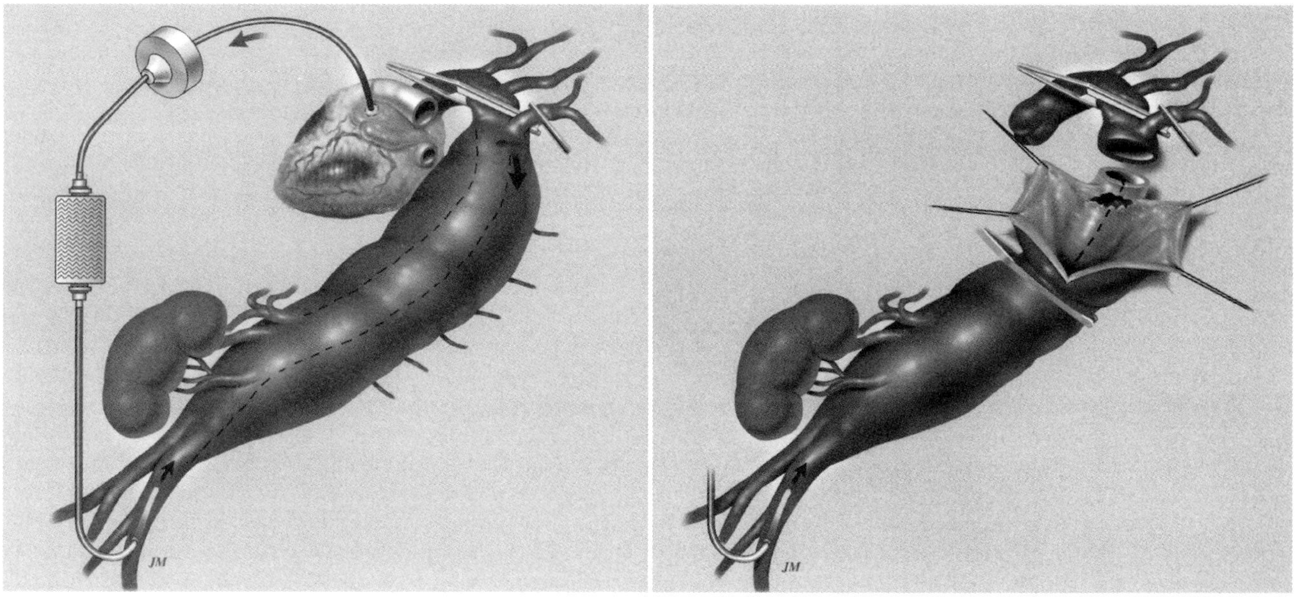

A B

Figure 69B–11 **A,** Sequence in repairing a thoracoabdominal aneurysm with first insertion of an atriofemoral bypass circuit with a heat exchange and cooling the patient systemically and then clamping of the distal aortic arch and subclavian artery. **B,** Transection of the aorta beyond the subclavian artery after clamping the mid-descending aorta.

(Continued)

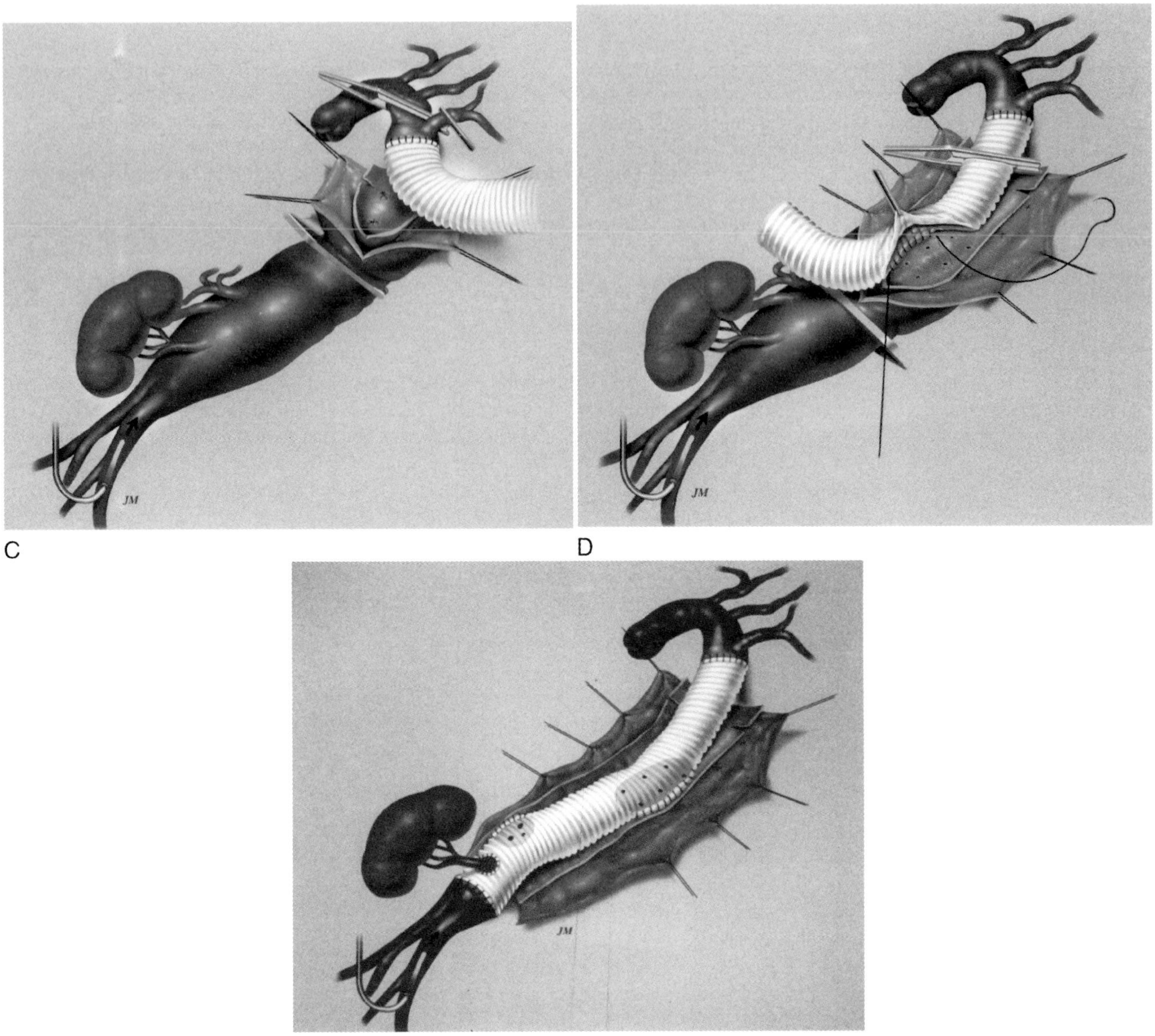

C D E

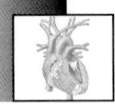

Figure 69B–11 cont'd **C,** Completion of the proximal anastomosis and oversewing of the intercostal arteries in the proximal segment to T6. **D,** Moving of the clamp to below the anastomosis and reattachment of the intercostal arteries after clamping immediately above the celiac artery. **E,** Completion of the repair with reattachment of the visceral arteries as a single Carrel patch except for the left kidney, which has been reattached as an ostial button; the patient is then rewarmed through the femoral artery.

ual grafts to the visceral vessels. This can be done using the grafts with multiple branch vessels that are available or by suturing a bifurcated graft to the new aortic graft and then performing a side-to-side anastomosis to the celiac artery and end-to-end anastomosis to the superior mesenteric artery. The right renal artery can be reattached directly to the graft or with an interposition graft. The left renal artery is managed by mobilizing the renal artery as a button and reattaching it directly to the aorta graft or by placing an interposition graft.[38,43] In patients in whom an 8-mm graft or saphenous vein graft is used for reattaching intercostal or lumbar arteries, we have noted on postoperative CT scans that these have often clotted off. To maintain greater flow and perfusion, we, therefore, attach the distal end of these grafts to either the left or right renal artery.

A clamp is then placed below the visceral segment and the visceral vessels are reperfused, carefully deairing the grafts prior to establishing blood flow to the segment. The infrarenal segment is replaced by placing a clamp at the aortic bifurcation or, more often, by clamping the left common iliac artery and opening the rest of the aorta. The lumbar arteries in this segment are usually preserved as much as possible by beveling the distal anastomosis, particularly in patients with aortic dissection. How this segment should be managed, however, with respect to the lumbar arteries has not been answered satisfactorily in patients with extensive Crawford type II thoracoabdominal aneurysms. Based on spinal motor-evoked potential monitoring, it appears some of these vessels may be critical to maintaining spinal cord blood flow during extensive aortic replacements. This may

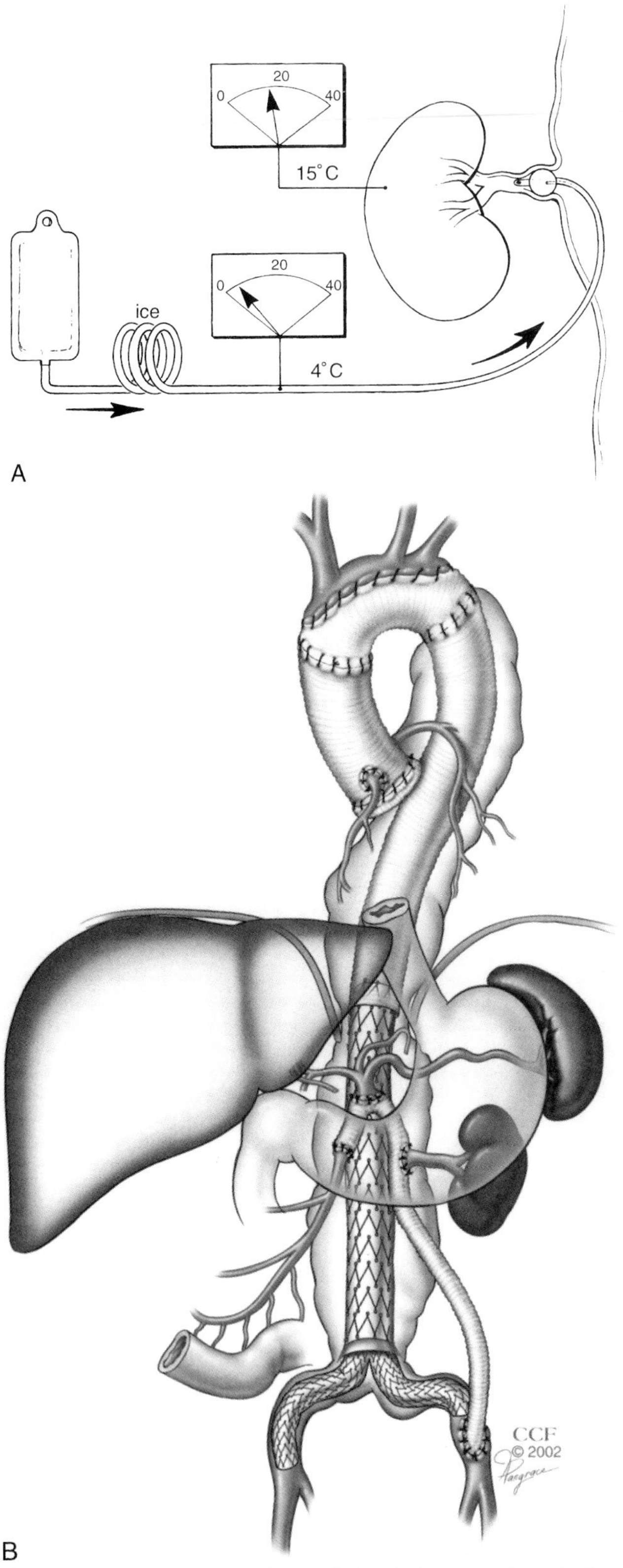

Figure 69B–12 **A,** Cooling of the kidneys with a balloon catheter placed in the origin of the renal artery and perfusion of the kidney with cold solution. We currently use three 60-ml syringes to cool the kidney and have found this cools the kidney to approximately 15° C. **B,** Bypass graft placed from the left iliac artery to the left kidney celiac artery and superior mesenteric artery. The remaining part of the aorta is stented with stent grafts from the elephant trunk down to the iliac arteries. Illustration of completed repair. Not shown is a femero-femoral bypass.

be because of the iliolumbar radicular artery that supplies the distal lumbar spinal cord and cauda equina.[41] Once the distal anastomosis has been performed, the patient is rewarmed and taken off the atriofemoral bypass circuit. It is important that the patient is not excessively warmed as this may increase the risk of spinal cord injury.[50] The aneurysm sac is then wrapped around the graft and the atriofemoral bypass circuit removed. The patient is closed in layers.[38,44,50]

Sometimes, in addition to placing bypass grafts to the visceral vessels, in patients with extensive atherosclerosis, particularly calcification, the aorta needs to be endarterectomized to do the repair.[38,43] Furthermore, endarterectomies of the visceral artery origins frequently need to be performed.[43] If the stenosis extends further into the vessel, bypass grafts to further down on the vessels should be performed with end-to-end anastomoses. The right renal artery in this situation can be difficult to mobilize beyond the first half inch or so. To deal with more distal right renal artery stenoses, an alternative is to open the peritoneum and mobilize the duodenum. A graft is then sewn to the renal artery end to side near the renal hiatus and brought down in the right lateral peritoneal gutter down to the common iliac artery and sewn to the right iliac artery. To do this, the thoracoabdominal incision must be extended down to the pubic bone to get adequate exposure. If the external iliac has to be used, a right inguinal incision at the pelvic crease has to be made and the iliac artery exposed intraperitoneally or extraperitoneally where it exits the pelvis.[38] Not shown is a femoro-femoral bypass.

In some patients an aorta bifemoral graft needs to be placed and this is sewn into position end to end to the distal aortic graft and then tunneled in the standard manner to the femoral arteries. Anastomoses to the femoral arteries are performed to the left and right sides as required. This is, as a rule, a rare procedure.[38]

Thoracic and Thoracoabdominal Stent Grafts

The field of thoracic aortic stent grafting is rapidly expanding and developing, despite the withdrawal of one stent graft system because of wire fractures. During the last 4 years ending in December of 2003, we performed 313 thoracic stent graft procedures. The indications were distal acute dissections with leakage or ischemia, descending thoracic saccular aneurysms, penetrating ulcers, descending aneurysm in high-risk patients, second-stage elephant trunk procedures in high-risk patients, and high-risk thoracoabdominal aneurysms. In the latter patients, before stenting, through a flank incision, bypasses are placed from the left iliac artery to the patent visceral arteries. The aorta, or elephant trunk proximally, is then stented down to the iliac arteries. (Figure 69B-12). The results have been good.[14]

Replacement of an Entire Aorta during a Single Operation

Fortunately, most patients with extensive aneurysms can be managed with two-stage elephant trunk procedures (see Chapter 69A). Sometimes, however, patients present with huge aneurysms where both the ascending aorta and thoracoabdominal aorta are symptomatic or the patient has severe coronary artery disease with a symptomatic thoracoabdominal aneurysm or where there is no neck in the aortic arch in which to sew the distal elephant trunk anastomosis into position without tearing the aorta.[54] In most patients, if there is a narrowing to approximately 4–5 cm in the arch, the aorta can be tailored down to a size 30 graft. If the aorta is larger than this, however, a replacement of the entire thoracic aorta or the entire aorta from the aortic valve to the aortic bifurcation must be considered.[54] One option is to do this through the left chest and, if the pulmonary artery is cut, the aortic valve also can be replaced (see above) (Figure 69B-12). However, using both a mediastinal and thoracoabdominal incision may be preferable. To replace the entire thoracic aorta or the entire aorta from aortic valve down to the aortic bifurcation, the positioning of the patient is critical (Figure 69B-13). The patient's right arm is placed alongside the chest and the left arm is elevated on an anesthesia screen support. A pillow is placed behind the left shoulder and the patient tilted to approximately 30° to the table. It is important that there is a gap between the table and the chest wall below the left shoulder blade so the incision can be carried behind the shoulder blade. The right femoral artery and vein may also be required and should be prepped into the field. Similarly, the right subclavian artery should be within the sterile field. In most patients, the right subclavian artery will be used for arterial inflow and a two-stage vena cava cannula for venous drainage. Nevertheless, we have had occasion to use both superior and inferior vena cava cannulas in patients with atrial septal defects that have been repaired at the same time or to use the right femoral vein with a long cannula into the right atrium for reoperations, particularly when using the minimally invasive "J" incisions for the reoperations.

Once the subclavian and femoral arteries have been exposed, the thoracoabdominal incision is then performed from behind the scapula across the costal margin down to the umbilicus as far as the pubic bone, if necessary. The aorta is then exposed and the retractor inserted. Once the entire aortic aneurysm has been exposed satisfactorily, the anterior retractor blades are relaxed so that the incision is allowed to come together again. The mediastinal incision is performed by a minimally invasive "J" incision or a complete mediastinal incision depending on what cardiac procedures are required (see Chapter 69A). Once the pericardium is opened and stay sutures placed, the patient is heparinized and cannulated in the standard manner. The patient is cooled for deep hypothermic circulatory arrest. During this period, if the aortic valve needs to be either repaired or replaced or coronary artery bypass grafts are required or the mitral valve or other lesions need to be dealt with, then this can be done while the patient is being cooled. In some patients, a composite valve graft has been inserted while the patient is being cooled.

After the patient has been sufficiently cooled (see Chapter 69A), circulation is arrested and the ascending aorta and the aortic arch opened. The tube graft is fed into the descending aorta for the repair through the thoracoabdominal incision. Because commercially available grafts are invariably not long enough, two 60-mm grafts are usually sutured together prior to placing these into the descending aorta. A side hole is made for the aortic arch. The greater vessel anastomosis is performed with sufficient length proximally to perform the proximal anastomosis to a composite valve graft or to the sinotubular ridge. The anastomosis for the greater vessels is usually quick and easy. For example, the anastomosis takes 10–15 min compared to the lengthier elephant trunk technique where a distal circumferential and aortic arch anastomoses are required.

A clamp is then placed on the graft beyond the greater vessels and proximal to the greater vessels. Perfusion of the greater vessels and brain is restarted. If the right subclavian artery is used, this is easily performed without any additional side grafts. If the femoral artery is used (which we try to avoid in most of these patients), a side graft has to be sutured to the aortic graft and connected to an arterial cannula to perfuse the brain. The proximal anastomosis is then performed and the heart is reperfused. If there is any possibility of left ventricular distention, the left ventricle has to be decompressed. We have found that it is sometimes better to maintain cardioplegic perfusion to the heart without unclamping the aorta if continued arrest of blood flow to the distal aorta and visceral vessels will continue for some time.

The retractor in the mediastinum is partially closed and the retractor in the left chest spread open again with the surgeon moving to the left side of the patient. The descending aorta is opened where the previously placed tube graft is located. A clamp is placed on the graft and the clamp on the

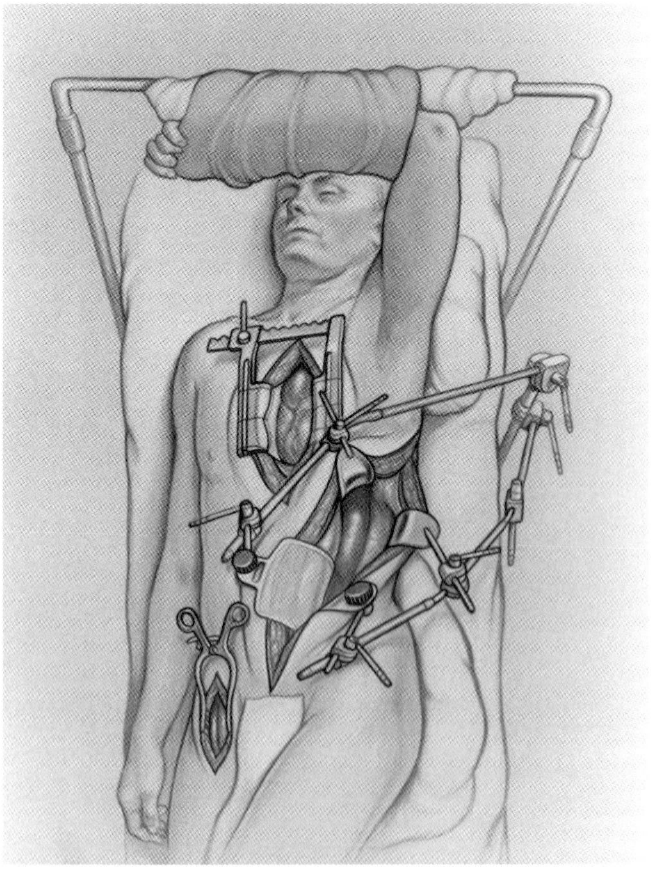

A

Figure 69B–13 **A,** Positioning patients for repairing both the ascending aorta and the aortic arch through the mediastinum and the descending and thoracoabdominal aorta through a left thoracoabdominal incision.

(Continued)

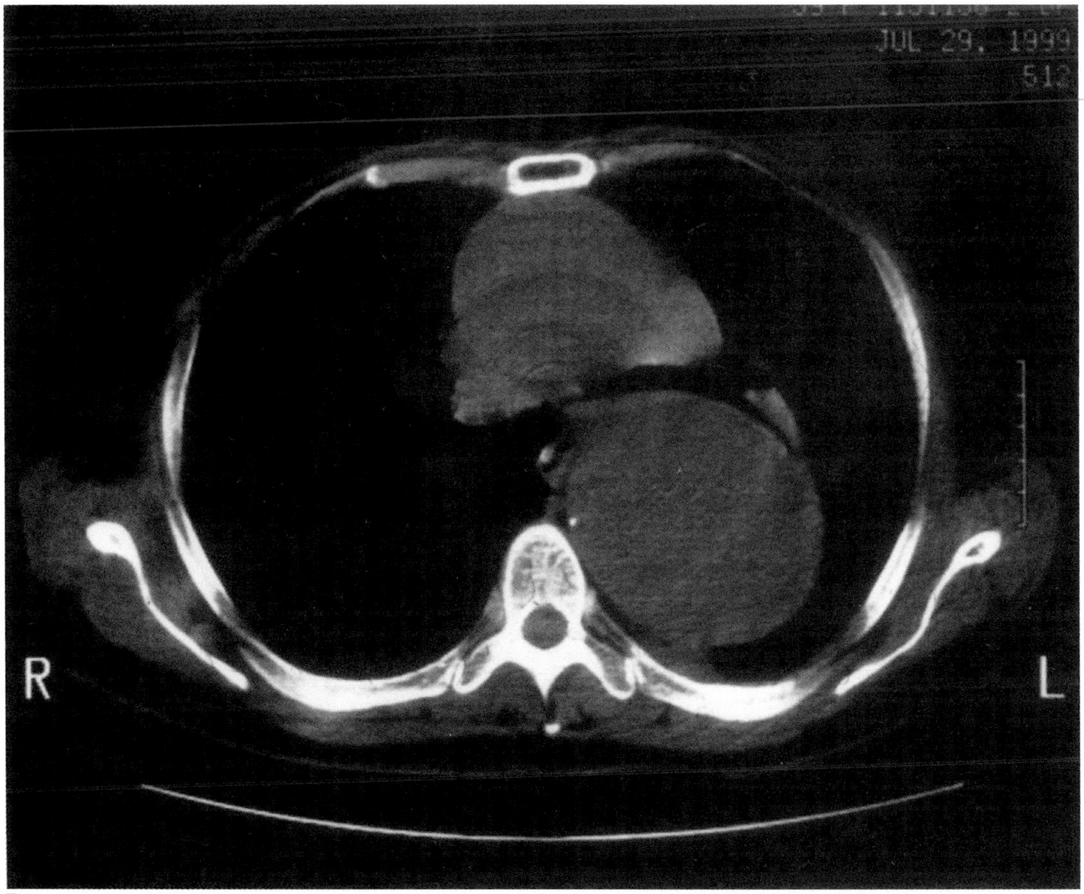

B1

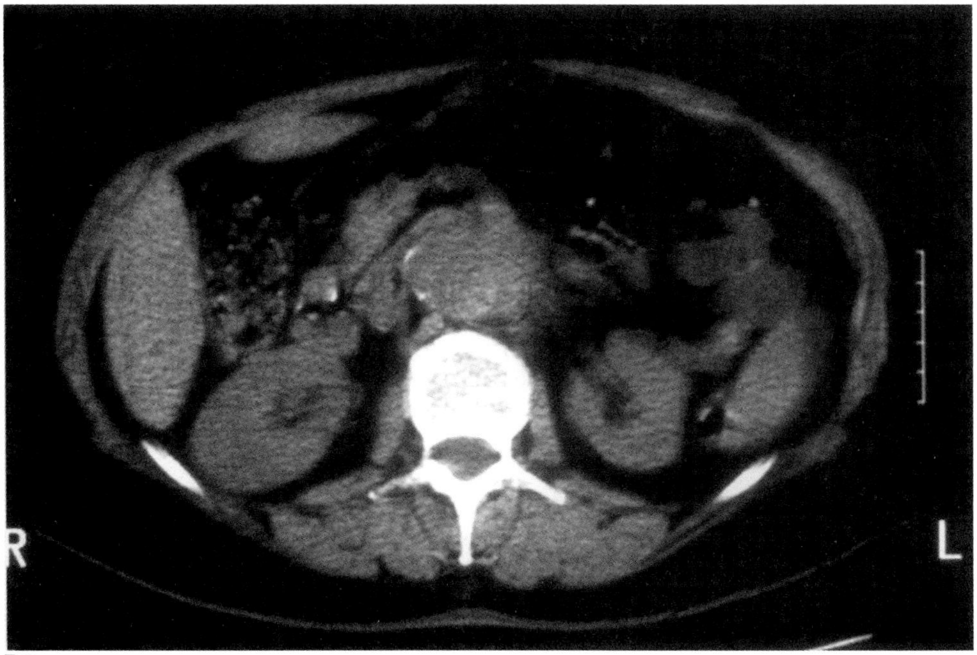

B2

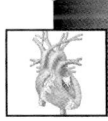

Figure 69B–13 cont'd B, (1) CT of nurse with large ascending and descending (2) thoracoabdominal aneurysm.

(Continued)

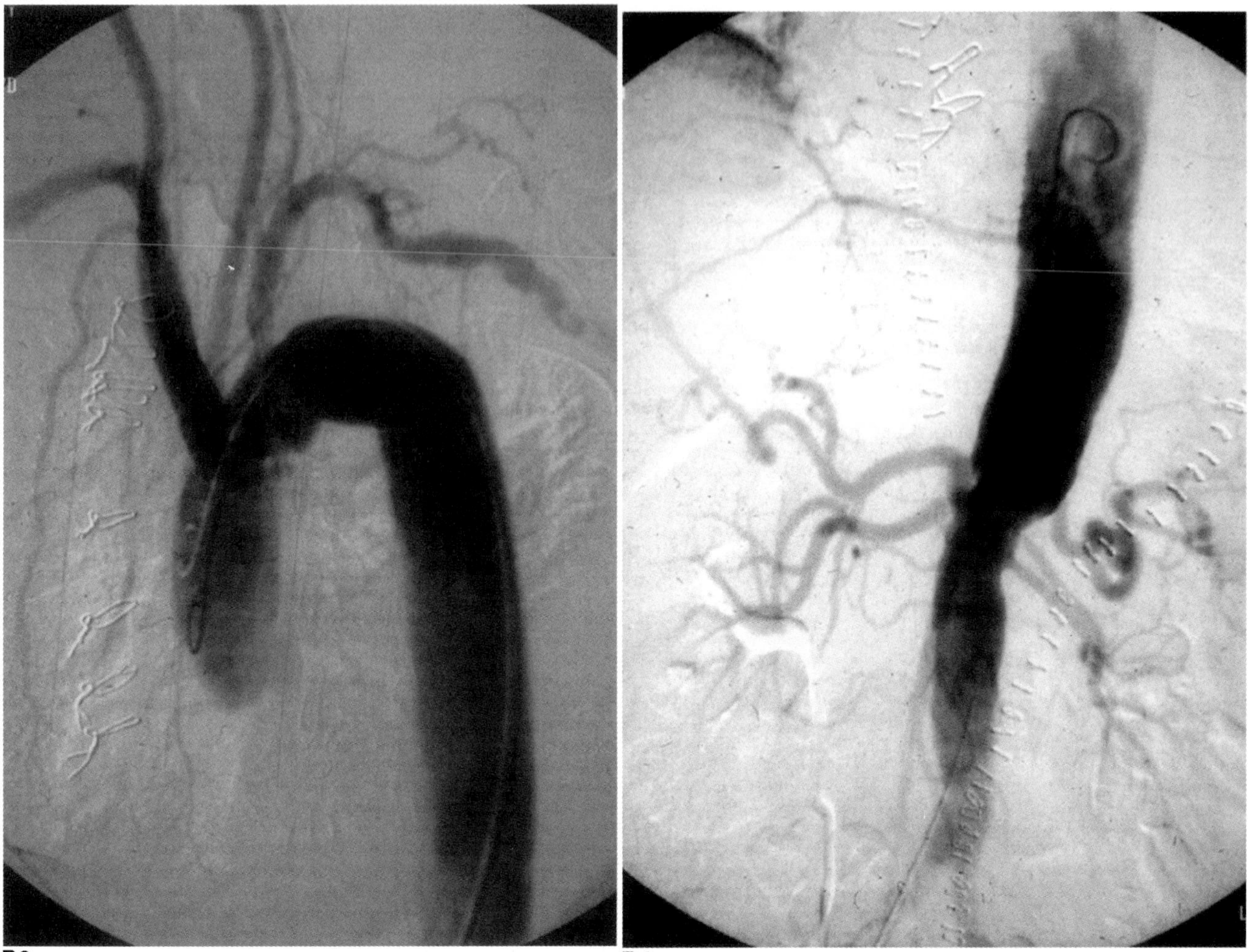

Figure 69B–13 cont'd (3) Postoperative angiogram of the thoracic aorta and (4) abdominal aorta after replacement of the entire thoracic aorta and down to the renal arteries.

graft beyond the left subclavian artery in the mediastinum is removed. By doing this, there is less likelihood of twisting the graft in the segment between the left subclavian artery and the clamp on the descending graft. The aorta is then opened down to the visceral segments and beyond as needed. Because the patient is still cold from circulatory arrest, no further cold solution is given to perfuse the kidneys. Next, the intercostal arteries are reattached as are the visceral vessels. These arteries and vessels are reperfused by removing the clamp from the graft in the descending segment. With a clamp on the graft below the visceral vessels, the anastomosis is completed at the aortic bifurcation. Once the visceral vessels have been reperfused, the patient is rewarmed. Hemostasis is ensured throughout and the aneurysm sac wrapped around the graft as described previously. Once satisfactory cardiac rhythm is established and hemostasis is ensured, the patient is closed in the standard fashion. We have noted that this long graft may produce significant impedance to the heart because of lack of elasticity of the graft. The patient, therefore, usually requires inotropes the first few days after surgery when this procedure has been performed. In addition, most patients require 2 weeks of ventilation prior to being removed from the ventilator. The shortest period that a patient was on the ventilator was 5 days and this was in a patient who was a young nurse. This is a formidable operation that has taken us a minimum of 6 h to perform with minimum circulatory arrest time of 60 min for visceral segments. Fortunately, this is an operation that is seldom required.

OUTCOMES

The results of descending and thoracoabdominal aneurysm surgery have improved considerably.* In a series of 832 patients, for patients operated since 1986, the survival rate was 98% with a 5% risk of paraplegia/paraparesis.[45] In an extensive review of 1509 historical thoracoabdominal aneurysm repairs, the mortality rate was 8% and the risk of

*References 4–13, 15–23, 26, 37, 40, 42–45, 47–50, 54, 57, 58.

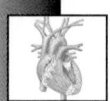

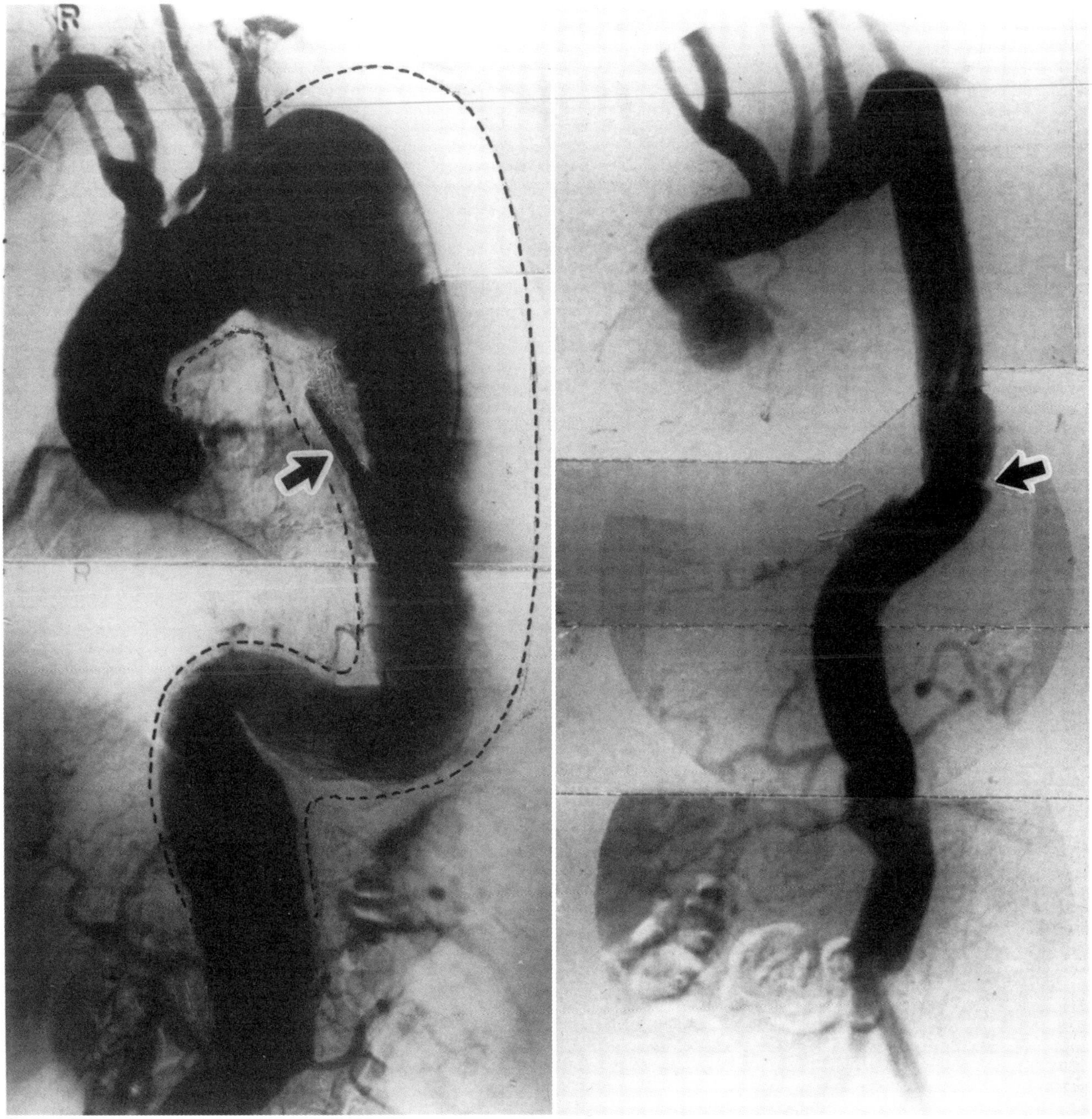

Figure 69B–13 cont'd C, (1) Patient with a large aneurysm involving the entire aorta with lifting of clot in the descending aorta (*black arrows*). The descending aorta diameter was 17 cm. (2) The postoperative angiogram and the joined grafts (*black arrow*).

(*Continued*)

paraplegia/paraparesis was 16%.[44] The highest risk was thoracoabdominal type II aneurysms at 31%. These results have improved over time with the introduction of new techniques as described above. In our most recent analysis of 132 complicated and high-risk descending or thoracoabdominal aneurysm repairs, the mortality rate was 8% and the permanent paraplegia/paraparesis rate was 3.8%.[50] This group of patients, also, included those who had the entire aorta or entire thoracic aorta replaced using both a mediastinal and thoracoabdominal incision and 20% underwent emergency operation for aortic rupture or dissection.[50] In patients who did not have cardiopulmonary bypass as part of the operative procedure, the mortality rate was 6%. In other series, results for mortality and the risk of paraplegia/paraparesis have improved. The Crawford type II thoracoabdominal aneurysms continue to have a high risk of mortality

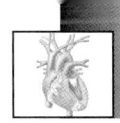

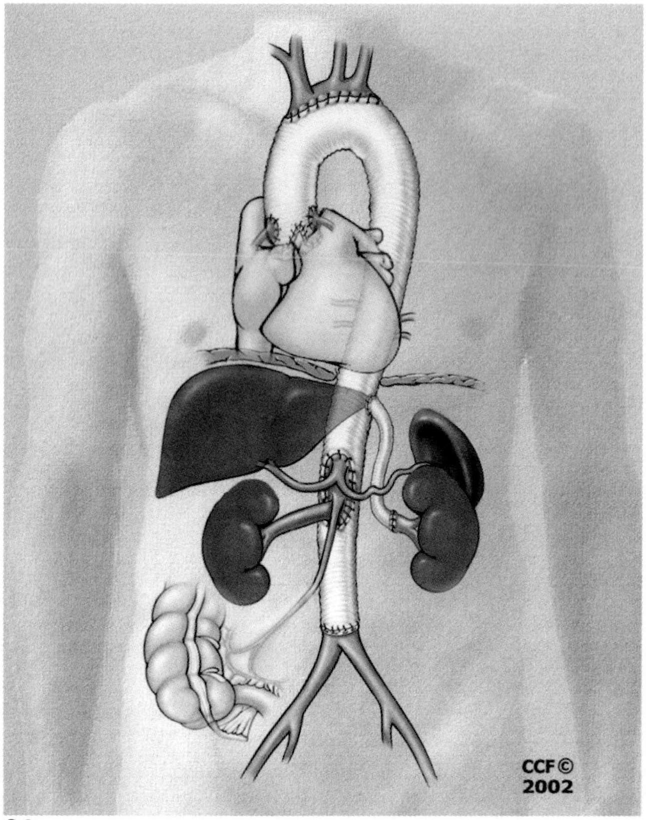

C3

Figure 69B–13 cont'd (3) Replacement of the entire aorta.

and increased risk of paraplegia/paraparesis,[6] although in our most recent analysis, extent was not as significant a factor as in the past with improved techniques.[50] Nevertheless, these operations can be unpredictable for outcome after surgery despite a seemingly uneventful and well-performed operation.

In the long-term follow-up of patients who have had aortic surgery, whether ascending, aortic arch, descending, thoracoabdominal or abdominal, or for aortic dissection, the 5-year survival has been 60%[38] (Figure 69B-14). Two thirds of late deaths were due to cardiac disease.[38,44,45] To improve long-term survival, evidence of cardiac disease needs to be aggressively sought and, if found, treated before or at the time of surgery.

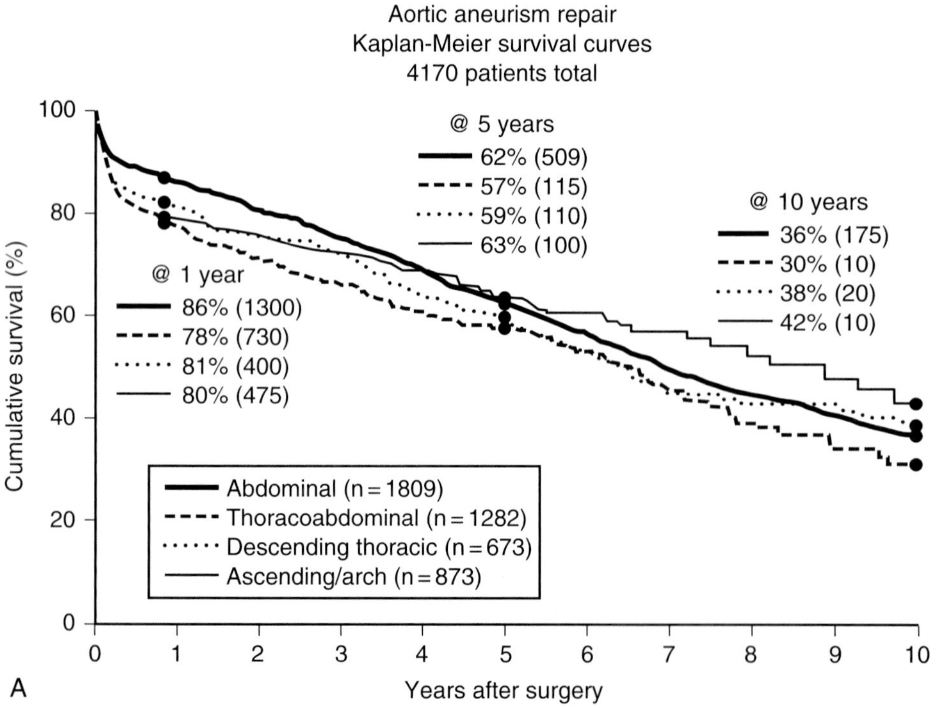

A

Figure 69B–14 **A,** Long-term survival for patients undergoing aortic repair. This stresses the importance of screening for and treating coronary artery disease.

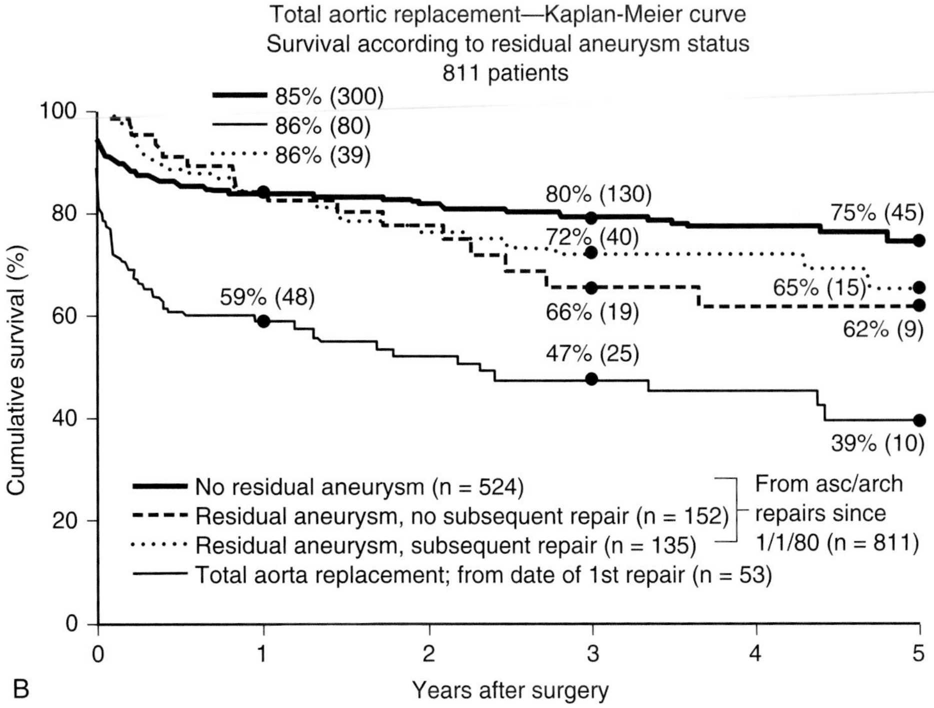

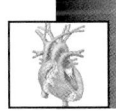

Figure 69B–14 cont'd B, Influence on long-term survival of residual aneurysms and whether they are repaired or not after the first aortic procedure.

REFERENCES

1. Acher CW, Wynn MM, Hoch JR, et al: Combined use of spinal fluid drainage and naloxone reduces risk of neurologic deficit in the repair of thoracoabdominal aneurysms. J Vasc Surg 19:236–248, 1994.
2. Acosta-Rua GJ: Treatment of traumatic paraplegic patients by localized cooling of the spinal cord. J Iowa Med Soc 60:326–328, 1970.
3. Biglioli P, Spirito R, Roberto M, et al: The anterior spinal artery: the main arterial supply of the human spinal cord—a preliminary anatomic study. J Thorac Cardiovasc Surg 119:376–379, 2000.
4. Cambria RP, Davison JK, Zanetti S, et al: Clinical experience with epidural cooling for spinal cord protection during thoracic and thoracoabdominal aneurysm repair. J Vasc Surg 5:234–243, 1997.
5. Cooley DA, Baldwin RT: Technique of open distal anastomosis for repair of descending thoracic aortic aneurysms. Ann Thorac Surg 54:932–936, 1992.
6. Coselli JS, LeMaire SA, Conklin LD, et al: Morbidity and mortality after extent II thoracoabdominal aortic aneurysm repair. Ann Thorac Surg 73:1107–1115; discussion 1115–1116, 2002.
7. Coselli JS, LeMaire SA, Koksoy C, et al: Cerebrospinal fluid drainage reduces paraplegia after thoracoabdominal aortic aneurysm repair: results of a randomized clinical trial. J Vasc Surg 35:631–635, 2002.
8. Coselli JS, LeMaire SA, Poli de Figueiredo L, Kirby RP: Paraplegia after thoracoabdominal aortic aneurysm repair: is dissection a risk factor? Ann Thorac Surg 63:28–36, 1997.
9. Cox GS, O'Hara PJ, Hertzer NR, et al: Thoracoabdominal aneurysm repair: a representative experience. J Vasc Surg 15:780–787, 1992.
10. Crawford ES, Svensson LG, Hess KR, et al: A prospective randomized study of cerebrospinal fluid drainage to prevent paraplegia after high-risk surgery on the thoracoabdominal aorta. J Vasc Surg 13:36–45, 1991.
11. de Haan P, Kalkman CJ, de Mol BA, et al: Efficacy of transcranial motor-evoked myogenic potentials to detect spinal cord ischemia during operations for thoracoabdominal aneurysms. J Thorac Cardiovasc Surg 113:87–101, 1997.
12. Fabian TC, Richardson JD, Croce MA, et al: Prospective study of the blunt aortic injury: Multicenter Trial of the American Association for the Surgery of Trauma. J Trauma 42:374–380; discussion 380–383, 1997.
13. Gilling-Smith GL, Worswick L, Knight PF, et al: Surgical repair of thoracoabdominal aortic aneurysm: 10 years' experience. Br J Surg 82:624–629, 1995.
14. Greenberg R, Harthun N: Endovascular repair of lesions of descending thoracic aorta: aneurysms and dissections. Curr Opin Cardiol 16:225–230, 2001.
15. Griepp RB, Ergin MA, Galla JD, et al: Looking for the artery of Adamkiewicz: a quest to minimize paraplegia after operation for aneurysms of the descending thoracic and thoracoabdominal aorta. J Thorac Cardiovasc Surg 112: 1202–1215, 1996.
16. Hollier LH, Money SR, Naslund TC, et al: Risk of spinal cord dysfunction in patients undergoing thoracoabdominal aortic replacement. Am J Surg 164:210–214, 1996.
17. Kieffer E, Richard T, Chiras J, et al: Preoperative spinal cord arteriography in aneurysmal disease of the descending thoracic and thoracoabdominal aorta: preliminary results in 45 patients. Ann Vasc Surg 3:34–46, 1989.
18. Kieffer E, Sabatier J, Plissonnier D, Knosalla C: Prosthetic graft infection after descending thoracic/thoracoabdominal aortic aneurysmectomy: management with in situ arterial allografts. J Vasc Surg 33:671–678, 2001.
19. Kieffer E: Surgical treatment of aneurysms of the thoracoabdominal aorta. Rev Prat 41:1793–1797, 1991.
20. Kouchoukos NT, Daily BD, Rokkas CK, et al: Hypothermic bypass and circulatory arrest for operations on the descending thoracic and thoracoabdominal aorta. Ann Thorac Surg 60:67–77, 1995.
21. Lawrie GM, Earle N, DeBakey ME: Evolution of surgical techniques for aneurysms of the descending thoracic aorta:

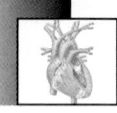

twenty-nine years experience with 659 patients. J Card Surg 9:648–661, 1994.

22. Maughan LR, Svensson LG: Elephant trunk reconstruction for aberrant right subclavian and aortic aneurysm. Ann Thorac Surg 64:547–548, 1997.
23. Nadolny EM, Svensson LG: Hypothermic arrest for descending aortic rupture in reoperative patients. Ann Thorac Surg 71:2027–2030, 2001.
24. Parmley LF, Mattingly TW, Manion WC, Jahnke EJJ: Nonpenetrating traumatic injury of the aorta. Circulation 17:1086–1102, 1958.
25. Robinson BL, Nadolny EM, Entrup MH, Svensson LG: Management of right-sided aortic arch aneurysms. Ann Thorac Surg 72:1764–1765, 2001.
26. Safi HJ, Bartoli S, Hess KR, et al: Neurologic deficit in patients at high risk with thoracoabdominal aortic aneurysms: the role of cerebral spinal fluid drainage and distal aortic perfusion. J Vasc Surg 20:434–443, 1994.
27. Safi HJ, Miller CC 3rd, Carr C, et al: Importance of intercostal artery reattachment during thoracoabdominal aortic aneurysm repair. J Vasc Surg 28:570–571, 1998.
28. Saltman AE, Svensson LG: Chronic traumatic aortic pseudoaneurysm: resolution with observation. Ann Thorac Surg 67:240–241, 1999.
29. Sugiyama S, Ishizaki M, Uchida H: Spinal epidural oxygen partial pressure and evoked spinal cord potential in relation to the severity of spinal ischemia during cross clamping of the thoracic aorta. Acta Med Okayama 47:369–376, 1993.
30. Sun J, Hirsch D, Svensson LG: Spinal cord protection by papaverine and intrathecal cooling during aortic crossclamping. J Cardiovasc Surg (Torino) 39:839–842, 1998.
31. Svensson LG: Management of acute aortic dissection associated with coarctation by a single operation. Ann Thorac Surg 58:241–243, 1994.
32. Svensson LG: Management of thora co abdominal graft infections. In Calligaro K, Veith FJ, editors: Management of Infected Arterial Grafts. St. Louis: Quality Medical Publishing, Inc., 1994, pp. 65–81.
33. Svensson LG: Intraoperative identification of spinal cord blood supply during descending and thoracoabdominal aortic repairs. J Thorac Cardiovasc Surg 112:1455–1461, 1996.
34. Svensson LG: Management of graft infection of the ascending aorta and aortic arch. In Kieffer E, editor: Arterial Infections (French). Paris: Expansion Scientifique Francaise, 1997.
35. Svensson LG: New and future approaches for spinal cord protection. Semin Thorac Cardiovasc Surg 9:206–221, 1997.
36. Svensson LG: Management of segmental intercostals and lumbar arteries during descending and thoracoabdominal aneurysm repairs. Semin Thorac Cardiovasc Surg 10:45–49, 1998.
37. Svensson LG, Crawford ES: Aortic dissection and aortic aneurysm surgery: clinical observations, experimental investigations and statistical analyses. Part III. Curr Probl Surg 30:1–172, 1993.
38. Svensson LG, Crawford ES: Cardiovascular and Vascular Disease of the Aorta. Philadelphia: W. B. Saunders, 1997.
39. Svensson LG, Loop FD: Prevention of spinal cord ischemia in aortic surgery. In Bergan JJ, Yao JST, editors: Arterial Surgery: New Diagnostic and Operative Techniques. New York: Grune & Stratton, 1988, pp. 2273–2285.
40. Svensson LG, Antunes MD, Kinsley RH: Traumatic rupture of the thoracic aorta. A report of 14 cases and a review of the literature. S Afr Med J 67:853–857, 1985.
41. Svensson LG, Klepp P, Hinder RA: Spinal cord anatomy of the baboon: comparison with man and implications on spinal cord blood flow during thoracic aortic cross clamping. S Afr J Surg 24:32–34, 1986.
42. Svensson LG, Coselli JS, Safi HJ, et al: Appraisal of adjuncts to prevent acute renal failure after surgery on the thoracic or thoracoabdominal aorta. J Vasc Surg 10:230–239, 1989.
43. Svensson LG, Crawford ES, Hess KR, et al: Thoracoabdominal aortic aneurysms associated with celiac, superior mesenteric, and renal artery occlusive disease: methods and analysis of results in 271 patients. J Vasc Surg 16:378–389; discussion 389–390, 1992.
44. Svensson LG, Crawford ES, Hess KR, et al: Experience with 1509 patients undergoing thoracoabdominal aortic operations. J Vasc Surg 17:357–370, 1993.
45. Svensson LG, Crawford ES, Hess KR, et al: Variables predictive of outcome in 832 patients undergoing repairs of the descending thoracic aorta. Chest 104:1248–1253, 1993.
46. Svensson LG, Crawford ES, Patel V, et al: Spinal cord oxygenation, intraoperative blood supply localization, cooling and function with aortic clamping. Ann Thorac Surg 54:74–79, 1992.
47. Svensson LG, Hess KR, Coselli JS, et al: A prospective study of respiratory failure after high-risk surgery on the thoracoabdominal aorta. J Vasc Surg 14:271–282, 1991.
48. Svensson LG, Hess KR, Coselli JS, Safi HR: Influence of segmental arteries, extent, and atrio-femoral bypass on postoperative paraplegia after thoracoabdominal aortic aneurysm repairs. J Vasc Surg 20:255–262, 1994.
49. Svensson LG, Hess KR, D'Agostino RS, et al: Reduction of neurologic injury after high-risk thoracoabdominal aortic operation. Ann Thorac Surg 66:132–138, 1998.
50. Svensson LG, Khitin L, Nadolny EM, Kimmel WA: Influence of systemic temperature on paralysis after complete thoracoabdominal and descending aortic operation. Arch Surg 138:175–179; discussion 180, 2003.
51. Svensson LG, Patel V, Coselli JS, Crawford ES: Preliminary report of localization of spinal cord blood supply by hydrogen during aortic operations. Ann Thorac Surg 49:528–535, 1990.
52. Svensson LG, Patel V, Robinson MF, et al: Influence of preservation or perfusion of intraoperatively identified spinal cord blood supply on spinal motor evoked potentials and paraplegia after aortic surgery. J Vasc Surg 13:355–365, 1991.
53. Svensson LG, Rickards E, Coull A, et al: Relationship of spinal cord blood flow to vascular anatomy during thoracic aortic crossclamping and shunting. J Thorac Cardiovasc Surg 91:71–78, 1986.
54. Svensson LG, Shahian DM, Davis FG, et al: Replacement of entire aorta from aortic valve to bifurcation during one operation. Ann Thorac Surg 58:1164–1166, 1994.
55. Svensson LG, Stewart RW, Cosgrove DM, et al: Intrathecal papaverine for the prevention of paraplegia after operation on the thoracic or thoracoabdominal aorta. J Thorac Cardiovasc Surg 96:823–829, 1988.
56. Svensson LG, Von Ritter CM, Groenveld HT, et al: Cross clamping of the thoracic aorta: influence of aortic shunts, laminectomy, papaverine, calcium channel blockers, allopurinol, and superoxide dismutase on spinal cord blood flow and paraplegia in baboons. Ann Surg 204:38–47, 1986.
57. van Dongen EP, Schepens MA, Morshuis WJ, et al: Thoracic and thoracoabdominal aortic aneurysm repair: use of evoked potential monitoring in 118 patients. J Vasc Surg 34:1035–1040, 2001.
58. Von Oppell DO, Dunne TT, DeGroot MK, Zilla P: Traumatic aortic rupture: twenty-year metaanalysis of mortality and risk of paraplegia. Ann Thorac Surg 58:585–593, 1994.
59. Williams GM, Perler BA, Burdick JF, et al: Angiographic localization of spinal cord blood supply and its relationship to postoperative paraplegia. J Vasc Surg 13:23–33, 1991.

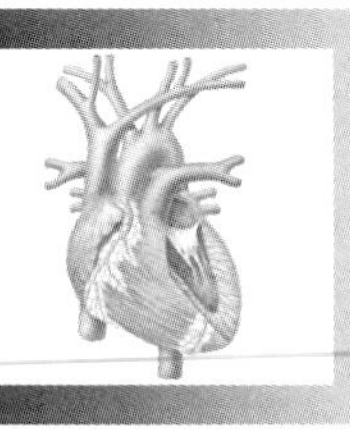

CHAPTER 69C

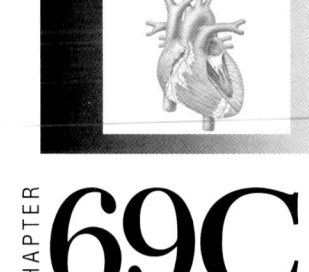

Surgery of the Aortic Arch, Descending Thoracic and Thoracoabdominal Surgery, and Aortic Dissection

Type A Aortic Dissection

Philippe Demers and D. Craig Miller

INTRODUCTION

Acute aortic dissection is one of the most common catastrophes involving the aorta. Dissection of the aorta is characterized by the separation of the aortic media from the adventitia by pulsatile blood, with variable extents of proximal and distal extension along the aorta and its branches. The process of dissection creates a *false lumen* (FL) in the aortic wall that parallels the aortic *true lumen* (TL). In the majority of cases, a *primary intimal tear* (PIT) initiates the dissection and allows communication between the true and false lumina, which are separated by a dissection *flap* or *septum*. Because this acute event is rarely associated with the presence of an aneurysm and the aortic intima (true lumen) is actually smaller than normal, the older term "dissecting aneurysm" is misleading and inappropriate. A thorough understanding of the pathophysiology of aortic dissection is critical for prompt diagnosis and effective management in the acute setting. On the other hand, aortic dissection in its chronic phase is responsible for a substantial proportion of thoracic aortic pathology and rupture due to false aneurysmal degeneration and enlargement of the false lumen. Numerous advances in diagnostic modalities, medical and surgical treatment, and long-term management have dramatically changed the prognosis for patients with this lethal condition. This chapter summarizes our current knowledge about the diagnosis and treatment of aortic dissection.

Historical Note

The observations by Morgagni in 1761 were followed by multiple early anatomical and postmortem reports describing aortic dissection, including the famous autopsy report on King George II of England in 1776.[104] In 1802, Maunoir describing this disease used the term "dissection."[111] Almost 20 years later, Rene Laennec coined the term "*Aneurysme Dissequant*," or dissecting aneurysm, believing that this entity represented the early stage of a saccular aneurysm.[99] Later, in 1863, Peacock published a comprehensive review of 80 cases of aortic dissection.[142] Until the last half of the twentieth century, the diagnosis of aortic dissection was almost exclusively an autopsy finding. Antemortem diagnosis was made in only 6 of the 300 cases reviewed by Shennan in 1934.[162] The use of contrast angiography for the diagnosis of aortic dissection was reported by Paullin and James.[141] The first attempt to treat this condition was described in 1935 by Gurin et al who used iliac artery fenestration to relieve lower extremity ischemia.[72] Although quickly abandoned, cellophane wrapping of the dissected aorta was also attempted to prevent rupture.[3] In 1955, DeBakey and associates launched the modern era of surgical management with graft replacement of the dissected aorta.[39] Subsequently, the same group introduced the use of cardiopulmonary bypass during clamping of the descending thoracic aorta.[60] The first large clinical series of aortic dissection was published in 1958 by Hirst et al; analysis of the findings in 505 cases allowed these authors to emphasize the high mortality rate and the infrequency of antemortem diagnosis at that time.[78] The modern medical approach to aortic dissection using pharmacological agents to diminish aortic *dP/dt* ("antiimpulse therapy") was introduced by Wheat and Palmer and associates in 1965.[188] The venerable DeBakey classification of aortic dissection was described the same year, while the simplified Stanford classification system (type A or type B) based on pathophysiological characteristics and treatment factors was proposed in 1970 by Daily, Shumway, and colleagues.[33,40] These developments were followed by other important advances such as less invasive and more accurate diagnostic modalities, improved anesthetic methods, safer extracorporeal perfusion techniques, the advent of profound hypothermic circulatory arrest for thoracic aortic arch surgery by Griepp et al from Stanford in 1975,[70] improved and safer prosthetic vascular grafts, and refinement of cardiovascular surgical techniques.

CLASSIFICATION

It is important to understand and apply accurately the classification of aortic dissection in order to treat patients most appropriately and to assess the results of various medical and surgical therapeutic interventions reported from different institutions. Considerable confusion has arisen in the past in classifying aortic dissections. Numerous systems have been proposed, beginning in 1955 with the nine categories initially suggested by DeBakey and associates.[39] The more widely used DeBakey type I, II, and III classification scheme was introduced in 1965[40] and modified in 1982[41] to comply with the Stanford A/B functional criteria. Despite the fact that different labels are used, a consensus has emerged concerning the essential elements of a common functional classification system of aortic dissection. The central element of all classification systems used today is the presence or absence of involvement of the ascending aorta, regardless of the location of the primary intimal tear and irrespective of the distal extension of the dissection process.[115] The Stanford classification approach as proposed by Daily and associates in 1970[33] has gained broad acceptance over the past 30 years. If the dissection involves the ascending aorta, it is a *Stanford type A*, which corresponds to a DeBakey type I[41]; University of Alabama "ascending"[6]; Massachusetts General Hospital "proximal"[46]; and Najafi "anterior" dissection.[120] Both DeBakey type I and II dissections involve the ascending aorta, but type I extends beyond the innominate artery while type II is confined just to the ascending aorta. If the ascending aorta proximal to the innominate artery is *not involved* in the process, then the dissection is called *Stanford type B*, DeBakey type III, descending, distal, or posterior, respectively (Figure 69C-1). A subtype of dissections where the PIT is located in the descending aorta or even farther distal yet the dissection process propagates backward to involve the arch and ascending aorta was originally termed "DeBakey type III-D" by Reul et al in 1975,[149] but now is simply termed "retro-A." Retro-A dissections constitute about 6% of all type A dissections.[102]

This functional classification approach is consistent with the pathophysiology of aortic dissection, considering that involvement of the ascending aorta is the principal predictor of the biological behavior of the disease process, including the most common fatal complications. Moreover, it simplifies diagnosis since it is easier to identify involvement of the ascending aorta accurately than to determine the exact site of the primary intimal tear (or tears) or the total extent of propagation of the dissection process. Furthermore, the Stanford classification system facilitates the clinical decision-making process and definitive patient management. Patients presenting with acute *Stanford type A* dissections should be treated surgically in essentially all cases, and individuals with *Stanford type B* dissections can be treated medically, either with early surgical intervention, or with an endovascular stent-graft, depending on the presence or absence of major complications. More specifically, patients with type A dissections require a

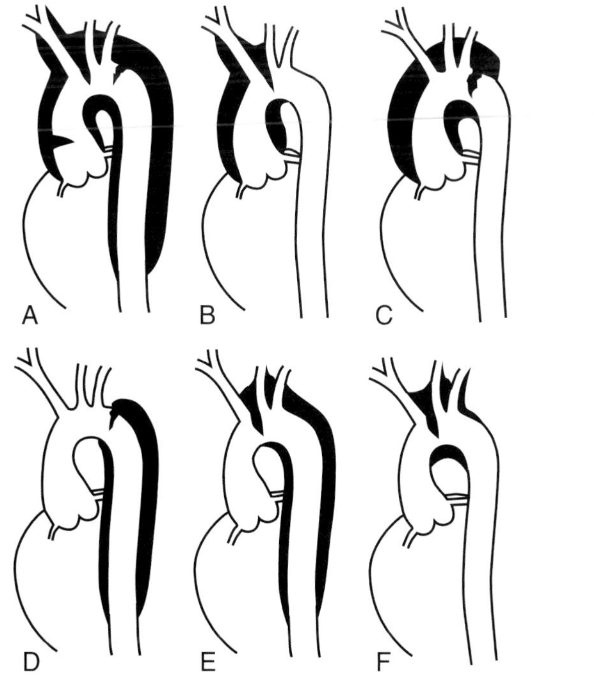

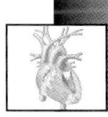

Figure 69C–1 Schematic illustration of the Stanford classification system of aortic dissections. The three examples in the top row are all type A aortic dissections because the ascending aorta is involved. The primary intimal tear can be located in the ascending aorta (**A**), in the transverse arch (**B**), or in the descending thoracic aorta (**C**). This last example is now called a "retro-A dissection" and is equivalent to what Reul et al termed a type III-D dissection. The dissections in (**D**) and (**E**) are type B dissections; whether the tear is in the descending thoracic aorta or the arch, the ascending aorta is not involved. The last example (**F**) is an isolated arch dissection without retrograde or antegrade propagation; these are rare.
(From Miller DC: Surgical management of aortic dissections: indications, perioperative management, and long-term results. In Doroghazi RM, Slater EE, editors: Aortic Dissection. New York: McGraw-Hill, 1983, p. 196; with permission.)

median sternotomy, total cardiopulmonary bypass (CPB), and profound hypothermic circulatory arrest (PHCA) to complete the repair; those with type B dissections are approached surgically using a left posterolateral thoracotomy, total CPB with PHCA, or partial CPB (or isolated left heart bypass).

Aortic dissections diagnosed within 14 days of the onset of presenting symptoms are defined as *acute*; those diagnosed more than 14 days after onset are classified as *chronic* dissections.[43,73,164] According to the *International Registry of Acute Aortic Dissection* (IRAD) investigators,[73] the cumulative mortality following acute type A and type B dissection treated medically reached a plateau after the fourteenth day following presentation, demonstrating the prognostic importance of this venerable arbitrary 14-day time distinction (Figure 69C-2). DeBakey and colleagues introduced the term "subacute" to describe dissections between 2 weeks and 2 months old, but this term is rarely used today.[41]

Over the past decade, advances in vascular imaging technology have led to increasing recognition of *intramural hematoma* (IMH) and *penetrating aortic ulcers* (PAU) as distinct pathological variants of classic aortic dissection.[151,171] Both are characterized by the absence of the classical intimal flap dividing the aorta into true and false channels. Intramural hematoma can be precipitated by an atherosclerotic ulcer penetrating into the internal elastic lamina or can occur spontaneously without any intimal disruption. Intramural hematoma can involve the ascending aorta (type A IMH) as well as the descending aorta (type B IMH). In rare cases, IMH can evolve suddenly into a classic aortic dissection with blood flow in both lumens.[136] Penetrating atherosclerotic ulcers occur most commonly in the descending thoracic aorta. Distinguishing IMH (with or without a PAU) or PAU from classic aortic dissection is critical since the pathophysiology, clinical behavior, prognosis, and management of these lesions can differ,[27,65] depending on which segment of the aorta is involved and the patient's symptoms.

EPIDEMIOLOGY

Aortic dissection is seen in all age groups, although the majority of the cases occurs between the ages of 50 and 69 years.[78] Typically, patients with type B dissection are older than those with type A dissection.[60,73] Dissection in patients younger than 40 years typically is an acute type A dissection; special importance should be given to patients who have Marfan syndrome or other associated connective tissue disorders and pregnant women during the last trimester or labor and delivery who present with sudden chest pain. In all studies, there is a clear male predominance with an estimated male-to-female ratio ranging from 2:1 to 3:1. Hirst et al found a higher incidence of aortic dissection in African-Americans,[78] which might be related to more hypertension rather than any intrinsic racial pathological weakness of the aorta increasing the probability of aortic dissection.

The exact incidence of aortic dissection has been difficult to determine since many patients die without the correct diagnosis being made antemortem. It is not widely appreciated that acute aortic dissection is the most common clinical catastrophe involving the aorta; moreover, its incidence may be increasing in the industrialized world. In a 1964 Danish study of 6480 autopsies covering 90% of a regional population, the incidence of acute aortic dissection was 5.2 per million population per year, higher than the incidence of ruptured abdominal aortic aneurysm (3.6 per million population per year), and more than four times the prevalence of ruptured thoracic aortic aneurysm (1.2 per million population per year).[170] In the seminal 1958 pathological series by Hirst and associates, acute aortic dissection was found in 1–2% of autopsies.[78] More recently, it was estimated that the incidence of acute aortic dissection in an urban population in the southeastern United States might be as high as 10–20 cases per million population per year,[139] or approximately 2000 to 4500 new cases each year.[13] Two thirds of aortic dissections involve the ascending aorta (Stanford type A). It is important to realize that these prevalence figures undoubtedly underestimate the real prevalence, since they do not consider patients who die suddenly from a complication of aortic dissection who are presumed to have succumbed to coronary disease or an arrhythmic event in the absence of a postmortem examination. Most physicians tend to think that ruptured abdominal aortic aneurysms (AAAs) are more common; this misconception comes from the fact that ruptured AAAs are diagnosed correctly more often than are acute aortic dissections.

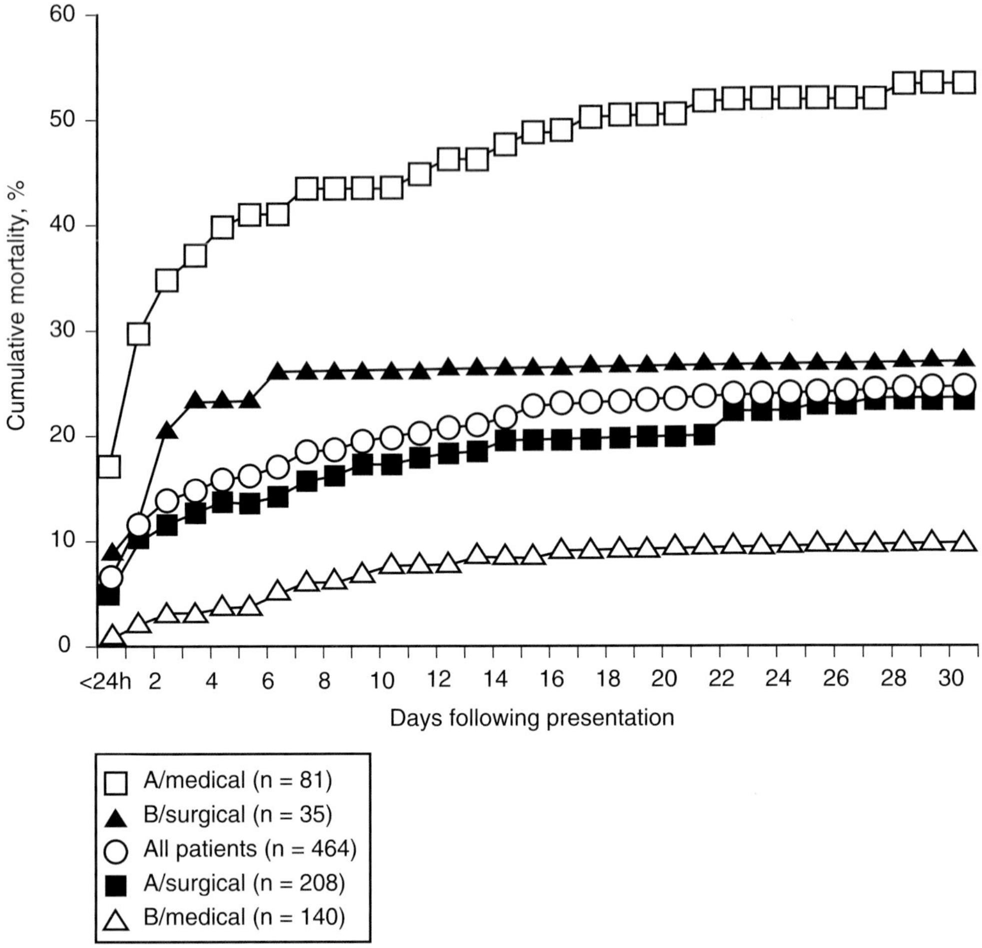

Figure 69C–2 **Thirty-day mortality according to dissection type and management in the International Registry of Acute Aortic Dissection (IRAD).** *(From Hagan PG, Nienaber CA, Isselbacher EM, et al: The international registry of acute aortic dissection [IRAD]. New insights into an old disease. JAMA 283:897–903, 2000, with permission.)*

NATURAL HISTORY

According to the historical autopsy analyses, untreated acute aortic dissection is a highly lethal event. In the study by Shennan published in 1934,[162] 40% of patients with dissection involving the ascending aorta died immediately, 70% died within the first 24 h, 94% within the first week, and 100% within 5 weeks. In 1967, Lindsay and Hurst reported that one third of patients sustaining an acute aortic dissection died within 24 h, 50% within 48 h, 80% within 7 days, and 95% within the first month.[105] In patients presenting with chronic dissection, only 15% were still alive after 5 years. In patients with dissection involving the descending thoracic aorta (Stanford type B), 75% were alive 1 month after onset. Later, Anagnostopoulos et al, in a large collected series of 963 cases of untreated aortic dissection of all types, reported a cumulative mortality of 70% at 1 week and 90% at 3 months.[4]

Most patients with untreated acute type A dissection die of intrapericardial rupture culminating in cardiac tamponade; other causes of death include acute aortic valvular regurgitation resulting in left ventricular failure, coronary compromise causing acute myocardial ischemia, occlusion of aortic branches supplying the cerebral or visceral circulation, and free rupture. Patients with untreated acute type B dissection usually die of aortic rupture or of occlusion of major aortic branches resulting in ischemic injury to vital abdominal organs (or "thoracoabdominal malperfusion").[43] In the Stanford experience, lower extremity ischemia at presentation did not significantly increase surgical mortality risk, whereas occlusion of major abdominal tributaries resulting in renal or splanchnic ischemia was associated with very high mortality rates.[76,167]

Only 10% of acute dissections are estimated to "heal," eventually becoming chronic dissections; in nearly all cases, distal reentry sites are found, allowing decompression of the false lumen.[44,59] After acute aortic dissection, the false lumen usually remains patent, but very rarely may thrombose, largely depending on the presence and site of distal reentry sites. When the false lumen remains patent, it will eventually be prone to progressive expansion over time, resulting in the formation of a false aneurysm.

PREDISPOSING FACTORS

Arterial Hypertension

In patients with aortic dissection, the prevalence of arterial hypertension varies between 45 and 80%,[43,59,60,73] being highest in patients with acute type B dissection. Untreated arterial hypertension promotes smooth muscle degeneration and other changes in the aortic wall, which may increase the susceptibility for aortic dissection.[20] Although there is no evidence to suggest that hypertension per se initiates the actual process, it is a major risk factor.

Connective Tissue Disorders

Heritable connective tissue disorders such as Marfan and Ehlers–Danlos syndromes are associated with an increased risk of aortic dissection. Marfan syndrome (MFS), described initially by Antoine-Bernard Marfan in 1896, is inherited as an autosomal dominant trait and is characterized by mutations of the *FBN1* gene, situated on the long arm of chromosome 15 and encoding for the glycoprotein *fibrillin-1*, which is a major component of elastic fibers of the cellular matrix in various organs.[147,173] In addition to cardiovascular manifestations, including mitral valve prolapse, progressive aortic dilatation, aortic valve regurgitation, and aortic dissection, these patients can have several other ocular and musculoskeletal abnormalities, tegument and pulmonary features, as well as dural ectasia. Because the genetic testing available is still unreliable and very complex (families of different "fibrillinopathies"), the diagnosis of Marfan syndrome today is made on clinical grounds according to the revised *Ghent criteria* (major and minor), which characterize the involvement of different organ systems.[42] When a patient presents with the classic MFS phenotype, the diagnosis is rarely in doubt; however, phenotypic expression of MFS can be extremely variable and many patients have only some of the characteristic features, including aortic root dilatation or *annuloaortic ectasia* with or without aortic valve regurgitation, the so-called *forme fruste* of MFS.[147] Aortic-related complications, including acute dissection and rupture, are the leading cause of death in patients with MFS.[109] If the patient with MFS has a family history of aortic dissection, the risk of dissection or rupture is considerably higher.[146,173] The prevalence of MFS in large clinical series of aortic dissection ranges between 5 and 12%.[60,73]

Patients with Ehlers–Danlos syndrome (EDS), particularly those with type IV EDS, which is transmitted in most cases as an autosomal dominant trait, have frequent arterial weakness of all large and muscular arteries; type IV EDS is characterized by a procollagen type III abnormality and an increased risk of aortic dissection or spontaneous rupture of peripheral arteries or a hollow abdominal viscus.[12] Aortic rupture has also been reported in patients with EDS type I and VI. Extremely fragile arteries are found in patients with EDS and vascular procedures, including simple arterial puncture, can be fraught with complications.[25] Familial clusters of aortic dissection linked to an autosomal dominant trait have also been reported, and could also be related to a mutation in the gene coding for type III procollagen.[93,180]

Congenital Valvular Abnormalities

Congenital heart problems such as bicuspid aortic valve (BAV), coarctation of the aorta, and Turner's syndrome are associated with an increased risk of aortic dissection compared to the general population. In an analysis of 186 autopsies of patients who died of type A aortic dissection, it was found that the prevalence of unicuspid and bicuspid aortic valves was 9%.[152] The risk of perioperative and late postoperative dissection is also increased in patients with a BAV undergoing any type of cardiac surgery, especially in patients with dilatation of the ascending aorta.[127,145] Aortic dissection predominantly involves the ascending aorta in patients with coarctation,[2] and the dissection may not propagate beyond the aortic isthmus. Simultaneous management of an acute type A aortic dissection in patients with uncorrected aortic coarctation is challenging and may require modification of the CPB arterial cannulation tactics, and occasionally the use of an extraanatomical conduit to bypass the coarctation.[28,175]

Iatrogenic Injury

Aortic dissection is a rare complication of cardiac catheterization and other percutaneous diagnostic and therapeutic interventional techniques involving manipulation of catheters inside the thoracic aorta. These are usually self-limited, localized subintimal dissections that only rarely require surgical intervention. Life-threatening iatrogenic dissections can also occur during surgical procedures; among 7000 cardiac operations, iatrogenic aortic dissection complicated 0.3% of cases.[128] These can be related to ascending aortic cannulation, retrograde dissection after femoral artery cannulation, aortic cross-clamp or partial occluding clamp injury, and intimal injury at the site of a proximal bypass graft anastomosis.[67] Surprisingly, the incidence of iatrogenic perioperative type A aortic dissection was noted to be increasing in patients undergoing off-pump coronary artery bypass, which was attributed to multiple ascending aortic manipulations for proximal anastomoses[22]; various proximal vein graft mechanical connectors have also been associated with dissection.

Pregnancy

In women under the age of 40 years, approximately 50% of dissections occur during the third trimester or during labor and delivery; only half of these patients have an identifiable heritable connective tissue disorder, such as MFS.[160] The hemodynamic and hormonal alterations of pregnancy, culminating in the third trimester, are thought to be the causes of dissection in susceptible individuals. These episodes can tragically result in the deaths of both the mother and the fetus.

Drug Related

One of the cardiovascular complications of cocaine use, particularly crack cocaine inhalation, is acute aortic dissection.[47,156] Aortic dissection in this setting occurs presumably as a consequence of abrupt, severe hypertension and catecholamine release, and this diagnosis should be considered in cocaine users presenting with chest pain.

Associations

Aortic dissections also occur more frequently in patients with Turner's syndrome, Noonan's syndrome, coarctation of the aorta, or BAV disease. Infrequent associations include giant cell aortitis, systemic lupus erythematosus, Cushing's syndrome, pheochromocytoma, polycystic kidney disease, familial hypercholesterolemia, and relapsing polychondritis.[44,59]

PATHOPHYSIOLOGY AND PATHOLOGICAL FINDINGS

Medial Degeneration

Erdheim was the first to describe, more than 70 years ago, what he called *cystic medial necrosis*, a nonspecific

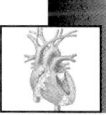

pathological process involving medial smooth muscle cell loss, elastic lamellar disruption, and acid mucopolysaccharide accumulation within the aortic media.[52] This abnormal architecture is believed to lead to changes in the distribution of both circumferential wall stress and shear stress in the aortic media, potentially leading to an intimal tear.[38] It is now known that the word *"cystic"* is a misnomer, since these medial lesions do not form true cysts (they are not lined by epithelial cells). The term "necrosis" is also misleading. In young patients (particularly those with a heritable connective tissue disorder) the elastic elements of the aortic media are disrupted and disorganized; in older individuals, it is the smooth muscular elements of the aortic media that are abnormal because of aging and hypertension[130,131] and probably represent changes associated with repeated aortic wall injury and repair. Thus, "cystic medial necrosis" should be replaced by more specific terms relating to alterations of the elastic fibers ("elastic type") and/or smooth muscle cells ("smooth muscle type") in the media. In patients with inherited connective tissue disorders, such as MFS, pathological examination of the aortic wall frequently revealed pronounced medial degeneration, with severe loss of elastic lamellae and accumulation of mucoid substance within the media. These young patients typically present with an acute type A dissection. On the other hand, in older individuals, type B dissections are more common and are associated with medial degeneration characterized by loss of smooth muscle cells.

Primary Intimal Tear

Most authors believe that the initiating event in aortic dissection is a tear or rent in the intima allowing blood to enter the aortic wall and culminating in progressive separation of the medial layers of the aorta and propagation of the dissecting hematoma. The primary intimal tear—or "PIT"—allows communication between the true aortic lumen and the false lumen. Only 2–4% of aortic dissections do not have an identifiable PIT and are usually confined to the descending thoracic aorta.[78] Rarely, an intimal disruption can be present without extensive undermining of the intima and without any false lumen,[176] or what we colloquially call "intimal stretch marks." If associated with localized hematoma within the wall, they have a "mushroom cap" appearance. Whether an intimal tear is the precipitating event in all aortic dissections is still debated.[38] IMH due to rupture of the *vasa vasorum* is another potential but infrequent initiating event leading to frank dissection. Rupture of the intima usually happens at points of maximal wall stress along the thoracic aorta. Intimal tears are usually transverse in orientation and typically involve one half to two thirds of the aortic circumference. In rare circumstances, total disruption of intimal continuity with a complete circumferential tear may lead to *intimointimal intussusception* and mechanical obstruction of blood flow[177] due to gross prolapse of the circumferential intima. In type A dissections, the majority of intimal tears (60–70%) are located in the ascending aorta, usually just distal to the sinotubular junction[54,78,114] (Figure 69C-3). The second most common site is the proximal third of the descending aorta, near the aortic isthmus, while in 10–20% the intimal tear is located is the aortic arch, usually on the lesser curvature.[31,193] In less than 5% of cases, the intimal tear can be located in the abdominal aorta and the dissection either will be confined to the abdominal aorta or will propagate in a retrograde fashion to involve the thoracic aorta.[61,153]

Propagation and Reentry

Within the aortic wall, the false lumen is situated between the inner two thirds and the outer one third of the aortic media. Pathoanatomically, the aortic pathology is that of a false aneurysm because the aortic intima containing the true lumen is not dilated, and actually is smaller than normal. Once initiated, aortic dissections usually propagate antegrade or "down stream," but may also extend in the retrograde

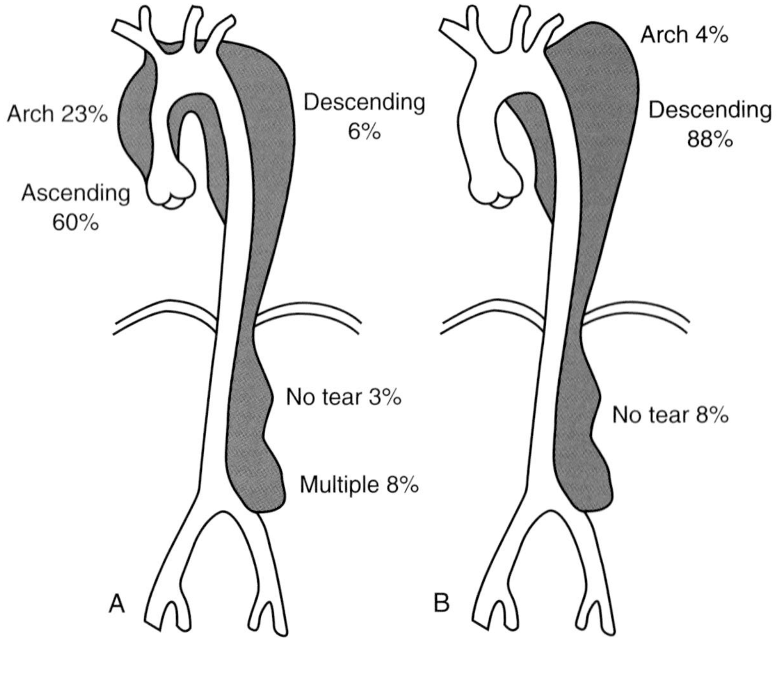

Figure 69C–3 Location of the primary intimal tear in a series of 168 patients who underwent operative repair of acute type A aortic dissection (n = 169) (A) and of acute type B aortic dissection (n = 29) (B).
(From Lansman SL, McCullough JN, Nguyen KH, et al: Subtypes of acute aortic dissection. Ann Thorac Surg 67:1975–1978, 1999, with permission.)

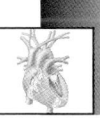

direction. The dissection often proceeds in a spiral fashion along the aorta. Propagation of the dissection depends on several factors, including rate of increase of aortic systolic pressure, or aortic *dP/dt*, magnitude of aortic diastolic elastic recoil, mean arterial pressure, and the aortic wall integrity and strength.[44,59,79,154] The mainstay of medical treatment of aortic dissection, as described by Wheat and Palmer in 1965, is directed at reducing aortic *dP/dt*.[188] In the ascending aorta, the false lumen usually occupies the right anterior portion; in the arch, the false lumen usually is located along the greater curvature and may extend into the innominate, left carotid, or left subclavian arteries. In the descending and abdominal the false lumen most often runs along the anterior and lateral aortic walls, frequently including the left renal artery.[78] Distal progression of the dissection may be limited by extensive atherosclerosis or anatomical constraints such as aortic coarctation or infrarenal AAA.[2] Otherwise, in young individuals, the dissection almost always involves the entire thoracic and abdominal aorta, and extends into the iliac arteries. In patients surviving the acute episode, the false lumen will usually remain patent, but rarely may thrombose spontaneously. The presence of distal reentry sites contributes to persistent patency of the false lumen. Partial or complete thrombosis of the false lumen may allow "healing" of the aorta; conversely, if the false lumen reenters distally and stays patent, it is prone to progressive false aneurysmal enlargement. Persistent patency of the distal false lumen is observed in up to 90% of patients after surgical repair of acute type A dissections, and may be an adverse prognostic factor associated with a higher incidence of late false aneurysmal degeneration.[51,53] Reentry sites are usually multiple, and frequently occur at the ostia of sheared-off branches, such as the intercostal, visceral, renal, or iliac arteries. Reentry into the true lumen, described by Peacock in 1843 as "an imperfect natural cure of the disease,"[104] allows decompression of the false lumen and is the rationale behind surgical and percutaneous flap fenestration techniques.[49,165]

Intramural Hematoma

In 1920, Krukenberg first described aortic intramural hematoma as a "dissection without intimal tear."[96] IMH is believed to originate from rupture of *vasa vasorum* within the outer third of the media, resulting in the circumferential accumulation of blood, as illustrated in Figure 69C-4, with no apparent intimal defect visualized on imaging studies.[27] IMH may occur spontaneously in predisposed individuals (e.g., elderly and hypertensive patients) or may be a secondary phenomenon occurring after the rupture of an atheromatous plaque through the internal elastic lamina and the formation of a penetrating atherosclerotic ulcer allowing extravasation of blood in the aortic wall, as shown in Figure 69C-4.[171] The natural history of these lesions was not well characterized until recently. The evolution of IMH may either be benign, with a stable clinical course and eventual "healing," or be a progressive, often fatal disease, with extension, evolution into classic aortic dissection, aneurysmal degeneration, or aortic rupture.[27,65,136] In recent years, it was recognized that IMH involving the ascending (type A IMH) or descending aorta (type B IMH) may have a different clinical course than patients with a classic aortic dissection, especially if detected incidentally in asymptomatic patients.

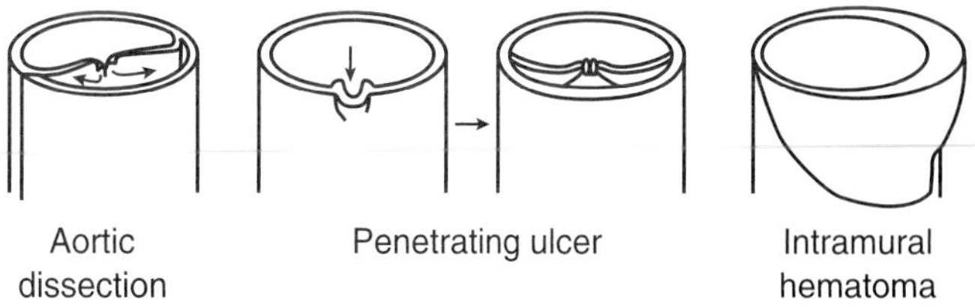

Figure 69C–4 Schematic illustration of classic aortic dissection with a distinct intimal flap separating the true and false lumina (left); penetrating atherosclerotic ulcer with a localized intimal lesion burrowing into the media and leading in some cases to localized dissection (middle); and intramural hematoma without intimal lesion (right). *(From Coady MA, Rizzo JA, Elefteriades JA: Pathologic variants of thoracic aortic dissections. Penetrating atherosclerotic ulcers and intramural hematomas. Cardiol Clin 17:637–657, 1999, with permission.)*

Conversely, those presenting with acute severe chest pain are more prone to disease progression and aortic rupture, especially in the presence of an associated deep penetrating ulcer.[65,151,179] We believe that IMH of the ascending aorta usually has a malignant prognosis comparable to that of acute type A aortic dissection, and should be treated accordingly.

Aortic Branch Compromise

Peripheral branch vessel ischemia or *malperfusion* arises when the dissection process compromises blood flow to various aortic tributaries. Acute aortic dissection may result in aortic branch compromise because of several mechanisms, including extrinsic compression of the true lumen by the pressurized false lumen (particularly a false lumen that does not reenter), an intimal flap compromising the orifice of the branch artery (Figure 69C-5), or occlusion of the tributary distally due to false lumen extrinsic compression of the true lumen. A useful pathophysiological classification of aortic branch compromise was proposed by Williams and associates: *Static obstruction* when the dissection flap extends into a branch vessel resulting in mechanical compromise of flow, and *dynamic obstruction* when the dissection flap narrows the aortic true lumen above the branch due to a large false lumen or when the flap prolapses into the vessel origin.[189] As the dissection often progresses in a spiral fashion along the aorta, some aortic branches may be spared and continue to be perfused by the true lumen, while other arteries may be perfused exclusively from the false lumen after being sheared off; in this latter scenario, the affected branch subsequently becomes permanently dependent on the false lumen for perfusion after healing of the ostial intimal flap. In some cases, compression by the false lumen may almost eliminate the entire aortic true channel ("true lumen collapse or obliteration") with resultant severe distal thoracoabdominal malperfusion.[166,189] The pattern of branch artery involvement and the degree of compromise of perfusion determine the clinical presentation, which may be enormously variable and often leads to delay before the correct diagnosis is established. In a large autopsy series, the most commonly affected aortic branches were (in descending order) the iliac arteries, followed by the innominate, left common carotid, left subclavian, coronary, renal, superior mesenteric, and the celiac axis.[78]

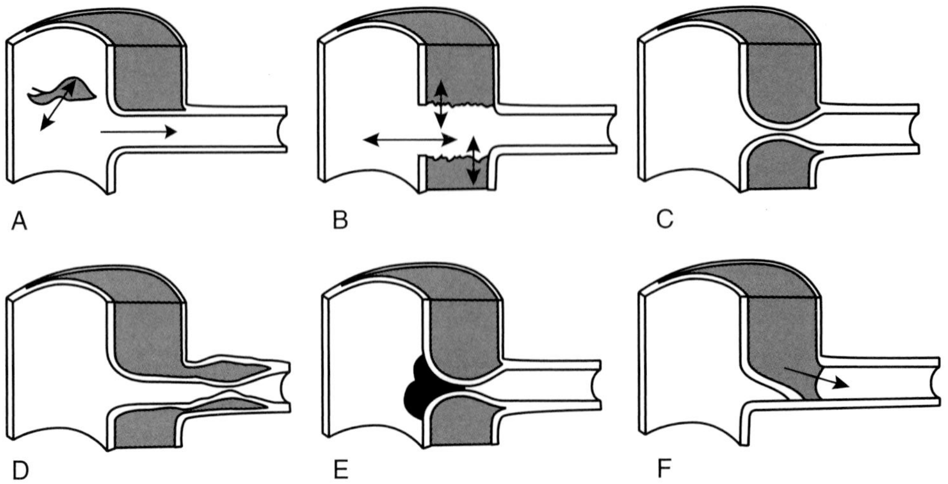

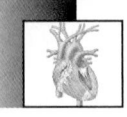

Figure 69C–5 Examples of branch artery involvement in aortic dissection. Continued adequate perfusion of an aortic tributary is illustrated in **A, B,** and **F**; however, perfusion is from the true lumen in **A** and **B** and through the false lumen in **F**. Obstruction of an aortic tributary due to extrinsic compression is shown in **C** and **D,** whereas compromise of the ostium of the true lumen with secondary thrombosis is shown in **E**. In **F,** reentry of the dissection into the branch vessel has created an intimal flap. This may become a permanent situation if the flap heals to the opposite wall of the artery in the chronic phase, thus rendering this branch solely dependent on false lumen perfusion.
(From Miller DC: Surgical management of aortic dissections: indications, perioperative management, and long-term results. In Doroghazi RA, Slater EE, editors: Aortic Dissection. New York: McGraw-Hill, 1983, with permission.)

CLINICAL MANIFESTATIONS

Patient Characteristics

Patients with type A dissections are usually younger, including those with MFS and other inherited connective tissue disorders or congenital aortic valve disease, whereas type B dissection is usually seen in middle-aged and elderly men. Either type of dissection may occur in women, particularly in young pregnant women, but is exceptionally rare in children and teenagers.[60,73] Older patients usually have coexisting conditions including hypertension and generalized arteriosclerosis, as well as associated medical comorbidities such as cerebrovascular, cardiac, pulmonary, and renal disease.

Acute Type A Dissections

Pain

The most common presenting symptom of aortic dissection is severe chest pain usually originating in the anterior chest or in the interscapular region, which correlates with the location of the dissection. The onset of pain is typically abrupt and the pain is severe at onset, described as sharp or tearing-like, and is thought to be due to stretching of the aortic adventitial nerve fibers by the dissection. Persistence or migration of the pain suggests continuing expansion within the chest or extension more distally. Differentiation of the chest pain associated with acute aortic dissection from other causes such as acute myocardial ischemia, pulmonary embolism, or pericarditis is critical in the initial evaluation of these patients to allow prompt management. In some patients, the initial pain will disappear either spontaneously or with institution of medical treatment; recurrence of pain thereafter is an ominous sign suggesting impending aortic rupture or continuing downstream extension of the dissection.[113] Occasionally, acute dissection can be painless. A high clinical index of suspicion is required to suspect aortic dissection as its manifestations can mimic any other acute medical or surgical illness. In a report from IRAD, pain of abrupt onset was the presenting symptom in 85% of patients, and the most common site was the chest. It was located anteriorly in 71% of patients with type A dissection, but 47% and 22%, respectively, of these patients reported back pain and abdominal pain.[73]

Systemic Manifestations

One third to one half of all patients with acute aortic dissection will demonstrate signs and symptoms secondary to cardiac and other organ system involvement.[18,44,57,59,60,73] Aortic branch compromise, aortic rupture or leak, and compression of adjacent organs by an expanding false lumen are the most common mechanisms responsible for systemic complications of aortic dissection.

Cardiovascular Manifestations

Patients with acute aortic dissection appear pale and poorly perfused peripherally, but generally have elevated blood pressure due to preexistent arterial hypertension, high circulating levels of catecholamines, and/or renal artery compromise by the dissection. Blood pressure should be recorded in both upper extremities, and a thorough evaluation of all peripheral pulses is essential. Hypotension in patients with acute dissection suggests cardiac tamponade[82] or impending

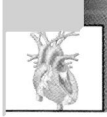

rupture; shock is usually due to intrapericardial rupture with tamponade, intrathoracic rupture, or acute left ventricular failure secondary to myocardial ischemia or acute, severe aortic valve regurgitation. Aortic rupture is the most frequent cause of death in the acute setting[78]; the most common site of rupture is near the site of the PIT.[154] Ascending aorta and arch involvement can cause rupture into the pericardial cavity or the mediastinum; however, rupture of a more distal aortic segment is also possible with exsanguination into the left pleural space or rarely the retroperitoneum. Aortic valve regurgitation is present in 20–50% of patients with acute type A dissection.[43,60,73,164] Extension of the dissection retrograde into the aortic root with shearing off of one or more aortic valve commissures causes diastolic prolapse of the leaflets. A murmur of aortic regurgitation is heard in 25–45% of patients and may be associated with an S3 gallop and pulmonary rales.[44,73] Acute, severe aortic regurgitation leading to refractory left ventricular failure is the second most common cause of death in patients with type A dissection, after aortic rupture. Less commonly, proximal extension of the dissection into the coronary artery ostia can impair coronary perfusion, and cause myocardial ischemia or infarction. In this situation, involvement of the right coronary artery (RCA) is more common than involvement of the left main coronary artery, and the ECG findings may include changes consistent with acute inferior myocardial infarction. Contained or frank aortic rupture or, more commonly, transudation of fluid through the intact false lumen into the pericardial cavity can lead to pericardial effusion and cardiac tamponade, associated with jugular venous distension, paradoxical pulse, and/or a pericardial friction rub. Cardiac tamponade is reported in 10–20% of patients with acute type A dissection, and mandates emergency surgical intervention.[82] More rarely, the expanding false lumen may compress surrounding structures, such as the pulmonary artery or the superior vena cava, or rupture into one of the cardiac chambers resulting in an aortoatrial or aortoventricular fistula.[106,107] Heart block can be seen in cases with involvement of the membranous and interatrial septum by a dissection-related hematoma.[190]

Peripheral Vascular Complications

Systemic arterial manifestations of aortic dissection are the result of the propagation of the dissection process leading to aortic branch compromise and ischemia or infarction of various end organs. Approximately 30% of patients present initially with symptoms related to acute peripheral arterial compromise or will develop such complications.[16,18,41,57,103] Clinical manifestations include stroke, paraplegia, upper or lower extremity ischemia, or anuria and/or abdominal pain due to renal or mesenteric ischemia.

In a review of the Stanford University experience with the management of aortic dissection associated with peripheral vascular complications by Fann and associates,[57] 31% (85 of 272 patients) of patients with all types of dissection had one or more peripheral arterial manifestations. One-hundred and twenty-eight had an acute type A dissection and 40 had an acute type B dissection: among these 168 patients, 4% presented with acute carotid occlusion and stroke, 5% had acute paraplegia secondary to spinal cord ischemia, 33% sustained loss of one or more peripheral pulses, 11% had impaired renal perfusion demonstrated angiographically, and 6% had compromised visceral perfusion by angiography. The prevalence of these complications according to type of dissection and the operative mortality following definitive intrathoracic surgical management are summarized in Table 69C-1. Those with advanced intraabdominal ischemia or infarction have a dismal prognosis, but simple loss of a peripheral pulse is not a portent of high postoperative mortality or morbidity.

Acute stroke or transient ischemic attack with hemiplegia is the most common neurological manifestation. This results from cerebral hypoperfusion secondary to aortic arch involvement or obstruction of the true lumen in a carotid artery. Stroke or transient ischemic attack usually occurs in patients with an acute type A dissection, and the reported incidence ranges from 3 to 7% in large series.[18,41,56,103] Besides stroke, altered cerebral perfusion may lead to altered or fluctuating mental status and syncope in upward of 12% of patients.[73] Extensive dissection can compromise perfusion of the spinal cord by shearing off critical intercostals arteries, thereby interrupting flow to the radicularis magna artery and causing paraplegia or paraparesis in 2–6% of cases.[18,41,57] Symptoms related to involvement of peripheral nerves, such as paresthesia or Horner's syndrome, are due to peripheral ischemic neuropathy or to direct compression of a nerve by the expanding false lumen. In rare circumstances, stroke, paraplegia or syncope without chest pain may be the only manifestation in cases of aortic dissection.[66]

The incidence of renal ischemia due to acute dissection varies from 5 to 25%.[18,57,59,103] This wide variability is probably related more to methods of detection (ultrasonography and angiography versus autopsy) than true population differences. Dissection resulting in renal artery compromise may be asymptomatic and remain undetected unless diagnostic

Table 69C–1

Peripheral Vascular Complications and Associated Operative Mortality Rates in a Series of 128 Patients with Acute Type A Aortic Dissection[a]

Vascular complication	*Prevalence (n)*	*Operative mortality (n)*
Stroke	6 ± 3% (7)	14 ± 14% (1)
Paraplegia	6 ± 3% (7)	43 ± 19% (3)
Pulse loss	38 ± 5% (48)	25 ± 6% (12)
Renal ischemia	12 ± 4% (15)	53 ± 13% (8)
Visceral ischemia	6 ± 3% (8)	50 ± 18% (4)

Data from Fann JI, Sarris GE, Mitchell RS, et al: Treatment of patients with aortic dissection presenting with peripheral vascular complications Ann Surg 212:705–713, 1990.

[a]Prevalence and operative mortality ±70% confidence limits; *n*, number of patients.

imaging studies are performed, but commonly is associated with oliguria or anuria and worsening renal function. Other clinical manifestations of impaired renal perfusion include refractory arterial hypertension, flank pain, and hematuria. In contrast to previous reports observing that the left renal artery is more frequently involved,[78] the right renal artery was more often compromised in our experience[57]; nonetheless, the left renal artery is more frequently fed by the aortic false lumen than the true lumen.

Aortic dissection involving the visceral arteries leads to mesenteric ischemia or infarction and is a highly lethal complication. Compromised splanchnic perfusion clinically is relatively uncommon, occurring in less than 5% of cases, although autopsy studies suggest that dissection involvement of the celiac or superior mesenteric arteries is present in more than 10% of patients.[57,78] At Stanford, the incidence of angiographically documented visceral ischemia was 6% in patients with acute type A dissection. Visceral ischemia portends a grave prognosis, with mortality rates reported as high as 88%,[18,57] but can have various clinical presentations, ranging from asymptomatic angiographic evidence of visceral hypoperfusion to frank gut infarction. Abdominal pain out of proportion to the findings on physical examination should prompt consideration of bowel ischemia.

Peripheral pulse loss occurs in 30–50% of patients with acute type A dissection and 25% of all patients irrespective of dissection type.[57] The clinical course of peripheral limb ischemia is highly variable[18]; therefore, frequent comprehensive pulse examinations are important. In the Massachusetts General Hospital experience, one third of these patients experienced either spontaneous resolution of the pulse deficit or a fluctuating clinical picture.[18] This phenomenon is thought to be related to redirection of flow into the true lumen from the false lumen through a spontaneous flap reentry site when the false lumen previously was nonreentering and occluded the true lumen. Alternatively, loss of a peripheral pulse can be asymptomatic, especially in the upper extremities. Rarely, proximal aortic occlusion, or what is termed "true lumen collapse" or dynamic "true lumen obliteration," and ischemia of the entire lower body are present.[166]

Chronic Type A Dissection

Patients surviving the initial acute phase of acute dissection, surgically treated or not, will be at risk of developing complications in the chronic phase of the disease. Most patients with chronic type A dissection are asymptomatic until they develop problems related to progressive expansion of the false lumen and aneurysmal degeneration, or development of severe aortic valve regurgitation. Up to one fourth of patients will develop an aneurysm and require operation within 10 years after an acute dissection, emphasizing the importance of comprehensive follow-up care and serial imaging studies.[41,51] Some patients who had an asymptomatic acute dissection may have a thoracic aortic aneurysm discovered incidentally on chest X-ray or a computed tomographic (CT) scan done for unrelated problems. Progressive expansion of the false lumen may eventually produce compression, obstruction, or erosion into adjacent mediastinal structures. Therefore, symptoms related to aortic aneurysmal enlargement can include chest pain, dyspnea, wheezing or stridor, hoarseness, dysphagia, superior vena cava syndrome, hemoptysis (aortobronchial fistula), and hematemesis (aortoesophageal fistula). Signs and symptoms of heart failure may result if the degree of aortic regurgitation becomes severe. Rarely, late thrombosis of the false lumen may compromise flow in a critical branch perfused solely by the false lumen, resulting in late complications such as paraplegia, lower extremity ischemia, new-onset renal failure, refractory arterial hypertension, or abdominal angina (visceral ischemia). Late aortic rupture can occur into the pericardium, bronchi, esophagus, or pleural cavity, causing tamponade in the former and exsanguination in the other cases.

DIAGNOSTIC MODALITIES

Prompt and accurate diagnosis of acute aortic dissection is crucial to determine the optimal treatment strategy for patients presenting with clinical manifestations suggesting acute dissection. The initial step in the diagnosis of aortic dissection is exercising a high degree of clinical suspicion, which is especially important considering that aortic dissection has been referred to as "the great clinical masquerader." For many years, aortography was considered the gold standard for the diagnosis of acute and chronic dissections, but developments in imaging during the past 20 years have greatly expanded the spectrum of modalities available for evaluation of thoracic aortic pathology. More specifically, CT angiographic scans, transesophageal echocardiography (or TEE), and magnetic resonance imaging (MRI) have been shown to be both more accurate and less invasive to diagnose aortic dissection. Angiography is very seldom used today, unless a catheter interventional procedure is being carried out.

In selecting which imaging study is best, the clinician should keep in mind what information is needed in patients with suspected acute aortic dissection. As a general rule, the best initial diagnostic imaging study is the one that can be performed most rapidly in any particular hospital.[24,50,181] This procedure of choice is TEE in most hospitals today, which can reliably confirm or refute the suspected diagnosis at the bedside. Then, the imaging modality should determine conclusively whether the dissection involves the ascending aorta (Stanford type A) or is restricted to the descending thoracic aorta (Stanford type B). Determination of the severity of aortic valve regurgitation and identification of a significant pericardial effusion are also important information, which reinforces the clinical utility of TEE. Lastly, localization of the PIT and determination of the extent of the dissection process as well as the presence or absence of aortic branch compromise are additional pathoanatomical features that should be identified. Interestingly, in a recent report by the IRAD investigators, two thirds of the 628 patients with acute aortic dissection enrolled in the registry required two or more imaging studies to obtain a definitive diagnosis and characterize the associated pathoanatomic features of the dissection process before commencing definitive management.[124]

Although chest radiography is neither sensitive nor specific for the diagnosis of aortic dissection, some findings may be suggestive. Widening of the mediastinal silhouette can be present in up to 50% of cases; other findings may include displacement of intimal calcification, a localized hump on the ascending aorta or arch, widening of the aortic knob, a double aortic shadow, and/or a pleural effusion.[48] Similarly,

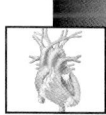

ECG findings, such as ST-segment or T-wave changes, are very nonspecific, and an abnormal ECG can be observed in up to two thirds of patients.[73]

Aortography

Historically, after the introduction of retrograde catheter aortography through the femoral artery in 1953 by Seldinger, this technique rapidly became the diagnostic method of choice for the diagnosis of acute dissection of the aorta.[161,172] Diagnosis of aortic dissection relies on the detection of direct and/or indirect angiographic signs. Direct signs include evidence of a double lumen or an intimal flap; indirect signs are suggestive of acute dissection and include compression of the true lumen by the expanding false lumen, thickening of the aortic wall, aortic regurgitation, ulcer-like projections in the aortic wall, and abnormal position of the guidewire or catheter in the aorta.[24,77] Biplane angiographic studies of the thoracic aorta are mandatory since single-plane aortography can miss the diagnosis. The reported sensitivity and specificity of aortography in the evaluation of aortic dissection range between 80 and 90% and 85 and 95%, respectively.[24,59] An aortic root injection can also detect coexistent coronary artery disease. In emergency situations, selective coronary angiography is not recommended unless the patient has undergone previous coronary bypass grafting or has a compelling clinical history suggesting severe native coronary artery disease. Aortography, however, is an invasive technique and requires the use of iodinated contrast agents, which is another reason why today catheter aortography is of historical interest only. Aortography can be time-consuming and is not an innocuous technique; moreover, concerns have been raised about the risk of iatrogenic propagation of the dissection proximally during manipulation of a guidewire or catheter within the aorta.[75]

Computed Tomography

Harris et al were the first to report on the use of CT scanning in the diagnosis of aortic dissection in 1979.[74] CT scanning is noninvasive, easy and rapid to perform, and can usually be obtained without delay in emergency situations as CT scanners are now available in most hospitals. Because of major technological advances, acquisition of a large number of thin-slice images is possible within minutes during one breath-hold using ultrafast multidetector helical CT scanners. Furthermore, computer technology now allows complex reconstruction of high-quality two-dimensional, three-dimensional, or even four-dimensional "angiographic" images (CT angiogram, or CTA). The definitive diagnosis of aortic dissection requires the identification of two distinct lumens separated by an intimal flap[24]; suggestive signs include compression of the true lumen by the false lumen, displaced intimal calcification, a thombosed false lumen or IMH, or ulcer-like projection (ULP) of contrast material within the aortic wall consistent with a penetrating aortic ulcer.[68] CT scanning is very helpful to determine accurately the transverse diameter of most aortic segments, can detect pericardial effusions, and provides information regarding extent of dissection, arch involvement, and perfusion of all major aortic branches. The new ECG-gated spiral CTA images usually visualize the proximal coronary arteries well. CT scanning can also help identify other causes of acute chest pain. In the evaluation of patients with suspected aortic dissection, contrast-enhanced CT scanning has a sensitivity of 82–100% and a specificity varying between 90 and 100%.* Disadvantages (besides the requirement for intravenous contrast material administration) of CT include the occasional inability to localize accurately the PIT, not being able to determine the severity of aortic regurgitation, and some limitations in demonstrating rapidly moving flaps in an acutely dissected aorta due to relatively slow temporal resolution.

Magnetic Resonance Imaging

The initial description of the use of MRI in the diagnosis of acute aortic dissection was made in 1983. MRI also is noninvasive and unlike aortography and CT scanning does not require the mandatory use of contrast material [newer MR angiography (MRA) techniques use intravenous administration of gadolinium]. MRI relies on the hydrogen ion concentration of blood and tissues to generate images.[181] When placed in an external magnetic field, alignment of the hydrogen atoms with the external field happens first; then this is followed by relaxation of the hydrogen ions such that the signal emitted during the relaxation phase is used to generate images. MRI can produce high-quality images of the aorta in the transverse, coronal, sagittal, and oblique planes allowing excellent delineation of the entire aorta, accurate diameter measurement, and excellent assessment of associated pathoanatomical features such as extent, localization of the PIT, branch artery involvement, and presence of a pericardial effusion. Dynamic imaging using ECG-gated sequences and cine-MRI modes can provide information regarding severity of aortic valve regurgitation and flow patterns within the aortic false and true lumens.[24,181] As with CT scanning, the criteria used for the diagnosis of acute aortic dissection with MRI is the identification of two lumens separated by an intimal flap. Similarly, identification of indirect signs, as described above for CT imaging, is suggestive but not diagnostic of dissection.[24] Several studies have shown that MRI is associated with sensitivity and specificity rates in the range of 95–100%.† Immediate availability of MRI in urgent circumstances is not always present; another shortcoming of MRI is that it cannot be performed safely in patients with pacemakers, defibrillators, or other ferrous metallic implants.[23] In the context of acute aortic dissection, MRI has many other limitations due to the relatively long time necessary for image acquisition and the inability to monitor and treat severely ill, hemodynamically unstable patients while in the magnet; these factor make MRI not the first choice in patients with acute type A aortic dissection.

Echocardiography

Echocardiography is an attractive technique for the evaluation of suspected aortic dissection because it is widely available, noninvasive, easily performed at the bedside, and does not necessitate the use of contrast material.[24,181] Initially, only M-mode TTE was available, but the introduction of two-dimensional echocardiography and color-flow Doppler studies

*References 24, 50, 59, 68, 124, 135, 168, 181.

†References 24, 59, 124, 135, 168, 181.

greatly improved visualization of the heart and the ascending aorta and permitted accurate assessment of valvular abnormalities and aortic flow patterns.[24,44,80,183] TTE has a very limited role because of suboptimal accuracy compared to other modern imaging modalities.[135,140,181] Development of transesophageal echocardiography (TEE), however, overcame the technical limitations of TTE in the evaluation of aortic dissection. High-resolution imaging of the heart and the thoracic aorta is possible with TEE because of the close proximity of the esophagus to the aorta. In addition, TEE provides information regarding aortic valve function, flow characteristics within the true and false lumens, and left ventricular size and systolic function; furthermore, TEE can also frequently image the ostia of the main coronary arteries to rule out proximal coronary disease or involvement by the dissection. A limitation of TEE using first-generation monoplane probes was limited visualization of the distal portion of the ascending aorta and the proximal arch because of the interposition of the trachea and left bronchus[50]; this limitation no longer exists using biplane and multiplane TEE probes. TEE can be performed in the emergency room, intensive care unit, or operating room under light sedation and topical anesthesia. Ideally, TEE should be performed after a fasting period of 1 h or more to minimize the risk of aspiration, but in emergency situations this risk is accepted. Close monitoring of vital signs is important during TEE. Contraindications to TEE include esophageal stricture or severe coagulopathy.[181] In the evaluation of suspected aortic dissection the most important diagnostic finding is the identification and locations of an intimal flap, ideally seen in more than one view, undulating independently from the motion of the aortic wall or other cardiac structures.[24,50,55,135,183] Visualization of different flow patterns in the true and false lumina and central displacement of intimal calcifications in case of thrombosis of the false lumen are other findings that suggest dissection or one of its variants, such as IMH or penetrating atherosclerotic ulcer with or without IMH.[121,126] TEE for assessment of suspected aortic dissection has a sensitivity rate between 97 and 100% and a specificity rate between 68 and 98%.* False-positive tests, accounting for the relatively low specificity, were usually the result of reverberations from surrounding cardiac structures or the aortic wall itself, producing echo images that were misinterpreted as an intimal flap in the ascending aorta.[24,135] M-mode echocardiography can distinguish between a genuine intimal flap in the ascending aorta and reverberation artifact.[55] The main limitations of TEE in the evaluation of suspected aortic dissection pivot on operator experience to interpret the findings accurately and the inability to assess branch vessel involvement (other than the coronary arteries) and extent of the dissection below the celiac axis level.

▶ DIAGNOSTIC STRATEGY AT STANFORD UNIVERSITY AND SPECIAL DIAGNOSTIC CONSIDERATIONS

Stanford Diagnostic Strategy

TEE is currently the initial diagnostic procedure of choice for patients with suspected acute type A dissection because of its accuracy, safety, and convenience. Patients with clear-cut TEE diagnostic findings are taken directly to the operating room for repair, while patients with inconclusive TEE findings require additional diagnostic studies (CTA scan or MRI). Patients transferred from outlying hospitals with suspected dissection have usually already undergone a contrast-enhanced CT scan, and are taken directly to the operating room where the diagnosis is confirmed using TEE. In patients presenting with symptoms of branch artery compromise, a thin-slice CT angiogram is the preferred diagnostic modality to evaluate both ascending aortic involvement and perfusion of major aortic branches in the chest and the abdomen. If malperfusion persists despite proximal aortic repair, another emergency CTA is performed immediately to delineate the mechanism of persistent branch vessel compromise before appropriate endovascular interventions are attempted to restore distal perfusion.[103,165,167] On the other hand, CT or MRI is the best modality today to plan surgical intervention in patients with chronic type A dissection, as well as to follow patients postoperatively.

Intramural Hematoma

Criteria for the diagnosis of IMH involving the ascending aorta are displaced intimal calcification, a crescent nonopacified area along the aortic wall of more than 5 mm thickness, increased aortic wall diameter, and no evidence of aortic intimal disruption or flap.[121,192] TEE, CT, and MRI can all detect IMH accurately and are capable of assessing progression or regression of the process during follow-up.[137] In this setting, MRI can help estimate the age of the hematoma based on the degradation of hemoglobin into methemoglobin after the acute event, resulting in high-intensity signals within the aortic wall on both T1- and T2-weighted images.[136]

Coronary Angiogram

The need for a selective coronary angiogram before surgical repair of acute aortic dissection is very rare today and confined solely to special circumstances. The incidence of significant coronary artery disease (at least one stenosis ≥50%) in patients with acute type A dissection is between 10 and 35%.[32,118] Ideally, stable patients with an acute type A aortic dissection presenting with a history of chronic angina or prior myocardial infarction, or a known history of coronary artery disease (CAD) or previous coronary artery bypass grafting should undergo coronary angiography preoperatively.[67,118,143] On the other hand, coronary angiography should not be performed in patients who are unstable, which is most often the case. The drawbacks of coronary angiography include the obligate delay, technical difficulties, risk, and potential for false positive findings. The Cleveland Clinic group recently reported that preoperative coronary angiogram before emergency aortic surgery did not reduce perioperative mortality and did not affect the proportion of patients requiring coronary artery bypass grafting at the time of ascending aortic repair, since 74% of coronary bypass grafts were performed due to coronary dissection and not intrinsic coronary artery disease.[143] An earlier study from the Brigham and Women's Hospital indicated that coronary angiography was a surrogate for preoperative delay, which actually increased risk.[150]

*References 24, 50, 55, 124, 133, 135, 163, 168, 181.

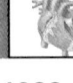

MANAGEMENT

Acute Type A Dissection

The aim of therapy in patients with acute aortic dissection is to prevent death and irreversible end-organ damage. A high clinical index of suspicion is mandatory in patients presenting with suggestive signs and symptoms, followed by prompt confirmation of the diagnosis to determine the definitive management strategy. All patients with acute type A aortic dissections should be considered for emergency surgical repair of the ascending aorta to prevent life-threatening complications such as aortic rupture or tamponade.* Operation on the ascending aorta should precede percutaneous or vascular surgical interventions addressing peripheral vascular complications of the dissection, since "proximal" or "central" repair will generally obviate the need for such revascularization procedures. Exceptions to early operative intervention in patients with acute type A dissection are few, including those with an irreversible stroke,[56,60,115] those with advanced, debilitating systemic diseases that limit life expectancy or preclude meaningful rehabilitation, and perhaps those over 80 years of age who present with multiple major complications. The presence of new-onset hemiplegia should not be considered an absolute contraindication to early surgical intervention,[56] since a majority of patients presenting with a stroke may experience partial or complete neurological recovery after graft replacement of the ascending aorta. Individuals presenting with paraplegia should also not be denied emergency operation, but the chances of the spinal cord deficit improving is low. In most centers, including Stanford, patients presenting with acute type A IMH are managed identically to those with an acute type A aortic dissection because of the high mortality risk unoperated patients with acute type A IMH face.[136,151] The rationale is to prevent aortic rupture and cardiac tamponade as well as to avoid the rapid evolution of IMH into a classic dissection.[65,121,136,137,151] This approach has been challenged by some, who propose intensive medical therapy for selected patients with uncomplicated acute type A IMH where the ascending aorta is not excessively large.[84,122,169] If a patient with acute type A IMH is treated medically, frequent serial imaging studies are mandatory since these patients can progress to overt dissection or aortic rupture within a short period of time.

As soon as the diagnosis of acute type A aortic dissection is suspected, comprehensive monitoring of the neurological status, arterial blood pressure, electrocardiogram, urine output, and peripheral pulses is initiated. An arterial line, central venous catheter, and a urinary catheter should be inserted. Intensive "antiimpulse" treatment (lowering mean arterial pressure and aortic dP/dt) is an integral part of the surgical management of patients with acute type A dissection before and after surgical repair to minimize propagation of the dissection, decrease the risk of aortic rupture, and control pain.[188] Intravenous antihypertensive and negative inotropic therapy should be started emergently as soon as acute aortic dissection is suspected using a β-blocker or calcium antagonist initially; if necessary, a short-acting arterial vasodilator, such as sodium nitroprusside, can then be added.[91,115] Hemodynamic instability suggests free aortic rupture, intrapericardial rupture with tamponade, or acute left ventricular failure secondary to severe aortic valve regurgitation or coronary artery compromise. In patients with severe hypotension and evidence of tamponade, pericardiocentesis should be attempted to resuscitate the patient only if immediate surgical intervention is not possible, with the goal of aspirating only enough fluid to allow the patient's blood pressure to rise to the lowest acceptable level, so as to minimize the risk of frank aortic rupture.[82]

*References 40, 41, 43, 44, 59, 73, 76, 105, 114–116, 120, 139.

Surgical Principles

The primary goal of surgical treatment for patients with acute type A dissection is to replace the ascending aorta to prevent aortic rupture or proximal extension of the process with resultant tamponade. The PIT if located in the ascending aorta or the arch should ideally be completely resected, and the dissected aortic layers reconstituted proximally and distally using fine continuous sutures with or without reinforcement to obliterate the false lumen. Aortic blood flow is redirected into the true aortic lumen distally, increasing the likelihood of reperfusion of aortic branches previously compromised by static or dynamic obstruction. When aortic valve regurgitation is present, aortic valve competence is achieved by reconstructing the sinuses of Valsalva and aortic root and with resuspension of the valve commissures, which is possible in the majority of cases.[58] If the aortic root is severely damaged by the dissection process, the patient has MFS or other connective tissue disorder, severe annuloaortic ectasia is present, or the valve needs to be replaced for other reasons (such as severe aortic stenosis), then complete aortic root replacement with reimplantation of the coronary ostia is indicated using either a composite valve-graft or a valve-sparing technique, as advocated by Yacoub and David.[36,69,191] The older technique of separate aortic valve replacement and supracoronary aortic graft (SVG) replacement has been abandoned for the most part for patients with acute type A aortic dissections.

Technical Considerations

Satisfactory hemostasis remains one of the technical challenges in surgery for acute type A aortic dissection because of the friable dissected aortic tissue and the coagulopathy that may be present preoperatively. In the past, inclusion-wrap repair and ringed intraluminal grafts were used in an attempt to minimize bleeding; however, these techniques were associated with high failure rates and late problems including perigraft leakage and false aneurysm formation with the former technique, and migration, erosion, and stenosis with the latter.[1,64,94] Most surgical authorities believe today that replacement of the dissected aorta includes complete transection of the aorta both proximally and distally and use of full-thickness aorta-to-graft anastomoses to minimize the risks of late complications.[19,94,117] A precise anastomotic technique is critical; deep but very closely spaced (1–2 mm) suture bites should be used, using a continuous 4-0 polypropylene suture with a fine (SH-1 or RB-1) needle. The needle must be advanced very carefully on its full curve through the aortic tissue so that needle hole tears are avoided, which can cause troublesome bleeding or even anastomotic disruption. When necessary, reinforcement of the dissected aortic layers is facilitated by reapproximation of the dissection flap to the aortic wall using strips of Teflon felt or bovine pericardium. European surgeons in the 1980s pioneered the use of gelatin-resorcin-formalin (GRF) biological glue to reapproximate the dissected aortic layers and strengthen the aortic tissue to facilitate anastomosis.[71] Despite wide use and good early results in many centers around the world,[8] concerns have been raised about the potential toxicity of the formalin component of GRF glue and the risk of late aortic wall necrosis leading to false aneurysm formation, anastomotic dehiscence, or redissection, especially in the aortic root.[89,97] As an alternative to GRF glue, a new biological glue composed of purified bovine serum albumin and 10% glutaraldehyde was recently approved in the United States (BioGlue, CryoLife Inc, Kennesaw, GA). This surgical adhesive is easy to use, facilitates the aortic repair, and decreases blood loss,[148] but it is necessary to be cautious. Do not use excessive amounts of Bioglue (just a 2-mm-thick layer extending only 2 cm into the false lumen is recommended), to avoid the coronary ostia, and do not apply the glue far downstream where is may inadvertently enter the true lumen through a flap fenestration. Long-term results after the use of BioGlue are not yet available, but we already have seen cases where use of a large amount of glue has resulted in false aneurysms, graft dehiscence, and full-thickness aortic necrosis 6–12 months later. Technical problems seen in earlier years with very stiff woven vascular grafts have been eliminated because of the advent of soft woven, double velour Dacron grafts that are presealed with collagen impregnation (Hemashield, Boston Scientific Corp., Natick, MA), which are now routinely used for thoracic aortic surgery.[186] Satisfactory woven vascular grafts presealed with other types of biological sealants also exist now.

In the past decade, PHCA allowing careful inspection of the aortic arch and performance of an "open" distal aortic anastomosis has been used increasingly in patients with acute type A dissection.[37,108,193] Careful inspection of the arch during PHCA minimizes the possibility of leaving unrecognized intimal tears in the arch, which are present in up to 20–30% of patients[102,182] and may increase the risk of late distal aortic reoperation. A "hemiarch" replacement is usually done sewing obliquely from the ligamentum arteriosus on the lesser curve of the arch to the innominate artery on the greater curve of the arch, which eliminates more dissected aorta. Moreover, careful construction of a sound, completely hemostatic distal anastomosis is technically easier in the absence of an aortic cross-clamp, which itself can also traumatize the fragile dissected aortic tissue and tear the intima. A recent analysis of all acute type A dissection repairs performed with or without PHCA at Stanford University using propensity score analysis methodology demonstrated that aortic repair with circulatory arrest was associated with comparable early complication and survival rates. Even though the long-term survival and late distal aortic complications were not improved after the use of PHCA,[100] most surgeons at Stanford use PHCA routinely today in these patients based on the technical advantages and theoretical potential merit of PHCA and an open distal aortic anastomosis.

Operative Technique

General anesthesia is induced with intravenous midazolam, fentanyl, and pancuronium. After intubation, anesthesia is maintained with inhaled isoflurane and intravenous fentanyl or other short-acting narcotic. α-Aminocaproic acid (Amicar), an antifibrinolytic agent, is used routinely.[125] Some surgeons use aprotinin to reduce bleeding, but we try to avoid it when PHCA is employed. Electrocardiogram, pulse oximetry, radial or femoral arterial pressure, central venous pressure, as well as bladder (or nasopharyngeal) and both tympanic membrane temperatures are monitored throughout the operation. TEE is used in all patients to assess the dissected aorta, aortic valve competency, and left ventricular size and systolic function.

A midline sternotomy incision is used for repair of acute type A dissection. Simultaneous exposure of the right axillary artery is made for arterial cannulation. The axillary artery is used preferentially in acute type A dissection to provide antegrade blood flow during CPB perfusion and cooling[132,157]; this technique is safe, simple to perform, and avoids retrograde femoral arterial perfusion, which can lead to false lumen pressurization and thoracoabdominal or cerebral malperfusion as well as cerebral embolization from debris in an atherosclerotic abdominal or descending aorta. Arterial cannulation is performed using a short 6-mm Dacron graft anastomosed end to side to the right axillary artery. If the artery is dissected, cannulation of the true lumen is essential to allow safe perfusion. Two venous cannulas are inserted into the superior and inferior vena cavae. The CPB circuit used for the surgical management of acute type A aortic dissection is illustrated in Figure 69C-6. Cardiopulmonary bypass is established slowly with continuous TEE monitoring of the flow pattern within the ascending and descending aorta to detect any evidence of malperfusion, which is suspected if the true lumen becomes very small or even obliterated.[98] If this occurs, direct cannulation of the aortic true lumen in the arch either using TEE guidance[119] or passing a long arterial cannula through the left ventricular apex and across the aortic valve into the true lumen,[63,155,185] or conversion to femoral CPB cannulation is carried out immediately. If severe aortic regurgitation is present, a sump vent is inserted into the left ventricle through the right superior pulmonary vein or the ventricular apex to prevent distension. Watching both tympanic temperatures and myocardial temperature, systemic cooling is initiated, avoiding gradients of more than 10° C between the patient and the arterial perfusate temperature, and continued for at least 30 min or until a tympanic or nasopharyngeal temperature under 24° C is reached. During cooling, the aortic root and ascending aorta are carefully dissected away from the right and left atria, RVOT myocardium, pulmonary valve annulus, and main and right pulmonary arteries. The ascending aorta is not clamped during cooling except when severe aortic valve insufficiency mandates aortic clamping as low as possible on the ascending aorta to prevent left ventricular dilatation. Dexamethasone (8–12 mg) and thiopental (7–15 mg/kg) are administered during cooling to enhance cerebral and spinal cord protection. The field is flooded with CO_2 flowing at 5–10 liters/min. Mannitol (0.3–0.4 g/kg) and furosemide (40–80 mg) are given prior to circulatory arrest to preserve renal function. The head is packed in ice. After reducing CPB flow to 200–400 ml/min, intermittent retrograde cold blood cardioplegia and a Daily cooling jacket (Daily Medical Products, San Diego, CA) are used for myocardial protection. The ascending aorta is opened to locate the PIT and to evaluate the aortic valve and sinuses, and then the arch and proximal descending thoracic aorta are inspected. After confirming CPB pump flow entering the arch from the true lumen of the innominate artery, the innominate artery is clamped and CPB flow through the axillary cannula is increased to 5 ml/kg; subsequently, back bleeding down the left common carotid and left subclavian arteries is seen indicating patency of the circle of Willis. The aortic segment containing the intimal tear is resected and the aortic arch is trimmed circumferentially in an oblique fashion in preparation for hemiarch replacement. Reapproximation of the aortic layers is accomplished with the anastomotic suture line or, alternatively, using biological glue between the dissected layers. Occasionally, the older technique of suturing two strips of Teflon felt (one inside the false lumen and one externally) using a separate 4-0 polypropylene suture line to form a solid full-thickness distal aortic cuff is still used. An end-to-end aortic anastomosis is then carried out using an appropriately sized and beveled woven double velour Dacron graft and running 4-0 polypropylene suture (Figure 69C-7A). The Griepp method of rotating the beveled end of the graft 180° such that the "toe" of the graft actually apposes the greater curve of the arch near the innominate artery is used, which tightly tucks the completed graft into the natural curve of the arch and prevents excessive angulation of the graft rightward. When completing the hemiarch anastomosis, the innominate clamp is removed and the arch and great vessels are deaired. CPB flow is resumed in an antegrade fashion using the original axillary artery cannula, the graft is clamped, and flow in the descending aorta is quickly assessed using TEE. After 5 min of cold CPB reperfusion, gradual rewarming of the patient to 36° C is initiated. Then, the aortic root and valve are evaluated. If aortic root replacement is not necessary, then the ascending aorta is transected immediately above the sinotubular junction. Valvular regurgitation secondary to commissural detachment can be corrected by resuspension of the valve at the level of the sinotubular junction using a continuous 4-0 polypropylene suture (with or without glue) to approximate the dissected layers of the sinuses of Valsalva; this is possible in 70–80% of patients.[58,129] The graft is then anastomosed to the reconstructed proximal aortic cuff in an end-to-end fashion using a running 4-0 SH-1 polypropylene suture (Figure 69C-7B). A needle vent to coronary suction is inserted in the graft for deairing and the cross-clamp is released. TEE rapidly confirms if the aortic valve is competent, and the anastomoses are inspected. Cardiopulmonary bypass is discontinued, and protamine sulfate is administered after all anastomoses are judged to be technically satisfactory with minimal bleeding. Platelets, fresh frozen plasma, and cryoprecipitate are used only if diffuse hemorrhage from suture lines and raw surfaces is evident after a normal activated clotting time (ACT) is achieved.

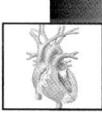

Management of the Aortic Root

Patients with dissection-related destruction of the aortic root, individuals with MFS (or other connective tissue disorder), and those with markedly dilated sinuses of Valsalva or annuloaortic ectasia should undergo composite valve graft (CVG) root replacement, or valve-sparing aortic root replacement using the David reimplantation method with complete excision of the sinuses of Valsalva (see Chapter 68), rather than resuspension of the aortic valve and preservation of the sinuses. A conservative approach limited just to the tubular part of the ascending aorta in these cases is associated with suboptimal long-term results and a high likelihood of late aortic or aortic valve problems requiring reoperation.[19,194] If the aortic valve is markedly abnormal or cannot be satisfactorily repaired, separate valve and supracoronary aortic graft (SVG) replacement is a reasonable alternative in selected, elderly patients, but this techniques is seldom used today.[194] Direct extension of the dissection into the coronary ostia is not common, but can be challenging. Usually the proximal main coronary artery can be glued together in the proximal reconstruction. Occasionally, the safest solution is root replacement with reimplantation of reconstituted coronary artery ostia as Carrel buttons into the graft, either directly or with a short interposition saphenous vein graft as introduced by Zubiate and Kay.[195] Alternative techniques include the "Cabrol-II" moustache coronary reconstruction using a small synthetic graft,[17] or in exceptional circumstances, suture ligation of the coronary ostia and bypass grafting to all coronary territories using the saphenous vein.[15]

Management of the Aortic Arch

In up to 20–30% of patients, the PIT is found in the aortic arch, which has been associated with a poorer prognosis.[31,102,182,193] Most tears are located on the lesser curve of the arch near the innominate artery, permitting complete resection of the tear using the hemiarch technique with a single suture line, as described above. In cases in which the PIT is located more distally in the arch or when arch rupture or a preexistent arch aneurysm is encountered, a more extensive resection is required, but perioperative mortality (between 21 and 55%) and morbidity are higher, especially in elderly patients.[7,31,101,193] Failure to include the arch in the repair may increase the probability of requiring subsequent "downstream" distal aortic reoperation and reduce long-term survival.[193] Improvements in surgical techniques and brain protection during PHCA using selective antegrade cerebral perfusion (SACP)[9,96] have made concomitant arch replacement a reasonable option in selected, low-risk younger patients. In these circumstances, total arch replacement is performed using the elephant trunk technique, as described originally by Borst (see Chapter 69A),[14] or a modification of this technique, using an aortic arch branched graft.[86,88] More recently, radical operations such as ascending and total arch replacement using a branched graft and hybrid procedures involving arch replacement as well as deployment of a stent-graft[81] into the descending thoracic aorta have been proposed as a primary strategy, even in the absence of arch tear, to obliterate flow in the residual distal aortic false lumen and minimize the likelihood of late distal reoperation.[5,62,81,110] Although these approaches have theoretical merit, the limited amount of evidence available today demonstrating real long-term clinical benefit of these more aggressive and radical procedures does not justify their widespread adoption at this time.

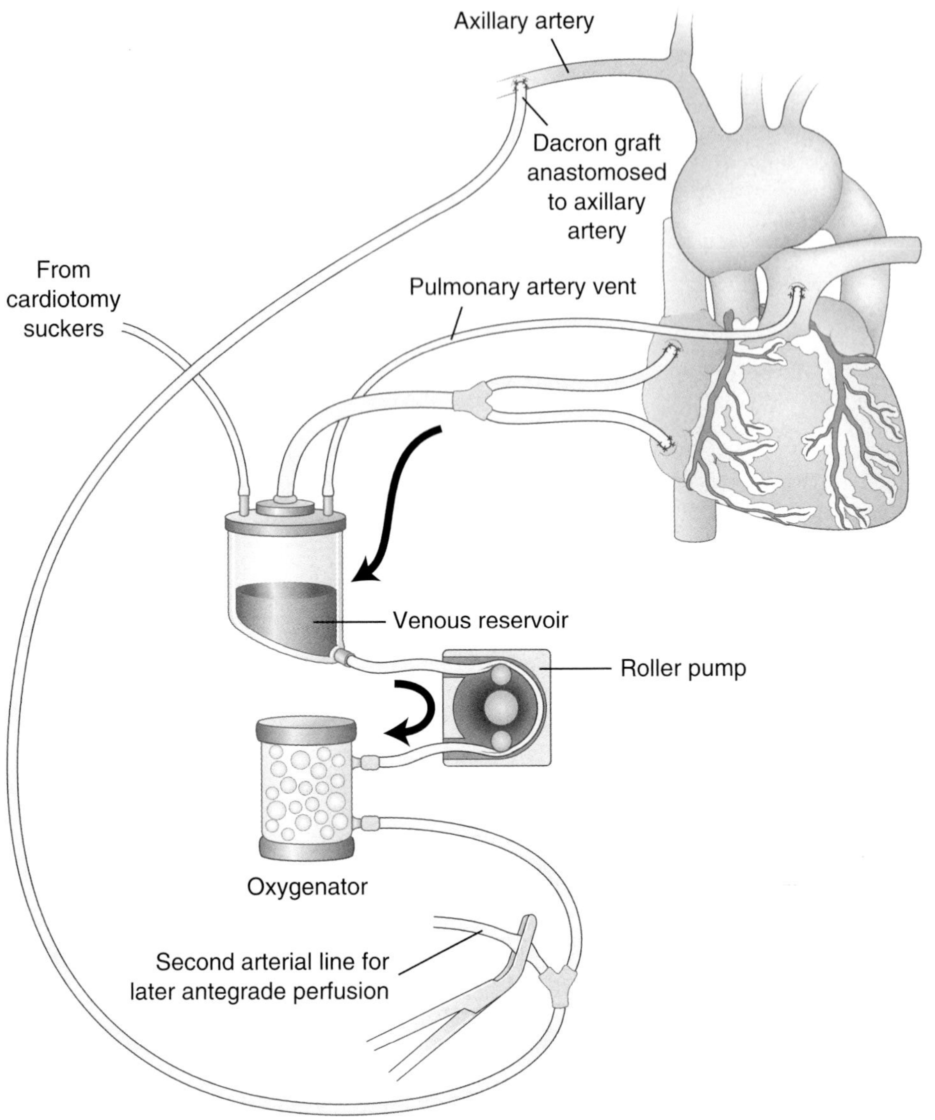

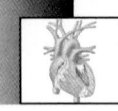

Figure 69C–6 Schematic of the CPB circuit for repair of an acute type A aortic dissection with an open distal anastomosis during a period of hypothermic circulatory arrest and selective antegrade cerebral perfusion. Arterial cannulation is performed using a short 6-mm Dacron graft anastomosed end to side to the right axillary artery.

Special Situations

Thoracoabdominal or Cerebral Malperfusion

Malperfusion can occur spontaneously or may develop during operation in up to 13% of patients, most commonly during CPB if femoral arterial CPB (retrograde) perfusion is used.[98] In addition to monitoring of arterial pressure, preferably in both arms and one leg, as well as bilateral tympanic membrane, myocardial, and bladder temperatures, TEE is used continuously to assess the size and shape of the two lumens in the thoracic aorta, and the flow pattern within the true and false lumens. Immediate detection of this potentially lethal complication while commencing CPB is crucial; CPB flow predominately in the false lumen can result in pressurization of the false lumen causing obliteration of the true lumen. If CPB malperfusion occurs, rapid action is necessary to avoid irreversible neurological or abdominal or spinal cord injury. CPB is briefly interrupted, and a separate arterial cannula is inserted into the aortic true lumen using one of the methods described above (including cannulating the ascending aorta across the aortic valve using a long cannula inserted through the left ventricular apex),[178] and CPB is resumed.

Primary Intimal Tear in the Descending Thoracic Aorta ("Retro-A Dissection")

In 5–10% of cases, acute type A aortic dissection is due to retrograde extension of the dissecting process from a PIT located in the descending thoracic aorta, a situation that Reul et al termed DeBakey type III-D dissection.[115,149] We prefer the simpler term "retro-A dissection," as introduced by the Mt. Sinai group. Patients with this subtype of acute type A dissection were thought to have a poor prognosis due to intraoperative troubles,[102,115] hemorrhage from the distal aortic anastomosis, or rupture of the descending aortic false lumen.[87,102] To prevent these complications, single-stage resection of the PIT in the descending aorta and replacement of the ascending aorta and entire arch through a

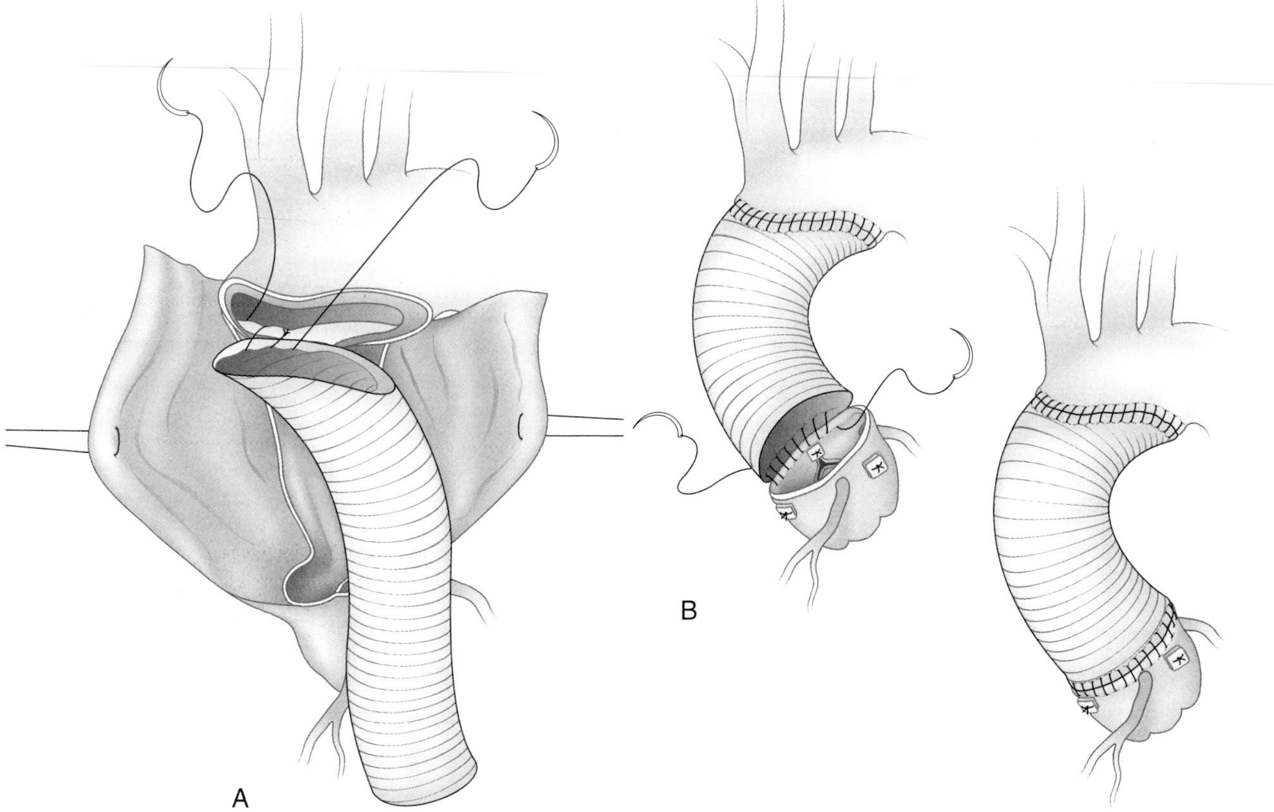

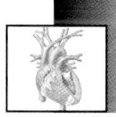

Figure 69C–7 **A,** An open distal anastomosis is always employed to avoid intimal damage with a clamp and to allow inspection of the aortic arch. The aorta is transected immediately proximal to the innominate artery and distally toward the lesser curvature to the level of the left subclavian artery. An appropriately sized graft is beveled and anastomosed using 4-0 polypropylene suture. The Griepp method of rotating the beveled end of the graft 180° such that the "toe" of the graft actually apposes the greater curve of the arch near the innominate artery is used, which tucks the completed graft into the natural curve of the arch and prevents excessive angulation of the graft. Most commonly, the false lumen is obliterated with the anastomotic suture line without reinforcing material. **B,** Following aortic root reconstruction and valve commissures resuspension, the graft is anastomosed to the reconstructed proximal aortic cuff in an end-to-end fashion using a running 4-0 SH-1 polypropylene suture.

median sternotomy or "L" thoracosternal incision has been proposed in selected patients with a patent false lumen in the ascending aorta, aortic regurgitation, cardiac tamponade, or dilatation of the ascending aorta.[87]

In patients in whom the false lumen of the ascending aorta has thrombosed and no dilatation of the ascending aorta is present, medical therapy is perhaps reasonable,[184] but our philosophy usually calls for more aggressive surgical treatment, meaning at least graft replacement of the ascending aorta and usually the arch in suitable operative candidates. Recently, endovascular stent-grafting has been applied for these challenging patients with favorable mid-term results, either as an isolated procedure designed to cover the entry site in the descending aorta[34,85] or in conjunction with extended surgical replacement of the ascending aorta and arch.[81]

Type A Dissection and Coarctation

Acute aortic dissection in the presence of an untreated aortic coarctation is a rare problem, with few reported cases in adults.[2,175] Simultaneous repair through a median sternotomy incision is advocated by most authors. Retrograde femoral arterial perfusion through the coarctation for cardiopulmonary bypass may be problematic in this situation, with resultant cerebral hypoperfusion; this potential problem is avoided with right axillary artery CPB cannulation, with or without simultaneous femoral CPB perfusion if the obstruction at the coarctation is very severe. In addition to standard ascending aortic and arch dissection repair, the coarctation is treated using a primary aortic graft or if necessary an extraanatomical bypass from the ascending aortic graft to the distal descending aorta, through the posterior pericardium.[28,175]

Postoperative Thoracoabdominal or Cerebral Malperfusion

Assiduous surveillance postoperatively is needed to detect persistent or new malperfusion before infarction of important end organs. Management of branch vessel compromise is discussed in detail in Chapters 71A and 71B.

Chronic Type A Dissections

Indications for Operative Intervention

Operation for patients with chronic type A dissection is indicated if symptoms related to the aortic false aneurysm or progressive aortic enlargement are present. Symptoms of congestive heart failure or evidence of left ventricular dysfunction or dilatation due to moderate or severe aortic valve insufficiency are also indications for operation. In asymptomatic patients, surgical intervention is generally recommended when the diameter of the ascending aorta is greater than 55 mm (50 mm in patients with MFS) or if the documented rate of expansion is greater than 5–10 mm over 1 year.[26,35] It should be remembered that thoracic aortic dissections rupture at a smaller size than do degenerative or atherosclerotic aneurysms.[83] Careful judgment is important, as the expected benefits of graft replacement of the aorta in asymptomatic patients must be weighed against the estimated operative risk, taking into account comorbidities that may increase surgical risk or otherwise limit life expectancy, which paradoxically are also the same risk factors that predispose to a higher risk of aortic rupture (e.g., MFS, other connective tissue disorders, uncontrolled hypertension, increasing age, and presence of chronic obstructive pulmonary disease).[26,35] Lastly, expansion of the size of the false lumen in the distal aorta after successful proximal aortic repair or local complications of previous operation such as sinus of Valsalva aneurysm, anastomotic false aneurysm, or worsening aortic regurgitation are other indications for operation in a patient with a chronic type A aortic dissection.

Surgical Technique

Extensive resection and complex aortic reconstruction are generally necessary in patients with chronic type A dissections. Preservation of the aortic valve and sinuses of Valsalva is seldom possible in these circumstances and may not be a durable solution; insertion of a composite valve graft is generally required. In highly selected young patients, a valve-sparing aortic root replacement may be an attractive alternative to avoid long-term anticoagulation, if feasible (see Chapter 68).[36,191] Similarly, because of frequent involvement of the aortic arch and descending thoracic aorta in the setting of chronic dissection, total arch replacement plus a distal dangling elephant trunk graft is often necessary to facilitate staged replacement of the entire thoracic aorta (see Chapter 69A).[14,30,159] Alternatively, a single-stage approach to operative repair of chronic type A dissection, using a bilateral anterior thoracotomy or clamshell incision, has been proposed by Kouchoukos et al, with reasonable early results, considering the magnitude of this operative procedure. This technique involves replacement of the transverse arch first under deep hypothermic circulatory arrest to minimize cerebral ischemic time, followed by distal and proximal aortic replacement.[95]

In contrast to patients with acute dissection, perfusion of downstream vital organs may depend solely on a patent false lumen in the chronic phase of dissection; maintenance of antegrade flow in both the true and the false lumina is important to avoid iatrogenic malperfusion following aortic repair. To achieve this goal, flap septectomy with or without distal flap fenestration is performed to allow graft flow to enter both the distal aortic true and false lumens. The distal anastomosis is sewn to the adventitial layer of the chronically dissected distal aorta.

RESULTS

Early Survival

Several reports have documented improved surgical outcome in patients with aortic dissection more recently, with perioperative mortality rates decreasing from 30–60% in the 1960s to 5–30%, in the last decade.* These lower early mortality rates were attributed to progressive advances in diagnostic modalities, improved surgical, myocardial protection, and cardiopulmonary bypass techniques, perioperative management, and increased surgical experience. Other factors, such as patient referral patterns and selection bias, must also be considered when comparing results from various eras and different institutions. Even in the current era, however, early mortality risk in surgically treated patients with acute type A dissection remains relatively high; according to the IRAD report incorporating 289 patients with acute type A dissections treated in 12 specialized referral centers in several countries between 1996 and 1999, in-hospital mortality following operative repair was 26%, as illustrated in Figure 69C-2.[73]

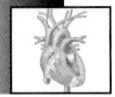

At Stanford University between 1963 and 1992, the overall operative mortality rate was 26% in 174 consecutive patients undergoing surgical repair for acute type A aortic dissection, decreasing from 38% in the 1963–1976 period, to 27% in the 1988–1992 era.[60] In this 30-year experience, the independent determinants of early mortality were earlier operative year, older age, hypertension, preoperative cardiac tamponade, and renal dysfunction. More recently, the early mortality rate decreased to 17% in a series of 151 patients presenting with an acute type A aortic dissection operated between 1993 and 1999,[100] as illustrated in Figure 69C-7. This is consonant with other large contemporary series of surgical treatment of patients with acute type A dissections.† In the entire cohort of patients from Stanford, the independent risk factors for early death were again earlier operative year, older age, preoperative tamponade, and renal dysfunction. Overall, it appears that patient-specific factors and not treatment strategies (such as the use of profound hypothermic circulatory arrest) were the main determinants of adverse outcome. Moreover, the only potentially modifiable factors were cardiac tamponade and renal dysfunction, which might theoretically be lower if the diagnosis is made earlier. Interestingly, site of intimal tear, pulmonary disease, and arterial hypertension, which were significant in earlier analyses,[116] were not risk factors for death in the later years of this 37-year series.

These observations parallel findings in other contemporary reports from centers with expertise in thoracic aortic surgery. According to analyses by Crawford and colleagues, earlier operative date, severe symptoms, presence of coro-

*References 11, 21, 31, 37, 41, 54, 59, 60, 73, 90, 94, 100, 105, 112, 114, 116, 134, 138, 158, 174.

†References 11, 21, 37, 54, 90, 138, 158.

nary artery disease, diabetes mellitus, reoperation for bleeding, postoperative stroke, and cardiac complications were independent risk factors for early death after surgical treatment of type A dissection.[31,174] In the Cleveland Clinic experience with 135 acute and 73 chronic type A dissections, independent predictors of early mortality were earlier operative year, hemodynamic instability, nonuse of PHCA, longer PHCA time, composite valve graft for aortic root replacement, and concomitant coronary artery bypass grafting.[158] Increasing age, hemodynamic compromise, and absence of hypertension were identified as risk factors for hospital death in the recent Mount Sinai Medical Center experience,[54] while renal or mesenteric ischemia and preoperative shock predicted early deaths in Kazui's experience in Japan.[90] In the subgroup of patients with acute type A dissection in the IRAD registry, predictors of early death were older age, abrupt onset of pain, hemodynamic compromise, renal failure, pulse deficit, and abnormal ECG findings,[112] again emphasizing the importance of patient-specific and dissection-related factors in terms of surgical outcome.

Early mortality risk following surgical treatment of patients with chronic type A dissection is generally lower than that for patients with acute dissections. In the 1995 summary of the Stanford 30-year experience, early mortality rate was 17% in 106 patients with chronic type A dissections, and only 6% in the subgroup of patients with MFS.[60] These early results were obtained even though concomitant aortic valve replacement was necessary in 45% of the cases, aortic root replacement with a composite valve graft in 10%, and total arch replacement in 10% of these patients. In an analysis of 690 patients with aortic dissections over a 33-year period, Crawford and colleagues observed a 30-day mortality rate of 12% in patients with chronic type A dissections operated before 1986, and only 8% in those operated after 1986.[174] Independent determinants of survival were severity of symptoms, previous aortic surgery, concomitant coronary artery disease, use of intraaortic balloon pump, cardiac complications, and postoperative stroke. Similarly, Sabik and associates reported an early mortality rate of 11% in 73 patients with chronic type A dissections treated surgically, which was not significantly lower than 16% in patients with acute A dissections.[158]

Late Survival

In DeBakey's seminal 1982 report on long-term results in 527 surgically treated patients with aortic dissection (type A or B, acute or chronic), overall survival 5, 10, and 20 years after surgery was 57, 32, and 5%, respectively.[41] In patients with type A dissections, 29% of late deaths were attributed to complications related to rupture of an aneurysm in a remote aortic location, emphasizing the long-term life-threatening nature of aortic dissection and the need for better long-term imaging surveillance and medical care.

In the 30-year Stanford experience, the overall survival rates (including hospital deaths) for patients with acute type A dissections at 1, 5, 10, and 15 years were 67, 55, 37, and 24%, respectively.[60] For patients with chronic type A dissections, their figures, respectively, were 76, 65, 45, and 27%. For patients with acute type A dissections, late survival for discharged patients was 91, 75, 51, and 32% at 1, 5, 10, and 15 years, respectively, compared to 93, 79, 54, and 33% for those with chronic type A dissections. One third of the late deaths were cardiac related, and at least 15% of deaths were due to complications related to or extension of the dissection. Multivariable analysis identified older age and previous cardiovascular operation to be significant risk factors for late death; interestingly, previous stroke, remote myocardial infarction, chronic renal dysfunction, and earlier operative date, which were independent predictors of adverse late outcome in the 1985 Stanford analysis,[76] no longer emerged as risk factors in the larger series. In the more recent report from Stanford on acute type A dissections, independent determinants of late death were increasing age, previous sternotomy, prior stroke, hypertension, liver disease, tamponade, arch involvement, and earlier year of operation; interestingly, the use of PHCA or resection of the intimal tear was not a significant predictor of late death.[100] Actuarial survival after surgical repair of acute and chronic type A aortic dissections in the patients operated at Stanford University Medical Center between 1963 and 2000 is shown in Figures 69C-8 and 69C-9.

In Crawford's 1990 report, survival at 1, 5, and 10 years in patients with proximal dissections (acute or chronic) was 78, 63, and 55%, respectively[174]; life expectancy was significantly worse in patients with acute dissections (67% for acute versus 81% for chronic at 1 year, and 51% versus 68% at 5 years). Independent predictors of late death in all patients included severity of symptoms, New York Heart Association (NYHA) functional class, distal extent of resection, unresected residual aneurysm, postoperative complications, and earlier year of operation. In his 1992 updated series focusing only on acute type A aortic dissections,[31] Crawford reported survival estimates at 5, 10, and 20 years after surgical repair of 56, 46, and 30%, respectively. Determinants of mortality in this series were earlier year of operation, inclusion of the arch in the repair, NYHA functional class, diabetes, and concomitant coronary artery by pass grafting (CABG). In the Cleveland Clinic series, long-term survival was comparable between those with acute or chronic type A dissections,[158] and older age, higher blood urea nitrogen (BUN), aortic arch replacement, and earlier date of operation were incremental risk factors for late death.

Reoperation

Despite successful intervention in the acute or chronic phase of aortic dissection, aneurysmal degeneration of the false lumen in other segments of the aorta may occur in a substantial proportion of patients, which may lead to late aortic rupture and death, or require reoperation. Late reoperation for aortic dissection is technically challenging and usually requires extensive aortic reconstruction, and reoperation in the past decades has been associated with high early mortality rates.[19,60,95] In the Stanford 30-year experience, freedom from late reoperation for patients with acute type A dissections at 1, 5, 10, and 15 years was 94, 83, 65, and 65%,respectively.[60] For chronic type A dissections, these freedom estimates were 96, 88, 65, and 52%, respectively. Younger age was the only significant, independent risk factor portending a higher likelihood of reoperation. In the more recent Stanford report focusing on acute type A dissections, male gender, MFS, coronary artery disease, peripheral pulse deficit, and arch involvement were associated with a higher likelihood of late distal aortic reoperation.[100] Freedom from proximal or

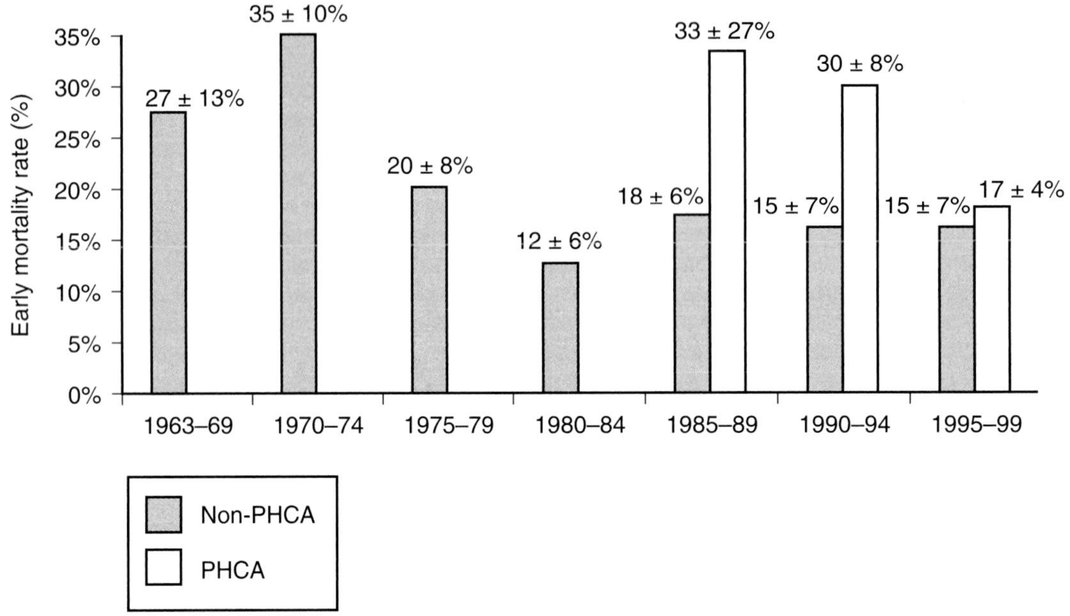

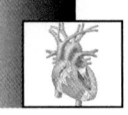

Figure 69C–8 Operative mortality rates as a function of time for patients with acute type A dissection operated between 1963 and 1999 at Stanford University and broken down according to treatment method. Non-PHCA, no circulatory arrest; PHCA, profound hypothermic circulatory arrest. *(From Lai DT, Robbins RC, Mitchell RS, et al: Does profound hypothermic circulatory arrest improve survival in patients with acute type A aortic dissection? Circulation 106:I-218–228, 2002, with permission. Copyright American Heart Association, 2002.)*

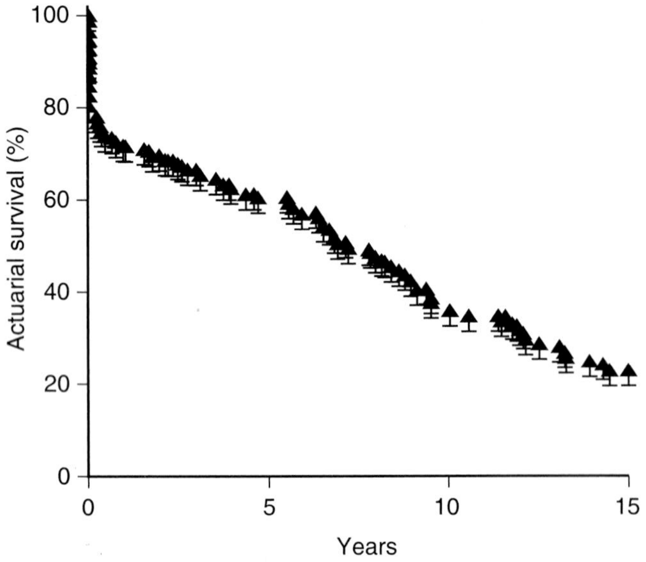

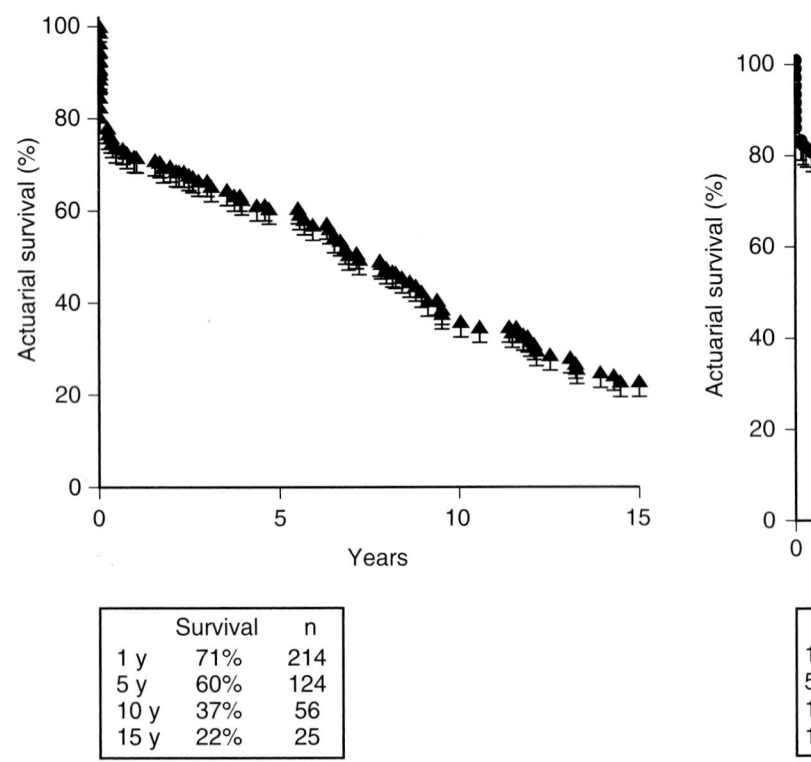

	Survival	n
1 y	71%	214
5 y	60%	124
10 y	37%	56
15 y	22%	25

Figure 69C–9 Actuarial survival after operative repair of acute type A aortic dissection in 323 consecutive patients operated between 1963 and 2000 at Stanford University Medical Center.

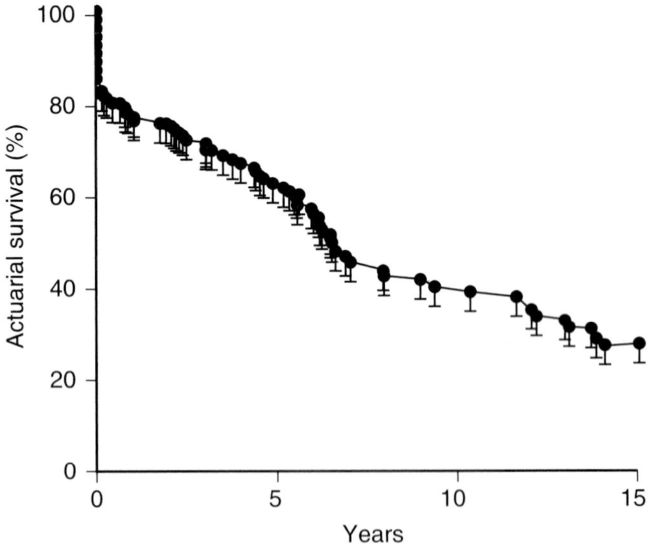

	Survival	n
1 y	77%	122
5 y	62%	71
10 y	40%	34
15 y	27%	19

Figure 69C–10 Actuarial survival after operative repair of chronic type A aortic dissection in 165 consecutive patients operated between 1964 and 2000 at Stanford University Medical Center.

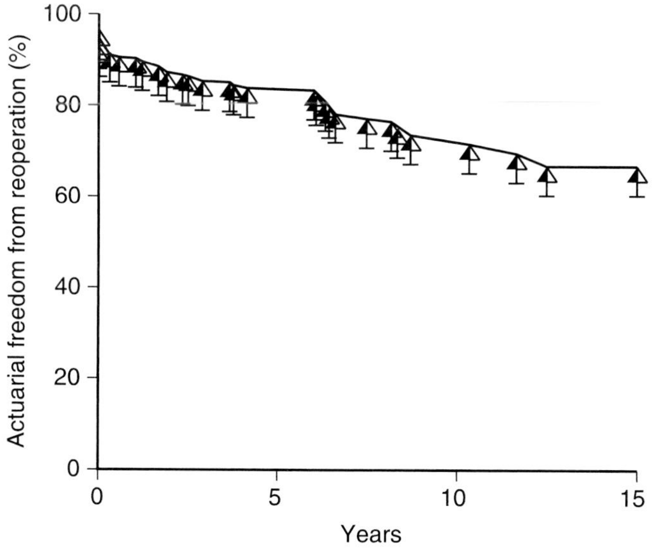

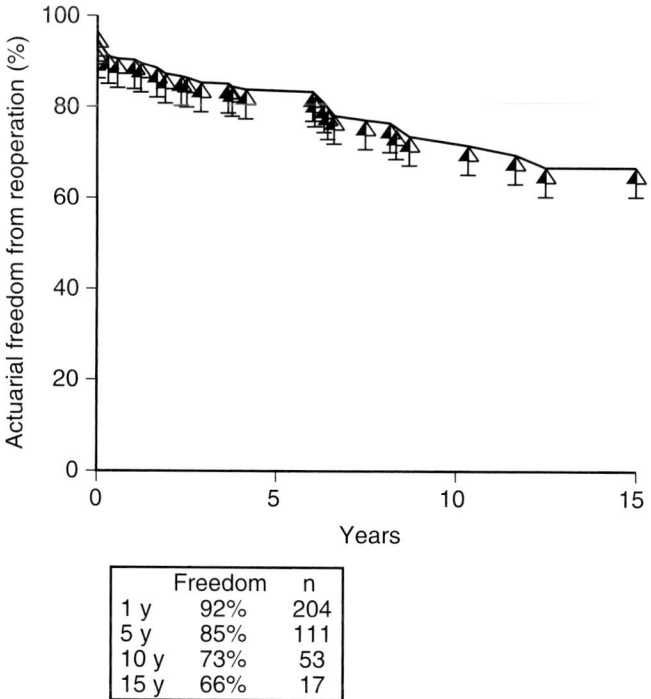

	Freedom	n
1 y	92%	204
5 y	85%	111
10 y	73%	53
15 y	66%	17

Figure 69C–11 Actuarial freedom from proximal or distal aortic reoperation after operative repair of acute type A aortic dissection in 323 patients operated between 1963 and 2000 at Stanford University Medical Center.

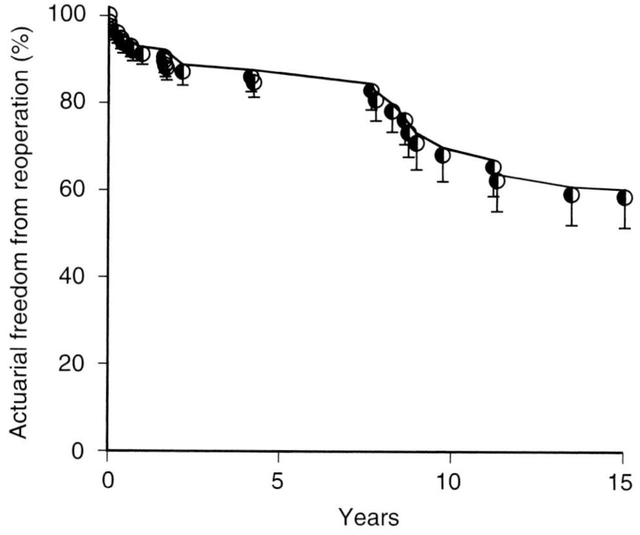

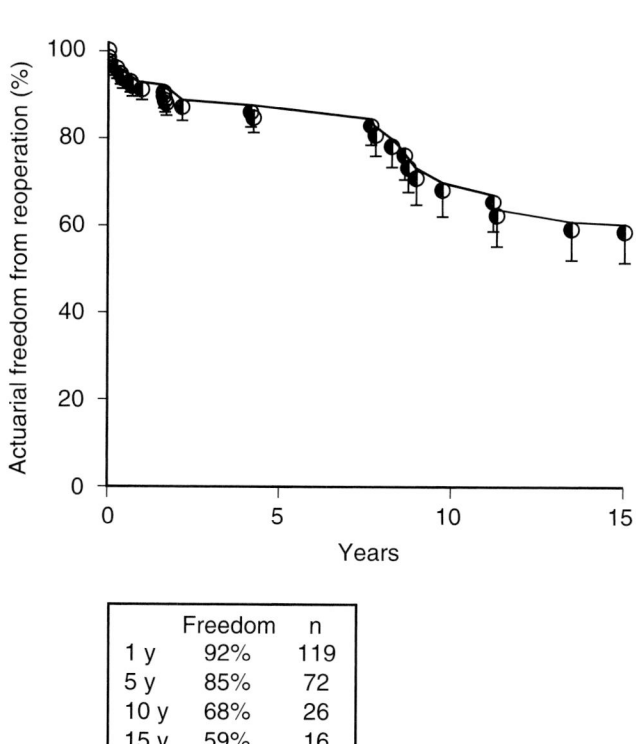

	Freedom	n
1 y	92%	119
5 y	85%	72
10 y	68%	26
15 y	59%	16

Figure 69C–12 Actuarial freedom from proximal or distal aortic reoperation after operative repair of chronic type A aortic dissection in 165 patients operated between 1964 and 2000 at Stanford University Medical Center.

distal aortic reoperations after surgical repair of acute and chronic type A aortic dissections in the patients operated at Stanford University Medical Center between 1963 and 2000 is shown in Figures 69C-10, 69C-11, and 69C-12.

In the Baylor experience, overall freedom from reoperation for patients with all types of dissections was 96, 91, and 78% at 1, 5, and 10 years, respectively.[174] In the Cleveland Clinic series, these respective freedom from reoperation estimates were 98, 91, and 85% for patients with type A dissections.[158] On the other hand, freedom from reoperation after repair of acute type A dissection was 66, 58, 52, and 43% at 1, 5, 10, and 15 years, respectively, in the recent report by Loisance and colleagues.[92] More severe aortic valve regurgitation at the time of the initial operation has been identified by different authors as a risk factor portending a higher probability of proximal reoperation on the aortic root and valve.[92,144] MFS has also been demonstrated to be associated with a higher risk of recurrent problems in the aortic root as well as distally,[10,21,123] suggesting that a more radical approach in patients with connective tissue disorders might be justified to reduce the incidence of late reoperation. The wisdom of using GRF or fibrin glue has also been questioned recently because it has been associated with late complications involving the aortic root.[21,89,97] Younger age at the initial operation, failure to excise the PIT, unresected residual aneurysm, and persistent patency of the false lumen have also been linked to a higher incidence of late distal aortic reoperations.[53,90,92,123,158]

FOLLOW-UP

Close medical follow-up and careful periodic imaging surveillance are mandatory for patients with aortic dissections on an indefinite basis. Following operative repair, serial CT or MRI scans of the thoracic and abdominal aorta are essential to detect complications related to the aortic dissection; these scans should be performed at 3-to 6-month intervals during the first year, and then every 12 months indefinitely. A transthoracic echocardiogram should also be performed annually to evaluate the aortic root and aortic valve function. Strict long-term arterial blood pressure control is essential for these patients. A combination of conventional antihypertensive agents and negative inotropic medications, such as oral β-blockers or calcium antagonists, is usually required and must be continued indefinitely.

REFERENCES

1. Ablaza SG, Gosh SC, Grana VP: Use of a ringed intraluminal graft in the surgical treatment of dissecting aneurysms of the thoracic aorta: a new technique. J Thorac Cardiovasc Surg 76: 390–396, 1978.
2. Abbott ME: Coarctation of the aorta of the adult type II. Am Heart J 3:574–618, 1928.
3. Abbott OA: Clinical experiences with application of polythene cellophane upon aneurysms of thoracic vessels. J Thorac Surg 18:435, 1949.
4. Anagnostopoulos CE, Prabhakar MJS, Vittle CF: Aortic dissections and dissecting aneurysms. Am J Cardiol 30: 263–273, 1972.

5. Ando M, Nakajima N, Adachi S, et al: Simultaneous graft replacement of the ascending aorta and total aortic arch for type A aortic dissection. Ann Thorac Surg 57:669–676, 1994.
6. Applebaum A, Karp RB, Kirklin JW: Ascending vs. descending aortic dissections. Ann Surg 183:296–300, 1976.
7. Bachet J, Teodori G, Goudot B, et al: Replacement of the transverse aortic arch during emergency operations for type A acute aortic dissection. Report of 26 cases. J Thorac Cardiovasc Surg 96:878–886, 1988.
8. Bachet J, Goudot B, Teodori G, et al: Surgery of type A acute aortic dissection with gelatine-resorcine-formol biological glue: a twelve-year experience. J Cardiovasc Surg (Torino) 31: 263–273, 1990.
9. Bachet J, Guilmet D, Goudot B, et al: Cold cerebroplegia. A new technique of cerebral protection during operations on the transverse aortic arch. J Thorac Cardiovasc Surg 102:85–93, 1991.
10. Bachet JE, Termignon JL, Dreyfus G, et al: Aortic dissection: prevalence, cause, and results of late reoperations. J Thorac Cardiovasc Surg 108:199–206, 1994.
11. Bachet J, Goudot B, Dreyfus GD, et al: Surgery for acute type A aortic dissection: the Hopital Foch Experience (1977–1998). Ann Thorac Surg 67:2006–2009, 1999.
12. Beighton P, DePaepe A, Danks D, et al: International nosology of heritable disorders of connective tissue, Berlin, 1986. Am J Med Genet 29:581–594, 1988.
13. Bickerstaff LK, Pairolero PC, Hollier LH, et al: Thoracic aortic aneurysms: a population-based study. Surgery 92: 1103–1108, 1982.
14. Borst HG, Frank G, Schaps D: Treatment of extensive aortic aneurysms by a new multiple-stage approach. J Thorac Cardiovasc Surg 95:11–13, 1988.
15. Borst HG, Laas J, Heinemann M: Type A aortic dissection: diagnosis and management of malperfusion phenomena. Sem Thorac Cardiovasc Surg 3:238–241, 1991.
16. Bossone E, Rampoldi V, Nienaber CA, et al: Usefulness of pulse deficit to predict in-hospital complications and mortality in patients with acute type A aortic dissection. Am J Cardiol 89:851–855, 2002.
17. Cabrol C, Pavie A, Mesnildrey P, et al: Long-term results with total replacement of the ascending aorta and reimplantation of the coronary arteries. J Thorac Cardiovasc Surg 91:17–25, 1986.
18. Cambria RP, Brewster DC, Gertler J, et al: Vascular complications associated with spontaneous aortic dissection. J Vasc Surg 7:199–202, 1988.
19. Carrel T, Pasic M, Jenni R, et al: Reoperations after operation on the thoracic aorta: etiology, surgical techniques, and prevention. Ann Thorac Surg 56:259–268, 1993.
20. Carlson RG, Lillehei CW, Edwards JE: Cystic medial necrosis of the ascending aorta in relation to age and hypertension. Am J Cardiol 25:411–415, 1970.
21. Casselman FP, Tan MES, Vermeulen FEE, et al: Durability of aortic valve preservation and root reconstruction in acute type A aortic dissection. Ann Thorac Surg 70:1227–1233, 2000.
22. Chavanon O, Carrier M, Cartier R, et al: Increased incidence of acute ascending aortic dissection with off-pump aorto-coronary bypass surgery? Ann Thorac Surg 71:117–121, 2001.
23. Chellock FG, Curtis JS: MR imaging and biomedical implants, materials and devices: an updated review. Radiology 180:541–550, 1991.
24. Cigarroa JE, Isselbacher EM, DeSanctis RW, et al: Diagnostic imaging in the evaluation of suspected aortic dissection. N Engl J Med 328:35–43, 1993.
25. Cikrit DF, Miles JH, Silver D: Spontaneous arterial perforation: the Ehler-Danlos specter. J Vasc Surg 8:470–475, 1987.
26. Coady MA, Rizzo JA, Hammond GL, et al: What is the appropriate size criterion for resection of thoracic aortic aneurysms? J Thorac Cardiovasc Surg 113:476–491, 1997.
27. Coady MA, Rizzo JA, Hammond GL, et al: Penetrating ulcer of the thoracic aorta: what is it? How do we recognize it? How do we manage it? J Vasc Surg 27:1006–1016, 1998.
28. Connolly HM, Schaff HV, Izhar U, et al: Posterior pericardial ascending-to-descending aortic bypass: an alternative approach for complex coarctation of the aorta. Circulation 104(Suppl. I):I-133–137, 2001.
29. Cooley DA, DeBakey ME, Morris GC Jr: Controlled extracorporeal circulation in surgical treatment of aortic aneurysm, Ann Surg 146:473, 1957.
30. Crawford ES, Coselli JS, Svensson LG, et al: Diffuse aneurysmal disease (chronic aortic dissection, Marfan, and mega aorta syndromes) and multiple aneurysm: treatment by subtotal and total aortic replacement emphasizing the elephant trunk operation. Ann Surg 211:521–537, 1990.
31. Crawford ES, Kirklin JW, Naftel DC, et al: Surgery for acute dissection of ascending aorta: should the arch be included? J Thorac Cardiovasc Surg 104:46–59, 1992.
32. Creswell L, Kouchoukos N, Cox JL, et al: Coronary artery disease in patients with type A dissection. Ann Thorac Surg 59:585–590, 1995.
33. Daily PO, Trueblood HW, Stinson EB, et al: Management of acute aortic dissections. Ann Thorac Surg 10:237–247, 1970.
34. Dake MD, Kato N, Mitchell RS, et al: Endovascular stent-graft placement for the treatment of acute aortic dissection. N Engl J Med 340:1546–1552, 1999.
35. Dapunt OE, Galla JD, Sadeghi AM, et al: The natural history of thoracic aortic aneurysms. J Thorac Cardiovasc Surg 107:1323–1333, 1994.
36. David TE, Feindel CM: An aortic valve-sparing operation for patients with aortic incompetence and aneurysm of the ascending aorta. J Thorac Cardiovasc Surg 103:617–621, 1992.
37. David TE, Armstrong S, Ivanov J, et al: Surgery for acute type A aortic dissection. Ann Thorac Surg 67:1999–2001, 1999.
38. Davies MJ, Treasure T, Richardson PD: The pathogenesis of spontaneous arterial dissection. Heart 75:434–435, 1996.
39. DeBakey ME, Cooley D, Creech O Jr: Surgical considerations of dissecting aneurysm of the aorta. Ann Surg 142:586–612, 1955.
40. DeBakey ME, Henry WS, Cooley DA, et al: Surgical management of dissecting aneurysms of the aorta. J Thorac Cardiovasc Surg 49:130–149, 1965.
41. DeBakey ME, McCollum CH, Crawford ES, et al: Dissection and dissecting aneurysms of the aorta: twenty-year follow-up of five hundred and twenty-seven patients treated surgically. Surgery 92:1118–1134, 1982.
42. DePaepe A, Deitz HC, Devereux RB, et al: Revised diagnosis criteria for the Marfan syndrome. Am J Med Genet 4:1799–1809, 1996.
43. DeSanctis RW, Doroghazi RM, Austen WG, et al: Aortic dissection. N Engl J Med 317:1060–1067, 1987.
44. DeSanctis RW, Eagle KA: Aortic dissection. Curr Probl Cardiol 14:227–278, 1989.
45. Dietz HC, Cutting GR, Pyeritz RE, et al: Defects in the fibrillin gene cause the Marfan syndrome; linkage evidence and identification of a missense mutation. Nature 352:337–339, 1991.
46. Doroghazi RM, Slater EE, DeSanctis RW, et al: Long-term survival of patients with treated aortic dissections. J Am Coll Cardiol 3:1026–1034, 1984.
47. Eagle KA, Isselbacher EM, DeSanctis RW: Cocaine-related aortic dissection in perspective. Circulation 105:1529–1530, 2002.
48. Earnest F, Muhm JR, Sheedy PF: Roentgenographic findings in thoracic aortic dissection. Mayo Clin Proc 54:43–50, 1979.
49. Elefteriades JA, Hammond GL, Gusberg RJ, et al: Fenestration revisited. A safe and effective procedure for descending aortic dissection. Arch Surg 125:786–790, 1990.
50. Erbel R, Engbergbing R, Daniel W, et al: Echocardiography in the diagnosis of aortic dissection. Lancet 1:457–461, 1989.

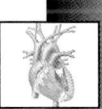

51. Erbel R, Oelert H, Meyer J, et al: Effect of medical and surgical therapy on aortic dissection evaluated by transesophageal echocardiography: implications for prognosis and therapy. Circulation 87:1604–1615, 1993.
52. Erdheim J: Medionecrosis aortae idiopathica cystica. Virchows Arch Pathol Anat 276:187–229, 1930.
53. Ergin MA, Phillips RA, Galla JD, et al: Significance of distal false lumen after type A dissection repair. Ann Thorac Surg 57: 820–824, 1994.
54. Erhlich MP, Ergin MA, McCullough JN, et al: Results of immediate surgical treatment of all acute type A dissections. Circulation 102 (Suppl. III):III-248–252, 2000.
55. Evangelista A, Garcia-del-Castillo H, Gonzalez-Alujas T, et al: Diagnosis of ascending aortic dissection by transesophageal echocardiography: utility of M-mode in recognizing artifacts. J Am Coll Cardiol 27:102–107, 1996.
56. Fann JI, Sarris GE, Miller DC, et al: Surgical management of acute aortic dissection complicated by a stroke. Circulation 80(Suppl. I):I-257–263, 1989.
57. Fann JI, Sarris GE, Mitchell RS, et al: Treatment of patients with aortic dissection presenting with peripheral vascular complications Ann Surg 212:705–713, 1990.
58. Fann JI, Glower DD, Miller DC, et al: Preservation of the aortic valve in patients with type A aortic dissection complicated by aortic valvular regurgitation. J Thorac Cardiovasc Surg 102:62–75, 1991.
59. Fann JI, Miller DC: Aortic dissection. Ann Vasc Surg 9: 311–323, 1995.
60. Fann JI, Smith JA, Miller DC, et al: Surgical management of aortic dissection during a 30-year period. Circulation 92(Suppl. II):II-113–121, 1995.
61. Farber A, Wagner WH, Cossman DV, et al: Isolated dissection of the abdominal aorta: clinical presentation and therapeutic options. J Vasc Surg 36:205–210, 2002.
62. Fleck T, Hutschala D, Czerny M, et al: Combined surgical and endovascular treatment of acute aortic dissection type A: preliminary results. Ann Thorac Surg 74:761–765, 2002.
63. Flege JB, Aberg T: Transventricular aortic cannulation for repair of aortic dissection. Ann Thorac Surg 72:955–956, 2001.
64. Galloway AC, Colvin SB, Grossi EA, et al: Surgical repair of type A aortic dissection by the circulatory arrest-graft inclusion technique in sixty-six patients. J Thorac Cardiovasc Surg 105:781–788, 1993.
65. Ganaha F, Miller DC, Sugimoto K, et al: Prognosis of aortic intramural hematoma with and without penetrating atherosclerotic ulcer. A clinical and radiologic analysis. Circulation 106:342–348, 2002.
66. Gerber O, Heyer EJ, Vieux U: Painless dissections of the aorta presenting as acute neurologic syndromes. Stroke 17:644–647, 1986.
67. Gillinov AM, Lytle BW, Kaplon RJ, et al: Dissection of the ascending aorta after previous cardiac surgery: differences in presentation and management. J Thorac Cardiovasc Surg 117:252–260, 1999.
68. Godwin JD, Herfkens RL, Skioldebrand CG, et al: Evaluation of dissections and aneurysms of the thoracic aorta by conventional and dynamic CT scanning. Radiology 136:135–139, 1980.
69. Graeter TP, Langer F, Nikoloudakis N, et al: Valve-preserving operation in acute aortic dissection type A. Ann Thorac Surg 70:1460–1465, 2000.
70. Griepp RB, Stinson EB, Hollingsworth JF, et al: Prosthetic replacement of the aortic arch. J Thorac Cardiovasc Surg 70:1051–1063, 1975.
71. Guilmet D, Bachet J, Goudet B: Use of biological glue in acute aortic dissection: preliminary results with a new surgical technique. J Thorac Cardiovasc Surg 77:516–521, 1979.
72. Gurin D, Bulmer JW, Derby R: Dissecting aneurysm of the aorta: diagnosis and operative relief of acute arterial obstruction due to this cause. NY State J Med 35:1200–1202, 1935.
73. Hagan PG, Nienaber CA, Isselbacher EM, et al: The international registry of acute aortic dissection (IRAD). JAMA 283:897–903, 2000.
74. Harris RD, Usselman JA, Vint VC, et al: Computerized tomographic diagnosis of aneurysms of the thoracic aorta. J Comput Assist Tomogr 3:81–91, 1979.
75. Hart WL, Berman EJ, LaCom RJ: Hazard of retrograde aortography in dissecting aneurysm. Circulation 27: 1140–1142, 1963.
76. Haverich A, Miller DC, Scott WC, et al: Acute and chronic aortic dissections—determinants of long-term outcome for operative survivors. Circulation 72(Suppl. II):II-22–34, 1985.
77. Hayashi K, Meaney TF, Zelch JV, et al: Aortographic analysis of aortic dissection. Am J Roentgenol 122:769–782, 1974.
78. Hirst AE, Johns VJ, Krime SJ: Dissecting aneurysm of the aorta: a review of 505 cases. Medicine 37:217–279, 1958.
79. Hirst AE, Gore I: Is cystic medionecrosis the cause of dissecting aortic aneurysm? Am Heart J 53:915–916, 1976.
80. Iliceto S, Nanda NC, Rizzon P, et al: Color Doppler evaluation of aortic dissection. Circulation 75:748–755, 1987.
81. Ishihara H, Uchida N, Yamasaki C, et al: Extensive primary repair of the thoracic aorta in Stanford type A acute aortic dissection by means of a synthetic vascular graft with a self-expandable stent. J Thorac Cardiovasc Surg 123:1035–1040, 2002.
82. Isselbacher EM, Cigarroa JE, Eagle KA: Cardiac tamponade complicating proximal aortic dissection. Is pericardiocentesis harmful? Circulation 90:2375–2378, 1994.
83. Juvonen T, Ergin MA, Galla JD, et al: Risk factors for rupture of chronic type B dissections. J Thorac Cardiovasc Surg 117:776–786, 1999.
84. Kaji S, Akasaka T, Horibata Y, et al: Long-term prognosis of patients with type A aortic intramural hematoma. Circulation 106(Suppl. I):I-248–252, 2002.
85. Kato N, Shimono T, Hirano T, et al: Transluminal placement of endovascular stent-grafts for the treatment of type A aortic dissection with an entry tear in the descending thoracic aorta. J Vasc Surg 34:1023–1028, 2001.
86. Kazui T, Inoue N, Yamada O, et al: Selective cerebral perfusion during operation for aneurysm of the aortic arch: a reassessment. Ann Thorac Surg 53:109–114, 1992.
87. Kazui T, Tamiya Y, Tanaka T, et al: Extended aortic replacement for acute type A dissection with the tear in the descending aorta. J Thorac Cardiovasc Surg 112:973–978, 1996.
88. Kazui T, Washiyama N, Muhammad BA, et al: Extended total arch replacement for acute type A aortic dissection: experience with seventy patients. J Thorac Cardiovasc Surg 119:558–565, 2000.
89. Kazui T, Washiyama N, Bashar AH, et al: Role of biologic glue repair of proximal aortic dissection in the development of early and midterm redissection of the aortic root. Ann Thorac Surg 72:509–514, 2001.
90. Kazui T, Washiyama N, Bashar AHM, et al: Surgical outcome of acute type A aortic dissection: analysis of risk factors. Ann Thorac Surg 74:75–82, 2002.
91. Khan IA, Nair CK: Clinical, diagnostic and management perspectives of aortic dissection. Chest 122:311–328, 2002.
92. Kirsch M, Soustelle C, Houel R, et al: Risk factor analysis for proximal and distal reoperations after surgery for acute type A aortic dissection. J Thorac Cardiovasc Surg 123:318–325, 2002.
93. Kontusaari S, Tromp G, Kuivaniemi H, et al: A mutation in the gene for type III procollagen (COL3A1) in a family with aortic aneurysms. J Clin Invest 86:1465–1473, 1990.
94. Kouchoukos NT, Wareing TH, Murphy SF, et al: Sixteen-year experience with aortic root replacement. Results of 172 operations. Ann Surg 214:308–318, 1991.

95. Kouchoukos NT, Masetti P, Rokkas CK, et al: Single-stage reoperative repair of chronic type A aortic dissection by means of the arch-first technique. J Thorac Cardiovasc Surg 122:578–582, 2001.
96. Krukenberg E: Beitrage sur frage des aneurysma dissecans. Beitr Pathol Anat Allg Pathol 67:329–351, 1920.
97. Kukunaga S, Karck M, Harringer W, et al: The use of gelatin-resorcin-formalin glue in acute aortic dissection type A. Eur J Cardiothorac Surg 15:564–569, 1999.
98. Kyo S, Takamoto S, Omoto R, et al: Intraoperative echocardiography for diagnosis and treatment of aortic dissection. Utility of color flow mapping for surgical decision making in acute stage. Herz 17:377–389, 1992.
99. Laennec RTH: De l'auscultations mediate, ou traité du diagnostic des maladies des poumons et du coeur, fondé principalement sur ce nouveau moyen d'exploration. Paris: Brosson & Chaude, 1819.
100. Lai DT, Robbins RC, Mitchell RS, et al: Does profound hypothermic circulatory arrest improve survival in patients with acute type A aortic dissection? Circulation 106(Suppl. 1):I-218–228, 2002.
101. Lansman SL, Raissi S, Ergin MA, et al: Urgent operation for acute transverse aortic arch dissection. J Thorac Cardiovasc Surg 97:334–341, 1989.
102. Lansman SL, McCullough JN, Nguyen KH, et al: Subtypes of acute aortic dissection. Ann Thorac Surg 67:1975–1978, 1999.
103. Lauterbach SR, Cambria RP, Brewster DC, et al: Contemporary management of aortic branch compromise resulting from acute aortic dissection. J Vasc Surg 33:1185–1192, 2001.
104. Leonard JC: Thomas Bevill Peacock and the early history of dissecting aneurysm. BMJ 2:260–262, 1979.
105. Lindsay J Jr, Hurst JW: Clinical features and prognosis in dissecting aneurysms of the aorta: a re-appraisal. Circulation 35:880–888, 1967.
106. Lindsay J Jr: Aorto-cameral fistula: a rare complication of aortic dissection. Am Heart J 126:441–443, 1993.
107. Link MD, Pietrzak MP: Aortic dissection presenting as superior vena cava syndrome. Am J Emerg Med 12:326–328, 1994.
108. Livesay JJ, Cooley DA, Duncan JM, et al: Open aortic anastomosis: improved results in the treatment of aneurysms of the aortic arch. Circulation 66:1122–1127, 1982.
109. Marselese DL, Moodie DS, Vacant M, et al: Marfan syndrome: natural history and long-term follow-up of cardiovascular involvement. J Am Coll Cardiol 14:422–428, 1989.
110. Massimo CG, Presenti LF, Marranci P, et al: Extended and total aortic resection in the surgical treatment of acute type A aortic dissection: experience with 54 patients. Ann Thorac Surg 46:420, 1988.
111. Maunoir JP: Memoires physiologiques et pratiques sur l'-aneurysme et la ligature des arteres. Geneva: J.J. Paschoud, 1802.
112. Mehta RH, Suzuki T, Hagan PG, et al: Predicting death in patients with acute type A aortic dissection. Circulation 105:200–206, 2002.
113. Meszaros I, Morocz J, Szlavi J, et al: Epidemiology and clinicopathology of aortic dissection. Chest 117:1271–1278, 2000.
114. Miller DC, Stinson EB, Oyer PE, et al: Operative treatment of aortic dissections. Experience with 125 patients over a sixteen-year period. J Thorac Cardiovasc Surg 78:365–382, 1979.
115. Miller DC: Surgical management of aortic dissections: indications, perioperative management, and long-term results. In Doroghazi RM, Slater EE, editors: Aortic Dissection. New York: McGraw-Hill, 1983, pp. 193–243.
116. Miller DC, Mitchell RS, Oyer PE, et al: Independent determinants of operative mortality for patients with aortic dissections. Circulation 70(Suppl. I):I-153–164, 1984.
117. Miller DC: Surgical treatment of aortic dissections. In Jamieson SW, Shumway NE, editors: Operative Surgery—Cardiac Surgery. London: Butterworths, 1986, pp. 526–537.
118. Miller J, Lemaire SA, Coselli JS: Evaluating aortic dissection: when is coronary angiogram indicated? Heart 83:615–616, 2000.
119. Minatoya K, Karck M, Szpakowski E, et al: Ascending aortic cannulation for Stanford type A acute aortic dissection: another option. J Thorac Cardiovasc Surg 125:952–953, 2003.
120. Ming RL, Najafi H, Javid H, et al: Acute ascending aortic dissection: surgical management. Circulation 64(Suppl. II): II-231–234, 1981.
121. Mohr-Lahaly S, Erbel R, Kearney P, et al: Aortic intramural hemorrhage visualized by transesophageal echocardiography: findings and prognostic implications. J Am Coll Cardiol 23:658–664, 1994.
122. Moizumi Y, Komatsu T, Motoyoshi N, et al: Management of patients with intramural hematoma involving the ascending aorta. J Thorac Cardiovasc Surg 124:918–924, 2002.
123. Moon MR, Sundt TM, Pasque MK, et al: Does the extent of proximal or distal resection influence outcome for type A dissections? Ann Thorac Surg 71:1244–1249, 2001.
124. Moore AG, Eagle KA, Bruckman D, et al: Choice of computed tomography, transesophageal echocardiography, magnetic resonance imaging, and aortography in acute aortic dissection: International Registry of Acute Aortic Dissection (IRAD). Am J Cardiol 89:1235–1238, 2002.
125. Mora-Mangano CT, Neville MJ, Hsu PH, et al: Aprotinin, blood loss, and renal dynfunction in deep hypothermic circulatory arrest. Circulation 104(Suppl. I):I-276–281, 2001.
126. Movskowitz HD, David M, Movskowitz C, et al: Penetrating atherosclerotic ulcers: the role of transesophageal echocardiography in diagnosis and clinical management. Am Heart J 126:745–747, 1993.
127. Muna WF, Spray TL, Morrow AG, Roberts WC: Aortic dissection after aortic valve replacement in patients with valvular aortic stenosis. J Thorac Cardiovasc Surg 74:65–69, 1977.
128. Murphy DA, Craver JM, Jones EL, et al: Recognition and management of ascending aortic dissection complicating cardiac surgical operations. J Thorac Cardiovasc Surg 85:247–256, 1983.
129. Najafi H, Dye WS, Javid H, et al: Acute aortic regurgitation secondary to aortic dissection: surgical management without valve replacement. Ann Thorac Surg 14:474–482, 1972.
130. Nakashima Y, Kurozumi T, Sueishi K, et al: Dissecting aneurysm: a clinicopathologic and histopathologic study of 111 autopsied cases. Hum Pathol 21:291–296, 1990.
131. Nakashima Y, Shiokawa Y, Sueishi K: Alterations of elastic architecture in human aortic dissecting aneurysm. Lab Invest 62:751–760, 1990.
132. Neri E, Masseti M, Capannini G, et al: Axillary artery cannulation in type A aortic dissection operations. J Thorac Cardiovasc Surg 118:324–329, 1999.
133. Nienaber CA, Spielmann RP, von Kodolitsch Y, et al: Diagnosis of thoracic aortic dissection. Magnetic resonance imaging versus transesophageal echocardiography. Circulation 85: 434–447, 1992.
134. Nienaber CA, von Kodolitsch Y: Meta-analysis of the prognosis of thoracic aortic dissection: changing mortality in the last four decades. Herz 17:298–416, 1992.
135. Nienaber CA, von Kodolitsch Y, Petersen B, et al: The diagnosis of thoracic aortic dissection by noninvasive imaging procedures. N Engl J Med 328:1–9, 1993.
136. Nienaber CA, von Kodolitsch Y, Petersen B, et al: Intramural hemorrhage of the aorta: diagnostic and clinical implications. Circulation 92:1465–1472, 1995.
137. O'Gara PT, DeSanctis RW: Acute aortic dissection and its variants: toward a common diagnostic and therapeutic approach. Circulation 92:1376–1378, 1995.

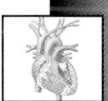

138. Pansini S, Gagliardotto PV, Pompei E, et al: Early and late risk factors in surgical treatment of acute type A aortic dissection. Ann Thorac Surg 66:779–884, 1998.
139. Pate JW, Richardson RL, Eastridge CE: Acute aortic dissections. Am Surgeon 42:395–404, 1976.
140. Patel S, Alam M, Rosman H: Pitfalls in the echocardiographic diagnosis of aortic dissection. Angiology 48:939–946, 1997.
141. Paullin JE, James DF: Dissecting aneurysm of aorta. Postgrad Med 4:291, 1948.
142. Peacock TB: Report on cases of dissecting aneurysms. Trans Pathol Soc Lond 14:87, 1863.
143. Penn MS, Smedira N, Lytle B, et al: Does coronary angiography before emergency aortic surgery affect in-hospital mortality? J Am Coll Cardiol 35:889–894, 2000.
144. Pessoto R, Santini F, Pugliese P, et al: Preservation of the aortic valve in acute type A aortic dissection complicated by aortic regurgitation. Ann Thorac Surg 67:2010–2013, 1999.
145. Pieters F, Widdenshoven J, Gerardy A, et al: Risk of aortic dissection after aortic valve replacement. Am J Cardiol 72:1043–1047, 1993.
146. Pyeritz RE: Marfan syndrome: current and future clinical and genetic management of cardiovascular manifestations. Semin Thorac Cardiovasc Surg 5:11–16, 1993.
147. Pyeritz RE: The Marfan syndrome. Annu Rev Med 51:481–510, 2000.
148. Raanani E, Latter DA, Errett LE, et al: Use of Bioglue in aortic surgical repair. Ann Thorac Surg 72:638–640, 2001.
149. Reul GJ, Cooley DA, Hallman GL, et al: Dissecting aneurysm of the descending aorta. Improved surgical results in 91 patients. Arch Surg 110:632–640, 1975.
150. Rizzo RJ, Aranki SF, Aklog L, et al: Rapid noninvasive diagnosis and surgical repair of acute ascending aortic dissection. Improved survival with less angiography. J Thorac Cardiovasc Surg 108:567–574, 1994.
151. Robbins RC, MacNamus RP, Mitchell RS, et al: Management of patients with intramural hematoma of the thoracic aorta. Circulation 88(Suppl. II):II1–10, 1993.
152. Roberts C, Roberts W: Dissection of the aorta associated with congenital malformation of the aortic valve. J Am Coll Cardiol 17:712–716, 1991.
153. Roberts CS, Roberts WC: Aortic dissection with the entrance tear in abdominal aorta. Am Heart J 121:1834–1835, 1991.
154. Roberts WC: Aortic dissection: anatomy, consequences, and cause. Am Heart J 101:195–214, 1981.
155. Robiscek F: Apical aortic cannulation: application of an old method with new paraphernalia. Ann Thorac Surg 51:330–332, 1991.
156. Rushid J, Eisenberg MJ, Topol EJ: Cocaine-induced aortic dissection. Am Heart J 132:1301–1304, 1996.
157. Sabik JF, Lytle BW, McCarthy PM, et al: Axillary artery: an alternative site of arterial cannulation for patients with extensive aortic and peripheral vascular disease. J Thorac Cardiovasc Surg 109:885–890, 1995.
158. Sabik JF, Lytle BW, Blackstone EH, et al: Long-term effectiveness of operations for ascending aortic dissections. J Thorac Cardiovasc Surg 119:946–962, 2000.
159. Safi HJ, Miller CC, Estrera AL, et al: Staged repair of extensive aortic aneurysms. Morbidity and mortality in the elephant trunk technique. Circulation 104:2938–2942, 2001.
160. Schnitker MA, Bayer CA: Dissecting aneurysm of the aorta in young individuals, particularly in association with pregnancy; with report of a case. Ann Intern Med 20:486–511, 1944.
161. Seldinger SI: Catheter replacement of the needle in percutaneous arteriography: a new technique. Acta Radiol 39:368–376, 1953.
162. Shennan T: Dissecting Aneurysms. Special report Medical Research Council series No. 193. London: His Majesty's Stationary Office, 1934.
163. Simon P, Owen AN, Havel M, et al: Transesophageal echocardiography in the emergency surgical management of patients with aortic dissection. J Thorac Cardiovasc Surg 103:1113–1118, 1992.
164. Slater EE: Aortic dissection: presentation and diagnosis. In Doroghazi RM, Slater EE, editors: Aortic Dissection. New York: McGraw-Hill, 1983, pp. 61–70.
165. Slonim SM, Nyman URO, Semba CP, et al: Aortic dissection: percutaneous management of ischemic complications with endovascular stents and balloon fenestration. J Vasc Surg 23:241–253, 1996.
166. Slonim SM, Nyman UR, Semba CP, et al: True lumen obliteration in complicated aortic dissection: endovascular treatment. Radiology 201:161–166, 1996.
167. Slonim SM, Miller DC, Mitchell RS, et al: Percutaneous balloon fenestration and stenting for life-threatening ischemic complications in patients with acute aortic dissection. J Thorac Cardiovasc Surg 117:1118–1126, 1999.
168. Sommer T, Fehske W, Holzknecht N, et al: Aortic dissection: a comparative study of diagnosis with spiral CT, multiplanar transesophageal echocardiography and MR imaging. Radiology 199:347–352, 1996.
169. Song JK, Kim HS, Somg JM, et al: Outcomes of medically treated patients with aortic intramural hematoma. Am J Med 113:181–187, 2002.
170. Sorenson HR, Olsen H: Ruptured and dissecting aneurysms of the aorta. Incidence and prospects of surgery. Acta Chir Scand 128:644, 1964.
171. Stanson AW, Kazmier FJ, Hollier LH, et al: Penetrating atherosclerotic ulcers of the thoracic aorta: natural history and clinicopathologic correlations. Ann Vasc Surg 1:15–23, 1986.
172. Stein HL, Steinberg I: Selective aortography, the definitive technique for diagnosis of dissecting aneurysm of the aorta. Am J Roentgenol 102:333–348, 1968.
173. Svensson LG, Crawford ES, Coselli JS, et al: Impact of cardiovascular operation on survival in the Marfan patient. Circulation 80(Suppl. I):I-233–242, 1989.
174. Svensson LG, Crawford ES, Hess KR, et al: Dissection of the aorta and dissecting aortic aneurysms. Improving early and long-term surgical results. Circulation 82(Suppl. IV): IV-24–38, 1990.
175. Svensson LG: Management of acute dissection with coarctation of the aorta in a single operation. Ann Thorac Surg 58:241–243, 1994.
176. Svensson LG, Labib SB, Eisenhauer AC, et al: Intimal tear without hematoma: an important variant of aortic dissection that can elude current imaging techniques. Circulation 99:1331–1336, 1999.
177. Symbas PN, Kelly TF, Vlasis SE, et al: Intimo-intimal intussusception and other unusual manifestations of aortic dissection. J Thorac Cardiovasc Surg 79:926–932, 1980.
178. Tanaka T, Kawamura T, Ohara K, et al: Transapical aortic perfusion with a double-barreled cannula. Ann Thorac Surg 25:209–214, 1978.
179. Tittle SL, Lynch RJ, Cole PE, et al: Midterm follow-up of penetrating ulcer and intramural hematoma of the aorta. J Thorac Cardiovasc Surg 123:1051–1059, 2002.
180. Toyama M, Amano A, Kameda T: Familial aortic dissection: a report of rare family cluster. Br Heart J 61:204–207, 1989.
181. Urban BA, Bleumke DA, Johnson KM, et al: Imaging of thoracic aortic disease. Cardiol Clin 17:659–682, 1999.
182. Van Arsdell GS, David TE, Butany J: Autopsies in acute type A aortic dissection. Surgical implications. Circulation 98(Suppl. II):II-299–302, 1998.
183. Victor MF, Mintz GS, Kotler MN, et al: Two dimensional echocardiographic diagnosis of aortic dissection. Am J Cardiol 48:1155–1159, 1981.

184. von Segesser LK, Killer I, Ziswiler M, et al: Dissection of the descending thoracic aorta extending into the ascending aorta: a therapeutic challenge. J Thorac Cardiovasc Surg 108: 755–761, 1994.
185. Wada J, Komatsu S, Nakae S, et al: A new cannulation method for isolated mitral valve surgery—"apicoaortic-PA" cannulation. Thoraxchir Vask Chir 24:204–212, 1976.
186. Westaby S, Parry A, Giannopoulos N, et al: Replacement of the thoracic aorta with collagen-impregnated Dacron grafts. Early results. J Thorac Cardiovasc Surg 106:427–433, 1993.
187. Westaby S, Saito S, Katsumata T: Acute type A dissection: conservative methods provide consistently low mortality. Ann Thorac Surg 73:707–713, 2002.
188. Wheat MW, Palmer RF, Bantley TD, et al: Treatment of dissecting aneurysms of the aorta without surgery. J Thorac Cardiovasc Surg 50:364–373, 1965.
189. Williams DM, Lee DY, Hamilton BH, et al: The dissected aorta: percutaneous treatment of ischemic complications—principles and results. J Vasc Interv Radiol 8:605–625, 1997.
190. Yacoub MH, Schottenfeld M, Kittle CF: Hematoma of the interatrial septum with heart block secondary to dissecting aneurysm of the aorta: a clinicopathologic entity. Circulation 46:537–545, 1972.
191. Yacoub MH, Gehle P, Chandrasekaran V, et al: Late results of a valve-preserving operation in patients with aneurysms of the ascending aorta and root. J Thorac Cardiovasc Surg 115:1080–1090, 1998.
192. Yamada T, Takamiya M, Naito H, et al: Diagnosis of aortic dissection without intimal rupture by x-ray computed tomography. Nippon Acta Radiol 45:699–710, 1985.
193. Yun KL, Glower DD, Miller DC, et al: Aortic dissection resulting from tear of transverse arch: is concomitant arch repair warranted? J Thorac Cardiovasc Surg 102:355–368, 1991.
194. Yun KL, Miller DC, Fann JI, et al: Composite valve graft versus separate aortic valve and ascending aortic replacement: is there still a role for the separate procedure? Circulation 96(Suppl. II):II-368–375, 1997.
195. Zubiate P, Kay JH: Surgical treatment of aneurysm of the ascending aorta with aortic insufficiency and marked displacement of the coronary ostia. J Thorac Cardiovasc Surg 71:415–421, 1976.

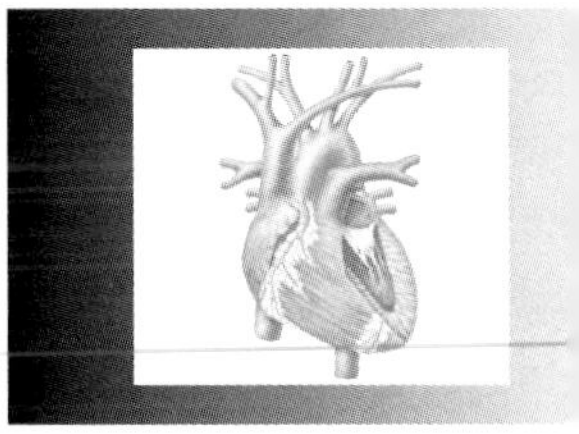

CHAPTER 69D

Surgery of the Aortic Arch, Descending Thoracic and Thoracoabdominal Surgery, and Aortic Dissection

Type B Aortic Dissection

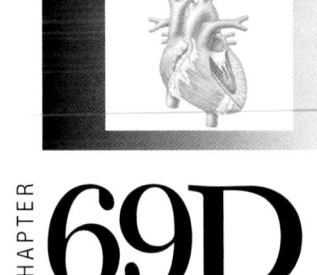

Philippe Demers and D. Craig Miller

INTRODUCTION

More so than ruptured abdominal aortic aneurysm, aortic dissection is one of the most common catastrophes involving the aorta. Because major aortic branch occlusion can complicate the clinical presentation of patients with acute dissection and thus mimic many other acute medical and surgical problems, a high clinical index of suspicion is necessary to diagnose this life-threatening condition early. The lethal nature of acute aortic dissection mandates prompt medical and/or surgical intervention. In the chronic phase, aortic dissection involving the descending thoracic aorta is responsible for a substantial proportion of aneurysms of the thoracic and thoracoabdominal aorta.

Although a consensus exists today regarding the need for emergency surgical treatment for essentially all patients with acute type A aortic dissection, the optimal management of patients with aortic dissection involving the descending thoracic aorta—medical only versus surgical plus medical—remains controversial.[77] The majority of patients with acute type B dissections are treated medically.* A complication-specific approach is favored by many centers, reserving surgical replacement of the descending thoracic aorta for patients with complicated dissections, including rupture, ischemia of vital organs, persistent pain, uncontrollable arterial hypertension, or sizable dilatation of the false lumen.[10,20,49] On the other hand, we and other groups have also advocated consideration of early surgical treatment for carefully selected patients with acute type B dissection who are young and are otherwise good surgical candidates (irrespective of the presence or absence of complications, including those with Marfan syndrome or other connective tissue disorders) in an attempt to lower the long-term risk of dissection-related complications and aortic reoperation.[38,48,66]

Historical Note

One of the first attempts to treat acute aortic dissection was described in 1935 by Gurin et al, who used surgical iliac artery fenestration to treat dissection-related lower extremity ischemia.[29] In 1955, DeBakey and colleagues initiated the modern era of surgical management of aortic dissection by introducing graft replacement of the dissected aortic segment.[14] Subsequently, the same group introduced the use of cardiopulmonary bypass during clamping of the descending thoracic aorta.[7] Wheat and associates recommended in 1965

*References 10, 17, 20, 23, 27, 49.

medical treatment using pharmacological antihypertensive drugs for aortic dissection involving the descending thoracic aorta.[79,80] The introduction of percutaneous interventional techniques in the early 1990s, e.g., flap fenestration and stenting, to alleviate dissection-induced branch vessel involvement (or malperfusion) modified the traditional indications for surgical treatment, with more patients now being treated medically and interventionally despite the presence of complications that in the past would have prompted operation.[70] The recent advent of successful endovascular stent-grafting in patients with acute type B aortic dissections has been associated with very promising early results.[13,58] Until the effectiveness and the durability of stent-grafting are confirmed in prospective trials and compared with standard medical and surgical therapy, the exact role of this new modality in the treatment of acute type B dissections remains to be determined.

NOMENCLATURE

As described in Chapter 69C, various classification methods have been applied to aortic dissection. Over the past 35 years, a functional approach based on whether the ascending aorta is involved, regardless of the site of primary intimal tear, has gained broad acceptance. If only the descending thoracic aorta is involved, the dissection is termed a Stanford type B, DeBakey type III, University of Alabama "descending," Massachusetts General Hospital "distal," or Najafi "posterior" dissection.[2,11,16,51,67] Examples of various types and extents of dissections are illustrated in Figure 69C-1 of Chapter 69C. This consensus has made it easier to interpret and compare outcomes of various therapeutic strategies reported from various institutions. Aortic dissections diagnosed within 14 days of the onset of presenting symptoms are termed acute; those diagnosed more than 14 days after onset are classified as chronic dissections.[17,23,49,67] *Intramural hematoma* (IMH) and *penetrating aortic ulcers* (PAUs) are now recognized as distinct pathological variants of classic aortic dissection.[60,72] These lesions are characterized by the absence of an intimal flap dividing the aorta into true and false lumens and more commonly involve the descending thoracic aorta. Distinguishing IMH and PAU from classic type B aortic dissection is important, but these entities form a continuum of pathophysiology that can evolve rapidly. Furthermore, management of these lesions can differ in certain clinical circumstances.[6,26]

EPIDEMIOLOGY AND NATURAL HISTORY

Epidemiology

Acute type B aortic dissection more commonly affects middle-aged to elderly men. Aortic dissection is seen in all age groups, although the peak incidence is found between the ages of 50 and 69 years.[32] Typically, patients with type B dissections are older than those with type A dissections.[24,30] In the Stanford 30-year experience with aortic dissection, the mean age of patients with acute type B dissection was 64 years, compared to 56 years in those with acute type A dissections.[24] The estimated male-to-female ratio is between 2:1 and 3:1. The prevalence of arterial hypertension ranges from 45–80% and is highest in patients with type B dissections.[17,18,23,24,30] Associated atherosclerotic disease is also found more frequently in patients with type B dissections.[30] Between 2 and 4% of patients presenting with acute type B dissections have Marfan syndrome.

The incidence of aortic dissection is estimated to be between 5 and 20 cases per million population per year, which is higher than the incidence of ruptured abdominal aortic aneurysms or ruptured thoracic aortic aneurysms.[1,41] Approximately two-thirds of all acute aortic dissections involve the ascending aorta (Stanford type A), with one-third limited to the descending aorta (Stanford type B).[24,30,32] In large autopsy series, acute aortic dissection was observed in 1–2% of cases.[32]

Natural History

Untreated, acute aortic dissection can be highly lethal. In the 1967 report by Lindsay and Hurst, one third of the patients suffering from acute aortic dissection died within 24 h, 50% within 48 h, 80% within 7 days, and 95% within the first month.[41] In patients presenting with chronic dissection, only 15% were still alive after 5 years. Patients with dissection involving the descending thoracic aorta (Stanford type B), however, had a less ominous prognosis: 75% were alive 1 month after onset. Anagnostopoulos et al, in a large collected series of 963 cases of patients with untreated aortic dissection (type A or B, acute or chronic), reported a cumulative mortality of 70% at 1 week and 90% at 3 months.[1]

Patients with untreated type B dissection usually die from aortic rupture in the left chest or from occlusion of major distal aortic branches resulting in ischemic injury to vital organs.[17] An autopsy study by Roberts and Roberts of 40 patients with acute or chronic type B dissections illustrated that the dissection per se or its vascular complications caused at least 84% of deaths in the 31 patients who were treated medically.[61] Some fortunate individuals with acute dissections survive untreated; in nearly all these cases, distal reentry sites are found, allowing decompression of the false lumen.[18,23] The false lumen remains prone to progressive expansion over time, resulting in the formation of a false aneurysm.

PATHOPHYSIOLOGY

The typical pathological lesion found in elderly patients with type B aortic dissection is smooth muscle degeneration within the aortic media, which represents a normal manifestation of the aging process.[64] These findings are distinct from the elastic tissue degeneration observed in younger patients presenting with type A dissection, which is usually an inherited connective tissue disorder.[65]

The initial event in aortic dissection is tearing of the intima.[23,65] Type B dissections can infrequently also arise from rupture of an atherosclerotic plaque,[39] but this usually represents a localized dissecting process producing a characteristic "mushroom cap" appearance on computed tomography (CT) scans; this is a different process from classic type B dissection, which frequently involves most or all of the descending and abdominal aorta. After a primary intimal tear (PIT) occurs, blood flow within the aortic wall separates the layers of the media and creates the false channel. Propagation of the dissection occurs within the outer third of the aortic media usually in an antegrade direction, but it may also propagate proximally to involve the transverse arch. As in type A dissections, distal reentry sites are usually multiple and are located in regions of sheared-off ostia of arterial branches. Factors influencing dissection propagation include the rate of increase of aortic systolic pressure, or aortic *dP/dt*, aortic diastolic elastic recoil pressure, mean arterial pressure, and aortic wall integrity.[23,33,63] In the descending aorta as well as in the abdominal aorta, the false lumen often runs along the left posterolateral wall, with the dissection frequently extending into the left renal artery.[32] The false lumen ordinarily remains patent, especially if reentry fenestrations are present, but it may occasionally thrombose. This latter situation is usually associated with a "nonreentering" false lumen, which can then extrinsically compromise aortic true lumen blood flow distally. In the chronic phase of dissection, progressive dilatation of the false lumen results in overall enlargement of the aorta and formation of a false aneurysm. This usually is a diffuse process involving the entire length of the dissection.

In aortic dissections involving the descending thoracic aorta, the PIT is located in the proximal descending thoracic aorta near the origin of the left subclavian artery in approximately 80% of cases, as illustrated in Figure 69C-3 of Chapter 69C.[45,77] In 10–20% of patients, the PIT is located in the transverse aortic arch, and the dissection extends in an antegrade direction to involve variable lengths of the descending aorta, or in a retrograde fashion to involve the ascending aorta (when it is termed a "retro-A," type A, or DeBakey type III-D dissection). In fewer than 5% of aortic dissections, a distinct PIT cannot be identified; these dissections are usually confined to the descending thoracic aorta.[32] Very rarely, the dissection can be limited to the aortic arch without either antegrade or retrograde propagation ("isolated arch dissection"). It is also estimated that 2–4% of aortic dissections may originate in the abdominal aorta.[25,62]

Intramural hematoma originates from spontaneous rupture of the *vasa vasorum* within the outer third of the aortic media, allowing accumulation of blood within the aortic wall in the absence of a large intimal defect.[26,60] Alternatively, IMH can occur following rupture of an atheromatous plaque through the internal elastic lamina, leading to the formation of a PAU, with subsequent extravasation of blood in the aortic wall.[6,26,72] In the past decade, major advances in cardiovascular imaging techniques have led to increasing recognition of IMH with or without associated PAU in patients with acute aortic syndromes. Several investigators reported that these lesions can stabilize with medical therapy, but IMH with or without associated PAU can also rupture or progress quickly to a classic dissection. It is now recognized that IMH involving the descending aorta (i.e., type B IMH) may have a different natural history from classic aortic dissection and a higher propensity for aortic rupture, especially in patients with severe symptoms or when the IMH is associated and a deep or large PAU.[6,26,76]

Aortic branch vessel involvement or thoracoabdominal malperfusion results when the dissection compromises blood flow to important downstream aortic tributaries. As illustrated in Figure 69C-4 of Chapter 69C, the most common mechanisms producing aortic branch compromise are extrinsic compression of the aortic true lumen by the false lumen or an intimal flap compromising the orifice of the branch artery. As defined by Williams and associates, *"static" branch compromise* is extension of the dissection flap into a branch vessel with subsequent mechanical obstruction of flow; conversely, *"dynamic" branch compromise* is when the dissection flap prolapses into the vessel origin or the true lumen is narrowed above it due to the bulk of flow being in the aortic false lumen.[81] Compression by the large false lumen can result in near obliteration of the true channel, or true lumen collapse.[68] With extension of the dissection, some aortic tributaries may be spared and continue to be perfused by the true lumen, while others may be perfused exclusively from the false lumen (after being sheared off) and eventually become permanently dependent on the false lumen. Thus, clinical presentation is dependent on which aortic branches are involved and the severity of compromised perfusion, which can be variable and which may potentially delay correct diagnosis. Simultaneous occurrence of a variety of acute clinical problems without a readily apparent unifying etiology should prompt consideration of acute aortic dissection.

CLINICAL MANIFESTATIONS

Patients with acute type B dissection can present with symptoms and physical findings that suggest almost any other acute medical or surgical disease process.[18,67] These numerous, nonspecific manifestations are the main reason that the rapid, correct diagnosis of aortic dissection remains such a formidable clinical challenge.[46,49] Indeed, aortic dissection occurs more frequently than ruptured abdominal aortic aneurysm, but sadly is diagnosed correctly less frequently *antemortem*.[17,67]

Most commonly, the clinical hallmark of acute type B aortic dissection is the acute onset of severe, lancinating chest or back pain.[18,23,49,67] The initial pain can be in any location, but it usually originates in the interscapular region with later migration to the lower back or abdomen. Pain in acute dissection is thought to be secondary to stretching of the aortic adventitia caused by the dissecting hematoma. Abrupt onset of symptoms and description of sharp, ripping, or tearing pain are also characteristic of acute dissection. Persistence or further migration of pain suggests continuing expansion or distal extension of the dissecting process. Rarely, acute dissection can be painless; vigilance is essential to recognize other manifestations of aortic dissection in these cases. In the International Registry of Acute Aortic Dissection (IRAD) summary report, 98% of 175 patients with acute type B dissection reported some pain; pain was of sudden onset in 84%; 63% reported chest pain (anterior in 44%, posterior in 41%), which was significantly different from acute type A dissection (chest pain in 79% and anterior in 71%). Back pain was observed in 64% of cases and abdominal pain in 43% of patients with acute type B dissections, much more frequently than in patients with type A dissection.[30] Moreover, the pain was described as the "worst ever" in 90% of patients, sharp in 68%, and tearing in 52%. Radiating pain was observed in 30% of cases, while migration was reported in only 19%.

Despite evidence of poor peripheral perfusion, elevated blood pressure is usually observed. In the IRAD report, 70% of patients with acute type B dissection were hypertensive at initial presentation; only 4% were hypotensive or in frank shock, compared to 25% of patients with acute type A dissection. If the patient is hypotensive, aortic rupture should be suspected. Cardiac tamponade is very rare in acute type B dissection; only 2% of patients with acute type B dissection in the 30-year Stanford experience had tamponade, which was thought to be due to leakage of blood and fluid into the pericardial sac from a large, high-pressure mediastinal hematoma.[24]

The constellation of other symptoms and signs relates largely to which distal aortic branches are involved in the dissection. Approximately 25% of patients present with symptoms related to aortic branch compromise or develop such symptoms early in the course of their illness; alternatively, loss of a peripheral pulse may be clinically asymptomatic. In a review of the Stanford experience with peripheral vascular complications of aortic dissection by Fann et al, 31% (85/272) of patients with all types of dissections sustained one or more peripheral vascular complications, while 20% of patients with type B dissections had such complications (Figure 69D-1).[22] Others have reported similar figures, with the prevalence of peripheral vascular manifestations ranging from 30–50%.[3,16,23,40] Of the 85 patients with a vascular complication, 18 individuals (21%) suffered two complications, and 7 (8%) had three or more vascular problems.[22] Among the 40 patients with acute type B dissection, no patient presented with a stroke, 3% had acute paraplegia at presentation, 20% sustained loss of one or more peripheral pulses, 8% had impaired renal perfusion (demonstrated angiographically), and 5% had compromised visceral perfusion by angiography. The incidence of these complications with the attendant operative mortality rate following surgical graft replacement of the descending thoracic aorta is summarized in Table 69D-1. The distribution of specific sites of peripheral pulse loss in these patients is summarized in Table 69D-2.

The clinical course of peripheral limb ischemia may vary; up to one-third of patients may experience spontaneous resolution of the pulse deficit or a fluctuating course, often due to reentry of flow into distal true lumen from the false lumen.[3] Stroke and transient ischemic attack can complicate acute type A dissection, but are seen only rarely in patients with type B dissections. Neurological findings can vary from minor sensory deficits to frank paraplegia resulting from spinal cord ischemia due to interruption of intercostal artery blood supply.[18,67] Abdominal pain out of proportion to the physical findings can reflect mesenteric ischemia or infarction.[3] Oliguria or anuria suggests renal perfusion compromise; flank pain or hematuria due to renal malperfusion or infarction can mimic symptoms usually associated with ureteral colic or kidney stones.

Physical examination of patients with suspected aortic dissection should include measurement of blood pressure in both upper and both lower extremities. A complete evaluation of peripheral pulses is imperative, in addition to a comprehensive neurological examination. Examination should be repeated periodically because new vascular or neurological deficits may appear. The remainder of the physical examination is often normal.

The majority of patients with chronic type B dissection are asymptomatic, but progressive enlargement of the aortic false lumen may eventually produce compression, obstruction, or erosion into adjacent thoracic structures, producing symptoms such as chest pain, dyspnea, wheezing, hoarse-

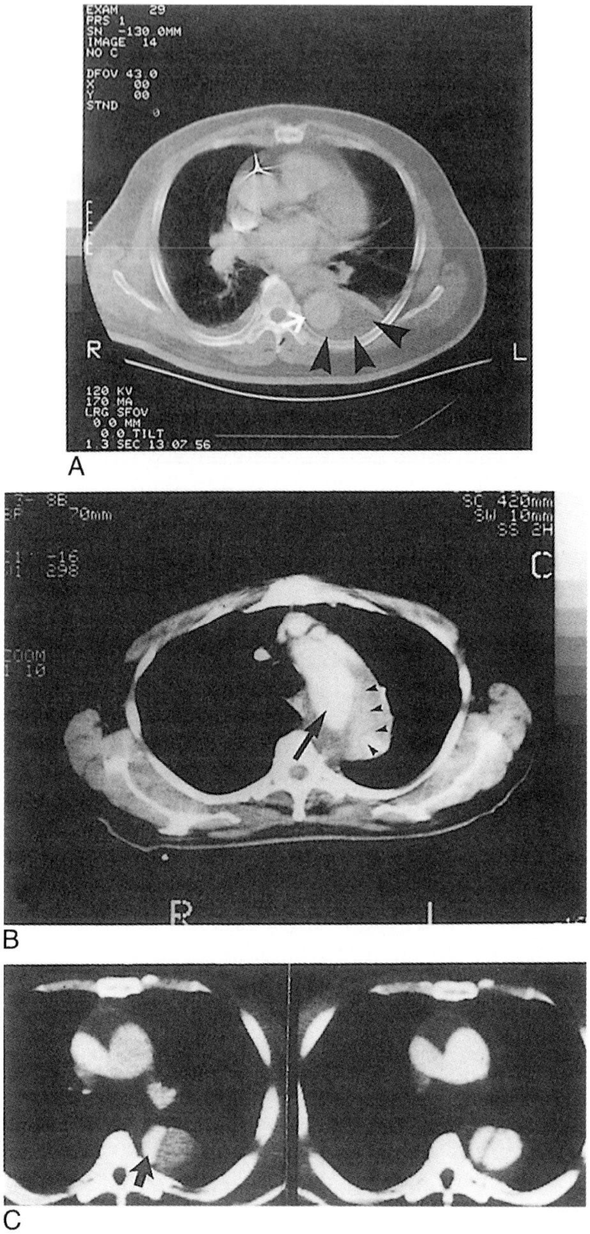

Figure 69D–1 **Examples of diagnostic CT scans. A,** The CT shows the linear flap (*black lucency, white arrow*) between the two aortic lumens in the descending thoracic aorta that is characteristic of aortic dissection. In addition, a relatively large hematoma surrounding the aorta is seen (*arrowheads*), representing recent hemorrhage contained in the posterior mediastinum. Despite this ominous appearance, this patient did well with medical therapy for more than 1 year until progressive enlargement of a localized false aneurysm prompted referral for operation. **B,** CT scan from a different patient with an acute type B dissection illustrating a false aneurysm involving the distal arch and proximal descending thoracic aorta. The false lumen (*arrowheads*) is partially thrombosed; therefore, it opacifies only faintly compared with the contrast seen in the true lumen (*arrow*). **C,** Although this patient had a type A dissection (note the deformed true lumen in the large ascending aorta), this CT demonstrates differential opacification of the true and false lumens in the descending thoracic aorta. The true lumen (*arrow*) is completely opacified in the left panel; later in the cardiac cycle (*right panel*), both the true and the false lumens are equally opacified.
(From Miller DC: Acute dissection of the descending thoracic aorta. Chest Surg Clin North Am 2:347–378, 1992; with permission.)

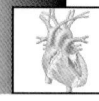

Table 69D-1

Peripheral Vascular Complications and Associated Operative Mortality Rates in a Series of 40 Patients with Complicated Acute Type B Aortic Dissection[a]

Vascular complication	*Prevalence (n)*	*Operative mortality (n)*
Stroke	0% (0)	—
Paraplegia	3 ± 3% (1)	100% (1)
Pulse loss	20 ± 8% (8)	50 ± 18% (4)
Renal ischemia	8 ± 4% (3)	67 ± 28% (2)
Visceral ischemia	5 ± 3% (2)	50 ± 37% (1)

[a]Data from Fann JI, Sarris GE, Mitchell RS, et al: Treatment of patients with aortic dissection presenting with peripheral vascular complications. Ann Surg 212:705–713, 1990.

Table 69D-2

Location of Peripheral Pulse Deficits in 56 of 168 Patients with Acute Type A or Type B Aortic Dissection[a]

	Type A (n = 128)	*Type B (n = 40)*
Right carotid	6	0
Left carotid	6	0
Right arm	25	0
Left arm	10	2
Right leg	21	4
Left leg	14	3
Total	82	9

[a]Data from Fann JI, Sarris GE, Mitchell RS, et al: Treatment of patients with aortic dissection presenting with peripheral vascular complications. Ann Surg 212:705–713, 1990.

ness, dysphagia, hemoptysis (aortobronchial fistula or erosion into the lung), hematemesis (aortoesophageal fistula), and/or symptoms secondary to compromised flow in an important distal aortic branch.

DEFINITIVE DIAGNOSIS

Definitive diagnostic procedures should be performed as expeditiously as possible to confirm or rule out the diagnosis of acute type B aortic dissection. Before the widespread availability of newer imaging techniques, the diagnosis was generally made by conventional catheter aortography. Today, better options include computed tomographic angiographic (CTA) scanning, transesophageal echocardiography (TEE), and magnetic resonance angiography (MRA). Chest radiography is neither sensitive nor specific. The imaging modality chosen should determine the type of dissection, its extent, the localization of the PIT, and the presence or absence of aortic branch compromise. More than one imaging study may be necessary to confirm the diagnosis or to identify additional pathoanatomical details; in the IRAD registry, an average of 2.2 imaging studies were carried out in patients with acute type B dissection before definitive treatment.[30]

CTA scanning has markedly facilitated the rapid and accurate diagnosis of acute aortic dissection in most hospitals. In the majority of cases, a thin-slice spiral CTA with intravenous contrast can determine rapidly and noninvasively the dissection type (type A or B), as illustrated in Figure 69D-1. The extent of dissection, perfusion status of individual aortic branches, and size of the true and false lumens in all aortic segments can also be assessed accurately. Identification of two distinct lumens in the descending thoracic aorta separated by an intimal flap confirms the diagnosis of type B aortic dissection.[4] Other important signs include compression of the true lumen by the false lumen, displaced intimal calcification, a thrombosed false lumen, a nonopacified crescent-shaped area along the aortic wall (IMH), or an ulcer-like projection (ULP) of contrast material within the aortic wall, indicating a PAU.[28] The sensitivity and specificity of CTA in making the diagnosis of acute type B aortic dissection are between 82 and 100% and 89 and 100%, respectively.[*] In the 1993 study by Nienaber et al that prospectively evaluated noninvasive modalities in 110 patients with suspected acute dissection, the sensitivity and specificity of CT scanning were 96% and 89% in patients with type B dissection, while the positive and negative predictive values were 80% and 98%, respectively.[56] A drawback associated with CT scanning is the requirement for administration of intravenous contrast material.

In most centers worldwide, TEE is currently considered to be the initial diagnostic modality of choice in patients with suspected type B aortic dissection, and many patients do not require additional corroborative studies.[4,21,23,49,56] TEE is rapid, convenient, and noninvasive and can be performed in the emergency room, in the intensive care unit, or in the operating room with minimal risk. Undesirable blood pressure elevation is a potential risk of TEE, mandating adequate patient sedation. Multiplanar TEE with color flow imaging can accurately demonstrate flow in both aortic channels and the flap

[*]References 4, 23, 28, 49, 52, 56, 71, 78.

separating the true and false lumens. The most important finding is identification of an intimal flap, ideally seen in more than one view, oscillating independently of the motion of the aortic wall.[4,21,56,78] Frequently, the PIT and secondary fenestrations can also be identified. Overall, the sensitivity and specificity of TEE in the evaluation of suspected type B aortic dissection are between 97 and 100% and 94 and 98%, respectively.* Limitations of TEE include dependence on an experienced interpretation of the findings and limited capability to assess abdominal branch vessel involvement and extent of the dissection below the diaphragm.

Currently, MRA scanning does not play a major diagnostic role in patients with acute dissection because these individuals are often critically ill and connected to various monitoring devices, infusion pumps, or respirators.[18,49] In the acute setting, limited 24 h a day availability of MRA, the relatively long time necessary for image acquisition, and limited access to the patient during the procedure make MRA less practical than other diagnostic modalities. Nevertheless, MRA noninvasively can delineate the entire thoracoabdominal aorta and demonstrate the intimal flap, both aortic channels, and involvement of major aortic branches. As with CTA, the most important criteria used for the diagnosis of acute aortic dissection with MRA is the identification of two distinct flow lumens separated by an intimal flap.[4] Many investigators have reported that MRA is associated with high sensitivity and specificity in the evaluation of suspected aortic dissection, both in the range of 95–100%.† For suspected acute type B dissection, Nienaber et al observed that MRA was associated with a sensitivity of 97% and a specificity of 100%.[56] Today, magnetic resonance (MR) scans are most useful for serial, long-term follow-up of patients with chronic aortic dissections, including postoperative patients and those initially treated medically.

Contrast aortography historically was the gold standard in the diagnosis of aortic dissection (Figure 69D-2).[73] Angiography, however, is invasive, time consuming, and necessitates the use of contrast; moreover, it is not infallible, and the technique carries a risk of morbidity and mortality,[4,18,47] but can provide detailed information regarding perfusion status of important aortic branches. Angiographic diagnosis of acute dissection requires identification of a double lumen or an intimal flap; indirect signs that are suggestive of an acute dissection include compression of the true channel by an expanding false lumen, thickening of the aortic wall, ULP in the aortic wall (in cases of penetrating atherosclerotic ulcer), and abnormal position of the guidewire or catheter in the aorta.[4,6,26,73] Biplane angiographic studies of the thoracic aorta are mandatory because single-plane aortography can miss subtle findings; false-negative results can also occur when the false lumen is thrombosed and in cases of IMH.[4,23,26] The sensitivity and specificity of aortography in the evaluation of aortic dissection range between 80 and 90% and 85 and 95%, respectively.[4,23,49] Currently, aortography is reserved for patients with acute type B dissection presenting with clinical evidence of malperfusion or those with persistent peripheral vascular complications after proximal aortic repair, to delineate the mechanism of aortic branch vessel compromise before appropriate endovascular interventions are carried out to restore distal perfusion.[4,13,40,70]

*References 4, 21, 23, 49, 56, 71, 78.
†References 4, 21, 23, 49, 55, 56, 71, 78.

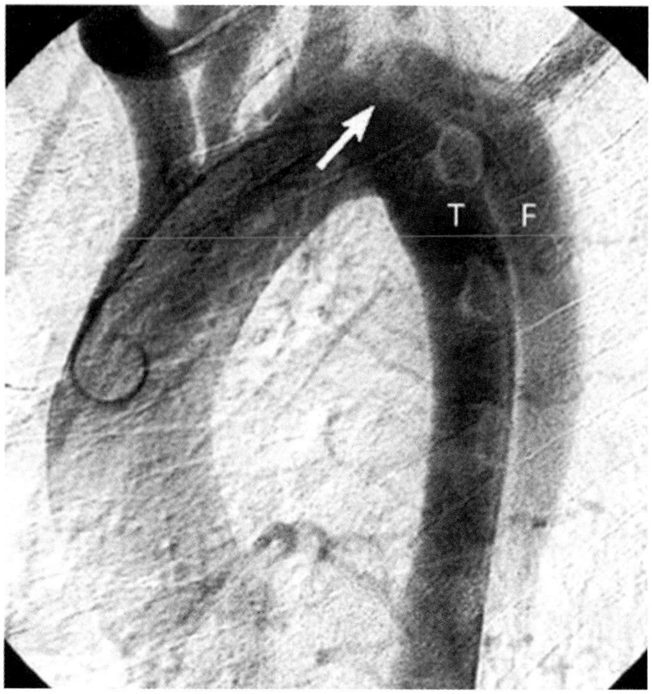

Figure 69D–2 Aortographic findings in acute type B aortic dissection. The true aortic lumen (T) is extrinsically narrowed by the false lumen (F). The true lumen is characteristically smaller and located medially. Note that the pigtail angiographic catheter has been passed up the true lumen from below. The primary intimal tear (*arrow*) is located just distal to the left subclavian artery.

MANAGEMENT

Strategy

The aim of therapy in patients with aortic dissection is to prevent death and irreversible end-organ damage. As discussed in Chapter 69C, almost all patients with acute type A dissection should be considered for emergency surgical repair of the ascending thoracic aorta.[10,17,23,49] In contrast, the optimal treatment strategy for patients with acute type B dissection continues to be debated.* In 1965, Wheat et al recommended medical "anti-impulse" therapy for acute aortic dissection,[79] but in 1970 Daily and colleagues from Stanford concluded that there was no major difference in early outcome between patients treated medically or surgically.[11] The rationale behind medical management is based on three observations. (1) Medical therapy prevents early death in the majority of patients.† (2) Operative mortality for patients with acute type B dissections has been relatively high.[27,30,45,49] (3) Long-term outcome has been similar between patients treated medically or surgically.‡ Today, most groups favor a complication-specific approach for patients with acute type B dissections (see Box 69D-1), reserving surgical replacement of the descending

*References 10, 11, 13, 17, 18, 20, 23, 27, 31, 37, 38, 42, 48–50, 54, 58, 66, 77.
†References 19, 23, 27, 30, 49, 77.
‡References 10, 17, 19, 27, 49, 77.

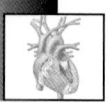

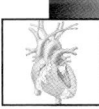

Box 69D–1. Firm or Relative Indications for Surgical Intervention in Patients with Acute Type B Aortic Dissection.

Persistent pain
Refractory arterial hypertension
Progression/expansion of dissection
Aortic rupture or impending rupture
Evidence of impaired distal organ perfusion
Sizable localized false aneurysm
Marfan syndrome

aorta for those with persistent pain, refractory hypertension, thoracoabdominal malperfusion, impending rupture, or other life-threatening complications.* Other conditions that should prompt consideration of early operation include extensive aortic arch involvement, expectations of poor medical compliance, and Marfan syndrome.[23,49] On the other hand, we and some other groups have advocated consideration of early surgical intervention for selected patients with acute type B dissections who are younger and otherwise good operative candidates, irrespective of the presence or absence of complications; this includes patients with connective tissue disorders such as Marfan syndrome.[31,38,48,49] If operation is successful, these patients theoretically should be at lower risk of sustaining late dissection-related complications or requiring aortic reoperation.

The Stanford aortic dissection classification concept has also been applied to intramural hematoma because the prognostic impact of the location and its treatment have been considered comparable to those for classic dissection.[26,57] It is generally accepted that patients with IMH involving the descending thoracic aorta (type B IMH) can be managed conservatively with aggressive blood pressure control in the absence of disease progression.[24,26,57,60] However, several groups recently reported that the prognosis of highly symptomatic patients with penetrating ulcers located in the descending thoracic aorta and type B IMH coexistent with a deep PAU was worse than that of those with classic aortic dissection, due to a higher incidence of aortic rupture.[6,26,76] In these cases, early surgical treatment should be considered, especially if persistent pain, increasing pleural effusion and/or a large, deep PAU are present.[26]

Initial Medical Treatment

As soon as acute aortic dissection is suspected, emergency medical therapy should be initiated and continued while the diagnostic procedures are performed.[18,23,49] The cornerstone of modern medical therapy, as originally described by Wheat and collaborators,[79,80] is reduction of mean, peak, and diastolic recoil arterial pressure and the rate of rise of arterial pressure, or aortic dP/dt (not left ventricular dP/dt) to the lowest acceptable level while maintaining adequate cerebral, coronary, and renal perfusion.[23,49] The goal of medical treatment is to relieve pain, control blood pressure, and limit extension of the dissection. Intensive, continuous patient monitoring in an intensive care unit is important, including electrocardiogram (ECG) and insertion of indwelling radial or femoral arterial and central venous lines. A urinary bladder catheter and a pulse oximeter are used. Intravenous β-blockers (e.g., esmolol, metoprolol, labetalol, propranolol) are administered in small boluses or as a continuous intravenous infusion along with an intravenous vasodilator infusion, most commonly sodium nitroprusside. Labetalol, an α_1-adrenergic and nonspecific β-adrenergic antagonist, is a good alternative to a combination of agents. Parenteral calcium channel antagonists like diltiazem or nifedipine that lower arterial blood pressure and left ventricular dP/dt can also be used. Because sodium nitroprusside and angiotensin-converting enzyme (ACE) inhibitors (e.g., enalapril, lisinopril) are pure arteriolar vasodilators, these agents actually increase aortic dP/dt; therefore, concomitant administration of a negative inotropic agent is essential. If surgical intervention or percutaneous endovascular techniques are carried out, antihypertensive and negative inotropic therapy are continued during anesthetic induction, intraoperatively, and postoperatively.

Definitive Long-Term Medical Management

Whether the patient is initially treated medically or surgically, the intravenous antihypertensive and negative inotropic drugs are gradually transitioned to oral agents during the hospitalization. Oral β-blockers (e.g., labetalol, metoprolol, atenolol) and calcium channel antagonists are preferentially used and continued indefinitely, complimented by oral ACE inhibitors, such as lisinopril. Hydralazine should probably be avoided since it is incorporated into mucopolysaccharides of the media and may weaken the aortic wall.[49]

Operative Approach

The goal of surgical treatment of patients with acute type B aortic dissection is graft replacement of a segment of the descending thoracic aorta, preferably including the site of the PIT.[49] At Stanford University, after induction of general anesthesia, insertion of a double-lumen endobronchial tube, and often a lumbar intrathecal catheter for cerebrospinal fluid drainage,[8,47,49] patients with acute type B dissections are explored through a left posterolateral thoracotomy. Full cardiopulmonary bypass (CPB) with antegrade perfusion is preferred using a long right femoral venous catheter advanced into the right atrium and an arterial CPB cannula inserted in either the left subclavian artery (LSCA), a short 6-mm graft anastomosed end to side to the LSCA, the undissected ascending aorta, the descending aortic true lumen (using TEE guidance), the left ventricular apex and across the aortic valve,[75] the left common carotid artery,[53] or, if absolutely necessary, the femoral artery on the side that is perfused by the distal aortic true lumen (usually the one with the reduced or absent pulse). Occasionally, if a venous cannula cannot be passed from below, an angled venous cannula can be placed through the pulmonary artery into the right ventricle to augment venous CPB return. Moderate hypothermia (25–28° C) is generally employed such that an open proximal anastomosis (OPA) can be performed in the distal arch during a brief period of hypothermic circulatory arrest (HCA); HCA is also employed in most cases of chronic type B dissection.[9,36] The patient is placed in a steep Trendelenburg position and uncontrolled venous retroperfusion at 400–500 ml/min is

*References 10, 20, 23, 27, 42, 49, 50, 66, 77.

used during HCA to keep the left heart and ascending aorta free of air. No preliminary proximal or distal aortic dissection is done, and no aortic cross-clamps are applied either proximally or distally. When the pump is turned down, the proximal aorta is opened and transected after mobilization of the phrenic, vagus, and recurrent laryngeal nerves. An OPA is performed on the full-thickness aortic cuff (thereby reapproximating the aortic intima and adventitia and obliterating any proximal false lumen) at the distal arch level. A 6.5-mm metal angled arterial perfusion cannula is then inserted into the graft, and after arch deairing, CPB perfusion to the head and the heart is resumed and systemic warming started. Proximal intercostal arteries are oversewn. A conservative segment of descending aorta containing the intimal tear and the most severe associated injury is replaced with a woven double velour Dacron graft using continuous 4-0 polypropylene sutures with a fine needle using deep, but closely spaced suture bites,[49] again taking care to incorporate both aortic layers and obliterate the false lumen. Before the anastomosis, the distal aorta can be reinforced using strips of Teflon felt or bovine pericardium, or alternatively biological glue, such as BioGlue (CryoLife, Inc., Kennesaw, GA), if necessary. The proximal cross-clamp is released, air is evacuated, and the anastomoses are checked for hemostasis. After warming to 35–36° C, CPB is discontinued.

Postoperative patient management involves intensive monitoring, including serial abdominal, neurological, and pulse examinations, as well as strict blood pressure control. Cerebrospinal fluid (CSF) is drained continuously to keep CSF pressure lower than 10 mm Hg. In patients without spinal cord injury, the drain is removed on the second or third postoperative day. Using partial CPB (without HCA) and confining the extent of resection to a short aortic segment, the incidence of new postoperative paraplegia in our earlier experience was 4% in patients with acute type B dissections.[45]

Management of Peripheral Vascular Complications

The Stanford approach in patients presenting with aortic dissection complicated by ischemic peripheral vascular complications prior to the advent of stent-grafting was to proceed initially with surgical repair of the thoracic aorta, since central aortic repair usually obviated the need for peripheral revascularization procedures.[22,49] The operative mortality rate for patients with all types of peripheral vascular compromise was no higher that that for those without such complications; however, visceral ischemia and impaired renal perfusion were associated with a very high risk of death. If persistent mesenteric, renal, or limb ischemia is detected following thoracic aortic repair, traditionally surgical fenestration of the distal descending thoracic aorta or suprarenal abdominal aorta or direct revascularization was attempted as a life-saving maneuvers.[3,22,49] Today, percutaneous endovascular techniques are the preferred initial intervention in cases of postoperative malperfusion, and also in high-risk patients with complicated acute type B dissections who are not undergoing operation[40,68,69,81] (see Chapter 70). Catheter-based bare stenting of the collapsed true lumen in the aorta or one of its branches and/or flap fenestration of the dissection septum (to increase flow in the distal true lumen by decompressing the false lumen) can successfully reestablish end-organ perfusion in most cases.[69,81] These endovascular approaches are described in detail in Chapter 70. More recently, endovascular stent-grafts have been used in patients with *complicated* acute type B dissections to cover the PIT in the thoracic aorta and restore blood flow in the distal aortic true lumen, which can be "obliterated" or "collapsed"; this successfully relieved distal ischemia in 76% of all compromised aortic branches (and 100% of those with "dynamic" obstructions), which was very encouraging.[12,13]

Endovascular Stent-Grafts

Since 1996, endovascular stent-grafts have been employed in selected patients with acute type B aortic dissections at Stanford.[13] The Stanford University and MIT combined series showed that endovascular stent-graft repair in patients with acute type B dissections who had life-threatening complications was associated with an early mortality rate of 16%. The long-term effectiveness and durability of this new therapeutic approach, however, remain unknown. Rigorous prospective comparison of this interventional approach with conventional surgical treatment (for *complicated* type B dissections) and with medical therapy (for *uncomplicated* type B dissections) is needed and important. This topic is discussed further in Chapter 70.

Chronic Type B Dissections

Surgical intervention for patients with chronic type B dissection is considered if symptoms related to the dissection (e.g., pain, symptoms secondary to compression of adjacent anatomical structures, renovascular hypertension [with or without renal dysfunction], mesenteric ischemia, claudication) or documented expansion of the false lumen occurs. Asymptomatic patients with large aortic dissections (exceeding 50–60 mm in diameter) are also offered surgical graft replacement if they are reasonable surgical candidates; in addition to maximal aortic diameter and symptoms, consideration of other risk factors that modulate the expected risk of aortic rupture, viz., increasing age, connective tissue disorders, uncontrolled hypertension, and chronic obstructive pulmonary disease, is also important to determine the optimal timing for operation.[5,34]

RESULTS

Comparison of Results of Surgical and Medical Treatment

Historical Perspective

The controversy regarding the optimal therapy for aortic dissections dates back to the 1960s, when DeBakey and colleagues reported results in 179 patients treated surgically with an early mortality of 21% and a 5-year survival rate of 50%.[15] DeBakey concluded that all patients with aortic dissection should undergo surgical intervention. Importantly, careful inspection of this paper subsequently revealed a very skewed patient population: only 38% of the patients had an acute dissection, and the majority had a DeBakey type III (Stanford type B) dissection. Wheat and associates then proposed a selective approach to the management of patients with acute dissection, arguing for medical treatment using a combination of agents that decreased arterial blood pressure and also the rate of rise of aortic pressure (aortic *dP/dt*).[79,80] In 1970, Daily et al introduced the Stanford type A/B dissection classification system and observed that there was no major difference in early outcome in patients with type B dissections treated medically or surgically. In a 1979 Stanford paper, the early results from 11 studies published in the 1970s were analyzed. The overall mortality rate in this era was 33% in medically treated patients (range 21–67%), while the average operative mortality rate for patients with acute type B dissections treated surgically was 36%.[43] Of course, the patient cohorts differed considerably, which confounded critical comparison of outcomes. Thereafter, the consensus opinion has been that most patients with acute type B dissections be treated medically, unless life-threatening dissection-related complications are present.*

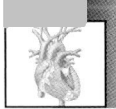

Contemporary Comparative Studies of Surgical versus Medical Treatment

No prospective, controlled trials comparing surgical with medical management of patients with acute type B dissections have been carried out; however, comprehensive, comparative retrospective analyses, including a 2002 report from Stanford, have been published.[27,65,77] Strict interpretation of the results of these two treatment modalities is difficult because of a marked disparity in risk factors between the medical and surgical cohorts, leading to a pronounced selection bias; in most series, patients with *uncomplicated* acute type B dissections were treated medically, while those presenting with life-threatening complications or developing complications while being treated medically are frequently treated surgically while *in extremis*.

A 1984 report from the Massachusetts General Hospital concluded that early survival in patients presenting with an acute type B dissection was determined primarily by the number and severity of presenting complications due to the dissection, irrespective of mode of treatment.[65] In the 1989 Stanford and Duke University study, 136 patients with acute and chronic type B dissections between 1975 and 1988 were treated medically (63%) or surgically (37%); patients treated medically tended to have more comorbidities or renal disease, while those in the surgical cohort were more likely to have aortic rupture or arch involvement.[27,50] Sequential analyses were performed to adjust for differences in baseline patient characteristics to separate patients with acute dissections into three subgroups: all patients (subset I), patients presenting without compelling indications for emergency operation (subset II), and those individuals from subset II who did not have severe comorbidities (subset III). This last cohort represented *low-risk, uncomplicated* patients who could have been treated either medically or surgically. For all patients, the significant determinants of overall mortality were aortic rupture, other dissection-related complications, increasing age, and cardiac disease. Treatment method was not a significant predictor of outcome in any subset. Moreover, in the low-risk subset of patients (subset III), early mortality rate was similar between the medically and surgically treated patients (16% versus 9%), as was long-term survival. More recently, a 36-year review of the Stanford experience including 189 patients with acute type B dissections used propensity score analysis to identify subsets of patients treated either medically or surgically who were at similar risks of death; the impact of mode of treatment on survival, reoperation, and late aortic complications or death was then determined in these more homogeneous cohorts.[77] This statistical analysis identified 142 well-matched patients who did not have any compelling emergency surgical indications (111 were treated medically and 31 underwent operation.). As illustrated in Figure 69D-3, long-term survival was similar for both groups. Freedom from reoperation and from late aortic complications or death were also comparable between the medically treated and surgical subsets. In all patients, multivariable analyses did not identify mode of treatment to be a significant predictor of outcome; instead, patient-related factors and dissection-specific complications determined the prognosis.

*References 2, 10, 17–19, 44, 46, 47, 59, 74.

Current Results

Early Survival

Over the past 30 years, advances in diagnostic imaging modalities, medical critical care, anesthetic expertise, and surgical techniques have allowed clinicians to make the definitive diagnosis more quickly and have improved early survival rate of patients with acute type B aortic dissection.* In the 2002 Stanford paper, the early mortality rate for patients treated medically did not change significantly between 1970 and 1999, ranging from 10 to 19% (Figure 69D-4). On the other hand, the early mortality rate for patients treated surgically decreased from 57% in the 1960s to 27% in the 1990s.[77] In the 2000 IRAD report of 175 patients with acute type B dissections treated in 12 centers between 1996 and 1998, 30-day mortality was 11% in medically treated patients and 31% in patients who underwent surgery[30]; of course, the two patient cohorts were markedly different. Crawford and associates and the Mount Sinai group also demonstrated that low operative mortality and morbidity

*References 20, 23, 24, 38, 49, 50, 66, 74.

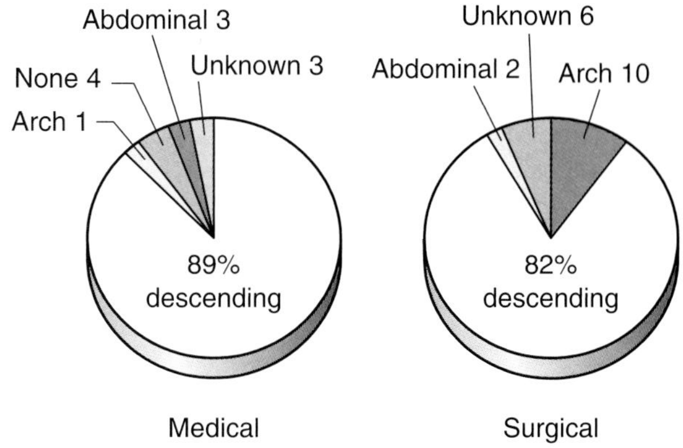

Figure 69D–3 **Site of primary intimal tear in 189 patients with acute type B aortic dissection treated at Stanford between 1963 and 1999, broken down into medical and surgical subgroups.**
(From Umana JP, Lai DT, Mitchell RS, et al: Is medical therapy still the optimal treatment strategy for patients with acute type B aortic dissections? J Thorac Cardiovasc Surg 124:896–910, 2002; with permission.)

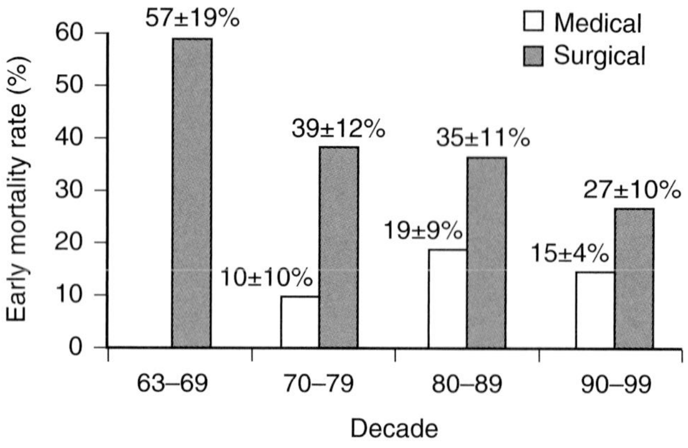

Figure 69D–4 Early (30-day) mortality rates illustrated as a function of time (decades) and broken down into medical and surgical subgroups in the overall Stanford experience. *(From Umana JP, Lai DT, Mitchell RS, et al: Is medical therapy still the optimal treatment strategy for patients with acute type B aortic dissections? J Thorac Cardiovasc Surg 124:896–910, 2002; with permission.)*

rates can be achieved in the current era in selected patients with acute type B dissections.[28,66,74] In an earlier Stanford study, multivariable analysis revealed that the independent determinants of operative risk in patients with type B dissections (acute or chronic) were renal or visceral ischemia, aortic rupture, and older age.[45] Acute type B dissection due to an intimal tear located in the arch, whether the patient was treated medically or surgically, was associated with high early mortality rates in a subsequent Duke–Stanford cooperative report.[27] In Crawford's surgical experience, the independent risk factors portending operative death were earlier year of operation, surgery within 24 h of onset of symptoms, and chronic obstructive pulmonary disease.[74]

Late Survival

In the 36-year Stanford experience, overall actuarial survival for the entire patient cohort was 71, 60, 35, and 17% at 1, 5, 10, and 15 years, respectively.[77] As illustrated in Figure 69D-5A, there was no significant difference in survival between the medical and surgical patients. Multivariable analyses identified shock, visceral ischemia, arch involvement, aortic rupture, stroke, previous sternotomy, pulmonary disease, and female gender as significant, independent predictors of overall death. In the Baylor University series, actuarial survival after surgical repair of type B dissections was 76, 54, and 35% at 1, 5, and 10 years[74]; independent determinants of late death were earlier year of operation, older age, severe symptoms, higher New York Heart Association functional class, extent of aorta replaced, type of procedure, residual aneurysmal disease, and postoperative complications. Congestive heart failure, renal failure, stroke, and cancer accounted for almost 50% of the late deaths in patients with acute type B dissection in the Stanford series, emphasizing the importance of patient-specific factors in determining the long-term prognosis.[77] Rupture of a contiguous or remote segment of the aorta was responsible for 16% of late deaths in this Stanford series, compared to 29% of late deaths in the 20-year long-term follow-up study from DeBakey et al.[16] This sobering figure should be amenable to improvement if more diligent serial patient follow-up imaging is provided.

Freedom from Aortic Reoperation

The actuarial freedom from late aortic reoperation and late aortic-related complications after acute type B dissection in the overall Stanford experience is shown in Figures 69D-5B–D. Surprisingly, there was no significant difference in reoperation rate between patients treated medically and those treated surgically.[77] After 5 years, reoperation was necessary in 14% of the medical group and 13% of the surgical patients; at 10 years, reoperation was necessary in 17% of both groups. The only independent predictor of late aortic reoperation was Marfan syndrome, underscoring the fragility of the dissected aorta in these patients. In Crawford's 1990 study analyzing a 33-year experience with surgical management of aortic dissection (type A or B, acute or chronic), 22% of patients required aortic reoperation 10 years later and 88% were free from aortic rupture.[74] Residual aneurysmal disease, no cardioplegia (probably indicative of improved surgical techniques over time), and preoperative New York Heart Association functional class were the determinants of late aortic rupture; a higher likelihood of reoperation was significantly linked to earlier year of operation, previous proximal aortic procedure, aortic cross-clamp time, and more limited surgical procedures (e.g., primary repair, aortoplasty, patch repair). More recently, Marui and associates in a retrospective analysis of 101 patients with uncomplicated acute type B dissections treated medically reported that a persistently patent false lumen during the acute phase and aortic diameter exceeding 40 mm were predictors of late aneurysm formation; these authors recommended that such patients be considered for early operation.[42]

FOLLOW-UP

In patients with acute type B aortic dissection—whether they initially were treated medically or surgically—an early predischarge CTA or MRI scan is mandatory to rule out early complications and to serve as a baseline imaging study. During the first few weeks, these patients require close outpatient medical care; attention should be focused on arterial blood pressure control and cerebral, cardiac, and renal function.[49] Periodic imaging studies of the entire thoracic and abdominal aorta are essential indefinitely to detect aortic complications, such as aneurysmal degeneration of the false lumen, before rupture or death. The interval between imaging studies is gradually increased from 3 to 6 months over the first year following the acute event if no worrisome changes are detected, and then annually thereafter. Lifelong rigorous arterial blood pressure control and negative inotropic therapy are also critical. In DeBakey's 1982 report, late aneurysmal formation occurred in 45% of patients with poor blood pressure control, compared to 17% of those with well-controlled hypertension.[16] A combination of conventional antihypertensive agents and negative inotropic medications, such as oral β-blockers or calcium antagonists, is usually required and needs to be continued indefinitely, even in normotensive patients.

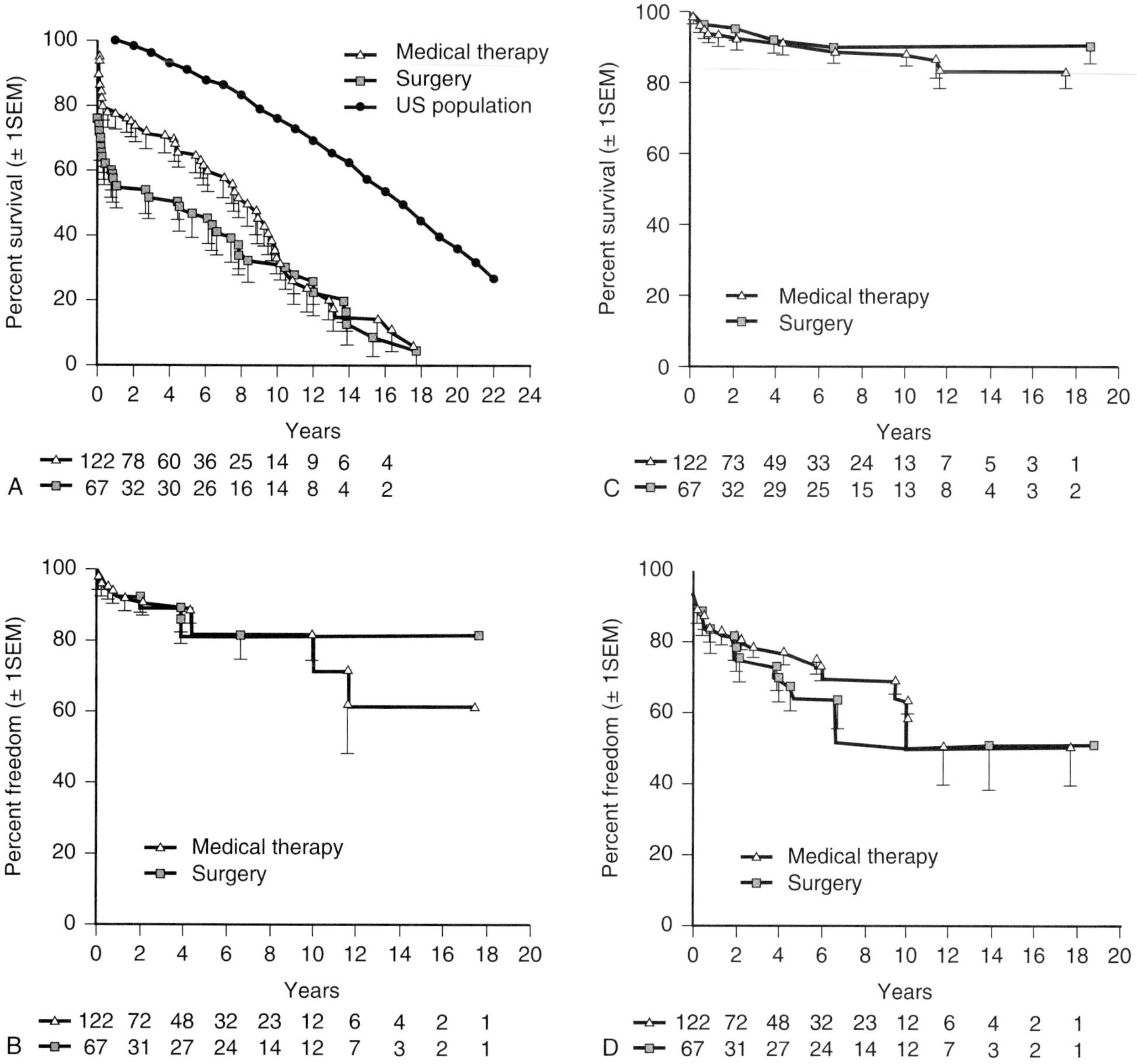

Figure 69D–5 **A,** Actuarial survival for all patients with acute type B dissections subdivided according to initial treatment method. There was no statistically significant difference in survival between those treated surgically and those treated medically. For perspective, this graph also portrays the survival curve for age- and gender-matched U.S. population; this indicates that only 35% of patients this age can be expected to be alive 20 years later. **B,** Actuarial freedom from late aortic reoperation (defined as surgical procedures related to the aorta or to complications of the dissection) subdivided according to initial treatment. There was no statistically significant difference between treatment modalities. **C,** Freedom from reoperation for all patients, expressed in actual (or observed cumulative frequency) terms. **D,** Actuarial freedom from late aortic-related complications or death for all 189 patients.

(From Umana JP, Lai DT, Mitchell RS, et al: Is medical therapy still the optimal treatment strategy for patients with acute type B aortic dissections? J Thorac Cardiovasc Surg 124:896–910, 2002; with permission.)

REFERENCES

1. Anagnostopoulos CE, Prabhakar MJS, Vittle CF: Aortic dissections and dissecting aneurysms. Am J Cardiol 30: 263–273, 1972.
2. Applebaum A, Karp RB, Kirklin JW: Ascending vs. descending aortic dissections. Ann Surg 183:296–300, 1976.
3. Cambria RP, Brewster DC, Gertler J, et al: Vascular complications associated with spontaneous aortic dissection. J Vasc Surg 7:199–202, 1988.
4. Cigarroa JE, Isselbacher EM, DeSanctis RW, et al: Diagnostic imaging in the evaluation of suspected aortic dissection. N Engl J Med 328:35–43, 1993.
5. Coady MA, Rizzo JA, Hammond GL, et al: What is the appropriate size criterion for resection of thoracic aortic aneurysms? J Thorac Cardiovasc Surg 113:476–491, 1997.
6. Coady MA, Rizzo JA, Hammond GL, et al: Penetrating ulcer of the thoracic aorta: What is it? How do we recognize it? How do we manage it? J Vasc Surg 27:1006–1016, 1998.

7. Cooley DA, DeBakey ME, Morris GC Jr: Controlled extracorporeal circulation in surgical treatment of aortic aneurysm. Ann Surg 146:473, 1957.
8. Coselli JS, Lemaire SA, Koksoy C, et al: Cerebrospinal fluid drainage reduces paraplegia after thoracoabdominal aortic aneurysm repair: results of a randomized clinical trial. J Vasc Surg 35:631–639, 2002.
9. Crawford ES, Coselli JS, Safi HJ: Partial cardiopulmonary bypass, hypothermic circulatory arrest, and posterolateral exposure for thoracic aneurysm operation. J Thorac Cardiovasc Surg 94:824–827, 1987.
10. Crawford ES: The diagnosis and management of aortic dissection. JAMA 264:2537–2541, 1990.
11. Daily PO, Trueblood HW, Stinson EB, et al: Management of acute aortic dissections. Ann Thorac Surg 10:237–247, 1970.
12. Dake MD, Semba CP, Razavi MK, et al: Endovascular procedures for the treatment of aortic dissection: techniques and results. J Cardiovasc Surg 39(Suppl. 1):45–52, 1998.
13. Dake MD, Kato N, Mitchell RS, et al: Endovascular stent-graft placement for the treatment of acute aortic dissection. N Engl J Med 340:1546–1552, 1999.
14. DeBakey ME, Cooley D, Creech O Jr: Surgical considerations of dissecting aneurysm of the aorta. Ann Surg 142:586–612, 1955.
15. DeBakey ME, Henly WS, Cooley DA, et al: Surgical management of dissecting aneurysms of the aorta. J Thorac Cardiovasc Surg 49:130–149, 1965.
16. DeBakey ME, McCollum CH, Crawford ES, et al: Dissection and dissecting aneurysms of the aorta: twenty-year follow-up of five hundred and twenty-seven patients treated surgically. Surgery 92:1118–1134, 1982.
17. DeSanctis RW, Doroghazi RM, Austen WG, Buckley MJ: Aortic dissection. N Engl J Med 317:1060–1067, 1987.
18. DeSanctis RW, Eagle KA: Aortic dissection. Curr Probl Cardiol 14:227–278, 1989.
19. Doroghazi RM, Slater EE, DeSanctis RW, et al: Long-term survival of patients with treated aortic dissections. J Am Coll Cardiol 3:1026–1034, 1984.
20. Elefteriades JA, Lovoulos CJ, Coady MA, et al: Management of descending aortic dissection. Ann Thorac Surg 67:2002–2005, 1999.
21. Erbel R, Engbergbing R, Daniel W, et al: Echocardiography in the diagnosis of aortic dissection. Lancet 1:457–461, 1989.
22. Fann JI, Sarris GE, Mitchell RS, et al: Treatment of patients with aortic dissection presenting with peripheral vascular complications. Ann Surg 212:705–713, 1990.
23. Fann JI, Miller DC: Aortic dissection. Ann Vasc Surg 9:311–323, 1995.
24. Fann JI, Smith JA, Miller DC, et al: Surgical management of aortic dissection during a 30-year period. Circulation 92(Suppl. II):II-113–121, 1995.
25. Farber A, Wagner WH, Cossman DV, et al: Isolated dissection of the abdominal aorta: clinical presentation and therapeutic options. J Vasc Surg 36:205–210, 2002.
26. Ganaha F, Miller DC, Sugimoto K, et al: Prognosis of aortic intramural hematoma with and without penetrating atherosclerotic ulcer. A clinical and radiologic analysis. Circulation 106:342–348, 2002.
27. Glower DD, Fann JI, Speier RH, et al: Comparison of medical and surgical therapy for uncomplicated descending aortic dissection. Circulation 82(Suppl. IV):39–46, 1990.
28. Godwin JD, Herfkens RL, Skioldebrand CG, et al: Evaluation of dissections and aneurysms of the thoracic aorta by conventional and dynamic CT scanning. Radiology 136:135–139, 1980.
29. Gurin D, Bulmer JW, Derby R: Dissecting aneurysm of aorta: Diagnosis and operative relief of acute arterial obstruction due to this cause. NY State J Med 35:1200–1202, 1935.
30. Hagan PG, Nienaber CA, Isselbacher EM, et al: The international registry of acute aortic dissection (IRAD). JAMA 283:897–903, 2000.
31. Haverich A: Letter to Hans Georg Borst. J Thorac Cardiovasc Surg 124:891–893, 2002.
32. Hirst AE, Johns VJ, Krime SJ: Dissecting aneurysm of the aorta: a review of 505 cases. Medicine 37:217–279, 1958.
33. Hirst AE, Gore I: Is cystic medionecrosis the cause of dissecting aortic aneurysm? Am Heart J 53:915–916, 1976.
34. Juvonen T, Ergin MA, Galla JD, et al: Risk factors for rupture of chronic type B dissections. J Thorac Cardiovasc Surg 117:776–786, 1999.
35. Khan IA, Nair CK: Clinical, diagnostic, and management perspectives of aortic dissection. Chest 122:311–328, 2002.
36. Kouchoukos NT, Massetti P, Rokkas CK, et al: Safety and efficacy of hypothermic cardiopulmonary bypass and circulatory arrest for operations on the descending thoracic and thoracoabdominal aorta. Ann Thorac Surg 72:699–708, 2001.
37. Lansman SL, McCullough JN, Nguyen KH, et al: Subtypes of acute aortic dissection. Ann Thorac Surg 67:1975–1978, 1999.
38. Lansman SL, Hagl C, Fink D, et al: Acute type B aortic dissection: surgical therapy. Ann Thorac Surg 74:S1833–S1835, 2002.
39. Larson EW, Edwards WD: Risk factors for aortic dissection: a necropsy study of 161 cases. Am J Cardiol 53:849–855, 1984.
40. Lauterbach SR, Cambria RP, Brewster DC, et al: Contemporary management of aortic branch compromise resulting from acute aortic dissection. J Vasc Surg 33:1185–1192, 2001.
41. Lindsay J Jr, Hurst JW: Clinical features and prognosis in dissecting aneurysms of the aorta: a re-appraisal. Circulation 35:880–888, 1967.
42. Marui A, Mochizuki T, Mitsui N, et al: Toward the best treatment of uncomplicated patients with type B acute aortic dissection. A consideration for sound surgical intervention. Circulation 100(Suppl. II):II-275–280, 1999.
43. Miller DC, Stinson EB, Oyer PE, et al: Operative treatment of aortic dissections. J Thorac Cardiovasc Surg 78:365–382, 1979.
44. Miller DC: Surgical management of aortic dissections: indications, perioperative management, and long-term results. In Doroghazi RM, Slater EE, editors: Aortic Dissection. New York: McGraw-Hill, 1983, pp. 193–243.
45. Miller DC, Mitchell RS, Oyer PE, et al: Independent determinants of operative mortality for patients with aortic dissections. Circulation 70(Suppl. I):I-153–164, 1984.
46. Miller DC: Acute dissection of the aorta—continuing need for earlier diagnosis and treatment. Modern Concepts Cardiovasc Dis 54:51–55, 1985.
47. Miller DC: Surgical treatment of aortic dissections. In Jamieson SW, Shumway NE, editors: Operative Surgery—Cardiac Surgery. London: Butterworth, 1986, pp. 526–537.
48. Miller DC: Surgical management of acute aortic dissection: new data. Semin Thorac Cardiovasc Surg 3:225–237, 1991.
49. Miller DC: Acute dissection of the descending thoracic aorta. Chest Surg Clin North Am 2:347–378, 1992.
50. Miller DC: The continuing dilemma concerning medical versus surgical management of patients with acute type B dissections. Sem Thorac Cardiovasc Surg 5:33–46, 1993.
51. Ming RL, Najafi H, Javid H, et al: Acute ascending aortic dissection: surgical management. Circulation 64(Suppl. II): II-231–234, 1981.
52. Moore AG, Eagle KA, Bruckman D, et al: Choice of computed tomography, transesophageal echocardiography, magnetic resonance imaging, and aortography in acute aortic dissection: International Registry of Acute Aortic Dissection (IRAD). Am J Cardiol 89:1235–1238, 2002.
53. Neri E, Massetti M, Barabesi L, et al: Extrathoracic cannulation of the left common carotid artery in thoracic aorta

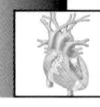

operations through a left thoracotomy: preliminary experience in 26 patients. J Thorac Cardiovasc Surg 123:901–910, 2002.
54. Neya K, Omoto R, Kyo S, et al: Outcome of Stanford type B dissection. Circulation 86(Suppl. II):II-1–7, 1992.
55. Nienaber CA, Spielmann RP, von Kodolitsch Y, et al: Diagnosis of thoracic aortic dissection. Magnetic resonance imaging versus transesophageal echocardiography. Circulation 85:434–447, 1992.
56. Nienaber CA, von Kodolitsch Y, Petersen B, et al: The diagnosis of thoracic aortic dissection by noninvasive imaging procedures. N Engl J Med 328:1–9, 1993.
57. Nienaber CA, von Kodolitsch Y, Petersen B, et al: Intramural hemorrhage of the thoracic aorta: diagnostic and therapeutic implications. Circulation 92:1465–1472, 1995.
58. Nienaber CA, Fattori R, Lund G, et al: Nonsurgical reconstruction of thoracic aortic dissection by stent-graft placement. N Engl J Med 340:1539–1545, 1999.
59. Reul GJ, Cooley DA, Hallman GL, et al: Dissecting aneurysm of the descending aorta. Arch Surg 110:632–640, 1975.
60. Robbins RC, MacNamus RP, Mitchell RS, et al: Management of patients with intramural hematoma of the thoracic aorta. Circulation 88(Suppl. II):II1–10, 1993.
61. Roberts CS, Roberts WC: Aortic dissection with entrance tear in the descending thoracic aorta: analysis of 40 necropsy patients. Ann Surg 231:356–368, 1991.
62. Roberts CS, Roberts WC: Aortic dissection with the entrance tear in abdominal aorta. Am Heart J 121:1834–1835, 1991.
63. Roberts WC: Aortic dissection: anatomy, consequences, and cause. Am Heart J 101:195–214, 1981.
64. Schlatmann TJM, Becker AE: Histologic changes in the normal aging aorta. Implications for dissecting aortic aneurysm. Am J Cardiol 39:13–20, 1977.
65. Schlatmann TJM, Becker AE: Pathogenesis of dissecting aneurysm of the aorta. Comparative histopathologic study of significance of medial changes. Am J Cardiol 39:21–26, 1977.
66. Schor JS, Yerlioglu E, Galla JD, et al: Selective management of acute type B aortic dissection: long-term follow-up. Ann Thorac Surg 61:1339–1341, 1996.
67. Slater EE: Aortic dissection: presentation and diagnosis. In Doroghazi RM, Slater EE, editors: Aortic Dissection. New York: McGraw-Hill, 1983, pp. 61–70.
68. Slonim SM, Nyman UR, Semba CP, et al: True lumen obliteration in complicated aortic dissection: endovascular treatment. Radiology 201:161–166, 1996.
69. Slonim SM, Nyman URO, Semba CP, et al: Aortic dissection: percutaneous management of ischemic complications with endovascular stents and balloon fenestration. J Vasc Surg 23:241–253, 1996.
70. Slonim SM, Miller DC, Mitchell RS, et al: Percutaneous balloon fenestrating and stenting for life-threatening ischemic complications in patients with acute aortic dissection. J Thorac Cardiovasc Surg 117:1118–1127, 1999.
71. Sommer T, Fehske W, Holzknecht N, et al: Aortic dissection: a comparative study of diagnosis with spiral CT, multiplanar transesophageal echocardiography and MR imaging. Radiology 199:347–352, 1996.
72. Stanson AW, Kazmier FJ, Hollier LH, et al: Penetrating atherosclerotic ulcers of the thoracic aorta: natural history and clinicopathologic correlations. Ann Vasc Surg 1:15–23, 1986.
73. Stein HL, Steinberg I: Selective aortography, the definitive technique for diagnosis of dissecting aneurysm of the aorta. Am J Roentgenol 102:333–348, 1968.
74. Svensson LG, Crawford ES, Hess KR, et al: Dissection of the aorta and dissecting aneurysms: improving early and long-term surgical results. Circulation 82(Suppl. 4):24–38, 1990.
75. Tanaka T, Kawamura T, Ohara K, et al: Transapical aortic perfusion with a double-barreled cannula. Ann Thorac Surg 25:209–214, 1978.
76. Tittle SL, Lynch RJ, Cole PE, et al: Midterm follow-up of penetrating ulcer and intramural hematoma of the aorta. J Thorac Cardiovasc Surg 123:1051–1059, 2002.
77. Umana JP, Lai DT, Mitchell RS, et al: Is medical therapy still the optimal treatment strategy for patients with acute type B aortic dissections? J Thorac Cardiovasc Surg 124:896–910, 2002.
78. Urban BA, Bleumke DA, Johnson KM, et al: Imaging of thoracic aortic disease. Cardiol Clin 17:659–682, 1999.
79. Wheat MW, Palmer RF, Bantley TD, et al: Treatment of dissecting aneurysms of the aorta without surgery. J Thorac Cardiovasc Surg 50:364–373, 1965.
80. Wheat MW, Harris PD, Malm JR, et al: Acute dissecting aneurysms of the aorta: results of treatment in 64 patients. J Thorac Cardiovasc Surg 58:344–351, 1969.
81. Williams DM, Lee DY, Hamilton BH, et al: The dissected aorta: percutaneous treatment of ischemic complications—principles and results. J Vasc Interv Radiol 8:605–625, 1997.
82. Yun KL, Glower DD, Miller DC, et al: Aortic dissection resulting from tear of transverse arch: is concomitant arch repair warranted? J Thorac Cardiovasc Surg 102:355–368, 1991.

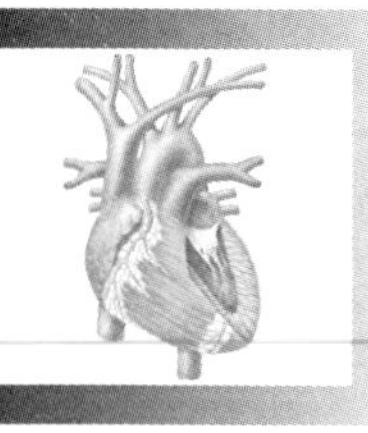

CHAPTER 70

Endovascular Therapy for the Treatment of Thoracic Aortic Aneurysms and Dissections

Susan D. Moffatt-Bruce and R. Scott Mitchell

INTRODUCTION

The treatment of thoracic aorta pathology is problematic because of a population that is often elderly, frail, and without physiological reserve. Associated cardiovascular disease, renal insufficiency, and pulmonary disease make operative intervention hazardous, frequently resulting in significant morbidity and mortality. Successful operative treatment of the thoracic aorta was initially reported in the 1950s when Swan, Lam, and DeBakey used segmental resection for a thoracic aneurysm; DeBakey and Cooley subsequently reported the successful repair of an ascending aortic aneurysm using cardiopulmonary bypass.[12,23,48,80] Over the ensuing 50 years, advances in diagnostic imaging coupled with improvement in surgical technique and perioperative care have improved thoracic aortic surgical outcomes. Additionally, the pathophysiology and natural history of thoracic aortic disease have slowly been elucidated, allowing more appropriate surgical timing and management.[2,31,34] The treatment of thoracic aortic disease remains, nonetheless, a highly specialized field requiring a multidisciplinary team approach.

In an effort to reduce the morbidity and mortality associated with surgical repair of the thoracic aorta, surgeons and interventional radiologist have united forces to develop, and subsequently introduce, endovascular stent-grafting.[5,64,69,85] Endovascular techniques were initially designed for high-risk surgical patients, but successful outcomes have allowed the expansion of this technology to use in younger, healthier patients.* Originally described by Parodi et al[64] for use in abdominal aortic aneurysms, endovascular stent-graft technology is steadily being developed and applied to the treatment of various thoracic aortic pathologies including descending aneurysms, acute and chronic dissections, intramural hematomas, penetrating atherosclerotic ulcers (giant penetrating ulcers), and traumatic injuries.* "Home-made" stent-grafts, limited by their large size and limited conformability, have been significantly improved upon by engineering advances made possible by commercial design and manufacture. Worldwide embracement of the technology has allowed ongoing refinement of surgical indications, and experience continues to grow rapidly. As commercial devices become more available and the technology more pervasive, a greater appreciation of the indications and limitations of these devices should result in improved outcomes.

NATURAL HISTORY AND SURGICAL OUTCOMES OF THORACIC AORTIC DISEASES

Thoracic Aortic Aneurysms

Aneurysms of the aorta are abnormal dilations that have undergone progressive expansion. Histological examination reveals fragmentation of elastic fibers in the media of the aorta and loss of structural integrity of the adventitia. These changes render the aorta less elastic, with significant loss of structural integrity.[9]

The incidence of thoracic aortic aneurysm has been estimated as 489 per 100,000 men and 437 per 100,000 women with a median age of 77.7 and 85.3 years, respectively.[9] In their original report, Pressler and McNamara noted a 78% mortality rate at 5 years for untreated symptomatic aneurysms.[65] More recently, Clouse et al reported a 3-fold increase in the incidence of thoracic aortic aneurysms, but reported a less ominous natural history.[6] For aneurysms less than 6 cm in greatest diameter, rupture occurred in only

*References 1, 3, 4, 13, 18–21, 26–28, 35, 36, 42, 43, 45, 47, 50–54, 57, 58, 60, 62, 63, 66, 70, 73–75, 78, 82, 84, 87, 88, 90–92.

16% of patients at 5 years, a figure that increased to 30% for aneurysms over 6 cm.

The natural history is related to the specific location and the underlying cause of the aortic aneurysm disease.[8,10,15,17,22,33] For patients with Marfan syndrome, dilation of the aortic root is most prevalent and the risk of aortic rupture or dissection is related to the size of the root. Elective replacement of the root is associated with morbidity and mortality rates under 1%. The elimination of ongoing aortic dilation, dissection, or rupture therefore neutralizes a potentially lethal event, and simplifies long-term management.[8,10] Juvonem et al from Mount Sinai in New York have identified clinical variables that affect the risk for rupture, the most important being increasing age, presence of chronic obstructive pulmonary disease (COPD), maximal thoracic and abdominal aneurysm diameter, and the presence of pain.[38]

The Yale group has recently published data that permit calculation of yearly rates of rupture or other complications.[22] They found that the mean yearly rate of rupture or dissection is 2% for small aneurysms, 3% for aneurysms 5.0–5.9 cm, and 6.9% for aneurysms 6.0 cm or greater in size. Using proportional hazards regression, the odds ratio for rupture is more than 25 times higher in patients with aneurysms of 6.0 cm or greater than in patients with aneurysms between 4.0 and 4.9 cm. Symptomatic states, organ compression, concomitant aortic insufficiency, and acute ascending aortic dissection are widely accepted as general indications for surgical intervention regardless of aortic size. Size-appropriate guidelines are now 5.5 cm for ascending aortic aneurysm (5.0 cm for Marfan syndrome) and 6.5 cm for descending aortic aneurysm (6.0 cm for Marfan syndrome).

Experience reveals that of all those that do undergo surgery for thoracic aneurysms, 70% are alive at 2 years and 59% are alive at 5 years. This emphasizes the fact that the natural course of thoracic aortic aneurysm disease can be favorably altered by appropriate surgical intervention.[79] The preoperative and postoperative variables predictive of a fatal outcome include increasing age, preoperative renal insufficiency, concurrent proximal aortic aneurysm, coronary artery disease, COPD, and total aortic clamp time.[16,32,79]

Aortic Dissections

Dissection of the aorta is the entry of blood into the aortic media causing the layers of the aorta to be torn apart, creating a false lumen that runs parallel to the true lumen.[15] Intimal tears typically occur at either the right lateral wall of the ascending aorta (Stanford type A dissection) or just distal to the ligamentum arteriosum (Stanford type B dissection) representing the points of greatest hemodynamic stress. Type A dissections represent two thirds of all dissections.[15] The majority of deaths from all types of aortic dissections are due to rupture of the aorta into the pericardial or pleural cavity, and branch vessel occlusion can also result in significant morbidity and mortality.[24,25,49] Aneurysmal dilation of the aorta can subsequently develop since the integrity of the aorta is greatly compromised by the dissection. The prevalence of aortic dissections ranges from 0.2 to 0.8% of the population, and usually males are affected more often than females with ratios similar to that of aortic aneurysms.[49] Hypertension is the most important risk factor, and other factors known to predispose the aorta to dissection include inborn errors of metabolism (Marfan disease), bicuspid aortic valve, aortic coarctation, pregnancy, and surgical manipulation of the thoracic aorta.

Type A dissections are treated surgically immediately upon diagnosis to avert the high risk of death due to cardiac tamponade, aortic regurgitation, or myocardial infarction. Untreated type A dissections are associated with a mortality rate of 1–2%/h during the first 24–48 h. The Stanford experience reveals that the operative mortality for acute type A dissections is as high as 26% and 17% for chronic type A dissections. Overall, the 5 year actuarial survival rate for discharged patients is 78%.[29]

The preferred treatment for type B dissection is less well defined, but in general aggressive blood pressure management is the first line of therapy. Surgical treatment is reserved for intractable pain, rupture or impending rupture, malperfusion syndromes, and early expansion to a diameter greater than 5 cm.[24,25,71,87] Marfan syndrome, the presence of a sizable localized false aneurysm in the proximal descending thoracic aorta, arch involvement, and poor medical compliance may prompt early surgical intervention.[29,71,87]

Penetrating Atherosclerotic Ulcer and Intramural Hematoma of the Thoracic Aorta

Penetrating atherosclerotic ulcer (PAU) and intramural hematoma (IMH) are distinct pathological entities that are now being diagnosed with increasing frequency.[7,11,59,76,83] PAU is a lesion of the intima that penetrates into the aortic media, resulting in a variable amount of intramural hematoma (Figure 70-1). Although distinct, it has been associated with both aortic dissection and aneurysm formation. It is most often found in the distal descending thoracic aorta but can occur anywhere throughout the thoracic and abdominal aorta.[7,11,83]

Often thought of as a variant form of aortic dissection, IMH was originally described as a dissection without an intimal tear. The cause of IMH may be a spontaneous rupture of an aortic vasa vasorum or an intimal fracture of an atherosclerotic plaque that initiates aortic wall disintegration leading to dissection.[7] Hypertension and PAU have been proposed as prerequisites for IMH. Circumferential thickening of the aortic wall in the absence of an intimal flap, and without enhancement after contrast injection, is considered diagnostic of IMH using computed tomographic angiography (CTA) (Figure 70-2).[7,59,76]

Neither IMH nor PAU results in branch vessel occlusion or organ ischemia as seen in classic aortic dissections. PAU may be an indolent process, however; among those not treated surgically, an ulcer with surrounding IMH may evolve quite rapidly, with the formation of saccular or fusiform pseudoaneurysms.[7,76] Management strategies for IMH of the descending thoracic aorta involves aggressive blood pressure control and good follow-up (Figure 70-3). The treatment of ascending IMH is less clear, as 20–30% of these will progress to overt type A aortic dissection in the first 2–4 weeks. For younger, good-risk surgical patients, a more aggressive surgical approach may be warranted.[59,76] Coady et al reported that the overall incidence of acute rupture for PAU is 42% as opposed to 35% for IMH, 7.5% for type A dissections, and 4.1% for type B dissections with all

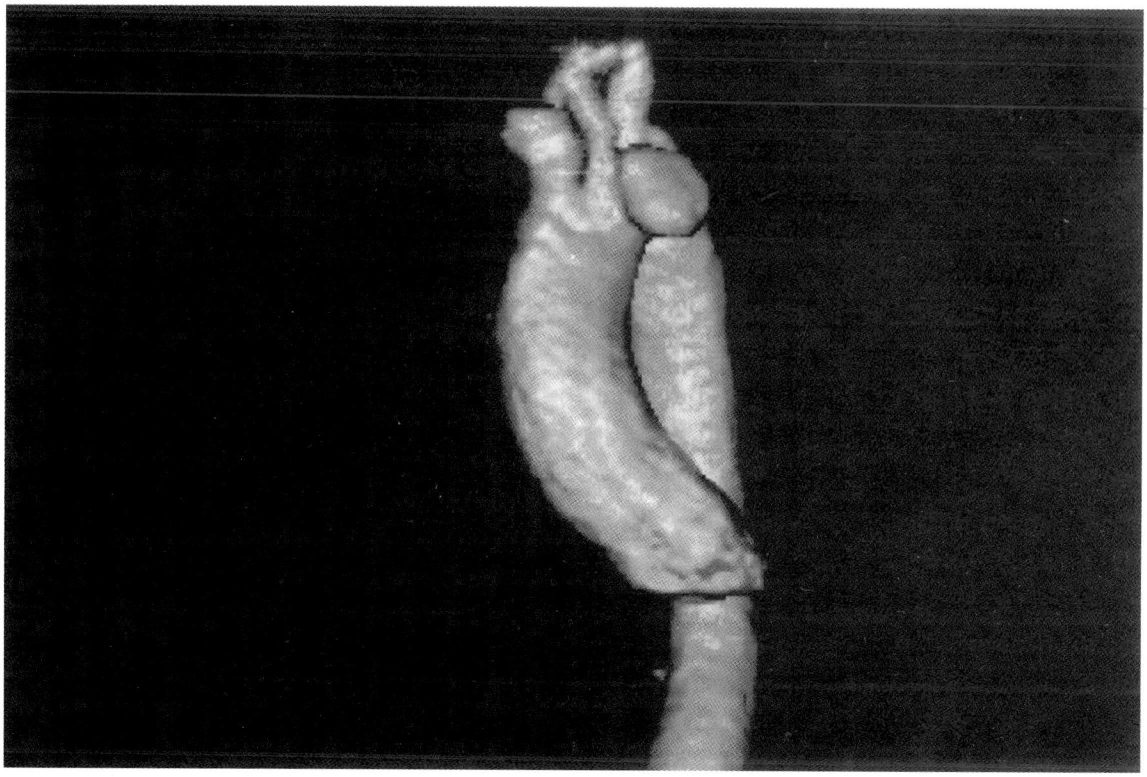

Figure 70–1 Shaded surface display of enlarging pseudoaneurysm from mid-aortic arch resulting from a giant penetrating ulcer.

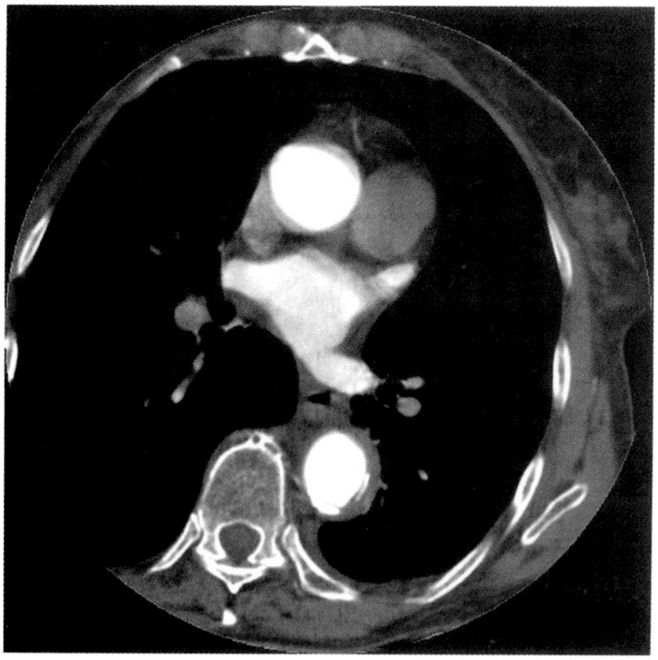

Figure 70–2 Intramural hematoma of the proximal descending thoracic aorta with multiple intimal irregularities.

ruptures occurring upon initial presentation or during the initial hospitalization.[7]

Thoracic Aortic Trauma

Blunt trauma of the thoracic aorta is commonly a catastrophic injury leading to death with most victims suffering a single rupture.[67,81] Mortality following admission to the hospital ranges from 39–73% and frequently is the result of other major injuries.[67] Suspected primary initiators of aortic injury have included deceleration or acceleration loads and crushing of the aorta against the spinal column.[67] The high associated morbidity and mortality are due to difficulty or delay in diagnosis, associated head and visceral injuries, and the immediacy of operative intervention. Aggressive medical treatment with β-blockers and vasodilators is required in the interval before operative intervention.

ENDOVASCULAR THERAPY OF THE THORACIC AORTA

Technical Development

Close collaboration between cardiovascular surgeons and interventional radiologists has allowed the introduction of endovascular stent-grafts for the treatment of aortic aneurysms, dissections, IMHs, and PAUs (giant penetrating ulcers).* This technology promises to be less invasive and may substantially reduce surgical morbidity and mortality. The obvious advantages of this technology include introduction of the stent-graft from a peripheral site, situation using radiographic guidance, elimination of a thoracotomy, minimal operative time, and avoidance of aortic cross-clamping.

Parodi et al were the first to introduce endovascular technology when they described the concept of balloon-expandable stents attached to the end of a vascular graft for

*References 1, 3, 4, 13, 18–21, 26–28, 35, 36, 42, 43, 45, 47, 50–54, 57, 58, 60, 62, 63, 66, 70, 73–75, 78, 82, 84, 87, 88, 90–92.

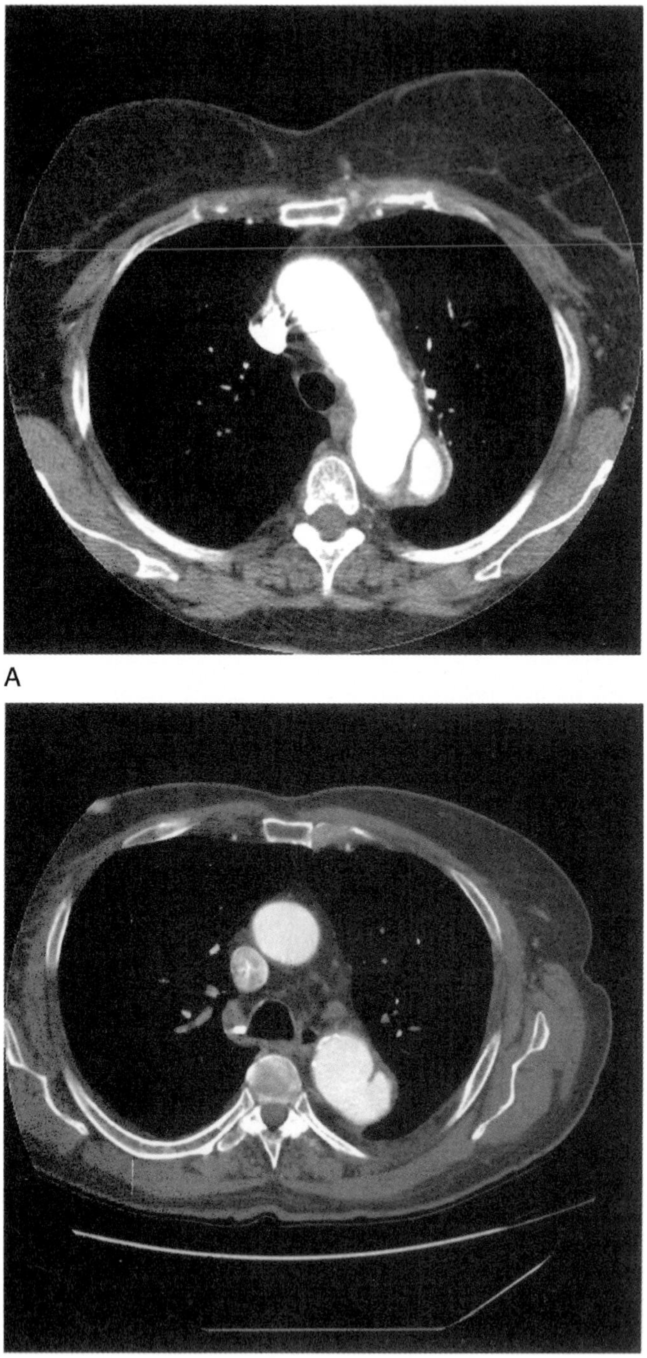

A

B

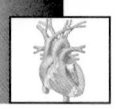

Figure 70–3 **A,** Proximal extent of Type B aortic dissection with a fairly thick dissection septum. **B,** Enlarging pseudoaneurysm of proximal descending thoracic aorta evolving from a penetrating ulcer into extensive IMH. Note the similarity between these two entities.

the repair of an abdominal aortic aneurysm.[64] The balloon catheters consisted of a 9F polyethylene shaft and one nylon balloon that was 3.5 cm in length and 30, 25, or 16 mm in inflated diameter. Mounted on the deflated balloon was a balloon-expandable stent and a thin-walled, crimped, knitted Dacron graft was sutured to the stent overlapping one half of its length. Similarly, at Stanford, uncovered endovascular stents were initially applied to animal models of aortic dissection. A covered stent was developed, and clinical trials were initiated as an integrated surgical and interventional approach.[21] A "first-generation" stent-graft was tailored for each patient using self-expanding 2.5-cm Gianturco Z stents (Cook Co., Bloomington, IN) that were fastened together and then covered with a woven Dacron graft (Meadox-Boston Scientific, Natick, MA). An internal review board (IRB) approval was initially obtained for a study in high-risk nonsurgical candidates and "first-generation" stents were used between 1992 and 1998.[20,53,54] The endografts were deployed using a 28 French sheath with a graduated dilator that was inserted over a stiff guide wire under fluoroscopic control. The stent was then placed into the delivery capsule, advanced through the sheath using a pusher rod, and finally deployed by withdrawing the external sheath.

Contrast-enhanced computed tomography (CT) with three-dimensional reconstruction was the primary diagnostic tool in these initial Stanford patients and remains our diagnostic modality of choice today. Using CT studies, aneurysm size or dissection extent was evaluated, as well as relationship to critical side branches. Digital subtraction angiography was used if necessary to clarify the affected anatomy, and intraoperative transesophageal echocardiography was invaluable for differentiating true from false lumens. Endovascular stent-grafts were oversized by approximately 10–15% based on the CT cross-sectional diameter in an effort to obtain sufficient radial force to achieve an endoseal and prevent stent-graft migration. Landing zones of normal aorta 2 cm or greater distal to the subclavian and proximal to the celiac were required to ensure adequate fixation; access to femoral and iliac arteries at least 8 mm in size was also necessary. Digital fluoroscopy and transesophageal echocardiography were used for graft positioning and deployment, and contrast angiography and transesophageal echocardiography were used at the conclusion of the operative procedure to ensure the absence of type I endoleaks. All patients received a CT angiogram prior to discharge and on follow-up.[20,21,53,54]

This new technology is associated with new terminology. "Endoleaks," that is, the failure to exclude the aneurysm sac from the bloodstream, are classified as types I through IV.* Type I endoleaks occur at the proximal or distal attachment sites and signify a failure to achieve a hemostatic seal at these implantation sites. Type II endoleaks denote a communication between a branch vessel and the excluded aneurysm sac. These usually occur from back bleeding of the inferior mesenteric artery in the abdomen or intercostal arteries in the chest. Both an entry and exit vessel is usually required for prolonged patency. Type III endoleaks originate from the midgraft sections and are usually caused by disruption of graft-to-graft overlaps or by leakage through the graft itself. Finally, type IV endoleaks are characterized by an increase in the size of the aneurysm sac in the absence of an identifiable patent branch vessel, variously ascribed to as "endotension."

In an effort to improve the "first-generation" stent-grafts in terms of maneuverability, size, and reliability of deployment, the medical device industry began to develop more technologically advanced stent-grafts. In 1998, a smaller, more flexible commercial endograft became available and was referred to as the "Excluder" (Gore "Excluder," WL Gore, Flagstaff, AZ).[84,85] This device, constructed from a

*References 20, 21, 51, 53, 54, 84, 85.

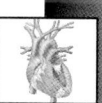

temperature-sensitive nitinol exoskeleton attached to a polytetrafluoroethylene (PTFE) graft, has been used at Stanford and has facilitated endovascular stenting in many ways. The smaller introducer sheath (20–24 French) need only reach the abdominal aorta. Lower device profile renders the stent more flexible allowing easier vascular passage. Increased conformability allows the stent-graft to be rapidly and precisely deployed. Unfortunately, wireform fractures precluded Food and Drug Administration (FDA) consideration. Currently in the United States, there are no commercially available endovascular stent-grafts specifically manufactured for the thoracic aorta. The "Talent" endograft by Medtronic is being used clinically under compassionate use permits, and a second-generation Gore "Excluder" will soon be available for FDA trials. It is hoped that patient outcomes will be improved with this advanced technology. One would anticipate fewer embolic strokes because of less manipulation within the aortic arch and an increase in applicability and utility because of increased arch conformability.

Stanford's initial experience involving endovascular stent placement was performed in the operating room with cardiac nurses and anesthesiologists. The chest, abdomen, and groins were prepped and a full vascular operative set was available. Double lumen endotracheal tubes and Swan–Ganz catheter monitoring were used. With increased experience and few if any urgent conversions to open procedures, endovascular stent procedures have transitioned to the interventional radiology suite with improved diagnostic imaging capabilities.

Thoracic Aortic Aneurysms

Descending thoracic aortic aneurysms constitute 31% of thoracic aortic pathology, whereas aneurysms of the ascending and transverse arch collectively contribute 40%.[9] Descending thoracic aortic aneurysms with relatively straight anatomical orientation are favorable for endovascular intervention. Many centers have reported the feasibility of stent-grafts in the descending aorta, and some agreement now exists regarding anatomical, constraints of the procedure.* The Stanford experience with the "first-generation" patients found that adequate landing zones were available in approximately 60% of patients, usually with relatively straight segments and no critical side branches.[20,21,53,54] Acute angulation of the distal arch was frequently associated with a proximal endoleak resulting from the nonconformability of the 2.5-cm-long articulating Z stents. Balloon inflation was occasionally effective in straightening the endograft and eliminating these endoleaks.

In the first 103 Stanford patients using Z stents, 60% were nonoperative candidates on the basis of severe medical comorbidities. The resulting early mortality, as defined by death during the same hospitalization, was 9% and was significantly associated with preoperative cerebrovascular accident or myocardial infarction. Actuarial survival was 81% at 1 year and 73% at 2 years.[54] Embolic strokes occurred in seven patients, likely because of atheroemboli dislodged during guide wire and sheath manipulation within the aortic arch. As noted previously, design modifications have eliminated the necessity for passing the introducer sheath into the aortic arch, with subsequent reduction in the incidence of this complication. Spinal cord injury was another unknown risk because critical intercostal arteries in the T8 to T12 distribution were frequently covered, with no possibility for maintaining their perfusion. Paraplegia occurred in three patients, all of whom had concomitant abdominal aortic aneurysm repair. Other authors have reported an incidence of up to 2%, and involved the rather perplexing delayed onset of paraplegia, 12–28 hours following the procedure.[35,58] Type I endoleaks proved to be the most prevalent complication with a reported incidence of 24% in the Stanford series requiring five patients to undergo late operative therapy.[54]

Open surgery using adjunctive endovascular stent-grafting is a hybrid procedure that may allow surgical repair of more extensive aneurysms. The addition of a stent-graft placed into the descending thoracic aorta after ascending or arch repair has both theoretical and practical appeal. However, as Miyairi et al have recently reported, extension below the T6 level may result in an unacceptably high incidence of paraplegia.[55]

Patients with multilevel aneurysmal aortic disease can present yet another formidable challenge for which stent-grafting is uniquely suited.[14,57] In patients with abdominal aortic aneurysms, 5% also have a descending thoracic aneurysm; in patients with a descending thoracic aneurysm, 13–29% have abdominal involvement.[65] Repair is usually performed sequentially and during that interval, the second aneurysm can rupture. Crawford found that 30% of early postoperative deaths after isolated repair of a descending thoracic aneurysm were caused by rupture of an untreated infrarenal aneurysm.[15,17] In asymptomatic patients, it is recommended that the thoracic aorta be repaired initially with close monitoring of the abdominal aneurysm while awaiting the second operation because the abdominal aorta is not associated with such unpredictable rupture rates as the thoracic aorta.[15] Among the Stanford patients, simultaneous repair of the abdominal and thoracic aorta was successfully undertaken in 18 patients. A retroperitoneal approach to the abdominal aorta was used combined with an endovascular repair of the thoracic aortic aneurysm inserted through a 10-mm side limb attached to the abdominal graft.[54,57] Thoracotomy was therefore avoided and complete aneurysm exclusion was achieved in 94% of patients. Although there was only a single mortality, paraplegia, as previously mentioned, occurred in three patients.[54] This application of endovascular repair may be a useful addition to the surgical management of multilevel aortic disease taking into account its limitations.

Aortic Dissections

Stanford Type A Aortic Dissection

Acute aortic dissection is the most common catastrophe affecting the aorta.[49] For Stanford type A dissections, open surgical repair is the traditional treatment. Replacement of the ascending aorta, including coronary sinuses if abnormally dilated, reimplantation of the coronary ostia, resuspension of the regurgitant aortic valve, and resection of the primary aortic tear in the ascending aorta or arch are associated with successful outcomes. Left untreated, 90% of patients with type A dissections are dead at 3 months.[9,49] As more aggressive repairs of acute type A dissections are undertaken, endovascular techniques to minimize late

*References 4, 20, 21, 27, 35, 51, 53, 54, 58, 90.

aneurysmal complications may be used.[30,37,46,56,68] In younger patients, and particularly those afflicted with Marfan disease, aneurysmal complications are more likely to develop late in the course of a chronic type A dissection. In an effort to minimize these late complications, Kazui et al have advocated ascending and arch replacement with a distal elephant trunk for young patients, with acceptably low mortality rates.[46] Other authors have advocated using a stent-graft through the open arch and down into the true lumen of the descending aorta in an effort to promote thrombosis of the false lumen, thus eliminating the risk of late aortic dilation.[30,37,56,68] This therapy allows for replacement of the affected ascending aorta, eliminates the need for a thoracotomy, and yet theoretically protects the patient from further descending thoracic aorta pathology. The safety and long-term benefits are undefined, yet several groups worldwide are reporting success using this combined surgical and endovascular treatment of type A aortic dissections.[30,37,41,56,68] At present, for young, good-risk, and marfanoid patients, it would seem appropriate to include an arch repair with elephant trunk so that any further aneurysmal changes of the thoracic aorta can be managed through a left thoracotomy approach.

Stanford Type B Aortic Dissection

Dissections of the descending aorta, referred to as Stanford type B, present the greatest challenge in terms of management decisions. Historically, surgical repair has been advocated for patients with rupture or impending rupture, intractable pain, early expansion to a diameter greater than 5 cm, and patients with branch vessel compromise.[24,25,44,86] In the absence of these complications, medical "antiimpulse" therapy is usually elected, even though it is associated with a hospital mortality of 10%. Surgical procedures are associated with a mortality of 20–30% and may be as high as 60% if there is preoperative visceral ischemia.[24,25,29,71] Furthermore, with medical management, it is estimated that approximately 70% of patients will have a persistently patent false lumen, and 20–30% of these will become aneurysmal.[9,25,71] If a minimally invasive, relatively safe procedure could be performed that would minimize the risk of rupture as well as late aneurysmal complications, one could significantly reduce short- and long-term morbidity from this catastrophic disease process. Stent-grafts have proven safe and effective therapy for the acute management of type B aortic dissections and will likely decrease the incidence of late aneurysm formation, as the false lumen is eliminated in 80% of patients (Figure 70-4).[4,18,61] Certainly an aggressive surgical approach, possibly involving endovascular therapy, can be justified for all patients with the complications mentioned above and even for younger good-risk patients without them.[86] Proving this hypothesis is difficult, however, because of the heterogeneity of the patient population, referral biases, and continuous evolution of therapeutic options.

Visceral malperfusion is a major indication for operative intervention in type B dissections. Successful management of vascular occlusion secondary to aortic dissection depends on the ability to predict which of the affected vascular beds will respond to restoration of true lumen flow and which will require further intervention to reestablish visceral perfusion. "Dynamic obstructions" result from true lumen compression and are not the result of a separate intimal tear at branch vessel ostia. Endovascular graft coverage of the primary intimal tear will redirect flow into the true lumen, which reverses distal ischemia secondary to true lumen collapse.[18,84] "Static obstructions" result from intimal tears at or near the branch vessel ostium, with obstruction to flow from the intimal intussusception. These require endovascular stenting of branch vessel orifices alone or in combination with fenestration of the dissection septum. Stent-graft coverage of the primary tear redirects flow into the true lumen, which will not only provide end-organ protection by eliminating obstructions but also provide protection from rupture and aneurysmal dilation.[19,28,84] This would therefore appear to be a desirable procedure for restoring visceral perfusion and much less morbid than a central aortic operation involving visceral arteries. Moreover, the stent-graft need not be overly long and it rarely extends distal to T6, thus minimizing the risk for paraplegia.

In a previously reported Stanford series, 12 of 15 complicated type B dissections were successfully repaired with this approach, with an early mortality rate of 20% and restoration of a single true lumen in 79% of patients.[18] Palma and associates have similarly reported a series of 70 patients with type B dissections repaired with stent grafts.[61] Procedural success was achieved in 92% of patients (65 patients) using the femoral artery to introduce the stent under general anesthesia. Surgical conversion was required in the remaining five patients because the proximal endoleak could not be controlled. Two patients required emergent surgical conversion because of aneurysm expansion and/or rupture at the time of presentation, and three other patients underwent elective surgical repair to eliminate large proximal endoleaks. Residual flow in the false lumen below the diaphragm persisted in 20% of patients because of more distal fenestrations. Survival was reported as 91% at a mean follow-up of 29 months, with no late aortic events. Kato and associates have reported a 100% success rate in placement of endovascular stent-grafts of 15 patients with chronic type B dissections.[44] No procedure-related complications were observed except for postimplantation syndrome manifested by transient fever and leukocytosis. The diameter of the true lumen was significantly increased and the diameter of the aorta was significantly decreased. There were no deaths and no instances of aortic rupture during the 24-month follow-up. When they included the treatment of acute type A and type B dissections using endovascular stents, their early and late complication rate, however, rose to 33% and 36%, respectively, but with a 0% mortality. They caution that although endovascular stents are useful, appropriate patient selection and good follow-up are essential.

Other interventional therapies are available to correct malperfusion abnormalities. Localized obstruction to flow at the branch vessel orifice, usually secondary to intussusception of the torn intima, may be stented open with an uncovered stent.[74] If the only communication to the branch vessel is from the aortic false lumen, which is poorly perfused, a fenestration of the dissection flap can be performed with a catheter-based needle (Rorsch-Uchida, Cook, Bloomington, IN), crossed with a guidewire and balloon dilated to increase the flow into the false lumen. This technique is especially applicable at the distal aorta with pseudoocclusion of an iliac artery. In a series reported by the Stanford group, 40 patients with acute aortic dissections (10 type A and 30 type B) were treated for extremity, renal, or

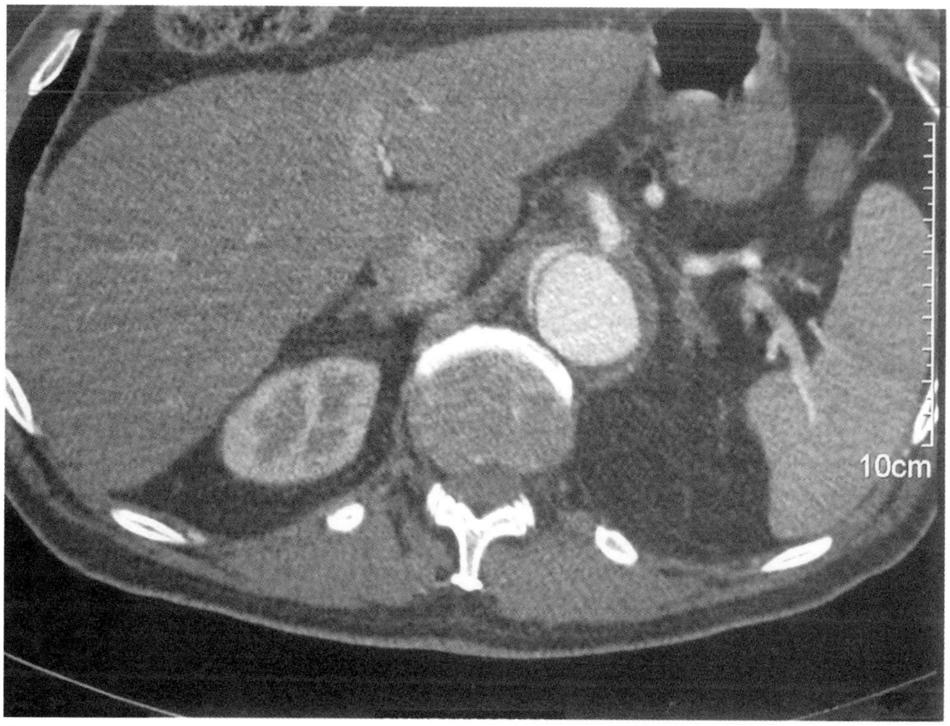

A

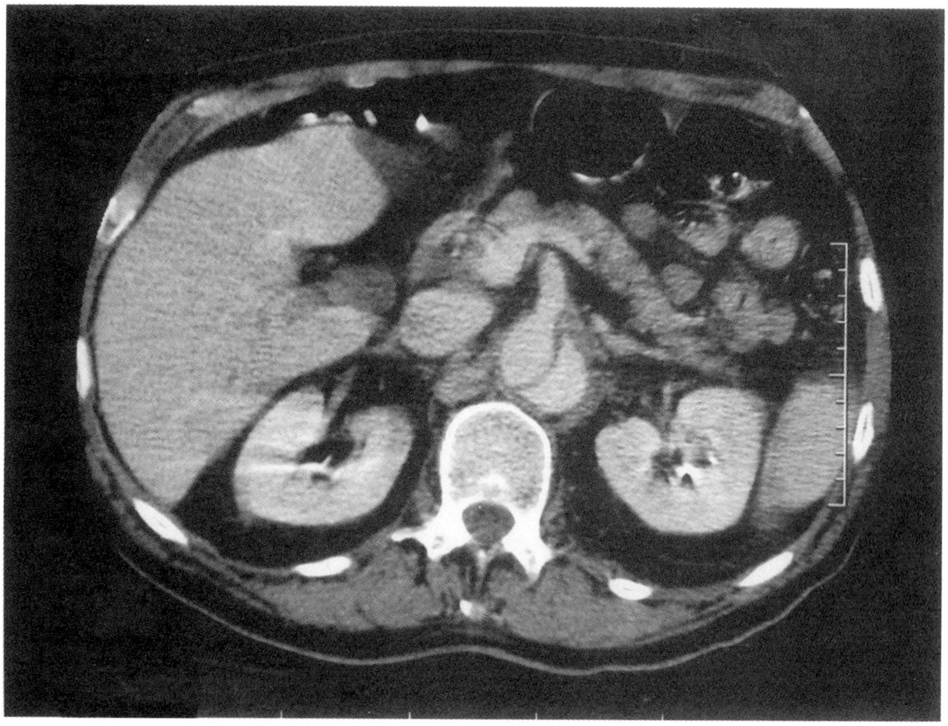

B

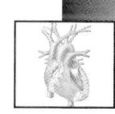

Figure 70–4 **A,** True lumen collapse (dynamic obstruction) of an acute dissection at the level of the celiac axis. **B,** Same patient after partial coverage of the primary intimal tear just distal to the left subclavian artery. Note increased size of the true lumen with increased flow and resolution of symptoms of intestinal angina and hypertension.

mesenteric ischemia appearing within 14 days of the onset of symptoms with a diagnosis established on clinical, laboratory, and angiographic findings.[74] Any arterial anatomical abnormality resulting from the dissection and related to the region suspected of being ischemic was treated. Thirty patients had renal, 22 had lower extremity, 18 had mesenteric, and one had upper extremity ischemia. Nine patients with type A dissections underwent surgical replacement of the ascending aorta prior to percutaneous intervention, whereas only one of the type B dissections required aortic replacement prior to percutaneous intervention. Successful revascularization was achieved in 93% (63) of patients. Nine patients had procedure-related complications. The 30-day mortality rate was 25% (10 to 40 patients), often related to irreversible ischemia of intraabdominal organs that was present before the procedure. Of the remaining 30 patients, 5 died and the remaining 25 continued to have relief of ischemic symptoms at a mean follow-up of 29 months.

Endovascular therapy is not without its possible complications.[63,92] In the acute phase of aortic dissection, the outer adventitial layer of the aorta is thin and friable and its perforation, even with a guide wire, could be disastrous. Similarly, the dissection septum is fragile and may provide an insufficient distal anchor for a stent-graft. There are some examples (M.D. Dake, personal communication) of septal perforations at the distal stent-graft fixation site, suggesting the susceptibility of the acute dissection septum to repetitive erosive trauma. Additionally, there are now reports of false aneurysm formation in the distal arch secondary to erosion from uncovered stent-graft wireforms.[41] The primary intimal tear may also be quite extensive and extend proximal to the left subclavian artery orifice. Effective exclusion of false lumen perfusion in these instances may be very difficult, requiring implanting the stent-graft adjacent to the left carotid artery, and covering the left subclavian orifice. Although it has been reported that the subclavian artery can be sacrificed with impunity, which may pertain in arteries free of occlusive disease, the Stanford approach has been to create a left carotid to subclavian bypass and then ligate the left subclavian proximal to the vertebral artery take-off so as to eliminate the possibility of retrograde filling of the aneurysm sac from the left subclavian stump.[18,27] Another possibility advocated by Inoue et al of Japan is to use a single branched stent-graft to ensure perfusion to the left subclavian artery.[36]

New strategies for the treatment of dissection of the descending aorta that extends back into the ascending aorta (type B with retrograde dissection of the ascending aorta) have been proposed by several groups.[45,72,89] Replacement of the arch with a variable portion of ascending aorta via median sternotomy is recommended in patients with an enlarged aortic diameter, pericardial effusion, and/or aortic insufficiency.[45] A predominantly distal dissection with an almost intact small ascending aorta, a small aortic arch, and a thrombosed false lumen of the ascending aorta is treated in the same manner as type B dissection where stent-graft repair is an alternative to conventional surgery.[72] Kato et al recently described their experience in 10 type A aortic dissections with the entry tears located in the descending aorta. Z stents were placed in the true lumen of the proximal descending thoracic aorta in 9 of 10 patients and in the mid-descending thoracic aorta in the remaining patient.[43] Complete closure of the entry tear was achieved at the end of the procedure in all patients, and complete thrombosis of the false lumen of the ascending aorta was observed in all patients. No procedure-related complications were reported, and after a 20-month follow-up, no aortic rupture or aneurysm formation was reported. They therefore concluded that endovascular stent-graft repair of type A aortic dissections with an entry tear in the descending thoracic aorta is a safe and effective method and may serve as an alternative to surgical graft placement in highly selected patients.

Many unanswered questions remain with respect to endovascular treatment of aortic dissections. For chronic dissections, thickening and fibrosis of the septum, the origin of critical branch vessels from both true and false lumens, as well as the presence of multiple true lumen to false lumen communications would seemingly limit the utility of this stent-graft technology. Furthermore, the presence of critical side branches, especially low intercostal arteries or critical visceral arteries arising from the false lumen, has tempered the enthusiasm for endograft insertion into the true lumen, because of the risk for ischemic injury. However, should the motivation for stent-graft repair become compelling, stent-grafting into the true lumen could be performed, and then false lumen flow could be ensured by angioplasty and stenting of septal perforations.

Penetrating Atherosclerotic Ulcers of the Thoracic Aorta

Penetrating atherosclerotic ulcers present perhaps one of the most appealing clinical indications for endovascular stent-graft technology.[70] Often presenting in an elderly population with multiple comorbidities, these diffusely diseased aortas present significant challenges for conventional repair. Poor tissue integrity combined with a high likelihood for intraoperative thromboembolism is a prime setting for severe complications.[11] Additionally, because of the diffuse nature of this process, representing end-stage atherosclerotic disease, it is difficult to limit the extent of surgical resection. Stent-graft coverage of the penetrating ulcer can limit the progression of IMH and allow healing to occur. Unfortunately, even with successful stent-graft implantation, retrograde aortic dissection and new ulcer formation have been noted in a significant percentage of patients, further amplifying the diffuse and severe nature of the aortic disease.[7]

Intramural Hematoma of the Thoracic Aorta

The natural history of IMH is progression according to one of two probable mechanisms: ulcerations penetrating into the aortic media that allow a high pressure jet into the medial layers, or hemorrhage within the media, which may arise spontaneously from the vasa vasorum during hypertension.[7,83] Although pure IMH of the thoracic aorta is not amenable to stent-graft repair, any secondary intimal defect could be covered and thereby perhaps limit progression of the disease.[7]

Thoracic Aortic Trauma

Traumatic aortic rupture is most often confined to the descending aorta at the isthmus, often referred to as the "classic" site, or it may occur in the ascending aorta proximal to the origin of the brachiocephalic artery.[67] Almost invariably, there are multiple other injuries that severely limit operative approaches, namely hepatic and splenic fractures, pulmonary contusions, and closed head injuries. All operations involving the descending thoracic aorta pose some risk of ischemic injury to the spinal cord, a dreaded complication in a predominately young population. And, finally, the immediacy of the operation may require nonexperienced surgeons to deal with complex pathology.[81]

The application of endovascular stents for treatment of acute traumatic aortic transactions has been enthusiastically received. In addition to its less invasive nature, stent-grafts avoid the peril of heparin anticoagulation, decrease the respiratory compromise of a thoracotomy, and reduce episodic hypotension that is particularly injurious to patients with head injuries. Multiple reports of successful intervention have emerged from Japan, Europe, and the Americas (Figure 70-5A and B).[39,40,77] However, unlike their counterparts with atherosclerotic disease, these younger patients have smaller access vessels, mandating low-profile devices,

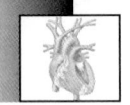

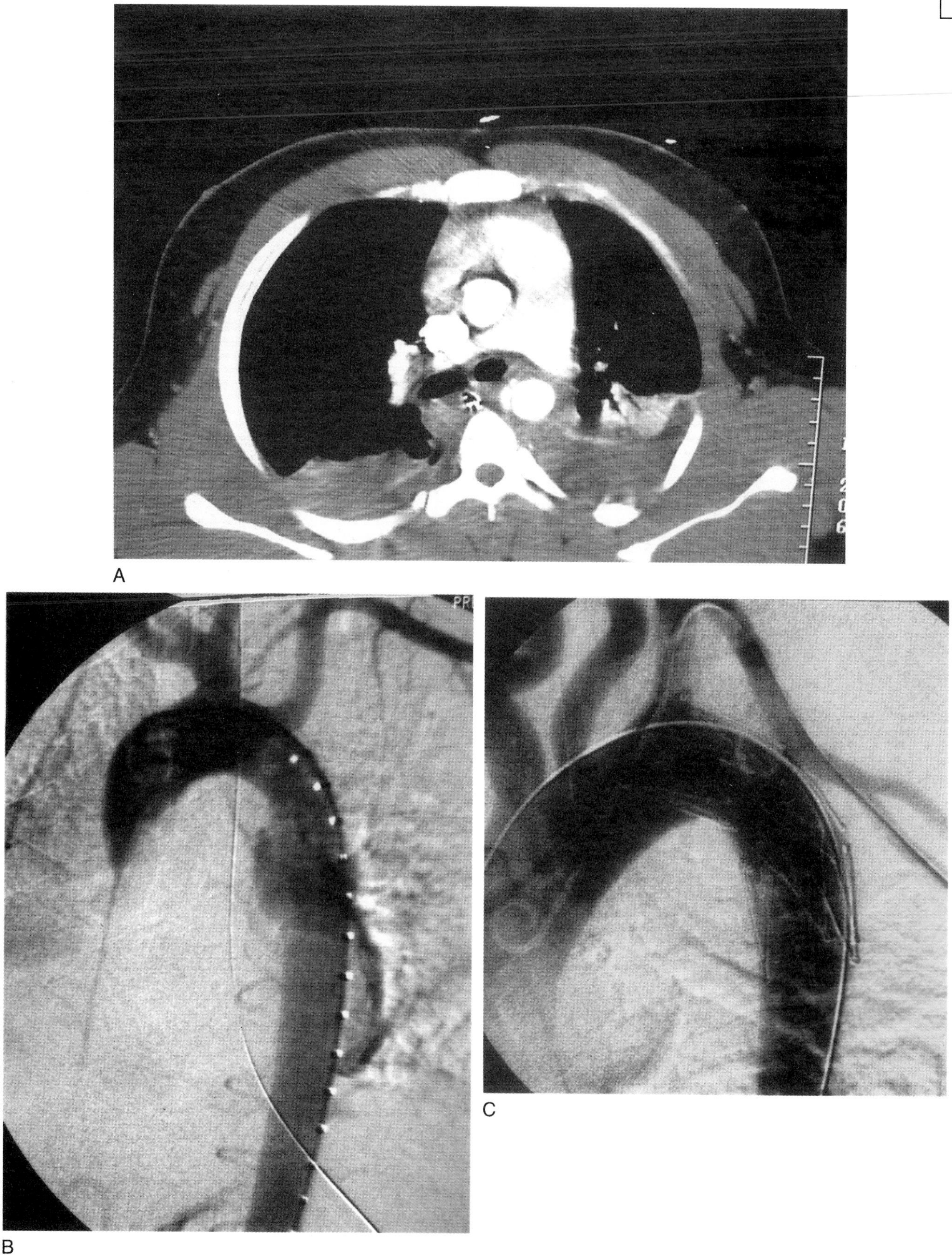

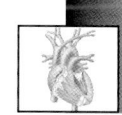

Figure 70–5 **A,** CT scan demonstrating traumatic tear in the proximal descending thoracic aorta. **B,** Thoracic aortogram confirming same pathology at the time of endograft repair. **C,** Thoracic aortogram after successful endograft repair of traumatic transection.

and smaller aortas, requiring smaller diameter grafts than usually required. Successful outcomes, however, will hopefully prompt further applications in trauma victims.

SUMMARY

Ten years of experience with endovascular abdominal aortic aneurysm repair have yielded important information regarding the relationship between stent-graft design and stent-graft performance.[3,5,60,63,92] For example, tapered, flexible, over-the-wire delivery systems of less than 20F diameter rarely fail to traverse tortuous iliac arteries. Hooks at the proximal stent-graft appear to provide the most secure means of proximal attachment, and column strength has been found to be of little value. Although modular stent-grafts are more versatile than unibody stent-grafts, graft-to-graft attachments and overlaps produce unusual stresses, and are prone to late failure. In addition, thoracic stent-grafts, because of their length, angulation, and tortuosity, are subjected to even more severe stresses than their abdominal counterparts. Frequent wireform fractures secondary to fatigue have unfortunately already been noted for all the commercially manufactured stent-grafts. Any movement between the stent body and the overlying fabric will lead to graft erosion. The Eurostar registry has revealed that up to 10% of patients per year may require secondary procedures to ensure exclusion of the aneurysm sac.[92] The evolution of the aneurysm sac is a dynamic process that requires monitoring over years; failure of the sac to stabilize and/or shrink in size suggests that protection from rupture has not been conferred. Other limitations include anatomical constraints, such as adequate proximal and distal aortic necks, the presence of critical aortic branches in the diseased aorta, and the fact that only relatively straight segments of aorta can be easily managed. Placement of the stent-graft close to the distal arch appears to be associated with a higher incidence of strokes, presumably due to catheter manipulation in the ascending aorta and arch. Guide wire manipulation within the severely atherosclerotic transverse arch poses some finite risk for atheroembolism and stroke, rendering this a very challenging clinical entity. Long-term follow-up of all these stent-graft patients will be mandatory until their long-term performance is better characterized.

There are currently no FDA approved devices for the thoracic aorta commercially available in the United States. Devices under evaluation include the Medtronic "Talent" and a new iteration of the Gore "Excluder." Other manufacturers are in various stages of stent-graft development as the utility of these grafts in the management of thoracic aneurysms, dissections, and traumatic disruptions has been appreciated. In Japan, where the technology has been more widely applied, the vast majority of the stents are individually constructed at the respective centers. The improvements in second- and third-generation stent-grafts to come will feature lower profiles, greater flexibility, increased conformability, and greater ease of insertion and deployment. Whether the perceived advantages of reduced operative time, blood loss, hospital stay, and overall complications will be confirmed await further study. The Phase II FDA study of the Gore "Excluder" is the first study to include a surgical control arm that may facilitate the comparison of outcomes in similar patient populations with aortic diseases. Certainly, for high-risk patients, these grafts will prove invaluable and will represent a welcome addition to our armamentarium of treatment options for an ever more aged and frail population.

REFERENCES

1. Bavaria JE, Brinster DR, Gorman RC, et al: Advances in the treatment of acute type A dissection: an integrated approach. Ann Thorac Surg 74:S1848–1852, 2002.
2. Bickerstaff LK, Pairolero PC, et al: Thoracic aortic aneurysms: a population-based study. Surgery 92:1103–1108, 1992.
3. Blum U, Voshage G, Lammer J, et al: Endoluminal stent-grafts for infrarenal abdominal aortic aneurysms. N Engl J Med 336: 13–20, 1997.
4. Buffolo E, da Fonseca JHP, de Souza JAM, Alves CMR: Revoluntionary treatment of aneurysms and dissections of descending aorta: the endovascular approach. Ann Thorac Surg 74:S1815–1817, 2002.
5. Chuter TAM: Stent-graft design: the good, the bad and the ugly. Cardiovasc Sur 10(1):7–13, 2002.
6. Clouse WD, Hallett JW, Schaff HV, et al: Improved prognosis of thoracic aortic aneurysms: a population-based study. JAMA 280(22):1926–1929, 1998.
7. Coady MA, Rizzo JA, Elefteriades JA: Pathologic variants of thoracic arotic dissections. Penetrating atherosclerotic ulcers and intramural hematomas. Cardiol Clin North Am 17(4): 637–657, 1999.
8. Coady MA, Rizzo JA, Elefteriades JA: Developing surgical intervention criteria for thoracic aortic aneurysms. Cardiol Clin North Am 17(4):827–839, 1999.
9. Coady MA, Rizzo JA, Goldstein LJ, Elefteriades JA: Natural history, pathogenesis, and etiology of thoracic aortic aneurysms and dissections. Cardiol Clin North Am 17(4):615–635, 1999.
10. Coady MA, Rizzo JA, Hammond GL, et al: What is the appropriate size criterion for resection of thoracic aortic aneurysms? J Thorac Cardiovasc Surg 113(3):476–491, 1997.
11. Coady MA, Rizzo JA, Hammond GL, et al: Penetrating ulcer of the thoracic aorta: what is it? How do we recognize it? How do we manage it? J Vasc Surg 27(6):1006–1016, 1998.
12. Cooley DA, DeBakey ME: Resection of entire ascending aorta in fusiform aneurysm using cardiac bypass. JAMA 162: 1158–1159, 1956.
13. Coselli JS, Conklin LD, LeMaire SA: Thoracoabdominal aortic aneurysm repair: review and update of current strategies. Ann Thorac Surg 74:S1881–1884, 2002.
14. Crawford ES: Aortic aneurysm: a multifocal disease. Arch Surg 117:1393–1414, 1982.
15. Crawford ES, Crawford JS: Diseases of the Aorta. Baltimore: Williams & Wilkins, 1984.
16. Crawford ES, Crawford JL, Safi HJ, et al: Thoracoabdominal aortic aneurysm: preoperative and intraoperative factors determining immediate and long-term results of operations in 605 patients. J Vasc Surg 3:389–404, 1986.
17. Crawford ES, DeNatale RW: Thoracoabdominal aortic aneurysm: observations regarding the natural course of the disease. J Vasc Surg 3:578–582, 1986.
18. Dake MD, Kato NK, Mitchell RS, et al: Endovascular stent-graft placement for the treatment of acute aortic dissection. N Engl J Med 340:1546–1552, 1999.
19. Dake MD, Kato N, Slonim SM, et al: Endovascular stent-graft placement to obliterate the entry tear: a new treatment for acute aortic dissection. Circulation 98:67, 1998.
20. Dake MD, Miller DC, Mitchell RS, et al: The "first generation" of endovascular stent-grafts for patients with

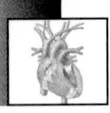

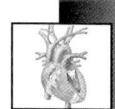

aneurysms of the descending thoracic aorta. J Thorac Cardiovasc Surg 116:689–704, 1998.
21. Dake MD, Miller DC, Semba CP, et al: Transluminal placement of endovascular stent-grafts for the treatment of descending thoracic aortic aneurysms. N Engl J Med 331(26): 1729–1734, 1994.
22. Davies RR, Goldstein LJ, Coady MA, et al: Yearly rupture or dissection rates for thoracic aortic aneurysms: simple prediction based on size. Ann Thorac Surg 73:17–28, 2002.
23. DeBakey ME, Cooley DA: Successful resection of aneurysm of thoracic aorta and replacement by graft. JAMA 152: 673–676, 1953.
24. Elefteriades JA, Hartleroad J, Gusberg RJ, et al: Long-term experience with descending aortic dissection: the complication-specific approach. Ann Thorac Surg 53:11–21, 1992.
25. Elefteriades JA, Lovoulos CJ, Coady MA, et al: Management of descending aortic dissection. Ann Thorac Surg 67: 2002–2005, 1999.
26. Estrera AL, Miller C, Porat EE, et al: Staged repair of extensive aortic aneurysms. Ann Thorac Surg 74:S1803–1805, 2002.
27. Fann JI, Miller DC: Endovascular treatment of descending thoracic aortic aneurysms and dissection. Surg Clin North Am 79:551–574, 1999.
28. Fann JI, Sarris GE, Mitchell RS, et al: Treatment of patients with aortic dissection presenting with peripheral vascular complications. Ann Surg 61:705–710, 1990.
29. Fann JI, Smith JA, Miller DC, et al: Surgical management of aortic dissection during a 30-year period. Circulation 92(9 Suppl.):II-113–121, 1995.
30. Fleck T, Hutschala D, Czerny M, et al: Combined surgical and endovascular treatment of acute aortic dissection type A: preliminary results. Ann Thorac Surg 74:761–766, 2002.
31. Gillum RF: Epidemiology of aortic aneurysm in the United States. J Clin Epidemiol 48(11):1289–1298, 1995.
32. Griepp RB, Ergin MA, Galla JD, et al: Minimizing spinal cord injury during repair of descending thoracic and thoracoabdominal aneurysms: the Mount Sinai approach. Sem Thorac Cardiovasc Surg 10(1):25–28, 1998.
33. Griepp RB, Ergin MA, Lansman SL, et al: The natural history of thoracic aortic aneurysms. Sem Thorac Cardiovasc Surg 3(4):258–265, 1991.
34. Hagan PG, Nienaber CA, Isselbacher EM, et al: The international registry of acute aortic dissection. New insights into an old disease. JAMA 283:897–903, 2000.
35. Heijmen RH, Deblier IG, Moll FL, et al: Endovascular stent-grafting for descending thoracic aortic aneurysms. Eur J Cardiothorac Surg 21:5–9, 2002.
36. Inoue K, Sata M, Iwase T, et al: Clinical endovascular placement of branched graft for type B aortic dissection. J Thorac Cardiovasc Surg 112:1111–1113, 1996.
37. Ishihara H, Uchida N, Yamasaki C, et al: Extensive primary repair of the thoracic aorta in Stanford type A acute aortic dissection by means of a synthetic vascular graft with a self-expandable stent. J Thorac Cardiovasc Surg 123:1035–1040, 2002.
38. Juvonem T, Ergin MA, Galla JD, et al: Prospective study of the natural history of thoracic aortic aneurysms. Ann Thorac Surg 63:1533–1545, 1999.
39. Kasirajan K, Marek J, Langsfeld M: Endovascular management of acute traumatic thoracic aneurysm. J Trauma 52: 357–390, 2002.
40. Kato N, Dake MD, Miller DC, et al: Traumatic thoracic aortic aneurysm: treatment with endovascular stent-grafts. Radiology 205(3):657–662, 1997.
41. Kato N, Hirano T, Kawaguchi T, et al: Aneurysmal degeneration of the aorta after stent-graft repair of acute aortic dissection. J Vasc Surg 34(3):513–518, 2001.
42. Kato N, Hirano T, Shimono T, et al: Treatment of chronic aortic dissection by transluminal endovascular stent-graft placement: preliminary results. J Vasc Interv Radiol 12:835–840, 2001.
43. Kato N, Shimono T, Hirano T, et al: Transluminal placement of endovascular stent-grafts for the treatment of type A aortic dissection with an entry tear in the descending thoracic aorta. J Vasc Surg 34:1023–1028, 2001.
44. Kato N, Shimono T, Hirano T, et al: Midterm results of stent-graft repair of acute and chronic aortic dissection with descending tear: the complication-specific approach. J Thorac Cardiovasc Surg 124:306–312, 2002.
45. Kazui T, Tamiya Y, Tanaka T, Komatsu S: Extended aortic replacement for acute type A dissection with the tear in the descending aorta. J Thorac Cardiovasc Surg 112:973–978, 1996.
46. Kazui T, Yamashita K, Washiyama N, et al: Impact of an aggressive surgical approach on surgical outcome in type A aortic dissection. Ann Thorac Surg 74:S1844–1847, 2002.
47. Kouchoukos NT, Masetti P, Rokkas CK, Murphy SF: Single-stage reoperative repair of chronic type A aortic dissection using the arch-first technique. Ann Thorac Surg 74: S1800–1802, 2002.
48. Lam CR, Aram HH: Resection of a descending thoracic aorta for aneurysm: a report of the use of a homograft in a case and an experimental study. Ann Surg 134:743–752, 1951.
49. Lansman SL, McCullough JN, Nguyen KH, et al: Subtypes of acute aortic dissection. Ann Thorac Surg 67:1975–1978, 1999.
50. Lauterback SR, Cambria RP, Brewster DC, et al: Contemporary management of aortic branch compromise resulting from acute aortic dissection. J Vasc Surg 33: 1185–1192, 2001.
51. Mitchell RS: Endovascular solution for diseases of the thoracic aorta. Cardiol Clin North Am 17(4):815–825, 1999.
52. Mitchell RS: Stent grafts for the thoracic aorta: a new paradigm? Ann Thorac Surg 74:S1818–1820, 2002.
53. Mitchell RS, Dake MD, Semba CP, et al: Endovascular stent-graft repair of thoracic aortic aneurysms. J Thorac Cardiovasc Surg 111(5):1054–1062, 1996.
54. Mitchell RS, Miller CD, Dake MD, et al: Thoracic aortic aneurysm repair with an endovascular stent graft: the "first generation." Ann Thorac Surg 67:1971–1974, 1999.
55. Miyairi T, Kotsuka Y, Ezure M, et al: Open stent-grafting for aortic arch aneurysm is associated with increased risk of paraplegia. Ann Thorac Surg 74:83–89, 2002.
56. Miyairi T, Ninomiya M, Munemoto E, et al: Conventional repair and operative stent-grafting for acute and chronic aortic dissection. Ann Thorac Surg 73:1621–1623, 2002.
57. Moon MR, Mitchell RS, Dake MD, et al: Simultaneous abdominal aortic replacement and stent-graft placement for multilevel aortic disease. J Vasc Surg 25(2):332–340, 1997.
58. Nienaber CA, Fattori R, Lund G, et al: Nonsurgical reconstruction of thoracic aortic dissection by stent-graft placement. N Engl J Med 340:1539–1545, 1999.
59. Nienaber CA, von Kodolitsch Y, Petersen B, et al: Intramural hemorrhage of the thoracic aorta: diagnostic and therapeutic implications. Circulation 92(6):1465–1472, 1995.
60. Ohki T, Veith FJ, Shaw P, et al: Increasing incidence of midterm and long-term complications after endovascular graft repair of abdominal aortic aneurysms: a note of caution based on a 9-year experience. Ann Surg 234(3):323–335, 2001.
61. Palma JH, de Souza JAM, Alves CMR, et al: Self-expandable aortic stent-grafts for treatment of descending aortic dissections. Ann Thorac Surg 73:1138–1142, 2002.
62. Palma JH, Miranda F, Gasques AR, et al: Treatment of thoracoabdominal aneurysm with self-Expandable aortic stent grafts. Ann Thorac Surg 74:1685–1687, 2002.
63. Parodi JC, Ferreria LM: Ten-year experience with endovascular therapy in aortic aneurysms. J Am Coll Surg 194: S58–S66, 2002.

64. Parodi JC, Palmaz JC, Barone HD: Transfemoral intraluminal graft implantation for abdominal aortic aneurysms. Ann Vasc Surg 5:491–499, 1991.
65. Pressler V, McNamara JJ: Thoracic aortic aneurysm. J Thorac Cardiovasc Surg 79:489–498, 1980.
66. Razavi MK, Nishimura E, Slonim S, et al: Percutaneous creation of acute type B aortic dissection. An experimental model for endoluminal therapy. J Vasc Interv Radiol 9: 626–632, 1996.
67. Richens D, Field M, Neale M, Oakley C: The mechanism of injury in blunt traumatic rupture of the aorta. Eur J Cardiothorac Surg 21:288–293, 2002.
68. Roux D, Brouchet L, Concina P, et al: Type-A acute aortic dissection: combined operation plus stent management. Ann Thorac Surg 73:1616–1618, 2002.
69. Ruiz CE, Zhang HP, Douglas JT, et al: A novel method for treatment of abdominal aortic aneurysms using percutaneous implantation of a newly designed endovascular device. Circulation 91:2470–2477, 1995.
70. Sailer J, Peloschek P, Rand T, et al: Endovascular treatment of aortic type B dissection and penetrating ulcer using commercially available stent-grafts. Am J Roentgenol 177:1365–1369, 2001.
71. Schor JS, Yerlioglu E, Galla JD, et al: Selective management of acute type B aortic dissection: long-term follow-up. Ann Thorac Surg 61:1339–1341, 1996.
72. Shimono T, Kato N, Tokui T, et al: Endovascular stent-graft repair for acute type A aortic dissection with an intimal tear in the descending aorta. J Thorac Cardiovasc Surg 116(1): 171–173, 1998.
73. Shimono T, Kato N, Yasuda F, et al: Transluminal stent-graft placements for the treatments of acute onset and chronic aortic dissections. Circulation 106(Suppl. I):I241–247, 2002.
74. Slonim SM, Miller DC, Mitchell RS, et al: Percutaneous balloon fenestration and stenting for life-threatening ischemic complications in patients with acute aortic dissection. J Thorac Cardiovasc Surg 117:1118–1127, 1999.
75. Slonim SM, Nyman U, Semba Charles P, et al: Aortic dissection: percutaneous management of ischemic complications with endovascular stents and balloon fenestration. J Vasc Surg 23(2): 241–253, 1996.
76. Song JK, Kim HS, Kang DH, et al: Different clinical features of aortic intramural hematoma versus dissection involving the ascending aorta. J Am Coll Cardiol 37:1604–1610, 2001.
77. Sueda T, Orihashi K, Watari M, et al: Endovascular stent-grafting for traumatic aortic aneurysms with the use of a fenestrated stent-graft. J Thorac Cardiovasc Surg 122:144–146, 2001.
78. Suzuki T, Shimono T, Kato N, et al: Extended total arch replacement by means of the open stent-grafting method to treat intimal tears after transluminal stent-graft placement for a ruptured acute type B aortic dissection. J Thorac Cardiovasc Surg 123:354–356, 2002.
79. Svensson LG, Crawford ES, Hees KR, et al: Experience with 1509 patients undergoing thoracoabdominal aortic operations. J Vasc Surg 17:357–370, 1993.
80. Swan H, Maaske C, Johnson M, Grover R: Arterial homografts II. Resection of thoracic aortic aneurysm using a stored human arterial transplant. Arch Surg 61:732–737, 1950.
81. Tatou E, Steinmetz E, Jazayeri S, et al: Surgical outcome of traumatic rupture of the thoracic aorta. Ann Thorac Surg 69:70–73, 2000.
82. Tokui T, Shimono T, Kato N, et al: Less invasive therapy using endovascular stent graft repair and video-assisted thoracoscopic surgery for ruptured acute aortic dissection. J Thorac Cardiovasc Surg 48:603–606, 2000.
83. Troxler M, Mavor AID, Homer-Vanniasinkam S: Penetrating atherosclerotic ulcers of the aorta. Br J Surg 88(9):1169–1177, 2001.
84. Umana JP, Mitchell RS: Endovascular treatment of aortic dissections and thoracic aortic aneurysms. Sem Vasc Surg 13(4):290–298, 2000.
85. Umana JP, Mitchell RS: Thoracic aortic stent-grafts. Coron Artery Dis 13:103–111, 2002.
86. Umana JP, Lai DT, Mitchell RS, et al: Is medical therapy still the optimal treatment strategy for patients with acute type B aortic dissections? J Thorac Cardiovasc Surg 124:896–910, 2002.
87. Umana JP, Miller DC, Mitchell RS: What is the best treatment for patients with acute type B aortic dissections—medical, surgical, or endovascular stent-grafting? Ann Thorac Surg 74:S1840–1843, 2002.
88. Vlahakes GJ: Catheter-based treatment of aortic dissection. N Engl J Med 340:1584–1586, 1999.
89. von Segesser LK, Killer I, Ziswiler M, et al: Dissection of the descending thoracic aorta extending into the ascending aorta. Thorac Cardiovasc Surg 108:755–761, 1994.
90. Won JY, Lee DY, Shim WH, et al: Elective endovascular treatment of descending thoracic aortic aneurysms and chronic dissections with stent-grafts. J Vasc Interv Radiol 12:575–582, 2001.
91. Yoshida, H, Yasuda K, Tanabe T: New approach to aortic dissection: development of an insertable aortic prosthesis. Ann Thorac Surg 58:806–810, 1994.
92. Zarins CK, White RA, Moll FL, et al: The AneuRx stent graft: four-year results and worldwide experience 2000. J Vasc Surg 33:S135–145, 2001.

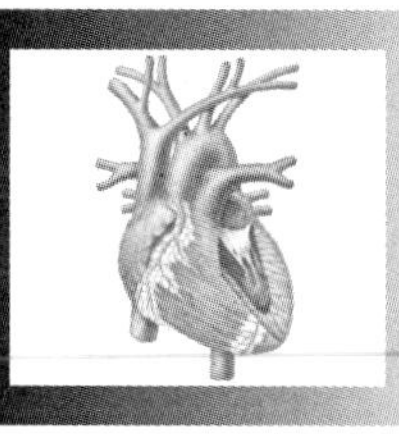

CHAPTER 71A

Occlusive Disease of Branches of the Thoracic Aorta and Peripheral Angiography Intervention

Occlusive Disease of the Supraaortic Trunk and Management of Simultaneous Surgical Carotid/Coronary Disease

Jeffrey S. Veluz and Ralph De La Torre

INTRODUCTION

Branch disease of the supraaortic trunk (SAT) manifests as a diverse series of clinical syndromes related to ischemia or embolism in the affected distribution. Since it was first described in 1856 many investigators have reported varying manifestations of arch vessel aortoocclusive disease.[41] In the not so distant past many of these lesions were thought incurable. As surgical technique, anesthetic management, and critical care have progressed, many of these lesions are treatable with low morbidity and mortality. Although most authors agree on the absolute indications for surgical intervention, such as life-limiting limb ischemia and neurological manifestations of disease, these indications continue to be expanded. With an aging population beset with atherosclerosis, concomitant branch disease presenting as incidental or secondary diagnoses during more routine cardiac surgery is becoming increasingly common. In particular, the increase in concomitant coronary and carotid occlusive disease has raised questions regarding proper timing of intervention. Treatment algorithms, whether it be simultaneous repair, staged repair, preoperative stenting, or medical treatment of carotid occlusive disease in the setting of concurrent surgical coronary disease, seem to be center dependent with ostensibly similar outcomes.

ATHEROSCLEROTIC DISEASE OF THE AORTA AND ARCH VESSELS

Occlusive disease affecting the primary branches of the aortic arch is thought to account for only 3–15% of surgically corrected extracranial lesions with the large majority of lesions being carotid bifurcation disease.[10,34] Although the left subclavian artery is the most common arch vessel occluded by atherosclerotic damage, multifocal stenoses affecting the innominate, left common carotid, or left subclavian arteries, are the rule, with large series reporting 65–84% multifocal disease.[3,13,24] In addition, while primary ostial occlusion of aortic arch branches does occur, the most common cause of common carotid occlusion is retrograde thrombosis emanating from carotid bifurcation occlusion.[44] Occlusive lesions of the innominate and subclavian arteries, however, are though to emanate from lesions occurring near their origin. The pertinent risk factors in aortic arch occlusive disease are those of atherosclerosis: smoking, hypertension, diabetes, and hyperlipidemia.

Clinical Pathophysiology

Atherosclerotic change usually affects the greater curvature of the aorta and the three branches. Alternatively, isolated ostial disease has also been reported. In 10% of patients, anomalous anatomy may coexist, with bovine anatomy (common trunk of innominate and left common carotid arteries) and left vertebral artery origin from the aortic arch proximal to the left subclavian the most common.[4] Clinical presentation of symptomatic aortic arch disease due to atherosclerosis usually falls into three distinct categories: ischemia due to (1) vessel thrombosis, (2) embolism/sudden vessel occlusion, or (3) hypoperfusion/steal syndrome. Neurological symptoms depend on the particular cervicocephalic vessel involved and can present as transient ischemic attacks, amaurosis fugax, hemiparesis, hemisensory loss, speech difficulty, gait difficulty, visual impairment, or vertigo depending on whether the anterior (carotid) or posterior (vertebrobasilar) circulation is affected. Thrombotic events predominantly occur in patients with multifocal disease. Embolic phenomena due to ulcerative ostial disease of the aortic arch are uncommon relative to carotid bifurcation atherosclerosis. However, with regard to embolic phenomena, the possibility of primary embolism from the atherosclerotic aortic arch as well as from a cardiogenic source must also be considered. Aside from cervicocephalic arterial occlusions, emboli may also lodge in the distal extremities resulting in pain, ischemia, or frank gangrene. Steal syndromes classically are related to severe stenosis or complete occlusion of the subclavian artery proximal to the vertebral artery takeoff, with ipsilateral retrograde perfusion of the affected limb via the vertebral artery. Patients are usually asymptomatic because of the rich network of collateral vessels, although syncope, vertigo, cranial nerve impairment, claudication, or rest pain of the upper extremity may occur in severe cases. Combinations of the three syndromes of course may also occur, with treatment directed at the amalgamation of findings.

Diagnosis

Physical examination with particular attention to the vascular and neurological findings is the first step in diagnosis. Comparison of blood pressures in each brachium should be obtained. A careful history can usually distinguish posterior versus anterior circulation symptomatology. Although several significant advances have been made in vascular radiology, angiography remains the diagnostic gold standard. Advances in endovascular therapies also allow for treatment at the time of study. Although ultrasound has been well established in the assessment of carotid bifurcation disease and should be performed on all patients being evaluated for aortic arch disease, limitations exist in the evaluation of aortic branch disease because of skeletal constraints. Transthoracic, or transesophageal, echocardiography (TEE) has been used to obtain reliable adjunctive information, but again is limited by depth of penetration of the ultrasonic signal. In particular, TEE is limited in its ability to assess the branches of the aortic arch primarily because of shadowing from the airway.[12,19] Endovascular ultrasound is an emerging technology without widespread use at this time. Computed tomography (CT) and magnetic resonance imaging (MRI) are becoming increasingly utilized adjunctively or in lieu of angiography. Recent application of spiral CT acquisition timed to contrast injectate with three-dimensional reconstruction (CTA) provides detailed information of the intrathoracic and extrathoracic circulation.[25] Similar information can be obtained using timed contrast-enhanced MRI with reconstruction (MRA). MRA, in particular, since it is not contrast dependent, may yield useful information in occluded vessels reconstituted via collaterals.[26] MRI also obtains definitive information of any intracranial lesions and delineates patterns of perfusion/diffusion abnormalities that may suggest the vascular etiology (e.g., embolic versus small vessel thrombotic versus hypoperfusion). It has been reported, however, that MRA tends to overestimate the degree of stenosis.[29]

Treatment

Because of the rarity of this disease, natural history data for the treatment of asymptomatic disease are lacking, with some centers advocating treatment for severe stenosis (>80%) or presence of ulceration with significant (>50%) stenosis.[34] Treatment for symptomatic aortic branch disease, whether it be cerebrovascular or upper extremity symptoms, remains the most common indication for surgical intervention. The treatment of aortic arch branch disease is constructed to address the sources of pathophysiology: restore pulsatile blood flow and exclude sources of embolic debris. Techniques used most commonly are bypass grafting and endarterectomy, although arterial transposition can be utilized for selected cases with similar results in selected patients.[7]

Innominate Artery

The innominate artery is seldom the only vessel requiring revascularization. Ruel et al found that patients undergoing revascularization for innominate artery symptoms required at least one other vessel intervened 60% of the time.[34] Early studies evaluating treatment of innominate atherosclerotic disease favored an extrathoracic approach because of the high morbidity and mortality of intrathoracic repair.[13] Advances in surgical technique and anesthesia, however, have resulted in equivalent results.[3] Direct repair or bypass via an intrathoracic approach appears to be simple and well tolerated, with the extrathoracic approach reserved for patients in whom transthoracic repair is contraindicated.[6,11] Relative contraindications to intrathoracic revascularization include a heavily diseased or calcified arch, a reoperative chest, and advanced age or poor medical condition. Others have advocated isolated single branch disease repair via a transcervical approach citing less morbidity and excellent long-term results.[7]

When revascularization of isolated innominate disease is contemplated two transthoracic options exist, endarterectomy or bypass. Endarterectomy has been well described with excellent results for isolated branch disease.[11] The vessel is approached via a partial or complete sternotomy with extension into the neck as necessary. Relative contraindications include inability to clamp the innominate, severe arch atherosclerosis, proximal left common carotid artery origin (including a common brachiocephalic trunk), or transmural arteritis. The endarterectomy proceeds as described in Figure 71A-1. Care should be taken not to injure the aorta while obtaining proximal control of the innominate origin, as atherosclerotic disease of the arch is common. Intraoperative epiaortic ultrasound may prove of benefit prior to clamping. Shunting is unnecessary unless critical multivessel disease is present. The vessel can be closed primarily or by patch angioplasty if narrowing the vessel is of concern. Surprisingly, postoperative neurological complications are rare, even in the setting of multivessel disease. Unless multivessel disease involving one or both carotids is encountered, EEG monitoring or shunting is usually unnecessary. Alternatively, bypass grafting using synthetic prosthetic graft material has been used with excellent results and has become the procedure of choice, primarily because of ease of performance rather than differences in outcome

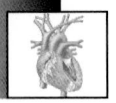

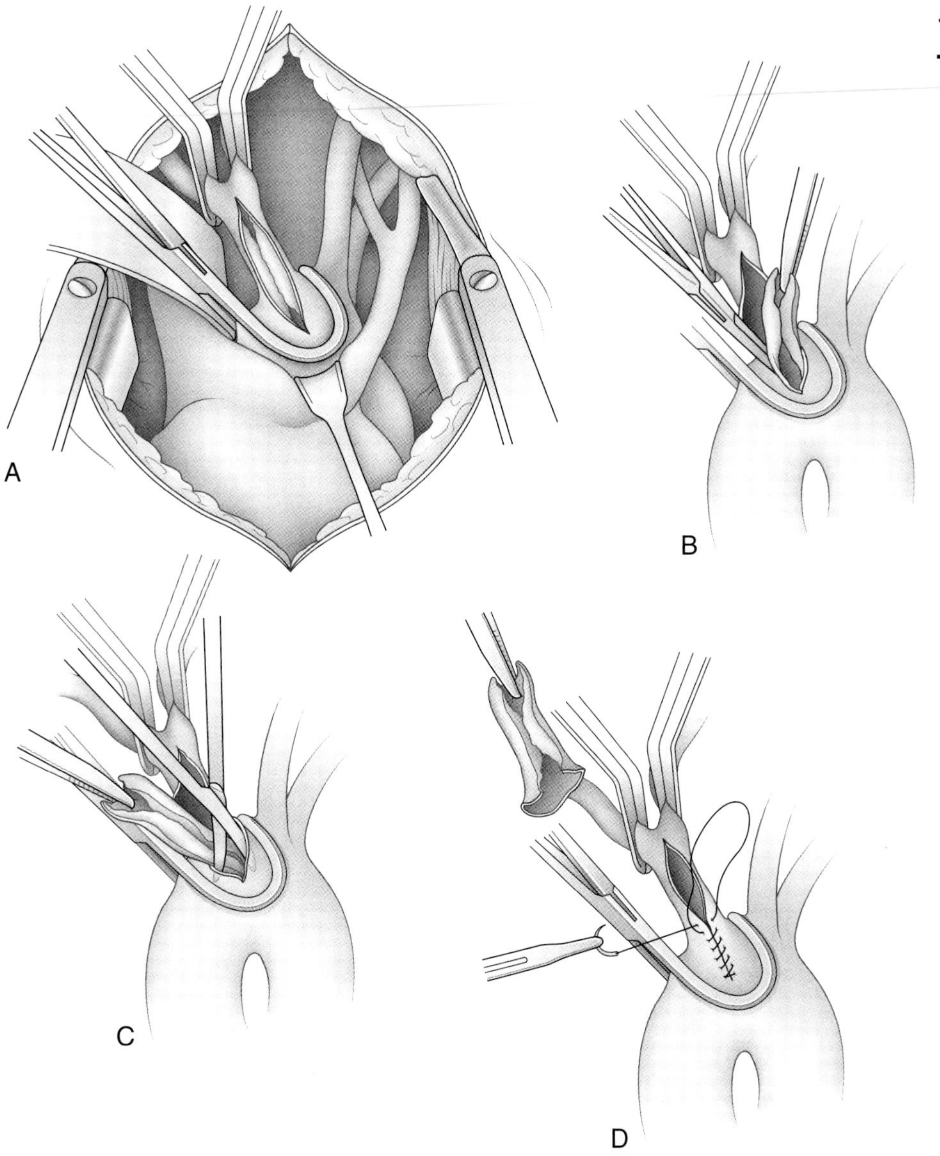

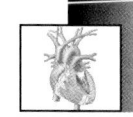

Figure 71A–1 A–D, A full-length sternotomy and upper cutaneous incision are used for an innominate artery endarterectomy. A J-shaped clamp is used to occlude the side of the aorta adjacent to the innominate orifice, and the endarterectomy is completed. *(Modified from Carlson RE, Ehrenfeld WK, Stoney RJ, et al: Innominate artery endarterectomy. Arch Surg 112:1389–1393, 1977. Copyright 1977, American Medical Association.)*

(Figure 71A-2). As with endarterectomy, epiaortic ultrasound is often useful in selecting the site of the proximal anastomosis. If at all possible the proximal anastomosis should be constructed toward the right lateral aspect of the ascending aorta to avoid potential compression from the sternum. Care should be taken when constructing the bevel and the orientation to avoid kinking of the graft. The distal anastomosis is constructed in an end-to-side fashion unless emboli are suspected to have originated from the diseased portion. In that situation the surgeon should consider excluding the diseased segment. Some centers advocate endarterectomy for specific situations including simultaneous or previous coronary artery bypass grafting (CABG), small thoracic outlet, or prior tracheostomy.

Common Carotid Artery (CCA)

Multiple surgical approaches to common carotid occlusions include carotid bifurcation endarterectomy along with retrograde endarterectomy, proximal CCA transection with endarterectomy and transposition to subclavian, carotid subclavian bypass, and aorta to CCA bypass with tube graft (Figure 71A-3). CCA disease concurrent with other lesions of the SAT is best approached by a transsternal repair utilizing a bypass graft. Isolated CCA disease can be effectively treated via a transcervical approach without sternotomy in the majority of cases. This approach also allows for simultaneous repair of ipsilateral carotid bifurcation stenosis. Contralateral carotid bifurcation occlusion is usually repaired at a later date.

Subclavian Artery

Relief of vertebrobasilar insufficiency is the most common indication for repair of the subclavian artery. Four surgical options exist: subclavian–carotid bypass with graft, subclavian–carotid transposition, transposition of the vertebral to common carotid artery, and extraanatomical axillary tube graft bypass. Symptoms prompting repair for isolated disease include upper extremity claudication, hand ischemia, or recurrent angina congestive heart failure (CHF) in patients with previous left internal mammary artery coronary bypass graft. Repair for isolated asymptomatic subclavian stenosis is generally not indicated. Multivessel disease again is best

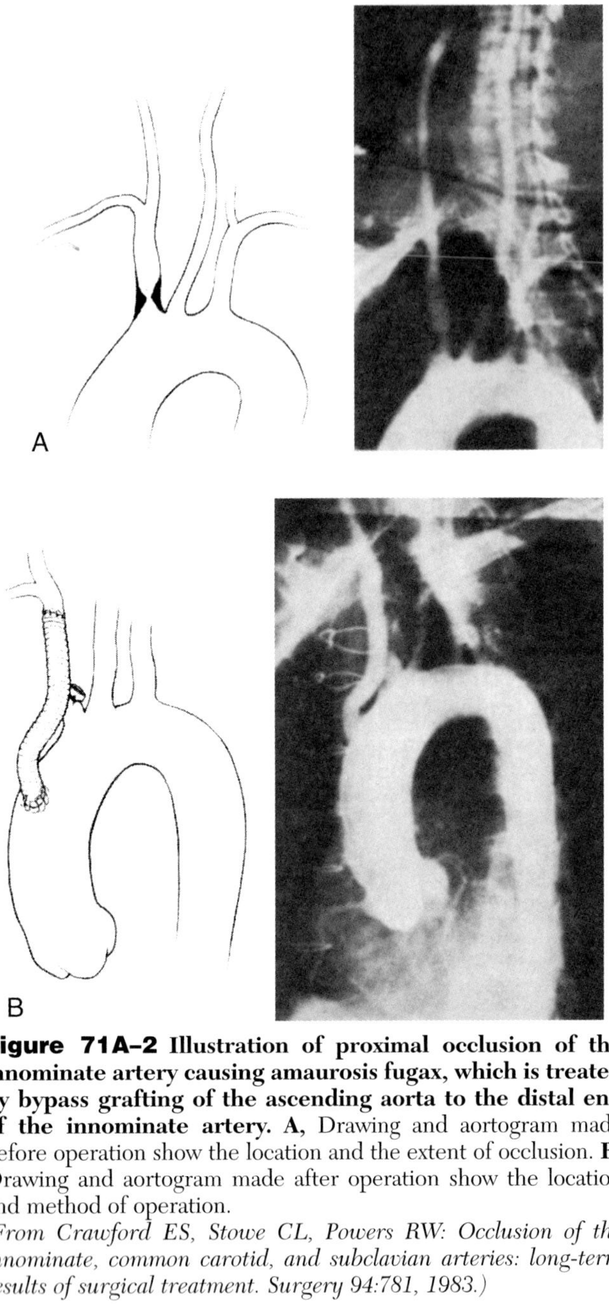

Figure 71A–2 Illustration of proximal occlusion of the innominate artery causing amaurosis fugax, which is treated by bypass grafting of the ascending aorta to the distal end of the innominate artery. A, Drawing and aortogram made before operation show the location and the extent of occlusion. **B,** Drawing and aortogram made after operation show the location and method of operation.
(From Crawford ES, Stowe CL, Powers RW: Occlusion of the innominate, common carotid, and subclavian arteries: long-term results of surgical treatment. Surgery 94:781, 1983.)

approached by transthoracic repair with branched prosthetic graft bypass.

Multivessel Disease

Most large series as mentioned previously indicate that patients with atherosclerotic stenosis of the SAT usually have multivessel disease. Although reports show successful repair of multivessel disease via transthoracic endarterectomy, these repairs are technically more challenging and less versatile. Transsternal aortobranch bypass appears most suited in these situations. Options include multiple grafts originating from the aorta to individual vessels versus single trunk tube graft with additional side branch grafts (Figure 71A-4). Because concomitant atherosclerotic aortic disease is present in many patients, avoidance of multiple proximal anastomoses appears prudent. A single large "parent" tube graft from the aortic arch with individual small-diameter tube grafts appropriate to branch sizes provides adequate flow with the flexibility of conduit positioning. Care should be taken in the placement of the proximal anastomosis as torsion, external compression from surrounding structures, and kinking may occur. We generally prefer originating the proximal tube graft to the right of midline along the greater curvature of the aortic arch in such a way as to avoid undue compression. Again, epiaortic ultrasound can assist the placement of grafts to avoid embolization of atheromatous plaque.

Results

Reports from high-volume centers utilizing either transthoracic or extrathoracic reconstruction of the SAT have steadily improved over the past several decades. Berguer et al recently report in two successive series a 5- and 10-year primary patency rate of 94 and 88% for an intrathoracic approach versus 91 and 82% via an extrathoracic approach, respectively.[6,7] Perioperative morbidity ranges from 8–25%, including a 0–6% risk for myocardial infarction (mostly nonfatal) and stroke rate ranging from 3 to 8%, with the remaining morbidity mostly respiratory. Perioperative mortality for transthoracic repair has been reported from 0 to 8%. Long-term mortality is primarily due to death from myocardial infarction or cerebrovascular accident.[6,11,32,34,44]

▸ CONCURRENT CAROTID AND CORONARY ATHEROSCLEROSIS

Much controversy exists over the management of patients with surgical disease of both carotid and coronary arteries. Stroke following CABG is perhaps the most devastating nonfatal complication. It is estimated that 3–14% of CABG patients have significant carotid disease.[22,37] There are of course many other factors contributing to the risk of stroke after CABG including age, female sex, prior stroke or transient ischemic attack (TIA), left main disease, low ejection fraction, diabetes, renal failure, smoking history, severe peripheral vascular disease, carotid bruit, ascending aortic arch atherosclerosis, and duration of cardiopulmonary bypass, and these etiologies should be considered prior to consideration of simultaneous repair of both coronary and carotid disease.[39]

Faggioli et al reported an almost 10-fold increase in the risk of perioperative stroke in CABG patients undergoing surgery with greater than 75% carotid stenosis if left uncorrected.[16] These findings, as well as others, have prompted aggressive preoperative screening of CABG patients in order to stratify and treat patients at increased risk. Confounding this dilemma is the finding that many perioperative strokes after CABG in patients with carotid stenosis do not actually occur in the ischemic brain territory ipsilateral to the carotid lesion. The majority of recent studies clearly agree that the cause of post-CABG stroke is multifactorial, with emboli from aortic and cardiac origin

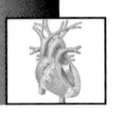

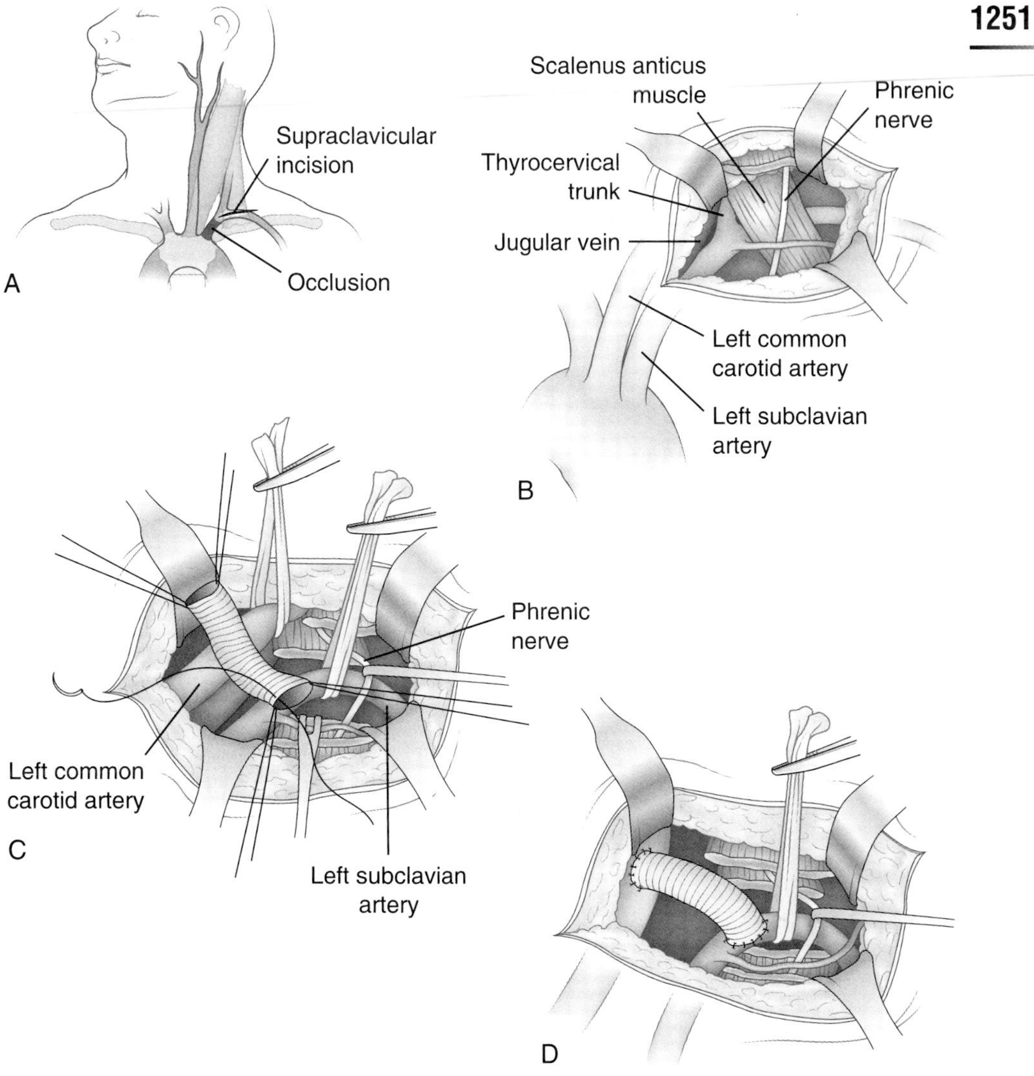

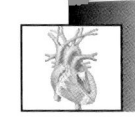

Figure 71A–3 **A,** Demonstration of the placement of the supraclavicular incision. It is centered over the clavicular head of the sternomastoid muscle. **B,** After division of the clavicular head of the sternomastoid muscle, the relationships of the phrenic nerve, scalenus anticus, and subclavian artery are shown. **C,** After mobilization of the carotid and subclavian arteries, preparation is made for a graft connection. **D,** Completion of the subclavian–carotid artery bypass is shown and denotes the proximity of the two arteries and the short length of graft that is required.
(Modified from Moore WS, Malone JM, Goldstone J: Extrathoracic repair of branch occlusions of the aortic arch. Am J Surg 132:249, 1976.)

accounting for a large majority of debris.[8] Barnes et al indicated that *long-term* outcome of neurological function is poor provided significant carotid disease remains uncorrected after CABG.[5] This conclusion would of course corroborate the long-term benefits derived from surgical repair of symptomatic carotid stenosis and well as treatment for asymptomatic severe carotid occlusion noted in the landmark NASCET and ACAS studies, respectively.[15,30] The indication for carotid intervention clearly must exist on its own merits irrespective of the indication for CABG. Of note, the benefit of carotid endarterectomy (CEA) for the asymptomatic patient with significant carotid stenosis relied upon a low surgical morbidity and mortality in the ACAS study.[15] The significance of this contingency as it applies to the treatment of combined carotid/coronary disease remains to be elucidated. The primary question that remains both unanswered and quite controversial, however, is the timing of carotid surgery relative to CABG when both disease entities have independent indication for operative repair. Strategies to address concomitant surgically correctable carotid and coronary disease include staged repair (CEA then CABG) "reversed" staged repair (CABG then CEA), combined approach (CABG and CEA), or no treatment of the carotid disease (CABG alone).

Several centers have reported their outcomes after combined repair with overall combined stroke and death rates averaging 10.3%.* Advocates for combined repair cite acceptable stroke rates, single anesthesia, lowered costs, and overall lower incidence of myocardial infarction over reversed staged repair. Akins et al at the Massachusetts General Hospital reported a series of 200 consecutive patients treated with concurrent CEA and CABG with overall stroke rate of 4% and mortality of 3.5.[1] It should be noted that the centers reporting the lowest stroke and death rates using a combined approach tended to have relatively high volume experience with this approach. In the only prospective trial involving partial randomization, Hertzer et al from the Cleveland Clinic divided patients into those with stable and unstable cardiac disease.[21] Those with stable cardiac disease (8.7%) underwent CEA followed by CABG as a staged procedure with a stroke rate of 4.8%. Those with unilateral *asymptomatic* carotid stenosis (46.9%) were then prospectively randomized to either combined operative repair or reversed

*References 1, 8, 14, 21, 23, 27, 35, 38, 47.

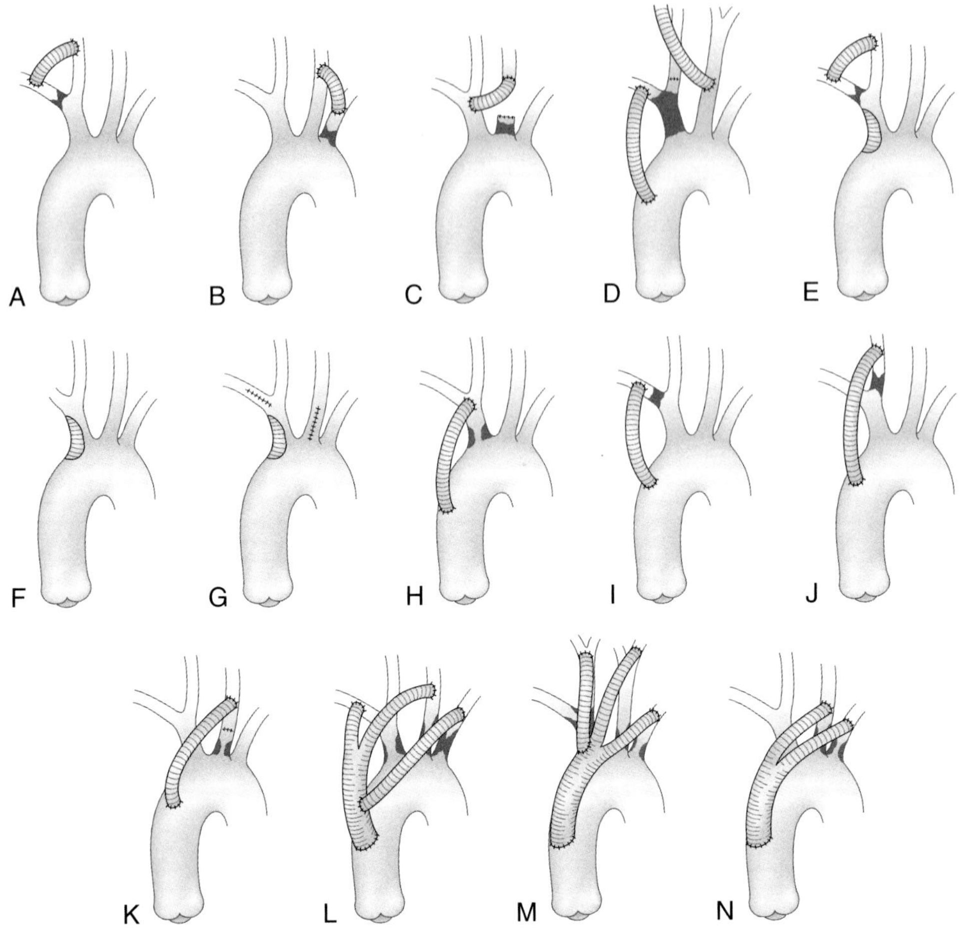

Figure 71A–4 Various brachiocephalic reconstruction techniques and approaches. (**A–F**) Extrathoracic bypass. (**E–G**) Transthoracic endarterectomy. (**D** and **H–N**) Transthoracic bypass. *(Modified from Takach TJ, et al: Concomitant occlusive disease of the coronary arteries and great vessels. Ann Thorac Surg 65:79–84, 1998.)*

staged repair (CABG followed later by CEA). Patients undergoing reversed staged repair had a stroke rate of 14% (half during CABG and half during CEA) with a mortality of 5.3%. Combined repair of carotid/coronary disease resulted in a much lower stroke rate of 2.8% with a mortality of 4.2%. A final nonrandomized group of patients in this cohort had either symptomatic carotid disease or significant bilateral disease and were treated individually. In this high-risk group, stroke occurred in 7.1% of patients and 6.1% died.

Of particular importance, it was observed in this study that patients in the reversed staged repair who received CEA after CABG during the same hospital admission had a stroke rate of 11% versus 2.2% in patients discharged home to receive CEA at least 2 weeks after their CABG. It is therefore possible that close proximity of CEA after CABG increases the overall risk of neurological events. As mentioned previously, CABG utilizing cardiopulmonary bypass involves multiple risk factors beyond carotid stenosis, most notably atheroemboli from the heart and aorta. In fact, studies show that intracranial flow and velocity do not show significant changes in patients with high-grade carotid stenosis during CABG, suggesting that the presence of carotid stenosis may be a marker for atherosclerotic disease and its attendant risks rather than the etiological factor in stroke after CABG in some cases.[48] In an elegant study by Bilfinger et al, 2071 nonrandomized patients underwent preoperative screening for carotid stenosis over a 4-year period.[8] Patients with asymptomatic stenosis greater than 80% underwent combined repair. The incidence of stroke in the combined group was 4.7% with a mortality of 5.9%. The CABG alone group who by definition had less than 80% stenosis had a stroke rate of 1.7% with a mortality of 2.0%, confirming the findings of others that a combined procedure carries an increased risk of combined stroke/death rate. Of particular interest, CABG-alone patients who did develop a perioperative cerebrovascular accident (CVA) had a mortality of 26.4%, while no deaths occurred in the combined group who developed a stroke. Symptomatic carotid patients were not studied.

The lowest report of the staged repair of concomitant carotid/coronary disease comes from the Texas Heart Institute with overall stroke rates of 1.9%.[45] Indeed the definition of "high-risk" CEA has undergone some revision in recent years with reports in the vascular surgery literature with high-volume centers reporting low stroke and death rates (1.3%) in patients with previously accepted "high-risk" factors for complication (elderly population, myocardial infarction [MI] within 6 months, NYHA Class III/IV, CHA Class III/IV, CHF, COPD, renal dysfunction).[20] Advances in anesthesia, in surgical technique, as well as in intraoperative monitoring for cerebral ischemia also have resulted in low morbidity/mortality including the use of CEA under local anesthesia.

Another possible confounding variable in the combined treatment for coronary/carotid disease is the institution itself. A recent retrospective review of 10,561 randomly selected Medicare patients who underwent CABG in 10 U.S. states showed a significantly worse outcome in the combined treatment CABG patients compared to published results with a combined stroke and death rate of 17.8% and overall stroke rate of 12%.[9] It seems there is a wide discrepancy in outcome between academic and community-based centers as well as between high- and low-volume centers. It would appear that until a large multicenter prospectively randomized trial is initiated, answers as to preferred treatment algorithms will remain unanswered. At the present time it appears that superior outcomes utilizing the combined CABG/CEA approach remain center dependent.

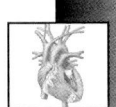

Recently, several clinical trials have investigated the use of carotid angioplasty and/or stenting as primary treatment for carotid stenosis.[31] Although results of carotid stenting await long-term validation, short-term results appear equivalent. Recent advances in technology, including covered stents, drug-eluting stents, cerebral protection devices, and novel antiplatelet therapy, have aided in refining treatment.[17] The advantages of stenting include avoidance of a general anesthetic, especially in high-risk groups with multiple comorbidities, including CABG patients. Disadvantages include unproven durability and lack of any randomized controlled trials, technician variability, and risk of stroke. Our preliminary experience at preoperative carotid stenting of high-risk CABG patients has been favorable (unpublished). Although experimental at this time, carotid stenting as an adjunct to CABG may represent the preferred treatment strategy in a patient population at high risk for morbidity and mortality.

INFLAMMATORY OCCLUSIVE DISEASE OF THE THORACIC AORTA

Vasculitis syndromes are characterized by inflammation of blood vessels with subsequent healing response. Many believe the process of inflammatory-mediated vascular damage centers on immune complex deposition with a subsequent vasculitis that resembles the process seen in serum sickness.[18] This hypothesis, however, has not been proven. Vasculitis syndromes can take many forms, having varying inciting agents or events, and affecting a variety of blood vessels. Furthermore, vasculitis syndromes can lead to aneurysm formation, stenosis, occlusion, or a combination thereof. Within the scope of this chapter, only one vasculitis syndrome commonly leads to occlusive disease of the thoracic aorta and its branches, Takayasu's arteritis.

Takayasu's arteritis was first described by a Japanese ophthalmologist and was thought to be a disease of young Asian women.[46] Although the incidence in women is clearly higher (4:1), it is now recognized as a vasculitis affecting both sexes and all cultures. Takayasu's arteritis is an inflammatory disease whose point of attack is the medial elastic fibers of the affected vessel. Scarring and destruction of the media and internal elastic lamina with concomitant intimal proliferation are commonly seen. Given its strong predilection for elastic fibers it is easy to understand why the aortic arch and its branches are so commonly affected.[42]

Clinical Pathophysiology

Takayasu's arteritis remains primarily a disease of the young (<40 years) with a strong predilection for women. The first presentation usually occurs during the acute phase of the disease process. The typical presentation involves malaise (83%), fever (62%), syncope or dizziness (47%), and chest pain (33%). A physical examination reveals bruits (89%), hypertension (58%), absent pulses (49%), abnormal funduscopic examination (41%), and aortic insufficiency (19%). On further investigation one commonly finds further symptoms of organ malperfusion and cardiac failure. Cardiac failure and cardiomegaly are usually secondary to hypertension and aortic insufficiency. At this stage the clinical course can vary from a fulminant rapidly progressing course to an indolent chronic course.[42]

The treatment of Takayasu's arteritis remains a combination of immunosuppressive therapy and percutaneous and surgical interventions. The first line of medical therapy remains glucocorticoids with methotrexate or cyclophosphamide reserved for the 30–40% of cases that do not respond appropriately to steroids. Surgical interventions are used in those cases with organ ischemia. The addition of percutaneous and surgical intervention in the treatment of Takayasu's arteritis has brought a substantial reduction of mortality and major morbidity.[2,43]

Diagnosis

Tissue diagnosis showing fragmentation and necrosis of smooth muscles and elastic fibers with fibrosis and arterial wall contraction with resultant intimal proliferation is usually not obtainable. Instead, the diagnosis of Takayasu's arteritis is usually suspected from the history and clinical presentation as described above.[2] The diagnosis is supported with specific serological tests and angiographic findings. Typically patients may be found to have an elevated erythrocyte sedimentation rate (ESR), eosinophilia, elevated VDLR, elevated globulin level, elevated C-reactive protein, elevated fibrinogen, and elevated leukocyte count.[42] Angiographic studies demonstrate a characteristic pattern of stenosis, poststenotic dilatation, aneurysm formation, and occlusion with collateral formation. On angiogram the disease is often localized to the aorta and the proximal aspect of its branches, although a complete body angiogram is often needed to establish a diagnosis.[32,49] Various groups have sought to classify Takayasu's arteritis based on the locale of the disease and its extent. Although helpful in establishing trends and comparing the disease across geographical locations, these classifications do not appear to aid in diagnosis or prognosis.

Treatment

Patients with stenotic lesions warrant surgical intervention when symptoms develop. In general, the principles of surgical bypass grafting as described above apply with a few notable exceptions. Surgical intervention should be undertaken, if possible, while Takayasu's arteritis is in its chronic or fibroocclusive stage. Some authors advocate deferring surgery during the acute phase of the disease until the patient can be treated with steroids or antimetabolites.[2,43]

Furthermore, innominate artery stenosis should be dealt with through distal grafting and not endarterectomy. The panarteritis and fibrosis yield an inconsistent plane for endarterectomy, and the adventitia that reconstitutes the vessel is often affected.[11]

Other principles in the surgical treatment of Takayasu's arteritis also need to be considered. When constructing proximal and distal anastomoses, sites free of disease should be chosen.[40] Although microscopic disease is most likely still present, the absence of macroscopic disease is felt by some surgeons to decrease the likelihood of recurrent stenosis or aneurysm formation. Although this has not been borne out in every study it seems a prudent measure. Also, anastomosis performed on the ascending aorta should be made large and widely patent. This will decrease the likelihood that progression of the disease will lead to recurrent occlusive disease. In the case of vein grafts originating from the ascending aorta, a Dacron patch is first placed on the aorta with the vein graft originating from this patch.[28,40,43]

In the construction of an anastomosis in the setting of Takayasu's arteritis, subsequent aneurysm formation also needs to be taken into account. In addition to operating during a quiescent stage and choosing a disease-free site, many authors advocate treating the patient with perioperative steroids. Other recommended technical maneuvers include liberal use of felting material, the use of multiple horizontal mattress sutures, and the incorporation of large amounts of tissue with each suture.

Results

The aggressive use of percutaneous and surgical interventions in combination with steroids and antimetabolites has significantly decreased mortality. A disease entity that previously carried a 10–40% mortality is now thought to carry a 5–10% mortality. Furthermore, using the aforementioned techniques, 10-year graft patencies on the order of 70% can be maintained.[36]

REFERENCES

1. Akins CW, Moncure AC, Daggett WM, et al: Safety and efficacy of concomitant carotid and coronary artery operations. Ann Thorac Surg 60(2):311–317, 1995; discussion 318.
2. Ando M, Sasako Y, Okita Y, et al: Surgical considerations of occlusive lesions associated with Takayasu's arteritis. Jpn J Thorac Cardiovasc Surg 48:173–179, 2000.
3. Azakie A, McElhinney DB, Higashima R, et al: Innominate artery reconstruction: over 3 decades of experience. Ann Surg 228(3):402–410, 1998.
4. Azakie A, McElhinney DB, Messina LM, Stoney RJ: Common brachiocephalic trunk: strategies for revascularization. Ann Thorac Surg 67(3):657–660, 1999.
5. Barnes RW, Nix ML, Sansonetti D, et al: Late outcome of untreated asymptomatic carotid disease following cardiovascular operations. J Vasc Surg 2(6):843–849, 1985.
6. Berguer R, Morasch MD, Kline RA: Transthoracic repair of innominate and common carotid artery disease: immediate and long-term outcome for 100 consecutive surgical reconstructions. J Vasc Surg 27(1):34–41; discussion 42, 1998.
7. Berguer R, Morasch MD, Kline RA, et al: Cervical reconstruction of the supra-aortic trunks: a 16-year experience. J Vasc Surg 29(2):239–246; discussion 246–248, 1999.
8. Bilfinger TV, Reda H, Giron F, et al: Coronary and carotid operations under prospective standardized conditions: incidence and outcome. Ann Thorac Surg 69(6):1792–1798, 2000.
9. Brown KR, Kresowik TF, Chin MH, et al: Multistate population-based outcomes of combined carotid endarterectomy and coronary artery bypass. J Vasc Surg 37(1):32–39, 2003.
10. Carlson RE, Ehrenfeld WK, Stoney RJ, Wylie EJ: Innominate artery endarterectomy. A 16-year experience. Arch Surg 112(11):1389–1393, 1977.
11. Cherry KJ Jr, McCullough JL, Hallett JW Jr, et al: Technical principles of direct innominate artery revascularization: a comparison of endarterectomy and bypass grafts. J Vasc Surg 9(5):718–723; discussion 723–724, 1989.
12. Chu VF, Chow CM, Stewart J, et al: Transesophageal echocardiography for ascending aortic dissection: is it enough for surgical intervention? J Card Surg 13(4):260–265, 1998.
13. Crawford ES, De Bakey ME, Morris GC Jr, Howell JF: Surgical treatment of occlusion of the innominate, common carotid, and subclavian arteries: a 10 year experience. Surgery 65(1):17–31, 1969.
14. Dunn EJ: Concomitant cerebral and myocardial revascularization. Surg Clin North Am 66(2):385–395, 1986.
15. [No authors listed] Endarterectomy for asymptomatic carotid artery stenosis. Executive Committee for the Asymptomatic Carotid Atherosclerosis Study. JAMA 273(18):1421–1428, 1995.
16. Faggioli GL, Curl GR, Ricotta JJ: The role of carotid screening before coronary artery bypass. J Vasc Surg 12(6):724–729; discussion 729–731, 1990.
17. Fattori R, Piva T: Drug-eluting stents in vascular intervention. Lancet 361(9353):247–249, 2003.
18. Fauci: Vascolitis syndroms. In Harrison, editor: Principles of Internal Medicine, 13th ed.
19. Fayad ZA, Nahar T, Fallon JT, et al: In vivo magnetic resonance evaluation of atherosclerotic plaques in the human thoracic aorta: a comparison with transesophageal echocardiography. Circulation 101(21):2503–2509, 2000.
20. Gasparis AP, Ricotta L, Cuadra SA, et al: High-risk carotid endarterectomy: fact or fiction. J Vasc Surg 37(1):40–46, 2003.
21. Hertzer NR, Loop FD, Beven EG, et al: Surgical staging for simultaneous coronary and carotid disease: a study including prospective randomization. J Vasc Surg 9(3):455–463, 1989.
22. Hirotani T, Kameda T, Kumamoto T, et al: Stroke after coronary artery bypass grafting in patients with cerebrovascular disease. Ann Thorac Surg 70(5):1571–1576, 2000.
23. Jones EL, Craver JM, Michalik RA, et al: Combined carotid and coronary operations: when are they necessary? J Thorac Cardiovasc Surg 87(1):7–16, 1984.
24. Kieffer E, Sabatier J, Koskas F, Bahnini A: Atherosclerotic innominate artery occlusive disease: early and long-term results of surgical reconstruction. J Vasc Surg 21(2):326–336; discussion 336–337, 1995.
25. Ledbetter S, Stuk JL, Kaufman JA: Helical (spiral) CT in the evaluation of emergent thoracic aortic syndromes. Traumatic aortic rupture, aortic aneurysm, aortic dissection, intramural hematoma, and penetrating atherosclerotic ulcer. Radiol Clin North Am 37(3):575–589, 1999.
26. Meduri A, Natale L, Marano P: Imaging of aortic atherosclerosis. Rays 26(4):237–245, 2001.
27. Minami K, Gawaz M, Ohlmeier H, et al: Management of concomitant occlusive disease of coronary and carotid arteries using cardiopulmonary bypass for both procedures. J Cardiovasc Surg (Torino) 30(5):723–728, 1989.
28. Miyata T, Sato O, Deguchi J, et al: Anastomotic aneurysms after surgical treatment of Takayasu's arteritis: a 40-year experience. J Vasc Surg 27(3):438–445, 1998.
29. Nederkoorn PJ, Elgersma OE, Mali WP, et al: Overestimation of carotid artery stenosis with magnetic resonance angiography compared with digital subtraction angiography. J Vasc Surg 36(4):806–813, 2002.

30. [No authors listed] Beneficial effect of carotid endarterectomy in symptomatic patients with high-grade carotid stenosis. North American Symptomatic Carotid Endarterectomy Trial Collaborators. N Engl J Med 325(7):445–453, 1991.
31. Oesterle SN, Whitbourn R, Fitzgerald PJ, et al: The stent decade: 1987 to 1997. Stanford Stent Summit faculty. Am Heart J 136(4 Pt 1):578–599, 1998.
32. Park JH: Conventional and CT angiographic diagnosis of Takayasu arteritis: a 40-year experience. Int J Cardiol 54(Suppl.):S165–171, 1996.
33. Pazakie A, McElhinnev DB, Messina LM, Stoney RJI.: Common brachiocephalic trunk: strategies for revascularization. Ann Thorac Surg 67(3):657–660, 1999.
34. Reul GJ, Jacobs MJ, Gregoric ID, et al: Innominate artery occlusive disease: surgical approach and long-term results. J Vasc Surg 14(3):405–412, 1991.
35. Reul GJ Jr, Cooley DA, Duncan JM, et al: The effect of coronary bypass on the outcome of peripheral vascular operations in 1093 patients. J Vasc Surg 3(5):788–798, 1986.
36. Rhodes JM, Cherry KJ Jr, Clark RC, et al: Aortic-origin reconstruction of the great vessels: risk factors of early and late complications. J Vasc Surg 31(2):260–269, 2000.
37. Ricotta JJ, Faggioli GL, Castilone A, Hassett JM: Risk factors for stroke after cardiac surgery: Buffalo Cardiac-Cerebral Study Group. J Vasc Surg 21(2):359–363; discussion 364, 1995.
38. Rizzo RJ, Whittemore AD, Couper GS, et al: Combined carotid and coronary revascularization: the preferred approach to the severe vasculopath. Ann Thorac Surg 54(6):1099–1108; discussion 1108–1109, 1992.
39. Roach GW, Kanchuger M, Mangano CM, et al: Adverse cerebral outcomes after coronary bypass surgery. Multicenter Study of Perioperative Ischemia Research Group and the Ischemia Research and Education Foundation Investigators. N Engl J Med 19;335(25):1857–1863, 1996.
40. Robbs JV, Human RR, Rajaruthman P: Operative treatment of nonspecific aortoarteritis. Takayasu's arteritis. J Vasc Surg 3:605–616, 198.
41. Savory WS: Case of a young woman in whom the main arteries of both upper extremities and of the left side of the neck were throughout completely obliterated. Med Chir Trans London 39:205–219, 1856.
42. Sheikhzadeh A, Tettenborn I, Noohi F, et al: Occlusive thromboaortopathy (Takayasu disease): clinical and angiographic features and a brief review of literature. Angiology 53(1):29–40, 2002.
43. Sparks SR, Chock A, Seslar S, et al: Surgical treatment of Takayasu's arteritis: case report and literature review. Ann Vasc Surg 14(2):125–129, 2000.
44. Stoney RJ, Messina LM, Azakie A, Cherry KJ: Surgical diseases of the great vessels. Curr Probl Surg 37(2):71–161, 2000.
45. Takach TJ, Reul GJ Jr, Cooley DA, et al: Is an integrated approach warranted for concomitant carotid and coronary artery disease? Ann Thorac Surg 64(1):16–22, 1997.
46. Takayasu M: Case of queer changes in central blood vessels of retina. Acta Soc Ophthal Tap 12:2552, 1908.
47. Vermeulen FE, Hamerlijnck RP, Defauw JJ, Ernst SM: Synchronous operation for ischemic cardiac and cerebrovascular disease: early results and long-term follow-up. Ann Thorac Surg 53(3):381–389; discussion 390, 1992.
48. von Reutern GM, Hetzel A, Birnbaum D, Schlosser V: Transcranial Doppler ultrasonography during cardiopulmonary bypass in patients with severe carotid stenosis or occlusion. Stroke 19(6):674–680, 1988.
49. Yamada I, Nakagawa T, Himeno Y, et al: Takayasu arteritis: evaluation of the thoracic aorta with CT angiography. Radiology 209(1):103–109, 1998.

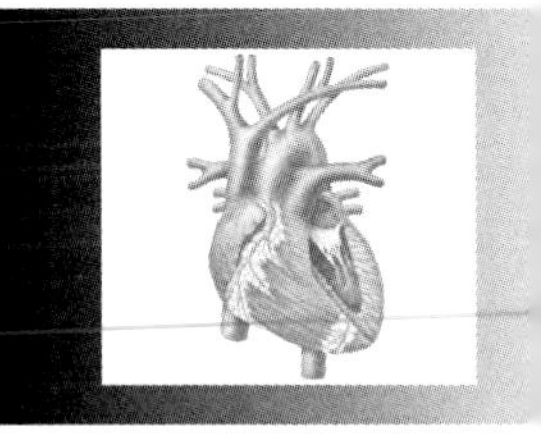

CHAPTER 71B

Occlusive Disease of Branches of the Thoracic Aorta and Peripheral Catheter-Based Intervention

Peripheral Angiography and Percutaneous Intervention

Lawrence A. Garcia

INTRODUCTION

Peripheral arterial occlusive disease (PAD) is a major cause of disability, loss of work, and lifestyle changes. The natural history of PAD is one of a slow progression in symptoms over time.[14,24,63,73,89] Although the symptoms of 70% of patients with PAD will remain stable over time or improve, 30% of patients will require intervention, and ultimately approximately 10% will require amputation. Limb loss is the tragic final outcome of PAD and is associated with disability and a poor prognosis. The increase in the population's age, continued tobacco use, high-fat diets, and sedentary lifestyles parallel the increasing prevalence of PAD. The estimated prevalence of PAD among people aged 65 and over may be 20% or greater given the potentially asymptomatic nature of the disease. In keeping with the rising prevalence of PAD, many cardiovascular specialists have adopted a strategy of "global vascular management" for their patients. In this strategy, the evaluation, care, and intervention plan is more comprehensive in its scope and includes the management of vascular disease in all of its manifestations and anatomical locations. To this end, we review here the general aspect of peripheral vascular disease with particular emphasis on the angiography and percutaneous interventions following medical evaluation.

Since the first catheter was placed in the vascular tree by Forsmann,[27] techniques to achieve vascular access have developed rapidly. Sones performed the first selective diagnostic coronary catheterization in 1956.[74,75] Later, Gruentzig performed the first coronary angioplasty in 1977.[35,36] Subsequently, the placement of intravascular stents has become the predominant form of catheter-based intervention in all major vascular beds.

INDICATIONS

The purpose of peripheral angiography is to define the vascular anatomy and to identify significant arterial narrowing requiring revascularization (either percutaneously or surgically). The appropriateness of peripheral angiography is dependent upon the risk versus benefits involved in obtaining peripheral imaging. This risk–benefit ratio should be evaluated prior to angiography to identify those patients that might fully benefit from imaging.[12,34,37]

Lower extremity claudication is classified according to the level of debilitation and/or restriction in activities. It is important to select the appropriate patients for angiography given that the morbidity from vascular access may be as high as 2.9% in patients with significant peripheral occlusive disease. The current scale used to group patients

Table 71B–1

The Rutherford–Baker Scale

Grade	*Category*	*Clinical description*	*Objective criteria*
0	0	Asymptomatic	Normal treadmill test
	1	Mild claudication	Ankle pressure after exercise <50 mm Hg but >25 mm Hg less than brachial
I	2	Moderate claudication	More moderate symptoms
	3	Severe claudication	Does not complete treadmill test Ankle pressure after exercise <50 mm Hg
II	4	Ischemic rest pain	Resting ankle pressure <60 mm Hg, decreased pulse volume recording (PVR)
	5	Minor tissue loss Nonhealing ulcers	Resting ankle pressure <40 mm Hg, PVR moderately decreased
III	6	Major tissue loss Loss above the metatarsal limb no longer salvageable	As noted in category 5

Adapted from Rutherford RB, Flanigan DP, Guptka SK, J Vasc Surg 4:80–94,1986.

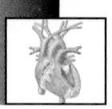

is the Rutherford–Baker scale, a 7-point scale (Table 71B-1) from 0 to 6. Classic claudicants usually fall within Rutherford scales 2 or 3 whereas more debilitated patients with more rest symptoms are in Rutherford 4 to 5. Patients with major tissue loss are Rutherford scale 6. Generally, patients with Rutherford scale 2 and higher and positive noninvasive studies would benefit from angiography and revascularization. Also, patients with nonhealing ulcers, a change in their lower extremity status following catheterization, acute limbs, or patients for limb salvage would benefit from lower extremity imaging. Finally, any patient with life-changing or limiting extremity claudication should undergo angiography to fully define the anatomy with an eye toward revascularization.

Angiography is indicated in the patient with an acute limb. Patients with acute onset of a cool pulseless extremity after catheterization or trauma require angiography to define the anatomy and site of occlusion. Angiography also allows the infusion of thrombolytic agents or mechanical rheolytic thrombectomy directly at the time of angiography.*

Angiography is indicated among patients with an abdominal aortic aneurysm or thoracic aneurysms in order to fully delineate the anatomy, particularly if endovascular repairs are contemplated. However, given current noninvasive imaging techniques (e.g., magnetic resonance angiography, [MRA]), it is unlikely that angiography is necessary to define thoracic or abdominal aneurysms. Only if angiography provides particular information (angle of the aneurysm neck) that cannot be adequately provided with a noninvasive study should angiography be pursued. MRA is also a particularly useful test in the evaluation of coarctation of the aorta. When angiography is needed then anterior-posterior (AP) and lateral images are the most useful for unoperated coarct patients. The angiography usually confirms the anatomic coarctation invariably seen, just distal to the origin of the left subclavian artery. Further, if the head and neck vessels are imaged with the thoracic aorta then an idea of collateral flows may be inferred as well (e.g., carotid or mammary).

Renal angiography is indicated in patients who have a positive noninvasive test such as an MRA or other noninvasive test (e.g., nuclear scan/Doppler). Further, new uncontrolled hypertension in patients under age 30 or over age 55, refractory hypertension, rising creatinine (specifically after the institution of angiotensin-converting enzyme [ACE] inhibitor therapy), or unexplained pulmonary edema is also considered an indication for renal angiography. The prevalence of renal vascular hypertension may be as high as 5% in the general population and 30% among patients with coronary artery disease or other PAD.

Because of the dual supply to the upper extremity, which can be derived from both the subclavian and the vertebral arteries, upper extremity claudication is rare. The most common cause of upper extremity claudication symptoms is a significant obstructive lesion. Upper extremity claudication symptoms include an inability to do activities with the affected limb, (e.g., general activities of daily living [ADLs], such as combing hair, brushing teeth, or repeated lifting). Another constellation of symptoms indicating obstructive disease in the upper extremity includes posterior circulation symptoms. In this condition, there is a reversal of flow from the vertebral artery in a patient with disease in the ipsilateral carotid leading to posterior circulation symptoms (dizziness or difficult gait).[3,11,72,77] Also, among patients who have undergone coronary artery bypass grafting (CABG) surgery with use of the internal mammary artery, persistent angina and anterior

*References 4, 39, 48, 52, 62, 80.

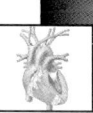

ischemia on noninvasive testing may suggest left subclavian stenosis as the cause of coronary ischemia.* Therefore, any patient with symptoms of upper extremity claudication, anterior ischemia following coronary artery bypass with the use of the left internal mammary artery, or posterior circulation events and the presence of a difference in upper extremity blood pressures should be evaluated for the possibility of subclavian stenosis and undergo angiography.

Indications for carotid or cerebral angiography are patients who have noninvasive testing that suggests critical stenosis of one or both carotid arteries or who have symptomatic disease (transient ischemic attack [TIA], cerebrovascular accident [CVA]) and a critical stenosis identified on noninvasive testing.

CONTRAINDICATIONS

The principal contraindications to peripheral angiography include bleeding diathesis, renal failure (true or impending), fever, ongoing infection, or severe anemia (Box 71B-1).

COMPLICATIONS

Complications of peripheral angiography primarily involve vascular access site complications, catheter manipulation within atherosclerotic vessels, emboli, clot formation, stroke, myocardial infarction, worsening renal function, or congestive heart failure (Table 71B-2). A particularly devastating complication of catheter manipulation within the arterial tree is atheroembolic distal emboli. In its most severe form to the lower extremities it may cause loss of limb or digits. Likewise, emboli to the renal circulation may lead to acute renal decompensation or failure requiring dialysis.[38,51,86] Pseudoaneurysm or vascular access complications may be as high as 3% in patients with severe peripheral occlusive disease.[7,47]

CATHETERS

There are a variety of preshaped catheters that are used for peripheral angiography. Catheters that are straight, curved, soft tipped, flush, or lubricious can be used to engage various vascular structures throughout the vascular tree. Each catheter has its own specific properties that make it useful in various setting in peripheral angiography.

*References 5, 19, 26, 72, 76, 85.

Box 71B–1. Relative Contraindications to Catheterization and Angiography.

1. Bleeding diathesis or inability to take aspirin, ADP inhibitor
2. Concurrent febrile illness
3. Severe renal insufficiency or anuria without dialysis planned
4. Severe allergy to contrast agents
5. Severe hypokalemia or digitalis toxicity
6. Severe hypertension or ongoing unstable coronary syndrome

Table 71B–2

Possible Complications of Peripheral Catheterization

Complication	%
Vascular access dissection or perforation	0.1–0.2
Bleeding/hematoma	1.5–2.0
Allergic reaction	0.5–2.0
Vasovagal events	1.0–2.0
Death	0.1–0.2

PERIPHERAL IMAGING IN GENERAL

There are several important differences in imaging peripheral vascular structures from coronary arteries. Peripheral angiography commonly employs a larger image intensifier field (14 inch or 36 cm) to encompass larger regions of interest. Digital (not film based) angiography allows online display of acquired images as well as advanced processing techniques to enhance brightness, contrast, or shift of underlying bony structures to enhance the final image (Figure 71B-1). Frequently, digital subtraction angiography (DSA) is used. With this imaging method a "mask" or baseline background image is obtained immediately prior to contrast injection to "subtract" any bone, calcifications, air, or soft tissues from the final image leading to the best image quality with the most definition regarding anatomy. Another advantage of DSA is that it may reduce the volume of contrast and imaging acquisition time required.

IMAGING SPECIFIC PERIPHERAL REGIONS

Aorta

Thoracic Aorta

Thoracic aortography is used to define the anatomical relation of the aortic arch and the great vessels, to determine the diameter of the thoracic aorta, to obtain evidence of dissection (Figure 71B-2), and to evaluate trauma or other vascular injuries. The optimal view of the aortic arch is obtained in the lateral anterior oblique (LAO) projection at 30–40° oblique. The injection of 30–40 ml of contrast at 20–30 ml/s generally opacifies the vessels for adequate imaging. If DSA angiography is used, patients should be instructed to hold their breath to avoid artifacts due to

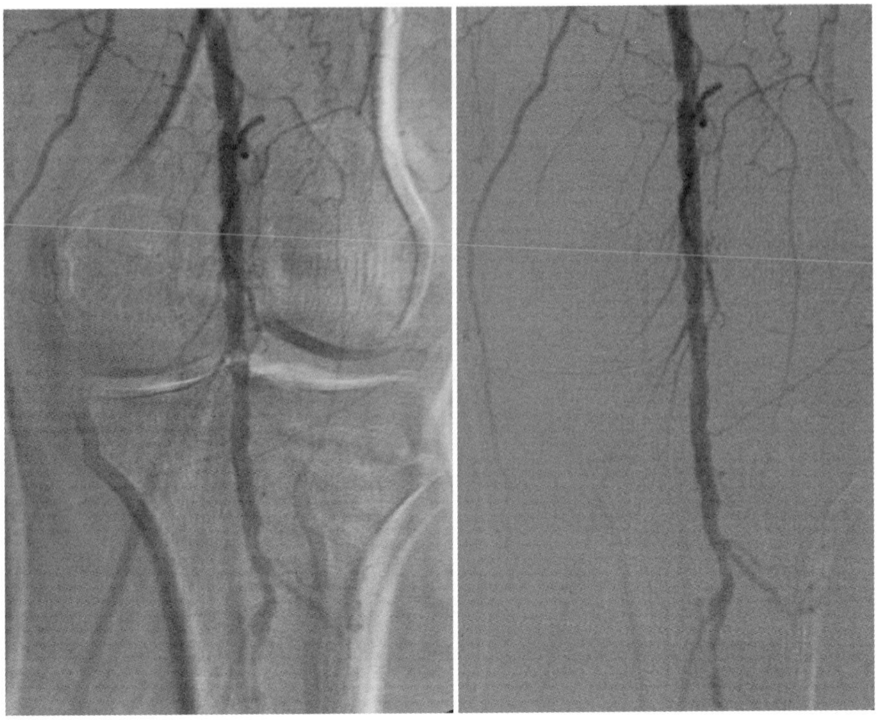

Figure 71B–1 Digital subtraction angiography (DSA) of the popliteal artery with moderate patient motion confounding the popliteal evaluation. Following "shifting" of the image to remask the underlying bony structures and allow direct evaluation of the angiographic anatomy.

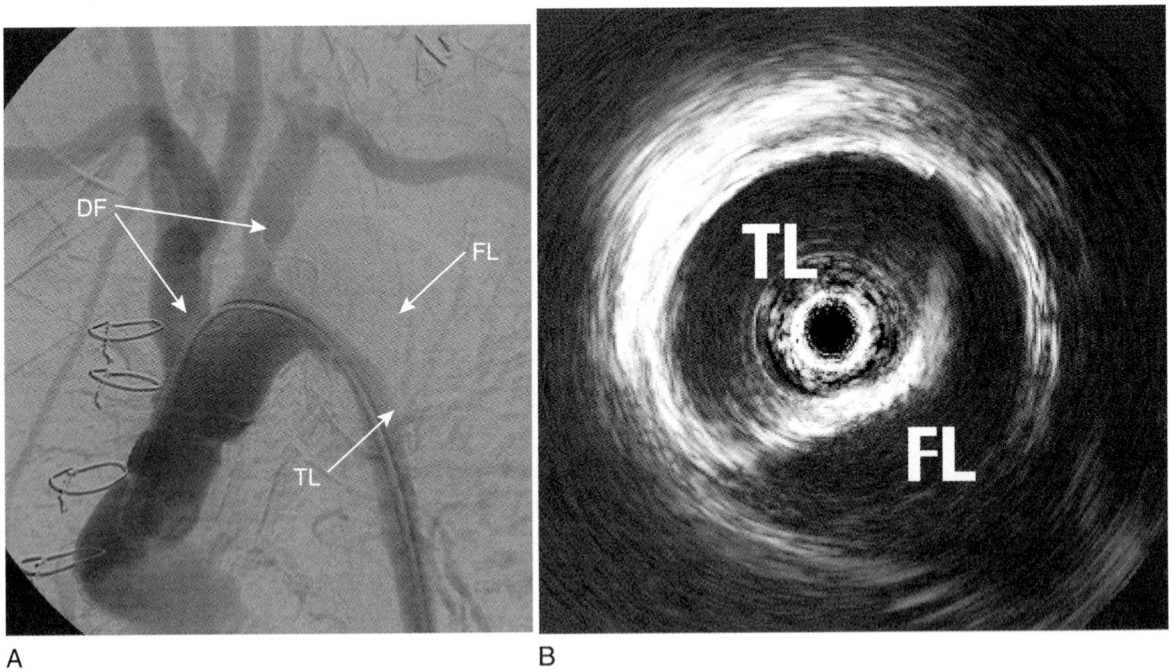

Figure 71B–2 (A) Angiogram and (B) intravascular ultrasound (IVUS) of a patient with type A dissection of the aortic arch. The false lumen (FL) and true lumen (TL) are evident from the IVUS images. The arrows on the angiogram correlate with the site of the IVUS image.

motion or breathing. Three principal vessels originate from the arch: first, the brachiocephalic (innominate), leading ultimately to the right subclavian and right carotid arteries, Second, the left common carotid, and third, the left subclavian artery (Figure 71B-3). The most common normal variant of this anatomy is the so-called bovine arch where the left common carotid artery originates from the brachiocephalic trunk. This normal variant occurs in 10% of patients.[47]

Abdominal Aorta

The abdominal aorta should be angiographically imaged for evaluation of abdominal aortic aneurysm (AAA), dissection,

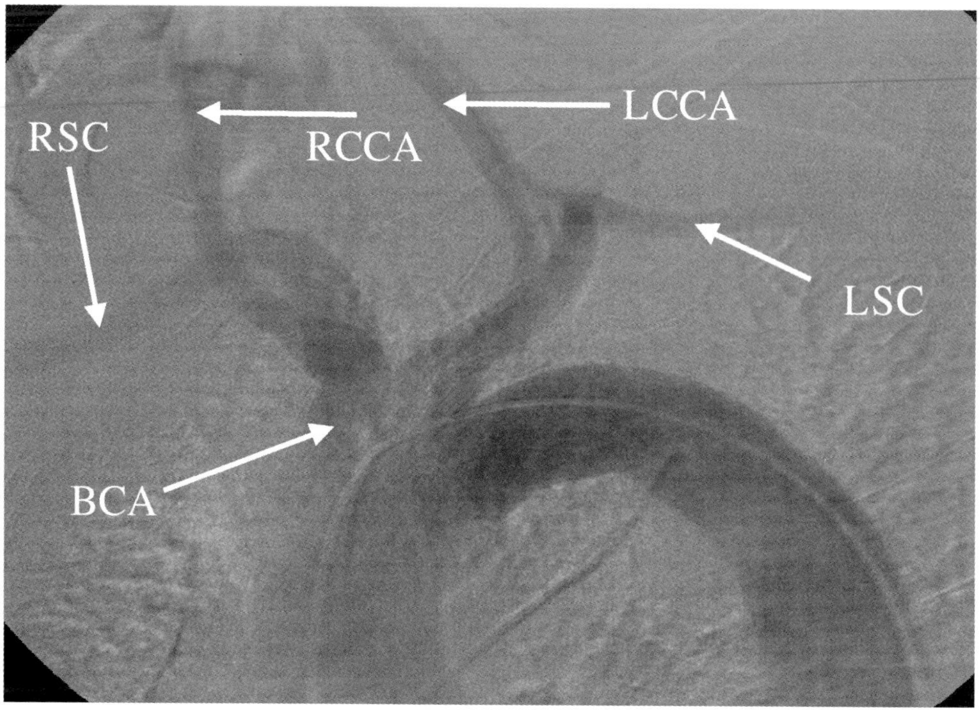

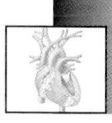

Figure 71B–3 **DSA of the thoracic arch and great vessels.** BCA, brachiocephalic artery; RSC, right subclavian artery; RCCA, right common carotid artery; LCCA, left common carotid artery; LSC, left subclavian artery.

lower extremity claudication, mesenteric ischemia, and renal vascular disease. The abdominal aorta begins at the level of the diaphragm (i.e., T_{12}). The principal vessels are, in descending order, the celiac artery at the level of L_1, the superior mesenteric artery (SMA) at the level of L_2–L_3, the renal arteries at the level of L_2–L_3 just caudal to the SMA, and finally the inferior mesenteric artery at the level of L_4. The abdominal aorta terminates at the bifurcation and the origin of the iliac arteries.

In general 20–40 ml of contrast injected at 15–30 ml/s will adequately opacify the vessels to define the anatomy. Again, as in the thoracic aorta, it is critical to fully opacify the lumen and the vessels of interest. Anterior-posterior and lateral imaging (Figure 71B-4) of the abdominal aorta are usually sufficient to delineate all anatomical areas of interest in the abdominal aorta and mesenteric vessels. If selected conduits require further visualization, then a soft tipped catheter (e.g., SosOmni, RDC, Cobra, or hockey stick) may provide selective angiography without requiring large contrast loads to fully define the anatomy.

Head and Neck Angiography

The three primary branches radiating from the aortic arch are the brachiocephalic, left common carotid, and left subclavian arteries. The right subclavian and carotid arteries are branches

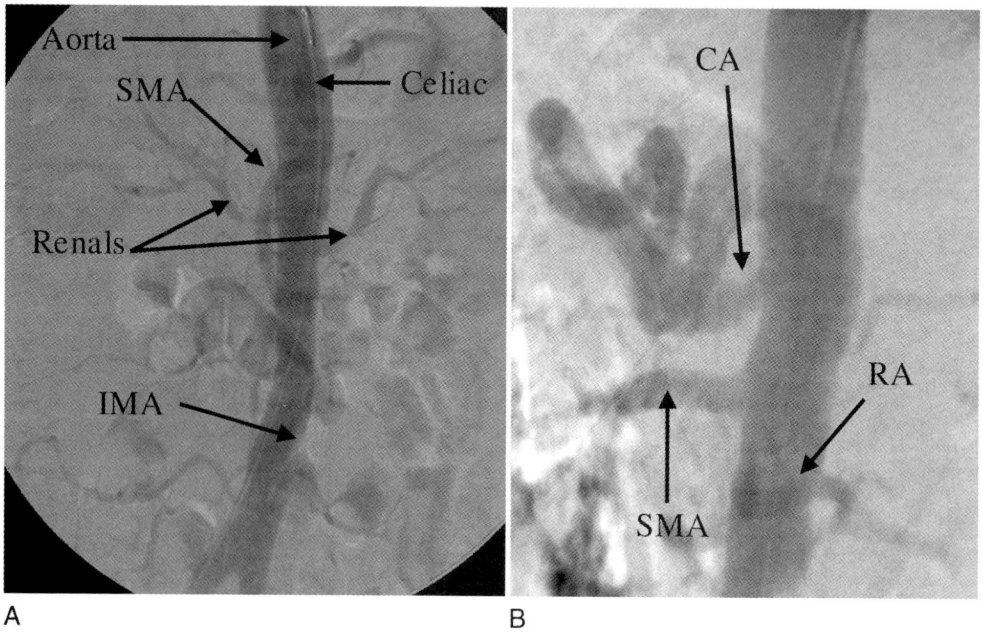

Figure 71B–4 (**A**) AP view of DSA of the abdominal aorta and major branches. SMA, superior mesenteric artery; IMA, inferior mesenteric artery. (**B**) Lateral DSA of the abdominal aorta and major branches. CA, celiac artery; RA, renal artery; SMA, superior mesenteric artery.

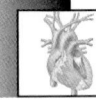

off the brachiocephalic trunk. As noted above, the most common variant of this anatomy is the "bovine" arch, where the left carotid and brachiocephalic arteries share a common origin, which occurs in 10% of the general population.[47]

Subclavian artery disease, stenosis, and occlusion are common. Symptoms are rare given the dual supply to the upper extremity via the subclavian and vertebral arteries. The presence of upper extremity claudication is rare but is manifested by upper extremity discomfort while engaging in activity with the upper extremity or activities of daily living. More common subclavian stenosis or occlusion is manifested by either posterior circulation events (flow is reversed in the ipsilateral vertebral artery with upper extremity activity), which are rare, or anterior ischemia (coronary steal syndrome) in the patient who has been treated with left internal mammary artery (LIMA) bypass grafting and continues to experience ischemia despite surgery[5,8,19,26,76,85] (Figure 71B-5).

Subclavian artery angiography is optimally performed using both AP and ipsilateral oblique views. Selective angiography can be performed with any straight or slightly angulated catheters (multipurpose, JR4, or IMA). As in thoracic angiography, nonselective angiography in general requires 30–40 ml of contrast injected at 20–30 ml/s to adequately opacify all vessels in the arch. Selective angiography can be performed with hand injections through the above-named catheters. The vessels are usually accessed with the use of the guidewire as a rail and then the catheter is advanced over the wire. Access to the brachiocephalic, carotid, or subclavian arteries usually requires a counterclockwise movement of the catheter in the ascending aorta for it to engage the vessel of interest. The "J" wire is then advanced into the vessel and ultimately the catheter is advanced over the wire. Once the wire has been removed and the catheter flushed, angiography can be performed safely. There is usually some shoulder and neck discomfort with moderate contrast injections and the patient should be forewarned of the "warm" feeling that will follow injections. Discomfort can be minimized if necessary with the use of half-diluted contrast. Excessively vigorous injections should be avoided to prevent subintimal injection or dye staining into the intima of the subclavian artery.

Atherosclerosis of the subclavian artery is generally proximal at the origin or within the first few millimeters from the aortic origin. The origin of the IMA is usually spared atherosclerosis. The origin of the vertebral artery may be involved with atherosclerotic lesions but the need for intervention is low because of the dual blood supply to the posterior circulation that arises from both the contralateral vertebral and ipsilateral carotid arteries.

The carotid arteries generally bifurcate at the level of the fourth cervical vertebra into the internal and external carotid arteries (Figure 71B-6A). The internal carotid usually has no major branches and becomes tortuous below the petrous bone, called the carotid siphon. Once the vessel enters the petrous bone it is considered the intracranial internal carotid artery. Once the vessel exits the petrous bone it bifurcates early into the anterior and middle cerebral arteries. The external carotid artery has several branches that supply the face.

Carotid atherosclerosis is common.[20,57] Intervention in the internal carotid artery is performed either percutaneously or surgically. Annually, there are 600,000 strokes in the United States,[2] of which 500,000 are first attacks. Among these strokes, 160,000 are fatal.[2] Cerebral occlusive disease encompasses CVA, TIA, and posterior circulation (vertebral-basilar) events. Several studies have evaluated the efficacy of various revascularization strategies in preventing future events.[23,25,61] The National Heart, Lung and Blood

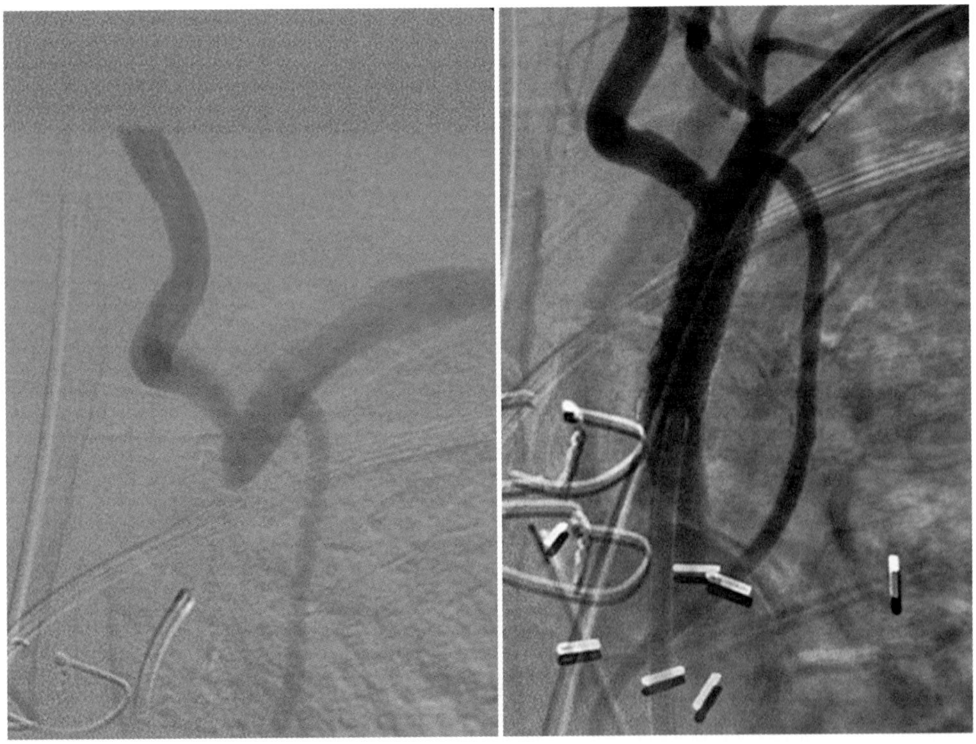

A B

Figure 71B–5 **DSA of the left subclavian artery preintervention and postintervention. A,** The LSC is occluded. After crossing in a retrograde fashion from the left brachial artery the subclavian artery is stented with the final angiographic result noted (**B**).

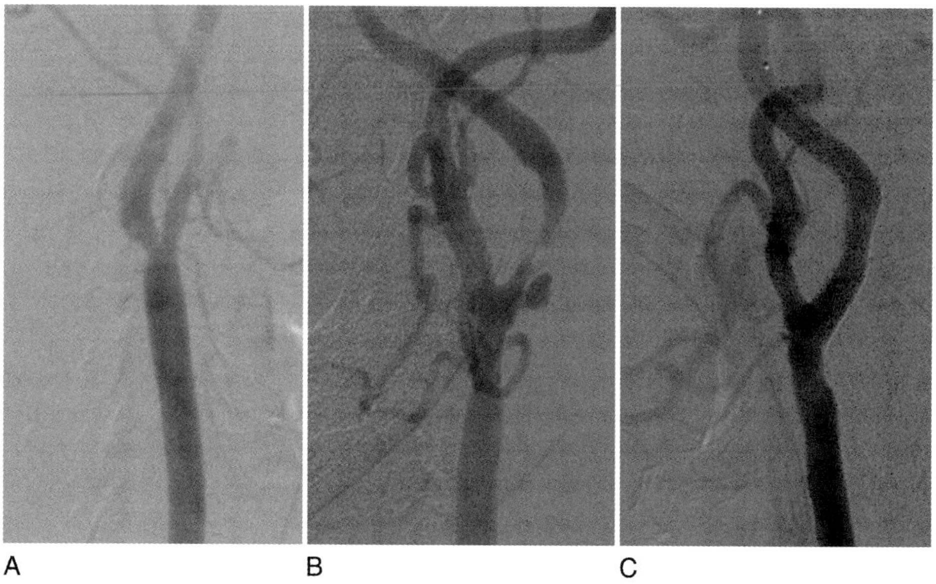

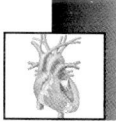

Figure 71B–6 (**A**) Angiography of a normal carotid artery and its bifurcation. (**B**) Abnormal angiography with an ulcerated left internal carotid artery in a patient several weeks after a transient ischemic attack. (**C**) Final angiography following angioplasty and stenting.

Institute's Atherosclerosis Risk in Communities study[69] revealed that 83% of all strokes were ischemic, 40% were lacunar, and 14% were thromboembolic. Most patients with extracranial carotid artery disease are asymptomatic.

Independent risk factors for the presence and progression of carotid artery disease are similar to those of coronary artery disease. These include diabetes mellitus (both type 1 and type 2), hypertension, hyperlipidemia, and family history. The presence of a bruit may aid in identifying patients with carotid stenoses. Obviously carotid bruits can be transmitted sounds from the heart, and as such, may result in the "false positive" identification of carotid disease. For example, in one study,[16] only 37% of 330 patients referred to a neurology clinic with a cervical bruit had a high-grade carotid artery lesion noted with duplex imaging. The presence of a carotid bruit may be associated with subsequent risk of stroke. The Framingham Heart Study demonstrated that asymptomatic patients with a carotid bruit have twice the risk of stroke.[91] In asymptomatic patients, risk of stroke was 2.5% if the stenosis was over 75%. These risks are higher for patients with symptoms (3.3%).[1,60,70]

Angiography of the carotid artery is generally performed in the AP and lateral views. Selective angiography should be performed with care to ensure adequate position of the catheter and distance from the bifurcation. Generally, a soft-tipped catheter such as a Berenstein, VTEK, Head hunter, or JR4 catheter is advanced over a wire into the common carotid artery for angiography.

Renal Vascular Imaging

The prevalence of renal vascular disease is high in patients with coronary artery disease or other anatomical peripheral disease (up to 50%).[41,71] Renal vascular disease is a cause of secondary hypertension in 0.5–5% of the general population.[18,68] Although other noninvasive and functional studies such as Doppler ultrasound, Captopril nuclear studies, or MRA remain vital screening tools, contrast angiography remains the gold standard. The renal arteries have a more posterior take-off from the abdominal aorta. Nonselective angiography can be obtained with a "tennis racket" or pigtail catheter positioned at the level of T_{12}. Contrast injection of 15–20 ml at 30 ml/s should opacify the intended vessels adequately. Selective angiography with a soft-tipped catheter (SosOmni, Cobra, RDC) can be performed with hand injections.

An improvement in blood pressure control is one goal of percutaneous revascularization of renal arteries.[10,21,84] Another potential benefit of renal artery revascularization is preservation of renal function.[42,64,71,88]

Lower Extremity Angiography

Iliac

The iliac vessels originate at the termination of the abdominal aorta, usually at the L_4–L_5 level. They remain retroperitoneal throughout their course until they cross the inguinal ligament and become the common femoral artery. The principal bifurcation in the iliac artery is the terminal bifurcation of the common iliac into the internal and external iliac arteries (Figure 71B-7).

Angiography of the iliac arteries is best achieved in the AP and oblique positions (LAO for the right iliac artery and RAO for the left iliac artery). The imaging catheter, usually a pigtail or flush catheter, is positioned just above the aortic bifurcation to allow the best opacification of the iliac arteries. In general, 15–30 ml of contrast injected at 20–30 ml/s is sufficient to provide adequate opacification.

In patients with lower extremity claudication, noninvasive testing with ankle-brachial indices (ABIs) with duplex and Doppler imaging is critical. Evaluation with and without exercise, either 5 min at 1.5 miles/h or 40 calf raises,[56] is often necessary to provoke symptoms and, more importantly, to determine the level of stenosis. Doppler imaging is vital in the evaluation of the lower extremities. Normal flow patterns are triphasic or biphasic (Figure 71B-8). When a critical lesion is present the waveform becomes monophasic

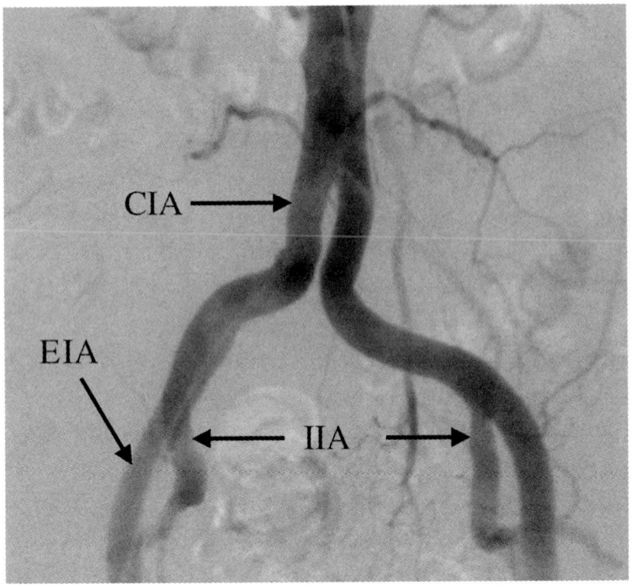

Figure 71B–7 DSA in the AP projection of the terminal abdominal aortic bifurcation. CIA, common iliac artery; EIA, external iliac artery; IIA, internal iliac artery.

(Figure 71B-8). Furthermore, during exertion resting triphasic/biphasic waveforms become monophasic distal to a critical stenosis. The location of the transition in the waveform pattern indicates the level of critical disease and can allow for more directed and focused lower extremity angiography. Because the lower extremity arterial tree is relatively superficial, occasionally the anatomy can be directly visualized noninvasively with duplex imaging. Here the anatomy may be defined and the level and extent of disease may be delineated without vascular access.

Techniques

Lower extremity angiography can be performed many ways. There has been an increase in the use of digital angiography and bolus chase techniques, where the table "steps" at various points of the run to mask the image then returns to the same location and follows the original bolus of contrast throughout the course. These methods allow for a single contrast injection and delineation of the anatomy without the need for multiple injections. The principal problem with this technique occurs when there is significant patient motion from the mask to the contrast "bolus-chase," and the images are out of register and of poor quality. Small motion from the patient may be digitally "shifted" in the final angiogram without much difficulty to remove the underlying bony structures and enhance the final angiographic image (Figure 71B-1). In general, contrast volumes for the lower extremity bolus-chase technique range from 30–40 ml at 8–10 ml/s. Other techniques include static images or older "cut-film" changers. In the static image technique a focal area is evaluated with single bolus contrast injections of 15–30 ml at 8–10 ml/s or by hand injection.

One unique aspect of peripheral angiography is the antegrade puncture of the femoral artery. The common femoral artery is entered as with standard retrograde access but it is entered in the antegrade (in the direction of blood flow to the leg) direction. The entry is less steep (about 45 degrees), but should enter the common femoral artery over the femoral head and below the inguinal ligament. This access allows direct intervention for the infrainguinal vessels.

Infrainguinal Vessels

The arterial tree below the inguinal ligament begins with the common femoral artery. This vessel bifurcates early at the level of the femoral head into the profunda femoral artery (PFA) and the superficial femoral artery (SFA) (Figure 71B-9A). The SFA is the principal vessel supplying the lower extremity. It courses anteriorly through the proximal 60% of its length and then begins to course posteriorly entering the adductor canal (Hunter's canal), a musculofascial canal bounded by the sartorius muscle anteriorly, vastus medialis muscle laterally, and adductor longus and magnus muscles posteriorly. This canal exits posteriorly and the artery becomes the popliteal artery when it exits. The popliteal artery then terminates at the level of the tibial plateau into the anterior tibial (AT) artery and tibial-peroneal trunk (TPT) vessels. The TPT then terminally bifurcates into the posterior tibial (PT) artery and the peroneal artery (Figure 71B-9). The PT and AT usually are the principal vessels to the foot. The PT supplies the medial and lateral plantar vessels and the AT supplies the dorsalis pedal (DP) artery. The distal plantar arteries along with the DP artery often communicate to form the plantar arch of the foot.

PERCUTANEOUS INTERVENTION TO SPECIFIC PERIPHERAL REGIONS

Thoracic and Abdominal Aorta

Intervention to the thoracic and abdominal aorta is usually performed for dissection, coarctation, or aneurysm and is discussed in full detail in Chapter 70. Furthermore, interventional issues regarding pediatric coarctation are not discussed here. For adults with coarctation they represent previously corrected (surgically), undiagnosed, or prior angioplasty with recurrence patients.

Intervention via a percutaneous route with stenting has become the primary method of correction of coarctation.[*] Success rates for percutaneous interventions are 70–80% with a reduction of peak gradient under 20 mm Hg. Most of the patients are seen within a pediatric population, and as such, adult disease is rarely seen as unoperated coarctation. Percutaneous intervention to postoperative coarctation is feasible and limits the risk of patients for second operation.[29] Here the bypass conduits or the primary coarctation may be revascularized through a percutaneous route[29] (Figure 71B-10).

In general, there is a greater degree of atherosclerosis in the aorta after it crosses the diaphragm into the abdomen. The consequence of this is either lower extremity claudication or mesenteric ischemia. The abdominal aorta can have intervention for lower extremity claudication (Figure

*References 13, 17, 22, 29, 30, 40, 43, 45, 50, 54, 66, 67, 83.

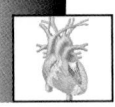

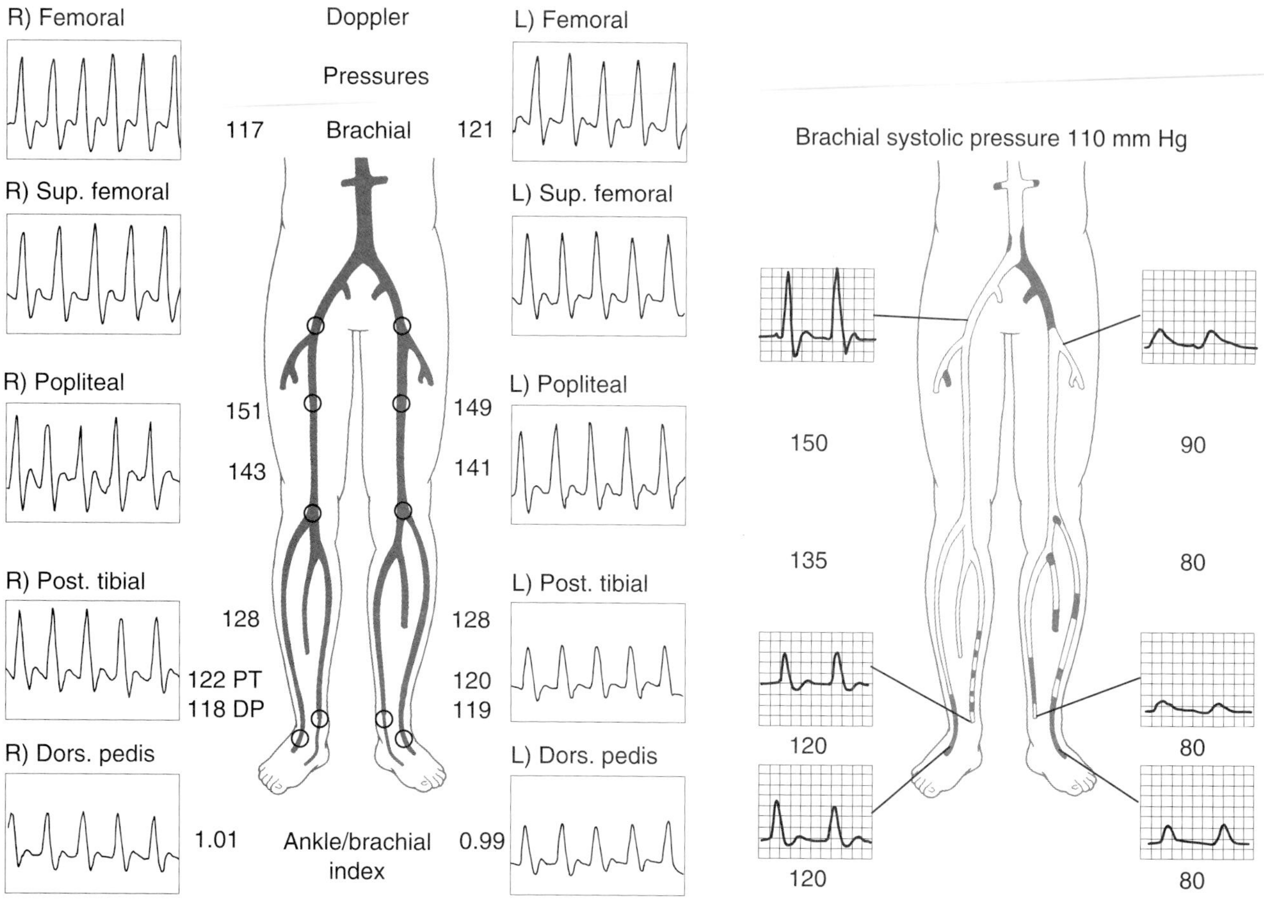

Figure 71B–8 Doppler waveforms in both a normal and abnormal lower extremity. Note the triphasic waveform in the normal patient and an attenuated, wide-based waveform consistent with a monophasic (abnormal) wave consistent with upstream stenosis or occlusion.

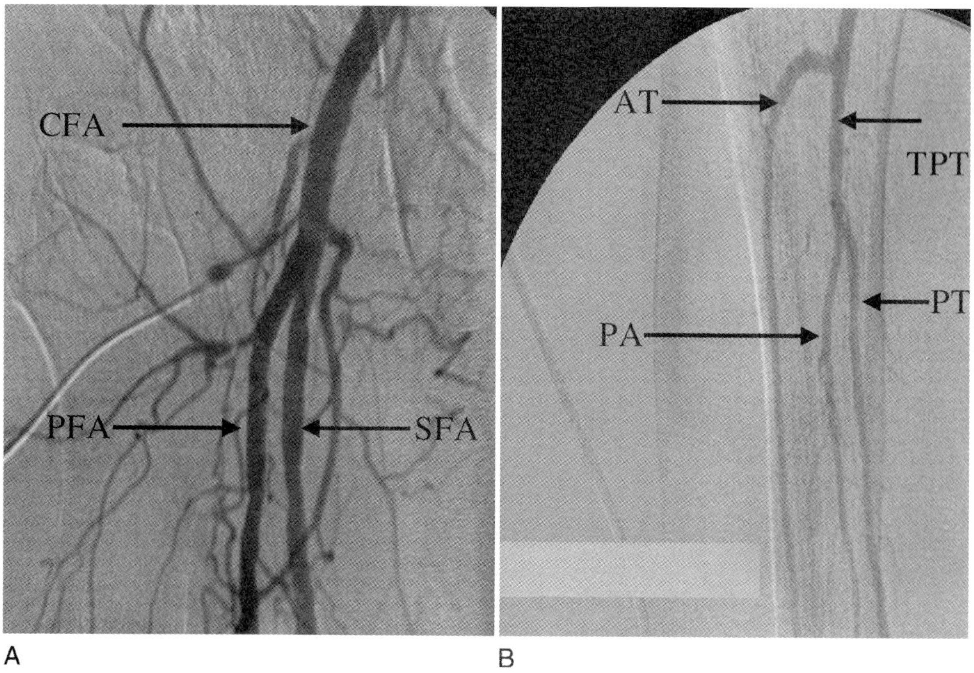

Figure 71B–9 A, DSA in the AP projection of the right common femoral artery. CFA, common femoral artery; PFA, profunda femoral artery; SFA, superficial femoral artery. **B,** Infrapopliteal DSA in the AP projection. AT, anterior tibial artery; TPT, tibial-peroneal trunk; PT, posterior tibial artery; PA, peroneal artery.

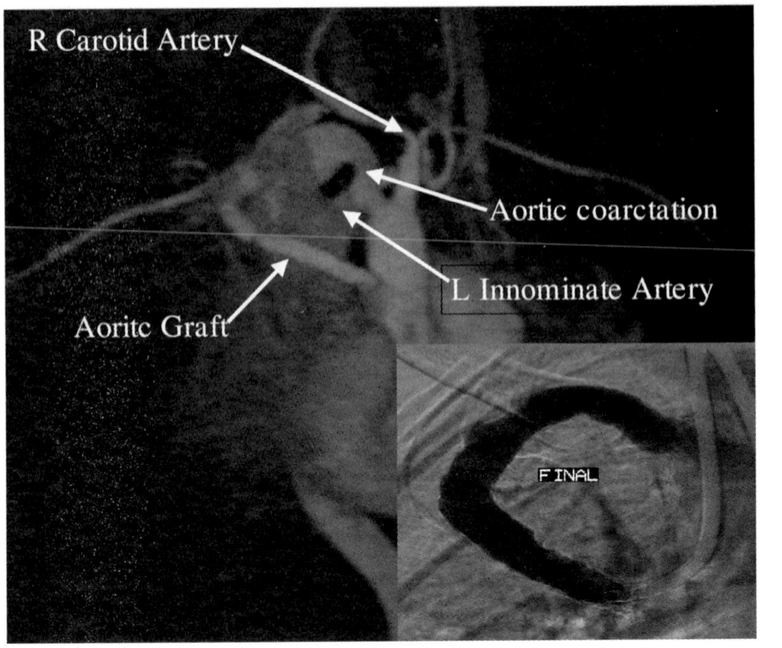

Figure 71B–10 MRA AP view of a hypoplastic (coarctation) aortic arch. The anatomy of this right-sided arch is as shown: first right carotid then right subclavian (not shown) followed by left brachiocephalic off the descending aorta with intervening aortic–aortic graft. Inset shows completed stenting to the aortic–aortic graft.

71B-11). Here it is important to determine the significance of the lesion and the possibility of intervention. Once the lesion characteristics are defined and percutaneous intervention pursued, the key elements are to gain access in each femoral artery. One access point will serve as the primary intervention for the aorta (Figure 71B-11) and the other vessel will then cross the aortic stent with further intervention to the iliac arteries performed in a "kissing" manner (Figure 71B-11). In this the distal abdominal aorta and iliac arteries can be revascularized without central abdominal surgery.

Mesenteric ischemia is a condition that given the redundant circuitry of the intestines' true ischemia is uncommon. If mesenteric ischemia is suspected and revascularization warranted a percutaneous procedure could afford less risk to the patient than from a central abdominal procedure. Stenting of the mesenteric vessels is performed usually from the common femoral artery. The catheter usually used is a hockey stick or other angled catheter to engage the ostium of the stenotic vessel. Once engaged, the vessel is primarily stented and dilated to the reference vessel diameter. Long term, there is a 10–15% restenosis rate after several years. Care should be taken when advancing the catheter or other devices through the lesion as they are generally friable "tongues" of aortic atherosclerosis and are likely to embolize downstream into the vessel to be revascularized.

Head and Neck Vessels

Although some patients may have significant stenoses without any signs or symptoms, those patients who are symptomatic face a higher risk of future events.[23,61] The North American Symptomatic Carotid Endarterectomy Trial (NASCET) demonstrated that the risk for ipsilateral stroke at 2 years was 26% for medical therapy versus 9% with surgery[61] among patients with a lesion >70% noted by angiography. Likewise, the European Symptomatic Carotid Trial (ECST)[40] showed that in symptomatic patients with all levels of stenosis, patients treated with medical therapy had a 17% rate of stroke compared with 2.8% when treated with surgical revascularization.[40] Thus, in symptomatic patients with high-grade stenoses (>70%), carotid endarterectomy (CEA) appears to be beneficial.

Percutaneous transluminal angioplasty (PTA) and stenting of the extracranial carotid artery have been performed for nearly 10 years now[72] (Figure 71B-6B and C). The Global Utilization Report by Wholey et al[90] showed that at 30 days the rate of TIA was 2.6%, minor stroke 2.5%, major stroke 1.4%, and mortality 0.8%. These values compare favorably with the surgical literature. The Carotid and Vertebral Artery Transluminal Angioplasty Study (CAVATAS)[73] compared, in a nonrandomized trial, carotid PTA and stenting with CEA. Overall, the combined stroke and mortality rate was similar between groups at 10% and 9.9% by 30 days. At 3 years these data remained the same.[9,31,65,93] Currently, there is only one randomized trial comparing percutaneous revascularization with surgical carotid revascularization, the CREST (carotid revascularization endarterectomy versus stent trial) trial comparing traditional CEA with stent-assisted carotid angioplasty for treatment of carotid artery stenosis. It is currently on hold to allow for distal protection devices to be used with the carotid intervention. The previous SAPPHIRE (stenting and angioplasty with protection in patients at high risk for endarterectomy) trial has completed randomization and preliminary results presented in 2002 revealed a reduction of combined end point events with stenting compared with surgery of stroke, death, or myocardial infarction from 12.6% with surgery to 5.8% ($p < .05$) with stenting. Removing the myocardial infarction events from the cohort with stenting, the composite end point was 3.8% compared with 5.3% for the surgical group. The results for the symptomatic patients were 4.2% in the stenting group compared

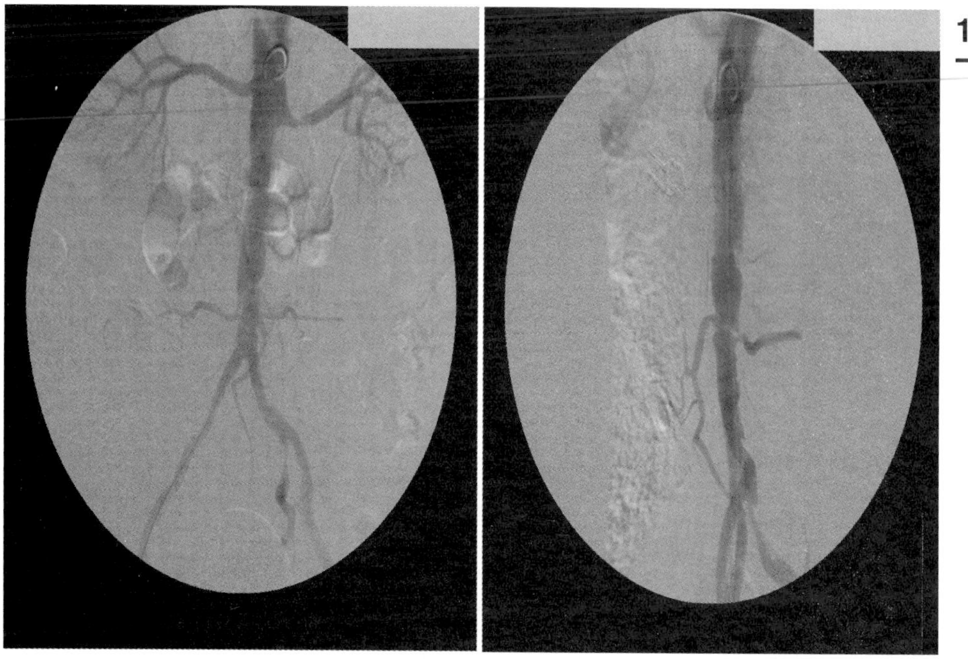

A

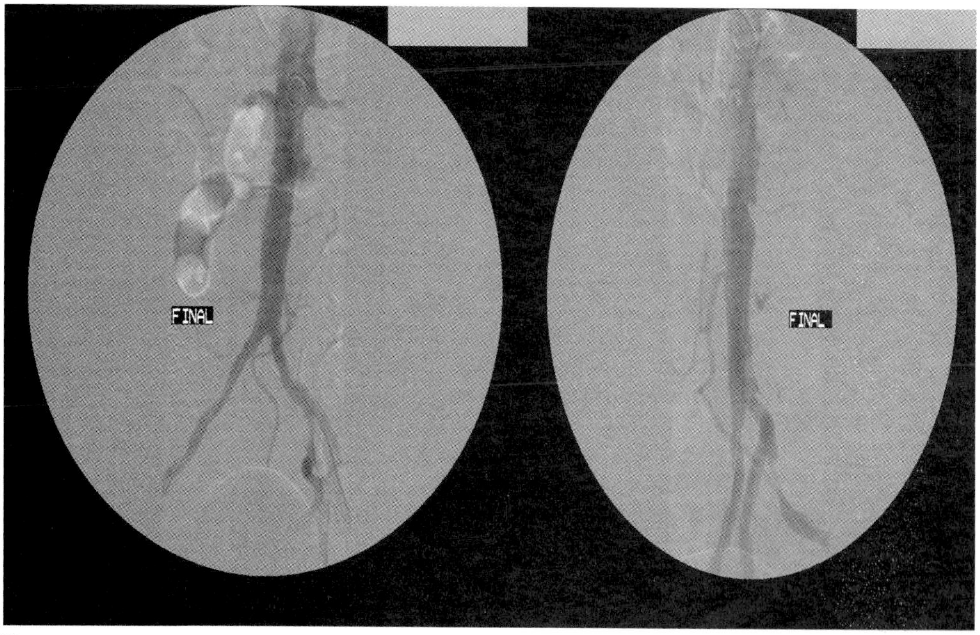

B

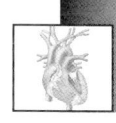

Figure 71B–11 **A,** AP and lateral DSA distal abdominal aorta showing a distal lesion at the level of the inferior mesenteric artery. **B,** Following angioplasty and stenting of the distal abdominal aorta revealing a widely patent vessel.

with 15.4% in the surgical group. Again, if the myocardial infarctions were removed, the event rate on the composite end point of death and stroke was 2.1% for the stent group compared with 10.3% for the surgical group. In the asymptomatic patient population the event rates were 6.7% in the stenting group compared with 11.2% in the surgical group. Removing the myocardial infarctions in both groups, the composite end point was 5.8% in the stenting group compared with 6.1% in the surgical group. Therefore, in this high-risk patient population the benefit of stenting was evident at all major end points but, more importantly, was evident in both the randomized population as well as the registry patients. The event rates were not statistically different except the composite end point of stroke, death, or myocardial infarction in the randomized patients. The statistical significance was driven primarily from the myocardial infarction rate periprocedure. Clearly, in a high-risk population, percutaneous revascularization of carotid stenoses will be the preferred method of revascularization. Whether or not this paradigm shifts to the general (non-high-risk) patient population is nuclear.

Following angiography, the decision to perform either percutaneous or surgical revascularization is dependent on several key factors. First, if the contralateral carotid artery is stenotic or occluded then the benefit of revascularization noted from the ACAS (Asymptomatic Carotid

Atherosclerosis Study) investigators is lost.[25] Recall, in ACAS, the patients had only a 60% or greater stenosis and were referred for surgery or medical therapy.[25] The overall benefit of surgical revascularization was a 53% reduction in events when compared with medical therapy alone. Furthermore, the symptomatic patients in NASCET had a higher complication rate with regards to TIA and strokes.[61] In these patients the use of PTA/stenting has shown a result similar to surgical literature in outcomes.

Percutaneous outcomes may be improved with the use of distal protection devices (Figure 71B-12) such as the balloon occlusion, GuardWire (PercuSurge, Inc, Sunnyvale, CA), or filter device Angioguard (Cordis, Warren, NJ) or EPI filter (EPI, Inc, Boston, MA). Such distal protection devices have been shown to capture distal emboli that may be liberated with catheter manipulation, balloon inflations, or stenting in the carotid arteries (Figure 71B-13). The major difference between these two devices is that the balloon occlusion device interrupts flow distally whereas the filter devices allow flow to continue but capture the debris. All current studies regarding percutaneous carotid revascularization employ some form of distal protection, either balloon occlusion or filter device as listed previously.

Renal Vascular

van Jaarsveld et al compared angioplasty alone with medical therapy in the control of hypertension in 100 patients.[84] Angioplasty alone did not improve blood pressure control when compared with aggressive medical therapy. This study had several limitations. No gradients were measured across the lesions treated (just visual assessment of percent diameter narrowing was used to guide management). In addition, nearly 50% of medical therapy patients crossed over to angioplasty by 3 months of follow-up. Creatinine clearance was significantly improved in the angioplasty group at the 3-month interval and continued, though not statistically significant, through 12 months. A second study demonstrated that blood pressure control was stable and creatinine/renal function improved over a 4-year period in a nonrandomized cohort of patients.[21]

Recent efforts have focused on the development of risk stratification tools to identify patients who would benefit from intervention. A normal resistive index (<80) is associated with a benefit from revascularization, whereas an index >80 is not associated with a benefit from revascularization.[64] Although assessment of the pressure gradient is critical in selecting appropriate patients for revascularization, it should be noted that the presence of a catheter in a diseased ostium may falsely elevate the "true" gradient. Figure 71B-14 shows our technique to ensure that the pressure gradient is not falsely elevated. As the figure details, when a catheter (4 or 5 French) is placed across a lesion and the pressure difference measured with the central aortic pressure the small catheter contributes significantly to the overall gradient, which falsely elevates the "true" gradient as measured with

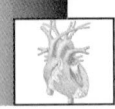

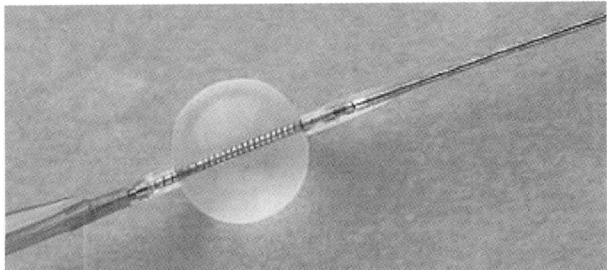

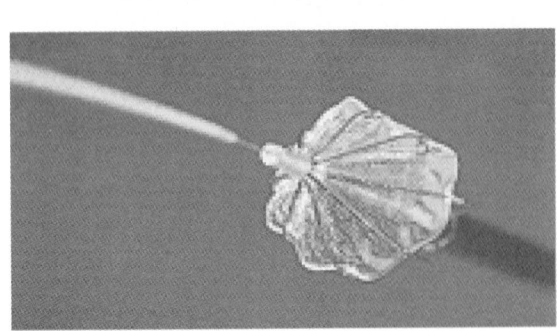

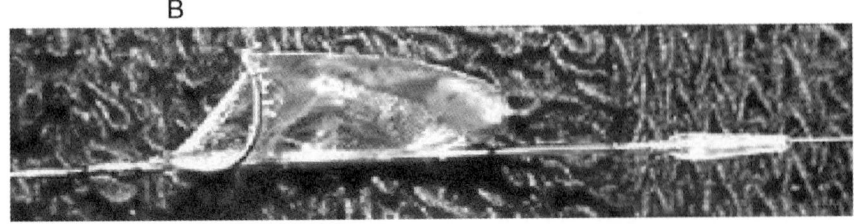

Figure 71B–12 **Distal protection devices:** GuardWire (PercuSurge, Inc., Sunnyvale, CA) **(A),** Angioguard (Cordis, Warren, NJ) **(B),** and EPI filter (EPI, Inc, Boston, MA) **(C).** (See color plate.)

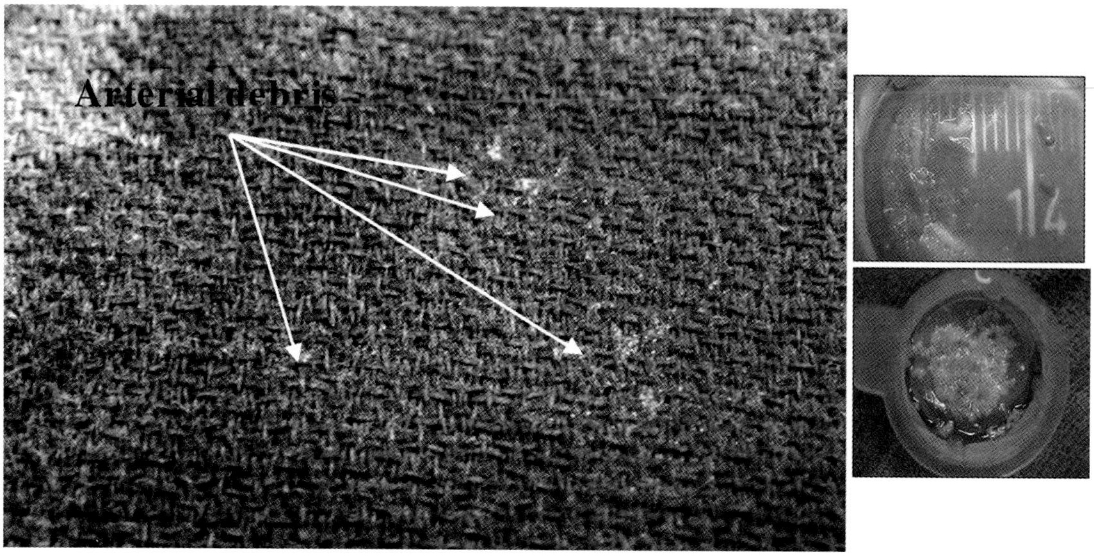

Figure 71B–13 Distal macroscopic emboli captured with the use of the GuardWire (PercuSurge, Inc., Sunnyvale, CA) in an ulcerated left internal carotid lesion following predilatation with angioplasty prior to stenting. (See color plate.)

a pressure wire alone. In this way, more "physiological" gradients are measured and may help in revascularizing more appropriate lesions in the renal vasculature.

Lower Extremity

Iliac

Once a lesion is identified on angiography, its functional significance and suitability for intervention can be further assessed using pressure wire measurements. Currently, a mean gradient of more than 10 mm Hg at rest or after hyperemia following vasodilatation with some form of vasodilator (trinitroglycerol, papaverine) is considered significant. The presence of symptoms, positive noninvasive studies, a significant stenosis on angiography, and a gradient of this magnitude indicate that the lesion likely merits revascularization.

Various revascularization techniques are available. Intravascular stenting has been associated with improved long-term patency compared with conventional balloon angioplasty,* and clinical outcomes following stent placement appear to be similar to long-term outcomes following vascular surgery,[6,78] although direct comparative data are lacking.

Infrainguinal Vessels

Percutaneous interventions to the infrainguinal vessels remain associated with poor long-term patency.[55,59,82]

*References 44, 58, 79, 81, 87, 92.

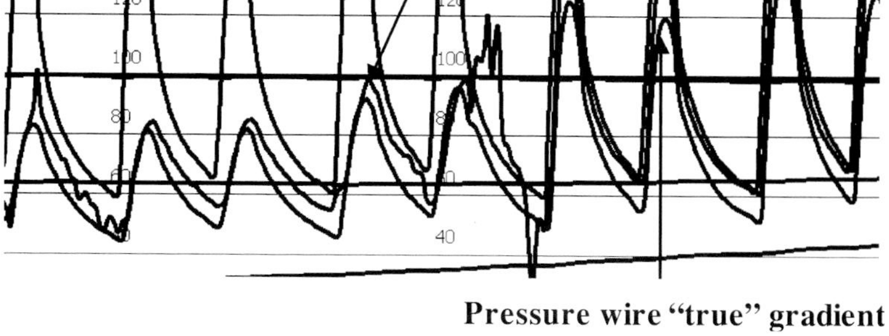

Figure 71B–14 Pressure measurements across a renal artery lesion using a 4-French multipurpose catheter and an 0.014-inch pressure wire (RADI corporation), revealing a "false" gradient and a more physiological gradient after the catheter is removed from the lesion. (See text.)

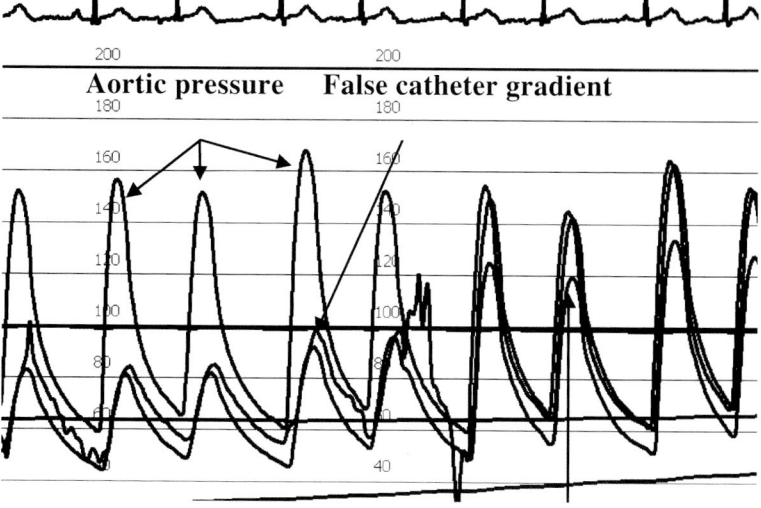

Generally, lesions in the SFA are best treated percutaneously if the lesion is focal and less than 3 cm.[22,46,53] As the lesion length increases, there is an increase in restenosis following angioplasty.[15,28,46,53,59] Stenting of the SFA has not been associated with improved patency.[32,33] With percutaneous intervention of the infrapopliteal arteries it is more difficult to maintain patency given the small diameter of the vessels and their dynamic properties at the level of the lower extremity.

REFERENCES

1. Allaqaband S, Tumuluri R, Goel AK, et al: Diagnosis and management of carotid artery disease: the role of carotid artery stenting. Curr Prob Cardiol 26:495–548, 2001.
2. American Heart Association: 2002 Heart and Stroke Statistical Update. Dallas, TX: American Heart Association, 2001.
3. Azakie A, McElhinney DB, Dowd CF, Stoney RJ: Percutaneous stenting for symptomatic stenosis of aberrant right subclavian artery. J Vasc Surg 27(4):756–758, 1998.
4. Baguneid M, Dodd D, Fulford P, et al: Mangement of acute nontraumatic upper limb ischemia. Angiology 50(9):715–720, 1999.
5. Belz M, Marshall JJ, Cowley MJ, Vetrovec GW: Subclavian balloon angioplasty in the management of the coronary-subclavian steal syndrome. Cathet Cardiovasc Diagn 25(2):161–163, 1992.
6. Bonn J: Percutaneous vascular intervention: value of hemodynamic measurements. Radiology 201:18–20, 1996.
7. Braunwald E, Swan HJC, Gorlin R, McIntosh HD: Cooperative study on cardiac catheterization. Circulation 37(Suppl.):1, 1968.
8. Brown AH: Coronary steal by internal mammary graft with subclavian stenosis. J Thorac Cardiovasc Surg 73:690–693, 1997.
9. Brown M: Results of the Carotid and Vertebral Artery Transluminal Angioplasty Study (CAVATAS) [abstract]. Cerebrovasc Dis 8(Suppl. 4):21, 1998.
10. Bush RL, Nahibi S, MacDonald J, Lin PH, et al: Endovascular revascularization of renal artery stenosis: technical and clinical results. J Vasc Surg 33:1041–1049, 2001.
11. Chang JB, Stein TA, Liu JP, Dunn ME: Long-term results with axillo-axillary bypass grafts for symptomatic subclavian artery insufficiency. J Vasc Surg 25(1):173–178, 1997.
12. Cohn PF, Goldberg S: Cardiac catheterization and coronary arteriography. In Cohn PF, editor: Diagnosis and Therapy of Coronary Artery Disease. Boston: Martinus Nijhoff, 1985, p. 219.
13. Cooper SG, Sullivan ID, Wren C: Treatment of recoarctation: balloon dilation angioplasty. J Am Coll Cardiol 14:413, 1989.
14. Criqui MH, Langer RD, Fronek A, et al: Mortality over a period of 10 years in patients with peripheral arterial disease. N Engl J Med 326:381–386, 1992.
15. Currie IC, Wakeley CJ, Cole SE, et al: Femoropopliteal angioplasty for severe limb ischemia. Br J Surg 81:191–193, 1994.
16. Davies KN, Humphrey PR: Do carotid bruits predict disease of the internal carotid arteries? Postgrad Med J 70:433–435, 1994.
17. de Giovanni JV: Covered stents in the treatment of aortic coarctation. J Interv Cardiol 14(2):187–190, 2001.
18. Derkx FH, Schalekamp MA: Renal artery stenosis and hypertension. Lancet 344:237–239, 1994.
19. Diethrich EB, Cozacov JC: Subclavian stent implantation to alleviate coronary steal through a patent internal mammary artery graft. J Endovasc Surg 2(1):77–80, 1995.
20. Dormandy J, Heeck L, Vig S: Lower extremity arteriosclerosis as a reflection of systemic process: implications for concomitant coronary and carotid disease. Semin Vasc Surg 12:118–122,1999.
21. Dorros G, Jaff M, Mathiak L, et al: Four year follow up of Palmaz-Schatz stent revascularization as treatment for atherosclerotic renal artery stenosis. Circulation 98:642–647, 1998.
22. Duke C, Qureshi SA: Aortic coarctation and recoarctation: to stent or not to stent? J Interv Cardiol 14(3):283–298, 2001.
23. European Carotid Surger Trialists (ECST) Collaterative Group: MRC European Carotid Surgery Trial: interim results for symptomatic patients with severe (70–90%) or mild (0–29%) stenosis. Lancet 337:1235–1243, 1991.
24. European Working Group on Critical Leg Ischemia: Second European consensus document on chronic critical leg ischemia. Circulation 84(Suppl. IV):IV-1, 1991.
25. Executive Committee for the Asymptomatic Carotid Atherosclerosis Study: Endarterectomy for asymptomatic carotid artery stenosis: Executive Committee for the Asymptomatic Carotid Athersclerosis Study. JAMA 273:1421–1428, 1995.
26. Fisher CM: A new vascular syndrome—"The subclavian steal." N Engl J Med 265:912, 1961.
27. Forssman W: Die Sondierung des rechten Herzens. Klin Wochenschr 8:2085, 1929.
28. Gallino A, Mahler F, Probst P, Nachbur B: Percutaneous transluminal angioplasty of the arteries of the lower limbs: a 5 year follow-up. Circulation 70:619–623, 1984.
29. Garcia LA, Carrozza JP Jr: Percutaneous revascularization of surgically corrected coarctation with graft restenosis. J Invasive Cardiol 14(7):400–403, 2002.
30. Gibbs JL: Treatment options for coarctation of the aorta. Heart 84(1):11–13, 2000.
31. Gollege J, Mitchell A, Greenhalgh RM, Davies AH: Systemic comparison of the early outcome of angioplasty and endarterectomy for symptomatic carotid artery disease. Stroke 31:1439–1443, 2000.
32. Gray BH, Olin JW: Limitations of percutaneous transluminal angioplasty with stenting for femoropopliteal arterial occlusive disease. Semin Vasc Surg 10:8–16, 1997.
33. Gray BH, Sullivan TM, Childs MB, et al: High incidence of restenosis/reocclusion of stents in the percutaneous treatment of long-segment superficial femoral artery disease after suboptimal angioplasty. J Vasc Surg 25:74–83, 1997.
34. Grossman W: In Baim DS, Grossman W, editors: Cardiac Catheterization, Angiography and Intervention, 6th ed. Philadelphia: Lippincott, Williams & Wilkins, 2000, p. 6.
35. Gruentzig AR: Perkutane Dilatation von Coronarstenosen-Beschreibung eines neuen Kathetersystems. Klin Wochenschr 54:543, 1976.
36. Gruentzig AR, Turina MI, Schneider JA: Experimental percutaneous dilatation of coronary artery stenosis. Circulation 54:81, 1976.
37. Guidelines for coronary angiography. A report of the American College of Cardiology/American Heart Association Task Force on Assessment of Diagnostic and Therapeutic Cardiovascular Procedures. Circulation 76:963A, 1987.
38. Haas M, Spargo BH, Wit EJ, Meehan SM: Etiologies and outcome of acute renal insufficiency in older adults: a renal biopsy study of 259 cases. Am J Kidney Dis 35(3):433–447, 2000.
39. Hall TB, Matson M, Belli AM: Thrombolysis in the peripheral vascular system. Eur Radiol 11(3):439–445, 2001.
40. Hamdan MA, Maheshwari S, Fahey JT, Hellenbrand WE: Endovascular stents for coarctation of the aorta: initial results and intermediate-term follow-up. J Am Coll Cardiol 38(5):1518–1523, 2001.

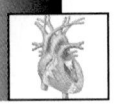

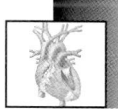

41. Hansen KJ: Prevalence of ischemic nephropathy in the atherosclerotic population. Am J Kidney Dis 24:615–621, 1994.
42. Harden PN, MacLeod MJ, Rodger RSC, et al: Effect of renal artery stenting on progression of renovascular renal failure. Lancet 349:1133–1136, 1997.
43. Harrison Da, McLaughlin PR, Lazzam C, et al: Endovascular stents in the management of coarctation of the aorta in the adolescent and adult: one year follow up. Heart 85(5):561–566, 2001.
44. Henry M, Amor M, Ethevenot G, et al: Palmaz stent placement in iliac and femoropopliteal arteries: primary and secondary patency in 310 patients with 2–4 year follow-up. Radiology 197:167–174, 1995.
45. Hornung TS, Benson LN, McLaughlin PR: Interventions for aortic coarctation. Cardiol Rev 10(3):139–148, 2002.
46. Johnston KW: Femoral and popliteal arteries: re analysis of results of balloon angioplasty. Radiology 183:767–771, 1992.
47. Kadir S: Regional anatomy of the thoracic aorta. In Kadir S, editor: Atlas of Normal and Variant Angiographic Anatomy. Philadelphia: W.B. Saunders, 1991, p. 19.
48. Kasirajan K, Gray B, Beavers FP, et al: Rheolytic thrombectomy in the management of acute and subacute limb-threatening ischemia. J Vasc Interv Radiol 12(4):413–421, 2001.
49. Keith DS, Markey B, Schiedler M: Successful long-term stenting of an atypical descending aortic coarctation. J Vasc Surg 35(1):166–167, 2002.
50. Koerselman J, de Vries H, Jaarsma W, et al: Balloon angioplasty of coarctation of the aorta: A safe alternative for surgery in adults: immediate and mid-term results. Catheter Cardiovasc Interv 50(1):28–33, 2000.
51. Kolh PH, Torchiana DF, Buckley MJ: Atheroembolization in cardiac surgery. The need for preoperative diagnosis. J Cardiovasc Surg 40(1):77–81, 1999.
52. Korn P, Khilnani NM, Fellers JC, et al: Thromolysis for native arterial occlusions of the lower extremities: clinical outcome and cost. J Vasc Surg 33(6):1148–1157, 2001.
53. Krepel VM, van Andel GJ, van Erp WF, Breslau PJ: Percutaneous transluminal angioplasty of the femoropopliteal artery: initial and long term results. Radiology 156:325–328, 1985.
54. Magee AG, Blauth CI, Qureshi SA: Interventional and surgical management of aortic stenosis and coarctation. Ann Thorac Surg 71(2):713–715, 2001.
55. Matsi PJ, Manninen HI, Vanninen RL, et al: Femoropopliteal angioplasty in patients with claudication: primary and secondary patency in 140 limbs with 1–3 year follow-up. Radiology 191:727–733, 1994.
56. McPhail IR, Spittell PC, Weston SA, Bailey KR: Intermittent claudication: An objective office based assessment. J Am Coll Cardiol 37:1381–1385, 2001.
57. Mukherjee D, Yadav JS: Carotid and cerebrovascular disease. Cardiol Rev 8:322–332, 2000.
58. Murphy TP, Webb MS, Lambiase RE, et al: Percutaneous revascularization of complex iliac artery stenoses and occlusions with the use of Wallstent: three year experience. J Vasc Interv Radiol 7:21–27, 1996.
59. Murray JG, Apthorp LA, Wilkins RA: Long segment (>10 cm) femoropopliteal angioplasty: improved technical success and long-term patency. Radiology 195:158–162, 1995.
60. Norris JW, Zhu CZ, Bornstein NM, Chambers BR: Vascular risks of asymptomatic carotid stenosis. Stroke 22:1485–1490, 1991.
61. North American Symptomatic Carotid Endarterectomy Trial (NASCET) Collaboration: Beneficial effect of carotid endarterectomy in symptomatic patients with high grade carotid stenosis. N Engl J Med 325:445–453, 1991.
62. Oureil K, Veith FJ, Sasahara AA: A comparison of recombinant urokinase with vascular surgery as initial treatment for acute arterial occlusion of the legs. Thrombolysis or Peripheral Arterial Surgery (TOPAS) Investigators. N Engl J Med 338:1105–1111, 1998.
63. Pentacost MJ, Criqui MH, Dorros G, et al: Guidelines for peripheral percutaneous transluminal angioplasty of the abdominal aorta and lower extremity vessels. Circulation 89:511–531, 1994.
64. Radermacher J, Chavan A, Bleck J, et al: Use of Doppler ultrasonography to predict the outcome of therapy for renal artery stenosis. N Engl J Med 344:410–417, 2001.
65. Ramee SR, Dawson R, McKinley K, et al: Provisional stenting for symptomatic intracranial stenosis using a multidisciplinary approach: acute results, unexpected benefit, and one year outcome. Cathet Cardiovasc Intervent 52:457–467, 2001.
66. Rao PS: Which aortic coarctations should we dilate? Am Heart J 117:987, 1989.
67. Recto MR, Elbl F, Austin E: Use of the new IntraStent for the treatment of transverse arch hypoplasia/coarctation of the aorta. Catheter Cardiovasc Interv 53(4):499–503, 2001.
68. Rimmer JM, Gennari FJ: Atherosclerotic renovascular disease and progressive renal failure. Ann Intern Med 118:712–719, 1993.
69. Rosamond WD, Folsom AR, Chambless LE, et al: Stroke incidence and survival among middle-aged adults: 9 year follow up of the Atherosclerosis Risk in Communities (ARIC) cohort. Stroke 30:736–743, 1999.
70. Sacco RL: Identifying patient populations at high risk for stroke. Neurology 51:S27–30, 1998.
71. Safian RD, Textor SC: Renal artery stenosis. N Engl J Med 344(6):431–442, 2001.
72. Schwend RB, Hambsch K, Baker L, et al: Carotid steal syndrome: a case study. J Neuroimaging 5(3):195–197, 1995.
73. Smith GD, Shipley MJ, Rose G: Intermittent claudication, heart disease risk factors, and mortality: The Whitehall Study. Circulation 82:1925–1931, 1990.
74. Sones FM Jr, Shirey EK: Cine coronary arteriography. Mod Concepts Cardiovasc Dis 31:735–738, 1962.
75. Sones FM Jr, Shirey EK, Proudfit WL, Wescott RN: Cine coronary arteriography. Circulation 20:773, 1959.
76. Stagg SJ 3rd, Abben RP, Chaisson GA, et al: Management of the coronary-subclavian steal syndrome with balloon angioplasty. A case report and review of the literature. Angiology 45(8):725–731, 1994.
77. Tan TY, Lien LM, Schminke U, et al: Hemodynamic effects of innominate artery occlusive disease on anterior cerebral artery. J Neuroimaging 12(1):59–62, 2002.
78. Tetteroo E, Haaring C, van der Graf Y, et al: Intraarterial pressure gradients after randomized angioplasty and stenting of iliac artery lesions. Dutch Iliac Stent Trial Group. Cardiovasc Intervent Radiol 19:411–417, 1996.
79. Tetteroo E, van der Graaf Y, Bosch JL, et al: Randomised comparison of primary stent placement versus primary angioplasty followed by selective stent placement in patients with iliac artery occlusive disease. Dutch Iliac Stent Trial Study Group. Lancet 351:1153–1159, 1998.
80. Thromobysis in the management of lower limb peripheral arterial occlusion—a consensus document. Working Party on Thrombolysis in the Management of Limb Ischemia. Am J Cardiol 81(2):207–218, 1998.
81. Treatment of intermittent claudication. Society of Vascular Surgery TASC paper. J Vasc Surg 31(part 2):S1–127, 2000.
82. Treatment of intermittent claudication. Society of Vascular Surgery TASC paper. J Vasc Surg 31(part 2):29–34, 2000.
83. Tynan M, Finley JP, Fontes V, et al: Balloon angioplasty for the treatment of native coarctation: results of valvuloplasty and angioplasty of congenital anomalies registry. Am J Cardiol 65:790, 1990.

84. van Jaarsveld BC, Pieta K, Pieterman H, et al: The effect of ballon angioplasty on hypertension in atherosclerotic renal artery stenosis. N Engl J Med 342(14):1007–1014, 2000.
85. Van Son JA, Aengevaeren WR, Skotnicki SH, et al: Diagnosis and management of the coronary subclavian steal syndrome. Eur J Cardiothorac Surg 3(6):565–567, 1989.
86. Vassalotti JA, Delgado FA, WheltonA: Atheroembolic renal disease. Am J Ther 3(7):544–549, 1996.
87. Vorwerk D, Gunther RW, Schurmann K, et al: Primary stent placement for chronic iliac artery occlusions: follow-up results in 103 patients. Radiology 194:745–749, 1995.
88. Watson RS, Hadjipetrou P, Cox SV, et al: Effect of renal artery stenting on renal artery stenting on renal function and size in patients with atherosclerotic renovascular disease. Circulation 201:1671–1677, 2000.
89. Weitz JI, Byrne J, Clagett P, et al: Diagnosis and treatment of chronic arterial insufficiency of the lower extremities: a critical review. Circulation 94:3026–3049, 1996.
90. Wholey MH, Wholey M, Mathias K, et al: Global experience in cervical carotid artery stent placement. Cathet Cardiovasc Interv 50:160–167, 2000.
91. Wolf PA, Kannel WB, Sorlie P, McNamara P: Asymptomatic carotid bruit and risk of stroke: the Framingham study. JAMA 245:1442–1445, 1981.
92. Wolf YG, Schatz RA, Knowles HJ, et al: Initial experience with the Palmaz stent for aortoiliac stenoses. Ann Vasc Surg 7:254–261, 1993.
93. Yadav JS, Roubin GS, Iyer S, et al: Elective stenting of the extracranial carotid arteries. Circulation 95:376–381, 1997.

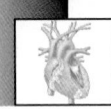

Surgical Management of Valvular Heart Disease

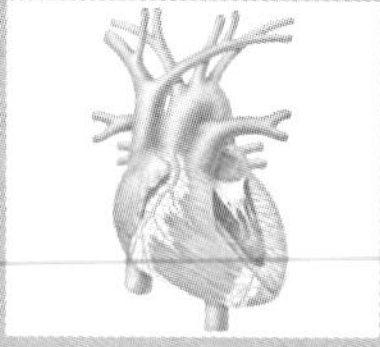

CHAPTER 72

Valve Replacement Therapy: History, Options, and Valve Types

Edwin C. McGee, Jr., Gus J. Vlahakes, and Ralph De La Torre

INTRODUCTION: THE IDEAL VALVE

Many acceptable substitutes exist today for the replacement of diseased human heart valves. The ideal valvular prosthesis, as described by Harken,[38] remains the Holy Grail of cardiac surgery. The ideal valve would be durable with a longevity approaching that of a native valve. Thrombogenicity would be nonexistent, and there would be no need for supplemental anticoagulation. In addition, the ideal replacement valve would have no inherent gradient in and of itself and would allow for unimpeded outflow. It also would be easily implanted and readily available. Finally, growth commensurate with that of the recipient would be possible.

HISTORY

The first human heart valve operation was a digital valvotomy of a stenotic aortic valve performed by Tuffier in 1914. Cutler, Souttar, Brock, Swan, and Harken refined valvotomies and commissurotomies over the ensuing decades. The need for a replacement valve arose out of the quest for an effective treatment of valvular insufficiency. In 1950 Hufnagel developed a ball valve, designed to be placed in the descending thoracic aorta. He was the first to implant a prosthetic valve in a human when he implanted his valve in the descending thoracic aorta of a patient with severe aortic insufficiency.[41] In 1956 Gordon Murray implanted an aortic homograft in the descending thoracic aorta of a patient with severe aortic regurgitation.[18] With the introduction of cardiopulmonary bypass, open valve replacement became a possibility. In 1960 Braunwald and Harken successfully performed mitral and aortic valve replacements with valves made of polyurethane.[26] In 1961 Albert Starr, a surgeon, and

Lowell Edwards, an engineer, developed a caged ball valve with which they achieved long-term survival.[63] Caged ball valves worked well in many patients, but their high profile made their use difficult in patients with small ventricular chambers and small aortic roots. High inherent gradients, along with a less favorable thromboembolic profile, made caged ball valves less desirable as new prostheses were introduced.

To overcome these limitations, several investigators designed disk valves, which functioned by having a disk pivot into an open or closed position as dictated by flow across the valve. The first of these tilting disk valves was the Wada hingeless valve introduced by the Japanese surgeon Jura Wada, in 1966.[68] The Lillihei–Kaster valve was a hingeless valve, with a freely rotating pivoting disk retained by struts, which was introduced in 1967 by C. Walton Lillehei and Robert L. Kaster.[46] Viking Björk, working with Shiley Laboratories, developed a similar version of a hingeless pivoting disk valve. Although the hemodynamic profile was improved when compared to the caged ball valves, these early pivoting disk valves were subject to occasional thrombosis. The 60° Convexo-Concave Björk–Shiley disk valve was prone to catastrophic structural failure secondary to fracture of its welded struts; the resultant strut fracture led to escape of the occluder disk, which led to its eventual withdrawal from the market.[10] Seeking to improve on the problems of durability and thrombogenicity seen with these initial pivoting disk valves, Karl-Victor Hall, along with Woien and Kaster and the Medtronic Corporation, introduced the Medtronic–Hall valve in 1977.

The St. Jude Medical bileaflet mechanical prosthesis was also introduced in 1977. It has gone through several refinements and is currently the most commonly used mechanical valve prosthesis.[29] Structural failure is no longer a source of significant morbidity with mechanical prostheses, but thromboembolism and anticoagulant-associated hemorrhage remain significant sources of morbidity.

Independently, in 1969 Carpentier and Hancock developed the first porcine xenografts.[15,57] Ionescu developed the first glutaraldehyde-preserved bovine pericardial valve in 1971. Limited long-term durability secondary to leaflet calcification and subsequent perforation plagued these early bioprostheses. Significant progress has been made with the latest generation bioprostheses using state-of-the-art fixation and preservation methods to achieve extended durability. Stentless xenografts were introduced in 1986 as a way to counteract the inherent gradient found with stented bioprostheses. To date, long-term durability of bioprosthetic valves does not approach that of mechanical bioprostheses.

Ross introduced the use of aortic homografts in 1962.[71] Barrett-Boyes popularized the subcoronary implantation technique. Methods of preservation have ranged from antibiotic sterilization to cryopreservation with liquid nitrogen. Valve failure results from extensive calcification and occurs more rapidly in younger patients in a mode similar to xenograft bioprostheses.

Donald Ross introduced the use of a pulmonary autograft to replace the aortic valve in 1967. It is now most commonly used in the pediatric population. As is true in all areas of surgery, minimally invasive approaches to valve replacement are gaining in interest. Percutaneous delivery of valves has been reported, but has yet to be achieved in any reproducible manner.

HEMODYNAMIC ASSESSMENT OF CARDIAC VALVES

The normal valve area is 3.0–4.0 cm^2 for the aortic valve and 4.0–5.0 cm^2 for the mitral valve. Stented bioprostheses and mechanical prostheses have inherent gradients because the actual valve is supported by a stent and housing material. The effective orifice area (EOA) refers to the true cross-sectional area of the prosthetic valve orifice through which blood must flow. The gold standard for measuring valve area is the Gorlin formula, which uses data derived from catheterization and applies hydraulic formulas for fixed orifice systems to heart valves.[36] The formula is as follows:

$$A = Q/\,(44.3 \times \sqrt{\Delta p})$$

Where A is the cross-sectional area of the valve (cm^2), Q is the flow across the valve (ml/sec), and Δp is the pressure gradient across the valve (mmHg). 44.3 is a derived coefficient.

The continuity equation uses echo Doppler-acquired data to calculate EOA. Both a standard and a simplified equation exist. The standard equation is as follows:

$$EOA = SV/VTI = \Sigma\ (t)\ dt/\Sigma\ V\ (t)\ dt$$

Where SV is the stroke volume (derived from flow measurement) and VTI is the velocity time integral across the prosthesis (also measured by Doppler).

The simplified equation is EOA = Qp/Vp, where Qp is peak flow (ml/sec) and Vp (ml/sec × cm^2) is the peak flow velocity across the valve.

The continuity equation has been shown to be accurate for bioprostheses.[60] When applied to bileaflet valves such as the St. Jude Medical prosthesis, it has been shown to underestimate valve area because of localized high-velocity jets.[8]

Although valve manufacturers have often used the geometrical cross-sectional area of prostheses to describe their size, the parameter that is clinically important is the functional orifice of the valve: the EOA. In general, EOA is proportional to valve size for a given type of prosthesis, and the EOA is generally always less than the cross-sectional area of a patient's valve annulus. Accordingly, some degree of obstruction is always imparted by prostheses, and this is particularly important in the case of the aortic valve. Many surgeons believe that particularly for aortic valve replacement, the EOA of an implanted aortic prosthesis must be matched to the size of the patient to provide sufficient gradient relief. This is particularly the case during exercise. Although the concept of patient–prosthesis mismatch makes intuitive sense, its impact on patient morbidity and mortality in the short or long term remains unclear and is the subject of numerous studies. Some authors have suggested that patient–prosthesis mismatch can be avoided when the ratio of EOA to patient body surface area exceeds 0.85 cm^2/m^2. It should be emphasized that the manufacturer's labeled valve size does not delineate the true internal or external diameter of a given valve

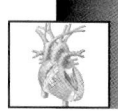

and often does not belie the true EOA. Indeed, labeling of the valve sizes is arbitrary, and as such it cannot be used to compare values among different manufacturers and is not a true indicator of EOA.[16]

MORBIDITY AND MORTALITY GUIDELINES FOR VALVE OPERATIONS

Clinical studies are crucial for determining outcomes after cardiac valve operations, and precise definitions of outcomes are critical when comparing prostheses. To address this need, the councils of the Society of Thoracic Surgeons (STS) and the American Association for Thoracic Surgery (AATS) formulated the Ad Hoc Liaison Committee for Standardizing Definitions of Prosthetic Heart Valve Morbidity. The initial report of this committee was issued in 1988[17,37] with an update following in 1996.[27] The report strictly defines types of morbidity and mortality that can occur after valvular operations. An understanding of these definitions is crucial for interpreting studies dealing with valvular prostheses.

The guidelines distinguish two types of mortality: hospital mortality and 30-day mortality. Hospital mortality refers to death occurring at any time before discharge during a patient's initial hospital stay. Thirty-day mortality, also referred to as operative mortality, is death that occurs at any time or place within 30 days of operation. There are several precise definitions of valve-related morbidity. Structural valve deterioration refers to "...any change in function (a decrease of one New York Heart Association functional class or more) of an operated valve resulting from an intrinsic abnormality of the valve that causes stenosis or regurgitation."[27] It includes "...changes intrinsic to the valve, such as wear, fracture, poppet escape, calcification, leaflet tear, stent creep, and suture line disruption of components...of an operated valve."[27] Thrombotic or infectious causes of valve dysfunction are not included.

Nonstructural dysfunction includes nonthrombotic and noninfectious causes of valvular stenosis or regurgitation that are not intrinsic to the valve itself. "Examples...include entrapment by pannus, tissue, or suture; paravalvular leak; inappropriate sizing or positioning; residual leak or obstruction from valve implantation or repair; and clinically important hemolytic anemia."[27] Morbid events are often reported as the composite linearized rate, or the number of events divided by the number of patient years of follow-up (events/pt yrs). The composite linearized rate for nonstructural dysfunction of the commonly available mechanical valves is 0.2–0.8 (events/pt yrs) for the aortic position and 0.3–1.4 (events/pt yrs) for the mitral position.[2]

Valve thrombosis is defined as thrombus in or about the valve that is not associated with infection and that interferes with valve function or obstructs blood flow through it. The composite linearized rate of thrombosis of mechanical valves is 0-0.2 (events/pt yrs) for the aortic position and 0.4-0.8 (events/pt yrs) for the mitral position.[2]

Embolism refers to any embolic event not associated with endocarditis that occurs after the immediate perioperative period and after the emergence from anesthesia. Embolic events are further delineated into neurological events and peripheral embolic events. The composite linearized rate of thromboembolism ranges from 1.4–2.5 (events/pt yrs) for the aortic position to 1.8–3.6 (events/pt yrs) for the mitral position.[2]

A bleeding event refers to any clinically significant bleed requiring hospitalization or transfusion or causing death. A patient does not have to be taking an anticoagulant to sustain a bleeding event. Composite linearized rates vary from 0.8–2.5 (events/pt yrs) for the aortic position to 1.2–2.2 (events/pt yrs) for the mitral position.[2]

Endocarditis involving an operated valve is designated as operated valvular endocarditis. "Morbidity associated with active infection, such as valve-thrombosis, thrombotic embolus, bleeding event, or paravalvular leak, is included under this category and is not included in other categories of morbidity."[27] Composite linearized rates for prosthetic valve endocarditis range from 0.4–0.7 (events/pt yrs) for both the aortic and mitral positions.[2]

Consequences of morbid events are also defined by the guidelines. A reoperation is any operation on "...a previously operated valve."[27] The composite linearized rate for reoperation ranges from 0.3–1.8 (events/pt yrs) for the aortic position to 0.6–1.6 (events/pt yrs) for the mitral position.[2]

Valve-related mortality is any death after a valve operation caused by a morbid event that is not related to progressive heart failure in patients with functioning valves. Unexplained deaths are just that and should be listed as such. Cardiac deaths include valve-related deaths, sudden deaths, and non–valve-related cardiac deaths. Total deaths refer to any and all deaths after a valve operation. "Permanent valve-related" impairment refers to any "...permanent neurologic or functional deficit..."[27] caused by a morbid event.

CURRENT FDA-APPROVED PROSTHETIC HEART VALVES

The following is a brief description of valves currently approved by the United States Food and Drug Administration (FDA). Discussion is by valve type and manufacturer (Box 72-1).

Mechanical Prostheses

Caged Ball Prostheses

Starr–Edwards Silastic Ball Valve Prosthesis

The Starr–Edwards ball valve prosthesis (Edwards Lifesciences, Inc, Irvine, CA) was introduced in 1966. The model currently available is constructed of a cage made from a single piece of titanium that encloses a silastic ball. Although the valve is very durable and has a notable history, indications for its use today are limited because its hemodynamic and thromboembolic profiles do not match more modern designs (Figure 72-1).[2]

Tilting Disk Prostheses

Medtronic–Hall Mechanical Heart Valve

The Medtronic–Hall tilting disk valve (Medtronic, Inc., Minneapolis, MN) came on the market in 1977 (Figure 72-2).

Box 72–1. Current FDA-Approved Prosthetic Heart Valves.

Mechanical

Alliance Medical Technologies Monostrut Cardiac Valve Prosthesis
ATS Medical Open Pivot Bileaflet Heart Valve
Edwards Lifesciences Starr–Edwards Silastic Ball Heart Valve Prosthesis
Medical Carbon Research Institute On-X Prosthetic Heart Valve
Medical CV Omniscience Cardiac Valve Prosthesis
Medical CV Omnicarbon Cardiac Valve Prosthesis
Medtronic–Hall Prosthetic Heart Valve
St. Jude Medical Mechanical Heart Valve
Sulzer CarboMedics Prosthetic Heart Valve

Bioprosthetic

Edwards Lifesciences Carpentier–Edwards Duraflex Low Pressure Mitral Bioprosthesis
Edwards Lifesciences Carpentier–Edwards Standard Porcine Bioprosthesis
Edwards Lifesciences Carpentier–Edwards Supra-Annular Porcine Bioprosthesis
Edwards Lifesciences Carpentier–Edwards PERIMOUNT Pericardial Bioprosthesis
Edwards Lifesciences Carpentier–Edwards PERIMOUNT Plus Pericardial Bioprosthesis
Edwards Lifesciences Prima Plus Stentless Bioprosthetic Valve
Edwards Lifesciences Carpentier–Edwards Supra-Annular Valve (CE-SAV) Bioprosthesis
Medtronic Hancock I Porcine Bioprosthesis
Medtronic Hancock II Bioprosthetic Heart Valve
Medtronic Hancock Modified Orifice (MO) Porcine Bioprosthesis
Medtronic Freestyle Aortic Root Bioprosthesis
Medtronic Mosaic Porcine Bioprosthesis
St. Jude Medical Toronto SPV Valve

The previous list does not include various specific models of the previous valves (involving aortic versus mitral models, rotatable sewing cuffs, supraannular or subannular sewing cuffs, or differences in sewing cuff size [e.g., reduced or expanded] or material [e.g., standard or Teflon] or valved grafts [valved conduits]).

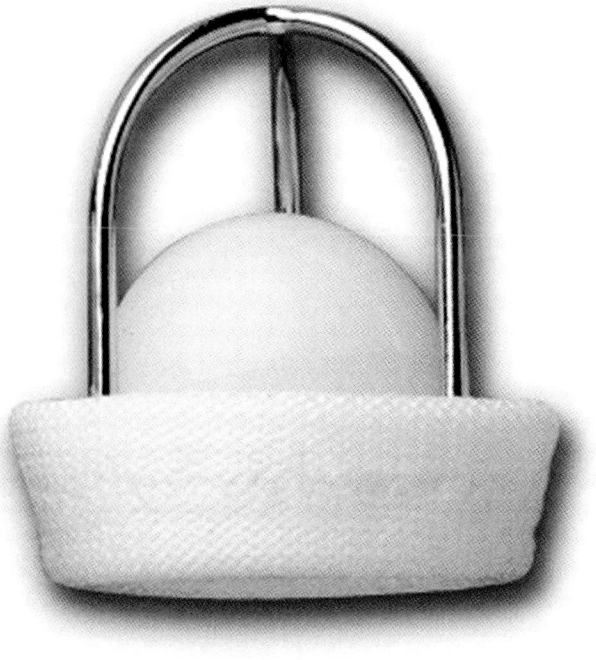

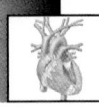

Figure 72–1 **Starr–Edwards Silastic Ball Valve Prosthesis.** *(Courtesy Edwards Lifesciences, Inc., Irvine, CA)*

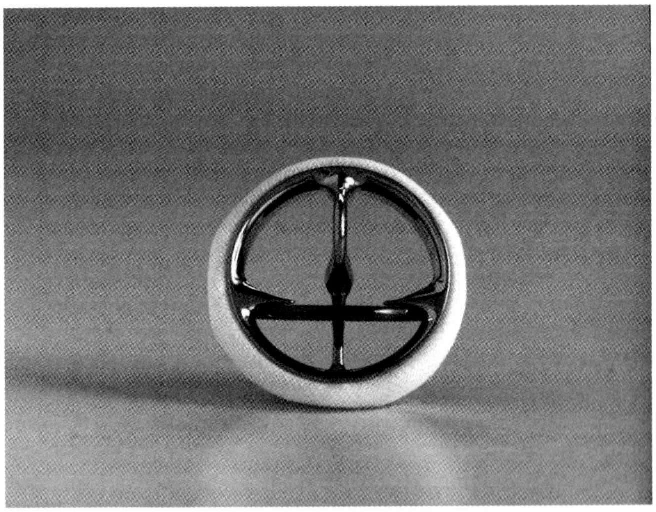

Figure 72–2 **Medtronic–Hall Mechanical Heart Valve.** *(Courtesy Medtronic, Inc., Minneapolis, MN)*

The valve housing is constructed from one piece of titanium alloy with no introduced welds or bends. The round central disk is made from tungsten-impregnated graphite with a pyrolytic carbon coating and has a central hole that allows the disk to be retained by a curved central guide strut that is part of the housing. It was hoped that its design would be an improvement on previous tilting disk valves in terms of durability, hemodynamic performance, and reduced thrombogenicity. Its design incorporated several new features designed to decrease thrombogenicity. Areas of low flow across the valve are reduced by a relatively larger minor orifice and a disk that lifts out of the housing and rotates with opening, which improves the ability of the valve to wash itself.[13] Loss of structural integrity has not been reported. The valve can be rotated after implantation and has a low inherent transvalvular gradient. It has a moderately high profile in the open position. Occluder impingement is possible because its position at the equator of the valve housing makes it susceptible to obstruction from retained valve elements or sutures cut too long.

Aortic prostheses are available in sizes from 20–31 mm. The optimal orientation is with the larger orifice of the aortic prosthesis facing the greater curvature of the aorta. Mitral prostheses are available in sizes from 23–33 mm. Low incidences of valve-related morbidity and mortality have been demonstrated by several studies. Most recently Butchart et al,[13] from the University Hospital of Wales, reported their 20-year experience with 1766 Medtronic–Hall valve replacements. Akins,[3] at the Massachusetts General Hospital, also recently reported his extensive experience with the Medtronic–Hall valve, with favorable results.

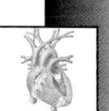

Omnicarbon Cardiac Valve Prosthesis

The Omnicarbon valve prosthesis (Medical CV, Inc., Inver Grove Heights, MN) is a low-profile tilting disk valve introduced in 1984. It is an evolution in design of the Lillehei–Kaster tilting disk valve and was introduced as an improvement over the Omniscience valve that was discontinued in 2000 primarily secondary to concerns with high rates of thrombosis and reoperation. Whereas the Omniscience valve had titanium housing, both the housing ring and tilting disk of the Omnicarbon valve are made of pyrolytic carbon. It can be rotated after implantation and has no fixed pivot grooves or recesses. The Omniscience design minimized diastolic regurgitation, which Edwards et al,[28] from the Wake Forest School of Medicine, postulated as the etiology of the valve's thromboembolic problems because of its inability to wash itself. The Omnicarbon valve is available in sizes from 19–33 mm in both aortic and mitral models. Studies in Japan and Europe[1,66] have shown diminished complication rates when compared with the Omniscience valve, and morbidity rates that are comparable to other mechanical prostheses on the market today.

Monostrut Cardiac Valve Prosthesis

The Monostrut cardiac valve prosthesis (Alliance Medical Technologies, Inc., Irvine, CA) is a third-generation tilting disk valve that is a descendant of the ill-fated 60 degrees Convexo-Concave Björk–Shiley tilting disk valve. Construction consists of a cobalt-based alloy orifice ring with an integral, nonwelded, monostrut retainer with a polytetrafluoroethylene (PTFE) sewing ring, a pyrolytic carbon disk occluder, and a 70° nominal opening angle.[23] Aris et al,[5] in the 10-year report of the Spanish Monostrut Group, demonstrated 100% freedom from structural deterioration and a low rate of valve-related complications. FDA approval occurred in 1997. The Monostrut is available in aortic sizes from 17–33 mm and mitral sizes from 27–33 mm. It is used in the Thoratec ventricular assist device.

Bileaflet Prostheses

St. Jude Medical Mechanical Heart Valve

The St. Jude Medical (SJM) valve prosthesis (St. Jude Medical, Inc., Minneapolis, MN) is the most commonly used bileaflet mechanical valve in the United States today (Figure 72-3). The FDA approved it in 1977, and over 1 million valves have been implanted. It is constructed of pyrolytic carbon and has proven to be extremely durable, with only 20 instances of structural integrity loss being reported.[2] The standard SJM valve is available in sizes from 19–31 mm for aortic valves and sizes from 19–33 mm for mitral valves. The SJM Masters series valves employ the same basic design as the standard series, but are designed to allow rotation after implantation. Several reports over the years have chronicled different institutions experiences with the valve. Most recently Lund et al,[51] from Copenhagen University in Denmark, reported a series of up to 694 patients who underwent aortic valve replacement with the standard SJM prosthesis with up to 18-year follow-up. Survival was 58%, 39%, and 37% at 10, 15, and 18 years, respectively. Thromboembolism (1.18%/pt yr) and anticoagulant-related bleeding (2.24%/pt yr) were the most common complications. No mechanical failures occurred, and two patients sustained valve thrombosis (0.04%/pt yr).

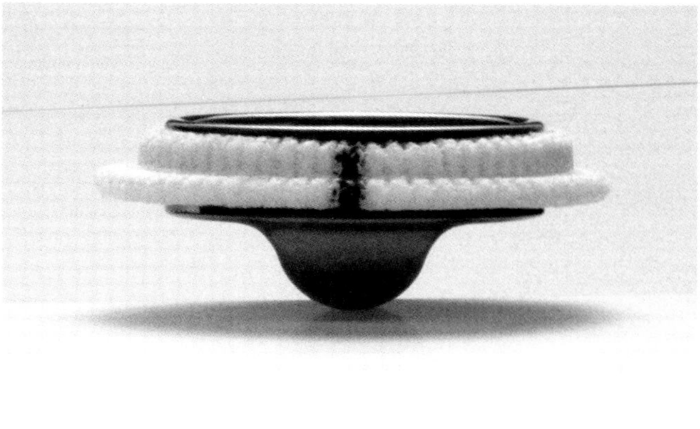

Figure 72–3 **St. Jude Medical Mechanical Heart Valve.** *(Courtesy St. Jude Medical, Inc., Minneapolis, MN)*

Zellner et al,[70] from the Medical University of South Carolina, reported their 17-year experience in 710 valve replacements carried out from 1979 to 1996. At least 418 aortic valve replacements (AVR) and 292 mitral valve replacements (MVR) were reported; 157 patients had associated coronary artery bypass grafts. Thirty-day mortality was 5.3% (AVR) and 5.1% (MVR), and follow-up was 96.9% complete with a total of 2376 (AVR) and 1868 (MVR) patient years reported. For the AVR patients, survival was 78%, 58%, and 37% at 5, 10, and 15 years, respectively. New York Heart Association (NYHA) functional class improved from 3 to 1.7. In the MVR group, survival was 79%, 60%, and 49% at 5, 10, and 15 years, respectively. NYHA class improvement improved from 3.3 to 1.8. Fifty-five and 64 thromboembolic events were reported in the AVR and MVR groups, respectively; 51 AVR and 23 MVR patients had anticoagulant-related bleeding. No mechanical failures were reported.[70] The authors concluded that function of the SJM valve is excellent and that much of valve replacement morbidity and mortality is secondary to patient comorbidities.

Baudet et al,[7] from France, reported their experience with up to 14-year follow-up of the 9-year implantation period from 1978 to 1987 with 1244 SJM valve replacements. At least 773 aortic valve replacements, 207 mitral valve replacements, and 132 double valve replacements with 8988 patient years were reported. Overall actuarial survival was 68% at 14 years. Other notable findings were as follows: thromboembolism (1.09%/pt yr), anticoagulant hemorrhage (0.94%/pt yr), prosthetic valve endocarditis (0.32%/pt yr), valve thrombosis (0.33%/pt yr), and paravalvular leak (0.19%/pt yr). The authors concluded that the SJM valve is one of the best performing mechanical prosthesis currently available.

To address the issue of inherent gradient in smaller-sized valves and the issue of patient–prosthesis size mismatch, the SJM Hemodynamic Plus (HP) series was developed. It was developed with the small aortic annulus in mind, with the sewing cuff redesigned to allow for supraannular placement. In 2001 Vitale et al[67] reported the results from the Italian Multicenter Study Group for the SJM HP aortic valve prosthesis. In this prospective randomized study, patients with 21- and 23-mm annulus diameters were randomized to receive either the standard cuff SJM valve or the HP valve. Postoperatively and at 6 months, echocardiographic hemodynamic variables such as ejection fraction, cardiac output, peak gradient, mean gradient, EOA, EOA index, and performance index were calculated. Data were available for 125 of 140 patients initially enrolled in the study. Decreased peak and mean gradients, increased EOA, EOA indexes, and performance indexes were found for the HP valves.[67] The authors concluded that utilization of HP valves may allow for implantation of smaller prostheses without patient–prosthesis mismatch and avoidance of the additional morbidity associated with root enlargement procedures. Ismeno et al,[42] from the Second University of Naples, reported similar results when comparing 19-mm standard and HP prostheses. At total of 119 patients (68 standard, 51 HP) were followed up for 5 years. The patients who received HP valves had statistically significantly better hemodynamics with lower peak and mean gradients and larger effective orifice areas. There was no difference in terms of 5-year survival, late complications, or left ventricular mass reduction between the groups.[42] The HP series is available in aortic sizes from 17–27 mm and mitral sizes from 17–27 mm.

The SJM Regent prosthesis is the latest evolution of the HP design. It achieves increased luminal orifice area with a modification of the orifice housing geometry. Preliminary in vivo experiences in Europe show encouraging hemodynamics.[34]

On-X Prosthetic Heart Valve

The On-X prosthetic valve (Medical Carbon Research Institute, Austin, TX) is a bileaflet valve constructed completely of pyrolytic carbon. The valve's manufacturer claims that the lack of silicon doping in the valve's carbon construction decreases its thrombogenicity. The manufacturer also points to a tall flared inlet that increases orifice area and decreases the ability of retained valve tissue to interfere with valve opening and closing. The design of the valve's pivots also allows the valve to wash itself. Aortic valves are available in sizes from 19–29 mm, and mitral valves are available in sizes from 23–33 mm. A Conform X model is available with a more flexible sewing ring. The valve was introduced in 1996 and received FDA approval in May 2001. It is not yet known if this valve will be less thrombogenic than other mechanical valves.

ATS Medical Open Pivot Mechanical Heart Valve

The ATS Medical Open Pivot mechanical heart valve (ATS Medical, Inc., Minneapolis, MN) is a bileaflet valve. It is available in sizes from 19–31 mm for the aortic position and from 19–33 mm for the mitral position.

CarboMedics Prosthetic Heart Valve

The CarboMedics prosthetic heart valve (Sulzer CarboMedics, Inc., Austin, TX), introduced in 1986, was the first rotatable bileaflet mechanical valve. Standard aortic and mitral prostheses are available in sizes from 19–31 mm and from 23–33 mm, respectively. Pediatric/small adult valves are available in smaller sizes: aortic: 16–18 mm; mitral: 16–21 mm. The Top Hat Supra-Annular aortic valve (Figure 72-4) is designed to maximize effective orifice area by having the sewing cuff of the valve sit above the annulus. A potential advantage over the SJM HP valve comes from the fact that the pivot guards of the Top Hat are completely supraannular. Top Hat valves are available in sizes from 19–27 mm. Concerns over valve thrombosis, particularly in the mitral position, have been raised by observational studies comparing the CarboMedics prosthetic heart valve with the SJM prosthesis.[59] Other studies,[30,61] including a randomized prospective trial from the Bristol Heart Institute in England, have not substantiated this concern and describe a similar pattern of morbidity and mortality for the two bileaflet mechanical valves.[50] The Optiform mitral prosthesis (Figure 72-5) is designed for supraannular, intraannular, or subannular placement and is available in sizes from 23–33 mm.

Bioprosthetic Valves

Bioprosthetic Valve Fixation

Durability remains the Achilles' heel of bioprosthetic valves. Over the years since the first valve replacement using a porcine xenograft was reported by Binet and colleagues in 1965,[9] tissue fixation methods have concentrated on improving durability. First-generation bioprosthetic valves were treated with glutaraldehyde fixation. It soon became evident that glutaraldehyde fixation led to calcification of xenograft tissue.[15] The pathophysiology of calcification is not completely understood. It is partly related to the affinity that calcium has for aldehyde groups that are generated by glutaraldehyde,[33] and partly due to the affinity of calcium for collagen in the extracellular matrix of cells exposed to glutaraldehyde. Damage caused by shear stress–induced

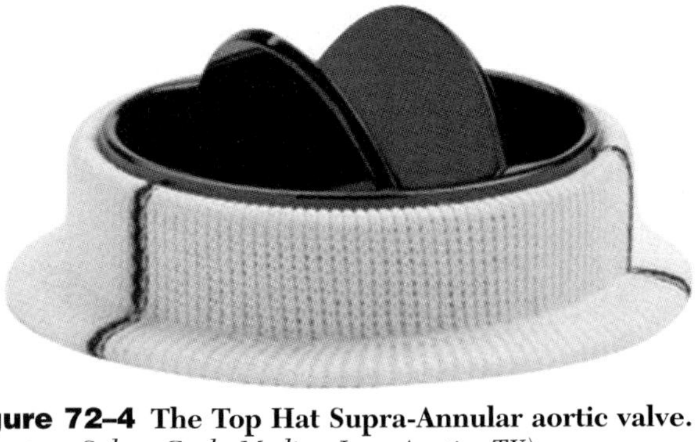

Figure 72–4 The Top Hat Supra-Annular aortic valve. *(Courtesy Sulzer CarboMedics, Inc., Austin, TX)*

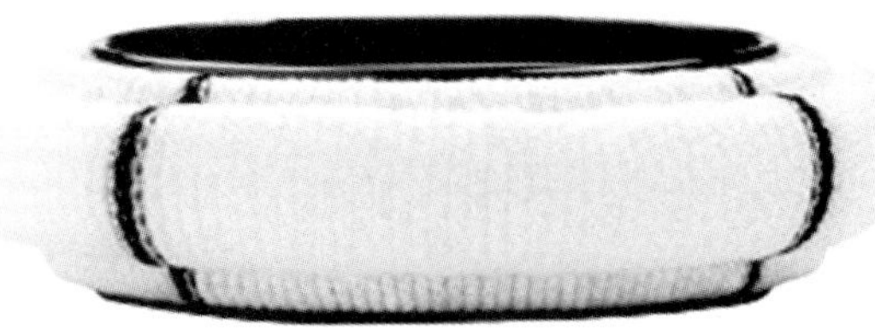

Figure 72–5 The Optiform mitral valve. *(Courtesy Sulzer CarboMedics, Inc., Austin, TX)*

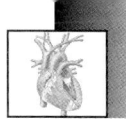

turbulence is also a contributing factor leading to calcification.[65] Amino-oleic acid treatment of tissue valves prevents calcium from binding to collagen.[35] High-pressure (60–80 mm Hg) glutaraldehyde fixation was used to prepare the first-generation bioprosthetic valves. Low (<2 mm Hg) and zero pressure glutaraldehyde fixation have been shown to maintain a more natural collagen alignment and are currently the strategies used in the latest generation of stented bioprostheses.[31,40] The ideal method of xenograft tissue preservation has yet to be found.

Stented Bioprostheses

Stented Porcine Bioprostheses

Hancock Porcine Bioprosthesis

The Hancock Standard, Hancock II, and the Hancock Modified Orifice II (Medtronic, Inc.) are porcine bioprostheses offered by Medtronic. They have a proven track record and have been shown to be safe in numerous studies.[12,19] The Hancock II aortic and mitral prostheses are constructed with a lower-profile flexible stent with a reduced sewing cuff to increase orifice area. In addition, the muscle shelf on the right coronary leaflet of the aortic Hancock II is reduced, leading to a larger orifice area. The aortic valve is designed for suprannular placement. The Modified Orifice II valve incorporates the noncoronary cusp from a second porcine valve into its design, which eliminates the bulk of the right coronary muscle shelf found in native porcine valves altogether and further increases the EOA.

Medtronic Mosaic Porcine Bioprosthesis

The Mosaic prosthesis (Medtronic, Inc.) is the latest generation of bioprostheses offered by Medtronic. It undergoes zero-pressure glutaraldehyde fixation to maintain collagen crimp morphology and leaflet flexibility and antimineralization treatment with α-amino oleic acid. It also has a low-profile semiflexible stent, and its porcine aortic root is predilated to 40 mm Hg in an attempt to maximize valve orifice area. Early performance results were reported from a multicenter nonrandomized prospective international clinical trial.[32] At least 1626 patients from 17 centers were included, with 1262 undergoing an aortic valve replacement and 366 undergoing a mitral valve replacement. Follow-up for AVR recipients was up to 6.2 years with a mean of 2.9 years. Follow-up for MVR recipients was 6.1 years with a mean of 2.4 years. Mortality for aortic valve replacement was 3.3%. There was only one event of structural valve dysfunction at 51 months, and the etiology of this was uncertain, because only minimal calcification was noted. Five events of nonstructural valve dysfunction were reported, with one case attributed to leaflet dysfunction and four attributed to patient–prosthesis mismatch. The early mortality for mitral valve replacement was 4.1%. There were no cases of structural or nonstructural valve dysfunction. This study demonstrated the safety of the Mosaic bioprostheses for up to 5 years. Continued follow-up is required to demonstrate the effectiveness of the Mosaic preparation techniques (Figure 72-6).

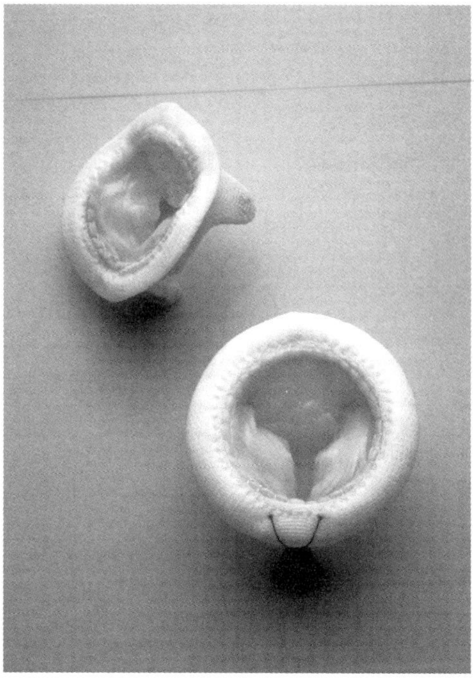

Figure 72–6 **The Medtronic Mosaic Porcine Bioprosthesis.** *(Courtesy Medtronic, Inc.)*

Carpentier–Edwards Porcine Bioprosthesis

The Carpentier–Edwards Standard valve (Edwards Lifesciences, Inc.) was introduced in 1975 (Figure 72-7). The following three main problems have been noted: (1) calcification, (2) fatigue lesions, and (3) transvalvular gradients. The Carpentier–Edwards Supra-Annular Valve (CE-SAV) was introduced in 1982 as a second- generation valve with modifications aimed at improving the durability and hemodynamics of the first-generation Carpentier–Edwards Standard valve. Both valves have a flexible stent and employ the surfactant polysorbate-80 as an antimineralization agent. The CE-SAV undergoes low-pressure glutaraldehyde fixation at 2 mm Hg, whereas the Standard valve is fixed with glutaraldehyde at 60 mm Hg. The Standard valve is an intraannular prosthesis, whereas

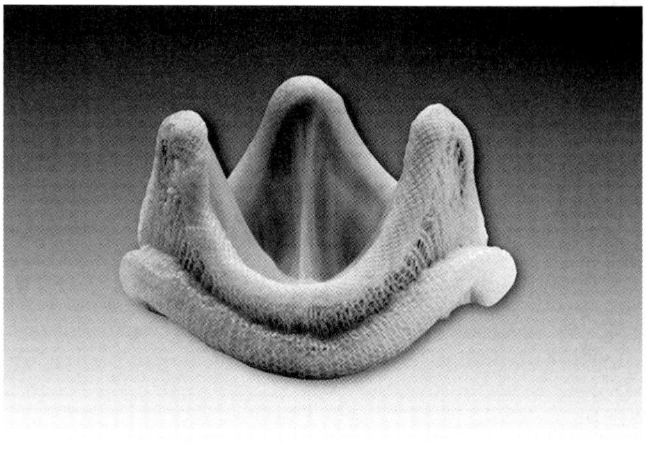

Figure 72–7 **The Carpentier–Edwards Porcine Bioprosthesis.** *(Courtesy Edwards Lifesciences, Inc.)*

the supraannular design allows for maximization of EOA in the CE-SAV. The mitral prosthesis also has a reduced strut height to limit intrusion into the ventricle. The CE-SAV Aortic Bioprosthesis is available in sizes from 21–27 mm. The Carpentier–Edwards Duraflex Low Pressure Mitral Bioprosthesis is available in sizes from 27–35 mm. Jamieson et al[43] concluded that the advancements made to reduce the incidence of structural valve deterioration in the second-generation supraannular prosthesis have not been successful. In their comparison of standard and supraannular bioprostheses with up to 15 years of follow-up, they showed that freedom from structural valve deterioration differed significantly only in the 21–40-year age group, where there was a 68% freedom from structural valve deterioration at 15 years with the CE-SAV as compared with a 31% freedom from structural valve deterioration with the standard prosthesis.

Pericardial Bioprostheses

Carpentier–Edwards PERIMOUNT Pericardial Bioprosthesis

The Carpentier–Edwards PERIMOUNT Prosthesis (Edwards Lifesciences, Inc.) (Figure 72-8) is a stented bovine pericardial aortic bioprosthesis. Its leaflets are mounted inside the support frame. It is manufactured using low-pressure fixation and undergoes treatments to remove phospholipids so as to lessen calcification. Aortic valves are available in Standard and Reduced Sewing Ring models in sizes from 19–29 mm. A number of studies have demonstrated durability exceeding that of other bioprostheses. Most recently Banbury et al,[6] from the Cleveland Clinic Foundation, have shown maintenance of hemodynamics at up to 17 years of follow-up. As with other bioprosthetic valves, the durability of these tissue valves is a function of age, with patients under age 65 showing diminished valve durability when compared with older cohorts. The Cleveland Group has shown that the durability of these valves approaches and in some cases exceeds that of homografts. Dellgren et al,[22] from the Toronto General Hospital,

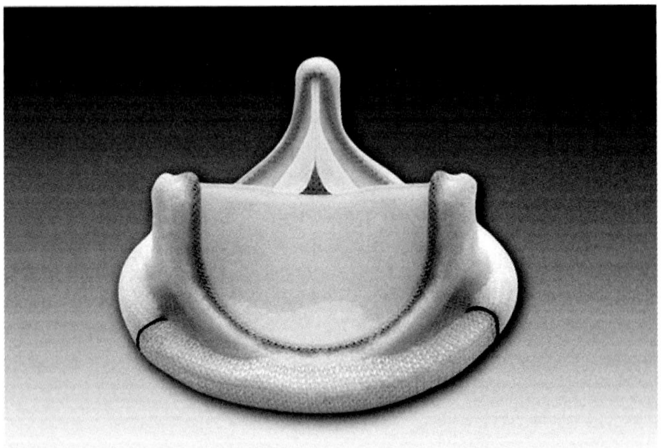

Figure 72-8 The Carpentier–Edwards PERIMOUNT Pericardial Bioprosthesis.
(Courtesy Edwards Lifesciences, Inc.)

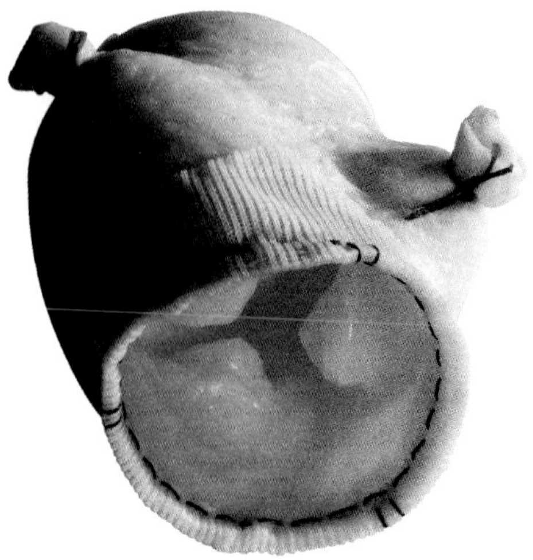

Figure 72-9 The Medtronic Freestyle valve.
(Courtesy Medtronic, Inc.)

have demonstrated similar results. The PERIMOUNT Plus valve is designed for the mitral position and is available in sizes from 27–33 mm.

Stentless Bioprostheses

The first use of a nonallograft stentless valve was in 1986 by David, at the Toronto General Hospital. Because these prostheses have no rigid metal stent, there is little inherent gradient across the valve. These valves are supported by the aortic root of the patient when implanted using the subcoronary or inclusion cylinder technique. Certain stentless valves also can be implanted as stand-alone aortic root replacement prostheses similar to the technique used with a homograft. Because no metal stent is employed and minimal inherent gradient exists, there is less chance for patient–prosthesis mismatch. Studies also have shown that there is also more favorable ventricular remodeling after implantation as compared with stented prostheses.[45] However, the implantation techniques required for stentless valves are more complex and are associated with longer cross-clamp times; long-term durability is also a question FDA-approved stentless valves on the market today are the Toronto Stentless SPV, the Medtronic Freestyle, and the Edwards Prima Plus.

Toronto SPV Valve

The Toronto Stentless SPV is offered by St. Jude Medical, Inc. It is a glutaraldehyde-preserved porcine valve available in sizes from 21–29 mm. It is covered with polyester for ease of handling and is designed for subcoronary implantation.

Medtronic Freestyle Stentless Aortic Bioprosthesis

The Freestyle valve (Figure 72-9) is available in sizes from 19–27 mm. It can be used as a freestanding aortic root prosthesis or can be trimmed and implanted with a subcoronary technique. Riley et al,[58] from Wake Forest University, demonstrated lower transvalvular gradients and less aortic insufficiency with the Freestyle prosthesis implanted as a

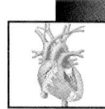

root replacement when compared with the subcoronary Toronto SPV valve. The Wake Forest group has also demonstrated excellent durability and freedom from aortic insufficiency at up to 8 years.[48]

Edwards Prima Plus Stentless Bioprosthesis

The Prima Plus is a stentless bioprosthesis that can be implanted either as a full root or with the subcoronary technique. It undergoes low-pressure fixation and is available in sizes from 21–29 mm. It has a helpful trim guide that facilitates subcoronary implantation. It has proven durability and hemodynamic performance at up to 8 years of follow-up.[44]

ALLOGRAFT VALVE REPLACEMENT

The first use of an allograft for aortic valve replacement was described in 1962 by Ross et al, in 1964 by Barrett-Boyes et al, and in 1968 by Engell et al. Since these early reports, multiple storage and preservation techniques have developed. Initially, freshly harvested allografts were treated for 24 hours in an antibiotic solution (30 mg/ml penicillin, 50 mg/ml streptomycin, and 10 mg/ml Fungizone) and stored at 4° C. This process evolved to the use of various antimicrobials, the elimination of Fungizone, and a decrease in treatment time to 6 hours.[54] Driving these changes was the observation that leaflet thinning and damage led to early failure.[47,54] In the mid-1970s the cryopreservation of allografts replaced prior methods. This technique, first described by O'Brien, was soon corroborated by Kirklin and others[47] using cryopreserved allografts; many authors saw improved functional results. O'Brien, for example, reported 75% freedom from moderate to severe aortic regurgitation for cryopreserved valves at 15–20 years versus 35% for antibiotic/4°C preserved valves. Despite this progress, many allografts show deterioration after 15 years. Theoretical explanations for deterioration of cryopreserved allografts include immunological rejection, ischemia of leaflets, chemical stress, and endothelial activation in response to tissue injury.[55] This process, however, has not been clearly elucidated.

The last 2 decades also have seen a refinement of surgical techniques. Early on, most allograft valve implantation was performed using a subcoronary technique.[25,47,53-55,64] This technique proved difficult for various reasons. Initially, undersizing of valves led to early valvular insufficiency. As this was corrected, other anatomical factors played increasing roles. Orientation of commissural posts, varying commissural heights, and varying sinus dimensions made creating a proper anatomical fit difficult.[25,64] Over time most surgeons adopted the technique of aortic root replacement with coronary implantation.

Initially surgeons avoided total root replacement because of the increased operative morbidity and mortality. With the advancement of cardiac surgical techniques, most centers reported operative risk roughly equivalent to aortic valve replacement.[14,53,69]

Thus refinement in allograft preservation and surgical techniques has led to increased success in the use of allografts. Current data indicate 80–90% freedom from significant structural deterioration at 15 years, with low operative mortality (0.6–2%).[14,55,63,69] Unfortunately, the rate of structural deterioration for allografts depends on recipient age. O'Brien, for example, reported that patients between 40 and 59 years of age at implant have a 65% freedom from significant SVD at 15 years.[54] Other studies have shown similar results.[64,69] This phenomenon, coupled with the increased complexity of reoperative root replacement (often but not always required) and advancements made in bioprosthetic valves, has made the use of allografts for isolated aortic valve replacement controversial.

Allografts, however, continue to be the treatment of choice for infective endocarditis and mixed valvular or aortic root pathology in patients who cannot tolerate anticoagulation. Many centers have shown a decrease in the rate of reinfection when aortic valve endocarditis is treated with the use of allografts.[21] This appears to especially hold true in complex endocarditis where the root or left ventricular outflow tract is affected or in cases of active endocarditis. Although it is higher risk than standard aortic valve replacement, root replacement for endocarditis has achieved acceptable mortality and morbidity.[24,39,56] The topic of complex aortic root reconstruction is discussed in a later chapter.

Allografts have also seen increased use in patients who require total aortic root replacement in whom anticoagulation is contraindicated.[62] Lewis et al[49] demonstrated acceptable risk with a 90% survival in elderly patients undergoing total root replacement for critical valvular disease and concomitant aneurysm disease. This cohort of patients has in the past has often been treated with tissue valves sewn to Dacron grafts. This mechanism has clear disadvantages. The dynamic of valve leaflets within the confines of nondistensible prosthetic material has not been investigated. It is irresponsible to assume that data generated from the study of tissue valves in the aortic position are applicable. Furthermore, allografts that suffer from valve failure can often be treated at a later date by simple reoperative valve replacement. Patients treated with a composite tissue valve/Dacron graft necessitate reoperative total root replacement.

FUTURE TRENDS

Percutaneous approaches to valve replacement have been described, but are still highly experimental. Such techniques currently seem most feasible for patients who require pulmonary valve replacement.[11] Recently aortic valve replacement with a percutaneous approach has also been described.[20] Undoubtedly this will be an area of much interest in the years to come.

There is a great deal of interest in the field of tissue engineering and its application to the field of valvular prostheses.[52] A valve cultured from a patient's own cells with the capacity for growth would go a long way toward fulfilling many of Harken's criteria of the ideal valve. Much work needs to be done, but the field of tissue engineering holds great promise for the future of valvular prostheses.

CHOICE OF VALVE REPLACEMENT

A favorite question in conferences and rounds is "What valve would you use for patient X? Would you use a homograft, a mechanical prosthesis, a bioprosthesis, or the Ross procedure?" Numerous studies show that there are many safe choices and that the operation has to be individualized to the patient. Factors such as patient lifestyle, age, need for or contraindication to anticoagulation, and potential for longevity must be taken into account. A mechanical prosthesis would likely be the best choice for a middle-aged adult who wants the greatest chance at avoiding a future operation and who does not mind the required changes in lifestyle mandated by anticoagulation. A pericardial bioprosthesis would be attractive for a similarly aged patient who does not want to sacrifice lifestyle for anticoagulation. A patient with an aortic root abscess or prosthetic valve endocarditis would be best treated with a homograft. An elderly patient with a small left ventricular cavity would be unlikely to accommodate a bioprosthetic mitral valve with a high-profile stent and would be best served with a mechanical prosthesis. Bioprosthetic valves are a reasonable choice in patients with concomitant coronary artery disease because their long-term survival is diminished compared with age-matched controls and avoiding anticoagulation decreases morbidity.[4]

REFERENCES

1. Abe T, Kamata K, Kuwaki K, et al: Ten years' experience of aortic valve replacement with the Omnicarbon valve prosthesis. Ann Thorac Surg 61:1182–1187, 1996.
2. Akins CW: Results with mechanical cardiac valvular prostheses. Ann Thorac Surg 60:1836–1844, 1995.
3. Akins CW: Long-term results with the Medtronic-Hall valvular prosthesis. Ann Thorac Surg 61:806–813, 1996.
4. Akins CW, Hilgenberg AD, Vlahakes GJ, et al: Results of bioprosthetic versus mechanical aortic valve replacement performed with concomitant coronary artery bypass grafting. Ann Thorac Surg 74:1098–1106, 2002.
5. Aris A, Igual A, Padro J: The Spanish Monostrut Study Group: A ten-year experience with 8599 implants. Ann Thorac Surg 62:40–47, 1996.
6. Banbury MK, Cosgrove DM, Thomas JD, et al: Hemodynamic stability during 17 years of the Carpentier-Edwards aortic pericardial bioprosthesis. Ann Thorac Surg 73:1460–1465, 2002.
7. Baudet EM, Puel V, McBride JT, et al: Long-term results of valve replacement with the St. Jude Medical prosthesis. J Thorac Cardiovasc Surg 109:858–870, 1995.
8. Baumgartner H, Khan SS, DeRobertis M, et al: Doppler assessment of prosthetic valve orifice area: An in vitro study. Circulation 85:2275–2283, 1992.
9. Binet JP, Duran CG, Carpentier A, Langlois J: Heterologous aortic valve transplantation. Lancet 2:1275, 1965.
10. Björk VO, Lindblom D: The Monostrut Björk-Shiley heart valve. J Am Coll Cardiol 6:1142–1148, 1985.
11. Bonhoeffer P, Boudjemline Y, Saliba Z, et al: Percutaneous insertion of the pulmonary valve. J Am Coll Cardiol 39: 1664–1669, 2002.
12. Burdon TA, Miller DC, Oyer PE, et al: Durability of porcine valves at fifteen years in a representative North American patient population. J Thorac Cardiovasc Surg 103:238–252, 1992.
13. Butchart EG, Hui-Hua L, Payne N, et al: Twenty years of experience with the Medtronic-Hall valve. J Thorac Cardiovasc Surg 121:1090–1100, 2001.
14. Byrne J, Karavas A, Mihalieuij T: Rode of the cryopreserved homograft in isolated elective aortic valve replacement. Am J Cardiol 91:616–619, 2003.
15. Carpentier A, Lemaigre G, Robert L, Carpentier S: Biological factors affecting long-term results of valvular heterografts. J Thorac Cardiovasc Surg 58:467–483, 1969.
16. Christakis GT, Buth KJ, Goldman BS, et al: Inaccurate and misleading valve sizing: A proposed standard for valve size nomenclature. Ann Thorac Surg 66:1198–1203, 1998.
17. Clark RE, Edmunds LH Jr, Cohn LH, et al: Guidelines for reporting morbidity and mortality after cardiac valvular operations. Eur J Cardiothorac Surg 2:293–295, 1988.
18. Clarke DR: Value, viability and valves. J Thorac Cardiovasc Surg 124:1–6, 2002.
19. Cohn LH, Collins JJ, DiShea VJ, et al: Fifteen-year experience with 1678 Hancock porcine bioprosthetic heart valve replacements. Ann Surg 210:435–443, 1989.
20. Cribier A, Eltchaninoff H, Bash A, et al: Percutaneous transcatheter implantation of an aortic valve prosthesis for calcific aortic stenosis: First human case description. Circulation 106:3006–3008, 2002.
21. Dearani JA, Orszulak TA, Schaff HV, et al: Results of allograft aortic valve replacement for complex endocarditis. J Thorac Cardiovasc Surg 113:285–291, 1997.
22. Dellgren G, David TE, Raanani E, et al: Late hemodynamic and clinical outcomes of aortic valve replacement with the Carpentier-Edwards Perimount pericardial bioprosthesis. J Thorac Cardiovasc Surg 124:146–154, 2002.
23. Dewall RA, Qasim N, Carr L: Evolution of mechanical heart valves. Ann Thorac Surg 69:1612–1621, 2000.
24. Donaldson RM, Ross DM: Homograft aortic root replacement for complicated prosthetic valve endocarditis. Circulation 70:I178–I181, 1984.
25. Doty D, Michidon G, Wang ND: Replacement of the aortic valve with cryopreserved aortic allograft. Ann Thorac Surg 56:228–236, 1993.
26. Edmunds LH: Evolution of prosthetic heart valves. Am Heart J 141:849–855, 2001.
27. Edmunds LH Jr, Clark RE, Cohn LH, et al: Guidelines for reporting morbidity and mortality after cardiac valvular operations. The American Association for Thoracic Surgery, Ad Hoc Liaison Committee for Standardizing Definitions of Prosthetic Heart Valve Morbidity. Ann Thorac Surg 62:932–935, 1996.
28. Edward MS, Russell GB, Edwards AF, et al: Results of valve replacement with omniscience mechanical prostheses. Ann Thorac Surg 74:665–670, 2002.
29. Emery RW, Palmquist WE, Mettler E, Nicoloff DM: A new cardiac valve prosthesis: In vitro results. Trans Am Soc Artif Int Organs 24:550–556, 1978.
30. Fiane AE, Geiran OR, Svennevig JL: Up to eight years' follow-up of 997 patients receiving the CarboMedics prosthetic heart valve. Ann Thorac Surg 66:443–448, 1998.
31. Flomembaum MA, Schoen FJ: Effects of fixation back pressure and antimineralization treatment on the morphology of porcine aortic bioprosthetic valves. J Thorac Cardiovasc Surg 105:154, 1993.
32. Fradet GJ, Bleese N, Burgess J: Mosaic valve international clinical trial: Early performance results. Ann Thorac Surg 71:S273–S277, 2001.
33. Gang G, Ling Z, Seifter E, et al: Aldehyde tanning: The villain in bioprosthetic calcification. Eur J Cardiothorac Surg 5:288, 1991.
34. Gelsomino S, Morocutti G, Paolo DC, et al: Preliminary experience with the St. Jude Medical Regent mechanical heart valve in the aortic position: Early in vivo hemodynamic results. Ann Thorac Surg 73:1830–1836; discussion 1836, 2002.
35. Girardot MN, Torrianni M, Giradot JM: Effect of AOA on glutaraldehyde-fixed bioprosthetic heart valve cusps and walls: Binding and calcification studies. Artif Organs 17: 76, 1994.

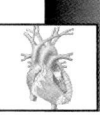

36. Gorlin R, Gorlin SG: Hydraulic formula for the calculation of area of the stenotic mitral valve, other cardiac valves and central circulatory shunts. Am Heart J 41:1–29, 1951.
37. Guidelines for reporting morbidity and mortality after cardiac valvular operations. Ann Thorac Surg 46:257–259, 1988.
38. Harken DE. Heart valves: Ten commandments and still counting. Ann Thorac Surg 48(suppl 3):S18–S19, 1989.
39. Haydock D, Barratt-Boyes B, Macedo T, et al: Aortic valve replacement for active infectious endocarditis in 108 patients: A comparison for freehand allograft valves with mechanical prothesis and bioprostheses. J Thorac Cardiovasc Surg 103:130–139, 1992.
40. Hilbert SL, Barrick MK, Ferrans VJ: Porcine aortic valve bioprostheses: A morphologic comparison of the effects of fixation pressure. J Biomed Mater Res 24:773–787, 1990.
41. Hufnagel CA, Harvey WP, Rabil PJ, et al: Surgical correction of aortic insufficiency. Surgery 35:673–683, 1954.
42. Ismeno G, Renzulli A, De Feo M, et al: Standard versus hemodynamic plus 19-mm St. Jude Medical aortic valves. J Thorac Cardiovasc Surg 121:723–728, 2001.
43. Jamieson WRE, Burr LH, Janusz MT, et al: Carpentier-Edwards standard and supraannular porcine bioprostheses: Comparison of technology. Ann Thorac Surg 67:10–17, 1999.
44. Jin XY, Ratnatunga C, Pillai R: Performance of Edwards Prima stentless valve over eight years. Semin Thorac Cardiovasc Surg 13(4 suppl 1):163–167, 2001.
45. Jin XY, Zhang A, Gibson DG, et al: Changes in left ventricular function and hypertrophy following aortic valve replacement using aortic homograft, stentless, or stented valve. Ann Thorac Surg 62:683–690, 1996.
46. Kaster RL, Lillehei CW: A new cageless free-floating pivoting disk prosthetic valve: Design development and evaluation. Digest 7th Internat Conf M Engineering, p. 387. Stockholm, 1967.
47. Kirklin JK, Smith D, Novick W: Long-term function of cryopreserved aortic homografts. J Thorac Cardiovasc Surg 106: 154–166; discussion 165–166, 1993.
48. Kon ND, Riley RD, Adair SM, et al: Eight-year results of aortic root replacement with the freestyle stentless porcine aortic root bioprosthesis. Ann Thorac Surg 73:1817–1821; discussion 1821, 2002.
49. Lewis ME, Jones TJ, Ranasinghe AM, et al: Homograft aortic root with prosthetic extension as treatment for aneurysm of proximal aorta in elderly patients. J Thorac Cardiovasc Surg 123:573–575, 2002.
50. Lim KH, Caputo M, Ascione R, et al: Prospective randomized comparison of CarboMedics and St. Jude Medical bileaflet mechanical heart valve prostheses: An interim report. J Thorac Cardiovasc Surg 123:21–32, 2002.
51. Lund O, Nielsen SL, Arildsen H: Standard aortic St. Jude valve at 18 years: Performance profile and determinants of outcome. Ann Thorac Surg 69:1459–1465, 2000.
52. Mayer JE: In search of the ideal valve replacement device. J Thorac Cardiovasc Surg 122:8–9, 2001.
53. O'Brien MF, Harrocks S, Stafford G: Allograft aortic root replacement in 418 patients over a span of 15 years: 1985 to 2000. Semin Thorac Cardiovasc Surg 13(4 suppl 1):180–185, 2001.
54. O'Brien MF, McGiffin DC, Stafford EG, et al: Allograft aortic valve replacement: Long-term comparative clinical analysis of viable cryopreserved and antibiotic stored 4°C stored valves. J Card Surg 6:534–543, 1991.
55. Palka P, Harrocks S, Lange A: Primary aortic valve replacement with cryopreserved aortic allograft. Circulation 105:61–66, 2002.
56. Petrou M, Wong K, Albertucci M, et al: Evaluation of unstented aortic valve endocarditis. Circulation 90:II198–II204, 1994.
57. Reis RL, Hancock WD, Yarbrough JW, et al: The flexible stent: A new concept in the fabrication of tissue heart valve prostheses. J Thorac Cardiovasc Surg 6:683–689, 1971.
58. Riley RD, Hammon JW, Adair SM, et al: Stentless aortic valve replacement with freestyle or Toronto SPV: An early comparison. Ann Thorac Surg 70:48–52, 2000.
59. Rosengart TK, O'Hara M, Lang SJ, et al: Outcome analysis of 245 CarboMedics and St. Jude valves implanted at the same institution. Ann Thorac Surg 66:1684–1691, 1998.
60. Rothbart RM, Castriz JL, Harding LV, et al: Determination of aortic valve area by two-dimensional and Doppler echocardiography in patients with normal and stenotic bioprosthetic valves. J Am Coll Cardiol 15:817–824, 1990.
61. Soga Y, Okabayashi H, Nishina T: Up to 8-year follow-up of valve replacement with CarboMedics valve. Ann Thorac Surg 73:474–479, 2002.
62. Stahle A: Homograft—The optimal aortic valve substitute? Eur Heart J 21:1644–1647, 2000.
63. Starr A, Edwards ML, McCord CW, Griswold HE: Aortic replacement: Clinical experience with a semirigid ball-valve prosthesis. Circulation 27:779–783, 1963.
64. Takkenberg JM, VanHerwerden LA, Eilkomans MJC: Evolution of allograft aortic valve replacement over 13 years: Results of 275 procedures. Eur J Cardiothorac Surg 21:683–691, 2002.
65. Thubrikar MJ, Deck JD, Aouad J, Nolan SP: Role of mechanical stress in calcification of aortic bioprosthetic valves. J Thorac Cardiovasc Surg 86:115, 1983.
66. Torregrosa S, Gomez-Plana J, Valara FJ, et al: Long-term clinical experience with the Omnicarbon prosthetic valve. Ann Thorac Surg 68:881–886, 1999.
67. Vitale N, Caldarera I, Muneretto C, et al: Clinical evaluation of St. Jude Medical Hemodynamic Plus versus standard aortic valve prostheses: The Italian multicenter, prospective, randomized study. J Thorac Cardiovasc Surg 122:691–698, 2001.
68. Wada J: Knotless suture method and Wada hingeless valve. Jpn J Thorac Surg 15:88, 1967.
69. Yacoub M, Rasmi N, Sundt T: Fourteen-year experience with homovital homografts for aortic valve replacement. J Thorac Cardiovasc Surg 110:186–194, 1995.
70. Zellner JL, Kratz JM, Crumbley AJ 3rd, et al: Long-term experience with the St. Jude Medical valve prosthesis. Ann Thorac Surg 68:1210–1218, 1999.
71. Gunning AJ: Ross' first homograft replacement of the aortic valve. Ann Thorac Surg 54:809–810, 1992.

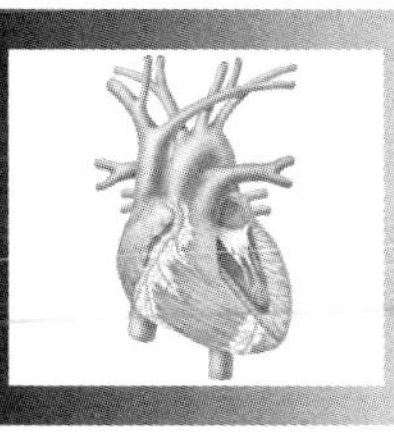

CHAPTER 73

Acquired Aortic Valve Disease

Michael K. Banbury

NORMAL AORTIC VALVE ANATOMY

The aortic valve is the last valve in the heart through which the blood is pumped before it goes to the body. The purpose at the aortic valve is to prevent backflow of blood from the aorta into the left ventricle. This function must be performed while providing no significant obstruction to the forward flow of the ejected blood. The normal aortic valve is tricuspid, with left coronary, right coronary, and noncoronary leaflets each attached just beneath one of three sinuses of Valsalva. The aortic valve is supported by a fibrous skeleton with a shallow U-shaped configuration at each leaflet, and this skeleton is continuous with the anterior leaflet of the mitral valve. The atrioventricular conduction system passes through the interventricular septum below the noncoronary cusp near the right noncoronary commissure. The valve leaflets themselves consist of fibrous tissue lined with endothelium and without a specific vascular supply. The nodular thickening at the central portion of the free edge of each leaflet is called the nodule of Arantius. During systole, each of the three leaflets is pushed aside by the flow of blood, but the bulbar contour of the sinuses prevents occlusion of the coronary ostia and prevents contact between the leaflet and the sidewall of the aorta. During diastole, all three leaflets meet at the center with 1–2 mm of coaptation at the free edge of each of the leaflets.

AORTIC STENOSIS

The most common cause of aortic stenosis is degenerative valve calcification. Some degree of collagen disruption and small calcific deposits are common in patients without clinically evident aortic valve disease. Significant aortic valve calcification is rarely present before the age of 30 years. Calcification is progressive and thought to be due to atherosclerotic processes. It is more common in bicuspid than in tricuspid valves. Frequently the calcification extends into the annulus and down into the interventricular septum and ventricular side of the anterior leaflet of the mitral valve. This calcification can usually be removed at operation (Figure 73-1).

Rheumatic heart disease is much less common in industrialized nations than it was a century ago; however, rheumatic valvular aortic stenosis is still seen. The early stage of rheumatic valvulitis produces edema, lymphocytic infiltration, and neovascularization of the leaflets. Later this process turns into thickening, commissural fusion, and rolled scarred leaflet edges. Late valvular calcification is common, but the annulus is often spared.

Bicuspid aortic valves are present in approximately 2% of the general population. Bicuspid valves are prone to calcification and eventual aortic stenosis (Figure 73-2).

Pathophysiology

The primary effect of aortic stenosis is to elevate left ventricular afterload, with secondary impairment of the left

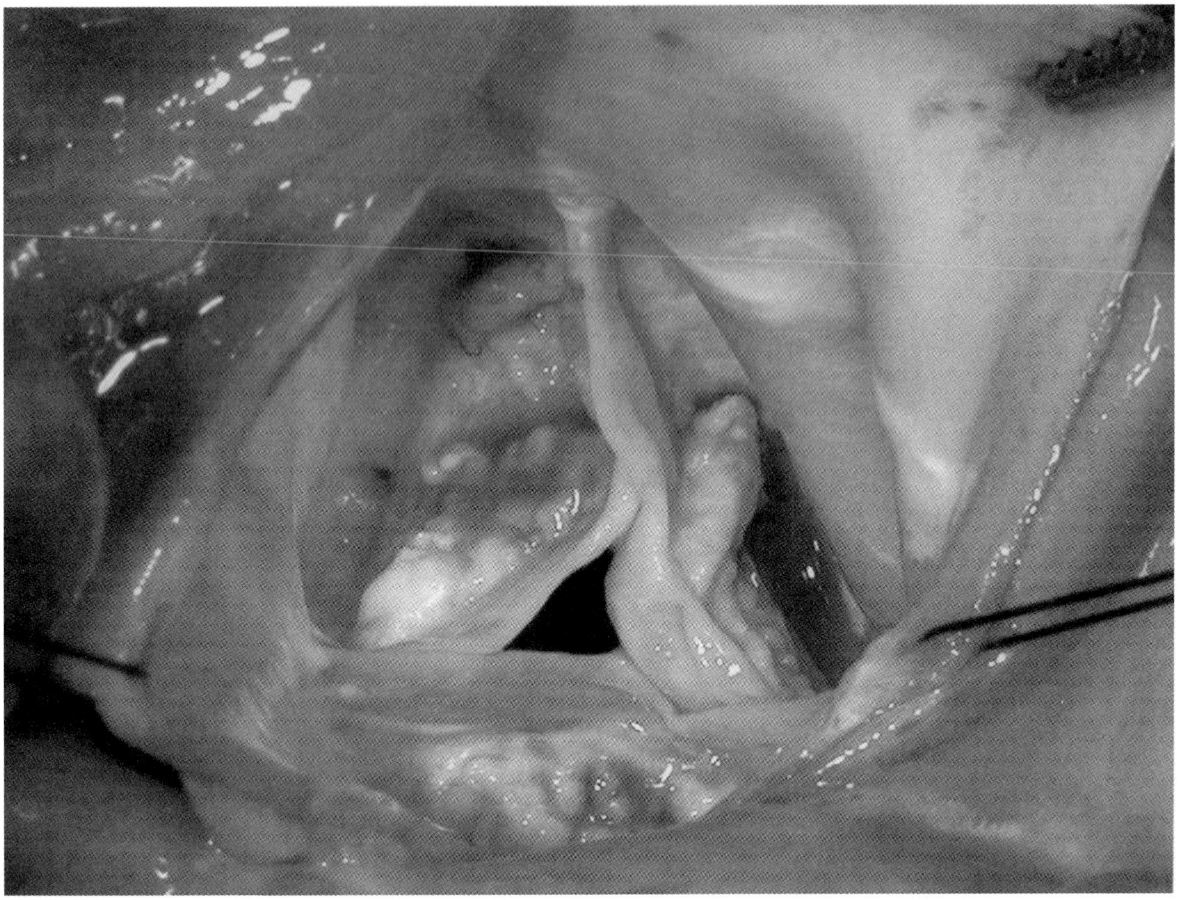

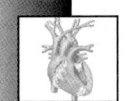

Figure 73–1 Calcific tricuspid aortic stenosis.

ventricular emptying during systole. The normal aortic valve has an undetectable gradient during systole, whereas stenotic valves are considered severe with a peak gradient over 40 mm Hg. Gradients can become as high as 100 mm Hg in well-compensated patients. Aortic stenosis is quantified by measuring the systolic pressure gradient across the valve or by calculating the effective orifice area using the Gorlin formula.[18]

$$AVA = \frac{AVF}{44.5\sqrt{AVG}}$$

where AVF = mean systolic aortic valve flow and AVG = mean systolic aortic valve gradient. A simpler estimate of aortic valve area may be calculated as

$$AVA = \frac{CO}{\sqrt{AVG}}$$

where CO = cardiac output (1/min). The normal aortic valve cross-sectional area is 2–4 cm^2, and an aortic valve area of 0.8 cm^2 (0.5 cm^2/m^2 of body surface area) or a mean aortic valve gradient over 40 mm Hg typically corresponds to severe aortic stenosis.

As a result of the pressure gradient across the aortic valve, left ventricular pressure must rise in order to maintain a normal perfusion pressure in the ascending aorta. This increase in left ventricular pressure (P) increases left ventricular wall stress (T) during systole by Laplace's law:

T = Pr/2h, where r = left ventricular radius and h = left ventricular wall thickness. In turn, increased wall stress is thought to be the stimulus for left ventricular hypertrophy, which ultimately normalizes wall stress by increasing wall thickness. Severe left ventricular hypertrophy may increase left ventricular mass from 150 g/m^2 to over 300 g/m^2. Left ventricular hypertrophy resulting from aortic stenosis tends to be concentric (i.e., the left ventricular cavitary volume tends to be normal or decreased despite significant increases in left ventricular wall mass). More recent studies of patients with aortic stenosis have suggested that concentric hypertrophy is predominant in women, whereas men are more likely than women to develop eccentric left ventricular hypertrophy, or some degree of left ventricular dilation along with increased left ventricular wall mass.[8] If left ventricular hypertrophy is insufficient to normalize ventricular wall stress by increased wall thickness (a condition termed afterload mismatch), chronic elevation of wall stress may produce left ventricular failure with decreased ventricular contractility and progressive left ventricular dilatation. Ventricular dilatation, in turn, increases wall stress by Laplace's law and may further accentuate left ventricular failure.

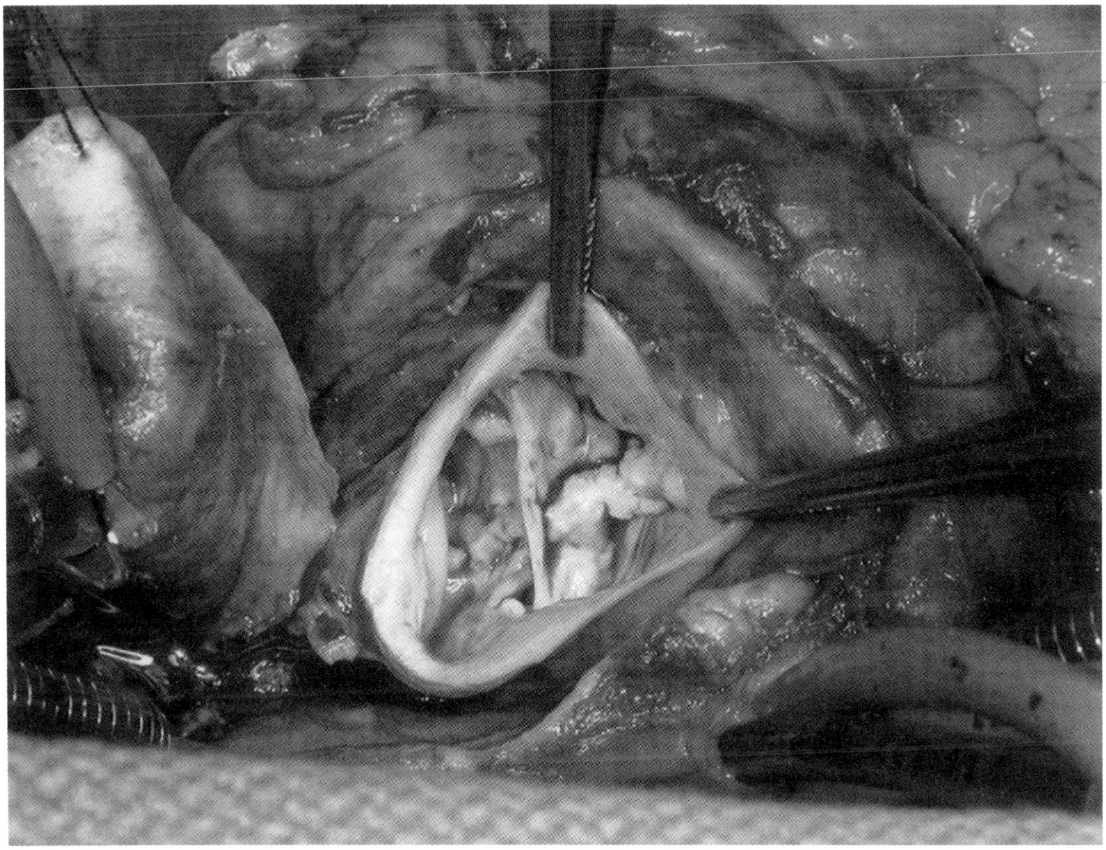

Figure 73–2 Calcific bicuspid aortic stenosis.

The compensated phase of aortic stenosis with progressive left ventricular hypertrophy may leave the patient asymptomatic for decades. As the left ventricle becomes less compliant because of hypertrophy, atrial systole becomes more important for left ventricular filling and maintaining cardiac output. The onset of atrial fibrillation in aortic stenosis may suddenly worsen clinical symptoms. In the early phases of left ventricular decompensation, left ventricular ejection fraction may fall rather markedly, owing to both loss of left ventricular contractility and the fact that ejection fraction falls with elevation of afterload, even without any change in contractility. Thus the patient with a mildly depressed ejection fraction and severe aortic stenosis may actually have well-preserved left ventricular contractility. Once symptomatic congestive heart failure develops, left ventricular dysfunction may progress rapidly toward death.

Symptoms of congestive heart failure generally reflect elevated pulmonary venous pressure at rest or with exercise. Aortic stenosis may produce pulmonary venous hypertension as a direct effect of afterload elevation or because of decreased left ventricular diastolic compliance, which in turn may result from a combination of left ventricular hypertrophy and dilatation. In addition to congestive heart failure, patients may experience exertional angina related to an impairment of subendocardial blood flow with increased left ventricular pressure. Syncope also is common, owing either to arrhythmia or to exercise-induced vasodilatation resulting from abnormal baroreceptor activity and sudden changes in left ventricular pressure.

Correction of aortic stenosis immediately improves left ventricular ejection fraction, left ventricular end-diastolic volume, and capillary wedge pressure caused by reduced left ventricular afterload.[21,31] Left ventricular hypertrophy from aortic stenosis tends to resolve over 6–12 months after aortic valve replacement, but may not totally normalize.[41] The relationship between ejection fraction and wall stress has not helped to predict outcome from valve replacement in aortic stenosis because patients with low ejection fraction and low wall stress often do well after valve replacement.[46,52]

Clinical Findings

Whereas patients with early aortic stenosis may be asymptomatic for many years, those with symptoms generally display exertional dyspnea, angina, or syncope. On physical examination the most prominent finding of aortic stenosis is a systolic ejection murmur best heard in the second intercostal space to the right of the sternum with radiation into both carotid arteries. In severe aortic stenosis, the murmur may peak in late systole, with a palpable thrill often being present, but severe left ventricular failure with decreased cardiac output may actually diminish the systolic murmur of aortic stenosis. The left ventricular impulse may be delayed and sustained by aortic stenosis, and the ventricular impulse may be laterally displaced in patients with left ventricular dilatation. In severe aortic stenosis, the second heart sound may be less prominent, and an associated murmur of aortic insufficiency may also be present.

The electrocardiogram generally shows left ventricular hypertrophy with strain, but may also demonstrate atrial fibrillation or intraventricular conduction defects, such as left or right bundle-branch block or atrioventricular nodal block. Chest radiograph may demonstrate calcification of the aortic valve, left ventricular enlargement, dilation of the ascending aorta, and occasionally, pulmonary edema associated with left ventricular failure.

Diagnosis

Doppler echocardiography is an invaluable noninvasive means to diagnose aortic stenosis. Doppler echocardiography can estimate the peak systolic gradient across the aortic valve (AVG) using the modified Bernoulli equation AVG (mm Hg) = $4V^2$ where V = peak blood velocity distal to the valve (m/sec). Doppler echocardiography may also detect and quantitate aortic regurgitation. Two-dimensional (2D) echocardiography may estimate the degree of stenosis using the planimetry technique. Valve thickening, calcification, and immobility, along with left ventricular ejection fraction and volume, may also be assessed by 2D echocardiography.

Cardiac catheterization is useful in the diagnosis of aortic stenosis. The gradient across the aortic valve may be measured directly, aortic regurgitation may be demonstrated on aortic root injection, and left ventricular function may be assessed from the left ventriculogram. Unlike echocardiography, cardiac catheterization can also evaluate the coronary artery anatomy through coronary arteriography. Given the availability of Doppler echocardiography, the current indications for cardiac catheterization in aortic stenosis are age over 40 years, the presence of risk factors for coronary disease, or borderline degree of stenosis seen through Doppler echocardiography, especially in the presence of impaired left ventricular function.

Natural History

Patients with mild aortic stenosis may remain asymptomatic for decades because of compensatory left ventricular hypertrophy. The rate at which mild aortic stenosis progresses to severe stenosis is probably variable.[47] However, most patients with moderate to severe aortic stenosis ultimately do develop symptoms of angina, congestive heart failure, or syncope. Studies by Ross and Braunwald[49] concluded that the average survival was 3–5 years after onset of angina, 3 years after syncope, and 1.5–2 years after onset of congestive heart failure. Recent studies have shown survival at 1, 2, and 3 years to be roughly 50%, 30%, and 20%, respectively, in patients with symptomatic aortic stenosis managed medically, regardless of whether symptoms were syncope, angina, or congestive heart failure.[33] Most patients with untreated aortic stenosis die of congestive heart failure, but many die of sudden death presumably associated with ventricular arrhythmias. Occasionally, balloon valvuloplasty is used to delay the need for surgery so a patient may recover from an intercurrent illness or to allow for preoperative rehabilitation. It may also be used to judge the symptomatic effect of increasing the aortic valve area in patients with complex medical comorbidities.

Percutaneous balloon aortic valvuloplasty has a very limited role to palliate severe aortic stenosis in patients otherwise too ill to undergo aortic valve replacement.[51] Studies now show that balloon aortic valvuloplasty may improve aortic valve area by up to 50% with some improvement in symptoms, although most hemodynamic or symptomatic benefits from balloon aortic valvuloplasty are lost 6 months after the procedure.[12] Patients treated with balloon aortic valvuloplasty alone have a markedly shorter survival than those treated with balloon aortic valvuloplasty followed by aortic valve replacement (Figure 73-3, A). Event-free survival after balloon aortic valvuloplasty alone is also dismal.[33,34]

Management

Medical therapy has a limited role in the treatment of symptomatic aortic stenosis. Diuretics to minimize symptoms of congestive heart failure and digoxin or antiarrhythmics to control atrial fibrillation may provide some symptomatic benefit, probably without altering the unfavorable natural history of symptomatic aortic stenosis. Afterload reduction therapy may excessively reduce coronary perfusion pressure and is relatively contraindicated in aortic stenosis. Cardiopulmonary resuscitation (CPR) in an arrested patient with aortic stenosis is rarely successful because of the small valve area and small ventricular chamber. Any symptoms of angina, congestive heart failure, or syncope constitute indications for aortic valve replacement. In relatively asymptomatic patients, a peak aortic gradient of 40 mm Hg or an aortic valve area of 0.8 cm^2 or 1.2 cm^2/m^2 indicates the need for aortic valve replacement. Similarly, any evidence of impaired left ventricular function (such as decreased ejection fraction, left ventricular dilatation, or significantly elevated left ventricular diastolic pressure at rest or with exercise) are an indication for aortic valve replacement with or without any clinical symptoms. Aortic valve repair for aortic stenosis has yielded relatively poor long-term results in comparison with aortic valve replacement.[10,29]

Treatment for low-gradient aortic stenosis has been controversial in the past. Recent reports indicate improved outcomes for patients with low ejection fraction (<30%) and a small aortic valve area (Figure 73-4).[46]

AORTIC REGURGITATION

Cause

The cause of aortic regurgitation overlaps significantly with that of aortic stenosis, and mixed aortic stenosis and regurgitation occur frequently. Degenerative calcific aortic valve disease may cause aortic insufficiency because of leaflet fixation that prevents full closure of the leaflets during diastole. Similarly, rheumatic heart disease may cause fibrosis of the aortic valve leaflets with retraction and rolling of the edges and secondary failure of the leaflets to fully approximate during diastole. Congenital bicuspid aortic valve disease may produce some degree of aortic valve regurgitation because of progressive fibrosis and calcification of the leaflets or because of distortion of the leaflets.

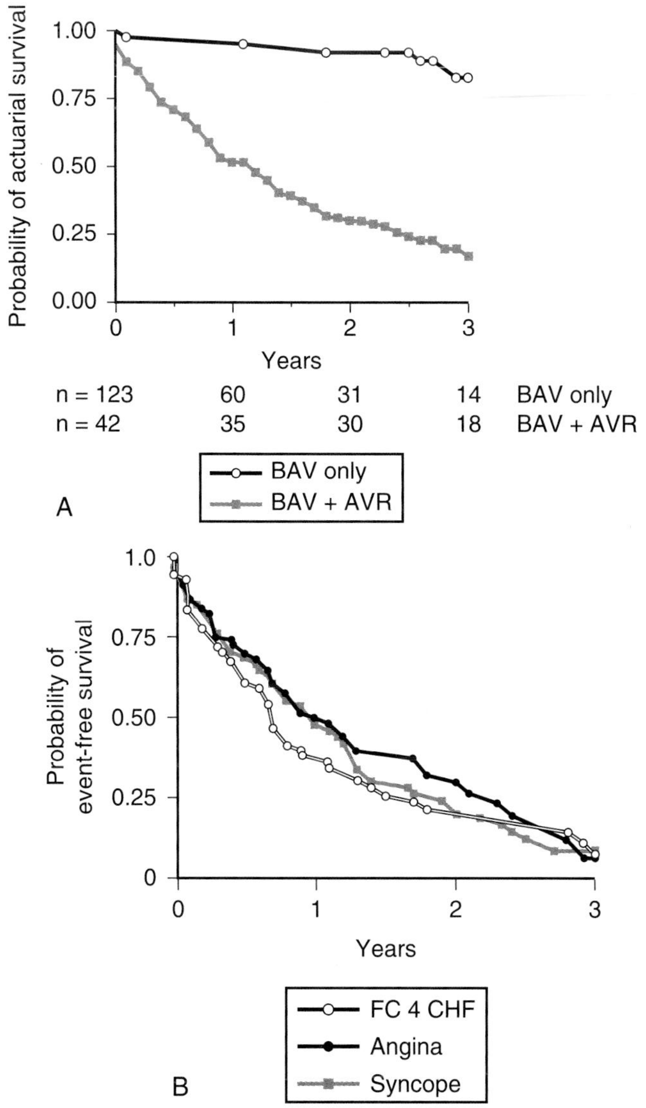

Figure 73–3 (**A**) Actuarial survival from the date of balloon aortic valvuloplasty in patients who subsequently underwent aortic valve replacement (BAV + AVR) and those treated by balloon aortic valvuloplasty alone (BAV only). (**B**) Event-free survival after balloon aortic valvuloplasty is similar for patients with syncope, angina, and New York Heart Association (NYHA) functional class IV congestive heart failure (FC 4 CHF). Patients with congestive heart failure tended to have events earliest.

(Reproduced with permission from Lieberman EB, Bashore TM, Hermiller JB, et al: Balloon aortic valvuloplasty in adults. J Am Coll Cardiol 26:1522–1528, 1995.)

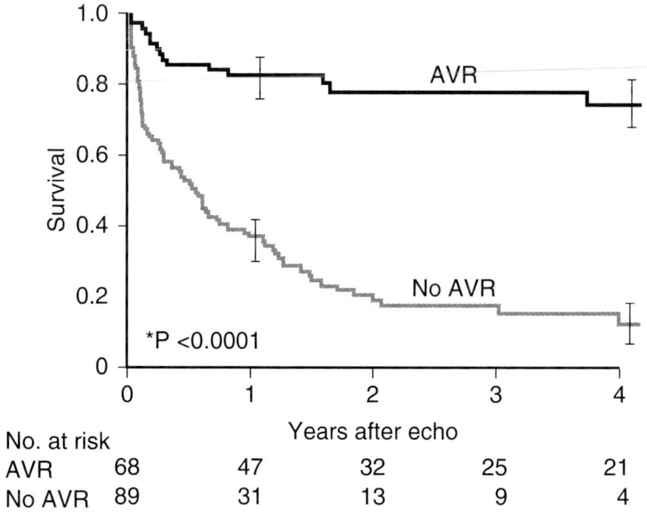

Figure 73–4 Patients with low gradient aortic stenosis still fare better with aortic valve replacement (AVR) than those who are treated medically (no AVR).

(Modified from Pereira JJ, Lauer MS, Bashir M, et al: Survival after aortic valve replacement for severe aortic stenosis with low transvalvular gradients survival. J Am Coll Cardiol 39:1356–1363, 2002. Courtesy of CarboMedics Inc.)

Aortic regurgitation may result from annuloaortic ectasia, defined as abnormal dilatation of the aortic valve annulus and aortic root. Cystic medial necrosis of the aortic wall is a frequent histological finding in annuloaortic ectasia and is characterized by degeneration of elastic bands in the aortic wall, abnormal organization of smooth muscle bundles, increased collagen, and cystic vacuoles in the aortic media. Defects in the genes that encode the production of the extracellular matrix of the aortic root have been implicated with the occurrence of bicuspid aortic valves and dilated aortic roots.[17]

Other causes of aortic regurgitation include myxoid degeneration of the aortic valve leaflets with progressive leaflet thinning, prolapse, and failure to coapt during diastole. Aortic dissection may produce aortic regurgitation as a result of detachment of the aortic valve apparatus from the aortic wall with prolapse of the leaflets inward toward the left ventricle. Bacterial endocarditis may account for 12% of patients with aortic regurgitation and typically produces aortic regurgitation by perforation or rupture of the aortic valve leaflets. Although endocarditis can occur on a previously normal valve, endocarditis commonly affects patients with underlying aortic valve disease. Other inflammatory conditions, such as rheumatoid arthritis, ankylosing spondylitis, and Reiter's syndrome, have been associated with aortitis and aortic regurgitation. Finally, blunt or penetrating chest trauma may produce aortic regurgitation by either rupture or puncture of the aortic valve leaflets.[45]

Pathophysiology

Aortic regurgitation causes volume overload of the left ventricle. Although left ventricular hemodynamics are relatively normal during systole, significant aortic regurgitation causes left ventricular diastolic filling from both the left atrium and the ascending aorta. Because a certain fraction of the forward cardiac output during systole returns to the left ventricle during diastole, cardiac output is increased by autonomic reflexes to maintain a normal net forward cardiac output. As a result of the increased left ventricular diastolic filling and the increased stroke volume necessary to maintain forward cardiac output, aortic regurgitation immediately increases left ventricular diastolic filling pressure. This increased diastolic filling pressure, in turn, raises left ventricular diastolic volume and diastolic wall stress, which causes long-term progressive left ventricular dilatation. The increased left ventricular wall stress caused by elevated filling pressure and increased radius of curvature produces eccentric hypertrophy.[53] With progressive left ventricular dilatation, massive enlargement of the left ventricle may occur, prompting the term cor bovinum.

Although increased circulating catecholamines may maintain ventricular performance in early aortic regurgitation, progressive left ventricular dilatation and increased wall stress subsequently lead to progressive fall in left ventricular contractility and ejection fraction, until forward cardiac output can no longer be maintained and the patient expires from progressive congestive heart failure. Symptoms of congestive heart failure derive from the increased pulmonary venous pressure at rest or with exercise resulting from increased left ventricular diastolic pressure. The onset of atrial fibrillation may be highly symptomatic in aortic regurgitation as a result of loss of the atrial systole that is normally so critical to filling a dilated, hypertrophied, and noncompliant left ventricle. Subendocardial ischemia may occur as a result of decreased diastolic coronary perfusion pressure, increased diastolic ventricular pressure, and left ventricular workload. Left ventricular afterload reduction may significantly improve forward cardiac output in aortic regurgitation (unlike aortic stenosis) by decreasing the pressure gradient across the aortic valve during diastole and thereby reducing the amount of regurgitation.

Aortic valve replacement has a more variable effect on postoperative left ventricular function in aortic regurgitation than in aortic stenosis. Correction of aortic regurgitation tends to normalize left ventricular ejection fraction, systolic and diastolic volumes, wall stress, and wall mass over a period of weeks to years.[5,7] However, a preoperative combination of abnormal ventricular chamber performance and abnormal myocardial function evidenced by the relationship between ejection fraction and end-systolic stress increases the likelihood of persistent or even progressive left ventricular dysfunction postoperatively.[53] Patients with persistent left ventricular dilatation 6 months after aortic valve replacement are much more likely to die early of cardiac disease.[4]

Clinical Findings

The most frequent symptoms in aortic regurgitation are those of congestive heart failure: dyspnea, orthopnea, and paroxysmal nocturnal dyspnea. Angina may occur in less than half of patients, and syncope is relatively unusual in aortic regurgitation. Physical examination may demonstrate lateral displacement of the left ventricular apical impulse. Because of increased systolic stroke volume and decreased diastolic aortic pressure to 60 mm Hg or less, the aortic pulse pressure may be markedly increased to over 50 mm Hg with aortic regurgitation. As a result, peripheral pulses may be dramatically pulsatile and have a "water hammer" character. Cardiac auscultation reveals an early diastolic decrescendo murmur radiating toward the left ventricular apex. In the presence of severe aortic regurgitation, a mid-diastolic Austin Flint murmur may occur at the left ventricular apex as a result of the regurgitant aortic jet fluttering the anterior mitral valve leaflet. A third heart sound may be present in association with left ventricular dilatation, decreased left ventricular compliance, and more rapid diastolic filling of the left ventricle.

Diagnosis

The chest radiograph in aortic regurgitation may be normal or may demonstrate left ventricular enlargement, enlargement of the ascending aorta, pulmonary edema, or pulmonary venous engorgement. Left ventricular hypertrophy with strain may be present on electrocardiogram.

Doppler echocardiography readily demonstrates diastolic regurgitation of blood flow across the aortic valve, which may be quantified on a 1+ to 4+ scale. Two-dimensional echocardiography may also detect associated aortic valve pathology, such as leaflet thickening, calcification, or stenosis; left ventricular dilatation or hypertrophy and impaired ejection fraction are also easily visualized.

Cineradiography can quantify diastolic regurgitation of dye across the aortic valve, using a similar scale of 1+ to 4+. Left ventriculography and aortography may demonstrate left ventricular dilatation, impaired left ventricular ejection fraction, and dilatation of the ascending aorta. Coronary arteriography is necessary to delineate coronary anatomy, and this should be performed in patients over the age of 40 years or with risk factors for coronary artery disease.

Natural History

As with aortic stenosis, aortic regurgitation may be present for many years before symptoms develop, and clinical symptoms may appear even 3–10 years after onset of severe aortic regurgitation. The onset of symptoms correlates with elevation of left ventricular end-diastolic pressure, left ventricular dilatation, and depressed left ventricular contractility, and generally follows within 3–6 months of detectable left ventricular dilatation in patients with asymptomatic aortic regurgitation. Survival may be 81% at 5 years in medically treated patients with aortic regurgitation, no symptoms, and normal left ventricular function.[6] Once symptoms develop, left ventricular performance may fall rapidly; mean survival is 5 years after onset of angina and 2 years after onset of heart failure with medical therapy.[22] Acute onset of severe aortic regurgitation resulting from aortic valve endocarditis may accelerate clinical deterioration with decompensated heart failure or even death within days or weeks.

Management

Because of the likelihood of death is low, patients with asymptomatic aortic regurgitation and normal left ventricular function may be managed medically. Diuretics or afterload reduction, or both, may improve early symptoms until surgical correction can be performed. Although the intraaortic balloon pump may be a useful means of afterload reduction in other critically ill patients, it is relatively contraindicated in patients with aortic regurgitation because the balloon pump increases aortic diastolic pressure and actually worsens aortic regurgitation.

The indications for aortic valve repair or replacement for aortic regurgitation from 3+ to 4+ include the presence of symptoms or any impairment of left ventricular function,

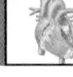

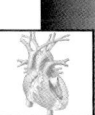

left ventricular dilatation, or significant elevation of left ventricular end-diastolic pressure.

Imaging

Cardiac Catheterization

Cardiac catheterization has been the traditional tool for the diagnosis of valvular heart disease. Catheterization offers the advantage that coronary angiography can be done at the same time, and this is necessary for operative candidates. The disadvantages to catheterization include the intravenous dye load, discomfort with arterial access, and the limited amount of information available.

Echocardiography

Echocardiography has revolutionized the diagnosis and management of valvular heart disease. This tool allows real-time monitoring of ventricular performance and valvular performance in a noninvasive manner. There is no appreciable risk to the patient who undergoes these studies. Valvular function and size can be carefully measured and evaluated. In addition, the size and quality of the ascending aorta can be determined. Intraoperative transesophageal echocardiography has become routine for valvular heart surgery. This technique allows immediate evaluation of the repaired or replaced valve and is an invaluable addition for the surgeon.

Magnetic Resonance Imaging

Magnetic resonance imaging (MRI) has helped in the diagnosis of valvular heart disease and heart disease in general. It gives very specific information about myocardial function and valvular function and allows the quantitation of regurgitant flow and degree of obstruction in stenosis. The disadvantages of MRI are the claustrophobic effect that many patients feel and the strong magnetic field. Patients with pacemakers or internal defibrillators are not candidates for MRI evaluation.

Ultra-high-speed computed tomography (CT) has also shown great promise in the evaluation and diagnosis of heart disease, specifically valvular heart disease.

SURGICAL TECHNIQUES

Aortic valve replacement requires cardiopulmonary bypass. Access to the aortic valve can be through a minimally invasive incision or traditional sternotomy (Figure 73-5). A number of minimally invasive approaches have been used, but the most common for aortic valve surgery is a partial sternotomy dividing the sternum from the sternal notch down to the fourth interspace and off toward the right chest. Once exposure of the cardiac structures has been achieved, patients are heparinized and cannulated in a traditional fashion. Cardiopulmonary bypass is instituted, the aorta is cross-clamped, and the heart is arrested with antegrade and retrograde cold-blood cardioplegia. Intermittent doses of cardioplegia are given throughout the case. In patients with significant aortic insufficiency, antegrade cardioplegia is often not completely effective and arrest can be initiated with retrograde cardioplegia followed by direct injection of cardioplegia down the coronary ostia. Access to the aortic valve can be through either an oblique or a transverse aortotomy. With the aortic valve exposed, the leaflets are resected and the annulus is débrided of calcium. Several suturing techniques have been employed, but the most common uses horizontal pledgeted sutures with pledges on the ventricular aspect of the annulus (Figure 73-6). The sutures are then passed through the sewing ring of the prosthesis, which is tied down in the supraannular position. Supraannular valves allow for a larger orifice area and tend to seat well on the annulus. Once the prosthesis has been tied into place, the aortotomy is closed with a running polypropylene suture. After release of the cross-clamp, transesophageal echocardiography is used to access the position of the prosthesis and to evaluate for the possibility of paravalvular leak. Intraventricular air volume can also be accessed. If a significant quantity of air remains in the ventricle, this can be aspirated using a needle in the ventricular apex. After recovery of a suitable heart rhythm, the patient is weaned from cardiopulmonary bypass with transesophageal echocardiography used as a monitor for ventricular function and valvular function. Cannulas are removed, heparin is reversed with protamine, and the patient is closed.

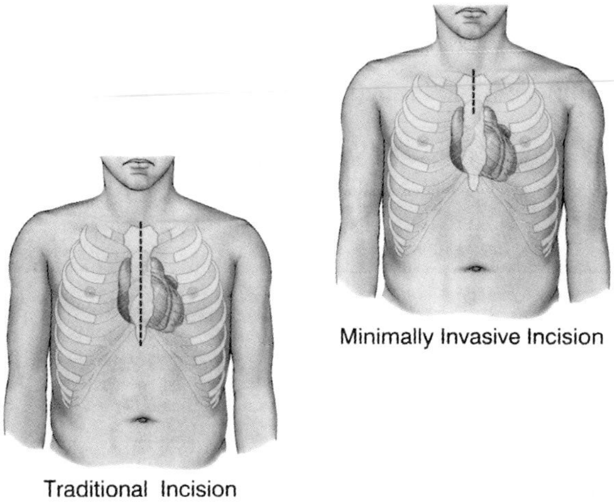

Figure 73–5 **Traditional incision compared with minimally invasive incision.**
(Courtesy of CarboMedics Inc.)

In the case of minimally invasive surgery, the limited exposure still allows direct cannulation of the ascending aorta and right atrium. Peripheral cannulation can also be used to allow satisfactory exposure of the intrapericardial structures.

Valve Selection

Bioprosthetic

Bioprosthetic valves (pericardial or porcine) have several distinct advantages. They are typically easy to implant and easy to replace should that become necessary. Neither pericardial nor porcine valves require anticoagulation. The valves are silent. A disadvantage is their limited durability when compared with mechanical valves.[19,24,25] Patients often choose the

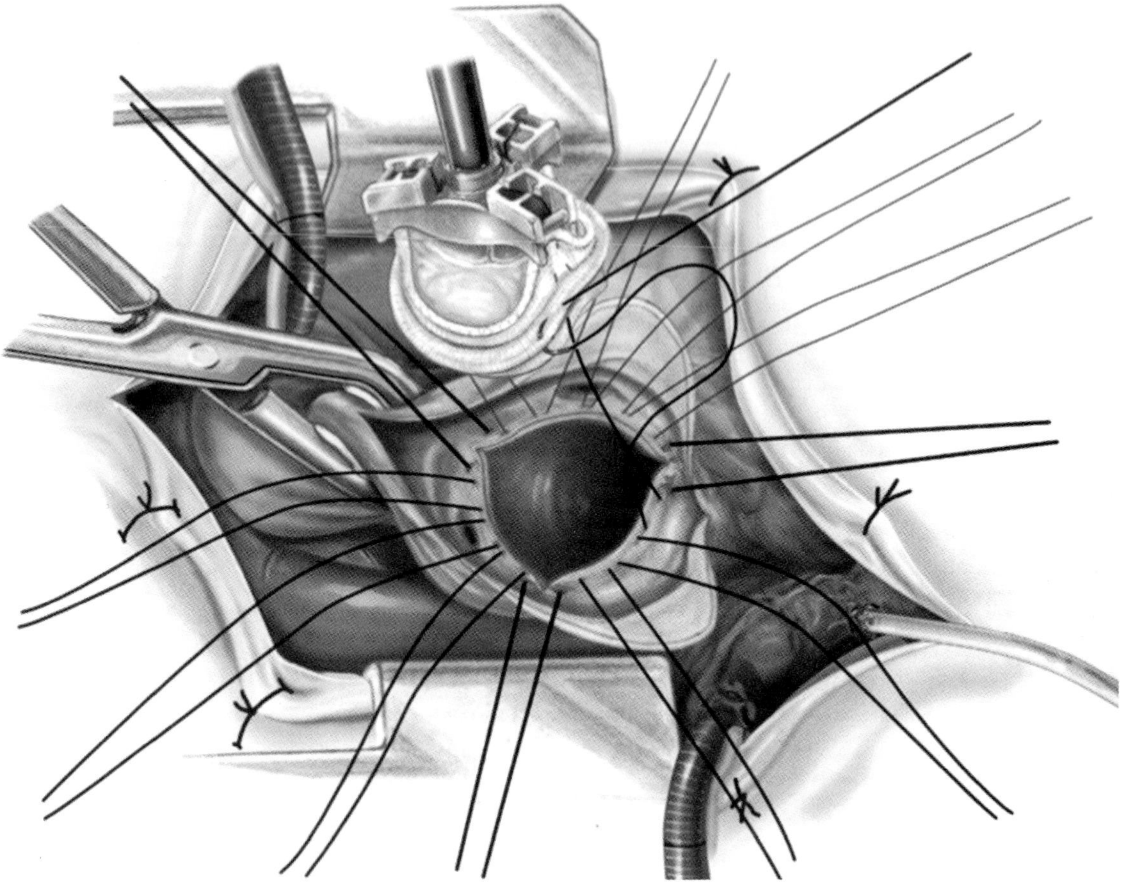

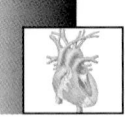

Figure 73–6 **Minimally invasive aortic valve replacement using a supraannular bioprosthetic and pledgeted horizontal mattress sutures.**

possibility of reoperation in the future so that they may avoid the need for lifelong anticoagulation (Figure 73-7).

Mechanical

Mechanical valves (bileaflet or tilting disk) have the advantages that they are easy to implant and easy to replace should that become necessary. They also have the advantage of durable structural function.[54] The disadvantages are a soft ticking sound that the patients can hear and a need for lifelong anticoagulant therapy, typically with warfarin.[50]

Stentless

Stentless valves were designed in the hope that their lower transvalvular gradients would provide improved left ventricular mass regression in patients with severe ventricular hypertrophy. It was also thought that stentless valves would be easier to implant in patients with a small aortic root. In general, stentless valves are more difficult to implant than stented valves. They require no anticoagulation, and they are silent. The long-term durability of stentless valves is unknown, but it appears that they may offer no durability benefit over traditional bioprosthetic valves.[9]

Allograft

Allograft aortic valves (homografts) have the advantage that they are more resistant to endocarditis than prosthetic valves. However, they are more difficult to implant than stented valves.[23] Reoperation and replacement of an aortic allograft is more difficult than reoperation in patients with traditional aortic prosthetic valves. Despite early enthusiasm for allograft aortic valves, it appears that their durability is no better than that of bioprosthetic aortic valves (Figure 73-8).

Ross Procedure

Aortic valve replacement with a pulmonary autograft enjoyed significant popularity in the 1990s; however, it has become less common in recent years.[48] This procedure involves replacing the aortic valve with the pulmonary valve and then implanting a pulmonary homograft in the pulmonary position. Advantages of this procedure include the living character of the pulmonary autograft, allowing growth and development of this valve in the aortic position. This benefit is most appealing for younger patients. Structurally the pulmonary autograft begins to leak in approximately

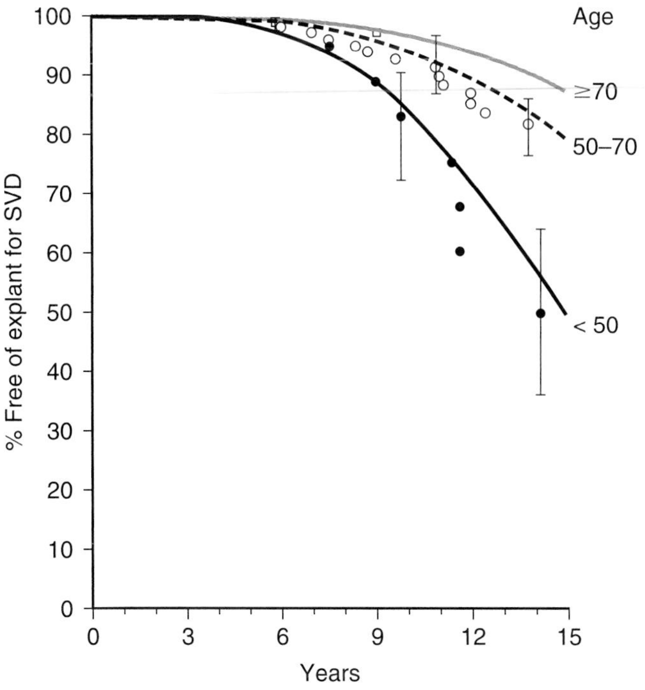

Figure 73–7 Impact of age on structural valve dysfunction (SVD). The patients have been stratified into broad age groups. *(Modified from Banbury MK, Cosgrove DM 3rd, White JA, et al: Age and valve size effect on the long-term durability of the Carpentier-Edwards aortic pericardial bioprosthesis. Ann Thorac Surg 72:753–757, 2001.)*

10% of patients by 10 years. The pulmonary homograft also has a tendency to develop supravalvular pulmonary stenosis.

Aortic Valve Repair

Aortic valve repair is only useful for patients with aortic insufficiency. Calcification of the aortic valve and aortic stenosis often damage the aortic valve leaflets, preventing adequate repair of stenotic lesions. Patients with bicuspid aortic valves often have insufficiency because one of the leaflets is longer than the other, allowing for prolapse (Figure 73-9). By plicating the elongated leaflet, the two leaflets then coapt uniformly (Figure 73-10). Repair for tricuspid aortic insufficiency has been less successful than that for bicuspid aortic insufficiency (Figure 73-11). This technique involves plication of the commissures to remove redundancy in one or more of the aortic leaflets (Figure 73-12). Patients in whom leaflet perforation is the mechanism of aortic insufficiency can be repaired with a pericardial patch. This is most common for cases of endocarditis and healed endocarditis where the infection has caused perforation in the belly of one of the cusps.[14] Traumatic rupture of the aortic valve is uncommon; however, it often requires immediate operative intervention. Aortic insufficiency from acute aortic dissection is well described. Prolapse of the commissure is the most common mechanism of aortic insufficiency, and this can be repaired by resuspension of the commissures at the time of ascending aortic replacement for dissection.[16]

RESULTS OF SURGICAL THERAPY

Operative Mortality

The in-hospital or 30-day mortality for isolated aortic valve replacement in large recent series has varied from 2–5%.[38] Mortality is increased to 6–15% by a prior median sternotomy,[39] increased to 6% by the addition of concurrent coronary bypass grafting,[35,37,42] and increased to 10% by the addition of mitral valve replacement. Mortality for patients over the age of 80 years with aortic stenosis has been 9%.[32] Other significant predictors of increased mortality in a series of 1689 primary isolated aortic valve replacements were increased age, decreased left ventricular function, poor preoperative functional status, renal insufficiency, and atrial fibrillation. The most common causes of operative mortality were cardiac failure or infarction in 58% of deaths, hemorrhage in 11%, infection in 7%, arrhythmia in 5%, and stroke in 4%.[38]

In-Hospital Complications

The most common serious complications after aortic valve operation include stroke in 1–2% of patients, mediastinal bleeding requiring reoperation in 5–11%, wound infection in 1–2%, heart block requiring a permanent pacemaker in less than 1%, renal failure requiring dialysis in 0.7%, prolonged ventilation in 3%, and perioperative myocardial infarction in 2%.[38] These risks are similar for all aortic valve operations. Strokes may be embolic or related to atherosclerosis, and strokes are best avoided by meticulous removal of air and potential embolic debris from the heart. The somewhat higher incidence of bleeding after aortic valve replacement relative to coronary bypass grafting suggests that meticulous hemostasis at the aortotomy and in previously operated fields is indicated.

Late Complications

The most frequent late complications from aortic replacement are thromboembolism and anticoagulant-related hemorrhage. The incidence of each of these is related to the valve prosthesis implanted, patient age, the presence of atrial fibrillation, and the degree of anticoagulation employed. For most bioprosthetic valves, incidence of thromboembolism is roughly 0.2–1.3% per patient year for isolated aortic valve replacement. For mechanical aortic valves, the rate of thromboembolism increases to 1.5–2.0% per patient year. The rate of anticoagulant-related hemorrhage is 0.3% for bioprostheses[26] and 2–3% per patient year for mechanical valves requiring warfarin anticoagulation.[13,15] Whether anticoagulant-related hemorrhage is more likely in elderly patients remains controversial.

Endocarditis is another late complication occurring after aortic valve operation with an incidence of roughly 0.5–1.0% per patient year after the first 6 months.[38] Most data currently available suggest that the type of aortic prosthesis has little effect on the incidence of prosthetic endocarditis.[19] The type of prosthesis does affect the incidence of aortic root abscess in patients developing prosthetic endocarditis, with the incidence of aortic root abscess being 65% for infected mechanical valves, 36% for porcine valves, and 20% for unstented homografts.[40]

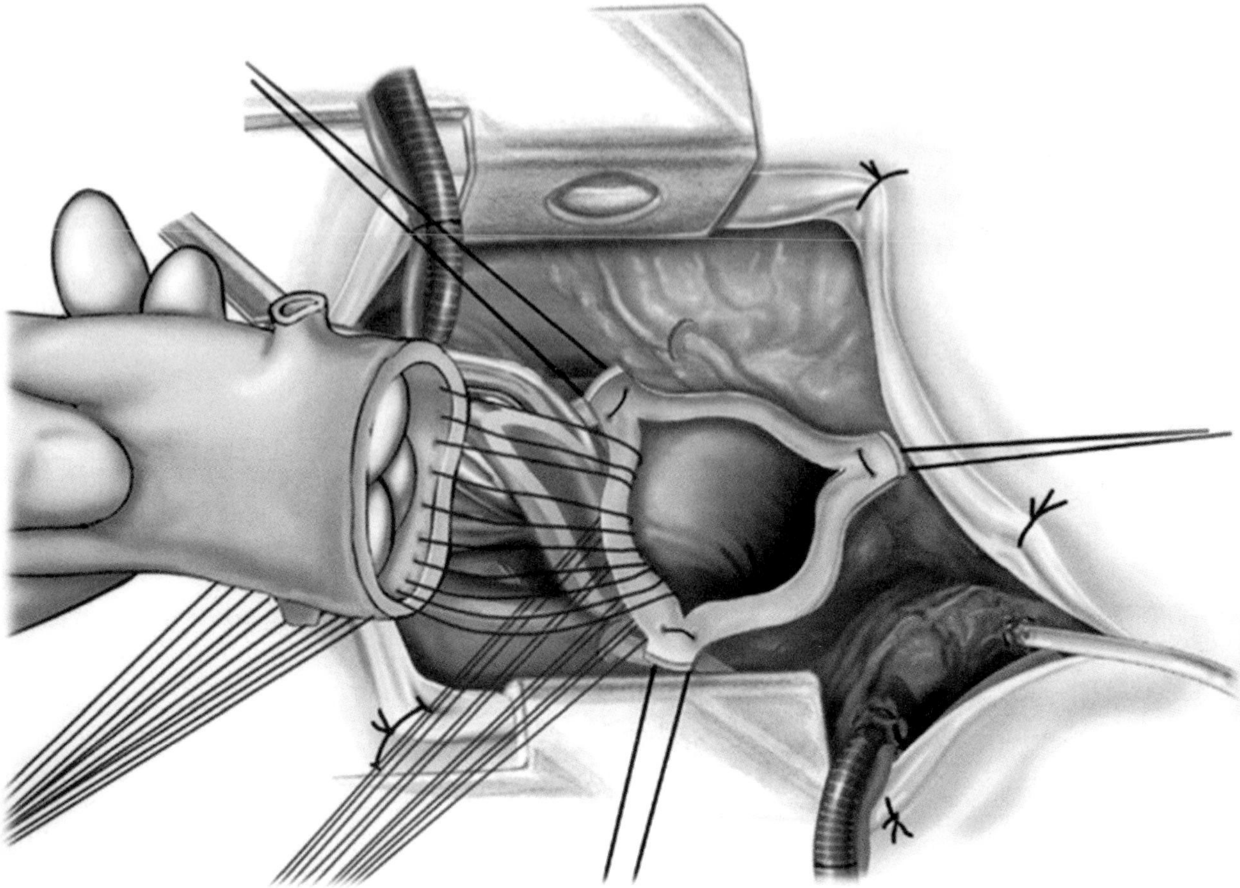

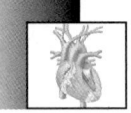

Figure 73–8 Aortic valve replacement using the allograft root technique.

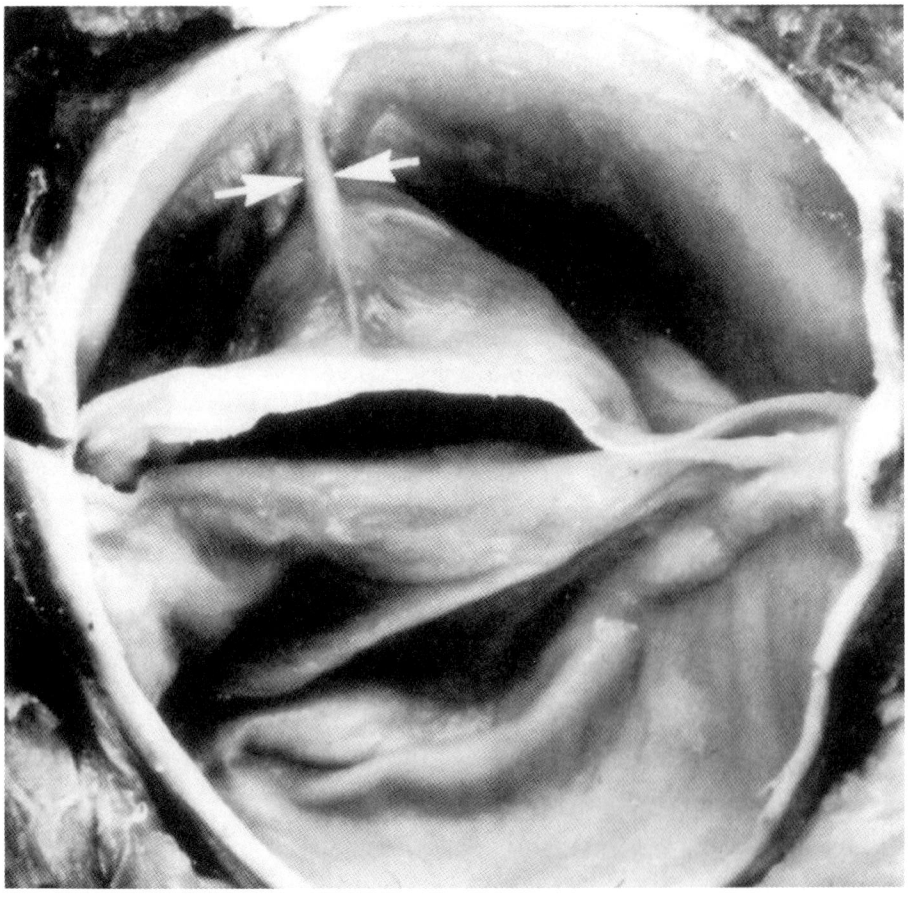

Figure 73–9 Bicuspid aortic valve. Arrows show raphe of conjoined leaflets. *(Courtesy of Medtronic Inc.)*

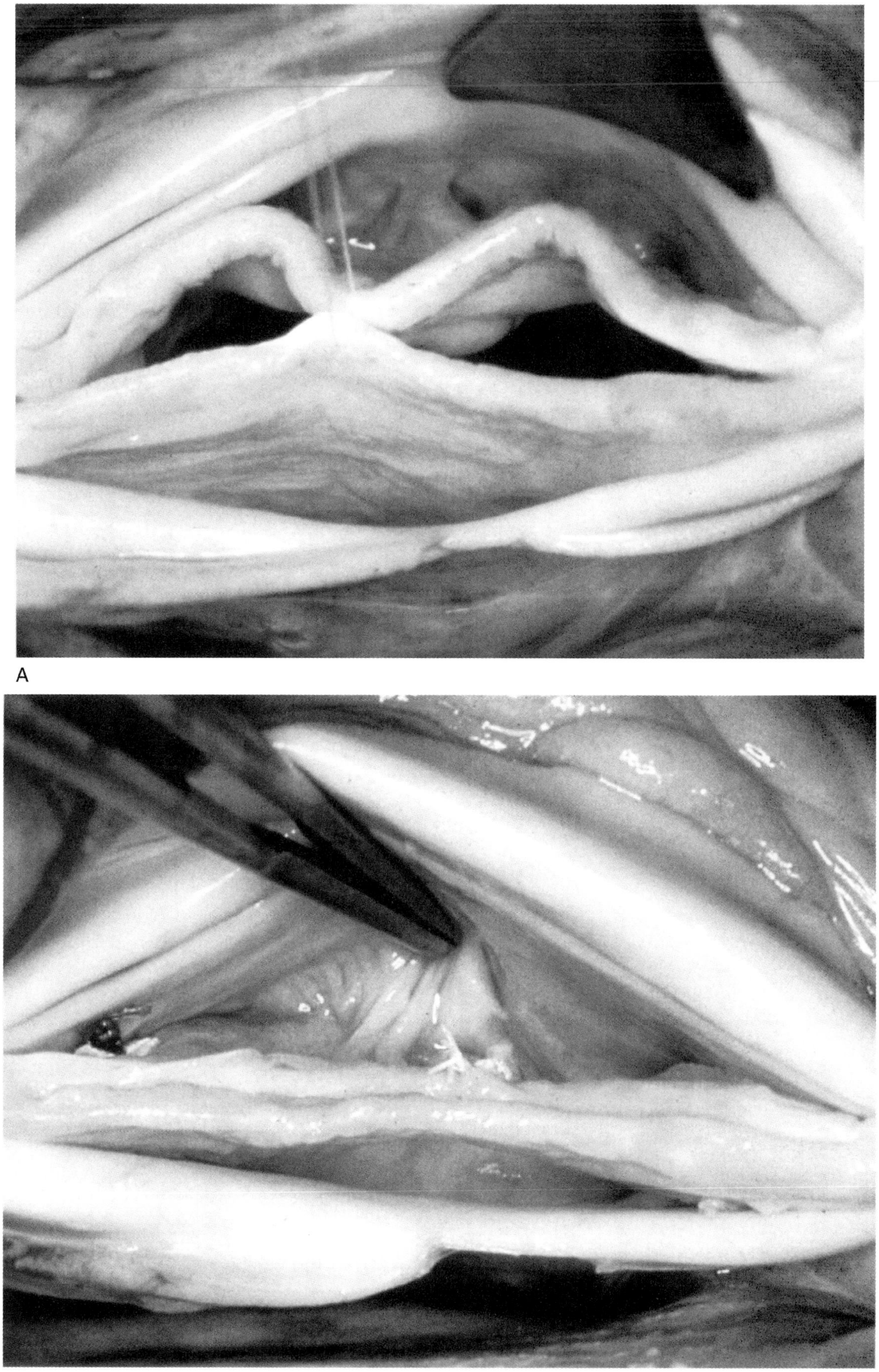

Figure 73–10 (**A**) Bicuspid aortic valve before repair. Note the redundant leaflet. (**B**) Bicuspid aortic valve after repair.

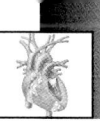

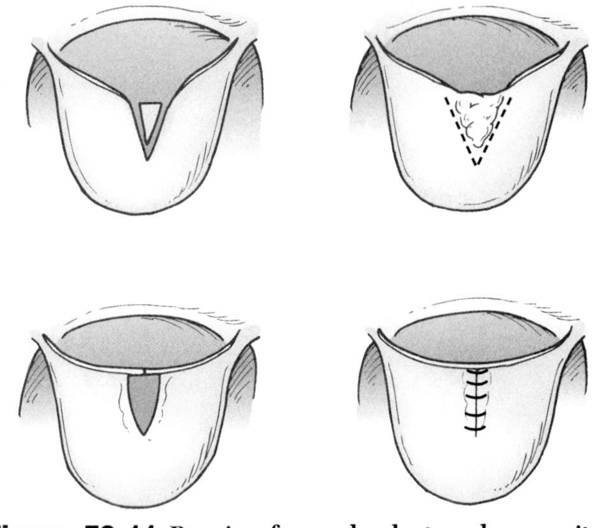

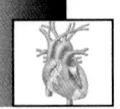

Figure 73–11 **Repair of a redundant and regurgitant aortic valve leaflet.**

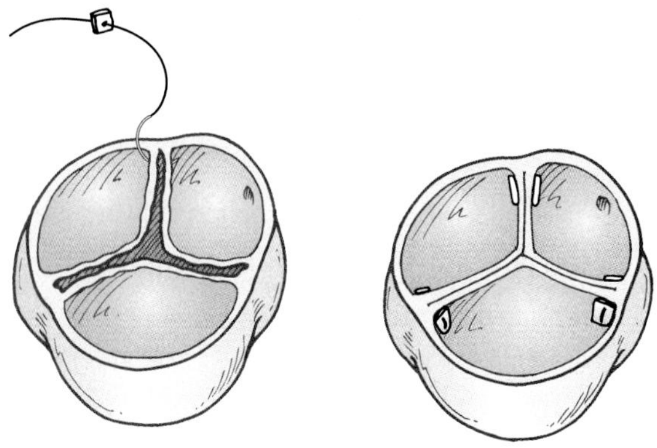

Figure 73–12 **Tricuspid aortic valve repair by commissure plication.**

Clinically significant hemolysis is unusual, and hemolysis is generally related to perivalvular leak and occasionally results from prosthetic dysfunction or small mechanical valve sizes. The incidence of perivalvular leak is 0.2–0.5% and is associated with infection in a significant number of cases.[38] Although some perivalvular leaks may be present at the time of operation, sterile perivalvular leak may occur weeks or even years after valve replacement. Risk factors for perivalvular leak may include endocarditis, prior operation, and large valve size.

Prosthetic dysfunction is an important late complication after aortic valve replacement, especially for biological prostheses.[2] Risk factors for prosthetic dysfunction may include the valve model and patient age.[3] Additional risk factors for aortic allografts include greater donor age and valve preparation technique.[30,43,44] False aneurysm or aortic dissection at the aortotomy site are extremely rare and probably related to aortic tissue characteristics and technical details of aortic closure. Complications from patient–prosthesis mismatch appear to have little clinical significance.[20,27,28]

Long-Term Survival

Long-term survival after aortic valve replacement is decreased by many factors, including older patient age, impaired left ventricular function, coronary artery disease, renal insufficiency, and other comorbidities.[1,11,38] Typical survival 10 years after aortic valve replacement is 60–70%, with primary causes of death including cardiac failure or sudden death in 42–83% of patients and hemorrhage (4%), infection (5%), thromboembolism (6%), and other noncardiac causes in the remainder.[36,38]

Symptomatic Relief

Most patients with aortic valve replacement for aortic valve disease notice fairly immediate improvement in preoperative symptoms. This improvement persists in the long term, with 96% of patients belonging to New York Heart Association (NYHA) functional class I or II 6 years after operation. In many patients, especially those with normal preoperative left ventricular function or with mildly depressed ejection fraction as a result of aortic stenosis, postoperative exercise capacity may be relatively normal.

REFERENCES

1. Akins CW, Hilgenberg AD, Vlahakes GJ, et al: Results of bioprosthetic versus mechanical aortic valve replacement performed with concomitant coronary bypass grafting. Ann Thorac Surg 74:1098–1106, 2002.
2. Banbury MK, Cosgrove DM, Thomas JD, et al: Hemodynamic stability during 17 years of the Carpentier-Edwards aortic pericardial bioprosthesis. Ann Thorac Surg 73:1460–1465, 2002.
3. Banbury MK, Cosgrove DM 3rd, White JA, et al: Age and valve size effect on the long-term durability of the Carpentier-Edwards aortic pericardial bioprosthesis. Ann Thorac Surg 72:753–757, 2001.
4. Bonow RO, Borer JS, Rosing DR, et al: Preoperative exercise capacity in symptomatic patients with aortic regurgitation as a predictor of postoperative left ventricular function and long-term prognosis. Circulation 62:1280–1290, 1980.
5. Bonow RO, Dodd JT, Maron BJ, et al: Long-term serial changes in left ventricular function and reversal of ventricular dilatation after valve replacement for chronic aortic regurgitation. Circulation 78:1108–1120, 1988.
6. Bonow RO, Rosing DR, McIntosh CL, et al: The natural history of asymptomatic patients with aortic regurgitation and normal left ventricular function. Circulation 68:509–517, 1983.
7. Borer JS, Herrold EM, Hochreiter C, et al. Natural history of left ventricular performance at rest and during exercise after aortic valve replacement for aortic regurgitation. Circulation 84:III133–139, 1991.
8. Carroll JD, Carroll EP, Feldman T, et al: Sex-associated differences in left ventricular function in aortic stenosis of the elderly. Circulation 86:1099–1107, 1992.
9. Cohen G, Christakis GT, Joyner CD, et al: Are stentless valves hemodynamically superior to stented valves? A prospective randomized trial. Ann Thorac Surg 73(3):767–775; discussion 775–778, 2002.
10. Craver JM: Aortic valve debridement by ultrasonic surgical aspirator: A word of caution. Ann Thorac Surg 49:746–752, 1990.

11. David TE, Ivanov J, Armstrong S, et al: Late results of heart valve replacement with the Hancock II bioprosthesis. J Thorac Cardiovasc Surg 121:268–278, 2001.
12. Davidson CJ, Harrison JK, Leithe ME, et al: Failure of balloon aortic valvuloplasty to result in sustained clinical improvement in patients with depressed left ventricular function. Am J Cardiol 65:72–77, 1990.
13. DiSesa VJ, Collins JJ, Cohn LH: Hematological complications with the St. Jude valve and reduced-dose Coumadin. Ann Thorac Surg 48:280–283, 1989.
14. Dreyfus G, Serraf A, Jebara VA, et al: Valve repair in acute endocarditis. Ann Thorac Surg 49:706–711, 1990.
15. Edmunds LH Jr: Thrombotic and bleeding complications of prosthetic heart valves. Ann Thorac Surg 44:430–445, 1987.
16. Fann JI, Glower DD, Miller DC, et al: Preservation of aortic valve in type A aortic dissection complicated by aortic regurgitation. J Thorac Cardiovasc Surg 102:62–73, 1991.
17. Fedak PWM, Verma S, David TE, et al: Clinical update: Clinical and pathophysiological implications of a bicuspid aortic valve. Circulation 106:900–904, 2002.
18. Gorlin R, Gorlin SG: Hydraulic formula for calculation of the area of the stenotic mitral valve, other valves, and central circulatory shunts. Am Heart J 41:1–29, 1951.
19. Hammermeister KE, Sethi GK, Henderson WG, et al: A comparison of outcomes in men 11 years after heart-valve replacement with a mechanical valve or bioprosthesis. N Engl J Med 328:1289–1296, 1993.
20. Hanayama N, Christakis GT, Mallidi HR, et al: Patient prosthesis mismatch is rare after aortic valve replacement: Valve size may be irrelevant. Ann Thorac Surg 73:1822–1829, 2002.
21. Harpole DH, Jones RH: Serial assessment of ventricular performance after valve replacement for aortic stenosis. J Thorac Cardiovasc Surg 99:645–650, 1990.
22. Hegglin R, Scheu H, Rothlin M: Aortic insufficiency. Circulation 38:77–92, 1968.
23. Hopkins RA: Cardiac Reconstructions with Allograft Valves. New York: Springer-Verlag, 1989.
24. Ionescu MI, Pakrashi BC, Holden MP, et al: Results of aortic valve replacement with frame-supported fascia lata and pericardial grafts. J Thorac Cardiovasc Surg 64:340–353, 1972.
25. Ionescu MI, Tandon AP: Long-term clinical and hemodynamic evaluation of the Ionescu-Shiley pericardial xenograft heart valve. Thoraxchir Vask Chir 26:250–258, 1978.
26. Jamieson WRE, Allen P, Miyagishima RT, et al: The Carpentier-Edwards standard porcine bioprosthesis. J Thorac Cardiovasc Surg 99:543–561, 1990.
27. Kallis P, Sneddon JR, Simpson IA, et al: Clinical and hemodynamic evaluation of the 19-mm Carpentier-Edwards supra-annular aortic valve. Ann Thorac Surg 54:1182–1185, 1992.
28. Khan SS, Mitchell RS, Derby GC, et al: Differences in Hancock and Carpentier-Edwards porcine xenograft aortic valve hemodynamics: Effect of valve size. Circulation 82:IV117–IV124, 1990.
29. King RM, Pluth JR, Giuliani ER, Piehler JM: Mechanical decalcification of the aortic valve. Ann Thorac Surg 42:269–272, 1986.
30. Kirklin JW, Barratt-Boyes BG: Cardiac Surgery, 2nd ed. New York: Churchill Livingstone, 1993.
31. Kirklin JW, Mankin HT: Open operation in the treatment of calcific aortic stenosis. Circulation 21:578–586, 1960.
32. Levinson JR, Akins CW, Buckley MJ, et al: Octogenarians with aortic stenosis. Outcome after aortic valve replacement. Circulation 80:I49–I56, 1989.
33. Lieberman EB, Bashore TM, Hermiller JB, et al: Balloon aortic valvuloplasty in adults: Failure of procedure to improve long-term survival. J Am Coll Cardiol 26:1522–1528, 1995.
34. Lieberman EB, Wilson JS, Harrison JK, et al: Aortic valve replacement in adult after balloon aortic valvuloplasty. Circulation 90:II205–II208, 1994.
35. Lund O, Neilson TT, Pilegaard HK, et al: The influence of coronary artery disease and bypass grafting on early and late survival after valve replacement for aortic stenosis. J Thorac Cardiovasc Surg 100:327–337, 1990.
36. Lund O, Pilegaard HK, Magnussen K, et al: Long-term prosthesis-related and sudden cardiac-related complications after valve replacement for aortic stenosis. Ann.Thorac Surg 50:396–406, 1990.
37. Lytle BW, Cosgrove DM, Gill CC, et al: Aortic valve replacement combined with myocardial revascularization. Late results and determinants of risk for 471 in-hospital survivors. J Thorac Cardiovasc Surg 95:402–414, 1988.
38. Lytle BW, Cosgrove DM, Taylor PC, et al: Primary isolated aortic valve replacement: Early and late results. J Thorac Cardiovasc Surg 97:675–694, 1989.
39. Lytle BW, Cosgrove DM, Taylor PC, et al: Reoperations for valve surgery: Perioperative mortality and determinants of risk for 1000 patients, 1958–1984. Ann Thorac Surg 42:632–643, 1986.
40. Miller DC: Predictors of outcome in patients with prosthetic valve endocarditis (PVE) and potential advantages of homograft aortic root replacement for prosthetic ascending aortic valve-graft infections. J Card Surg 5:53–62, 1990.
41. Monrad ES, Hess OM, Murakami T, et al: Time course of regression of left ventricular hypertrophy after aortic valve replacement. Circulation 77:1345–1355, 1988.
42. Mullaney CJ, Elveback LR, Frye RL, et al: Coronary artery disease and its management: Influence on survival in patients undergoing aortic valve replacement. J Am Coll Cardiol 10:66, 1987.
43. O'Brien MF, Stafford EG, Gardner MA, et al: A comparison of aortic valve replacement with viable cryopreserved and fresh allograft valves, with a note on chromosomal studies. J Thorac Cardiovasc Surg 94:812–823, 1987.
44. Okita Y, Franciosi G, Matsuki O, et al: Early and late results of aortic root replacement with antibiotic-sterilized aortic homograft. J Thorac Cardiovasc Surg 95:696–704, 1988.
45. Ovil Y, Wahi R, Liu P, et al: Aortic valvuloplasty for traumatic aortic insufficiency: A two-year follow-up. Ann Thorac Surg 49:143–144, 1990.
46. Pereira JJ, Lauer MS, Bashir M, et al: Survival after aortic valve replacement for severe aortic stenosis with low transvalvular gradients and severe left ventricular dysfunction. J Am Coll Cardiol 39:1356–1363, 2002.
47. Roger VL, Tajik AJ, Bailey KR, et al: Progression of aortic stenosis in adults: New appraisal using Doppler echocardiography. Am Heart J 119:331, 1990.
48. Ross DN: Replacement of the aortic valve with a pulmonary autograft: The "switch" operation. Ann Thorac Surg 52:1346–1350, 1991.
49. Ross J Jr, Braunwald E: Aortic stenosis. Circulation 38:61–67, 1968.
50. Saour JN, Sieck JO, Mamo LAR, Gallus AS: Trial of different intensities of anticoagulation in patients with prosthetic heart valves. N Engl J Med 332:428–432, 1990.
51. Smedira NG, Ports TA, Merrick SH, Rankin JS: Balloon aortic valvuloplasty as a bridge to aortic valve replacement in critically ill patients. Ann Thorac Surg 55:914–916, 1993.
52. Smucker ML, Manning SB, Stuckey TD, et al: Preoperative left ventricular wall stress, ejection fraction, and aortic valve gradient as prognostic indicators in aortic valve stenosis. Catheter Cardiovasc Diagn 17:133–143, 1989.
53. Starling MR, Kirsch MM, Montgomery DG, Gross MD: Mechanisms for left ventricular systolic dysfunction in aortic regurgitation: Importance for predicting the functional response to aortic valve replacement. J Am Coll Cardiol 17:887–897, 1991.
54. Swanson JS, Starr A: The ball valve experience over three decades. Ann Thorac Surg 48:S51–52, 1989.

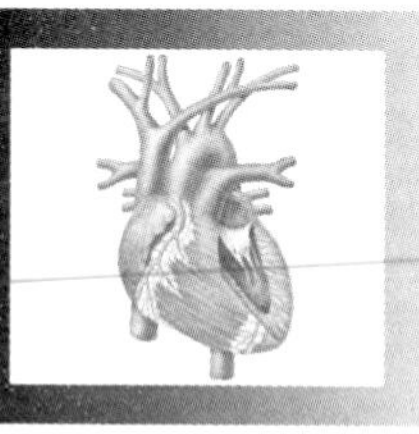

Acquired Disease of the Mitral Valve

Farzan Filsoufi, Sacha P. Salzberg, Lishan Aklog, and David H. Adams

CHAPTER 74

HISTORY

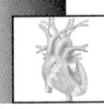

Early attempts to surgically correct mitral valve disease began at the end of the nineteenth century. In 1902 Brunton suggested that stenotic lesions of the mitral valve "might be susceptible of surgical intervention."[159] Eliott Cutler at the Peter Bent Brigham Hospital in Boston was the first to perform a mitral valvulotomy through the left ventricular apex for mitral stenosis in 1923.[51] This procedure was developed in close collaboration with Sam Levine, a renowned cardiologist from the same institution. In 1925 Souttar[171] performed the first-ever closed commissurotomy using his finger. In 1946 Bailey[12] used the same technique to split open a heavily calcified mitral valve, but in view of the very high restenosis rate, he later developed a technique for closed incisional commissurotomy. Despite good early results in some patients, mitral regurgitation and recurrent mitral stenosis remained two important complications of these procedures. At the same time an increasing number of patients with rheumatic disease were displaying symptoms of predominant mitral regurgitation. In the 1950s several techniques of repair for mitral regurgitation without the use of cardiopulmonary bypass were attempted. In 1954 Bailey et al[13] reported the correction of mitral regurgitation by using a pericardial graft. Davila et al[63] described the concept of annular size reduction by circumferential suture of the mitral annulus in 1955. In 1956 Nichols[160] reported his technique of annular plication at the posteromedial commissure using transatrial sutures. After the first successful use of cardiopulmonary bypass by Gibbon in 1953, the entire field of cardiac surgery entered a new era. It was Lillehei et al[140] in 1957 who reported the first suture mitral annuloplasty by placing heavy silk sutures in the dilated area of the mitral annulus. In 1959 Merendino et al[148] reported the concept of posteromedial annuloplasty. Subsequently, Kay et al,[134] Wooler et al,[190] and Reed and associates[165] described other techniques of annuloplasty, but none provided good long-term results and were therefore abandoned. In 1960 McGoon and associates[78] from the Mayo Clinic reported the resection–plication of the posterior leaflet for the treatment of mitral valve insufficiency.

Development of valve prosthesis was the next step in the development of mitral surgery. Nina Brunwald implanted a polyurethane prosthesis in the mitral position in 1959 at the National Institutes of Health. In 1960 Starr and Edwards[173] were the first to successfully implant a caged ball valve with good long-term results. During the following 2 decades, significant technological advances were made in the development of different types of reliable prostheses, such as porcine valves, tilting disk valves, and bileaflet mechanical valves. However, because of limited durability of the bioprosthetic material and the high rate of thromboembolic and hemorrhagic events associated with mechanical valves, Carpentier et al[33] and Duran and Ubago[73] focused their interest on the development of new repair techniques. In 1968 Carpentier performed the first remodeling annuloplasty with a prosthetic ring. Additional repair techniques were developed to broaden the application of reconstructive surgery in patients with valvular disease during the following 2 decades.[31,36]

In the mid-1990s research efforts further focused on the development of minimally invasive cardiac procedures. In 1996 Carpentier et al[35] performed the first videoscopic mitral valve repair through a right minithoracotomy. In 1998 it was Carpentier et al[34] and Mohr et al[155] who performed the first mitral valve repair using robotic assistance.

ANATOMY

The mitral valvular apparatus is an assembly of complex independent elements that constitute a functional entity. The mitral valve is composed of leaflets (valve tissue), mitral annulus, chordae tendineae, papillary muscles, and the left ventricle. The chordae tendineae and papillary muscles form the subvalvular apparatus.

Valvular Tissue

Anterior and posterior leaflets, as well as the commissures (posteromedial and anterolateral), constitute the valvular tissue (Figure 74-1). They are inserted on the entire circumference of the mitral annulus.

Commissures

Commissures are identified using two anatomical landmarks: the axis of corresponding papillary muscles and the commissural chordae, which has a specific configuration. Eight millimeters of valvular tissue separate the free edge of the commissures from the annulus. During an open commissurotomy, the surgical incision should respect this interval. Otherwise, its extension to the annulus may cause mitral regurgitation.

Leaflets

The anterior leaflet (aortic leaflet) has a semicircular shape and is attached to two fifths of the annular circumference. Its free edge does not present any indentations. There is continuity between the anterior leaflet of the mitral valve and the left and noncoronary cusps of the aortic valve. The anterior leaflet defines an important boundary between the inflow and outflow tracts of the left ventricle.

The posterior leaflet (mural leaflet) has a quadrangular shape and is attached to three fifths of the annular circumference. Posterior leaflet height is reduced when compared with the anterior leaflet; however, both leaflets have similar surface areas.

The mitral valve is separated into eight segments (Figure 74-2).[36] Anterolateral and posteromedial commissures are

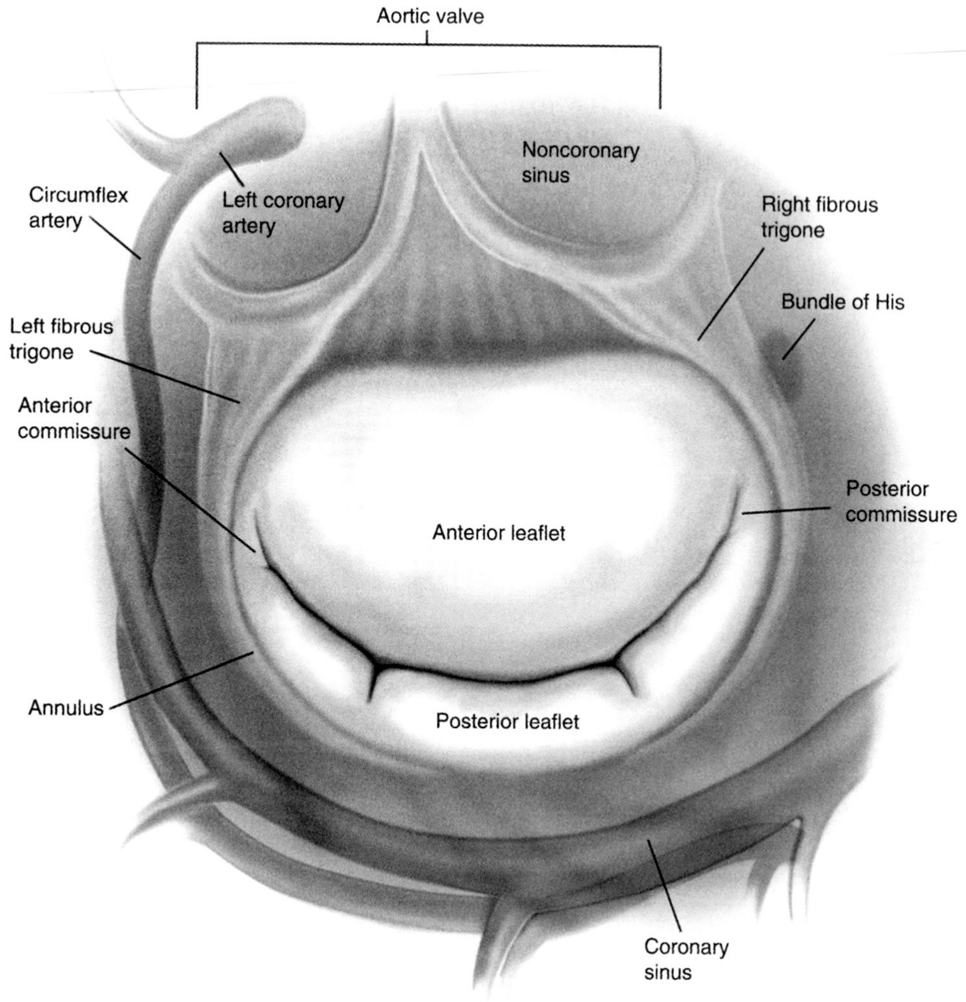

Figure 74–1 **Surgical anatomy of the mitral valve with important structures surrounding the annulus.**

two segments. Two indentations on the posterior leaflet divide this structure into three anatomically individualized scallops. The three scallops of the posterior leaflet are identified as P_1 (anterior scallop), P_2 (middle scallop), and P_3 (posterior scallop). The three corresponding segments of the anterior leaflet are A_1 (anterior segment), A_2 (middle segment), and A_3 (posterior segment). This anatomical nomenclature is the basis of segmental valve analysis, allowing a precise location of valve pathology (leaflet prolapse or restriction), which is of critical importance while performing reconstructive surgery.

On the atrial surface of the leaflets are two zones, one peripheral smooth zone and one central rough zone. A curved line, called the coaptation line, separates these two areas. The rough zone represents the coaptation surface of the valve. This zone is the insertion site of most of the chordae tendineae.

Mitral Annulus

The mitral annulus constitutes the junction between the ventricle and the left atrium, and an insertion site for the valvular tissue. The mitral annulus is attached to the fibrous trigones. The right fibrous trigone is a dense junctional area between the mitral, tricuspid, and noncoronary cusps of the aortic annuli and the membranous septum. The left fibrous trigone is situated at the junction of both left fibrous borders of the aortic and the mitral valve.

The mitral annulus is particularly thin at the insertion site of the posterior leaflet. This segment is not attached to any rigid structures, and it is at this area that annular dilation occurs predominantly. However, more recent studies have demonstrated that moderate annular dilation can also occur at the anterior portion of the mitral annulus between both trigones.[126] The mitral annulus is surrounded by several important anatomical structures, which are highlighted in Figure 74-1.

Chordae Tendineae

The chordae tendineae form the connection between the papillary muscles and the leaflets. They are classified according to the site of insertion between the free margin and the base of leaflets (Figure 74-3). Marginal chordae (primary chordae) are inserted on the free margin of the leaflets and function to limit leaflet prolapse. Intermediate chordae (secondary chordae) are inserted on the ventricular surface of the leaflets and relieve the valvular tissue of

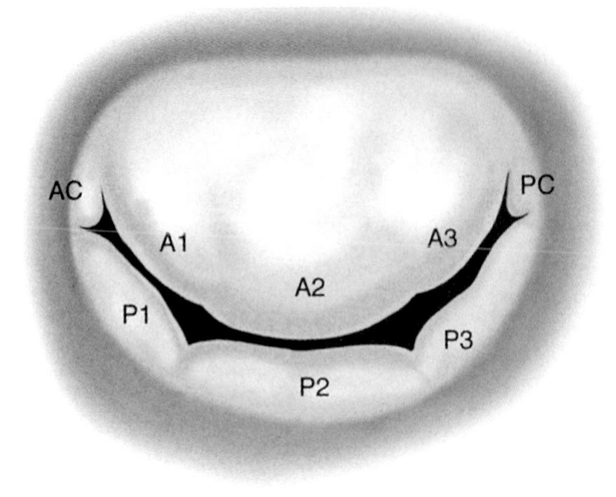

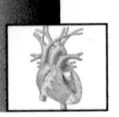

Figure 74–2 Segmental description of the valvular tissue. The mitral valve is divided into eight segments. Anterolateral and posteromedial commissures and posterior and anterior leaflets are divided into P_1, P_2, and P_3 and A_1, A_2, and A_3 segments, respectively. AC, anterolateral commissure; PC, posteromedial commissure.

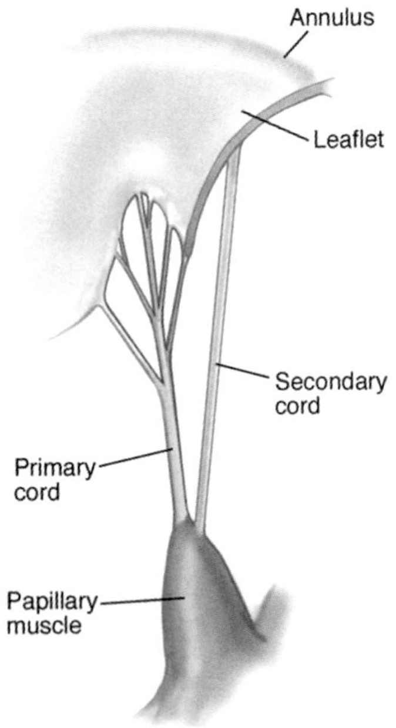

Figure 74–3 Subvalvular apparatus. Primary (marginal) chordae are attached to the free margin of the leaflet. Secondary chordae are attached to the ventricular side of the leaflet.

excess tension. Basal chordae (tertiary chordae) are limited to the posterior leaflet. They are attached to the leaflet base and connect it to the mitral annulus and the surrounding myocardial tissue.

Papillary Muscles and Left Ventricular Wall

There are two papillary muscles arising from the area between the apical and middle thirds of the left ventricular wall: The anterolateral is often composed of one body and the posteromedial is composed of two bodies. Each papillary muscle provides chordae to both leaflets. The anterolateral papillary muscle vasculature is supplied by the left anterior descending and the diagonal or a marginal branch of the circumflex artery. Left circumflex or right coronary arteries provide the blood supply to the posteromedial papillary muscle. Because of its single system of blood supply, the posteromedial papillary muscle is most commonly affected in ischemic cardiomyopathy. The attachment of the papillary muscles to the lateral wall of the left ventricle makes it part of the mitral valve complex. This structure plays a major role in the pathogenesis of mitral regurgitation in patients with ischemic cardiomyopathy.

MITRAL STENOSIS

Pathophysiology

The normal mitral valve area (MVA) is 4–6 cm^2. Mitral stenosis is considered mild when the area is less than 2 cm^2. It is considered critical when the valve area is less than 1 cm^2. This reduction in MVA causes an increase in atrioventricular gradient, which may exceed 20 mm Hg in critical stenosis. This elevation in left-sided pressures secondarily leads to pulmonary hypertension, reflected clinically by dyspnea. Several mechanisms are involved in the pathogenesis of pulmonary hypertension. They include retrograde transmission of the elevated left atrial pressure, pulmonary arteriolar constriction, and pulmonary interstitial edema. When the pulmonary artery systolic pressures increase, both right ventricular end-diastolic pressure and volume rise gradually, leading to right ventricular dilatation, which can further be complicated by tricuspid valve regurgitation. The left ventricular diastolic pressure is often normal in isolated mitral stenosis. Left ventricular dysfunction occurs in about one fourth of patients with severe, chronic mitral stenosis and may be a consequence of prolonged reduction of preload and/or extension of scarring from the valve into the adjacent myocardium.

Etiology

Rheumatic fever is the predominant cause of mitral valve disease in developing countries and the principal cause of mitral stenosis. Approximately 25% of all patients with rheumatic heart disease have pure mitral stenosis. However, the combination of mitral stenosis and regurgitation remains the most common form of this condition.[26] Rheumatic disease causes a fibroretractive transformation of the valve. Fibrosis is a slow process affecting all segments of the mitral apparatus. Valvular lesions include leaflet thickening, chordal thickening and fusion, and commissural fusion. In mitral stenosis, thickening of the valvular tissue restricts leaflet motion during diastole. In advanced stages of the disease, calcifications are present, especially at the commissural edges, producing a "fish mouth"–like single central opening. Lesions, which reduce the coaptation area (leaflet retraction) or restrict leaflet mobility (chordal shortening), are often present in patients with combined mitral regurgitation and stenosis. Other etiologies such as malignant carcinoid and systemic lupus rarely affect the mitral valve, causing varying degrees of mitral stenosis.

Diagnosis

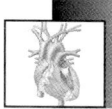

The diagnosis of mitral stenosis should be made on the basis of the medical history, physical examination, chest X-ray, electrocardiogram (ECG), and echocardiography. Patients may be asymptomatic, with abnormal findings from physical examination. Although some patients may show symptoms of fatigue, dyspnea, or hemoptysis, in others the initial manifestation of mitral stenosis is the onset of atrial fibrillation or an embolic event.

Auscultatory findings include a loud first heart sound, a diastolic murmur, and an opening snap in some patients. The diastolic murmur is a low-pitched rumble, which is heard at the apex of the heart. The opening snap can be heard in patients with preserved leaflet mobility. The chest X-ray may be normal; however, an enlarged left atrium is frequently seen. In patients with severe mitral stenosis and pulmonary hypertension, the right atrium and ventricle are often enlarged. ECG may be normal, but often demonstrates P-wave abnormalities, revealing left atrial enlargement, atrial fibrillation, and/or right ventricular hypertrophy.

The diagnostic tool of choice in the evaluation of patients with mitral stenosis is two-dimensional (2D) echocardiography Doppler.[135] This examination evaluates the appearance and mobility of the mitral valve leaflets, commissures, and the subvalvular apparatus, as well as the presence of calcifications. It also allows determining the severity of mitral stenosis by measuring the MVA, the transmitral gradient, and pulmonary artery pressures. Transthoracic echo also studies other valves to rule out any associated aortic or tricuspid regurgitation and evaluate right and left ventricular function.

Cardiac catheterization is usually not necessary for diagnosis of mitral stenosis, but it becomes necessary in patients older than 40 years if surgical correction is indicated.

Indication for Surgery

During the last decade the percutaneous mitral valvulotomy has become the first-line therapy for many patients with mitral stenosis. This procedure is ideally indicated in symptomatic patients (New York Heart Association [NYHA] class II, III, and IV) with isolated moderate to severe mitral stenosis (MVA <1.5 cm^2) and favorable valve morphology.[23] Asymptomatic patients with moderate to severe mitral stenosis and pulmonary hypertension at rest (pulmonary artery systolic pressure >50 mm Hg) may also be considered for percutaneous mitral valvulotomy. However, percutaneous valvulotomy is contraindicated in the setting of left atrial thrombus, at least moderate mitral regurgitation, and inadequate valve morphology (important valvular calcifications, subvalvular fusion). Percutaneous mitral valvulotomy is associated with a finite incidence of recurrent mitral stenosis, especially in patients undergoing repeat procedures and iatrogenic mitral regurgitation in patients with high valve scores.[97]

Therefore surgery is indicated in symptomatic patients (NYHA class III or IV) with moderate to severe mitral stenosis (MVA <1.5 cm^2) who are not appropriate for, or who have failed balloon valvulotomy.[23,43] There is also a subset of asymptomatic patients with severe mitral stenosis and severe pulmonary hypertension with no favorable morphology for percutaneous balloon valvulotomy. Mitral valve surgery is recommended in this subgroup of patients in order to prevent right ventricular failure.

In patients with mild asymptomatic mitral stenosis (valve area >1.5 cm^2 and mean gradient <5 mm Hg), no further evaluation is required after the initial workup. These patients usually remain stable for years and should be treated medically with a close follow up.

MITRAL REGURGITATION

Pathophysiology

Mitral insufficiency is defined as a retrograde regurgitation of blood from the left ventricle to the left atrium during systole. This regurgitant volume creates a volume overload in the left chambers. The effect of this volume overload on left ventricular performance depends on the severity and the duration of the regurgitation. In the early stage of mitral regurgitation, the left ventricle is able to compensate according to the Starling curve. Over time, however, the volume overload leads to myocardial remodeling. The two most important compensatory mechanisms are left ventricular dilatation and left ventricular hypertrophy caused by increased wall stress. Left atrial enlargement is another consequence of chronic mitral regurgitation. This enlargement can lead to atrial fibrillation, which in turn decreases ventricular filling. Both regurgitant flow and atrial fibrillation are very important in the onset of pulmonary hypertension. Initially the increased pulmonary vascular resistances are reversible, but eventually, fixed pulmonary hypertension may occur in untreated patients with severe chronic regurgitation. In most patients, chronic mitral regurgitation can cause left ventricular dysfunction. The occurrence of this complication impacts negatively survival regardless of the treatment modality.[80,82,85]

Carpentier's Functional Classification

The understanding of valve pathology is facilitated by the use of the "pathophysiological triad" first described by Carpentier (Table 74-1). This triad is composed of etiology (cause of the disease), valve lesions (resulting from the disease), and valve dysfunction (resulting from the lesion) (Figure 74-4). These distinctions are relevant because long-term prognosis depends on etiology, whereas treatment strategy and surgical techniques depend on valve dysfunctions and lesions, respectively.[2]

Carpentier's functional classification is used to describe the mechanism of mitral regurgitation.[31] This classification is based on the opening and closing motions of the mitral leaflets. Patients with type I dysfunction have normal leaflet motion. Mitral regurgitation in these patients is due to annular dilatation or leaflet perforation. There is an increased leaflet motion in patients with type II dysfunction, with the free edge of the leaflet overriding the plane of the annulus during systole (leaflet prolapse). The most common lesions responsible for type II dysfunction are chordal elongation or rupture and papillary muscle elongation or rupture. Patients with type IIIA dysfunction have a restricted leaflet motion during both diastole and systole. The most common lesions are leaflet thickening/retraction, chordal thickening/shortening or fusion, and commissural fusion. Mitral regurgitation is most often associated with some degree of mitral stenosis.

Table 74–1

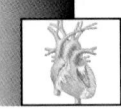

Pathophysiological Triad

Dysfunction	*Lesions*	*Etiology*
Type I		
Normal leaflet motion	Annular dilatation Leaflet perforation	Ischemic CMP (basal MI), DCMP Endocarditis
Type II		

Increased leaflet motion (leaflet prolapse)	Elongation/rupture of chordae	Degenerative mitral disease
		  Fibroelastic deficiency
		  Barlow's disease
		  Marfan's syndrome
		Endocarditis
		Rheumatic
		Trauma

	Elongation/rupture of papillary muscle	Ischemic CMP
Type IIIA		
Restricted leaflet motion (systole and diastole)	Leaflet thickening/retraction Chordal thickening/retraction/fusion Commissural fusion	Rheumatic disease Carcinoid disease
Type IIIB		
Restricted leaflet motion (systole)	PM displacement Leaflet tethering	Ischemic CMP DCMP

CMP, Cardiomyopathy; MI, myocardial infarction; DCMP, dilated cardiomyopathy; PM, papillary muscle.

The mechanism of mitral regurgitation in type IIIB dysfunction is restricted leaflet motion during systole. Left ventricular enlargement with apical papillary muscle displacement causes this type of valve dysfunction.

Etiology

Degenerative Disease

Degenerative mitral valve disease is the most common cause of mitral regurgitation in Western countries. The main mechanism of mitral insufficiency is type II dysfunction (leaflet prolapse).[31,47,56,102,157] However, type I dysfunction with isolated annular dilatation has also been reported. Etiologies of degenerative mitral valve disease include fibroelastic deficiency, Barlow's disease, and Marfan's syndrome.[32,37] In some cases the exact etiology remains undetermined.

Fibroelastic deficiency is most common in elderly patients with a relatively short history of mitral regurgitation. Valve analysis typically shows transparent leaflets with no excess tissue except in the prolapsing segment, and elongated, thin, frail, and often ruptured chordae. The annulus is often dilated and may be calcified.[32]

Barlow's disease appears early in life, and patients typically have a long history of a systolic murmur. The valve is billowing with typically thick leaflets and with marked excess tissue. The chordae are thickened and elongated, and may be ruptured. Papillary muscles are also occasionally elongated. The annulus is dilated and sometimes calcified. Histologically there is extensive myxoid degeneration with destruction of the normal three-layer leaflet tissue architecture.[32]

Marfan's syndrome with mitral regurgitation is characterized by excess leaflet tissue, which may be thickened (without myxoid degeneration), and a dilated annulus that is rarely calcified.[94]

Rheumatic Heart Disease

The mechanism of mitral regurgitation is often type IIIA dysfunction.[40,41,54] Leaflet thickening/retraction, and chordal shortening/fusion are common lesions. These lesions significantly reduce leaflet motion during diastole and systole, leading to combined mitral regurgitation and mitral stenosis. In addition, lesions such as commissural fusion, and leaflet thickening may decrease the opening of the valve during diastole and cause some degree of mitral stenosis. Occasionally chordal elongations are observed on the anterior leaflet, causing type II dysfunction. Anterior leaflet prolapse and posterior leaflet restriction (type II anterior, type III posterior) is one of the most common

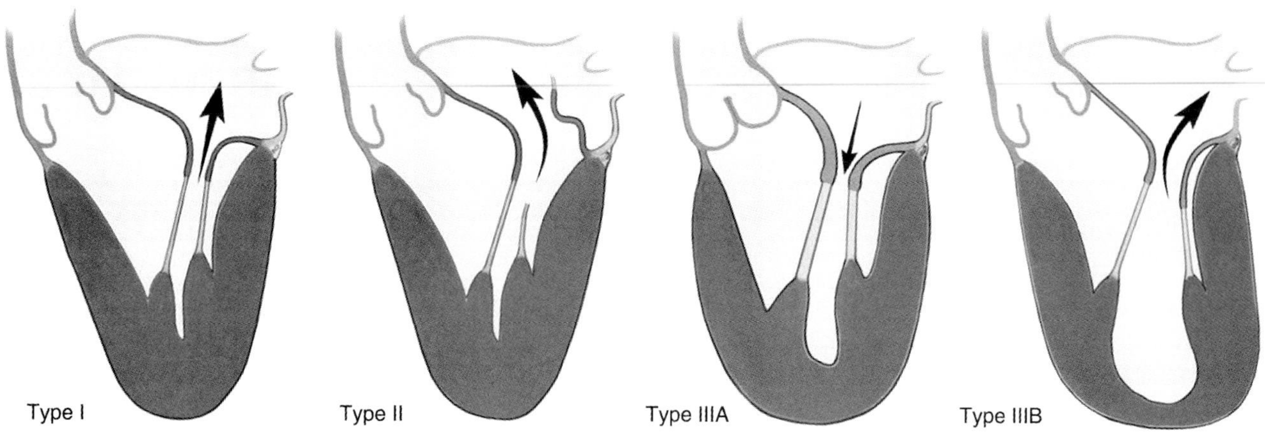

Figure 74–4 Carpentier's functional classification. Type I: Normal leaflet motion; type II: increased leaflet motion (leaflet prolapse); type III: restricted leaflet motion. A: During diastole and systole; B: during systole only. The arrow shows the direction of the jet in type I, II, and IIIB. It shows the association of some degrees of mitral stenosis in type IIIA.

mechanisms of mitral regurgitation in young rheumatic patients.[40]

Endocarditis

Mitral valve endocarditis usually occurs in patients with a structurally abnormal valve (degenerative, rheumatic valve disease), but certain organisms such as *Staphylococcus aureus* are capable of infecting completely normal valves. The principal organisms involved in native endocarditis are *Streptococcus viridans*, *Streptococcus bovis*, and *Staphylococcus aureus*.[90] Primary native mitral endocarditis may cause several types of lesions, including vegetations, chordal rupture, leaflet abscess or perforation, and annular abscess.[10,57,68,121,158] Aortic valve endocarditis may also cause native mitral valve endocarditis by extension of the infective process.[104] In some cases an aortic annular abscess can locally extend to the intervalvular fibrous body and the mitral annulus. The infection can further spread to the anterior leaflet of the mitral valve. Furthermore, the diastolic jet of aortic regurgitation resulting from aortic endocarditis may also cause secondary mitral endocarditis with vegetations or leaflet perforation on the ventricular surface of the anterior leaflet. These so-called kissing lesions occur in 15% of patients with aortic endocarditis.

Trauma

Mitral regurgitation is rarely due to blunt or penetrating chest trauma. Chordal rupture is the most common lesion. Percutaneous mitral valvulotomy can also be complicated by leaflet injury, and by chordal rupture, causing traumatic mitral regurgitation.[1,87]

Ischemic Cardiomyopathy

Ischemic cardiomyopathy causes mitral regurgitation by several mechanisms. Type I dysfunction with annular dilatation occurs in basal myocardial infarction. Type II dysfunction results from papillary muscle rupture, which usually involves the posteromedial papillary muscle.[107,114,179] In some instances the necrotic papillary muscle may not be ruptured and becomes fibrotic. The fibrotic papillary muscle is usually elongated and causes leaflet prolapse, particularly in the commissural area. Carpentier's type IIIB dysfunction is the most common form of ischemic mitral regurgitation.[*] Several anatomical and physiological changes are associated with the pathogenesis of this complex process, such as left ventricular remodeling after myocardial infarction, left ventricular wall motion abnormalities, papillary muscle infarction, and mitral annulus dilatation. After myocardial infarction, left ventricular remodeling converts the ventricular shape from ellipsoidal to spherical. This process leads to papillary muscle displacement, which causes a restriction of posterior leaflet motion during the systole (tethering effect), which reduces the leaflet coaptation surface area and leads to the onset of mitral regurgitation.[136,149] In some patients, further ventricular remodeling and dilatation causes annular dilatation, which may worsen mitral regurgitation. Ischemic mitral regurgitation is extensively discussed in Chapter 82.

Dilated Cardiomyopathy

Dilated cardiomyopathy is one of the most common causes of end-stage heart failure. The exact etiology of this disease remains unknown, even though multiple factors such as immunological abnormalities, viral infections, and excessive alcohol consumption have been incriminated. Natural history of dilated cardiomyopathy is often complicated by secondary or so-called functional mitral regurgitation, which has a negative impact on survival.[18,131] The mechanism of mitral regurgitation is type IIIB dysfunction.[19,30,136,137,186]

Calcifying Disease of the Annulus

Calcification is due to a degenerative process involving the base of the leaflets. Calcifications are localized at the posterior part of the annulus and may extend toward the base of the left ventricle. This process is often seen in elderly patients.[37,76,88,113] The mechanisms of mitral regurgitation are

*References 8, 20, 49, 67, 110, 122.

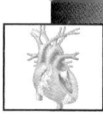

the loss of annular contraction and the restricted motion of the posterior leaflet.

Endomyocardial Fibrosis

Endomyocardial fibrosis is characterized by a progressive fibrosis of the ventricular endocardium, resulting in a restrictive cardiomyopathy. The exact etiology of this disease is undetermined. Mitral insufficiency is related to the invasion of the posterior leaflet and the subvalvular apparatus by the fibrotic process.[150,187] Posterior leaflet restriction in the opening position is the most frequently encountered valve dysfunction (type IIIA).

Diagnosis

Patients with mitral regurgitation may remain asymptomatic for long periods of time. However, they often display signs of fatigue, decreased exercise capacity, shortness of breath, or more advanced symptoms of heart failure. Supraventricular arrhythmias such as atrial fibrillation are a frequent finding in these patients.

The auscultatory findings are a high-pitched systolic murmur at the apex that irradiates to the axilla. Isolated late systolic murmur is in favor of mild mitral regurgitation. Chest X-ray may show left atrial and ventricular dilatation in patients with severe chronic mitral regurgitation. Prominence of the pulmonary vessels is an evidence of pulmonary hypertension. In the acute setting, pulmonary edema may be present. ECG may be normal; however, in most patients, evidence of left atrial enlargement with P-wave abnormalities is present. ECG may also show atrial fibrillation and signs of left and right ventricular hypertrophy in patients with chronic valve disease.

2D echocardiography Doppler is essential in determining the mechanism and the severity of mitral regurgitation.[176] Carpentier's functional classification can be used to exactly describe the underlying mechanisms of mitral regurgitation. The precise location of valve dysfunction can further be defined using segmental valve analysis. During echocardiography the transgastric view best visualizes the different segments of the valve.

Semiquantitative assessment of regurgitant flow using maximal jet length, area, and ratio of jet to left atrial area has been used to assess the severity of mitral regurgitation. The degree of mitral regurgitation is determined by assessing jet geometry and area in multiple views. The severity of mitral regurgitation is graded on a scale from 1+ to 4+ (1+, trace; 2+, mild; 3+, moderate; and 4+ severe mitral regurgitation with flow reversal in the pulmonary veins). The direction of the jet is a good indicator of the mechanism of mitral regurgitation. In type II dysfunction (prolapse) the direction of the jet is opposite to the prolapsing leaflet. With restricted leaflet motion the direction of the jet is either central, or toward the restricted leaflet.

More recently, quantitative Doppler methods have been developed allowing quantitative grading of mitral regurgitation.[110,184] This quantitative grading is based on the calculation of regurgitant volume (the difference between the mitral and aortic stroke volumes) and effective regurgitant orifice (ratio of regurgitant volume to regurgitant time velocity integral). Table 74-2 shows the relationship between the semiquantitative and quantitative grading of mitral regurgitation in degenerative mitral disease.

Table 74–2

Selected Ranges for Grading Severity of Mitral Regurgitation in Patients with Degenerative Disease

Grade	*Rvol (ml)*	*RF (%)*	*ERO (mm²)*
1	<30	<30	<20
2	30–44	30–39	20–29
3	45–59	40–49	30–39
4	≥60	≥50	≥40

From Enriquez-Sarano M, Tajik AJ, Schaff HV, et al: Echocardiographic prediction of survival after surgical correction of organic mitral regurgitation. Circulation 90:830–837, 1994.

Rvol, Regurgitant volume; RF, right ventricular ejection fraction; ERO, effective regurgitant orifice.

Transesophageal echocardiography (TEE) should be considered in a selected group of patients (e.g., complex degenerative disease, native valve endocarditis).[163] TEE has a significantly higher sensitivity and specificity for detection of perivalvular infection and vegetations. The indications for cardiac catheterization are similar to those reported for mitral stenosis.

In the future, three-dimensional (3D) echocardiography and cardiac magnetic resonance imaging (MRI) will play a role in the determination of the mechanism and severity of mitral regurgitation.[108,178]

Indication of Surgery

The very low operative mortality and excellent results of mitral valve repair have dramatically changed the indications of surgery during the last decade. Several factors such as severity of mitral regurgitation, left ventricular function, symptoms, etiology, overall surgical risk (age, comorbid risk factors), and the likelihood of valve repair should be taken into consideration for the decision making in regard to the indication of surgery (Table 74-3).[*]

Patients with severe symptomatic mitral regurgitation should undergo mitral valve surgery. Left ventricular dysfunction is no longer a contraindication for mitral valve repair. Even if the operative risk is significantly higher in this subgroup of patients, long-term results remain significantly better compared with medical treatment. Enriquez-Sarano et al[79,84] from the Mayo Clinic have demonstrated that in patients with degenerative mitral valve disease undergoing mitral valve surgery, preoperative left ventricular function was the most powerful predictor of late survival. Patients with ejection fraction (EF) <60% displayed an excess mortality when compared with those with EF >60% (Figure 74-5). More interestingly in the group of patients with EF >60%, the late observed survival was excellent and similar to the expected survival.

---

[*]References 45, 79, 80, 81, 84, 85, 185.

Table 74–3

Timing of Surgery in Organic Mitral Regurgitation

	Prompt mitral surgery decision
Severe mitral regurgitation	
Symptoms or LV dysfunction present	Yes
No symptoms and no LV dysfunction	
AAF, VT, or PHTN	Yes
No AF, no VT, no PHTN	
Repairable = No	
Massive MR (regurgitant volume ≥100 ml)	Possibly yes
Pronounced left atrial enlargement	
Repairable = Yes	
Low risk	Usually yes
High risk or severe comorbidity	Usually no
Not severe mitral regurgitation	
Regurgitant volume <45 ml	No
Regurgitant volume 45–60 ml	Usually no
VT, AF, or LV dysfunction ad repairable = Yes	Possibly yes
Other cardiac operation scheduled and repairable = Yes	Possibly yes

Modified from Enriquez-Sarano M, Tajik AJ, Schaff HV, et al: Echocardiographic prediction of survival after surgical correction of organic mitral regurgitation. Circulation 90:830–837, 1994.

LV, Left ventricle; AF, atrial fibrillation; VT, ventricular tachycardia; PHTN, pulmonary hypertension; MR, mitral regurgitation.

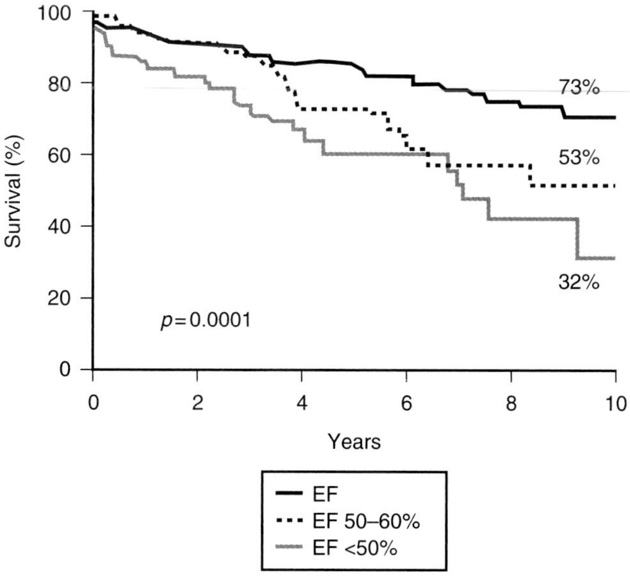

Figure 74–5 Graph of late survival of operative survivors according to preoperative echocardiographic ejection fraction (EF).

Furthermore, Tribouilloy et al[185] have shown that with preoperative functional NYHA class III or IV, the surgical results are associated with excessive short- and long-term postoperative mortality. They have also reported that the late observed survival was the same as the expected survival in patients with preoperative functional NYHA class I or II (Figure 74-6).

These data suggest that in patients with severe mitral regurgitation, surgical treatment should be considered early, even in the absence of symptoms, before left ventricular dysfunction occurs, especially if valve repair is feasible and the patient does not present additional comorbid risk factors.

Because repair is less likely in patients with rheumatic heart disease and the risk of reoperation is higher than in degenerative disease, surgical treatment should only be considered in patients with severe mitral regurgitation when symptoms or early signs of left ventricular dysfunction develop.

Finally, in asymptomatic patients with moderate mitral regurgitation (Rvol 45–60 ml, 3+ mitral regurgitation), surgery can be considered in the presence of left ventricular dysfunction and supraventricular arrhythmias if the valve is repairable, especially in patients with degenerative disease.

Surgical intervention is indicated in specific circumstances for native mitral valve endocarditis.* They include the following: (1) significant mitral regurgitation with or without symptoms of congestive heart failure; (2) uncontrolled sepsis despite proper antibiotic therapy; (3) presence of an antibiotic resistant organism; (4) fungal, *S. aureus*, or gram-negative bacilli endocarditis; (5) evidence of mitral annular abscess; (6) extension of infection to intervalvular fibrous body; (7) formation of intracardiac fistulas; (8) onset of a new conduction disturbance; (9) large vegetations (>1 cm), particularly those that are mobile and located on the anterior leaflet, at high risk for embolic complications; and (10) multiple emboli after appropriate antibiotic therapy. Surgical therapy has dramatically improved both morbidity and mortality in the previous settings.[10,158] The timing of surgery is also a critical issue in the appropriate management of this condition. Patients should be taken to the operating room regardless of the duration of antimicrobial therapy when there is an indication for surgery. However, surgery should be delayed when recent neurological injuries are present (at least 2 weeks for ischemic injury and 4 weeks for hemorrhagic lesions).[75]

*References 45, 79, 80, 81, 84, 85, 185.

SURGERY

Perioperative Management

Standard techniques of monitoring (e.g., arterial line, central venous access, Foley catheter) are used in patients undergoing mitral valve surgery. A Swan-Ganz catheter should be placed in cases of complex mitral valve reconstructive surgery, multivalve surgery, combined mitral and coronary artery bypass graft (CABG) surgery, and in patients with increased operative risk (e.g., left ventricular dysfunction, pulmonary hypertension, reoperation). Initially a TEE should be performed in all patients.[93] TEE is a key element to determine the mechanism and severity of mitral regurgitation, and to assess left ventric-

*References 10, 57, 68, 90, 121, 158.

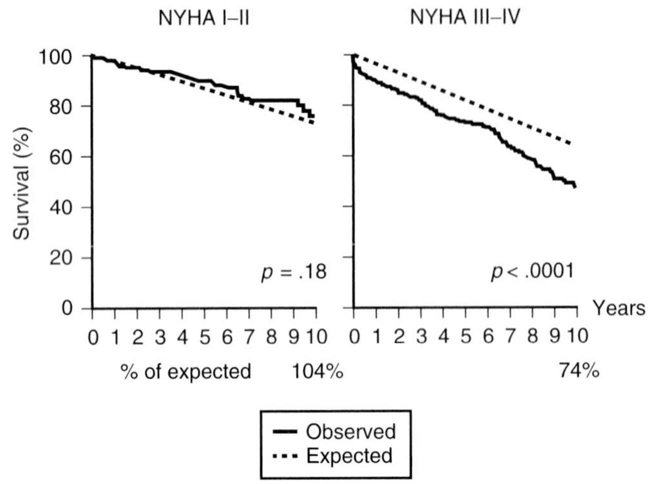

Figure 74–6 Comparison of observed with expected survival after surgery in patients in NYHA classes I–II *(left)* and classes III–IV *(right)*. Numbers underneath indicate percentage of expected survival achieved.
(Modified from Tribouilloy CM, Enriquez-Sarano M, Schaff HV, et al: Impact of preoperative symptoms on survival after surgical correction of organic mitral regurgitation: Rationale for optimizing surgical indications. Circulation 99:400–405, 1999.)

ular function, quality of repair, and de-airing of the cardiac cavities at the completion of the procedure (Figure 74-7). An external defibrillator is placed in redo operations and minimally invasive procedures for subsequent defibrillation. A double-lumen endotracheal tube is inserted in right thoracotomy approaches. An epiaortic scan of the ascending aorta is recommended in elderly patients with associated atherosclerotic risk factors, and in those undergoing a combined mitral valve and CABG surgery before arterial cannulation.

Surgical Approaches/Cardiopulmonary Bypass

Median Sternotomy

Median sternotomy is the most commonly used surgical approach in mitral valve surgery (Figure 74-8). It provides excellent access to all cardiac structures, allowing for central cannulation using the ascending aorta and the superior and inferior vena cava. It remains the surgical approach of choice in patients undergoing complex mitral valve, multivalve, combined mitral and CABG, and reoperative surgery.

During the last decade the population of patients being referred for reoperative mitral surgery has increased. The most common clinical scenarios include failed bioprosthetic mitral valves and ischemic mitral regurgitation after prior CABG or after prior aortic valve replacement.[4,93,125] The choice of cannulation sites and the indications for peripheral bypass before sternotomy are important determinants to avoid any major complications during reoperative surgery. Femoral vessel exposure is recommended for possible severe mediastinal adhesions (e.g., recent reoperation, multiple previous sternotomies, mediastinitis, mediastinal radiation) and in patients with patent grafts. Femoral vessel cannulation with peripheral bypass at the time of sternotomy may be indicated in patients with patent left internal mammary artery (LIMA) graft, dilated ascending aorta, and severe right ventricular dilation.

Right Anterolateral Thoracotomy

The patient is rotated 30 degrees to the left side, and a 12- to 15-cm right anterolateral thoracotomy is performed through the fourth intercostal space.[48,128,174,182,183] This surgical approach is useful in patients with prior CABG and patent internal thoracic grafts[27,28] and prior aortic valve replacement undergoing isolated reoperative mitral surgery. Because the right thoracotomy approach does not require extensive mediastinal dissection, it is also an interesting alternative if dense mediastinal adhesions are suspected. Right thoracotomy is contraindicated in patients with previous right-sided chest surgery, severe chronic obstructive pulmonary disease (COPD), and moderate to severe aortic insufficiency.

Direct cannulation of the ascending aorta and percutaneous femoral vein and superior vena cava cannulation are performed whenever possible. If the ascending aorta is not suitable for cannulation (because of inaccessibility and inadequate exposure, presence of multiple venous grafts, or calcification), femoral and axillary[16] arteries are other alternatives for arterial cannulation. Cardiopulmonary bypass is instituted using vacuum-assisted drainage. Mitral valve exposure occasionally can be difficult with this approach.

Minimally Invasive Mitral Valve Surgery

Since the 1990s, a variety of minimally invasive surgical approaches have been described to perform mitral valve surgery. These procedures were developed to decrease operative morbidities associated with the conventional approaches (e.g., postoperative pain, infection, transfusion requirements), as well as to reduce length of hospital stay and accelerate patient recovery.[48,117,142] According to their increased difficulty, minimally invasive approaches are divided into four categories: limited incision with direct vision (level 1), video-assisted (level 2), video-directed and robot-assisted (level 3), and robotic telemanipulation (level 4).[89]

Currently, minimally invasive direct vision mitral surgery is performed through the partial upper or lower hemisternotomy.[29,100,109] The right parasternal approach is abandoned because of a high rate of pulmonary herniation.[7] A 6-cm skin incision is performed in both cases. The sternum is partially divided from the sternal notch to the left fourth intercostal space (upper hemisternotomy) and from the xiphoid to the second right intercostal space (lower hemisternotomy). Central arterial and venous cannulation is often possible with these approaches. Video-directed[38,112] and robotic mitral valve surgeries[89,155,161] are performed through a right minithoracotomy at the fourth intercostal space. Multiport access is obtained by additional keyhole incisions. Peripheral vessels are used to initiate cardiopulmonary bypass. Additional adjunctive techniques such as port access instrumentation, endoaortic balloon, Chitwood aortic cross-clamp, CO_2 insufflation, and vacuum-assisted venous drainage are commonly used to facilitate these surgical procedures.

Myocardial Management

Mitral valve surgery is classically performed with cardioplegic arrest. Alternative techniques such as beating heart and ventricular fibrillatory arrest are available in a selected group of

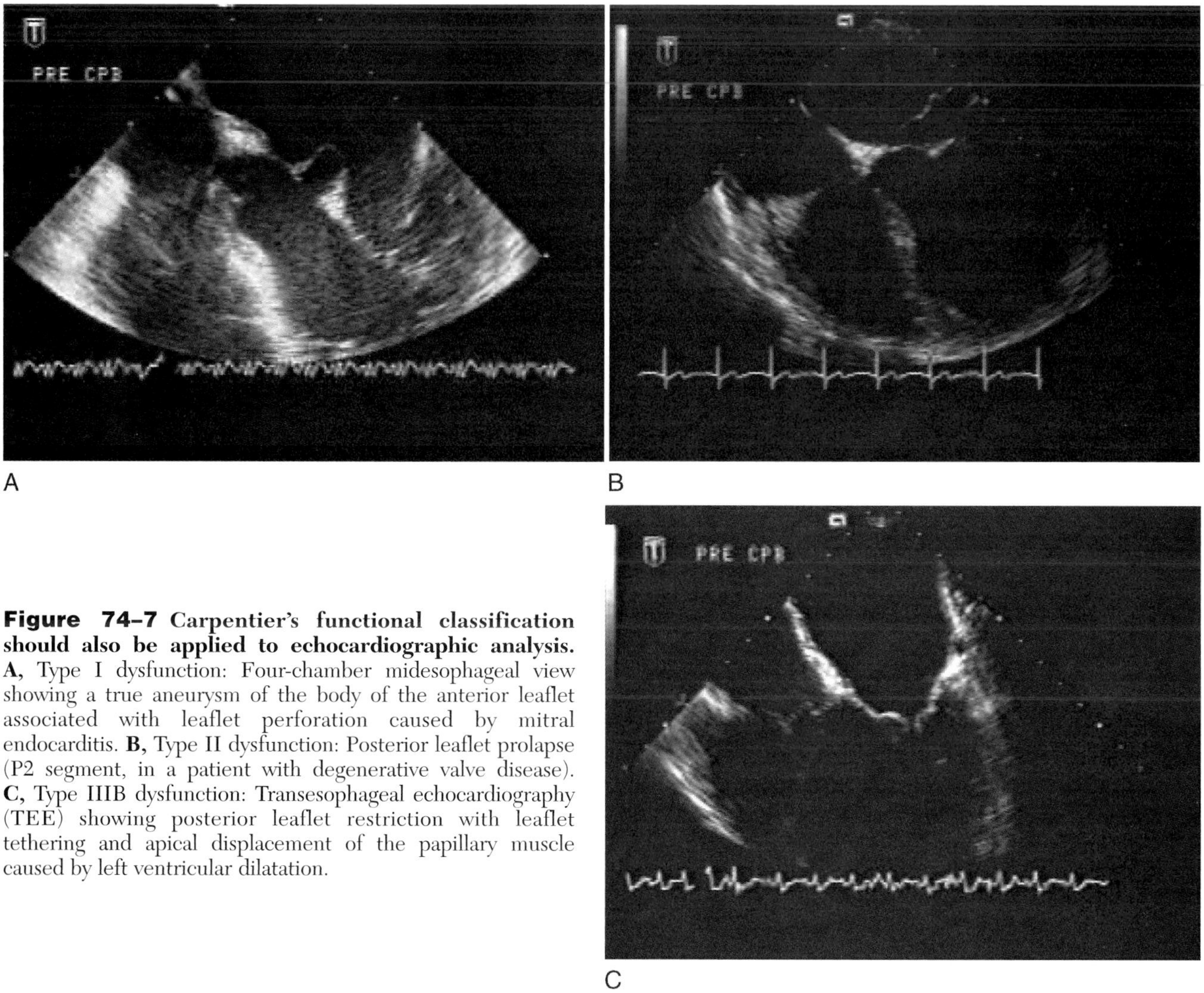

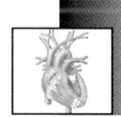

Figure 74–7 Carpentier's functional classification should also be applied to echocardiographic analysis. **A,** Type I dysfunction: Four-chamber midesophageal view showing a true aneurysm of the body of the anterior leaflet associated with leaflet perforation caused by mitral endocarditis. **B,** Type II dysfunction: Posterior leaflet prolapse (P2 segment, in a patient with degenerative valve disease). **C,** Type IIIB dysfunction: Transesophageal echocardiography (TEE) showing posterior leaflet restriction with leaflet tethering and apical displacement of the papillary muscle caused by left ventricular dilatation.

patients. However, the quality of myocardial protection provided by these techniques is not as optimal as cardioplegic arrest. The cardioplegic arrest requires the use of cold-blood, high-potassium cardioplegia for myocardial protection. This is achieved with intermittent antegrade infusion or a combined antegrade and retrograde infusion. Further myocardial protection can be obtained by moderate systemic hypothermia between 28–30° C and local hypothermia with topical ice.

In reoperative mitral valve surgery, specifically through a right anterolateral thoracotomy, it is often difficult to cross-clamp the ascending aorta. Therefore other types of myocardial management such as beating heart and moderate to deep hypothermia and fibrillatory arrest should be considered as long as there is no more than trace to mild aortic regurgitation.[29,46,125,182] These noncardioplegic techniques are particularly useful in patients with prior CABG and patent internal thoracic grafts. In other clinical circumstances, such as in patients with severely depressed left ventricular function (beating heart) and severe atherosclerotic disease of the ascending aorta (beating heart or ventricular fibrillatory arrest), these techniques present an interesting alternative. Despite the potential advantages provided in the preceding clinical scenarios, de-airing of the cardiac chambers can be more challenging. The beating heart technique is performed with the patient placed in the Trendelenburg position and rotated to elevate the left atrium relative to the ventricle. Both the Trendelenburg position and active aortic venting minimize the risk of cerebral air embolization. At the end of the procedure, further deairing is performed by filling the heart with blood while the mitral valve is made incompetent. The ventricular fibrillatory arrest technique requires institution of cardiopulmonary bypass with moderate to deep hypothermia. Once the patient is in the Trendelenburg position, ventricular fibrillation is induced either by an electrical cable or a brief cold myocardial perfusion. Active aortic venting should be maintained throughout the entire procedure to minimize the risk of air emboli.

Exposure of the Mitral Valve

Perfect exposition of the mitral valve is essential before undertaking any type of mitral valve surgery. Three approaches have been described (Figure 74-9).

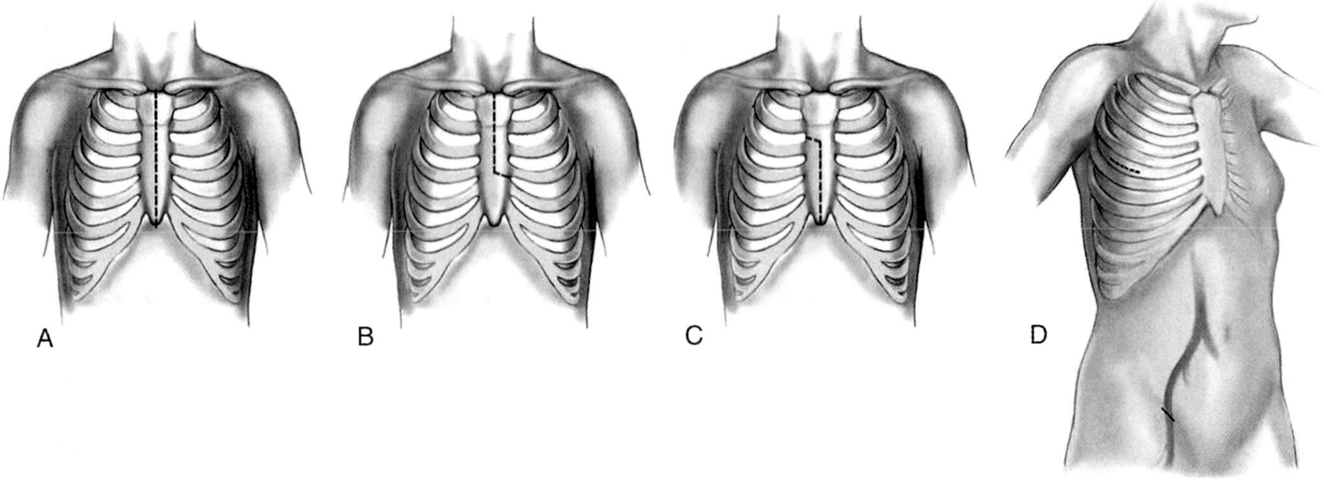

Figure 74–8 **Surgical incisions. A,** Limited skin incision and full sternotomy. **B,** Upper hemisternotomy. **C,** Lower hemisternotomy. **D,** Right minithoracotomy, groin incision for peripheral cannulation.

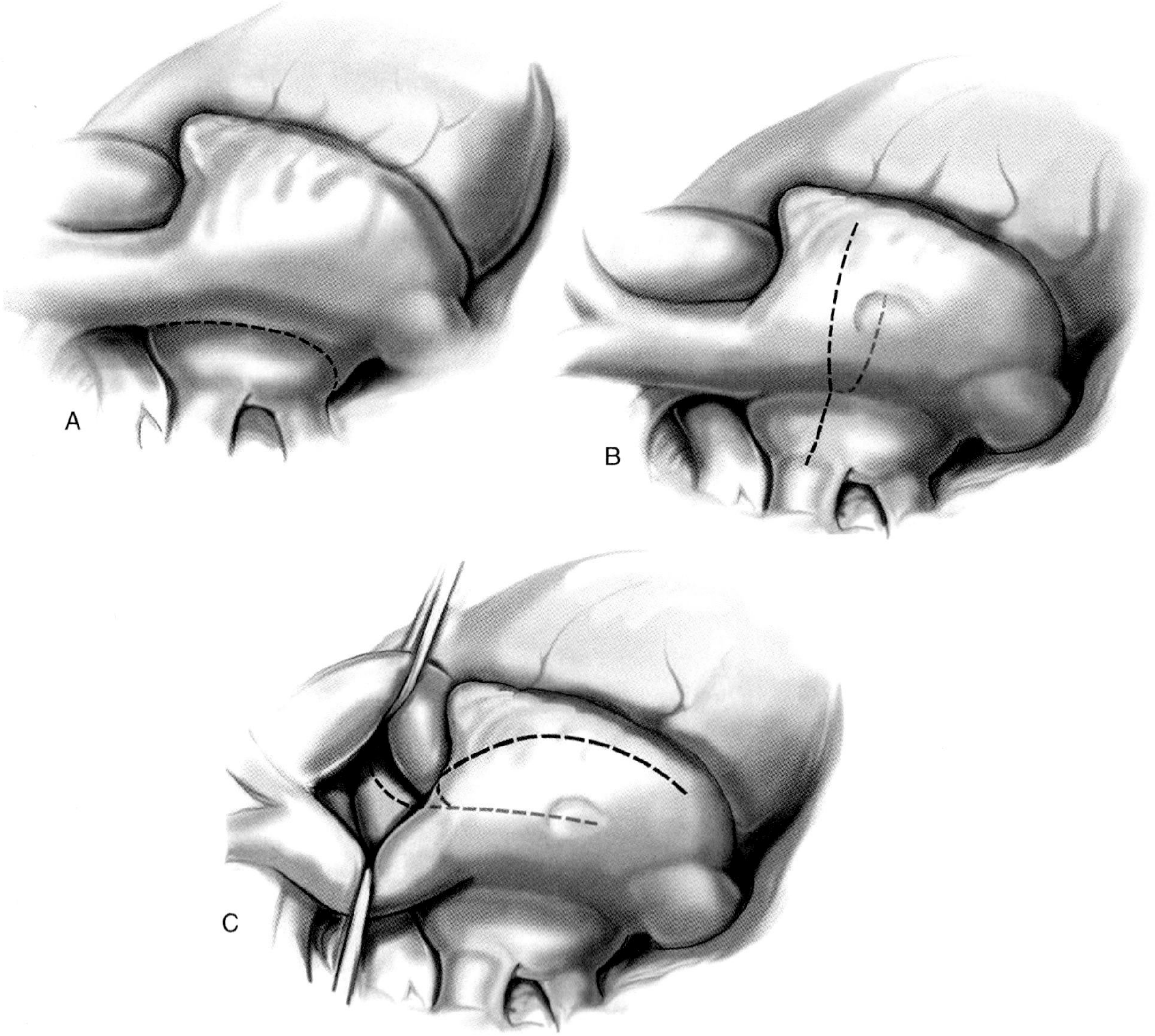

Figure 74–9 **Left atrial incisions. A,** Interatrial approach through the Sondergaard's groove; the extension of the left atrial incision between the right inferior pulmonary vein and inferior vena cava improves valve exposure. **B,** Horizontal biatrial transseptal approach. **C,** Superior biatrial transseptal approach.

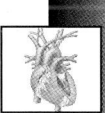

Interatrial Approach Through the Sondergaard's Groove

This is the most commonly used approach to expose the mitral valve. The interatrial groove is incised, and the two atria are dissected and divided up to the fossa ovalis. This dissection exposes the roof of the left atrium, which is opened close to the mitral valve.[36] In patients with a small left atrium, the inferior extension of the left atrial incision between the right inferior pulmonary vein and the inferior vena cava optimizes the mitral valve exposure.

Horizontal Biatrial Transseptal

The incision is started at the level of the right atrial appendage 2 cm posterior to the atrioventricular groove. Then it is extended horizontally to the right superior pulmonary vein; at this point both atria are opened. The interatrial septum at the fossa ovalis is incised and extended posteriorly and laterally to meet the inferior edge of the previous incision.[64,69] The septal component of this incision should not be extended inferiorly in order to avoid injury to the bundle of His and the tricuspid annulus.

Superior Biatrial Transseptal

The right atrium is incised longitudinally at a distance from the atrioventricular groove. The interatrial septum is opened at the inferior limit of the fossa ovalis and extended superiorly about 2 cm. The right atriotomy is prolonged further superiorly between the right atrial appendage and the atrioventricular sulcus. When the right atriotomy incision meets the septal incision, the roof of the left atrium can then be opened effectively by continuation of the joined incision. The left atriotomy can be further extended to the left at a distance from the aortic root to improve valve exposure.[120] Transseptal approaches, particularly the superior biatrial approach, are useful in minimally invasive direct mitral valve surgery (upper and lower hemisternotomy),[100,109] in reoperative mitral surgery after prior aortic valve replacement,[4] and in patients with a small left atrium.

Deairing Process

Careful deairing at the end of the procedure is essential. Carbon dioxide insufflation at 6 liters/min is used in all patients to reduce intracardiac air. Before the aortic cross-clamp is removed, both lungs are inflated to dislodge any air bubbles in the pulmonary veins, and the left atrial appendage is inverted. Blood and air are expelled through the left atriotomy incision, with the blood being returned to the patient through the cardiotomy suction. The next step is air removal from the left ventricle by active suction in the ascending aorta while manually mobilizing the left ventricle. A small vent should be left across the mitral valve to facilitate deairing after closure of the left atrium. When most of the air is expelled from the heart, the aortic cross-clamp is removed safely. Additional deairing is performed during the rewarming period. The aortic vent is maintained on suction until the patient is totally weaned from cardiopulmonary bypass and complete air removal is confirmed by TEE.

Open Commissurotomy for Mitral Stenosis

Mitral commissurotomy is indicated in pure mitral stenosis with commissural fusion, and preserved leaflet mobility and nonfused subvalvular apparatus. Commissural fusion is usually more intense at the posteromedial commissure than at the anterolateral commissure.

Locating the site of the commissures can be difficult in the presence of advanced rheumatic lesions.[31] Traction on the free edge of the anterior leaflet toward the center of the mitral orifice is helpful to identify the commissural groove. Commissurotomy is started along this groove while leaving a 3-mm tissue ridge from the annulus and is directed toward the center of the orifice. When fused chordae beneath the commissure are identified, they should be fenestrated using a triangular wedge resection. The incision can be extended to the papillary muscle to increase its mobility (Figure 74-10). Calcified nodules in the commissural area should be excised. However, extensive commissural tissue resection is not recommended, because it is very difficult to reconstruct a new commissure. Advanced leaflet thickening or retraction, subvalvular fusion, and commissural calcification are contraindications to mitral commissurotomy, and valve replacement becomes necessary.

Mitral Valve Repair

Mitral valve repair is the procedure of choice for correction of severe mitral regurgitation. The goals of valve repair[31] include preserving leaflet mobility, restoring a large surface of coaptation, and stabilizing the results with a remodeling annuloplasty. Current surgical techniques allow surgeons to perform reconstructive surgery in almost all patients with mitral regurgitation, provided there is an adequate amount of pliable and mobile leaflet tissue. A systematic approach to reconstructive surgery includes the determination of the exact mechanism of mitral regurgitation by intraoperative inspection and valve analysis; meticulous application of standard techniques of repair, including remodeling annuloplasty; and evaluation of the quality of repair by saline test and TEE.

Fundamentals of Reconstructive Surgery

Valve Analysis

The entire mitral valve apparatus must be carefully examined to confirm the mechanism of mitral regurgitation, to assess the feasibility of repair, and to plan the exact operative technique. The endocardium of the left atrium is examined for jet lesions, which indicate opposite leaflet prolapse. The mitral annulus is examined to assess the severity of annular dilatation, which can be asymmetrical. The valvular apparatus is examined with a nerve hook to assess tissue pliability and to identify leaflet prolapse or restriction according to segmental valve analysis.[36] The anterior paracommissural scallop of the posterior leaflet (P_1) is often intact and rarely prolapsing in patients with degenerative disease. The P_1 segment constitutes the reference point. Applying traction to the free edge of other valvular segments and comparing them with P_1 determines the extent of leaflet prolapse or restriction (Figure 74-11).

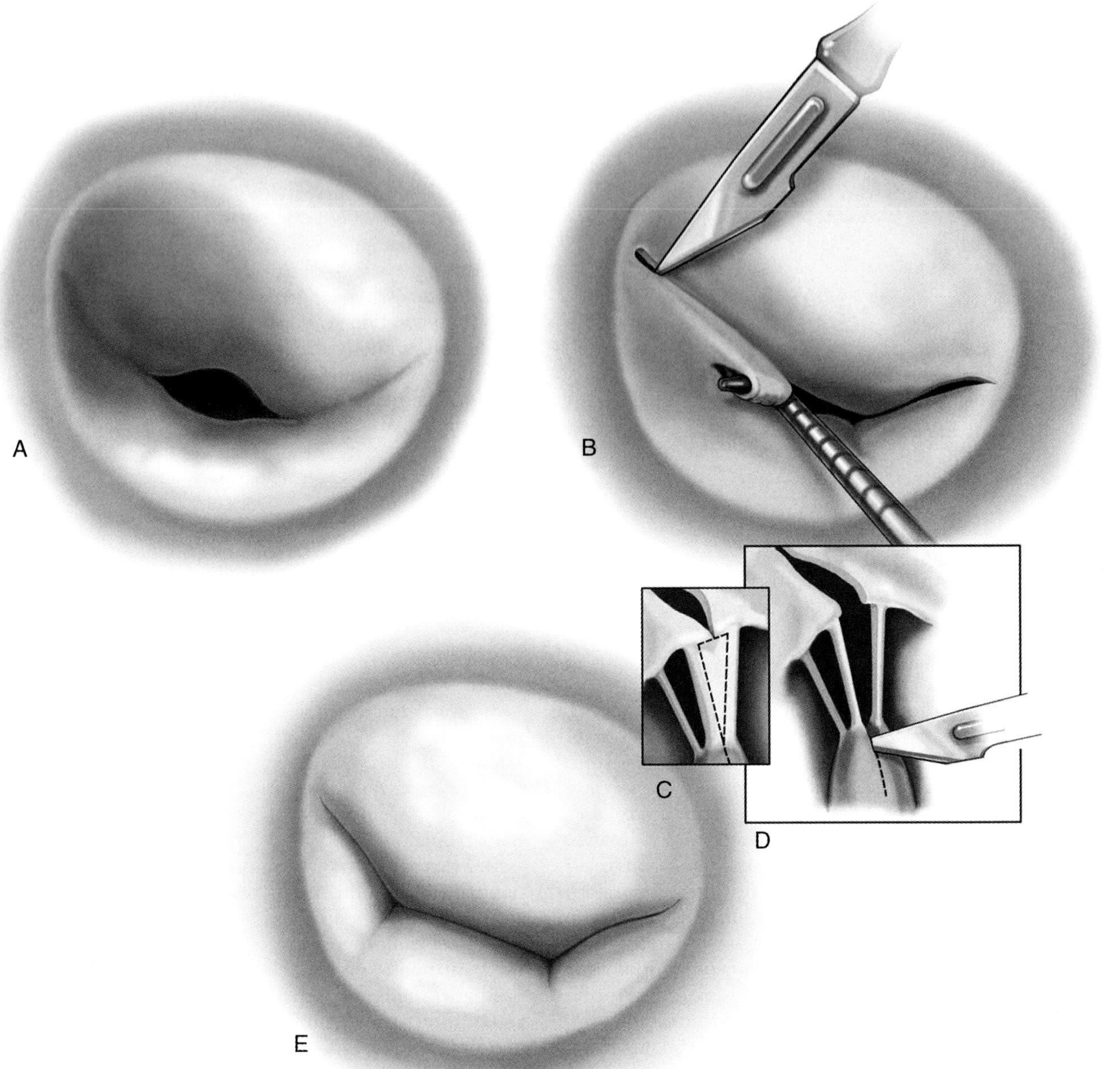

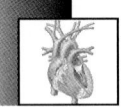

Figure 74–10 **Open commissurotomy. A,** "Fish mouth" opening of a stenotic mitral valve. **B,** Traction on the free edge of the anterior leaflet improves the identification of the commissural area. Commissurotomy is started at 3 mm from the annulus and extends toward the center of the valve. **C,** Triangular wedge resection of fused chordae, which increases subvalvular and leaflet mobility. **D,** Occasionally the incision is extended to the papillary muscle to increase its mobility. **E,** Final aspect of the valve after anterolateral and posteromedial commissurotomies.

Remodeling Ring Annuloplasty

In patients with a normal mitral valve, the ratio between anteroposterior (septolateral) and transverse diameter of the mitral annulus is 3:4 during systole. This ratio is inverted in patients with annular dilatation (Figure 74-12).[36] Regardless of the type of valvular dysfunction, all patients with chronic mitral regurgitation display some degree of annular dilatation, and benefit from a complete remodeling annuloplasty. The remodeling ring annuloplasty restores the physiological ratio with maximal orifice area during systole. Therefore the prosthetic ring restores not only the size, but also the shape of the annulus. Remodeling annuloplasty provides increased leaflet coaptation area without causing any mitral stenosis. Furthermore, it prevents late annular dilatation and preserves leaflet mobility. Appropriate ring sizing is based on the intercommissural distance and the surface area of the anterior leaflet, measured with an obturator (Figure 74-13). Sutures are placed circumferentially through the mitral annulus. These sutures are equally spaced in the area between the two commissures and the corresponding segment of the prosthetic ring. In the remaining portion of the

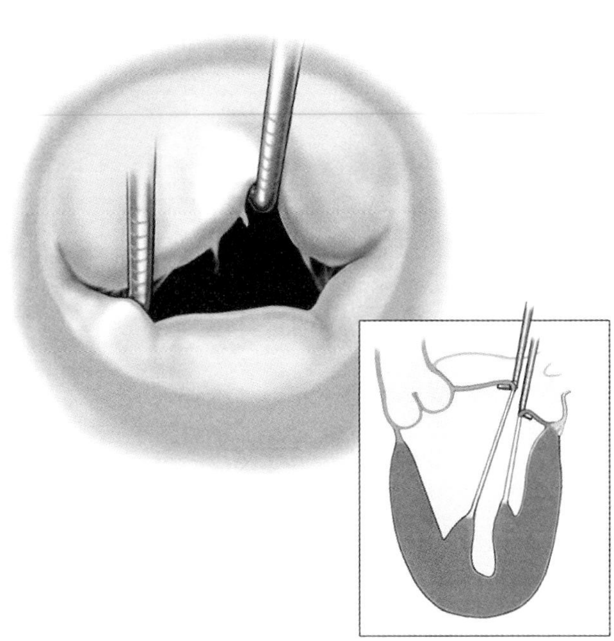

Figure 74–11 Intraoperative segmental valve analysis. P_1 is used as the reference point. Traction on the free edge of P_1 and A_2 reveals prolapse of A_2.

annulus, the spacing is set to conform the annulus to the shape and size of the prosthetic ring.

Assessment of Repair

The quality of the repair must be evaluated at the completion of the repair and before tying the ring to the annulus with a saline test. Saline is injected into the ventricular cavity through the mitral valve with a syringe while the aortic root is vented in order to prevent the presence of air emboli in the coronary arteries. A symmetrical line of coaptation, parallel to the posterior part of the ring, and at a distance from the left ventricular outflow tract, indicates a satisfactory repair. An asymmetrical line of coaptation indicates the presence of residual leaflet prolapse or restricted leaflet motion, which must be corrected. At the completion of cardiopulmonary bypass, the quality of repair is assessed by TEE (see also failure after repair section).[132]

Valve Repair in Type I Dysfunction

Patients with type I dysfunction may have two different types of lesions. Annular dilatation is the most common lesion, which should be corrected with a remodeling annuloplasty. The second type of lesion is leaflet perforation (see considerations in endocarditis section).

Valve Repair in Type II Dysfunction

Posterior Leaflet Prolapse

Posterior leaflet prolapse is treated by a quadrangular resection of the prolapsed area. Stay sutures are placed around the normal chordae to determine the prolapsed area. The prolapsed segment is then removed by performing a perpendicular incision to the free edge toward the annulus, thereby excising a quadrangular portion of the leaflet. Plication sutures are placed along the posterior annulus in the resected area. Finally, direct sutures of the leaflet remnants restore valve continuity (Figure 74-14).

When excessive posterior leaflet tissue is present, such as in Barlow's disease, it is important to reduce the height of the posterior leaflet to avoid postoperative systolic anterior motion (SAM).[129] A sliding leaflet technique is performed after quadrangular resection. The P_1 and P_3 segments are detached from the annulus; compression sutures are then placed in the posterior segment of the annulus. A sliding plasty of the P_1 and P_3 segments is performed, and the gap between the two scallops is closed with interrupted sutures (Figure 74-15). Sliding plasty is also indicated if a large segment of the posterior leaflet is excised. Plication of a large segment of the posterior annulus must be avoided because of the increased risk of circumflex artery kinking.

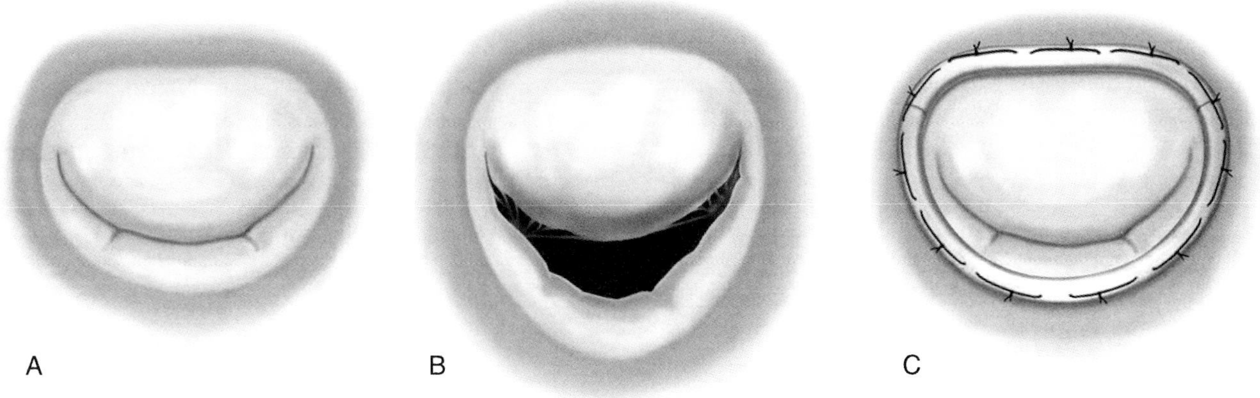

Figure 74–12 Concept of remodeling annuloplasty. A, Normal mitral annulus: The transverse diameter is superior to the anteroposterior (septo lateral) diameter during systole (ratio 3:4). **B,** Dilated mitral annulus (ratio is inverted in mitral regurgitation). **C,** Remodeling prosthetic annuloplasty restores the physiological ratio with maximum orifice area.

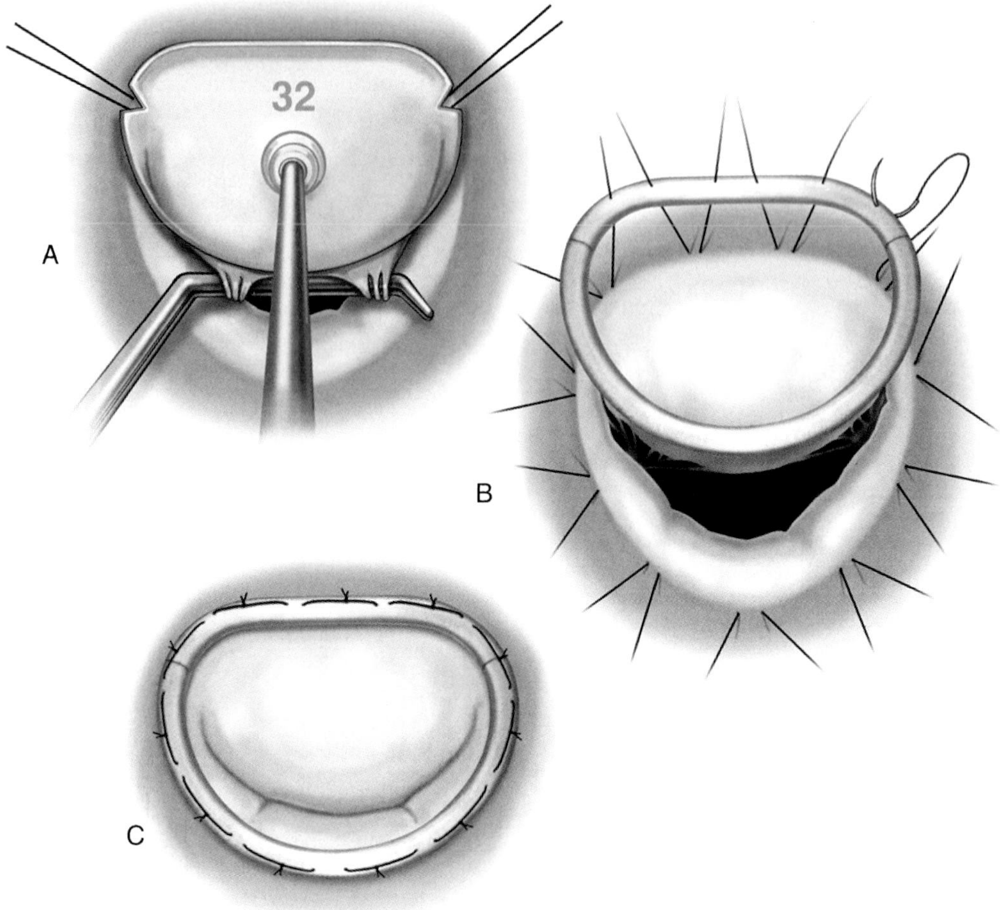

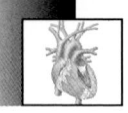

Figure 74–13 **Annuloplasty ring implantation. A,** Ring selection is based on measurements of the intercommissural distance, as well as the height of the anterior leaflet. **B,** Sutures are placed carefully around the annulus and through the ring. **C,** Final result after remodeling annuloplasty.

Anterior Leaflet Prolapse

Several techniques are available to correct anterior leaflet prolapse.

Triangular Resection

Limited prolapse of the anterior leaflet with excess tissue can be treated by a small triangular resection of the prolapsed area, followed by direct closure with interrupted polypropylene sutures.[115] The triangular resection must not be extended to the body of the anterior leaflet. Large resection of the anterior leaflet reduces the coaptation area considerably and is incriminated as a risk factor for repair failure.

Chordal Transfer

Chordal transfer from the secondary position to the free margin of the anterior leaflet is the most preferable technique. A strong and normal secondary chorda adjacent to the prolapsing area is identified. This chorda is detached at 2 mm from its origin on the body of the anterior leaflet. If the chorda is cut at its base, this will likely cause leaflet perforation. It is then attached to the free margin of the anterior leaflet in the prolapsed area with a figure-of-eight suture (Figure 74-16). In case of a large prolapsed area, several secondary chordae should be transferred to the free margin every 5 mm.

Chordal Transposition

In the absence of normal secondary chordae, chordal transposition should be considered. If marginal chordae of the posterior segment opposite to the prolapsed area of the anterior leaflet are normal, they can be used for chordal transposition. This small segment is then detached and reattached to the free margin of the anterior leaflet at the site of prolapse. Interrupted sutures close the defect in the posterior leaflet.

Artificial Chordoplasty

This technique should be used if the previous options are not available. One of the difficulties associated with this technique is the determination of the exact height of the artificial chorda (the distance between the base of the papillary muscle and the free margin of the leaflet) in order to

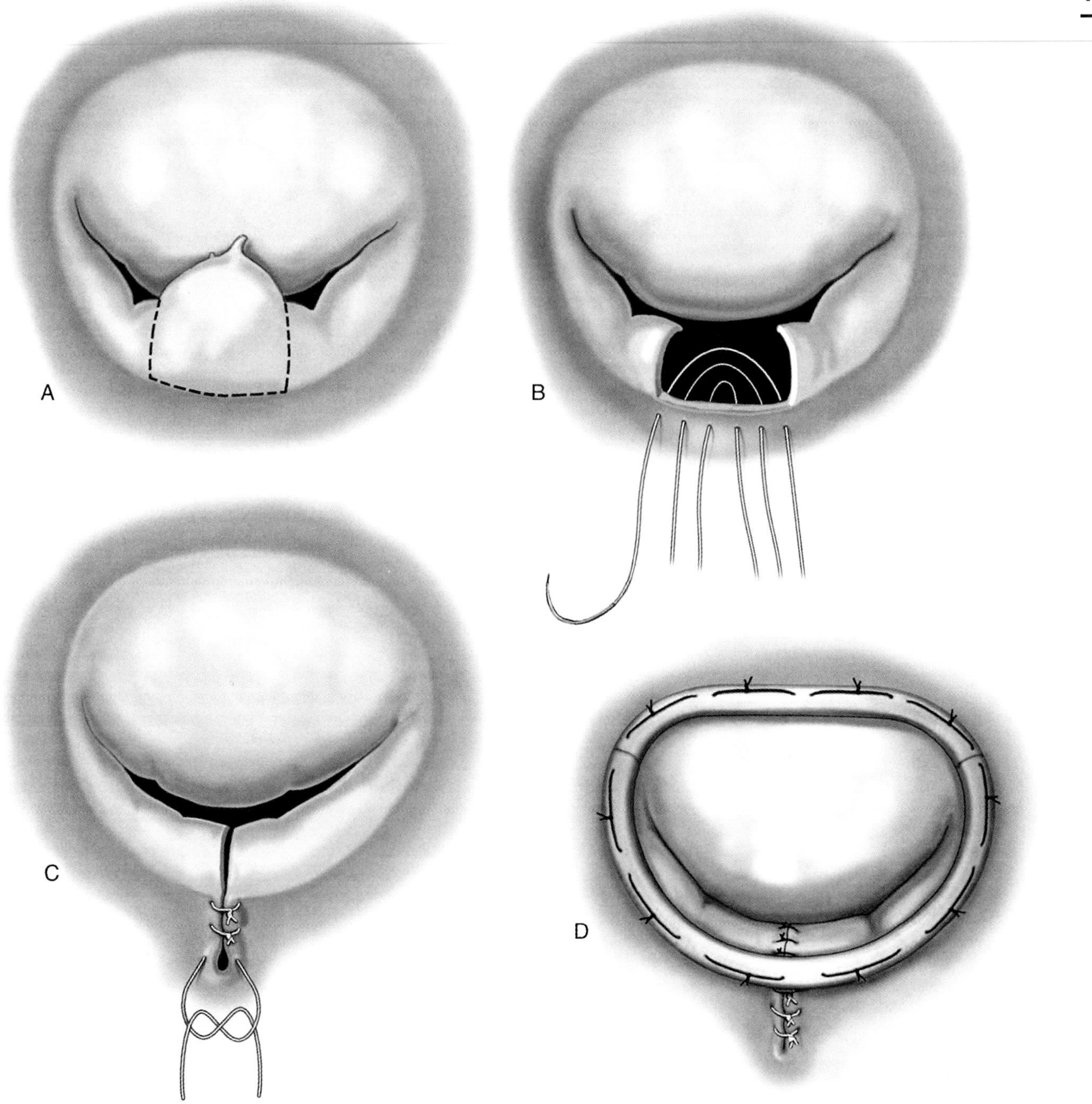

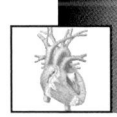

Figure 74–14 Posterior leaflet quadrangular resection. A, Initially the limits of the resection are identified and quadrangular resection is performed as indicated. **B–C,** Several sutures are used to plicate the posterior annulus. **D,** The gap between P_1 and P_3 is closed, and a remodeling annuloplasty is performed.

correct leaflet prolapse without causing leaflet restriction. Several techniques of implantation are described to overcome this hurdle. We use a "functional approach" to determine the exact height of the artificial chorda.[5] According to the extent of leaflet prolapse, one or more 4-0 Gore-Tex sutures without pledgets are placed into the head of the papillary muscle. The Gore-Tex suture is now left aside while the leaflet reconstruction is performed. After ring annuloplasty, symmetrical leaflet apposition limits leaflet incompetence caused by the prolapsing anterior leaflet segment. Now both arms of the previously placed Gore-Tex suture are passed through the margin of the prolapsing leaflet segment. Passing the suture through the free edge of the cusp twice, and starting with a surgeon's knot, are useful techniques to prevent overaggressive sliding of knots when tying the Gore-Tex suture. Optimal chordal height is achieved by intermittently testing valve competency with ventricular saline injections (Figure 74-17).

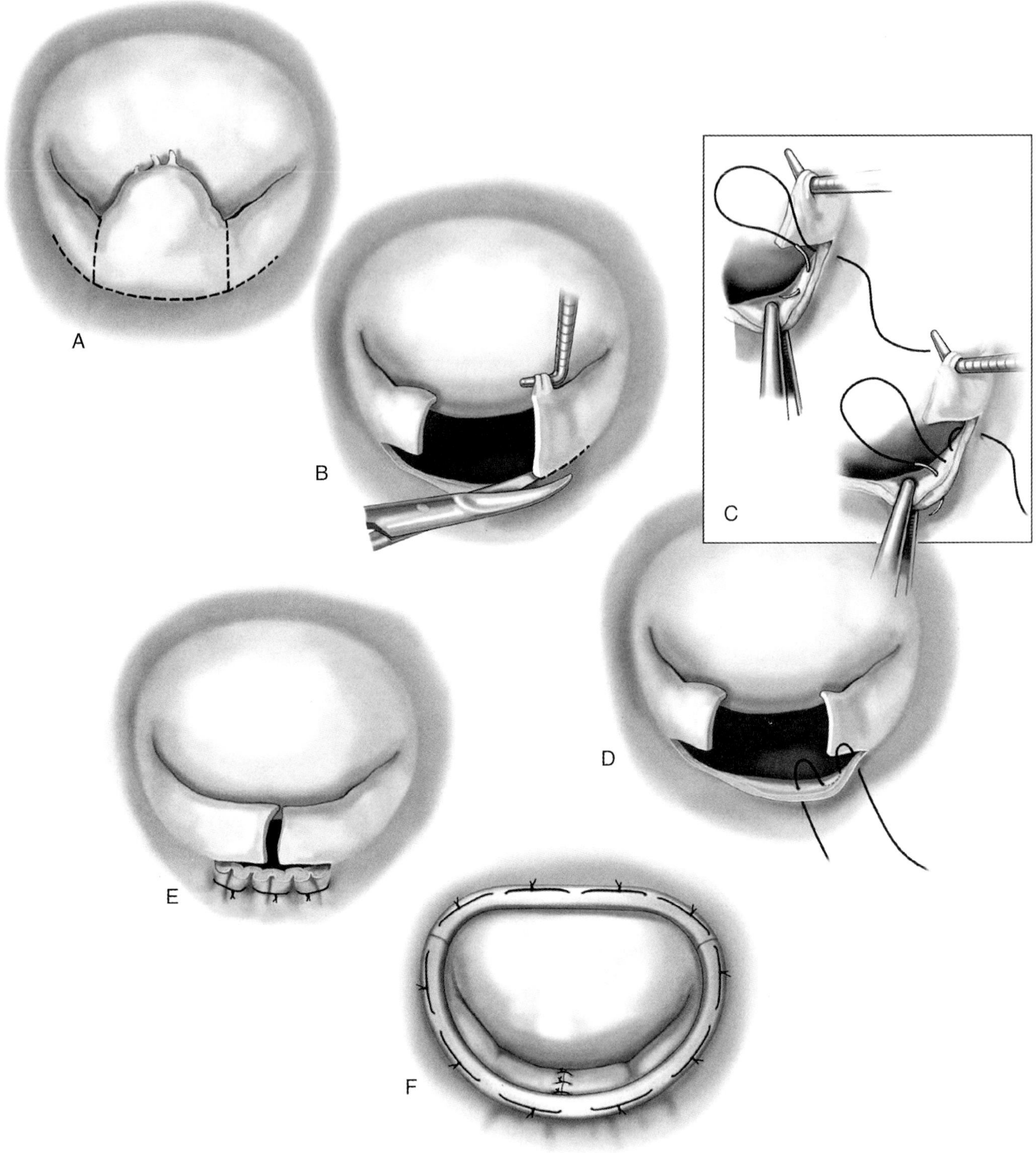

Figure 74–15 **Quadrangular resection and sliding plasty. A–B,** Quadrangular resection is performed. P_1 and P_3 are partially detached from the annulus. **C–E,** Multiple compression sutures are placed. **F,** P_1 and P_3 are translated medially to close the gap. Both segments are reapproximated to restore leaflet continuity, and a remodeling annuloplasty is performed.

Papillary Muscle Sliding Plasty

This technique is convenient for anterior leaflet prolapse caused by elongation of multiple chordae arising from a papillary muscle. The portion of the papillary muscle supporting the elongated chordae is split longitudinally and sutured at a lower level toward its base.

Papillary Muscle Shortening

Papillary muscle elongation or chordal elongation involving a group of chordae can also be treated by papillary muscle shortening. A triangular wedge at the base of the papillary muscle is resected. This defect is then closed by direct suture, resulting in a reduced height of the papillary muscle

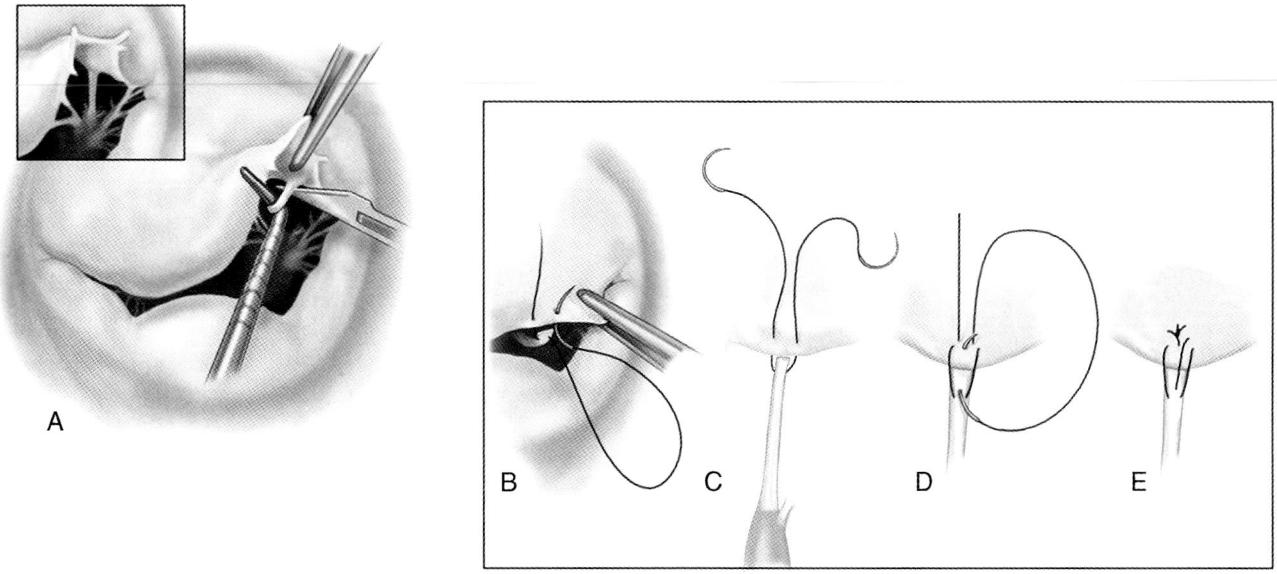

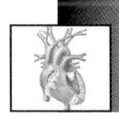

Figure 74–16 **Chordal transfer. A,** A solid secondary chorda is identified adjacent to the prolapsing area of the anterior leaflet. The chorda is detached at 2 mm from its origin of the body of the leaflet. **B–E,** The secondary chorda is reattached to the free margin of the anterior leaflet with a figure-of-eight 6-0 polypropylene suture.

and correction of chordal length. Papillary muscle shortening not only corrects the leaflet prolapse, but also considerably reduces the billowing of the leaflet body. This procedure is typically indicated in Barlow's disease with bileaflet prolapse.

Commissural Prolapse

Commissural prolapse is best treated by resection of the prolapsed area and sliding plasty of the paracommissural area (e.g., A_1 and P_1 sliding plasty for anterolateral commissural prolapse). Additional inverting sutures should be placed in the newly created commissure to avoid residual minimal regurgitation. Occasionally a patient may have a papillary muscle with two heads. The rupture of one head can lead to commissural prolapse, which can be corrected by reattachment of the latter head to the remnant of papillary muscle. If extensive commissural and paracommissural prolapse are present, papillary muscle sliding plasty or papillary muscle shortening are valuable options.

Mitral Valve Repair in Type IIIA Dysfunction

In type IIIA dysfunction, correction of mitral regurgitation and adequate leaflet mobilization can be achieved by treating each type of lesion. Leaflet restriction is often due to chordal thickening, retraction, and fusion. Resection of the secondary chordae, particularly on the posterior leaflet, may increase leaflet mobility. The fusion of marginal chordae is best treated by chordal fenestration with removal of a triangular wedge of fibrous tissue; this maneuver not only improves leaflet mobility, but also reduces the subvalvular stenosis. Leaflet retraction can also be treated by pericardial patch enlargement. Severe retraction of the posterior leaflet is a common finding in patients with type IIIA dysfunction. The posterior leaflet is detached from the mitral annulus, and the secondary chordae are removed. Inserting a diamond-shaped segment of autologous glutaraldehyde-fixed pericardial patch between the posterior leaflet and the annulus restores posterior leaflet integrity.[41] In the presence of commissural fusion, additional commissurotomy as previously described is necessary.

Mitral Valve Repair in Type IIIB Dysfunction

Remodeling annuloplasty using an undersized ring is the technique of choice in type IIIB dysfunction.[3] The typical size of the ring is between 24–28 mm. The insertion of an undersized prosthetic ring in a severely dilated annulus may cause excessive tension on the sutures, leading to ring dehiscence. Placing multiple sutures around the annulus, which overlap each other, prevents this complication. This overlapping is particularly important at the level of the posteromedial commissure and the P_3 segment, in ischemic mitral regurgitation. Other adjunct techniques, such as posterior leaflet extension with a patch of autologous pericardium and resection of secondary chordae, are indicated in a selected group of patients. The first procedure increases the coaptation surface of the posterior leaflet, whereas the second improves its mobility. For further description, see Chapter 82.

Annular Decalcification and Annular Reconstruction

Mitral reconstructive surgery is difficult in the presence of annular calcification. In this setting, valve replacement carries a greater risk of atrioventricular disruption, perivalvular leak, and valve dehiscence. In most cases it is necessary to remove annular calcification before valve repair or replacement. Annular decalcification is performed by detachment of the leaflet, followed by en bloc excision of the calcifications.[15,37]

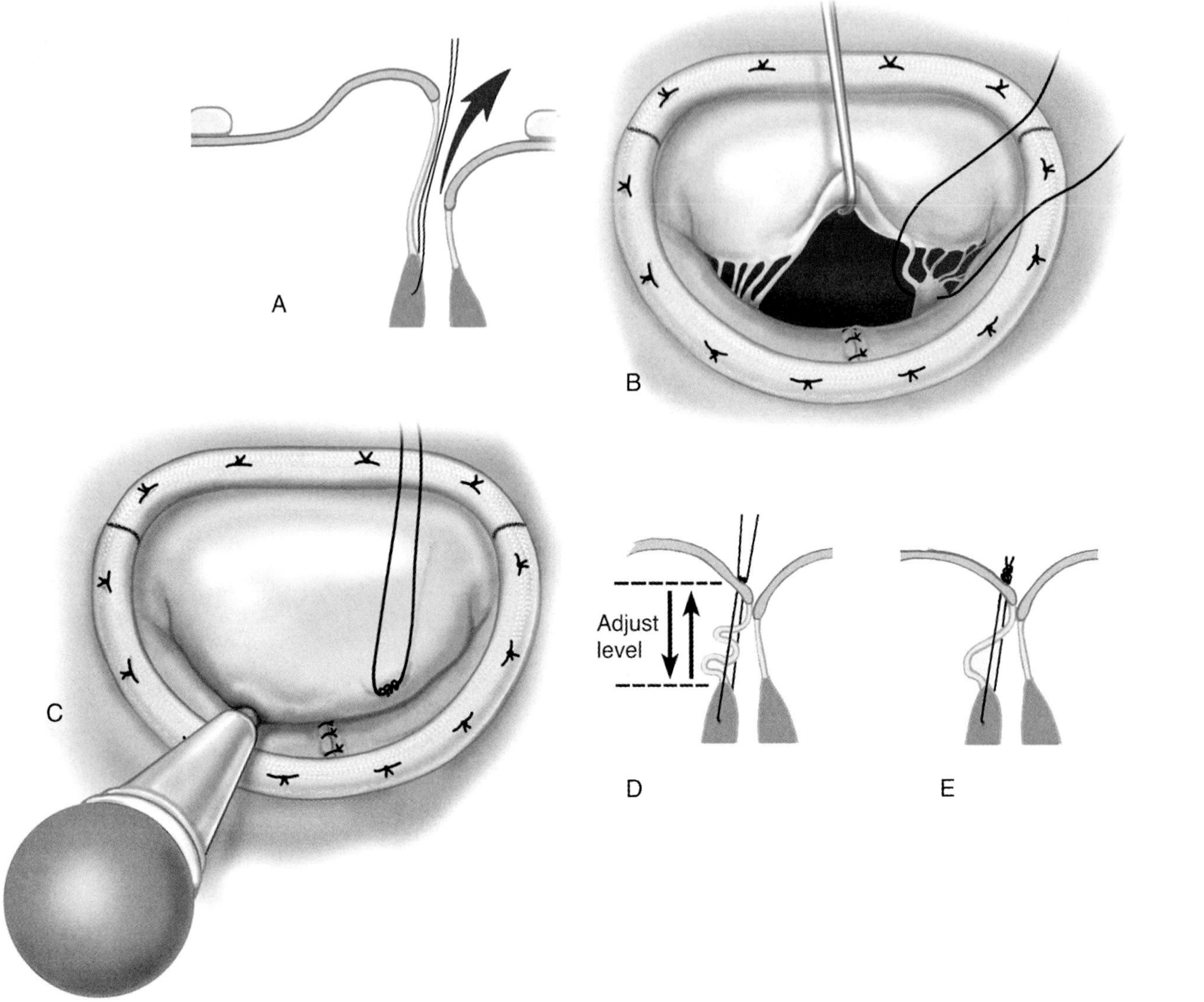

Figure 74–17 Artificial chordoplasty. A, The artificial Gore-Tex chorda is placed into the head of the papillary muscle at the initial phase of the repair, before remodeling annuloplasty and is left aside while the leaflet reconstruction is performed. **B,** After remodeling annuloplasty, systemic leaflet apposition limits valve incompetence to the prolapsing anterior leaflet segment. Also, both arms of the Gore-Tex suture are passed through the margin of the prolapsing segment. **C–E,** Optimal artificial chordal height is determined by intermittently testing valve competency by injecting saline into the ventricle.

This procedure may lead to localized atrioventricular disjunction, which requires annular reconstruction.

An annular abscess can complicate native endocarditis or prosthetic endocarditis.[57,61] After annular débridement, annular reconstruction may become necessary. Carpentier and David have described different techniques for mitral annular reconstruction.

Mitral annular reconstruction using autologous or glutaraldehyde-fixed bovine pericardium is known as the David technique.[59,60] Posterior annular reconstruction is accomplished using a semicircular-shaped pericardial patch. While ensuring that the patch is large enough to completely cover the defect, one side of the patch is sutured to the endocardium of the left ventricle and the other side is used to secure the prosthetic valve. In patients with complete destruction of the annulus, a circumferential patch is tailored for annular reconstruction.

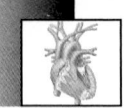

Mitral annular reconstruction using figure-of-eight atrial and ventricular sutures is known as the Carpentier technique.[37] With this technique the atrioventricular junction is constructed by a series of figure-of-eight 2-0 braided sutures placed into the atrial and ventricular edges. These sutures are then brought out on the atrial side. The ventricular bites of theses sutures should only involve one third of the thickness of the myocardial wall and be as wide as possible, taking advantage of any fibrous tissue present on the surface of the myocardium. Exerting traction on these sutures reduces the size of the annulus and closes the atrioventricular groove without injury to the circumflex vessels. The closure of the atrioventricular groove is facilitated by downward displacement of the atrial edge toward the ventricular edge with forceps. By means of this technique, the circumflex vessels and surrounding fat are displaced outward and the atrioventricular junction is restored as a firm fibrous structure available for valve replacement. If the infectious process involves the ventricular myocardium, the atrial edge is dissected free to mobilize an atrial flap (sliding atrium technique), which is used to cover the destroyed area. The fat and connective tissue surrounding the circumflex vessels are left attached to the ventricular side. Figure-of-eight sutures, as described earlier, are used to reconstruct the annulus and cover the ventricular area. After mitral annular reconstruction, valve repair or replacement is performed using the standard technique. In patients undergoing valve replacement, the presence of pliable annular tissue significantly decreases the risk of valve dehiscence and perivalvular leak.

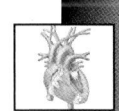

Considerations in Endocarditis

The first step of mitral valve surgery for endocarditis is the radical resection of all infected and necrotic tissues within a 1–2-mm margin of normal tissue without any concern about the possibility of repair. The feasibility of mitral valve repair depends on the availability of healthy tissue after débridement. In the event of entire leaflet involvement or extensive destruction of subvalvular apparatus, prosthetic valve replacement is required. However, mitral valve repair can be achieved safely in multiple anatomical presentations, provided sufficient tissue remains to allow valvular reconstruction without excessive tension on the suture lines.[68,121,158,175] Leaflet perforation with normal leaflet motion (type I dysfunction) is a typical lesion in acute endocarditis, which often affects the anterior leaflet. After débridement, the leaflet defect is repaired with a patch of glutaraldehyde-fixed preserved autologous pericardium. The patch is sewn to the remaining leaflet with polypropylene suture. Other standard techniques of repair such as leaflet resection and sliding plasty, chordal transposition, and so on, are commonly applicable according to specific lesions. The implantation of a prosthetic ring remains controversial. In patients with a dilated annulus, prosthetic ring annuloplasty should be used, whereas in absence of annular dilatation, its implantation can be avoided. Alternatively, a glutaraldehyde-fixed pericardial strip can be used to fashion a posterior annuloplasty.[158]

Mitral Valve Replacement

Mitral valve replacement should be performed in patients who are not suitable for mitral valve repair (extensive leaflet destruction resulting from endocarditis, heavy calcification of leaflets, and subvalvular apparatus resulting from rheumatic disease). Chordal-sparing mitral valve replacement is the preferred technique whenever possible.[53,55] This technique preserves postoperative left ventricular function, contributing to improved long-term survival of these patients.[24,62,189,192]

A traction suture is placed in the midportion of the anterior leaflet. Traction on the suture toward the center of the orifice improves leaflet exposure. An incision is made in the center of the anterior leaflet parallel to and 2 mm from the annulus. The incision is continued in both directions toward the commissures. Detachment of the anterior leaflet improves visualization of the subvalvular apparatus. The underlying fused chordae are resected. In most cases the posterior leaflet and its chordae are left intact to preserve ventriculoannular continuity. Therefore only the anterior leaflet is completely excised. If the subvalvular apparatus of the posterior leaflet is severely fused and retracted, a partial excision of the subvalvular apparatus may be necessary. Partial preservation of the anterior leaflet and its subvalvular apparatus should be considered if these structures are thin and mobile. A segment of A_1 and A_3 with their respective subvalvular apparatus are detached from their anatomical position and reattached with interrupted sutures to the corresponding commissures.[154]

Appropriate obturators are used to determine the exact size of valvular prosthesis. Mitral prostheses (mechanical or bioprosthesis) can be inserted with different suture techniques, including interrupted sutures and continuous running sutures. Everting pledgeted horizontal mattress sutures (pledgets on the atrial side) are favored by most surgeons (Figure 74-18). In the presence of annular calcification, noneverting pledgeted horizontal mattress sutures (pledgets on the ventricular side) become a valuable option. After the insertion of a bileaflet mitral prosthesis, opening and closing motions of both leaflets must be checked to rule out tissue impingement. When a bioprosthesis is used, the valve struts should be oriented away from the left ventricular outflow tract. In addition, it is essential to ensure that no suture is looping around a strut. A Foley catheter is usually placed through the mitral prosthesis to provide left ventricular decompression by maintaining the mitral prosthetic valve incompetent. The atrium is then closed in a standard fashion around the Foley catheter. After mitral valve replacement, cardiac manipulation should be minimized to avoid atrioventricular rupture.

RESULTS

Open Commissurotomy for Mitral Stenosis

Open commissurotomy for pure mitral stenosis carries an operative risk less than 0.5%.[43,111,123,124] The procedure is associated with good early and late outcome; however, mitral commissurotomy is not a definite procedure, and most patients will require another intervention (valve replacement is most likely) at some point in their life. The progression of the disease with advanced rheumatic lesions is the principal indication for reoperative mitral valve replacement. In a consecutive series of 339 young patients undergoing open mitral commissurotomy, Hickey et al[124] reported an overall survival of 95%, 87%, and 59% at 5, 10, and 20 years, respectively. Freedom from reoperation was 78% and 47% at 10 and 20 years, respectively. In the report by Herrera et al,[123] actuarial survival was 89% and 75% at 15 and 18 years, respectively. Freedom from reoperation at 18-year follow up was 92%.

Mitral Valve Repair for Mitral Regurgitation

Mortality and Late Survival

The operative mortality of mitral valve surgery has significantly decreased over the last 2 decades after both repair and replacement. These improved results are achieved despite referral of most complex patients secondary to advanced age and increased comorbidities, including left ventricular dysfunction. Several variables such as a better

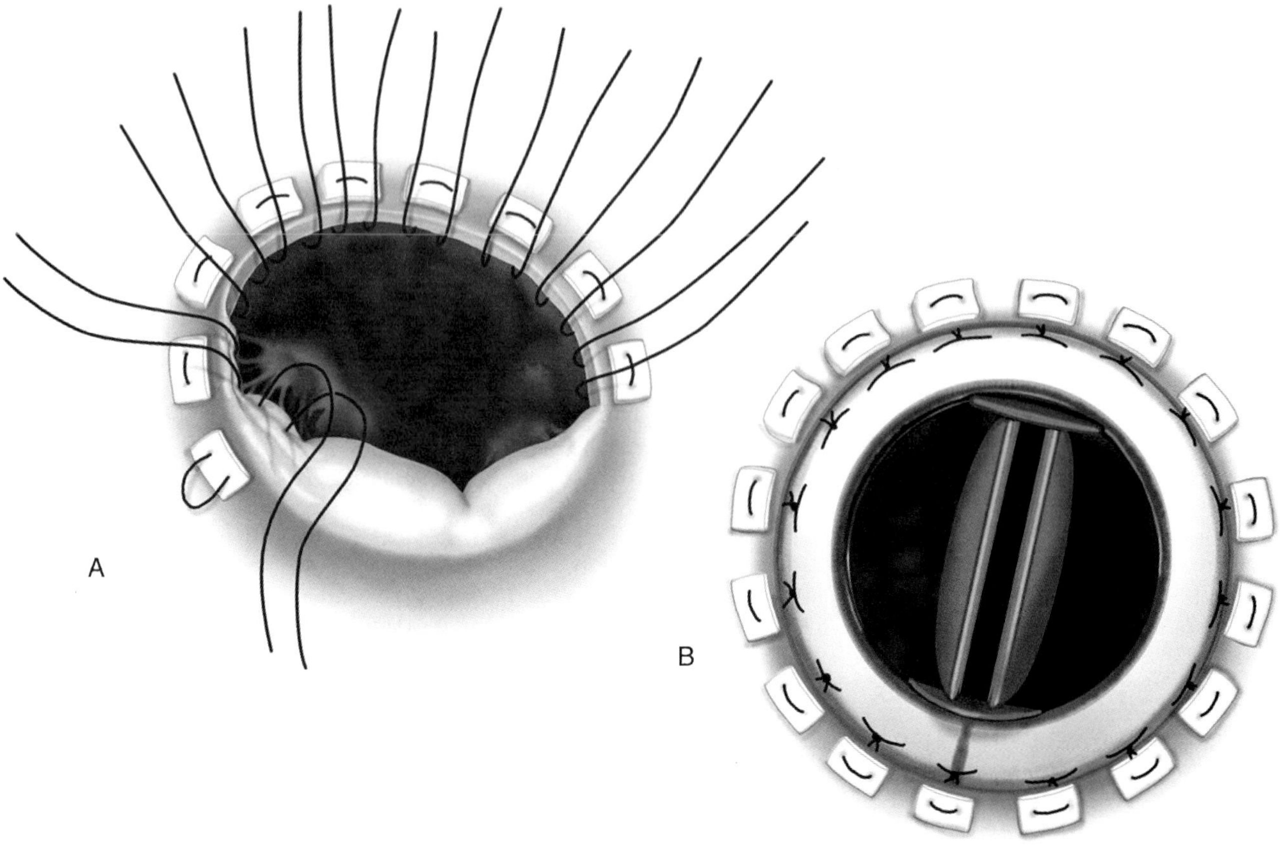

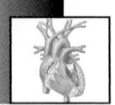

Figure 74–18 **Mitral valve replacement. A,** Suture placement: Everting pledgeted horizontal mattress sutures are placed around the annulus. **B,** Sutures are placed through the sewing ring of a bileaflet mechanical prosthesis, which is then secured in place.

understanding of the pathophysiology of mitral regurgitation, patient selection, intraoperative TEE, myocardial protection, and improved surgical techniques have all contributed to decrease operative mortality.[96]

Early clinical studies reported an operative mortality of 2–4% in patients with nonischemic mitral regurgitation after valve repair (Table 74-3). Currently in advanced centers the mortality of isolated elective mitral valve repair is less than 0.5% (Table 74-4).* Several studies have confirmed the superiority of mitral valve repair over mitral valve replacement (see Table 74-3).† The reduced mortality in the repair group is related to a better preservation of postoperative left ventricular function.[84] In a comparative study between mitral valve repair and replacement, Enriquez-Sarano et al[83] demonstrated that valve repair was an independent predictor of higher postoperative EF in multivariate analysis. Risk factors incriminated in early mortality include advanced age, functional class (NYHA class III–IV), and associated coronary artery disease.[83]

Long-term survival for mitral valve repair at 10 years ranges from 68–94% in nonischemic patients. In Braunberger's series,[25,79,181] 20-year survival after repair for degenerative mitral valve disease was 47%. It is important to notice that in patients with degenerative disease and normal preoperative left ventricular function and minimal symptoms (NYHA class I–II), the observed life expectancy after repair is similar to that of the general population at the same age.[25,79] The long-term survival after repair is also superior when compared with that of valve replacement (Figure 74-19; see Table 74-3). This survival benefit is maintained in all subgroup analyses regardless of the etiology (except ischemic mitral regurgitation) and age (see Table 74-3).

Congestive heart failure is the most common cause of late death.[82] This complication is often due to preoperative left ventricular dysfunction, best reflected by depressed EF (Figure 74-20). Several other factors such as preoperative symptoms, etiology of mitral regurgitation (ischemic versus nonischemic), and age also affect late survival.[156,157]

The feasibility and long-term results of mitral valve repair varies according to the primary etiology of valve disease. For example, with the current techniques, mitral valve repair can be performed in more than 95% of patients with degenerative valve disease, whereas the repair rate is about 70% in patients with rheumatic disease.[65] The prognostic value of etiology on long-term surgical outcome is also well demonstrated when comparing the reoperation rate between degenerative and rheumatic disease.[52] Moreover, the results of mitral valve repair are affected at a lesser

*References 70, 79, 105, 138, 169, 170.
†References 6, 83, 95, 105, 157, 191.

Table 74–4

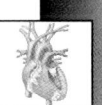

Clinical Series Comparing Mitral Valve Repair versus Replacement

Reference (year)	*Study period*	*Etiology of MR*	*Operative mortality (%) repair vs. replacement*	**Survival (%) repair versus replacement**		
				5 yr	*10 yr*	*15 yr*
Galloway et al (1989)	1976–1987	Mixed	2 vs. 8	81 vs. 73	—	—
Akins et al (1994)	1985–1992	Degenerative	3 vs. 12	89 vs. 61	—	
Enriquez-Sarano et al (1995)	1980–1989	Degenerative	2.6 vs. 10.3	83 vs. 69	68 vs. 52	—
Yau et al (2000)	1978–1995	Rheumatic	0.7 vs. 5.2[a] 5.6[b]	97 vs. 88[a] 83[b]	88 vs. 83[a] 73[b]	— —
Mohty et al (2001)	1980–1995	Degenerative	—	86 vs. 71	68 vs. 49	37 vs. 29
Gillinov et al (2003)	1973–1999	Degenerative and coronary artery disease[c]	3 vs. 6	79 vs. 70	59 vs. 37	—

MR, Mitral regurgitation.
[a]Mechanical valve.
[b]Bioprosthetic valve.
[c]Patients with true ischemic MR were excluded.

degree by the choice of repair techniques.[39,103] Refined analysis of surgical outcome after valve repair should therefore take these two parameters into consideration.

Results According to Etiology

Degenerative Valve Disease

Patients with degenerative valve disease are most suitable for reconstructive surgery. Long-term results of repair are excellent in this group (Table 74-4).* Carpentier's group has recently published their very long-term results (20 years) of mitral repair using his techniques.[25,77] This observational study of 162 consecutive patients operated on between 1970 and 1984 was mostly composed of patients with degenerative disease (90%). The main mechanism of mitral regurgitation was type II dysfunction. Posterior, anterior, and bileaflet prolapse were present in 93%, 28%, and 31% of patients, respectively. All patients underwent annuloplasty; valve resection was done in 126 patients, and shortening or transposition of the chordae was performed in 46 patients. The linearized rate of reoperation was 0.4% per patient year. Freedom from reoperation was 97%, 86%, and 83% for posterior, anterior, and bileaflet prolapse, respectively, at 20 years (Figure 74-21). Other studies have confirmed the increased freedom from reoperation for posterior leaflet prolapse compared with anterior leaflet.[102,157] These data confirm the increased difficulty of repair for anterior leaflet prolapse compared with posterior prolapse. The increased rate of early reoperation in the anterior leaflet prolapse group was attributed to technical failure. The widespread use of intraoperative TEE and improved surgical techniques (chordal transfer) have most likely contributed to reducing the incidence of early failure in recent years.[152,177] However, the freedom from reoperation was constant and identical at 10, 20, and 25 years of follow-up. These excellent and stable results confirm the predictability and durability of valve repair in the majority of patients with degenerative disease. Incremental risk factors for early and late failure are discussed in the reoperation section. Finally, it should be noted that several clinical studies have reported a similar reoperation rate after valve repair and replacement.[56,157]

*References 25, 47, 56, 102, 130, 157.

Rheumatic Disease

Mitral valve repair is more difficult and less durable in rheumatic patients compared with patients with degenerative valve disease (Table 74-5).* Patients with advanced rheumatic

*References 14, 40, 44, 72, 74, 141, 191.

Table 74–5

Results in Patients with Degenerative Mitral Valve Disease

Reference (year)	*Study period*	*Operative mortality (%)*	Survival (%)				Freedom from reoperation (%)				Freedom from TE complications (%)		Freedom from endocarditis (%)	
			5 yr	*10 yr*	*15 yr*	*20 yr*	*5 yr*	*10 yr*	*15 yr*	*20 yr*	*5 yr*	*10 yr*	*5 yr*	*10 yr*
David et al (1993)	1981–1992	0	91	88*	—	—	95	95*	—	—	87	82	100	100[a]
Cohn et al (1994)	1984–1993	2.3	89	—	—	—	88	—	—	—	92	—	97	—
Gillinov et al (1998)	1985–1997	0.3	93	81	—	—	97	93	—	—	96	88	99	99
Mohty et al (2001)	1980–1995	—	86	68	37	—	Post 97 Ant 89	92 82	97 86	97 86	—	—	—	—
Braunberger et al (2001)	1970–1984	1.9	—	74	—	47	Post 99 Ant 92	98 86	97 86	97 86	—	—	—	—

TE, Thromboembolic; Post, posterior leaflet prolapse; Ant, anterior leaflet prolapse.
[a]Survival at 8 years.

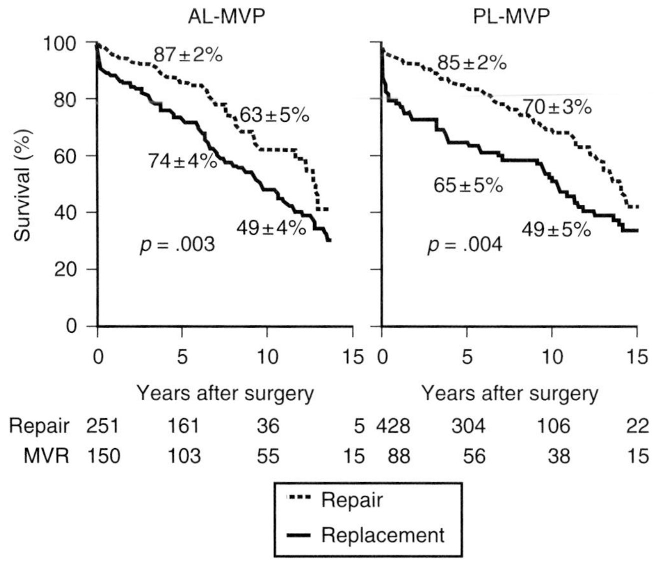

Figure 74–19 Long-term survival after surgical correction of mitral regurgitation (MR) resulting from mitral valve prolapse (MVP) (repair, dashed lines; replacement [MVR], solid lines) in patients with anterolateral MVP (AL-MVP) *(left)* and posterolateral MVP (PL-MVP) *(right)*. Numbers at bottom of each graph indicate number of patients at risk for the interval. Survival estimates (mean ± SE) are indicated at 5 and 10 years.
(Modified from Mohty D, Orszulak TA, Schaff HV, et al: Very long-term survival and durability of mitral valve repair for mitral valve prolapse. Circulation 104:I1–I7, 2001.)

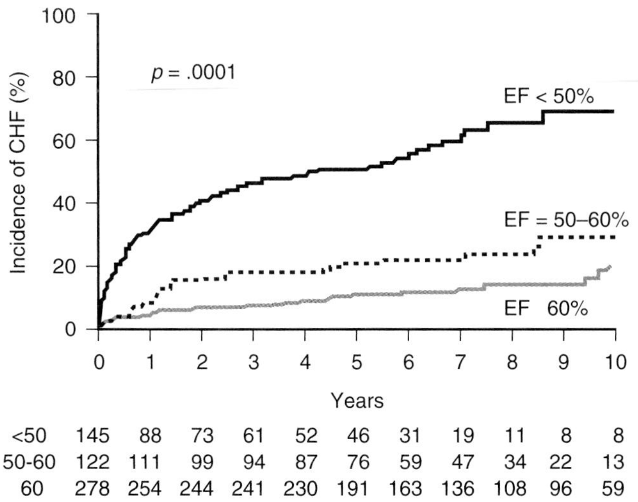

Figure 74–20 Graph showing incidence of congestive heart failure (CHF) according to the level of preoperative ejection fraction (EF). Numbers underneath show indicate the number of patients at risk for the interval.
(Modified from Enriquez-Sarano M, Schaff HV, Orszulak TA, et al: Congestive heart failure after surgical correction of mitral regurgitation. A long-term study. Circulation 92:2496–2503, 1995.)

disease (severe leaflet thickening or retraction, fusion of the subvalvular apparatus, and extensive leaflet calcification) are not ideal candidates for valve repair. These suboptimal outcomes are best reflected by a linearized rate of reoperation, which is 2–3% patient year. Chauvaud et al[40] studied 951 patients with rheumatic mitral regurgitation who underwent mitral surgery from 1970 to 1994. Type I, II, and IIIA valvu-

Table 74–6

Results of Mitral Valve Repair in Patients with Rheumatic Mitral Valve Disease

Reference (year)	*Study period*	*Operative mortality (%)*	Survival (%)				Freedom from reoperation (%)			
			5 yr	*10 yr*	*15 yr*	*20 yr*	*5 yr*	*10 yr*	*15 yr*	*20 yr*
Duran et al (1991)	1988–1990	1	94[a]	—	—	—	—	—	—	—
Bernal et al (1993)	1975–1999	2.7	—	—	84	—	—	—	89	—
Yau et al (2000)	1978–1995	0.7	97	88	—	—	87	72	—	—
Choudhary et al[b] (2001)	1988–1999	4	—	92	—	—	—	65	—	—
Chauvaud et al (2001)	1970–1994	2	—	89	—	82	—	82	—	55

[a]30 months follow-up.
[b]88% of patients with rheumatic etiology.

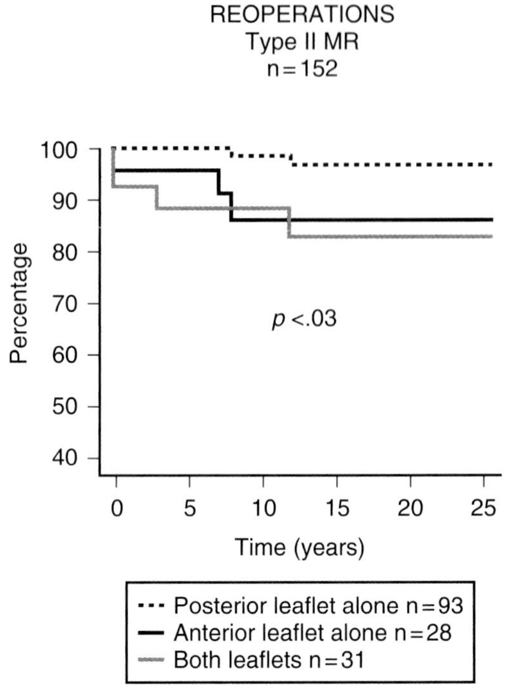

Figure 74–21 **Reoperations according to leaflet prolapse.** *(Modified from Braunberger E, Deloche A, Berrebi A, et al: Very long-term results (more than 20 years) of valve repair with Carpentier's techniques in nonrheumatic mitral valve insufficiency. Circulation 104:I8–I11, 2001.)*

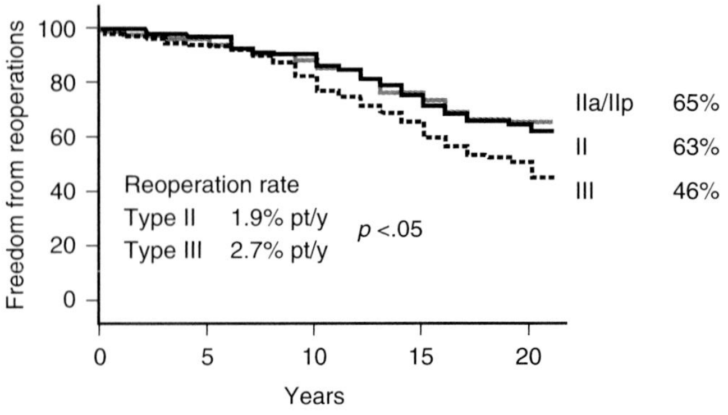

Figure 74–22 **Freedom from reoperation related to functional type.** *(Modified from Chauvaud S, Fuzellier JF, Berrebi A, et al: Long-term [29 years] results of reconstructive surgery in rheumatic mitral valve insufficiency. Circulation 104:I12–I15, 2001.)*

lar dysfunction were noted in 7%, 33%, and 36% of patients, respectively. The prolapse of anterior leaflet combined with restriction of the posterior leaflet (type II anterior, IIIA posterior) was present in 224 patients (24%). Valve repair was performed in 95% of patients. Freedom from reoperation was 82% and 55% at 10 and 20 years, respectively. Progression of the disease with advanced fibrosis of the mitral valve was the principal cause for reoperation (83% of cases). In this study the reoperation rate for type II dysfunction was 1.9% patient year, whereas it was 2.7% patient year for type IIIA dysfunction (Figure 74-22). The initial presence of leaflet thickening and commissural fibrosis had a negative impact on the late outcome. Finally, freedom from valve-related complications was 82% and 52%, respectively, at 10 and 20 years. Similarly, Yau et al[191] reported a series of 573 rheumatic patients who underwent mitral valve surgery (repair 25%, replacement 75%) from 1978 to 1995. At 10 years, freedom from reoperation for the repair group was 87%. Also in this study, advanced rheumatic valve disease, complex repair for mitral regurgitation, and combined lesions of mitral regurgitation with mitral stenosis were associated with a high reoperative rate.

Endocarditis

Clinical series from Broussais Hospital[68] and the Cleveland Clinic[121,158] have reported repair rates of 80% and 45%, respectively, in native mitral valve endocarditis. Historically the operative mortality of native mitral endocarditis has been high. Recent clinical series have documented outstanding results with valve repair in the setting of mitral endocarditis, with mortality rates up to 9%.[10,57,68,133,162] Preserving native mitral valve tissue by means of repair and avoiding valve prosthesis in the setting of active infection most likely accounts for this observation. The survival benefit for repair versus replacement has also been demonstrated in this condition. In a series of 146 patients from the Cleveland Clinic who underwent mitral valve surgery (repair 102 versus replacement 44) for mitral valve endocarditis, event-free survival rate after mitral valve repair versus replacement was 74% versus 24% at 6 years.[158,175]

Dilated Cardiomyopathy

In 1995 Bolling et al[21] first reported the correction of severe mitral regurgitation with prosthetic ring annuloplasty in the very high-risk group of patients with dilated cardiomyopathy. Limited data and only midterm results are currently available to assess the efficacy and the potential survival benefit of this procedure.[17,22,30,42,166] In 2002 Bolling[19] published his experience in a group of 140 patients with end-stage cardiomyopathy and refractory mitral regurgitation despite maximal medical therapy. All patients were in NYHA class III–IV, had severe left ventricular dysfunction (EF <25%), and underwent undersized flexible annuloplasty ring implantation. Operative mortality was 5%. Actuarial survival at 1, 2, and 5 years was 80%, 70%, and 57%, respectively. At 2-year follow up, all patients were in NYHA class I and II, and the mean cardiac output increased from 3.1 liters/min (preoperative) to 5.2 liters/min. These data suggest a survival benefit of mitral valve repair compared with medical treatment in advanced dilated cardiomyopathy with severe mitral regurgitation (57% versus 20% at 5 years). Randomized prospective trials are necessary to further confirm these encouraging results.

Calcifying Disease of the Annulus

In a series of 68 patients with extensive calcification of the annulus and severe mitral regurgitation, Carpentier et al[37] reported their experience with his technique of "en bloc" decalcification, annular reconstruction, and valve repair. Decalcification remains localized in 77% of the cases and involved more than one third of the annulus in 88%. The operative mortality was 3%. No cases of annulus dehiscence or early reoperation were reported. At 7 years the actuarial survival and freedom from reoperation were 93% and 83%, respectively. Freedom from valve-related complication at 9 years was 85%. Feindel et al[88] also reported a series of 54 patients undergoing mitral valve surgery for extensive annular calcification and severe mitral regurgitation. Annular decalcification and reconstruction with autologous pericardium was performed in all patients. Mitral valve repair and replacement were performed in 12 and 42 patients, respectively. In this series the 5-year survival rate was 73%, whereas 89% of patients remained free from reoperation at 5 years. The 5-year freedom from valve-related mortality and morbidity was 75%. None of these series reported any case of atrioventricular disruption.

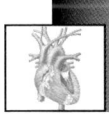

Results According to Operative Technique

Artificial Chordoplasty

The use of artificial chordoplasty in mitral valve repair remains controversial. Some surgeons use artificial chordoplasty as their primary technique for correcting anterior leaflet prolapse, whereas others reserve this technique to scenarios where chordal transfer or transposition is not feasible. David and associates[58] reported a series of 165 patients undergoing mitral repair by artificial chordoplasty with Gore-Tex, for anterior or bileaflet prolapse. Actuarial freedom from reoperation was 96% at 10 years. In a study reported by Cohn et al,[47] the freedom for reoperation rate was 85% at 5 years with the use of artificial chordoplasty. This technique is a valuable adjunct in selected patients with extensive anterior leaflet prolapse or when other techniques (e.g., chordal transfer, chordal transposition) cannot be performed.

Edge-to-Edge Repair

In the early 1990s Alfieri et al[9] popularized the concept of edge-to-edge repair, which was first described by Nichols[160] about 50 years ago. This simple technique of repair consists of suturing the edges of the leaflets at the site of regurgitation. This procedure can be applied at the paracommissural area (e.g., A_1–P_1 segments: paracommissural repair) or at the middle of the valve (e.g., A_2–P_2 segments: double-orifice repair).

Initially Alfieri applied the edge-to edge repair in patients regardless of the etiology of mitral regurgitation. These studies showed a high rate of failure in patients with rheumatic mitral regurgitation. They also showed that isolated edge-to-edge repair is associated with a high rate of failure and that a concomitant annuloplasty should be performed in every patient.

More recently he applied the double-orifice technique to patients with Barlow's disease and bileaflet prolapse.[144] Most patients with Barlow's disease have prolapse of multiple segments, not merely A_2 and P_2, resulting in more than one regurgitant jet. It is unclear why elimination of the central jet by an edge-to edge repair would lead to a satisfactory result. There are several additional specific fundamental concerns that need to be addressed with this technique. The edge-to edge repair, particularly the double-orifice technique, results in a significant decrease in mitral valve area. Thus the possibility of mitral stenosis should not be dismissed in patients with Barlow's disease, even if the risk is less than in those with other etiologies (e.g., ischemic, rheumatic). Even without physiological mitral stenosis, the decrease in orifice area increases flow velocities and turbulence, which can lead to fibrosis and calcification of the functioning (A_1P_1, A_3P_3) valve segments. This will likely impact the long-term durability of this repair. Another factor, which may impact the long-term durability of the edge-to-edge technique, is the increased stress on the subvalvular apparatus of all segments. For example, in a patient with isolated A_2 prolapse, suturing A_2 to P_2 clearly increases the stress on the latter. In contrast, decreasing the stress on a still diseased subvalvular apparatus is one of the key principles behind Carpentier's repair techniques and is the likely explanation for the excellent long-term results. In Alfieri's series the 5-year freedom of reoperation was 86% in patients with Barlow's disease, which is significantly lower than that of the standard Carpentier's techniques reported earlier. Present data do not support the routine use of the edge-to-edge technique for the treatment of type II mitral regurgitation.

Systolic Anterior Motion

Left ventricular outflow obstruction may occur occasionally after mitral valve reconstructive surgery for degenerative disease with excess leaflet tissue (Barlow's disease).[129,153] The extra amount of valve tissue displaces the line of coaptation and anterior leaflet toward the left ventricular outflow tract (LVOT), which leads to obstruction.[151] This systolic anterior motion (SAM) may produce important mitral regurgitation despite a large surface of coaptation. SAM should be suspected intraoperatively when patients develop borderline hemodynamics after discontinuation of cardiopulmonary bypass.[118] Intraoperative TEE confirms the diagnosis by demonstrating systolic anterior motion of the anterior leaflet, with left ventricular outflow tract obstruction and mitral regurgitation. Pressure measurements typically reveal an increased ventriculoaortic gradient.

Occasionally SAM is diagnosed postoperatively by the presence of a systolic murmur. It was first thought that the use of a rigid prosthetic ring might explain SAM. However, this complication has also been reported after flexible ring annuloplasty. Incremental risk factors for SAM include excess tissue (Barlow's disease, enlarged posterior leaflet), small ring, hyperkinetic heart, septum bulging, small ventricle, and reduced aortomitral angle (<120 degrees). In patients with Barlow's disease, SAM can be prevented by quadrangular resection of the posterior leaflet followed by a sliding plasty and insertion of a large prosthetic ring, hence displacing the closure line away from the LVOT.

The first step in the management of patients with intraoperative SAM is to discontinue all inotropic support and to optimize filling pressures. These hemodynamic optimizations often lead to the resolution of SAM and normalization of the ventriculoaortic gradient with disappearance of mitral regurgitation. Despite these maneuvers, moderate residual ventriculoaortic pressure gradients (<30 mm Hg) may persist, but often normalize within 6 months to 1 year, resulting from left ventricular remodeling. However, if these initial measures remain ineffective (persistence of SAM with a high ventriculoaortic gradient and mitral regurgitation), a second run of cardiopulmonary bypass is initiated and mitral valve reexploration with additional repair is required (reduction of posterior leaflet height, ring removal with insertion of a larger ring). It is important to emphasize that the insertion of an undersized prosthetic ring in patients with ischemic and dilated cardiomyopathy (absence of excess tissue) does not cause SAM.

Reoperations

Failure after repair can be classified as immediate failure (intraoperative), early failure (<2 years), and late failure (>2 years). Immediate and early failures are often related to technique, whereas late failure is due to the progression of the disease (Table 74-6). Degenerative etiology is significantly more prevalent in those patients with immediate and early failure, whereas late failure is often seen in patients with rheumatic etiology.[39,103]

Immediate failures are explained by suture dehiscence, interscallop leakage (e.g., incomplete closure of the gap between P_1 and P_3 after P_2 resection), systolic anterior motion, and inadequate surface of coaptation (e.g., extensive anterior leaflet resection, absence of annuloplasty, improperly sized or implanted ring, residual prolapse).[147] The incidence of immediate failure can be minimized by an accurate determination of the mechanism of mitral regurgitation (e.g., intraoperative TEE, direct valve analysis), meticulous application of standardized repair techniques, and careful assessment of repair (saline test that should demonstrate a symmetrical line of coaptation far from the outflow tract, large surface of coaptation, and no residual prolapse). An imperfect immediate result must lead the surgeon to reexplore the valve and to recognize the anomaly and correct it. Several studies have shown that residual mitral regurgitation is associated with a high reoperation rate (Figure 74-23).[157,167,170] The patient should not leave the operating room with more than a trace to minimal regurgitation.

Early failure is defined as the recurrence of mitral regurgitation after an initially satisfactory result. It is often related to a variety of technical issues and occurs mostly in patients with degenerative disease. The predominant causes of early failure are mitral valve repair without annuloplasty ring,[32,34,36] ring dehiscence (improper suture placement, incorrect ring sizing), suture line dehiscence (improper suture placement, excess tension on the leaflet after extensive tissue resection), and rupture of repaired chords (chordal abrasion after improper chordal shortening). Late failures (>2 years) are often related to the progression of the disease, with new prolapsing areas in patients with degenerative valve disease and progression of the fibrotic progress in rheumatic patients. Several clinical series have reported a re-repair rate of 15–20% (see Table 74-21).

Thromboembolic Events and Endocarditis

Thromboembolic (TE) events and endocarditis are rare complications after mitral valve repair. Studies have shown that the freedom of TE events varies from 87–96% at 10 years. The linearized rate of TE and bleeding events as low as 0.2 and 0.1% per patient year, respectively, have been reported in a clinical study with very long-term follow up.[25] Long-term observational studies have also shown high rates of freedom for endocarditis (99–100%) at 10 years after valve repair.[49,60,105]

Mitral Valve Replacement

Mortality and Late Survival

The operative mortality of mitral valve replacement ranges from 4–7% in recent clinical series.[145,180] This improvement in results is most likely related to the preservation of the posterior leaflet (decreasing the incidence of left ventricular disrupture) and chordal sparing valve replacement.* The preservation of ventriculoannular continuity is the major

*References 24, 53, 66, 71, 139, 164, 189.

Table 74–7

Reoperation after Mitral Valve Repair

Reference (year)	*Study interval (years)*	*No. of patients*	*Interval to reoperation (years, mean)*	*Technical failure (%)*	*Disease progression (%)*	*Replacement (%)*	*Re-repair (%)*	*Operative mortality (%)*
Chauvaud et al (1986)	16	72	5	28	72	85	15	1.4
Cerfolio et al (1996)	18	49	2.4	35	65	84	16	4
Gillinov et al (1997)	8	81	1.3	58	38	79	21	3

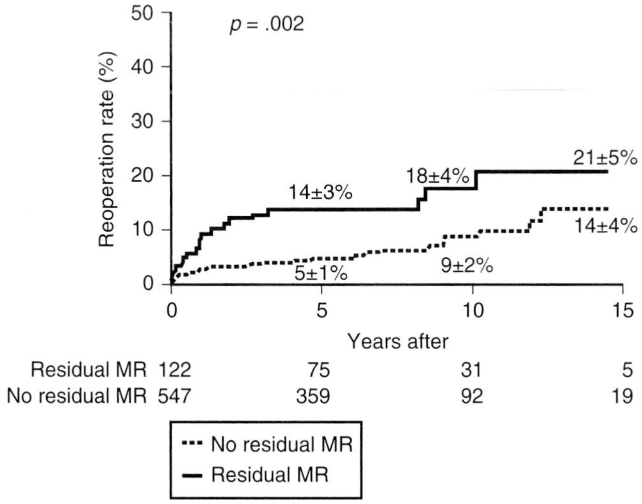

Figure 74–23 Reoperation rate after repair, according to presence or not of residual mitral regurgitation (MR) at end of surgery, as judged by double sampling dye curves and/or transesophageal echocardiography (TEE). *(Modified from Mohty D, Orszulak TA, Schaff HV, et al: Very long-term survival and durability of mitral valve repair for mitral valve prolapse. Circulation 104:I1–I7, 2001.)*

factor contributing to the conservation of postoperative ventricular function. In a series published by Jamieson et al[128] on 13,936 patients (STS National Database) undergoing isolated mitral valve replacement, operative mortality was found to be 6.4%. Independent predictors of operative mortality include age, urgent/emergent of the operation, renal failure (dialysis and non–dialysis-dependent), functional classification, multiple reoperation, previous myocardial infarction, and associated coronary disease. In Jamieson's study the addition of CABG more than doubled the operative mortality. The survival rate after mitral valve replacement is about 50–60% at 10 years. The long-term survival is almost identical between different types of mechanical valves and tissue valves.[45,98,143,168] As for patients with valve repair, congestive heart failure is the most common mode of death. Preoperative left ventricular dysfunction and all other predictors of operative mortality also affect late survival.

Valve-Related Complications

Valve-related complications include structural valve deterioration, thromboembolic and hemorrhagic events, endocarditis, perivalvular leaks, and hemolysis. Structural valve deterioration (SVD) is the most common complication of bioprosthetic valves.[11,86,119,188] The prevalence of this complication is higher in the mitral position than in the aortic position because of the increased hemodynamic stress during systole. The rate of SVD is related to the age of the patients at implantation. In a study by Marchand et al[146] on the durability of the Carpentier–Edwards pericardial valve, the freedom from reoperation at 11 years was 78%, 89%, and 100% in patients <60 years of age, between 61 and 70 years of age, and >70 years of age, respectively.[146] The linearized rate of TE complications is 1–3% per patient year and is identical with mechanical or tissue valves. However, major bleeding is more common with mechanical than with biological valves, with a linearized rate of 2–4% per patient year. The actuarial cumulative incidence of prosthetic valve endocarditis is estimated to be from 1.4–3.1% at 1 year and 3.2–5.7% at 5 years. The risk is greatest during the first 6 months after surgery. However, it is identical between tissue and mechanical valve. The rate of late prosthetic endocarditis is estimated to be between 0.2–0.35% per patient year and is slightly higher with mechanical valves. Perivalvular leak is a rare complication of valve replacement; it is often seen in the setting of mitral valve surgery for infective endocarditis, and in the presence of annular calcification.[99,106] Perivalvular leak can cause moderate to severe regurgitation according to the extent of valvular dehiscence, as well as hemolysis. The incidence of this complication can considerably be reduced by proper placement of the sutures around the annulus using Teflon pledgets.

Left Ventricular Rupture

Left ventricular rupture is a catastrophic complication, occurring in less than 1% of patients undergoing mitral valve replacement.[50] Posterior leaflet preservation and chordal-sparing techniques in valve replacement have dramatically reduced the incidence of this complication.[189] Underlying risk factors include advanced age, annular calcification, annular destruction in endocarditis, complete resection of the mitral valve apparatus, deep sutures placed inside the ventricle, and insertion of an oversized valve in a small ventricle. Pathological findings consist of a dissection pathway from the annulus or endocardial surface of the left ventricle through the myocardium with an exit point at a distance from the entry point. Several types of ventricular ruptures have been described according to the entry point.[172] Type I ruptures occur at the level of the annulus. Type II ruptures originate at the base of an excised papillary muscle. This type of rupture is very rare, because the technique of papillary muscle excision has been abandoned. Type III (midventricular rupture) originates at the mid-distance between the stumps of papillary muscles and the annulus. Type I ruptures are best treated by the removal of the valve prosthesis, with reconstruction of the annulus, and subsequent valvular reimplantation. Surgical attempts to repair type II and III ruptures using endocardial or epicardial approaches have been reported. Anecdotic cases of successful repair for type III rupture with mattress sutures, oriented transversally to the long axis of the ventricle, have been reported. However, the overall mortality of this condition remains in excess of 50%.

Minimally Invasive Mitral Valve Surgery

There are only a limited number of studies on minimally invasive mitral valve surgery. Among these different approaches, the most frequently used is the minimally invasive direct vision technique.[116] These series often include a cohort of young patients with degenerative mitral valve disease and preserved left ventricular function. Most of these procedures require a learning curve explaining the initial increase in ischemic and perfusion times. However, with increased experience, ischemic times similar to those obtained with conventional mitral valve surgery are possible.

Greelish et al[109] described their experience in a series of 413 patients undergoing minimally invasive direct vision mitral valve repair, using a variety of surgical approaches (lower hemisternotomy, right parasternal, and right minithoracotomy in 50%, 47%, and 3%, respectively). The etiology was degenerative in 91% of patients. Posterior leaflet prolapse, anterior leaflet prolapse, and bileaflet prolapse were present in 74%, 6%, and 20% of patients, respectively. Operative mortality was 0% in this series. Blood transfusions were necessary in 25% of patients. Mean length of stay was 6 days. Twenty-one patients required late reoperation for failed repair. At 5 years, freedom from reoperation was 92%. Finally, survival at 5 years was 95%. Gillinov et al[101] from the Cleveland Clinic used the upper hemisternotomy in 827 patients. Aortic valve surgery and mitral valve surgery were performed in 365 and 462 (repair 87%, replacement 13%) patients. The operative mortality of this cohort was 0.8%. Conversion rate to a full sternotomy was 2.4%. Grossi et al[112] reported their experience with minimally invasive mitral valve surgery in over 700 consecutive patients from 1995 to 2001. They used a right anterior minithoracotomy in nearly all patients (97%). Arterial cannulation was femoral in 79% of patients, and endoaortic balloon occlusion was used in 83%. Overall hospital mortality was 4.2% (repair 1.1%, replacement 5.8%). On follow-up echocardiography, either trace or no residual mitral regurgitation was present in 90% of patients. Casselman, Vanermen, and colleagues[38] reported a series of 187 patients undergoing totally endoscopic mitral valve repair. The etiology of mitral regurgitation was degenerative in 83.4% of patients. Isolated posterior leaflet prolapse (type II dysfunction) was noted in 90% of patients. Only 17% of patients displayed anterior or bileaflet prolapse. Intraoperative conversion to a median sternotomy was necessary in two patients. There was one early death and six late mitral reoperations. After a mean follow-up period of 14 months, 48 patients (27%) had 1+ mitral regurgitation and 14 patients (7.9%) still had 2+ or 3+ mitral regurgitation. Chitwood et al[89] reported the results of the phase II United States Food and Drug Administration (FDA) trial with mitral valve repair in 112 patients. After a 1-month follow-up period, nine patients (8%) had 2+ mitral regurgitation and six (5.4%) underwent reoperation for recurrent mitral regurgitation. Operative mortality was 0% in that series. Mohr et al[155] used the da Vinci robotic system in 17 patients who underwent mitral valve repair for degenerative disease. The majority of these patients displayed posterior leaflet prolapse. Mitral valve repair was successful in 14 patients. Three patients were converted to a standard endoscopic procedure. At 3 months one patient underwent reoperation for recurrent mitral regurgitation.

These advanced techniques of mitral valve repair (level 3–4) are currently under clinical investigation. Accurate evaluations of these new procedures are ongoing to assess their effectiveness and to define their role in the armamentarium of mitral valve surgery.

REFERENCES

1. Acar C, Jebara VA, Grare P, et al: Traumatic mitral insufficiency following percutaneous mitral dilation: Anatomic lesions and surgical implications. Eur J Cardiothorac Surg 6(12):660–663; discussion 663–664, 1992.
2. Adams DH, Filsoufi F: Another chapter in an enlarging book: Repair degenerative mitral valves. J Thorac Cardiovasc Surg 125(6):1197–1199, 2003.
3. Adams DH, Filsoufi F, Aklog L: Surgical treatment of the ischemic mitral valve. J Heart Valve Dis 11(suppl 1):S21–S25, 2002.
4. Adams DH, Filsoufi F, Byrne JG, et al: Mitral valve repair in redo cardiac surgery. J Card Surg 17(1):40–45, 2002.
5. Adams DH, Kadner A, Chen RH: Artificial mitral valve chordae replacement made simple. Ann Thorac Surg 71(4):1377–1378; discussion 1378–1379, 2001.
6. Akins CW, Hilgenberg AD, Buckley MJ, et al: Mitral valve reconstruction versus replacement for degenerative or ischemic mitral regurgitation. Ann Thorac Surg 58(3):668–675; discussion 675–676, 1994.
7. Aklog L, Adams DH, Couper GS, et al: Techniques and results of direct-access minimally invasive mitral valve surgery: A paradigm for the future. J Thorac Cardiovasc Surg 116(5):705–715, 1998.
8. Aklog L, Filsoufi F, Flores KO, et al: Does coronary artery bypass grafting alone correct moderate ischemic mitral regurgitation? Circulation 104(12 suppl 1):I68–I75, 2001.
9. Alfieri O, Maisano F, De Bonis M, et al: The double-orifice technique in mitral valve repair: A simple solution for complex problems. J Thorac Cardiovasc Surg 122(4):674–681, 2001.
10. Aranki SF, Adams DH, Rizzo RJ, et al: Determinants of early mortality and late survival in mitral valve endocarditis. Circulation 92(suppl 9): II143–II149, 1995.
11. Aupart M, Babuty D, Neville P, et al: Influence of age on valve-related events with Carpentier-Edwards pericardial bioprosthesis. Eur J Cardiothorac Surg 11(5):929–934, 1997.
12. Bailey C: Surgical repair of mitral insufficiency. Dis Chest 19(2):125–137, 1951.
13. Bailey CP, Jamison WI, Bakst AE, et al: The surgical correction of mitral insufficiency by the use of pericardial grafts. J Thorac Surg 28(6):551–603, 1954.
14. Bernal JM, Rabasa JM, Vilchez FG, et al: Mitral valve repair in rheumatic disease. The flexible solution. Circulation 88(4 pt 1):1746–1753, 1993.
15. Bichell DP, Adams DH, Aranki SF, et al: Repair of mitral regurgitation from myxomatous degeneration in the patient with a severely calcified posterior annulus. J Card Surg 10(4 pt 1):281–284, 1995.
16. Bichell DP, Balaguer JM, Aranki SF, et al: Axilloaxillary cardiopulmonary bypass: A practical alternative to femorofemoral bypass. Ann Thorac Surg 64(3):702–705, 1997.
17. Bishay ES, McCarthy PM, Cosgrove DM, et al: Mitral valve surgery in patients with severe left ventricular dysfunction. Eur J Cardiothorac Surg 17(3):213–221, 2000.
18. Blondheim DS, Jacobs LE, Kotler MN, et al: Dilated cardiomyopathy with mitral regurgitation: Decreased survival despite a low frequency of left ventricular thrombus. Am Heart J 122(3 pt 1):763–771, 1991.
19. Bolling SF: Mitral reconstruction in cardiomyopathy. J Heart Valve Dis 11(suppl 1):S26–S31, 2002.
20. Bolling SF, Deeb GM, Bach DS: Mitral valve reconstruction in elderly, ischemic patients. Chest 109(1):35–40, 1996.
21. Bolling SF, Deeb GM, Brunsting LA, et al: Early outcome of mitral valve reconstruction in patients with end-stage cardiomyopathy. J Thorac Cardiovasc Surg 109(4):676–682; discussion 682–683, 1995.
22. Bolling SF, Pagani FD, Deeb GM, et al: Intermediate-term outcome of mitral reconstruction in cardiomyopathy. J Thorac Cardiovasc Surg 115(2):381–386; discussion 387–388, 1998.
23. Bonow RO, Carabello B, de Leon AC, et al: ACC/AHA Guidelines for the Management of Patients with Valvular Heart Disease. Executive Summary. A report of the

American College of Cardiology/American Heart Association Task Force on Practice Guidelines (Committee on Management of Patients with Valvular Heart Disease). J Heart Valve Dis 7(6):672–707, 1998.
24. Borger MA, Yau TM, Rao V, et al: Reoperative mitral valve replacement: importance of preservation of the subvalvular apparatus. Ann Thorac Surg 74(5):1482–1487, 2002.
25. Braunberger E, Deloche A, Berrebi A, et al: Very long-term results (more than 20 years) of valve repair with Carpentier's techniques in nonrheumatic mitral valve insufficiency. Circulation 104(12 suppl 1):I8–I11, 2001.
26. Braunwald Z, Libby P: Heart Disease, 6th ed. Philadelphia: W.B. Saunders, 2001.
27. Byrne JG, Aranki SF, Adams DH, et al: Mitral valve surgery after previous CABG with functioning IMA grafts. Ann Thorac Surg 68(6):2243–2247, 1999.
28. Byrne JG, Karavas AN, Adams DH, et al: The preferred approach for mitral valve surgery after CABG: Right thoracotomy, hypothermia and avoidance of LIMA-LAD graft. J Heart Valve Dis 10(5):584–590, 2001.
29. Byrne JG, Mitchell ME, Adams DH, et al: Minimally invasive direct access mitral valve surgery. Semin Thorac Cardiovasc Surg 11(3):212–222, 1999.
30. Calafiore AM, Gallina S, Di Mauro M, et al: Mitral valve procedure in dilated cardiomyopathy: Repair or replacement? Ann Thorac Surg 71(4):1146–1152; discussion 1152–1153, 2001.
31. Carpentier A: Cardiac valve surgery—the "French correction." J Thorac Cardiovasc Surg 86(3):323–337, 1983.
32. Carpentier A, Chauvad S, Fabiani JN, et al: Reconstructive surgery of mitral valve incompetence: Ten-year appraisal. J Thorac Cardiovasc Surg 79(3):338–348, 1980.
33. Carpentier A, Deloche A, Dauptain J, et al: A new reconstructive operation for correction of mitral and tricuspid insufficiency. J Thorac Cardiovasc Surg 61(1):1–13, 1971.
34. Carpentier A, Loulmet D, Aupecle B, et al: Computer-assisted cardiac surgery. Lancet 353(9150):379–380, 1999.
35. Carpentier A, Loulmet D, Carpentier A, et al: [Open heart operation under videosurgery and minithoracotomy. First case (mitral valvuloplasty) operated with success]. C R Acad Sci III 319(3):219–223, 1996.
36. Carpentier AF, Lessano A, Relland JY, et al: The "physio-ring": An advanced concept in mitral valve annuloplasty. Ann Thorac Surg 60(5):1177–1185; discussion 1185–1186, 1995.
37. Carpentier AF, Pellerin M, Fuzellier JF, et al: Extensive calcification of the mitral valve anulus: Pathology and surgical management. J Thorac Cardiovasc Surg 111(4):718–729; discussion 729–730, 1996.
38. Casselman FP, Van Slycke S, Dom H, et al: Endoscopic mitral valve repair: Feasible, reproducible, and durable. J Thorac Cardiovasc Surg 125(2):273–282, 2003.
39. Cerfolio RJ, Orszulak TA, Pluth JR, et al: Reoperation after valve repair for mitral regurgitation: Early and intermediate results. J Thorac Cardiovasc Surg 111(6):1177–1183; discussion 1183–1184, 1996.
40. Chauvaud S, Fuzellier JF, Berrebi A, et al: Long-term (29 years) results of reconstructive surgery in rheumatic mitral valve insufficiency. Circulation 104(12 suppl 1):I12–I15, 2001.
41. Chauvaud S, Jebara V, Chachques JC, et al: Valve extension with glutaraldehyde-preserved autologous pericardium. Results in mitral valve repair. J Thorac Cardiovasc Surg 102(2):171–177; discussion 177–178, 1991.
42. Chen FY, Adams DH, Aranki SF, et al: Mitral valve repair in cardiomyopathy. Circulation 98(suppl 19):II124–II127, 1998.
43. Choudhary SK, Dhareshwar J, Govil A, et al: Open mitral commissurotomy in the current era: Indications, technique, and results. Ann Thorac Surg 75(1):41–46, 2003.
44. Choudhary SK, Talwar S. Dubey B, et al: Mitral valve repair in a predominantly rheumatic population. Long-term results. Tex Heart Inst J 28(1):8–15, 2001.
45. Christakis GT, Kormos RL, Weisel RD, et al: Morbidity and mortality in mitral valve surgery. Circulation 72(3 pt 2):II120–II128, 1985.
46. Cohn LH, Adams DH, Couper GS, et al: Minimally invasive cardiac valve surgery improves patient satisfaction while reducing costs of cardiac valve replacement and repair. Ann Surg 226(4):421–426; discussion 427–428, 1997.
47. Cohn LH, Couper GS, Aranki SF, et al: The long-term results of mitral valve reconstruction for the "floppy" valve. J Card Surg 9(suppl 2):278–281, 1994.
48. Cohn LH, Peigh PS, Sell J, et al: Right thoracotomy, femorofemoral bypass, and deep hypothermia for re-replacement of the mitral valve. Ann Thorac Surg 48(1):69–71, 1989.
49. Cohn LH, Rizzo RJ, Adams DH, et al: The effect of pathophysiology on the surgical treatment of ischemic mitral regurgitation: Operative and late risks of repair versus replacement. Eur J Cardiothorac Surg 9(10):568–574, 1995.
50. Craver JM, Jones EL, Guyton RA, et al: Avoidance of transverse midventricular disruption following mitral valve replacement. Ann Thorac Surg 40(2):163–171, 1985.
51. Cutler E: The current status of the surgical procedures in chronic valvular disease of the heart. Arch Surg 403–416, 1923.
52. Dahlberg PS, Orszulak TA, Mullany CJ, et al: Late outcome of mitral valve surgery for patients with coronary artery disease. Ann Thorac Surg 76(5):1539–1487; discussion 1547–1548, 2003.
53. David TE: Mitral valve replacement with preservation of chordae tendineae: Rationale and technical considerations. Ann Thorac Surg 41(6):680–682, 1986.
54. David TE: The appropriateness of mitral valve repair for rheumatic mitral valve disease. J Heart Valve Dis 6(4):373–374, 1997.
55. David TE, Armstrong S, Sun Z: Left ventricular function after mitral valve surgery. J Heart Valve Dis 4(suppl 2):S175–S180, 1995.
56. David TE, Armstrong S, Sun Z, et al: Late results of mitral valve repair for mitral regurgitation due to degenerative disease. Ann Thorac Surg 56(1):7–12; discussion 13–14, 1993.
57. David TE, Bos J, Christakis GT, et al: Heart valve operations in patients with active infective endocarditis. Ann Thorac Surg 49(5):701–705; discussion 712–713, 1990.
58. David TE, Bos J, Rakowski H: Mitral valve repair by replacement of chordae tendineae with polytetrafluoroethylene sutures. J Thorac Cardiovasc Surg 101(3):495–501, 1991.
59. David TE, Feindel CM: Reconstruction of the mitral anulus. Circulation 76(3 pt 2):III102–III107, 1987.
60. David TE, Feindel CM, Armstrong S, et al: Reconstruction of the mitral anulus. A ten-year experience. J Thorac Cardiovasc Surg 110(5):1323–1332, 1995.
61. David TE, Kuo J, Armstrong S: Aortic and mitral valve replacement with reconstruction of the intervalvular fibrous body. J Thorac Cardiovasc Surg 114(5):766–771; discussion 771–772; 1997.
62. David TE, Uden DE, Strauss HD: The importance of the mitral apparatus in left ventricular function after correction of mitral regurgitation. Circulation 68(3 pt 2):II76–II82, 1983.
63. Davila JC, Glover RP, Trout RG, et al: Circumferential suture of the mitral ring; a method for the surgical correction of mitral insufficiency. J Thorac Surg 30(5):531–560; discussion 560–563, 1955.
64. Deloche A, Acar C, Jebara V, et al: Biatrial transseptal approach in case of difficult exposure to the mitral valve. Ann Thorac Surg 50(2):318–319, 1990.
65. Deloche A, Jebara VA, Relland JY, et al: Valve repair with Carpentier techniques. The second decade. J Thorac

Cardiovasc Surg 99(6):990–1001; discussion 1001–1002, 1990.
66. Dilip D, Chandra A, Rajashekhar D, et al: Early beneficial effect of preservation of papillo-annular continuity in mitral valve replacement on left ventricular function. J Heart Valve Dis 10(3):294–300; discussion 300–301, 2001.
67. Dion R, Benetis R, Elias B, et al: Mitral valve procedures in ischemic regurgitation. J Heart Valve Dis 4(suppl 2):S124–S129; discussion S129–S131, 1995.
68. Dreyfus G, Serraf A, Jebara VA, et al: Valve repair in acute endocarditis. Ann Thorac Surg 49(5):706–711; discussion 712–713, 1990.
69. Dubost C, Guilmet D, de Parades B, et al: [New technic of opening of the left auricle in open-heart surgery: The transseptal bi-auricular approach]. Presse Med 74(30):1607–1608, 1966.
70. Dujardin KS, Seward JB, Orszulak TA, et al: Outcome after surgery for mitral regurgitation. Determinants of postoperative morbidity and mortality. J Heart Valve Dis 6(1):17–21, 1997.
71. Duran CG, Pomar JL, Revuelta JM, et al: Conservative operation for mitral insufficiency: Critical analysis supported by postoperative hemodynamic studies of 72 patients. J Thorac Cardiovasc Surg 79(3):326–337, 1980.
72. Duran CG, Revuelta JM, Gaite L, et al: Stability of mitral reconstructive surgery at 10–12 years for predominantly rheumatic valvular disease. Circulation 78(3 pt 2): I91–I96, 1988.
73. Duran CG, Ubago JL: Clinical and hemodynamic performance of a totally flexible prosthetic ring for atrioventricular valve reconstruction. Ann Thorac Surg 22(5):458–463, 1976.
74. Duran CM, Gometza B, De Vol EB: Valve repair in rheumatic mitral disease. Circulation 84(suppl 5):III125–III132, 1991.
75. Eishi K, Kawazoe K. Kuriyama Y, et al: Surgical management of infective endocarditis associated with cerebral complications. Multi-center retrospective study in Japan. J Thorac Cardiovasc Surg 110(6):1745–1755, 1995.
76. el Asmar B, Acker M, Couetil JP, et al: Mitral valve repair in the extensively calcified mitral valve annulus. Ann Thorac Surg 52(1):66–69, 1991.
77. el Asmar B, Perier P, Couetil JP, et al: Failures in reconstructive mitral valve surgery. J Med Liban 39(1):7–11, 1991.
78. Ellis FH Jr, Frye RL, McGoon DC: Results of reconstructive operations for mitral insufficiency due to ruptured chordae tendineae. Surgery 59(1):165–172, 1966.
79. Enriquez-Sarano M: Timing of mitral valve surgery. Heart 87(1):79–85, 2002.
80. Enriquez-Sarano M, Nkomo V, Mohty D, et al: Mitral regurgitation: Predictors of outcome and natural history. Adv Cardiol 39:133–143, 2002.
81. Enriquez-Sarano M, Schaff HV, Frye RL: Early surgery for mitral regurgitation: The advantages of youth. Circulation 96(12):4121–4123, 1997.
82. Enriquez-Sarano M, Schaff HV, Orszulak TA, et al: Congestive heart failure after surgical correction of mitral regurgitation. A long-term study. Circulation 92(9):2496–2503, 1995.
83. Enriquez-Sarano M, Schaff HV, Orszulak TA, et al: Valve repair improves the outcome of surgery for mitral regurgitation. A multivariate analysis. Circulation 91(4):1022–1028, 1995.
84. Enriquez-Sarano M, Tajik AJ, Schaff HV, et al: Echocardiographic prediction of left ventricular function after correction of mitral regurgitation: Results and clinical implications. J Am Coll Cardiol 24(6):1536–1543, 1994.
85. Enriquez-Sarano M, Tajik AJ, Schaff HV, et al: Echocardiographic prediction of survival after surgical correction of organic mitral regurgitation. Circulation 90(2):830–837, 1994.
86. Eric Jamieson WR, Marchand MA, Pelletier CL, et al: Structural valve deterioration in mitral replacement surgery: Comparison of Carpentier-Edwards supra-annular porcine and Perimount pericardial bioprostheses. J Thorac Cardiovasc Surg 118(2):297–304, 1999.
87. Farb A, Galloway JR, Davis RC, et al: Mitral valve laceration and papillary muscle rupture secondary to percutaneous balloon aortic valvuloplasty. Am J Cardiol 69(8):829–830, 1992.
88. Feindel CM, Tufail Z, David TE, et al: Mitral valve surgery in patients with extensive calcification of the mitral annulus. J Thorac Cardiovasc Surg 126(3):777–782, 2003.
89. Felger JE, Chitwood WR Jr, Nifong LW, et al: Evolution of mitral valve surgery: Toward a totally endoscopic approach. Ann Thorac Surg 72(4):1203–1208; discussion 1208–1209, 2001.
90. Filsoufi A, Adams DH: Surgical treatment of mitral valve endocarditis. In Cohn LH, Edmunds LH Jr: editors: Cardiac Surgery in the Adult, pp. 987–997. New York: McGraw-Hill, 2003.
91. Fiore AC, Barner HB, Swartz MT, et al: Mitral valve replacement: randomized trial of St. Jude and Medtronic Hall prostheses. Ann Thorac Surg 66(3):707–712; discussion 712–713, 1998.
92. Fix J, Isada L, Cosgrove D, et al: Do patients with less than `echo-perfect' results from mitral valve repair by intraoperative echocardiography have a different outcome? Circulation 88(5 pt 2):II39–II48, 1993.
93. Freeman WK, Schaff HV, Khandheria BK, et al: Intraoperative evaluation of mitral valve regurgitation and repair by transesophageal echocardiography: Incidence and significance of systolic anterior motion. J Am Coll Cardiol 20(3):599–609, 1992.
94. Fuzellier JF, Chauvaud SM, Fornes P, et al: Surgical management of mitral regurgitation associated with Marfan's syndrome. Ann Thorac Surg 66(1):68–72, 1998.
95. Galloway AC, Colvin SB, Baumann FG, et al: Long-term results of mitral valve reconstruction with Carpentier techniques in 148 patients with mitral insufficiency. Circulation 78(3 pt 2):I97–I105, 1988.
96. Galloway AC, Colvin SB, Baumann FG, et al: A comparison of mitral valve reconstruction with mitral valve replacement: Intermediate-term results. Ann Thorac Surg 47(5):655–662, 1989.
97. Garbarz E, Iung B, Cormier B, et al: Echocardiographic Criteria in Selection of Patients for Percutaneous Mitral Commissurotomy. Echocardiography 16(7 pt 1):711–721, 1999.
98. Garcia Andrade I, Cartier R, Panisi P, et al: Factors influencing early and late survival in patients with combined mitral valve replacement and myocardial revascularization and in those with isolated replacement. Ann Thorac Surg 44(6):607–613, 1987.
99. Genoni M, Franzen D, Tavakoli R, et al: Does the morphology of mitral paravalvular leaks influence symptoms and hemolysis? J Heart Valve Dis 10(4):426–430, 2001.
100. Gillinov AM, Banbury MK, Cosgrove DM: Hemisternotomy approach for aortic and mitral valve surgery. J Card Surg 15(1):15–20, 2000.
101. Gillinov AM, Cosgrove DM: Minimally invasive mitral valve surgery: Mini-sternotomy with extended transseptal approach. Semin Thorac Cardiovasc Surg 11(3):206–211, 1999.
102. Gillinov AM, Cosgrove DM, Blackstone EH, et al: Durability of mitral valve repair for degenerative disease. J Thorac Cardiovasc Surg 116(5):734–743, 1998.
103. Gillinov AM, Cosgrove DM, Lytle BW, et al: Reoperation for failure of mitral valve repair. J Thorac Cardiovasc Surg 113(3):467–473; discussion 473–475, 1997.

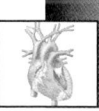

104. Gillinov AM, Diaz R, Blackstone EH, et al: Double valve endocarditis. Ann Thorac Surg 71(6):1874–1879, 2001.
105. Gillinov AM, Faber C, Houghtaling PL, et al: Repair versus replacement for degenerative mitral valve disease with coexisting ischemic heart disease. J Thorac Cardiovasc Surg 125(6):1350–1362, 2003.
106. Gillinov AM, Faber CN, Sabik JF, et al: Endocarditis after mitral valve repair. Ann Thorac Surg 73(6):1813–1816, 2002.
107. Gillinov AM, Wierup PN, Blackstone EH, et al: Is repair preferable to replacement for ischemic mitral regurgitation? J Thorac Cardiovasc Surg 122(6):1125–1141, 2001.
108. Glockner JF, Johnston DL, McGee KP: Evaluation of cardiac valvular disease with MR imaging: Qualitative and quantitative techniques. Radiographics 23(1):e9, 2003.
109. Greelish JP, Cohn LH, Leacche M, et al: Minimally invasive mitral valve repair suggests earlier operations for mitral valve disease. J Thorac Cardiovasc Surg 126(2):365–371; discussion 371–373, 2003.
110. Grigioni F, Enriquez-Sarano M, Zehr KJ, et al: Ischemic mitral regurgitation: Long-term outcome and prognostic implications with quantitative Doppler assessment. Circulation 103(13):1759–1764, 2001.
111. Gross RI, Cunningham JN Jr, Snively SL, et al: Long-term results of open radical mitral commissurotomy: Ten year follow-up study of 202 patients. Am J Cardiol 47(4):821–825, 1981.
112. Grossi EA, Galloway AC, LaPietra A, et al: Minimally invasive mitral valve surgery: A 6-year experience with 714 patients. Ann Thorac Surg 74(3):660–663; discussion 663–664, 2002.
113. Grossi EA, Galloway AC, Steinberg BM, et al: Severe calcification does not affect long-term outcome of mitral valve repair. Ann Thorac Surg 58(3):685–687; discussion 688, 1994.
114. Grossi EA, Goldberg JD, LaPietra A, et al: Ischemic mitral valve reconstruction and replacement: Comparison of long-term survival and complications. J Thorac Cardiovasc Surg 122(6):1107–1124, 2001.
115. Grossi A, LaPietra A, Galloway AC, et al: History of mitral valve anterior leaflet repair with triangular resection. Ann Thorac Surg 72(5):1794–1795, 2001.
116. Grossi EA, LaPietra A, Galloway AC, et al: Videoscopic mitral valve repair and replacement using the port-access technique. Adv Card Surg 13:77–88, 2001.
117. Grossi EA, LaPietra A, Ribakove GH, et al: Minimally invasive versus sternotomy approaches for mitral reconstruction: Comparison of intermediate-term results. J Thorac Cardiovasc Surg 121(4):708–713, 2001.
118. Grossi EA, Steinberg BM, LeBoutillier M 3rd, et al: Decreasing incidence of systolic anterior motion after mitral valve reconstruction. Circulation 90(5 pt 2):II195–II197, 1994.
119. Grunkemeier G, Wu Y, Jin R: Statistical analysis of heart valve outcomes. J Heart Valve Dis 11(suppl)1:S2–S7, 2002.
120. Guiraudon GM, Ofiesh JG, Kaushik R: Extended vertical transatrial septal approach to the mitral valve. Ann Thorac Surg 52(5):1058–1060; discussion 1060–1062, 1991.
121. Hendren WG, Morris AS, Rosenkrantz ER, et al: Mitral valve repair for bacterial endocarditis. J Thorac Cardiovasc Surg 103(1):124–128; discussion 128–129, 1992.
122. Hendren WG, Nemec JJ, Lytle BW, et al: Mitral valve repair for ischemic mitral insufficiency. Ann Thorac Surg 52(6):1246–1251; discussion 1251–1252, 1991.
123. Herrera JM, Vega JL, Bernal JM, et al: Open mitral commissurotomy: Fourteen- to eighteen-year follow-up clinical study. Ann Thorac Surg 55(3):641–645, 1993.
124. Hickey MS, Blackstone EH, Kirklin JW, et al: Outcome probabilities and life history after surgical mitral commissurotomy: Implications for balloon commissurotomy. J Am Coll Cardiol 17(1):29–42, 1991.
125. Holman WL, Goldberg SP, Early LJ, et al: Right thoracotomy for mitral reoperation: Analysis of technique and outcome. Ann Thorac Surg 70(6):1970–1973, 2000.
126. Hueb AC, Jatene FB, Moreira LF, et al: Ventricular remodeling and mitral valve modifications in dilated cardiomyopathy: New insights from anatomic study. J Thorac Cardiovasc Surg 124(6):1216–1224, 2002.
127. Izhar U, Daly RC, Dearani JA, et al: Mitral valve replacement or repair after previous coronary artery bypass grafting. Circulation 100(suppl 19):II84–II89, 1999.
128. Jamieson WR, Edwards FH, Schwartz M, et al: Risk stratification for cardiac valve replacement. National Cardiac Surgery Database. Database Committee of The Society of Thoracic Surgeons. Ann Thorac Surg 67(4):943–951, 1999.
129. Jebara VA, Milaileanu S, Acar C, et al: Left ventricular outflow tract obstruction after mitral valve repair. Results of the sliding leaflet technique. Circulation 88(5 pt 2):II30–I34, 1993.
130. Jebara VA, Dervanian P, Acar C, et al: Mitral valve repair using Carpentier techniques in patients more than 70 years old. Early and late results. Circulation 86(suppl 5):II53–II59, 1992.
131. Junker A, Thayssen P, Nielsen B, et al: The hemodynamic and prognostic significance of echo-Doppler-proven mitral regurgitation in patients with dilated cardiomyopathy. Cardiology 83(1-2):14–20, 1993.
132. Kalman JM, Jones EF. Lubicz S, et al: Evaluation of mitral valve repair by intraoperative transoesophageal echocardiography. Aust N Z J Med 23(5):463–469, 1993.
133. Karavas AN, Filsoufi F, Mihaljevic T, et al: Risk factors and management of endocarditis after mitral valve repair. J Heart Valve Dis 11(5):660–664, 2002.
134. Kay EB, Nogueira C, Head LR, et al: Surgical treatment of mitral insufficiency. J Thorac Surg 36(5):677–690, 1958.
135. Klein AL, Bailey AS, Cohen GI, et al: Effects of mitral stenosis on pulmonary venous flow as measured by Doppler transesophageal echocardiography. Am J Cardiol 72(1):66–72, 1993.
136. Kono T, Sabbah HN, Stein PD, et al: Left ventricular shape as a determinant of functional mitral regurgitation in patients with severe heart failure secondary to either coronary artery disease or idiopathic dilated cardiomyopathy. Am J Cardiol 68(4):355–359, 1991.
137. Kwan J, Shiota T, Agler DA, et al: Geometric differences of the mitral apparatus between ischemic and dilated cardiomyopathy with significant mitral regurgitation: Real-time three-dimensional echocardiography study. Circulation 107(8):1135–1140, 2003.
138. Lee EM, Shapiro LM, Wells FC: Superiority of mitral valve repair in surgery for degenerative mitral regurgitation. Eur Heart J 18(4):655–663, 1997.
139. Lee KS, Stewart WJ, Savage RM, et al: Systolic anterior motion of mitral valve after the posterior leaflet sliding advancement procedure. Ann Thorac Surg 57(5):1338–1340, 1994.
140. Lillehei CW, Gott VL, Dewall RA, et al: The surgical treatment of stenotic or regurgitant lesions of the mitral and aortic valves by direct vision utilizing a pump-oxygenator. J Thorac Surg 35(2):154–191, 1958.
141. Ling LH, Enriquez-Sarano M, Seward JB, et al: Early surgery in patients with mitral regurgitation due to flail leaflets: A long-term outcome study. Circulation 96(6):1819–1825, 1997.
142. Loulmet DF, Carpentier A, Cho PW, et al: Less invasive techniques for mitral valve surgery. J Thorac Cardiovasc Surg 115(4):772–779, 1998.
143. Magovern JA, Pennock JL, Campbell DB, et al: Risks of mitral valve replacement and mitral valve replacement with

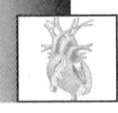

coronary artery bypass. Ann Thorac Surg 39(4):346–352, 1985.
144. Maisano F, Schreuder JJ, Oppizzi M, et al: The double-orifice technique as a standardized approach to treat mitral regurgitation due to severe myxomatous disease: Surgical technique. Eur J Cardiothorac Surg 17(3):201–205, 2000.
145. Marchand M, Aupart M, Norton R, et al: Twelve-year experience with Carpentier-Edwards PERIMOUNT pericardial valve in the mitral position: A multicenter study. J Heart Valve Dis 7(3):292–298, 1998.
146. Marchand MA, Aupart M, Norton R, et al: Fifteen-year experience with the mitral Carpentier-Edwards PERIMOUNT pericardial bioprosthesis. Ann Thorac Surg 71(suppl 5):S236–S239, 2001.
147. Marwick TH, Stewart WJ, Currie PJ, et al: Mechanisms of failure of mitral valve repair: An echocardiographic study. Am Heart J 122(1 pt 1):149–156, 1991.
148. Merendino KA, Thomas GI, Jesseph JE, et al: The open correction of rheumatic mitral regurgitation and/or stenosis; with special reference to regurgitation treated by posteromedial annuloplasty utilizing a pump-oxygenator. Ann Surg 150(1):5–22, 1959.
149. Messas E, Guerrero JL, Handschumacher MD, et al: Paradoxic decrease in ischemic mitral regurgitation with papillary muscle dysfunction: Insights from three-dimensional and contrast echocardiography with strain rate measurement. Circulation 104(16):1952–1957, 2001.
150. Metras D, Coulibaly AO, Ouattara K: The surgical treatment of endomyocardial fibrosis: Results in 55 patients. Circulation 72(3 pt 2):II274–II279, 1985.
151. Mihaileanu S: Outflow tract obstruction and failed mitral repair. Circulation 90(2):1107–1108, 1994.
152. Mihaileanu S, el Asmar B, Acar C, et al: Intra-operative transoesophageal echocardiography after mitral repair—specific conditions and pitfalls. Eur Heart J 12(suppl B):26–29, 1991.
153. Mihaileanu S, Marino JP, Chauvaud S, et al: Left ventricular outflow obstruction after mitral valve repair (Carpentier's technique). Proposed mechanisms of disease. Circulation 78(3 pt 2):I78–I84, 1988.
154. Miki S, Kusuhara K, Ueda Y, et al: Mitral valve replacement with preservation of chordae tendineae and papillary muscles. Ann Thorac Surg 45(1):28–34, 1988.
155. Mohr FW, Falk V, Diegeler A, et al: Computer-enhanced "robotic" cardiac surgery: Experience in 148 patients. J Thorac Cardiovasc Surg 121(5):842–853, 2001.
156. Mohty D, Enriquez-Sarano M: The long-term outcome of mitral valve repair for mitral valve prolapse. Curr Cardiol Rep 4(2):104–110, 2002.
157. Mohty D, Orszulak TA, Schaff HV, et al: Very long-term survival and durability of mitral valve repair for mitral valve prolapse. Circulation 104(12 suppl 1):I1–I7, 2001.
158. Muehrcke DD, Cosgrove DM 3rd, Lytle BW, et al: Is there an advantage to repairing infected mitral valves? Ann Thorac Surg 63(6):1718–1724, 1997.
159. Murray G: Reconstruction of the valves of the heart. Can Med Assoc J 38(4):317–319, 1938.
160. Nichols HT: Mitral insufficiency: Treatment by polar cross-fusion of the mitral annulus fibrosus. J Thorac Surg 33(1):102–122, 1957.
161. Nifong LW, Chu VF, Bailey BM, et al: Robotic mitral valve repair: Experience with the da Vinci system. Ann Thorac Surg 75(2):438–442; discussion 443, 2003.
162. Pagani FD, Monaghan HL, Deeb GM, et al: Mitral valve reconstruction for active and healed endocarditis. Circulation 94(suppl 9):II133–II138, 1996.
163. Pu M, Vandervoort PM, Griffin BP, et al: Quantification of mitral regurgitation by the proximal convergence method using transesophageal echocardiography. Clinical validation of a geometric correction for proximal flow constraint. Circulation 92(8):2169–2177, 1995.
164. Reardon MJ, David TE: Mitral valve replacement with preservation of the subvalvular apparatus. Curr Opin Cardiol 14(2):104–110, 1999.
165. Reed GE, Tice DA, Clauss RH: Asymmetric exaggerated mitral annuloplasty: Repair of mitral insufficiency with hemodynamic predictability. J Thorac Cardiovasc Surg 49:752–761, 1965.
166. Romano MA, Bolling SF: Mitral valve repair as an alternative treatment for heart failure patients. Heart Fail Monit 4(1):7–12, 2003.
167. Saiki Y, Kasegawa H, Kawase M, et al: Intraoperative TEE during mitral valve repair: Does it predict early and late post-operative mitral valve dysfunction? Ann Thorac Surg 66(4):1277–1281, 1998.
168. Scott WC, Miller DC, Haverich A, et al: Operative risk of mitral valve replacement: Discriminant analysis of 1329 procedures. Circulation 72(3 pt 2):II108–II119, 1985.
169. Smolens IA, Pagani FD, Deeb GM, et al: Prophylactic mitral reconstruction for mitral regurgitation. Ann Thorac Surg 72(4):1210–1215; discussion 1215–1216, 2001.
170. Sousa Uva M, Dreyfus G, Rescigno G, et al: Surgical treatment of asymptomatic and mildly symptomatic mitral regurgitation. J Thorac Cardiovasc Surg 112(5):1240–1248; discussion 1248–1249, 1996.
171. Souttar H: The surgical treatment of mitral stenosis. Br Med J 2:603, 1925.
172. Spencer FC, Galloway AC, Colvin SB: A clinical evaluation of the hypothesis that rupture of the left ventricle following mitral valve replacement can be prevented by preservation of the chordae of the mural leaflet. Ann Surg 202(6):673–680, 1985.
173. Starr A, Edwards ML: Mitral replacement: Clinical experience with a ball-valve prosthesis. Ann Surg 154:726–740, 1961.
174. Steimle CN, Bolling SF: Outcome of reoperative valve surgery via right thoracotomy. Circulation 94(suppl 9):II126–II128, 1996.
175. Sternik L, Zehr KJ, Orszulak TA, et al: The advantage of repair of mitral valve in acute endocarditis. J Heart Valve Dis 11(1):91–97; discussion 97–98, 2002.
176. Stewart WJ, Currie PJ, Salcedo EE, et al: Evaluation of mitral leaflet motion by echocardiography and jet direction by Doppler color flow mapping to determine the mechanisms of mitral regurgitation. J Am Coll Cardiol 20(6):1353–1361, 1992.
177. Stewart WJ, Griffin B, Thomas JD: Multiplane transesophageal echocardiographic evaluation of mitral valve disease. Am J Card Imaging 9(2):121–128, 1995.
178. Sugeng L, Spencer KT, Mor-Avi V, et al: Dynamic three-dimensional color flow Doppler: An improved technique for the assessment of mitral regurgitation. Echocardiography 20(3):265–273, 2003.
179. Tavakoli R, Weber A, Vogt P, et al: Surgical management of acute mitral valve regurgitation due to post-infarction papillary muscle rupture. J Heart Valve Dis 11(1):20–25; discussion 26, 2002.
180. Thourani VH, Weintraub WS, Craver JM, et al: Influence of concomitant CABG and urgent/emergent status on mitral valve replacement surgery. Ann Thorac Surg 70(3):778–783; discussion 783–784, 2000.
181. Thourani VH, Weintraub WS, Guyton RA, et al: Outcomes and long-term survival for patients undergoing mitral valve repair versus replacement: Effect of age and concomitant coronary artery bypass grafting. Circulation 108(3):298–304, 2003.
182. Tribble CG, Killinger WA Jr, Harman PK, et al: Anterolateral thoracotomy as an alternative to repeat median sternotomy

for replacement of the mitral valve. Ann Thorac Surg 43(4):380–382, 1987.
183. Tribble CG, Nolan SP, Kron IL: 1987: Anterolateral thoracotomy as an alternative to repeat median sternotomy for replacement of the mitral valve. Updated in 1995. Ann Thorac Surg 59(1):255–256, 1995.
184. Tribouilloy CM, Enriquez-Sarano M, Capps MA, et al: Contrasting effect of similar effective regurgitant orifice area in mitral and tricuspid regurgitation: A quantitative Doppler echocardiographic study. J Am Soc Echocardiogr 15(9):958–965, 2002.
185. Tribouilloy CM, Enriquez-Sarano M, Schaff HV, et al: Impact of preoperative symptoms on survival after surgical correction of organic mitral regurgitation: Rationale for optimizing surgical indications. Circulation 99(3):400–405, 1999.
186. Trichon BH, Felker GM, Shaw LK, et al: Relation of frequency and severity of mitral regurgitation to survival among patients with left ventricular systolic dysfunction and heart failure. Am J Cardiol 91(5):538–543, 2003.
187. Uva MS, Jebara VA, Acar C, et al: Mitral valve repair in patients with endomyocardial fibrosis. Ann Thorac Surg 54(1):89–92, 1992.
188. van Doorn CA, Stoodley KD, Saunders NR, et al: Mitral valve replacement with the Carpentier-Edwards standard bioprosthesis: Performance into the second decade. Eur J Cardiothorac Surg 9(5):253–258, 1995.
189. Wasir H, Choudhary SK, Airan B, et al: Mitral valve replacement with chordal preservation in a rheumatic population. J Heart Valve Dis 10(1):84–89, 2001.
190. Wooler GH, Nixon PG, Grimshaw VA, et al: Experiences with the repair of the mitral valve in mitral in competence. Thorax 17:49–57, 1962.
191. Yau TM, El-Ghoneimi YA, Armstrong S, et al: Mitral valve repair and replacement for rheumatic disease. J Thorac Cardiovasc Surg 119(1):53–60, 2000.
192. Yun KL, Sintek CF, Miller DC, et al: Randomized trial comparing partial versus complete chordal-sparing mitral valve replacement: Effects on left ventricular volume and function. J Thorac Cardiovasc Surg 123(4):707–714, 2002.

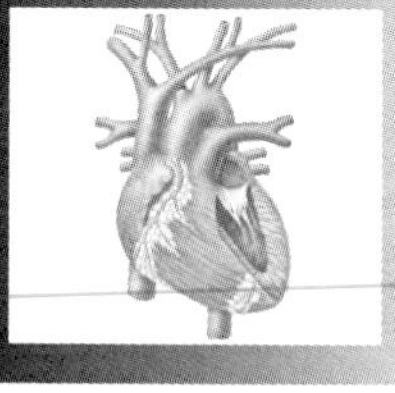

CHAPTER 75

Acquired Disease of the Tricuspid Valve

Carlos M. G. Duran

INTRODUCTION

The tricuspid valve is often ignored by cardiologists and surgeons because of its unique characteristics: (1) With the exception of infective endocarditis, it is rarely affected in isolation. Most often, the prominent impact of other diseased valves minimizes its importance. (2) Located at the entrance of the heart, its symptomatology is primarily extracardiac and is often silent. (3) Its behavior is closely related to the function of the right ventricle. In most cases, tricuspid regurgitation is secondary to right ventricular failure. (4) It follows the dictates of the mitral valve. Resolution of the mitral problem is often followed by improvement in the degree of tricuspid regurgitation. (5) Because it works in a low-pressure system, it is difficult to evaluate its preoperative importance and assess the value of different surgical techniques. These characteristics of the tricuspid valve cause cardiologists and surgeons to often ignore it with apparent impunity. However, recent developments in diagnostic tools and in two-dimensional (2D) color Doppler echocardiography in particular have increased the awareness of this valve, which has been defined as the "Cinderella" of cardiac valves.

SURGICAL ANATOMY

Situated at the base of the heart, the tricuspid valve separates the right atrium from the right ventricle. It has traditionally been accepted that the tricuspid valve consists of three very thin leaflets attached to the tricuspid annulus.

The Tricuspid Annulus

The base of the anterior and posterior leaflets is attached to the free wall of the right ventricle, but the septal leaflet is inserted into the base of the interventricular septum. This line of leaflet attachment, known as the tricuspid annulus, is more a landmark than an actual fibrous ring. The absence of an encircling fibrotic structure explains the large changes in the tricuspid orifice during the cardiac cycle and its easy dilation in disease. The mobility and size of the tricuspid orifice are dependent on the transversely oriented myocardial fibers, which surround the atrioventricular valves. Torrent-Guasp et al[90] described the macroscopic structure of the heart as a single muscular band that starts at the base of the pulmonary root and ends at the base of the aortic root. This band forms a basal loop that surrounds the tricuspid and mitral orifices and then descends toward the left ventricular apex in a spiral helix to form the apical loop (Figure 75-1). Contraction of the basal loop reduces the atrioventricular valve orifices. In a canine model, Tsakiris and associates[91] found that the size of the tricuspid orifice changed continuously during the cardiac cycle. Under control conditions, the tricuspid orifice area reduction from its maximal diastolic size varied between 20% and 39%. Most of the contraction occurred during the end of atrial contraction and throughout ventricular contraction. Approximately two thirds of the total decrease in annulus size occurred before the onset of systole (Figure 75-2). Tricuspid orifice narrowing was caused by shortening of the free wall portions of the annulus, with the anteroposterior commissure moving toward the septum. During ventricular contraction, most of the narrowing was due to bulging of the septum. In our laboratory in an ovine model, we analyzed the changes in the tricuspid orifice during the cardiac cycle as detected by changes in the distance between ultrasound crystals placed around the line of insertion of the leaflets. The degree of annulus reduction was 12.1% in the segment corresponding to the septal leaflet, 15.3% in the anterior, and 16.6% in the posterior segment. The generally accepted notion that the

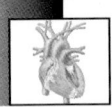

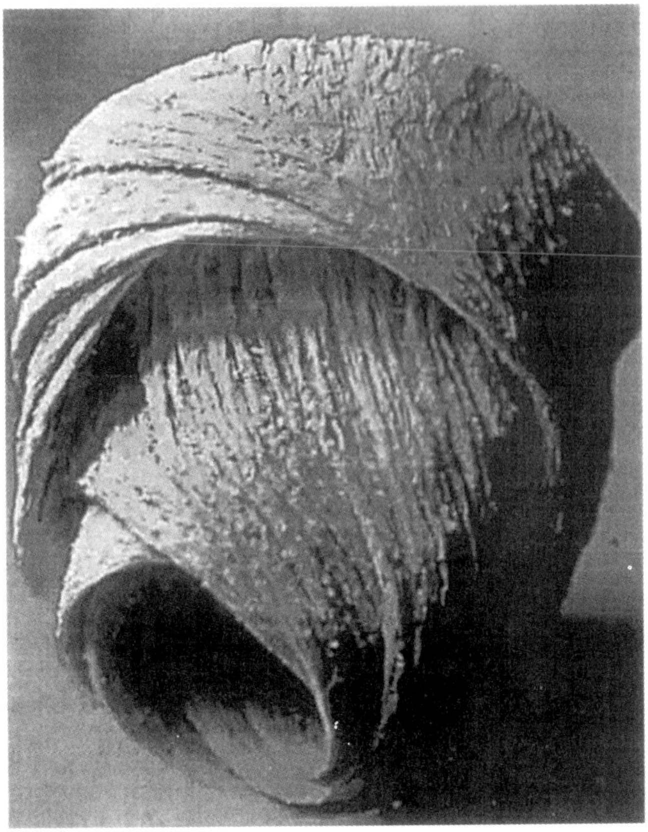

Figure 75–1 Relationship between the transverse layers of the right ventricular free wall formed by the basal loop and the obliquely oriented fibers of the apical loop that forms the septum.
(Reproduced with permission from Torrent-Guasp F, Buckberg GD, Clemente C, et al: The structure and function of the helical heart and its buttress wrapping. I. The normal macroscopic structure of the heart. Semin Thorac Cardiovasc Surg 13[4]: 301–319, 2001.)

septal portion of the annulus hardly changes during the cardiac cycle obviously needs revision. Tei and associates[88] have echocardiographically confirmed these continuous changes in the tricuspid orifice area in the human.

As in the case of the mitral valve, the "annulus" or line of leaflet insertion is not in a single plane. In fact, the tricuspid annulus is saddle shaped, with its horn or pommel corresponding to the area of the anteroseptal commissure and its cantle to the midpoint of the base of the posterior leaflet (Figure 75-3). This saddle shape, or hyperbolic parabola, which is well known to architects as an ideal design to reduce building tension, has been shown to significantly reduce peak leaflet stress in the mitral valve.[84] Rigid structures, such as stented prostheses or rigid annuloplasty rings, destroy this configuration and probably negatively impact the function of the right ventricle.

The Leaflets

Although the number of tricuspid leaflets varies according to the author,[96] it is generally accepted that the tricuspid valve consists of three leaflets (septal, anterior, and posterior), which are separated by three clefts or commissures—the anteroseptal, anteromedial, and posteroseptal (Figures 75-4 and 75-5A). These clefts do not reach the annulus but delineate small "commissural leaflets." This is an important surgical point because in cases of fused commissures, their incision should not extend all the way to the annulus, which destroys the commissural leaflets. The anterior leaflet is largest, followed by the posterior leaflet, and the septal leaflet is the smallest. The contribution of each leaflet to the closure of the tricuspid valve has been studied in normal dogs by Higashidate at al,[47] who showed that resection of the septal leaflet did not result in valve insufficiency (provided no pulmonary hypertension was present). The anterior and posterior leaflets were sufficient for the full closure of a valve without annular dilation.

The Chordae Tendineae and Papillary Muscles

The leaflets are held down by marginal and basal chords that arise from three papillary muscles. The marginal chords are inserted into the leaflet's free margin, and the basal chords are inserted into the ventricular surface of the leaflets. Elongation or rupture of the marginal chords results in leaflet prolapse. The tricuspid basal chords, although far less prominent than the mitral basal chords, probably play a similar role in maintaining the valve and ventricular geometry. In most cases, three tricuspid papillary muscles are found and are identified as anterior, posterior, and septal. Although the anterior and posterior muscles are practically always present, the septal muscle might be absent in 20% of patients. The anterior papillary muscle is the longest; it most often has a single head, and it sustains the highest number of chordae.[70]

Anatomical Relationships

The area corresponding to the anteroseptal commissure is very close to the noncoronary sinus of the aortic valve (Figure 75-6). This has important surgical implications because placing the anchoring sutures of a prosthetic device can be difficult at this level if a prosthetic aortic valve is already present. Because tears at this level can be difficult to repair, when a concomitant aortic valve replacement is planned, it is preferable to place the tricuspid sutures before the aortic valve replacement.

The right coronary artery runs parallel to the segment of the annulus corresponding to the right ventricular free wall. Despite this proximity, injury to this vascular structure when performing a valve replacement or annuloplasty is extremely rare. The ostium of the coronary sinus is situated above the posteroseptal commissure. Because of its distance from the conducting system (close to the right trigone), it is safe to place a pursestring suture around the ostium of the coronary sinus to hold a retrograde cardioplegia cannula.

PHYSIOPATHOLOGY

Tricuspid valve lesions have traditionally been classified into two groups. These groups have an important impact on the type of surgery performed and the long-term postoperative results. In organic lesions, the valve apparatus is macroscopically abnormal (Figure 75-5B). Functional lesions are insuf-

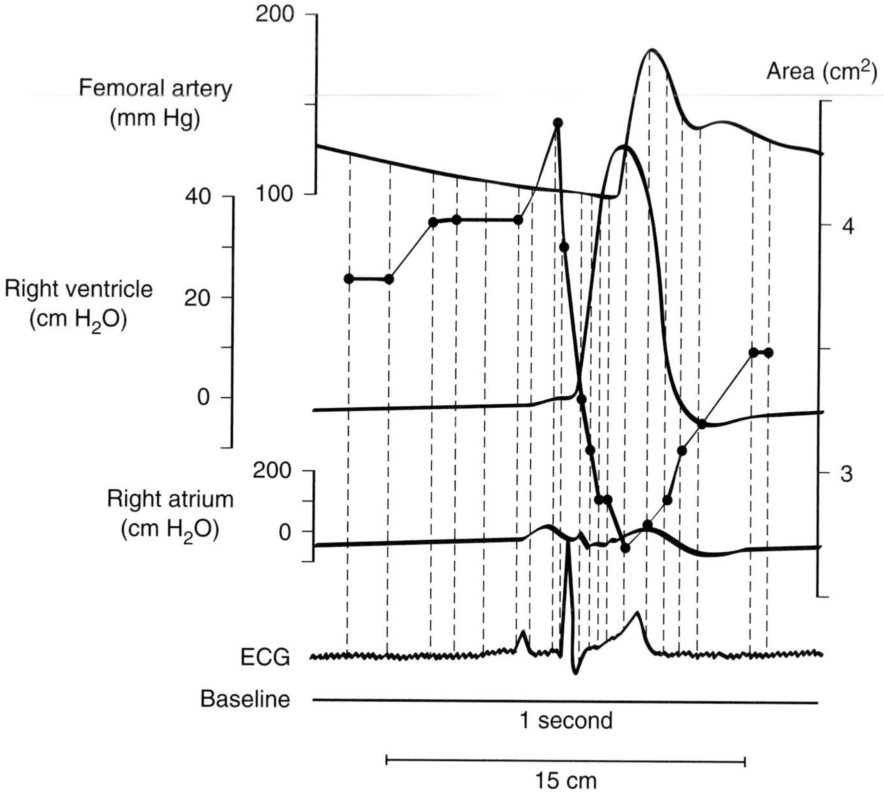

Figure 75–2 Changes in tricuspid annulus area *(solid line connecting solid circles).* Vertical lines indicate times of measurement. The area of the tricuspid annulus is reduced during atrial and ventricular contraction.
(Reproduced with permission from Tsakiris AG, Mair DD, Seki S, et al: Motion of the tricuspid valve annulus in anesthetized intact dogs. Circ Res 36:45, 1975.)

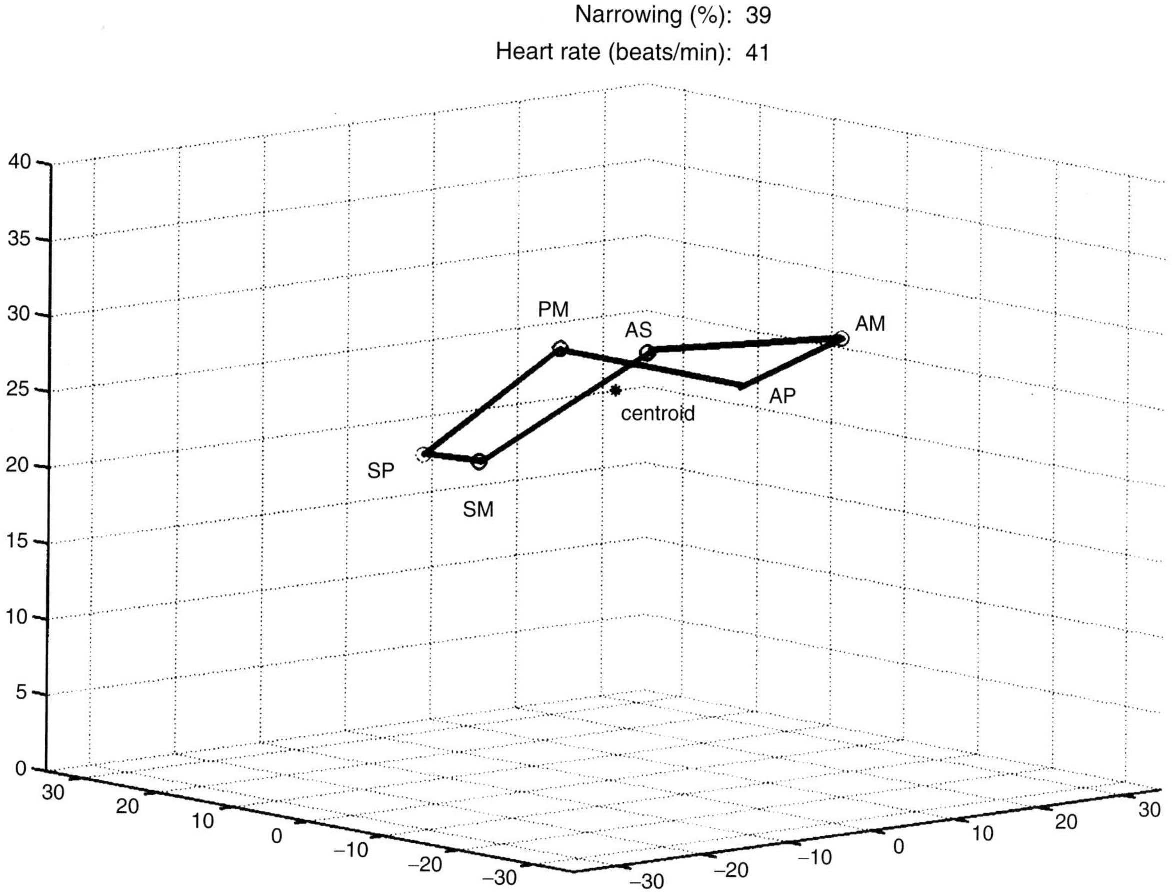

Figure 75–3 Saddle shape of the tricuspid annulus delineated by six ultrasound crystals placed on the annulus. The horn of the saddle corresponds to the anteroseptal commissure. AS, anteroseptal commissure; AM, midpoint base anterior leaflet; AP, anteroposterior commissure; PM, midpoint base of posterior leaflet; SP, posteroseptal commissure; SM, midpoint base of septal leaflet.

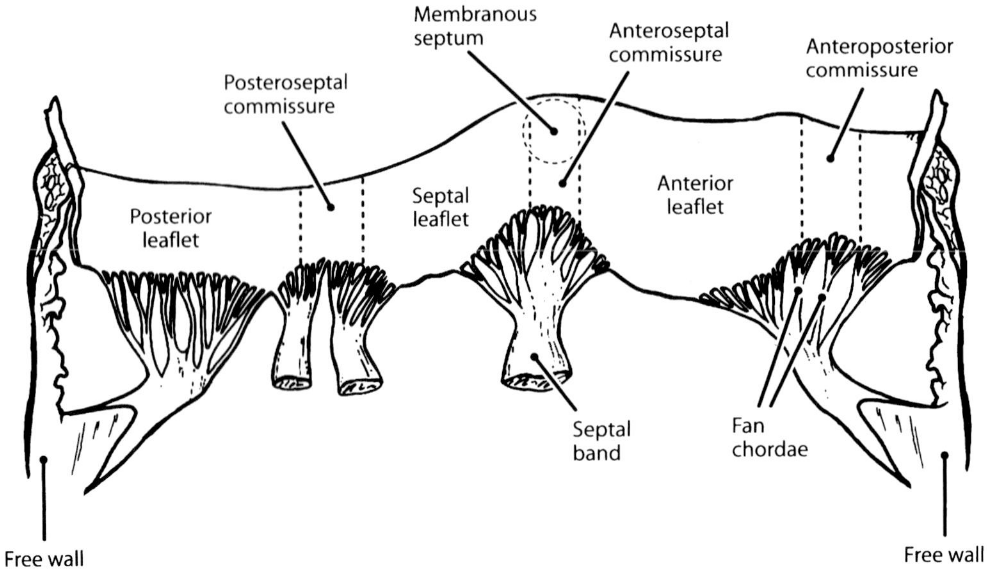

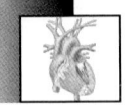

Figure 75–4 Tricuspid valve sectioned through the right ventricular free wall. Note that the clefts or commissures do not reach the annulus.
(Reproduced with permission from Duran CMG: Duran ring annuloplasty of the tricuspid valve. Op Tech Thorac Cardiovasc Surg 8: 201–212, 2003.)

ficiencies in which only a dilation of the annulus reduces coaptation of otherwise normal leaflets and subvalvular apparatus (Figure 75-5C). A different classification has been proposed by Carpentier,[14] who distinguished three main pathologies according to the mobility of the tricuspid leaflets: type I—normal leaflet motion with annular dilation; type II—increased leaflet movement due to leaflet prolapse secondary to chordal rupture or elongation; and type III—reduced leaflet motion due to leaflet thickening, fused commissures, or leaflet tethering.

Organic Tricuspid Valve Disease

A variety of etiologies can induce organic tricuspid regurgitation, but the most frequent cause of organic tricuspid disease in urban populations today is infective endocarditis (Box 75-1). Tricuspid endocarditis used to be relatively rare, with an incidence of only 5–10% of patients with infective endocarditis. Presently, its frequency has dramatically increased with the spread of intravenous drug abuse. In some institutions, right-sided endocarditis now constitutes more than half of all infectious cases.[75] In this population, the tricuspid valve usually has no preexisting pathology. Roberts and Buchbinder[81] reported that virtually all cases of right-sided endocarditis exhibited anatomically normal valves at autopsy except for evidence of the current infection. Minor valvular alterations might still be a substrate for the infection. Several animal studies have shown a relationship between repetitive particulate matter and bacterial endocarditis.[4,45] The anatomical location of the tricuspid valve at the entrance to the heart before the lung filter explains why tricuspid endocarditis is far more common in this population than involvement of the mitral or aortic valves. The lesions vary from isolated vegetations to total destruction of the valve and the annulus. Contrary to similar pathology in the mitral valve, the vegetations in the tricuspid valve tend to grow on the free edge of the leaflets, which facilitates conservative surgery of these lesions. *Staphylococcus aureus* remains the most common organism found in drug addicts,[16] followed by gram negatives and *Candida*.[18] Fungal infections are also increasing because of the longer periods of invasive monitoring of patients with multiorgan failure in intensive care units.[37]

In the developing world, rheumatic disease is the main cause of organic valvular disease. Typical lesions show varying degrees of leaflet thickening and (most often) commissural fusion. In severe cases, the thickened leaflets become diaphragm-like, with a central circular orifice (Figures 75-5B and 75-7). The subvalvular apparatus is seldom affected, and calcifications are very rare. Although tricuspid stenosis is the classic lesion, predominant insufficiency is just as common. In a series of 253 mostly rheumatic patients who underwent tricuspid surgery, we found that organic involvement was present in 45% of the cases, and 45% also had annulus dilation.[78] In a classic study of 100 postmortem hearts with rheumatic disease, Gross and Friedberg[40] found microscopic evidence of rheumatic inflammation in the tricuspid valve as frequently as in the mitral valve. Because the early acute rheumatic attack involves the annulus of all four valves,[40] rheumatic tricuspid disease is always associated with rheumatic mitral or mitroaortic lesions. The incidence of rheumatic tricuspid disease associated with rheumatic mitral disease varies widely: from 6% in an echocardiographic study by Daniels et al[25] to 33% in the anatomical series of Aceves and Carral[1] and 11% in our series of 1052 patients undergoing rheumatic valvular surgery.[78] These differences in incidence are obviously related to whether the study was based on postmortem, echocardiographic, or surgical findings. In a study from the Mayo Clinic[45] of the surgical pathology of excised tricuspid valves at the time of valve replacement, postinflammatory etiology was responsible for 53% of the 363 valves studied. However, this frequency had diminished

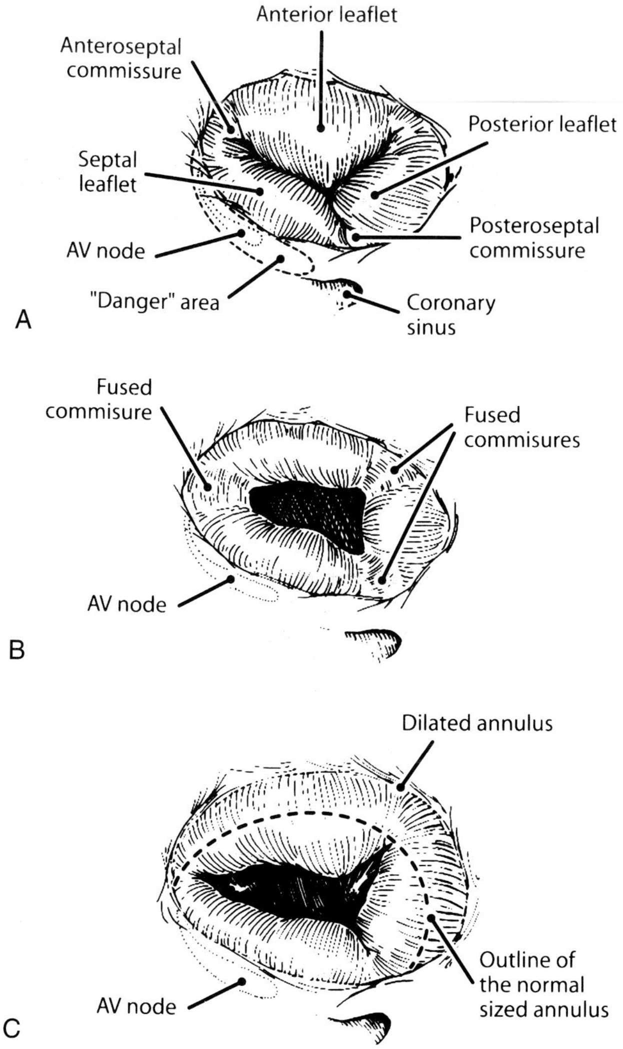

Figure 75–5 Atrial view of the (A) normal, (B) stenotic, and (C) insufficient tricuspid valve.
(Reproduced with permission from Duran CMG: Duran ring annuloplasty of the tricuspid valve. Op Tech Thorac Cardiovasc Surg 8:201-212, 2003.)

from 79% during the period 1963–1967 to only 24% during 1983–1987, reflecting the reduction in the incidence of rheumatic fever in the United States.

Leaflet tears and total or partial avulsion of a papillary muscle head may also occur after closed chest trauma. They are occasionally found at surgery and often confirmed postoperatively as traumatic by the patient who recalls an old accident (when prompted by the surgeon).[44,95] An occasional cause of traumatic tricuspid regurgitation is that induced by the bioptome when performing a right myocardial biopsy in transplanted patients. Leaflet tears or chordal avulsion result in severe regurgitation that requires urgent surgery.[100]

Myxomatous tricuspid regurgitation associated with mitral valve prolapse has been increasingly observed. This double-valve lesion is particularly frequent in Marfan syndrome[98] as manifestation of a fibrillopathy that also involves the aortic valve and ascending aorta. The frequency of tricuspid involvement among patients with myxomatous mitral disease diagnosed with echocardiography[71] or angiography[39] varies between 21% and 52%. Chen and associates[19] reported an incidence of tricuspid prolapse in 40% of patients studied with contrast echocardiography. Contrary to our opinion, these regurgitations are usually considered well tolerated and are generally ignored surgically.

Less common etiologies include organic tricuspid lesions secondary to carcinoid syndrome and appetite suppressant drugs.[22] In both cases, the leaflets are encased by a fibrous sheath that reduces their mobility, resulting in stenotic and regurgitant lesions. Other rare etiologies are listed in Box 75-1.[43,58,63]

Functional Tricuspid Regurgitation

Functional tricuspid insufficiency exclusively due to annulus dilation and/or dysfunction is the most frequent cause of tricuspid disease (Figure 75-8). The leaflets, chords, and papillary muscles are otherwise normal. In a necropsy study of patients with pure insufficiency, Waller et al[97] reported that 47% of all cases of tricuspid regurgitation were functional. In one of our studies,[78] 54% of 253 mostly rheumatic patients who underwent tricuspid surgery had functional

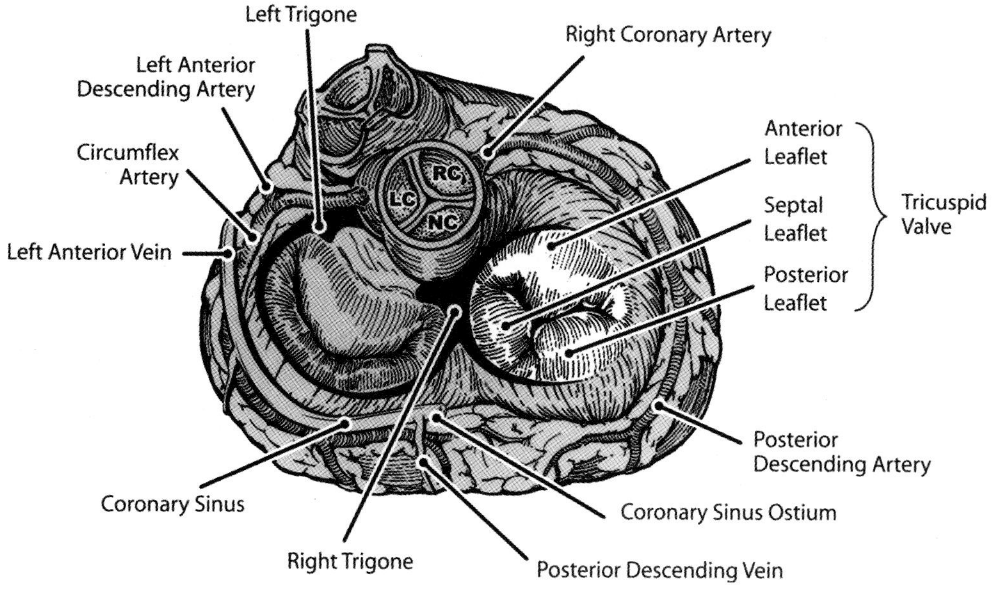

Figure 75–6 Base of the heart showing the relationships of the tricuspid valve.
(Reproduced with permission from Duran CMG: Duran ring annuloplasty of the tricuspid valve. Op Tech Thorac Cardiovasc Surg 8:201-212, 2003.)

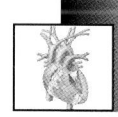

Box 75–1. Etiologies of Organic Tricuspid Disease.

Infective endocarditis
Rheumatic fever
Degenerative (myxomatous)
Traumatic
Postinfarction
Carcinoid
Appetite suppressing drugs
Endocardial fibroelastosis
Lupus erythematosus
Tumors (myxoma)
Mediastinal fibrosis

tricuspid disease, but 30% of these cases with organic disease also had a concomitant annular dilation. Because of the lack of an anatomical fibrous annulus, the tricuspid annulus follows the dilation of the right cavities and of the right ventricle in particular. The total perimeter of the normal annulus is approximately 100–120 mm. In cases of functional tricuspid regurgitation, the circumference of the annulus can reach 150–170 mm.[94,97] This annulus dilation is nonhomogeneous. In a postmortem study that included normal controls and hearts with rheumatic or myxomatous tricuspid disease, Carpentier and colleagues[15] showed that the anterior and posterior segments of the annulus dilated far more than the septal portion (Figure 75-9). This report forms the basis for all annuloplasties that selectively reduce the whole annulus except at the level of the septum. Classically, the most frequent cause of this annular dilation is right ventricular pressure overload secondary to mitral disease. However, the absence of functional insufficiency in many congenital patients with severe pulmonary hypertension refutes this oversimplified view.[28] We prefer to understand functional tricuspid regurgitation as an expression of right ventricular failure. This view might explain the different clinical outcomes after surgery for organic and functional tricuspid disease. Although surgery can successfully abolish functional tricuspid regurgitation, it cannot resolve the right ventricular dysfunction. Furthermore, recent awareness of the presence of functional tricuspid regurgitation in patients with ischemic and dilated cardiomyopathies raises another physiopathological mechanism where septal dilation/dysfunction might well be the cause.

Ischemic tricuspid regurgitation secondary to a right heart infarction, although frequent, is rarely referred to the surgeon.[64] Recently, we reviewed the preoperative transthoracic echocardiograms of 110 patients who had undergone revascularization and ring annuloplasty for ischemic mitral regurgitation. Twenty percent of them had significant (≥ 2+) tricuspid regurgitation. In congestive heart failure, the presence of functional tricuspid regurgitation is a predictor of poor survival[51] and may be an independent risk factor for the development of cardiac cachexia and protein-loosing enteropathy.[2] Koelling et al[59] studied a total of 1436 patients with left ventricular systolic dysfunction (ejection fraction <35%). Mitral regurgitation was very common; it was moderate in 30% and severe in 19% of patients. Although less common, tricuspid regurgitation was also significant, including moderate regurgitation in 23% and severe in 12% of the

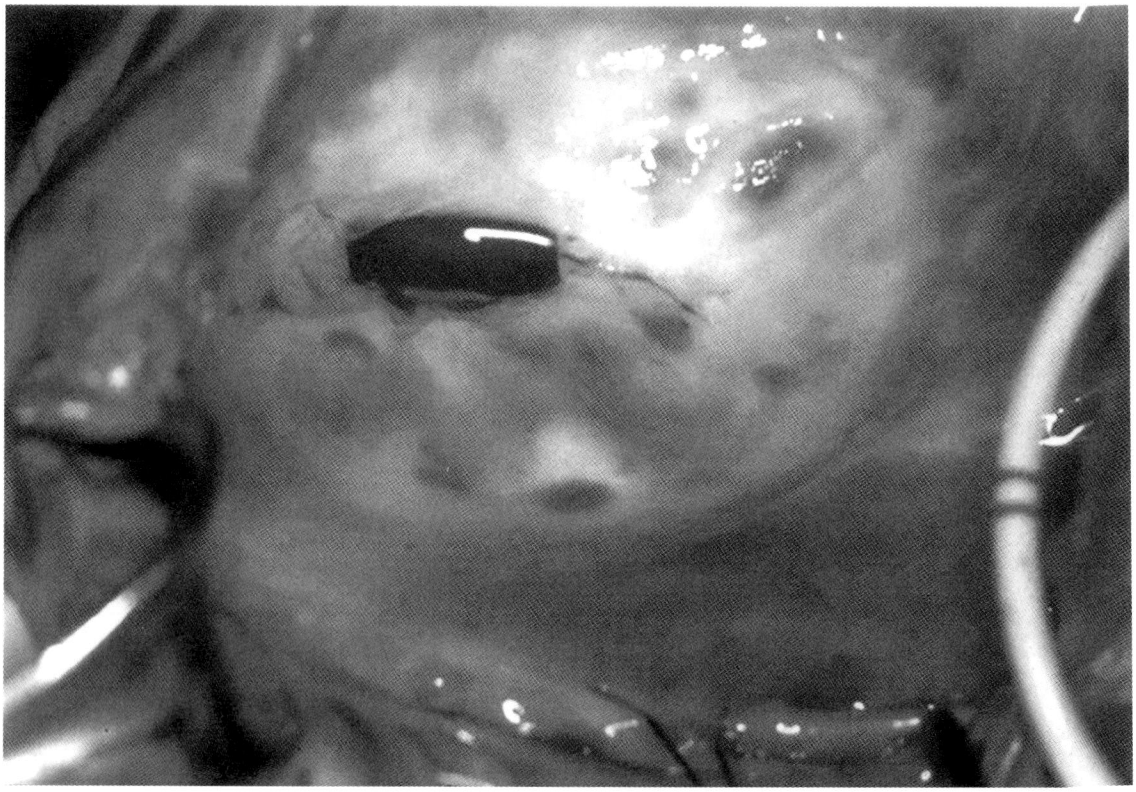

Figure 75–7 Operative photograph of the diseased tricuspid valve as a diaphragm.

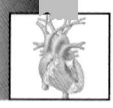

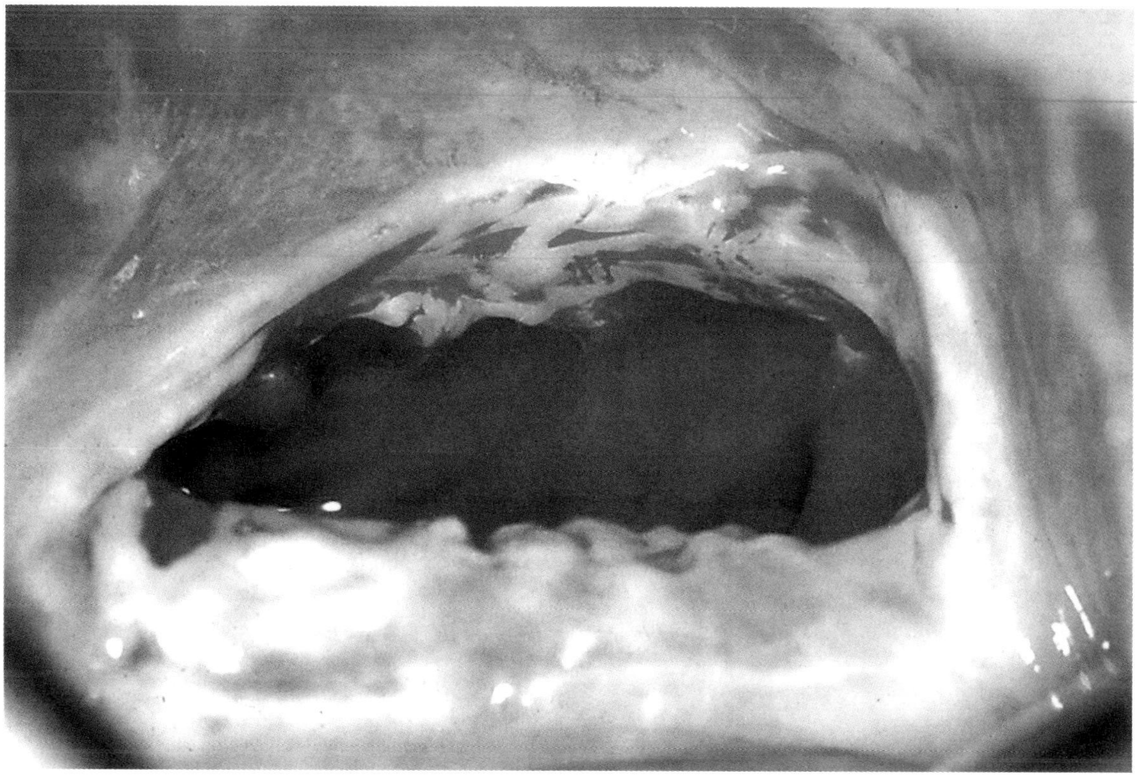

Figure 75–8 **Operative photograph of tricuspid insufficiency resulting from annulus dilation.**

patients. Patients with severe mitral regurgitation were also more likely to have tricuspid regurgitation. Severe tricuspid regurgitation was an independent predictor of mortality.

Tricuspid insufficiency after cardiac transplantation is a frequent early finding that usually decreases with time.[9,46] It may be due to distortion of the tricuspid valve but is more frequently attributed to chronic rejection and ventricular failure. Angermann et al[3] reported an incidence of 85% in long-term survivors, and Yankah et al[100] described a prevalence of 20% among 647 patients followed between 31 days and 13 years. The regurgitation was mild in 14.5% and severe in 2.5% of the patients.

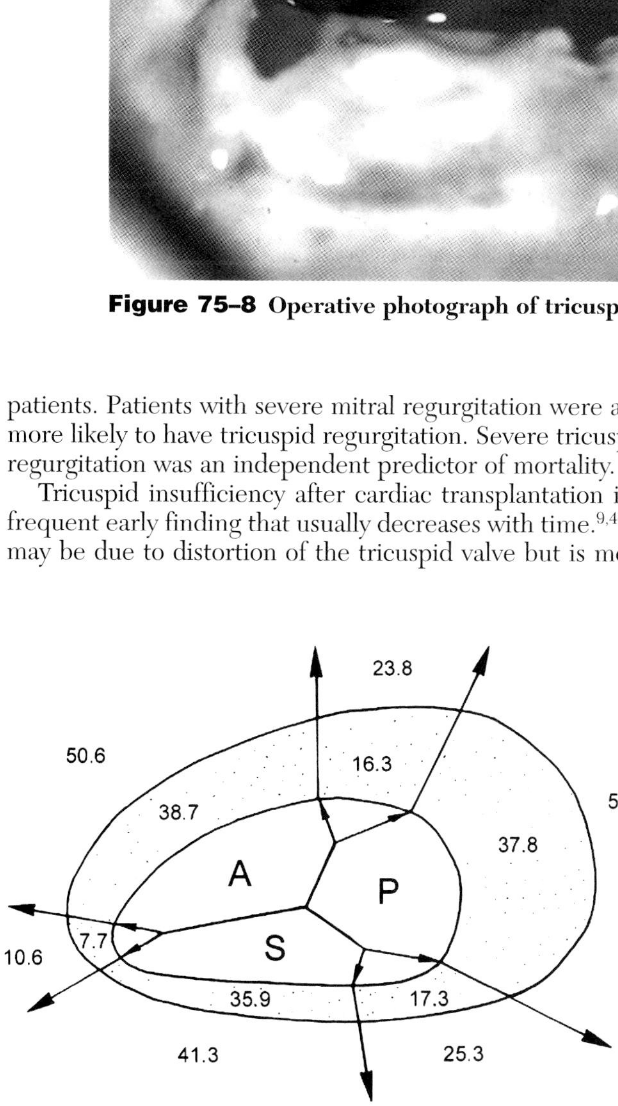

Figure 75–9 **Diagram of the tricuspid valve annulus showing the normal *(inner ellipse)* and myxomatous *(outer ellipse)* valve.** Figures in centimeters. S, septal leaflet; A, anterior leaflet; P, posterior leaflet.
(From Carpentier A, Deloche A, Hanania G, et al: Surgical management of acquired tricuspid valve disease. J Thorac Cardiovasc Surg 67:55, 1974, with permission from Excerpta Medica, Inc.)

DIAGNOSIS

Very little precise clinical criteria exist to determine the presence and degree of tricuspid disease. The well-known clinical signs of tricuspid disease are unmistakable, but their absence does not exonerate the surgeon from suspecting and treating it. Clinical experience has repeatedly shown that although tricuspid regurgitation regresses spontaneously after correction of left-sided lesions in some patients, other patients require reoperation only to repair a previously ignored tricuspid valve. The symptomatology of the patient with tricuspid disease is usually minimal and overshadowed by the more apparent left-sided symptoms. Because the tricuspid valve is situated at the entrance of the heart, tricuspid symptoms are extracardiac. With the exception of advanced cardiomyopathy, it is now rare to encounter a patient with the classic symptoms of venous engorgement (such as peripheral edema, hepatomegaly, and ascites). Tricuspid disease is mostly silent; the patient complains only of asthenia at most.

Until recently, diagnosis of tricuspid disease was considered difficult. Because of the unreliability of the available preoperative diagnostic methods, the surgeon used to digitally explore the tricuspid valve through the right atrium and decide whether to treat or ignore the lesion according to the intensity of the regurgitant jet. This method has been completely abandoned because of its subjectivity and inability to detect moderate degrees of insufficiency. Right heart catheterization and ventriculography, which were considered the gold standards for the study of all cardiac valves, have been superseded by 2D color Doppler echocardiography. The reasons for this shift are the reliability and noninvasive nature of Doppler echo compared with the invasiveness of catheterization and the unreliability of right ventriculography (which crosses the tricuspid valve with a catheter that induces PVCs and false positive regurgitations because it interferes with the closing of the valve). Even if the right ventriculogram is properly performed with a malleable pulmonary balloon catheter trapped in the inflow trabeculae, it is far more cumbersome than a noninvasive echocardiographic study.[93]

Because of its noninvasiveness, reliability, and visual impact, 2D Doppler echocardiography is the best tool for determining the presence, degree, and etiology of tricuspid disease (Figures 75-10, and 75-11). Although transesophageal echocardiography (TEE) provides invaluable anatomical information at the time of surgery, transthoracic echocardiography (TTE) remains the most important examination. Besides the better window obtained with TTE, the main reason for its superiority is the notorious temporal variability in degree of tricuspid regurgitation. This is particularly important in functional insufficiencies where changes in blood volume secondary to diuretic administration or vascular tone under general anesthesia can severely reduce the degree of regurgitation. A lack of awareness of these facts and exclusively relying on intraoperative TEE examination very often result in ignoring significant tricuspid regurgitations.

From a surgical point of view, the essential preoperative information needed includes (1) whether or not the patient has tricuspid valve disease; (2) whether it is organic, functional, or mixed; (3) quantification of the degree of regurgitation and direction of the regurgitant jet; (4) pulmonary artery peak and mean pressures; (5) presence and quantification of transvalvular pressure gradients; (6) maximum and minimum tricuspid annulus diameter and systolic shortening; (7) anatomical features of the valve, such as leaflet thickness, mobility, billowing of the leaflet body, and location of the prolapsing free edge toward the right atrium; and (8) absence of a patent foramen ovale.

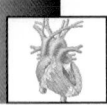

Color Doppler echo has been repeatedly shown to have a reasonably good correlation with angiography.[87] Although the technique is semiquantitative, the maximal area of the jet can be imaged. Remember that the image represents velocity flow and not volume flow (which we are used to seeing in angiography). We are not truly imaging the regurgitant volume. We must also be aware that under estimation and over estimation of the regurgitant jet area are possible because of changes in gain, filter settings, angle, and distance of the transducer. Experience is required to have a three-dimensional concept of the direction, location, size, and number of regurgitant jets.[20] Color Doppler can even discover minimal regurgitations in 60–100% of the normal population.[101] These "physiological"

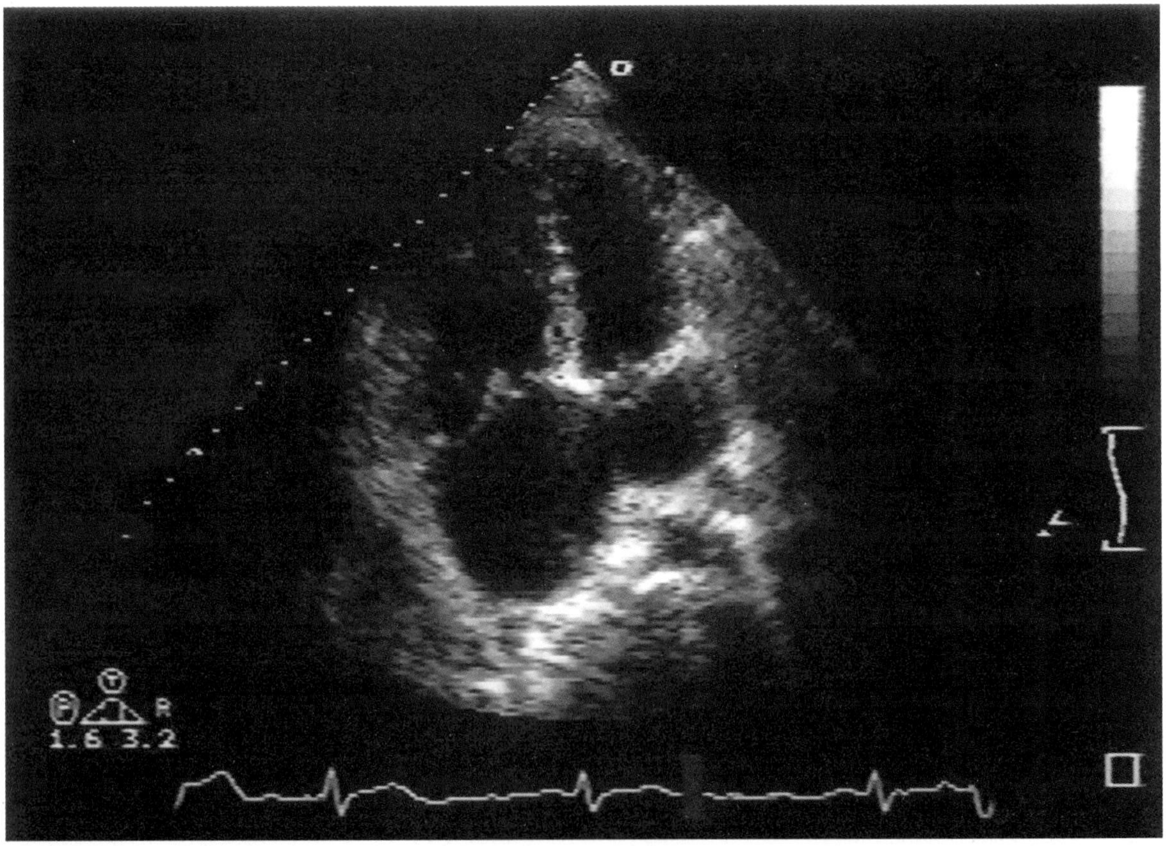

Figure 75–10 Apical four-chamber transthoracic echocardiogram. A normal tricuspid annulus is shown on the left and normal mitral valve is shown on the right.

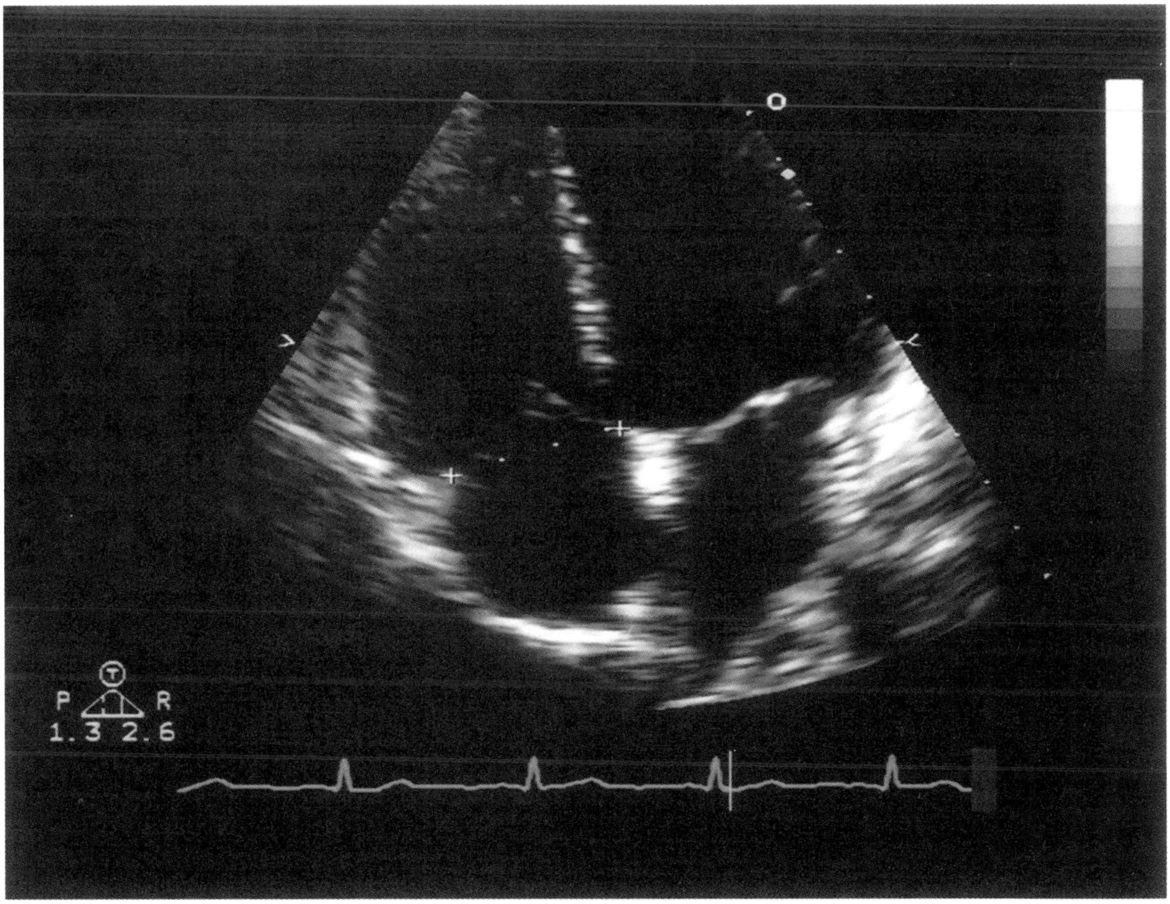

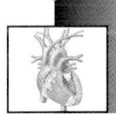

Figure 75–11 Apical four-chamber transthoracic echocardiogram. Dilated tricuspid annulus in a 45-year-old patient with a long-standing dehiscence of a closed atrial septal defect operated as a child.

regurgitations are useful to evaluate the right ventricular and pulmonary pressures.[8] Contrast echocardiography is a very reliable method for the detection of tricuspid regurgitation[24] and the presence of a patent foramen ovale. It involves injecting saline with microbubbles in a peripheral vein while observing for the presence of the bubbles in the right atrium during systole. Goldman and associates[38] evaluated the value of intraoperative contrast echocardiography to determine the presence and quantification of tricuspid regurgitation in 50 patients undergoing cardiac surgery. Five milliliters of dextrose or saline was injected into the right ventricle to generate echogenic "contrast." In patients with tricuspid regurgitation, systolic reflux into the right atrium was found that could be semiquantified in a scale of 0 to 4+. The correlation with the preoperative echo study for the presence or absence of tricuspid regurgitation had a sensitivity of 0.90 and specificity of 1.00.

Knowledge of the tricuspid annulus diameter is important for the surgeon, but its echocardiographic measurement is difficult because the annulus is not circular; therefore, small variations in the orientation of the ultrasound beam can provide very different figures. Based on the idea that the cause of functional regurgitation is the lack of leaflet coaptation due to annulus dilation, measurement of the tricuspid orifice diameter can provide a useful method to determine the importance of the regurgitation. The search for a "critical annulus diameter" beyond which the tricuspid valve should not be ignored by the surgeon has been ongoing. Ubago and associates[94] showed that among patients without regurgitation, the indexed mean maximum diameter (measured in a right ventriculogram) was 21 mm/m^2. Among those with mild regurgitation, it was 31 mm/m^2 and among those with moderate or severe regurgitation, it was 37 mm/m^2. The authors suggested 27 mm/m^2 as the "critical diameter" above which functional regurgitation always appeared (Figure 75-12). Using TTE of 11 consecutive patients with clinically severe tricuspid regurgitation, Come and Riley[21] reported a mean diastolic annulus diameter of 51 mm in the four-chamber view and 54 mm in the short axis view. Among 15 controls, the mean annulus diameter was 34 mm in the four-chamber view and 33 mm in the short axis view. Using intraoperative epicardial echocardiography, Goldman et al[38] measured the largest tricuspid annulus diameter from the base of the septal leaflet to the insertion of the anterior leaflet in the free right ventricular wall: Among the 36 patients with no or mild regurgitation (0 to 2+), the annulus length was 26 mm; in the 14 patients with moderate or severe regurgitation (3 to 4+), the annulus length was 39 mm. Although the authors did not find a difference between the lengths in systole and diastole, they suggested 30 mm as the cut-off point between absent/mild regurgitation and moderate/severe regurgitation. Additionally, the tricuspid annulus diameter as measured in the right ventricular inflow view

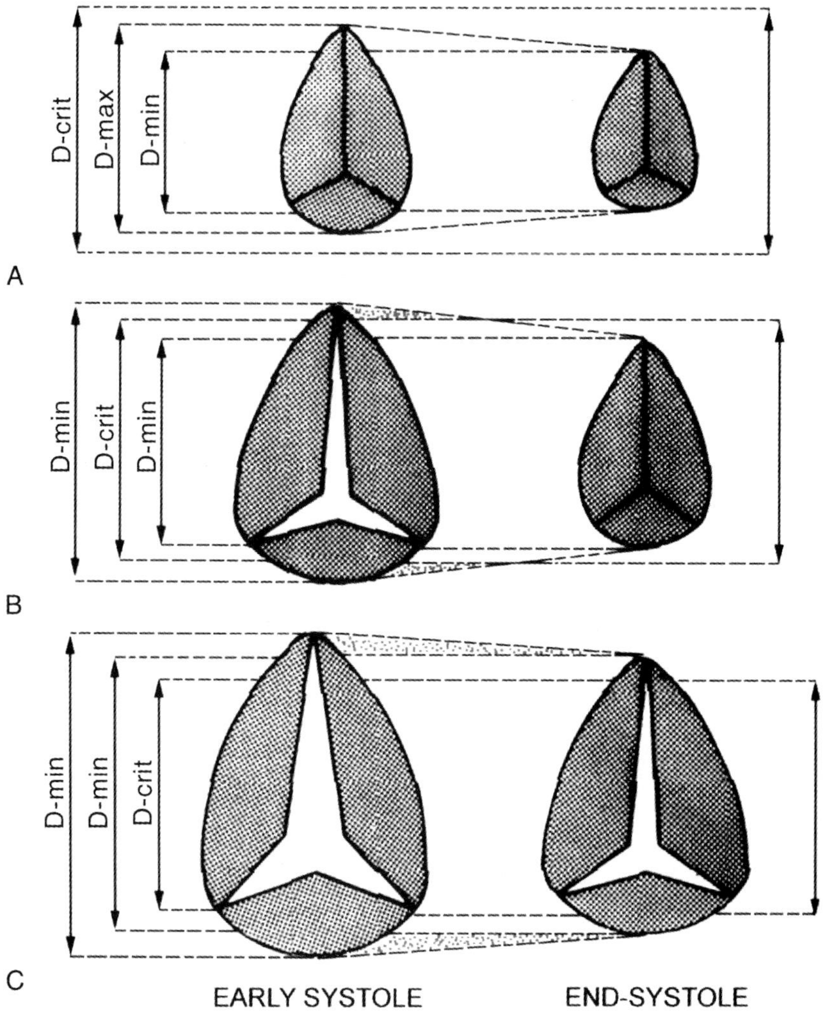

Figure 75–12 Diagram of the tricuspid valve. (**A**) Patients without regurgitation. Both maximal early systolic (D-max) and minimal late end systolic (D-min) are below the critical diameter (D-crit) of 27 mm/m^2. (**B**) Patients with mild regurgitation. D-max is larger, but D-min is smaller than D-crit. No cusp apposition occurs during early and mid-systole. (**C**) Patients with severe regurgitation. D-max and D-min are above D-crit. Pansystolic regurgitation
(From Ubago JL, Figueroa A, Ochoteco A, et al: Analysis of the amount of tricuspid valve annular dilatation required to produce functional tricuspid regurgitation. Am J Cardiol 52:157, 1983, with permission from Exerpta Medica, Inc.)

correlated better with the severity of tricuspid regurgitation than the mean pulmonary artery pressure.

The preoperative differentiation between organic and functional tricuspid disease is also possible. The presence of transvalvular gradients, leaflet irregularities, thickening, and doming is a clear indication of organic disease. Transvalvular gradients calculated with continuous wave Doppler echocardiography have been shown to correlate well with cardiac catheterization.[69] Annulus dilation is most often present in both organic and functional lesions, but it is larger in functional regurgitation. In a necropsy study, Waller et al[97] showed that patients with functional regurgitation had a much larger annulus than patients with organic disease. We studied the preoperative data of 206 patients who underwent tricuspid surgery to search for possible hemodynamic and angiographic differentiating characteristics of organic and functional lesions as defined at surgery by the surgeon.[92] We found no significant differences in right atrial, ventricular, and pulmonary pressures and pulmonary resistances between organic and functional lesions. However, the mean end-diastolic annulus diameter was significantly different between the patients with organic and functional lesions. In the organic lesions, the mean annulus diameter measured 39 ± 7 mm; in the functional lesions, it was 45 ± 7 mm. Although the amount of annulus dilation did not correlate with the degree of functional regurgitation, it did correlate in the organic patients (Table 75-1).

SURGICAL INDICATIONS

The vast majority of diseased tricuspid valves can be easily repaired. However, unless very severe, most lesions are usually ignored based on the wrong assumption that tricuspid disease is rare and, in most cases, irrelevant to the patient's outcome after the problem that brings the patient to surgery has been solved. However, the regression of tricuspid regurgitation after repair of the left side valve is unpredictable at best. Severe lesions are usually treated, but real or erroneously labeled moderate lesions are ignored. The problem often lies in the absence of a detailed preoperative search for tricuspid disease. Intraoperative decision making is unreliable unless the lesion is severe. A preoperative TTE specifically interrogating the tricuspid valve is an absolute requirement. Unfortunately, this is not always available to the surgeon who has to rely on the intraoperative TEE.

Ignoring Tricuspid Disease

Notwithstanding the concern for leaving behind sufficient tricuspid regurgitation that would require a later second

Table 75–1

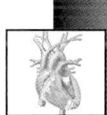

Relation between Tricuspid Annulus and Degree of Tricuspid Regurgitation (TR)

Degree TR	*Functional TR (mm)*	*Organic TR (mm)*	*p value*
I	46 ± 4	35 ± 6	<.01
II	44 ± 6	39 ± 7	<.01
III	46 ± 8	42 ± 8	Not significant
Global	45 ± 7	39 ± 7	<.01

Modified from Ubago JL, Figueroa A, et al: Diagnostico hemodinamico de afectacion organica de la valvular tricuspide. Rev Esp Cardiol 33:515–523, 1980.

operation, the immediate postoperative well being of the patient (starting with the ability to be weaned from cardiopulmonary bypass) is at issue.[41] A widely cited report suggested that tricuspid regurgitation can resolve after the diseased mitral valve has been replaced.[53] This conservative approach was based on the well-known postoperative regression of pulmonary hypertension, which would reduce the tricuspid regurgitation and obviate the need for a combined mitral and tricuspid surgery. A significant and growing body of evidence suggests that ignoring a diseased tricuspid valve at the time of surgery for left-sided pathology will interfere with the eventual outcome of the patient. King and associates[56] reported that 66% of patients returning for tricuspid valve surgery late after mitral valve replacement had only mild tricuspid valve insufficiency at the time of the initial operation. It must be noted that in some patients, this course of events was related to failure of the mitral operation (as evidenced by the fact that concomitant mitral surgery was necessary in half of the patients). Porter et al[76] studied a group of 65 patients with rheumatic heart disease who underwent mitral valve replacement without tricuspid surgery and were followed for up to 30 years (mean 11.3 years). Echocardiography revealed significant tricuspid regurgitation in 67% of the patients. In 34% of them, the lesion was organic and therefore present and presumably undiagnosed at the time of the initial surgery. Groves et al[41] reported persistence of the tricuspid regurgitation in 38% of the patients with isolated mitral replacement. We studied a group of 150 patients with mitral repair and concomitant tricuspid disease who underwent a preoperative and postoperative right heart catheterization and ventriculography.[34] The diseased tricuspid valve was repaired in 119 patients, and it was ignored in 31. The tricuspid insufficiency persisted in all patients with ignored organic lesions and persisted in 53% of those with ignored functional lesions. Recent experience with balloon dilation of stenotic mitral valves in patients with an associated tricuspid lesion that is necessarily ignored throws further light on this issue. Sagie et al[83] found a lack of resolution of tricuspid regurgitation 1 year after surgical mitral valvotomy in 34.8% of the patients.

Specific Surgical Indications

The surgical indications for tricuspid valve disease should be determined by the severity of the lesion and its repairability. Severe lesions demand surgery regardless of whether the valve is expected to be replaced or repaired. Moderate lesions should be treated if repair is expected. This principle emphasizes the importance of a precise preoperative diagnosis.

1. Tricuspid disease associated with left-sided valvular lesions should not be ignored, even if mild to moderate (≥ 2+). It should be treated at the time of surgery for the other valves.
2. Organic lesions should be always treated. In cases of rheumatic polyvalvular lesions, ignoring the tricuspid lesion on the basis of the small gradient present before surgery is dangerous because it is likely to become significant postoperatively (because of the increase in cardiac output after repair of the left-sided lesions). If regurgitation is present, the persistence of right ventricular preload will further affect the right ventricle and further promote functional regurgitation. In our previously mentioned study,[92] independent of satisfactory mitral repair, the right ventricular end diastolic volume improved after tricuspid repair but did not change when the tricuspid regurgitation persisted.
3. Traumatic insufficiencies are usually always amenable to repair. In chronic cases, the common finding is a leaflet prolapse due to a fibrotic and elongated papillary muscle head. Repair by plication of the elongated head is easy and successful. Acute tears of a leaflet or avulsion of a chord are more difficult to repair because resuturing the torn leaflet is seldom successful. A resection of the unsupported leaflet with reapproximation of its edges followed by selective reduction of the annulus with an annuloplasty ring has a better chance of success. Recently, the use of Gore-Tex sutures to replace the torn chord has simplified this problem.
4. In infective endocarditis, the traditional attitude to operate only those cases with bacteriological resistance or hemodynamic compromise should be revised. The rate of successful repair is directly related to the degree of valve destruction. Although early, still localized lesions can be easily repaired, a destroyed valve requires replacement. It is worth pointing out that although mitral repair demands excellent competence, imperfect tricuspid repairs are well tolerated because of the low pressure system. An imperfect, native tricuspid valve is superior to prosthesis.
5. Functional tricuspid regurgitations should also be surgically treated. Severe lesions are obvious candidates for repair. The old argument that the sudden increase in afterload after valve replacement would result in ventricular failure known as the "pop off" mechanism must be abandoned. This principle has repeatedly been shown to be wrong in the mitral valve. The original argument was based on the severe drop in ejection fraction after mitral replacement with severance of the subvalvular apparatus. When mitral repair was performed (and therefore the annulopapillary continuity was retained), the ejection fraction was preserved. The same argument should apply to the right ventricle.

Mild-to-moderate regurgitations are still under discussion. Adding a short ischemic time to perform a simple annuloplasty is worthwhile when it is known that spontaneous regression is unpredictable. In rheumatic cases, if the decision is based on one (or preferably more) well-performed, preoperative TTE studies, mild degrees of regurgitation can be ignored. This decision is reinforced if the pulmonary pressure is low. Mild regurgitations in the presence of high pulmonary resistances should also be treated prophylactically. Despite the well-known reduction in regurgitation under anesthesia, a useful intraoperative indicator for repair is the TEE measurement of the end-systolic tricuspid annulus. A maximum tricuspid diameter above 30 mm should constitute an indication for repair.

6. A special subset of patients with functional tricuspid insufficiency is appearing after heart transplantation. Possible causes of tricuspid regurgitation after transplantation include (a) distortion of the geometry of the tricuspid annulus due to the right atrial anastomosis[3]; it has been shown that the change in surgical technique from biatrial to bicaval anastomosis significantly reduces the incidence of immediate regurgitation; (b) size mismatch of the donor heart and the pericardial cavity[46]; and (c) ischemic right ventricular failure and global heart failure secondary to ongoing rejection.[100]

   In a small number of patients, we performed a tricuspid double resorbable suture annuloplasty ("Vanishing DeVega") in the donor heart immediately prior to transplantation. We had previously shown in sheep that a 2/0 polydioxanone suture (PDS) used to perform a DeVega tricuspid annuloplasty disappeared completely in 5 months and the tricuspid orifice returned to its original size.[32,33]

7. Congestive heart failure secondary to ischemic or idiopathic cardiomyopathy with mitral regurgitation is currently treated with "overcorrection" using a reducing ring annuloplasty.[60] In our opinion, tricuspid annuloplasty should be added because in many cases, a tricuspid regurgitation is already present. It also avoids the inexorable progression of the tricuspid annulus dilation. Additionally, a double-ring annuloplasty might have a contention effect on the base of the heart. This is a far simpler surgery than the new procedures directed toward passively restraining the heart's diastolic expansion.[65,74] Radovanovic et al[79] reported significant echocardiographic benefits immediately after a double mitral and tricuspid reducing annuloplasty in 222 patients with ischemic (152) or dilated (70) cardiomyopathy. The overall hospital mortality was 2.3%, and the ejection fraction and fractional shortening increased while the left ventricular diastolic and systolic volumes were reduced. Although this is a single center report without any follow-up, the concept of reducing and securing the base of the heart warrants further study.

TRICUSPID VALVE SURGERY

Because of the lower incidence of tricuspid compared with mitral valve disease, its surgery has lagged behind and followed the surgical techniques used in mitral valve surgery. Practically no specific tricuspid valve surgery has been developed. Both the reconstructive techniques and valve prostheses used in the tricuspid are similar to those designed for the mitral position. Recent awareness of the suboptimal long-term results of ignoring its importance and the realization of its unique characteristics should stimulate the development of new and specific approaches to the tricuspid valve.

Surgical Approaches to the Tricuspid Valve

The approach to the tricuspid valve is easy because of its anatomical location. It can be visualized through a midsternotomy or a right thoracotomy. Unless an isolated tricuspid lesion is contemplated, the type of thoracotomy and incision is dictated by the concomitant surgery. A standard or minimally invasive approach can be safely used. To establish cardiopulmonary bypass, the superior caval cannula is inserted through the right appendage, and the inferior cannula is inserted through the lateral wall of the right atrium close to the entrance of the inferior vena cava. The right atrial incision is started close to the appendage and directed toward the posterior aspect of the atrium between the right inferior pulmonary vein and the inferior vena cava (Figure 75-13). This incision minimizes the problem when an accidental tear of the lower extremity of the incision occurs from overretraction. Instead of being directed toward the inferior vena cava, the tear will extend into the posterior wall of the atrium. Although tricuspid valve surgery can be easily performed in the beating heart, the surgeon most often prefers an arrested heart. If retrograde cardioplegia is planned, the coronary sinus is located above the posteroseptal commissure and can-

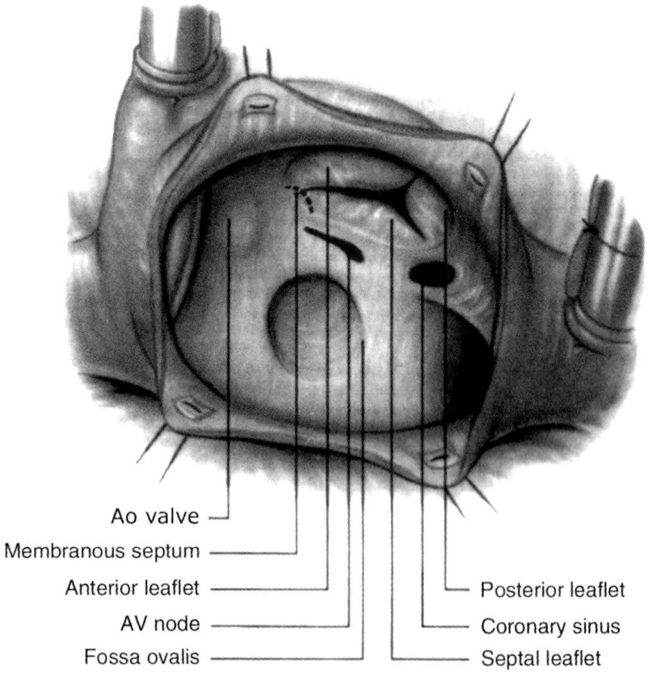

Figure 75–13 Surgical view of the tricuspid valve through a standard right atriotomy. The "danger" area corresponding to the atrioventricular node is located near the anterior half of the base of the septal leaflet.
(Reproduced with permission from Duran CMG: Reoperations on the mitral and tricuspid valves. In Sabiston Jr. DC, Stark J, Pacifico A, Courtney M, editors: Reoperations in Cardiac Surgery. New York: Springer-Verlag, 1989, p. 346.)

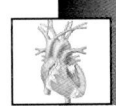

nulated. To ensure the maximum distribution of cardioplegia to the whole heart, a pursestring is placed around the coronary ostium. After the retrograde cannula is in place, the pursestring is tightened, the balloon is inflated, and the catheter is pulled outwardly until arrested by the pursestring.

When a simultaneous mitral valve surgery is required, most surgeons approach both valves through separate incisions. An alternative is the use of the extended transatrial septal incision described by Guiraudon et al.[42] The right atriotomy is performed parallel to and as close as possible to the atrioventricular groove to avoid damage to the sinus node and it is stopped at the junction of the right and left atria. A vertical incision is started at the fossa ovalis, continued until it joins the right atriotomy, and prolonged along the roof the left atrium. Practically no retractors are needed to obtain an excellent view of both the tricuspid and mitral valves. This is an attractive alternative in cases of small left atria. Although a higher incidence of junctional rhythms occurs in the immediate postoperative period, no rhythm differences have been found several months later.[62]

Tricuspid Commissurotomy

The first closed tricuspid commissurotomy was performed in 1952 by Charles Bailey.[6] Although significantly improving desperately sick patients, these early procedures, which used valve dilators, were soon replaced by the more precise open commissurotomy after cardiopulmonary bypass became available. Today, percutaneous balloon dilation has replaced closed commissurotomy. The results are similar with both techniques because they are based on the same principle of splitting the commissures through distending pressure exercised on the leaflets.

The results of tricuspid balloon dilation are considerably inferior to mitral balloon dilation because of the difference between the mitral and tricuspid leaflet's resistance to tears. Tricuspid balloon dilation is now reserved for patients for whom its minimal invasiveness compensates for its mediocre results. Also, the low pressure in the right cavities minimizes the importance of the frequent residual gradients and iatrogenic regurgitations. Today, most tricuspid valve lesions are treated surgically because they accompany more florid mitral problems that demand surgery.

When performing an open tricuspid commissurotomy, the valve should be inspected carefully because in severe cases, it appears as a diaphragm with a central circular orifice and fibrotic edges. In these extreme cases, it is difficult to identify the commissures. The subvalvular apparatus is often fairly intact; therefore, a conservative procedure is still possible (although the result will most likely be suboptimal). Valve hooks are placed on either side of the commissure to explore the "fan" chordae that are always present at the commissures. The incision must ensure that the two edges of the incision are supported by chordae. When the chords are not clearly seen, a dental mirror is used to observe the commissural subvalvular apparatus. It is often easier to start the incision 4–5 mm from the annulus rather than at the edge of the fused leaflets (Figure 75-14). A better view

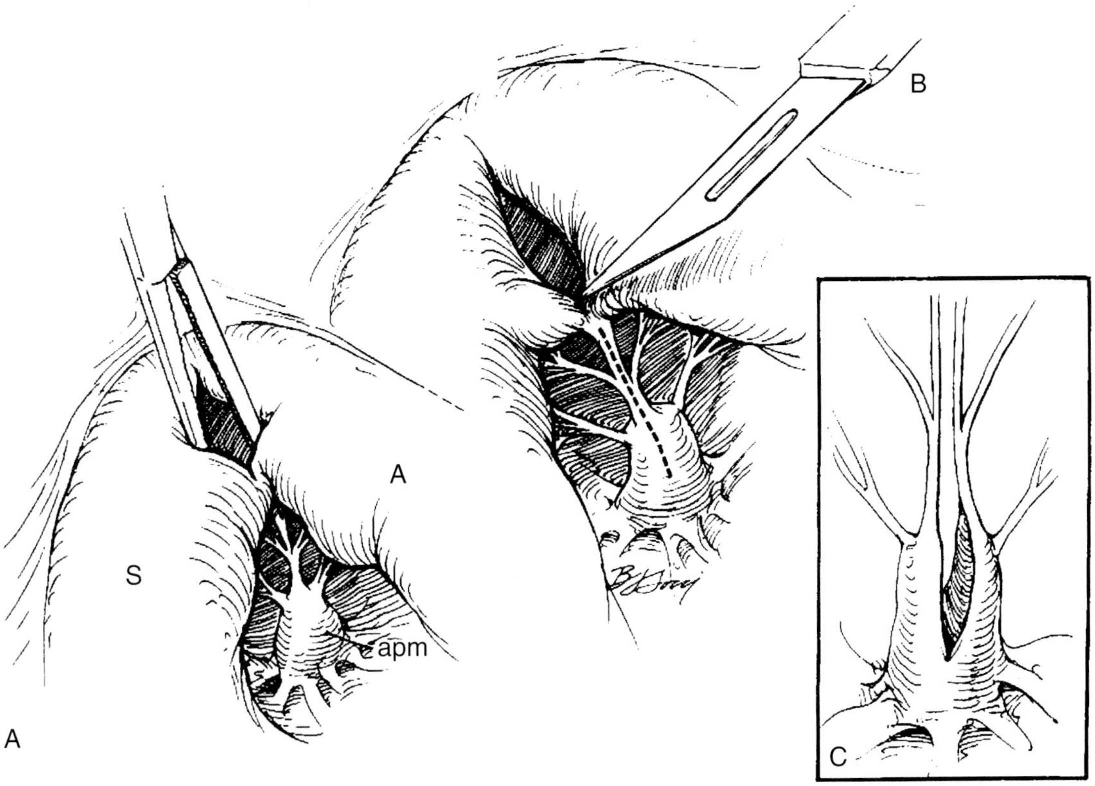

Figure 75–14 Tricuspid valve commissurotomy. The anteroseptal commissure is opened distal to the free edge to identify the fused chords.
(From Revuelta JM, Garcia-Rinalda R, Duran CMG: Tricuspid commissurotomy. Ann Thorac Surg 39:489–491, 1985, with permission from Society of Thoracic Surgeons.)

of the chords through that gap will direct the incision toward the free edge. In most cases, two "fanlike," thin chords are fused. This incision is then prolonged apically into the papillary muscle. This papillotomy should extend for at least 1 cm. The purpose of this essential maneuver is not only to slow down the ongoing fibrotic process but to increase leaflet mobility. At present, these very severe forms of commissural fusion are rare. However, lesser degrees of fusion are frequently present and missed unless a careful inspection of the valve is done. Often only one or two commissures are affected, with the anteroseptal being the most frequently fused. In the vast majority of cases, a tricuspid annuloplasty must accompany the commissurotomy because of a lack of leaflet tissue or because an annular dilation is also present.

Repair Maneuvers

Because most tricuspid regurgitations are functional, repair maneuvers other than annuloplasty are less often needed than in mitral valve repair. However, in nonrheumatic cases, they are often required. In acute infective endocarditis, the vegetation(s) must be excised. The vegetation is resected a few millimeters beyond its base in the leaflet. This resection should be in healthy tissue (which is easily identified because of its normal coloration compared with the reddish color of the inflamed area). A triangular resection with its base at the free edge of the leaflet is most often the best solution. The gap is closed with 5-0 polypropylene sutures. Unless this resection is small, an annuloplasty must follow. Leaflet perforations present in healed endocarditis can be closed with sutures or, if extensive, with a patch of glutaraldehyde-treated autologous pericardium. Important destructions can be reconstructed with pericardium supported by Gore-Tex neochords.

Tricuspid Annuloplasty

The principle behind all tricuspid annuloplasties is to selectively reduce the length of the tricuspid annulus and, consequently, the tricuspid orifice. The lack of leaflet coaptation is compensated by the induced smaller tricuspid orifice. The earliest annuloplasties consisted of plicating the annulus at the level of the base of the posterior leaflet. This approach, borrowed from the early mitral annuloplasties, was described by Wooler et al[99] and Kay et al[55] (Figure 75-15). Both have been abandoned because of the difficulty of determining the amount of plication necessary and the lack of support of the remaining annulus. Cabrol[12] and DeVega[27] independently described a partial encircling suture to narrow the annulus. The extremities of a double suture that runs along the base of the anterior and posterior leaflets are anchored with pledgets at the anteroseptal and posteroseptal commissures (Figure 75-16). The partial pursestring is tied over an obturator of the desired size. This technique has been popular because of its simplicity and low cost, but it is rarely used today because of late recurrence of incompetence resulting from the sutures cutting through or breaking (which gives a guitar string appearance at reoperation).[57] Among 80 surviving patients receiving a DeVega annuloplasty, Holper et al[48] reported a recurrence of tricuspid regurgitation rated as moderate in

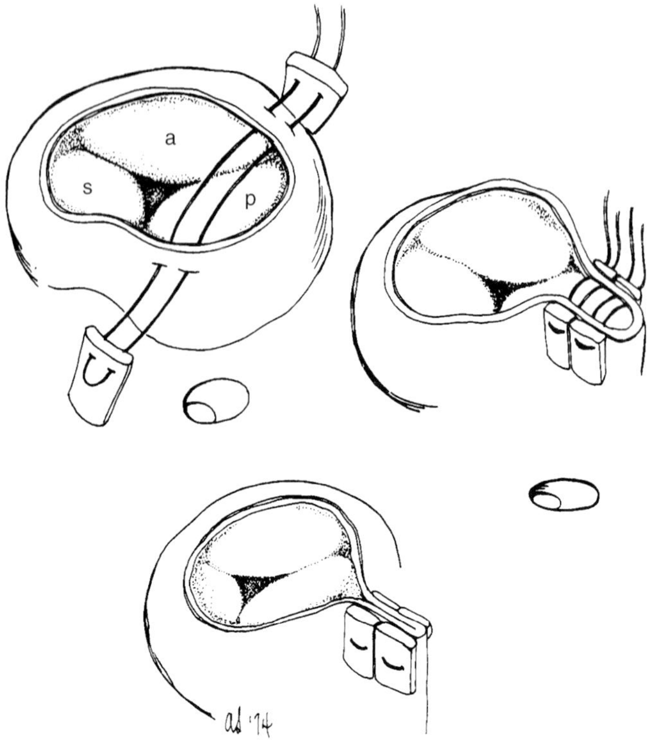

Figure 75–15 **Tricuspid valve annuloplasty.** Posterior annulus plication or Kay procedure.
(From Boyd AD, Engelman RM, Isom OW, et al: Tricuspid annuloplasty. Five and one-half years' experience with 78 patients. J Thorac Cardiovasc Surg 68:347, 1974, with permission from Excerpta Medica, Inc.)

15% and severe in 19%. De Paulis et al[26] reported a residual insufficiency in 12% and severe insufficiency in 4% among the 136 hospital survivors. Carpentier's[13] description of a measured, rigid prosthetic ring that selectively reduced the annulus opened the era of modern mitral and tricuspid annuloplasty. The ring has the systolic shape of the tricuspid annulus and is open at the level of the anteroseptal commissure to avoid passing the anchoring sutures close to the conducting system. Awareness of the continuous changes in size and shape of the normal tricuspid annulus during the cardiac cycle[88,91] led us to the development of a totally flexible ring.[31]

The surgical technique for implanting a tricuspid ring is very similar for all types of rings. The selection of the appropriate ring size is based on the length of the septal segment of the annulus (Figure 75-17). Large U sutures are placed around the annulus and through the ring (Figure 75-18). The ring is brought down, and the sutures are tied, reducing the overall perimeter of the tricuspid annulus (Figure 75-19). More recently, open bands that selectively reduce the posterior mitral annulus have been developed and applied to the tricuspid valve where the annulus contention is limited to the base of the anterior and posterior leaflets.[23] The advantage of these bands is to avoid placing sutures at the level of the septal leaflet. On the other hand, the correct implantation of a band is more critical. Anchoring the extremities of the band beyond both septal commissures will result in a larger tricuspid annulus than intended. Additionally, the septal area of the

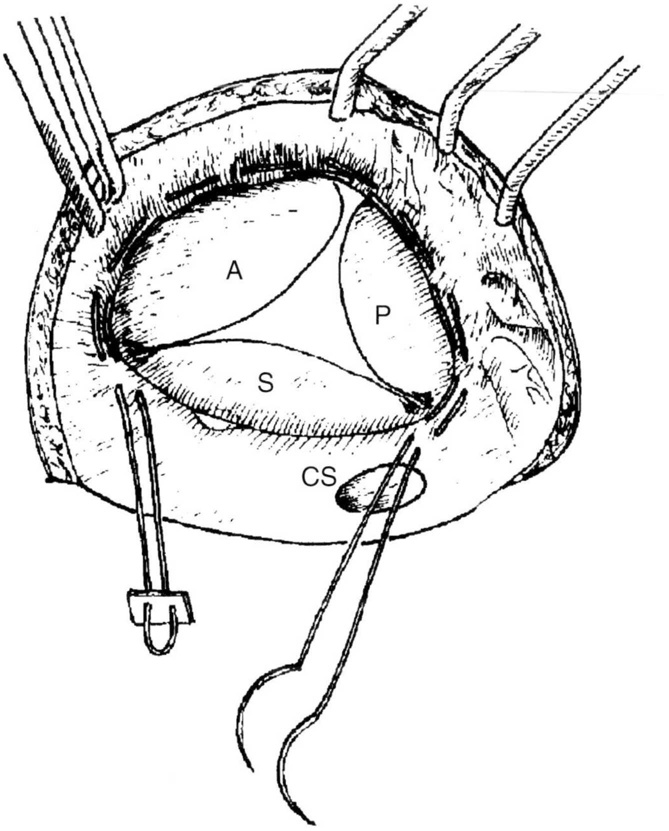

Figure 75–16 Tricuspid valve annuloplasty. DeVega semicircular suture annuloplasty.
(From Inamura E, Ohteki H, Koyanagi H: An improved DeVega tricuspid annuloplasty. Ann Thorac Surg 34:710, 1982, with permission from Society of Thoracic Surgeons.)

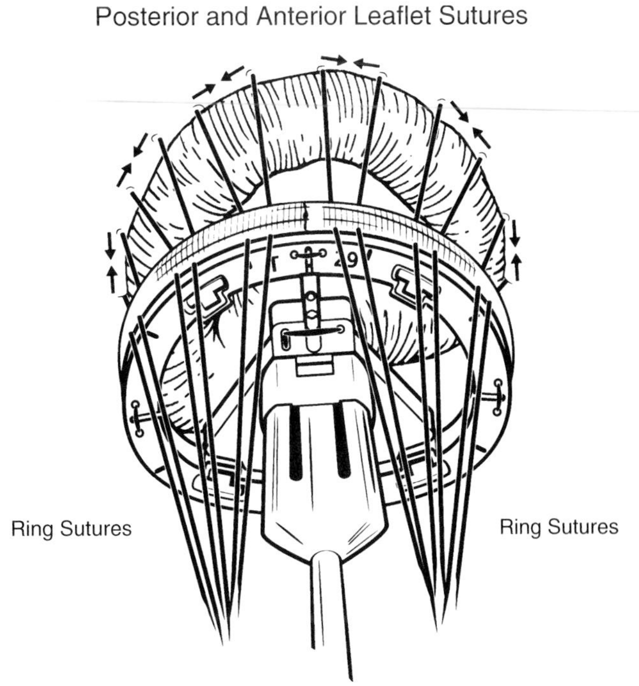

Figure 75–18 Tricuspid valve flexible ring annuloplasty. Passing the anterior and posterior annulus sutures through the ring held in the ring holder.
(Reproduced with permission from Duran CMG: Duran ring annuloplasty of the tricuspid valve. Op Tech Thorac Cardiovasc Surg 8:201–212, 2003.)

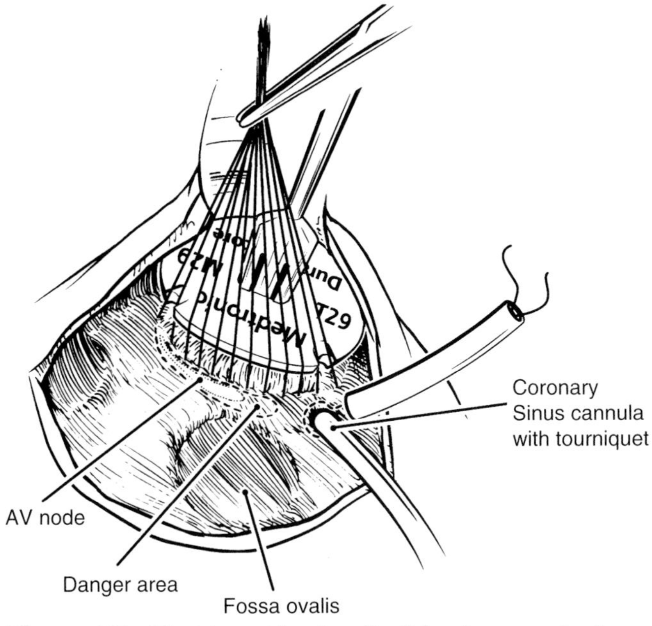

Figure 75–17 Tricuspid valve flexible ring annuloplasty. Determining the appropriate ring size.
(Reproduced with permission from Duran CMG: Duran ring annuloplasty of the tricuspid valve. Op Tech Thorac Cardiovasc Surg 8:201–212; 2003.)

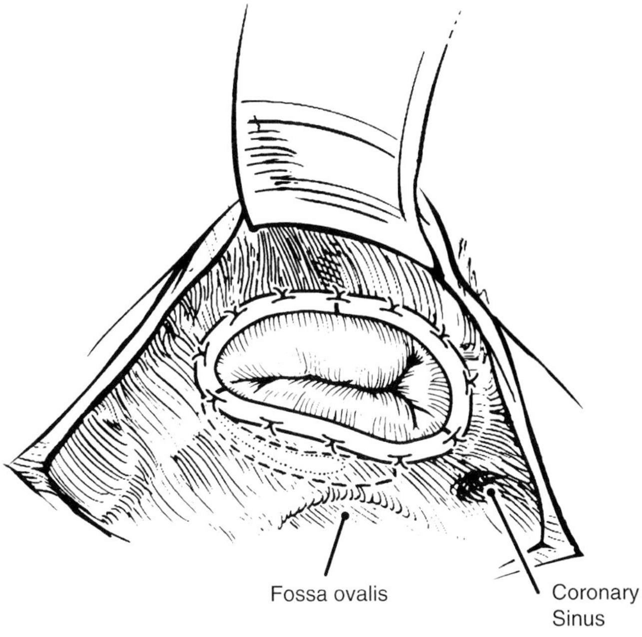

Figure 75–19 Tricuspid flexible ring annuloplasty. Ring in place. The ring sutures have been tied with the ring holder in place, which makes the ring temporarily rigid and therefore avoids plication.
(Reproduced with permission from Duran CMG: Duran ring annuloplasty of the tricuspid valve. Op Tech Thorac Cardiovasc Surg 8:201–212, 2003.)

tricuspid annulus is not protected from the further dilation that occurs in ischemic and dilated cardiomyopathies (Figure 75-20).

Tricuspid Replacement

Although the majority of tricuspid lesions can be repaired, in some cases, the degree of valve destruction is such that the valve must be excised. The alternatives are

1. excision of the valve without replacement;
2. the use of mitral or tricuspid homografts;
3. replacement with stented porcine or pericardial valves; and
4. replacement with a mechanical prosthesis.

The recent epidemic increase in endocarditis caused by drug abuse and the poor rehabilitation of these patients stimulated Arbulu and Holmes[5] to propose complete excision of the tricuspid valve without replacement. They reported the long-term results of tricuspid valvulectomy in 53 patients and 2 further cases where both the tricuspid and the pulmonary valves were excised without valve replacement. The duration of the patients' intravenous drug addiction averaged 9 years. Six (11%) died within 6 weeks and 10 (18%) died between 6 months and 13 years after surgery. Nine of the 10 deaths were related to continued drug abuse. Six patients required late prosthetic implantation. At 22 years, follow-up, the actuarial survival was 64%. This radical approach has several advantages. It avoids placing a foreign body into a potentially infected area, reduces the risk of recurrent infection of the prosthesis, and reduces cost in a population with a high degree of recurrent addiction.[36] Although the absence of a tricuspid valve is apparently well tolerated, the fact that these patients are very young and have normal pulmonary artery pressures must be emphasized. It has been suggested that this approach could be applied first, and if the patient is rehabilitated, a second surgery for valve replacement should then be undertaken.

The recent increase in infective endocarditis and the higher resistance to infection of the aortic homografts have rekindled an interest in the use of atrioventricular homografts. The first experimental replacements with atrioventricular homografts were done in 1951 by Robicksec,[82] who used a tricuspid, and in 1965 by Hubka et al[50] who used a tricuspid and a mitral. These techniques were followed by isolated, intermittent, and mostly unsuccessful clinical cases until 1993 when Pomar and Mestres[75] reported a successful tricuspid replacement with a mitral homograft followed for up to 20 months, and di Summa et al[29] reported the use of a fresh tricuspid homograft. Because of its technical difficulty, limited experience, and doubtful results in the mitral position, this procedure should still be considered experimental.[61]

In the vast majority of cases, severe tricuspid lesions are treated with a standard mechanical or a stented, glutaraldehyde-treated porcine or pericardial valve. The arguments between the proponents of either alternative are based on the problem of permanent anticoagulation required with a mechanical prosthesis versus the limited durability of the bioprosthesis. Standard bioprostheses in the mitral and aortic positions are known to fail due to leaflet tears and calcification with an incidence of approximately 25% 10 years after implantation. However, such complications are rare in the low-pressure pulmonary and tricuspid position.[35] Ohata et al[72] reported a comparative study between patients with the Carpentier–Edwards bioprosthesis in the mitral and in the tricuspid position. The actuarial freedom from structural deterioration and reoperation at 13 years was 78% for the mitral versus 100% for the tricuspid. Although these findings would favor the tissue valve, several studies do not show significant differences between mechanical valves and bioprostheses. Carrier and associates[17] recently reported a series of 97 patients with tricuspid replacement who were followed for up to 25 years. The overall hospital mortality was 17.5%. Because of their acknowledged preference for the bioprosthesis, the authors compared two unequal groups of 81 patients with bioprosthesis versus 15 with a mechanical valve operated between 1977 and 2002. No significant differences were found in survival and reoperation rates between both groups. The 5-year actuarial survival was 56% in the bioprosthesis group and 60% in the mechanical group. The freedom from reoperation at 5 years was 97% and 91%, respectively. Studying 435 patients in the United Kingdom heart valve registry, Ratnatunga and colleagues[80] showed similar survival and

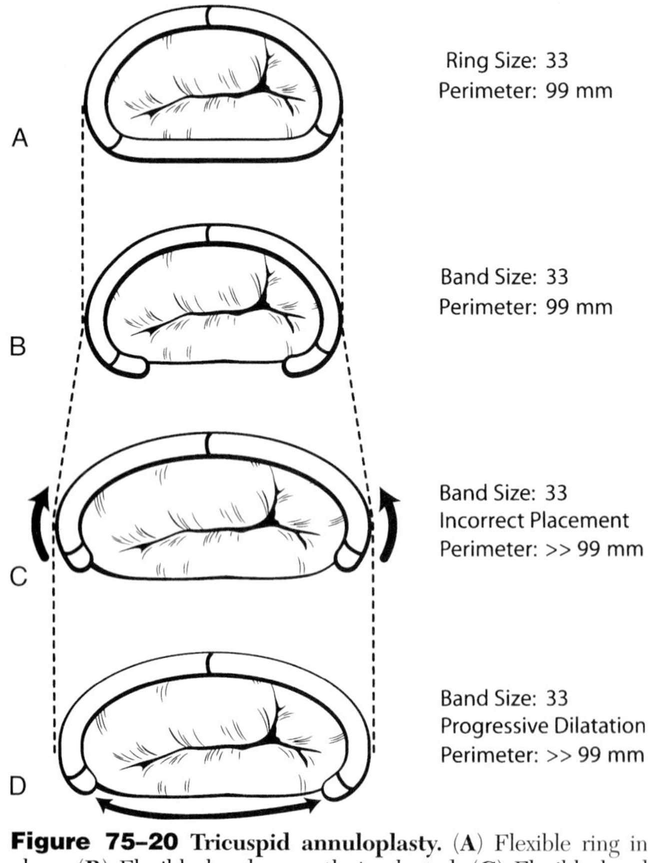

Figure 75–20 Tricuspid annuloplasty. (**A**) Flexible ring in place. (**B**) Flexible band correctly implanted. (**C**) Flexible band incorrectly implanted, resulting in a larger tricuspid orifice than planned. (**D**) Flexible band correctly implanted does not protect against further dilation of the septal annulus.
(Reproduced with permission from Duran CMG: Duran ring annuloplasty of the tricuspid valve. Op Tech Thorac Cardiovasc Surg 8:201–212, 2003.)

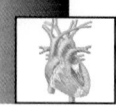

reoperation rates between patients with biological and mechanical prostheses. Kaplan and associates[52] also reported similar results among 122 patients averaging 35 years of age at the time of tricuspid replacement. Although prosthetic thrombosis and pulmonary embolism occurred in 10 patients, the authors recommended the use of low-profile, bileaflet prostheses. The problem of mechanical valve thrombosis is highlighted by Kawano and colleagues,[53] who reported thrombosis in 6 of 23 patients with a St. Jude Medical valve. Rarely, bioprostheses will also thrombose but also pannus formation can result in progressive stenosis requiring reoperation. Kawashi et al[54] reported a small series of 23 patients aged 9 to 53 years who underwent tricuspid replacement with a standard Hancock bioprosthesis. All patients were followed for up to 16 years. The actuarial freedom from structural degeneration was 94% at 10 years. At present, the danger of prosthetic thrombosis and the need for a stringent anticoagulation regimen when a mechanical valve is used together with the satisfactory performance of tissue valves in the tricuspid position have tilted the balance toward the bioprosthesis in the majority of centers. As in the case of the mitral valve, a pressing need exists for a more anatomical and, consequently, more physiological new atrioventricular prosthesis.

In most cases of tricuspid valve replacement, the entire tricuspid valve can be retained. Interrupted, pledgeted "U" sutures are passed along the annulus incorporating the leaflets. Care must be taken to avoid damaging the atrioventricular node with the septal sutures close to the anteroseptal commissure. In this region, the pledgeted "U" sutures should be passed at the base of the leaflet, avoiding myocardial tissue. These riff sutures not only increase the holding power of the stitches but maintain continuity between the annulus and papillary muscles (which has been shown in the mitral to be essential for ventricular function).

Results

Irrespective of the etiology and type of surgery, results of tricuspid surgery have been rather poor. The published series of tricuspid replacement tend to report few patients and to increase their number, they span for a very long time, which dilutes the improvements that have occurred in cardiac surgery. These reports include very different tricuspid pathologies and often include reoperations. Furthermore, only the very severe tricuspid lesions were treated in poor risk and evolved patients. Moderate lesions were often not diagnosed or ignored by the surgeon's attention directed toward the other valvular pathologies that condition the prognosis. Also, the majority of lesions operated are functional regurgitations that represent severe left side impairment, pulmonary hypertension, and right ventricular failure. The poor results of tricuspid surgery are therefore not surprising.

Most published series that include all tricuspid surgeries report hospital mortalities between 15% and 20%.[17,66–68] When only tricuspid replacement is reported, the hospital mortality went up to 39% in the series of Poveda et al,[77] which included patients operated between 1974 and 1993. If the replacement was subsequent to previous open heart surgery, Hornick et al[49] reported a hospital mortality of 50% in patients operated between 1985 and 1993.

A more recent experience of 34 patients undergoing isolated tricuspid surgery after prior left heart surgery between 1980 and 1997 reported by Staab et al[86] showed a hospital mortality of 8.8%. However, at 5 years, the event-free actuarial survival was only of 41%. As can be expected, predictors of poor outcome were the age of the patient, number of previous surgeries and preoperative functional class, congestive heart failure, and pulmonary artery pressure.[49,77] In our experience[30] with 306 patients, where tricuspid surgery was aggressively treated and therefore applied to patients in better condition, the hospital mortality was 7.5% with an actuarial survival rate of 77% at 48 months. The published late mortalities are close to 50%,[17,66,67] with survivals of 70% at 3 years for Sanfelippo et al,[85] 47% at 10 years for Thorburn et al,[89] and 41% at 8 years for Kratz et al.[60] In most series that stretch back to the 1970s, insignificant differences in the overall results are found between tricuspid replacement with mechanical and tissue prostheses.

During the 1980s, the superiority of repair over replacement became clearly established. It was shown that repair was possible in the vast majority of cases,[7,60] including organic lesions. In our series,[78] more than 90% of patients had a repair with satisfactory results. The absence of valve thrombosis, no need for permanent anticoagulation, and a low reoperation rate have reduced valve replacement to the exceptional case.[60,73] These findings are inducing a more aggressive surgical attitude toward the tricuspid valve and, consequently, earlier indications are made in lower risk patients. However, it is still necessary to alert the cardiologist and surgeon to the much higher incidence of tricuspid pathology than previously thought. We must be aware that beyond the classic rheumatic lesions, the myxomatous and, even more frequently, the ischemic and cardiomyopathic tricuspid regurgitations need to be treated. The superior diagnostic tools and surgical techniques available today will enlarge the field of tricuspid surgery.

ACKNOWLEDGMENTS

The author would like to thank Pete Dolan, Senior Medical Illustrator, Medtronic, Inc. (Minneapolis, MN) for providing the majority of the illustrations for this chapter and Jill Roberts for her editorial assistance.

REFERENCES

1. Aceves S, Carral R: The diagnosis of tricuspid valve disease. Am Heart J 34:114–130, 1947.
2. Ajayi AA, Adigun AQ, Ojofeitimi EO, et al: Anthropometric evaluation of cachexia in chronic congestive heart failure: the role of tricuspid regurgitation. Int J Cardiol 71:79–84, 1999.
3. Angermann CE, Spes CH, Tammen A, et al: Anatomic characteristics and valvular function of the transplanted heart: transthoracic versus transesophageal echocardiographic findings. J Heart Transplant 9:331–338, 1990.
4. Angrist AA, Oka M: Pathogenesis of bacterial endocarditis. JAMA 183–117, 1963.
5. Arbulu A, Holmes RJ: Surgical treatment of intractable right-sided infective endocarditis in drug addicts: 25 years experience. J Heart Valve Dis 2:129–137, 1993.

6. Bailey CP: Tricuspid stenosis. In Bailey CP, editor: Surgery of the Heart. Philadelphia: Lea & Febiger, 1955, pp. 846–861.
7. Baughman KL, Kallman CH, Yurchak PM, et al: Predictors of survival after tricuspid valve surgery. Am J Cardiol 54: 137–141, 1984.
8. Berger M, Haimovitz A, Van Tosh A, et al: Quantitative assessment of pulmonary hypertension in patients with tricuspid regurgitation using continuous wave Doppler ultrasound. J Am Coll Cardiol 6:359–365, 1985.
9. Bhatia SJ, Kirshenbaum JM, Shemin RJ, et al: Time course of resolution of pulmonary hypertension and right ventricular remodeling after orthotopic cardiac transplantation. Circulation 76:819–826, 1987.
10. Bolling SF, Pagani FD, Deeb GM, et al: Intermediate-term outcome of mitral reconstruction in cardiomyopathy. J Thorac Cardiovasc Surg 115:381–386, 1998.
11. Braunwald NS, Ross J, Morrow AG: Conservative management of tricuspid regurgitation in patients undergoing mitral valve replacement. Circulation 35(4 Suppl):163–169, 1967.
12. Cabrol C: Annuloplastie valvulaire. Nouv Presse Med I:1366, 1972.
13. Carpentier A: La valvuloplasty reconstitutive. Une nouvelle technique de valvuloplastie mitrale. Presse Med 7:251–253, 1969.
14. Carpentier A: Cardiac valve surgery—the French correction. J Thorac Cardiovasc Surg 88:323–327, 1983.
15. Carpentier A, Deloche A, Hanania G, et al: Surgical management of acquired tricuspid valve disease. J Thorac Cardiovasc Surg 67(1):53–65, 1974.
16. Carrel T, Schaffner A, Vogt P, et al: Endocarditis in intravenous drug addicts and HIV-infected patients: possibility and limitations of surgical treatment. J Heart Valve Dis 2:140–147, 1993.
17. Carrier M, Heber Y, Pellerin M, et al: Tricuspid valve replacement: an analysis of 25 years of experience at a single center. Ann Thorac Surg 75:47–50, 2003.
18. Chan P, Ogilby D, Segal B: Tricuspid valve endocarditis. Am Heart J 117:1140–1145, 1988.
19. Chen CC, Morganroth J, Mardelli TJ, et al: Tricuspid regurgitation in tricuspid valve prolapse demonstrated with contrast cross-sectional echocardiography. Am J Cardiol 46: 983–987, 1980.
20. Child JS: Improved guides to tricuspid valve repair: two-dimensional echocardiographic analysis of tricuspid annulus function and color flow imaging of severity of tricuspid regurgitation (editorial). J Am Coll Cardiol 14:1275–1277, 1989.
21. Come PC, Riley MF: Tricuspid anular dilatation and failure of tricuspid leaflet coaptation in tricuspid regurgitation. Am J Cardiol 55:599–601, 1985.
22. Connolly HM, Crary JL, McGoon MD, et al: Valvular tricuspid disease associated with fenfluoramine-phentermine. N Engl J Med 337:581–588, 1997.
23. Cosgrove DM, Arcidi JM, Rodriguez L, et al: Initial experience with the Cosgrove-Edwards annuloplasty system. Ann Thorac Surg 60:499–504, 1995.
24. Curtius JM, Thyssen M, Breuer HW, et al: Doppler versus contrast echocardiography for diagnosis of tricuspid regurgitation. Am J Cardiol 56:333–336, 1985.
25. Daniels SJ, Mintz GS, Kotler MN: Rheumatic tricuspid valve disease: two-dimensional echocardiographic, hemodynamic, and angiographic correlations. Am J Cardiol 51:492–496, 1983.
26. De Paulis R, Bobbio M, Ottino G, et al: The DeVega tricuspid annuloplasty. Perioperative mortality and long-term follow-up. J Cardiovasc Surg 31:512–517, 1990.
27. DeVega NG: La anuloplastia selective, regulable y permanente. Rev Esp Cardiol 25:555–560, 1972.
28. Dickerman SA, Rubler S: Mitral and tricuspid valve regurgitation in dilated cardiomyopathy. Am J Cardiol 63: 621–631, 1989.
29. di Summa M, Donegani E, Zattera GF, et al: Successful orthotopic transplantation of a fresh tricuspid valve homograft in a human. Ann Thorac Surg 56:1407–1408, 1993.
30. Duran CMG: Tricuspid valve revisited. J Card Surg 9(Suppl):242–247, 1994.
31. Duran CG, Ubago JL: Clinical and hemodynamic performance of a totally flexible prosthetic ring for atrioventricular valve reconstruction. Ann Thorac Cardiovasc Surg 22:458–463, 1976.
32. Duran CMG, Balasundaram, Bianchi S, et al: The vanishing tricuspid annuloplasty. J Thorac Cardiovasc Surg 104:796–801, 1992.
33. Duran CMG, Kumar N, Prabhakar G, et al: Vanishing DeVega annuloplasty for functional tricuspid regurgitation. J Thorac Cardiovasc Surg 106:609–613, 1993.
34. Duran CMG, Pomar JL, Colman T, et al: Is tricuspid valve repair necessary? J Thorac Cardiovasc Surg 80:849–860, 1980.
35. Fleming WH, Sarafian LB, Moulton AL, et al: Valve replacement in the right side of the heart in children: Long-term follow-up. Ann Thorac Surg 48:404–408, 1989.
36. Frater RWM: Editor's comment to surgical treatment of intractable right-sided infective endocarditis in drug addicts: 25 years' experience. J Heart Valve Dis 2:138–139, 1993.
37. Garrison PK, Freeman LR: Experimental endocarditis in rabbits resulting from placement of a polyethylene catheter in the right side of the heart. Yale J Biol 42:39, 1970.
38. Goldman ME, Guarino T, Fuster V, et al: The necessity for tricuspid valve repair can be determined intraoperatively by two-dimensional echocardiography. J Thorac Cardiovasc Surg 94:542–550, 1987.
39. Gooch AS, Maranhao V, Scampardonis G, et al: Prolapse of both mitral and tricuspid leaflets in systolic murmur-click syndrome. N Engl J Med 287:1218–1222, 1972.
40. Gross L, Friedberg CK: Lesions of cardiac valve rings in rheumatic fever. Am J Pathol 12:469, 1936.
41. Groves PH, Ikrams S, Ingold U, et al: Tricuspid regurgitation following mitral valve replacement: an echocardiographic study. J Heart Valve Dis 2:273–278, 1993.
42. Guiraudon GM, Ofiesh AG, Kushk R: Extended vertical transatrial septal approach to the mitral valve. Ann Thorac Surg 53:1058–1062, 1991.
43. Harley JB, McIntosh CL, Kirklin JJ, et al: Atrioventricular valve replacement in the idiopathic hypereosinophilic syndrome. Am J Med 73:77–78, 1982.
44. Hashiro Y, Sugimoto S, Takagi N, et al: Native valve salvage for post-traumatic tricuspid regurgitation. J Heart Valve Dis 10: 275–278, 2001.
45. Hauck AJ, Freeman DP, Ackerman, DP, et al: Surgical pathology of the tricuspid valve: a study of 363 cases spanning 25 years. Mayo Clin Proc 63:851–853, 1988.
46. Haverich A, Albes JM, Fahrenkamp G, et al: Intraoperative echocardiography to detect and prevent tricuspid valve regurgitation after heart transplantation. Eur J Cardiothorac Surg 5:41–45, 1991.
47. Higashidate M, Tamiya K, Kurosawa H, et al: Role of septal leaflet in tricuspid valve closure. J Thorac Cardiovasc Surg 104:1212–1217, 1992.
48. Holper K, Haehnel JC, Augustin N, et al: Surgery for tricuspid insufficiency: long-term follow up after DeVega annuloplasty. Thorac Cardiovasc Surg 41:1–8, 1993.
49. Hornick P, Harris PA, Taylor KM: Tricuspid valve replacement subsequent to previous open heart surgery. J Heart Valve Dis 5:20–25, 1996.
50. Hubka M, Siska K, Brozman M, et al: Replacement of the mitral and tricuspid valves by mitral homografts. J Thorac Cardiovasc Surg 51:195–294, 1966.
51. Hung J, Koelling T, Semigran MJ, et al: Usefulness of echocardiographic determined tricuspid regurgitation in predicting event-free survival in severe heart failure secondary to

idiopathic-dilated cardiomyopathy or ischemic cardiomyopathy. Am J Cardiol 82:1301–1303, 1998.
52. Kaplan M, Kut MS, Demirtas MM, et al: Prosthetic replacement of tricuspid valve: bioprosthesis or mechanical? Ann Thorac Surg 73:467–473, 2001.
53. Kawano H, Oda T, Fukunaga S, et al: Tricuspid valve replacement with the St. Jude Medical valve. Eur J Cardiothoracic Surg 18:565–569, 2000.
54. Kawashi Y, Tominaga R, Hisahara M, et al: Excellent durability of the Hancock porcine bioprosthesis in the tricuspid position. J Thorac Cardiovasc Surg 104:1561–1566, 1992.
55. Kay JH, Maselli-Campagna G, Tsuji KK: Surgical treatment of tricuspid insufficiency. Ann Surg 162:53–58, 1965.
56. King RM, Schaff HV, Danielson GK, et al: Surgery for tricuspid late after mitral valve replacement. Circulation 70 (3 Suppl II):I193–I197, 1984.
57. Kirklin J, Barrat-Boyes B: Cardiac Surgery. New York: John Wiley & Sons, 1986.
58. Knight CJ, Sutton GC: Complete heart block and severe tricuspid regurgitation after radiotherapy. Case report and review of the literature. Chest 108:1748–1751, 1995.
59. Koelling TM, Aaronson KD, Cody RJ, et al: Prognostic significance of mitral regurgitation and tricuspid regurgitation in patients with left ventricular systolic dysfunction. Am Heart J 144:524–529, 2002.
60. Kratz JM, Crawford FA, Stoud MR, et al: Trends and results in tricuspid surgery. Chest 88:837–840, 1985.
61. Kumar AS, Chaudhary SK, Mathur A, et al: Homograft mitral valve replacement: Five years' results. J Thorac Cardiovasc Surg 120:450–458, 2000.
62. Kumar N, Saad E, Prabahkar, et al: Extended transeptal versus conventional atriotomy. Early postoperative study. Ann Thorac Surg 60:426–430, 1995.
63. Lauper J, Frand M, Milo S: Valve replacement for severe tricuspid regurgitation caused by Libman-Sacks endocarditis. Br Heart J 48:294–297, 1982.
64. McAllistair RG, Friesinger GC, Sinclair-Smith BC: Tricuspid regurgitation following inferior myocardial infarction. Arch Intern Med 136:95–99, 1976.
65. McCarthy PM: New surgical options for the failing heart. J Heart Valve Dis 8:472–475, 1999.
66. McGrath AB, Gonzalez-Lavin L, Bailey BM, et al: Tricuspid valve operations in 530 patients. Twenty-five-year assessment of early and late phase events. J Thorac Cardiovasc Surg 99:124–133, 1990.
67. Munro AI, Jamieson WRE, Tyers GFO, et al: Tricuspid valve replacement: porcine bioprosthesis and mechanical prosthesis. Ann Thorac Surg 59:S470–S471, 1995.
68. Nakano K, Eishi K, Kosakai Y, et al: Ten-year experience with the Carpentier-Edwards pericardial xenograft in the tricuspid position. J Thorac Cardiovasc Surg 111:605–612, 1996.
69. Nanna M, Chandraratna PA, Reid C, et al: Value of two-dimensional echocardiography in detecting tricuspid stenosis. Circulation 67:221–224, 1983.
70. Nigri GR, Di Dio LJA, Baptista CAC: Papillary muscles and tendinous chords of the right ventricle of the human heart: morphologic characteristics. Surg Radiol Anat 23:45–49, 2001.
71. Ogawa S, Hayashi J, Sasaki H, et al: Evaluation of combined valvular prolapse syndrome by two-dimensional echocardiography. Circulation 65:174–180, 1982.
72. Ohata T, Kigawa I, Tohda E, et al: Comparison of durability of bioprosthesis in tricuspid and mitral position. Ann Thorac Surg 71:S240–S243, 2001.
73. Onada K, Yasuda F, Takao M, et al: Long-term follow-up after Carpentier-Edwards ring annuloplasty for tricuspid regurgitation. Ann Thorac Surg 70:796–799, 2000.
74. Oz MC: Passive ventricular constraint for the treatment of congestive heart failure. Ann Thorac Surg 71:S185–S187, 2001.
75. Pomar JL, Mestres CA: Tricuspid valve replacement using a mitral homograft. Surgical technique and initial results. J Heart Valve Dis 2:125–128, 1993.
76. Porter A, Shapira Y, Wurzel M, et al: Tricuspid regurgitation late after mitral valve replacement: clinical and echocardiographic evaluation. J Heart Valve Dis 8:57–62, 1999.
77. Poveda JJ, Bernal JM, Matorras P, et al: Tricuspid valve replacement in rheumatic disease: preoperative predictors of hospital mortality. J Heart Valve Dis 5:26–30, 1996.
78. Prabhakar G, Kumar N, Gometza B, et al: Surgery for organic rheumatic disease of the tricuspid valve. J Heart Valve Dis 2:561–566, 1993.
79. Radovanovic N, Petrovic L, Kovac M, et al: Change in left ventricular morphology and function in end-stage dilated cardiomyopathy after reductive annuloplasty of double mitral and tricuspid orifices: TEE study. World Symposium on Heart Valve Disease, London, 1999 (abstract P94).
80. Ratnatunga CP, Edwards MD, Dore CJ, et al: Tricuspid valve replacement: UK heart valve registry mid-term results comparing mechanical and biological prosthesis. Ann Thorac Surg 66:1940–1947, 1998.
81. Roberts WC, Buchbinder NA: Right-sided valvular endocarditis: a clinicopathologic study of twelve necropsy patients. Am J Med 53–57, 1972.
82. Robicksec F: Cardiac valve transplantation. Acta Med Hung 1–2:81–91, 1954.
83. Sagie A, Schwammenthal E, Palacios I, et al: Significant tricuspid regurgitation does not resolve after percutaneous balloon mitral valvotomy. J Thorac Cardiovasc Surg 108:727–735, 1994.
84. Salgo IS, Gorman JH III, Gorman RC, et al: Effect of annular shape on leaflet curvature in reducing mitral leaflet stress. Circulation 106:711–717, 2002.
85. Sanfelippo PM, Giuliani ER, Danielson GK, et al: Tricuspid valve prosthetic replacement. J Thorac Cardiovasc Surg 71: 445–446, 1976.
86. Staab ME, Nishimura RA, Dearani JA: Isolated tricuspid valve surgery for severe tricuspid regurgitation following prior left heart surgery: analysis of outcome in 34 patients. J Heart Valve Dis 6:567–574, 1999.
87. Suzuki Y, Hirofumi K, Kazunori K, et al: Detection and evaluation of tricuspid regurgitation using a real-time, two-dimensional, color-coded Doppler imaging system: comparison with contrast two-dimensional echocardiography and right ventriculography. Am J Cardiol 57:811–815, 1986.
88. Tei C, Pilgrim JF, Shah PM, et al: The tricuspid valve annulus: study in size and motion in normal subjects and in patients with tricuspid regurgitation. Circulation 66:665–671, 1982.
89. Thorburn CW, Morgan JJ, Shanahan MX, et al: Long-term results of tricuspid valve replacement and the problem of tricuspid valve thrombosis. Am J Cardiol 51:1128–1132, 1985.
90. Torrent-Guasp F, Buckberg GD, Clemente C, et al: The structure and function of the helical heart and its buttress wrapping. I. The normal macroscopic structure of the heart. Semin Thorac Cardiovasc Surg 13:301–319, 2001.
91. Tsakiris AG, Mair DD, Seki S, et al: Motion of the tricuspid valve annulus in anesthetized intact dogs. Circulation Res 36: 43–48, 1975.
92. Ubago JL, Figueroa A, et al: Diagnostico hemodinamico de afectacion organica de la valvular tricuspide. Rev Esp Cardiol 33:515–523, 1980.
93. Ubago JL, Figueroa A, Colman T, et al: Right ventriculography as a valid method for the diagnosis of tricuspid insufficiency. Cath Cardiovasc Diag 7:433–44, 1981.
94. Ubago JL, Figueroa A, Ochoteco A, et al: Analysis of the amount of tricuspid valve annular dilatation required to produce functional tricuspid regurgitation. Am J Cardiol 52: 155–158, 1983.

95. van Son JA, Danielson GK, Schaff HV, et al: Traumatic tricuspid insufficiency. Experience in 13 patients. J Thorac Cardiovasc Surg 108:893–898, 1994.
96. Victor S, Nayak VM: The tricuspid valve is bicuspid. J Heart Valve Dis 3:27–36, 1994.
97. Waller BF, Moriarty AT, Eble JN, et al: Etiology of pure tricuspid regurgitation based on annulus circumference and leaflet area: analysis of 45 necropsy patients with clinical and morphologic evidence of pure tricuspid regurgitation. Am J Cardiol 7: 1063–1074, 1986.
98. Werner JA, Schiller NB, Prasquier R: Occurrence and significance of echocardiographically demonstrated tricuspid valve prolapse. Am Heart J 96:180–186, 1978.
99. Wooler GH, Nixon PGF, Grimshow VA, et al: Experiences with the repair of the mitral valve in mitral incompetence. Thorax 17:49–57, 1962.
100. Yankah AC, Musci M, Weng Y, et al: Tricuspid valve dysfunction after orthotopic cardiac transplantation. Eur J Cardiothorac Surg 17:343–348, 2000.
101. Yoshida K, Yoshikawa J, Shakudo M, et al: Color Doppler evaluation of valvular regurgitation in normal subjects. Circulation 78:840–847, 1988.

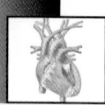

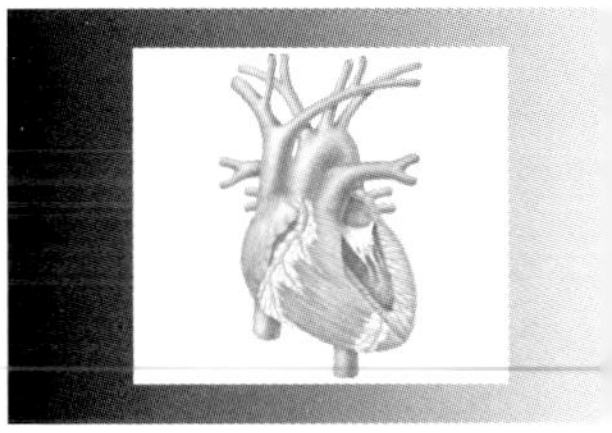

Prosthetic Valve Endocarditis

David A. Fullerton and Frederick L. Grover

CHAPTER 76

INTRODUCTION

Prosthetic valve endocarditis (PVE) is one of the most devastating complications of valve replacement. It is associated with a very high rate of morbidity and mortality and usually requires reoperation. As the number of patients in the population with prosthetic valves continues to increase, the number of cases of PVE continues to rise.[50] In most large series, the incidence of PVE is reported to be 2–4%.[70] For unclear reasons, prosthetic valves are more likely to become infected in the aortic position than in the mitral position.[18] This is in contradistinction to native valve endocarditis, wherein the mitral valve is more likely to become infected. In patients undergoing simultaneous aortic and mitral valve replacements, the incidence of prosthetic valve infection is greater, but the likelihood of either prosthesis becoming infected is probably equal[7] (Figure 76-1).

HISTORICAL NOTE

Not long after the initial reports of valve replacements by Starr and Harken, the first reports of PVE appeared in the literature. Before the routine use of prophylactic antibiotics, Geraci and associates (1963)[36] and Stein and co-workers (1966)[82] reported incidences of early PVE of 10% and 12%, respectively. Routine prophylactic antibiotics markedly reduced the incidence of this devastating complication. In a consecutive series of 288 patients receiving preoperative antibiotics, the incidence of PVE was reduced to 0.2%.[82] From the outset, the surgical management of PVE was a formidable challenge. Particularly in the 1960s and 1970s, surgery for PVE was associated with an extremely high mortality rate. Discouraged by such early surgical experience, cardiac surgeons understandably made efforts to avoid operation for PVE. Although it was recognized that antibiotic treatment alone for PVE frequently produced fatal results, surgery for PVE was still reserved for the worst cases, and the surgical results were predictably poor. Hence, a vicious cycle developed in which surgery was avoided for fear of poor surgical outcomes, and poor surgical outcomes were achieved in very high-risk cases.

In 1972, Ross successfully performed aortic root replacement for PVE using an aortic homograft.[75] His report stressed the surgical principles still true today: complete surgical debridement of all infected tissue, the use of a homograft for reconstruction, and minimal use of foreign material in the infected area. In 1977 Olinger and Maloney[64] reported replacement of an infected aortic prosthesis and external felt buttressing for correction of aortic ventricular discontinuity. The following year, Frantz et al.[35] reported repair of ventricular–aortic discontinuity from endocarditis and abscess formation by aortic root replacement using a synthetic valved conduit. In 1974, Danielson and associates[20] described a technique for treating extensive periannular abscess formation in native aortic valve endocarditis by translocation of a prosthetic aortic valve into the ascending aorta and saphenous vein coronary artery bypass grafting. In 1981, Reitz and co-workers[73] successfully applied this technique to treatment of prosthetic aortic valve endocarditis. In 1982, Symbas and colleagues[83] combined aortic valve replacement with patch repair of periannular abscess cavity. In 1987, David and Feindel[22] described techniques to reconstruct the mitral annulus with pericardium after debridement for PVE.

Surgical treatment of PVE remains a significant challenge, but outcomes improved in the 1990s. Several factors contributed to these improved outcomes including (1) widespread use of transesophageal echocardiography in making an early, accurate diagnosis. (2) An appreciation that like surgical infections elsewhere, surgery for PVE requires radical debridement of infected and devitalized tissue. (3) Improvements in myocardial protection, including routine use of retrograde cardioplegia, permitted longer and safer

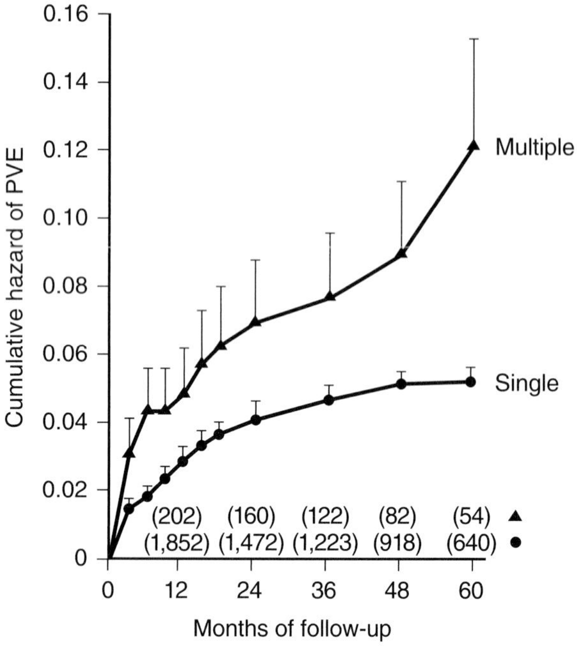

Figure 76–1 Cumulative hazard curve of prosthetic valve endocarditis (PVE) in single- and multiple-valve recipients. *(Modified from Calderwood SB, Swinski LA, Waternaux CM, et al: Risk factors for the development of prosthetic valve endocarditis. Circulation 72:31–37, 1985.)*

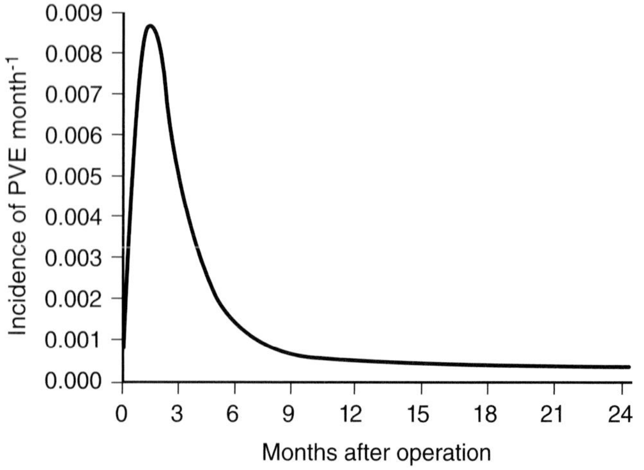

Figure 76–2 Hazard function curve for prosthetic valve endocarditis (PVE) for patients undergoing single-valve replacement. *(Modified from Ivert TSA, Dismukes WE, Cobbs CG, et al: Prosthetic valve endocarditis. Circulation 69:223–232, 1984.)*

cardiac operations. (4) Cryopreserved homografts became more widely available. Combined with their resistance to reinfection, homografts provided flexibility in the reconstruction of the heart. Currently, most surgeons consider homograft root replacement the procedure of choice for treatment of aortic PVE.[76]

RISK

The risk of prosthetic valve infection to the patient is lifelong. However, as assessed by hazard function analysis, the risk of infection appears to be greatest at approximately 5 weeks following valve implantation and thereafter declines. By 12 months after valve implantation, the risk reaches a low, constant level[14,15,44] (Figure 76-2). For a given patient, the risk is approximately 3% during the first year after valve implantation and 1% per year thereafter.[50]

By clinical convention, PVE that is diagnosed within 60 days of valve implantation is called "early" PVE, whereas PVE diagnosed beyond 60 days of valve implantation is called "late".[28] The incidence of PVE appears to be evenly distributed between early and late, each occurring with an incidence of approximately 1 to 2%.[18] This distinction of early from late PVE is clinically valuable in providing insight into the acquisition of the infection, the clinical course of the patient, and management of the disease.

This definition distinguishing "early" from "late" endocarditis was made somewhat arbitrarily. More recently, some authorities have suggested that 1 year post-valve implantation should define the timeframe for early as opposed to late PVE.[50,68] Regardless of the specific time used to define early PVE, it is assumed that the infection derived from perioperative contamination of the valve. On the other hand, late PVE is an infection acquired at a time remote from the perioperative period. As such, the bacteriology of early PVE differs from that of late PVE.

Early Prosthetic Valve Endocarditis

Early PVE is believed to arise from perioperative contamination of the valve. In a review of nearly 1500 consecutive patients undergoing valve replacement, Ivert and co-workers[44] identified the following as risk factors for early PVE: valve replacement for native valve endocarditis, black race, male gender, and prolonged cardiopulmonary bypass time.

Perioperative bacteremia, perhaps arising from infections such as wound infections, mediastinitis, and pneumonia, increases the risk of early prosthetic valve contamination. Fortunately, such perioperative bacteremias do not invariably cause PVE. Parker and co-workers[65] reported that 32 of 890 patients had documented bacteremia in the early postoperative period following valve replacement. Surprisingly, of these 32 bacteremic patients, only 2 (6%) developed PVE, but both died. In a multiinstitutional review, Fang and colleagues[33] determined that 18 of 115 patients (16%) with prosthetic heart valves developed PVE following bacteremia. The most common portals of bacterial entry were indwelling catheter infections (33%) and skin/wound infections (28%).

Fungal infections account for between 2% and 10% of PVE, and are usually lethal.[59] Unfortunately, fungemia has become more common in hospitalized patients. Nasser and colleagues[59] found that 9% of patients with prosthetic heart valves developed fungal endocarditis following documented candidemia. Of note, the mean time between candidemia and the clinical diagnosis of prosthetic fungal endocarditis was 232 days. Hence, patients with candidemia must be aggressively treated in the acute setting and carefully followed long term.

Replacing a native valve in the setting of bacterial contamination may well increase the risk of PVE. For that reason, many surgeons routinely culture excised valve leaflets to be certain the new valve is not contaminated at implantation.

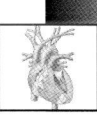

Campbell and colleagues[16] examined this practice and found that 32 of 222 patients (14%) who underwent elective valve replacement procedures had positive valve cultures. None of these patients had clinical evidence of infection. Only 1 of these 32 (3%) developed PVE. The authors concluded that most positive valve cultures were false positives. Nonetheless, PVE is such a terrible complication that the practice of culturing excised valve tissue for unsuspected bacteria may well be justified. Positive cultures should be treated.

The most likely source of early infection is intraoperative contamination. Cardiac surgical procedures are extremely complex and entail numerous operating room personnel, multiple intravascular monitoring devices, and the circuit of the heart–lung machine. Given this complexity of cardiac surgical procedures, the incidence of positive intraoperative cultures is high. Kluge and co-workers[47] reported that 71% of cardiac surgical patients had positive intraoperative cultures taken from a variety of sampling sites such as intravenous and intraarterial catheters and urinary bladder drainage catheters. Likewise, Ankeney and Parker[4] reported that 19% of cardiac surgical patients had positive intraoperative blood cultures. In the latter study, 3 of the 12 patients with positive intraoperative blood cultures who did not receive preoperative prophylactic antibiotics developed early PVE.

The heart–lung bypass circuit has been implicated in several studies as a source of intraoperative contamination. The suction devices of the circuit in particular are believed to return bacteria from the air over the operative field and from the operative field directly into the blood of the pump circuit. Intraoperative use of autologous transfusion via red blood cell recycling devices has increased markedly in recent years. Of particular interest is the very high incidence of positive cultures in these blood-recycling circuits. Bland and associates[11] reported that in 30 of 31 cases (97%), bags of recycled blood yielded positive cultures.

The choice of suture materials used to implant the prosthesis may influence the risk. In a laboratory study designed to examine sutures commonly used to implant valves, Shuhaiber and colleagues[81] used gram-positive bacteria labeled with [^{3}H]leucine to demonstrate that adherence of bacteria was least to monofilament polypropylene suture, 3 times higher to braided polyester, and 10 times higher to braided polyester coated with polybutilate. Invasive monitoring devices such as intraarterial catheters, central venous catheters, pulmonary arterial catheters, thermodilution cardiac output measurement systems, and urinary bladder catheters all carry the risk of perioperative infection. Although difficult to quantitate, the risk clearly rises the longer these devices are in place. In fact, by 72 h after insertion, the incidence of central venous line infection is estimated to be 12%, and this incidence rises daily thereafter.[17] Therefore, every effort should be made to remove these monitoring devices as early as possible in the perioperative period.

Considering the high frequency of positive intraoperative cultures, it is surprising that early prosthetic valve infection does not occur more frequently. Prophylactic antibiotic administration is standard practice, although the data supporting the efficacy of such therapy must be inferred from observational studies. These show that use of prophylactic antibiotics has been associated with a significantly lower incidence of PVE than in historical control subjects. Stein and co-workers[82] noted a reduction in the incidence of early PVE from 12% to nearly 0% with use of preoperative prophylactic antibiotics. Ankeney and Parker[4] noted that 3 of 12 patients not receiving prophylactic antibiotics but who were bacteremic perioperatively developed PVE, whereas no bacteremic patients receiving antibiotics developed PVE.

Late Prosthetic Valve Endocarditis

Late PVE is believed to arise either from infection acquired after the perioperative period or from insidious infection acquired during the operation, but that is not clinically evident until more than 60 days following valve implantation.

As with any patient with valvular heart disease, patients with prosthetic valves should receive prophylactic antibiotics before any procedure that may produce bacteremia.[9,13] Such bacteremias are common with dental procedures and any procedures involving the genitourinary or gastrointestinal tracts. The prophylactic regimens recommended by the American Heart Association are listed in Table 76-1.

Type of Prosthesis

Most large series have found the incidence of PVE to be the same whether a mechanical or bioprosthetic valve is used.[18,39,76] However, the risk of early as opposed to late PVE may differ as a function of the type of prosthesis. Calderwood and colleagues[15] found that the overall incidence of PVE at 5 years was not different between mechanical and bioprosthetic valves. However, the incidence of early PVE was higher in the mechanical group, whereas the incidence of late PVE was higher in the bioprosthetic group (Figure 76-3).

Table 76–1

Standard Prophylactic Antibiotic Regimen for Heart Valves[a]

Antibiotic administered	*Time of administration*
Standard regimen: ampicillin, 2.0 g intravenously or intramuscularly, *plus* gentamicin, 1.5 mg/kg intravenously or intramuscularly (not to exceed 120 mg)	Within 30 min before the procedure
For patients allergic to amoxicillin/ampicillin: vancomycin, 1.0 g intravenously over 1–2 h, *plus* gentamicin, 1.5 mg/kg intravenously or intramuscularly (not to exceed 120 mg)	Within 30 min before the procedure

[a]Modified from the American Heart Association.

The hazard function of PVE for homografts differs from that of other prosthetic devices. Unlike data pertaining to mechanical and bioprosthetic valves, which demonstrate the risk of PVE to be highest in the early postoperative period, data from several series suggest that the incidence of endocarditis following homograft valve implantation is both low and constant[43,52,64] (Figure 76-4).

Operation for Native Endocarditis

Valve replacement in the setting of native valve endocarditis might logically be expected to increase the incidence of PVE. Surprisingly, many large studies have demonstrated the incidence to be approximately 4%, which is not higher than the overall reported incidence of PVE.[1,5,18,26,40] However, several investigators have found patients to be at increased risk for PVE following valve replacement for native endocarditis. Ivert and associates[44] found a 5-fold increase in PVE when valve replacement was performed for active native valve endocarditis. Alexiou et al[3] reported a 6.7% incidence and Wantanabe and colleagues[91] reported an 11% incidence. In an extensive analysis, Moon and colleagues[55] reported the linearized rate of recurrent or residual endocarditis during the first 5 years after valve replacement for native endocarditis was 2.1% per patient-year. After the first 5 years, the rate fell to 0.9% per patient-year.

Some investigators have historically suggested that mechanical valves may pose a greater risk of recurrent infection than biological valves when placed in active native valve endocarditis. For this reason, attempts were made to reduce the risk of mechanical valve infection by incorporating silver into the sewing ring. Although silver is an effective antimicrobial, a silver-coated sewing ring on mechanical prosthetic valves was not shown to offer an advantage over conventional valves.[80] When comparing the influence of the type of valve implanted in the setting of native valve endocarditis, Moon and colleagues[55] reported the linearized rate of recurrent or residual endocarditis to be 1.5% per patient-year, and this was not different for mechanical or biological valves.

Use of an aortic homograft in native valve endocarditis offers the theoretical advantage of placing minimal foreign material in the setting of infection. In a series of 78 patients undergoing aortic valve replacement with an aortic homograft for active native aortic endocarditis, 8 patients (10%) developed endocarditis in the homograft valve.[43] McGiffin and associates[52] reported a nonrandomized series that examined the influence of replacement valve type for active aortic endocarditis. In this series, the incidence of both early and late endocarditis in the replacement device was 5% (2 of 40 patients) if a homograft was used and 10.8% (4 of 37 patients) if a bioprosthetic device was used. Finally, Okita and associates[62] reported a 4.4% reinfection rate with the use of an aortic homograft for aortic root replacement to treat severe periannular abscess, which is virtually the same as reports of procedures using mechanical bioprostheses.

Most authorities recommend use of a mechanical or biological valve to replace "simple" native valve endocarditis.[55] The available data suggest acceptably low rates of PVE in the replacement device. If significant tissue destruction is found at operation, and particularly in the setting of *Staphylococcus aureus* infection, a homograft root replacement may be required.

MICROBIOLOGY

Early prosthetic valve infections are believed to result from perioperative contamination, and such contamination is

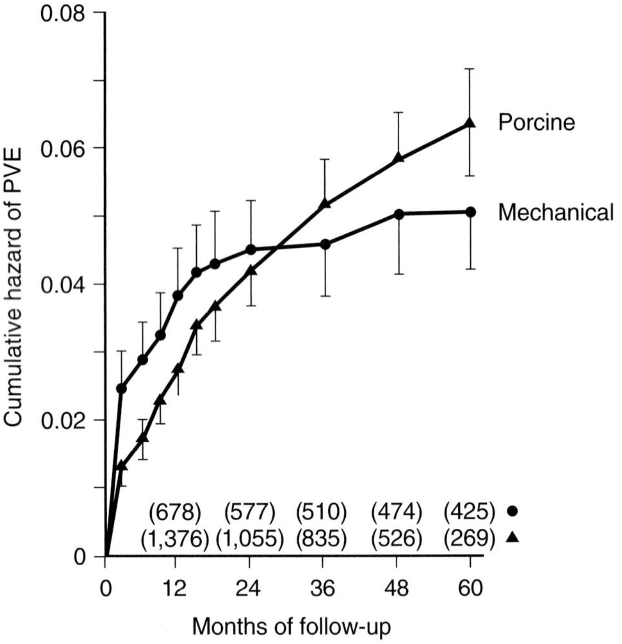

Figure 76-3 Cumulative hazard curve of prosthetic valve endocarditis (PVE) in recipients of mechanical prostheses and porcine prostheses.
(Modified from Calderwood SB, Swinski LA, Waternaux CM, et al: Risk factors for the development of prosthetic valve endocarditis. Circulation 72:31–37, 1985.)

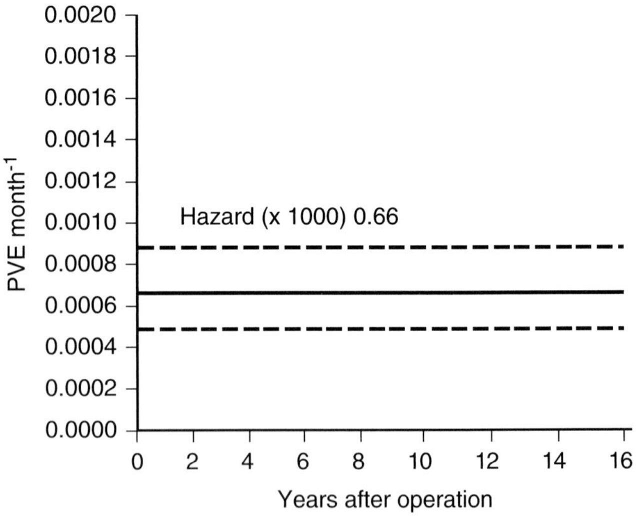

Figure 76-4 Hazard function curve for homograft endocarditis (PVE). The hazard function is constant.
(Modified from O'Brien MR, Stafford EG, Garner MAH, et al: A comparison of aortic valve replacement with viable cryopreserved and fresh allograft valves, with a note on chromosomal studies. J Thorac Cardiovasc Surg 94:812–823, 1987.)

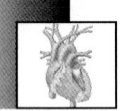

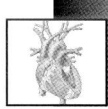

reflected in the microbiology of early PVE. In most series, staphylococcal species account for at least 50% of early infections, whereas streptococcal and diphtheroid species together account for another 20–25%. A variety of gram-negative organisms account for approximately 20% of early infections; fungal infections account for about 10% of cases.[18]

On the other hand, the microbiology of late PVE is quite similar to that of native valve endocarditis[31] (Table 76-2). This reflects the fact that late PVE is acquired under circumstances similar to native valve endocarditis. Gram-positive cocci also dominate the microbiology of late PVE. But unlike early PVE, in which staphylococcal species predominate, streptococci, particularly non-Group D streptococci, are the most prevalent organisms, accounting for at least 30% of cases of late PVE. *Staphylococcus epidermidis* also accounts for approximately 30% of late cases.[18] *S. aureus*, gram-negative bacilli, and fungi each account for 10% or less of cases. Thus, the bacteriology of late PVE is more favorable to successful antibiotic treatment than is early PVE.

Although uncommon, patients may have the clinical picture of PVE yet have negative blood cultures. In this setting, the diagnosis of endocarditis due to fastidious organisms must be considered. In particular, microorganisms in the HACEK group may account for up to 3% of cases. The HACEK group is made of species from the *Haemophilus, Actinobacillus, Cardiobacterium, Eikenella*, and *Kingella* families.[10] Along with nutritionally variant streptococci, the HACEK group is considered normal upper respiratory tract flora and may cause endocarditis in the setting of poor dentition.

PATHOLOGY

A feature common to all prosthetic valves is the sewing ring. This foreign material markedly reduces the inoculum of bacteria required to produce infection, and the valve sewing ring therefore becomes the primary focus of infection. Thus the pathological hallmark of PVE is an abscess involving the valve ring and surrounding tissue. The incidence of paravalvular abscess in PVE is between 50% and 100%[12] and occurs more frequently in the aortic position than in the mitral position.[6] With abscess formation, the surrounding tissue may be progressively destroyed. With such destruction, valve dehiscence begins, and a paravalvular leak is produced. Likewise, the infection may destroy tissue between adjacent cardiac structures, creating a fistula. Extensive destruction of surrounding tissue may lead to pseudoaneurysm formation, and indeed, disruption of the aorta from the ventricle.[50]

If the paravalvular abscess extends into the conduction system, conduction from the atrium to the ventricle is delayed, and the electrocardiographic (P-R) interval will lengthen. Ultimately, complete atrioventricular block may occur. Historically, the development of complete heart block has been a clinical sign associated with an abscess.

The infectious pathology differs somewhat between mechanical and bioprosthetic valves. Mechanical valve infection is virtually always focused in the sewing ring, and therefore paravalvular abscess formation occurs in the vast majority of mechanical valve infections.[68] On the other hand, infections of tissue valves may involve the leaflets alone, the sewing ring alone, or both.[34] Unlike infection of mechanical valves,

Table 76–2

Bacteriology of Prosthetic Valve Endocarditis

Early PVE		Late PVE	
Organism	***Percentage***	***Organism***	***Percentage***
Streptococci	10	Streptococci	40
		S. viridans	30
		Group D, *S. pneumoniae*	10
Staphylococci	45	Staphylococci	35
S. epidermidis	25	*S. epidermidis*	25
S. aureus	20	*S. aureus*	10
Gram-negative organisms	20	Gram-negative organisms	10
Fungi	10	Fungi	5
Diphtheroids	10	Diphtheroids	5
Other	5	Other	5

From Cowgill LD, Addonizio VP, Hopeman AR, Harken AH: Prosthetic valve endocarditis. In O'Rourke RA, Crawford MJ, editors: Current Problems in Cardiology. Chicago: Year Book, 1986, p. 617.

paravalvular abscess formation is therefore not a uniform finding in infected biological valves. In some series, fewer than 20% of infected biological valves had abscess formation.[34] Infections of the bioprosthetic valve leaflets may also cause stenosis of the infected tissue valve from vegetations in 28% and valve leaflet destruction and perforation in 36% of cases.[18] Because the incidence of abscess formation is lower in tissue valve infection, success of antibiotic therapy alone has been reported to be greater in treatment of infected tissue valves.[2,87]

DIAGNOSIS

Clinical Findings

PVE, particularly early PVE, may be difficult to diagnose. Fever is the most common clinical finding and is virtually always present.[18] However, in the postoperative period, there are many potential sources of fever, making this a nonspecific finding. Nonetheless, the diagnosis of PVE must be considered in any patient with a prosthetic valve and fever.

Other physical findings include a new regurgitant murmur or a changing murmur, frequently caused by valve dehiscence. This occurs in approximately 56% of patients[18] and is therefore not found in close to one half of patients with PVE.

One of the classic physical findings of native valve endocarditis is splenomegaly, and it is present in 25% of early PVE cases and 44% of late PVE cases.[92] However, other physical signs that are classically associated with native valve endocarditis, such as petechiae, Roth's spots, Osler's nodes, and Janeway lesions, are found only rarely with PVE.

Most laboratory data are very nonspecific in the diagnosis of PVE. Despite the presence of fever, leukocytosis with a white blood cell count of greater than 12,000/mm^3 is present in only one-half of patients.[18] As in native valve endocarditis, anemia (hematocrit less than 34%) is present in more than 70% of patients, particularly with late PVE.[18] Again, however, anemia is a very nonspecific finding in patients following cardiac surgery. As in native valve endocarditis, hematuria is common and is found in 57% of patients.[18]

The diagnosis of PVE is confirmed by positive blood cultures. Two blood cultures drawn from separate venipuncture sites will be positive in at least 99% of patients with bacterial endocarditis.[93] However, infection by very fastidious organisms or fungus may not create positive cultures for several weeks; cultures should therefore be kept for at least 3 weeks before being considered negative.

Echocardiography

The diagnosis is made by echocardiography; an echocardiogram should be performed in all patients suspected of having PVE. The echocardiographic features consistent with PVE include vegetations in the valve, a paravalvular leak, and a paravalvular abscess.

Transthoracic echocardiography (TTE) is readily available and noninvasive. However, the image quality of TTE may be operator dependent. Further, its images may be compromised by structures such as lung parenchyma, chest wall deformities, pericardial adipose tissue, etc. It is approximately 50% sensitive and 90% specific for PVE.[82]

Transesophageal echocardiography (TEE) is the diagnostic modality of choice and offers more precise information than TTE. In making the diagnosis of PVE, TEE is approximately 100% sensitive and 100% specific.[82] It is particularly valuable in visualizing a paravalvular abscess or an intracardiac fistula resultant to the infection.

Duke Criteria

Because endocarditis may be difficult to diagnose, the Duke criteria system has been proposed to help increase the certainty of the diagnosis. Initially put forth to help in the diagnosis of native valve endocarditis (NVE),[30] the Duke criteria have proven accurate in the diagnosis of PVE as well.[66] It is both sensitive and specific. As shown in Boxes 76-1 and 76-2, it combines clinical, echocardiographic, and microbiological data. The system permits the clinician to characterize the likelihood of PVE as definite, probable, possible, or rejected.

Conduction Abnormalities

Cardiac conduction abnormalities are common in patients with endocarditis, especially PVE. The electrocardiogram should be monitored on a regular basis. Among 1390 patients with endocarditis, 47% of patients with PVE and 23% of patients with NVE had conduction abnormalities.[54] Complete atrioventricular (AV) block was noted 13%. The presence of conduction abnormalities strongly suggests paravalvular abscess formation. Perhaps because it is associated with more extensive infection, the presence of conduction abnormalities was associated with 2-fold higher mortality rate.[54]

MANAGEMENT

The management of PVE is challenging.[86] Patients should be hospitalized, at least for the initiation of therapy, and monitored for cardiac dysrhythmias. As in the management of NVE, the mainstay of medical therapy is antibiotic therapy. As reviewed by Cowgill and co-workers,[18] the following guidelines should be followed: (1) bactericidal antibiotics should be used, (2) therapy should include two drugs that have synergistic bactericidal efficacy against the pathogen, (3) *in vitro* susceptibility testing should be performed to ensure that bactericidal drug levels are achieved, and (4) antibiotic therapy should be administered for 6–8 weeks.

The first objective of medical therapy is to sterilize the blood. After antibiotic therapy is initiated, blood cultures should be drawn every 3–4 days to ensure blood sterilization.[18] Once cultures are consistently negative, they should be drawn weekly or whenever the patient experiences fever or other clinical change. Blood cultures should become negative within 3–5 days of initiation of antibiotic therapy. Blood cultures should continue to be negative for at least 1 month after completion of antibiotic therapy. Failure of blood cultures to become negative after starting antibiotic therapy has been discontinued is an indication for surgical intervention.

Although controversial, anticoagulation should be started in patients with PVE. The infection may serve as a nidus for thrombus formation with subsequent embolization, and

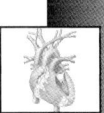

Box 76–1. Definitions of Terminology Used in the Duke Criteria.

Major criteria
Positive blood cultures for infective endocarditis
Typical microorganism for infective endocarditis from two separate blood cultures: *Viridans* streptococci, *Streptococcus bovis*, and HACEK group or community-acquired *Staphylococcus aureus* or enterococci in the absence of a primary focus or
Persistently positive blood cultures, defined as recovery of a microorganism consistent with infective endocarditis from
Blood cultures drawn >12 h apart or
All of three or most of four or more separate blood cultures, with the first and last drawn at least 1 h apart
Evidence of endocardial involvement
Positive echocardiogram for infective endocarditis
Oscillating intracardiac mass on valve or supporting structures or in the path of regurgitant jets or on implanted material in the absence of an alternative anatomical explanation or abscess or new partial dehiscence of prosthetic valve or new valvular regurgitation (increase or change in preexisting murmur not sufficient)
Minor criteria
Predisposition: predisposing heart condition or intravenous drug use
Fever: temperature ≥38° C (100.4° F)
Vascular phenomena: major arterial emboli, septic pulmonary infarcts, mycotic aneurysm, intracranial hemorrhage, conjunctival hemorrhages, and Janeway lesions
Immunological phenomena: glomerulonephritis, Osler nodes, Roth spots, rheumatoid factor
Microbiological evidence: positive blood culture but not meeting major criterion as noted previously or serological evidence of active infection with organism consistent with infective endocarditis
Echocardiogram: consistent with infective endocarditis but not meeting major criterion as noted previously

Modified from Perez-Vasquez A, Farinas MC, Garcia-Palomo JD, et al: Evaluation of the Duke criteria in 93 episodes of prosthetic valve endocarditis. Arch Intern Med 160:1185–1191, 2000.

Box 76–2. Proposed New Criteria (Additional Minor Criteria for Duke Classification Only for Prosthetic Valve Endocarditis).

Major criteria
As in the Duke criteria
Minor criteria
Predisposition: predisposing heart condition or intravenous drug use
Fever: temperature ≥38°C (100.4°F)
Vascular phenomena: major arterial emboli, septic pulmonary infarcts, mycotic aneurysm, intracranial hemorrhage, conjunctival hemorrhages, and Janeway lesions
Immunological phenomena: glomerulonephritis, Osler nodes, Roth spots, rheumatoid factor
Microbiological evidence: positive blood culture but not meeting major criterion as noted previously or serological evidence of active infection with organism consistent with infective endocarditis
Echocardiogram: consistent with infective endocarditis but not meeting major criterion as noted previously
New-onset heart failure
New conduction disturbances

Modified from Perez-Vasquez A, Farinas MC, Garcia-Palomo JD, et al: Evaluation of the Duke criteria in 93 episodes of prosthetic valve endocarditis. Arch Intern Med 160:1185–1191, 2000.

cerebral embolization is a major cause of death among these patients. Neurological complications of PVE are common, and both early and late PVE are associated with a 25–40% incidence of neurological complication.[56] Among patients with PVE who do not undergo anticoagulation, the incidence of embolic stroke has been reported to be 25–60%, which anticoagulation reduces to 3–14%.[21] Davenport and Hart[21] estimate that the daily stroke rate is 1–9%. Of note, most emboli occur with uncontrolled infection, and the incidence is markedly decreased with initiation of antibiotics. Although the risk of embolization is reduced by antibiotic therapy, it is not eliminated. Vilacosta et al[88] found that after the initiation of antibiotics, systemic embolism occurred in about 15% of patients with left-sided PVE. Two thirds of these embolic events occurred within the first 2 weeks of antibiotic therapy. Beyond the first 2 weeks after the infection is controlled with antibiotics, recurrent embolization is rare.[78] Therefore, if recurrent embolization does occur, it should be inferred that the infection is not controlled; recurrent embolization may be considered a relative indication for surgery.

The majority of patients with PVE require surgery, and the challenge for the surgeon is determining the appropriate timing for operation.[62] As reviewed by Cowgill et al[18] as well as Olaison et al,[63] the indications for replacement of the infected prosthesis all stem from failure of medical management. They include heart failure, ongoing sepsis or relapse of infection, valve obstruction, new onset of heart block (which implies a myocardial abscess), valve dehiscence, fungal infection, and recurrent systemic embolism. Of these surgical indications, congestive heart failure is probably the most significant prognostic factor.

Prognosis: Medical Treatment

Medical treatment of PVE is associated with a high mortality rate. A review of several major series demonstrates that the overall mortality rate is approximately 60%.[18,39,56] Early PVE is particularly lethal and carries a mortality rate of 74%. Although somewhat better, the mortality rate with late PVE is also substantial at 43%. Factors contributing to the higher mortality rate of early PVE include a predominance of virulent (nonstreptococcal) organisms, postoperative debilitation of patients, and involvement of a freshly implanted, nonendothelialized valve and sewing ring.

The infecting organism has a significant relationship to prognosis. Nonstreptococcal organisms have a significantly higher mortality rate than streptococcal organisms. The mortality rate associated with fungi is 93%, *S. aureus* 86%, diphtheroids, 64%; and gram-negative bacilli 60%. On the other hand, streptococcal infections have a mortality rate of 32%.[18]

Other factors that significantly affect prognosis include congestive heart failure, which is the leading prognostic factor; its presence is associated with a mortality rate exceeding 75%. Likewise, renal dysfunction and systemic emboli are associated with a significant increase in mortality rate.[57]

Most patients with PVE will require surgery. However, some highly selected patients may be successfully treated with antibiotics alone. In such patients, infection with less virulent organisms is essential, such as with coagulase negative *Staphylococcus* species or *Streptococcus viridans*.[2] Even without periannular abscess formation, PVE with *S. aureus* should have early operation. Clinically, such patients must at least remain stable, but preferably show clinical improvement on antibiotics alone. Accurate echocardiographic evaluation is needed, and TEE is essential.[38] There must be no evidence of paravalvular abscess or valve dehiscence. Infection limited to the leaflets of a bioprosthetic valve, particularly with late PVE, is favorable.

Using these guidelines for conservative treatment with antibiotics alone, Akowuah and colleagues[2] reported a 29% in-hospital mortality rate, which was not different from a surgically treated cohort. Truninger and colleagues[87] however, reported no in-hospital mortality as compared with 15% in surgically treated controls. Provided patients are successfully treated with antibiotics alone, careful longitudinal follow-up is required. Patients may exhibit subsequent valve dysfunction or recurrent infection, and require operation at a later time.[2]

Surgery

Historically, outcomes following surgical therapy for PVE were poor and associated with a mortality rate of 20–50%.[19,39,45,49] It is noteworthy that the mortality rates associated with surgical treatment of PVE have fallen in the past decade.[50,76] Several factors have contributed to improved surgical outcomes, including more effective antibiotics, improvements in myocardial protection and perioperative management, as well as an appreciation for earlier surgical intervention. Perhaps the most important contribution to improved outcomes is an understanding of the need to radically excise infected cardiac tissue and the ability of surgeons to reconstruct it.

Aortic PVE

Regardless of the type of infected valve (mechanical of bioprosthetic), extensive tissue destruction may complicate PVE. Approximately 80% of operated patients with aortic PVE have periannular abscess formation. A significant number may have intracardiac fistula formation and complete aortoventricular discontinuity has been reported in as many as 40% of surgical cases of aortic PVE.[76] Without surgery, these patients will die of sepsis or heart failure.

Extension of the infection into the annular and periannular structures is a major determinant of both early and late surgical results. The presence of periannular destruction relates to both the virulence of the organism and the duration of infection. Varying degrees of annular involvement are a constant feature of PVE. Abscess formation that begins at the sewing ring often extends into the aortic annulus, commonly in the region of aortic–mitral valvar continuity. The spectrum of periannular infection ranges from a simple localized abscess to larger subannular aneurysms, with or without perforation into other cardiac chambers. Likewise, the infection may extend into the pericardial space, create total disruption of ventriculoaortic continuity, or disrupt the mitral–aortic trigone.

When operating for paravalvular abscess, the surgeon must (1) ensure complete debridement of all grossly infected structures and nonviable tissue, (2) reestablish valve competency with elimination of any external or intracardiac defects, and (3) exclude attenuated areas from high pressure. These principles sometimes require radical cardiac debridement. Without adherence to these principles, the patient is at significant risk for recurrent infection, valve dehiscence, or both.[32]

Surgical reconstruction must be determined by the particular situation after complete debridement. In the majority of instances, an aortic root replacement is indicated. Aortic root replacement excludes attenuated regions from high pressure and permits suturing to noninfected, viable structures. If necessary, transmural sutures may be used to secure the conduit to the interventricular crest. Surgical principals dictate minimal use of synthetic materials in the infected area. Nonetheless, Hagl and associates[41] reported good results using prosthetic valved conduits for surgical treatment of aortic PVE. Among 28 patients operated on between 1988 and 2000, they reported an operative mortality of 11% and a 4% risk of recurrent endocarditis or reoperation up to 5 years postoperatively.

Nonetheless, the procedure of choice for aortic PVE is reconstruction and aortic root replacement with a cryopreserved homograft. Data from laboratory animals[48] and humans[89,90] have confirmed that homograft vascular tissue is significantly more resistant to infection than prosthetic material. Aortic root replacement using a homograft minimizes placement of prosthetic material into the area of infection, thereby minimizing the risk of recurrent infection.[25,53] Use of a homograft offers much greater flexibility in reconstruction of the debrided areas. They may be implanted in such a way as to exclude an abscess cavity by sewing the proximal anastomosis of the homograft to the inferior border of the abscess cavity. Use of an aortic homograft with its attached anterior mitral leaflet is particularly valuable in this regard[22,76] (Figure 76-5).

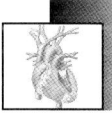

In 32 patients with aortic PVE, Dossche and associates[29] found 81% had periannular abscess formation and 34% had ventricular–aortic discontinuity. Homograft aortic root replacement was associated with an operative mortality of only 9.4% and 96% were free of reinfection at 5 years. Sabik and colleagues[76] found a very similar incidence of periannular abscess formation (78%) and ventricular–aortic discontinuity (40%) in 103 patients with aortic PVE. Despite these advanced infections, excellent surgical results were achieved. Following radical cardiac debridement of all infected and nonviable tissue, reconstruction with a cryopreserved aortic homograft was associated with a hospital mortality of 3.9% (Figure 76-6). Only 4 patients underwent reoperation for recurrent endocarditis; 95% were free of infection at 2 years.

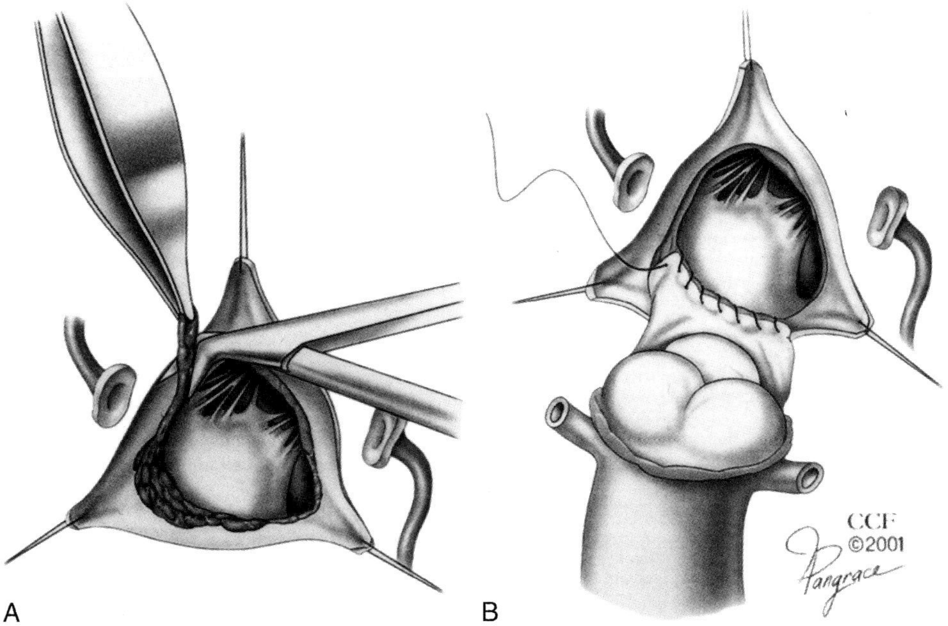

A B

Figure 76–5 Technique of aortic root replacement and homograft reconstruction. A, The infected valve is excised, and all infected and necrotic tissue is radically debrided. The coronary ostia are preserved as buttons. **B,** The defect is reconstructed by suturing the homograft mitral valve leaflet below the level of the infection.
(From Sabik JF, Lytle BW, Blackstone EH, et al: Aortic root replacement with cryopreserved allograft for prosthetic valve endocarditis. Ann Thorac Surg 74:650–659, 2002.)

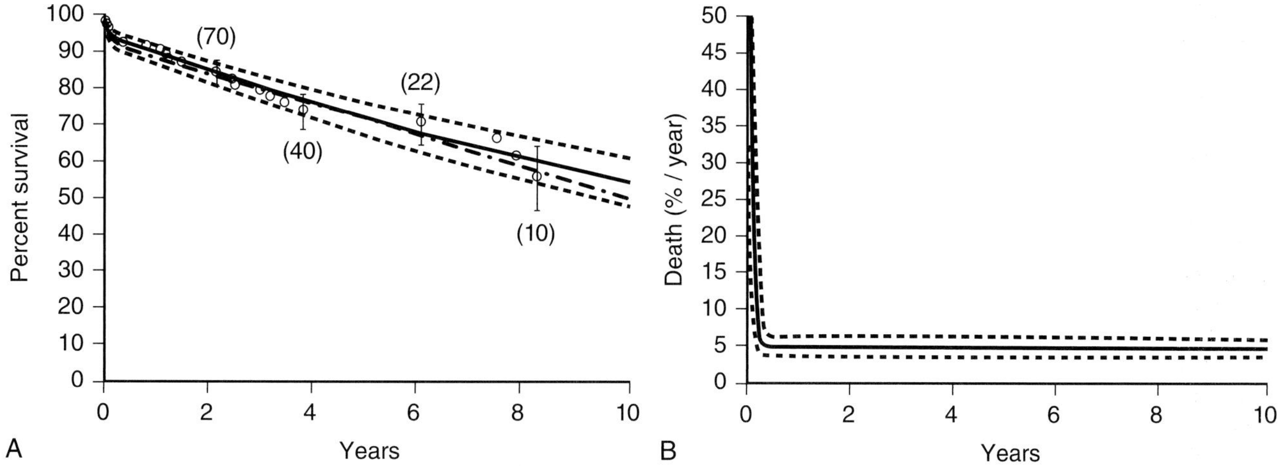

Figure 76–6 Survival after homograft aortic root replacement for prosthetic valve endocarditis (PVE). A, Survival. The dot-dash-dot line represents survival predicted after aortic valve rereplacement for indications other that PVE for patients with similar characteristics. **B,** Hazard function for death.
(Modified from Sabik JF, Lytle BW, Blackstone EH, et al: Aortic root replacement with cryopreserved allograft for prosthetic valve endocarditis. Ann Thorac Surg 74:650–659, 2002.)

Following its application in the treatment of NVE, the Ross procedure has been used in the treatment of aortic PVE.[60,69] While the Ross procedure may minimize the use of prosthetic material, in the setting of PVE it is a more complex procedure and performed in critically ill patients. It should therefore be used very selectively in PVE. Likewise, aortic root replacement with a stentless porcine valve has also been used in aortic PVE.[58,77] Used to replace the aortic root, a stentless valve does offer flexibility in reconstruction of the debrided myocardium. It does, however, place prosthetic material into the infected area and a homograft is preferred.

Aortic PVE in patients who have previously undergone aortic root replacement with composite valve-conduit poses an even greater surgical challenge.[71] The surgical principles remain the same, however, and extensive surgical debridement is required to remove the infected prosthetic material. The aortic root should be replaced with a homograft.

Two particular surgical challenges must be overcome to replace an infected composite valve-conduit. The first is reimplantation of the coronary artery ostia into the homograft. Scarring from the initial procedure may make it difficult to effectively mobilize the left and right main coronary ostia for anastomosis to the homograft without undue tension. Raanani and colleagues found it might be necessary to extend the main coronary arteries with a short length of saphenous vein in 52% of patients undergoing rereplacement of the aortic root.[70] Second, it may be necessary to employ deep hypothermia and circulatory arrest to achieve adequate resection and debridement of the distal graft-to-aorta anastomosis.[51,79] Further, a homograft may not have sufficient length to reach the distal aortic anastomosis. Lytle and colleagues[51] have used a second homograft to effectively bridge the distance between the first homograft and the aorta (Figure 76-7).

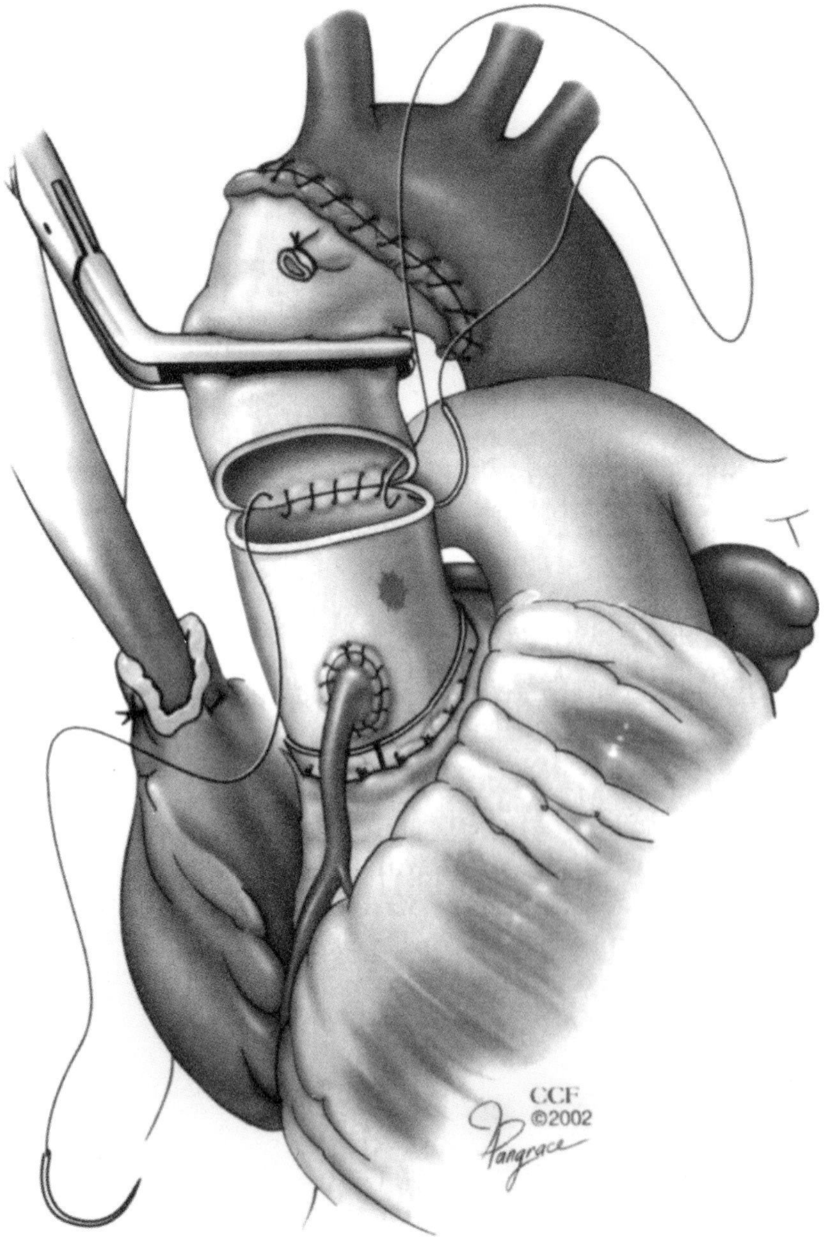

Figure 76–7 Reconstruction after resection and debridement of an infected valve-conduit may require two homografts to provide sufficient length to reach the distal aortic anastomosis.
(From Lytle BW, Sabik JF, Blackstone BH, et al: Reoperative cryopreserved root and ascending aorta replacement for acute aortic prosthetic valve endocarditis. Ann Thorac Surg 74:S1754–1757, 2002.)

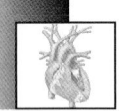

Despite the complexity of replacement of the infected composite valve-conduit, radical surgical debridement has achieved excellent surgical results. Using these techniques, operative mortality rates of 3–6.6% have been achieved.[51,70,79] In the experience of Lytle and colleagues,[51] the actuarial survival was 56% at 5 years, and no patients had reinfection.

Mitral PVE

Endocarditis is rare following mitral valve repair.[37,46] But when it happens, the principles of its management are the same. If surgery is necessary, the annuloplasty ring should be removed, as well as all infected and devitalized tissue. The valve should usually be replaced.

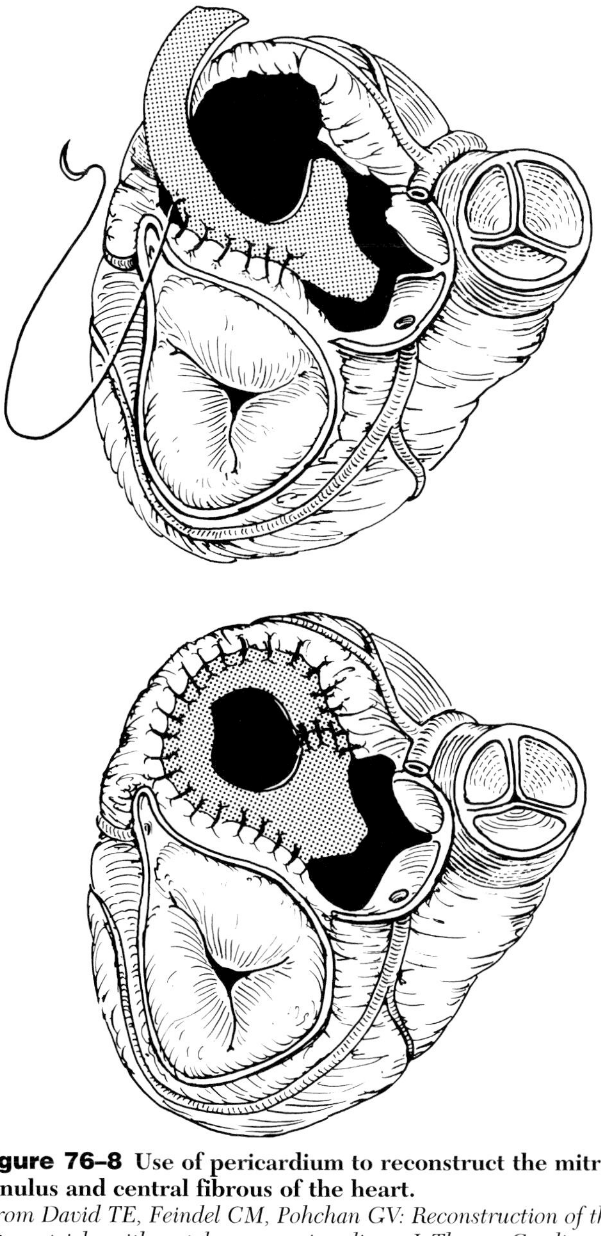

Figure 76–8 **Use of pericardium to reconstruct the mitral annulus and central fibrous of the heart.**
(From David TE, Feindel CM, Pohchan GV: Reconstruction of the left ventricle with autologous pericardium. J Thorac Cardiovasc Surg 94:710–714, 1987.)

Fortunately, destruction of the mitral annular region is much less common than periaortic annular destruction[24]; debridement and reconstruction of the mitral annulus are much more difficult than in the aortic region. The mitral annulus may be reconstructed with autologous pericardium following debridement, as described by David and Feindel[22] and by David and associates[22,23] (Figure 76-8). If the posterior mitral annular region requires reconstruction, this may be done using pericardium, following which, if necessary, the new mitral prosthesis may be translocated onto either the atrial or the ventricular side of the annulus. If it is technically possible, ventricular translocation can prevent exposure of the attenuated area to high pressure.[32,74] Although uncommon, repair of aortic–mitral discontinuity is particularly difficult to reconstruct. This trigonal region may be reconstructed using a modification of the technique described by Rastan and associates.[72] The material used in the reconstruction should be a sandwich of pericardium exposed to the blood side and synthetic material for stability (Figure 76-9).

Operation with Recent Stroke

As noted earlier, neurological complications are common with PVE. The mechanisms of neurological injury include pyogenic arteritis, hemorrhagic transformation of embolic infarction, rupture of intracranial mycotic aneurysms, and ischemic stroke secondary to embolization of clot or septic material.[42,78] Systemic embolization occurs in up to 50% of cases of left-sided endocarditis, and more than half are to the brain.[8] Such neurological events are associated with significant morbidity and mortality. Intracranial hemorrhage in the setting of PVE carries a mortality rate as high as 28–69%.[21]

In 211 patients with left-sided endocarditis, Vilacosta and colleagues[88] found the risk of systemic embolization to be the same for PVE and native valve endocarditis. Further, the risk of embolization was about the same for aortic and mitral endocarditis.

The most common neurological complication is ischemic stroke.[8,21] From the surgical perspective, the main concern is the transformation of an ischemic infarct into a hemorrhagic infarct as a consequence of the anticoagulation required during cardiopulmonary bypass. This is particularly important because up to 32% of cerebral infarctions in patients with endocarditis may be asymptomatic.[84]

Ting and colleagues[84] found that patients with intracranial hemorrhage secondary to endocarditis who then underwent valve replacement suffered a perioperative stroke, which was associated with a significantly increased mortality rate. On the other hand, patients with a preoperative ischemic infarct (without hemorrhage) secondary to endocarditis who underwent valve replacement had no perioperative strokes. Nonetheless, DiSesa[27] has documented the risk of transforming an ischemic infarct into a hemorrhagic one. Thus, before undergoing a valve replacement, patients with PVE should undergo a careful neurological evaluation, including computed tomography of the head. If a small ischemic infarct is identified, the risk of making this worse with valve replacement appears to be low. However, if a large ischemic infarct or intracranial hemorrhage is identified, the risk of a significant perioperative neurological

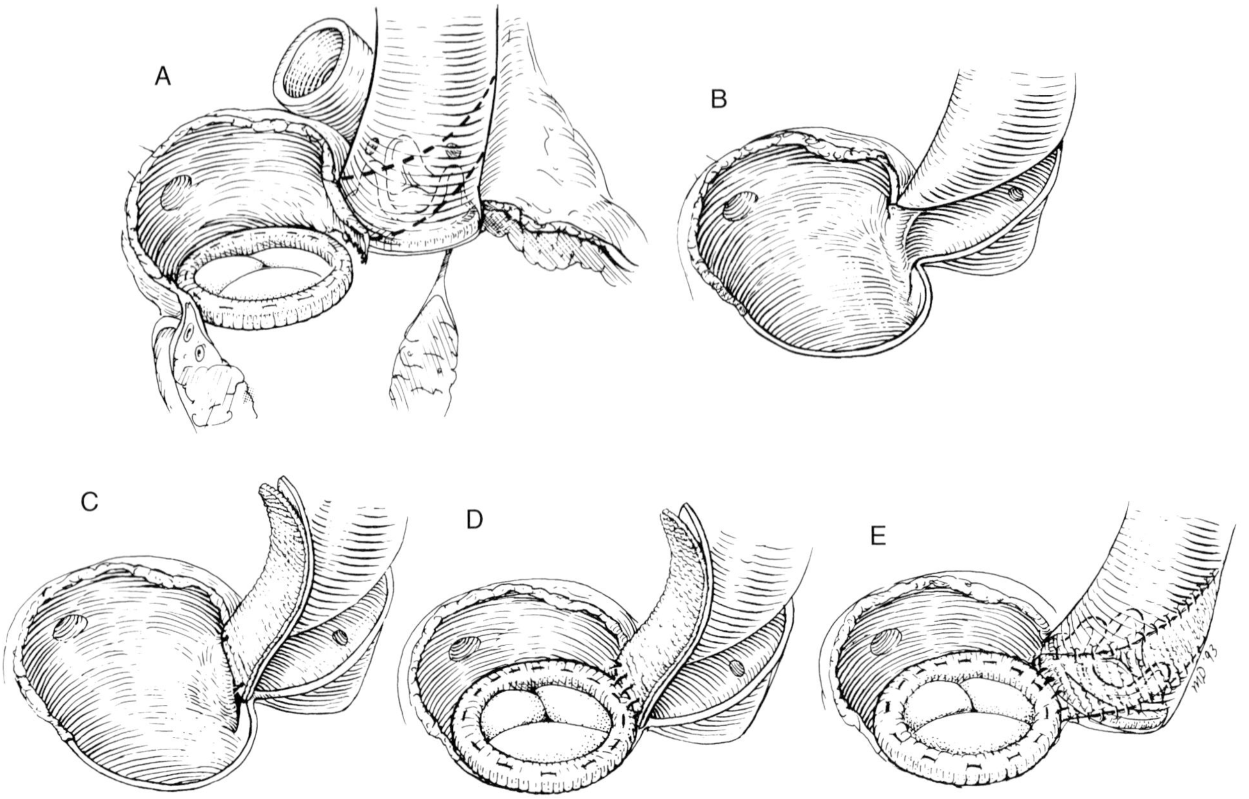

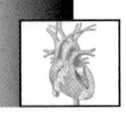

Figure 76–9 (**A–E**) Steps in reconstruction of extensive destruction of the left fibrous trigone with a composite patch. *(From Ergin MA, Raissi S, Follis F, et al: Annular destruction in acute bacterial endocarditis: surgical techniques to meet the challenge. J Thorac Cardiovasc Surg 97:755–763, 1989.)*

event is high. In such patients, the need for valve replacement should be balanced against high neurological risk. If possible, operation should be delayed as long as possible to allow healing of the brain injury.

REFERENCES

1. Aagaard J, Andersen PV: Acute endocarditis treated with radical debridement and implantation of mechanical of stented bioprosthetic devices. Ann Thorac Surg 71:100–104, 2001.
2. Akowauh EF, Davies W, Oliver S, et al: Prosthetic valve endocarditits: early and late outcomes following medical of surgical treatment. Heart 89:269–272, 2003.
3. Alexiou C, Langley SM, Stafford H, et at: Surgery for active culture-positive endocarditis: determinants of early and late oucome. Ann Thorac Surg 69:1448–1454, 2000.
4. Ankeney JL, Parker RF: Staphylococcal endocarditis following open heart surgery related to positive intraoperative blood cultures. In Brewer L, editor: Prosthetic Heart Valves. Springfield, IL: Charles C Thomas, 1969, p. 719.
5. Bauernschmitt R, Jakob HG, Vahl C-F, et al: Operation for infective endocarditis: results after implantation of mechanical valves. Ann Thorac Surg 65:359–364, 1998.
6. Baumgartner FJ, Omari BO, Robertson JM, et al: Annular abscesses in surgical endocarditis: anatomic, clinical and operative features. Ann Thorac Surg 70:442–447, 2000.
7. Baumgartner WA, Miller DC, Rietz BA, et al: Surgical treatment of prosthetic valve endocarditis. Ann Thorac Surg 35:87–104, 1983.
8. Bayer AS, Bolger AF, Taubert KA, et al: Diagnosis and management of infective endocarditis and its complications. Circulation 98:2936–2948, 1998.
9. Bayer AS, Nelson FJ, Slama TG: Current concepts in prevention of prosthetic valve endocarditis. Chest 97: 1203–1207, 1990.
10. Berbari EF, Cockerill FR, Steckelberg JM: Infective endocarditis due to unusual or fastidious microorganisms. Mayo Clin Proc 72:532–542, 1997.
11. Bland LA, Villarino ME, Ardnino JJ, et al: Bacteriologic and endotoxin analysis of salvaged blood used in autologous transfusions during cardiac operation. J Thorac Cardiovasc Surg 103:582–588, 1992.
12. Blumberg EA, Karalis AD, Chandrasekaran K, et at: Endocarditis-associated paravalvular abscesses. Do clinical parameters predict the presence of abscess? Chest 107: 898–903, 1995.
13. Bonow RO, Carabello B, De Leon AC, et al: ACC/AHA guidelines for the management of patients with valvular heart disease. Circulation 98:1949–1984, 1998.
14. Calderwood SB, Swinski LA, Waternaux CM, et al: Risk factors for the development of prosthetic valve endocarditis. Circulation 72:31–37, 1985.
15. Calderwood SB, Swinski LA, Karchmer AW, et al: Prosthetic valve endocarditis. Analysis of factors affecting outcome of therapy. J Thorac Cardiovasc Surg 92:776–783, 1986.
16. Campbell WN, Tsai W, Mispireta LA: Evaluation of the practice of routine culturing of the native valves during replacement surgery. Ann Thorac Surg 69:548–550, 2000.
17. Corona ML, Peters SG, Narr BJ, Thompson RL: Infections related to central venous catheters. Mayo Clin Proc 65: 979–986, 1990.

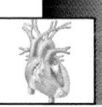

18. Cowgill LD, Addonizio VP, Hopeman AR, Harken AH: A practical approach to prosthetic valve endocarditis. Ann Thorac Surg 43:450–457, 1987.
19. Danchin N, Retournay G, Stchepinsky O, et al: Comparison of long term outcome in patients with or without aortic ring abscess treated surgically for aortic valve infective endocarditis. Heart 81:177–181, 1999.
20. Danielson GK, Titus JL, DuShane JWL: Successful treatment of aortic valve endocarditis and aortic root abscesses by insertion of prosthetic valve in ascending aorta and placement of bypass grafts to coronary arteries. J Thorac Cardiovasc Surg 67:443–449, 1974.
21. Davenport J, Hart RG: Prosthetic valve endocarditis 1976–1987. Stroke 21:993–999, 1990.
22. David TE, Feindel CM: Reconstruction of the mitral annulus. Circulation 76(Suppl. III):III102–III107, 1987.
23. David TE, Feindel CM, Pohchan GV: Reconstruction of the left ventricle with autologous pericardium. J Thorac Cardiovasc Surg 94:710–714, 1987.
24. David TE, Komeda M, Brofman PR: Surgical treatment of aortic root abscess. Circulation 80(Suppl. I):I269–I274, 1989.
25. Dearani JA, Orszulak TA, Schaff HV, et al: Results of allograft aortic valve replacement for complex endocarditis. J Thorac Cardiovasc Surg 113:285–291, 1997.
26. Delay D, Pellerin M, Carrier M, et al: Immediate and long-term results of valve replacement for native and prosthetic valve endocarditis. Ann Thorac Surg 70:1219–1223, 2000.
27. DiSesa VJ: Art and science in the management of endocarditis. Ann Thorac Surg 51:6–7, 1991.
28. Dismukes WE, Karchmer AW, Buckly MJ, et al: Prosthetic valve endocarditis: an analysis of 38 cases. Circulation 48:365–377, 1973.
29. Dossche KM, Defauw JJ, Ernst SM, et al: Allograft aortic root replacement in prosthetic aortic valve endocarditis: a review of 32 patients. Ann Thorac Surg 63:1644–1649, 1997.
30. Durack DT, Lukes AS, Bright DK: New criteria for diagnosis of infective endocarditis: utilization of specific echocardiographic findings. Am J Med 96:200–209, 1994.
31. Dyson, C, Barnes RA, Harrison GAJ: Infective endocarditis: an epidemiological review of 128 episodes. J Infect 38:87–93, 1999.
32. Ergin MA, Raissi, S, Follis F, et al: Annular destruction in acute bacterial endocarditis: surgical techniques to meet the challenge. J Thorac Cardiovasc Surg 97:755–763, 1989.
33. Fang G, Keys TF, Gentry LO, et al: Prosthetic valve endocarditis resulting from nosocomial bacteremia. Ann Intern Med 119:560–567, 1993.
34. Fernicola DJ, Roberts W: Frequency of ring abscess and leaflet infection in active infective endocarditis involving bioprosthetic valves. Am J Cardiol 72:314–323, 1993.
35. Frantz PT, Murray GF, Wilcox BR: Surgical management of left ventricular-aortic discontinuity complicating bacterial endocarditis. Ann Thorac Surg 29:1–7, 1978.
36. Geraci JE, Dale AJD, McGoon DC, et al: Bacterial endocarditis and endarteritis following cardiac operations. Wis Med J 62:302–305, 1963.
37. Gillinov AM, Faber CN, Sabik JF, et al: Endocarditis after mitral valve repair. Ann Thorac Surg 73:1813–1816, 2002.
38. Graupner C, Vilacosta I, San Roman A, et al: Periannular extension of infective endocarditis. J Am Coll Cardiol 39:1204–1211, 2002.
39. Grover FL, Cohen DJ, Oprian C, et al: Determinants of the occurrence of and survival from prosthetic valve endocarditis. Experience of the Veterans Affairs Cooperative Study on Valvular Heart Disease. J Thorac Cardiovasc Surg 108: 207–214, 1994.
40. Guerra JM, Tornos MP, Permanyer-Miralda G, et al: Long term results of mechanical prosthesis for treatment of active infective endocarditis. Heart 86:63–68, 2001.
41. Hagl C, Galla JD, Lansman SL: Replacing the ascending aorta and aortic valve for acute prosthetic valve endocarditis: is using prosthetic material contraindicated? Ann Thorac Surg 74: S1781–S1785, 2002.
42. Hart RG, Kagan-Hallet K, Joerns SE: Mechanisms of intracranial hemorrhage in infective endocarditis. Stroke 18:1048–1056, 1987.
43. Haydock D, Barrat-Boyes B, Macedo, T, et al: Aortic valve replacement for active infectious endocarditis in 108 patients. J Thorac Cardiovasc Surg 103:130–139, 1992.
44. Ivert TSA, Dismukes WE, Cobbs CG, et al: Prosthetic valve endocarditis. Circulation 69:223–232, 1984.
45. Jones JM, O'Kane H, Gladstone DJ, et al: Repeat heart valve surgery: risk factors for operative mortality. J Thorac Cardiovasc Surg 122:913–918, 2001.
46. Karavas AN, Filsoufi, F, Mihaljevic T, et al: Risk factors and management of endocarditis after mitral valve repair. J Heart Valve Dis 11:660–664, 2002.
47. Kluge RM, Calia FM, McLaughlin JA, et al: Source of contamination in open heart surgery. JAMA 230:1415–1418, 1974.
48. Koskas F, Goeau-Brissonniere O, Nicolas M-H, et al: Arteries from human beings are less infectible by Staphylococcus aureus than polytetrafluoroethylene in an aortic dog model. J Vasc Surg 23:472–476, 1996.
49. Larbalestier RI, Kinchla NM, Aranki SF, et al: Acute bacterial endocarditis. Optimizing surgical results. Circulation 86 (Suppl. II):II-68–II-74, 1992.
50. Lytle BW, Priest BP, Taylor PC, et al: Surgical treatment of prosthetic valve endocarditis. J Thorac Cardiovasc Surg 111:198–210, 1996.
51. Lytle BW, Sabik JF, Blackstone BH, et al: Reoperative cryopreserve root and ascending aorta replacement for acute aortic prosthetic valve endocarditis. Ann Thorac Surg 74: S1754–1757, 2002.
52. McGiffin DC, Galbraith AJ, McLachlan GJ, et al: Aortic valve infection. Risk factors for death and recurrent endocarditis after aortic valve replacement. J Thorac Cardiovasc Surg 105: 511–520, 1992.
53. Meine TJ, Nettles RE, Anderson DJ, et al: Cardiac conduction abnormalities in endocarditis defined by the Duke criteria. Am Heart J 142:280–285, 2001.
54. Miller DC: Predictors of outcome in patients with prosthetic valve endocarditis (PVE) and potential advantages of homograft aortic root replacement for prosthetic ascending aortic valve-graft infections. J Cardiovasc Surg 5:53–62, 1990.
55. Moon MR, Miller DC, Moore KA, et al: Treatment of endocarditis with valve replacement: the question of tissue versus mechanical prosthesis. Ann Thorac Surg 71:1164–1171, 2001.
56. Moon MR, Stinson EB, Miller DC: Surgical treatment of endocarditis. Prog Cardiovasc Dis 40:239–274, 1997.
57. Mullany CJ, McIsaacs AL, Rowe MH, Hale GS: The surgical treatment of infective endocarditis. World J Surg 13:132–136, 1989.
58. Muller LC, Chevtchik O, Bonatti JO, et al: Treatment of destructive aortic valve endocarditis with the freestyle aortic root bioprosthesis. Ann Thorac Surg 75:453–456, 2003.
59. Nasser RM, Melgar GR, Longworth KL, Gordon SM: Incidence and risk of developing fungal prosthetic valve endocarditis after nosocomial candidemia. Am J Med 103: 25–32, 1997.
60. Niwaya K, Knott-Craig CJ, Santangelo K, et al: Advantages of autograft and homograft valve replacements for complex aortic endocarditis. Ann Thorac Surg 67:1603–1608, 1999.
61. O'Brien MR, Stafford EG, Garner MAH, et al: A comparison of aortic valve replacement with viable cryopreserved and fresh allograft valves, with a note on chromosomal studies. J Throac Cardiovasc Surg 94:812–823, 1987.

62. Okita Y, Franciosi G, Matsuki O, et al: Early and late results of aortic root replacement with antibiotic-sterilized aortic homograft. J Thorac Cardiovasc Surg 95:696–704, 1988.
63. Olaison L, Pettersson G: Current best practices and guidelines. Indications for surgical intervention in infective endocarditis. Infect Dis Clin N Am 16:453–475, 2002.
64. Olinger GN, Maloney JV Jr: Repair of left ventricular-aortic discontinuity complicating endocarditis from an aortic valve prosthesis. Ann Thorac Surg 23:576–577, 1977.
65. Parker FB, Greiner-Hayes C, Tomar RH, et al: Bacteremia following prosthetic valve replacement. Ann Thorac Surg 197:147–151, 1983.
66. Perez-Vasquez A, Farinas MC, Garcia-Palomo JD, et al: Evaluation of the Duke criteria in 93 episodes of prosthetic valve endocarditis. Arch Intern Med 160:1185–1191, 2000.
67. Petrou M, Wong K, Albertucci M, et al: Evaluation of unstented aortic homografts for the treatment of prosthetic aortic valve endocarditis. Circulation 90(Suppl. II):II 198–II 204, 1994.
68. Piper C, Korfer R, Horstkotte D: Prosthetic valve endocarditis. Heart 85:590–593, 2001.
69. Prat A, Saez de Ibarra JI, Vincentelli A, et al: Ross operation for active culture-positive aortic valve endocarditis with extensive paravalvular involvement. Ann Thorac Surg 72:1492–1496, 2001.
70. Raanani E, Davie TE, Dellgren G, et al: Redo aortic root replacement: experience with 31 patients. Ann Thorac Surg 71:1460–1463, 2001.
71. Ralph-Edwards A, Davie TE, Bos J: Infective endocarditis in patients who had replacement of the aortic root. Ann Thorac Surg 58:429–433, 1994.
72. Rastan A, Atai M, Hadi H, et al: Enlargement of mitral valvular ring. New technique for double valve replacement in children or adults with small mitral annulus. J Thorac Cardiovasc Surg 81:106–111, 1981.
73. Reitz BA, Stinson EB, Watson DE, et al: Translocation of the aortic valve for prosthetic valve endocarditis. J Thorac Cardiovasc Surg 81:212–218, 1981.
74. Rochiccioli C, Chastre J, Lecompte Y, et al: Prosthetic valve endocarditis. J Thorac Cardiovasc Surg 92:784–789, 1986.
75. Ross DN: Allograft root replacement for prosthetic endocarditis. J Cardiovasc Surg 5:68–73, 1990.
76. Sabik JF, Lytle BW, Blackstone EH, et al: Aortic root replacement with cryopreserved allograft for prosthetic valve endocarditis. Ann Thorac Surg 74:650–659, 2002.
77. Sakaguchi T, Sawa Y, Ohtake S, et al: The Freestyle Stentless bioprosthesis for prosthetic valve endocarditis. Ann Thorac Surg 67:533–555, 1999.
78. Salgado AV, Furlan AJ, Keys TF, et al: Neurological complications of endocarditis: a 12 year experience. Neurology 39: 173–178, 1989.
79. Schepens MAAM, Dossche KM, Morchuis J: Reoperations on the ascending aortic and aortic root: pitfalls and results in 134 patients. Ann Thorac Surg 68:176–180, 1999.
80. Seipelt RG, Vazques-Jimenez JF, Seipelt IM, et al: The St Jude "Silzone" valve: midterm results in treatment of active endocarditis. Ann Thorac Surg 72:758–763, 2001.
81. Shuhaiber H, Chugh T, Burns G: In vitro adherence of bacteria to sutures in cardiac surgery. J Thorac Cardiovasc Surg 30:749–753, 1989.
82. Stein PD, Harken DE, Dexter L: The nature and prevention of prosthetic valve endocarditis. Am Heart J 71:393–407, 1966.
83. Symbas PN, Vlais SE, Zacharopuolos L, Lutz JF: Acute endocarditis: surgical treatment of aortic regurgitation and aortic-left ventricular discontinuity. J Throac Cardiovasc Surg 84:291–296, 1982.
84. Ting W, Silverman N, Levitsky S: Valve replacement in patients with endocarditis and cerebral septic emboli. Ann Thorac Surg 51:18–21, 1991.
85. Tong JS: Role of echocardiography in the diagnosis and management of infective endocarditis. Curr Opin Cardiol 17:478–485, 2002.
86. Tornos P: Management of prosthetic valve endocarditis: a clinical challenge. Heart 89:245–246, 2003.
87. Truninger K, Attenhofer CH, Seifert B: Long term follow up of prosthetic valve endocarditis: what characteristic identify patient who were treated successfully with antibiotics alone? Heart 82:714–720, 1999.
88. Vilacosta I, Graupner C, San Romn JA, et al: Risk of embolization after institution of antibiotic therapy for infective endocarditis. J Am Coll Cardiol 39:1489–1495, 2002.
89. Vogt PR, Brunner-La Rocca H-P, Carrel T, et al: Cryopreserved arterial allografts in the treatment of major vascular infection: a comparison with conventional surgical techniques. J Thorac Cardioavsc Surg 116:965–972, 1998.
90. Vogt PR, Turino MI: Management of infected aortic grafts: development of less invasive surgery using cryopreserved homografts. Ann Thorac Surg 67:1986–1989, 1999.
91. Wantanabe GO, Haverich A, Speier R, et al: Surgical treatment of active infective endocarditis with paravalvular involvement. J Thorac Cardiovasc Surg 107:171–177, 1994.
92. Watanakunakorn C: Prosthetic valve infective endocarditis: a review. Prog Cardiovasc Dis 22:181–192, 1979.
93. Weinstein MP, Rell LB, Murphy JR, et al: The clinical significance of positive blood cultures: a comprehensive analysis of 500 episodes of bacteremia and fungemia in adults: I. Laboratory and epidemiology observations. Rev Infect Dis 5:35–53, 1983.

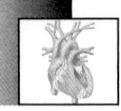

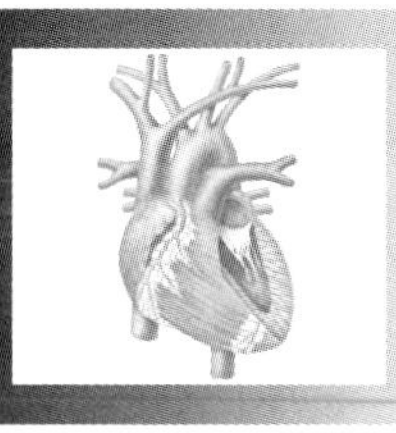

CHAPTER 77

Thrombosis and Thromboembolism of Prosthetic Cardiac Valves and Extracardiac Prostheses

David N. Campbell and Frederick L. Grover

ARTIFICAL SURFACES, COAGULATION CASCADES, THROMBOSIS, AND LYSIS

Intravascular placement of a foreign body with its nonendothelial surface activates the clotting mechanism leading toward thrombus formation. One possible exception is, of course, an aortic allograft valve or an allograft pulmonary valved conduit. The exposure of blood to the synthetic surface leads rapidly to deposition of a fine layer of plasma components, mostly protein, followed by platelet deposition. The intrinsic coagulation cascade is initiated along with the extrinsic coagulation cascade: the inflammatory response, including leukocyte activation, the complement system, and fibrinolysis.

Fibrinogen is one of the major plasma proteins, often the first, that is deposited on these artificial surfaces. Once the layer of fibrinogen is absorbed onto the surface, platelets can adhere to the fibrinogen. Although surfaces vary greatly in their tendency to promote thrombosis, the reactivity of most materials to blood can be significantly increased if they are first exposed to fibrinogen.[106] Other proteins also are deposited, including fibronectin (a surface protein of many cells), von Willebrand's factor (a glycoprotein essential for the adhesion of platelets to subendothelial tissue), thrombospondin (a platelet protein secreted by activated platelets), and Factor XII (Hageman's factor, the primary activator of the intrinsic coagulation system).

Once platelets attach to the protein layer and spread out on the artificial surface, materials present in the platelet intracellular granules are secreted, including β-thromboglobulin, which inhibits prostacyclin production, platelet Factor IV, which neutralizes heparin sulfate in the endothelium, serotonin, adenosine triphosphate (ATP), and adenosine diphosphate (ADP). Synthesis of prostaglandins E and F is evident as well, suggesting that endoperoxide metabolism has taken place along with formation of thromboxane A_2 from platelet arachidonic acid. Serotonin, thromboxane A_2, and endoperoxide are potent vasoconstrictors and platelet stimulatory factors.[82] Finally, platelet aggregation follows platelet adhesion, probably by ADP and serotonin secretion from the adherent platelets. Fibrinogen and thromboxane A_2 are key in this step.

The coagulation cascade is initiated either by reaction of plasma proteins with the artificial surface to form enzymatically active components such as Factor XII (intrinsic system) or by introduction of thromboplastin via exposure of subendothelial tissue to the surface (extrinsic system). Figure 77-1 is a schematic diagram of the clotting cascade. Activation of Factors XIIa and XIa initiate the intrinsic system leading to activated Factor Xa. Platelets provide the phospholipid surface for this reaction. Activated Factor XIIa also initiates the kininogen–kallikrein system and kallikrein provides positive feedback for the contact activation. Kallikrein cleaves Factor XII to convert it to Factor XIIa, thereby accelerating contact activation. Bradykinin is also released when kallikrein cleaves high-molecular-weight kininogen (HMWK). Activated HMWK can then bind more prekallikrein and Factor XI to the activating surface, which further increases the reaction. In the final common pathway, prothrombin is converted to thrombin, and fibrinogen is converted to fibrin. Thrombin recruits more platelets, creating more adhesion and aggregation. A fibrin platelet clot is formed, and thrombosis occurs.

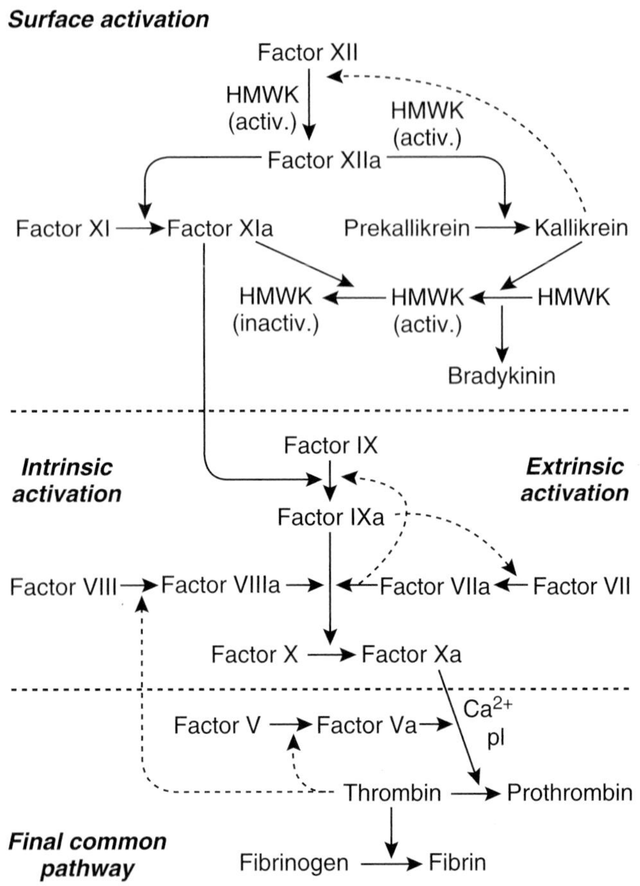

Figure 77–1 The coagulation cascade from surface activation to the final common pathway. HMWK, high-molecular-weight kininogen.
(From Ware JA, Lewis J, Salzman EW: Antithrombotic therapy. In Rutherford RB, editor: Vascular Surgery, 3rd ed. Philadelphia: Saunders, 1989.)

Activation of the clotting cascade on the surface or an artificial device occurs similarly whether on the cardiac valve, cardiopulmonary bypass system, vascular graft, extracorporeal membrane oxygenation (ECMO) circuit, mechanism assist device, or vascular catheter. It will produce thrombus formation; macroscopic and microscopic platelet-fibrin emboli occur commonly as well. Factor XII, kallikrein, and plasmin activate the complement system and activate neutrophils, and kinin formation mediates vasodilatation, vascular permeability, and white blood cell migration. Normally, a delicate balance is maintained between these two systems, so that uncontrolled clotting or hemorrhage does not occur. The coagulation cascade is initiated, Factor XII and kallikrein initiate clot lysis with conversion of plasminogen to plasmin. Antiplasmins in the circulating blood, particularly α_2-antiplasmin, rapidly neutralize most of the circulating plasmin; however, plasmin also is incorporated into the clot during clot formation. The fibrin meshwork protects plasmin form antiplasmin once the plasmin is activated to plasmin, allowing fibrin degradation in the clot. In fact, many natural inhibitors offset activated procoagulant protein. Protein C, heparin, antithrombin III, protein S, thrombomodulin, prostacyclin, and plasmin all counter steps in the coagulation cascade.[25]

ANTICOAGULATION THERAPY

Clinically useful drugs that block the clotting cascade fall into four primary groups: orally administered vitamin K antagonists, natural anticoagulants such as the heparin–antithrombin III system, antiplatelet drugs, and fibrinolytic agents.

Warfarin sodium remains the most popular orally administered vitamin K antagonist used today in the United States. It blocks the formation of the four vitamin K-dependent clotting factors—prothrombin, VII, IX, and X—creating a buildup of their precursors. Warfarin sodium blocks the vitamin K cycle at the regeneration of reduced vitamin K, which is the active form of vitamin K (Figure 77-2).

Heparin's anticoagulant effect is fairly complex and not completely understood. Heparin sulfate is a glycosaminoglycan that binds to antithrombin III and activates this serine protease inhibitor. Heparin and antithrombin III occur naturally in humans, are secreted by endothelial cells, and are both required to produce their anticoagulant effect. Antithrombin III binds to thrombin and blocks the enzymes of the intrinsic coagulation cascade, including thrombin and Factors IXa, Xa, XIa, and XIIa.

The various antiplatelet drugs have different mechanisms of action, making them more or less useful as therapeutic anticoagulation agents. Figure 77-3 is a schematic diagram of the actions of antiplatelet drugs. Aspirin inhibits platelet aggregation by *irreversible* acetylation of platelet cyclooxygenase, hence blocking the synthesis of prostaglandins and thromboxane A_2. Asprin *will* prolong the bleeding, time, and its effect lasts for about 10 days (the life of the platelet). Dipyridamole, on the other hand, is a *reversible* platelet agent, a weak vasodilator, and a weak inhibitor of the enzyme phosphodiesterase, which degrades cyclic adenosine monophosphate (AMP) to 5′ AMP. With this block, more cyclic AMP is available to inhibit platelet aggregation. Sulfinpyrazone appears to *reversibly* block platelet prostaglandin synthesis and is another fairly weak anticoagulant. Low-molecular-weight dextran prevents platelet adhesion and aggregation by a mechanism that also is poorly understood. At clinical dosages, neither dipyridamole nor sulfinpyrazone prolongs the bleeding time.

Finally, fibrinolytic therapy has a small but definite place in the management of thrombosis of artificial devices. Streptokinase (SK) and urokinase (UK) act similarly and induce rapid thrombolysis by activating plasminogen and subsequently forming plasmin. Plasmin causes degradation of the fibrin, reducing thrombus size. Unfortunately, SK and UK also induce a generalized plasma proteolytic state as well as local fibrin degradation in the thrombus, and this can lead to uncontrolled hemorrhage. Newer agents (second-generation plasminogen activators) such as recombinant tissue plasminogen activator were developed to prevent induction of this generalized plasma proteolytic state by making these agents fibrin specific. However, this function appears to depend on the dose, and clinical use has not confirmed the decrease in potential for hemorrhage that was hoped for with these drugs.

In clinical practice, anticoagulant therapy for artificial devices placed in the bloodstream, particularly artificial valves, is based primarily on the orally administered vitamin K antagonist (warfarin sodium). Warfarin therapy is managed

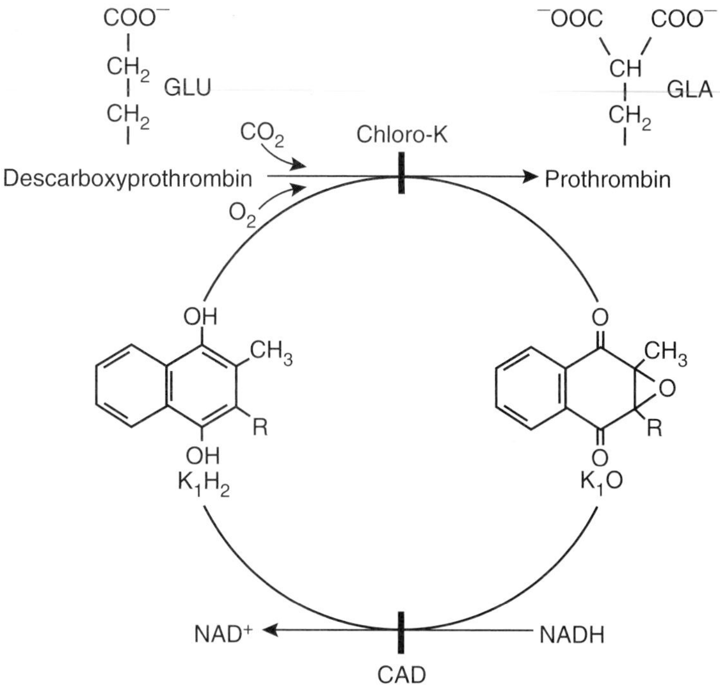

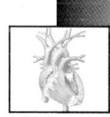

Figure 77–2 The vitamin K cycle in the formation of the vitamin K-dependent clotting factors. Vitamin K enters the body and is reduced to vitamin K_1H_2. K_1H_2 and carboxylase convert vitamin K-dependent clotting factor precursor proteins into active factors, while epoxidase converts vitamin K_1H_2 to vitamin K_1-epoxide (K_1O). Reduced vitamin K_1H_2 is regenerated by reduced nicotinamide-adenine dinucleotide (NAD) (NADH) and is the warfarin-sensitive step. CAD, coumarin-type anticoagulant drugs.
(From O'Reilly RA: Therapeutic modalities for thrombotic disorders: vitamin K antagonists. In Colman RW, Hirsh J, Marder VJ, et al, editors: Hematosis and Thrombosis: Basic Principles and Clinical Practice, 2nd ed. Philadelphia: Lippincott, 1987.)

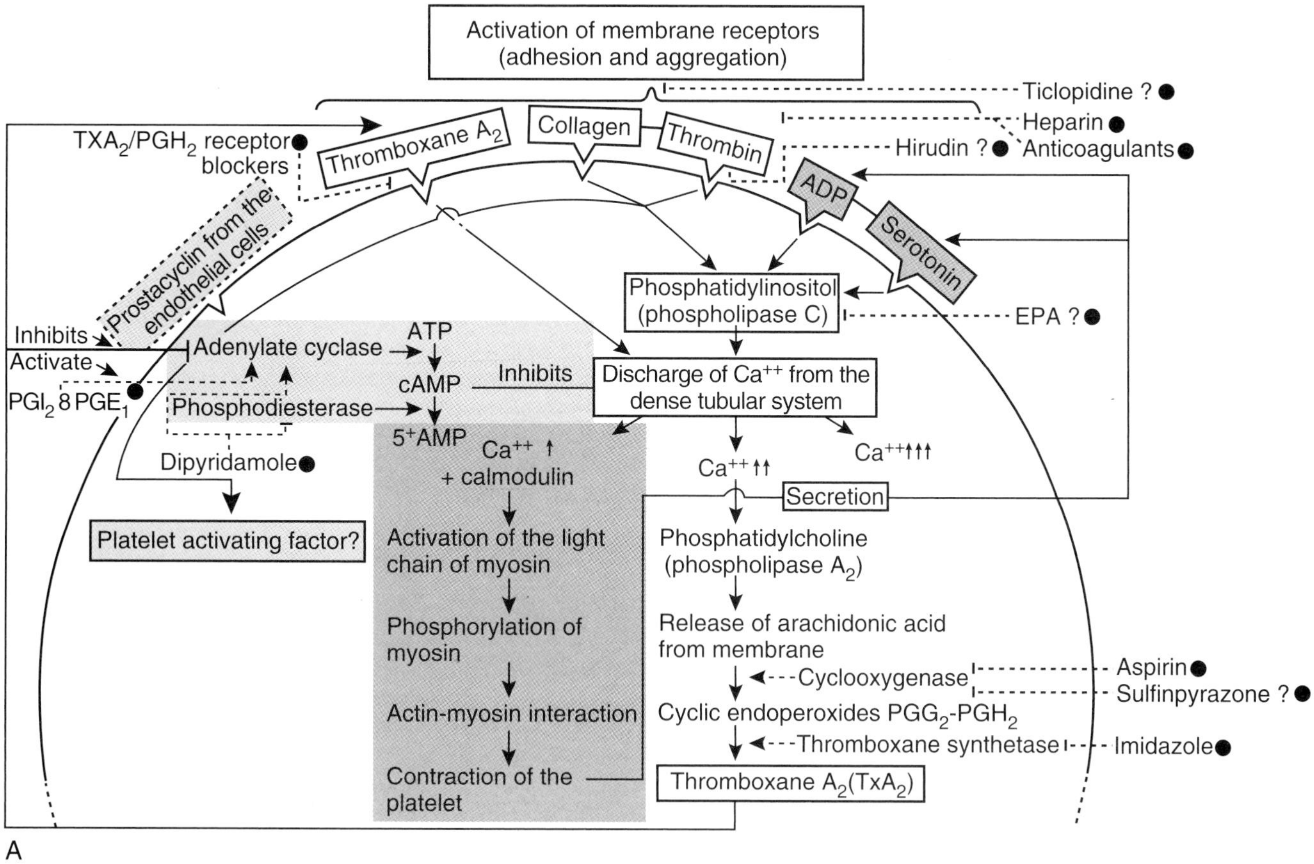

Figure 77–3 **A,** Presumed sites of action of various platelet inhibitors. Cyclic adenosine monophosphate (cAMP) inhibits calcium mobilization from the dense tubular system. Asterisks indicate a platelet inhibitor drug. Dashed lines indicate the presumed site of action of the drug.
(From Stein B, Fuster V, Israel DH, et al: Platelet inhibitor agents in cardiovascular disease: an update. J Am Coll Cardiol 14:813–836, 1989. Reprinted with permission from the American College of Cardiology.)

(Continued)

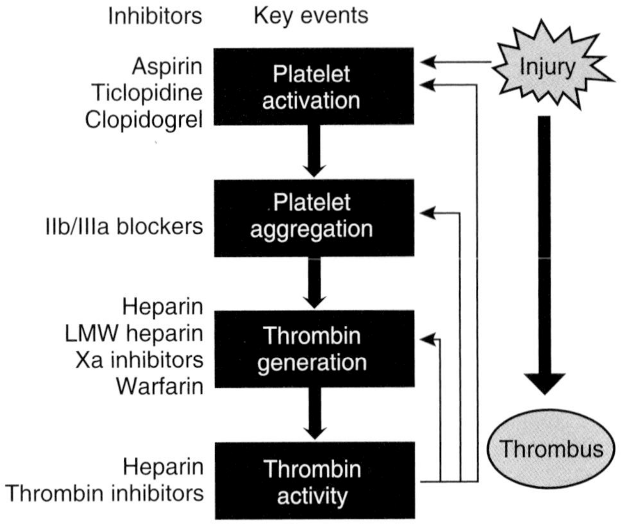

B

Figure 77–3 cont'd **B,** Key events in thrombosis formation and inhibitors that can prevent specific steps in the process. *(Reprinted with permission from the Institute for Continuing Healthcare Education. The Rationale for Extended Antithrombotic Therapy for Patients With Post-Acute Coronary Syndromes CME Monograph.)*

by following the International Normalized Ratio (INR) and maintaining it in a therapeutic range of 2–3.5 INR.[17,25] The INR is determined by comparing an individual clinical laboratory thromboplastin against an international reference thromboplastin. The reported International Standardized Index (ISI) is used along with the patient's ProTime (PT) and the control PT to calculate the INR. This removes the significant variability between individual laboratories. The better the anticoagulation control the better the outcome,[15] but many things affect the level, including foods high in vitamin K (such as broccoli), liver disease, gut absorption, and albumin binding. Therefore, 30–50% of all measured values in patients with prosthetic valves may be outside the therapeutic range,[17,51] and close follow-up of all patients is necessary. Recent studies demonstrate the best methods for anticoagulation management involve either anticoagulation services (i.e., an anticoagulation clinic) or a self-management program.[7] This is true for both adults and children.[86] Several studies with prosthetic valves[3,115] have shown the benefit of adding antiplatelet therapy to warfarin.

It is well recognized that with artificial devices, particularly prosthetic heart valves, platelet survival time is decreased significantly and correlates closely with increased platelet activation and deposition.[127] Addition of an antiplatelet drug (aspirin, dipyridamole, or sulfinpyrazone) normalizes platelet survival time, indicating a block in the thrombotic process.[127] Several studies document a decrease in the incidence of thromboembolism in patients receiving both orally administered vitamin K antagonist anticoagulation and aspirin. However, the risk of gastrointestinal bleeding was significantly higher with the concomitant use of aspirin.[17,21] Therefore, aspirin should be used with caution with warfarin because of possible excessive bleeding complications.[69]

Use of antiplatelet agents alone is strongly discouraged with mechanical valves, except possibly for a St. Jude valve placed in the aortic position in a child. Verrier and associates[120] reported that children with mechanical aortic valves in normal sinus rhythm can be treated safely with antiplatelet agents alone with little or no risk of thrombotic events, including valve thrombosis or valve failure. Rao and colleagues[99] found that aspirin plus dipyridamole was adequate for mechanical aortic valves in children, but warfarin was necessary with double valves or a valve in the mitral position. Robbins and associates[100] had similar findings. Sade et al initially indicated that the St. Jude valve could be placed in children without anticoagulation, but, after 7 years of follow-up, they reported an excessive thromboembolic rate when no anticoagulation was used.[104] Yet Sade et al were unable to answer the question of whether it was necessary to provide full anticoagulation with warfarin sodium or whether use of antiplatelet agents alone was adequate. Other studies have suggested that antiplatelet agents alone in adults and children provide adequate anticoagulation,[56,74] but most patients with mechanical valves should undergo anticoagulation with warfarin unless they are at high risk for bleeding.

For tissue bioprostheses, the decision of whether to use anticoagulation is more difficult. In the initial 3- to 6-month period following implantation, the risk of thrombus formation on the sewing ring is increased, so anticoagulation is usually recommended. Most centers use warfarin sodium, but aspirin alone has been used if the patients tend to bleed.[88,109] Warfarin sodium often is continued indefinitely if the patient is older, has atrial fibrillation, poor ventricular function, a history of emboli, or a valve placed in the mitral position. Results of a multicenter study suggest that left atrial dimension is not independently related to the development of systemic embolism in patients undergoing valve replacement.[14] Edmunds[25] believes that neither warfarin nor antiplatelet drugs are justified from the time of bioprosthetic valve replacement unless *more* than one of the mentioned risk factors for systemic embolization are present.

Full anticoagulation with heparin is used for cardiopulmonary bypass, intraaortic balloon assist devices, ECMO circuits, and mechanical assist devices. During bypass, activated clotting times (ACTs) are employed. The ACT should be maintained above 400 s because clot has been shown to form below this value.[129] If a mechanical assist device is to remain in a patient for a prolonged period, the patient may be switched to orally administered anticoagulation with warfarin sodium. A notable exception to this is the HeartMate VAD system. Antiplatelet therapy alone is used with this device.[33] The addition of antiplatelet therapy in this group of patients, particularly those on cardiopulmonary bypass or ECMO circuits, has had significant theoretical support, but *no* clear clinical advantage. Cardiopulmonary bypass requires that the blood come into extensive contact with the tubing, heat exchanger, reservoir, and oxygenator, either bubble or membrane. Platelets become activated, form aggregates, and release thromboxane A_2. However, membrane oxygenators are much less likely to cause severe damage to the blood than bubble oxygenators, and 20-μm millipore filters[123] are usually employed to remove the platelet aggregates that may form to prevent microemboli, particularly to the brain.

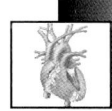

Initially, thrombosis is the major problem, but in time hemorrhage becomes the more significant complication as heparin is continued; platelet function is severely disturbed; thrombocytopenia occurs secondary to dilution, consumption, and sequestration of the platelets in the reticuloendothelial cell system; and fibrinolysis is initiated. For this reason, inhibition of platelet activation while the patient is on cardiopulmonary bypass has been tried with infusion of prostaglandin E_1 and prostacyclin PGE_2. These agents block platelet adhesion and aggregation by increasing platelet cyclic AMP. However, hypotension from vasodilation has been a significant problem, and several studies have shown no true benefit.[32,75] New studies using aprotinin with cardiopulmonary bypass are more promising. Aprotinin is a serine protease inhibitor that has been shown to be a powerful antithrombolytic agent and is being used with increasing frequency to reduce perioperative and postoperative blood loss during open-heart surgery. Aprotinin may also have some antiplatelet effect, which preserves platelet function during cardiopulmonary bypass and adds to the ability to clot postoperatively, thereby decreasing blood loss. Mohr and associates[84] suggested that aprotinin has a known antifibrinolytic effect and may protect postoperative platelet aggregation by inhibiting the high deleterious plasmin levels. This probably occurs through preservation of the glycoprotein Ib and glycoprotein IIb–IIIa receptors.

Though no study has shown significant improved patient outcome, a meta-analysis by Levi et al[68] of the use of aprotinin in adult cardiac surgery demonstrated decreased surgical blood loss, decreased blood transfusion requirement, and a nearly 2-fold decrease in operative mortality. Equally important, aprotinin may have an important role in blocking the inflammatory response secondary to the initiation of cardiopulmonary bypass.[66] However, aprotinin is quite expensive (up to $1000.00 per procedure) and concerns are still raised about increased risk of myocardial infarction, renal dysfunction, and graft occlusion.[4] No clear evidence exists that it is beneficial in pediatric cardiac surgery at the present time.[42]

Finally, fibrinolytic therapy has been used to declot valves to avoid high-risk emergency operations. All prosthetic valves, including bioprostheses, are subject to thrombosis.[9,67] Some authors recommend that patients who are stable and less critically ill undergo surgery to either declot or remove the valve and replace it with another valve.[76] In the case of a mechanical valve, this has usually meant replacement with a bioprosthesis. However, fibrinolytic therapy as the primary and sole method of treatment for both left- and right-sided thrombosed valves has gained considerable support.[103,110]

Complications of Anticoagulants

Warfarin Sodium

Bleeding is obviously the most common and most significant complication encountered with the use of warfarin, and therefore close monitoring of the prothrombin time is mandatory. Excessive amounts of warfarin that increase the prothrombin time beyond 2.5 times control and the INR >5 will increase bleeding complications four to eight times.[51] The gastrointestinal tract is the site of most bleeding complications and is often associated with preexisting disease states such as peptic ulcer, gastritis, genitourinary lesions, cancer, and hypertension. Another significant complication of *initial* warfarin therapy is skin necrosis. This is secondary to a temporary hypercoagulable state induced in the capillaries when the concentration of protein C (a natural vitamin K-dependent and warfarin sodium-sensitive anticoagulant that circulates in the blood) falls before warfarin's inhibition of factors II, IX, and X becomes effective and the desired hypocoagulable state occurs. The activated form of protein C is a powerful inactivator of Factors V and VIII. Why this is limited to the skin is unknown.[20] When used in pregnant women, warfarin can cause embryopathy in 4–8% of fetuses exposed in the first trimester, and exposure to warfarin in the second and third trimester causes central nervous system abnormalities in 3% of pregnancies. Finally, prematurity, fetal hemorrhage, and stillbirth are increased in babies exposed to warfarin.[58,72] For this reason, bioprostheses or allografts should always be placed, when possible, in women of childbearing age.

Heparin Sulfate System

Again, the most common complication of heparin therapy is bleeding. Hemorrhagic complications occur in 10–20% of patients with normal hemostasis and in up to 50% of patients with thrombocytopenia or uremia.[124] Thrombocytopenia has been reported in up to 31% of patients and can cause significant morbidity and mortality when associated with platelet clumping and thrombosis. Heparin-induced thrombocytopenia (HIT I) occurs in about 5% of patients receiving heparin, is usually mild, occurs about 1 week after heparin therapy, and is not antibody mediated. Heparin-induced thrombocytopenia II (HIT II) or heparin-induced thrombotic thrombocytopenia (HITT) is antibody mediated, occurs in fewer than 1% of patients with HIT, and can be lethal if heparin is not stopped. The IgG antibodies form a complex against platelet Factor IV–heparin, which binds to the platelet Fc receptor leading to platelet aggregation and release of prothrombotic microparticules. If further anticoagulation becomes necessary, such as cardiac reoperation, one may wait for the antibodies to become undetectable and reuse heparin.[98] However, this may take up to 40 days. Other alternatives include the use of nonheparin anticoagulants such as danaparoid sodium, lepirudin, and argatroban.[34] Platelet inhibition with GPIIb/IIIa antagonists followed by unfractionated heparins has also been used successfully.[65]

Interestingly, fractions of heparin that display this effect have the least anticoagulant activity, so the use of low-molecular-weight heparin with high anticoagulant effect and low ability to lead to platelet clumping has become clinically more important.

Antiplatelet Agents

Aspirin

Use of aspirin with orally administered anticoagulants should be avoided because of the reports of excessive bleeding. However, aspirin does not cause a generalized bleeding abnormality except in patients with an underlying hemostatic defect, such as hemophilia or uremia. In fact, aspirin may uncover a mild hemorrhagic disorder or vascular defect by inducing bleeding when used therapeutically.

BPIIb/IIIa Agents

With the increasing use of GPIIb/IIIa agents in the catheterization laboratory, cardiac surgeons are faced with the necessity to operate emergently on some of these patients. Though the clinical safety and efficiency of agents such as abciximab (Reopro; Eli Lily; Indianapolis, IN) have been shown through clinical trials of percutaneous transluminal coronary angioplasty (PTCA) and stent placement, there is little question that increased bleeding occurs when these patients require early (within 12 h) cardiac surgical intervention.[35] Large quantities of exogenous platelets will likely be necessary, but may not entirely reverse the severe coagulopathy.

PROSTHETIC HEART VALVES

Edmunds and co-workers,[26,27] and Cohn[19] have detailed the need for standardized reporting of thrombotic complications, including uniform definitions, stratification of the data to include the severity of the event including death, and careful complete long-term follow-up. Without this standardization, it is difficult to make accurate statements about results, complications, and appropriate anticoagulation therapy. Likewise, it is difficult to compare valves placed in the 1960s and 1970s and their associated complications with valves placed in the 1980s and 1990s and their complications.

Through the years, bioengineering advances have led to fewer thrombogenic materials, such as carbon pyrolite for the St. Jude valve, and a better mechanical valve design has decreased the incidence of valve thrombosis and thromboembolism through greater central flow characteristics. However, more effective anticoagulation has been the most important factor for the decreased incidence of thrombotic in the 1980s and 1990s as compared with the 1960s and 1970s, particularly with mechanical valves.[15] Bioprosthetic valves have less inherent thrombogenicity, but this is due to better central flow characteristics, flexible leaflets, and sinusoidal washout more than to true thromboresistance of the preserved tissue.[73] At present, two stinted porcine xenograft valves are used: the Hancock and the Carpentier–Edwards Glutaraldehyde Preserved Valves. Several pericardial valves also have been used. These include the Ionescu–Shiley Pericardial Valve and the Hancock Pericardial Valve, both of which have been withdrawn from use in the United States. The Carpentier–Edwards Pericardial Valve is the only remaining pericardial valve being implanted today in the United States, though three other valves are marketed internationally. The major problem with the former two pericardial xenograft valves was their durability. Both valves developed tearing of the cusps secondary to stress after only a few years of use. The pericardial valves used today are much better and tend to fail by calcification.[10]

Most prosthetic valves have a sewing ring that is covered with a Dacron or Teflon cloth. When this is exposed to the blood, an adherent layer of thrombus is laid down and serves as a blood-compatible coating. It is initially thin and delicate, but later comes invaded by well-vascularized fibrous tissue. This resists further formation of thrombus. However, if the flow pattern is abnormal, this tissue ingrowth can creep into the orifice from below the valve-sewing ring, forming an *obstructive pannus*. "Stentless" insertion of xenografts[6,22] including placement of porcine xenografts in the aortic root with either a cylinder of xenograft tissue or a thin Dacron support cylinder has shown excellent early hemodynamic results without any evidence of thromboembolic events in a large number of patients. These results are encouraging, but a much longer follow-up is needed. Finally, as mentioned earlier, allograft aortic valves and pulmonary valved conduits have almost normal platelet survival time and do not form thrombi.

All prosthetic valves, including bioprostheses, may develop thrombotic occlusion, but the incidence is higher for the mechanical valve, specifically the ball-caged valve, and the tilting disk valve. The thrombosis is usually more acute, presenting as "sudden" valve dysfunction with clinical shock, pulmonary edema, and loss of valve click sounds in mechanical valves and muffled sounds in bioprostheses. The diagnosis is made by fluoroscopy or two-dimensional echocardiography, or both. Mortality is high without either fibrinolytic therapy or reoperation. The incidence of this complication is less than 0.3 per 100 patient-years, except for the Omniscience Tilting Disk Valve placed in the mitral position, which has significantly higher incidence of thrombosis.[25]

The incidence of all thrombotic complications, including thromboembolic events for a mechanical aortic prosthesis, is about 1–2% per patient-year, whereas the rate for bioprosthetic valves in the aortic position is about half that of the mechanical prostheses.[25] The risk of bleeding complication is, however, significantly higher for the mechanical valves because of the use of anticoagulants, particularly warfarin sodium.

The incidence of thrombotic complications for a prosthetic mitral valve is similar in mechanical and bioprosthesis, except for the Omniscience valve. There is little difference between the two valve positions (aortic and mitral) and between the use of a mitral prosthesis alone or a combined aortic and mitral prosthesis. However, fatal thrombotic events occur two to four times more often in patients with mechanical valves.[25] Hammermeister and the Veterans Affairs Cooperative Study on Valvular Heart Disease[43] concluded that after 11 years, the rates of survival and freedom from all valve-related complications were similar for patients who received mechanical heart valves and for those who received bioprostheses. Structural failure, however, was observed only with the bioprosthetic valves, and bleeding complications were statistically more frequent among patients who received mechanical valves. Hammond and associates,[44] in another study of 1012 adult patients who underwent placement of either a mechanical valve or a bioprosthesis with a follow-up of 4814 patient-years, found little direct evidence to strongly support the generalized use of one type of valve over another.

Unfortunately, bioprostheses have a very high failure rate in children, probably because of accelerated calcium metabolism, and there is currently a renewed interest in the use of both fresh and commercially available frozen allograft valves for children and young adults to prevent anticoagulation. The risk of thrombotic or thromboembolic events using allograft aortic valves in the subcoronary position, as a free sewn graft or using the root replacement technique in which a cylinder including the valve is placed by the technique of Ross,[113] is nearly zero *without anticoagulation*. Matsuki and co-workers[78] reported on 555 consecutive hospital survivors who underwent isolated aortic valve replacement using a free-sewn allograft. The incidence of thromboembolism was 0.034% per patient-year, or 1 patient of the 555 studied. Results with the aortic root replacement in 108 patients reported by Okita and associates[92] showed no incidence of thromboembolism in 180 patient-years of follow-up. Penta and colleagues[97] likewise found no incidence of thrombosis or thromboemboli in 140 consecutive patients who underwent homograft replacement of the aortic valve and were followed for a minimum of 10 years. Many of these valves were either fresh or antibiotic-preserved valves. O'Brien and associates[91] reported on a comparison of aortic valve replacements with viable cryopreserved and fresh allograft valves. The freedom from thromboembolism for both groups was 97% at 10 years and 96% at 15 years; the reoperation rate for valve failure was much greater in the fresh valves. O'Brien initially believed that cryopreserved valves were superior because fibroblastic cell viability is preserved, providing durability. However, recent developments have pointed toward an immunological basis for valve deterioration with live cells. Decellularized homografts (Synergraft, CryoLife, Inc., Kennesaw, Georgia) may offer better long-term results,[90] but they are not approved and are temporarily unavailable.

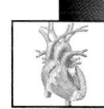

The fate of the aortic valve or pulmonary valve used as a conduit to reconstruct the right ventricular outflow tract is not so clear. Bull and associates[13] reported on 249 patients who received extracardiac conduits in the right side of the heart. Of the 173 patients who survived 30 days, 72 underwent placement of xenograft conduits of various types, and 4 underwent placement of valveless tubes. The complication and reoperation rates for both valved conduit groups were similar. Calcification of the allograft tube occurred commonly, but, interestingly, the obstruction tended to be at the proximal portion of the conduit where Dacron extensions, which are circumferential, were commonly placed. The development of the neointimal peel in this position led to the obstruction in over two thirds of patients.

If a *noncircumferential* proximal hood is used, thrombus and neointimal peel formation is minimal, and obstruction is markedly decreased. Livi and associates[70] have shown that the valve of choice for right ventricular outflow tract reconstruction is, in fact, the pulmonary allograft rather than the aortic allograft. Finally, Matsuki and associates[77] have used the pulmonary autograft valve (the patient's own pulmonary valve) to replace the aortic valve with excellent results (Ross procedure). However, this requires the reconstruction of the right ventricular outflow tract with a pulmonary or aortic allograft, essentially giving the patient disease of two valves rather than one-valve disease the patient had originally. Despite this, Matsuki and associates[77] have shown excellent results with this technique.

Finally, the Contegra bovine valves jugular vein seems to be a good alternative for pediatric right ventricular outflow tract reconstruction. Several general rules make some clinically applicable sense out of all of these sometimes conflicting data. For children, aortic valve replacement should be carried out either with a mechanical valve such as the St. Jude Bileaflet Valve, or with the pulmonary autograft technique to replace the aortic valve as described by Ross in 1967.[102] This has become the method of choice for aortic valve replacement in children. For mitral valve replacement in children, mechanical valves are required, and these patients should undergo full anticoagulation with warfarin. Xenograft bioprostheses should not be used because of the rapid calcification and degeneration that occurs with these valves in children. Similar guidelines should be followed for young adults. For women who are of childbearing age or wish to have children, mechanical valves should be strongly discouraged. The complications of anticoagulation, particularly with warfarin sodium and heparin, place the young woman and unborn child at too great a risk. For nonchildbearing women and for men under 60 years of age, individual differences in the patients and their desired lifestyle following valve replacement should be strongly considered in choosing the valve. Finally, probably for patients over the age of 60, but definitely for those over the age of 70, the use of xenograft bioprostheses (stinted or "stintless") or aortic allografts should be strongly considered in view of the decreased degeneration rate of these valves in older patients and the higher risk of anticoagulation in this patient population.

INTRAAORTIC BALLOON ASSIST DEVICES

Placement of the intraaortic balloon assist device (known as the IABP, the "intraaortic balloon pump") remains the first-line therapy for medically refractory angina or cardiac failure either preoperatively or postoperatively, and approximately 70,000 balloons are placed each year.[61] Initially, the intraaortic balloons were placed directly in the femoral artery with graft extensions, but more recently they have been placed by the femoral or subclavian percutaneous method or with a direct cutdown to the artery and use of the Seldinger technique through the arterial wall, with no graft. A few balloons were placed transthoracically (at the time of open-heart surgery) if a balloon could not be placed by one of the former techniques. The need for this has all but disappeared with the placement of a guidewire percutaneously, preoperatively in high-risk patients.

The risk of vascular complications, including bleeding, ischemia, thrombosis, and central and peripheral embolism, remains significant, anywhere from 2.5% to 30% in the high-risk patients, particularly females and diabetics. Most reports have found the risk to be greater when the balloon is placed percutaneously.[38,95] However, a recent report by Naunheim and co-workers[89] found no difference overall between the two techniques. Also the vascular complication rate has significantly decreased over the last two decades, probably because of the smaller (No. 9.5 French) diameter devices, use of a guidewire, and liberal use of direct visualization of the artery. It is difficult to be sure whether vascular complications are due to preexisting atherosclerotic vascular disease in these patients, vascular occlusion due to thrombosis, or, more likely, a combination of both. In the report of Naunheim and colleagues, 3.6% of patients required IABP removal, and 3.6% required thrombectomy. Four patients (0.7%) required amputation. Other groups have reported similar thromboembolic complications despite anticoagulation, primarily because of the severity of the atherosclerotic disease. Spinal paralysis, renal failure, and bowel infarction have all been reported. Management of limb ischemia, when it occurs, remains a difficult problem. If the IABP can be removed safely with the patient remaining stable, this should be the procedure of choice. Concomitant thrombectomy may be necessary. Evans[28] has suggested that simple withdrawal of the sheath from the femoral artery may sometimes be enough to reestablish distal flow, so the balloon does not have to be removed. If an IABP is required, it can be removed after a second is placed in the opposite leg. Other authors have suggested femoral–femoral bypass to relieve the ischemia in the leg receiving the balloon. More recently, placement of the balloon via the subclavian artery into the thoracic aorta has been suggested so that patients can be mobile while waiting for heart transplantation. Percutaneous removal should be accomplished with temporary manual occlusion of the distal femoral artery while the balloon is removed. The arterial puncture site is not occluded, and blood flow is allowed to flush out the arterial debris for a few seconds. This will often prevent distal emboli and obviate the need for arterial embolectomy.

Anticoagulation is necessary and is usually accomplished using full-dose heparin or low-molecular-weight dextran if bleeding is a major problem. Clinical reports have shown that endothelial damage occurs secondary to trauma from the balloon and that platelet counts drop to below 50% of the baseline over several days,[126] probably because of mechanical trauma, adhesion and aggregation, and sequestration. Hoover and associates[53] have demonstrated that despite this drop in platelets, prostacyclin levels are significantly elevated, and levels of thromboxane A_2 are decreased. The exact significance of this is unknown.

CARDIOPULMONARY BYPASS CIRCUITS

The harmful effects of cardiopulmonary bypass result from the large surface interface of blood with the artificial material in the circuitry, including the tubing, the oxygenator, the heat exchanger, the cardiotomy reservoir, and the blood suction system. Although technological advances such as the hollow-fiber membrane oxygenator have removed a few of these negative effects, major hemological complications continue to contribute to significant operative and postoperative morbidity and mortality. Respiratory distress, postoperative bleeding, paradoxic thrombosis, increased susceptibility to infection, and multiorgan failure have been linked to the thrombocytopenia, platelet dysfunction, leukopenia and leukocyte activation, complement activation, and other changes in plasma proteins, particularly during routine periods of hypothermia during cardiopulmonary bypass. All the components of the humoral amplification system are activated by the bypass circuitry, including the coagulation cascade, the fibrinolytic system, the kallikrein system, the complement system, and the leukocyte inflammatory system.[63]

In blood, only Factor XII (Hageman's factor) and platelets are directly activated by initial contact with foreign surfaces. On the other hand, prekallikrein, HMWK, and Factor XI—the three other primary proteins of the contact activation system—are rapidly activated after Factor XII is activated. This system initiates the inflammatory response, which includes the coagulation system, complement activation, fibrinolysis, kinin formation, and neutrophil activation. Blood component trauma occurs throughout the circuitry as the blood passes through the silicon rubber or polyurethane tubing and is exposed to high sheer stress, turbulence, and complex hydrolytic stresses while it is constantly deformed by the passage of the components through the roller pump, the heat exchanger, and the gas exchange device. Centrifugal pump devices such as the Medtronic Bio-Medicus are less traumatic to the blood, but still lead to hemostatic dysfunction.

Abnormal bleeding after cardiopulmonary bypass is a problem in about 2–5% of patients.[45] This is significantly increased for ECMO because of the greater time the circuitry is required, anywhere from several hours to several weeks in duration. Platelet numbers are reduced, platelet function is markedly impaired, platelet release products from platelet granules appear in the plasma, and excessive fibrinolysis may occur. Platelet numbers are decreased primarily because of hemodilution, but also because some activated platelets are damaged and are removed by the reticuloendothelial system. Other activated platelets adhere to the foreign surfaces through membrane receptor links with fibrinogen, platelet adhesive receptors (glycoprotein Ib), and aggregating receptors (glycoprotein complex IIb/IIIa).

The most important of these platelet factors is platelet dysfunction. Platelet dysfunction occurs very early during the first pass of blood through the cardiopulmonary bypass circuit.[117] The platelets are activated, and contractile platelet elements cause a sequence of typical morphological alterations called the "platelet shape change." Interestingly, the platelet morphology returns to normal although the stimulus of cardiopulmonary bypass continues. Most platelets return to the blood milieu, with only a few passing through adhesion to irreversible "secondary" aggregation with release of their specific granules. "Alpha granules" release platelet Factor IV, β-thromboglobulin, and fibrinogen, whereas "dense granules" release ADP, ATP, serotonin, and calcium. During bypass, these platelets become less responsive to soluble agonists with time, which indicates this increased platelet dysfunction.

Wenger and associates[128] have suggested that as bypass begins, platelets are activated by ADP released from hemolyzed red cells or release of human neutrophil elastase by activation of the contact pathway. The *fibrinogen receptors* (glycoprotein IIb/IIIa) of the activated platelets are exposed, and the platelets adhere to the surface of absorbed fibrinogen. Some pull away, have fewer glycoprotein IIb/IIIa receptors, and hence are not fully functional. Van Oeveren and co-workers[117] found no change in the platelet membrane glycoprotein-aggregating complex IIb/IIIa between a control group and a group given aprotinin. However, there was a significant decrease in the platelet membrane adhesive Ib glycoproteins in the control group, suggesting that this occurs routinely with bypass. Von Willebrand factor (vWF) is required in platelet adhesion, and the platelet glycoprotein Ib receptor is the primary target for vWF. This theory is supported by improvement in hemostasis after bypass with desmopressin acetate, which increases levels of vWF.[107]

Heparin is the primary anticoagulant that blocks formation of thrombin and fibrin deposition, but several other

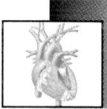

agents have been used during cardiopulmonary bypass along with heparin to decrease the deleterious effects of activation of blood components, particularly platelets. These include the antiplatelet agents dipyridamole and desmopressin acetate, prostanoids including prostaglandin E_1, prostacyclin, and iloprost, aprotinin, and ε-aminocaproic acid (EACA). Interestingly, heparin by itself can inhibit platelet function.[59]

Unfortunately, aspirin increases postcardiotomy bleeding in patients undergoing cardiopulmonary bypass when given preoperatively because of its irreversibility.[39] However, dipyridamole has been shown to preserve platelet counts by reducing platelet activation, aggregation, and depletion through inhibition of platelet phosphodiesterase activity and increasing cyclic AMP concentration. Clinically, this has reduced postoperative blood loss.[49] Results of studies with desmopressin acetate, as mentioned earlier, have shown shortened bleeding time and increased plasma levels of vWF.

The results with the use of prostanoids have been mixed. Addonizio and associates[2] demonstrated that prostacyclin preserved platelet function during *simulated* cardiopulmonary bypass and ECMO. However, hypotension was a problem. Fish and colleagues[32] studied prostacyclin in a randomized, double-blind study of patients undergoing coronary bypass operations. Prostacyclin preserved platelet numbers, decreased granule release, reduced the bleeding time, and reduced early blood loss. However, hypotension caused by vasodilation, a significant side effect, tempered the authors' enthusiasm for its routine use. Malpass and colleagues[75] and DiSesa and associates,[23] however, found no platelet-sparing effect of prostacyclin. More recent studies with cardiopulmonary bypass and ECMO circuits with iloprost, a prostacyclin analogue, have been more encouraging.[1]

Aprotinin is a serum protease inhibitor that is effective against trypsin, chymotrypsin, plasmin, and kallikreins. By blocking plasmin, it blocks a major activator of the fibrinolytic system. Its more important effect, however, may be in blocking kallikreins. Kallikreins act as plasminogen activators leading to plasmin formation and can be activated by Factor XIIa (activated by contact with the artificial tubing in the bypass circuit). They can in turn activate more Factor XII. Kallikrein also accelerates the "cold-dependent" activation of Factor VII, leading to activation of the extrinsic pathway during hypothermia used commonly with cardiopulmonary bypass. Finally, kallikrein activates the kinin and complement systems and activates leukocytes. Blocking the kallikrein system with aprotinin, therefore, may block all five systems, including the coagulation system, complement system, fibrinolysis system, kinin system, and inflammatory system.[125] The primary effect of aprotinin is probably to stabilize platelet function through a preserved adhesive capacity of platelets.[84,117] One explanation is that plasmin is generated during cardiopulmonary bypass and activates platelets. These activated platelets become nonreactive, and lower temperatures probably enhance this effect. Aprotinin blocks the plasmin and hence adhesion and aggregation of the platelets. A few believe that aprotinin's major effect is on the prevention of hyperfibrinolysis and not on platelets.[54] Concern about renal dysfunction and coronary graft thrombosis has been raised with aprotinin, but this may be unwarranted, because the incidence of reported renal dysfunction is quite low, and when it occurs it is usually mild.[12] However, care must be taken when aprotinin is used during cardiopulmonary bypass. For now it probably should be used only in high-risk groups, particularly those undergoing reoperation or those with endocarditis. It should be remembered that aprotinin prolongs the ACT independently of heparin and is a procoagulant. Therefore, ACTs need to be maintained around 750 s or greater to prevent clotting.[55]

It is also clear that excessive fibrinolysis can occur during cardiopulmonary bypass, but its occurrence is uncommon with adequate heparinization. Van der Lei and colleagues[118] have suggested the routine use of EACA, a clotting agent, following cardiopulmonary bypass. However, consumption coagulopathy (secondary disseminated intravascular coagulation) is more likely to occur than primary fibrinolysis, because platelets aggregate during cardiopulmonary bypass, and this may be accelerated by complement activation. Clinically important primary fibrinolysis for which EACA should be used is uncommon following cardiac surgery, and administration of EACA in a routine situation would only make platelet consumption worse. Therefore, its routine use cannot be recommended.

EXTRACORPOREAL MEMBRANE OXYGENATION SYSTEMS

Use of ECMO circuitry (more appropriately called extracorporeal life support [ECLS]) has had renewed interest over the last decade. Initial reports by Hill and co-workers[50] have led to its use in over 6000 patients since 1972. The survival rate is high for infants treated for respiratory failure (80–90%), particularly when meconium aspiration or blood aspiration is involved (90–100%). These results are less impressive for sepsis, persistent primary pulmonary hypertension, and respiratory distress syndrome. Initially, venoarterial access was employed, but more recently Gattinoni and associates[36] and Sinard and Bartlett[111] favored the use of venovenous access if cardiac function is normal. This eliminates the need for constant mechanical ventilation and prevents overventilation and distention of the alveoli by providing low continuous positive pressure inflation.

Following excellent results in neonates, ECLS has been employed in nearly 200 children for respiratory failure and in over 200 pediatric patients for cardiac failure (often secondary to cardiac surgery and the inability bypass). This experience has not been as rewarding, with only 44% of pediatric pulmonary patients successfully weaned off ECMO and 43% successfully weaned off ECMO for cardiac failure.[83] More adults are also being placed on ECLS for a variety of indications, including both pulmonary and cardiac failure. Early experience with such use has shown a similarly recovery rate of 40%.[5]

Complications with ECMO or ECLS are similar to those with cardiopulmonary bypass but are amplified because of the prolonged time required for support. Heparin is required to maintain the ACT at 180–200 s, though some centers have recommended ACTs as high as 250–300 s. Platelet counts often are markedly decreased, and significant bleeding complications occur in 10–75% of patients. Platelet counts should be maintained well above 50,000 with several centers recommending well above 100,000. If counts drop below 50,000–100,000, platelet transfusions should be given. Application of biological glue to the neck cannula sites has decreased the bleeding in neonates at the surgical site. However, intracranial bleeding remains a significant problem. Mediastinal hemorrhage in patients placed on ECLS for cardiac failure is likewise a significant problem.

Reports of the successful clinical use of nitric oxide (endothelial-derived relaxing factor) by Roberts and associates[101] and Kinsella and colleagues[62] have markedly decreased the need for ECMO in neonates. Nitric oxide directly stimulates cyclic AMP in vascular smooth muscle, causing relaxation. When given by inhalation, it selectively dilates the pulmonary vascular bed.

VENTRICULAR ASSIST DEVICES

Ventricular assist devices (VADs) include (1) systems that can be used for separate left-sided heart assist, right-sided heart assist, or both, and (2) the total artificial heart. These systems include pulsatile *external* pneumatic assist devices, such as the Pierce-Donachy VAD and the Abiomed BVS System 5000; *totally implantable* devices, such as the pneumatically or electrically driven HeartMate LVAD and the electrically driven Novacor LVAD; intravascular continuous flow pumps, such as the hemopump; and nonpulsatile centrifugal VADS, such as the Medtronic Bio-Medicus system. Early experience with these devices included a very high complication rate, particularly with bleeding, mediastinitis, and neurological deficit.[96] However, differences in implantation technique, inexperience with these devices, lack of uniform anticoagulation regimen, poor patient selection, delayed implantation, and lack of biventricular support were primarily responsible for the high complication rate. More recently, as experience has been gained, use of VADs, either total or partial, as a bridge to transplantation has yielded a much lower incidence of bleeding and thromboembolism.[122] These patients are all desperately ill and often have some degree of hypotension preimplant. It is thus quite difficult to know whether neurological complications are due to embolic phenomena or to prolonged hypotension. Walenga and co-workers[121] studied specific blood markers in patients who underwent placement of the Jarvick 7 total artifical heart and found significant hemostatic abnormalities, including a marked hypercoagulable state, platelet activation even though the platelet count was normal, and excessive fibrinolytic activation. Low levels of protein C and antithrombin III contributed to the hypercoagulable state. It appears that these devices, left in contact with the bloodstream for a long time, disturbed the delicate balance between clotting and lysis. Patients placed on mechanical assist or the total artificial heart should be anticoagulated initially with low-molecular-weight dextran, particularly if they have recently undergone cardiotomy. Then when bleeding is slowed, heparin should be started. Use of an antiplatelet agent, later switching those patients to warfarin sodium, appears to reduce the incidence of thromboembolism, but these patients must be followed closely for excessive bleeding.

Finally, the use of newer biomaterials for the blood sac may decrease thrombus formation even further. A new-segmented polyurethane elastomer coated with a 1% concentration of high-molecular-weight polymeric, surface-modifying additive is now being used in the Pierce-Donachy VAD. The surface activity of this additive causes it to migrate to the blood-contacting surface to reduce interfacial energy while still bound to the base polymer.[30] The HeartMate has used the design of a textured polyurethane lining rather than the smooth lining in the Pierce-Donachy device. The rationale for this has been to encourage formation of a thin, adherent pseudointima. Experience with this lining is encouraging with evidence of thromboembolism in only 34 patients out of 280 patients who had the vented electric ventricular assist system placed. Seventeen events (6%) were deemed device related.[33]

VALVED AND NONVALVED VASCULAR PROSTHESES IN THE THORACIC AORTA

Prosthetic vascular grafts used in the thorax are for the most part large-diameter conduits with high–low and low-resistant characteristics. Thrombosis and thromboembolism rarely occur, and 5- to 10-year patency rates of 80–90% are common.[18] Smaller conduits using Dacron or polytetrafluoroethylene (PTFE), particularly for coronary revascularization wherein the diameter is 4 mm or smaller, have a much poorer patency rate. Most reports indicate less than 67% patency at 1 year.[57,87] Coronary grafts using autologous saphenous vein have a significantly better patency rate than synthetic materials, but because of damage of the endothelium with preparation (high potassium flush, devascularization, rapid distention, arterial pulsatile flow), platelet deposition occurs, followed by thrombus formation. The reported 1-year patency rate is 80%, and the 10-year patency rate is 40%, considerably worse than the internal mammary artery graft, which has a 10-year patency rate of 85–90%. This appears to be due to much greater progression of atherosclerosis in the vein graft compared with the arterial graft, because the vein graft is not designed by nature to handle high-pressure flow as well as the artery.[71]

Large grafts made out of low-porosity woven or velour-knitted Dacron are often preclotted with albumin, platelets, plasma, or unheparinized blood. If a composite valved conduit is used, the mechanical valve is protected from the preclotting solution, and the graft is autoclaved at 270°F for 5 min. A knitted graft must be preclotted because the fabric weave is very porous. Woven grafts are much less porous, and preclotting is optional but still a good idea. PTFE grafts are not very low porous and do not require preclotting. However, both Dacron and PTFE similarly form an internal neointimal layer.

Following implantation of the prosthesis, a fibrin-platelet thrombus is rapidly deposited on the surface, indicated by a rapid decrease in platelet survival time.[46] Over the first year, the platelet survival normalizes[79] but the graft does not become endothelialized at the anastomotic sites,[108] where fibrous intimal hyperplasia may lead to late graft obstruction and thrombosis. Instead, the surface is covered with a compacted fibrin layer overlying a collagenous matrix (Figure 77-4). With Dacron grafts, fibroblasts are dispersed sporadically throughout this matrix, secondary to ingrowth through the interstices of the porous graft wall. The PTFE graft has a similar neointima except that fibroblasts are not present, because the interstices are much less porous. Roughened velour material has been implemented to promote fibroblastic infiltration through the more porous knitted Dacron interstices, enhance growth of the neointima, and decrease thrombogenicity. However, the roughness of the velour surface may, in fact, promote thrombosis because of increased platelet adhesion. Whether the internal velour lining is an advantage to help decrease thrombogenicity is still controversial.

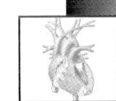

PTFE also has been used intrathoracically for construction of aortopulmonary shunts, right ventricular outflow tract nonvalved conduits, and patch repair and interposition graft replacement for coarctation repairs in children with complex coarctation of the thoracic aorta. Gazzaniga and colleagues[37] first described the use of PTFE for construction of aortopulmonary shunts, and since then multiple reports have shown excellent palliation with greater than 89% patency at 2 years.[24,93] However, complications such as thrombosis, infection, cardiac failure, shunt stenosis, and deformity of the pulmonary arteries occur with the use of PTFE grafts, particularly the grafts that are 4 mm in diameter. The use of 5-mm and 6-mm grafts is encouraged to decrease thrombosis.

Chronic anticoagulation has not been proved necessary and therefore is not used in large thoracic vascular grafts. Mechanical valve aortic conduits require the same anticoagulation regimen that isolated aortic valve replacement with a mechanical valve requires (usually warfarin alone). However, a review by Peigh and co-workers[94] reported a significantly higher incidence of neurological and ophthalmological phenomena after aortic valve conduit surgery. In that study, 27 patients undergoing valved conduit replacement were compared with 21 patients who underwent combined aortic valve replacement and ascending aortic graft replacement, but not as a combined valved conduit. Among the 20 surviving valved conduit patients, 50% experienced repetitive neurological and visual signs (felt to be embolic), whereas no patient who underwent aortic valve replacement plus ascending aortic graft experienced any events. These authors recommended the addition of antiplatelet therapy, which, in their population, seemed to help decrease the incidence with the addition of dipyridamole.

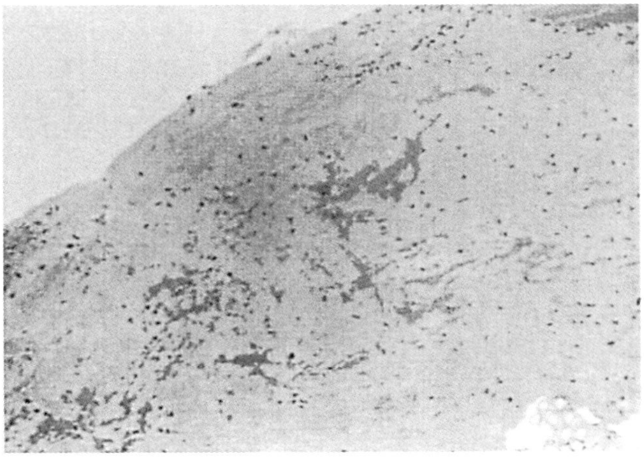

Figure 77–4 Photomicrograph of a thick, compacted, fibrin-lined surface of a Dacron double-velour prosthesis after 4 weeks of canine implantation. Note the absence of any endothelial cells.
(Courtesy of Michael B. Herring, M.D.)

PTFE should be used in aortocoronary procedures only when no autologous vein or intrinsic arterial graft is available. Antiplatelet therapy is advisable,[46] although Kohler and coworkers,[64] in a double-blind, prospective, randomized study of aspirin (325 mg) and dipyridamole (75 mg) three times a day, found no beneficial effect in lower-extremity PTFE grafts. PTFE is used extensively for aortopulmonary shunts without anticoagulation primarily because it is a temporary step. Long-term patency usually is not required, and therefore it is important to avoid the effects of overanticoagulation. Use of 325 mg of aspirin and 75 mg of dipyridamole three times a day has been shown to improve saphenous vein graft patency for aortocoronary conduits,[16] especially when it is started preoperatively, but it is probably most important in the first year following surgery.[80]

VASCULAR CATHETERS

Catheters placed for arterial or venous access, including Swan-Ganz catheters, arterial cannulas to monitor blood pressure, central venous lines often for chronic access, and umbilical artery and venous catheters in neonates, all have a high rate of thrombogenicity, approaching 90–100%. The major determinants to thrombus formation, however, are size of the vessel in relation to the cannula, flow characteristics of the blood, high flow versus low flow, duration of catheter placement, trauma to the vessel during implantation, and stiffness of the catheter. Microthrombus formation on the catheter may cause infection, which then causes thrombosis of the major vessel.

Radial artery cannulation produces partial or complete thrombosis in up to 25% of patients. However, hand ischemia is uncommon if the ulnar blood supply is adequate.[112] Umbilical artery lines in sick, unstable neonates may lead to aortic thrombosis, visceral ischemia, paraplegia, and lower-extremity ischemia in 1–2% of cases.[81] Local infection occurs in 20% of cases, and sepsis occurs about 4–5% of the time.[11]

Use of smooth-surface, pliable infusion catheters for chronic indwelling central venous lines, such as the Hickman-Broviac catheters and the Groshong catheters,[48] has decreased the incidence of major venous thrombosis and thromboembolism, but these condition still occur in 8% of patients in whom these techniques are used.[114] Major venous thrombosis may be tolerated well by children when isolated, but when both superior and inferior venae cavae are occluded or when the occlusion occurs in neonates or infants, major complications may occur, including pulmonary embolus, congestive heart failure, sepsis, and death.[85]

Use of percutaneous placement, careful sterile technique, routine care of the catheter by experience personnel, and removal of the cannulas and catheters as soon as possible help keep the thrombus rate low. For chronic indwelling catheters, proper placement in high-flow areas, sterile technique, and careful monitoring for infection are necessary.

Finally, the use of heparin bonding in catheters such as the Swan-Ganz catheter has decreased the incidence of venous thrombosis.[52] Reports of successful declotting of infected catheters with thrombolytic therapy may decrease the up to 20% incidence of catheter removal for continued infection and thrombus formation in these often very ill, very small children.[60] In these patients, vascular access is often required for a long period, immunocompromise is common, and repeated implantation of these catheters leads to a higher complication rate.

THROMBORESISTANT SURFACES

No artificial material today resembles living endothelium in its freedom from activation of the thrombotic process. Research in the past has centered on development of inert materials such as polyurethane and silicone rubber. However, such research may be misdirected, because the role of products of endothelial metabolism, including prostacyclin, the heparin–antithrombin III system, and the thromodulin system, in preventing platelet activation on endothelial surface is well known.[106] Inert materials alone, *in vivo*, may always require pharmacological manipulation.

Properties such as surface wettability and surface charge have been thought to be very important. Hydrophilic (wettable) surfaces appear to resist thrombosis better than hydrophobic (nonwettable) surfaces, and materials that combine polyurethane and silicone rubber, taking advantage of this chemical property, appear to be among the most thromboresistant materials made today. Attempts at designing a negatively charged surface that will resist the negatively charged platelets and plasma proteins have not as yet been clinically successful. On the other hand, covalent, heparin-bonded surfaces have been used clinically since Gott first introduced the idea in 1961,[40] but the exact mechanism by which the heparin confers thromboresistance to the artificial surface is not clear. One theory is that it is desorbed from the surface and provides a thin film of anticoagulated blood just above the surface. A second theory is that it stays bonded in the material and forms a complex with plasma antithrombin III, providing an anticoagulant effect. However, heparin-bonded surfaces still may not affect platelet deposition, and this whole mechanism of clotting may not be addressed. Despite this, the Gott shunt, which combines a graphite lining with heparin bonding, has been used clinically with great success for many years in repair of thoracic and thoracoabdominal aneurysms. Recent *experimental* work has shown heparin-bonded (Carmedia Bio-Active surface) cardiopulmonary bypass, ventricular assist, and ECMO circuitry to be thromboresistant. This material prevents activation of the complement system and preserves platelet count and function without systemic heparinization.[105] Recent *clinical* reports have demonstrated a 45% reduction in complement activation, decreased blood loss, and reduced transfusion requirements, with 25% lower heparin use and with the ACT maintained around 200 s.[8,41]

It is doubtful that any bioprosthetic material can be made to act like endothelium. Therefore, a major thrust of experimental development of vascular grafts has been to develop truly endothelialized grafts. One approach has been to use selective *biodegradable* vascular grafts using Dacron coated

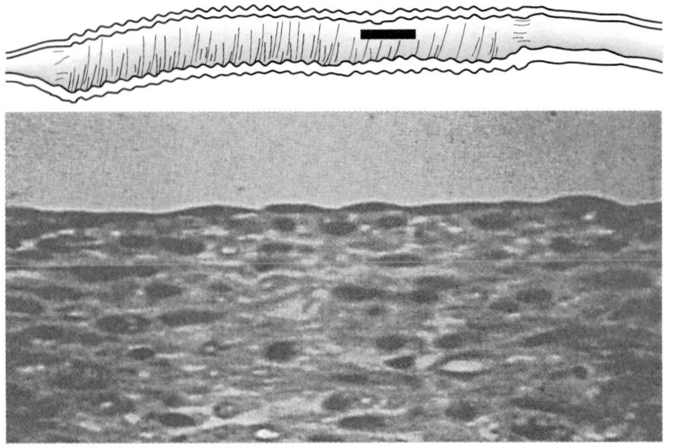

Figure 77–5 Photomicrograph of a seeded Dacron arterial prosthesis after 4 weeks following implantation in the abdominal aorta of a dog. Distinct lining cells are seen on the luminal surface. These cells have a high nuclear-to-cytoplasmic ratio consistent with endothelium. There is excellent sublining cellularity and organization. The top portion shows where the preparation was obtained from the graft.
(Courtesy of Michael B.Herring, M.D.)

with either polyethylene oxide polylactic acid[116] or completely biodegradable grafts of polyurethane and poly-L-lactic acid.[118] With this technique, a neointima is developed that contains true endothelial cells and smooth muscle cells that migrate from the anastomoses. As the biodegradable lattice disintegrates, fibroblasts migrate inward from the perigraft tissue anchoring the vascular neointima, essentially forming a neoartery.

A second approach has been direct endothelial cell seeding of freshly harvested or cultured cells onto a synthetic graft. Herring and associates[47] first described a single-state technique for seeding vascular grafts with autologous endothelium (Figure 77-5). However, many endothelial cells are necessary to seed the graft, and most patients who require these grafts have little or no saphenous vein. In clinical trials, results were inconclusive. Zilla and co-workers[130] and Fasol and colleagues[31] found no difference in overall results between seeded and nonseeded grafts.

An alternative to the single-stage seeding has been the two-stage approach using the cell culture technique. The advantage of this technique is that it provides a uniformly endothelialized graft immediately after implantation.[131] Results of early clinical trials appear favorable.[131] This technique also holds great promise for mechanical heart devices, particularly with polyurethane sacks and with bioprosthetic heart valves when the toxic aldehydes are neutralized by L-glutamic acid and a collagenous precoating is used.[29]

REFERENCES

1. Addonizio VP, Fisher CA, Jenkin BK, et al: Iloprost (2K36374), a stable analogue of prostacyclin, preserves platelets during simulated extracorporeal circulation. J Thorac Cardiovasc Surg 89:926, 1985.
2. Addonizio VP, Strauss JF III, Macarak EJ, et al: Preservation of platelet number and function with prostaglandin E, during

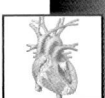

total cardiopulmonary bypass in Rhesus monkeys. Surgery 85: 619, 1978.

3. Altman R, Rouvier J, Gurfinkel E, et al: Comparison of high-dose with low-dose aspirin in patients with mechanical heart valve replacement treated with oral anticoagulant. Circulation 94:2113–2116, 1996.
4. Alvarez JM, Jackson LR, Chatwin C, Smolich JJ: Low-dose postoperative aprotinin reduces mediastinal drainage and blood product use in patients undergoing primary coronary artery bypass grafting who are taking aspirin. A prospective, double-blind, placebo-controlled study J Thorac Cardiovasc Surg 122:457–463, 2001.
5. Anderson HL III, Delius RE, Sinard JM, et al: Early experience with adult extracorporeal membrane oxygenation in the modem era. Ann Thorac Surg 53:553, 1992.
6. Angell WW, Pupello DF, Bessone LN, Hiro SP: University method for insertion of unstented aortic autografts, homografts, and xenografts. J Thorac Cardiovasc Surg 103: 642, 1992.
7. Ansell J, Hirsh J, Dalen J, et al: Managing oral anticoagulant therapy. Chest 119:225–385, 2001.
8. Aranki SF, Adams DH, Rizzo RJ, et al: Femoral veno-arterial extracorporeal life support with minimal or no heparin. Ann Thorac Surg 56:149, 1993.
9. Baciewicz PA, del Rio C, Concalves MA, et al: Catastrophic thrombosis of porcine aortic bioprostheses. Ann Thorac Surg 50:817, 1990.
10. Banbury MK, Cosgrove DM III, Lytle BW, et al: Long-term results of the Carpentier-Edwards pericardial aortic valve: a 12-year follow-up. Ann Thorac Surg 66:573–576, 1998.
11. Band JD, Maki DG: Infections caused by arterial catheters used for hemodynamic monitoring. Am J Med 67:735, 1979.
12. Blauhut B, Gross C, Necek S, et al: Effects of high-dose aprotinin on blood loss, platelet function, fibrinolysis, complement, and renal function after cardiopulmonary bypass. J Thorac Cardiovasc Surg 101:958, 1991.
13. Bull C, Horvath P, Merrill W, et al: Evaluation of long term results of homograft and heterograft valves in extracardiac conduits. J Thorac Cardiovasc Surg 94:12, 1987.
14. Burchfiel CM, Hammermeister KE, Krause-Steinrauf H, et al: Left atrial dimension and risk of systemic embolization in patients with a prosthetic heart valve. J Am Coll Cardiol 15:32, 1990.
15. Butchart EG, Payne N, Li HH, et al: Better anticoagulation control improves survival after valve replacement. J Thorac Cardiovasc Surg 123:715–723, 2002.
16. Chesebro JH, Fuster V, Elveback LR, et al: Effect of dipyridamole and aspirin on late vein-graft patency after coronary bypass operations. N Engl J Med 310:209, 1984.
17. Chesebro JH, Fuster V, Elveback LR, et al: Trial of combined warfarin plus dipyridamole or aspirin therapy in prosthetic heart valve replacement: danger of aspirin compared with dipyridamole. Am J Cardiol 51:1537, 1983.
18. Clagett GP: Artificial devices in clinical practice. In Coleman RW, Hirsh J, Marder VJ, Salzman EW, editors: Hemostasis and Thrombosis, 2nd ed. Philadelphia: Lippincott, 1987.
19. Cohn LH: Statistical treatment of valve surgery outcomes: an influence on the evaluation of devices as well as practice. J Am Coll Cardiol 15:574, 1990.
20. Crouse LH, Comp PC: The regulation of hemostasis: the protein C system. N Engl J Med 314:1298, 1986.
21. Dale J, Myhre E, Loew, D: Bleeding during acetylsalicylic acid and anticoagulant therapy in patients with reduced platelet reactivity after aortic valve replacement. Am Heart J 99:746, 1980.
22. David JE, Pollick C, Boss J: Aortic valve replacement with stentless porcine aortic bioprosthesis. J Thorac Cardiovasc Surg 99:113, 1990.
23. DiSesa VJ, Huval W, Lelcuk S, et al: Disadvantages of prostacyclin infusion during cardiopulmonary bypass. A double-blind study of 50 patients having coronary revascularization. Ann Thorac Surg 38:514, 1984.
24. Donahoo, JS, Gardner TJ, Zahka K, Kidd BSL: Systemic pulmonary shunts in neonates and infants using microporous expanded polytetrafluoroethylene: immediate and late results. Ann Thorac Surg 30:146, 1980.
25. Edmunds LH: Thrombotic and bleeding complications of prosthetic heart valves. Ann Thorac Surg 44:430, 1987.
26. Edmunds LH, Clark RE, Cohn LH, et al: Guidelines for reporting morbidity and mortality after cardiac valvular operations. J Thorac Cardiovasc Surg 112:708, 1996.
27. Edmunds LH, Clark RE, Cohn LH, et al: Guidelines for reporting morbidity and mortality after cardiac valvular operations. J Thorac Cardiovasc Surg 96:351, 1988.
28. Evans RW: Incidence and management of limb ischemia with percutaneous wire-guided intra-aortic ballon catheters. J Am Coll Cardiol 9:524, 1987.
29. Eybl E, Grimm M, Grabenwoger M, et al: Endothelial cell lining of bioprosthetic heart valve materials. J Thorac Cardiovasc Surg 104:763, 1992.
30. Farrar DJ, Litwak P, Lawson JH, et al: In vivo evaluations of new thrombo-resistant polyurethane for artificial heart blood pumps. J Thorac Cardiovasc Surg 95:191, 1988.
31. Fasol R, Zilla P, Deutsch M, et al: Human endothelial cell seeding: evaluation of its effectiveness by platelet parameters after one year. J Vasc Surg 9:432, 1989.
32. Fish KJ, Sarnguist FH, van Steennis C, et al: A prospective, randomized study of the effects of prostacyclin on platelets and blood loss during coronary bypass operations. J Thorac Cardiovasc Surg 91:436, 1986.
33. Frazier OH, Rose EA, Oz MC, et al: Multicenter clinical evaluation of the HeartMate vented electrical left ventricular assist system in patients awaiting heart transplantation. J Thorac Cardiovasc Surg 122:1186–1194, 2001.
34. Furukawa K, Ohteki H, Hirahara K, et al: The use of argatroban as an anticoagulant for cardiopulmonary bypass in cardiac operations. J Thorac Cardiovasc Surg 122:1255–1256, 2001.
35. Gammie JS, Zenati M, Kormos RL, et al: ABCIXIMAB and excessive bleeding in patients undergoing emergency cardiac operations. Ann Thorac Surg 65:465–469, 1998.
36. Gattinoni L, Pesenti A, Mascheroni D, et al: Low frequency positive pressure ventilation with extracorporeal CO_2 removal in severe acute respiratory failure: clinical results. JAMA 256:881, 1986.
37. Gazzaniga AB, Lamberti JJ, Siewers RD, et al: Arterial prosthesis of microporous expended polytetrafluoroethylene for construction of aorto-pulmonary shunts. J Thorac Cardiovasc Surg 72:357, 1976.
38. Goldberg MJ, Rubenfire M, Kantrowitz A, et al: Intra-aortic balloon pump insertion: a randomized study comparing percutaneous and surgical techniques. J Am Coll Cardiol 9:515, 1987.
39. Goldman S, Copeland J, Murtiz T, et al: Starting aspirin therapy after operation: effects on early graft patency. Circulation 84: 520, 1991.
40. Gott VL, Koepke DE, Daggett RL, et al: The coating of intravascular plastic prostheses with colloidal graphite. Surgery 50:382, 1961.
41. Gu YJ, van Oeveren W, Akkerman C, et al: Heparin coated circuits reduce the inflammatory response to cardiopulmonary bypass. Ann Thorac Surg 55:917, 1993.
42. Guay J, Rivard GE: Mediastinal bleeding after cardiopulmonary bypass in pediatric patients. Ann Thorac Surg 62:1955–1960, 1996.

43. Hammermeister KE, Sethi GK, Henderson WG, et al: A comparison of outcomes in men 11 years after heart-valve replacement with a mechanical valve or bioprosthesis. N Engl J Med 328:1289, 1993.
44. Hammond GL, Geha AS, Kopf GS, Hashim SW: Biological versus mechanical valves. J Thorac Cardiovasc Surg 93:182, 1987.
45. Harker LA, Malpass TN, Branson HE, et al: Mechanism of abnormal bleeding in patients undergoing cardiopulmonary bypass: acquired transient platelet dysfunction associated with selective granule release. Blood 56:824, 1980.
46. Harker LA, Slichter SJ, Sauvage LR: Platelet consumption by arterial prostheses: the effects of endothelialization and pharmacologic inhibition of platelet function. Ann Surg 186:594, 1977.
47. Herring M, Gardner A, Glover J: A single-staged technique for seeding vascular grafts with autogenous endothelium. Surgery 84:498, 1978.
48. Hickman RO, Buckner CD, Clift RA, et al: A modified right atrial catheter for access to the venous system in marrow transplant recipients. Surg Gynecol Obstet 148:871, 1979.
49. Hicks G, Jensen LA, Norsen LH, et al: Platelet inhibitors and hydroxyethyl starch: safe and cost-effective interventions in coronary artery surgery. Ann Thorac Surg 39:422, 1985.
50. Hill JD, O'Brien JG, Murray JJ, et al: Prolonged extracorporeal oxygenation for acute post-traumatic respiratory failure (shock lung syndrome). N Engl J Med 286:629, 1972.
51. Hirsh J, Dalen JE, Anderson DR, et al: Oral anticoagulants: mechanism of action, clinical effectiveness, and optimal therapeutic range. Sixth ACCP Consensus Conference on Antithombotic Therapy. Chest 119:85–215, 2001.
52. Hoar PF, Wilson RM, Mangano DT, et al: Heparin bonding reduces thrombogenicity of pulmonary artery catheters. N Engl J Med 305:993, 1981.
53. Hoover EL, Kharma B, Ross M, et al: The temporal relationship in arterial and venous prostacyclin and thromboxane activity during 24 hours of IABP in dogs. Ann Thorac Surg 46:661, 1988.
54. Huang H, Ding W, Su K, et al: Mechanism of the preserving effect of aprotinin on platelet function and its use in cardiac surgery. J Thorac Cardiovasc Surg 106:11, 1993.
55. Hunt BJ, Segal H, Yacoub M: Aprotinin and heparin monitoring during cardiopulmonary bypass. Circulation 86(Suppl. 11):410, 1992.
56. Ilbawi MN, Lockhart CG, Idriss FS, et al: Experience with the St. Jude Medical valve prosthesis in children: a word of caution regarding right sided placement. J Thorac Cardiovasc Surg 93:73, 1987.
57. Islam MN, Zikria EA, Sullivan ME, et al: Aortocoronary Gore-Tex graft: 18 month patency. Ann Thorac Surg 31:569, 1981.
58. Iturbe-Alessio I, Fonseca M, Mutchinik O, et al: Risks of anticoagulant therapy in pregnant women with artificial heart valves. N Engl J Med 315:1390, 1986.
59. John LCH, Rees GM, Kovacs IB: Inhibition of platelet function by heparin: an etiologic factor in post bypass hemorrhage. J Thorac Cardiovasc Surg 105:816, 1993.
60. Jones GR, Konsler GX, Dunaway RP, et al: Prospective analysis of urokinase in the treatment of catheter sepsis in pediatric hematology-oncology patients. J Pediatr Surg 28:350, 1993.
61. Kantrowitz A: Origins of intra-aortic balloon pumping. Ann Thorac Surg 50:672, 1990.
62. Kinsella JP, Neish SR, Shaffer E, Abman SH: Low dose inhalational nitric oxide in persistent pulmonary hypertension of the newborn. Lancet 340:819, 1992.
63. Kirklin JK, Wostaby S, Blackstone EH, et al: Complement and the damaging effects of cardiopulmonary bypass. J Thorac Cardiovasc Surg 86:845, 1983.
64. Kohler TR, Kaufman JL, Kacoyanis G, et al: Effect of aspirin and dipyridamole on the patency of lower extremity bypass grafts. Surgery 96:461, 1984.
65. Koster A, Meyer O, Fischer T, et al: One-year experience with the platelet glycoprotein IIb/IIIa antagonist tirofiban and heparin during cardiopulmonary bypass in patients with heparin-induced thrombocytopenia type II. J Thorac Cardiovasc Surg 122:1254–1255, 2001.
66. Laffey JG, Boylan JF, Cheng DCH: The systemic inflammatory response to cardiac surgery: implications for the anesthesiologist. Anesthesiology 97:215–252, 2002.
67. Lesnefsky E, Woelfel GF, Dauber IM, et al: Early thrombosis of a porcine aortic valve. Am J Cardiol 5:1120, 1986.
68. Levi M, Cromheecke ME, DeJorge E, et al: Pharmacological strategies to decrease excessive blood loss in cardiac surgery: a meta-analysis of clinically relevant endpoints. Lancet 354: 1940–1947, 1999.
69. Levine MN, Raskob G, Landefeld S, Kearon C: Hemorrhagic complications of anticoagulant treatment. Chest 119:108s–121s, 2001.
70. Livi U, Abdulla AK, Parker R, et al: Viability and morphology of aortic and pulmonary homografts. A comparative study. J Thorac Cardiovasc Surg 93:755, 1987.
71. Loop FD, Lytle BW, Cosgrove DM, et al: Influence of the internal mammary artery graft on 10-year survival and other cardiac events. N Engl J Med 314:1, 1986.
72. Lutz DJ. Noller KL, Spittell JA, et al: Pregnancy and its complications following cardiac valve prostheses. Am J Obstet Gynecol 131:460, 1978.
73. Magilligan DJ Jr, Oyama C, Klein S, et al: Platelet adherence to bioprosthetic cardiac valves. Am J Cardiol 53:945, 1984.
74. Makhlouf AEL, Friedli B, Oberhansli I, et al: Prosthetic heart valve replacement in children: results and follow-up of 273 patients. J Thorac Cardiovasc Surg 93:80, 1987.
75. Malpass TW, Amory DW, Harker LA, et al: The effect of prostacyclin infusion on platelet hemostatic function in patients under going cardiopulmonary bypass. J Thorac Cardiovasc Surg 87:550, 1984.
76. Martinell J, Jimenez A, Rabago G, et al: Mechanical cardiac valve thrombosis: is thrombectomy justified? Circulation 84(Suppl. 111):70, 1991.
77. Matsuki O, Okita Y, Almoida RS, et al: Two decades experience with aortic valve replacement with pulmonary autograft. J Thorac Cardiovasc Surg 95:705, 1988a.
78. Matsuki O, Robles A, Gibbs S, et al: Long-term performance of 555 aortic homografts in the aortic position. Ann Thorac Surg 46:187, 1988b.
79. McCollum CN, Kester RC, Rajah SM, et al: Arterial graft maturation: the duration of thrombotic activity in Dacron aorto-bifemoral grafts measured by platelet and fibrinogen kinetics. Br J Surg 68:61, 1981.
80. McEnany MT, Salzman EW, Mundth ED, et al: The effect of antithrombotic therapy on patency rates of saphenous vein coronary artery bypass grafts. J Thorac Cardiovasc Surg 83:81, 1982.
81. Mcfadden PM, Ochsner JL: Neonatal aortic thrombosis: complication of umbilical artery cannulation. J Cardiovasc Surg 24:1 1983.
82. Mehta P, Mehta J: Effects of aspirin in arterial thrombosis: why don't animals behave the way humans do? J Am Coll Cardiol 21:511, 1993.
83. Meliones JN, Custer JR, Snedecor S, et al: Extracorporeal life support for cardiac assist in pediatric patients. Review of ELSO registry data. Circulation 84(Suppl. 111):168, 1991.
84. Mohr R, Goor DA, Lusky A, Lavee J: Aprotinin prevents cardiopulmonary bypass-induced platelet dysfunction: a scanning electron microscope study. Circulation 86(Suppl. 11):405, 1992.

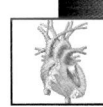

85. Mollitt DL, Golladay ES: Complications of TPN catheter-induced vena caval thrombosis in children less than one year of age. J Pediatr Surg 18:462, 1983.
86. Monagle P, Michelson AD, Bovill E, et al: Antithrombotic therapy in children. Chest 119:344–370, 2001.
87. Murtra M, Mostres CA, Igual A: Long-term patency of PTFE vascular grafts in coronary artery surgery. Ann Thorac Surg 39:86, 1985.
88. Myers ML, Lawrie GM, Crawford ES, et al: The St. Jude valve prostheses: Analysis of the clinical results in 815 implants and the need for systemic anticoagulation. J Am Coll Cardiol 13:57, 1989.
89. Naunheim KS, Swartz MT, Pennington DG, et al: Intra-aortic balloon pumping in patients requiring cardiac operations. Risk analysis and long term follow-up. J Thorac Cardiovasc Surg 104:1654, 1992.
90. O'Brien MF, Goldstein S, Walse S, et al: The Synergraft® valve: A new acellular (nonglutaraldehyde-fixed) tissue heart valve for autologous recellularization first experimental studies before clinical implantation. Sem Thorac Cardiovasc Surg II (Suppl. 1):194–200, 1999.
91. O'Brien MF, Stafford EG, Gardner MAH, et al: A comparison of aortic valve replacement with viable cryopreserves and fresh allograft valves with a note on chromosome studies. J Thorac Cardiovasc Surg 94:812, 1987.
92. Okita Y, Franciosi G, Matsuki O, et al: Early and late results of aortic root replacement with antibiotic sterilized aortic homograft. J Thorac Cardiovasc Surg 95:696, 1988.
93. Opie JC, Traverse L, Hayden RI, et al: Experience with polytetrafluoroethylene grafts in children with cyanotic congenital heart surgery. Ann Thorac Surg 41:164, 1986.
94. Peigh PS, DiSesa VJ, Cohn LH, Collins JJ Jr: Neurological and ophthalmological phenomena after aortic conduit surgery. Circulation 82(Suppl. IV):47, 1990.
95. Pennington DG, Swartz M, Codd JE, et al: Intra-aortic balloon pumping in cardiac surgical patients: a nine year experience. Ann Thorac Surg 36:125, 1983.
96. Pennington DG, Kanter KR, McBride LR, et al: Seven years' experience with the Pierce-Donachy ventricular assist device. J Thorac Cardiovasc Surg 96:901, 1988.
97. Penta A, Qureshi S, Radley-Smith R, Yacoub MH: Patient status 10 or more years after "fresh" homograft replacement of the aortic valve. Circulation 70(Suppl. 1):182, 1984.
98. Potzsch B, Klovekorn WP, Madlener K: Use of heparin-induced thrombocytopenia. N Engl J Med 343:515, 2000.
99. Rao PS, Solymar L, Mardini MK, et al: Anticoagulant therapy in children with prosthetic valves. Ann Thorac Surg 47:589, 1989.
100. Robbins RC, Bowman FO, Maim JR: Cardiac valve replacement in children: a twenty year series. Ann Thorac Surg 45:56, 1988.
101. Roberts JD Jr, Polaner DM, Todres ID, et al: Inhaled nitric oxide (NO): a selective pulmonary vasodilator for the treatment of persistent pulmonary hypertension of the newborn. Circulation 84:A-1279, 1991.
102. Ross DN: Replacement of aortic and mitral valves with a pulmonary autograft. Lancet 2:956, 1967.
103. Roudaut R, Labbe T, Lorient-Roudaut MF, et al: Mechanical cardiac valve thrombosis: is fibrinolysis justified? Circulation 86(Suppl. 11):8, 1992.
104. Sade RM, Crawford FA Jr, Fyfe DA, Stroud MR: Valve prostheses in children: a reassessment of anticoagulation. J Thorac Cardiovasc Surg 95:553, 1988.
105. Saito A, Hayashi J, Eguchi S: Mechanical circulatory assist using heparin coated tube and roller pump system. Ann Thorac Surg 53:659, 1992.
106. Salzman EW, Merrill EW: Interaction of blood, with artificial surfaces. In Coleman RW, Hirsh J, Marder VJ, Salzman EW, editors: Hemostasis and Thrombosis. Philadelphia: Lippincott, 1987.
107. Salzman EW, Weinstein MJ, Weintraub RM, et al: Treatment with desmopressin acetate to reduce blood loss after cardiac surgery: a double-blind randomized study. N Engl J Med 314:1402, 1986.
108. Sauvage LR, Berger K, Beilin LB, et al: Presence of endothelium in an axillary-femoral graft of knitted Dacron with an external velour surface. Ann Surg 182:749, 1975.
109. Schaffer MS, Clarke DR, Campbell DN, et al: The St. Jude Medical cardiac valve in infants and children: role of anticoagulant therapy. J Am Coll Cardiol 9:235, 1987.
110. Silber H, Khan SS, Matloff JM, et al: The St. Jude valve thrombolysis as the first line of therapy for cardiac valve thrombosis. Circulation 87:30, 1993.
111. Sinard JM, Bartlett RH: Extracorporeal life support in critical care medicine. J Crit Care 5:165, 1990.
112. Slogoff S, Keats AS, Arlund C: On the safety of radial artery cannulation. Anesthesiology 59:42, 1983.
113. Sommerville J, Ross D: Homograft replacement of the aortic root with reimplantation of coronary arteries. Br Heart J 47: 473, 1982.
114. Thomas JH, MacArthur RI, Pierce GE, et al: Hickman-Broviac catheters: indications and results. Am J Surg 140:791, 1980.
115. Turpie AG, Gent M, Laupacis A, et al: A comparison of aspirin with placebo in patients treated with warfarin after heart-valve replacement. N Engl J Med 329:524–549, 1993.
116. Uretzky G, Appelbaum Y, Younes H, et al: Long term evaluation of a new selectively biodegradable vascular graft coated with polyethylene oxide-polylactic acid for right ventricular conduit: an experimental study. J Thorac Cardiovasc Surg 100:769, 1990.
117. van Oeveren W, Harder MP, Roozendaal KJ, et al: Aprotinin protects platelets against the initial effect of cardiopulmonary bypass. J Thorac Cardiovasc Surg 99:788, 1990.
118. van der Lei B, Wildevuur CRH, Dijk F, et al: Sequential studies of arterial wall regeneration in microporous, compliant, biodegradable small caliber vascular grafts in rats. J Thorac Cardiovasc Surg 93:695, 1987.
119. Van der Salm TJ, Ansell JE, Okike ON, et al: The role of epsilon aminocaproic acid in reducing bleeding after cardiac operation: a double-blind randomized study. J Thorac Cardiovasc Surg 95:538, 1988.
120. Verrier ED, Tranbaugh RF, Soifer SJ, et al: Aspirin anticoagulation in children with mechanical aortic valves. J Thorac Cardiovasc Surg 92:1013, 1986.
121. Walenga JM, Hopponsteadt D, Fareed J, Pifarre R: Hemostatic abnormalities in total artificial heart patients as detected by specific blood markers. Ann Thorac Surg 53:844, 1992.
122. Wampler RK, Frazier OH, Lansing AM, et al: Treatment of cardiogenic shock with the hemopump left ventricular assist device. Ann Thorac Surg 52:506, 1991.
123. Ware JA, Scott MA, Horak JK, et al: Platelet aggregation during and after cardiopulmonary bypass: effect of two different cardiotomy filters. Ann Thorac Surg 34:204, 1982.
124. Ware JA, Lewis J, Salzman EW: Antithrombic therapy. In Rutherford RB, editor: Vascular Surgery. Philadelphia: Saunders, 1989.
125. Wachtfogel YT, Kucick U, Hack CE, et al: Aprotinin inhibits the contact, neutrophil, and platelet activation systems during simulated extracorporeal perfusion. J Thorac Cardiovasc Surg 106:1, 1993.
126. Weber KT, Janicki JS: Intra-aortic balloon counterpulsation: a collective review. Ann Thorac Surg 17:602, 1974.
127. Weily HS, Steele PP, Davies H, et al: Platelet survival in patients with substitute heart valves. N Engl J Med 290:534, 1974.

128. Wenger RK, Lukasiewicz H, Mikuta BS, et al: Loss of platelet fibrinogen receptors during clinical cardiopulmonary bypass. J Thorac Cardiovasc Surg 97:235, 1989.
129. Young JA, Kisker CT, Doty DB: Adequate anticoagulation during cardiopulmonary bypass determined by activated clotting time and the appearance of fibrin monomer. Ann Thorac Surg 26:231, 1978.
130. Zilla P, Fasol R, Deutsch M, et al: Endothelial cell seeding of polytetrafluoroethylene vascular grafts in humans: a preliminary report. J Vasc Surg 6:535, 1987.
131. Zilla P, von Oppell U, Deutsch M: The endothelium: a key to the future. J Cardiovasc Surg 8:32, 1993.

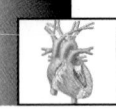

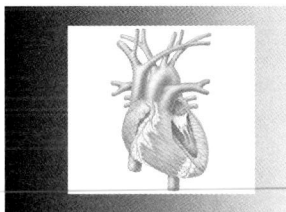

Robotic and Novel Visualization Systems

Alan P. Kypson, L. Wiley Nifong, and W. Randolph Chitwood, Jr.

CHAPTER 78

INTRODUCTION

Traditional cardiac surgery generally has been performed through a median sternotomy, which provides generous operative exposure and allows ample access to all cardiac structures and the great vessels. During the past decade, improvements in endoscopic technology and techniques have resulted in a substantial increase in the number of minimally invasive noncardiac surgical procedures performed. Nevertheless, because of the complex nature of cardiovascular procedures, most have required a median sternotomy and cardiopulmonary bypass. Only after closed-chest cardiopulmonary bypass and cardioplegic arrest methods were developed[38,44] did reductions in incision size become possible. Clearly, advances in cardiopulmonary perfusion, intracardiac visualization, instrumentation, and robotic telemanipulation have hastened a shift toward efficient and safe minimally invasive cardiac surgery. Today, cardiac surgery, particularly valve surgery done through small incisions, has become standard practice for many surgeons. Moreover, closed-chest coronary bypass surgery is in its early developmental phases.

Six degrees of freedom are required to allow free orientation in space. Thus, standard endoscopic instruments with only four degrees of freedom reduce dexterity significantly. When working through a fixed entry point, such as a trocar, the operator must reverse hand motions (fulcrum effect). At the same time instrument shaft shear, or drag, induces the need for higher manipulation forces, leading to hand muscle fatigue.[30] Also, human motor skills deteriorate with visual–motor incompatibility, which is associated commonly with endoscopic surgery. Computer-enhanced instrumentation systems have been developed to overcome these and other limitations. These systems provide both telemanipulation and micromanipulation of tissues in small spaces. The surgeon operates from a console, immersed in a three-dimensional view of the operative field, and through a computer interface, his or her motions are reproduced in scaled proportion through "microwrist" instruments that are mounted on robotic arms inserted through the chest wall. These instruments emulate human X–Y–Z axis wrist activity throughout seven full degrees of freedom.

ROBOTIC TELEMANIPULATION SYSTEMS

Clearly, telemanipulation systems have helped to overcome the limitations of conventional endoscopic instruments. These systems can be classified according to the tasks they help perform. The first group functions as an assisting tool that holds and positions instruments automatically during surgery. The Automated Endoscopic System for Optimal Positioning (AESOP 3000, Computer Motion, Inc., Santa Barbara, CA) is typically used to guide an endoscope, which is controlled using voice activation. The robot can be ordered either to hold a specific position or to reorient to a specific operative field, providing a clear and steady view without tremor. The second group consists of telemanipulators that were invented to facilitate fine manipulations done either under remote or hazardous conditions or both. An operator who works at some distance from a console controls these machines. Connected mechanically or electronically through a controller panel, the operator's motions direct the remote manipulator or end-effector. Tremor filtering and motion scaling enable dexterous manipulations to be done in confined spaces. For cardiac surgery there are two telemanipulation systems in current use, the da Vinci (Intuitive Surgical, Inc., Mountain View, CA) and the Zeus robotic system (Computer Motion, Inc., Santa Barbara, CA).

The da Vinci system is composed of three components: a surgeon console, an instrument cart, and a visioning platform (Figure 78-1). The operative console is removed physically

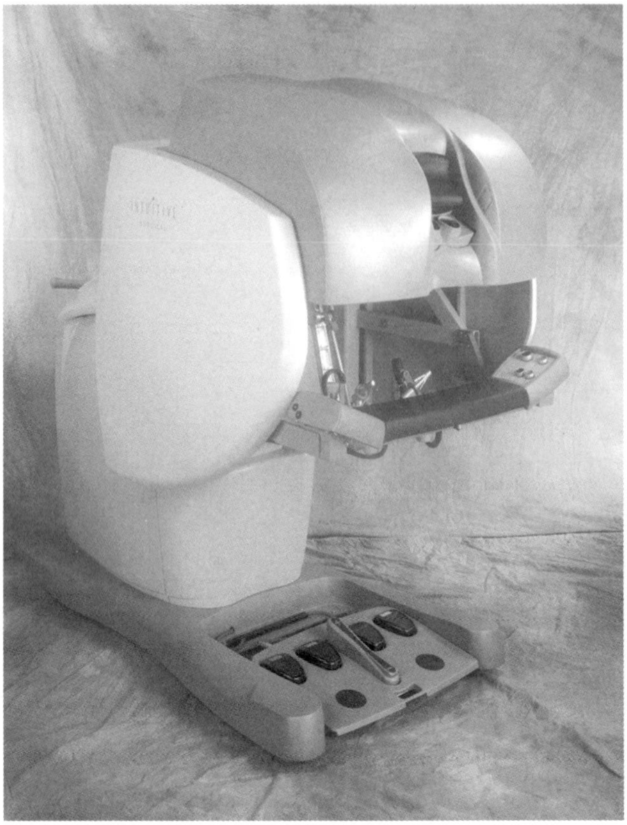

A

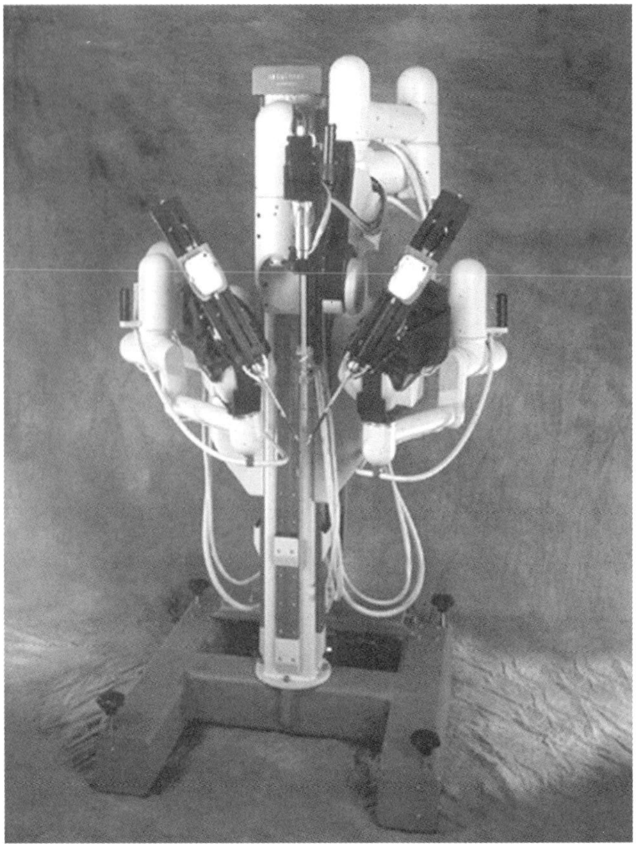

B

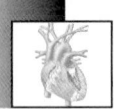

Figure 78–1 **da Vinci Robotic Telemanipulation System. A,** The operative console where the surgeon is seated. **B,** The instrument cart. It is placed on the left side of the tilted patient with arms entering the right thorax.

from the patient and allows the surgeon to sit comfortably, resting the arms ergonomically with the head positioned in a three-dimensional vision array. The surgeon's finger and wrist movements are registered digitally, through sensors, in computer memory banks, and then these actions are transferred efficiently to an instrument cart, which operates the synchronous end-effector instruments (Figure 78-2). Through 1-cm ports, instruments are positioned near cardiac operative sites in the thorax, and the camera is passed via a 4-cm working port used for suture and prosthesis passage (Figure 78-3). Every analog finger movement, along with inherent human tremor at 8–10 Hz/s, is converted to binary digital data, which are smoothed and filtered to increase microinstrument precision. Wrist-like instrument articulation emulates precisely the surgeon's actions at the tissue level, and dexterity becomes enhanced through combined tremor suppression and motion scaling. This allows both increased precision and dexterity with the surgeon becoming truly ambidextrous. A clutching mechanism enables readjustment of hand positions to maintain an optimal ergonomic attitude with respect to the visual field. This clutch acts very much like a computer mouse, which can be reoriented by lifting and repositioning it to reestablish unrestrained freedom of computer activation. The three-dimensional digital visioning system enables natural depth perception with high-power magnification (10×).

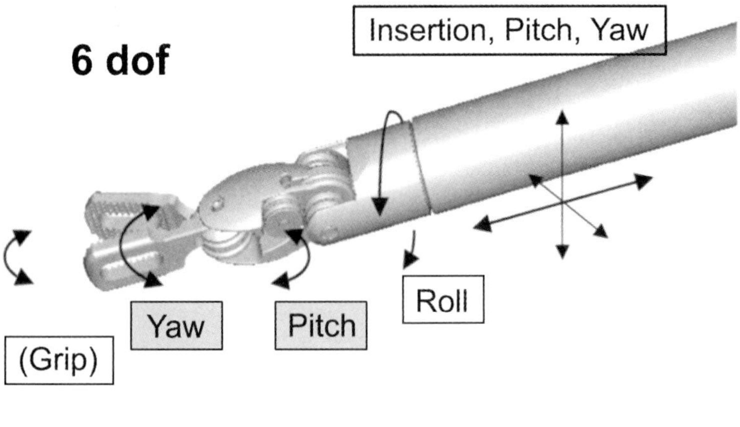

Figure 78–2 **da Vinci Robotic Telemanipulation System: The end-effector arms demonstrating all axis of motion.**

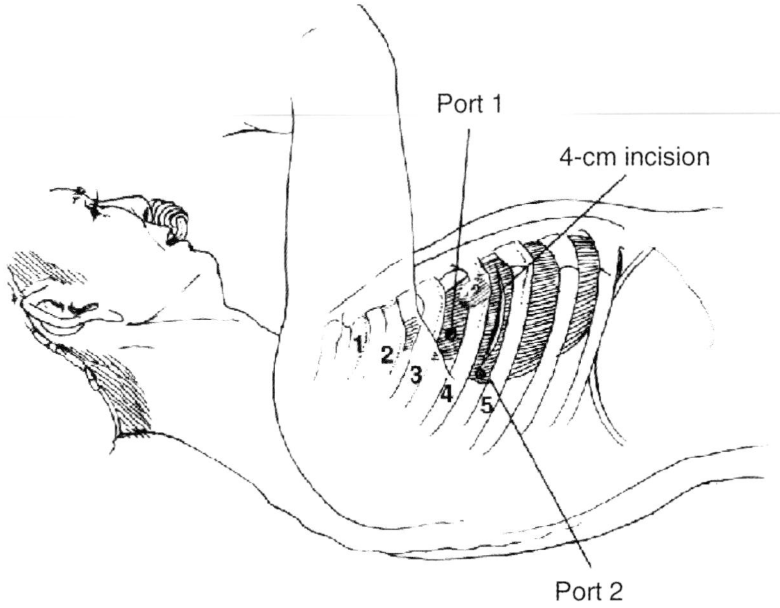

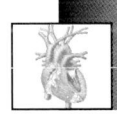

Figure 78–3 Schematic representation of a 4-cm working port site and two 1-cm port sites for the robotic arms.

Both 0- and 30-degree endoscopes can be manipulated electronically to look either "up" or "down" within the heart. Access to and visualization of the internal thoracic artery, coronary arteries, and mitral apparatus are excellent. The operator becomes ensconced in the three-dimensional operative topography and can perform extremely precise surgical manipulations, devoid of traditional distractions. Figure 78-4 shows the surgeon's operative field during a da Vinci mitral repair. Perfusion technology is the same as for video-assisted operations and a larger minithoracotomy.

The advantages of the da Vinci system include integrated three-dimensional visualization and a robotic wrist. This array provides articulated motion subtending seven degrees of movement freedom inside the chest cavity. The Zeus system is composed of three interactive arms, mounted directly on the operating table, compared with the da Vinci, which is positioned on the floor next to the patient. Although the Zeus system lacks a fully articulated wrist and allows only 4 degrees of freedom, the instrument diameter is only 3.9 mm compared with the 7-mm da Vinci arm. The basic Zeus visualization system is two dimensional; however, it can be used in combination with new and independently developed three-dimensional visualization systems.

Given the availability of these new telemanipulative systems, totally endoscopic robotic cardiac operations now have become possible. Minimally invasive robotic-assisted cardiac surgery has evolved through graded levels of difficulty with increasingly less exposure to a progressive reliance on video assistance. Distinct target levels have been set for surgeons in order to acquire maximal experience before progressing to smaller incisions, which require increasingly more video direction (Box 78-1). In this scheme, entry levels of technical complexity are mastered premonitory to advancing past small incision, direct-vision approaches (Level I), toward more complex video-assisted procedures (Levels II–III), and finally, to robotic valve operations (Level IV).

EVOLUTION OF ROBOTIC CARDIAC SURGERY

To perform the *ideal cardiac valve operation* (Box 78-2), surgeons will need to operate in restricted spaces through tiny incisions, which will require assisted vision and advanced instrumentation. Although this goal has not been widely achieved, minimally invasive cardiac surgery has continued to evolve toward video-assisted or video-directed operations. Both video-assisted and direct-vision limited access valve surgery is now within the reach of most cardiac surgeons. Moreover, robotic methods will now offer near endoscopic possibilities for the mitral valve surgeon.

Level I: Direct Vision and Miniincisions

Initially, minimally invasive cardiac valve surgery was based on modifications of previously used incisions and performed under direct vision. In 1996, ministernotomies, parasternal incisions, and minithoracotomies were used in the first truly minimally invasive aortic valve operations.[14,16,24] Surgeons also found that minimal access incisions provided adequate exposure of the mitral valve. Arom, Gundry, Cosgrove and co-workers[3,15,24,35] showed that mitral valve operations could be done with incisions other than a median sternotomy. Results with low surgical mortality (1–3%) and morbidity were comparable with those of conventional mitral surgery. In Cosgrove's first 50 minimally invasive aortic operations, operative times approximated conventional operations, and mortality was only 2%, with half of the patients being discharged by postoperative day 5.[16] Cohn et al, in 1997, presented their series of 41 minimally invasive aortic operations and demonstrated economic benefits.[14] Clearly, by employing familiar approaches and relying on direct vision, initial steps in minimally invasive mitral surgery became less daunting.

Since its introduction in 1996 at Stanford University,[38,44] Port-access (Cardiovations Inc., Ethicon, Somerville, NJ) technology has combined a minimal surgical approach

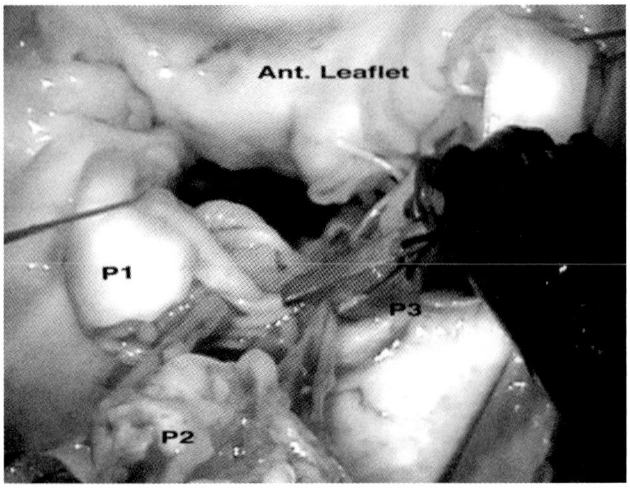

Figure 78–4 Typical da Vinci mitral valve repair. The P_2 segment of the posterior leaflet is being resected by robotic microscissors. The annulus is reduced, and both P_1 and P_3 are approximated.

Box 78–1. Minimally Invasive Cardiac Surgery.

Level I: Direct vision Mini (10–12 cm) incisions
Level II: Video-assisted Micro (4–6 cm) incisions
Level III: Video-directed and robot-assisted Micro or Port incisions (1 cm)
Level IV: Robotic telemanipulation Port incisions (1 cm)

Box 78–2. Ideal Cardiac Valve Operation.

Tiny incisions—endoscopic Ports
Central antegrade perfusion
Tactile feedback
Eye–brain-"like" visualization
Facile, secure valve attachment
Intracardiac access
Dexterous topographic access
  Valve and subvalvular
No instrument conflicts
Minimal
  Cardiopulmonary perfusion
  Blood product usage
  Ventilation and ICU care
  Hospitalization
Same or better quality
  Valve repairs in 60–80%
  Few reoperations (1–2%)
  Low mortality (1–2%)
Computerized surgical pathway memory
Instrument navigation systems

(avoidance of median sternotomy) with total cardiopulmonary bypass and an arrested heart providing for a still and bloodless field. The system provides extrathoracic cardiopulmonary bypass with a specialized set of endovascular cannulas and catheters that allow for antegrade or retrograde cardioplegic arrest, as well as ventricular decompression. Falk et al, at the University of Leipzig, reported on 24 mitral valve repairs performed through a miniincision with Port-access techniques.[18] By 1997, the New York University group had performed 27 Port-access mitral repairs/replacements with one death. There were no aortic dissections, and no repairs had residual regurgitation requiring reoperation.[43] Cosgrove et al reported 115 minimally invasive mitral valve operations using either a ministernotomy or parasternal incision with one death resulting from a stroke. Comparison with median sternotomy demonstrated reductions in both postoperative length of stay and direct hospital costs.[15] These encouraging results confirmed the feasibility and safety of these techniques and further advanced the next level of "minimal invasiveness."

Level II: Video-Assisted and Microincisions

Advances in videooptics initiated a wave of new endoscopic approaches in general, orthopedic, urological, and gynecological procedures. Cardiac surgery has lagged behind these specialties in utilizing the benefits of video assistance because fine coronary anastomoses and complex valve reconstructions are the centerpiece of contemporary adult cardiac surgery. Microincisions are considered as 4- to 6-cm skin incisions, and video assistance indicates that 50% or less of the operation is performed while viewing the operative field from a screen.

Video assistance was used first for closed chest internal mammary artery harvests and congenital heart operations.[1,5,34] Although Kaneko et al[25] first described the use of video assistance for mitral valve surgery done through a sternotomy, it was Carpentier et al who, in February 1996, performed the first video-assisted mitral valve repair via a minithoracotomy using ventricular fibrillation.[6] Three months later, our group at East Carolina University performed a mitral valve replacement using a microincision, videoscopic vision, percutaneous transthoracic aortic clamp, and retrograde cardioplegia.[8,9] In 1998, Mohr et al reported the Leipzig experience of 51 minimally invasive mitral operations using Port-access technology, a 4-cm incision, and three-dimensional videoscopy. Video technology was helpful for replacement and simple repair operations; however, complex reconstructions were still approached under direct vision.[29] Concurrently, our group reported 31 patients using video assistance with a two-dimensional 5-mm camera. Complex repairs were possible and included quadrangular resections, sliding valvuloplasties, and chordal replacements with no major complications and mortality less than 1%.[10]

Level III: Video-Directed and Port Incisions

In 1997, Mohr first used the AESOP voice-activated camera robot in minimally invasive videoscopic mitral valve surgery.[17] With the assistance of a voice-activated robot-driven camera, cardiac surgery entered the robotic age. With this device, a voice-controlled robotic arm allows hands-free camera manipulation. The surgeon commands camera movements verbally, providing a direct eye–brain action. This technology has enabled use of even smaller

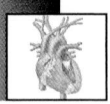

incisions with better valve and subvalvular visualization. Microincisions or Port incisions (1–2 cm) can be used at this level and video direction implies that most of the operation is done via secondary or assisted vision. Both Reichenspurner et al and Mohr et al have used three-dimensional systems successfully controlling image position with an AESOP robotic arm.[17,39] They noted that camera motion is smoother, more predictable, and requires less lens cleaning than during manual direction. In June 1998, our group performed the first video-directed mitral operation in the United States using the voice-controlled AESOP 3000 robotic arm and a Vista (Vista Cardiothoracic Systems, Inc., Westborough, MA) three-dimensional camera.[8,9] Visual accuracy was improved by voice manipulation of the camera by the operating surgeon. We now use the robotic arm, endoscope, and a conventional two-dimensional monitor routinely and have done over 250 videoscopic mitral operations successfully using this method. Image stability during complex surgical maneuvers remains crucial. Recently, we reported the use of this approach and compared the results to a cohort who underwent conventional sternotomy. Reduced bleeding, ventilator times, and hospital stays were shown for the minimally invasive cohort.[19] The addition of three-dimensional visualization, robotic camera control, and instrument tip articulation was the next essential step toward a totally endoscopic mitral operation where wrist-like instruments and three-dimensional vision could transpose surgical manipulations from outside the chest wall to deep within cardiac chambers.

Level IV: Video-Directed and Robotic Instruments

Innovations in computer-assisted, robotic mitral surgery have rapidly increased. In May 1998, Carpentier et al in Paris performed the first mitral valve repair using an early prototype of the da Vinci articulated intracardiac "wrist" robotic device.[7] The "microwrist" permits intraatrial instrument articulation with the seven full degrees of freedom offered by the human wrist. The operator becomes transported to the valvular topography affecting "telepresence" at all levels of vision, dexterity, access, and proprioception. Grossi et al of New York University partially repaired a mitral valve using the Zeus system.[23] In May 2000,[12] using the da Vinci system, our group performed the first complete repair of a mitral valve in North America. Using the articulated wrist instruments, a trapezoidal resection of a large P_2 was performed with the defect closed using multiple interrupted sutures, followed by implantation of a #28 Cosgrove annuloplasty band. Subsequently, we have performed 50 other mitral repairs as part of Food and Drug Administration (FDA)-approved trials. To date, more than 200 mitral operations have been done between Europe and North America using the da Vinci system. We have found that with da Vinci, complex mitral repairs can be done with reasonable cross-clamp and perfusion times as well as excellent midterm results. Repairs done to date have included annuloplasty band insertions, chordal replacements, sliding valvuloplasties, chordal transfers, and leaflet resections. Although a 4-cm incision is still used for assistant access, the advancements in three-dimensional video and robotic instrumentation have progressed to a point at which totally endoscopic mitral procedures are feasible. In fact, Lange and associates in Munich were the first to perform a totally endoscopic mitral valve repair using only the 1-cm ports with da Vinci.[27] Future refinements in these devices are needed to apply this new technology more widely.

CLINICAL APPLICATIONS/PATIENT SELECTION

Early in the development of any robotic mitral valve repair program, strict inclusion and exclusion criteria should be followed (Box 78-3). In our initial experience, all patients had isolated mitral insufficiency without either valvular or coronary artery disease that may have required operative intervention. Patients with a previous right thoracotomy were excluded from the da Vinci procedures; however, we now approach these patients with a video-assisted mitral valve operation. As mentioned in Box 78-3, patients with severely calcified mitral annulus are not candidates. Decalcification requires further instrument development as well as a reliable means to evacuate any calcium that may fall into the left ventricle. Patients with mitral valve stenosis were excluded in the early FDA trials; however, patients treatable by commissurotomy would be suitable candidates for robotic repair. The improved visualization of the valve and subvalvular apparatus along with the maneuverability of bladed microinstruments would facilitate performance of a commissurotomy. Recently our group performed a mitral valve replacement for the first time in a clinical setting.[37]

SURGICAL TECHNIQUES

Preoperative and postoperative surface and transesophageal echocardiographic (TEE) studies should be done in every patient. Patients are anesthetized and positioned (Figure 78-5), with the right chest elevated 30–40 degrees and with the right arm suspended, padded, and positioned over the patients' forehead.[8] Single left-lung ventilation is used for complete intrathoracic exposure.

Cardiopulmonary bypass is established at 26° C using femoral arterial inflow and kinetic venous drainage through a femoral (21–23 Fr) and right internal jugular vein (17 Fr) cannula in every case. If the femoral artery is too small

Box 78–3. Robotic Mitral Surgery Exclusion Criteria.

- Previous right thoracotomy
- Renal failure
- Liver dysfunction
- Bleeding disorders
- Pulmonary hypertension (PAS >60 torr)
- Significant aortic or tricuspid valve disease
- Coronary artery disease requiring surgery
- Recent myocardial ischemia (<30 days)
- Recent stroke (<30 days)
- Severely calcified mitral valve annulus
- A body mass index (BMI) >35 kg/m^2

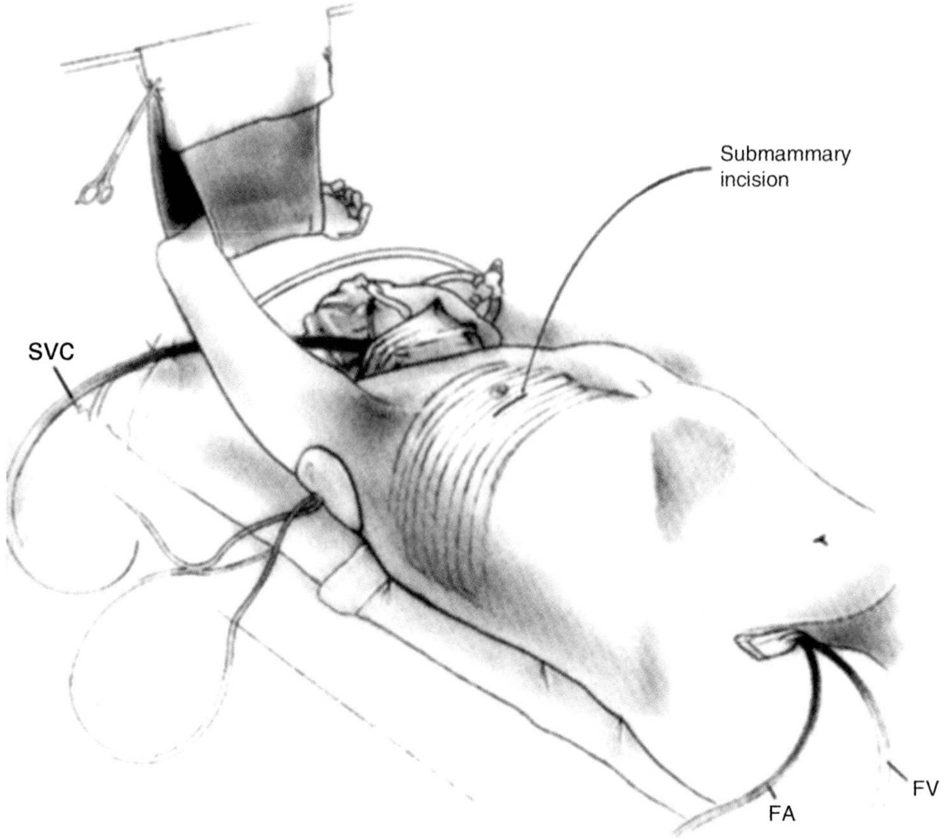

Figure 78–5 Appropriate patient position for robotic mitral surgery. Note that the right chest is elevated approximately 30–40 degrees with the right arm suspended. The 4-cm working site is shown, as are the arterial and venous cannulas. SVC, superior vena cava; FA, femoral artery; FV, femoral vein.

or atherosclerotic, either a Bio-Medicus (Medtronic, Minneapolis, MN) or Directflow (Cardiovations, Inc., Somerville, NJ) cannula can be placed through a second interspace port for antegrade aortic perfusion. A 4- to 5-cm inframammary incision is used and a subpectoral fourth intercostal space (ICS) minithoracotomy is developed to provide cardiac access. The pericardium is opened under direct vision 2 cm anterior to the phrenic nerve. Antegrade cardioplegia is given by an aortic needle/vent placed either under direct vision or videoscopically. To minimize intracardiac air entrainment, the thoracic cavity is flooded continuously with carbon dioxide at 1–2 liters/min via a 14-gauge plastic catheter. A transthoracic aortic cross-clamp (Scanlan International, Inc., Minneapolis, MN) is positioned in the midaxillary line via a 4-mm incision in the third ICS and intermittent antegrade cold blood cardioplegia maintains cardiac arrest and myocardial protection. Under video-assisted guidance, the posterior tine of the clamp is passed through the transverse sinus with care taken not to injure the right pulmonary artery, left atrial appendage, left main coronary, or aorta. After cardioplegic arrest, a transthoracic retractor is introduced and used to expose the mitral valve through a 3- to 4-cm left atriotomy made medially to the right superior pulmonary vein entrance (Figure 78-6). After valve inspection, positions for da Vinci left and right arm port incisions are determined. The right trocar is placed in the fourth ICS posterior-lateral to the incision and parallel to the right superior pulmonary vein. Occasionally, the fifth ICS provides a better angle for the right robotic arm. The left trocar generally is placed 6 cm cephalad and medial to the right trocar, ensuring internal clearance between arms to avoid both external and internal conflicts. Optimal robotic arm convergence avoids left atrial wall tearing during instrument manipulations. A "high-magnification" camera is used with a 30° (looking up), three-dimensional endoscope placed through the medial portion of the minithoracotomy. The remainder of the incision is used as a working port for the assistant.

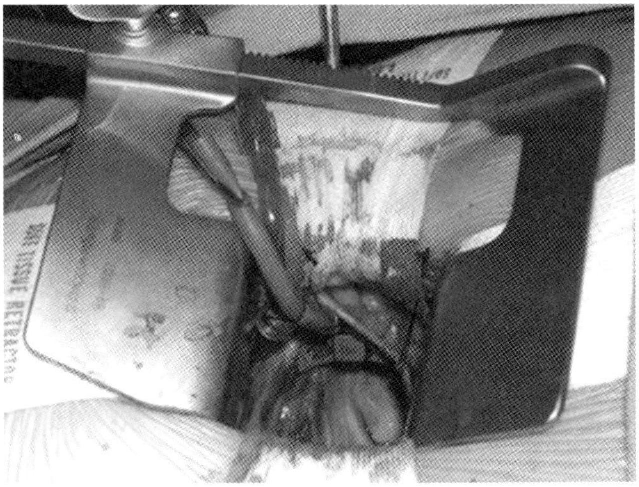

Figure 78–6 Operative view through the working port. Note the excellent view of the mitral valve apparatus with the left atrial retractor in place seen exiting through the chest wall.

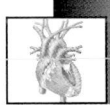

Needles are retrieved using a long magnetic device and suture remnants are removed from the surgical field using vacuum assistance.

Operative procedures are performed from the surgeon's console placed approximately 10 feet from the operating table but in the same operating room (Figure 78-7). The patient-side assistant changes instruments as well as supplies and retrieves operative materials. Most often an annuloplasty band (Edwards Lifesciences, LLC, Irvine, CA) has been used to support repairs or provide annular reduction. In video-assisted robotic cases, early placement of annuloplasty sutures facilitates exposure during complex repairs. Exposure of each new suture often becomes predicated on retraction of the previous one. Leaflet resections, papillary muscle reconstruction, and chord insertions or transpositions should be performed after annular sutures are completed and suspended. In da Vinci cases, each suture is placed and tied intracorporeal. Upon completion of the repair, robotic devices are removed, and the left atrium is closed under direct vision to decrease operative times. Standard deairing and weaning procedures are performed under TEE control. Intraoperative time metrics are collected and cataloged in spreadsheets. One month after discharge, all patients return for a follow-up visit and a transthoracic echocardiogram.

CLINICAL OUTCOMES

Currently, the world experience with robotic mitral valve surgery is mostly anecdotal, retrospective, and noncontrolled. Nevertheless, surgical results thus far have been encouraging and are hastening the way toward a completely endoscopic, robotic mitral valve operation.

In the year 2000, we completed and presented to the FDA our results from the first approved robotic mitral valve trial.[12] This trial consisted of 10 patients. With the flexibility of the da Vinci we successfully performed quadrangular leaflet resections, leaflet sliding plasties, chord transfers, polytetrafluoroethylene chord replacements, reduction annuloplasties, and annuloplasty band insertions. The mean total arrest time was 150 minutes with 52 minutes assigned to leaflet repairs. Of the total arrest time, a mean of 42 minutes was needed to place an average of 7.5 annuloplasty band sutures. Total operating room times averaged 4.8 hours. There were no device-related complications and only one reexploration for bleeding from an atrial pacing wire. The average postoperative stay was 4 days (range, 3–7 days). At 3-month follow-up echocardiography revealed nothing more that trace mitral regurgitation. All patients returned to normal activity by 1 month after surgery. On the basis of these results, an FDA extension of this safety and efficacy trial was granted at our institution.

In reviewing the Leipzig robotic mitral experience, Mohr et al described 17 patients who underwent robotic mitral valve repair.[30] Their cohort was relatively young (58 ± 9 years) and predominantly female (n = 9). Fourteen of the 17 patients underwent a successful mitral valve repair with the da Vinci system. In three patients, conversion to conventional endoscopic instruments became necessary. The average cross-clamp time was 89 ± 18 minutes. Following the repair, intraoperative TEE demonstrated no regurgitation in 13 patients and trace regurgitation in 3. One patient had a grade 2 leak requiring immediate endoscopic valve replacement. Postoperative results were notable for one failure of a repair requiring emergent valve replacement on postoperative day 3 secondary to a disrupted annuloplasty ring. As

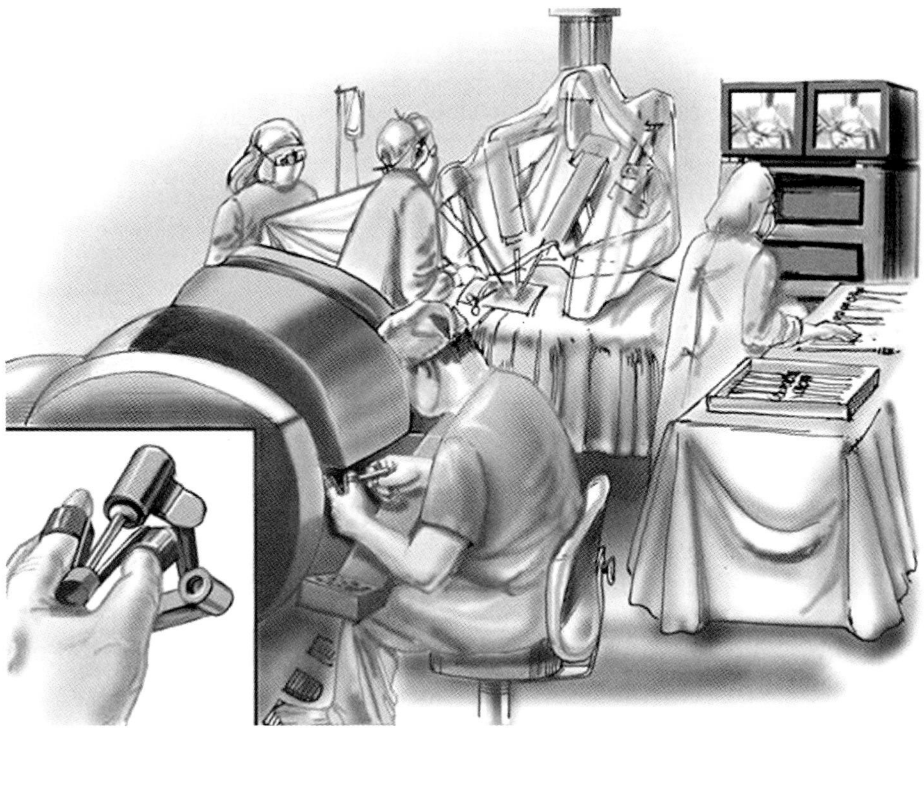

Figure 78–7 Robot-assisted mitral valve procedure. Note the surgeon seated at the operative console manipulating the robotic instruments and the instrument cart positioned over the patient. There is a patient-side surgeon, and video monitors allow the operative team to view the surgery. Inset: finger grips for the operating surgeon.

of January 2003, over 40 mitral valves have been successfully repaired with the da Vinci system in Leipzig.[31]

Recently, we published our results of the first 38 mitral repairs with the da Vinci system.[36] Total robot time represents the exact time of robot deployment after valve exposure and continues until the end of annuloplasty band placement. This time decreased significantly from 1.9 h in the first group of 19 patients to 1.5 h in the second group. At the same time, leaflet repair times fell significantly from 1.0 h to 0.6 h, respectively. Also, total operating times decreased significantly from 5.1 to 4.4 h in the second group of patients. Furthermore, both cross-clamp and bypass times decreased significantly with experience as well. For the entire group of 38 patients, the total length of stay was 3.8 days, with no difference between the two groups. Of all patients in the study, 84% demonstrated a grade 3 or greater reduction in mitral regurgitation at follow-up. In the entire series there were no device-related complications or operative deaths. One valve was replaced at 19 days because of hemolysis secondary to a leak that was directed against a prosthetic chord.

To date, we have completed a total of 50 robotic mitral valve repairs with the da Vinci system and trends noted above continue to be observed. For example, bypass and cross-clamp times between the first 25 patients and the second group of 25 patients continue to significantly decrease and are currently averaging 2.69 and 2.12 h, respectively. Suture placement time for annuloplasty rings has decreased significantly from 2.15 min per suture to 1.46 min in the second group. When P_2 robotic repair times were compared from the first group of 25 to the second, there was a significant decrease from 54.19 to 30.79 min. Interestingly enough, the average knot tying time did not change significantly with experience, averaging 1.78 min for the first group of 25 patients and 1.56 min for the second. This might indicate the inherent limitations of current robotic suturing methods. Maybe alternative and simpler suture technology might significantly impact this aspect of the procedure. Nevertheless, a multicenter da Vinci trial enlisting 112 patients has recently been completed and demonstrates efficacy and safety in performing these operations by multiple surgeons at various centers, thereby becoming the first robotic telemanipulation system to become FDA approved for mitral valve repair surgery.

LIMITATIONS

The early clinical experience with computer-enhanced telemanipulation system has defined many of the limitations of this approach despite rapid procedural success. The lack of force feedback is being addressed currently and a strain sensor is being incorporated into advanced robotic surgical tools and may soon allow more control of force applied at the robotic end-effector.[47] Furthermore, conventional suture and knot tying add significant time to each procedure. Technological advancements, such as the use of nitinol U-clips (Figure 78-8) (Coalescent Surgical Inc., Sunnyvale, CA) instead of sutures requiring manual knot tying, should decrease operative times significantly. In a series of experiments at East Carolina University, average suture/clip placement times and knot tying/deployment times significantly decreased to 2.6 min by using clips compared with suture placement times of 4.9 min. The main differences when implanting mitral annuloplasty bands were found to be clip deployments at 0.75 min versus 2.78 min for suture tying.[26] With further refinements and development of adjunctive technologies, computer-enhanced endoscopic cardiac surgery should evolve and promises to be beneficial for selected patients.

FUTURE/NOVEL VISUALIZATION TECHNIQUES

Technological advances are occurring at a rapid pace. In just a short span of 6 years, cardiac surgery has witnessed the incorporation of robotic telemanipulative systems into the mitral surgeon's armamentarium. Nevertheless, these systems will continue to evolve, not only in their technical capabilities, but also in their ability to visualize the operative field, collectively creating a new paradigm for the way cardiac surgery is performed in the twenty-first century. Furthermore, these systems can serve as educational tools and allow simulation training for the surgeon of tomorrow.

Current robotic systems are large and take up a lot of space in the operating room. As technology develops, systems will become smaller and less cumbersome. Miniaturization is an expanding field and surely will influence the way future robotic systems are developed. This will allow easier mobility resulting in decreased setup times. Furthermore, the miniaturization of these devices probably will become more widespread, enabling surgeons to move them more easily from one operating room to another. In addition, flexible arms may create a greater range of arm motion enhancing the flexibility of the device. At the National Center of Competence in Research in Zurich, Switzerland, projects are already underway in which current large robotic arms are being replaced by handheld instrument controllers, which provide more intuitive functionality than current surgical robots.[33] Furthermore, advancements in microchip and wireless technology may allow the development of ingestible cameras, implantable sensors, and surgical microrobots, as well as magnetically controlled implants that can be navigated remotely. For example, new technologies to facilitate minimally invasive surgery are being developed that deliver a 2-mm stereoscopic camera with a clear, high-quality image with the ability to visualize through blood and other body fluids.[32]

Currently, one of the more significant limitations of contemporary robotic systems remains the lack of haptic feedback. Improving surgical dexterity is critical to the continued evolution of robotic technology in minimally invasive surgery. The study of haptics is based on tactile feedback, which is transmitted through an electronic system to the operator contemporaneously from either a geographical target or an instrument action. Its perception is related intimately to both tissue modeling and the tissue–tool interactions. Nearly everything a surgeon does relates to force feedback. Organs and blood vessels respond to manipulation and the forces involved have been considered essential in identifying pathological areas, determining tissue boundaries, and assessing the quality of an operation. The level of fidelity required for an effective haptic response is an area of active research, especially as it pertains to the amount of

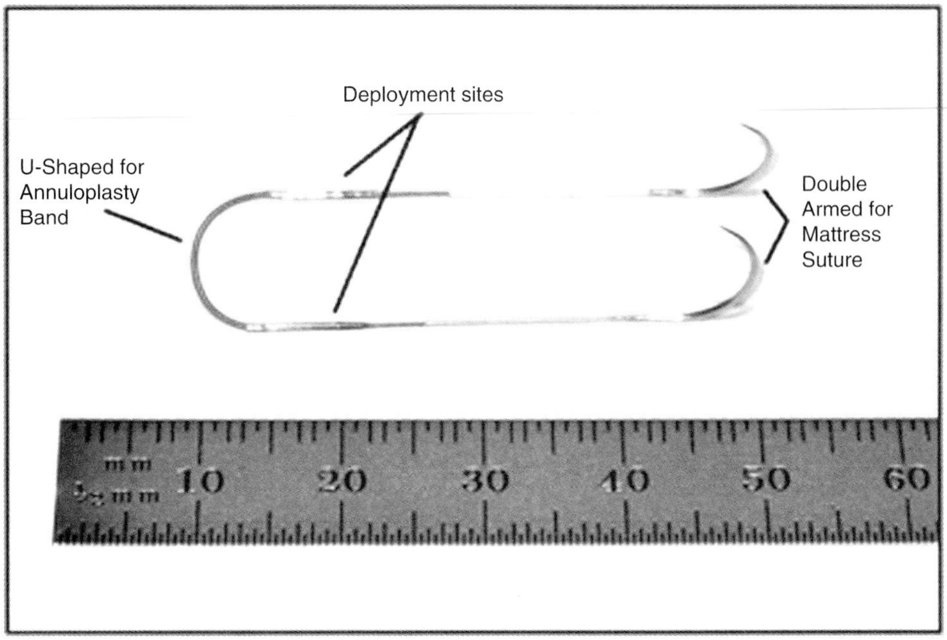

A

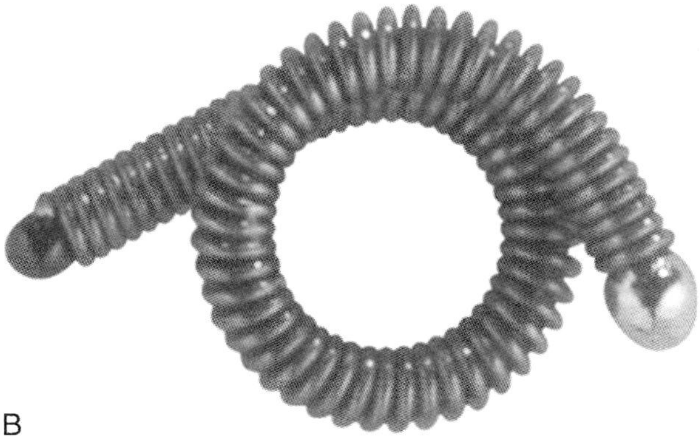

B

Figure 78–8 (A) Nitinol U-clip and (B) Nitinol U-clip, deployed.

feedback that needs to be apportioned between the visual aspects of the system and the "touch" of the system. Researchers at Pennsylvania State and Millersville Universities have developed a haptic suture simulator that gives a realistic feeling when handling and suturing tissue. Specialized software has been developed to simulate the impact of pushing, pulling, and cutting the skin and underlying tissue. A basic mass-spring model was developed in which the skin is approximated to a deformable surface made of a network of masses and springs. The skin deforms relative to the weight, or pressure, applied to the springs through the surgical tool. The software calculates contact forces in the soft tissue surrounding the wound and returns the appropriate forces to the user. The resistant forces change when the needle is inserted into the virtual skin and when it is pushed through the soft tissue.[46] Technology like this can be applied to robotics allowing the surgeon to "feel" through transmission via the robotic arms, enabling a more precise and realistic operation.

Besides advances in haptics, which will change the way surgeons "feel" with robotic telemanipulative systems, the way surgeons will "see" or visualize the operative field will change as well. The potential use of imaging techniques may include three-dimensional modeling and reconstruction from computerized tomography, magnetic resonance imaging, or ultrasound. These image-guided surgical technologies will provide real-time data acquisition of pathological characteristics, allowing one to assess better the delivery of percutaneous therapy remotely. Research being conducted at the National Research Institute in Computer Science and Control of France, in collaboration with Professor Carpentier, is focusing on simulating and planning robotic procedures. Computer modeling of organs, such as the heart, is generated from combined information from different imaging modalities. For example, dynamic models of the coronary arteries can be reconstituted from biplanar angiography, magnetic resonance imaging, and computed tomography. Once these data are acquired and combined (Figure 78-9), surgeons have a virtual platform to analyze and plan optimal topographic surface targets that would optimize port site placement.[2,4] Investigators at the University of Western Ontario are developing a three-dimensional guidance system with a virtual cardiac surgical planning platform for endoscopic cardiac procedures as well.[13] Preoperative three-dimensional images of the thorax are acquired by both computed tomography and electrocardiogram-gated magnetic resonance imaging and are imported into the planning platform. A surgeon may visualize and manipulate simulated objects interactively and once optimal access port placements are determined, the positions of the simulated tools

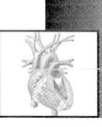

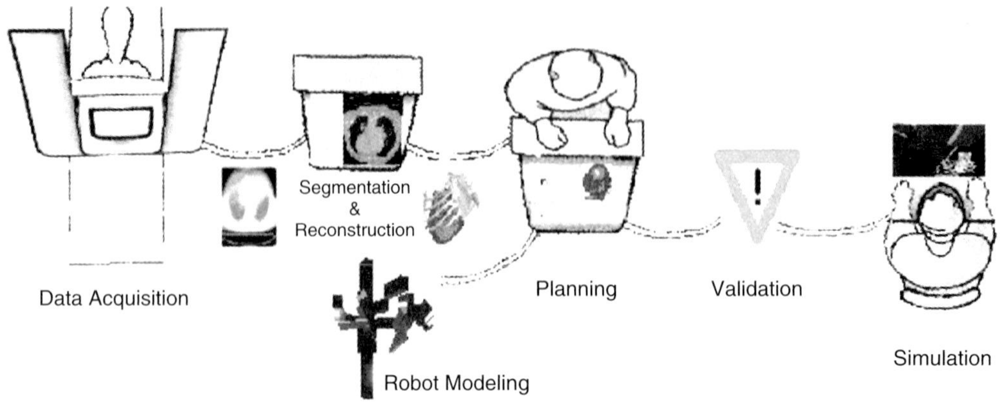

Figure 78–9 **A paradigm for planning and simulation of a robotic cardiac procedure.**

can be recorded and marked directly on the patient to specify positions for port incisions. They are also developing a virtual endoscope to simulate the endoscopic view observed by a surgeon during an operation. Such three-dimensional planning systems based on preoperative imaging data have already been introduced into other surgical specialties including craniomaxillofacial and orthopedic surgery.[45]

Augmented reality research at the University of North Carolina is showing that surgeons theoretically can see directly into a patient using combined computer graphic technology and real world images. They use ultrasonic echo graphic imaging, laparoscopic range imaging, a video see-through head-mounted display, and a high-performance graphics computer to create live images that combine computer-generated imagery with the live video image of a patient. An augmented reality system that displays real time ultrasound and/or thoracoscopic range data and registers this information with the anatomical part being scanned could be a powerful tool for guiding surgeons during closed-chest cardiac procedures. This technology has already been applied experimentally,[40] and results suggest that it could improve accuracy over traditional biopsy guidance methods. Clearly, technology such as this may have potential use in visualization and navigational systems that could be used to visualize the operative field in a minimal-access environment.

Ultimately, all of these technical advances will enable virtual reality to become an integral part of the operating room and in the training of surgeons, residents, and medical students. In health care, virtual reality can be viewed as an emergence of the three-dimensional visualization processes employed to cross-sectional data of digital imaging technologies, such as computed tomography, magnetic resonance imaging, and ultrasound scanning. The essential components are (1) the creation of a fully three-dimensional representation of an organ system or body region, (2) the ability to interact with that image as if it really existed, and (3) performing tasks such as organ or body slicing, flying-through, rotation, and manipulation. Future surgeons will be practicing their techniques through virtual reality goggles and feel the tension of moving through human tissue as they manipulate surgical tools in life-like situations. The teaching potential of such systems is enormous. These simulators already exist and have been stratified by the skills they emphasize. These systems already are proving to be of an educational benefit.[41] The principal aim of virtual reality technology is to present virtual objects or complete scans in a way identical to the natural counterpart. Recently, it has been shown that the use of virtual reality surgical stimulation in reaching a specific target significantly improves operating room performance of residents during a laparoscopic cholecystectomy.[42] Virtual reality training models already exist for the heart and can be used for heart surgery education.[20] Specifically, detailed cardiac anatomy, including valves and coronary arteries, can be used as an interactive, three-dimensional teaching tool. Techniques employing three-dimensional animation can be used to teach deployment of new endovascular connectors. It is conceivable that one day a system may exist that will allow surgeons to enter all preoperative imaging data on a patient, perform the operation on a virtual simulator, store it, and then transfer it to a robotic telemanipulation system that will perform the operation flawlessly. It will do so because if mistakes are made on the virtual simulator, they can be changed and never performed on the patient. Obviously, scenarios like this are years away, but the groundwork clearly has been laid for virtual surgery.

SUMMARY

A renaissance in cardiac surgery has begun and robotic technology has provided benefits to cardiac surgery. With improved optics and instrumentation, incisions are smaller. Inherent ergometric movements and simulated three-dimensional vision in new telemanipulation systems enhance surgeon hand–eye coordination. The placement of wrist-like articulations at the end of the instruments moves the pivoting action to the plane of the mitral annulus. This improves dexterity in tight spaces and allows for ambidextrous suture placement. Sutures can be placed more accurately because of tremor filtration and high-resolution video magnification. Furthermore, the robotic system may have potential as an educational tool. In the near future, surgical vision and training systems may be able to model most surgical procedures through immersive technology.[21,22,28] Thus, a "flight simulator" concept emerges in which it is possible to simulate, practice, and perform the operation without a patient. Already, effective curriculums for training teams in robotic surgery exist.[11]

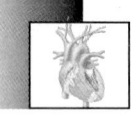

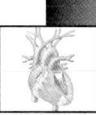

Nevertheless, certain constraints continue to limit the advancement to a totally endoscopic computer-enhanced mitral valve operation. The current size of the instruments, intrathoracic instrument collisions, and extrathoracic "elbow" conflicts still can limit dexterity. When smaller instruments are developed, these restraints may be resolved. Furthermore, a working port incision is still required for placement of an atrial retractor, as well as needle, suture, and specimen retrieval. With the development of specialized retractors and delivery/retrieval ports, a truly endoscopic approach should be reproducible and consistent.

Robotic cardiac surgery is an evolutionary process, and even the greatest skeptics must concede that progress has been made toward endoscopic cardiac valve operations. This new science is a trek and not a destination. Surgical scientists must continue to evaluate this technology critically in this new era of cardiac surgery. Despite enthusiasm, caution cannot be overemphasized. Surgeons must be careful as indices of operative safety, speed of recovery, level of discomfort, procedural cost, and long-term operative quality have yet to be defined. Traditional valve operations still enjoy long-term success with ever-decreasing morbidity and mortality, and remain our measure for comparison.

REFERENCES

1. Acuff TE, Landrenau RJ, Griffith BP, et al: Minimally invasive coronary artery bypass grafting. Ann Thorac Surg 61:135–137, 1996.
2. Adhami L, Coste-Maniere E: Postioning tele-operated surgical robots for collision-free optimal operation. Proceedings of the 2002 IEEE International Conference on Robotics and Automation, 2002.
3. Arom KV, Emery RW: Minimally invasive mitral operations [letter]. Ann Thorac Surg 63:1219–1220, 1997.
4. Blondel C, Vaillant R, Devernay F, et al: Automatic trinocular 3d reconstruction of coronary artery centerlines from rotational x-ray angiography. In Computer Assisted Radiology and Surgery 2002 Proceedings, 2002.
5. Burke RP, Wernovsky G, van der Velde M, et al: Video-assisted thoracoscopic surgery for congenital heart disease. J Thorac Cardiovasc Surg 109:499–507, 1995.
6. Carpentier A, Loulmet D, LeBret E, et al: Chirurgie à coeur ouvert par video-chirurgie et mini-thoracotomie-primer cas (valvuloplastie mitrale) opéré avec succès. CR Acad Sci: Sci vie 319:219–223, 1996.
7. Carpentier A, Loulmet D, Aupecle B, et al: Computer assisted open-heart surgery. First case operated on with success. CR Acad Sci II 321:437–442, 1998.
8. Chitwood WR, Elbeery JR, Chapman WHH, et al: Video-assisted minimally invasive mitral valve surgery: the "micro-mitral" operation. J Thorac Cardiovasc Surg 113:413–414, 1997.
9. Chitwood WR, Elbeery JR, Moran JM: Minimally invasive mitral valve repair: using a mini-thoracotomy and trans-thoracic aortic occlusion. Ann Thorac Surg 63:1477–1479, 1997.
10. Chitwood WR Jr, Wixon CL, Elbeery JR, et al: Video-assisted minimally invasive mitral valve surgery. J Thorac Cardiovasc Surg 114:773–780, 1997.
11. Chitwood WR, Nifong LW, Chapman WHH, et al: Robotic surgical training in an academic institution. Ann Surg 234: 475–486, 2001.
12. Chitwood WR Jr, Nifong LW, Elbeery JE, et al: Robotic mitral valve repair: trapezoidal resection and prosthetic annuloplasty with the da Vinci surgical system. J Thorac Cardiovasc Surg 120:1171–1172, 2000.
13. Chiu AM, Dey D, Drangova M, et al: 3-D image guidance for minimally invasive robotic coronary artery bypass. Heart Surg Forum 3:224–231, 2000.
14. Cohn LH, Adams DH, Couper GS, et al: Minimally invasive aortic valve replacement. Semin Thorac Cardiovasc Surg 9: 331–336, 1997.
15. Cosgrove DM, Sabik JF, Navia J: Minimally invasive valve surgery. Ann Thorac Surg 65:1535–1538, 1998.
16. Cosgrove DM, Sabik JF: Minimally invasive approach for aortic valve operations. Ann Thorac Surg 62:596–597, 1996.
17. Falk V, Walter T, Autschbach R, et al: Robot-assisted minimally invasive solo mitral valve operation. J Thorac Cardiovasc Surg 115:470–471, 1998.
18. Falk V, Walther T, Diegeler R, et al: Echocardiographic monitoring of minimally invasive mitral valve surgery using an endoaortic clamp. J Heart Valve Dis 5:630–637, 1996.
19. Felger JE, Chitwood WR Jr, Nifong LW, et al: Evolution of mitral valve surgery: toward a totally endoscopic approach. Ann Thorac Surg 72:1203–1209, 2001.
20. Friedl R, Preisack MB, Klas W, et al: Virtual reality and 3D visualizations in heart surgery education. Heart Surg Forum 5: E17–21, 2002.
21. Gorman PJ, Meir AH, Krummel TH: Simulation and virtual reality in surgical education: real or unreal. Arch Surg 134: 1203–1208, 1999.
22. Gorman PJ, Meir AH, Krummel TH: Computer-assisted training and learning in surgery. Comput Aided Surg 5: 120–130, 2000.
23. Grossi EA, LaPietra A, Applebaum RM, et al: Case report of robotic instrument-enhanced mitral valve surgery. J Thorac Cardiovasc Surg 120:1169–1171, 2000.
24. Gundry SR, Shattuck OH, Razzouk AJ, et al: Facile minimally invasive cardiac surgery via ministernotomy. Ann Thorac Surg 65:1100–1104, 1998.
25. Kaneko Y, Kohno T, Ohtsuka T, et al: Video-assisted observation in mitral valve surgery. J Thorac Cardiovasc Surg 111:279–280, 1996.
26. Maziarz DM, Chu VF, Conquest AM, et al: Use of nitinol U-clips decreases time for annuloplasty band placement in robotic mitral valve repairs. J Am Coll Surg 195(Suppl. 3):S22, 2002 (abstract).
27. Mehmanesh H, Henze R, Lange R: Totally endoscopic mitral valve repair. J Thorac Cardiovasc Surg 123:96–97, 2002.
28. Meir AH, Rawn CL, Krummel TM: Virtual reality: surgical application-challenge for the new millennium. J Am Coll Surg 192:372–384, 2001.
29. Mohr FW, Falk V, Diegler A, et al: Minimally invasive port-access mitral valve surgery. J Thorac Cardiovasc Surg 115: 567–576, 1998.
30. Mohr FW, Falk V, Diegler A, et al: Computer-enhanced "robotic" cardiac surgery: experience in 148 patients. J Thorac Cardiovasc Surg 121:842–853, 2001.
31. Mohr FW: Personal Communication, February 2003.
32. Morgenstern J: Improving visualization allows seeing into the unseen in Israel. High Tech Invest Rep 18:5–6, 2002.
33. Muller B: Robotics in cardiovascular surgery. Http//www.co-me.ch/projects/cardio.en.html, 2002.
34. Nataf P, Lima L, Regan M, et al: Minimally invasive coronary surgery with thoracoscopic internal mammary dissection: surgical technique. J Card Surg 11:288–292, 1996.
35. Navia JL, Cosgrove DM: Minimally invasive mitral valve operations. Ann Thorac Surg 62:1542–1544, 1996.
36. Nifong LW, Chu VR, Bailey BM, et al: Robotic mitral valve repair: experience with the da Vinci system. Ann Thorac Surg 75:438–443, 2003.
37. Nifong LW, Bolotin G, Kypson AP, et al: Robotic mitral valve replacement. Ann Thorac Surg (in press).

38. Pompili MF, Stevens JH, Burdon TA, et al: Port-access mitral valve replacement in dogs. J Thorac Cardiovasc Surg 112:1268–1274, 1996.
39. Reichenspurner H, Boehm DH, Gulbins H, et al: Three-dimensional video and robot-assisted port-access mitral valve surgery. Ann Thorac Surg 69:1176–1181, 2000.
40. Rosenthal M, Stake A, Lee J, et al: Augmented reality guidance for needle biopsies: an initial randomized, controlled trial in phantoms. Med Image Anal 6:313–320, 2002.
41. Satava RM: Surgical education and surgical simulation. World J Surg 25:1484–1489, 2001.
42. Seymour NE, Gallagher AG, Roman SA, et al: Virtual reality training improves operating room performance: results of a randomized, double-blinded study. Ann Surg 236:458–463, 2002.
43. Spencer FC, Galloway, AC, Grossi EA, et al: Recent developments and evolving techniques of mitral valve reconstruction. Ann Thorac Surg 65:307–313, 1998.
44. Stevens JH, Burdon TA, Peters WS, et al: Port-access coronary artery bypass grafting: a proposed surgical method. J Thorac Cardiovasc Surg 111:567–573, 1996.
45. Troulis MJ, Everett P, Seldin ED, et al: Development of a three-dimensional treatment planning system based on computed tomographic data. Int J Oral Maxillofac Surg 31:349–357, 2002.
46. Webster RW, Zimmerman DI, Mohler BJ, et al: A prototype haptic suturing simulator. Stud Health Technol Inform 81:567–569, 2001.
47. Zenati MA: Robotic heart surgery. Cardiol Rev 9:287–294, 2001.

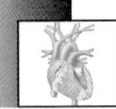

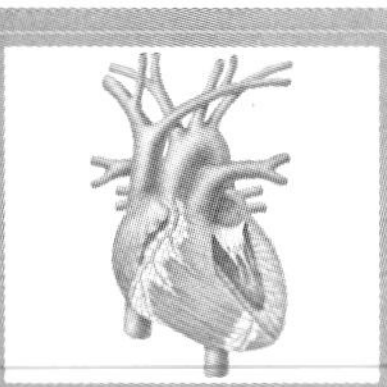

CHAPTER 79

Cardiac Devices for the Treatment of Bradyarrhythmias and Tachyarrhythmias

Lilian P. Joventino and Peter J. Zimetbaum

HISTORICAL PERSPECTIVE AND OVERVIEW

Paul Zoll, M.D., developed the first transcutaneous electronic pacemaker in 1952[33] for the treatment of life-threatening bradycardia. The first internal pacemaker was implanted in 1958 for the treatment of complete heart block[9] and in the management of Stokes–Adams seizures.[12] Early pacemaker models were simple, fixed-rate devices. Thoracic surgeons performed the majority of early implants by placing epimyocardial leads directly on the exposed heart; these leads were connected to an abdominally implanted pulse generator. Modern pacemakers have sophisticated microprocessors that apply diagnostic and therapeutic algorithms, which have dramatically increased their versatility.

The development of the implantable cardioverter defibrillator (ICD) was pioneered by Michel Mirowski.[20,21] The initial purpose of the ICD was to provide immediate, automatic defibrillation to ambulatory patients who were victims of a lethal ventricular arrhythmia. Dr. Mirowski performed the first human ICD implant in 1980.[22] First-generation ICDs were composed of large generators (>200 cm^3 volume) implanted in an abdominal pocket with epicardial defibrillator patches; these early ICDs were capable only of high-energy shocks. Current ICDs are small (<40 cm^3 volume), but contain all the advanced pacing functions of modern pacemakers as well as complex tachycardia treatment options (Figures 79-1 and 79-2). Despite their diminutive size, newer ICDs have become progressively superior in their sensing, detection, and treatment of arrhythmias. Over the last decade, ICDs have emerged as the single most effective life-saving intervention in modern medicine.[2,18,24,25]

With increased sophistication and miniaturization of pulse generators and the development of the much simpler and safer transvenous approach for implantation of cardiac devices, indications for cardiac pacing as well as for ICDs have dramatically expanded.[14,15] Nearly 350,000 cardiac devices are now implanted in the United States alone, and more than 970,000 worldwide.

The remainder of this chapter will focus on the description, implant techniques, indications, and complications of current implantable cardiac pacemakers and defibrillators.

INDICATIONS FOR IMPLANTATION OF CARDIAC DEVICES

The ACC/AHA/NASPE Guidelines for Implantation of Cardiac Pacemakers and Antiarrhythmia Devices were updated in November 2002.[14,15]

Temporary Pacemakers

Indications

Placement of a temporary pacemaker is indicated whenever hemodynamic compromise is present because of a bradyarrhythmia. Temporary pacemakers should also be placed prophylactically if high risk for development of hemodynamically important bradycardia is present. Specific guide-

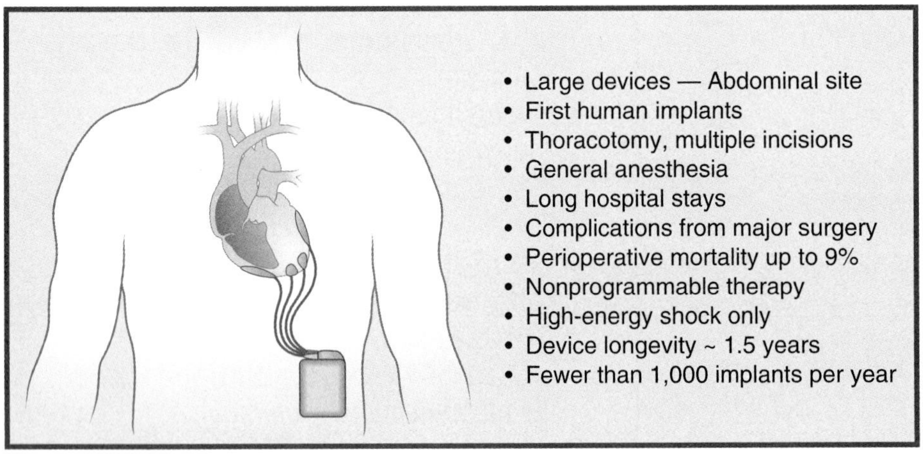
• Large devices — Abdominal site
• First human implants
• Thoracotomy, multiple incisions
• General anesthesia
• Long hospital stays
• Complications from major surgery
• Perioperative mortality up to 9%
• Nonprogrammable therapy
• High-energy shock only
• Device longevity ~ 1.5 years
• Fewer than 1,000 implants per year

Figure 79–1 Implantable cardioverter defibrillators in 1980. *(Courtesy of Medtronic, Inc.)*

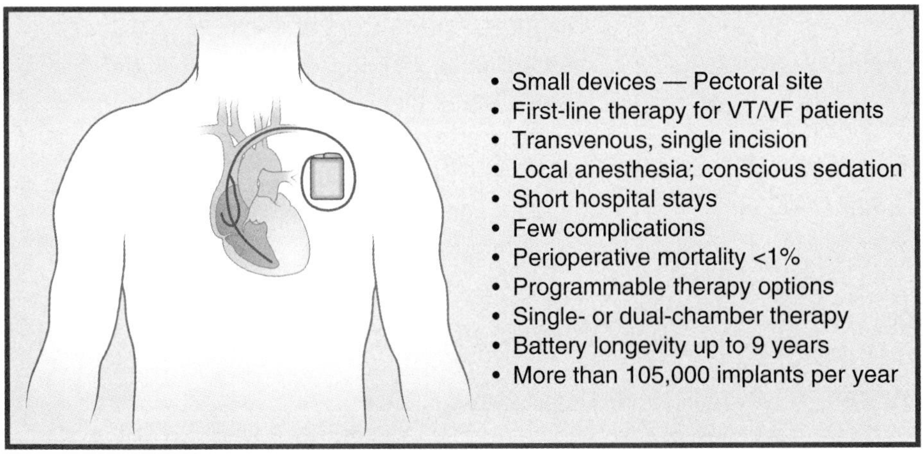
• Small devices — Pectoral site
• First-line therapy for VT/VF patients
• Transvenous, single incision
• Local anesthesia; conscious sedation
• Short hospital stays
• Few complications
• Perioperative mortality <1%
• Programmable therapy options
• Single- or dual-chamber therapy
• Battery longevity up to 9 years
• More than 105,000 implants per year

Figure 79–2 Implantable cardioverter defibrillators today. VT/VF, ventricular tachycardia/ventricular flutter. *(Courtesy of Medtronic, Inc.)*

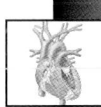

lines for placement of temporary pacemakers in the setting of acute myocardial infarction may be found in Box 79-1.[29]

Venous Access

Table 79-1 summarizes the different sites that can be used for insertion of a temporary pacemaker.[31] Careful consideration of the site to be used is important as it relates to the particular patient and advantages/disadvantages of each site. For instance, the internal jugular and subclavian veins may be chosen when need for stability and longer pacing requirement is anticipated. If a permanent pacemaker will be required in the future, the temporary pacemaker should be placed via a vein remote from the preferred site for permanent pacemaker implantation. Use of the antecubital veins minimizes bleeding in the coagulopathic patient. However, the risk of cardiac perforation or lead dislodgement is higher if the arm is not kept fully immobilized.

Permanent Pacemakers

Indications

Justifications for permanent pacemaker implantation include alleviation of symptoms and/or prevention of subsequent morbidity or mortality as a direct result of bradycardia. Bradycardia can result from a variety of disorders of the sinus node, the atrioventricular (AV) node, the His–Purkinje system, or a combination of these. Sinus node or AV nodal disease is often not life threatening, but may cause significant symptoms. On the other hand, disease of the His–Purkinje system may be asymptomatic until the development of severe adverse events.

Symptoms from bradycardia generally result from inappropriate cardiac output. Such symptoms may be vague and include fatigue, decreased exercise tolerance, dyspnea on exertion, lightheadedness, dizziness, congestive heart failure, presyncope, or syncope. Patient-triggered ambulatory cardiac monitoring is often helpful in establishing that symptoms, which may be nonspecific, are in fact the result of symptomatic bradycardia. Boxes 79-2 through 79-11 summarize the indications for permanent cardiac pacing published by the American College of Cardiology/American Heart Association (ACC/AHA) Task Force on Practice Guidelines in 2002.[14,15]

New Class I indications for permanent pacing in the 2002 guidelines include advanced second-degree AV block, heart failure as a major symptom from AV block-induced bradycardia, patients with neuromuscular disease with third-degree AV block (regardless of the presence of symptoms), alternating bundle-branch block (BBB), and congenital third-degree AV block with complex ventricular ectopy.

Indications for cardiac pacing in specific clinical conditions such as hypertrophic obstructive cardiomyopathy, dilated cardiomyopathy, and cardiac transplantation are outlined in Boxes 79-9 through 79-11.[14,15]

Contraindications

Active infection is a contraindication for placement of permanent pacemaker systems. If the need for pacing is urgent, a temporary transvenous pacemaker should be employed. In patients with recurrent or protracted infectious illnesses, temporary placement of a standard (screw-in) pacemaker

Box 79–1. Indications for Temporary Pacing in the Setting of Acute Myocardial Infarction.

Class I

1. Asystole.
2. Symptomatic bradycardia (includes sinus bradycardia with hypotension and type I second-degree AV block with hypotension not responsive to atropine).
3. Bilateral BBB (alternating BBB or RBBB with alternating LAFB/LPFB), of any age.
4. New or indeterminate-age bifascicular block (RBBB with LAFB, or LPFB, or LBBB) with first-degree AV block.
5. Mobitz type II second-degree AV block.

Class IIa

1. RBBB and LAFB or LPFB, new or indeterminate.
2. RBBB with first-degree AV block.
3. LBBB, new or indeterminate.
4. Incessant VT, for atrial or ventricular overdrive pacing.
5. Recurrent sinus pauses (greater than 3 s) not responsive to atropine.

Class IIb

1. Bifascicular block of indeterminate age.
2. New or age-indeterminate isolated RBBB.

Class III

1. First-degree heart block.
2. Type I second-degree AV block with normal hemodynamics.
3. Accelerated idioventricular rhythm.
4. BBB or fascicular block known to exist before AMI.

From Ryan TJ, Antman EM, Brooks NH, et al: ACC/AHA guidelines for the management of patients with acute myocardial infarction: Executive summary and recommendations. Circulation 100:1016–1030, 1999.

lead is suggested. The proximal end of the lead is externalized and connected to an external pulse generator and a sterile dressing is placed over the entry site. Such temporary systems may be left in place for weeks, and may serve as a bridge to implantation of a permanent pacemaker. Alternatively, an epicardial pacing system can be implanted.

Implantable Cardioverter Defibrillators

Indications

Current ACC/AHA/NASPE Practice Guidelines for ICD therapy are listed in Box 79-12.

New Class I indications for implantable cardioverter-defibrillator therapy in the guidelines include spontaneous sustained ventricular tachycardia (VT) in association with structural heart disease [new requirement for structural heart disease (SHD) to be present], nonsustained VT in patients with coronary artery disease (CAD), prior myocardial infarction (MI), left ventricular (LV) dysfunction, and inducible ventricular fibrillation (VF) or sustained VT at electrophysiological study (EPS) that is not suppressible by a Class I antiar-

Table 79–1

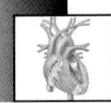

Sites for Placement of a Temporary Pacemaker

Site	*Advantages*	*Disadvantages*
Femoral vein	Easy access	Leg must remain immobilized High infection risk Fluoroscopy required for proper placement Patient must lie flat
Internal jugular vein	Good site for pacer placement (right better than left)	Risk of pneumothorax, inadvertent carotid artery puncture Patient must lie flat for access; Trendelenburg position preferred to avoid air embolism
Subclavian vein	Good site for pacer placement (left better than right)	Risk of pneumothorax, hemothorax with inadvertent subclavian artery puncture Patient must lie flat for access; Trendelenburg position preferred to avoid air embolism
Antecubital vein (basilic, median basilic or cephalic)	Access is low risk Good site for pacer placement (left better than right)	Risk of dislodgment; arm must remain immobilized Basilic or median basilic preferred (cephalic has tortuous course to central veins) Fluoroscopy required for pacer placement

From Baim DS, Grossman W, editors: Grossman's Cardiac Catheterization, Angiography, and Intervention, 6th ed. Philadelphia: Lippincott Williams & Wilkins, 2000.

Box 79–2. 2002 Recommendations for Permanent Pacing in Acquired Atrioventricular Block in Adults.

Class I

1. Third-degree and advanced second-degree AV block at any anatomical level, associated with any one of the following conditions:[a]
   a. Bradycardia with symptoms (including heart failure) presumed to be due to AV block. (*Level of Evidence: C*)[a]
   b. Arrhythmias and other medical conditions that require drugs that result in symptomatic bradycardia. (*Level of Evidence: C*)
   c. Documented periods of asystole greater than or equal to 3.0 s or any escape rate less than 40 beats per minute (bpm) in awake, symptom-free patients. (*Level of Evidence: B, C*)[a]
   d. After catheter ablation of the AV junction. (*Level of Evidence B, C*) There are no trials to assess outcomes without pacing, and pacing is virtually always planned in this situation unless the operative procedure is AV junction modification.[a]
   e. Postoperative AV block that is not expected to resolve after cardiac surgery. (*Level of Evidence: C*)[a]
   f. Neuromuscular diseases with AV block, such as myotonic muscular dystrophy, Kearns-Sayre syndrome, Erb's dystrophy (limb-girdle), and peroneal muscular atrophy, with or without symptoms, because there may be unpredictable progression of AV conduction disease. (*Level of Evidence: B*)[a]

Class IIa[a]

1. Asymptomatic third-degree AV block at any anatomical site with average awake ventricular rates of 40 bpm or faster especially if cardiomegaly or left ventricular (LV) dysfunction is present. (*Level of Evidence: B, C*)
2. Asymptomatic type II second-degree AV block with a narrow QRS. When type II second-degree AV block occurs with a wide QRS, pacing becomes a Class I recommendation (see next section regarding "Pacing for Chronic Bifascicular and Trifascicular Block"). (*Level of Evidence: B*)
3. Asymptomatic type I second-degree AV block at intra- or infra-His levels found at electrophysiological study performed for other indications. (*Level of Evidence: B*)
4. First- or second-degree AV block with symptoms similar to those of pacemaker syndrome. (*Level of Evidence: B*)

Class IIb

1. Marked first-degree AV block (more than 0.30 s) in patients with LV dysfunction and symptoms of congestive heart failure in whom a shorter AV interval results in hemodynamic improvement, presumably by decreasing left atrial filling pressure. (*Level of Evidence: C*)

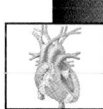

Box 79–2. 2002 Recommendations for Permanent Pacing in Acquired Atrioventricular Block in Adults—cont'd

2. Neuromuscular diseases such as myotonic muscular dystrophy, Kearns-Sayre syndrome, Erb's dystrophy (limb-girdle), and peroneal muscular atrophy with any degree of AV block (including first-degree AV block) with or without symptoms, because there may be unpredictable progression of AV conduction disease. (*Level of Evidence: B*)[a]

Class III

1. Asymptomatic first-degree AV block. (*Level of Evidence: B*) (See also "Pacing for Chronic Bifascicular and Trifascicular Block")
2. Asymptomatic type I second-degree AV block at the supra-His (AV node) level or not known to be intra- or infra-Hisian. (*Level of Evidence: B, C*)
3. AV block expected to resolve and/or unlikely to recur (e.g., drug toxicity, Lyme disease, or during hypoxia in sleep apnea syndrome in absence of symptoms). (*Level of Evidence: B*)[a]

[a]Portions of the guidelines that have been modified.

Box 79–3. 2002 Recommendations for Permanent Pacing in Chronic Bifascicular and Trifascicular Block.

Class I

1. Intermittent third-degree AV block. (*Level of Evidence: B*)
2. Type II second-degree AV block. (*Level of Evidence: B*)
3. Alternating bundle-branch block. (*Level of Evidence: C*)[a]

Class IIa

1. Syncope not demonstrated to be due to AV block when other likely causes have been excluded, specifically ventricular tachycardia (VT). (*Level of Evidence: B*)[a]
2. Incidental finding at electrophysiological study or markedly prolonged HV interval (greater than or equal to 100 ms) in asymptomatic patients. (*Level of Evidence: B*)
3. Incidental finding at electrophysiological study of pacing-induced infra-His block that is not physiological. (*Level of Evidence: B*)

Class IIb[a]

1. Neuromuscular diseases such as myotonic muscular dystrophy, Kearns-Sayre syndrome, Erb's dystrophy (limb-girdle), and peroneal muscular atrophy with any degree of fascicular block with or without symptoms, because there may be unpredictable progression of AV conduction disease. (*Level of Evidence: C*)

Class III

1. Fascicular block without AV block or symptoms. (*Level of Evidence: B*)
2. Fascicular block with first-degree AV block without symptoms. (*Level of Evidence: B*)

[a]Portions of the guidelines that have been modified.

Box 79–4. 2002 Recommendations for Permanent Pacing after the Acute Phase of Myocardial Infarction.

Class I

1. Persistent second-degree AV block in the His–Purkinje system with bilateral bundle-branch block or third-degree AV block within or below the His–Purkinje system after acute myocardial infarction (AMI). (*Level of Evidence: B*)
2. Transient advanced (second- or third-degree) infranodal AV block and associated bundle-branch block. If the site of block is uncertain, an electrophysiological study may be necessary. (*Level of Evidence: B*)
3. Persistent and symptomatic second- or third-degree AV block. (*Level of Evidence: C*)

Class IIb

1. Persistent second- or third-degree AV block at the AV node level. (*Level of Evidence: B*)

Class III

1. Transient AV block in the absence of intraventricular conduction defects. (*Level of Evidence: B*)
2. Transient AV block in the presence of isolated left anterior fascicular block. (*Level of Evidence: B*)
3. Acquired left anterior fascicular block in the absence of AV block. (*Level of Evidence: B*)
4. Persistent first-degree AV block in the presence of bundle-branch block that is old or age indeterminate. (*Level of Evidence: B*)

Box 79–5. 2002 Recommendations for Permanent Pacing in Sinus Node Dysfunction.

Class I

1. Sinus node dysfunction with documented symptomatic bradycardia, including frequent sinus pauses that produce symptoms. In some patients, bradycardia is iatrogenic and will occur as a consequence of essential long-term drug therapy of a type and dose for which there are no acceptable alternatives. (*Level of Evidence: C*)
2. Symptomatic chronotropic incompetence. (*Level of Evidence: C*)

Class IIa

1. Sinus node dysfunction occurring spontaneously or as a result of necessary drug therapy, with heart rate less than 40 bpm when a clear association between significant symptoms consistent with bradycardia and the actual presence of bradycardia has not been documented. (*Level of Evidence: C*)
2. Syncope of unexplained origin when major abnormalities of sinus node function are discovered or provoked in electrophysiological studies. (*Level of Evidence: C*)[a]

Class IIb

1. In minimally symptomatic patients, chronic heart rate less than 40 bpm while awake. (*Level of Evidence: C*)

Class III

1. Sinus node dysfunction in asymptomatic patients, including those in whom substantial sinus bradycardia (heart rate less than 40 bpm) is a consequence of long-term drug treatment.
2. Sinus node dysfunction in patients with symptoms suggestive of bradycardia that are clearly documented as not associated with a slow heart rate.
3. Sinus node dysfunction with symptomatic bradycardia due to nonessential drug therapy.

[a]Portions of the guidelines that have been modified.

rhythmic drug, and spontaneous sustained VT in patients who do not have SHD that is not amenable to other treatments.

In view of the recently published MADIT II study,[10] a new Class IIa indication for ICD therapy has emerged in the 2002 guidelines: patients with left ventricular ejection fraction (LVEF) of less than or equal to 30%, at least 1 month post-MI and 3 months post-coronary artery revascularization surgery. In addition, two new Class IIb indications for ICD therapy have been added to the guidelines: syncope of unexplained etiology or family history of unexplained SCD in association with typical or atypical right BBB and ST-segment elevations (Brugada syndrome) and syncope in patients with advanced SHD in which thorough invasive and noninvasive investigation has failed to define a cause.

Contraindications to ICD therapy

If VT/VF is a result of a reversible cause such as acute MI or serious electrolyte derangements, ICD implant/therapy

Box 79–6. Prevention and Termination of Tachyarrhythmias by Pacing.

2002 Recommendations for Permanent Pacemakers That Automatically Detect and Pace to Terminate Tachycardias

Class I

1. Symptomatic recurrent supraventricular tachycardia (SVT) that is reproducibly terminated by pacing after drugs and catheter ablation fail to control the arrhythmia or produce intolerable side effects. (*Level of Evidence: C*)
2. Symptomatic recurrent sustained VT as part of an automatic defibrillator system. (*Level of Evidence: B*)

Class IIa[a]

1. Symptomatic recurrent SVT that is reproducibly terminated by pacing in the unlikely event that catheter ablation and/or drugs fail to control the arrhythmia or produce intolerable side effects. (*Level of Evidence: C*)

Class IIb

1. Recurrent SVT or atrial flutter that is reproducibly terminated by pacing as an alternative to drug therapy or ablation. (*Level of Evidence: C*)

Class III

1. Tachycardias frequently accelerated or converted to fibrillation by pacing.
2. The presence of accessory pathways with the capacity for rapid anterograde conduction whether or not the pathways participate in the mechanism of the tachycardia.

2002 Pacing Recommendations to Prevent Tachycardia

Class I

1. Sustained pause-dependent VT, with or without prolonged QT, in which the efficacy of pacing is thoroughly documented. (*Level of Evidence: C*)

Class IIa

1. High-risk patients with congenital long-QT syndrome. (*Level of Evidence: C*)

Class IIb

1. AV reentrant or AV node reentrant supraventricular tachycardia not responsive to medical or ablative therapy. (*Level of Evidence: C*)
2. Prevention of symptomatic, drug-refractory, recurrent atrial fibrillation in patients with coexisting sinus node dysfunction. (*Level of Evidence: B*)

Class III

1. Frequent or complex ventricular ectopic activity without sustained VT in the absence of the long-QT syndrome.
2. Torsade de Pointes VT due to reversible causes.[a]

[a]Portions of the guidelines that have been modified.

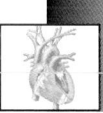

Box 79–7. 2002 Recommendations for Permanent Pacing in Hypersensitive Carotid Sinus Syndrome and Neurocardiogenic Syncope.

Class I

1. Recurrent syncope caused by carotid sinus stimulation; minimal carotid sinus pressure induces ventricular asystole of more than 3-s duration in the absence of any medication that depresses the sinus node or AV conduction. (*Level of Evidence: C*)

Class IIa

1. Recurrent syncope without clear, provocative events and with a hypersensitive cardioinhibitory response. (*Level of Evidence: C*)
2. Syncope of unexplained origin when major abnormalities of sinus node function or AV conduction are discovered or provoked in electrophysiological studies. (*Level of Evidence: C*)
3. Significantly symptomatic and recurrent neurocardiogenic syncope associated with bradycardia documented spontaneously or at the time of tilt-table testing. (*Level of Evidence: B*)[a]

Class IIb

1. Neurally mediated syncope with significant bradycardia reproduced by a head-up tilt with or without isoproterenol or other provocative maneuvers. (*Level of Evidence: B*)

Class III

1. A hyperactive cardioinhibitory response to carotid sinus stimulation in the absence of symptoms or in the presence of vague symptoms such as dizziness, lightheadedness, or both. (*Level of Evidence: C*)[a]
2. A hyperactive cardioinhibitory response to carotid sinus stimulation in the presence of vague symptoms such as dizziness, lightheadedness, or both.
3. Recurrent syncope, lightheadedness, or dizziness in the absence of a hyperactive cardioinhibitory response. (*Level of Evidence: C*)
4. Situational vasovagal syncope in which avoidance behavior is effective. (*Level of Evidence: C*)

[a]Portions of the guidelines that have been modified.

is not indicated. An ICD is not recommended for patients who have a terminal illness and whose life expectancy is less than 6 months. Patients who have severe psychiatric disorders whose illness may be exacerbated by ICD shocks or whose illness may preclude proper ICD follow-up may not be appropriate candidates for ICD implantation. Additionally, incessant VT/VF that is refractory to medications is also considered a contraindication for ICD implant until the arrhythmia is controlled by surgical or catheter ablation.

Similarly to implantation of permanent pacemakers, ICD implant is not recommended in patients with ongoing infection. Patients with infectious issues who have an indication for ICD therapy may undergo telemetry monitoring in an acute care or rehabilitation facility until their infection is cleared.

BASIC CONCEPTS OF PACING AND ANTITACHYCARDIA THERAPY

Permanent Pacemakers

Pulse Generator

Despite the many variations and designs of modern pacemakers, basic components are similar and include power source (battery), circuitry (output, sensing, telemetry, microprocessor, and memory), a metal shell (can), a ceramic feedthrough (a piece of wire surrounded by glass or sapphire) to provide an electric connection through the can, outlets through which pacing leads are connected to the header of the pacemaker, and sensors.[30] Most pacemaker batteries since 1975 are lithium iodide based. Lithium-based batteries have an ideal energy density that has allowed newer pacemakers to be of small volume yet possess longer battery life. In addition, as opposed to the original mercury-zinc cells, which develop a sudden decrease in voltage shortly prior to battery depletion, lithium iodide cells have a predictable and gradual decrease in battery voltage as they approach depletion.[30]

At the beginning of life (BOL), the lithium iodide battery has a voltage output of ~2.8 V. The initial decay is slow until the battery approaches depletion at which time the battery voltage decays more rapidly. When the battery voltage reaches 2.0–2.4 V the elective replacement indicator (ERI) is triggered, which may precipitate a change in pacing mode such as dual-chamber to single-chamber pacing, rate response to nonrate response, or a change in magnet rate behavior.[30] Once ERI is triggered, the device has about 3–6 months before it reaches its end of useful life (EOL).

The pulse generator is connected to one or two pacing leads and subsequently implanted into a subcutaneous or submuscular pocket (see implant techniques). The leads are placed under fluoroscopy at standard right atrial and/or right ventricular locations. The generator is programmed to sense and pace according to a chosen mode that addresses the individual patient's needs.

Pacemaker Leads

Pacing leads are the direct connection between the pulse generator and the myocardium. The distal end of pacing leads consists of one or two exposed metal electrodes that are linked to the pulse generator via insulated wires.

Leads may be *unipolar* or *bipolar*; these distinctions apply to both sensing and pacing functions. Unipolar leads have a single electrode incorporated into the lead (typically the cathode) and the other electrode (typically the anode) incorporated into the generator. Bipolar leads have both electrodes (the anode and the cathode) incorporated into the distal end of the lead. The potential difference sensed or created (to produce a pacing stimulus) by a bipolar lead occurs over a few millimeters, while the difference in

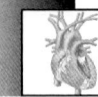

Box 79–8. 2002 Recommendations for Permanent Pacing in Children, Adolescents, and Patients with Congenital Heart Disease.

Class I

1. Advanced second- or third-degree AV block associated with symptomatic bradycardia, ventricular dysfunction, or low cardiac output. (*Level of Evidence: C*)[a]
2. Sinus node dysfunction with correlation of symptoms during age-inappropriate bradycardia. The definition of bradycardia varies with the patient's age and expected heart rate. (*Level of Evidence: B*)
3. Postoperative advanced second- or third-degree AV block that is not expected to resolve or persists at least 7 days after cardiac surgery. (*Level of Evidence: B, C*)[a]
4. Congenital third-degree AV block with a wide QRS escape rhythm, complex ventricular ectopy, or ventricular dysfunction. (*Level of Evidence: B*)[a]
5. Congenital third-degree AV block in the infant with a ventricular rate less than 50–55 bpm or with congenital heart disease and a ventricular rate less than 70 bpm. (*Level of Evidence: B, C*)
6. Sustained pause-dependent VT, with or without prolonged QT, in which the efficacy of pacing is thoroughly documented. (*Level of Evidence: B*)

Class IIa

1. Bradycardia–tachycardia syndrome with the need for long-term antiarrhythmic treatment other than digitalis. (*Level of Evidence: C*)
2. Congenital third-degree AV block beyond the first year of life with an average heart rate less than 50 bpm, abrupt pauses in ventricular rate that are two or three times the basic cycle length, or associated with symptoms due to chronotropic incompetence. (*Level of Evidence: B*)[a]
3. Long-QT syndrome with 2:1 AV or third-degree AV block. (*Level of Evidence: B*)
4. Asymptomatic sinus bradycardia in the child with complex congenital heart disease with resting heart rate less than 40 bpm or pauses in ventricular rate more than 3 s. (*Level of Evidence: C*)[a]
5. Patients with congenital heart disease and impaired hemodynamics due to sinus bradycardia or loss of AV synchrony. (*Level of Evidence: C*)[a]

Class IIb

1. Transient postoperative third-degree AV block that reverts to sinus rhythm with residual bifascicular block. (*Level of Evidence: C*)
2. Congenital third-degree AV block in the asymptomatic infant, child, adolescent, or young adult with an acceptable rate, narrow QRS complex, and normal ventricular function. (*Level of Evidence: B*)[a]
3. Asymptomatic sinus bradycardia in the adolescent with congenital heart disease with resting heart rate less than 40 bpm or pauses in ventricular rate more than 3 s. (*Level of Evidence: C*)[a]
4. Neuromuscular diseases with any degree of AV block (including first-degree AV block), with or without symptoms, because there may be unpredictable progression of AV conduction disease.[a]

Class III

1. Transient postoperative AV block with return of normal AV conduction. (*Level of Evidence: B*)[a]
2. Asymptomatic postoperative bifascicular block with or without first-degree AV block. (*Level of Evidence: C*)
3. Asymptomatic type I second-degree AV block. (*Level of Evidence: C*)
4. Asymptomatic sinus bradycardia in the adolescent with longest RR interval less than 3 s and minimum heart rate more than 40 bpm. (*Level of Evidence: C*)

[a]Portions of the guidelines that have been modified.

a unipolar lead spans the distance between the tip of the lead and the pulse generator across the chest. Bipolar leads possess significant advantages over their unipolar counterparts: no sensing of musculoskeletal potentials that may inappropriately inhibit pacing, less chance of "cross-talk" between the two leads of dual-chamber devices, less chance of interference with an ICD (ICDs should *not* be used in conjunction with unipolar leads), and less chance of pacing skeletal muscle. Additionally, most generators are compatible with unipolar pacing via a bipolar lead, if needed as a result of lead damage or high pacing thresholds.

Leads have fixation mechanisms that may be passive (e.g., tines, talons, and fins) or active (e.g., helical screws), both of which are depicted in Figure 79-3. Passive-fixation leads acquire stability by becoming entrapped in myocardial trabeculations. Active-fixation leads have distal screws that are deployed and penetrate the myocardial wall. Active mechanisms carry a lower risk of dislodgement and provide

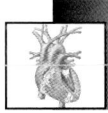

Box 79–9. 2002 Pacing Recommendations for Hypertrophic Cardiomyopathy.

Class I

1. Class I indications for sinus node dysfunction or AV block as previously described. (*Level of Evidence: C*)

Class IIba

1. Medically refractory, symptomatic hypertrophic cardiomyopathy with significant resting or provoked LV outflow obstruction. (*Level of Evidence: A*)

Class III

1. Patient who are asymptomatic or medically controlled.
2. Symptomatic patients without evidence of LV outflow obstruction.

Box 79–10. 2002 Pacing Recommendations for Dilated Cardiomyopathy.

Class I

1. Class I indications for sinus node dysfunction or AV block as previously described. (*Level of Evidence: C*)

Class IIa[a]

1. Biventricular pacing in medically refractory, symptomatic New York Heart Association (NYHA) class III or IV patients with idiopathic dilated or ischemic cardiomyopathy, prolonged QRS interval (greater than or equal to 130 ms), LV end-diastolic diameter greater than or equal to 55 mm and ejection fraction less than or equal to 35%. (*Level of Evidence: A*)

Class IIb

1. Symptomatic, drug refractory dilated cardiomyopathy with prolonged PR interval when acute hemodynamic studies have demonstrated hemodynamic benefit of pacing. (*Level of Evidence: C*)

Class III

1. Asymptomatic dilated cardiomyopathy.
2. Symptomatic dilated cardiomyopathy when patients are rendered asymptomatic by drug therapy.
3. Symptomatic ischemic cardiomyopathy when the ischemia is amenable to intervention.[a]

[a]Portions of the guidelines that have been modified.

Box 79–11. 2002 Pacing Recommendations after Cardiac Transplantation.

Class I

1. Symptomatic bradyarrhythmias/chronotropic incompetence not expected to resolve and other Class I indications for permanent pacing. (*Level of Evidence: C*)

Class IIb

1. Symptomatic bradyarrhythmias/chronotropic incompetence that, although transient, may persist for months and require intervention. (*Level of Evidence: C*)

Class III

1. Asymptomatic bradyarrhythmias after cardiac transplantation.

greater versatility in the choice of implantation sites, as their stability does not depend on the presence of trabeculations. However, active fixation leads generate a more extensive inflammatory response, which may lead to acute rises in pacing threshold after implantation. Steroid-eluting leads are now available to address the problem of acute rise in capture threshold. Such leads have a reservoir of steroid near the electrode that flows through the porous electrode into the myocardium, thereby reducing the inflammatory response and the rise in pacing threshold.[19,23,28]

Pacing

Effective cardiac pacing requires the timed introduction of an electrical impulse, which depolarizes nearby myocardium leading to propagation of an activation wave front. The term "capture" is used to indicate that successful pacing has occurred.[31] The minimum amount of energy required to produce successful myocardial depolarization and pacing is called the stimulation (or pacing) threshold. The pacing energy threshold is a function of the voltage (denoted in Volts) delivered by each electrical impulse and the duration over which the impulse is delivered (pulse width, denoted in milliseconds). For chronic pacing leads, a 2-fold pacing threshold voltage or 3-fold pacing threshold pulse width safety margin is generally provided.

Sensing

Sensing is required for the pacemaker to coordinate pacing with any intrinsic electric cardiac activity. The earliest pacemakers were not able to sense, and paced only in VOO mode (see pacing modes below). Pacing leads have a recording electrode and an indifferent electrode. As a wave of depolarization approaches the recording electrode and then proceeds away from it, it creates what is called an "intrinsic deflection," which is the transition from the approaching to the receding deflection. The slope of the intrinsic deflection is called the "slew rate." The pacemaker system has an amplifier that increases the signal from the recording electrode and a band pass filter to delete signals with frequencies too high or too low to represent an intrinsic deflection. The electrogram is "sensed" when the amplitude of the filtered signal exceeds the programmed sensing threshold. When sensing occurs, the programmed timing circuits of the pulse generator are reset. Generally, a 2- to 3-fold sensing safety margin is also incorporated in the pacemaker programming.

Box 79–12. 2002 Recommendations for Implantable Cardioverter-Defibrillator (ICD) Therapy.

Class I

1. Cardiac arrest due to ventricular fibrillation (VF) or VT not due to a transient or reversible cause. (*Level of Evidence: A*)
2. Spontaneous sustained VT in association with structural heart disease. (*Level of Evidence: B*)[a]
3. Syncope of undetermined origin with clinically relevant, hemodynamically significant sustained VT or VF induced at electrophysiological study when drug therapy is ineffective, not tolerated, or not preferred. (*Level of Evidence: B*)
4. Nonsustained VT in patients with coronary disease, prior myocardial infarction (MI), LV dysfunction, and inducible VF or sustained VT at electrophysiological study that is not suppressible by a Class I antiarrhythmic drug. (*Level of Evidence: A*)[a]
5. Spontaneous sustained VT in patients who do not have structural heart disease that is not amenable to other treatments. (*Level of Evidence: C*)[a]

Class IIa[a]

1. Patients with LV ejection fraction of less than or equal to 30%, at least 1 month post-myocardial infarction and 3 months post-coronary artery revascularization surgery. (*Level of Evidence: B*)

Class IIb

1. Cardiac arrest presumed to be due to VF when electrophysiological testing is precluded by other medical conditions. (*Level of Evidence: C*)
2. Severe symptoms (e.g., syncope) attributable to ventricular tachyarrhythmias in patients awaiting cardiac transplantation. (*Level of Evidence: C*)[a]
3. Familial or inherited conditions with a high risk for life-threatening ventricular tachyarrhythmias such as long-QT syndrome or hypertrophic cardiomyopathy. (*Level of Evidence: B*)
4. Nonsustained VT with coronary artery disease, prior MI, LV dysfunction, and inducible sustained VT or VF at electrophysiological study. (*Level of Evidence: B*)
5. Recurrent syncope of undetermined etiology in the presence of ventricular dysfunction and inducible ventricular arrhythmias at electrophysiological study when other causes of syncope have been excluded. (*Level of Evidence: C*)
6. Syncope of unexplained etiology or family history of unexplained sudden cardiac death in association with typical or atypical right bundle-branch block and ST-segment elevations (Brugada syndrome). (*Level of Evidence: C*)[a]
7. Syncope in patients with advanced structural heart disease in which thorough invasive and noninvasive investigation has failed to define a cause. (*Level of Evidence: C*)[a]

Class III

1. Syncope of undetermined cause in a patient without inducible ventricular tachyarrhythmias and without structural heart disease. (*Level of Evidence: C*)[a]
2. Incessant VT or VF. (*Level of Evidence: C*)
3. VF or VT resulting from arrhythmias amenable to surgical or catheter ablation; for example, atrial arrhythmias associated with the Wolff–Parkinson–White syndrome, right ventricular outflow tract VT, idiopathic left ventricular tachycardia, or fascicular VT. (*Level of Evidence: C*)
4. Ventricular tachyarrhythmias due to a transient or reversible disorder (e.g., AMI, electrolyte imbalance, drugs, or trauma) when correction of the disorder is considered feasible and likely to substantially reduce the risk of recurrent arrhythmia. (*Level of Evidence: B*)[a]
5. Significant psychiatric illnesses that may be aggravated by device implantation or may preclude systematic follow-up. (*Level of Evidence: C*)
6. Terminal illnesses with projected life expectancy less than 6 months. (*Level of Evidence: C*)
7. Patients with coronary artery disease with LV dysfunction and prolonged QRS duration in the absence of spontaneous or inducible sustained or nonsustained VT who are undergoing coronary artery bypass surgery. (*Level of Evidence: B*)
8. NYHA Class IV drug-refractory congestive heart failure in patients who are not candidates for cardiac transplantation. (*Level of Evidence: C*)

[a]Portions of the guidelines that have been modified.

Note that pacing intervals and cycle lengths are expressed in milliseconds, and pacing rates are denoted in beats per minute (bpm) or pulses per minute (ppm). Rate and cycle lengths are inversely related and easily converted into one another: rate in bpm (or ppm) may be obtained by dividing 60,000 by the cycle length (CL) in milliseconds; conversely, CL in milliseconds may be determined by dividing 60,000 by the rate in bpm (or ppm).

Basic Pacing Modes

A generic pacemaker code allows for the uniform functional classification of all pacing systems.[32]

The first three letters are the most widely used and refer to the pacing and sensing functions of the pacemaker. The first position denotes the cardiac chamber(s), which may be **paced** (i.e., the atrium [A], ventricle [V], both [D], or none

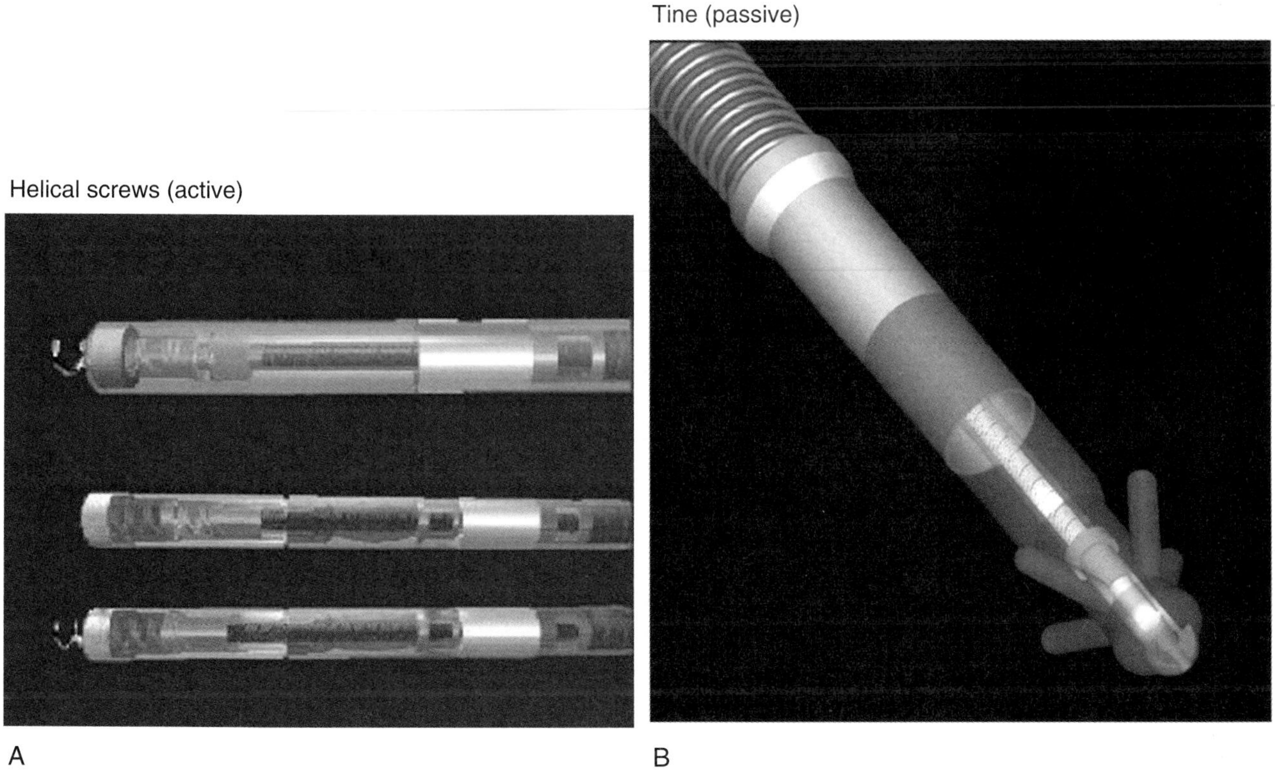

Figure 79–3 **Fixation mechanisms of pacing leads.**
(Courtesy of Medtronic, Inc.)

[O]). The second position refers to the chamber(s) being **sensed**. The third position is used to indicate the **response the pacemaker has to sensing**, or the action performed by the pacemaker (PM) in response to sensing of intrinsic electric activity. The response to sensing events by the PM may be *triggered* (T), *inhibited* (I), both (D), or none (O). In a *triggered* mode, a sensed event leads to delivery of a pacing stimulus. The triggered mode is used to prevent inappropriate inhibition by an incorrectly sensed event, such as skeletal muscle myopotentials. This function can be life saving in patients who are pacemaker dependent. The *inhibited* mode leads to inhibition of stimulus delivery in the designated chamber after sensing of intrinsic electrical activity. When the sensing response is *dual* (i.e., triggered *and* inhibited), pacing in the ventricle or atrium does not occur for a programmable period of time after intrinsic ventricular activity is sensed (i.e., pacing is *inhibited*). Additionally, when the sensing response is *dual*, sensing of intrinsic atrial activity leads to *inhibition* of an atrial pacing stimulus but it results in *triggering* of a ventricular pacing stimulus after the programmed AV delay.

The fourth position of the generic pacemaker code denotes the **programmability or rate modulation**. The possible functions at this position include simple programmable (P), multiprogrammable (M), communicating (C), rate modulation (R), or none (O). Simple programmable suggests that the programmability of the PM is limited to certain parameters, while multiprogrammable PMs are able to program a large number of parameters. The communicating function refers to the ability to exchange signals between the PM and a PM programming device. Rate modulation (R) is the most commonly denoted function in the fourth position. It denotes the capability of the PM to adjust the pacing rate according to a sensor device. Pacemaker manufacturers have designed a variety of sensors that attempt to match the individual's physical activity or metabolic demands by responding to different sources such as motion, temperature, and/or chest wall impedance (as an estimate of minute ventilation).

The fifth position in the pacemaker code relates to **antitachycardia therapies**: antitachycardia pacing (P), shock (S), dual (D = shock and pacing), or none (O). Since the advent of implantable cardioverter defibrillators, the fifth position is not generally used when referring to pacing systems.

Table 79-2 summarizes the most commonly used pacing modes, including advantages/disadvantages of each one as well as their clinical applications.[32] See Figure 79-4 for an example of DDD pacing mode on a 12-lead ECG.

Implantable Cardioverter Defibrillators

The guidelines for implantation of ICDs are reviewed earlier in this chapter. Despite the ongoing advancement in the development of today's defibrillators, their primary goal remains to deliver rapid and effective treatment of ventricular tachyarrhythmias.

Pulse Generator

The vast majority of ICD generators are currently implanted in the pectoral region. The pulse generator is composed of a

Table 79–2

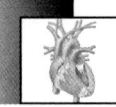

Commonly Encountered Pacing Modes

Mode	Advantages	Disadvantages	Clinical uses
AAI(R)	Requires only a single lead Simple	Slow ventricular rates may develop if AV block occurs	Sinus node dysfunction without AV node dysfunction
VVI(R)	Requires only a single lead Simple	During pacing, atrioventricular synchrony is not preserved	AV block in a patient with atrial fibrillation
DDD(R)	AV synchrony is maintained for patients with sinus node and AV node disease	Requires two leads More complex	Bradycardia caused by sinus node node disease or AV node disease
VDD(R)	AV synchrony is maintained for patients with AV node disease One specially designed lead can be used	AV synchrony is lost if the patient develops sinus bradycardia	Bradycardia caused by AV node disease
DDI(R)	AV synchrony is maintained during atrial pacing	AV synchrony is not maintained during atrial sensing	For patients with bradycardia and intermittent atrial tachycardias. Not used as a stand-alone pacing mode but as a mode switching pacing mode

From Wang PJ, et al: Modes of pacemaker function in cardiac pacing for the clinician. In Kusumoto M, Goldschlager N, editors: Cardiac Pacing for the Clinician. Philadelphia: Lippincott Williams & Wilkins, 2001.

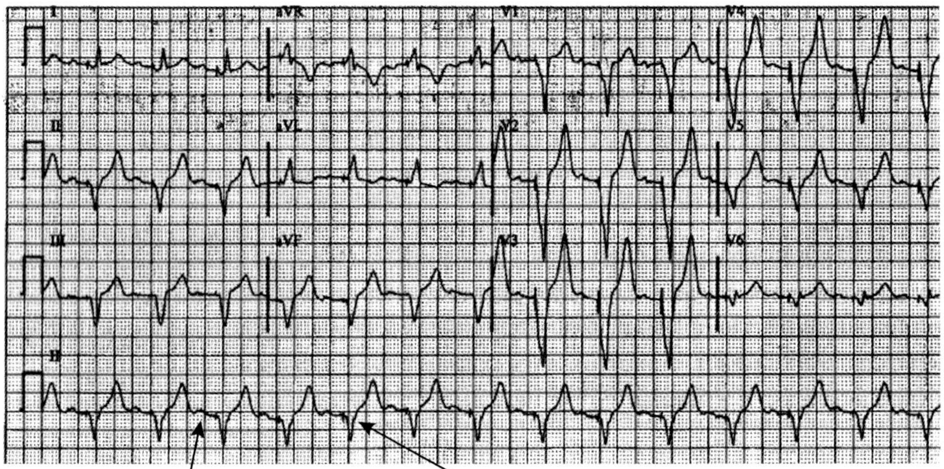

Figure 79–4 Example of DDD pacing mode on a 12-lead ECG.

lithium silver vanadium oxide battery and a capacitator. Whereas in 1989, generator volumes exceeded 200 cm^3, current generators are less than 40 cm^3.[10] Progressively smaller ICD generators have become viable as a result of continued progress in battery and capacitator technology. Essential functions that must be reliably performed by the ICD generator include monitoring of cardiac electrical activity through sense amplifiers, analyzing waveforms for the proper diagnosis of arrhythmias, and delivering appropriate therapy. The lifetime of the battery depends on the battery capacity and it is inversely related to the number of shocks and to the percentage of time spent in monitoring and pacing.

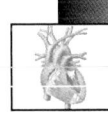

In addition to the battery and capacitator, the generator houses the operational circuitry of the device, which is comprised of low-power circuits (sensing, pacing, amplifiers, microprocessors) and high-power charging and output circuits.[10]

Leads

Early defibrillators used high-voltage epicardial (or pericardial) electrode patches for defibrillation. These electrode patches were also responsible for sensing, but frequent problems due to oversensing prompted the use of a separate sensing lead (epicardial or endocardial). With the development of transvenous defibrillators, electrode patches are now only rarely used.

Currently used endocardial leads are made of high-voltage conductors. At least one conductor is used as the defibrillation coil, which is generally found near the tip of the lead and placed along the posterior right ventricular wall. Some leads have two conductors (or two shocking coils). In such dual-coil leads, the distal coil is in the right ventricle (RV) and the proximal coil resides anywhere between the subclavian vein, superior vena cava (SVC), and right atrium. Separate single-coil leads may instead be implanted in the RV, SVC, coronary sinus (CS), or in a combination of these sites; subcutaneous tissue arrays may also be used. Leads placed in the RV are required to exhibit sensing and pacing capabilities, whereas such functions are not necessary in leads placed in the SVC or CS.

Generally, defibrillation using the pulse generator as one of the electrodes can be achieved using lower energies than defibrillation with a combination of leads. The defibrillation threshold (DFT) is the "lowest clinically obtained energy that can achieve defibrillation."[31] A combination of any three electrodes may be used, instead of two, in an attempt to lower the DFT.

Endocardial ICD leads perform sensing through a distal electrode at the tip of the lead. The same electrode may also be used for pacing. Unipolar ICD leads (normally placed in the SVC or CS) have a single high-voltage coil used for defibrillation and are not able to pace/sense. Bipolar ICD leads have two conductors, one of which is used for defibrillation and the other for sensing. Such leads sense intrinsic electric activity between the tip of the lead and anywhere along the extent of the shocking coil (*integrated bipolar sensing*). In contrast to true bipolar sensing, integrated bipolar sensing more often leads to oversensing because of noise and far field artifact as well as to undersensing after high-voltage defibrillation.[16] Newer defibrillator leads perform true bipolar sensing between the distal tip of the lead and a ring located approximately 1 cm proximally from the tip. Most recently, "quadripolar" leads are now available that perform true bipolar sensing (between the tip of the lead and the ring, as described above) and also incorporate two defibrillation coils.

Tachyarrhythmia Detection

Detection of tachyarrhythmias occurs when the device analyzes recent cycle lengths and R-wave morphologies in order to classify rhythms and determine appropriate programmed therapy.[10] Since some arrhythmias are unsustained, ICDs must effectively be able to detect the arrhythmia, confirm it prior to delivering therapy, and redetect the arrhythmia if the delivered therapy was unsuccessful. Current devices may be set to have multiple zones of detection (e.g., VT, fast VT, and/or VF zones) for which specific therapies can be individually programmed (*tiered therapy*).

Although arrhythmia detection by current ICDs is very reliable, inappropriate shocks may still occur even if the device is functioning properly. Such unnecessary shocks most commonly occur in the setting of atrial fibrillation (or other supraventricular tachycardia) or sinus tachycardia if the ventricular rate falls into one of the detection zones.[16] Newer and more sophisticated devices have built-in algorithms or additional detection parameters designed to prevent inappropriate shocks by increasing the specificity of VT detection. For safety reasons, these algorithms are available only in the lowest VT rate cutoff zones and include sudden onset and rate stability criteria as well as criterion based on electrogram morphology.

Tachyarrhythmia Therapy

Current devices can deliver a range of programmable therapies: high-energy defibrillation shocks, low-energy synchronized cardioversion, and antitachycardia pacing.

High-Energy Defibrillation

As previously described, the DFT is the lowest clinically obtained energy that can accomplish defibrillation. The patient's autonomic and metabolic state may alter the DFT such that an energy output previously able to achieve defibrillation at a particular time may fail at others. Therefore, after the DFT is determined, a safety margin of at least 10 J is recommended between the maximum output of the device and the DFT. Figure 79-5 depicts an episode of successful defibrillation of VF by a high-energy therapy delivered by an ICD.

It is important to note that antiarrhythmic drugs may alter the DFT. Amiodarone commonly raises the DFT while sotalol lowers it.[17,26] Procainamide and quinidine do not appear to affect DFT.[11]

Low-Energy Synchronized Cardioversions

Low-energy synchronized cardioversions can be delivered faster (shorter charging time) than high-energy defibrillation and may save device battery. Unlike VF, some VT can be terminated with very low energy therapies, which may cause less discomfort to the patient. Disadvantages of low-energy synchronized shocks include acceleration of VT to VF, which may delay definitive therapy.

Antitachycardia Pacing (ATP)

Multiple extra stimuli (with or without addition of premature stimuli to a train of extra stimuli) delivered during tachycardia may interact with the tachycardia circuit and thereby terminate it. ATP can be programmed in today's ICDs, and it is widely used as initial therapy to treat VT. Similarly to low-energy synchronized cardioversions, ATP carries the risk of accelerating VT to VF in which case a

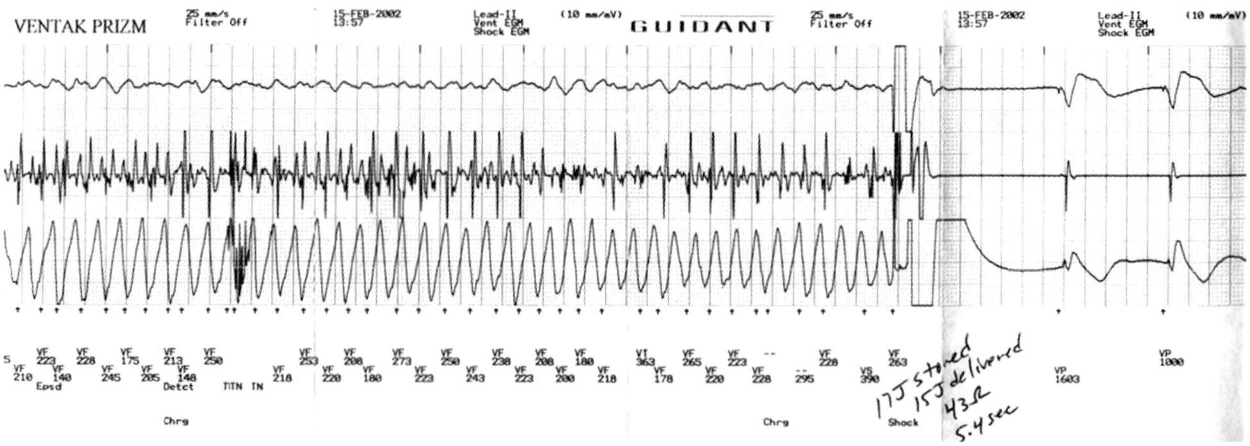

Figure 79–5 **High-energy defibrillation of ventricular fibrillation.**

high-voltage shock could be delivered to terminate VF. Advantages of ATP as initial therapy for VT include faster delivery time, less patient discomfort, and sparing of device battery (if successful). Figure 79-6 shows an example of successful termination of VT by ATP, while Figure 79-7 depicts a failed ATP attempt to terminate VT.

PREOPERATIVE EVALUATION PRIOR TO IMPLANTATION OF CARDIAC DEVICES

Clinical Considerations

A careful history and physical examination should be performed. Aspects that warrant special attention focus on the assessment of prior injury or pathology within the planned region for device implantation. A history of prior shoulder/chest injury, surgery, or radiation may alert the implanting physician of the potential for abnormal venous drainage, which may increase the technical complexity of the implant. Allergies to medications (including antibiotics, local anesthetic, and intravenous narcotics and benzodiazepines used for conscious sedation) and/or intravenous contrast should be identified and recorded. It is especially important to recognize and appropriately treat signs and/or symptoms of active infection prior to implantation of a permanent cardiac device. Prophylactic antibiotics are administered immediately prior to and for 48 h post-device implantation. Another essential consideration is the patient's respiratory status. Device implantations generally require that the patient lies flat for the duration of the procedure (up to 2–3 h). Therefore, oxygenation and volume status should be optimized prior to implant.

If the patient is being treated with warfarin, the medication should be held ~4 days prior to the implant date. In our institution, it is generally required that the INR be less than 1.8 prior to implant.

STANDARD TRANSVENOUS TECHNIQUE FOR IMPLANTATION OF CARDIAC DEVICES

Temporary Transvenous Pacemakers

Percutaneous venous access may be obtained via the internal jugular, subclavian, femoral, or antecubital veins. A lock-

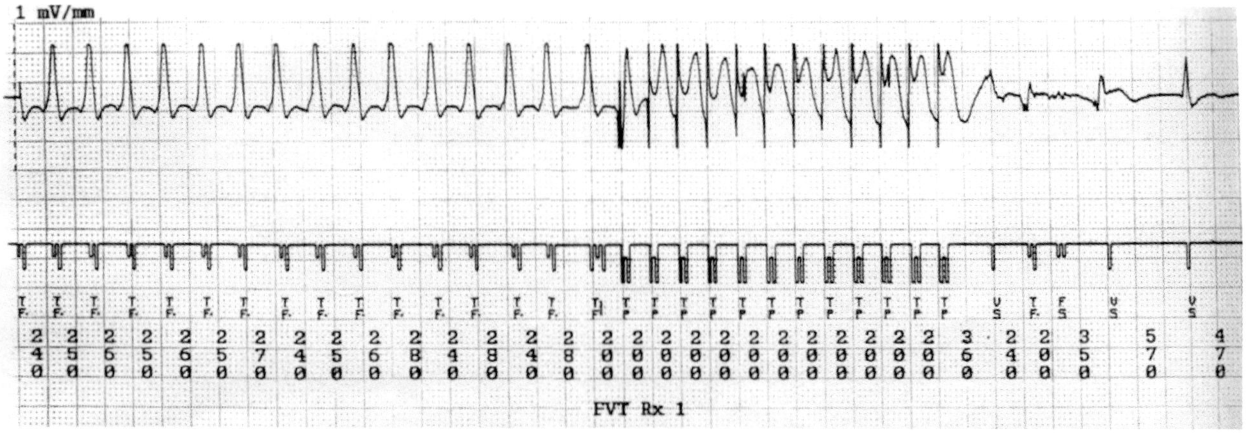

Figure 79–6 **Electrograms of antitachycardia pacing-induced termination of ventricular tachycardia (VT) stored by implantable cardioverter defibrillator.** 250 ms = 240 bpm; FVT, fast VT.

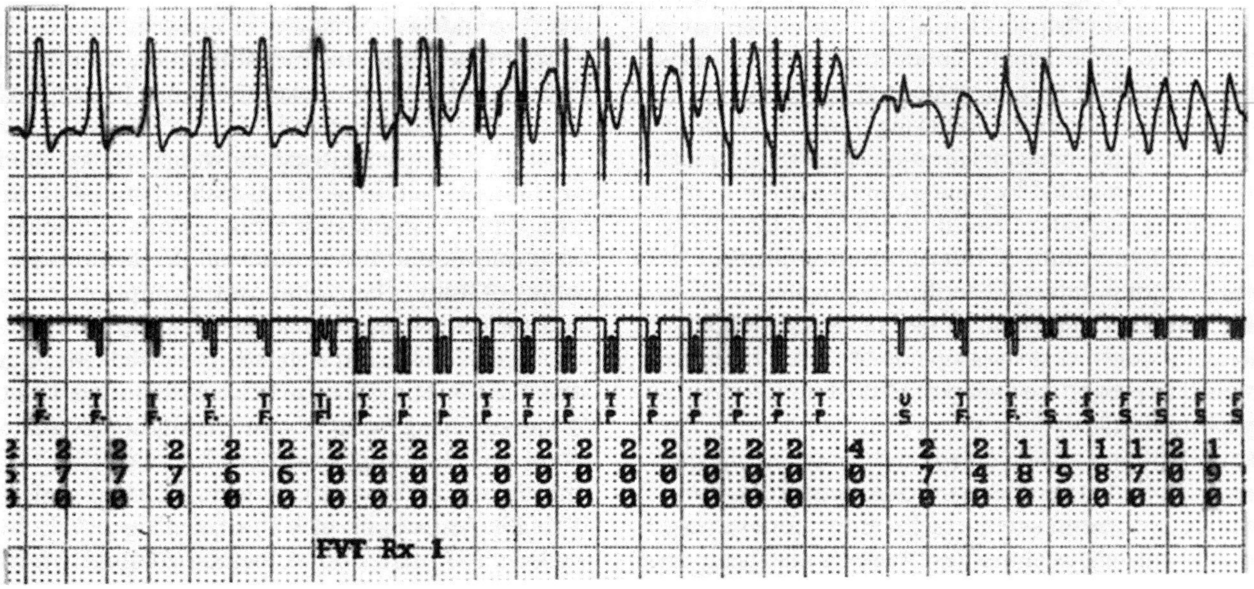

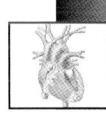

Figure 79–7 **Failed attempt by antitachycardia pacing to terminate ventricular tachycardia.**

down sheath should be introduced in the vein for better lead stability. Fluoroscopy should always be used to guide lead placement when the femoral or antecubital veins are used. The pacing catheter should be advanced to the right ventricle with care to avoid excessive force that could result in cardiac perforation. The ideal position for the catheter tip is the distal RV septum or inferoapex. The right ventricular free wall and outflow tract should be avoided because of the risk of catheter-induced ectopy and decreased lead stability. After placement of the lead, the sensing and pacing thresholds should be determined. An R-wave greater or equal to 5 mV and a pacing threshold of 1 mA or less are adequate. After acceptable placement of the lead has occurred, the sheath should be locked down around the lead. The sheath should then be sutured and the lead secured to the adjacent skin and covered with a dry sterile dressing. A postprocedure chest X-ray should be obtained to confirm lead position and rule out pneumothorax. At least twice daily sensing and pacing thresholds should be assessed.

If fluoroscopy is not available, a balloon-tipped catheter should be introduced via the internal jugular or subclavian veins. The distal electrode tip (generally negatively charged) should be connected to one of the precordial leads of a 12-lead ECG (generally V_1). The limb leads (e.g., lead II) should be recorded and the intracardiac electrogram (EGM) should be monitored as the balloon-tipped pacing catheter is slowly introduced. When the distal electrode on the tip of the catheter reaches the right atrium, a large atrial EGM (corresponding to the P wave seen on the limb leads) followed by a smaller ventricular EGM (corresponding to the QRS on the surface ECG) should be noted. As the catheter is advanced into the right ventricle, the ventricular EGM grows larger and the atrial signal becomes smaller. Once the tip of the pacing catheter comes in contact with the myocardium, an injury current (reminiscent of "ST elevation") will be recorded immediately following the ventricular EGM, and the catheter should not be advanced further. After the pacing catheter is positioned and secured, a 12-lead ECG should always be obtained to corroborate, based on the morphology of the paced QRS complexes, proper positioning of the catheter.

When asystole (or severe bradycardia) is present, the pacing electrode tips (distal and proximal) should be connected to an active pacing box (or generator) programmed to pace in VVI mode. Paced QRS complexes should emerge once contact of the catheter tip to myocardium occurs.

When temporary atrial (instead of ventricular) or AV sequential pacing is required, a temporary pacing catheter/lead can be placed in the right atrium (active fixation lead) or in the coronary sinus. The atrial pacing threshold is generally higher in the coronary sinus than in the right atrium.

Duration of temporary pacing should be limited to less than 72 h to minimize the risk of infection, cardiac perforation, and lead dislodgement. Active fixation leads connected to an externalized pacemaker generator may be left in place for longer periods of time.

Permanent Pacemakers

Most permanent transvenous pacemakers are placed in the right or left pectoral region via the cephalic, axillary, or subclavian veins. A peripheral intravenous catheter should be placed on the upper extremity ipsilateral to the planned implant in the event venography is necessary to define the anatomy and/or availability of access. Unless the patient is left-handed or the left side is inaccessible, the left pectoral region is preferable due to greater simplicity of lead placement and manipulation. Prophylactic antibiotics should be administered as described above and the pectoral region should be prepped and draped in sterile fashion.

Cephalic Vein (Cut Down Approach)

Local anesthetic is delivered to the pectoral region. An oblique incision is made over the deltopectoral groove and extended inward using blunt dissection. Alternatively, a horizontal incision 2 cm below the clavicle (with its lateral border extending over the deltopectoral groove) may be chosen. The cephalic vein runs in the deltopectoral groove, which can be identified by the presence of a fatty streak between the pectoralis and deltoid muscles. Once the cephalic vein is identified, it should be dissected free from the surrounding fat and connective tissue. An 0 silk suture is placed around the vein (but not tied) proximally and another one distally, and a 5 French (F) dilator is placed in the vein. Under fluoroscopic guidance, a guide wire is introduced into the 5F dilator and advanced to the inferior vena cava (IVC) via the subclavian vein, SVC, and the right atrium (RA); the 5F dilator is then removed. Venography may be necessary via the 5F introducer or via a peripheral line to establish patency of the vessels or define the venous anatomy, if difficulty in advancing the wire is encountered.

Axillary Vein Approach

The axillary vein can be cannulated via the same cut down location in the deltopectoral region. The axillary vein is accessed through a single wall puncture technique utilizing landmarks or direct visualization via venography.

Subclavian Vein Approach

The subclavian vein may also be accessed by using a single wall puncture technique. Figure 79-8 illustrates the anatomical location of the subclavian, axillary, and cephalic veins.

Regardless of the vein used for access, a guide wire is advanced to the IVC under fluoroscopy. The subclavian vein approach is generally the least desirable because of the risk of pneumothorax and the potential risk of crush injury to the pacing leads as they pass between the clavicle and first rib.

Once venous access has been secured and the guide wire positioned in the IVC, sheaths (or introducers) are utilized for sequential placement of atrial and ventricular leads. While a lead is being placed through the sheath, the patient should be instructed to transiently refrain from talking or breathing to avoid complication by air embolus via the introducer sheath. The fluoroscopic view for optimal placement of the RV lead is generally obtained from the right anterior oblique (RAO) position. This view allows for proper visualization of the full length of the RV (foreshortened in the anteroposterior view). Adequate lead position along the RV inferoseptum and apex should also be confirmed in the left anterior oblique (LAO) view. Ventricular ectopy may occur during lead placement, but it is generally transient. If there is persistent VT, the lead should be repositioned. If VT continues despite lead repositioning, the rhythm should be terminated by ATP or defibrillation.

Ventricular sensing and pacing thresholds should be checked, and the QRS morphology in lead V_1 should be assessed to confirm that pacing originates from the right ventricle (left bundle-branch block morphology should be present in lead V_1). When a right bundle-branch block (RBBB) morphology is present in lead V_1, pacing from the left ventricular endocardium (via an atrial or ventricular septal defect), from the coronary sinus, or from the LV epicardium (as a result of cardiac perforation) should be suspected. Occasionally, an RBBB morphology will be seen with pacing from the RV septum.

The atrial lead is generally placed in the right atrial appendage if present. However, any location in the RA is acceptable if stable, provided no excessive sensing of the ventricular electrogram is present.

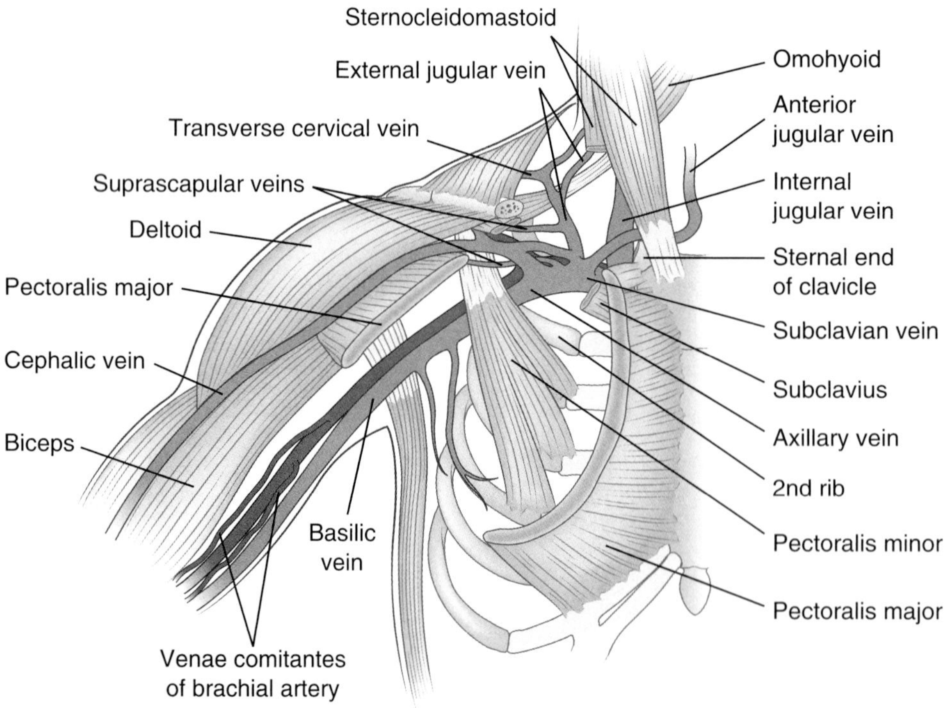

Figure 79–8 Anatomical illustration of the subclavian, axillary, and cephalic veins. *(Modified from Agur AMR, Lee MJ: Upper limb. In Grant's Atlas of Anatomy, 10th ed. Philadelphia: Lippincott Williams & Wilkins, 1999.)*

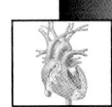

Once acceptable positions for both leads have been obtained, lead stability should be confirmed during coughing and deep breathing exercises. Lead locations should be confirmed from the RAO and LAO views. High output pacing should be performed from both leads to rule out diaphragmatic capture during pacing. Stylets and guide wire should be removed, and proper amount of slack in each lead should be ensured fluoroscopically. After optimal lead positions are confirmed, the leads should be secured to the pectoralis muscle using nonabsorbable suture tied around anchoring sleeves. Final sensing and pacing thresholds should be checked after the leads have been sutured to the pectoralis fascia.

After the leads are secured, local anesthesia is administered to the subcutaneous tissues medial to the deltopectoral groove in order to create a subcutaneous (or submuscular) pocket for the device generator. The pocket is created using blunt dissection and copiously irrigated. The leads are then connected to the pulse generator according to the indicated positions. The leads are coiled under the generator and the entire system is implanted into the pocket. Proper sensing and pacing by the device should be confirmed.

The subcutaneous tissues are closed with absorbable suture, and the skin is closed using a subcuticular layer of absorbable suture or staples. A dry sterile dressing should be placed over the wound.

Implantation of single-chamber devices is done using the same technique described above, except for placement of the second lead. Figure 79-9 depicts a chest X-ray with the expected lead position for a single-chamber transvenous pacemaker.

Implantable Cardioverter Defibrillators

Surgical techniques used to implant epicardial patches used in early ICDs will not be discussed in this chapter, which will concentrate on the transvenous implantation of current cardioverter defibrillators.

The left pectoral region is preferred for most ICD implants, whether the patient is right- or left-handed. The coil configuration obtained with a left-sided implant allows for a more effective field orientation for defibrillation, when one of the shocking electrodes lies within the pulse generator. The technique used to place modern transvenous ICDs is the same as the one described to implant transvenous permanent pacemakers (see previously), although the first transvenous ICDs required abdominal pulse generators because of their large size (transvenous leads were tunneled subcutaneously to the abdomen where the generator was implanted). Also, subcutaneous patches or arrays were often necessary in early ICDs in order to achieve acceptable DFT. In Figure 79-10, a postprocedure chest X-ray confirms appropriate lead positions in a dual-chamber transvenous ICD.

In addition to the technique described for transvenous pacemakers, the procedure for any ICD implant includes defibrillation testing to determine the DFT. Defibrillation testing is generally performed prior to wound closure, after the leads are connected to the pulse generator and after the system is implanted into the pocket.

The programmer is used to communicate with the device via a sterile wand placed over the pocket. Prior to VF induction and ICD testing, some operators deliver a low-energy synchronized shock to allow for confirmation of intact connections by checking the high-voltage lead impedance. External defibrillation hands-off pads are also placed and connected to an external biphasic defibrillator in the event of device failure to terminate VF. Testing is generally performed at the least sensitive device setting to

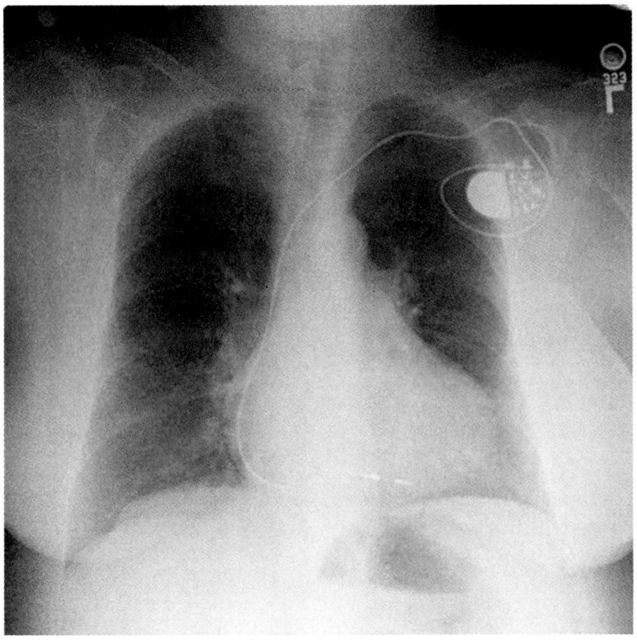

Figure 79–9 Posteroanterior chest X-ray showing appropriate lead position for a single-chamber transvenous pacemaker.

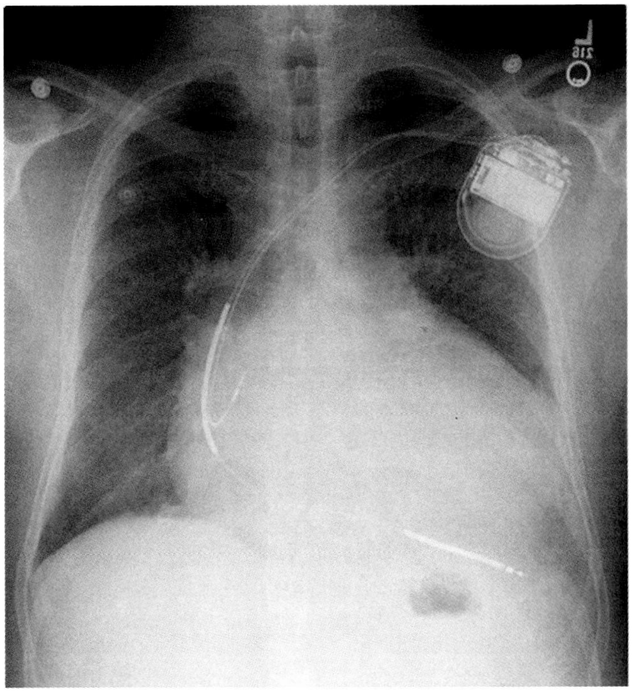

Figure 79–10 Posteroanterior chest X-ray showing appropriate lead positions for a dual-chamber transvenous implantable cardioverter defibrillator.

detect VF to ensure an adequate safety margin. After successful testing, the device is programmed at the most sensitive setting for VF detection. VF is most commonly induced by timed T wave shocks or by rapid-burst ventricular pacing at 50 Hz.

At our institution, initial testing is performed using a selected energy (~10 J lower than the maximum device output), which allows for an adequate safety margin between the tested energy and the maximum device output (margin-verification protocol). A second shock using a lower energy is often performed. Prior to testing, we generally set the second device therapy as a maximum output shock, which is delivered if the first tested energy fails and after VF is redetected. If a high-output shock via the device fails to terminate VF, a 360-J biphasic shock is externally delivered.

Normally, a 5-min "rest" period is provided between each induction of VF. Other important parameters evaluated during ICD testing include the high-voltage lead impedance and the charge time for delivery of high-voltage therapies.

If an adequate DFT is not obtained during testing, addition of extra defibrillation coils (including subcutaneous arrays or patches), reversing shock polarity, and/or repositioning of the RV lead may be necessary. A 7–10 J safety margin should be incorporated in the final therapy programming of the device. After an acceptable DFT is obtained, the wound is closed as described previously.

POSTIMPLANT CARE OF TRANSVENOUS CARDIAC DEVICES

Patients undergoing implantation of electrophysiological cardiac devices should be observed overnight in the hospital. Continuous telemetry monitoring should be performed during this time to allow for early diagnosis and treatment of lead malfunction and/or dislodgement (the most common complication in the early postoperative period). Bed rest is recommended overnight, and the arm ipsilateral to the implant is placed in a sling for 24 h. While the patient is allowed to move that arm after 24 h, lifting of objects weighing more than 5–10 pounds and raising the arm above shoulder level should be avoided for 6 weeks after the procedure. A posteroanterior and lateral chest X-ray should be obtained on the morning after implant to assess adequate lead and generator positions. If the subclavian vein was used for venous access, a portable chest X-ray is required immediately postimplant to rule out pneumothorax. Anticoagulation with intravenous heparin or low-molecular-weight heparin should be avoided for at least the first 8 h after implant. If anticoagulation must be started within the first week postimplant, it should be dosed cautiously to avoid overanticoagulation and bleeding complications. Since it may take days for warfarin to reach therapeutic levels, it may be started on the evening after the procedure. We recommend the use of prophylactic antibiotics as described previously.

The device should be interrogated on the day after implant to ensure proper device function and to fine-tune the device programming if necessary. The wound should be kept dry for at least 1 week postimplant. A follow-up appointment should be scheduled within 7–10 days of discharge for wound check and device reinterrogation. Marked changes in lead impedance and in pacing and sensing thresholds would be identified at that time and could indicate lead dislodgement and/or malfunction.

COMPLICATIONS OF IMPLANTABLE CARDIAC DEVICES

Serious complications of device implantation occur in less than 2% of patients undergoing the procedure. Procedural complications may be classified as *"early,"* which may include intraoperative, perioperative (within 24 h), or postoperative complications (after 24 h but within 30 days of the procedure), or *"late,"* occurring after 30 days from the procedure.

Examples of early complications are outlined in Box 79-13 and include bleeding, vascular injury, infection, pneumothorax, hemothorax, air embolus, cardiac perforation/ tamponade, rhythm abnormalities, deep vein thrombosis, pulmonary embolism, lead dislodgement/fracture/damage, and pocket hematoma. Late complications are also listed in Box 79-13 and may include lead fracture or insulation break, lead dislodgement, pocket skin erosion, infection, migration of generator possibly leading to lead twisting and fracture, and deep vein thrombosis/scarring. Figure 79-11 shows an example of skin erosion with subsequent infection of a device pocket.

EXTRACTION OF CHRONIC LEADS USED IN TRANSVENOUS CARDIAC DEVICES

Overview

Since the introduction of transvenous pacing electrodes in 1958 by Furman and Schwedel,[12] techniques to safely remove such leads have been developed and perfected over time. Earlier techniques focused on the simple use of trac-

Box 79–13. Early and Late Complications of Implantable Cardiac Devices.

Early	Late
Bleeding	Infection of device pocket or lead(s) (2.7%)
Infection	Pocket erosion/wound breakdown
Pneumothorax/hemothorax	Lead fracture/insulation damage (0.2%)
Cardiac perforation	Venous thrombosis
SVC perforation	Chronic pain
Lead migration/dislodgement (2%)	Tricuspid regurgitation
Air embolus	Left ventricular dysfunction
Venous thrombosis	Migration of pulse generator
Atrial tachyarrhythmias	Twisting and/or fracture of leads due to manipulation of generator (Twiddler's syndrome)
Ventricular tachycardia	
AV block by contact injury to the conduction system	
Pocket hematoma	

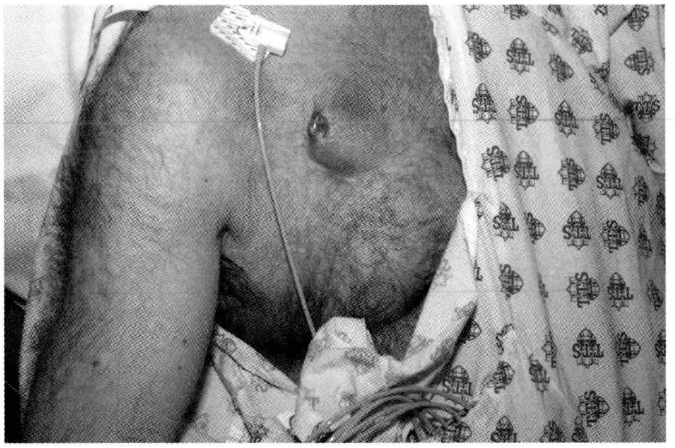

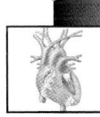

Figure 79–11 Example of skin erosion and subsequent infection of device pocket.

tion, which can be done safely and without the assistance of especially designed tools only in recently implanted leads (generally, <1-year-old implants) that have not developed significant fibrosis. For more chronic leads, complications preclude the use of simple traction, and surgical approaches that require sternotomy or thoracotomy were initially the only viable options. Since the mid-1980s,[3–6,8,13] safer transvenous methods for chronic lead extraction have continued to be developed.

Official definitions and guidelines for the practice of transvenously placed-lead extractions were published in 1999.[27] The term "lead extraction" is reserved only for the removal of a lead that requires specialized equipment, or from a route other than the implant vein, or of any lead implanted for more than 1 year. A complete summary of indications for lead extraction is provided in Box 79-14. Class 1 indications include serious illness caused by an infected lead, clinical need for a new transvenous cardiac device when all usable veins are obstructed, and malfunctioning, fractured, or suboptimally positioned leads that pose danger to the patient. Relative contraindications for transvenous lead extraction include lead calcification (detected on X-ray) involving the RA or the SVC, unavailability of suitable equipment, patient's clinical condition precludes emergent thoracotomy, or lead placed via unusual routes (e.g., subclavian artery, pericardial space). Because of the potentially serious complications of transvenous lead extractions, physicians properly trained in these techniques and adequately equipped institutions are absolute requirements for the performance of lead extractions.

Data from the United States Extraction Database for intravascular extraction of infected or problematic pacemaker leads from January 1994 to April 1996 were published in 1999.[7] In this series, success rate for complete removal of the

Box 79–14. Indications for Lead Removal/Extraction Using Transvenous Techniques.

Class 1	Class 2	Class 3
Sepsis (including endocarditis) due to documented infection of any intravascular part of the pacing system, or as a result of a device pocket infection when the intravascular portion of the lead system cannot be aseptically separated from the pocket Life-threatening arrhythmias secondary to a retained lead fragment	Localized pocket infection or erosion that does not involve the transvenous portion of the lead system, when the lead can be cut through a clean incision that is totally separate from the infected area	Any situation where the risk posed by removal of the lead is significantly higher than the benefit of removing the lead
	An occult infection for which no source can be found and for which the pacing system is suspected	A single nonfunctional transvenous lead in an older patient
A retained lead, lead fragment, or extraction hardware that poses an immediate or imminent physical threat to the patient	Chronic pain at the pocket or lead insertion site that causes significant discomfort for the patient, is not manageable by medical or surgical techniques A lead that may pose a nonimmediate or nonimminent threat to the patient if left in place A lead that interferes with the treatment of a malignancy	Any normally functioning lead that may be reused at the time of pulse generator replacement, provided the lead has a reliable performance history
Clinically significant thromboembolic events caused by a retained lead or lead fragment Obliteration or occlusion of all usable, veins with the need to implant a new transvenous pacing system A lead that interferes with the operation of another implanted device (e.g., pacemaker or defibrillator)	A traumatic injury to the entry site of the lead for which the lead may interfere with reconstruction of the site Leads preventing access to the venous circulation for newly required implantable devices Nonfunctional leads in a young patient	

From North American Society of Pacing and Electrophysiology Lead Extraction Conference Faculty: Love CJ, Wilkoff BL, Byrd CL, et al: NASPE policy statement. Recommendations for extraction of chronically implanted transvenous pacing and defibrillator leads: indications, facilities, training. Pacing Clin Electrophysiol 23(4): 544–551, 2000.

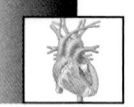

lead occurred in 93% of leads and for partial removal in 5% of leads; 2% failed. Major complications occurred in 1.4% (<1% in centers that performed >300 extractions) of patients and minor complications in 1.7% of patients. Major complications occurred more frequently in women. Predictors of incomplete lead removal or failure included longer implant duration, less experienced operators, ventricular lead location, noninfected leads, and younger patient age.

Tools Used in Chronic Lead Transvenous Extractions

Angiographic Catheters, Snares, Forceps, and Locking Stylets

Angiographic catheters that are commonly used to assist in lead extractions include the angled pigtail catheter, the Judkins right coronary catheter, the multipurpose coronary catheter, and the Amplatz catheter. These catheters are used in combination with common guide wires or tip-deflecting guide wires that loop around or hook onto the pacemaker lead in order to retrieve it. This approach may also be used to retrieve loose lead ends or free-floating lead remnants. Other tools used include the basket retriever catheter, the Dotter intravascular retriever (helical-loop basket) that gets irreversibly entrapped to the lead, and the Dormia basket.

Different types of snares are also available and are used in conjunction with catheters and guide wires to recover and extract chronic pacemaker leads. Examples of snares include the Curry snare (used to form a wire-loop system), the Amplatz gooseneck snare (loop at a right angle to the guide wire), and the Needle's Eye snare created by Cook Vascular, Inc. (consisting of a hoop-shaped loop and a locking slide threader) that provides a reversible system that is able to release the seized object.

Cook has also developed a "locking stylet" that is efficient in seizing and holding the lead while preventing the lead from stretching or uncoiling as it is being retrieved.[1]

Forceps (grasping forceps, alligator forceps, and myocardial bicep forceps) have also been used for lead extractions. This stylet intensifies the tensile power of the lead and directs the extraction force to the tip of the lead. The locking system is engaged and released by counterclockwise and clockwise rotation, respectively.

Byrd Dilator Sheaths

These sheaths were marketed by Cook Vascular, Inc. and may be used to assist with extractions performed via the implant vein. They consist of telescoping stainless steel sheaths with metal dilators that are advanced over the lead to sever through the thick fibrous adhesions found at the venous entry site and distal ends of chronic leads. Once entrance to the vein is attained, the metal dilators are exchanged for telescoping flexible plastic sheaths that are able to negotiate the turns.

Excimer Laser Sheaths

Excimer laser sheaths were developed by Charles Byrd and are used in association with the Spectranetics CVX-300 excimer laser system.[1] The laser sheath contains a ring of optical fibers at its distal tip able to emit pulses of ultraviolet light that destroy the surrounding fibrous tissues around the lead. Mild countertraction and counterpressure activate the laser. An advantage of the laser system is that tissue vaporization is achieved, as opposed to blunt tissue dissection and shredding. One disadvantage is that the system is not effective against calcifications, which are often encountered around older leads.

Electrosurgical Dissection Systems

The most recent advancement in lead extraction equipment includes the electrosurgical dissection system (EDS) developed by Cook Vascular, Inc. Such systems use radiofrequency (RF) energy (instead of laser or blunt dissection) to destroy the fibrous endovascular adhesions that anchor device leads to venous walls. The most recent RF-based system has a dual electrode scheme that performs a bipolar dissection while also functioning as a mechanical dissection sheath. The tip electrode spacing is such that it effectively localizes the disruptive energies to the specific regions interfering with extraction of the lead, as opposed to circumferentially obliterating the endovascular border.

Techniques of Chronic Lead Transvenous Extractions

Transvenous lead extractions should preferably be performed in a setting appropriate for emergent thoracotomy; a cardiothoracic surgeon should be promptly available. Prior to any transvenous extraction of chronic pacemaker leads, the patient should be prepped in advance for potential thoracotomy. Intraarterial blood pressure monitoring is recommended. Transthoracic and transesophageal echocardiography and a pericardiocentesis tray should be readily accessible to allow for expeditious diagnosis and treatment of possible complications. A temporary pacing wire should be placed via the femoral vein if the patient is pacemaker dependent.

Extraction via the Implant Vein

The generator should be removed and the leads completely freed from adhesions and sutures, and dissected down to the venous entry site. If the patient is pacemaker dependent, a temporary pacing wire (normally introduced via the femoral vein) should have been placed ahead of time. The proximal end of the lead, which includes the connector pin, should be cut and 1 cm of the lead inner coil should be exposed. A coil expander is used to remove any wire burs and to ensure patency of the lead lumen. A locking stylet should then be advanced into the lead inner coil until it reaches the distal tip of the lead. The locking mechanism is activated, and the outer lead insulation should be secured with a tie prior to introduction of the sheaths. If simple traction is not sufficient to free the lead from the myocardium once the locking stylet is in place, sheaths should be introduced to disrupt fibrous adhesions/scarring. Telescoping stainless steel sheaths (or other available sheaths including excimer laser sheaths and, most recently, electrosurgical dissection sheaths) should be advanced over the lead down to the venous entry site where they disrupt the scar tissue surrounding the lead. The sheaths should be advanced down under fluoroscopy to the distal tip of the lead as continuous traction is placed on the locking stylet system. The lead tip may then be pulled free by counterpressure and countertraction and the entire lead is extracted. If this method is unsuccessful, another technique (e.g., extraction via the femoral vein) may be used.

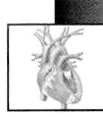

Extraction via the Femoral Vein

The femoral vein approach is the preferred technique used to extract lead remnants or broken/cut leads that are free-floating in the venous system, heart, or pulmonary artery.[1] It may also be used as a primary approach for transvenous extraction of permanent leads, especially if concern exists to push infected debris from the original entry site into the circulation. This approach engages angiographic catheters such as the angled pigtail catheter or a variety of snares (see previous page for different types of available snares) to grasp loose lead ends, or the deflecting wire and Dotter retriever if no freed ends are available. Traction is applied to pull the lead (or lead remnants) from the heart and the lead is then withdrawn from the body via the femoral vein sheath.

Complications

Serious complications may occur as a result of transvenous lead extractions. Complications may be intraoperative, perioperative (events that occur or are diagnosed within 24 h following the procedure), postoperative (events that occur or are diagnosed after 24 h but within 30 days of the procedure), or late (events that occur or are diagnosed at > 30 days from the procedure date). Box 79-15 summarizes major and minor complications related to transvenous lead extractions.

EMERGING APPLICATIONS OF CARDIAC DEVICES

Biventricular Pacing for the Treatment of Congestive Heart Failure

Over the past few years, biventricular (BiV) pacing or cardiac resynchronization therapy (CRT) has emerged as a new therapy for patients with advanced congestive heart failure (NYHA Class >II) due to systolic dysfunction (LVEF <35%) with intraventricular conduction delay (generally of the left bundle branch block [LBBB] type; QRS duration >120 ms) and mechanical desynchrony. The therapeutic intent is to improve the mechanical efficiency of the heart by simultaneously activating both ventricles with the use of an implantable pacemaker or pacemaker-defibrillator system.

Box 79–15. Major and Minor Complications Related to Transvenous Lead Extractions.

Major complications

- Death
- Cardiac avulsion or tear requiring thoracotomy, pericardiocentesis, chest tube, or surgical repair
- Vascular avulsion or tear requiring thoracotomy, pericardiocentesis, chest tube, or surgical repair
- Hemothorax or severe bleeding from any source requiring transfusion
- Pneumothorax requiring chest tube drainage
- Pulmonary embolism requiring surgical intervention
- Respiratory arrest
- Septic shock
- Stroke

Minor complications

- Pericardial effusion not requiring pericardiocentesis or surgical intervention
- Hemodynamically significant air embolism
- Pulmonary embolism not requiring intervention
- Vascular repair near the implant site or venous entry site
- Arrhythmia requiring cardioversion
- Hematoma at the pocket requiring drainage
- Arm swelling or thrombosis of implant veins resulting in medical intervention
- Sepsis in a previously nonseptic patient with infection
- Pacing system-related infection of a previously noninfected site

Observation

- Transient hypotension that responds to fluids or minor pharmacological intervention
- Nonsignificant air embolism
- Small pneumothorax not requiring intervention
- Ectopy not requiring cardioversion
- Arm swelling or thrombosis of implant veins without need for medical intervention
- Pain at cut-down site
- Myocardial avulsion without sequelae
- Migrated lead fragment without sequelae

From North American Society of Pacing and Electrophysiology Lead Extraction Conference Faculty: Love CJ, Wilkoff BL, Byrd CL, et al: NASPE policy statement. Recommendations for extraction of chronically implanted transvenous pacing and defibrillator leads: indications, facilities, training. Pacing Clin Electrophysiol 23(4):544–551, 2000.

Patients who have benefited from BiV pacing may have systolic dysfunction due to either coronary or noncoronary cardiomyopathies.

Simultaneous pacing of both ventricles is achieved by pacing the RV from a standard transvenous right ventricular apical lead while the left ventricle (LV) is paced by a transvenously placed coronary sinus lead. The preferred location for the coronary sinus (CS) lead is within the posterolateral CS vein where the activation delay is generally most pronounced because of the baseline LBBB-type intraventricular conduction delay. Figure 79-12 illustrates typical lead positions for a BiV pacing system.

MANAGEMENT OF CARDIAC DEVICES DURING AND AFTER SURGERY

Pacemakers

Application of a magnet over a pacemaker inhibits all sensing function of the pacemaker. The previously programmed pacing mode is subsequently transiently changed to DOO, VOO, or AOO until the magnet is removed. The magnet pacing rate varies according to the pacemaker manufacturer. The magnet may be used prophylactically prior to surgical procedures to avoid inappropriate sensing by the pacer due to noise artifact created by cautery. Other procedures during which there is a risk of inhibition of the pacer by inappropriate sensing of noise include electroconvulsive therapy, extracorporeal shockwave lithotripsy, and occasionally electric cardioversions.

Implantable Cardioverter Defibrillators

Unlike standard pacemakers, defibrillators with back-up pacing and pacemaker-defibrillators do not have their sensing function inhibited by a magnet. The magnet does, however, inhibit delivery of any antitachycardia therapy, such as ATP or high-energy defibrillation. Magnet inhibition of antitachycardia therapies prevents delivery of inappropriate ICD therapies during cautery or other procedures that could produce noise erroneously sensed by the lead as VT or VF. It is important to note that while a magnet is applied to an ICD causing inhibition of the programmed ICD therapies, the patient should be treated as any patient who does not have an ICD in the event that a tachyarrhythmia occurs. Alternatively, cautery (or other problematic procedures) may be transiently halted and the magnet removed from the ICD to allow for implementation and delivery of programmed ICD therapies. Additionally, if a patient is pacemaker dependent, a temporary pacing wire should be placed prior to potentially problematic procedures to avoid inappropriate sensing of noise and subsequent inappropriate inhibition of the pacing function of the ICD. Such inappropriate inhibition of pacing in a pacemaker-dependent patient could be catastrophic if not anticipated.

In general, ICDs should be interrogated following surgery to confirm proper functioning and parameter settings.

REFERENCES

1. Belott PH: Endocardial lead extraction. In Kusumoto FM, Goldschlager NF, editors: Cardiac Pacing for the Clinician. Philadelphia: Lippincott Williams & Wilkins, 2001, pp. 162–192.
2. Buxton AE, Lee KL, Fisher JD, et al: A randomized study of the prevention of sudden death in patients with coronary artery disease. N Engl J Med 341:1882–1890, 1999.
3. Byrd CL, Schwartz SJ, Hedin N: Intravascular techniques for extraction of permanent pacemaker leads. J Thorac Cardiovasc Surg 101:989–997, 1991.
4. Byrd CL, Schwartz SJ, Hedin NB: Lead extraction: Techniques and indications. In Barold SS, Mugica J, editors: New Perspectives in Cardiac Pacing. Mount Kisco, NY: Futura Publishing, 1993, pp. 29–55.
5. Byrd CL, Schwartz SJ, Ciraldo RJ, et al: Update on transvenous countertraction lead extraction experience (abstract). Pacing Clin Electrophysiol 10:443, 1987.
6. Byrd CL, Schwartz SJ, Hedin NB, et al: Intravascular lead extraction using locking stylets and sheaths. Pacing Clin Electrophysiol 13:1871–1875, 1990.

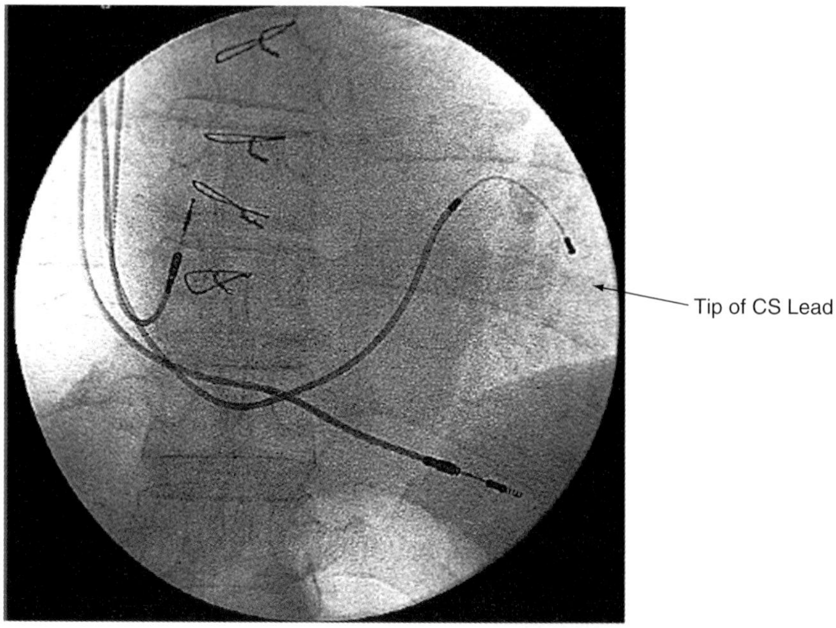

Figure 79–12 Fluoroscopic view of a biventricular pacing device. The tip of the coronary sinus (CS) lead is seen within the posterolateral CS vein.
(Courtesy of Medtronic, Inc.)

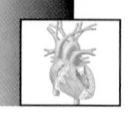

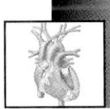

7. Byrd CL, Wilkoff BL, Love CJ, et al: Intravascular extraction of problematic or infected permanent pacemaker leads: 1994–1996. U.S. Extraction Database, MED Institute. Pacing Clin Electrophysiol 22(9):1348–1357, 1999.
8. Byrd CL, Schwartz SJ, Sivina M, et al: Experience with 127 pacemaker lead extractions (abstract). Pacing Clin Electrophysiol 9:282, 1986.
9. Chardack WM, Gage AA, Greatbach W: A transistorised, self-contained, implantable pacemaker for the long-term correction of complete heart block. Surgery 48:643–654, 1960.
10. Chen J, EL: Defibrillator function and implantation. In Kusumoto, FM, Goldschlager NF, editors: Cardiac Pacing for the Clinician. Philadelphia: Lippincott Williams & Wilkins, 2001, pp. 426–452.
11. Deeb GM, Hardesty RL, Griffith BP, et al: The effects of cardiovascular drugs on the defibrillation threshold and the pathological effects on the heart using an automatic implantable defibrillator. Ann Thorac Surg 35(4):361–366, 1983.
12. Furman S, Schwedel JB: An intracardiac pacemaker for Stokes-Adams seizures. N Engl J Med 261:943–948, 1959.
13. Goode LB, BC, Wilkoff BL, et al: Development of a new technique for explantation of chronic transvenous pacemaker leads: Five initial case studies. Biomed Instrument Technol 25: 50–53, 1991.
14. Gregoratos G, Abrams J, Epstein A, et al: ACC/AHA/NASPE 2002 guideline update for implantation of cardiac pacemakers and antiarrhythmia devices—summary article: A report of the American College of Cardiology/American Heart Association Task Force on Practice Guidelines (ACC/AHA/NASPE Committee to Update the 1998 Pacemaker Guidelines). J Am Coll Cardiol 40(9):1703–1719, 2002.
15. Gregoratos G, Abrams J, Epstein A, et al: ACC/AHA/NASPE 2002 guideline update for implantation of cardiac pacemakers and antiarrhythmia devices: summary article: A report of the American College of Cardiology/American Heart Association Task Force on Practice Guidelines (ACC/AHA/NASPE Committee to Update the 1998 Pacemaker Guidelines). Circulation 106(16):2145–2161, 2002.
16. Grimm W, Flores BF, Marchilinski FE: Electrocardiographically documented unnecessary, spontaneous shocks in 241 patients with implantable cardioverter defibrillators. Pacing Clin Electrophysiol 15:1667–1673, 1992.
17. Guarnieri T, Levine JH, Veltri EP, et al: Success of chronic defibrillation and the role of antiarrhythmic drugs with the automatic implantable cardioverter/defibrillator. Am J Cardiol 60:1061–1064, 1987.
18. The antiarrhythmics versus implantable defibrillators (AVID) investigators: A comparison of antiarrhythmic drug therapy with implantable defibrillators in patients resuscitated from near fatal ventricular arrhythmias. N Engl J Med 337: 1576–1583, 1997.
19. Kruse IM, Terpstra B: Acute and long-term atrial and ventricular stimulation thresholds with a steroid eluting electrode. Pacing Clin Electrophysiol 8:45–49, 1985.
20. Mirowski M: The automatic implantable cardioverter/defibrillator: an overview. J Am Coll Cardiol 6:461–466, 1985.
21. Mirowski M, Mower MM, Staewen WS, et al: Standby automatic defibrillator: an approach to prevention of sudden cardiac death. Arch Intern Med 126:158–161, 1970.
22. Mirowski M, Reid PR, Mower MM, et al: Termination of malignant ventricular arrhythmias with an implanted automatic defibrillator in human beings. N Engl J Med 303:322–324, 1980.
23. Mond H, Stokes K, Helland J, et al: The porous titanium steroid eluting electrode: a double blind study assessing the stimulation threshold effects of steroid. Pacing Clin Electrophysiol 11:214–219, 1988.
24. Moss AJ, Hall WJ, Cannom DS, et al: Improved survival with an implantable defibrillator in patients of coronary disease at high risk for ventricular arrhythmia. Multicenter Automatic Defibrillator Implantation Trial Investigators. N Engl J Med 335:1933–1940, 1996.
25. Moss AJ, Zareba W., Hall WJ, et al: Prophylactic implantation of a defibrillator in patients with myocardial infarction and reduced ejection fraction for the Multicenter Automatic Defibrillator Implantation Trial II Investigators. N Engl J Med 346:877–883, 2002.
26. Movsowitz C, Marchlinski FE: Interactions between implantable cardioverter-defibrillator and class III agents. Am J Cardiol 82:41I–48I, 1998.
27. North American Society of Pacing and Electrophysiology Lead Extraction Conference Faculty: Love CJ, Wilkoff BL, Byrd CL, et al: NASPE policy statement. Recommendations for extraction of chronically implanted transvenous pacing and defibrillator leads: indications, facilities, training. Pacing Clin Electrophysiol 23(4):544–551, 2000.
28. Pirzada FA, Moschitto LJ, Diorio D: Clinical experience with steroid-eluting unipolar electrodes. Pacing Clin Electrophysiol 11(Pt. 2):1739–1744, 1988.
29. Ryan TJ, Antman EM, Brooks NH, et al: 1999 update: ACC/AHA guidelines for the management of patients with acute myocardial infarction: executive summary and recommendations, a report of the American College of Cardiology/American Heart Association Task Force on Practice Guidelines (Committee on Management of Acute Myocardial Infarction). Circulation 100:1016–1030, 1999.
30. Sanders RS: The pulse generator. In Kusumoto, FM, Goldschlager NF, editors: Cardiac Pacing for the Clinician. Philadelphia: Lippincott Williams & Wilkins, 2001, pp. 41–62.
31. Smith TW, CJ, Epstein LM: Implantable devices for the treatment of cardiac arrhythmia. In Grossman W, Baim DS, editors: Grossman's Cardiac Catheterization, Angiography, and Intervention. Philadelphia: Lippincott Williams & Wilkins, 2000, pp. 489–543.
32. Wang PJ, MJ, Homoud MK, et al: Modes of pacemaker function. In Kusumoto FM, Goldschlager NF, editors: Cardiac Pacing for the Clinician. Philadelphia: Lippincott Williams & Wilkins, 2001, pp. 63–90.
33. Zoll PM: Resuscitation of the heart in ventricular standstill by external electrical stimulation. N Engl J Med 247:768–771, 1952.

Catheter Ablation of Arrhythmias

David Wrobleski and Mark E. Josephson

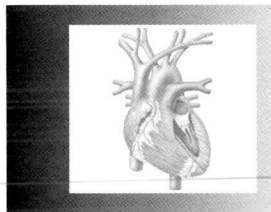

CHAPTER 80

INTRODUCTION

Over the past 30 years, cardiac electrophysiology has progressed from an esoteric research endeavor whose initial goals were the understanding of mechanisms of arrhythmia to an indispensable modality in the diagnosis and treatment of cardiac arrhythmias. An electrophysiology study (EPS) involves the percutaneous introduction of intracardiac catheters. These catheters have electrodes at varying interelectrode distances for recording the local electrical activity, delivering pacing impulses, and/or delivering energy to facilitate catheter-based ablation of cardiac arrhythmias.

INDICATIONS FOR EPS

The indications for EPS were most recently delineated by the American College of Cardiology and the American Heart Association (ACC/AHA) in 1995.[1] Class I recommendations involve conditions for which there is a general agreement among experts and evidence that EPS provides useful and important information for patient treatment. Class II recommendations involve conditions for which EP studies are frequently performed but there is less certainty about the usefulness of the information obtained. There is a dichotomy among experts as to the benefit of EPS in these patients. Class III recommendations involve conditions for which there is general consensus that EPS is not useful.

The ACC/AHA guidelines can be summarized as follows:

1. Sinus node function: patients with syncope or presyncope with sinus node dysfunction suspected but not demonstrated as the cause (class I). Patients with documented sinus node dysfunction (a) to evaluate for other arrhythmias (class II), (b) to evaluate the conduction system or susceptibility to arrhythmias to assist in selection of pacing modality (class II), (c) to attempt to determine the etiology of the bradyarrhythmia to assist in selecting therapeutic options (class II).
2. Acquired atrioventricular (AV) block: symptomatic patients with His–Purkinje block suspected but not demonstrated as the cause (class I) or patients with demonstrated AV block and a pacemaker implanted to exclude other arrhythmias as etiology of symptoms (class I). Patients with second- or third-degree AV block to elicit site of block to direct therapy or assess prognosis (class II), to rule out concealed junctional depolarizations as a cause of AV block (class II).
3. Chronic intraventricular conduction delay: patients with syncope or presyncope of unknown etiology (class I). Asymptomatic patients in whom pharmacological therapy that could exacerbate conduction abnormalities is contemplated (class II).
4. Narrow QRS tachycardia (QRS <120 ms): patients with frequent or poorly tolerated episodes nonresponsive to a pharmacological approach, to define the mechanism of the tachycardia to facilitate pharmacological treatment or to proceed with ablation (class I), or patients who prefer catheter-based ablation as first-line therapy (class I). Patients receiving medical treatment for the tachycardia for whom there is concern for adverse effects on conduction or for proarrhythmia (class II).
5. Wide QRS tachycardia (QRS ≥120 ms): patients in whom the diagnosis is uncertain and knowledge of the correct diagnosis is necessary for treatment (class I).
6. Prolonged QT interval: no indication for invasive EPS at this time.
7. Wolff–Parkinson–White syndrome: patients with arrhythmias being evaluated for ablative treatment (class I), patients with ventricular preexcitation and unexplained syncope (class I). Asymptomatic patients with a family history of sudden cardiac death (class II), who engage in high-risk occupations or activities (class II), or who are undergoing cardiac surgery for other reasons (class II).
8. Premature ventricular complexes and couplets: patients with highly symptomatic monomorphic premature ventricular complexes and couplets who are considered potential candidates for catheter ablation (class II).
9. Unexplained syncope: patients with known or suspected structural heart disease and unexplained syncope (class I). Patients with recurrent symptoms without structural heart disease and a negative head-up tilt test (class II).
10. Survivors of cardiac arrest: patients surviving cardiac arrest unrelated to acute myocardial infarction (MI) (class I) or occurring more than 48 h after the acute MI in the absence

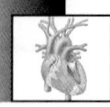

of a recurrent event (class I). Patients surviving a bradyarrhythmic cardiac arrest (class II).

11. Unexplained palpitations: patients with a pulse rate documented by medical personnel as inappropriately rapid without ECG recordings (class I) or palpitations preceding syncope (class I). Patients with significant palpitations, suspected to be of cardiac origin, but without any ECG documentation despite ambulatory monitoring (class II).
12. EPS to guide drug therapy: patients with atrioventricular nodal reentry tachycardia (AVNRT), AV reentrant tachycardia, or atrial fibrillation and an accessory pathway for whom chronic drug therapy is planned (class I). Of note, the guidelines list EPS-guided drug therapy for sustained ventricular tachycardia (VT) or cardiac arrest as class I as well, but this has been revised by the more recent MUSTT and AVID trials (detailed below).

Several important studies have been published since the release of these guidelines, which have expanded and refined the indications for EPS summarized above. The Antiarrhythmics Versus Implantable Defibrillators (AVID) trial[2] included patients who had been resuscitated from ventricular fibrillation or had been cardioverted from sustained symptomatic ventricular tachycardia with a left ventricular ejection fraction of ≤0.40. The patients were randomized to treatment with implantation of a cardioverter-defibrillator (ICD) or to treatment with class III antiarrhythmic drugs, primarily amiodarone. The ICD group had significant reductions in mortality compared to the medical group at 1-, 2-, and 3-year follow-up. This has led to a class I indication for ICD implantation in these patients, and EPS pre-ICD in the AVID population has become a class II indication, with many experts skipping EPS prior to implantation. Useful information can be gained from EPS pre-ICD implantation in this patient population, such as inducibility of VT and the ability to pace terminate it, which would be helpful in ICD programming and management, and EPS is still performed in the majority of these patients in our laboratory.

Two important trials have led to a refinement in the approach to patients with a prior MI and evidence of nonsustained ventricular tachycardia (NSVT; 3–30 beats). The Multicenter Automatic Defibrillator Trial (MADIT)[77] enrolled patients with a left ventricular ejection fraction ≤0.035, documented NSVT, New York Heart Association functional class I–III, and inducible, nonsuppressible VT by EPS. The patients were randomized to receive conventional medical therapy or an ICD. Antiarrhythmic drugs could be given to patients in either group. The ICD group had a significantly improved survival over an average follow-up of 27 months. This study created a new class I indication for EPS in these patients.

The second important study applicable to the population of patients with a prior MI and evidence of NSVT was the Multicenter Unsustained Tachycardia Trial (MUSTT).[5] The patients included in this trial had coronary artery disease with a left ventricular ejection fraction of ≤0.40, and documented NSVT. Patients with sustained ventricular tachyarrhythmias induced during EPS were randomized to antiarrhythmic therapy consisting of either ICD implantation or EPS-guided antiarrhythmic drug therapy, or no antiarrhythmic therapy. There was a significant mortality benefit in the antiarrhythmic therapy group over a mean follow-up of 39 months. Subgroup analysis revealed all of the mortality benefit in the antiarrhythmic therapy group came from the patients who had received ICD implantation, not EPS-guided drug therapy alone. This led to a class I indication for EPS in this patient population and contributed to the demise of EPS-guided antiarrhythmic drug therapy for VT.

Recently, the Multicenter Automatic Defibrillator Trial II (MADIT II) was published.[78] This trial randomized patients with a prior MI and a left ventricular ejection fraction of 0.30 or less to either an ICD implantation or conventional medical therapy. This trial specifically had no entry criteria of ventricular ectopy or electrophysiology study. There was a 31% reduction in the risk of death at any interval among patients in the ICD group. The indication to implant an ICD in this patient population is currently class II. There are concerns regarding this trial, however. The ICD group had a trend toward worsening heart failure. This may be due to increased right ventricular pacing in the ICD group,[19] findings that were supported in the recent DAVID trial.[17] Also, with an estimated three to four million patients with coronary heart disease and advanced left ventricular dysfunction in the United States, and 400,000 new cases annually, the cost of universal ICD implantation in this population would be substantial.[13,78] Approval for implantation with reimbursement is limited to those with a QRS greater than 120 mg. Further risk stratification with invasive EPS may still be warranted in some of these patients.

THE ELECTROPHYSIOLOGY STUDY

The electrophysiology study involves placing electrode catheters in various chambers of the heart for recording, stimulation, mapping, and ablation. Femoral veins and arteries are the most common sites of vascular access used for EPS. Less commonly used sites include the antecubital fossa and subclavian and jugular veins. Adequate local anesthesia is administered prior to vascular puncture. A 0.035-inch short J guide wire is placed via the percutaneous Seldinger technique into the femoral vein or artery just below the inguinal ligament. The needle is removed, and the protruding end of the guide wire is wiped with a saline moistened gauze. A second wire is placed 5–10 mm caudal to the first, up to three wires in a single vein. A single triple-headed vascular access device that can accommodate three catheters through a single access sheath is commercially available, but not utilized in our laboratory because of the large diameter of this device. 6F–8F hemostatic sheaths are placed over the guide wires, up to three in a single vein. If more than three catheters are required, another vein is utilized, typically the contralateral femoral vein.

For His bundle recordings, the femoral approach allows superior catheter stability. However, catheterization of the coronary sinus is more readily accomplished via the internal jugular, left subclavian, or left antecubital veins. The lateral antecubital veins that drain into the cephalic vein are avoided because of the right angle at which it enters the axillary vein, making catheter manipulation more difficult. In our laboratory, these nonfemoral sites are usually reserved for patients with inaccessible femoral access or difficult coronary sinus cannulation despite attempts via the femoral approach with a steerable catheter. Although accessing the coronary sinus through a femoral vein is generally more difficult, in experienced hands it can be readily accomplished either via a direct approach, often facilitated by bending the catheter in the hepatic vein to achieve a greater posterior angulation, or more indirectly by first forming a catheter loop within the right atrium.

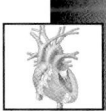

A diagnostic electrophysiology study typically requires at least three catheters, one in the high right atrium (HRA) near the sinus node, the His bundle area across the tricuspid valve, and the right ventricular apex (RVA). Depending on the type of study, additional catheters may be placed in the right ventricular outflow tract (RVOT), coronary sinus (CS), anterolateral right atrium (ALRA), interatrial septum, left atrium, pulmonary veins, and left ventricle.

Accessing the left ventricular cavity is accomplished either via the mitral valve from transseptal left atrial catheterization or via a retrograde aortic approach through the arterial system, typically the femoral artery. Although left ventricular catheterization is not a routine part of a diagnostic EPS, it may have importance in patients with VT and accessory pathway-mediated tachycardia. Detailed catheter mapping of the left ventricular endocardium may also have benefit in defining the myocardial substrate in patients with ventricular arrhythmias, depressed ventricular function, or prolonged intraventricular conduction and congestive heart failure. These utilizations of ventricular mapping are an area of active research.

CATHETER ABLATION

Catheter-based ablation techniques have been so successful in treating a variety of arrhythmias that they have virtually replaced surgical approaches. In a catheter-based ablation, energy is delivered to a precise area of the heart. This is typically on the endocardial surface of the heart, although closed-chest catheter ablation to the epicardial surface of the heart is an area of active interest.[101–103]

Knowledge of the precise area of the heart to be ablated is derived through mapping techniques. The most common approaches to mapping are activation mapping and pace mapping. Activation mapping involves manipulation of a roving mapping catheter during the arrhythmia (either a spontaneous or an induced arrhythmia). Areas of the heart with local electrical activity earliest compared to a reference point, such as onset of the QRS or an intracardiac electrogram from a fixed position reference catheter, are target areas for ablation of the arrhythmia.

Pace mapping is a mapping technique that can be employed when the patient is not in the arrhythmia.[47] It is often employed in conjunction with activation mapping as a second confirmatory test as to the accuracy of the selected site for ablation, but can be used as a stand-alone mapping technique if the documented clinical arrhythmia cannot be induced during EPS. Pace mapping entails pacing the suspected target area for ablation at a rate similar to the clinical arrhythmia, and comparing the 12-lead electrocardiogram to the ECG of the arrhythmia. A good pace map will have an exact QRS match in 12 out of 12 leads. When minor differences in ECG configuration and amplitude are sought, the spatial resolution of pace mapping can be as good as 5 mm.[50] Pace mapping also compares the intracardiac activation sequence seen on the EP catheters with the sequence observed during the arrhythmia; however, this additional information may not be available if the arrhythmia was not inducible in the laboratory.

Electrograms acquired during mapping techniques are either bipolar or unipolar. Bipolar electrograms reveal the local electrical activity of the heart between two designated electrodes on the catheter. This typically is over an interelectrode spacing ranging from 1 to 10 mm. Unipolar electrograms reveal the local electrical activity at a single catheter point (usually the distal tip) relative to an electrode placed at a distance from the heart. The advantages of utilizing unipolar mapping include a more precise measure of local activation as well as information about the direction of impulse propagation. The advantages of utilizing bipolar mapping include superior signal-to-noise ratio and less contribution from distant electrical activity ("far-field" activity). Frequently, accurate mapping involves utilizing both bipolar and unipolar electrograms at different points of the study.

There are also specialized computer systems to assist with mapping. Most commonly used are the CARTO system (Biosense-Cordis) and the ESI system (Endocardial Solutions, Inc.). The CARTO electroanatomical mapping system has been described in detail.[26] It allows three-dimensional electroanatomical mapping using a low-intensity magnetic field that allows localization of the mapping catheter with six degrees of freedom. The accuracy of this system has been described as 0.8 mm and five degrees. ESI is a noncontact mapping system that generates mathematically derived electrograms and places them on a map of a cardiac chamber defined by a second, roving contact catheter.[109] It utilizes a 64-electrode noncontact balloon catheter and computes 3360 virtual endocardial electrograms simultaneously.[29] The use of these systems or other localizing systems can greatly reduce the amount of fluoroscopy time and may contribute to eliminating the need for biplane systems.

After mapping techniques are utilized to identify the precise area to be ablated, an ablation catheter is positioned in the desired location and connected to an energy source. Radiofrequency energy (RF) is by far the modality most commonly used clinically, having replaced DC ablation because of superior safety and efficacy. Freezing the target area of the heart through a catheter-based system (cryoablation) is currently being explored as an alternative to RF energy.

Radiofrequency current is typically delivered in a unipolar configuration from the distal tip of the ablation catheter to a cutaneous grounding patch. The energy is generated as an alternating current with a frequency of 300–750 kHz.[42] These frequencies produce effective heating with negligible muscle stimulation. During RF ablation, the electrical energy is converted to thermal energy by resistive heating. Most of the heating is concentrated at the tip of the catheter secondary to the small surface area of the tip relative to the cutaneous patch. The heat that is generated is transferred to the adjacent cardiac tissue primarily by conduction and to a lesser extent by radiation, which decreases by the fourth power of the distance from the catheter tip. It has been demonstrated *in vitro* that at steady state the RF lesion size is proportional to the temperature measured at the tissue–catheter interface, as well as proportional to the RF power amplitude.[34]

RF ablation results in thermal injury with coagulation necrosis when tissue heating exceeds approximately 50° C for at least 10 s.[33,35,42,64] As heat is produced at the catheter–myocardial interface, the impedance drops. A drop of 5–10 Ω is a sign of conductive heating to the adjacent tissue. The time to electrophysiological effect after onset of RF current delivery is often shorter than would be anticipated for a pure thermal mechanism based upon the documented rate of tissue temperature rise contiguous to the electrode.[36] This raises the possibility that there is a contribution of a direct electrical effect in addition to the thermal effect of RF.

Cryoablation has been used in the surgical treatment of arrhythmias for over 20 years. Near transmural lesions can be produced intraoperatively at temperatures of –60° C in the presence of cold cardioplegia. The blood pool presents catheter-based cryoablation systems with a major impediment in achieving adequate temperature. However, a catheter-based closed coolant system has been developed, and has begun to see clinical use. The major advantage is the ability to induce a nonpermanent change in tissue conduction "ice mapping" followed by a permanent lesion if the ice mapping reveals a desirable location. This method has been used surgically[39] with temperatures of approximately 0° C producing transient loss of electrical function and 60° C producing irreversible damage. A closed-chest approach has to deal with the warming effect of the circulating blood pool, and mean temperatures of –27° C were needed to achieve transient altering of electrical function.[18] The temperature required for irreversible damage was similar to that needed in surgery, however (–58° C).

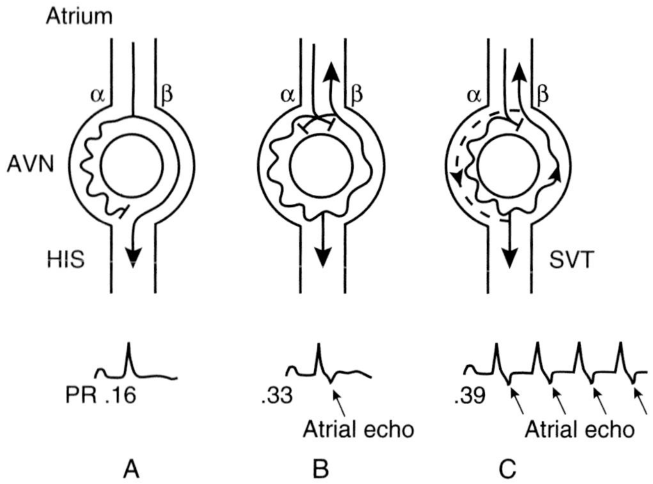

Figure 80–1 Schema of mechanism of AV rodal reentry. (**A–C**) The AV node has two functional pathways: an α (slow) and β (fast) pathway. The pathway has a longer refractory period than the more slowly conductive α pathway. As such, during sinus rhythm (**A**) the PR is short, refractory fast pathway conductions. **B,** A late APC blocks the β pathway, which leads to conduction down the slow pathway (longer PR interval) and an atrial echo beat. Antigrade block in the slow pathway prevents SVT. **C,** A critically timed APC produces enough delay in the α pathway, with retrograde conduction up the fast pathway with sequential activation over the α pathway to initiate SVT.

(Modified with permission from Josephson ME: Clinical Cardiac Electrophysiology. Philadelphia: Lippincott Williams & Wilkins, 2002.)

AV Nodal Reentrant Tachycardia

AVNRT is the most common form of supraventricular tachycardia.[49,122] Medically, this arrhythmia is often treated with AV nodal blocking agents as well as type IA antiarrhythmic agents. The ability to cure this arrhythmia with a safe, well-tolerated, and highly efficacious catheter ablation[92] has made this a viable option for first-line therapy of AVNRT.

The AV node lies within the triangle of Koch, an area confined by the septal leaflet of the tricuspid valve inferiorly, the tendon of Todaro superiorly, and the coronary sinus os posteriorly.[62] In 1956, Moe and colleagues described physiological evidence for a dual AV nodal pathway system.[75] These pathways were termed "slow" and "fast" based on their conduction time.[75] However, there are no anatomical-specific pathways that have been described that correlate with the fast and slow pathways. The functional dissociation of AV conduction into fast and slow pathways provides the substrate most often associated with AVNRT. The "fast" pathway normally lies at the apex of the triangle of Koch and the "slow" pathway at the base. However, there is often heterogeneity of atrial activation and these locations are not universal.

"Typical" or "common" AVNRT is usually initiated when a premature atrial impulse blocks in the fast pathway, conducts over the slow pathway, then reenters the fast pathway in a retrograde direction (Figure 80-1). This "slow–fast" AVNRT is responsible for approximately 90% of cases. The "atypical" or "uncommon" form of AVNRT utilizes the slow pathway retrogradely and the fast pathway anterogradely. Uncommonly, two relatively slow pathways constitute the reentry circuit ("slow–slow").

Initial catheter ablation of AVNRT targeted the fast pathway in the anterior interatrial septum.[65] Ablation at the apex of the triangle of Koch in the region of the fast pathway was >90% successful; however, it carried an unacceptably high risk of AV block (5–10%). Ablation of the slow pathway was proposed[43,93,117] as an alternative to fast pathway ablation. This is accomplished via a posterior approach, with the ablation catheter initially positioned near the coronary sinus os, at the base of the triangle of Koch (Figure 80-2). RF current in the slow pathway region is often accompanied by transient accelerated junctional rhythm with rapid retrograde atrial conduction. This rhythm also serves as a marker of a potentially successful ablation. Atrial pacing may be performed during the junctional rhythm to ensure 1:1 antegrade conduction. A rapid junctional tachycardia can be a marker for complete heart block, and ablation should be halted if it is seen.[70,112] It has been proposed that junctional tachycardia with a cycle length of less than 350 ms should prompt cessation of ablation.[70] Energy delivery should also be stopped if AV block or junctional rhythm with retrograde block is seen. Ablation should be performed under continuous fluoroscopic monitoring to ensure catheter stability. In approximately 40% of cases, dual pathways are still present postablation, but sustained ANVRT cannot be induced. Single AV nodal complexes ("echo beats") are observed in

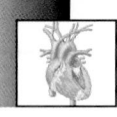

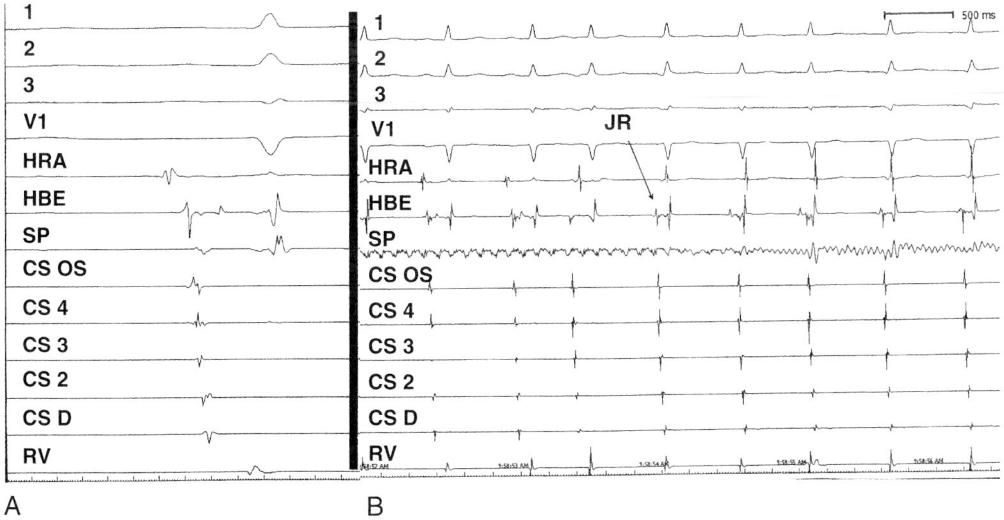

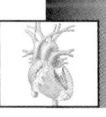

Figure 80–2 **Radiofrequency ablation of AV nodal reentry.** ECG leads 1, 2, 3, and V are shown with intracardiac electrograms from the high right atrium (HRA), His bundle (HBE), slow pathway (SP), coronary sinus (CS) from the os to the distal tip (D) of a decapolar catheter, and right ventricle (RV). The SP electrogram in sinus rhythm **(A)** is characterized by a multicomponent signal recorded after the atrium on the HBE, with an atrial/ventricular electrogram ratio of ≤1:3. **B,** Radiofrequency energy is delivered at the SP resulting in a junctional rhythm (JR), a good sign of a successful lesion.
(Modified with permission from Josephson ME: Clinical Cardiac Electrophysiology. Philadelphia: Lippincott Williams & Wilkins, 2002.)

three fourths of these patients with dual pathways postablation, with block always occurring antegradely in the slow pathway. The success rate using a slow pathway approach is in excess of 95%. Slow pathway ablation is preferred to fast pathway ablation because of the equivalent success rate and the much lower risk of complete heart block (1–2%).

Atrial Tachycardia

Catheter ablation therapy for atrial tachycardia had progressed from rate control via AV junction ablation to potentially curative therapy targeting the tachycardia foci.* Atrial tachycardias that are incessant and are due to abnormal automaticity or triggered activity are most amenable to ablation. The arrhythmias tend to be resistant to drug therapy.[28] Microreentrant atrial tachycardias are frequently easily managed pharmacologically, making ablation second-line therapy.

Incessant atrial tachycardias can occur from a variety of locations in the heart, but seem to have a propensity for the crista terminalis, both atrial appendages, the coronary sinus, the regions of the mitral and tricuspid annulae, and the pulmonary veins. It is unclear why these structures are prone to develop these rhythms. It has been postulated that regions such as the crista terminalis are sources of automatic atrial tachycardias because of relatively poor cell-to-cell coupling.[66] Fractionated electrograms at successful ablation sites may be markers of the nonuniformly anisotropic substrate because of poor coupling that allows focal automaticity to occur. In our experience, the crista terminalis, the tricuspid annulus, the pulmonary veins, and the left atrial appendage have been the major sources of arrhythmias.[48] In adults, they are somewhat more common in the right atrium, and multiple foci are present in 10–15% of patients.

Because the majority of incessant atrial tachycardias are focal in origin, the goal of catheter mapping is to find the earliest site of activation (Figure 80-3). If the tachycardias are not incessant, catecholamine infusion, such as isoproterenol 1–4 μg/min IV, or atropine 0.5–1.0 mg IV may be necessary to induce sustained arrhythmia. The initial localization of the arrhythmia focus is made by analysis of the P wave morphology and axis. Catheter mapping is performed by identifying the site of earliest atrial activation relative to the onset of the P wave. Once the catheter is positioned at what appears to be the earliest site of atrial activation, further evidence that it is the correct site of origin can be obtained by pace mapping. Pace mapping involves pacing at the early intracardiac site and comparing both the resultant paced P wave morphology with the tachycardia P wave morphology, as well as comparing the sequence of intracardiac atrial activation during pacing and during the tachycardia.[113] Pacing with higher output at the proposed site of ablation also helps confirm minimal risk of injury to the surrounding extracardiac structures. This is particularly important in the right atrium with the proximity of the phrenic nerve; however, left phrenic nerve damage has also been reported.[94] Pacing that results in diaphragmatic stimulation would preclude ablation at that site.

The success rate of atrial tachycardia is variable. When they are present incessantly, the success rate approaches 90%, although the recurrence rate may be as high as 25%.[21,53,57,67,113] Because the arrhythmia may not be reliably present or inducible at EPS (factors such as conscious sedation may serve to make them less inducible), a true success rate on an intention to treat basis would be lower than 90%.

Sinoatrial node reentrant tachycardia represents a distinct entity within the category of atrial tachycardias. Criteria for

*References 21, 52, 53, 57, 67, 113, 116.

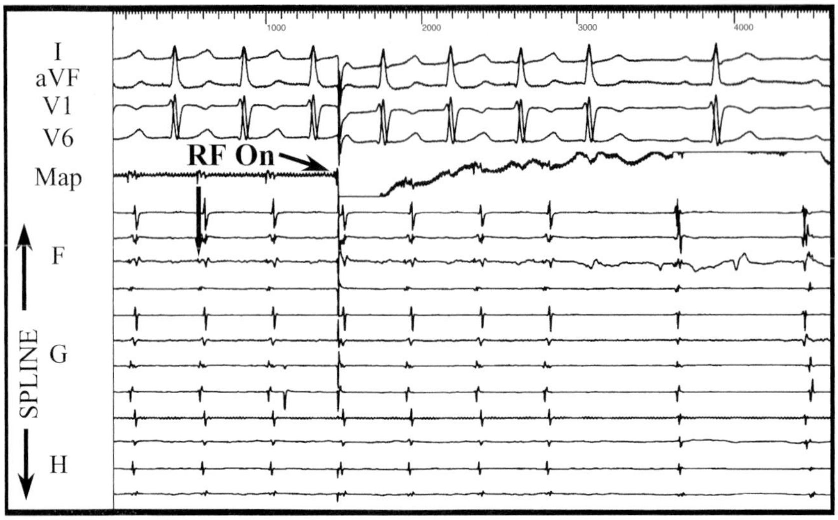

Figure 80–3 Ablation of atrial tachycardia. Atrial tachycardia is present. The ablation/mapping catheter is placed at the earliest electrogram recorded on a 64 pole basket catheter *(vertical arrow)*. Radiofrequency energy delivered at this site terminates the tachycardia.

the diagnosis are consistent atrial activation sequence and P wave morphology in sinus rhythm and tachycardia, consistent initiation and termination with programmed electrical stimulation, and termination of tachycardia with vagal maneuvers or with adenosine.[30,82,118] Catheter ablation can be accomplished with good results and a paucity of complications,[96] typically by ablating in the high posterolateral region of the right atrium at the "tail" of the sinus node.

Atrial Flutter

Typical atrial flutters are macroreentrant circuits involving the right atrium. The posterior barrier is formed by the crista terminalis and its continuation as the Eustachian ridge.[86] The anterior barrier in typical flutter is the tricuspid annulus.[54] Atrial flutter can be divided into counterclockwise ("common" or typical) and clockwise ("uncommon" or atypical), depending upon the direction of rotation in the frontal plane around the tricuspid annulus. Although clockwise flutter is the more common clinical entity, clockwise flutter can be initiated in most patients with typical atrial flutter.[55] The electrocardiogram can give clues to the pattern of the atrial flutter, but can be ambiguous or misleading. Counterclockwise flutter is characterized by a predominantly negative, sawtooth-like atrial pattern in the inferior leads, with positive atrial deflections in lead V1 and negative deflections in lead V6. Clockwise flutter is characterized by a predominantly positive, notched atrial pattern in the inferior lead, with negative atrial deflections in lead V1 and positive deflections in lead V6.

In a catheter ablation procedure, a 10-electrode catheter (decapolar catheter) is placed in the coronary sinus and in the ALRA, anterior to the crista terminalis. The ALRA catheter can help determine the direction of rotation, with atrial activation cranial–caudal in counterclockwise flutter and caudal–cranial in clockwise flutter (Figure 80-4).

Catheter ablation of atrial flutter is dependent upon the ability to interrupt the macroreentrant circuit at a critical narrow portion between barriers to conduction, termed the isthmus. In both counterclockwise and clockwise flutter, the isthmus targeted for ablation lies anterior to the inferior vena cava (IVC) and Eustachian ridge, and posterior to the tricuspid annulus. During flutter, this isthmus is a zone of slow conduction.[87] Pacing from within this area at a paced cycle length slightly shorter than the tachycardia will help demonstrate if the flutter utilizes this critical isthmus (i.e., isthmus dependent). If pacing in the isthmus at a rate slightly faster than the tachycardia entrains the tachycardia without alteration of the surface ECG flutter wave morphology with a local postpacing interval equal to the tachycardia cycle length, the tachycardia can be termed isthmus dependent. Non-isthmus-dependent flutters include macroreentry around the coronary sinus os, fossa ovalis, postoperative incisional scar tissue, and left atrial flutters such as reentry around pulmonary vein ostia.

Ablation of isthmus-dependent atrial flutter consists of creating a line of block across the right atrial isthmus. This has been described connecting the coronary sinus os to the tricuspid annulus; however, this approach can be prone to failure because of slow conduction through the Eustachian ridge, which may not necessarily be a fixed obstacle-producing block.[81] This can lead to a lower loop of reentry around the IVC, which meets the flutter loop going around the tricuspid annulus in a figure of eight manner.[10] Ablation between the tricuspid annulus and the IVC will eliminate lower loop reentry as well as isthmus-dependent flutter and is the preferred ablation method in our laboratory.

Usually the ablation is performed during atrial flutter. If flutter is not present at baseline, it can be induced with one or two atrial extrastimuli and/or rapid atrial pacing in 90% of atrial flutter patients and 95% of patients with isthmus-dependent flutter.[48] The flutter is typically terminated during RF application in the isthmus; however, termination does not necessarily mean that the line of block is complete. Lack of complete isthmus block has been described in more than 50% of cases when RF energy terminates flutter.[66] To increase the success of the procedure, bidirectional block must be demonstrated.[14,91,100] This is demonstrated by pacing the coronary sinus catheter, which is medial to the line of isthmus block. When the line of ablation is complete, there is no clockwise propagation through the isthmus, and activation is around the tricuspid annulus in a counterclockwise direction. This is seen on the ALRA catheter as

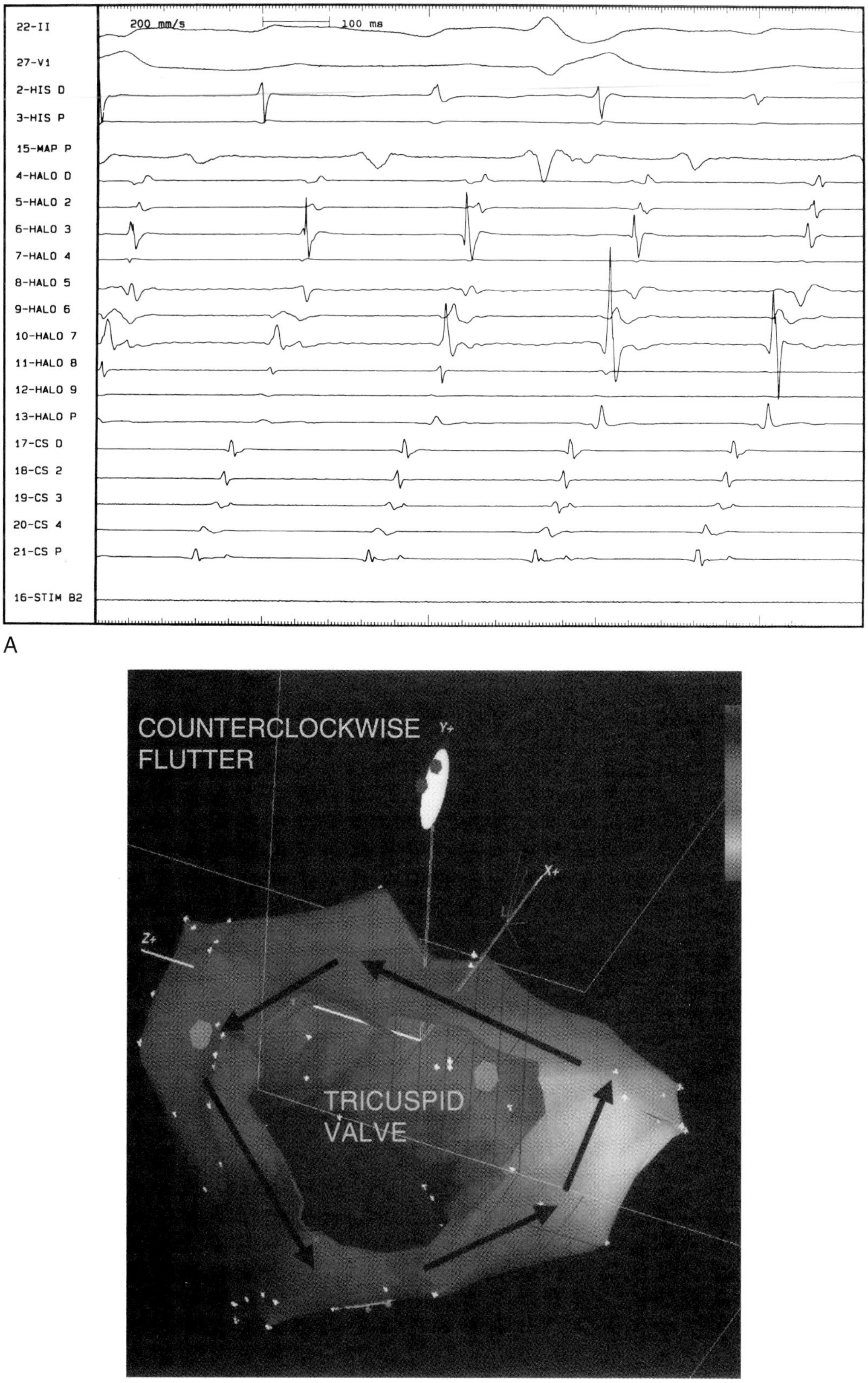

Figure 80–4 **A,** Atrial activation during counterclockwise flutter. ECG leads II and V_1 are shown with His bundle electrograms (His) and multiple poles of a halo catheter placed along the tricuspid ring. Halo is superior while Halo distal (D) is at the tricuspid isthmus. CSP is at the os of the CS with more distal bipolar pairs. Note atrial activation moves from high to low on the Halo and proximal to distal on the CS. This is typical for counterclockwise flutter. **B,** Three-dimensional isochromic map is shown above. Arrows point to the activation sequence.

(Modified with permission from Josephson ME: Clinical Cardiac Electrophysiology. Philadelphia: Lippincott Williams & Wilkins, 2002.)

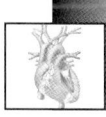

cranial–caudal activation during CS pacing. To verify the bidirectional nature of the block, pacing is performed from the distal ALRA catheter, which is lateral to the line of isthmus block. If the line of block is complete, there is no counterclockwise propagation through the isthmus, and activation is around the tricuspid annulus in a clockwise direction. In addition to bidirectional block, at the conclusion of the procedure split atrial potentials (>100 ms apart) or absence of atrial potentials (electrograms <0.05 mV) may be seen along the ablation line. If bidirectional block is demonstrated, the incidence of atrial flutter recurrence in our laboratory is 6%.[48]

Accessory Pathway-Mediated Tachycardia

Accessory AV connections ("accessory pathways," "bypass tracts") are part of a group of physiological connections producing preexcitation syndromes. This group includes AV,[120] nodoventricular,[45] nodofascicular, atriofascicular, and fasciculoventricular[71] connections. These pathways appear to represent developmental abnormalities, and it is not surprising that multiple types of accessory pathways may exist in any one patient. AV connections are responsible for the classic Wolff–Parkinson–White (WPW) syndrome. They may conduct antegradely leading to a preexcited ECG or may be concealed and conduct only retrogradely.

The clinical tachycardia most frequently associated with accessory AV pathways is atrioventricular reciprocating tachycardia (AVRT), circus movement tachycardia (CMT). AVRT is further classified as orthodromic or antidromic. Orthodromic tachycardia results from antegrade conduction down the AV node and retrograde up the accessory pathway, while antidromic is the opposite direction.

The initial step in an ablation procedure is careful inspection of the 12-lead ECG. The initial inspection is dependent upon a manifest pathway and the accuracy is enhanced the greater the degree of preexcitation. Although more complex schema have been proposed,[3,11,23,111] we believe a simpler approach is warranted due to variability in degree of preexcitation, variability in precordial lead placement, and variations in body shape/size, heart size, and position in the chest. This approach divides the location of accessory pathways into five regions[48]: anteroseptal, right free wall, posteroseptal, left posterior free wall, and left lateral free wall.

Full description of our approach to localizing pathways based on 12-lead ECG is well described elsewhere,[48] but in summary, left lateral bypass tracts are characterized by negative delta waves in leads I and AVL, and positive in inferior leads and precordial leads. Left posterior free wall tracts are characterized by positive delta waves in lead I, negative in inferior leads, and positive in right precordial leads. Posteroseptal tracts have a positive delta wave in leads I and AVL and negative in inferior leads (although lead II may be isoelectric or biphasic, the more negative the more leftward the location). Right free wall tracts generally have negative delta waves in lead V1, positive in I and II, and slightly negative in III. Anteroseptal tracts have a positive delta wave in lead I, positive in inferior leads (with lead II greater than III), and precordial leads with primarily negative or biphasic delta waves.

Analysis of retrograde P wave morphology during CMT is also helpful in localizing the atrial insertion site.[48] This is crucial for concealed accessory pathways, which have no ventricular preexcitation. Thus, left lateral insertion is associated with a negative P wave in lead I and AVL. A positive P wave in inferior leads arises from superiorly located accessory pathways, with a positive P wave in leads I and AVL if it is on the right and negative if it is on the left. A negative P wave in the inferior leads arises from posteroseptal and paraseptal sites.

In a catheter ablation procedure, a decapolar catheter is placed in the coronary sinus, and quadripolar catheters into the high right atrium, right ventricular apex, and His bundle region. The CS catheter should be advanced to the anterolateral mitral annulus, which will permit mapping of all left-sided pathways except possibly the most anterolateral pathways. If the accessory pathway is not concealed, a 12-lead ECG is obtained during atrial pacing at a rate slightly slower than the rate at which block is observed in the accessory pathway, producing a maximally preexcited ECG. This assists in the evaluation of the delta wave for a more accurate prediction of the accessory pathway location.

Left-sided accessory pathways can be performed via either a transseptal approach or a retrograde aortic approach. A manifest pathway is then maximally preexcited by atrial pacing, and the location of the shortest AV interval along the coronary sinus is noted. If the pathway is concealed, evaluation of retrograde conduction over the pathway is performed during ventricular pacing, or, preferably, during CMT, with analysis of the shortest ventriculoatrial electrogram interval (i.e., site of earliest atrial activation). If retrograde conduction over the pathway is intermittent or tenuous during the resting sedated state of EPS, isoproterenol can be administered. This may also facilitate initiation of CMT. If rapid retrograde conduction over the AV node during ventricular pacing makes localization difficult, verapamil can be administered to facilitate conduction over the pathway.

An ablation catheter is then advanced into position. The ventricular insertion of the pathway is best identified via the retrograde aortic approach. This is the technique typically used as the first-line approach in our laboratory. Alternatively, the atrial insertion site can be mapped via the transseptal approach or retrograde aortic approach with prolapse of the catheter across the mitral valve. Success rates at initial attempts at ablation appear to be similar in either approach.[68] Final localization of the pathway is then performed by mapping the AV groove with the ablation catheter, localizing the site of shortest AV interval in manifest pathways and VA interval in concealed pathways. Electrograms recorded at insertion sites of pathways are often fractionated, and occasionally a bypass tract potential can be recorded. This potential is seen as a discrete sharp spike between the atrial and ventricular electrograms, is not always present at sites of successful ablation, and does not guarantee successful ablation if seen.[4,6]

Factors that predict a successful ablation site for a pathway include a stable electrogram, catheter stability and catheter motion in conjunction with the CS catheter, presence of an accessory pathway potential, catheter position at the shortest recorded AV interval (or shortest ventriculoatrial interval if concealed), and activation of the local ventricular electrogram prior to the onset of the QRS if it is a manifest pathway.

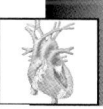

The mapping of right-sided pathways uses principles similar to those used for left-sided pathways. We prefer to use an atrial approach to right-sided accessory pathways. Right atrial pathway ablation can be more complicated because of (1) the presence of a "sack" of atrial myocardium folding over the tricuspid AV ring[22] making catheter manipulation more difficult, (2) possible circumferential tricuspid pathway location vs. only approximately 75% of the mitral annulus due to lack of pathways in the region of aortomitral continuity, and (3) lack of an AV groove reference catheter. Insertion of a small catheter in the right coronary artery to serve as a right-sided AV groove reference has been suggested by some investigators.[110] This may be useful in patients with Ebstein's anomaly or a history of multiple unsuccessful ablations of right-sided pathways, but needs to be used with extreme caution because there are potentially disastrous consequences as well as lack of long-term follow-up. A multipolar halo catheter can also be positioned around the tricuspid annulus to serve as an AV groove reference.

After adequately localizing the accessory pathway, RF current is delivered through the distal electrode of the ablation catheter for up to 60 s. Successful ablation typically results in loss of accessory pathway conduction within 10 s (Figure 80-5). The patient is then monitored for at least 20 min to watch for resumption of accessory pathway conduction, often in the presence of isoproterenol given intravenously. The overall success rate for ablation of all accessory pathways at our institution is 97%.

Ventricular Tachycardia Associated with Coronary Artery Disease

Sustained monomorphic VT in patients with coronary artery disease most frequently arises from scarred myocardial substrate from a prior MI. Reentrant circuits are prone to develop secondary to fibrosis from the prior infarction causing disruptions in cellular coupling leading to abnormal paths of conduction as well as zones of slow conduction. Surgical subendocardial resection of these areas has proven curative in selected patients,[24,32,73] but with unacceptable morbidity and mortality.[40] However, the high mortality rate comes from data from surgical series in the 1980s and could possibly be lower today with improved myocardial preservation techniques and additional methods to facilitate the procedure. Thus, surgical therapy for ventricular arrhythmias, particularly in conjunction with coronary artery bypass grafting surgery, is possibly underutilized today. Nevertheless, catheter-based VT ablation has supplanted surgical treatment in the majority of cases.

Approximately 95% of patients with a prior MI who present with sustained monomorphic VT will be able to have the clinical arrhythmia induced at EPS. Ideally, to be considered for ablation the VT should be hemodynamically tolerated to allow for careful left ventricular mapping during the arrhythmia. As will be discussed, newer techniques for VT ablation during sinus rhythm utilizing mapping of the scarred arrhythmogenic substrate are being explored, but most mapping techniques require hemodynamically tolerated inducible VT. If rapid rate of the VT is contributing to hemodynamic compromise, administration of agents such as procainamide can slow the VT to allow for adequate mapping during VT.

The "site of origin" of the VT is essentially the source of electrical activity producing the VT QRS. Although this is a discrete site in automatic and triggered rhythms, post-MI VT is typically a reentrant rhythm. During reentrant VT, the site of origin represents the exit site from the diastolic pathway to the myocardium giving rise to the QRS. The initial step in localization of the VT is examination of the ECG.[46,63,74] Our laboratory has reported on hundreds of such VTs, and these results are reported elsewhere,[46,48,74] but in summary approximately 59% of VTs can be localized

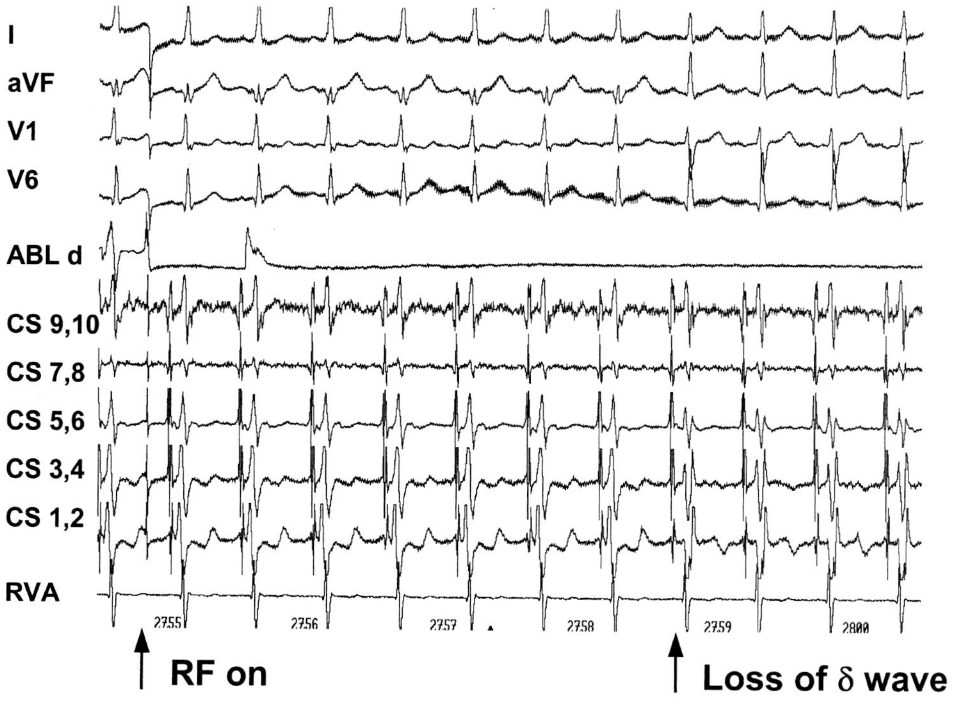

Figure 80–5 **Ablation in the Wolff–Parkinson–White syndrome.** ECG leads I, aVF, V1, and V6 and proximal (CS 9, 10) to distal (CS 1,2), and RV apical (RVA) recordings are shown. The bypass tract is a left posterior bypass tract. RF energy produces loss of the delta (δ) wave in 4 s. See text.

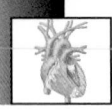

with 93% accuracy, with left bundle branch block VT morphology being more accurate than right bundle and VT from a prior inferior MI being more easy to localize than prior anterior MI.

During EPS, once the clinical VT is induced, a mapping-ablation catheter is advanced into the left ventricle after heparinization to an ACT >250 s. Either a transseptal or retrograde aortic approach is feasible, but for left ventricular VT ablations the retrograde aortic approach provides superior catheter maneuverability. Further mapping of the VT is then performed by examination of the electrograms obtained during the VT, as well as their response to pacing during the VT. Stevenson et al[106] have devised a scheme to help understand the various components of the reentry circuit, including the central common pathway or protected isthmus of myocardium that is the target site for ablation.

There is more than one approach to localizing the central common pathway, but the three major steps are as follows: (1) Activation mapping, consisting of finding the site of earliest activation closest to middiastole (or continuous electrical activity). These electrograms frequently are low-amplitude fractionated potentials. (2) Demonstration that this diastolic electrogram has a fixed relationship to the subsequent QRS despite pacing-induced oscillations in the VT cycle length. Finally, the goal is to establish whether such an early site is part of the reentry circuit vs. myocardium outside of the circuit activated passively ("bystander site"). (3) Performing entrainment mapping to demonstrate an entrained QRS morphology identical to the VT morphology ("concealed entrainment"), a stimulus to QRS duration within 10 ms of the electrogram to QRS duration during VT, and a postpacing interval within 10 ms of the tachycardia cycle length. In our experience, if all three criteria are met, there is a greater than 95% chance of terminating the VT with ablation at a single site[20] (Figure 80–6).

Entrainment mapping[20,59,84,105–107] consists of ventricular pacing at a cycle length slightly shorter then the VT cycle length and seeing if the above criteria are met. If pacing is carried out too rapidly, delays in conduction may occur such that the postpacing interval and the stimulus to QRS may be falsely long. We do not advocate using pace mapping as a primary mapping modality for post-MI VT. A pace map that appears similar to the VT would identify only the exit point for the critical isthmus and may be distant from the common pathway ablation target. Additionally, pacing during sinus rhythm activates the myocardium omnidirectionally, while the QRS during reentrant VT is the result of orthodromic activation of the myocardium by the cyclical depolarization front.

When the clinical VT cannot be hemodynamically tolerated after being induced during EPS, consideration can be given to mapping and ablation during sinus rhythm. Low-amplitude fractionated electrograms and late potentials have been demonstrated in areas of infarction using standard catheter techniques during sinus rhythm.[115] Although no specific electrogram characteristic could predict a VT site of origin with adequate specificity, 86% of ventricular tachycardias arose from areas with these abnormal electrograms.[115] It has also been shown that there are a smaller number of abnormal electrograms in cardiac arrest patients compared to patients with sustained VT.[9] Standard catheter techniques do not allow for precise three-dimensional localization of the abnormal electrograms. Endocardial voltage mapping using the CARTO electroanatomical mapping system in a chronic infarct model has been shown to accurately delineate infarcted myocardium compared to pathology.[8,121] Clinically, voltage mapping has been used in a small number of highly selected patients with VT producing multiple ICD shocks to effectively guide endocardial VT ablation.[72] Using bipolar voltage mapping, normal endocardial bipolar electrogram voltage using electroanatomic mapping was defined at >1.5 mV, based on mapping of six controls. Linear lesions were extended from areas of dense scar to areas of normal voltage myocardium, resulting in a 75% success rate in patients with drug refractory VT that was not hemodynamically tolerated during EPS (Figure 80–7).

Idiopathic Ventricular Tachycardia

VT occurs most often in the post-MI population; however, it is also seen in patients without definite structural heart disease, termed idiopathic VT. The most common type of idiopathic VT is due to triggered activity from delayed afterdepolarizations. It is typically catecholamine dependent, frequently brought on by exertion or emotional stress and can be terminated by vagal maneuvers, adenosine, calcium channel blockers, or sodium channel blockers. These tachycardias usually arise from the right ventricular outflow tract (RVOT),[79] but can also come from the left ventricular outflow tract (LVOT).[7,108] The characteristic ECG for RVOT VT is a left bundle, inferior axis, with either a right or left axis depending on the location in the outflow tract. For LVOT VT, the ECG typically is right bundle, right inferior axis. These VTs often require catecholamine infusion during EPS for induction. The approach to mapping and ablation for both RVOT and LVOT VTs is similar.[12,56,61,114] We advocate activation mapping using both bipolar and unipolar electrograms followed by confirmatory pace mapping. Because idiopathic VT occurs in the absence of structural heart disease and is focal in nature, pace mapping is a viable modality,[21] unlike in post-MI VT.

A second and less common variety of idiopathic VT arises from the left ventricle, is reentrant, and verapamil sensitive.[12,60,61] The characteristic ECG is right bundle, superior axis, which can be left superior if coming from the posterior third of the septum or right superior if coming from the apical third. Opinions regarding the optimal approach to ablation vary, but activation mapping the site of earliest ventricular activation along the septum, followed by pace mapping is generally a reasonable approach. Some authors advocate looking for a Purkinje potential preceding the onset of ventricular activation to target for ablation,[80] although using this method as a primary modality has been questioned by others.[119] Entrainment mapping has also been used successfully, but is difficult to achieve. We advocate ablation for this type of VT using as many mapping modalities as possible, with consideration of the Purkinje spike, concealed entrainment if attainable, activation mapping, and confirmatory pace mapping.

Atrial Fibrillation

Initially, ablation therapy for atrial fibrillation for patients who are refractory or intolerant to pharmacotherapy con-

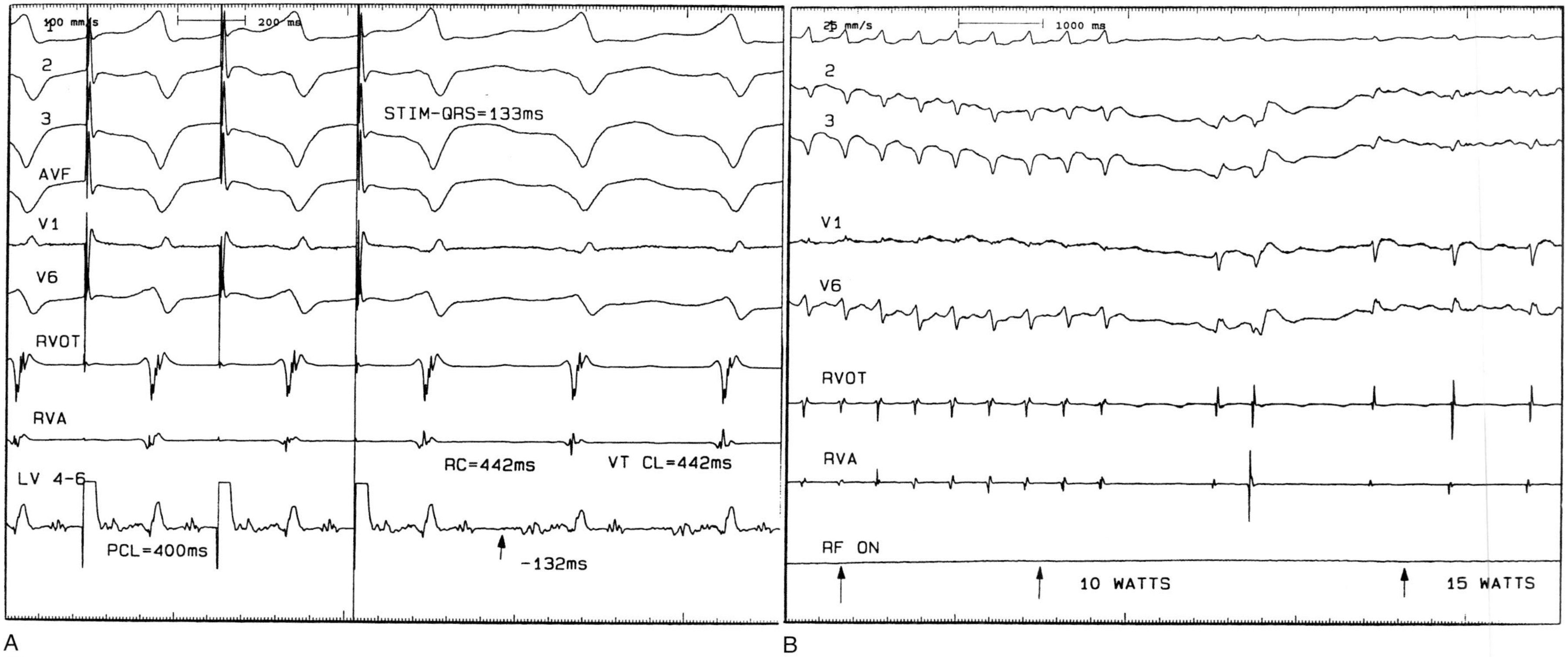

Figure 80–6 Mapping and ablation of ventricular tachycardia. A, ECG leads 1, 2, 3, aVF, V1, and V5 are shown during VT with electrograms from the RV outflow tract (RVOT), RVA, and site of earliest activity in the left ventricle (LV 4–6). Entrainment of VT from LV 4–6 produces a QRS identical to VT, a stimulus (stim)–QRS identical to the electrogram to QRS (arrow). Radiofrequency application at this site terminates VT (**B**).

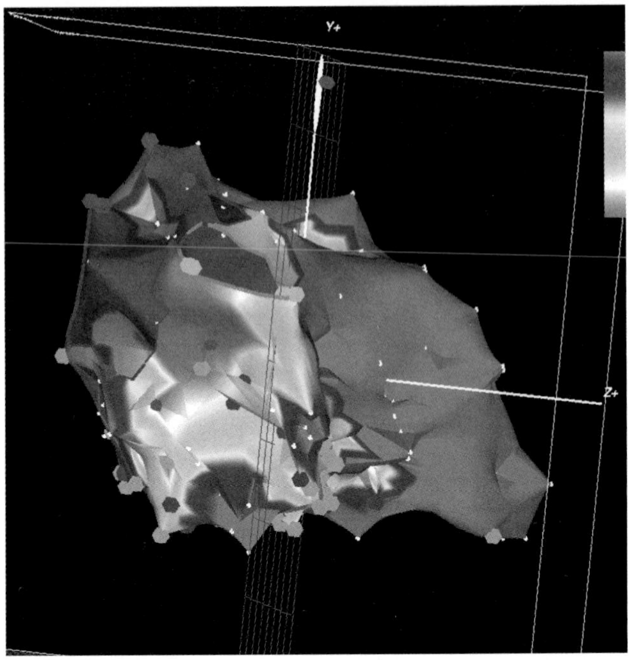

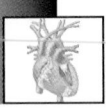

Figure 80–7 Substrate mapping guided ablation of untolerated VT. A voltage map demonstrates low voltage (*scar*) in the center of an old, inferior infarction. Induced unstable VT had morphology that was replicated by pacing the exit site at the border zone. RF lesions from exit site to center of scar abolished VT. (See text.) SP, split potential. (See color plate.)
(Reproduced with permission from Josephson, ME: Clinical Cardiac Electrophysiology. Philadelphia: Lippincott Williams & Wilkins, 2002.)

sisted of AV junction ablation, pacemaker implantation, and anticoagulation. Today, ablation therapy aimed at eliminating or reducing atrial fibrillation is also an option in some patients. Ablation of the AV junction was the first use of catheter ablation and utilized DC energy,[99] which has been supplanted by RF energy today.[76] An ablation catheter is positioned across the tricuspid valve and is positioned to achieve a large His bundle recording. The catheter is then withdrawn 2 cm, resulting in a large atrial electrogram; a very small His bundle recording may also be seen. This technique targets the distal portion of the AV node, allowing for an intact junctional escape pacemaker. Although this does not eliminate the need for pacemaker implantation, it provides backup in case of pacemaker malfunction or lead failure. Our laboratory has a >80% success rate of achieving selective AV nodal block. When this approach fails, the catheter is advanced and the His bundle is targeted directly. Should conduction persist despite repeated ablations in the His bundle area on the right side, ablations on the left side of the heart may prove successful.[51,104] The acute success rate for complete heart block has been reported as 97.6%, with a 3% recurrence of AV conduction.[98] In our laboratory, we monitor successful ablations in the procedure room, with catheters in place, for at least 20 min in the presence of isoproterenol for any resumption of conduction.

AV junction ablation has been associated with an increased risk of sudden cardiac death.[16,25,85] These ventricular arrhythmias are likely polymorphic and related to a phase of electrical instability due to an initial prolongation and then slow adaptation of repolarization caused by the change in heart rate and activation sequence.[85] This may cause prolongation of the QT and propensity for torsades de pointes. Structural heart disease, and other factors that predispose for the acquired long QT syndrome, seem to add to the risk. As a result, the implanted pacemaker should be programmed initially to 80 ppm, which is then typically lowered to 70 ppm at follow up.

Currently, there is increasing interest in the practice of using catheter ablation to eliminate or isolate potential triggers of atrial fibrillation in an effort to eliminate or reduce the amount of fibrillation. Most commonly, these triggers are spontaneous impulses from within the pulmonary veins. Other initiating sites outside of the pulmonary veins have been described, including the left atrial posterior free wall, superior vena cava, crista terminalis, ligament of Marshall, coronary sinus ostium, interatrial septum, and the atrial appendages.[37,48,69] Haissaguerre et al first described initiation of atrial fibrillation by repetitive pulmonary vein potentials (Figure 80-8).[37,44] This mechanism of focal fibrillation initiation is more likely in patients with multiple episodes of paroxysmal atrial fibrillation.

Sustained pulmonary vein (PV) potentials can be triggered mechanically by catheter placement within the vein. Thus, it is important to demonstrate spontaneous ectopic

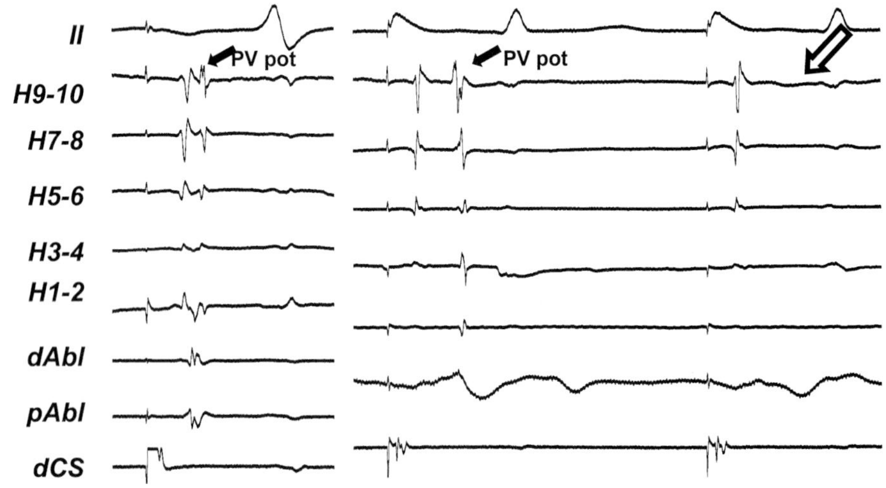

Figure 80–8 Pulmonary vein isolation for atrial fibrillation. Lead 2 and 5 bipolar pair of electrograms from a lasso catheter at the ostium of the left superior pulmonary vein is shown with the ablation catheter (Abl) and the distal coronary sinus (dCS). Pulmonary vein (PV) potentials are shown by arrow. Application of RF delays then isolates (*open arrow*) PV from left atrium (*right panel*). See text.

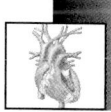

impulse formation in the PVs. The initial step in ascertaining if ectopic atrial activity comes from the PVs is analysis of the ECG P wave and intracardiac mapping catheters. The right and left superior pulmonary veins are the most common sites of ectopic foci.[37] An atrial impulse originating from the right superior PV will be anteriorly directed with a predominantly positive P wave in V1 and have an inferior axis (positive in lead II, III, AVF). It will be narrower than the sinus P wave. In contrast, impulses originating from the left superior PV will have a broad, notched P wave, completely positive in V1 and an inferior axis as well. Decapolar mapping catheters are positioned along the interatrial septum and in the coronary sinus. Right superior PV impulses will have early activation of the posterior septum and CS activation will be proximal to distal. In contrast, left superior PV impulses will show activation in the CS catheter before the interatrial septal catheter. Once the appearance of spontaneous PV foci is suggested, transseptal catheterization is performed. Although some authors advocate a single puncture followed by two wires and two transseptal sheaths, we use a double transseptal puncture to lessen the incidence of persistent atrial septal defect and femoral vein trauma.[31]

A mapping-ablation catheter and a multielectrode halo mapping catheter are then advanced into the left atrium after heparinization to an ACT >250 s, and the halo catheter is placed in the os of a PV. The initial method of ablation was to target the foci by activation mapping within the pulmonary veins,[37] and only in pulmonary veins displaying ectopic activity.[38] Focal ablation in the PV was associated with a high recurrence rate and often produced ablations deeper in the PV, increasing the risk of PV stenosis.[123] Thus, there is currently a move toward complete isolation of the arrhythmogenic myocardial sleeves of the PVs by placing lesions at the os of the PVs. This can be accomplished with a segmental approach, targeting the area of earliest PV activation on the halo catheter[88] or a complete circumferential approach. The segmental approach is possible because the myocardial connections between the PVs and left atrium are typically not fully circumferential around the PV os. A fully circumferential ablation approach can utilize multiple RF lesions around the PV ostia, guided by CARTO mapping[90] or a balloon catheter that wedges in the PV os and creates circumferential lesions with a single application of energy, utilizing either RF with a radiofrequency thermal balloon,[97] or ultrasound,[83] or other energy sources under investigation, such as diode laser.[58] In our laboratory, currently we try to achieve complete PV isolation of all veins with RF lesions placed at the PV os in a segmental manner utilizing the halo mapping catheter. Although the relative importance of isolation of the two superior PVs and the left inferior vein has been stressed[88] because of more prominent myocardial sleeves,[95] increased difficulty of cannulating the right inferior vein, and relative infrequency of PV foci originating from the right inferior vein,[37] we strive for electrical isolation of all PVs. We also often employ CARTO mapping to confirm the ostial location of the ablation and to reduce fluoroscopy time. End points are absence of PV electrical activity or constant dissociation of persistent PV activity. A confirmation test is pacing from each bipolar electrode pair from the halo catheter seated in the PV to ensure lack of atrial capture.

Complications of PV atrial fibrillation ablations include stroke, transient ischemic attack, perforation/tamponade, phrenic nerve injury, and PV stenosis. Although the incidence of PV stenosis has declined with the use of ostial locations for ablation, a very recent study cited a stenosis rate of 17.3%.[15] The majority of stenoses appear to be minimally symptomatic, although severe cases with accompanying hemoptysis and dyspnea have been described[15] and are usually referred for venous stenting. The reported success rate of atrial fibrillation ablation varies widely, but is typically in the order of 50–75%. Patients with paroxysmal atrial fibrillation and minimal structural heart disease can have success rates in excess of 80%.[88] There are some early data to suggest that atrial fibrillation ablation is associated with a reduction in morbidity and mortality compared to medical therapy, as well as an improvement in quality of life.[89]

The optimal therapy for atrial fibrillation must be tailored to each patient. Structural heart disease, sleep apnea, aging, and fibrosis all make catheter ablation less likely to be successful. Combination therapy is often needed, such as antiarrhythmic pharmacotherapy plus atrial fibrillation ablation, or so-called hybrid therapy, which involves patients in whom class I antiarrhythmic medication organizes the fibrillation to atrial flutter and then are treated with a flutter ablation.[41] Clearly, however, there is a subpopulation of patients in whom the pulmonary veins play a prominent role in the initiation of the arrhythmia and in whom isolation of the pulmonary veins or ablation of specific foci can be curative.

REFERENCES

1. ACC/AHA Task Force Report: Guidelines for clinical intracardiac electrophysiological and catheter ablation procedures. A report of the American College of Cardiology/American Heart Association task force on practice guidelines (Committee on Clinical Intracardiac Electrophysiologic and Catheter Ablation Procedures). Developed in collaboration with the North American Society of Pacing and Electrophysiology. J Am Coll Cardiol 26: 555–573, 1995.
2. Antiarrhythmics versus Implantable Defibrillators (AVID) Investigators: A comparison of antiarrhythmic-drug therapy with implantable defibrillators in patients resuscitated from near-fatal ventricular arrhythmias. N Engl J Med 337: 1576–1583, 1997.
3. Arruda MS, McClelland JH, Wang X, et al: Development and validation of an ECG algorithm for identifying accessory pathway ablation site in Wolff-Parkinson-White syndrome. J Cardiovasc Electrophysiol 9:2–12, 1998.
4. Bashir Y, Heald SC, Katritsis D, et al: Radiofrequency ablation of accessory atrioventricular pathways: predictive value of local electrogram characteristics for the identification of successful target sites. Br Heart J 69:315–321, 1993.
5. Buxton AE, Lee KL, Fisher JD, et al: A randomized study of the prevention of sudden death in patients with coronary artery disease. Multicenter Unsustained Tachycardia Trial Investigators. N Engl J Med 341:1882–1890, 1999.
6. Calkins H, Langberg J, Sousa J, et al: Radiofrequency catheter ablation of accessory atrioventricular connections in 250 patients. Abbreviated therapeutic approach to Wolff-Parkinson-White syndrome. Circulation 85:1337–1346, 1992.
7. Callans DJ, Menz V, Schwartzman D, et al: Repetitive monomorphic tachycardia from the left ventricular outflow

tract: electrocardiographic patterns consistent with a left ventricular site of origin. J Am Coll Cardiol 29:1023–1027, 1997.
8. Callans DJ, Ren JF, Michele J, et al: Electroanatomic left ventricular mapping in the porcine model of healed anterior myocardial infarction. Correlation with intracardiac echocardiography and pathological analysis. Circulation 100: 1744–1750, 1999.
9. Cassidy DM, Vassallo JA, Miller JM, et al: Endocardial catheter mapping in patients in sinus rhythm: relationship to underlying heart disease and ventricular arrhythmias. Circulation 73:645–652, 1986.
10. Cheng J, Cabeen WR, Scheinman MM: Right atrial flutter due to lower loop reentry: mechanism and anatomic substrates. Circulation 99:1700–1705, 1999.
11. Chiang CE, Chen SA, Teo WS, et al: An accurate stepwise electrocardiographic algorithm for localization of accessory pathways in patients with Wolff-Parkinson-White syndrome from a comprehensive analysis of delta waves and R/S ratio during sinus rhythm. Am J Cardiol 76:40–46, 1995.
12. Coggins DL, Lee RJ, Sweeney J, et al: Radiofrequency catheter ablation as a cure for idiopathic tachycardia of both left and right ventricular origin. J Am Coll Cardiol 23: 1333–1341, 1994.
13. Cohn JN, Bristow MR, Chien KR, et al: Report of the national heart, lung, and blood institute special emphasis panel on heart failure research. Circulation 95:766–770, 1997.
14. Cosio FG, Arribas F, Lopez-Gil M, Gonzalez HD: Radiofrequency ablation of atrial flutter. J Cardiovasc Electrophysiol 7:60–70, 1996.
15. Deisenhofer I, Schneider MA, Bohlen-Knauf M, et al: Circumferential mapping and electric isolation of pulmonary veins in patients with atrial fibrillation. Am J Cardiol 91: 159–163, 2003.
16. Dizon J, Blitzer M, Rubin D, et al: Time dependent changes in duration of ventricular repolarization after AV node ablation: insights into the possible mechanism of postprocedural sudden death. Pacing Clin Electrophysiol 23: 1539–1544, 2000.
17. Dual-chamber pacing or ventricular backup pacing in patients with an implantable defibrillator. JAMA 288: 3115–3123, 2002.
18. Dubac M, Khairy P, Rodriguez-Santiago A, et al: Catheter cryoablation of the atrioventricular node in patients with atrial fibrillation: a novel technology for ablation of cardiac arrhythmias. J Cardiovasc Electrophysiol 12:439–444, 2001.
19. Ellenbogen KA, Thames MD, Mohanty PK: New insights into pacemaker syndrome gained from hemodynamic, humoral and vascular responses during ventriculo-atrial pacing. Am J Cardiol 65:53–59, 1990.
20. El-Shalakany A, Hadjis T, Papageorgiou P, et al: Entrainment/mapping criteria for the prediction of termination of ventricular tachycardia by single radiofrequency lesion in patients with coronary artery disease. Circulation X 99: 2283–2289, 1990.
21. Feld GK: Catheter ablation for the treatment of atrial tachycardia. Prog Cardiovasc Dis 37:205–224, 1995.
22. Ferguson TB, Cox JL: Surgical treatment for the Wolff-Parkinson-White syndrome: the endocardial approach. In Zipes DP, Jalife J, editors: Cardiac Electrophysiology: From Cell to Bedside. Philadelphia: W.B. Saunders, 1990.
23. Fitzpatrick AP, Gonzales RP, Lesh MD, et al: New algorithm for the localization of accessory atrioventricular connections using a baseline electrocardiogram. J Am Coll Cardiol 23: 107–116, 1994.
24. Garan H, Nguyen K, McGovern B, et al: Perioperative and long-term results after electrophysiologically directed ventricular surgery for recurrent ventricular tachycardia. J Am Coll Cardiol 8:201–209, 1986.
25. Geelen P, Brugada J, Andries E, Brugada P: Ventricular fibrillation and sudden death after radiofrequency catheter ablation of the atrioventricular junction. Pacing Clin Electrophysiol 20:343–348, 1997.
26. Gepstein L, Hayam G, Ben-Haim SA: A novel method for nonfluoroscopic catheter-based electroanatomical mapping of the heart. In vitro and in vivo accuracy results. Circulation 95:1611–1622, 1997.
27. Gerstenfeld EP, Dixit S, Callans DJ, et al: Quantitative comparison of spontaneous and paced 12-lead electrocardiogram during right ventricular outflow tract ventricular tachycardia. J Am Coll Cardiol 41:2046–2053, 2003.
28. Gillette PC, Garson A: Electrophysiologic and pharmacologic characteristics of automatic ectopic atrial tachycardia. Circulation 56:571–575, 1977.
29. Gornick CC, Adler SW, Pederson B, et al: Validation of a new noncontact catheter system for electroanatomic mapping of left ventricular endocardium. Circulation 99:829–835, 1999.
30. Griffith MJ, Garratt CJ, Ward DE, Camm AJ: The effects of adenosine on sinus node reentrant tachycardia. Clin Cardiol 12:409–411, 1989.
31. Grifka RG, O'Laughlin MP, Nihill MR, Mullins CE: Double-transseptal, double-balloon valvuloplasty for congenital mitral stenosis. Circulation 85:123–129, 1992.
32. Haines DE, Lerman BB, Kron IL, DiMarco JP: Surgical ablation of ventricular tachycardia with sequential map-guided subendocardial resection: electrophysiologic assessment and long-term follow-up. Circulation 77:131–141, 1988.
33. Haines DE, Watson DD, Verow AF: Electrode radius predicts lesion radius during radiofrequency energy heating. Validation of a proposed thermodynamic model. Circ Res 67:124–129, 1990.
34. Haines DE, Watson DD: Tissue heating during radiofrequency catheter ablation: a thermodynamic model and observations in isolated perfused and superfused canine right ventricular free wall. PACE 12:962–976, 1989.
35. Haines DE: The biophysics of radiofrequency catheter ablation in the heart: the importance of temperature monitoring. Pacing Clin Electrophysiol 16:586–591, 1993.
36. Haines DE: The pathophysiology of radiofrequency lesion formation. In Zipes DP, editor: Catheter Ablation of Arrythmias. Armonk, NY: Futura, 1994.
37. Haissaguerre M, Jais P, Shah DC, et al: Spontaneous initiation of atrial fibrillation by ectopic beats originating in the pulmonary veins. N Engl J Med 339:659–666, 1998.
38. Haissaguerre M, Shah DC, Jais P, et al: Electrophysiological breakthroughs from the left atrium to the pulmonary veins. Circulation 102:2463–2465, 2000.
39. Harrison L, Gallagher JJ, Kasell J, et al: Cryosurgical ablation of the AV node His bundle: a new method for producing AV block. Circulation 55:463–470, 1977.
40. Horowitz LN, Harken AH, Kastor JA, Josephson ME: Ventricular resection guided by epicardial and endocardial mapping for treatment of recurrent ventricular tachycardia. N Engl J Med 302:589–593, 1980.
41. Huang DT, Monahan KM, Zimetbaum P, et al: Hybrid pharmacologic and ablative therapy: a novel and effective approach for the management of atrial fibrillation. J Cardiovasc Electrophysiol 9:462–469, 1998.
42. Huang SK, Graham AR, Lee MA, et al: Comparison of catheter ablation using radiofrequency versus direct current energy: biophysical, electrophysiologic and pathologic observations. J Am Coll Cardiol 18:1091–1097, 1991.
43. Jackman WM, Beckman KJ, McClelland JH, et al: Treatment of supraventricular tachycardia due to atrioventricular nodal reentry, by radiofrequency catheter ablation of slow-pathway conduction. N Engl J Med 327:313–318, 1992.

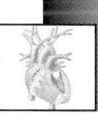

44. Jais P, Haissaguerre M, Shah DC, et al: A focal source of atrial fibrillation treated by discrete radiofrequency ablation. Circulation 95:572–576, 1997.
45. James TN: Morphology of the human atrioventricular node with remarks pertinent to its electrophysiology. Am Heart J 62:756, 1961.
46. Josephson ME, Horowitz LN, Waxman HL, et al: Sustained ventricular tachycardia: role of the 12-lead electrocardiogram in localizing site of tachycardia: role of the 12-lead electrocardiogram in localizing site of origin. Circulation 64:257–272, 1981.
47. Josephson ME, Waxman HL, Cain ME, et al: Ventricular activation during ventricular endocardial pacing. II. Role of pace-mapping to localize origin of ventricular tachycardia. Am J Cardiol 50:11–22, 1982.
48. Josephson ME: Clinical Cardiac Electrophysiology. Philadelphia, PA: Lippincott Williams & Wilkins, 2002.
49. Josephson ME: Paraxysmal supraventricular tachycardia: an electrophysiologic approach. Am J Cardiol 41:1123–1126, 1978.
50. Kadish AH, Childs K, Schmaltz S, Morady F: Differences in QRS configuration during unipolar pacing from adjacent sites: implications for the spatial resolution of pace-mapping. J Am Coll Cardiol 17:143–151, 1991.
51. Kalbfleisch SJ, Williamson B, Man KC, et al: A randomized comparison of the right-and left-sided approaches to ablation of the atrioventricular junction. Am J Cardiol 72:1406–1410, 1993.
52. Kall JG, Wilber DJ: Radiofrequency catheter ablation of an automatic atrial tachycardia in an adult. Pacing Clin Electrophysiol 15:280–287, 1992.
53. Kalman JM, Olgin JE, Karch MR, et al: "Cristal tachycardias": origin of right atrial tachycardias from the crista terminalis identified by intracardiac echocardiography. J Am Coll Cardiol 31:451–459, 1998.
54. Kalman JM, Olgin JE, Saxon LA, et al: Activation and entrainment mapping defines the tricuspid annulus as the anterior barrier in typical atrial flutter. Circulation 94: 398–406, 1996.
55. Kalman JM, Olgin JE, Saxon LA, et al: Electrocardiographic and electrophysiologic characterization of atypical atrial flutter in man: use of activation and entrainment mapping and implications for catheter ablation. J Cardiovasc Electrophysiol 8: 121–144, 1997.
56. Kamakura S, Shimizu W, Matsuo K, et al: Localization of optimal ablation site of idiopathic ventricular tachycardia from right and left ventricular outflow tract by body surface ECG. Circulation 98:1525–1533, 1998.
57. Kay GN, Chong F, Epstein AE, et al: Radiofrequency ablation for treatment of primary atrial tachycardias. J Am Coll Cardiol 21:901–909, 1993.
58. Keane D, Ruskin J: Pulmonary vein isolation for atrial fibrillation. Rev Cardiovasc Med 3:167–175, 2002.
59. Khan HH, Stevenson WG: Activation times in and adjacent to reentry circuits during entrainment: implications for mapping ventricular tachycardia. Am Heart J 127:833–842, 1994.
60. Klein GJ, Millman PJ, Yee R: Recurrent ventricular tachycardia responsive to verapamil. Pacing Clin Electrophysiol 7: 938–948, 1984.
61. Klein LS, Shih HT, Hackett FK, et al: Radiofrequency catheter ablation of ventricular tachycardia in patients without structural heart disease. Circulation 85:1666–1674, 1992.
62. Koch W: Euber das ultimem moriens des menslichen herzens. Beitr Pathol Anat Allg Pathol 42:203, 1907.
63. Kuchar DL, Ruskin JN, Garan H: Electrocardiographic localization of the site of origin of ventricular tachycardia in patients with prior myocardial infarction. J Am Coll Cardiol 13:893–903, 1989.
64. Langberg JJ, Gallagher M, Strickberger SA, Amirana O: Temperature-guided radiofrequency catheter ablation with very large distal electrodes. Circulation 88:245–249, 1993.
65. Lee MA, Morady F, Kadish A, et al: Catheter modification of the atrioventricular junction with radiofrequency energy for control of atioventricular nodal reentry tachycardia. Circulation 83:827–835, 1991.
66. Lesh MD, Kalman JM, Olgin JE: An electrophysiologic approach to catheter ablation of atrial flutter and tachycardia: from mechanism to practice. In Singer I, editor: Interventional Electrophysiology. Baltimore, MD: Williams & Wilkins, 1997.
67. Lesh MD, Van Hare GF, Epstein LM, et al: Radiofrequency catheter ablation of atrial arrhythmias. Results and mechanisms. Circulation 83:1074–1089, 1994.
68. Lesh MD, Van Hare GF, Scheinman MM, et al: Comparison of the retrograde and transseptal methods for ablation of left free wall accessory pathways. J Am Coll Cardiol 22:542–549, 1993.
69. Lin WS, Tai CT, Hsieh MH, et al: Catheter ablation of paroxysmal atrial fibrillation initiated by non-pulmonary vein ectopy. Circulation 107:3176–3183, 2003.
70. Lipscomb KJ, Zaidi AM, Fitzpatrick AP, Lefroy D: Slow pathway modification for atrioventricular node reentrant tachycardia: fast junctional tachycardia predicts adverse prognosis. Heart 85:44–47, 2001.
71. Mahain I: Kent's fibers and the AV paraspecific conduction through the upper connections of the bundle of His-Tawara. Am Heart J 33:651, 1947.
72. Marchlinski FE, Callans DJ, Gottlieb CD, Zado E: Linear ablation lesions for control of unmappable ventricular tachycardia in patients with ischemic and nonischemic cardiomyopathy. Circulation 101:1288–1296, 2000.
73. Miller JM, Kienzle MG, Harken AH, Josephson ME: Subendocardial resection for ventricular tachycardia: predictors of surgical success. Circulation 70:624–631, 1984.
74. Miller JM, Marchlinski FE, Buxton AE, Josephson ME: Relationship between the 12-lead electrocardiogram during ventricular tachycardia and endocardial site of origin in patients with coronary artery disease. Circulation 77: 759–766, 1988.
75. Moe GK, Preston JB, Burlington HJ: Physiologic evidence for a dual AV transmission system. Circ Res 4:357, 1956.
76. Morady F, Calkins H, Langberg JJ, et al: A prospective randomized comparison of direct current and radiofrequency ablation of the atrioventricular junction. J Am Coll Cardiol 21:102–109, 1993.
77. Moss AJ, Hall WJ, Cannom DS, et al: Improved survival with an implanted defibrillator in patients with coronary disease at high risk for ventricular arrhythmia. Multicenter Automatic Defibrillator Implantation Trial Investigators. N Engl J Med 335:1933–1940, 1996.
78. Moss AJ, Wojciech Z, Hall WJ, et al: Prophylactic implantation of a defibrillator in patients with myocardial infarction and reduced ejection fraction. N Engl J Med 346:877–883, 2002.
79. Movsowitz C, Schwartzman D, Callans DJ, et al: Idiopathic right ventricular outflow tract tachycardia: narrowing the anatomic location for successful ablation. Am Heart J 131: 930–936, 1996.
80. Nakagawa H, Beckman KJ, McClelland JH, et al: Radiofrequency catheter ablation of idiopathic left ventricular tachycardia guided by a Purkinje potential. Circulation 86: 2607–2617, 1993.
81. Nakagawa H, Lazzara R, Khastgir T, et al: Role of the tricuspid annulus and the eustachian valve/ridge on atrial flutter. Relevance to catheter ablation of the septal isthmus and a new technique for rapid identification of ablation success. Circulation 94:407–424, 1996.
82. Narula OS: Sinus node re-entry: a mechanism for supraventricular tachycardia. Circulation 50:1114–1128, 1974.

83. Natale A, Pisano E, Shewchik J, et al: First human experience with pulmonary vein isolation using a through-the-balloon circumferential ultrasound ablation system for recurrent atrial fibrillation. Circulation 102:1879–1882, 2000.
84. Nitta T, Schuessler RB, Mitsuno M, et al: Return cycle mapping after entrainment of ventricular tachycardia. Circulation 97:1164–1175, 1998.
85. Nowinski K, Gadler F, Jensen-Urstad M, Bergfeldt L: Transient proarrhythmic state following atrioventricular junction radiofrequency ablation: pathophysiologic mechanisms and recommendations for management. Am J Med 113: 596–602, 2002.
86. Olgin JE, Kalman JM, Fitzpatrick AP, Lesh MD: Role of right atrial endocardial structures as barriers to conduction during human type I atrial flutter. Activation and entrainment mapping guided by intracardiac echocardiography. Circulation 92:1839–1848, 1995.
87. Olshansky B, Okumura K, Hess PG, Waldo AL: Demonstration of an area of slow conduction in human atrial flutter. J Am Coll Cardiol 16:1639–1648, 1990.
88. Oral H, Knight BP, Tada H, et al: Pulmonary vein isolation for paroxysmal and persistent atrial fibrillation. Circulation 105: 1077–1081, 2002.
89. Pappone C, Rosanio S, Augello G, et al: Mortality, morbidity, and quality of life after circumferential pulmonary vein ablation for atrial fibrillation: outcomes from a controlled nonrandomized long-term study. J Am Coll Cardiol 42:185–197, 2003.
90. Pappone C, Rosanio S, Oreto G, et al: Circumferential radiofrequency ablation of pulmonary vein ostia: a new anatomic approach for curing atrial fibrillation. Circulation 102: 2619–2628, 2000.
91. Poty H, Saoudi N, Nair M, et al: Radiofrequency catheter ablation of atrial flutter. Further insights into the various types of isthmus block: application to ablation during sinus rhythm. Circulation 94:3204–3213, 1996.
92. Prystowsky EN: Atrioventricular node reentry: physiology and radiofrequency ablation. Pacing Clin Electrophysiol 20: 552–571, 1997.
93. Roman CA, Wang X, Friday KJ: Catheter technique with selective ablation of slow pathway and AV nodal reentrant tachycardia. PACE 13:498, 1990.
94. Rumbak MJ, Chokshi SK, Abel N, et al: Left phrenic nerve paresis complicating catheter radiofrequency ablation for Wolff-Parkinson-White syndrome. Am Heart J 132: 1280–1285, 1996.
95. Saito T, Waki K, Becker AE: Left atrial myocardial extension onto pulmonary veins in humans: anatomic observations relevant for atrial arrhythmias. J Cardiovasc Electrophysiol 11: 888–894, 2000.
96. Sanders WE, Sorrentino RA, Greenfield RA, et al: Catheter ablation of sinoatrial node reentrant tachycardia. J Am Coll Cardiol 23:926–934, 1994.
97. Satake S, Tanaka K, Saito S, et al: Usefulness of a new radiofrequency thermal balloon catheter for pulmonary vein isolation: a new device for treatment of atrial fibrillation. J Cardiovasc Electrophysiol 14:609–615, 2003.
98. Scheinman MM, Huang S: The 1998 NASPE prospective catheter ablation registry. Pacing Clin Electrophysiol 23: 1020–1028, 2000.
99. Scheinman MM, Morady F, Hess DS, Gonzalez R: Catheter-induced ablation of the atrioventricular junction to control refractory supraventricular arrhythmias. JAMA 248:851–855, 1982.
100. Schwartzman D, Callans DJ, Gottlieb CD, et al: Conduction block in the inferior vena caval-tricuspid valve isthmus: association with outcome of radiofrequency ablation of type I atrial flutter. J Am Coll Cardiol 28:1519–1531, 1996.
101. Sosa E, Scanavacca M, d'Avila A, et al: Endocardial and epicardial ablation guided by nonsurgical transthoracic epicardial mapping to treat recurrent ventricular tachycardia. J Cardiovasc Electrophysiol 9:229–239, 1998.
102. Sosa E, Scanavacca M, d'Avila A, et al: Nonsurgical transthoracic epicardial catheter ablation to treat recurrent ventricular tachycardia occurring late after myocardial infarction. J Am Coll Cardiol 35:1442–1449, 2000.
103. Sosa E, Scanavacca M, d'Avila A, Pilleggi F: A new technique to perform epicardial mapping in the electrophysiology laboratory. J Cardiovasc Electrophysiol 7:531–536, 1996.
104. Souza O, Gursoy S, Simonis F, et al: Right-sided versus left-sided radiofrequency ablation of the His bundle. Pacing Clin Electrophysiol 15:1454–1459, 1992.
105. Stevenson WG, Friedman PL, Sager PT, et al: Exploring postinfarction reentrant ventricular tachycardia with entrainment mapping. J Am Coll Cardiol 29:1180–1189, 1997.
106. Stevenson WG, Khan H, Sager P, et al: Identification of reentry circuit sites during catheter mapping and radiofrequency ablation of ventricular tachycardia late after myocardial infarction. Circulation 88:1647–1670, 1993.
107. Stevenson WG, Sager PT, Friedman PL: Entrainment techniques for mapping atrial and ventricular tachycardias. J Cardiovasc Electrophysiol 6:201–216, 1995.
108. Storey J, Iwasa A, Feld GK: Left ventricular outflow tract tachycardia originating from the right coronary cusp: identification of location of origin by endocardial noncontact activation mapping from the right ventricular outflow tract. J Cardiovasc Electrophysiol 13:1050–1053, 2002.
109. Strickberger SA, Knight BP, Michaud GF, et al: Mapping and ablation of ventricular tachycardia guided by virtual electrograms using a noncontact, computerized mapping system. J Am Coll Cardiol 35:414–421, 2000.
110. Swartz JF, Cohen AI, Fletcher RD, et al: Right coronary epicardial mapping inproves accessory pathway catheter ablation success. Circulation 80:II-431, 1989.
111. Tai CT, Chen SA, Chiang CE, et al: Electrocardiographic and electrophysiologic characteristics of anteroseptal, midseptal, and para-Hisian accessory pathways. Implication for radiofrequency catheter ablation. Chest 109:730–740, 1996.
112. Thakur RK, Klein GJ, Yee R, Stites HW: Junctional tachycardia: a useful marker during radiofrequency ablation for atrioventricular node reentrant tachycardia. J Am Coll Cardiol 22:1706–1710, 1993.
113. Tracy CM, Swartz JF, Fletcher RD, et al: Radiofrequency catheter ablation of ectopic atrial tachycardia using paced activation sequence mapping. J Am Coll Cardiol 22:910–917, 1993.
114. Varma N, Josephson ME: Therapy of "idiopathic" ventricular tachycardia. J Cardiovasc Electrophysiol 8:104–116, 1997.
115. Vassallo JA, Cassidy D, Simson MB, et al: Relation of late potentials to site of origin of ventricular tachycardia associated with coronary heart disease. Am J Cardiol 55:985–989, 1985.
116. Walsh EP, Saul JP, Hulse JE, et al: Transcatheter ablation of ectopic atrial tachycardia in young patients using radiofrequency current. Circulation 86:1138–1146, 1992.
117. Wathen M, Natale A, Wolfe K, et al: An anatomically guided approach to atrioventricular node slow pathway ablation. Am J Cardiol 70:886–889, 1992.
118. Weisfogel GM, Batsford WP, Paulay KL, et al: Sinus node reentrant tachycardia in man. Am Heart J 90:295–304, 1975.
119. Wellens HJ, Smeets JL: Idiopathic left ventricular tachycardia: cure by catheter ablation (editorial). Circulation 88:2978–2979, 1993.
120. Wood FC, Wolferth GC, Geckler GD: Histologic demonstration of accessory muscular connections between auricle and ventricle in a case of short PR interval and prolonged QRS complex. Am Heart J 25:454, 1943.

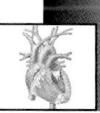

121. Wrobleski D, Houghtaling C, Josephson ME, et al: Use of electrogram characteristics during sinus rhythm to delineate the endocardial scar in a porcine model of healed myocardial infarction. J Cardiovasc Electrophysiol 14:524–529, 2003.
122. Wu D, Denes P, Amat-y-Leon F, et al: Clinical, electrocardiographic and electrophysiologic observations in patients with paroxysmal supraventricular tachycardia. Am J Cardiol 41:1045–1051, 1978.
123. Yu WC, Hsu TL, Tai CT, et al: Acquired pulmonary vein stenosis after radiofrequency catheter ablation of paroxysmal atrial fibrillation. J Cardiovasc Electrophysiol 12:887–892, 2001.

Surgical Treatment of Cardiac Arrhythmias

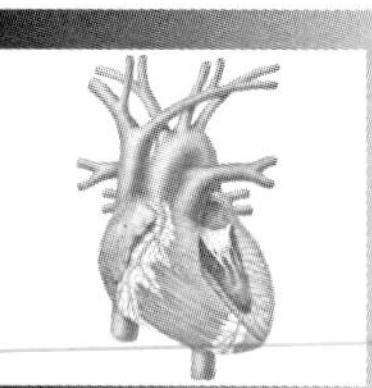

CHAPTER 81

Louis I. Astra and Robert E. Michler

INTRODUCTION

Arrhythmia surgery began in the late 1960s, when Sealy and colleagues performed the first successful surgical treatment of Wolff–Parkinson–White (WPW) syndrome.[121] Since that time, arrhythmia surgery has evolved to treat all types of arrhythmias. In more recent years, technology has enabled us to treat a number of arrhythmias with endocardial catheter techniques. Also, there has been a dramatic increase in treatment options that utilize implantable defibrillators and antitachycardia pacemakers. Over the years, the role of surgery has been steadily declining as the primary treatment of arrhythmias. However, it is important for surgeons to stay abreast of the various surgical techniques to treat arrhythmias since some patients may have failed other therapies or may require conventional cardiac surgery in addition to arrhythmia surgery. Moreover, the surgical treatment of atrial fibrillation is increasing in frequency. Surgical treatments are becoming less invasive and easier to perform, and, therefore, we may see a resurgence of many arrhythmia operations.

This chapter will review the fundamental concepts underlying the pathophysiology of cardiac arrhythmias followed by surgical treatment options, concluding with future directions of arrhythmia surgery.

BASIC ELECTROPHYSIOLOGY

To understand the treatment of arrhythmias, one must understand the mechanisms of arrhythmias as well as normal cardiac electrical conduction. We begin by examining the sequence of electrical events during a normal cardiac cycle.

Before the onset of mechanical activity, an electrical impulse is delivered to the myocardium. At the cellular level, the electrical impulse begins as a membrane depolarization followed by repolarization termed the action potential (AP). The AP is propagated throughout the heart via specialized pathways. The AP is generated and propagated through a series of coordinated conductance changes of sodium, calcium, and potassium ions. These conductance changes are enabled through variably gated ion channels located on the cellular membrane. The resting potential of approximately −80 to −90 mV is established by an Na-K-ATPase, which is an ATP-dependent pump designed to drive Na^+ out of the cell. The cardiac AP has five distinct phases (Figure 81-1). Phase 0, or depolarization, is a result of Na channels opening with subsequent rapid inward Na current. Phase 1 occurs immediately following depolarization, during which time the cells are absolutely refractory to further depolarization. Phase 2, the plateau phase, is a result of voltage-sensitive L-type (long-lasting) Ca channels opening and results in a slow, inward Ca current. The Ca ions are responsible for initiating the cell's contraction apparatus. Phase 3, or repolarization, is brought about by potassium efflux, which returns the voltage of the cell to baseline. Phase 4, the resting potential, is maintained by Na efflux and K influx through the ATPase mechanisms described above.

Anatomically, electrical activity normally begins at the sinoatrial (SA) node, located in the right atrium (RA) at the junction between the superior vena cavae (SVC), RA,

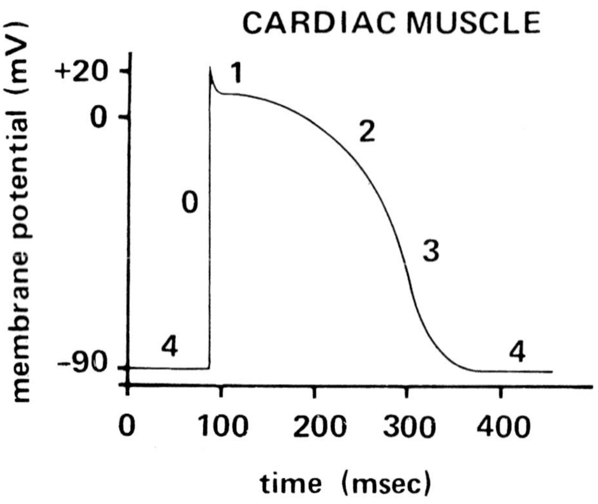

Figure 81–1 The cardiac action potential (shown here for Purkinje fiber) lasts more than 300 ms and consists of five phases, 0 through 4. Spontaneous Phase 4 depolarization is believed to be responsible for automatic arrhythmias.
(From Katz AM: The arrhythmias. II: Abnormal impulse formation and reentry, premature systoles, preexcitation. In Katz AM, editor: Physiology of the Heart. New York: Raven Press, 1977, p. 320.)

and right atrial appendage (RAA) (Figure 81-2). The signal then traverses both atria via specialized conduction tissue and converges at the atrioventricular (AV) node. The AV node is located in tissue between the interatrial and interventricular septa. From a surgical perspective, the node is located within the triangle of Koch. The tendon of Todaro, the tricuspid valve annulus, and the thebesian valve of the coronary sinus bound this region. The AV node is responsible for slowing the electrical impulse resulting in the normal conduction delay seen between the atria and ventricles. Once past the AV node, the impulse proceeds through both ventricles via the His bundle, which branches to form left and right bundles. The left and right bundles further branch and eventually form the Purkinje system fibers, which are the terminal branches innervating individual ventricular myocytes. The myocytes themselves also are able to conduct electrical activity via intercalated disks, which contain low-resistance gap junctions through which electrical current can easily travel.

The summation of all cardiac electrical signals gives rise to the surface electrocardiogram (ECG). The P-wave represents the electrical depolarization of the atria, the QRS complex represents the depolarization of the ventricles, and the T-wave represents the repolarization of the ventricles. The diagnosis of any arrhythmia begins with an analysis of the ECG. Because the treatment of arrhythmias depends upon the type of arrhythmia, all patients require an ECG demonstrating the arrhythmia prior to diagnosis and treatment. If the arrhythmia is paroxysmal, the patient may require continuous monitoring until the arrhythmia is documented and clearly defined.

The heart contains specialized cells that are capable of spontaneous depolarization called pacemaker cells. Pacemaker cells are located within the conducting fibers of the atria, the AV junction, and the His–Purkinje system. The dominant pacemaker system of the heart is located in the SA node. Cells located in the SA node region typically fire at a rate of between 60 and 100 beats/min. All other sites for pacemaker cells are referred to as ectopic sites. Ectopic pacemakers located in the AV junction (AV node and proximal His bundle) typically fire at a rate of 40–60 beats/min. Finally, His–Purkinje system pacemaker cells typically fire between 20 and 40 beats/min.

GENERAL MECHANISMS OF ARRHYTHMIAS

Arrhythmias result from one of three mechanisms: automatic, triggered, or reentry. Automaticity refers to spontaneous depolarization by ectopic pacemaker cells. During normal conduction, an "automatic" rhythm is generated by the sinus node. Arrhythmias occur if an ectopic pacemaker

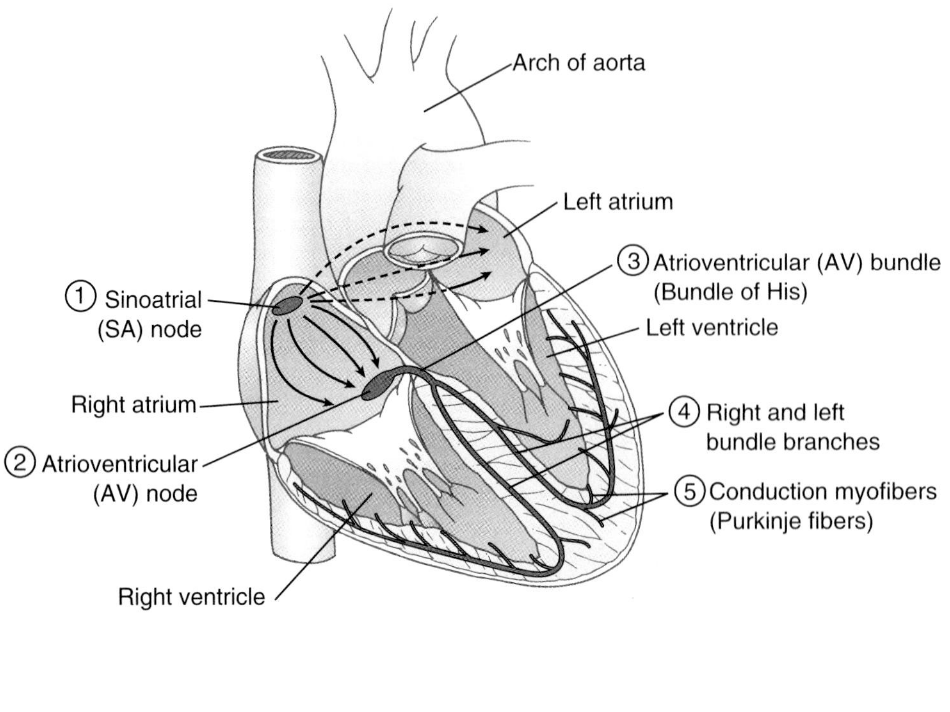

Figure 81–2 Illustration of the heart's conduction system. Impulses normally begin at the SA node (1), travel to the AV node (2), where a delay is present, and then travel to ventricles via bundle of His (3), which bifurcates to left and right bundle branches (4), and later, Purkinje fibers (5).

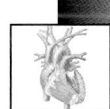

generates an automatic rhythm. This can occur if the intrinsic rate of the sinus node decreases, the intrinsic rate of the ectopic pacemaker increases, or the normal electrical path from the sinus node is blocked.

Triggered arrhythmias arise from "afterdepolarizations" that can occur early or late (after Phase 3 repolarization). During an early afterdepolarization, a positive deflection of sufficient magnitude in the AP during repolarization can lead to another depolarization. Repetitive afterdepolarizations can lead to tachycardias. A clinical example of repetitive afterdepolarizations is torsades de pointes. Repetitive afterdepolarizations can result from various electrolyte abnormalities, hypoxia, class IA or III antiarrhythmias, or congenital prolonged QT syndromes. Late afterdepolarizations are those that occur following Phase 3 repolarization. These can occur as a result of increased catecholamines, digitalis effect, or abnormally high intracellular calcium levels.

During normal conduction, each electrical impulse is extinguished by the tissue refractory period (Phase 4). If, however, an area of myocardium prevents electrical conduction, a unidirectional block may occur. This can result in an impulse that will travel in a continuous circuit, continually reactivating itself forming a reentry circuit (Figure 81-3). Reentry is the most clinically significant tachyarrhythmia. Mayer first described the mechanism of reentry in 1906.[91]

To appropriately treat any arrhythmia, one must accurately define the arrhythmia in terms of its type, mechanism, and location. The type of arrhythmia can usually be deduced from the ECG. However, the mechanism and location are not always easily deduced. Using sophisticated endocardial multisite electrical catheters, it is now possible to obtain accurate maps of electrical activity within the heart in three dimensions. These techniques have allowed for the evolution of electrophysiological cardiology. Indirect approaches have also evolved utilizing such tools as cardiac pacing, effects of selected drugs, and effects of radiofrequency ablation. The interventional treatment of an arrhythmia stems from either surgically removing the focus of the arrhythmia, or from creating a block so that the arrhythmogenic focus is unable to be transmitted to the remainder of the heart.

In assessing the benefit of interventional arrhythmia treatment, it is necessary to understand the severity of patient symptoms, the hemodynamic effects of the arrhythmia, and the potential for progression to more malignant arrhythmias. These factors must be weighed against the standard risks of surgical or catheter-based intervention, which must include the risk of interruption of normal conduction.

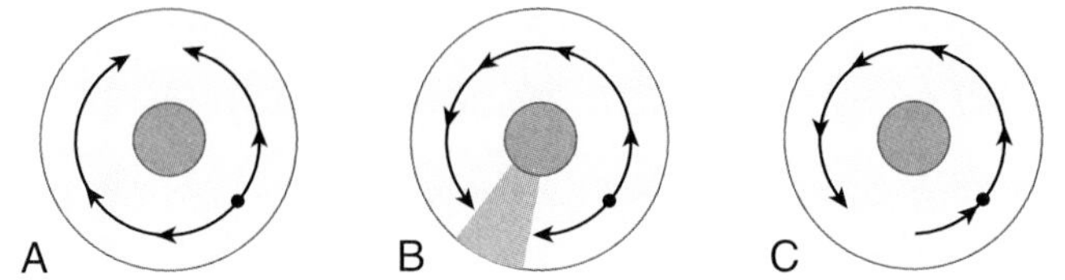

Figure 81-3 Schematic to illustrate the concept of reentry. Region with a central area of block. A, The impulse starts at the black dot and propagates in both directions until it collides; no reentry occurs. **B,** The impulse again starts at the black dot; however, it reaches an area of conduction block represented by the gray area. **C,** If the conduction block is relieved or if the conduction block a unidirectional, the impulse is able to return to the point of origin after the refractory period has ended, and the cycle starts again.

TREATMENT OF SUPRAVENTRICULAR ARRHYTHMIAS

Wolff–Parkinson–White Syndrome

The surgical treatment for WPW syndrome in 1968 marked the beginning of a new era in the treatment of arrhythmias.[121] WPW syndrome is a preexcitation syndrome resulting from accessory AV pathways or Kent bundles. When anomalous electrical accessory pathways exist that bypass the normal AV conducting system, the ventricles may become activated prematurely, without the normal delay produced by the AV node. The result is a shortened PR interval and a functional bundle branch block producing the characteristic delta wave.

Other types of accessory pathways can occur and may give rise to preexcitation syndromes similar to the WPW syndrome. For example, Mahaim pathways refer to bypass tracts arising in the AV node, the His bundle, or bundle branches that connect to the ventricle and bypass the compact AV node[7] (Table 81-1).

Accessory pathways exist normally in the human fetus, and rarely cause problems. During postnatal cardiac development, the pathways normally obliterate. It is understandable why accessory pathway arrhythmias such as WPW

Table 81-1

Names of Accessory Pathways Causing Ventricular Preexcitation Syndromes

Anatomic term for pathway	*Previous nomenclature*
Accessory AV bundle	Kent bundle (present in WPW syndrome)
Septal accessory AV bundle	Paladino tract
Compact nodoventricular bundle	Mahaim fiber
Atriofascicular bypass tract	AtrioHisian fibers
Fasciculoventricular connections	Mahaim fibers
Intranodal bypass tracts	James fibers

From Kottkamp H, Hindricks G, Shenasa H, et al: Variants of preexcitation: Specialized atriofascicular pathways, nodofascicular pathways, and fasciculoventricular pathways: Electrophysiologic findings and target sites for radiofrequency catheter ablation. J Cardiovasc Electrophysiol 7: 916–930, 1996.

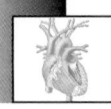

syndrome may be associated with other congenital heart defects including Ebstein's anomaly, mitral valve prolapse, and cardiomyopathy.

Clinical Presentation

WPW syndrome usually presents as paroxysmal tachycardia or paroxysmal atrial flutter/fibrillation. Occasionally, atrial tachycardias can give rise to ventricular tachycardias when the accessory pathway bypasses the normal delay imposed by the AV node.

Intermittent atrial tachycardias most commonly occur when a premature atrial impulse is conducted in the normal manner to the ventricles via the AV node, but then retrograde through an accessory pathway to the atrium, causing premature reexcitation of the atrium and completion of the continuous circuit (Figure 81-4). In some WPW patients, the accessory pathway can conduct only in retrograde fashion, thereby allowing for paroxysmal tachycardias, but not permitting ventricular preexcitation. These WPW patients have a "concealed pathway" and do not have the characteristic delta wave on an ECG.

Anatomical Basis

To interrupt the accessory pathways, a thorough knowledge is necessary of the anatomy of the AV junction. A detailed review can be found in a recent article describing the anatomy involved in ventricular preexcitation.[6] The AV junction comprises the points of coaptation between the three orifices of the mitral, tricuspid, and aortic valves, as well as the surrounding tissue where the ventricles meet the atria (Figure 81-5). The AV junction is composed of both fibrous and adipose tissue, which ordinarily insulate the ventricles from direct atrial electrical stimulation, resulting in normal electrical conduction through the AV node. When accessory pathways exist, muscular connections interrupt this fibroadipose tissue between the atria and ventricles. The locations of accessory pathways have been categorized into four distinct but arbitrary locations (Figure 81-5). In decreasing order of frequency, those locations are left free wall, posteroseptal, right free wall, and anteroseptal.[13,22] Interestingly, patients with WPW syndrome and Ebstein's anomaly more commonly have pathways located in the posteroseptal and right free wall locations.[22] Cox advocates that if a preoperative electrophysiological study reveals this combination of pathways, an ECG should be performed to rule out Ebstein's anomaly.[21] Posteroseptal pathways are also associated with coronary sinus diverticuli. The pathway is usually part of the diverticulum and surgical treatment to divide the neck of the diverticulum interrupts the pathway. Because of the fibrous tissue connection between the mitral and aortic valve leaflets, accessory pathways cannot exist between the right and left fibrous trigones (Figure 81-5).

Surgical Indications

Surgical treatment of WPW syndrome is rarely indicated today. Advances in catheter ablation techniques have resulted in the ability of the cardiac electrophysiologist to

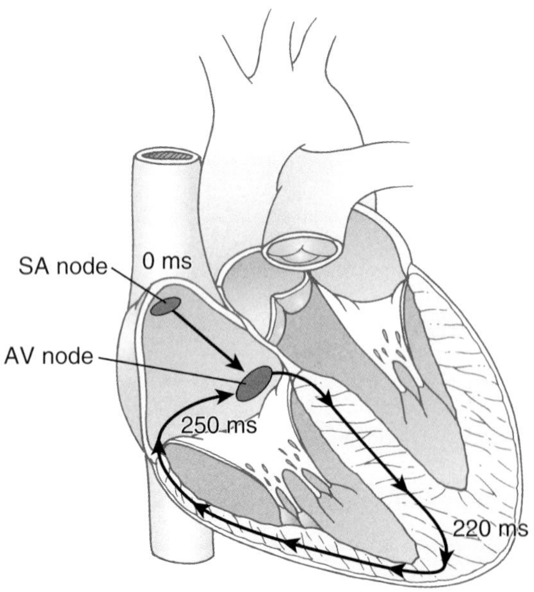

Figure 81–4 WPW reentrant circuit demonstrating normal antegrade conduction through the AV node, with retrograde conduction across the Kent bundle (accessory pathway) completing the circuit. Mapping reveals the timing of the circuit to be about 250 ms, which corresponds to a heart rate of about 200–250 beats/min. SA, sinoatrial; AV, atrioventricular. *(Modified from Lewis WH, editor: Gray's Anatomy: Anatomy of the Human Body. Philadelphia: Lea & Febiger, 1918.)*

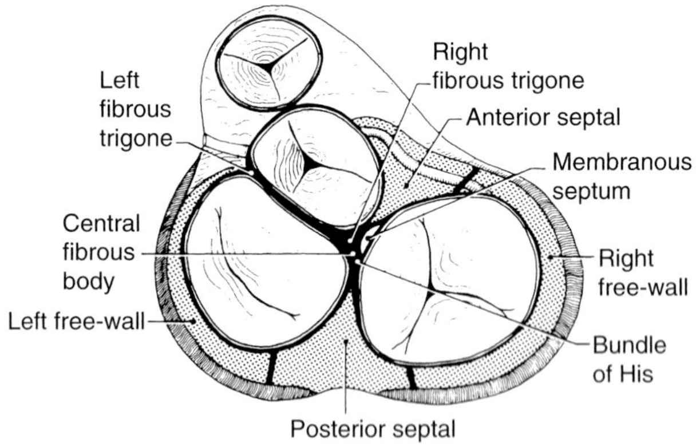

Figure 81–5 Diagram of the superior view of the heart with the atria cut away, demonstrating the boundaries of each of the four anatomical areas where accessory pathways can occur in the Wolff–Parkinson–White (WPW) syndrome. The boundaries of the left free wall space are the mitral valve annulus and the ventricular epicardial reflection extending from the left fibrous trigone to the posterior septum. The boundaries of the posterior septal space are the tricuspid annulus, the mitral valve annulus, the posterior superior process of the left ventricle, and the ventricular epicardial reflection. The boundaries of the right free wall space are the tricuspid valve annulus and the epicardial reflection extending from the posterior septum to the anterior septal space. All accessory atrioventricular (AV) connections must insert into the ventricle somewhere within these anatomical boundaries. *(From Cox JL, Gallagher JJ, Cain ME: Experience with 118 consecutive patients undergoing surgery for the Wolff-Parkinson-White syndrome. J Thorac Cardiovasc Surg 90:490–501, 1985.)*

less invasively cure most patients with WPW syndrome. At the present time, surgical treatment is limited to failed catheter ablation, usually due to complex anatomy or congenital heart lesions. Primary therapy for patients diagnosed with WPW syndrome is catheter ablation. Medical therapy is less efficacious, and is associated with greater side effects. Ablation therapy is indicated to prevent sudden death even in asymptomatic patients.

Surgical Technique

The surgical technique for treating WPW syndrome was first described by Sealy in 1969,[1] and later expanded upon by Sealy[114–118,120] and Cox.[22] This endocardial approach involves cardiopulmonary bypass and cardioplegic arrest. In an effort to make the surgical procedure simpler and potentially decrease morbidity, Guiraudon and colleagues[48] developed an epicardial approach, which they believe obviates the need for cardioplegic arrest and cardiopulmonary bypass. Cox contends that the Guiraudon epicardial approach still requires cardiopulmonary bypass to prevent significant hypotension associated with manipulation and elevation of the heart.[21]

The accessory pathways that were identified preoperatively should be confirmed at the time of operation by epicardial mapping. In the endocardial approach, the dissection depends upon localization of the accessory pathways. If the accessory pathways are located on the left free wall, an atriotomy is performed 2 mm behind the posterior mitral valve annulus. This is accomplished while on cardiopulmonary bypass with application of the aortic cross-clamp. Dissection is then carried out between the underlying fat pad in the AV groove and the top of the ventricle (Figure 81-6). The coronary artery and vein should be identified and preserved in the coronary sulcus. If accessory pathways exist in the posterior septal, anterior septal, or right free wall, a right atriotomy is performed. On the right side, the atriotomy is made posteriorly, just above the tricuspid valve annulus. Endocardial mapping should then be performed for two reasons. The first is to identify and avoid injuring the His bundle. The second is to better localize the accessory pathways since epicardial mapping on the right is not as precise as on

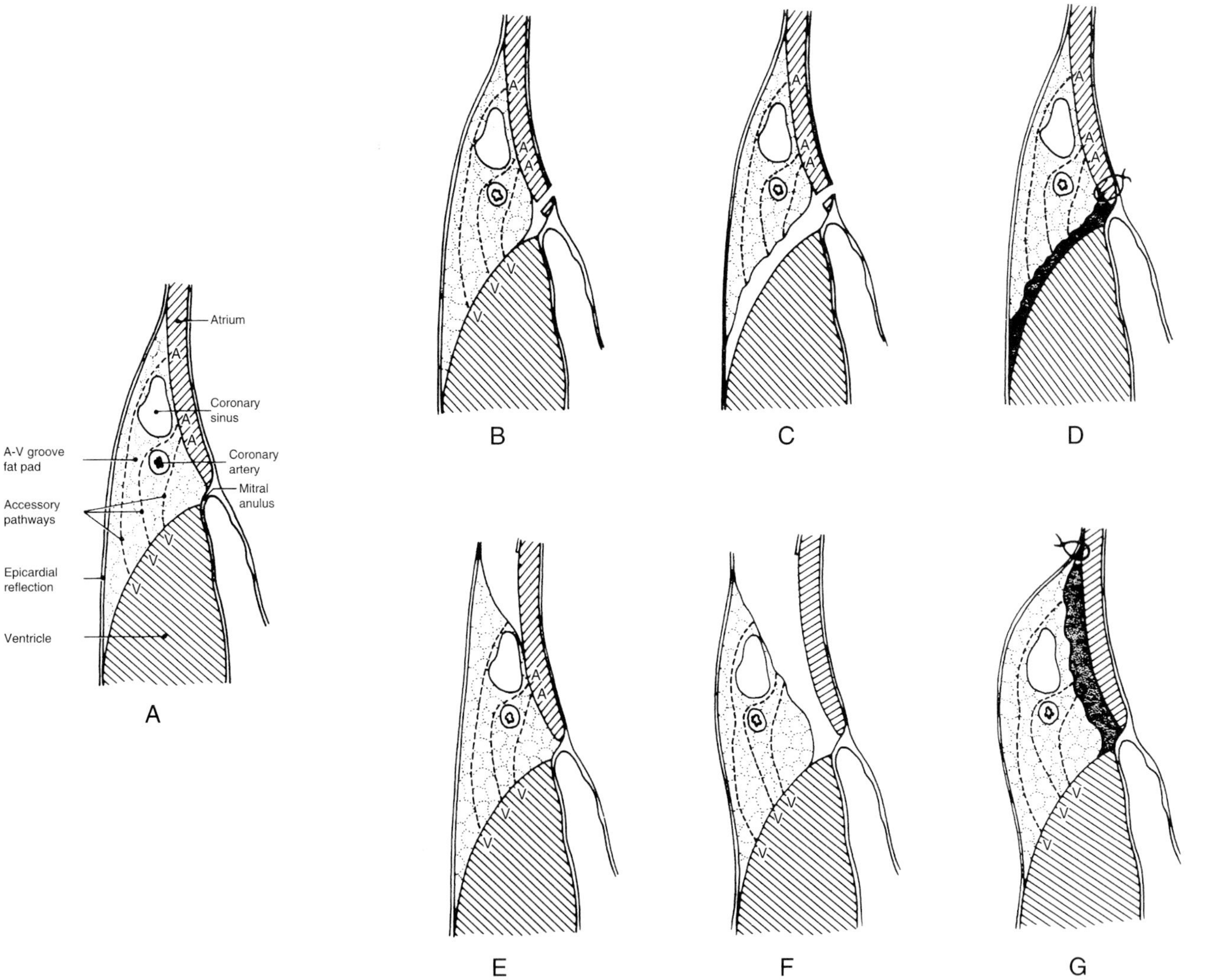

Figure 81–6 Diagrammatic representation of a cross section of the posterior left side of the heart showing the different depths that left free-wall pathways can be located in relation to the mitral annulus and epicardial reflection (**A**). The endocardial surgical technique is depicted **(B–D)** as well as the epicardial technique **(E–G)**.

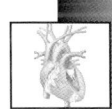

the left due to the thicker fat pad of the right ventricle. Care is taken to avoid injury to the proximal right coronary artery.

The epicardial technique combines dissection of the AV fat pad along with cryoablation of the mitral and/or tricuspid annulus.[49,52,53] In left free wall accessory pathways, exposure of the left coronary sulcus is accomplished with the use of a sling.[55] A sling made of a laparotomy sponge is passed around the ventricle in the transverse sinus and used to elevate the apex of the heart and expose the left AV junction. The epicardium along the ventricular side is incised and the fat pad is bluntly dissected avoiding injury to the coronary arteries. The obtuse cardiac vein may be divided for better exposure. After dissection, division of the accessory pathways should be confirmed with electrophysiological testing. If the pathways are still present, transmural cryoablation should be performed under normothermic cardiopulmonary bypass. Right free wall and anterior septal pathways are readily exposed and dissection along the AV fat pad is carried out in a fashion similar to posterior lesions. Atypical accessory pathways that are not located adjacent to the annulus (i.e., within the myocardial septum, within the membranous septum, or over the intervalvular trigone) can be ablated with discrete transmural cryoablation under cardiopulmonary bypass.[50,51,127]

Surgical Results

The surgical success of curing WPW syndrome is virtually 100%, with a mortality between 0 and 0.5% in elective cases.[22,49] The incidence of heart block is also very low. Prior catheter ablation has not increased the risk of the surgical procedure. Morbidity is similar to that associated with conventional cardiac surgery.

Treatment of Arrhythmias Secondary to Mahaim Pathways

As mentioned in the previous section, Mahaim pathways are accessory pathways that arise in the AV node, His bundle, or bundle branches and travel to the ventricular septum. These tracts may traverse either the anterior (anterior to the His bundle) or posterior septal space. Treatment is very similar to that of WPW syndrome. The treatment of choice is catheter ablation; however, treatment failures lead to surgical intervention. As with most arrhythmia surgery, preoperative localization is imperative. The surgical approach is fundamentally the same as described for WPW syndrome with pathways located in the anterior or posterior septal region. When the pathways are close to the His bundles, treatment includes a combination of dissection and discrete cryoablation. In some cases, the pathways are so close to the His bundles that ablation of the His bundles becomes necessary, resulting in the need for a permanent pacemaker.

Ectopic Atrial Tachycardias

Ectopic atrial tachycardias are classified as automatic arrhythmias with ectopic pacemakers. It is important to distinguish ectopic atrial tachycardias from multifocal atrial tachycardias. Multifocal arrhythmias are usually due to systemic abnormalities such as electrolyte abnormalities, drug side effects, and hyperthyroidism. The treatment of multifocal arrhythmias is medical with correction of the underlying cause.

Ectopic atrial tachycardias are rare in the adult population, comprising less than 1% of all supraventricular tachycardias (SVTs). In children, they are much more common, consisting of 10% of SVTs.[64,86] Between 10 and 50% of patients with ectopic atrial tachycardias have a positive family history of the arrhythmia.[86] Most commonly, they arise from the right atria, followed by the left atria, with a minority arising from the septum. These tachycardias are often incessant, and they may lead to a tachycardia-induced dilated cardiomyopathy.

Once diagnosed, patients should undergo curative therapy since these tachycardias can lead to cardiomyopathy. Once again, catheter-based ablation is the treatment of choice. Only if catheter ablation fails should the patient be referred for surgical intervention. Because these tachycardias are automatic, and not reentrant, they cannot be induced. Also, the tachycardia is frequently suppressed by general anesthesia. Surgical therapy relies on precise preoperative localization by the electrophysiologist.

Surgical Treatment

Surgical therapy consists of resection, ablation, and/or exclusion of the focus. Ablation is favored for septal locations. Exclusion is useful for left atrial lesions, where precise anatomical localization is often more difficult. Left atrial exclusion involves cardiopulmonary bypass and consists of a combination of a left atriotomy incision and two cryoablations[133] (Figure 81-7). The atriotomy disrupts all left atrioventricular connections, and the cryoablations disrupt the interatrial connections. It has been proposed that right atrial foci be treated with an isolation procedure, rather than resection or ablation.[21] Even though a focus can usually be localized on the right atrium, the recurrence rate due to a new focus arising is unacceptably high with ablation alone. The right atrial exclusion procedure is similar to that of the left and includes creation of a cryolesion[61,66] (Figure 81-8).

Paroxysmal Supraventricular Tachycardia

Most paroxysmal supraventricular tachycardias (PSVTs) arise from AV node reentry circuits. The circuit is confined to the AV node or perinodal tissues in the lower atrial septum. The abnormality leading to the reentrant circuit results from two separate conduction pathways through the AV node. There is a slow pathway with a short refractory period and a fast pathway with a long refractory period. During periods of SVT, antegrade conduction occurs through the slow pathway, followed by retrograde conduction in the fast pathway, thereby completing the circuit.

Unlike ectopic tachycardias, PSVT does not usually cause cardiomyopathy. Indications for treatment of these tachycardias are primarily intolerance of symptoms. Once again, treatment for PSVT is usually via catheter ablation. If catheter ablation fails, patients may then be referred for surgical treatment.

Surgical Treatment

The original surgical treatment consisted of division of the His bundle, resulting in complete heart block and implantation

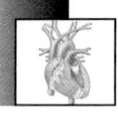

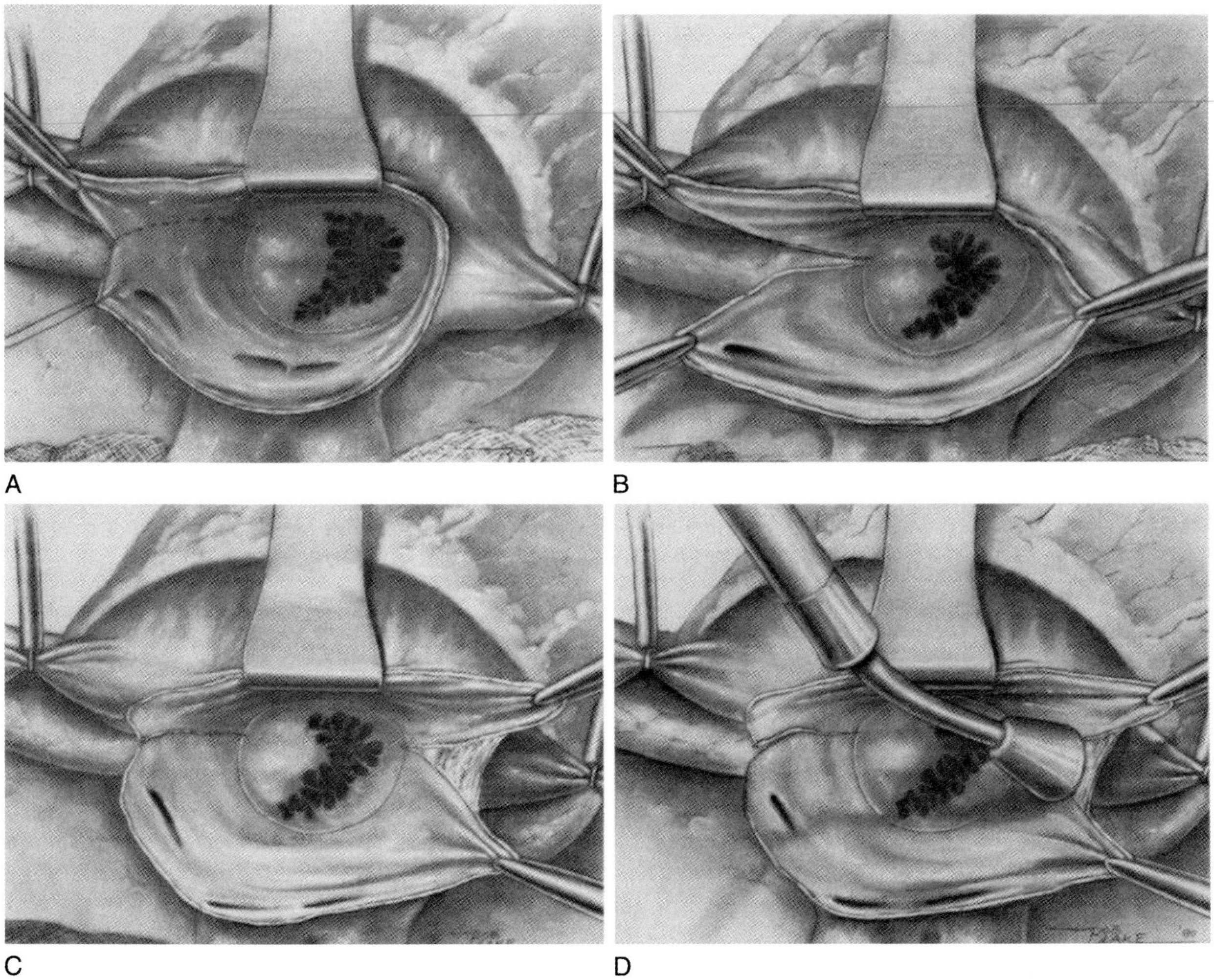

Figure 81–7 Left atrial isolation procedure. A, After a standard left atriotomy incision is made, the interatrial septum is retracted gently, and the atriotomy is extended anteriorly (*dashed line*) across Bachmann's bundle to the level of the mitral valve annulus just to the left of the right fibrous trigone. **B,** The anterior extension of the standard left atriotomy has been completed. The base of the aorta and its juxtaposition with the anterior leaflet of the mitral valve are demonstrated. Note that the anterior atriotomy extends across the mitral valve annulus. The main body of the left atrium has been separated anteriorly from the remainder of the heart. **C,** The transmural left atriotomy is extended posteriorly to the level of the coronary sinus. The remaining portion of the incision is made through the endocardium and extends across the mitral valve annulus posteriorly just to the left of the interatrial septum. At this point, electrical activity continues to be propagated in a 1:1 manner between the right and left atria because of the presence of interatrial muscular connections accompanying the coronary sinus. **D,** A cryoprobe is positioned over the endocardial aspect of the posterior atriotomy, and its temperature is decreased to –60° C for 2 min. This cryolesion ablates the endocardial interatrial fibers accompanying the coronary sinus. A similar cryolesion is created on the epicardial aspect of the AV groove on the opposite side of the coronary sinus to ablate all remaining interatrial epicardial connections. The left atriotomy is closed with a continuous 4–0 nonabsorbable suture.
(From Williams JM, Ungerleider RM, Lofland GK, Cox JL: Left atrial isolation: New technique for the treatment of supraventricular arrhythmias. J Thorac Cardiovasc Surg 80:373, 1980.)

of a ventricular pacemaker.[119] Subsequent realization that the circuit was not in the compact AV node led to the development of surgical treatments that would not result in heart block. Current therapies involve either discrete cryoablation lesions around the periphery of the AV node[24] or sharp dissection around the node.[54,70,90,111] Surgical therapy for PSVT has had excellent short- and long-term results. The reported mortality from the procedure is extremely low, with no operative deaths reported in the series cited. The incidence of complete heart block or recurrent PSVT is very low following surgical therapy.

Atrial Flutter

Pathophysiology

Atrial flutter is usually an unsustained tachycardia that has a characteristic sawtooth pattern on an ECG. Mechanistically, atrial flutter results from a macroreentry phenomenon.[131] The reentry circuit is usually based on an isthmus of tissue in the right atrium. Left atrial circuits have been reported, but have a much more variable location.[68] The isthmus for right atrial circuits is located at the base of the triangle of Koch, between the IVC orifice and tricuspid valve annulus

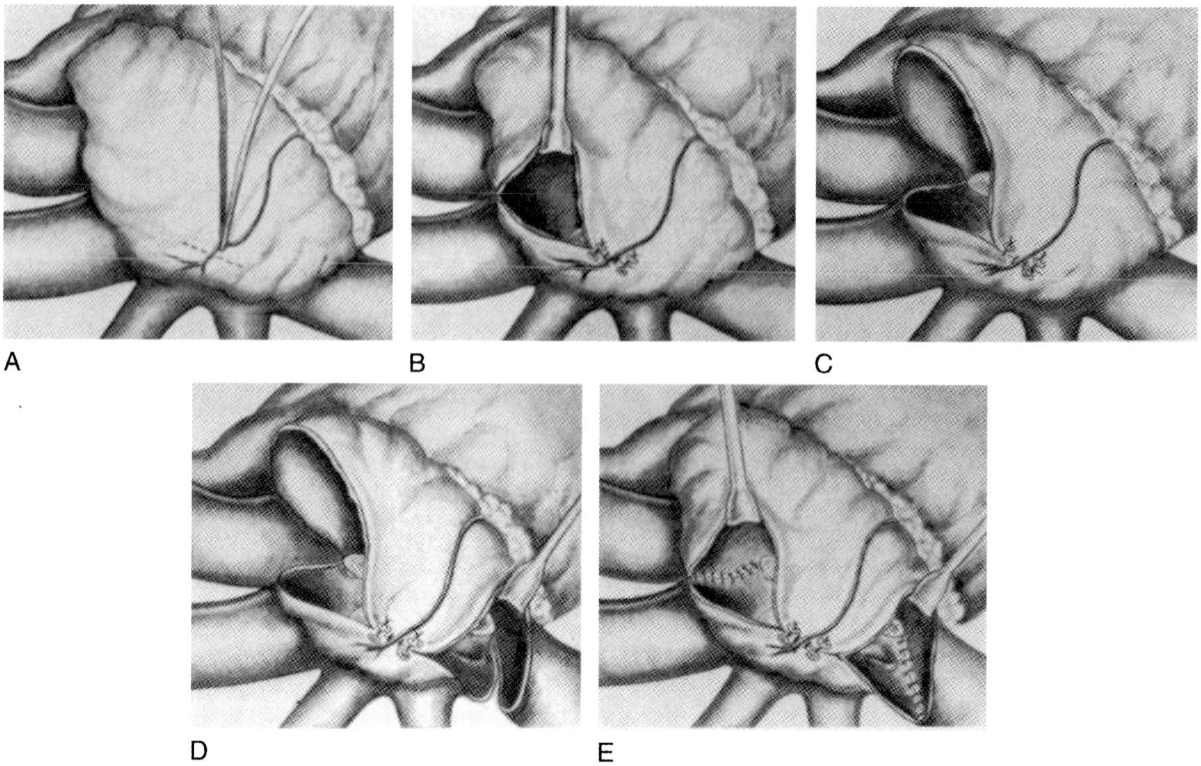

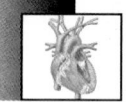

Figure 81–8 **Right atrial isolation. A,** Initially, the SA node artery is dissected free from the atrial tissue 5 mm anterior to the crista terminalis. A 2-cm incision parallel to the crista terminalis is placed beneath the artery. **B,** The incision beneath the SA node artery is closed with a continuous nonabsorbable 5–0 suture, taking care not to damage the artery. The small pledgets are used above and below the artery to reinforce the incision. The right atriotomy is then extended to a point anterior to the junction of the superior vena cava and the base of the right atrial appendage. **C,** The atriotomy is extended along the anterior limbus of the fossa ovalis to the anteromedial tricuspid valve annulus, just anterior to the membranous interatrial septum. **D,** Caudad extension of the right atriotomy around the posterior right atrial–inferior vena cava junction to the posterolateral tricuspid valve annulus. A cryolesion (−60° C for 2 min) is placed at the end of the incision to ensure complete interruption of connecting atrial muscle fibers between the body of the right atrium and the remainder of the heart. **E,** The atriotomy is closed with a continuous 4–0 nonabsorbable suture.
(From Harada A, D'Agostino JJ Jr, Boineau JP, Cox JL: Right atrial isolation: A new surgical treatment for supraventricular tachycardia. I: Surgical technique and electrophysiologic effects. J Thorac Cardiovasc Surg 95:643, 1988.)

(Figure 81-9). Within this area, conduction is slowed to allow for reactivation within the atrium, resulting in significant tachycardia.[35,75,108] The left atrium is involved in the flutter mechanism through interatrial connections.

Indications for Surgery

The indications are very limited for surgical treatment. Currently, patients will undergo catheter-based mapping and ablation, which are highly successful. If catheter-based treatment fails, then surgical therapy is an option. Indications for primary surgical treatment include patients with congenital cardiac disease that requires surgical treatment of the congenital lesion.[128]

Surgical Treatment

Surgical treatment involves ablating the tissue responsible for the reentrant circuit. Intraoperative mapping must be performed to confirm the location of the circuit. Ablation can be accomplished through cryoablation of the area of slow conductance. If epicardial ablation is unsuccessful, then an atriotomy is made and endocardial ablation is carried out. Results from surgical ablation are excellent. Almost all patients can expect long-term cure of the atrial flutter, with extremely low morbidity/mortality. Even though one can expect cure of the atrial flutter rhythm, the atrium is still vulnerable to developing atrial fibrillation. This has led surgeons to abandon performing ablations for atrial flutter, instead performing a right-sided Maze procedure.[32] Details for the Maze procedure are included in the next section describing treatment for atrial fibrillation.

Atrial Fibrillation

Atrial fibrillation (AF) is one of the most common arrhythmias, affecting approximately 2.2 million Americans, 5% of people over 69 years of age, and 0.4–2% of the general population. Yet it is one of the least understood arrhythmias. The prevalence of AF rises dramatically with age, affecting about 10% of the population over the age of 60. The mechanism for AF is quite complicated and does not involve a discrete focus, as in the previously described arrhythmias. Because there is no discrete focus, one cannot discretely

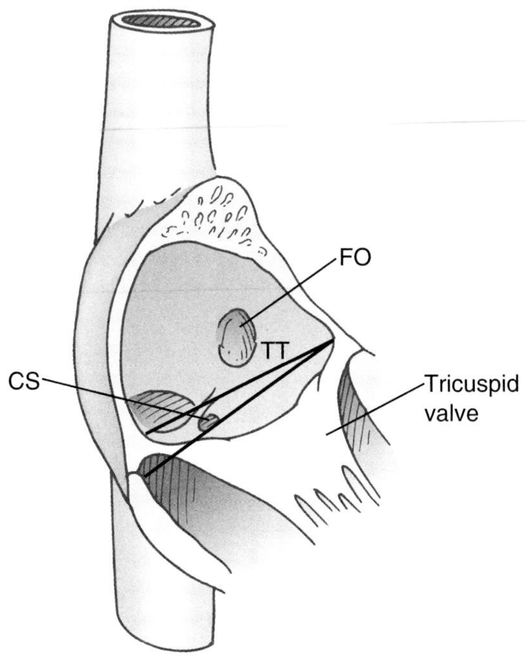

Figure 81–9 Depiction of the isthmus of tissue involved in the macroreentry circuit for atrial flutter. The isthmus is located in the right atrium and is bounded by the IVC, the tendon of Todaro, and the tricuspid valve. The coronary sinus divides the isthmus. TT, tendon of Todaro; CS, coronary sinus; FO, fossa ovales.

ablate the lesion. AF is a more stable type of arrhythmia. The chronicity of AF results in cardiac remodeling, adding to its resistance to medical treatment.[2,41,132]

Clinical Presentation and Pathophysiology

AF is an arrhythmia with no organized electrical or mechanical activity within either atrium. The ventricular rate is dependent upon the transmission of electrical activity through the AV node. Occasionally, the AV node does not sufficiently slow the impulses, resulting in significant tachycardias, though usually not as fast as seen with atrial flutter. Also, because the atrial impulses are completely chaotic, the ventricular responses follow an "irregularly irregular" pattern. Patients usually present in one of three ways: (1) feelings of discomfort or anxiety, (2) congestive heart failure, or (3) thromboembolic event. The discomfort or anxiety may result from having an irregular heartbeat, or from having episodes of significant, unexpected tachycardias. Congestive heart failure is much less common and results from loss of the "atrial kick," usually in a patient with other cardiac conditions. These patients depend upon atrial contraction for adequate filling of the ventricle. In addition, because the atria do not contract during atrial fibrillation, stasis of blood occurs in the atria. Stasis may lead to thrombus formation, which may lead to embolization and end-organ ischemia (stroke, bowel ischemia, limb ischemia, etc.). The goals of therapy are to control ventricular rate, restore sinus rhythm, and restore atrial mechanical function.

The mechanism of AF is complex and based on a pattern of macroreentry within the atrium. In 1962, Moe speculated that AF resulted from multiple simultaneous electrical wavelets.[99] Allessie and colleagues later confirmed this hypothesis experimentally.[4,5] In their model, approximately four to six intraatrial reentry circuits are randomly moving. These circuits are short-lived, with the average cycle length being 90–100 ms in the left atrium and 110–120 ms in the right. New wavelets are continually being generated from existing wavelets. Allessie and his group have suggested that there may be a background of "stable circuit" activity that could account for transitions from flutter to fibrillation.[3] Even though is it well accepted that AF is known not to be a focal process, evidence shows that there may exist focal sites for abnormal impulse generation.[57,67,82] Much investigative work has focused on the cuff of left atrial tissue surrounding the pulmonary veins as a source of impulse generation in many patients.[15,33,73,136] This has led to the development of new ablative techniques.[16,58,60,85,129]

Historical Perspectives on Surgical Therapy

Mapping studies of AF have not been able to demonstrate a discrete focus of activity that would permit focal ablation. Without a focus, early days of surgical treatment was limited to severe refractory disease, and included His bundle ablation and a permanent pacemaker. This therapy left the atria vulnerable to thrombus formation and did not allow for atrial contraction to assist in ventricular filling.

The current era of surgical treatment for AF, which began in the mid-1980s, is based largely on the work that was done at Washington University in the 1920s by Garrey[44] and Lewis.[84] They made the important observation that a critical mass of atrial tissue was necessary to support atrial fibrillation. In addition, Garrey stated: "Any sufficiently narrow bridge of cardiac muscle, whether auricular or ventricular, will suffice to prevent the spread of the fibrillary state, but will allow individual impulses to pass." In 1991, Cox postulated that a surgical procedure to cure AF would require eliminating all potential reentrant circuits around anatomical obstacles, subdivision of the atrium into segments smaller than the critical mass needed for AF, and preserving the continuity of each segment to allow for activation of the entire atria from an impulse at the SA node.[26] The Maze procedure (described in the next section) was developed by Cox and his colleagues and revolutionized the surgical treatment of AF.[19,25,27–30]

Almost contemporaneously, Guiraudon developed the Corridor operation.[47,83] Similar to His bundle ablation, the Corridor operation does not cure AF but effectively isolates the atria, permitting only SA node impulses to reach the ventricles. The concept for the Corridor operation stems from knowing that a narrow bridge of atrial muscle will prevent the spread of a fibrillary state. In this operation, a left atrial horseshoe incision is made that circumscribes a narrow corridor from the SA node to the AV node region. The end of the incision attaches onto the mitral valve annulus in the anterior and posterior commissure regions. Cryosurgical ablation at the annulus completes the isolation in the area of the AV node.

Maze Procedures

The original Maze I procedure was described in 1991 by Cox.[19] Two additional modifications have culminated in the Maze III procedure.[20] The Maze I procedure created a series of atriotomies in the left and right atria, resected both atrial appendages, and cryoablated the coronary sinus

(Figure 81-10). Even though the Maze I was very efficacious, it was associated with four significant adverse consequences[26]: (1) blunted chronotropic response to exercise, (2) 30% risk of no left atrial transport function, (3) 40% risk of requiring a pacemaker, and (4) technical difficulty, especially in patients with previous heart surgery.

These initial concerns led Cox to revise the atriotomy incisions. The Maze II procedure was designed to improve chronotropic function and improve left atrial contractility. However, the Maze II procedure was technically more difficult; it required transection of the SVC in order to gain exposure to the left atrium. Therefore, a third modification resulted in the Maze III procedure. The Maze III atriotomy lesions are now considered the "gold standard" for the surgical treatment of atrial fibrillation. The primary change incorporated in the Maze III lesion set is movement of the posterior septal incision more inferior to the orifice of the SVC, through the fossa ovalis, obviating the need to transect the SVC for left atrial exposure (Figure 81-11).

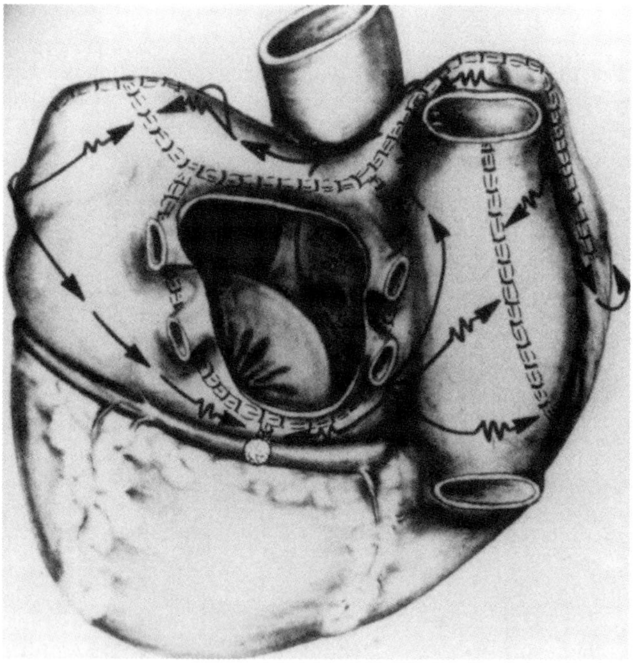

Figure 81–10 Three-dimensional depiction of the incisions used for performing the Maze I procedure. Note the presence of the transmural cryolesions *(white dot)* of the coronary sinus at the site of the posteroinferior left atriotomy. Both atrial appendages have been excised. The only completely isolated portions of the atrium are the orifices of the pulmonary veins. The impulse originates from the region of the SA node and can escape from that region only by passing inferiorly and anteriorly around the base of the right atrium. The impulse continues to propagate around the anterior right atrium onto the top of the interatrial septum. There, it bifurcates into two wave fronts, one passing through the septum in an anterior-to-posterior direction to activate the posteromedial right and left atria, and the other continuing around the base of the excised left atrial appendage to activate the posterolateral atrial wall. In this manner, all atrial myocardium, except the pulmonary vein orifices, is activated. The activation of this atrial myocardium is fundamental to the preservation of atrial transport function postoperatively.
(From Cox JL, Schuessler RB, D'Agostino HJ Jr, et al: The surgical treatment of atrial fibrillation. Development of a definite surgical procedure. J Thorac Cardiovasc Surg 101:569–583, 1991.)

Even though the Maze III procedure is highly effective in the treatment of atrial fibrillation, it is widely underutilized because of its technical complexity. To address this issue, many surgeons have converted from performing "incision and suture" atrial lesions to the creation of cryoablation atrial lesions. Cryoablation lesions are more quickly performed compared to the incision and suture technique and have been shown to be transmural lesions. This change in technique has been met with excellent clinical results equal to the incision and suture atrial lesions, resulting in a growing confidence by surgeons to offer the procedure to patients.

Recent evidence indicates that there does exist focal sources for the initiation of AF, primarily in the posterior left atrial wall near the pulmonary vein orifices. Focal ablation, or even isolation, of this area has led to cure of AF in some patients and improvement in atrial contraction. This has stimulated many groups to attempt less invasive ablative means of treatment. Electrophysiologists have attempted catheter-based ablations of pulmonary vein orifices with varying success and significant potential complications. Complications include pulmonary vein stenosis as well as long operative times secondary to technical difficulties.[39,56,59,106,110]

Surgeons have attempted various less-invasive modifications of the Maze procedure, including smaller incisions through which lesions are created using alternative ablative technologies such as radiofrequency (RF) waves, microwaves, and cryoablation.* In addition, procedural modifications have included fewer lesion sets, excluding right atrial lesions, and primarily focusing on pulmonary vein isolation. These modifications have paved the way for treating AF with minimally invasive techniques including robotic assistance. New devices are being developed that can create cryoablation, RF, microwave, and ultrasound lesions in a beating, closed-heart

*References 12, 38, 45, 65, 74, 78, 79, 93, 94, 100, 107, 124, 125.

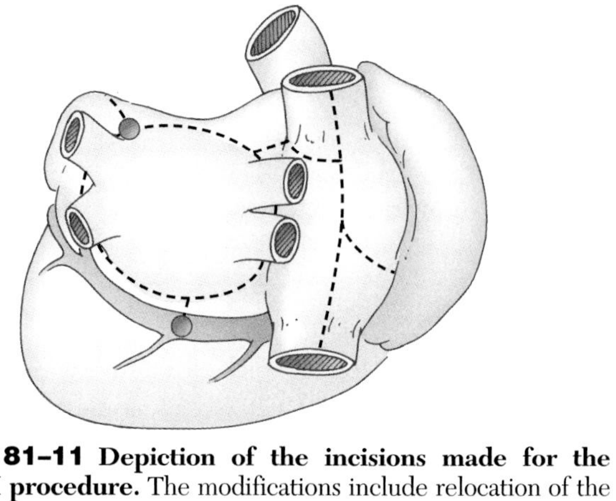

Figure 81–11 Depiction of the incisions made for the Maze III procedure. The modifications include relocation of the posterior septal incision away from the orifice of the superior vena cava (SVC) so that the SVC does not have to be transected, and the transverse atriotomy across the left atrium moves more posterior.
(From Cox JL, Schuessler RB, Lappas DG, Boineau JP: An 8 1/2-year clinical experience with surgery for atrial fibrillation. Ann Surg 224(3):267–273; discussion 273–275, 1996.)

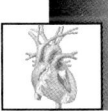

system. The ability to evaluate treatment efficacy and modify lesion sets while in the operating room is on the horizon.

Surgical Techniques in the Current Era

The cryoablation Maze procedure is the gold standard against which all techniques must be measured. The advent of less-invasive procedures has led to alternative techniques with fewer lesion sets. These technologies include cryoablation, RF ablation, microwave, ultrasound, and laser ablation.[130] The most widely studied minimally invasive surgical technique involves complete isolation of the pulmonary veins using RF ablation[79,95] (Figure 81-12). This approach is relatively straightforward technically, and it also appears to be efficacious, with cure rates of approximately 75%. Important factors when considering pulmonary vein isolation as a curative treatment include left atrial size, technique of ablation, and chronicity of AF. Patients with large left atria (>200 ml) appear to have much lower success rates for curing AF with pulmonary vein isolation.[95] At 6 months, the cure rates for those patients with large left atria and small left atria are 20 and 69%, respectively. The reasons for differences in cure rates are not completely understood but are suspected to be related to chronicity of AF, atrial remodeling, and the limited lesion set.

Technical considerations are very important to achieve success. With all ablation techniques, transmural lesions and the continuity of linear ablation lines are of the utmost importance. One of the major difficulties with catheter-based approaches has been obtaining transmural, continuous lesions. This appears to be less problematic with direct application of ablative technology.

The chronicity of AF impacts surgical success. Medical treatment and cardioversion are much more likely to fail in patients with long-standing AF. Chronic AF appears to be best treated with the lesion sets of the Maze III procedure. Minimally invasive ablative techniques appear to be more effective in treating paroxysmal or shorter-duration atrial fibrillation than chronic atrial fibrillation.

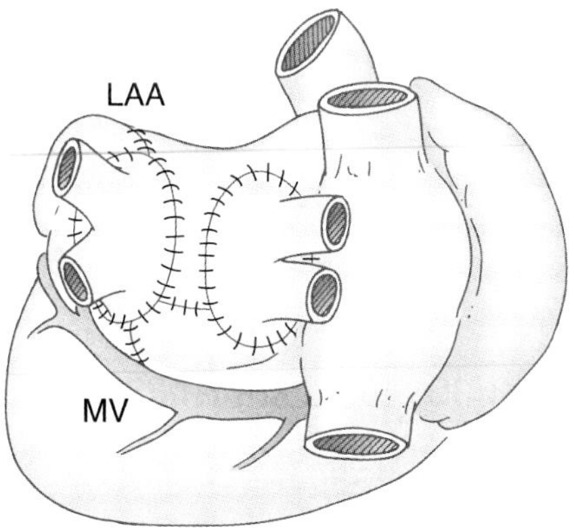

Figure 81–12 Depiction of the lesion set used to create complete pulmonary vein isolation. LAA, left atrial appendage; MV, mitral valve.

Microwave energy is not as well studied as RF; however, it does have some potential advantages (Table 81-2). It appears easier to handle in that it requires shorter application times, longer linear lesions with fewer applications, less scarring of the endocardium with reduced risk of thromboembolism, and the ability to penetrate areas of fibrosis.

Lasers may also have a role in creating linear ablative lesions; however, there is currently very limited clinical experience. Potential advantages include short application times, minimal lateral expansion of the lesion, and low tissue temperatures. However, the major concern with laser therapy is the potential for perforation. Due to the intensity of energy within the laser beam, it can easily penetrate tissues. Experimental studies have been able to minimize the risk of perforation by using lower energies and special diffusing fibers on the probes.

There is debate and an evolution in thinking regarding the number and locations of lesions necessary to cure atrial fibrillation. The Maze III lesion set remains the gold standard, however, this is not entirely practical for minimally

Table 81–2

Characteristics for Different Ablative Technologies Used to Treat Atrial Fibrillation

	Cryoablation	*Microwave*	*Radiofrequency*	*Laser*
Temperature	–60° C	>50° C	50–60° C	50° C
Duration	90–120 s	20–30 s	90–120 s	60–180 s, depending on energy level
Width–depth ratio	Low	Low	Very high	Very low
Risk of perforation	Low	Possible at higher energies, although it has not been seen clinically	Low	Low to high, depending on wavelength

invasive surgery. Which lesions can both be performed less invasively and result in the highest cure rate remains to be determined. The basis for all lesion sets is the isolation of the pulmonary veins. Some experts advocate right atrial lesions for chronic AF,[76] and others advocate basing the number of lesions on left atrial size.

It is unclear whether epicardial lesions are as effective as endocardial lesions. Recent reports suggest that epicardial lesions are probably as effective as endocardial lesions.[1,95]

Surgical Outcomes

The results of current surgical treatments for AF need to be compared with the Maze III procedure, which demonstrates a less than 2% incidence of recurrent AF, a 7–10% incidence of permanent pacemaker implantation, a 94% incidence of preserved left atrial function, and a less than 6% incidence of blunted SA node chronotropic function.*

The Maze III procedure is often performed concurrently with mitral valve surgery. David and associates have shown that when combined with open mitral valve surgery, the only significant differences for patients undergoing a Maze procedure were longer bypass times (120 vs. 83 min), longer cross-clamp times (100 vs. 66 min), and longer ICU stays (3.0 vs. 1.8 days).[109] The perioperative mortality, myocardial infarction, stroke, and bleeding rates were not significantly different between those that received the Maze and those that had mitral valve surgery alone. In long-term follow-up, 75% of the Maze patients were in sinus rhythm, compared to only 36% of the non-Maze patients. This translated to a 3-year thromboembolic rate of 0% in Maze vs. 27% non-Maze, despite anticoagulation in the non-Maze group.

Reported outcomes for less-invasive approaches to AF treatment are not as good compared with the conventional Maze III procedure. However, the less-invasive procedures carry advantages that make such procedures attractive to patients. These advantages include the absence of cardiopulmonary bypass, smaller and more easily tolerated incisions, and quicker return to full activity. A summary of recent reported results for less-invasive procedures can be found in Table 81-3. It is clear that at present, the cure rate for less-invasive procedures is less than that for the standard Maze III procedure and, therefore, patients must be carefully counseled on the advantages and disadvantages of each therapy. There is also significant momentum to develop new hand-held probes for performing minimally invasive AF surgery, which may allow for additional lesion sets to be performed, thus increasing cure rates.

SURGICAL TREATMENT OF VENTRICULAR ARRHYTHMIAS

Ventricular arrhythmia surgery is now very uncommon. Early surgical therapies for ventricular arrhythmias suffered from inaccurate intraoperative mapping techniques and a poor understanding of the mechanisms of ventricular arrhythmias. Treatments for ventricular arrhythmias generally were at the expense of decreasing left ventricular contractility. Unfortunately, most patients suffering from ventricular arrhythmias at that time already manifest poor left ventricular function. Poor left ventricular function led to poor surgical results and high recurrence rates. It was not until the advent of implantable defibrillators that the initial hypothesis for treating ventricular arrhythmias was confirmed. In other words, controlling ventricular arrhythmias in patients with significant left ventricular dysfunction could reduce mortality. The Multicenter Automatic Defibrillator Implantation Trial (MADIT) and Antiarrhythmics Versus Implantable Defibrillators (AVID) trials demonstrated a reduction in mortality of 30–39%.[17,104] Currently, operative mortality has decreased for the treatment of ventricular arrhythmias to less than 10%. This is the result of not only improved techniques but also improved patient selection criteria. With the advent of automatic implantable cardioverter-defibrillators (AICD), many high-risk surgical patients can now be deferred to AICD placement alone or CABG + AICD.

Treatment algorithms for patients with ventricular arrhythmias depend on the type of arrhythmia present. Patients considered for surgery generally have recalcitrant episodes of either ventricular tachycardia (VT) or ventricular fibrillation (VF). Patients with multiple episodes of primary VF benefit most from AICD implantation alone. However, it is important to determine whether the VF is preceded by a run of VT, since those patients usually respond to surgical therapy. When a patient first presents, medical therapy is primary therapy. If the arrhythmia is controlled with medical therapy, no further therapy is needed. In cases not adequately controlled on medication, patients should undergo electrophysiological mapping to localize the focus. If a focus is found, catheter ablation is attempted initially. If the patient is an acceptable surgical candidate, with good ventricular function, and catheter ablation has failed, surgery may be indicated. Alternatives include AICD implantation or, in severe cases, heart transplantation. AICD placement is not a cure for the arrhythmia. Although it is quite effective for reducing mortality, it may also be uncomfortable for the patient with frequent discharges. Those patients with an AICD with frequent discharges should be considered for surgical therapy.

As surgical techniques for the treatment of ventricular arrhythmias evolved, it became clear that electrophysiological mapping was necessary for optimum surgical treatment. Although the general area of the arrhythmogenic focus can be ascertained from the ECG, accurate intraoperative mapping is necessary for targeted therapy and the best results. Unfortunately, the time necessary for intraoperative mapping has added significantly to the cost of these procedures, questioning its necessity.[81,101,103] On the other hand, it is clear that complete mapping of the ventricular arrhythmia leads to improved outcomes.[96] Ventricular mapping is essential in those patients who lack visible pathology, such as those with a recent history of myocardial infarction.[11,34,97]

Even though the need for intraoperative mapping has significantly declined in recent years, the mapping systems continue to evolve, and those currently available have become quite sophisticated. Current systems contain an array of electrodes embedded in a Silastic, form-fitting mold that is placed within the ventricle via a ventriculotomy (Figure 81-13). Computer processing of all concurrent signals in real time can display three-dimensional

*References 31, 66, 77, 78, 92, 112.

Table 81–3

Surgical Results of Atrial Fibrillation Treatment

Reference	*Number of patients*	*Number of survivors*	*Mean follow-up*	*Lesion set*	*Modality*	*Free of AF (%)*	*Requiring pacemaker (%)*	*Patients in sinus with left atrial transport documented (%)*
Kress et al[80]	23	22	32 weeks	BPV, R-L PV, LAA-LPV	RF ablation	86	7	100
Chen et al[14]	12	10	10 months	Classic Maze	RF and cryo	80	N/A	30
Patwardhan et al[107]	18	15	5 months	Maze III	RF and cryo	80	N/A	75
Williams et al[134]	48	42	5 months	Endocardial PV isolation	RF	81	N/A	N/A
Sie et al[123]	122	110	39 months	Maze III	RF	78	6	77
Benussi et al[9]	40	39	11.6 months	BPV, R-L PV, MV-LIPV	RF	77	0	100
Maessen et al[87]	24	23	6.4 months	BPV isolation	MW	87	N/A	N/A
Gaita et al[42]	32	29	>9 months	BPV, MV-LIPV, LAA excision	Cryo ± RF	90	N/A	N/A

BPV, bilateral pulmonary vein isolation; R-L PV, connecting lesion between right and left pulmonary veins; LAA-LPV, connecting lesion between left atrial appendage and left pulmonary vein; MV-LIPV, connecting lesion between mitral valve and left inferior pulmonary vein; RF, radiofrequency; cryo, cryoablation; MW, microwave.

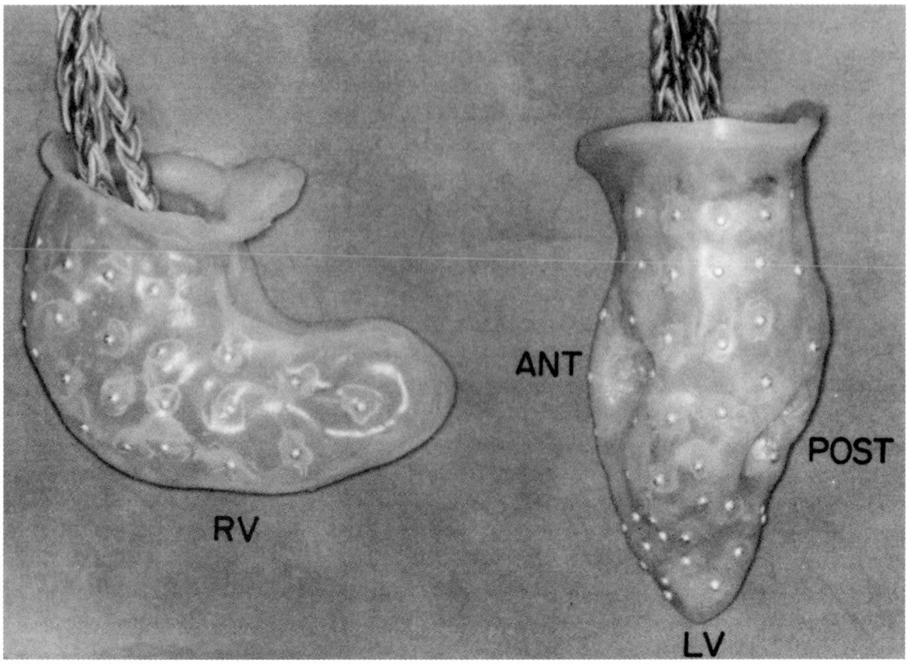

Figure 81–13 Endocardial electrodes used for recording both activation time maps and potential distribution maps in patients with ventricular tachycardia. The electrode templates are made of Silastic, and target-tipped bipolar electrodes are embedded in the wall of the Silastic templates. The templates are constructed over a form-fitting mold of the right ventricle (RV) and its outflow tract and of the left ventricle (LV). The indentations of the anterior (ANT) and posterior (POST) papillary muscles can be seen on the left ventricular template. These electrode templates are introduced into their respective ventricles via right and left atriotomies. The flanged portion of each template abuts the respective tricuspid or mitral valve annulus. A low-pressure balloon resides inside each of these templates that, when inflated, ensures excellent electrode contact with the endocardium of each ventricle.

functional mapping of ventricular activation. The mapping allows one to precisely localize the focus of the arrhythmia, which is used to exactly determine the operative approach.

The operative approach for ventricular tachycardias depends upon the cause for the arrhythmia. A distinction must be made between ischemic and nonischemic etiologies. In patients with no identifiable ischemic disease, an ECG and/or ventriculogram should be performed to evaluate myocardial contractility. Those with abnormal contractility are categorized to have either nonischemic cardiomyopathy or right ventricular dysplasia. If contractility is normal, the patient is categorized as having either normal or prolonged Q–T interval. In patients with ischemic ventricular tachycardia, therapy is dependent on whether a left ventricular aneurysm is present.

Fontaine initially described arrhythmogenic right ventricular dysplasia in 1979.[40,89] The lesions involve replacement and/or infiltration of the myocardium by adipose tissue. It is usually confined to the right ventricular free wall but occasionally can involve other areas. Patients typically present with large, bulging, dyskinetic areas over the infundibulum, apex, and basal portion of the right ventricular wall. Because the tachycardia originates from the right side, the ECG during the tachycardia usually shows a left bundle branch block. Surgical therapy involves a complete right free wall isolation procedure. This is accomplished by performing a transmural ventriculotomy extending anteriorly from the pulmonic valve annulus around the apex to the tricuspid valve posteriorly as shown (Figure 81-14). Good long-term results can be achieved with appropriate patient selection.[36,98] Patient selection is mostly determined by good left ventricular function.

In those patients with nonischemic cardiomyopathy and refractory VT, surgical therapy is guided by intraoperative localization of the origin. Once the arrhythmia origin is localized, a combination of isolation and ablation may be utilized. It is important to try to perform the surgery without arresting the heart. This will allow confirmation that the arrhythmia cannot be induced prior to leaving the operating room. If the heart is arrested, the cardioplegia may alter the reentry circuits, leading to failure of the operation. Similar therapy may be used for idiopathic VT, in which myocardial function is good and the Q–T interval is normal. Most of these patients have foci localized to the septum that can be cryoablated.

Patients who have VT in association with prolonged Q–T syndrome typically display torsades de pointes on ECG. The most common causes of this tachycardia are medication-induced and electrolyte abnormalities, which resolve once the medication is withdrawn and electrolytes are corrected. There is a congenital type that may have a genetic basis or infectious origin.[113] The mechanism in these patients is not completely understood, but it involves myocardial repolarization. Therapy usually involves medication and AICD placement. If the VT continues to be problematic, surgical therapy is aimed at altering sympathetic tone.[88,105,113] This can be accomplished by resection of the left stellate ganglion. However, results have shown early success and late failure.[8,10]

Patients with ischemic VT represent the majority of patients presenting for surgical treatment of their tachycardia. It is well known that hypoxic myocardial tissue is prone to arrhythmias. Most arrhythmias that are present acutely during ischemic conditions resolve spontaneously. After remodeling takes place and a scar develops, localized areas of tissue, especially on the periphery of the scar, may be arrhythmogenic. VT that occurs under these conditions can often be intractable and unresponsive to medical therapy. Surgical therapy should be considered in these patients.

Early therapies were directed toward resecting the scar or aneurysm associated with the infarction. Most of these therapies prior to 1969 were doomed with failures. It did not improve until good intraoperative mapping techniques

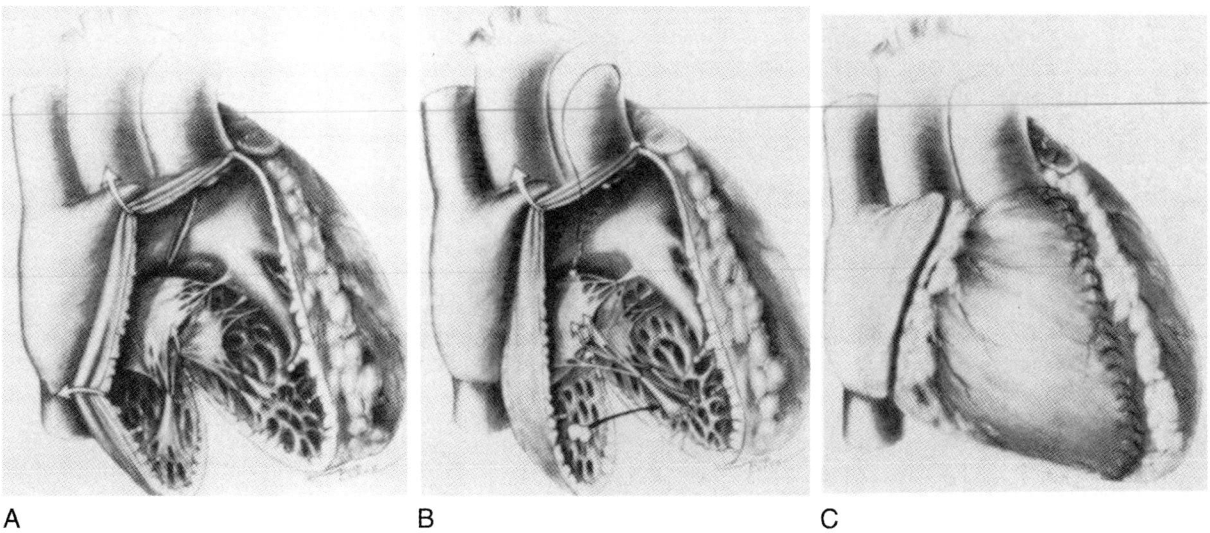

Figure 81–14 **Right ventricular disconnection procedure.** **A,** A transmural right ventriculotomy is placed parallel to and 5 mm from the interventricular septum extending from just across the pulmonic valve annulus anteriorly to the tricuspid valve posteriorly. It is necessary to divide several large infundibular muscular bundles and to divide the moderator band of the RV. Although the entire incision is transmural, special care must be taken to avoid injury to the right coronary artery lying in the AV groove at the posterior extent of this incision. After identification of the location of the His bundle and right bundle branch, a second transmural incision is placed from the posterior pulmonic valve annulus to the anterior medial tricuspid valve annulus, exposing the underlying aortic root. If the tricuspid portion of this incision is placed too far anteriorly, the bundle of His may be inadvertently divided. **B,** After completion of the two transmural incisions, the papillary muscle attached to the anterior leaflet of the tricuspid valve is divided at its base and reimplanted on the lower ventricular septum using interrupted 3–0 pledgeted Prolene sutures. Cryolesions are laced at each end of the anteroposterior ventriculotomy and at each end of the ventriculotomy between the posterior pulmonic valve annulus and the anterior medial suture followed by closure of the long free wall ventriculotomy with continuous 3–0 nonabsorbable sutures (**C**).
(Modified from Cox JL: Surgery for cardiac arrhythmias. In Harvey WP, editor: Current problems in cardiology, Vol. 8, No. 4. Chicago: Year Book Medical, 1983.)

allowed for more precise localization of the arrhythmogenic focus and better guided surgical approaches.[72] By the mid-1970s, surgeons began using intraoperative mapping to specifically guide ablation for VT.[43,135] In 1978, Guiraudon described the encircling endocardial ventriculotomy for treatment of VT.[46] Finally, in 1979, Harken and associates described endocardial resection,[63,71] which became the mainstay of treatment with some modifications up to the present time. In more recent times, two techniques for repair of left ventricular aneurysms have also shown great relief from VT.[37,69]

As in other arrhythmia surgery, the goal of surgery for ischemic VT is to isolate, ablate, or resect the arrhythmogenic focus. It remains important not to interfere much with ventricular function. Patients with ischemic VT already have decreased function, and if it is worsened with surgery, one can expect unacceptable levels of morbidity and mortality. The encircling endocardial ventriculotomy described by Guiraudon et al[46] involves making an endocardial incision around the border of the scar–myocardium interface. This procedure was quite effective for relieving the VT; however, ventricular function was often sacrificed and mortality was therefore quite high.[23] Limited endocardial resections of just the arrhythmogenic focus proved to be much more successful.[71] This involved mapping the focus and removing only that section of tissue. If the focus was located near valve annuli or papillary muscles, then cryoablation could be utilized instead.[18] A newer therapy employing a laser allows for ablation via an epicardial approach.[101,122,126]

Newer therapies directed at repairing left ventricular aneurysms have shown unexpectedly good results at treating ischemic VT. The procedure described by Dor et al[37] involves resecting the aneurysm, followed by repairing the defect utilizing a circular Dacron patch with interrupted, pledgeted, horizontal mattress sutures. This procedure usually leads to functional improvement as well as good control of the arrhythmia. Cure of VT with this technique is about 98%, with a mortality of only 2–3%.

SUMMARY

The development of arrhythmia surgery has been both challenging and exciting. Over time, many surgical approaches have been supplanted by catheter-based techniques. Today, the role of surgery is primarily limited to the treatment of atrial fibrillation. This is indeed a very exciting and engaging time for surgeons since atrial fibrillation is by far the most common arrhythmia and its clinical consequences can be devastating. The resurgence of interest and creativity in the surgical treatment of atrial fibrillation can only be of great benefit to our patients. Many questions remain to be answered, including the optimum lesion set, the preferred energy source, patient selection criteria, and minimally invasive lesion sets, to name but a few. It is clear that a new era has been born in the surgical treatment of arrhythmias and how it unfolds for the benefit of our patients will be limited only by the surgeon's imagination.

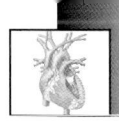

REFERENCES

1. Alfieri O, Benussi S: Mitral valve surgery with concomitant treatment of atrial fibrillation. Cardiol Rev 8(6):317–321, 2000.
2. Allessie MA: Atrial electrophysiologic remodeling: another vicious circle? J Cardiovasc Electrophysiol 9(12):1378–1393, 1998.
3. Allessie M, Chorro E, Wijffels M: What are the electrophysiological mechanisms of perpetuation of atrial fibrillation. In Raviele A, editor: Cardiac Arrhythmias. Berlin: Springer-Verlag, 1997, pp. 3–11.
4. Allessie M, Lammers W, Bonke F: Experimental evaluation of Moe's multiple wavelet hypothesis of atrial fibrillation. In Zipes D, Jalife J, editors: Cardiac Electrophysiology and Arrhythmias. New York: Grune & Stratton, 1985.
5. Allessie M, Rensma P, Brugada J: Pathophysiology of atrial fibrillation. In Zipes D, Jalife J, editors: Cardiac Electrophysiology. Philadelphia: W.B. Saunders, 1990. pp. 548–558.
6. Anderson RH, Ho SY: Anatomy of the atrioventricular junctions with regard to ventricular preexcitation. Pacing Clin Electrophysiol 20(8 Pt 2):2072–2076, 1997.
7. Anderson RH, Becker AE, Brechenmacher C, et al: Ventricular preexcitation. A proposed nomenclature for its substrates. Eur J Cardiol 3(1):27–36, 1975.
8. Benson DJ, Cox J: Surgical treatment of cardiac arrhythmias. In Roberts N, Gelband H, editors: Cardiac Arrhythmias in the Neonate, Infant, and Child. New York: Appleton-Century Crofts, 1982, pp. 341–366.
9. Benussi S, Pappone C, Nascimbene S, et al: A simple way to treat chronic atrial fibrillation during mitral valve surgery: the epicardial radiofrequency approach. Eur J Cardiothorac Surg 17(5):524–529, 2000.
10. Bhandari AK, Scheinman MM, Morady F, et al: Efficacy of left cardiac sympathectomy in the treatment of patients with the long QT syndrome. Circulation 70(6):1018–1023, 1984.
11. Bourke JP, Hilton CJ, McComb JM, et al: Surgery for control of recurrent life-threatening ventricular tachyarrhythmias within 2 months of myocardial infarction. J Am Coll Cardiol 16(1):42–48, 1990.
12. Brodman RF, Frame R, Fisher JD, et al: Combined treatment of mitral stenosis and atrial fibrillation with valvuloplasty and a left atrial maze procedure. J Thorac Cardiovasc Surg 107(2): 622–624, 1994.
13. Cain ME, Luke RA, Lindsay BD: Diagnosis and localization of accessory pathways. Pacing Clin Electrophysiol 15(5): 801–824, 1992.
14. Chen MC, Guo GB, Chang JP, et al: Radiofrequency and cryoablation of atrial fibrillation in patients undergoing valvular operations. Ann Thorac Surg 65(6):1666–1672, 1998.
15. Chen PS, Wu TJ, Hwang C, et al: Thoracic veins and the mechanisms of non-paroxysmal atrial fibrillation. Cardiovasc Res 54(2):295–301, 2002.
16. Chen SA, Hsieh MH, Tai CT, et al: Initiation of atrial fibrillation by ectopic beats originating from the pulmonary veins: electrophysiological characteristics, pharmacological responses, and effects of radiofrequency ablation. Circulation 100(18):1879–1886, 1999.
17. A comparison of antiarrhythmic-drug therapy with implantable defibrillators in patients resuscitated from near-fatal ventricular arrhythmias. The Antiarrhythmics versus Implantable Defibrillators (AVID) Investigators. N Engl J Med 337(22):1576–1583, 1997.
18. Cox JL: Anatomic-electrophysiologic basis for the surgical treatment of refractory ischemic ventricular tachycardia. Ann Surg 198(2):119–129, 1983.
19. Cox JL: The surgical treatment of atrial fibrillation. IV. Surgical technique. J Thorac Cardiovasc Surg 101(4):584–592, 1991.
20. Cox J: The Maze III procedure for treatment of atrial fibrillation. In Sabiston D, editor: Atlas of Cardiothoracic Surgery. Philadelphia: W.B. Saunders, 1995, pp. 460–475.
21. Cox JL: The surgical management of cardiac arrhythmias. In Sabiston DC, Spencer FC, editors: Surgery of the Chest. Philadelphia: W.B. Saunders, 1995, pp. 2043–2049.
22. Cox JL, Gallagher JJ, Cain ME: Experience with 118 consecutive patients undergoing operation for the Wolff–Parkinson–White syndrome. J Thorac Cardiovasc Surg 90(4): 490–501, 1985.
23. Cox JL, Gallagher JJ, Ungerleider RM: Encircling endocardial ventriculotomy for refractory ischemic ventricular tachycardia. IV. Clinical indication, surgical technique, mechanism of action, and results. J Thorac Cardiovasc Surg 83(6):865–872, 1982.
24. Cox JL, Holman WL, Cain ME: Cryosurgical treatment of atrioventricular node reentrant tachycardia. Circulation 76(6):1329–1336, 1987.
25. Cox JL, Schuessler RB, Boineau JP: The surgical treatment of atrial fibrillation. I. Summary of the current concepts of the mechanisms of atrial flutter and atrial fibrillation. J Thorac Cardiovasc Surg 101(3):402–405, 1991.
26. Cox J, Boineau J, Schuessler R, et al: A review of surgery for atrial fibrillation. J Cardiovasc Electrophysiol 2:541–561, 1991.
27. Cox JL, Boineau JP, Schuessler RB, et al: Successful surgical treatment of atrial fibrillation. Review and clinical update. JAMA 266(14):1976–1980, 1991.
28. Cox JL, Boineau JP, Schuessler RB, et al: Operations for atrial fibrillation. Clin Cardiol 14(10):827–834, 1991.
29. Cox JL, Canavan TE, Schuessler RB, et al: The surgical treatment of atrial fibrillation. II. Intraoperative electrophysiologic mapping and description of the electrophysiologic basis of atrial flutter and atrial fibrillation. J Thorac Cardiovasc Surg 101(3):406–426, 1991.
30. Cox JL, Schuessler RB, D'Agostino HJ Jr, et al: The surgical treatment of atrial fibrillation. III. Development of a definitive surgical procedure. J Thorac Cardiovasc Surg 101(4):569–583, 1991.
31. Cox JL, Schuessler RB, Lappas DG, Boineau JP: An 8 1/2-year clinical experience with surgery for atrial fibrillation. Ann Surg 224(3):267–273; discussion 273–275, 1996.
32. Dakik HA, Arnaout S, Khoury M, Obeid M: Cox-Maze procedure for treatment of atrial flutter associated with an atrial septal defect. Clin Cardiol 23(7):548–549, 2000.
33. Deen VR, Morton JB, Vohra JK, Kalman JM: Pulmonary vein paced activation sequence mapping: comparison with activation sequences during onset of focal atrial fibrillation. J Cardiovasc Electrophysiol 13(2):101–107, 2002.
34. DiMarco JP, Lerman BB, Kron IL, Sellers TD: Sustained ventricular tachyarrhythmias within 2 months of acute myocardial infarction: results of medical and surgical therapy in patients resuscitated from the initial episode. J Am Coll Cardiol 6(4):759–768, 1985.
35. Disertori M, Inama G, Vergara G, et al: Evidence of a reentry circuit in the common type of atrial flutter in man. Circulation 67(2):434–440, 1983.
36. Doig JC, Nimkhedkar K, Bourke JP, et al: Acute and chronic hemodynamic impact of total right ventricular disarticulation. Pacing Clin Electrophysiol 14(11 Pt 2):1971–1975, 1991.
37. Dor V, Saab M, Coste P, et al: Left ventricular aneurysm: a new surgical approach. Thorac Cardiovasc Surg 37(1):11–19, 1989.
38. Duru F, Hindricks G, Kottkamp H: Atypical left atrial flutter after intraoperative radiofrequency ablation of chronic atrial fibrillation: successful ablation using three-dimensional electroanatomic mapping. J Cardiovasc Electrophysiol 12(5): 602–605, 2001.
39. Ernst S, Schluter M, Ouyang F, et al: Modification of the substrate for maintenance of idiopathic human atrial fibrillation:

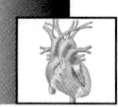

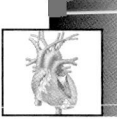

efficacy of radiofrequency ablation using nonfluoroscopic catheter guidance. Circulation 100(20):2085–2092, 1999.
40. Fontaine G, Guiraudon G, Frank R: Management of chronic ventricular tachycardia. In Os N, editor: Innovations in Diagnosis and Management of Cardiac Arrhythmias. Baltimore: Williams & Wilkins, 1979.
41. Franz MR, Karasik PL, Li C, et al: Electrical remodeling of the human atrium: similar effects in patients with chronic atrial fibrillation and atrial flutter. J Am Coll Cardiol 30(7): 1785–1792, 1997.
42. Gaita F, Gallotti R, Calo L, et al: Limited posterior left atrial cryoablation in patients with chronic atrial fibrillation undergoing valvular heart surgery. J Am Coll Cardiol 36(1): 159–166, 2000.
43. Gallagher JJ, Oldham HN, Wallace AG, et al: Ventricular aneurysm with ventricular tachycardia. Report of a case with epicardial mapping and successful resection. Am J Cardiol 35(5):696–700, 1975.
44. Garrey W: Auricular fibrillation. Physiology Rev 4:215–250, 1924.
45. Gregori F Jr, Cordeiro CO, Couto WJ, et al: Cox Maze operation without cryoablation for the treatment of chronic atrial fibrillation. Ann Thorac Surg 60(2):361–363; discussion 364, 1995.
46. Guiraudon G, Fontaine G, Frank R, et al: Encircling endocardial ventriculotomy: a new surgical treatment for life-threatening ventricular tachycardias resistant to medical treatment following myocardial infarction. Ann Thorac Surg 26(5):438–444, 1978.
47. Guiraudon G, Klein G, Guiraudon C, Yee R: Treatment of atrial fibrillation: preservation of sinoventricular impulse conduction (the corridor operation). In Olsson S, Allessie M, Campbell R, editors: Atrial Fibrillation: Mechanisms and Therapeutic Strategies. Armonk, NY: Futura Publishing, 1994.
48. Guiraudon GM, Klein GJ, Gulamhusein S, et al: Surgical repair of Wolff-Parkinson-White syndrome: a new closed-heart technique. Ann Thorac Surg 37(1):67–71, 1984.
49. Guiraudon GM, Klein GJ, Sharma AD, et al: Closed-heart technique for Wolff-Parkinson-White syndrome: further experience and potential limitations. Ann Thorac Surg 42(6): 651–657, 1986.
50. Guiraudon GM, Klein GJ, Sharma AD, et al: "Atypical" posteroseptal accessory pathway in Wolff-Parkinson-White syndrome. J Am Coll Cardiol 12(6):1605–1608, 1988.
51. Guiraudon GM, Klein GJ, Sharma AD, et al: Surgical approach to anterior septal accessory pathways in 20 patients with the Wolff-Parkinson-White syndrome. Eur J Cardio-thorac Surg 2(4):201–206, 1988.
52. Guiraudon GM, Klein GJ, Sharma AD, et al: Surgery for the Wolff-Parkinson-White syndrome: the epicardial approach. Semin Thorac Cardiovasc Surg 1(1):21–33, 1989.
53. Guiraudon GM, Klein GJ, Sharma AD, Yee R: Surgical alternatives for supraventricular tachycardias. Am J Cardiol 64(20):92J–96J, 1989.
54. Guiraudon GM, Klein GJ, van Hemel N, et al: Anatomically guided surgery to the AV node. AV nodal skeletonization: experience in 46 patients with AV nodal reentrant tachycardia. Eur J Cardiothorac Surg 4(9):461–464, 1990.
55. Guiraudon GM, Klein GJ, Yee R, et al: Surgical epicardial ablation of left ventricular pathway using sling exposure. Ann Thorac Surg 50(6):968–971, 1990.
56. Haissaguerre M, Jais P, Shah DC, et al: Right and left atrial radiofrequency catheter therapy of paroxysmal atrial fibrillation. J Cardiovasc Electrophysiol 7(12):1132–1144, 1996.
57. Haissaguerre M, Jais P, Shah DC, et al: Spontaneous initiation of atrial fibrillation by ectopic beats originating in the pulmonary veins. N Engl J Med 339(10):659–666, 1998.
58. Haissaguerre M, Jais P, Shah DC, et al: Electrophysiological end point for catheter ablation of atrial fibrillation initiated from multiple pulmonary venous foci. Circulation 101(12): 1409–1417, 2000.
59. Haissaguerre M, Shah DC, Jais P, Clementy J: Role of catheter ablation for atrial fibrillation. Curr Opin Cardiol 12(1):18–23, 1997.
60. Haissaguerre M, Shah DC, Jais P, et al: Electrophysiological breakthroughs from the left atrium to the pulmonary veins. Circulation 102(20):2463–2465, 2000.
61. Harada A, D'Agostino HJ Jr, Boineau JP, Cox JL: Right atrial isolation: a new surgical treatment for supraventricular tachycardia. II. Hemodynamic effects. J Thorac Cardiovasc Surg 95(4):651–657, 1988.
62. Harada A, D'Agostino HJ Jr, Schuessler RB, et al: Right atrial isolation: a new surgical treatment for supraventricular tachycardia. I. Surgical technique and electrophysiologic effects. J Thorac Cardiovasc Surg 95(4):643–650, 1988.
63. Harken AH, Josephson ME, Horowitz LN: Surgical endocardial resection for the treatment of malignant ventricular tachycardia. Ann Surg 190(4):456–460, 1979.
64. Hendry PJ, Packer DL, Anstadt MP, et al: Surgical treatment of automatic atrial tachycardias. Ann Thorac Surg 49(2):253–259; discussion 259–260, 1990.
65. Imai K, Sueda T, Orihashi K, et al: Clinical analysis of results of a simple left atrial procedure for chronic atrial fibrillation. Ann Thorac Surg 71(2):577–581, 2001.
66. Itoh T, Okamoto H, Nimi T, et al: Left atrial function after Cox's Maze operation concomitant with mitral valve operation. Ann Thorac Surg 60(2):354–359; discussion 359–360, 1995.
67. Jais P, Haissaguerre M, Shah DC, et al: A focal source of atrial fibrillation treated by discrete radiofrequency ablation. Circulation 95(3):572–576, 1997.
68. Jais P, Shah DC, Haissaguerre M, et al: Mapping and ablation of left atrial flutters. Circulation 101(25):2928–2934, 2000.
69. Jatene AD: Left ventricular aneurysmectomy. Resection or reconstruction. J Thorac Cardiovasc Surg 89(3):321–331, 1985.
70. Johnson DC, Nunn GR, Meldrum-Hanna W: Surgery for atrioventricular node reentry tachycardia: the surgical dissection technique. Semin Thorac Cardiovasc Surg 1(1): 53–57, 1989.
71. Josephson ME, Harken AH, Horowitz LN: Endocardial excision: a new surgical technique for the treatment of recurrent ventricular tachycardia. Circulation 60(7): 1430–1439, 1979.
72. Kaiser GA, Waldo AL, Harris PD, et al: New method to delineate myocardial damage at surgery. Circulation 39(5 Suppl 1):I83–I89, 1969.
73. Kantachuvessiri A: Pulmonary veins: preferred site for catheter ablation of atrial fibrillation. Heart Lung 31(4): 271–278, 2002.
74. Kawaguchi AT, Kosakai Y, Sasako Y, et al: Risks and benefits of combined Maze procedure for atrial fibrillation associated with organic heart disease. J Am Coll Cardiol 28(4):985–990, 1996.
75. Klein GJ, Guiraudon GM, Sharma AD, Milstein S: Demonstration of macroreentry and feasibility of operative therapy in the common type of atrial flutter. Am J Cardiol 57(8):587–591, 1986.
76. Knaut M, Spitzer SG, Karolyi L, et al: Intraoperative microwave ablation for curative treatment of atrial fibrillation in open heart surgery—the MICRO-STAF and MICRO-PASS pilot trial. MICROwave Application in Surgical Treatment of Atrial Fibrillation. MICROwave Application for the Treatment of Atrial Fibrillation in Bypass Surgery. Thorac Cardiovasc Surg 47(Suppl 3):379–384, 1999.
77. Kosakai Y, Kawaguchi AT, Isobe F, et al: Cox Maze procedure for chronic atrial fibrillation associated with mitral valve

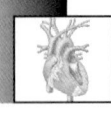

disease. J Thorac Cardiovasc Surg 108(6):1049–1054; discussion 1054–1055, 1994.
78. Kosakai Y, Kawaguchi AT, Isobe F, et al: Modified Maze procedure for patients with atrial fibrillation undergoing simultaneous open heart surgery. Circulation 92(9 Suppl): II359–II364, 1995.
79. Kottamp H, Hindricks G, Hammel D, et al: Intraoperative radiofrequency ablation of chronic atrial fibrillation: a left atrial curative approach by elimination of anatomic "anchor" reentrant circuits. J Cardiovasc Electrophysiol 10(6):772–780, 1999.
80. Kress DC, Sra J, Krum D, et al: Radiofrequency ablation of atrial fibrillation during mitral valve surgery. Semin Thorac Cardiovasc Surg 14(3):210–218, 2002.
81. Landymore RW, Kinley CE, Gardner M: Encircling endocardial resection with complete removal of endocardial scar without intraoperative mapping for the ablation of drug-resistant ventricular tachycardia. J Thorac Cardiovasc Surg 89(1):18–24, 1985.
82. Lau CP, Tse HF, Ayers GM: Defibrillation-guided radiofrequency ablation of atrial fibrillation secondary to an atrial focus. J Am Coll Cardiol 33(5):1217–1226, 1999.
83. Leitch JW, Klein G, Yee R, Guiraudon G: Sinus node-atrioventricular node isolation: long-term results with the "Corridor" operation for atrial fibrillation. J Am Coll Cardiol 17(4):970–975, 1991.
84. Lewis T, Drury A, Iliescu C: A demonstartion of circus movement in clinical flutter of the auricles. Heart 8:341–359, 1921.
85. Lin WS, Prakash VS, Tai CT, et al: Pulmonary vein morphology in patients with paroxysmal atrial fibrillation initiated by ectopic beats originating from the pulmonary veins: implications for catheter ablation. Circulation 101(11): 1274–1281, 2000.
86. Lowe JE, Hendry PJ, Packer DL, Tang AS: Surgical management of chronic ectopic atrial tachycardia. Semin Thorac Cardiovasc Surg 1(1):58–66, 1989.
87. Maessen JG, Nijs JF, Smeets JL, et al: Beating-heart surgical treatment of atrial fibrillation with microwave ablation. Ann Thorac Surg 74(4):S1307–S1311, 2002.
88. Malliani A, Schwartz PJ, Zanchetti A: Neural mechanisms in life-threatening arrhythmias. Am Heart J 100(5):705–715, 1980.
89. Marcus FI, Fontaine GH, Guiraudon G, et al: Right ventricular dysplasia: a report of 24 adult cases. Circulation 65(2):384–398, 1982.
90. Marquez-Montes J, Rufilanchas JJ, Esteve JJ, et al: Paroxysmal nodal reentrant tachycardia. Surgical cure with preservation of atrioventricular conduction. Chest 83(4):690–694, 1983.
91. Mayer A: Rhythmical pulsation in Scyphomedusae. Carnegie Institution of Washington, 1906.
92. McCarthy PM, Castle LW, Maloney JD, et al: Initial experience with the Maze procedure for atrial fibrillation. J Thorac Cardiovasc Surg 105(6):1077–1087, 1993.
93. Melo J, Adragao PR, Neves J, et al: Electrosurgical treatment of atrial fibrillation with a new intraoperative radiofrequency ablation catheter. Thorac Cardiovasc Surg 47(Suppl 3): 370–372, 1999.
94. Melo J, Adragao P, Neves J, et al: Surgery for atrial fibrillation using radiofrequency catheter ablation: assessment of results at one year. Eur J Cardiothorac Surg 15(6):851–854; discussion 855, 1999.
95. Melo J, Adragao P, Neves J, et al: Endocardial and epicardial radiofrequency ablation in the treatment of atrial fibrillation with a new intra-operative device. Eur J Cardiothorac Surg 18(2):181–186, 2000.
96. Miller J, Gottlieb C, Marchlinski F: Does ventricular tachycardia mapping influence the success of antiarrhythmic surgery? J Am Coll Cardiol 11:112A, 1988.
97. Miller JM, Marchlinski FE, Harken AH, et al: Subendocardial resection for sustained ventricular tachycardia in the early period after acute myocardial infarction. Am J Cardiol 55(8):980–984, 1985.
98. Misaki T, Watanabe G, Iwa T, et al: Surgical treatment of arrhythmogenic right ventricular dysplasia: long-term outcome. Ann Thorac Surg 58(5):1380–1385, 1994.
99. Moe G: On the multiple wavelet hypothesis of atrial fibrillation. Arch Int Pharmacodyn Ther 140:183, 1962.
100. Mohr FW, Fabricius AM, Falk V, et al: Curative treatment of atrial fibrillation with intraoperative radiofrequency ablation: short-term and midterm results. J Thorac Cardiovasc Surg 123(5):919–927, 2002.
101. Moosdorf R, Pfeiffer D, Schneider C, Jung W: Intraoperative laser photocoagulation of ventricular tachycardia. Am Heart J 127(4 Pt 2):1133–1138, 1994.
102. Moran JM, Kehoe RF, Loeb JM, et al: Extended endocardial resection for the treatment of ventricular tachycardia and ventricular fibrillation. Ann Thorac Surg 34(5):538–552, 1982.
103. Moran JM, Kehoe RF, Loeb JM, et al: Operative therapy of malignant ventricular rhythm disturbances. Ann Surg 198(4):479–486, 1983.
104. Moss AJ: Background, outcome, and clinical implications of the Multicenter Automatic Defibrillator Implantation Trial (MADIT). Am J Cardiol 80(5B):28F–32F, 1997.
105. Moss AJ, McDonald J: Unilateral cervicothoracic sympathetic ganglionectomy for the treatment of long QT interval syndrome. N Engl J Med 285(16):903–904, 1971.
106. Pappone C, Oreto G, Lamberti F, et al: Catheter ablation of paroxysmal atrial fibrillation using a 3D mapping system. Circulation 100(11):1203–1208, 1999.
107. Patwardhan AM, Dave HH, Tamhane AA, et al: Intraoperative radiofrequency microbipolar coagulation to replace incisions of Maze III procedure for correcting atrial fibrillation in patients with rheumatic valvular disease. Eur J Cardiothorac Surg 12(4):627–633, 1997.
108. Puech P, Gallay P, Grolleau R: Mechanism of atrial flutter in humans. In P. T, AL W, editors: Atrial Arrhythmias: Current Concepts and Management. St. Louis: Mosby-Year Book, 1990.
109. Raanani E, Albage A, David TE, et al: The efficacy of the Cox/Maze procedure combined with mitral valve surgery: a matched control study. Eur J Cardiothorac Surg 19(4): 438–442, 2001.
110. Robbins IM, Colvin EV, Doyle TP, et al: Pulmonary vein stenosis after catheter ablation of atrial fibrillation. Circulation 98(17):1769–1775, 1998.
111. Ross DL, Johnson DC, Denniss AR, et al: Curative surgery for atrioventricular junctional ("AV nodal") reentrant tachycardia. J Am Coll Cardiol 6(6):1383–1392, 1985.
112. Schaff HV, Dearani JA, Daly RC, et al: Cox-Maze procedure for atrial fibrillation: Mayo Clinic experience. Semin Thorac Cardiovasc Surg 12(1):30–37, 2000.
113. Schwartz PJ, Periti M, Malliani A: The long Q-T syndrome. Am Heart J 89(3):378–390, 1975.
114. Sealy WC: Effectiveness of surgical management of the Wolff-Parkinson-White syndrome. Am J Surg 145(6): 756–762, 1983.
115. Sealy WC: The evolution of the surgical methods for interruption of right free wall Kent bundles. Ann Thorac Surg 36(1):29–36, 1983.
116. Sealy WC: Kent bundles in the anterior septal space. Ann Thorac Surg 36(2):18, 1983.
117. Sealy WC: Surgical treatment of the two types of tachycardia caused by Kent bundles with only retrograde function. J Thorac Cardiovasc Surg 85(5):746–751, 1983.
118. Sealy WC, Gallagher JJ: The surgical approach to the septal area of the heart based on experiences with 45 patients

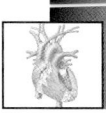

with Kent bundles. J Thorac Cardiovasc Surg 79(4):542–551, 1980.

119. Sealy WC, Gallagher JJ, Kasell J: His bundle interruption for control of inappropriate ventricular responses to atrial arrhythmias. Ann Thorac Surg 32(5):429–438, 1981.
120. Sealy WC, Gallagher JJ, Pritchett EL, Wallace AG: Surgical treatment of tachyarrhythmias in patients with both an Ebstein anomaly and a Kent bundle. J Thorac Cardiovasc Surg 75(6):847–853, 1978.
121. Sealy WC, Hattler BG Jr, Blumenschein SD, Cobb FR: Surgical treatment of Wolff-Parkinson-White syndrome. Ann Thorac Surg 8(1):1–11, 1969.
122. Selle JG, Svenson RH, Sealy WC, et al: Successful clinical laser ablation of ventricular tachycardia: a promising new therapeutic method. Ann Thorac Surg 42(4):380–384, 1986.
123. Sie HT, Beukema WP, Misier AR, et al: Radiofrequency modified Maze in patients with atrial fibrillation undergoing concomitant cardiac surgery. J Thorac Cardiovasc Surg 122(2):249–256, 2001.
124. Sueda T, Nagata H, Orihashi K, et al: Efficacy of a simple left atrial procedure for chronic atrial fibrillation in mitral valve operations. Ann Thorac Surg 63(4):1070–1075, 1997.
125. Sueda T, Nagata H, Shikata H, et al: Simple left atrial procedure for chronic atrial fibrillation associated with mitral valve disease. Ann Thorac Surg 62(6):1796–1800, 1996.
126. Svenson RH, Gallagher JJ, Selle JG, et al: Neodymium: YAG laser photocoagulation: a successful new map-guided technique for the intraoperative ablation of ventricular tachycardia. Circulation 76(6):1319–1328, 1987.
127. Teo WS, Guiraudon G, Klein GJ, et al: A unique preexcitation pattern related to an atypical anteroseptal accessory pathway. Pacing Clin Electrophysiol 15(11 Pt 1):1696–1701, 1992.
128. Theodoro DA, Danielson GK, Porter CJ, Warnes CA: Right-sided Maze procedure for right atrial arrhythmias in congenital heart disease. Ann Thorac Surg 65(1):149–153; discussion 153–154, 1998.
129. Tsai CF, Chen SA, Tai CT, et al: Bezold-Jarisch-like reflex during radiofrequency ablation of the pulmonary vein tissues in patients with paroxysmal focal atrial fibrillation. J Cardiovasc Electrophysiol 10(1):27–35, 1999.
130. Viola N, Williams MR, Oz MC, Ad N: The technology in use for the surgical ablation of atrial fibrillation. Semin Thorac Cardiovasc Surg 14(3):198–205, 2002.
131. Waldo AL: Pathogenesis of atrial flutter. J Cardiovasc Electrophysiol 9(8 Suppl):S18–S25, 1998.
132. Wijffels MC, Kirchhof CJ, Dorland R, Allessie MA: Atrial fibrillation begets atrial fibrillation. A study in awake chronically instrumented goats. Circulation 92(7):1954–1968, 1995.
133. Williams JM, Ungerleider RM, Lofland GK, Cox JL: Left atrial isolation: new technique for the treatment of supraventricular arrhythmias. J Thorac Cardiovasc Surg 80(3): 373–380, 1980.
134. Williams MR, Stewart JR, Bolling SF, et al: Surgical treatment of atrial fibrillation using radiofrequency energy. Ann Thorac Surg 71(6):1939–1943; discussion 1943–1944, 2001.
135. Wittig JH, Boineau JP: Surgical treatment of ventricular arrhythmias using epicardial, transmural, and endocardial mapping. Ann Thorac Surg 20(2):117–126, 1975.
136. Zhou S, Chang CM, Wu TJ, et al: Nonreentrant focal activations in pulmonary veins in canine model of sustained atrial fibrillation. Am J Physiol Heart Circ Physiol 283(3): H1244–H1252, 2002.

Surgical Treatment of Coronary Artery Disease and its Complications

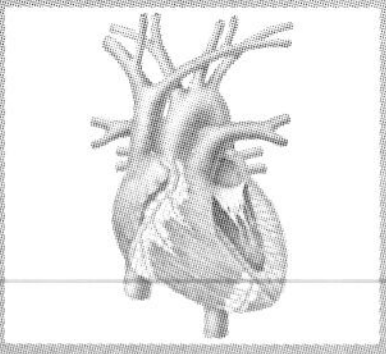

CHAPTER 82

Coronary Artery Bypass Grafting

Marc Ruel and Frank W. Sellke

INTRODUCTION

Coronary artery bypass grafting (CABG) is one of the procedures with the highest impact in the history of medicine. No other operation has led to more lives prolonged and been better characterized with respect to its short- and long-term outcomes. CABG constitutes the keystone of adult cardiac surgery, but its future is increasingly threatened by novel surgical, percutaneous, and medical alternatives. Yet CABG is constantly evolving and remains the most durable means of revascularization for patients with coronary artery disease (CAD). This chapter outlines the history, anatomical considerations, indications, techniques, postoperative care, and results of the CABG procedure as performed in the twenty-first century. Separate chapters on the coronary circulation, cardiac anatomy, cardiopulmonary bypass, myocardial protection, postoperative care, bypass conduits, off-pump grafting techniques, reoperations, and combined procedures are also found in this book and complement the text.

BACKGROUND

History

Surgical attempts at increasing blood flow to the ischemic myocardium originated a century ago when Alexis Carrel anastomosed a carotid artery segment between the descending aorta and the left coronary artery in a dog, for which he was later awarded the Nobel prize (Figure 82-1).[41] Three decades later, Arthur Vineberg started implanting the left internal thoracic artery (LITA) into the anterior myocardial territory of patients with CAD in order to increase arterial inflow and relieve angina,[293] with some experiencing prolonged symptomatic improvement.[221] Surgery on the coronary arteries was introduced clinically in 1958 by William Longmire, who reported on the use of endarterectomy in five patients operated without cardiopulmonary bypass (CPB).[172] That year also saw the invention of selective coronary angiography by Sones and Shirey in Cleveland, who accidentally injected contrast into the right coronary ostium instead of the aortic root and observed that this could be done safely.[262]

The first reported successful CABG operation took place in 1964 in Leningrad, where Kolesov grafted an LITA to the left anterior descending (LAD) artery without CPB.[156] The world's first CABG program started 3 years later in Cleveland, as Favaloro began to routinely use reversed saphenous veins for aortocoronary grafting.[82] The CABG procedure was then rapidly adopted and developed worldwide. LITA grafting of the LAD was introduced in the Western world by Green in 1968,[114] sequential grafting by Flemma in 1971,[94] bilateral internal thoracic grafting by Kay in 1972,[272] and radial artery grafts by Carpentier in 1973 and revived by Acar in 1989.[2,39]

Anatomical Considerations

Coronary artery anatomy and size vary widely from one person to another, with different impacts on myocardial perfusion. For instance, a nondiseased 1-mm LAD may perfectly meet the myocardial demands of an individual during exercise, but another person of identical body size may experience angina from a focal 60% stenosis on a 2.5-mm vessel. In health, basal arteriogenic processes match the distributive coronary anatomy of each human being to his or her needs without providing excess coronary blood supply; the development of CAD breaks this equilibrium. The result is either supply ischemia, responsible for myocardial infarction and most episodes of unstable angina, or demand ischemia, where coronary blood flow is insufficient only during periods of increased myocardial demands from exercise, tachycardia, hypertension, or emotion.[101] Basal arteriogenesis and collateral formation are enhanced when new coronary flow patterns and subclinical ischemia develop, but depend on the time course of CAD development and on genetic, environmental, and endothelial factors. It is the

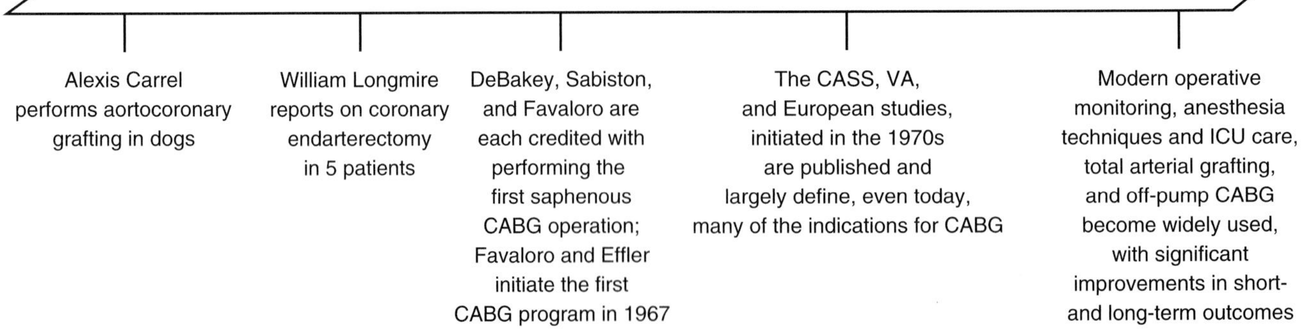

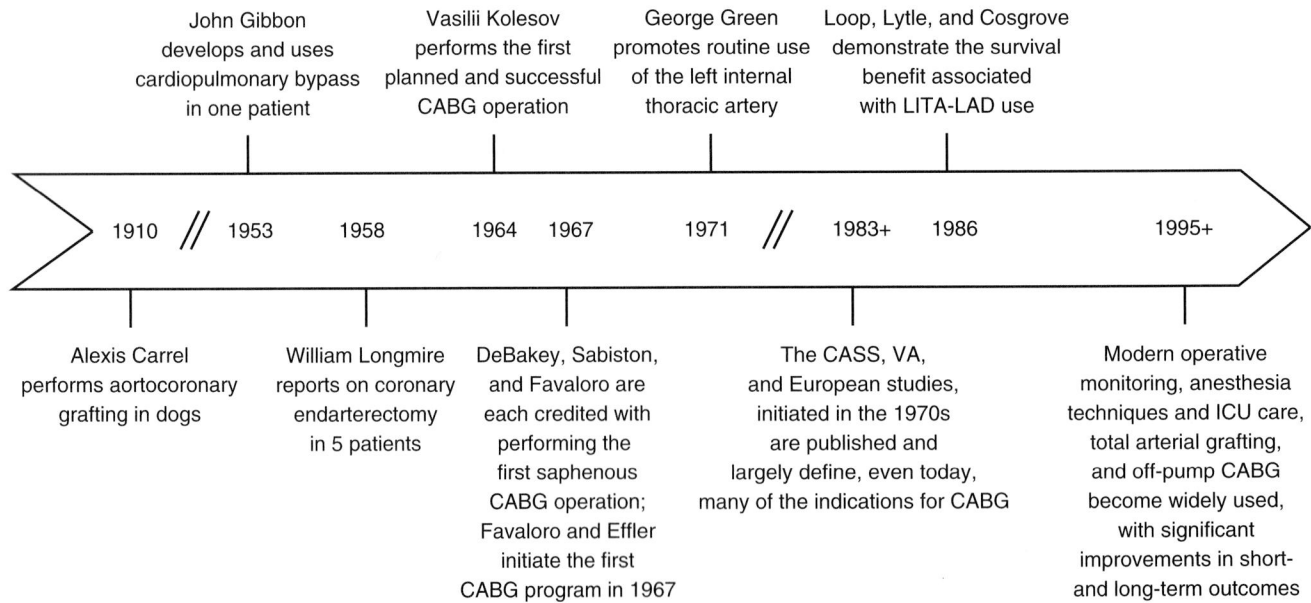

Figure 82–1 Landmark events in the history of coronary artery bypass grafting. CABG, coronary artery bypass grafting; CASS, Coronary Artery Surgery Study; LITA–LAD, left internal thoracic artery graft to the left anterior descending coronary artery; VA, Veterans Administration Coronary Artery Bypass Surgery Cooperative Study; ICU, intensive care unit.

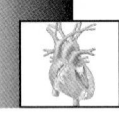

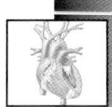

magnitude of this collateral development that determines the degree of ischemia experienced by a patient and the size of the subtended myocardial territory at risk for a given severity of coronary artery stenosis.

Depending on referral patterns, approximately 40–50% of patients who undergo coronary angiography have significant involvement of all three coronary arteries, and 5–10% have stenosis of the left main stem. Approximately 5% of patients have diffuse disease of one or more major coronary branches.[207] In patients with single- or double-vessel disease, the most frequently stenosed coronary artery is the right, followed closely by the LAD and least frequently by the circumflex.[152] In some patients, atherosclerosis may be mimicked by myocardial bridging of a coronary artery, which most often involves the LAD or circumflex in a segment almost always devoid of atherosclerosis. Bridging is not always benign, however, as it can result in ischemic symptoms during strenuous exercise and even trigger ventricular arrhythmias.[24]

Hypocontractile or noncontractile myocardium subtended by a diseased coronary artery may represent one of four pathologies: stunned myocardium, hibernating myocardium, nontransmural scar tissue, or transmural scar tissue. Clinical determination is based on the evaluation of contractile recruitment during dobutamine-stress echocardiography, or scintigraphic assessment of perfusion and glucose utilization on[201] Tl single-photon emission computerized tomography (SPECT) and ^{18}F-2-deoxyglucose (FDG) positron emission tomography (PET).[20] With PET, stunned myocardium appears as a hypocontractile segment with normal perfusion and glucose utilization at rest, and hibernating myocardium as a territory with decreased perfusion but preserved glucose utilization (Figure 82-2).[249] Scar tissue, unlikely to benefit from CABG, exhibits both reduced perfusion and glucose utilization, with a mild reduction in nontransmural scars and a severe reduction in transmural scars. Clinical PET findings have been shown to correlate with ultrastructural damage and myocardial fibrosis on histological examination.[182]

INDICATIONS FOR OPERATION

Chronic Stable Angina

Chronic stable angina is associated with lifestyle-limiting symptoms and an increased risk of major adverse cardiac events and death. From the point of view of providing a survival benefit alone, CABG is indicated in patients with chronic stable angina and left main coronary artery stenosis ≥50%, left main equivalent (i.e., proximal stenosis of at least 70% of the proximal LAD and circumflex), three-vessel disease (especially if left ventricular ejection fraction [LVEF] is less than 0.50), and one- or two-vessel disease with either a large myocardial area at risk on noninvasive testing or depressed LVEF (Table 82-1).[70,302]

CABG may also be indicated for symptomatic improvement in low-risk patients with significant CAD who do not fulfill the above criteria but experience disabling myocardial ischemia or unacceptable lifestyle restrictions on maximal medical therapy. CABG is not indicated in patients with one- or two-vessel disease not involving the proximal LAD and with only a small area of viable myocardium or no objective evidence of ischemia on noninvasive testing.

It is important to recognize that most of the indications for CABG in patients with chronic stable angina are, even today, derived from the survival benefit observed in patients randomized to CABG versus maximum medical therapy in the Coronary Artery Surgery Study (CASS),[49] Veterans Administration (VA) Coronary Artery Bypass Surgery Cooperative Study,[77] and European Coronary Surgery Study.[289] These trials were performed in the 1970s; almost exclusively used saphenous vein grafts (the exception being CASS in which a single LITA–LAD graft was used in 13% of patients); did not include women (with the exception of CASS); and did not use lipid-lowering therapy, postoperative aspirin, or angiotensin-converting enzyme (ACE) inhibitors. In addition, the mean age of randomized patients in the three major trials was 50.8 years, and only 19.7% of patients had an LVEF of 0.50 or less (no patient with an LVEF of 0.35 or less was enrolled).

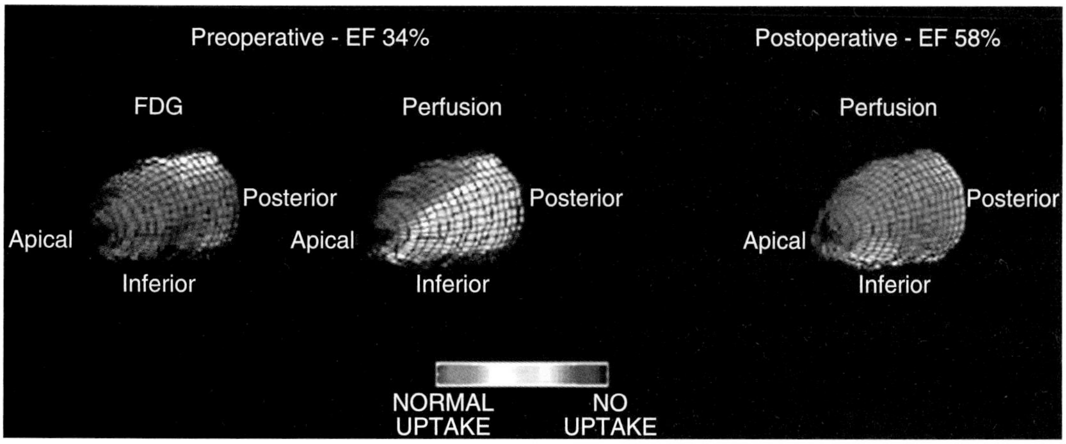

Figure 82–2 **Preoperative myocardial viability assessment.** This patient with CHF symptoms and inferior wall akinesis was evaluated prior to CABG with ^{18}F–2–deoxyglucose (FDG) positron emission tomography (PET) and perfusion scintigraphy. Depressed ejection fraction (EF), viable myocytes (indicated by the normal FDG uptake), and the presence of a large posteroinferior perfusion defect were identified preoperatively. After CABG the perfusion defect disappeared and the ejection fraction normalized. (See color plate.)
(Images courtesy of Robert S. Beanlands, MD, Division of Nuclear Cardiology, University of Ottawa Heart Institute.)

Table 82–1

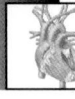

Indications for Coronary Artery Bypass Grafting

	Chronic stable angina	*Acute coronary syndromes*	*Complications of PCI*	*Asymptomatic CAD*	*Kawasaki disease*	*Trauma*
Definite indications	Left main coronary stenosis Left main equivalent Three-vessel disease (especially if LVEF <50%) Two-vessel disease with proximal LAD and either LVEF <50% or objective evidence of ischemia on noninvasive testing One- or two-vessel disease with a large area of viable myocardium at risk on noninvasive testing Disabling angina or unacceptable lifestyle restrictions despite optimal medical therapy, when surgery can be performed with a low risk	Unstable angina/non-Q wave MI Subacute period Same as for chronic stable angina Acute period Ongoing myocardial ischemia not responsive to maximal nonsurgical therapy ST-segment elevation (Q wave) MI Subacute period Same as for chronic stable angina Acute period (<12 h) None	Ongoing ischemia or threatened occlusion with significant myocardium at risk after failed PCI Hemodynamic compromise after failed PCI Coronary artery rupture with impending pericardial tamponade	Left main coronary stenosis Left main equivalent Three-vessel disease (especially if LVEF <50%) Two-vessel disease with proximal LAD and either LVEF <50% or objective evidence of ischemia on noninvasive testing	None	None
Probable indications	Proximal LAD disease without a large territory at risk or extensive ischemia One- or two-vessel disease not involving the LAD, with a moderate area of viable myocardium at risk on noninvasive testing	ST-segment elevation (Q wave) MI Acute period (<12 h) Intractable ischemia or cardiogenic shock after failed thrombolysis and PCI	Foreign body in crucial anatomical position Hemodynamic compromise in patients with coagulation impairment and without previous sternotomy	Proximal LAD stenosis with one- or two-vessel disease	Objective evidence of myocardial ischemia in the presence of (1) demonstrated coronary stenosis[es], (2) myocardial viability in the supplied area(s), and (3) at least one involved but graftable coronary artery	Demonstrated proximal coronary injury with objective evidence of ischemia on ECG or wall-motion anomaly on TEE

Table 82–1

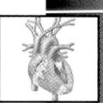

Indications for Coronary Artery Bypass Grafting—cont'd

	Chronic stable angina	*Acute coronary syndromes*	*Complications of PCI*	*Asymptomatic CAD*	*Kawasaki disease*	*Trauma*
Possible indications	Borderline coronary stenosis (50–60% diameter reduction in locations other than the left main coronary artery) with demonstrable ischemia despite maximal medical therapy	Progressive LV failure with coronary stenosis compromising viable myocardium outside the initial infarct area	Hemodynamic compromise in patients with coagulation impairment and with previous sternotomy	One- or two-vessel disease not involving the LAD	Asymptomatic giant coronary aneurysms subtending a large myocardial areas at risk (>8 mm)	Proximal coronary injury with no evidence of ischemia or wall-motion anomaly Distal coronary injury with evidence of ischemia on ECG or wall-motion anomaly on TEE
Not indications	One- or two-vessel disease not involving the LAD and with only a small area of viable myocardium at risk Borderline coronary stenosis (50–60% diameter reduction in locations other than the left main coronary artery) without demonstrable ischemia Insignificant coronary stenosis (<50% diameter reduction)	Primary CABG in the acute period of unstable angina, non–Q wave MI, or ST-segment elevation MI without attempts at maximal nonsurgical therapy	Emergency revascularization for no-reflow state or failed PCI resulting from unsuitable anatomy in otherwise stable patients	Same as for chronic stable angina	Small (<8 mm) asymptomatic coronary aneurysms without ischemia or significant coronary stenosis	Distal coronary injury with no evidence of ischemia or wall-motion anomaly (ligation only)

CABG, coronary artery bypass grafting; CAD, coronary artery disease; LAD, left anterior descending coronary artery; LV, left ventricle; LVEF, left ventricular ejection fraction; MI, myocardial infarction; PCI, percutaneous coronary interventions; TEE, transesophageal echocardiography; ECG, electrocardiogram.

Not only does today's "average" CABG patient not fit well in the groups studied in the CASS, VA, and European trials, but subsequent data indicating that the survival benefits of CABG over medical therapy may increase with age and left ventricular dysfunction suggest that the indications for revascularization in patients with chronic stable angina be extended beyond those derived from these trials.[70,113]

Acute Coronary Syndromes

Unstable Angina/Non–Q Wave MI

The indications for CABG in the setting of chronic stable angina similarly constitute basic indications for CABG after unstable angina or non–Q wave myocardial infarction (MI).

In addition, ongoing ischemia not responsive to maximal nonsurgical therapy may warrant CABG. Several studies have shown, however, that emergent surgery for relentless unstable angina or non–Q wave MI in the context of failed or unfeasible PCI is associated with an increase in perioperative mortality compared with semiurgent CABG,[4,52,98,163,177] although surgical revascularization may still be preferable to a conservative strategy.[96] Consequently, an attempt should be made at stabilizing these patients with maximal medical therapy (and in some cases the temporary use of an intraaortic balloon pump) to allow surgery to be performed on a nonemergent basis with a lower operative risk.

ST-Segment Elevation (Q Wave) MI

Intravenous thrombolytic therapy and primary percutaneous coronary interventions (PCI) have supplanted CABG as the first line of therapy for patients in the acute period of ST-segment elevation MI. As a result, residual ongoing ischemia and cardiogenic shock despite maximal nonsurgical therapy now constitute the main indication for emergent CABG in acute MI patients.[70] Other acute indications include failed thrombolysis and demonstration of a large myocardial territory at risk in combination with an unsuitable anatomy for PCI, a left main coronary stenosis, an LV failure with severe coronary stenosis outside the initial infarct area, significant valve disease, or a mechanical complication of MI.

In the subacute phase, the indications for CABG in the setting of chronic stable angina also apply to patients who have experienced an ST-segment elevation MI. Although surgery performed on an emergent basis during the first 24 h of MI has an increased mortality, the timing of the operation after that initial period has otherwise not been shown to determine operative risk.[52,163]

Complications of PCI

PCI may occasionally result in intractable coronary dissection or plaque hemorrhage, threatened proximal occlusion with a large myocardial area at risk, loss of a foreign body in a crucial anatomical position, or coronary rupture. These complications are indications for immediate surgical intervention, but in-hospital mortality is high in these patients (10–14%) because of unfavorable selection factors such as hemodynamic compromise and severe impairment of the coagulation system.[161,233] CABG should not be attempted on an emergency basis in stable patients in whom PCI has failed because of unsuitable anatomy or no-reflow state.[9,70]

Asymptomatic CAD

Indications for CABG in patients with asymptomatic CAD include left main coronary artery stenosis, left main equivalent, and three-vessel disease with LVEF <0.50, for which CABG results in increased survival compared to medical therapy.[70] In addition, patients with three-vessel disease and normal LV function and those with proximal LAD disease may benefit from revascularization.[69] These guidelines also apply to the majority of patients in whom asymptomatic CAD is discovered during preoperative evaluation prior to noncardiac surgery and may not be expanded if the noncardiac operation carries a high risk of MI and CABG can be performed with a low risk of mortality.

Kawasaki Disease

The indications and timing of operation in patients who had childhood Kawasaki disease, subsequently developed coronary aneurysms, and have coronary stenoses or thromboembolic events related to these aneurysms are unclear.[110,153] CABG and PCI have a complementary but poorly defined role in the management of these complications.[64,137,153,301] Arterial grafts have better long-term patency than saphenous veins grafts in patients with Kawasaki disease,[153] despite reports of very late patency and growth potential for vein grafts.[78,269] Transplantation has been used in patients with intractable ischemia or heart failure who exhibit diffuse distal coronary disease and transmural scarring. Occasionally aneurysms can become very large and prone to rupture, and have been managed with interposition saphenous vein grafting.[88]

Trauma

Penetrating cardiac trauma is an indication for immediate surgical intervention; in doubtful cases, transesophageal echocardiography may be helpful in determining whether penetration of the heart has taken place.[16] CABG is indicated if injury to a major coronary vessel or branch has occurred; in this regard, the most frequently affected coronary artery is the LAD, followed by the right, and the circumflex.[213] Concomitant injury to other cardiac structures, great vessels, or internal thoracic arteries is common. The diagnosis of coronary injury requires a high index of suspicion and may occasionally necessitate angiographic confirmation. Distal injuries with a small area of myocardium at risk are best treated with ligation alone, while proximal injuries and those associated with a large area of ischemia necessitate CABG.[145]

SURGICAL TECHNIQUE

Preoperative Preparation

Virtually all CABG patients have had a diagnosis of myocardial ischemia established by noninvasive testing, undergone a coronary angiogram, and been seen by a cardiologist prior to surgical referral. Yet examination of the patient by the surgeon and a thorough review of routine laboratory examinations, noninvasive cardiac tests, and coronary angiogram allow for confirmation of the surgical indication, determination of the operative risk, and optimal planning of the surgical strategy.

History and Physical Examination

Particular attention must be given to a possible misdiagnosis (especially when symptoms appear out of proportion to the angiographic severity of coronary stenoses), to comorbid conditions, and to the availability of conduits for revascularization (Table 82-2). For instance, patients with predominant symptoms of dyspnea may have concomitant valvular disease, cardiomyopathy, or pulmonary hypertension that has been missed and that a soft murmur, a loud P_2, signs of cardiomegaly, and subtle cyanosis or clubbing may unveil. Symptoms and signs of congestive heart failure (CHF) should be sought, since CHF may impact perioperative medical management, intraoperative planning (with respect, in some cases, to the choice of myocardial protection strategy and the selection of conduits), and short- and long-term prognosis after operation.[196] Patients with previous mediastinal irradiation should undergo preoperative echocardiography to rule out valve disease, pulmonary function testing, and carotid duplex examination.[121] Patients with a history of peptic ulcer disease should be identified as such and the use of perioperative nonsteroidal antiinflammatory agents avoided in them.

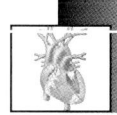

The peripheral vascular examination is of utmost importance. Brachial blood pressure should be measured in both arms to potentially unveil a hemodynamically significant subclavian artery stenosis; a difference of more than 10 mm Hg warrants Doppler examination and the use of a free internal thoracic artery (ITA) graft or alternate conduit if a stenosis is confirmed.[128,277] The lower extremities should be examined for the presence of varicose veins and incisions from previous saphenectomy or peripheral vascular procedures, and the patient should be asked whether sclerotherapy has ever been performed. Lower extremity arterial disease is associated with an increase in mortality risk of nearly 5-fold, regardless of the presence of symptoms.[33] These patients have the highest incidence of aortic calcification and perioperative stroke, and particular attention must be given to the ascending aorta when assessing the preoperative chest X-ray and reviewing the coronary angiogram.[169] Documentation of peripheral pulses is also

Table 82–2

History and Physical Examination Findings of Particular Importance before CABG

Finding	*Surgical implication*
Orthopnea and other symptoms of heart failure; third heart sound; increased jugular venous pressure; peripheral edema	Echocardiography to rule out severe left ventricular dysfunction, cardiomyopathy, right ventricular failure, valve disease; may warrant viability testing
Clubbing; loud pulmonary component of the second heart sound; right ventricular heave; cyanosis	Possible primary or secondary pulmonary hypertension; warrants right heart catheterization +/− pulmonary angiogram
Previous stroke, transient ischemic attack, or amaurosis fugax; carotid bruit	Warrants carotid duplex examination and echocardiography; magnetic resonance imaging angiography if symptoms of vertebrobasilar insufficiency
Diabetes mellitus; severe obesity; chronic obstructive pulmonary disease; oral steroid therapy; previous mediastinal irradiation	May contraindicate the use of bilateral internal thoracic arteries
Brachial blood pressure differential between the two arms	Warrants carotid and subclavian duplex examination; contraindicates the use of an *in situ* internal thoracic graft on the side of a subclavian stenosis
Claudication; decreased peripheral pulses; Leriche syndrome (claudication, decreased femoral pulses, impotence)	Increased risk of perioperative mortality; warrants echocardiographic assessment of the ascending aorta and arch; carotid duplex examination desirable; Leriche syndrome may contraindicate internal thoracic artery use
Varicose veins; previous saphenous vein harvesting or sclerotherapy	Must plan for alternate conduits
Raynaud's syndrome; absent ulnar pulse; slow refill on Allen test; previous ipsilateral radial-catheterization for coronary angiography	May warrant Doppler examination of the wrist circulation; contraindicates the use of a radial artery for revascularization in most cases
Abdominal pain after meals; previous upper abdominal surgery	May warrant celiac axis and mesenteric angiography; contraindicates the use of the gastroepiploic artery for revascularization

important if the use of an intraaortic balloon pump becomes necessary, and provides a rapid, albeit imperfect, baseline assessment for postoperative comparison if delayed hemodynamic compromise or tamponade is suspected after the patient has left the intensive care unit.

Absolute contraindications to the use of an ITA include previous damage from penetrating trauma or surgery, and documentation of the artery as a major source of collateral perfusion to a lower extremity in patients with Leriche syndrome (unless lower extremity revascularization is performed concomitantly).[13,125] ITA grafts are also best avoided in patients with previous mediastinal irradiation if other arterial conduits are available,[121] or the anterior myocardial territory should be revascularized with a second, redundant graft in addition to the ITA. Patients on chronic hemodialysis should have a free rather than an *in situ* ITA graft performed on the side of their arteriovenous fistula.[53] Severe obesity, chronic obstructive pulmonary disease (COPD), oral steroid therapy, and diabetes may contraindicate the use of bilateral ITAs, but this is controversial and ultimately depends on individual preferences.[219]

Previous upper abdominal surgery or symptoms suggestive of mesenteric angina contraindicate the use of a gastroepiploic artery. Radial artery harvest is avoided in patients with Raynaud's syndrome or on the side of a previous radial artery catheterization for coronary angiography. It is important to both feel for an ulnar pulse and perform the Allen test (using a cutoff of 3 s, which has a 100% sensitivity for inadequate collateral hand circulation)[139] before planning to use a radial artery, because the ulnar artery may exceptionally be congenitally absent and the Allen test still be normal, with potentially disastrous consequences if unrecognized.[220] Although the 3-s Allen test remains a controversial screening tool,[266] the routine use of Doppler ultrasound in every patient considered for radial artery harvest poses logistic and economic constraints that are not justifiable solely on the basis of yielding a lower false-positive rate.

Asymptomatic carotid bruits have unreliable predictive accuracy,[248] but their presence warrants consideration of carotid duplex examination if CABG is performed on a nonurgent basis.[197] Perioperative stroke risk is less than 2% in patients with carotid stenoses less than 50%, 10% when stenoses are 50–80%, and 11–19% in patients with stenoses of more than 80%.[246,296] However, the routine evaluation of asymptomatic carotid bruits with duplex examination and combined carotid endarterectomy/CABG surgery in patients with hemodynamically significant carotid lesions is of questionable advantage over initial treatment of the symptomatic coronary disease alone. A history of transient ischemic attack or stroke warrants a carotid duplex examination and echocardiogram to rule out a carotid stenosis, a cardiac embolic source, or a patent foramen ovale. If no source is found and symptoms suggestive of vertebrobasilar insufficiency are elicited, magnetic resonance imaging angiography of the arch vessels should be performed. Patients who had a recent stroke should ideally have a minimum interval of 4 weeks prior to undergoing CABG to minimize the possibility of neurological damage extension. Although the combined performance of CABG and carotid endarterectomy is controversial (associated with an increased risk of cardiovascular accident [CVA] in a meta-analysis in which confounding by indication may have biased against patients who received the combined procedure[27]) preoperative documentation of hemodynamically significant carotid stenoses allows for risk stratification, consideration of a staged procedure, special intraoperative neuromonitoring, and optimization of perioperative blood pressure management.

Medications

Aspirin and cardiac medications are continued up to the time of operation, with the exception of digoxin, which is discontinued 1 day prior to surgery. Warfarin is stopped several days before surgery in orally anticoagulated nonemergency patients, who are started on heparin when their international normalized ratio (INR) becomes 2.0 or less; emergent cases are reversed with fresh-frozen plasma. Management of the oral glycoprotein IIb/IIIa inhibitor clopidogrel varies according to personal preferences; our approach is to stop the medication 3 days to 1 week prior to operation in stable patients. Urgent cases having received clopidogrel may need to receive platelet transfusions and/or aprotinin to reduce bleeding. Patients started on an ACE inhibitor a few days or weeks prior to surgical referral should have the progression of their serum creatinine levels monitored; if a progressive elevation is noted the medication should be stopped and the serum creatinine levels allowed to normalize prior to operation.

Laboratory Tests

Complete blood counts, serum chemistries, liver function tests, coagulogram, ECG, chest X-ray, and urinalysis are routinely performed. Particular attention is given to a low platelet count (suggestive of possible heparin-induced thrombocytopenia in patients on heparin), an elevated serum creatinine (an independent predictor of increased operative mortality), and the presence of vascular calcification on the chest X-ray. Anterior Q waves with poor R wave progression on the ECG are indicative of transmural myocardial scarring and may warrant preoperative viability testing. Most patients have undergone preoperative nuclear scintigrams and echocardiography, which are reviewed to determine the functional significance of borderline coronary stenoses, and provide an assessment of valve function, left ventricular systolic wall motion, diastolic function, and right ventricular contractility.

A major improvement in the preoperative evaluation in patients with poor LV function and CHF has resulted from the availability of scintigraphic myocardial viability assessment. Viability is best assessed with PET; recovery of regional and global left ventricular function after surgical revascularization correlates with a higher preoperative blood flow and glucose uptake, indicative of less tissue fibrosis and a high proportion of viable cardiomyocytes in a dysfunctional area (Figure 82-2).[58,93] Results are best if both hibernating myocardium and angina symptoms are present and attributed to a myocardial territory subtended by a graftable vessel with a significant proximal stenosis; on the other hand, patients with no viability, no angina symptoms, and diffuse CAD are unlikely to derive a survival benefit with CABG, compared to medical therapy alone,[59] although this remains controversial.[76,196] If PET is not available, dobutamine stress echocardiography or magnetic resonance imaging may be used to identify reversible myocardial dysfunction; although not as sensitive as PET (i.e., More patients may inaccurately appear to have no viability.), dobutamine wall-motion indices are specific (i.e., If the segment does improve, it is likely viable.) in predicting postoperative improvement.[116,160]

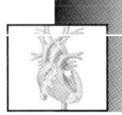

Coronary Angiogram

For nearly half a century, coronary angiography has been the road map used by surgeons and cardiologists to assess the severity of CAD and plan myocardial revascularization. As a general rule, vessels 1.5 mm or more on which a stenosis of at least 50% is observed should be grafted. Consideration is also given to smaller vessels if no other target is found in a coronary distribution where myocardial ischemia has been demonstrated on noninvasive testing. With modern techniques of cardiopulmonary bypass and myocardial protection, the planning of incomplete revascularization because of comorbid factors alone is justified only in exceptional circumstances and associated with suboptimal short- and long-term outcomes.[225,251] Failure to bypass a functionally significant and stenosed coronary artery should result from nongraftability, diffuse aortic calcification with inability to perform Y- or T-grafting, conduit shortage, or severe unexpected intraoperative problems.

An intramyocardial LAD can sometimes be a vexing problem. Because LITA–LAD grafting provides a survival benefit in CABG patients,[174] the failure to graft a stenosed LAD because of its intramyocardial location is clearly suboptimal. The situation can, however, be identified preoperatively by seeing the vessel going downward and, after several centimeters, upward on the angiogram, or by noticing that the LAD goes straight down to the apex without any curve (Figure 82-3). Several techniques can be used intraoperatively to find the LAD at its proximal or mid portion, such as the use of epicardial Doppler, retrograde probing of the LAD after performing a minute arteriotomy at its apical portion, or retrograde probing during construction of a graft to a diagonal branch. However, an alternative approach is to anastomose the ITA to a diagonal branch of the LAD and to place a vein graft to the distal LAD proper, especially if there is minimal obstructive disease between the LAD and diagonal branch.

Conduit Selection

Internal Thoracic Artery Grafts

The ITA is the best conduit available for CABG and provides short- and long-term survival benefits in all patients subgroups, including those 75 years of age or older.[84,174] Use of the LITA to graft the LAD (or a main target vessel on the left coronary circulation if the LAD is free of disease) should be performed except in exceptional circumstances such as preexisting or iatrogenic damage to the LITA, poor flow from severe spasm, injury, or dissection,[123] involvement of the LITA in providing collateral supply to the lower extremity, mediastinal irradiation (if other arterial conduits are available), and emergency CABG with cardiogenic shock. Previous concern regarding the development of a string sign when the LITA is used to graft a coronary with only moderate (i.e., 50–60%) stenosis has not been substantiated.[148]

The use of bilateral ITAs should be considered over single ITA grafting whenever possible in young patients, as they may lead to lower reoperation rates, decreased late PCI rates, and long-term survival benefits.[178] However, the actual benefit derived from the use of bilateral ITA grafts or multiple arterial grafts over the use of a single ITA graft to the LAD and placement of vein grafts to the other diseased arteries remains controversial. Relative contraindications to the use of bilateral ITAs include emergency operation, advanced age, diabetes mellitus, obesity, and severe COPD for which the patient requires systemic steroid therapy. After decades of debate, the use of bilateral ITAs in non-obese, non-diabetic patients has not shown to increase the incidence of deep sternal wound infection except in emergent cases and patients older than 70 years of age.[136] Excellent results have also been reported with the use of skeletonized bilateral ITAs in diabetic patients (with the exception of obese diabetic women who have an unacceptably high incidence of deep sternal would infection), and diabetes per se no longer constitutes a contraindication to bilateral ITA use.[130,131,192,219,288] Skeletonization provides more

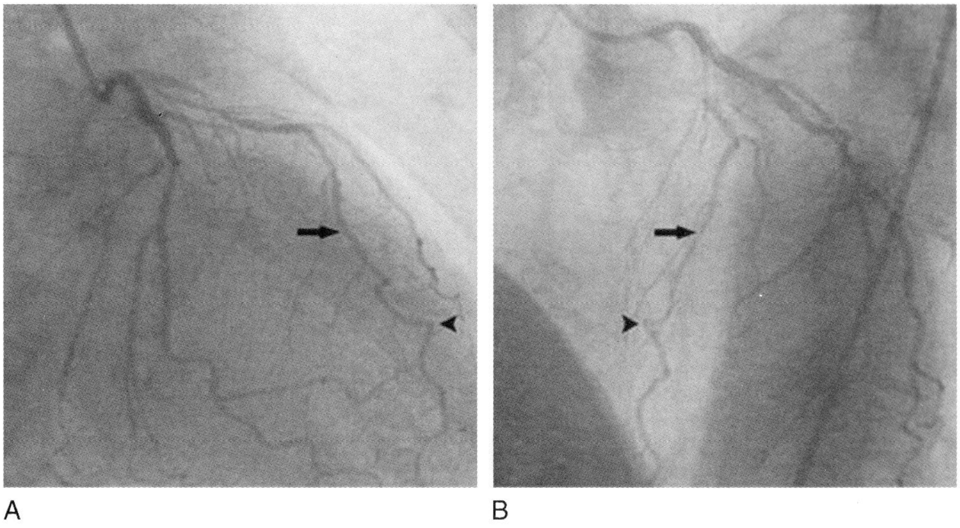

Figure 82–3 Intramyocardial left anterior descending artery (LAD). The LAD goes downward (*arrow*) and, after several centimeters, upward on the angiogram (*arrowhead*). **A,** Right anterior oblique projection. **B,** Left anterior oblique projection.

conduit length,[56] preserves sternal vascularity,[45] and has been associated with higher flows and larger anastomotic diameters.[279,299] Skeletonization does not appear to have a detrimental effect on vascular integrity and long-term patency.[37,247]

Whether a free or *in situ* ITA graft is performed makes little difference with respect to patency and endothelial function provided that a flawless anastomotic technique is employed.[157,174,280] The avoidance of grafts that are too short is unarguably more important, because insufficient graft length leads to angle distortion at one or more sites within the conduit with resultant compromise in flow and patency. An *in situ* ITA graft that appears too short is better cut proximally and repositioned onto the aorta or onto another ITA than left under tension.

In some patients, ITA flow may be very low (i.e., less than 20 ml/min) prior to construction of the anastomosis. This may be due to spasm, small size, or intraoperative injury such as an intimal dissection. If an area of injury is suspected, the ITA should be either converted to a free graft (if long enough), or transected a few millimeters above and below the injury site, the two stumps beveled, and an end-to-end anastomosis carried out using 8-0 polypropylene.[108] If no injury is apparent, the ITA may still be used for grafting, and this was shown not to result in an increased incidence of angiographic string sign or graft occlusion at 1 year postoperatively.[123] Unrecognized ITA intimal dissections may heal spontaneously with anticoagulation, antiplatelet therapy, and vasodilators alone.[200] If blood flow in the ITA is felt to be suboptimal, a second graft may be constructed to the LAD in addition to the ITA to ensure adequate perfusion.

Radial Artery Grafts

The radial artery likely constitutes, after the left and right ITA, the next best conduit for CABG. Results demonstrating its short- and long-term superiority over a saphenous vein graft have, however, not been published, and a multicenter trial is currently ongoing.[97] A case-matched study demonstrated marked short- and mid-term clinical benefits in patients who received a radial artery graft instead of a saphenous vein, but these benefits were of such magnitude early on that confounding by indication was possibly influential.[46,142] Radial grafts are highly versatile, can be used for virtually any type of grafting configuration (e.g., aortocoronary, Y, or T), but should not be used to graft coronaries with less than 70% stenosis because of reduced patency.[97,185,205]

Intraoperatively the radial artery may be treated immediately following harvest with a blood/phenoxybenzamine flush (100 mg of phenoxybenzamine mixed in 50 ml of heparinized blood) and left soaking in this mixture for 30 min. Phenoxybenzamine, a noncompetitive α_1-anatagonist agent, is nontoxic for endothelial cells and highly effective in preventing acute spasm of the radial artery.[62,291] It is important both to flush out the phenoxybenzamine from the radial artery and rinse the pedicle with plasmalyte prior to constructing the graft, because failure to do so could result in low systemic vascular resistances for 1–2 days postoperatively in otherwise normally convalescing patients. Alternatively, nitroglycerin can be used to dilate the radial artery prior to grafting.

Radial artery harvest is contraindicated in the presence of insufficient collateral supply to the hand or Raynaud's syndrome, in patients with high manual demands such as professional musicians, in the very elderly (who have a high prevalence of radial arteriosclerosis and are unlikely to derive a survival benefit from preferential use of the radial artery over a vein graft), during emergency operations, and in patients who are likely to require postoperative vasopressors such as those with very poor LV function. Radial artery use should be discussed during patient consent, because the incidence of postharvest neurological complications, which most often consist of decreased thumb strength and sensation abnormality, is approximately 30%.[57] Diabetes, peripheral vascular disease, elevated creatinine levels, and smoking are associated with an increased risk of these complications, which resolve with time in the vast majority of patients.[11]

Gastroepiploic Artery Grafts

The gastroepiploic artery is a conduit with a higher propensity for intraoperative problems and a lower postoperative patency than the radial artery. Although excellent results have been reported by several groups who have developed expertise with routine use of the gastroepiploic artery,[129,219] several factors make it a relatively difficult conduit: harvest elicits spasm, kinking and torsion may go unrecognized, and anastomotic problems are more likely to occur because of the small size of the vessel. Furthermore, use of the gastroepiploic artery to graft coronaries with moderate proximal stenosis or poor runoff should be avoided, as this results in decreased patency.[271] Its use as a free graft has also been associated with a lower patency than the *in situ* configuration.[198] For these reasons, we favor the use of other arterial conduits before selecting the gastroepiploic artery for primary revascularization.

Saphenous Vein Grafts

Because of lower short- and long-term patency than ITAs, saphenous veins have been known not to be the conduit of choice for CABG for nearly 20 years.[174] Nevertheless, saphenous veins are still used in the majority of CABG operations by a large number of surgeons for practicality reasons. They are also particularly useful for specific situations. They constitute the most readily available CABG conduit, provide immediate and reliable coronary flow with a low propensity for spasm or flow compromise during low-output states, and provide a time-honored means of coronary revascularization during emergency procedures or in patients with severe comorbidity and limited life expectancy in whom procedural simplicity, expeditiousness, and reliability are most desirable.

Other Conduits

The lesser saphenous vein and inferior epigastric artery constitute two additional available conduits that are rarely needed for primary revascularization, but which may be useful as a last resort in patients with severe conduit shortage.

Operative Preparation

Intraoperative preparation by the anesthesiologist includes the provision of peripheral intravenous and arterial access in

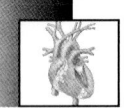

the arm contralateral to the side of radial artery harvest, induction of anesthesia, endotracheal intubation, central venous access, and placement of a pulmonary artery catheter. Intravenous antibiotics with gram-positive coverage are administered 30–60 min before skin incision and consist in most institutions of cefuroxime 1.5 g IV every 12 h or cefazolin 1–2 g IV every 8 h for 48 h. In patients with penicillin allergy, vancomycin 1 g IV every 12 h is given for at least two doses until all lines and tubes have been removed.[70,245] A nasogastric tube and transesophageal echocardiography probe (if available) are advanced in the esophagus. Baseline measurements of filling pressures, cardiac output, arterial blood gases, activated clotting time, hematocrit level, and electrolytes are obtained prior to surgical incision.

The patient is prepped and draped, and a midline skin incision is made from the manubrium of the sternum to the xiphoid process while the assistant starts harvesting the radial artery and/or saphenous vein. If the use of a gastroepiploic artery is planned, the median sternotomy skin incision is carried 2–3 inches below the xiphoid. Median sternotomy is performed through this incision by slightly mobilizing the subcutaneous fat in the upper portion of the wound away from the pectoralis muscle while an assistant retracts it superiorly, and by proceeding from bottom to top of the sternum with the saw. Meticulous hemostasis is ensured at all stages (unless the patient is acutely ischemic or hemodynamically unstable), as this prevents continuous oozing during the remainder of the operation, minimizes the use of the cardiotomy suction with its potential detrimental effects, prevents consumptive coagulopathy, and saves time before closure. Our preference is to open the pericardium before harvesting the ITAs, as this does not lengthen the procedure and allows for digital assessment of the aorta and performance of epiaortic scanning early in the operation (with the planning of alternate cannulation sites and no-touch Y-arterial grafting if aortic disease is discovered). Epiaortic scanning is a useful adjunct during CABG and may detect ascending aortic atherosclerosis in up to 30% of patients.[100,273] If epiaortic scanning is not available, routine preoperative carotid screening, intraoperative transesophageal echocardiography, and a tailored approach to revascularization that includes the use of alternate cannulation sites, fibrillatory arrest, and off-pump revascularization techniques are effective in minimizing the incidence of perioperative CVA. In a series of more than 6000 CABG patients in whom this approach was used, Trick et al reported a stroke incidence of less than 1% even in high-risk patients.[285]

The ITAs are harvested and transected distally only after intravenous heparin has been administered. There are two ways to perform this while minimizing bleeding during harvest of the second ITA: either a partial dose of heparin (e.g., 10,000 units) is given at completion and prior to transaction of the first ITA (with the remainder of the full heparin dose being administered prior to transaction of the second ITA), or both ITAs are transected at the same time after the second ITA has been harvested and the full dose of heparin given.

Cardiopulmonary Bypass and Cardioplegia

CPB is established with ascending aortic cannulation and placement of a single venous cannula, and carried out under mild hypothermia (32–34° C). Venting is performed via the proximal ascending aorta by using the antegrade cardioplegia delivery catheter, at a site that may later be used for a proximal anastomosis. Antegrade intermittent cold blood cardioplegia provides adequate myocardial protection for the majority of primary revascularization cases; consideration is given to the combination of antegrade and retrograde routes in severely ischemic patients or in those with an obstructed or severely stenotic LAD.[229] Topical cooling makes little or no difference in myocardial temperature and outcome when combined with antegrade cold blood cardioplegia, and may actually result in an increased incidence of hemidiaphragmatic paresis and pleural effusions postoperatively.[216,281]

Intraoperative transcranial Doppler scanning of the middle cerebral arteries, if available, is a useful adjunct for CPB cases and has in our experience helped design modifications in cannulation, perfusion, clamping, and venting techniques that have minimized the number of high-intensity transient cerebral signals.[239,268] Use of the cardiotomy suction is best avoided since it may result in clotting activation, micelle formation, and microembolism during CPB, and is adequately replaced by the use of a cell-saver device for routine cases. Moderate hypothermia and slow rewarming as well as meticulous control of blood glucose levels may also help decrease the incidence of postoperative neurocognitive deficits.[215,216]

Special Situations

Diffuse Aortic Disease

One of the most formidable obstacles that can be encountered during CABG is diffuse disease of the aorta and its branches. Mills and Everson described three types of aortic pathology, depicted in Figure 82-4.[199] Regardless of the type present, manipulation of a diseased aortic segment may lead to embolization and aortic disease constitutes the most important risk factor for stroke after CABG.[236] If the disease is focal and does not involve the distal third of the ascending aorta, the area can usually be avoided during cannulation, clamping, and construction of proximal anastomoses under single cross-clamping. Multifocal disease, diffuse disease, or disease involving the distal third of the ascending aorta, however, traditionally mandated the use of femoral or axillary artery cannulation, the relocation of proximal anastomoses to the proximal ascending aorta, brachiocephalic artery, or descending aorta, the use of hypothermic fibrillation or hypothermic circulatory arrest, and in some cases ascending aortic replacement. Fortunately, off-pump and Y-grafting techniques have widened the management options for patients with diffuse aortic disease. In most cases an off-pump aortic no-touch CABG operation with bilateral *in situ* ITAs or Y/T-arterial graft configuration can be performed with acceptably low risk, provided the patient is hemodynamically stable and not acutely ischemic.[211,284,298] If refractory hemodynamic instability develops, the patient may be managed with cannulation of the axillary or femoral artery,[244] establishment of CPB, hypothermic fibrillatory arrest during performance of distal anastomoses, and construction of the proximal anastomoses to the innominate artery or to a disease-free area of the ascending aorta during a short period of hypothermic circulatory arrest.[169]

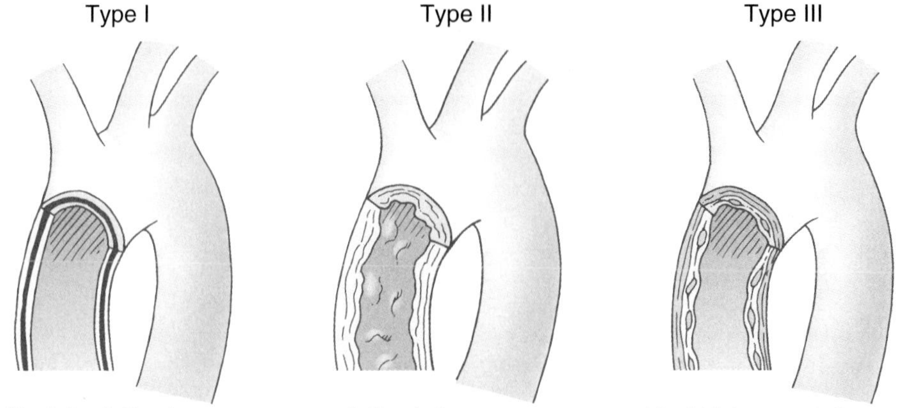

Figure 82–4 Patterns of diffuse ascending aortic atherosclerosis, described by Mills and Everson.[199] Type I: Circumferential medial calcification, known as "porcelain aorta." This type is the easiest to recognize clinically, either by the presence of aortic calcification on the coronary angiogram, computed tomography, or chest X–ray, or by digital palpation at surgery. Type II: Diffuse intimal thickening with ragged and friable edges. This type of pathology may sometimes be identified on angiography during root visualization by noting irregularities of the aortic lining. Visual and digital examination of the aorta at surgery is often normal. Type III: Intramural liquid debris constitutes the most difficult type of aortic pathology to detect, and may be missed even on transesophageal echocardiography.

Preoperative Cardiogenic Shock

Preoperative cardiogenic shock requires the immediate establishment of CPB, via either a femoral approach or sternotomy depending on patient characteristics (such as a history of previous aortobifemoral grafting) and individual surgeon preferences.[204] If time and hemodynamics allow, patients may benefit from insertion of an intraaortic balloon pump preoperatively.[83] Combined antegrade/retrograde cardioplegia delivery with warm induction and warm reperfusion techniques is indicated in these patients. Although consideration is given to the use of one ITA graft if the patient is relatively stable, the use of an all-saphenous vein operation is appropriate in most cases because of the high immediate myocardial demands and anticipated need for inotropes postoperatively.[263] Emergency revascularization entails the performance of at least one graft to each ischemic myocardial territory.

Medication-Related Coagulation Impairment

Whether the use of aprotinin or antifibrinolytics is beneficial during routine CABG cases remains controversial. Aprotonin is, however, indicated in patients with known coagulation impairment, such as resulting from the recent administration of thrombolytics or the use of clopidogrel.[74,132] Transfusion of platelets, fresh-frozen plasma, and cryoprecipitate may also be needed in these patients. Patients on abciximab may benefit from the routine administration of a single platelet transfusion after protamine administration, which may decrease the rate of reexploration for bleeding.[166,170]

Use of the reversible glycoprotein IIb/IIIa inhibitor eptifibatide before CABG may in fact be beneficial. In one large randomized study, the preoperative administration of eptifibatide versus placebo was associated with no adverse clinical effects, significantly decreased the incidence of perioperative MI, and resulted in higher platelet counts after CPB possibly because of a platelet-sparing effect.[68] Furthermore, these benefits persisted at 6-month follow-up in non-ST elevation MI patients operated emergently, with a significant reduction in MI rates and mortality in eptifibatide-treated patients.[189]

Previous Tracheostomy

The presence of a tracheal stoma in patients with previous total laryngectomy who require CABG is associated with an increased risk of wound complications, mediastinitis, tracheal injury, or stoma necrosis when a full sternotomy is used. In these patients, a manubrium-sparing sternotomy may be used, where the upper edge of the sternotomy does not extend beyond the top of the third rib. Slow progressive opening of the retractor allows for the operation to be conducted successfully while minimizing the possibility of manubrial fracture, bleeding, and patient discomfort.[234] An alternative approach is to incise the sternum transversely at the second intercostal space and complete the median sternotomy longitudinally down to the xiphoid process.[165]

Distal Anastomoses

Construction of distal coronary anastomoses begins after the first dose of cardioplegia has been delivered. With current methods of myocardial protection and the increased prevalence of diffuse CAD in CABG patients, there is little justification in performing proximal anastomoses first during on-pump CABG. Proximal anastomoses are constructed either sequentially (i.e., each distal followed by its proximal under single cross-clamping) or all at once after completion of distal anastomoses. One exception to this approach is during arterial Y- or T-grafting, where the surgeon may complete all proximal conduit anastomoses onto one to two pedicled ITAs prior to the establishment of CPB. This strategy minimizes unnecessary CPB time and allows for assessment of free flow in each ramus of the configuration prior to distal grafting.

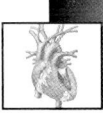

Although the order of revascularization is not of critical importance during on-pump CABG, the first graft performed is usually to the inferior circulation, followed by the lateral wall, the diagonal system, and the left anterior descending artery. Vessels that are completely occluded and for which a free graft is planned may benefit from construction of the distal anastomosis earlier in the revascularization sequence in order to directly deliver cardioplegia to the subtended myocardium.

Many conduit–graft configurations are possible, and these are planned on a case-by-case basis. The *in situ* LITA is usually grafted to the LAD, although the *in situ* RITA can also be used with success on the LAD and placed in the superior mediastinum to decrease the risk of injury during subsequent resternotomy.[167] The next best conduits (i.e., the second ITA, followed by the radial and saphenous vein[s]) are kept for other vessels according to their decreasing order of "importance." Poorly graftable coronary arteries do not necessarily only deserve a vein graft, as the short- and long-term patency of an ITA or radial graft to a diffusely stenotic vessel may be better than a vein. Conduit length problems are almost always solved by the use of arterial Y-grafting techniques, which should, however, be avoided with saphenous veins as differences in vein size and subsequent intimal hyperplasia formation may result in unpredictable flow patterns.

Exposure of the coronary branches is not problematic during on-pump CABG. The inferior wall may be exposed by packing a small sponge against the inferior vena cava at the right inferior aspect of the oblique sinus. The lateral wall may be exposed by gently twisting and folding the heart upon itself in the long axis and placing a sponge underneath to expose the marginal branches. The anterior wall is usually exposed with a single sponge placed under the left ventricle.

The most proximal disease-free portion of the coronary artery to be grafted (i.e., immediately after the most distal disease involvement) is selected for the anastomosis.[117] The epicardium is incised over the area of the coronary artery with a No. 15 blade or a special rounded blade.[152] The anterior surface of the artery is cleared by gentle transverse brushing with the scalpel. Even with cardioplegia, careful inspection of the artery will reveal a thin central line that is red or translucent, indicating the lumen. The anterior wall of the artery is opened longitudinally over this line by caressing gently with the scalpel so as to not damage the posterior wall. Administration of a small amount of cardioplegia to distend the coronary artery lumen may be used during this step, especially for small (1 mm or less) vessels. Occasionally, when the anterior wall of the artery cannot be placed under proper tension, it may be opened by stabbing it with a sharp-pointed scalpel. The blade must enter the artery obliquely and superficially, so as not to penetrate the back wall. The incision is enlarged with angled scissors to a length of 4–6 mm for end-to-side anastomoses and 3–5 mm for side-to-side anastomoses. The epicardial incision is extended beyond each angle of the arteriotomy to facilitate the anastomosis. The artery may be sized and proximal and distal patency assessed by passing measuring probes into it. Aortic root venting is used only as necessary so as not to introduce an excessive amount of air into the ascending aorta. The distal end of the conduit is incised longitudinally approximately 20% longer than the coronary arteriotomy; this, in conjunction with a slightly more distant spacing of suture bites on the conduit than on the coronary artery, creates the desired "cobra head" appearance (Figure 82-5).

Many anastomotic techniques exist, each with their advantages and disadvantages. For the sake of reliability under all circumstances, surgeons should probably focus on one main anastomotic technique that can be perfectly mastered and used for all conduit types, for end-to-side as well as side-to-side anastomoses, and during on-pump as well as off-pump CABG. General principles include the use of 7-0 or 8-0 polypropylene, the use of a no-touch technique in which the intima of the coronary and of the conduit are never grabbed, and compulsive attention to the geometric distribution of sutures as the anastomosis is performed, because an otherwise adequate but deformed anastomosis may be prone to thrombosis. Another more important point is that no impediment to native coronary flow should result from an anastomosis, therefore mandating flawless patency at both anastomotic angles such that if for some reason the conduit itself was to become nonfunctional, native coronary flow would potentially be the same as if a bypass graft had not been performed on this coronary artery.

Some surgeons prefer to use sequential grafts within a single coronary distribution only (e.g., for two marginal branches of the circumflex system) to avoid potential flow diversion from one myocardial territory to another. Other groups have

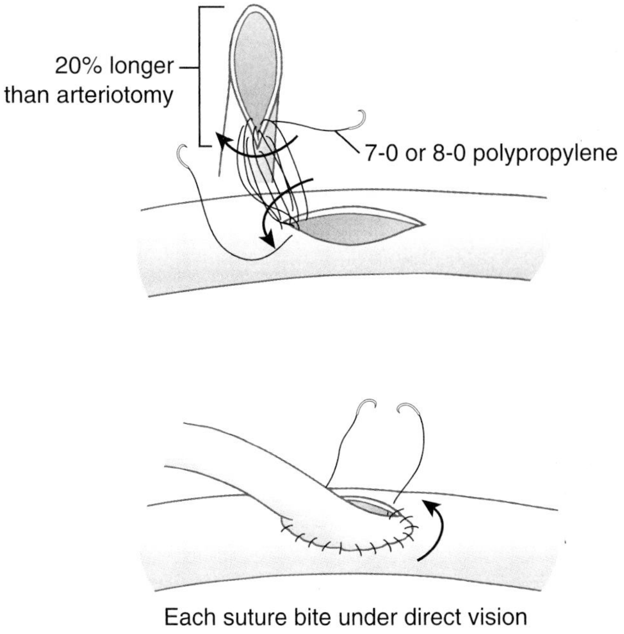

Figure 82–5 Technique of distal coronary anastomosis. An open anastomotic technique involving small suture bites taken under direct vision and where constant attention is given to the geometry of the anastomosis is desirable. Arrows indicate the direction of suture bites.

reported good results using a T-graft configuration that may bridge two or even three myocardial territories.[36,298] However, others feel that a separate graft to each artery lessens the chance of kinking and misjudgment of graft length and optimize long-term patency. This remains to be demonstrated. In general, sequential grafts allow for a greater number of arterial anastomoses and with vein grafts may actually contribute to an increased long-term patency.[36,294] Transverse sequential side-to-side anastomoses may be used for saphenous vein grafts, but are relatively contraindicated with arterial grafts. For the latter, a longitudinal or circular side opening created with a 2.7-mm punch may be used.[187] Perfect orientation of the sequential arterial anastomoses with respect to one another and avoidance of tension or excessive redundancy on the conduit are crucial. Because of the potential to jeopardize revascularization to two or more vessels, any sequential graft that appears technically unsatisfactory is best redone and replaced with individual grafts.

Coronary Endarterectomy

Coronary endarterectomy is a technique that preceded the invention of CABG.[172] It is now reserved for select cases of severe diffuse disease when no anastomotic site can be found on a coronary artery that supplies an ischemic and viable myocardial territory.[242] The use of coronary endarterectomy is exceptional when extreme care is given at the preoperative planning and intraoperative selection of target anastomotic sites. The procedure should not be used because of failure to find the true lumen as may occur when a diffusely diseased coronary artery is mistakenly incised laterally through a plaque. Arteries that are seen on coronary angiography do have a lumen, which can usually be found despite poor target site selection and extraluminal cutting into a plaque, by carefully extending the incision proximally and distally into the true lumen and performing a patch angioplasty by using the conduit as an onlay patch.[19] Endarterectomy should be used only on vessels with high-grade stenoses (>80%); vessels with a lesser degree of stenosis provide significant coronary flow and a massive myocardial infarction may ensue if the endarterectomized vessel thromboses. Endarterectomy is combined in most cases with a patch angioplasty of the endarterectomized vessel and a bypass graft. A possible exception may be when the vessel can be adequately endarterectomized through a small arteriotomy. When used in carefully selected situations, coronary endarterectomy is associated with a rate of perioperative myocardial infarction of 5% or less, a graft–coronary axis patency of 72% at 30 months, and a good functional outcome.[188,242] Although perioperative use of aprotinin has been linked to an increased incidence of coronary thrombosis in endarterectomized coronary segments,[107] a subsequent study found the use of tranexamic acid to be safe in coronary endarterectomy patients.[242]

Sutureless Distal Coronary Connectors

Significant advances have been made in the development of automated coronary connectors and self-closing U-clip distal anastomotic devices. Preliminary reports on the use of these devices in humans demonstrated geometrically adequate anastomoses, excellent immediate graft flows, and good patency at 3- and 6-month angiographic follow-up.[72,224]

Proximal Anastomoses

Most proximal anastomoses are constructed onto the ascending aorta, although alternative sites such as the brachiocephalic artery, axillary artery, and descending aorta can be used in special situations. Y- and T-grafting involves constructing the inflow anastomosis of a free arterial graft to an *in situ* arterial conduit, using either an end-to-side or a side-to-side configuration. General principles of proximal anastomosis construction include the ensurance of a perfect graft lie (i.e., without torsion, tension, or excessive redundancy) and the minimization of aortic manipulations.

Although personal preferences vary, the use of a side-biting tangential clamp is best avoided because of its association with increased cerebral microembolic load during CABG.[55] In our experience, however, several techniques can be used to reduce this embolic load to levels equal or below that of single aortic cross-clamp techniques. These consist of (1) using tangential side-biting clamps only in the presence of a nondiseased ascending aorta, (2) releasing the cross-clamp and applying the side clamp while the pump is momentarily stopped, (3) irrigating and suctioning the inside of the aorta after the punch holes are made, (4) displacing air prior to tying the last proximal anastomosis by saline instillation or by removal of the bulldog clamp on one of the free arterial grafts to backfill the aorta with blood, and (5) releasing the tangential clamp while the pump is momentarily stopped.

For a proximal anastomosis to be performed, a longitudinal slit, approximately 3 mm in length, is made with a No. 11 blade at the chosen sites on the aorta.[152] A punch of either 4.0 (for free arterial grafts) or 4.4 mm (for saphenous vein grafts) in diameter is slipped completely and freely through each slit and closed so as to punch out a circular piece of aorta at each site. Each conduit is irrigated intraluminally, and its orientation is determined under direct vision, measured so as to not prove too short or long once the heart fills (using the pericardium as a guide or pinching the venous line to fill the right heart is useful in evaluating this), occluded with a light bulldog clamp, spatulated at its proximal end and anastomosed to the aorta using 6-0 polypropylene. If an arterial conduit appears too short it is either anastomosed in an end-to-end fashion to a short segment of saphenous vein itself anastomosed to the aorta, or anastomosed side-to-side as a Y-graft onto another arterial graft.

Sutureless Proximal Coronary Connectors

Commercially available automated proximal aortic connectors have been used successfully by several groups with good patency rates (Figure 82-6).[71,73,75] Advantages of these connectors include the avoidance of aortic manipulations except at the anastomotic site and ease of use, especially for off-pump or robotic-assisted procedures. However, there have been reports of an increased incidence of proximal anastomotic vein stenosis when these devices are used.

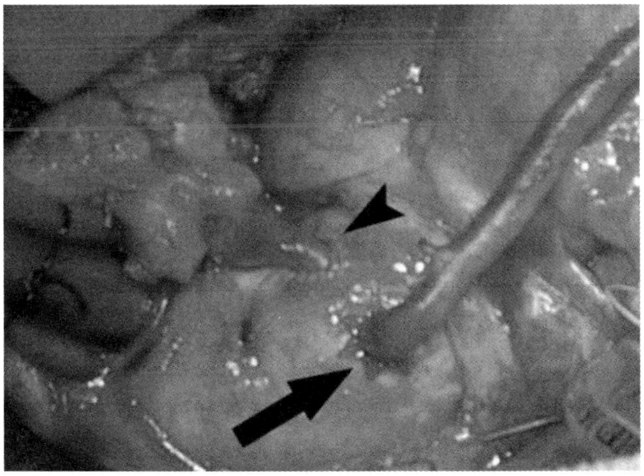

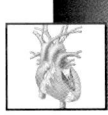

Figure 82–6 **Proximal anastomosis of a saphenous graft to the right coronary artery, constructed in a clampless fashion with an automated proximal aortic connector *(arrow)*.** A conventional, hand–sewn anastomosis of a right internal thoracic artery graft to the circumflex system is seen above and to the left *(arrowhead)*.
(Photo courtesy of Terrence M. Yau, MD, Division of Cardiac Surgery, Toronto General Hospital.)

Intraoperative Graft Assessment

The higher prevalence of small and diffusely diseased target vessels in CABG patients and the increasingly challenging surgical techniques used today (such as complex arterial grafting and off-pump procedures) may justify routine graft validation in the operating room (Table 82-3). Unfortunately, the gold standard of intraoperative angiography remains cumbersome and invasive, and entails additional risks when used in the intraoperative setting. One subjective method of assessment is to gently probe each anastomosis at critical points during construction to ensure proximal, distal, and conduit patency, and rule out a pursestring effect that may go unrecognized if too large or too few bites are taken around the anastomosis, if its geometric configuration is not perfect, or if the assistant pulls excessively on the suture when "following."

The most widely used modality of objective graft assessment is transit-time flow measurement (TTFM). With this tool, a diastolic-to-systolic perfusion pattern of at least 2:1 for grafts constructed to vessels on the left ventricle (such as the LAD and circumflex branches) is a good predictor of patency, but low absolute flow values can represent false positives that result from arterial spasm without anastomotic error.[54,259] TTFM is also imperfect in detecting less than critical stenosis, regardless of the use of spectral or fast Fourier transformation analysis.[155,278] Alternative modalities such as high-frequency epicardial echocardiography and power Doppler imaging have been described, but experience is limited.[270] Thermal imaging has poor image resolution and is largely unsuitable for off-pump or minimally invasive surgery.[202] Another approach is to use postoperative or intraoperative transesophageal echocardiography to assess regional wall motion when EKG changes suggest possible graft stenosis or thrombosis. When a new wall motion abnormality presents, coronary angiography may be

Table 82–3

Modalities of Intraoperative Graft Assessment during CABG

Modality	*Advantages*	*Disadvantages*
Antegrade, retrograde, and conduit probing during anastomotic construction	Simple and quick; allow for good lumen visualization at anastomotic angles	Subjective and unreliable; potentially damaging to the coronary endothelium; may cause embolization; does not prevent a purse-string effect during tying; cannot be done once the anastomosis is completed
Intraoperative angiography	Gold standard method; best anatomical accuracy	Invasive; special operating room bed and large cumbersome equipment required; risks of renal toxicity, embolization, and hematoma formation; experienced operator needed; anatomical modality
Transit time flow measurements	Simple, readily available, risk free; a physiological measurement	Low sensitivity to less than severe graft stenosis or occlusion; false positives if native coronary flow competition; interpretation difficult with sequential grafts
Fluorescent imaging	Noninvasive; simple to use; less cumbersome than angiography; good for sequential grafts	Imperfect anastomotic resolution; must retract heart to image posterior and inferior walls; primarily anatomic modality

indicated to assess graft patency even in the absence of hemodynamic instability.

Intraoperative fluorescent cardiac imaging is on alternative to TTFM that may prove clinically useful.[240] This modality uses a 0.5-ml injection of indocyanine green (ICG) and a portable imaging device to visualize coronary anatomy and grafts during conventional CABG, OP-CAB, or MIDCAB (Figure 82-7). Graft and coronary visualization is excellent, but anastomotic resolution is imperfect and overlying fat or muscle can obscure the penetration and detection of ICG fluorescence. The modality works best with skeletonized arterial grafts and saphenous vein grafts.

Weaning from Cardiopulmonary Bypass

Once the proximal anastomoses are completed, each vein graft is deaired with a #27-gauge needle prior to release of the bulldog clamp. Graft conduits are examined for adequateness of lie and hemostasis at each anastomotic site and side branch, while the mean arterial pressure is increased to >70 mm Hg. Distal anastomotic jet bleeding is repaired with a single stitch of 7-0 Prolene; if the toe or heel is involved, repair may compromise the anastomosis and consideration should be given to redoing it. It is often preferable to spend 10–15 min redoing an anastomosis that has a significant leak at or near the angle than to repair it with a potential for distortion or occlusion. The epicardium may be used to cover and repair small lateral anastomotic leaks but should not be used near an anastomotic angle.

Preparation of the patient for weaning from CPB involves a routine but thorough assessment of the cardiac, pulmonary, and metabolic systems (Table 82-4). The chosen temperature for weaning, a point of controversy, is reached by rewarming the patient.[215,216] Hematocrit level and metabolic and electrolyte balance are checked and corrected as necessary. The trachea is suctioned and the lungs are reexpanded by hand under direct vision and mechanically ventilated with 100% O_2. Respiratory monitors and alarms are reactivated. The pleural spaces are checked for the presence of fluid or pneumothorax. Atrial and ventricular epicardial pacing wires are affixed onto the heart and exteriorized on the chest, and heart rhythm and rate are optimized by using synchronized cardioversion or pacing as necessary. Sinus rhythm or atrial pacing at 75–95 beats/min is ideal for weaning, although patients with significant diastolic dysfunction from left ventricular hypertrophy or with incomplete revascularization benefit from a slower atrial rate in conjunction with a slightly prolonged atrioventricular interval. The ECG is examined for ST-segment changes suggestive of ischemia and if present consideration is given to reassessment and reconstruction of one or several grafts.

The perfusionist progressively clamps the venous line to provide preload to the ejecting right ventricle, which in turn results in left ventricular preload. Afterload is managed by the anesthesiologist by using either an α-agonist agent such as phenylephrine or in some cases a direct vasodilator such as nitroprusside. Contractility is assessed by observing right ventricular contraction and the evolution of pulmonary arterial pressures during the weaning process, which are reflective of left ventricular function (except in cases of pulmonary vascular hypertension or isolated right ventricular dysfunction).

The following procedures are carried out when weaning is difficult. First, each of the above steps is rechecked and corrected as necessary while CPB support is reestablished and a period of reperfusion on the empty beating heart is reinitiated. Second, consideration is given to ischemia or intracoronary air and grafts are objectively reassessed. Third, inotropic support and intraaortic balloon pump (IAPB) are used as necessary. Inotropic and IABP use in nonemergency patients with good left ventricular function preoperatively is abnormal and warrants questioning the adequacy of revascularization (i.e., nonfunctional grafts, plaque or cholesterol embolism during the construction of an anastomosis, grafting of the wrong coronary vessels or of a coronary vein, etc.), and may justify redoing or adding one or several grafts. Further attempts at weaning from CPB are taken after exhausting the above possibilities. If weaning is still unsuccessful after many attempts and clearly related to poor contractility, consideration is given to the use of extracorporeal membrane oxygenation or mechanical ventricular support as a bridge to recovery.

Once the patient is satisfactorily weaned from CPB, the venous cannula is removed and the atrial pursestring suture is snared. The scrub nurse sumps the venous line blood back to the perfusionist by using saline. The aortic line is checked for air that may have migrated up during cardiac ejection and the perfusionist transfuses aliquots of remaining pump blood according to the directives of the surgeon and anesthesiologist. Excessive right ventricular distention and pulmonary artery diastolic pressures of more than 22–25 mm Hg are avoided. If these develop and mean arterial pressure is satisfactory, IV nitroglycerine is used as a preload reducer and pulmonary venodilator.

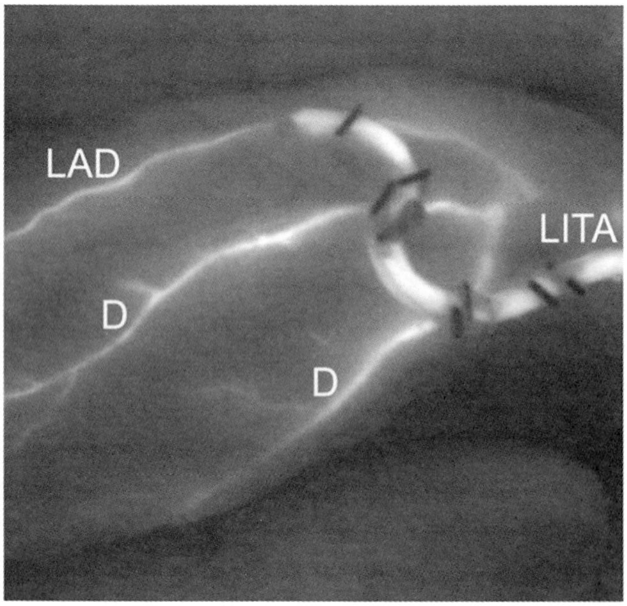

Figure 82-7 Intraoperative graft assessment using fluorescent imaging. After injection of 0.5 ml of indocyanine green and by using a low-intensity laser, visualization is obtained of a skeletonized double-sequential left internal thoracic graft (LITA) to each of two diagonal branches (D) and to the left anterior descending artery (LAD).

(Photo courtesy of Antonio M. Calafiore, MD, Department of Cardiac Surgery, G. D'Annunzio University, Chieti, Italy.)

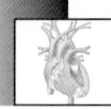

Table 82–4

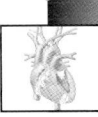

Problems during Weaning from Cardiopulmonary Bypass

Problems	*Presentation*	*Treatment*
Rate and rhythm	Ventricular arrhythmias	Defibrillate if temperature >30° C; correct K^+, Mg^{2+} deficits; rule out ischemia; consider lidocaine and amiodarone
	Atrial arrhythmias	Perform synchronized cardioversion; correct K^+, Mg^{2+} deficits; use overdrive atrial pacing; give amiodarone for treatment and prophylaxis; give calcium channel blockers or digoxin for rate control; if sinus tachycardia rule out hypercarbia, inadequate anesthesia, or ischemia
	Slow sinus or junctional rhythm; atrioventricular block	Use atrial or atrioventricular pacing at 76 to 95 beats/min if slow or atrioventricular block (if ischemia or diastolic dysfunction choose lower rate with longer AV interval; if limited stroke volume or systolic dysfunction choose higher rate)
Arterial blood pressure	Low afterload	Increase preload; use α-agonist agents: phenylephrine, noradrenaline, epinephrine, or dopamine (>5 μg/kg/min)
	High afterload	Use vasodilators (nitroprusside, nitroglycerine); deepen anesthesia; rewarm patient to 37° C
	Poor contractility; elevated pulmonary artery diastolic pressures; new onset ECG changes	Rule out persistent air, kinks, or forgotten clamps on grafts; reperfuse on CPB and rewarm patient to 37° C; optimize hematocrit (20–25%), oxygenation, preload, and coronary perfusion pressure; assess regional contractility with transesophageal echocardiography; correct acidosis and K^+; consider graft revision if ischemia is suspected; give inotropic support if no correctable cause is identified (use milrinone over catecholamines if ischemia or arrhythmias); insert IABP if ischemia persists despite confirmation of functional grafts
Oxygenation	Low oxygen saturation readings	Confirm probe readings with arterial blood gases; lavage and suction trachea; suction gastric tube; use 100% oxygen; give bronchodilators; inspect lungs for residual atelectasis; check pleural spaces for fluid and pneumothorax; consider the need for PEEP; rule out low cardiac output as a cause

AV, atrioventricular; CPB, cardiopulmonary bypass; IABP, intraaortic balloon pump; PEEP, positive end-expiratory pressure; ECG, electrocardiogram.

Protamine is administered once stable hemodynamics have been achieved and reestablishment of CPB appears unlikely. Chest tubes are inserted in the posterior pericardium, anterior mediastinum, and each pleural cavity that has been opened. Care is taken to ensure that chest tubes do not lie in proximity to a graft once the chest is closed; not only could they mechanically compress the graft and lead to distortion and thrombosis, but they may also damage the graft if entrapped into a side-hole of the tube.

The aortic cannula is removed after the first dose of protamine has been administered without untoward hemodynamic consequences. The purse-string sutures are securely tied and reinforced with 4-0 polypropylene pledgeted sutures as needed. Hemostasis is checked at each anastomotic site, along each conduit, at each cannulation site, and on the chest wall. If blood accumulation is still noted in the pericardium the left atrial appendage is examined, as it may have been damaged by the cardiotomy suction during CPB. Radioopaque markers are left around proximal vein graft anastomoses.[227] The pericardium is partially reapproximated over the anterior left ventricle but not closed to avoid adverse hemodynamic effects.[232] Routine closure of the sternotomy incision completes the operation.

SPECIAL FEATURES OF POSTOPERATIVE CARE

Early Postoperative Period

Patients with a radial, gastroepiploic, or inferior epigastric artery graft are started on intravenous nitroglycerin as soon as blood pressure parameters allow. Nitroglycerin has been shown to be more effective, cheaper, and safer (with a decreased incidence of bradycardia and negative inotropy) than intravenous diltiazem.[257,258] Nitroprusside is not used in patients with decreased creatinine clearance or intrapulmonary shunt. Aspirin 650 mg is given orally or via suppository within 6–24 h of operation and subsequently by mouth at a dose of 325 mg/day.[32,105,184] Most patients can be extubated within 4–6 h of CABG and discharged from the intensive care unit on the following morning.[226] Chest tubes are removed when draining less than 100 ml per 12 h if the chest X-ray shows no residual effusion. Most patients experience relatively little postoperative pain, which is managed initially with intravenous morphine and subsequently with oral codeine or hydromorphone. A short course of nonsteroidal antiinflammatory drugs combined with misoprostol is added as an adjuvant in patients with normal renal function, and without a history of peptic ulcer or CHF. β-Blockers and other antihypertensive medications are restarted at half-dose on the morning following the operation and progressively titrated back to the preoperative dose prior to hospital discharge. Patients with moderate left ventricular dysfunction (ejection fraction [EF] between 0.30 and 0.50) and normal renal function are started on enalapril or another ACE inhibitor.[154] Patients with radial or gastro-epiploic grafts should be placed on oral long-acting nitrates or on daily amlodipine, which is more effective than diltiazem and more specific than nifedipine in preventing arterial spasm.[26,35] Atrial fibrillation prophylaxis varies according to personal preferences; our approach consists in maximizing the use of β-blockers early postoperatively. Prophylactic regimens based on the administration of sotalol or amiodarone have been shown to be useful, but may not be cost-effective.* Discharge home occurs at a median of 5 days postoperatively and in some patients as early as the third postoperative day.

Late Postoperative Period

During the first 3–4 weeks after CABG, patients commonly have a poor appetite, insomnia, tiredness, lack of sexual desire, and a depressed mood. These phenomena are related to the postoperative state and are transient for the vast majority; reassurance from the surgeon is often all that is needed. Patients are encouraged to walk progressively more during their convalescence; from a minimum distance of 120 m when discharged from the hospital, patients should progressively increase their daily walking routine to 1 h or more by the end of the first postoperative month. Lifting is limited to 5 kg during the first postoperative month, which is increased to 10 kg during the second month. Some surgeons restrict lifting to 30 kg or less up to 6 months after the operation, whereas others remove limitations 2–3 months after operation. Structured cardiac rehabilitation programs are a useful adjunct, and patients are encouraged to join as soon as discharged from the hospital. Patients who have a normal convalescence can usually resume driving within 3 weeks of operation and return to work within 1–3 months. Patients who have a special occupation where recurrent cardiac events could put the lives of others at risk (such as bus drivers) must undergo noninvasive cardiac testing to rule out ischemia prior to resuming work.

CABG represents only one of many treatment interventions for patients with CAD, as coronary disease continues to progress. Aggressive secondary prevention is therefore essential: aspirin must be continued, smoking must never resume, second-hand smoke must be avoided, exercise must be encouraged, obesity must be addressed if present, the lipid profile optimized, and hypertension and diabetes strictly controlled. These factors have significant effect on the progression of saphenous vein graft atherosclerosis, and may also benefit arterial grafts.[38,65] Chronic oral anticoagulation with warfarin has no effect on long-term graft patency.

β-Blockers are progressively weaned 6 months following uncomplicated CABG in patients who have no arrhythmias, no angina, normal ventricular function, and in whom other medications are used for antihypertensive therapy. Amlodipine is discontinued after 1 year in patients with radial or gastroepiploic grafts.[175] Patients with moderate left ventricular dysfunction (EF between 0.30 and 0.50) and stable renal function are kept on enalapril or another ACE inhibitor indefinitely, as this may be associated with a reduced incidence of cardiac death, acute myocardial infarction, and clinical heart failure.[154,223]

RESULTS

Morbidity

The most common complications of CABG are postoperative bleeding, low cardiac output syndrome, postoperative renal dysfunction, neurological events, atrial arrhythmias, and deep sternal wound infection. These complications are discussed subsequently.

Postoperative Bleeding and Transfusion

Predisposing factors for transfusion after CABG include advanced age, female gender, lower preoperative hematocrit, priority of operation, lower body weight, recent thrombolytic therapy, duration of CPB, and lack of institutional guidelines for postoperative transfusions.[70,86,146,241] The incidence of transfusion during primary on-pump CABG ranges from near zero to 50%, with most centers transfusing approximately 20% of patients undergoing CABG.[126,146] In addition to well-known infectious risks, a significant untoward consequence of blood transfusions is their immunosuppressive effect, as perioperative transfusions were in a retrospective study independently associated with wound and remote infections in 4% of patients who received ≤2 units of packed blood cells, 7% of those transfused with 3–5 units, and 22% of those who received 6 or more units.[209]

The rate of reexploration for bleeding after CABG was 2.0% or less in a study of 12,555 consecutive patients from the Northern New England Study Group.[208] Despite higher-risk patients, routine use of aspirin up to the time of operation,[132,184] and technically more complex arterial grafting procedures, the use of antifibrinolytics and improved surgical techniques have contributed to keeping the overall incidence of this complication low.[8,241] Reexploration is indicated if bleeding exceeds 400 ml in 1 h, 300 ml/h for 2 h or more, 200 ml/h for more than 4 h, or at any time if pericardial tamponade is suspected.

Perioperative Myocardial Infarction and Low Cardiac Output Syndrome

Perioperative myocardial infarction after CABG is defined differently among various institutions. In general, new Q waves after CABG are reliable indicators of perioperative myocardial infarction. In addition, several enzymatic release

*References 66, 81, 95, 164, 182, 228.

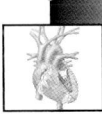

criteria involving creatine kinase MB fraction and troponin T or I have been used to define perioperative MI.[43,242,292] Underlying causes of perioperative MI may relate to incomplete or unsuccessful revascularization or inadequate myocardial protection. There is also an independent association between a hematocrit value on entry into the intensive care unit of 34% or more and an increased incidence of perioperative MI and LV dysfunction after CABG.[264] The rate of perioperative MI using both ECG and enzyme criteria at our institutions is less than 2%. In contrast to what was previously thought, the impact of enzyme-determined perioperative MI on survival is not negligible.[31,51] Brener et al,[31] in a study of nearly 4000 CABG patients, found that although mild to moderate elevation was not associated with a decreased midterm survival at 3 years, elevation above 10 times the upper limit value (encountered in 6% of their patients) was associated with a 30% decrease in survival at 3 years.

Low cardiac output syndrome is a clinical situation that may result from poor baseline ventricular function, inadequate myocardial protection, or perioperative ischemic injury. It is defined as the need for postoperative IABP or inotropic support for longer than 30 min in the intensive care unit to maintain the systolic blood pressure greater than 90 mm Hg and the cardiac index greater than 2.2 l/min/m^2.[231] Its incidence is 5–9% after CABG with a 17% mortality risk. Predictors include LVEF less than 0.20, emergency operation, female gender, diabetes, age older than 70 years, left main coronary artery stenosis, recent MI, and three-vessel disease.[231] Low cardiac output syndrome (LCOS) in the presence of ischemia requires an immediate and thorough assessment of potentially correctable causes, and consideration of immediate graft catheterization, PCI, or return to the operating room for CABG as indicated.[201] LCOS may require treatment with IABP and inotropic support, open chest management in some cases,[10] and consideration of left ventricular mechanical assistance if adrenaline requirements are higher than 0.5 μg/kg/min, left atrial pressure more than 15 mm Hg, urine output less than 100 ml/h, and mixed venous saturation less than 60% despite IABP support.[124]

Postoperative Renal Dysfunction

Postoperative renal dysfunction (PRD) after CABG is defined as a postoperative serum creatinine level of 177 μmol/l or more with a preoperative-to-postoperative increase of at least 62 μmol/l.[183] In a multicenter study of 2222 patients undergoing CABG, the incidence was 7.7%, with 1.4% overall requiring dialysis, and a mortality of 19% and 63%, respectively. Risk factors include age older than 70 years, CHF, type 1 diabetes, preoperative serum creatinine levels of 124–177 μmol/l, and CPB lasting 3 or more h. Most of these risk factors are nonmodifiable, but the use of off-pump CABG techniques may be associated with a lower incidence of PRD and complications in those with preexisting renal insufficiency.[14]

Neurological and Neurobehavioral Complications

Neurological derangement after CABG has been attributed to hypoxia, emboli, hemorrhage, and metabolic abnormalities, and has been subclassified into two types: type 1 deficits, which represent major focal neurological deficits, and type 2 deficits, which are characterized by deterioration of intellectual function or memory.[70] In one study involving 2108 CABG patients, the incidence of type 1 deficit was 3.1% and that of type 2 deficits was 3.0%.[236] A large registry found the incidence of type 1 deficit after CABG to be 1.4%, and the complication to be associated with a mortality of 25%.[141] Independent risk factors for both type 1 and type 2 deficits were age older than 70 years and hypertension. Type 1 alone was related to the presence of aortic atherosclerosis, a previous history of CVA, the presence of a carotid bruit, a history of hypertension, renal failure, smoking, diabetes mellitus, and the use of IABP.[141,194] Type 2 alone was related to a history of alcoholism, atrial fibrillation, peripheral vascular disease, CHF, and preoperative small cerebral infarctions on magnetic resonance imaging (MRI).[109,253] Aortic atherosclerosis was not a predictor of type 2 complications. Many controversies exist regarding the role of CPB in type 2 deficits after CABG.[274] After CABG most patients show some degree of cognitive decline across one or more domains tested,[193] but Taggart et al, in a small observational study, noted that the similar pattern of early decline and recovery of cognitive function at 3 months in patients undergoing CABG with and without CPB suggests that CPB may not be the major cause.[276] Ascione et al showed in a randomized study that there was no significant difference between the incidence of type 1 deficit in CABG versus OP-CAB patients.[15] Several groups are actively studying this controversial issue.

Atrial Arrhythmias

New-onset postoperative atrial fibrillation develops in approximately 20–40% of patients undergoing CABG, with the peak incidence on the second to third postoperative day.[95,99] It is associated with a 2- to 3-fold increase in the risk of postoperative stroke.[191] Predictors of postoperative atrial fibrillation include advanced age, prolonged cross-clamp time, COPD, and withdrawal of β-blockers. Patients who have had atrial fibrillation for 24 h or more should be anticoagulated with heparin prior to cardioversion. If atrial fibrillation persists, anticoagulation with warfarin is indicated.

Many prophylactic regimens for the prevention of atrial fibrillation have been examined in a randomized setting. Effective regimens include sotalol 80 mg twice daily for 9 days postoperatively (43% reduction),[228] intravenous amiodarone at a 150 mg bolus and 0.4 mg/kg/h maintenance dose for 3 days before and 5 days after operation (65% reduction),[164,182] restarting preoperative β-blocker therapy after CABG (55% reduction),[6] 4 days of biatrial pacing at a base rate of 80 bpm (65% reduction),[168] and sotalol 80 mg twice daily for 5 days in combination with magnesium supplementation 1.5 g daily for 6 days starting in the operating room just before CPB (95% reduction).[95] Intravenous magnesium 3 g daily for 4 days or intravenous diltiazem 0.1 mg/kg/h for 4 days was not found to be effective.[17,144]

Deep Sternal Wound Infection

Mediastinitis and deep sternal wound infection occur in 0.7–2.4% of patients after CABG and carries a mortality of nearly 15%.* Risk factors include use of pedicled

*References 28, 175, 192, 195, 235, 265.

bilateral ITAs in diabetic patients (which is associated with an incidence of more than 14%), obesity, diabetes, male sex, and advanced age. Control of preoperative[285] and perioperative glucose levels has been shown to reduce the incidence of postoperative deep sternal wound infection.[119,303] Its incidence can also be reduced by clipping rather than shaving the skin preoperatively,[5] by administering intravenous antibiotics before the skin incision,[44] by keeping perfusion and operative times to a minimum,[218] by avoiding the excessive use of electrocautery,[218] by using meticulous aseptic technique, and by favoring the use of skeletonized over pedicled ITAs in diabetic patients.[192] If deep sternal wound infection develops, aggressive surgical débridement and early vascularized muscle flap coverage are indicated in most patients and have a higher success rate than the combination of exploration, rewiring, and drainage.[230]

Mortality

The overall operative mortality of CABG (defined as all in-hospital deaths and all out-of-hospital deaths occurring within 30 days of the procedure) across North American centers that are part of the Society of Surgeons database is 3.0%, an improvement since 1990 despite an increase in the mean age of patients (65.1 years), the mean priority status, and the prevalence of comorbid conditions.[85] This figure is in accordance with that reported in several other studies.[12,80,104,136,206] In the 19,016 patients of the Northern New England Cardiovascular Disease Study Group who received an LITA during CABG, the overall 30-day mortality was 2.4%.[162]

A 30-day mortality of 1% or less can be predicted in patients undergoing elective CABG who are younger than 65 years of age and who have no severe LV dysfunction or CHF.[70] Risk factors for 30-day mortality include a high priority of operation, advanced age, female gender, diabetes mellitus, poor left ventricular function (especially in the presence of CHF symptoms),[12] high creatinine level, peripheral vascular disease, pulmonary disease, and left main coronary artery disease. Emergent CABG for extreme hemodynamic instability secondary to refractory ischemia has a mortality of nearly 30%, for which the nonuse of blood cardioplegia may constitute an independent risk factor.[283]

Long-term survival of patients after CABG may depend on the baseline characteristics of the population studied, on the geographic location of the cohort,[63] and on the surgical era, with the potential impact of secondary prevention and arterial revascularization techniques. Most long-term data, however, examined patients operated in the 1970s and 1980s. Kirklin et al reported that survival after CABG was 92% at 5 years and 81% at 10 years.[151] Long-term vital data of patients enrolled in the CASS registry (who were operated on between 1974 and 1979) have shown that survival after CABG in all comers is 96% at 1 year, 90% at 5 years, 74% at 10 years, and 56% at 15 years.[210] A surprising finding of this study, in which arterial grafts were used in only 13% of patients, is that the survival of patients 65–70 years or older exceeded that of a matched U.S. population.

Although elderly patients are at a higher risk of morbidity and stroke after CABG,[197] the benefits of CABG versus medical therapy in elderly patients were demonstrated in the APPROACH registry, a large clinical data collection and outcome monitoring initiative that captured all patients undergoing cardiac catheterization and revascularization in the province of Alberta, Canada between 1995 and 2000.[113] In 15,392 patients younger than 70 years of age examined in this registry, 4-year adjusted actuarial survival rates for CABG, PCI, and medical therapy were 95.0%, 93.8%, and 90.5%, respectively. Survival decreased to 87.3%, 83.9%, and 79.1% for patients 70–79 years of age after CABG, PCI, and medical therapy, respectively, and to 77.4%, 71.6%, and 60.3% for patients 80 years of age or older. CABG patients fared better than those who received PCI or medical therapy in all age groups. Absolute mortality risk reductions after CABG versus medical therapy were greatest for patients 80 years of age or older.

Despite the possibility of confounding by indication, evidence suggests that the use of bilateral over single ITA may be associated with improved long-term survival after CABG. Lytle et al reported a risk-adjusted survival of 94%, 84%, and 67% at 5, 10, and 15 postoperative years, respectively, in 2000 patients who received bilateral ITAs versus 92%, 79%, and 64% in 8100 patients who had a single ITA, and a even greater risk reduction was observed with respect to reoperation rates.[178] Other authors also found that single ITA grafting was a predictor of mortality, late myocardial infarction, or late reoperation when compared with bilateral ITA grafting.[34,79] Taggart et al showed in a meta-analysis of available observational studies that the use of bilateral versus single ITA resulted in a hazard ratio for death of 0.81.[275] No evidence of improved long-term survival exists regarding other arterial grafts such as the radial artery, but a multicenter trial is currently ongoing.[97]

Freedom from Cardiac Events

In addition to conferring a survival benefit, CABG may be indicated to alleviate symptoms of angina and reduce the incidence of nonfatal outcomes such as MI, CHF, and hospitalization. Most long-term studies, however, are limited in their generalizability by the rare use of arterial grafts and the lack of modern secondary prevention programs after CABG. Kirklin et al reported that freedom from angina was 83% at 5 years and 63% at 10 years after CABG performed exclusively or predominantly with vein grafts.[151] Yusuf et al demonstrated that CABG reduced the incidence of MI in the long-term in the CASS, VA, and European studies, but that the overall MI rate was not different than medically treated patients because of a relatively high incidence of perioperative MI in these early studies.[302] Sergeant et al reported on 9600 consecutive CABG patients operated on at the Cleveland Clinic between 1971 and 1992 and found that the freedom rate from return of angina was 94%, 82%, 61%, and 38% at 1, 5, 10, and 15 years, respectively, and that secondary prevention and management of noncardiac comorbidity had the most impact on delaying the return of angina.[254] It is conceivable that arterial grafting may lead to even better results: in a series of 256 patients with three-vessel disease who received three arterial grafts, freedom from MI and from angina was 97.3% and 85.7% at 7 years, respectively.[23]

Left Ventricular Function

The greatest survival benefit after CABG is seen in patients with three-vessel or left main CAD and depressed left ventricular function.[70,302] CABG often leads to improvement of

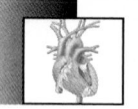

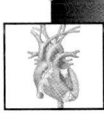

left ventricular function indices of 0.05–0.12 in patients with depressed LVEF preoperatively, because of the presence of stunned or hibernating myocardium.[236–238] In patients with severe CHF symptoms preoperatively, an expected mean gain of at least one NYHA class should persist for at least 4 years on average.[40] Bax et al used echocardiography to examine the time course of contractile recovery in stunned and hibernating myocardial PET segments after CABG and found that 61% of stunned segments had improved at 3 months, and an additional 9% had improved at 14 months.[20] In contrast, hibernating myocardium segments showed contractile improvement at 3 months in 31% of patients, with a further improvement at 14 months in an additional 61%. Five-year survival in patients with very low LVEF (less than 0.20) ranges from 70–73%, with significant improvements in heart failure and angina class among survivors.[29,147,196]

A recent anterior MI with residual wall-motion anomaly is associated with an intramural thrombus in 31% of patients.[149] In contrast, this is much less frequent after an inferior or lateral MI. For these reasons, patients having suffered a recent large anterior MI (including a perioperative MI) and with significant residual anterior or apical wall-motion abnormality should be anticoagulated for 3–6 months after CABG.[140]

Functional Status and Quality of Life

Quality of life is very good to excellent in the majority of patients after CABG and corresponds to that of a matched control population.[158,171,267] Risk factors for lower SF-36 scores include female sex, low socioeconomic status, recurrent symptoms of angina, hypertension, comorbid illnesses, smoking, and nonenrollment in a cardiac rehabilitation program.[171,260] Advanced age does not in itself preclude marked improvements in quality of life after CABG.[295] Postoperatively, a major improvement is usually seen by 3 months, with further improvement observed up to 2 years after surgery. In contrast to the overall improvement in quality of life and functional status, persistent sexual problems are, however, relatively common after CABG and are most prevalent in men, diabetics, and those with preoperative sexual problems.[261]

Graft Patency

In comparison with other forms of revascularization such as PCI, OP-CAB, MIDCAB, TMR, or angiogenic therapy, on-pump CABG has one advantage in that its long-term procedural outcome is well characterized. Multiple long-term angiographic studies have described the patency rates of different types of grafts, and factors associated with their premature closure. The pathology of graft failure has also been well characterized. Early closure (i.e., within 1–2 months) of a graft is usually due to thrombosis, which develops as a result of hemodynamic factors related to poor graft outflow or technical errors.[30] Once the early postoperative period is over, vein grafts start developing a disease complex of their own with intimal hyperplasia noted as early as 1 month after operation,[30,118,152,282] to which the ITA appears immune.[222,290] This process results in a diffuse concentric reduction in vein graft diameter on angiography, which usually matches that of the native coronary vessel by 1 year after implantation. Intimal hyperplasia is often most significant at suture lines, and may lead to anastomotic stenosis in up to 20% of vein grafts.[118] The radial and gastroepiploic arteries are less susceptible to intimal hyperplasia than vein grafts, which could translate into better long-term freedom from atherosclerosis and patency since intimal hyperplasia sites usually correspond to areas that later develop graft atherosclerosis.[103,243,290] Graft atherosclerosis may be observed in vein grafts as early as 3–4 years after operation. It is characterized by a noncapsulated lipid-rich core that is much more friable than native coronary artherosclerotic plaque.

Saphenous Vein Grafts

The angiographic long-term patency of saphenous vein grafts (in the preaspirin and prestatin era) has been extensively studied by FitzGibbon.[90–92] He and his colleagues found that vein graft patency was 88% early postoperatively, 81% at 1 year, 75% at 5 years, and 50% at 15 years; when stenosed grafts were excluded, the proportion of nondiseased grafts was 40% at 12.5 years. This corresponded to a vein graft occlusion rate of 2.1%/year after the initial postoperative period. Vein graft disease appeared by 1 year, involved 48% of grafts at 5 years, and 81% at 15 years. Goldman et al found that for a patient with patent vein grafts 7–10 days after the operation, 3-year graft patency was independently predicted by a lower serum cholesterol and a larger recipient coronary artery diameter.[106]

Sequential vein grafts may have a higher patency rate than individual vein grafts, with up to 76% at 7.5 years for sequential compared with 64.5% for individual grafts.[61] This may be the result of higher graft flow because of better runoff, and consequent decrease in intimal hyperplasia formation in sequential grafts. However, most surgeons believe that the patency of sequential versus individual saphenous vein grafts is similar if the anastomoses are technically flawless and no issue exists such as kinking or poor distal runoff.

Internal Thoracic Artery Grafts

ITA grafts rarely develop significant intimal hyperplasia or late atherosclerosis, and late attrition rates of patent ITA grafts are low. Long-term patency of LITA to LAD grafts is more than 98.7% early on,[21] 94% at 7 years,[180] and 88% at 11 years in the era prior to aspirin use and structured secondary prevention programs,[87,115,138,180,186] and may be even higher today. This patency rate is matched by no other myocardial revascularization modality. Furthermore, the ITA has a potential to grow up to 1.4 times its original size to match the diameter of the coronary artery to which it is anastomosed,[212] with more growth if the ITA is initially small.[190] Progression of native CAD after operation is more common in segments bypassed with venous grafts than with arterial grafts.[186] Free ITA grafts likely have comparable patency provided that a flawless anastomotic technique is used.[174,280] The RITA may have a patency similar to the LITA–LAD, regardless of whether it is used on the circumflex (through the transverse sinus or not),[285,286] the LAD,[7] or the right coronary artery.[87]

Radial Artery Grafts

Acar et al, who led to the revival of the radial artery as a bypass conduit, reported a patency of 83% at 5.6 years in 50 of 910 patients who received a radial artery, which included all patients with symptoms of myocardial ischemia.[3] Iaco et al reported a 96% 4-year patency in selected patients, with no difference in patency whether the radial was anastomosed to the aorta or to the ITA as a Y-graft.[135] Possati et al reported an impressive radial artery graft patency of 92% at a mean of 8.8 years after CABG.[226a] Moderate severity of the native target vessel stenosis (70% or less) is associated with lower patency rates.[185,226a] The effect of target vessel location and calcium channel blockers use on late patency remains controversial.

Gastroepiploic Artery Grafts

Late results of the gastroepiploic artery as a bypass graft are not as good as that of the ITA and radial artery. The 5-year angiographic patency was reported by Hirose et al to be 84%,[129] and 63% at 10 years by Suma et al.[271] Factors associated with premature closure include technical anastomotic factors, free graft configuration, and anastomosis to a less critically stenosed coronary artery.

CABG versus PCI

A detailed comparative analysis of the results of CABG versus those of percutaneous catheter interventions is beyond the scope of this chapter. However, a number of general observations can be made after appraisal of the literature available as of this writing. Conclusions drawn from past data are subject to change, however, as technical and technological advances benefit both CABG (arterial grafting, off-pump techniques, advances in perioperative management) and PCI (drug-eluting stents, intravascular ultrasound, brachytherapy). The winner of this ongoing debate is clearly the patient, who today can be offered surgical and percutaneous revascularization procedures that are safer and are associated with better short- and long-term outcomes than just 10 years ago.

Seventeen randomized clinical trials have compared CABG with PCI as of this writing.* Virtually each one of these trials, with the possible exception of BARI, which enrolled 1792 patients, was underpowered to show a significant difference in early survival between PCI and CABG groups. Patients in whom CABG was assumed to be clearly beneficial (such as those with three-vessel disease with depressed LV function or left main stenosis) were also generally excluded from the trials. Finally, these trials are limited with respect to the generalizability of their conclusions, because only approximately 5% of screened patients were actually enrolled.

A qualitative appraisal of these trials allows for the formulation of the following observations:

1. PCI is associated with a shorter hospital stay and is less morbid than CABG.*
2. In patients with one-, two-, or three-vessel disease and with normal ventricular function, there is generally no difference in midterm survival between nondiabetic patients randomized to PCI or CABG,[238,255,256] although two trials, including one in which stents were routinely employed, showed an event-free survival benefit for CABG in patients with three-vessel disease regardless of diabetic status.[42,49]
3. In patients with diabetes and three-vessel disease, CABG is superior to PCI.[49,255,256] In contrast to PCI, the clinical and angiographic efficacy of CABG is relatively unaffected by the presence of diabetes.[25,157,250,255]
4. Symptomatic improvement and freedom from repeat revascularization are better with CABG than PCI.[48,127,300]
5. CABG provides more complete revascularization than PCI, which correlates with a greater improvement in angina class.[18,300]
6. PCI may be safer and better than CABG in high-risk, acutely unstable patients, regardless of diabetic status.[252]
7. Initial procedural cost is higher with CABG,[1,255] but the two strategies tend to subsequently converge due to an increased need for repeat procedures with PCI.[127,297]
8. Patients with single-vessel proximal LAD disease treated with CABG or MIDCAB versus PCI have higher freedom from angina,[60,112,134] but no difference in freedom from major adverse cardiac events (MACE) is observed at 1-year follow-up.[60,112] Freedom from MACE at midterm and long-term follow-up may be better with CABG[67,134] (Table 82-5).

Although randomization protects against confounding and selection bias, the randomized studies of CABG versus PCI have poor generalizability due to the small proportion of screened patients who actually entered the studies (i.e., efficacy studies). The results of four large CABG/PCI registries, although susceptible to selection bias, may be more useful in comparing the effectiveness of the two modalities in a population-based, clinical practice setting. These registries are (1) the New York State PCI and CABG registries, which followed more than 60,000 patients[122]; (2) the Alberta Provincial Project for Outcomes Assessment in Coronary Heart Disease (APPROACH) registry, which examined nearly 16,000 patients after CABG or PCI[113]; (3) the Northern New England Cardiovascular Disease Study Group Registry, which reported on 2766 patients with diabetes and eligibility criteria compatible with BARI[217]; and (4) the Duke registry, which examined nearly 7000 patients who underwent CABG or PCI.[143] Caution must be exerted when interpreting the results of these registries, because as advances in PCI and CABG techniques since three of these registries were initiated may make it impossible to derive definitive conclusions from these data.[122,143,217] Taken together, their results nevertheless suggest the following:

1. Three-, four-, and five-year risk-adjusted survival after CABG may be superior to PCI for most patients with three-vessel disease, regardless of diabetic status or left ventricular function.[113,122,143]
2. Patients with high-grade proximal LAD stenosis may also derive a long-term survival benefit from undergoing CABG over PCI.[122,143]
3. The superiority of CABG over PCI in diabetic patients seems to be confirmed.[217]
4. Elderly patients with CAD may benefit the most from undergoing revascularization versus medical therapy, and the APPROACH registry demonstrated a small but statistically significant survival benefit in the elderly undergoing CABG versus PCI.[113]

*References 18, 42, 47–49, 60, 67, 89, 111, 112, 120, 133, 150, 237, 238, 252, 255.

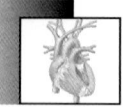

Table 82–5

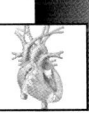

Randomized Trials of CABG versus PCI

Disease extent	*Use of stents*	*Trial name*	*Number of centers/number of patients*	*Follow-up duration (years)*	*Findings*	*Remarks*
Multivessel	Yes	SOS[49]	53/988	2	Survival: CABG better Angina: CABG better Freedom from TVR: CABG better	On-pump CABG
	Yes	ERACI II[22]	7/450	1.5	Survival, MACE: PCI better Angina: no difference Freedom from TVR: CABG better	High-risk patients; on-pump CABG
	No	ERACI 1[157]	1/127	3	MACE: CABG better Angina: CABG better Freedom from TVR: CABG better	On-pump CABG
	Yes	ARTS[1,255]	68/1205	1	Survival: no difference overall; CABG better in diabetics Angina: CABG better Freedom from TVR: CABG better	PCI less costly at 1 year; on-pump CABG
	No	BARI[47,118,250,300]	18/1792	5	Survival: CABG better (no difference of diabetics excluded) Angina: CABG better Freedom from TVR: CABG better	Largest randomized study of PCI versus CABG
	No	EAST[44,219]	1/392	Up to 8	Survival: trend for CABG better in diabetics and proximal LAD Angina: CABG better Freedom from TVR: CABG better	
	No	GABI-1[303]	8/359	1	Survival: no difference Angina: CABG better Freedom from TVR: CABG better	
	Yes	GABI-II[263]	8/136 stents, 177 CABG (historical controls)	1	Survival: no difference Angina: CABG better Freedom from TVR: CABG better	No actual randomization done; historical CABG control group derived from historical GABI-1 CABG patients
	No	Toulouse[250]	1/152	5	Survival, MACE: CABG better Angina: CABG better Freedom from TVR: CABG better	
	No	RITA[90,91]	16/1011	6.5	Survival, MACE: no difference Angina: CABG better Freedom from TVR: CABG better	

(Continued)

Table 82–5

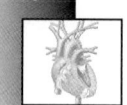

Randomized Trials of CABG versus PCI—cont'd

Disease extent	*Use of stents*	*Trial name*	*Number of centers/number of patients*	*Follow-up duration (years)*	*Findings*	*Remarks*
	No	CABRI[144,265]	26/1054	4	Survival, MACE: no difference Angina: CABG better Freedom from TVR: CABG better	
	No	AWESOME[193]	?/454	3	Survival, MACE: no difference	Diabetic patients with unstable angina and at high-risk for CABG only
Proximal LAD	Yes	Leipzig[60]	1/220	0.5	Survival, MACE: no difference Periprocedural events: PCI better Angina: CABG better Freedom from TVR: CABG better	All CABG were MIDCAB
	Yes	Groningen[60]	1/102	3	Survival, MACE: trend for CABG better Angina: CABG better Freedom from TVR: trend for CABG better	All CABG were off-pump
	Yes	SIMA (Lausanne II)[210]	1/121	2.4	Survival, MACE: no difference Angina: no difference Freedom from TVR: CABG better	On-pump CABG
	No	Lausanne[193]	1/134	2.5	Survival, MACE: no difference Angina: CABG better Freedom from TVR: CABG better	On-pump CABG
	No	MASS[193]	1/142	5	Survival, MACE: CABG better Angina: CABG better Freedom from TVR: CABG better	On-pump CABG

CABG, coronary artery bypass grafting; PCI, percutaneous coronary intervention; MACE, major adverse cardiac events; TVR, target vessel revascularization; LAD, left anterior descending (artery); MIDCAB, minimally invasive direct coronary artery bypass grafting.

SUMMARY

Coronary artery bypass grafting remains the most durable method of coronary revascularization available today. Its future will be influenced by the results of further research on the role of complete arterial revascularization, minimally invasive techniques, secondary prevention programs, adjunct pharmacological strategies, and hybrid procedures in conjunction with PCI. With advances in surgical techniques and secondary prevention, one ambitious but achievable goal for all cardiac surgeons should consist of making CABG a routinely infallible, permanent method of coronary revascularization associated with near zero risk for all patients.

REFERENCES

1. Abizaid A, Costa MA, Centemero M, et al: Clinical and economic impact of diabetes mellitus on percutaneous and surgical treatment of multivessel coronary disease patients: insights from the Arterial Revascularization Therapy Study (ARTS) trial. Circulation 104:533, 2001.

2. Acar C, Jebara VA, Portoghese M, et al: Revival of the radial artery for coronary artery bypass grafting. Ann Thorac Surg 54:652, 1992.
3. Acar C, Ramsheyi A, Pagny JY, et al: The radial artery for coronary artery bypass grafting: clinical and angiographic results at five years. J Thorac Cardiovasc Surg 116:981, 1998.
4. Albes JM, Gross M, Franke U, et al: Revascularization during acute myocardial infarction: risks and benefits revisited. Ann Thorac Surg 74:102, 2002.
5. Alexander JW, Fischer JE, Boyajian M, et al: The influence of hair-removal methods on wound infections. Arch Surg 118:347, 1983.
6. Ali IM, Sanalla AA, Clark V: Beta-blocker effects on postoperative atrial fibrillation. Eur J Cardiothorac Surg 11:1154, 1997.
7. Al-Ruzzeh S, George S, Bustami M, et al: Early clinical and angiographic outcome of the pedicled right internal thoracic artery graft to the left anterior descending artery. Ann Thorac Surg 73:1431, 2002.
8. Alvarez JM, Jackson LR, Chatwin C, Smolich JJ: Low-dose postoperative aprotinin reduces mediastinal drainage and blood product use in patients undergoing primary coronary artery bypass grafting who are taking aspirin: a prospective, randomized, double-blind, placebo-controlled trial. J Thorac Cardiovasc Surg 122:457, 2001.
9. Ambrosio G, Tritto I: Reperfusion injury: experimental evidence and clinical implications. Am Heart J 138:S69, 1999.
10. Anderson CA, Filsoufi F, Aklog L, et al: Liberal use of delayed sternal closure for postcardiotomy hemodynamic instability. Ann Thorac Surg 73:1484, 2002.
11. Anyanwu AC, Saeed I, Bustami M, et al: Does routine use of the radial artery increase complexity or morbidity of coronary bypass surgery? Ann Thorac Surg 71:555, 2001.
12. Argenziano M, Spotnitz HM, Whang W, et al: Risk stratification for coronary bypass surgery in patients with left ventricular dysfunction: analysis of the coronary artery bypass grafting patch trial database. Circulation 100:II119, 1999.
13. Arnold JR, Greenberg JD, Clements S: Internal mammary artery perfusing the Leriche's syndrome. Ann Thorac Surg 69:1244, 2000.
14. Ascione R, Nason G, Al-Ruzzeh S, et al: Coronary revascularization with or without cardiopulmonary bypass in patients with preoperative nondialysis-dependent renal insufficiency. Ann Thorac Surg 72:2020, 2001.
15. Ascione R, Reeves BC, Chamberlain MH, et al: Predictors of stroke in the modern era of coronary artery bypass grafting: a case control study. Ann Thorac Surg 74:474, 2002.
16. Attar S, Suter CM, Hankins JR, et al: Penetrating cardiac injuries. Ann Thorac Surg 51:711, 1991.
17. Babin-Ebell J, Keith PR, Elert O: Efficacy and safety of low-dose propranolol versus diltiazem in the prophylaxis of supraventricular tachyarrhythmia after coronary artery bypass grafting. Eur J Cardiothorac Surg 10:412, 1996.
18. Baldus S, Koster R, Kuchler R, et al: [Percutaneous revascularization of multivessel coronary disease using stents—a multicenter, prospective study]. Dtsch Med Wochenschr 127:547, 2002.
19. Barra JA, Bezon E, Mondine P, et al: Surgical angioplasty with exclusion of atheromatous plaques in case of diffuse disease of the left anterior descending artery: 2 years' follow-up. Eur J Cardiothorac Surg 17:509, 2000.
20. Bax JJ, Visser FC, Poldermans D, et al: Time course of functional recovery of stunned and hibernating segments after surgical revascularization. Circulation 104:I314, 2001.
21. Berger PB, Alderman EL, Nadel A, Schaff HV: Frequency of early occlusion and stenosis in a left internal mammary artery to left anterior descending artery bypass graft after surgery through a median sternotomy on conventional bypass: benchmark for minimally invasive direct coronary artery bypass. Circulation 100:2353, 1999.
22. Bergh C, Backstrom M, Jonsson H, et al: In the eye of both patient and spouse: memory is poor 1 to 2 years after coronary bypass and angioplasty. Ann Thorac Surg 74:689, 2002.
23. Bergsma TM, Grandjean JG, Voors AA, et al: Low recurrence of angina pectoris after coronary artery bypass graft surgery with bilateral internal thoracic and right gastroepiploic arteries. Circulation 97:2402, 1998.
24. Bestetti RB, Costa RS, Kazava DK, Oliveira JS: Can isolated myocardial bridging of the left anterior descending coronary artery be associated with sudden death during exercise? Acta Cardiol 46:27, 1991.
25. Bhatt DL, Topol EJ: Debate: PCI or CABG for multivessel disease? Viewpoint: no clear winner in an unfair fight. Curr Control Trials Cardiovasc Med 2:260, 2001.
26. Bond BR, Zellner JL, Dorman BH, et al: Differential effects of calcium channel antagonists in the amelioration of radial artery vasospasm. Ann Thorac Surg 69:1035, 2000.
27. Borger MA, Fremes SE, Weisel RD, et al: Coronary bypass and carotid endarterectomy: does a combined approach increase risk? A metaanalysis. Ann Thorac Surg 68:14, 1999.
28. Borger MA, Rao V, Weisel RD, et al: Deep sternal wound infection: risk factors and outcomes. Ann Thorac Surg 65:1050, 1998.
29. Bouchart F, Tabley A, Litzler PY, et al: Myocardial revascularization in patients with severe ischemic left ventricular dysfunction. Long term follow-up in 141 patients. Eur J Cardiothorac Surg 20:1157, 2001.
30. Bourassa MG, Campeau L, Lesperance J: Changes in grafts and in coronary arteries after coronary bypass surgery. Cardiovasc Clin 21:83, 1991.
31. Brener SJ, Lytle BW, Schneider JP, et al: Association between CK-MB elevation after percutaneous or surgical revascularization and three-year mortality. J Am Coll Cardiol 40:1961, 2002.
32. Buchanan MR, Brister SJ: Individual variation in the effects of ASA on platelet function: implications for the use of ASA clinically. Can J Cardiol 11:221, 1995.
33. Burek KA, Sutton-Tyrrell K, Brooks MM, et al: Prognostic importance of lower extremity arterial disease in patients undergoing coronary revascularization in the Bypass Angioplasty Revascularization Investigation (BARI). J Am Coll Cardiol 34:716, 1999.
34. Buxton BF, Komeda M, Fuller JA, Gordon I: Bilateral internal thoracic artery grafting may improve outcome of coronary artery surgery. Risk-adjusted survival. Circulation 98:II1, 1998.
35. Cable DG, Caccitolo JA, Pearson PJ, et al: New approaches to prevention and treatment of radial artery graft vasospasm. Circulation 98:II15, 1998.
36. Calafiore AM, Contini M, Vitolla G, et al: Bilateral internal thoracic artery grafting: long-term clinical and angiographic results of in situ versus Y grafts. J Thorac Cardiovasc Surg 120:990, 2000.
37. Calafiore AM, Vitolla G, Iaco AL, et al: Bilateral internal mammary artery grafting: midterm results of pedicled versus skeletonized conduits. Ann Thorac Surg 67:1637, 1999.
38. Campeau L, Hunninghake DB, Knatterud GL, et al: Aggressive cholesterol lowering delays saphenous vein graft atherosclerosis in women, the elderly, and patients with associated risk factors. NHLBI post coronary artery bypass graft clinical trial. Post CABG Trial Investigators. Circulation 99:3241, 1999.
39. Carpentier A, Guermonprez JL, Deloche A, et al: The aorta-to-coronary radial artery bypass graft. A technique avoiding pathological changes in grafts. Ann Thorac Surg 16:111, 1973.
40. Carr JA, Haithcock BE, Paone G, et al: Long-term outcome after coronary artery bypass grafting in patients with severe left ventricular dysfunction. Ann Thorac Surg 74:1531, 2002.

41. Carrel A: On the experimental surgery of the thoracic aorta and the heart. Ann Surg 52:83, 1910.
42. Carrie D, Elbaz M, Puel J, et al: Five-year outcome after coronary angioplasty versus bypass surgery in multivessel coronary artery disease: results from the French Monocentric Study. Circulation 96:II, 1997.
43. Carrier M, Pellerin M, Perrault LP, et al: Troponin levels in patients with myocardial infarction after coronary artery bypass grafting. Ann Thorac Surg 69:435, 2000.
44. Classen DC, Evans RS, Pestotnik SL, et al: The timing of prophylactic administration of antibiotics and the risk of surgical-wound infection. N Engl J Med 326:281, 1992.
45. Cohen AJ, Lockman J, Lorberboym M, et al: Assessment of sternal vascularity with single photon emission computed tomography after harvesting of the internal thoracic artery. J Thorac Cardiovasc Surg 118:496, 1999.
46. Cohen G, Tamariz MG, Sever JY, et al: The radial artery versus the saphenous vein graft in contemporary CABG: a case-matched study. Ann Thorac Surg 71:180, 2001.
47. Comparison of coronary bypass surgery with angioplasty in patients with multivessel disease. The Bypass Angioplasty Revascularization Investigation (BARI) Investigators. N Engl J Med 335:217, 1996.
48. Coronary angioplasty versus coronary artery bypass surgery: the Randomized Intervention Treatment of Angina (RITA) trial. Lancet 341:573, 1993.
49. Coronary artery bypass surgery versus percutaneous coronary intervention with stent implantation in patients with multivessel coronary artery disease (the Stent or Surgery trial): a randomised controlled trial. Lancet 360:965, 2002.
50. Coronary artery surgery study (CASS): a randomized trial of coronary artery bypass surgery. Survival data. Circulation 68:939, 1983.
51. Costa MA, Carere RG, Lichtenstein SV, et al: Incidence, predictors, and significance of abnormal cardiac enzyme rise in patients treated with bypass surgery in the arterial revascularization therapies study (ARTS). Circulation 104:2689, 2001.
52. Creswell LL, Moulton MJ, Cox JL, Rosenbloom M: Revascularization after acute myocardial infarction. Ann Thorac Surg 60:19, 1995.
53. Crowley SD, Butterly DW, Peter RH, Schwab SJ: Coronary steal from a left internal mammary artery coronary bypass graft by a left upper extremity arteriovenous hemodialysis fistula. Am J Kidney Dis 40:852, 2002.
54. D'Ancona G, Karamanoukian HL, Ricci M, et al: Graft revision after transit time flow measurement in off-pump coronary artery bypass grafting. Eur J Cardiothorac Surg 17:287, 2000.
55. Dar MI, Gillott T, Ciulli F, Cooper GJ: Single aortic cross-clamp technique reduces S-100 release after coronary artery surgery. Ann Thorac Surg 71:794, 2001.
56. Deja MA, Wos S, Golba KS, et al: Intraoperative and laboratory evaluation of skeletonized versus pedicled internal thoracic artery. Ann Thorac Surg 68:2164, 1999.
57. Denton TA, Trento L, Cohen M, et al: Radial artery harvesting for coronary bypass operations: neurologic complications and their potential mechanisms. J Thorac Cardiovasc Surg 121:951, 2001.
58. Depre C, Vanoverschelde JL, Gerber B, et al: Correlation of functional recovery with myocardial blood flow, glucose uptake, and morphologic features in patients with chronic left ventricular ischemic dysfunction undergoing coronary artery bypass grafting. J Thorac Cardiovasc Surg 113:371, 1997.
59. Di Carli MF, Maddahi J, Rokhsar S, et al: Long-term survival of patients with coronary artery disease and left ventricular dysfunction: implications for the role of myocardial viability assessment in management decisions. J Thorac Cardiovasc Surg 116:997, 1998.
60. Diegeler A, Thiele H, Falk V, et al: Comparison of stenting with minimally invasive bypass surgery for stenosis of the left anterior descending coronary artery. N Engl J Med 347:561, 2002.
61. Dion R, Glineur D, Derouck D, et al: Complementary saphenous grafting: long-term follow-up. J Thorac Cardiovasc Surg 122:296, 2001.
62. Dipp MA, Nye PC, Taggart DP: Phenoxybenzamine is more effective and less harmful than papverine in the prevention of radial artery vasospasm. Eur J Cardiothorac Surg 19:482, 2001.
63. Dockery DW, Pope CA 3rd, Xu X, et al: An association between air pollution and mortality in six U.S. cities. N Engl J Med 329:1753, 1993.
64. Dohmen G, Dahm M, Elsner M, et al: Coronary artery bypass grafting in adult coronary artery disease due to suspected Kawasaki disease in childhood. Ann Thorac Surg 70:1704, 2000.
65. Domanski MJ, Borkowf CB, Campeau L, et al: Prognostic factors for atherosclerosis progression in saphenous vein grafts: the postcoronary artery bypass graft (Post-CABG) trial. Post-CABG Trial Investigators. J Am Coll Cardiol 36:1877, 2000.
66. Dorge H, Schoendube FA, Schoberer M, et al: Intraoperative amiodarone as prophylaxis against atrial fibrillation after coronary operations. Ann Thorac Surg 69:1358, 2000.
67. Drenth DJ, Veeger NJ, Winter JB, et al: A prospective randomized trial comparing stenting with off-pump coronary surgery for high-grade stenosis in the proximal left anterior descending coronary artery: three-year follow-up. J Am Coll Cardiol 40:1955, 2002.
68. Dyke CM, Bhatia D, Lorenz TJ, et al: Immediate coronary artery bypass surgery after platelet inhibition with eptifibatide: results from PURSUIT. Platelet Glycoprotein IIb/IIIa in Unstable Angina: Receptor Suppression Using Integrelin Therapy. Ann Thorac Surg 70:866, 2000.
69. Eagle KA, Berger PB, Calkins H, et al: ACC/AHA guideline update for perioperative cardiovascular evaluation for noncardiac surgery—executive summary: a report of the American College of Cardiology/American Heart Association Task Force on Practice Guidelines (Committee to Update the 1996 Guidelines on Perioperative Cardiovascular Evaluation for Noncardiac Surgery). J Am Coll Cardiol 39:542, 2002.
70. Eagle KA, Guyton RA, Davidoff R, et al: ACC/AHA Guidelines for Coronary Artery Bypass Graft Surgery: A Report of the American College of Cardiology/American Heart Association Task Force on Practice Guidelines (Committee to Revise the 1991 Guidelines for Coronary Artery Bypass Graft Surgery). American College of Cardiology/American Heart Association. J Am Coll Cardiol 34:1262, 1999.
71. Eckstein FS, Bonilla LF, Englberger L, et al: Minimizing aortic manipulation during OPCAB using the symmetry aortic connector system for proximal vein graft anastomoses. Ann Thorac Surg 72:S995, 2001.
72. Eckstein FS, Bonilla LF, Englberger L, et al: First clinical results with a new mechanical connector for distal coronary artery anastomoses in CABG. Circulation 106:I1, 2002.
73. Eckstein FS, Bonilla LF, Englberger L, et al: The St Jude Medical symmetry aortic connector system for proximal vein graft anastomoses in coronary artery bypass grafting. J Thorac Cardiovasc Surg 123:777, 2002.
74. Efstratiadis T, Munsch C, Crossman D, Taylor K: Aprotinin used in emergency coronary operation after streptokinase treatment. Ann Thorac Surg 52:1320, 1991.

75. Eigel P, van Ingen G, Wagenpfeil S: Predictive value of perioperative cardiac troponin I for adverse outcome in coronary artery bypass surgery. Eur J Cardiothorac Surg 20:544, 2001.
76. Elefteriades J, Edwards R: Coronary bypass in left heart failure. Semin Thorac Cardiovasc Surg 14:125, 2002.
77. Eleven-year survival in the Veterans Administration randomized trial of coronary bypass surgery for stable angina. The Veterans Administration Coronary Artery Bypass Surgery Cooperative Study Group. N Engl J Med 311:1333, 1984.
78. El-Khouri HM, Danilowicz DA, Slovis AJ, et al: Saphenous vein graft growth 13 years after coronary bypass in a child with Kawasaki disease. Ann Thorac Surg 65:1127, 1998.
79. Endo M, Nishida H, Tomizawa Y, Kasanuki H: Benefit of bilateral over single internal mammary artery grafts for multiple coronary artery bypass grafting. Circulation 104:2164, 2001.
80. Estafanous FG, Loop FD, Higgins TL, et al: Increased risk and decreased morbidity of coronary artery bypass grafting between 1986 and 1994. Ann Thorac Surg 65:383, 1998.
81. Evrard P, Gonzalez M, Jamart J, et al: Prophylaxis of supraventricular and ventricular arrhythmias after coronary artery bypass grafting with low-dose sotalol. Ann Thorac Surg 70:151, 2000.
82. Favaloro RG: Saphenous vein graft in the surgical treatment of coronary artery disease: operative technique. J Thorac Cardiovasc Surg 58:178, 1969.
83. Ferguson JJ 3rd, Cohen M, Freedman RJ Jr, et al: The current practice of intra-aortic balloon counterpulsation: results from the Benchmark Registry. J Am Coll Cardiol 38:1456, 2001.
84. Ferguson TB Jr, Coombs LP, Peterson ED: Internal thoracic artery grafting in the elderly patient undergoing coronary artery bypass grafting: room for process improvement? J Thorac Cardiovasc Surg 123:869, 2002.
85. Ferguson TB Jr, Hammill BG, Peterson ED, et al: A decade of change—risk profiles and outcomes for isolated coronary artery bypass grafting procedures, 1990–1999: a report from the STS National Database Committee and the Duke Clinical Research Institute. Society of Thoracic Surgeons. Ann Thorac Surg 73:480, 2002.
86. Ferraris VA, Gildengorin V: Predictors of excessive blood use after coronary artery bypass grafting. A multivariate analysis. J Thorac Cardiovasc Surg 98:492, 1989.
87. Fiore AC, Naunheim KS, Dean P, et al: Results of internal thoracic artery grafting over 15 years: single versus double grafts. Ann Thorac Surg 49:202, 1990.
88. Firstenberg MS, Azoury F, Lytle BW, Thomas JD: Interposition vein graft for giant coronary aneurysm repair. Ann Thorac Surg 70:1397, 2000.
89. First-year results of CABRI (Coronary Angioplasty versus Bypass Revascularisation Investigation). CABRI Trial Participants. Lancet 346:1179, 1995.
90. FitzGibbon GM, Burton JR, Leach AJ: Coronary bypass graft fate: angiographic grading of 1400 consecutive grafts early after operation and of 1132 after one year. Circulation 57:1070, 1978.
91. FitzGibbon GM, Kafka HP, Leach AJ, et al: Coronary bypass graft fate and patient outcome: angiographic follow-up of 5,065 grafts related to survival and reoperation in 1,388 patients during 25 years. J Am Coll Cardiol 28:616, 1996.
92. FitzGibbon GM, Leach AJ, Kafka HP, Keon WJ: Coronary bypass graft fate: long-term angiographic study. J Am Coll Cardiol 17:1075, 1991.
93. Flameng WJ, Shivalkar B, Spiessens B, et al: PET scan predicts recovery of left ventricular function after coronary artery bypass operation. Ann Thorac Surg 64:1694, 1997.
94. Flemma RJ, Johnson WD, Lepley D Jr: Triple aorto-coronary vein bypass as treatment for coronary insufficiency. Arch Surg 103:82, 1971.
95. Forlani S, De Paulis R, de Notaris S, et al: Combination of sotalol and magnesium prevents atrial fibrillation after coronary artery bypass grafting. Ann Thorac Surg 74:720, 2002.
96. Fox KA, Poole-Wilson PA, Henderson RA, et al: Interventional versus conservative treatment for patients with unstable angina or non-ST-elevation myocardial infarction: the British Heart Foundation RITA 3 randomised trial. Randomized Intervention Trial of unstable Angina. Lancet 360:743, 2002.
97. Fremes SE: Multicenter radial artery patency study (RAPS). Study design. Control Clin Trials 21:397, 2000.
98. Fremes SE, Goldman BS, Christakis GT, et al: Current risk of coronary bypass for unstable angina. Eur J Cardiothorac Surg 5:235, 1991.
99. Frost L, Molgaard H, Christiansen EH, et al: Atrial fibrillation and flutter after coronary artery bypass surgery: epidemiology, risk factors and preventive trials. Int J Cardiol 36:253, 1992.
100. Fukuda I, Gomi S, Watanabe K, Seita J: Carotid and aortic screening for coronary artery bypass grafting. Ann Thorac Surg 70:2034, 2000.
101. Ganz P, Ganz W: Coronary blood flow and myocardial ischemia. In Libby P, editor: Heart Disease. Philadelphia: W.B. Saunders, 2001, p. 1087.
102. Gaudino M, Glieca F, Luciani N, et al: Clinical and angiographic effects of chronic calcium channel blocker therapy continued beyond first postoperative year in patients with radial artery grafts: results of a prospective randomized investigation. Circulation 104:164, 2001.
103. Gaudino M, Glieca F, Trani C, et al: Midterm endothelial function and remodeling of radial artery grafts anastomosed to the aorta. J Thorac Cardiovasc Surg 120:298, 2000.
104. Ghali WA, Rothwell DM, Quan H, et al: A Canadian comparison of data sources for coronary artery bypass surgery outcome "report cards." Am Heart J 140:402, 2000.
105. Goldman S, Copeland J, Moritz T, et al: Starting aspirin therapy after operation. Effects on early graft patency. Department of Veterans Affairs Cooperative Study Group. Circulation 84:520, 1991.
106. Goldman S, Zadina K, Krasnicka B, et al: Predictors of graft patency 3 years after coronary artery bypass graft surgery. Department of Veterans Affairs Cooperative Study Group No. 297. J Am Coll Cardiol 29:1563, 1997.
107. Goldstein J, Cooper E, Saltups A, Boxall J: Angiographic assessment of graft patency after coronary endarterectomy. J Thorac Cardiovasc Surg 102:539, 1991.
108. Gomes WJ, Santos PC, Branco JN, Buffolo E: Repair of damaged internal mammary artery. Ann Thorac Surg 74:906, 2002.
109. Goto T, Baba T, Honma K, et al: Magnetic resonance imaging findings and postoperative neurologic dysfunction in elderly patients undergoing coronary artery bypass grafting. Ann Thorac Surg 72:137, 2001.
110. Gotteiner N, Mavroudis C, Backer CL, et al: Coronary artery bypass grafting for Kawasaki disease. Pediatr Cardiol 23:62, 2002.
111. Goy JJ, Eeckhout E, Burnand B, et al: Coronary angioplasty versus left internal mammary artery grafting for isolated proximal left anterior descending artery stenosis. Lancet 343:1449, 1994.
112. Goy JJ, Kaufmann U, Goy-Eggenberger D, et al: A prospective randomized trial comparing stenting to internal mammary artery grafting for proximal, isolated de novo left anterior coronary artery stenosis: the SIMA trial. Stenting vs Internal Mammary Artery. Mayo Clin Proc 75:1116, 2000.
113. Graham MM, Ghali WA, Faris PD, et al: Survival after coronary revascularization in the elderly. Circulation 105:2378, 2002.

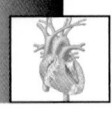

114. Green GE, Spencer FC, Tice DA, Stertzer SH: Arterial and venous microsurgical bypass grafts for coronary artery disease. J Thorac Cardiovasc Surg 60:491, 1970.
115. Grondin CM, Campeau L, Lesperance J, et al: Comparison of late changes in internal mammary artery and saphenous vein grafts in two consecutive series of patients 10 years after operation. Circulation 70:1208, 1984.
116. Gunning MG, Anagnostopoulos C, Knight CJ, et al: Comparison of 201TL1, 99mTc-tetrofosmin, and dobutamine magnetic resonance imaging for identifying hibernating myocardium. Circulation 98:1869, 1998.
117. Guo LR, Steinman DA, Moon BC, et al: Effect of distal graft anastomosis site on retrograde perfusion and flow patterns of native coronary vasculature. Ann Thorac Surg 72:782, 2001.
118. Guthaner DF, Robert EW, Alderman EL, Wexler L: Long-term serial angiographic studies after coronary artery bypass surgery. Circulation 60:250, 1979.
119. Guvener M, Pasaoglu I, Demircin M, Oc M: Perioperative hyperglycemia is a strong correlate of postoperative infection in type II diabetic patients after coronary artery bypass grafting. Endocr J 49:531, 2002.
120. Hamm CW, Reimers J, Ischinger T, et al: A randomized study of coronary angioplasty compared with bypass surgery in patients with symptomatic multivessel coronary disease. German Angioplasty Bypass Surgery Investigation (GABI). N Engl J Med 331:1037, 1994.
121. Handa N, McGregor CG, Danielson GK, et al: Coronary artery bypass grafting in patients with previous mediastinal radiation therapy. J Thorac Cardiovasc Surg 117:1136, 1999.
122. Hannan EL, Racz MJ, McCallister BD, et al: A comparison of three-year survival after coronary artery bypass graft surgery and percutaneous transluminal coronary angioplasty. J Am Coll Cardiol 33:63, 1999.
123. Hata M, Shiono M, Orime Y, et al: Clinical results of coronary artery bypass grafting with use of the internal thoracic artery under low free flow conditions. J Thorac Cardiovasc Surg 119:125, 2000.
124. Hausmann H, Potapov EV, Koster A, et al: Prognosis after the implantation of an intra-aortic balloon pump in cardiac surgery calculated with a new score. Circulation 106:1203, 2002.
125. Hayashida N, Kai E, Enomoto N, Aoyagi S: Internal thoracic artery as a collateral source to the ischemic lower extremity. Eur J Cardiothorac Surg 18:613, 2000.
126. Helm RE, Rosengart TK, Gomez M, et al: Comprehensive multimodality blood conservation: 100 consecutive CABG operations without transfusion. Ann Thorac Surg 65:125, 1998.
127. Henderson RA, Pocock SJ, Sharp SJ, et al: Long-term results of RITA-1 trial: clinical and cost comparisons of coronary angioplasty and coronary-artery bypass grafting. Randomised Intervention Treatment of Angina. Lancet 352:1419, 1998.
128. Hennen B, Markwirth T, Scheller B, et al: Impaired flow in left internal mammary artery grafts due to subclavian artery stenosis. Ann Thorac Surg 72:917, 2001.
129. Hirose H, Amano A, Takanashi S, Takahashi A: Coronary artery bypass grafting using the gastroepiploic artery in 1,000 patients. Ann Thorac Surg 73:1371, 2002.
130. Hirotani T, Kameda T, Kumamoto T, et al: Effects of coronary artery bypass grafting using internal mammary arteries for diabetic patients. J Am Coll Cardiol 34:532, 1999.
131. Hirotani T, Shirota S, Cho Y, Takeuchi S: Feasibility and suitability of the routine use of bilateral internal thoracic arteries. Ann Thorac Surg 73:511, 2002.
132. Hongo RH, Ley J, Dick SE, Yee RR: The effect of clopidogrel in combination with aspirin when given before coronary artery bypass grafting. J Am Coll Cardiol 40:231, 2002.
133. Hueb WA, Bellotti G, de Oliveira SA, et al: The Medicine, Angioplasty or Surgery Study (MASS): a prospective, randomized trial of medical therapy, balloon angioplasty or bypass surgery for single proximal left anterior descending artery stenoses. J Am Coll Cardiol 26:1600, 1995.
134. Hueb WA, Soares PR, Almeida De Oliveira S, et al: Five-year follow-up of the medicine, angioplasty, or surgery study (MASS): a prospective, randomized trial of medical therapy, balloon angioplasty, or bypass surgery for single proximal left anterior descending coronary artery stenosis. Circulation 100:II107, 1999.
135. Iaco AL, Teodori G, Di Giammarco G, et al: Radial artery for myocardial revascularization: long-term clinical and angiographic results. Ann Thorac Surg 72:464, 2001.
136. Ioannidis JP, Galanos O, Katritsis D, et al: Early mortality and morbidity of bilateral versus single internal thoracic artery revascularization: propensity and risk modeling. J Am Coll Cardiol 37:521, 2001.
137. Ishii M, Ueno T, Ikeda H, et al: Sequential follow-up results of catheter intervention for coronary artery lesions after Kawasaki disease: quantitative coronary artery angiography and intravascular ultrasound imaging study. Circulation 105:3004, 2002.
138. Ivert T, Huttunen K, Landou C, Bjork VO: Angiographic studies of internal mammary artery grafts 11 years after coronary artery bypass grafting. J Thorac Cardiovasc Surg 96:1, 1988.
139. Jarvis MA, Jarvis CL, Jones PR, Spyt TJ: Reliability of Allen's test in selection of patients for radial artery harvest. Ann Thorac Surg 70:1362, 2000.
140. Johannessen KA, Nordrehaug JE, von der Lippe G: Left ventricular thrombi after short-term high-dose anticoagulants in acute myocardial infarction. Eur Heart J 8:975, 1987.
141. John R, Choudhri AF, Weinberg AD, et al: Multicenter review of preoperative risk factors for stroke after coronary artery bypass grafting. Ann Thorac Surg 69:30, 2000.
142. Johnston SC: Identifying confounding by indication through blinded prospective review. Am J Epidemiol 154:276, 2001.
143. Jones RH, Kesler K, Phillips HR 3rd, et al: Long-term survival benefits of coronary artery bypass grafting and percutaneous transluminal angioplasty in patients with coronary artery disease. J Thorac Cardiovasc Surg 111:1013, 1996.
144. Kaplan M, Kut MS, Icer UA, Demirtas MM: Intravenous magnesium sulfate prophylaxis for atrial fibrillation after coronary artery bypass surgery. J Thorac Cardiovasc Surg 125:344, 2003.
145. Karin E, Greenberg R, Avital S, et al: The management of stab wounds to the heart with laceration of the left anterior descending coronary artery. Eur J Emerg Med 8:321, 2001.
146. Karkouti K, Cohen MM, McCluskey SA, Sher GD: A multivariable model for predicting the need for blood transfusion in patients undergoing first-time elective coronary bypass graft surgery. Transfusion 41:1193, 2001.
147. Kaul TK, Agnihotri AK, Fields BL, et al: Coronary artery bypass grafting in patients with an ejection fraction of twenty percent or less. J Thorac Cardiovasc Surg 111:1001, 1996.
148. Kawasuji M, Sakakibara N, Takemura H, et al: Is internal thoracic artery grafting suitable for a moderately stenotic coronary artery? J Thorac Cardiovasc Surg 112:253, 1996.
149. Keren A, Goldberg S, Gottlieb S, et al: Natural history of left ventricular thrombi: their appearance and resolution in the posthospitalization period of acute myocardial infarction. J Am Coll Cardiol 15:790, 1990.
150. King SB 3rd, Lembo NJ, Weintraub WS, et al: A randomized trial comparing coronary angioplasty with coronary bypass surgery. Emory Angioplasty versus Surgery Trial (EAST). N Engl J Med 331:1044, 1994.
151. Kirklin JW, Akins CW, Blackstone EH, et al: Guidelines and indications for coronary artery bypass graft surgery: a report of the American College of Cardiology/American Heart Association Task Force on Assessment of Diagnostic and

Therapeutic Cardiovascular Procedures (Subcommittee on Coronary Artery Bypass Graft Surgery). J Am Coll Cardiol 17:543, 1991.

152. Kirklin JW, Barratt-Boyes BG: Stenotic arteriosclerotic coronary artery disease. In Barratt-Boyes BG, editor: Cardiac Surgery. New York: Churchill Livingstone, 1993, p. 300.
153. Kitamura S, Kameda Y, Seki T, et al: Long-term outcome of myocardial revascularization in patients with Kawasaki coronary artery disease. A multicenter cooperative study. J Thorac Cardiovasc Surg 107:663, 1994.
154. Kjoller-Hansen L, Steffensen R, Grande P: The Angiotensin-converting Enzyme Inhibition Post Revascularization Study (APRES). J Am Coll Cardiol 35:881, 2000.
155. Koenig SC, VanHimbergen DJ, Jaber SF, et al: Spectral analysis of graft flow for anastomotic error detection in off-pump CABG. Eur J Cardiothorac Surg 16(Suppl. 1):S83, 1999.
156. Kolesov VI, Potashov LV: [Surgery of coronary arteries]. Eksp Khir Anesteziol 10:3, 1965.
157. Kurbaan AS, Bowker TJ, Ilsley CD, et al: Difference in the mortality of the CABRI diabetic and nondiabetic populations and its relation to coronary artery disease and the revascularization mode. Am J Cardiol 87:947, 2001.
158. Kurlansky PA, Traad EA, Galbut DL, et al: Coronary bypass surgery in women: a long-term comparative study of quality of life after bilateral internal mammary artery grafting in men and women. Ann Thorac Surg 74:1517, 2002.
159. Kushwaha SS, Bustami M, Tadjkarimi S, et al: Late endothelial function of free and pedicled internal mammary artery grafts. J Thorac Cardiovasc Surg 110:453, 1995.
160. La Canna G, Alfieri O, Giubbini R, et al: Echocardiography during infusion of dobutamine for identification of reversibly dysfunction in patients with chronic coronary artery disease. J Am Coll Cardiol 23:617, 1994.
161. Lazar HL, Jacobs AK, Aldea GS, et al: Factors influencing mortality after emergency coronary artery bypass grafting for failed percutaneous transluminal coronary angioplasty. Ann Thorac Surg 64:1747, 1997.
162. Leavitt BJ, O'Connor GT, Olmstead EM, et al: Use of the internal mammary artery graft and in-hospital mortality and other adverse outcomes associated with coronary artery bypass surgery. Circulation 103:507, 2001.
163. Lee DC, Oz MC, Weinberg AD, et al: Optimal timing of revascularization: transmural versus nontransmural acute myocardial infarction. Ann Thorac Surg 71:1197, 2001.
164. Lee SH, Chang CM, Lu MJ, et al: Intravenous amiodarone for prevention of atrial fibrillation after coronary artery bypass grafting. Ann Thorac Surg 70:157, 2000.
165. Legarra JJ, Sarralde JA, Lopez Coronado JL, Trenor AM: Surgical approach for cardiac surgery in a patient with tracheostoma. Eur J Cardiothorac Surg 14:338, 1998.
166. Lemmer JH Jr, Metzdorff MT, Krause AH Jr, et al: Emergency coronary artery bypass graft surgery in abciximab-treated patients. Ann Thorac Surg 69:90, 2000.
167. Lev-Ran O, Paz Y, Pevni D, et al: Bilateral internal thoracic artery grafting: midterm results of composite versus in situ crossover graft. Ann Thorac Surg 74:704, 2002.
168. Levy T, Fotopoulos G, Walker S, et al: Randomized controlled study investigating the effect of biatrial pacing in prevention of atrial fibrillation after coronary artery bypass grafting. Circulation 102:1382, 2000.
169. Leyh RG, Bartels C, Notzold A, Sievers HH: Management of porcelain aorta during coronary artery bypass grafting. Ann Thorac Surg 67:986, 1999.
170. Lincoff AM, LeNarz LA, Despotis GJ, et al: Abciximab and bleeding during coronary surgery: results from the EPILOG and EPISTENT trials. Improve Long-term Outcome with abciximab GP IIb/IIIa blockade. Evaluation of Platelet IIb/IIIa Inhibition in STENTing. Ann Thorac Surg 70:516, 2000.
171. Lindsay GM, Hanlon P, Smith LN, Wheatley DJ: Assessment of changes in general health status using the short-form 36 questionnaire 1 year following coronary artery bypass grafting. Eur J Cardiothorac Surg 18:557, 2000.
172. Longmire WP, Cannon JA, Kattus AA: Direct-vision coronary endarterectomy for angina pectoris. N Engl J Med 259:259, 1958.
173. Loop FD, Lytle BW, Cosgrove DM, et al: Free (aorta-coronary) internal mammary artery graft. Late results. J Thorac Cardiovasc Surg 92:827, 1986.
174. Loop FD, Lytle BW, Cosgrove DM, et al: Influence of the internal-mammary-artery graft on 10-year survival and other cardiac events. N Engl J Med 314:1, 1986.
175. Loop FD, Lytle BW, Cosgrove DM, et al: J. Maxwell Chamberlain memorial paper. Sternal wound complications after isolated coronary artery bypass grafting: early and late mortality, morbidity, and cost of care. Ann Thorac Surg 49:179, 1990.
176. Lorusso R, La Canna G, Ceconi C, et al: Long-term results of coronary artery bypass grafting procedure in the presence of left ventricular dysfunction and hibernating myocardium. Eur J Cardiothorac Surg 20:937, 2001.
177. Louagie YA, Jamart J, Buche M, et al: Operation for unstable angina pectoris: factors influencing adverse in-hospital outcome. Ann Thorac Surg 59:1141, 1995.
178. Lytle BW, Blackstone EH, Loop FD, et al: Two internal thoracic artery grafts are better than one. J Thorac Cardiovasc Surg 117:855, 1999.
179. Lytle BW, Loop FD, Cosgrove DM, et al: Long-term (5 to 12 years) serial studies of internal mammary artery and saphenous vein coronary bypass grafts. J Thorac Cardiovasc Surg 89:248, 1985.
180. Mack MJ, Osborne JA, Shennib H: Arterial graft patency in coronary artery bypass grafting: what do we really know? Ann Thorac Surg 66:1055, 1998.
181. Maes A, Flameng W, Nuyts J, et al: Histological alterations in chronically hypoperfused myocardium. Correlation with PET findings. Circulation 90:735, 1994.
182. Mahoney EM, Thompson TD, Veledar E, et al: Cost-effectiveness of targeting patients undergoing cardiac surgery for therapy with intravenous amiodarone to prevent atrial fibrillation. J Am Coll Cardiol 40:737, 2002.
183. Mangano CM, Diamondstone LS, Ramsay JG, et al: Renal dysfunction after myocardial revascularization: risk factors, adverse outcomes, and hospital resource utilization. The Multicenter Study of Perioperative Ischemia Research Group. Ann Intern Med 128:194, 1998.
184. Mangano DT: Aspirin and mortality from coronary bypass surgery. N Engl J Med 347:1309, 2002.
185. Maniar HS, Sundt TM, Barner HB, et al: Effect of target stenosis and location on radial artery graft patency. J Thorac Cardiovasc Surg 123:45, 2002.
186. Manninen HI, Jaakkola P, Suhonen M, et al: Angiographic predictors of graft patency and disease progression after coronary artery bypass grafting with arterial and venous grafts. Ann Thorac Surg 66:1289, 1998.
187. Marasco S, Esmore D: A novel method for performing sequential grafts with the radial artery. Ann Thorac Surg 74:1262, 2002.
188. Marinelli G, Chiappini B, Di Eusanio M, et al: Bypass grafting with coronary endarterectomy: immediate and long-term results. J Thorac Cardiovasc Surg 124:553, 2002.
189. Marso SP, Bhatt DL, Roe MT, et al: Enhanced efficacy of eptifibatide administration in patients with acute coronary syndrome requiring in-hospital coronary artery bypass grafting. PURSUIT Investigators. Circulation 102:2952, 2000.
190. Masuda T, Matsuda Y, Tanimoto Y, et al: Angiographic follow-up of internal thoracic artery for free bypass grafting. Ann Thorac Surg 65:731, 1998.

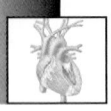

191. Mathew JP, Parks R, Savino JS, et al: Atrial fibrillation following coronary artery bypass graft surgery: predictors, outcomes, and resource utilization. MultiCenter Study of Perioperative Ischemia Research Group. JAMA 276:300, 1996.
192. Matsa M, Paz Y, Gurevitch J, et al: Bilateral skeletonized internal thoracic artery grafts in patients with diabetes mellitus. J Thorac Cardiovasc Surg 121:668, 2001.
193. McKhann GM, Goldsborough MA, Borowicz LM Jr, et al: Cognitive outcome after coronary artery bypass: a one-year prospective study. Ann Thorac Surg 63:510, 1997.
194. McKhann GM, Goldsborough MA, Borowicz LM Jr, et al: Predictors of stroke risk in coronary artery bypass patients. Ann Thorac Surg 63:516, 1997.
195. Medalion B, Katz MG, Lorberboym M, et al: Decreased sternal vascularity after internal thoracic artery harvesting resolves with time: an assessment with single photon emission computed tomography. J Thorac Cardiovasc Surg 123:508, 2002.
196. Mickleborough LL, Carson S, Tamariz M, Ivanov J: Results of revascularization in patients with severe left ventricular dysfunction. J Thorac Cardiovasc Surg 119:550, 2000.
197. Mickleborough LL, Walker PM, Takagi Y, et al: Risk factors for stroke in patients undergoing coronary artery bypass grafting. J Thorac Cardiovasc Surg 112:1250, 1996.
198. Mills NL, Everson CT: Right gastroepiploic artery: a third arterial conduit for coronary artery bypass. Ann Thorac Surg 47:706, 1989.
199. Mills NL, Everson CT: Atherosclerosis of the ascending aorta and coronary artery bypass. Pathology, clinical correlates, and operative management. J Thorac Cardiovasc Surg 102:546, 1991.
200. Mochizuki Y, Okamura Y, Iida H, et al: Healing of the intimal dissection of the internal thoracic artery graft. Ann Thorac Surg 67:541, 1999.
201. Mohl W, Simon P, Neumann F, et al: Analysis of left ventricular function after emergency coronary artery bypass grafting for life-threatening ischaemia following primary revascularization. Eur J Cardiothorac Surg 13:27, 1998.
202. Mohr FW, Falk V: As originally published in 1989: thermal coronary angiography: a method for assessing graft patency and coronary anatomy in coronary bypass surgery. Updated in 1997. Ann Thorac Surg 63:1506, 1997.
203. Monin JL, Garot J, Scherrer-Crosbie M, et al: Prediction of functional recovery of viable myocardium after delayed revascularization in postinfarction patients: accuracy of dobutamine stress echocardiography and influence of long-term vessel patency. J Am Coll Cardiol 34:1012, 1999.
204. Mooney MR, Arom KV, Joyce LD, et al: Emergency cardiopulmonary bypass support in patients with cardiac arrest. J Thorac Cardiovasc Surg 101:450, 1991.
205. Moran SV, Baeza R, Guarda E, et al: Predictors of radial artery patency for coronary bypass operations. Ann Thorac Surg 72:1552, 2001.
206. Mozes B, Olmer L, Galai N, Simchen E: A national study of postoperative mortality associated with coronary artery bypass grafting in Israel. ISCAB Consortium. Israel Coronary Artery Bypass Study. Ann Thorac Surg 66:1254, 1998.
207. Mukherjee D, Bhatt DL, Roe MT, et al: Direct myocardial revascularization and angiogenesis—how many patients might be eligible? Am J Cardiol 84:598, 1999.
208. Munoz JJ, Birkmeyer NJ, Dacey LJ, et al: Trends in rates of reexploration for hemorrhage after coronary artery bypass surgery. Northern New England Cardiovascular Disease Study Group. Ann Thorac Surg 68:1321, 1999.
209. Murphy PJ, Connery C, Hicks GL Jr, Blumberg N: Homologous blood transfusion as a risk factor for postoperative infection after coronary artery bypass graft operations. J Thorac Cardiovasc Surg 104:1092, 1992.
210. Myers WO, Blackstone EH, Davis K, et al: CASS Registry long term surgical survival. Coronary Artery Surgery Study. J Am Coll Cardiol 33:488, 1999.
211. Nakayama Y, Sakata R, Ura M: Bilateral internal thoracic artery use for dialysis patients: does it increase operative risk? Ann Thorac Surg 71:783, 2001.
212. Nakayama Y, Sakata R, Ura M: Growth potential of left internal thoracic artery grafts: analysis of angiographic findings. Ann Thorac Surg 71:142, 2001.
213. Narayan P, Caputo M, Roidl M, Casula R: The use of off pump surgery for management of penetrating coronary artery injury. Eur J Cardiothorac Surg 21:361, 2002.
214. Nathan HJ, Munson J, Wells G, et al: The management of temperature during cardiopulmonary bypass: effect on neuropsychological outcome. J Card Surg 10:481, 1995.
215. Nathan HJ, Wells GA, Munson JL, Wozny D: Neuroprotective effect of mild hypothermia in patients undergoing coronary artery surgery with cardiopulmonary bypass: a randomized trial. Circulation 104:185, 2001.
216. Nikas DJ, Ramadan FM, Elefteriades JA: Topical hypothermia: ineffective and deleterious as adjunct to cardioplegia for myocardial protection. Ann Thorac Surg 65:28, 1998.
217. Niles NW, McGrath PD, Malenka D, et al: Survival of patients with diabetes and multivessel coronary artery disease after surgical or percutaneous coronary revascularization: results of a large regional prospective study. Northern New England Cardiovascular Disease Study Group. J Am Coll Cardiol 37:1008, 2001.
218. Nishida H, Endo M, Koyanagi H, et al: Coronary artery bypass grafting with the right gastroepiploic artery and evaluation of flow with transcutaneous Doppler echocardiography. J Thorac Cardiovasc Surg 108:532, 1994.
219. Nishida H, Tomizawa Y, Endo M, et al: Coronary artery bypass with only in situ bilateral internal thoracic arteries and right gastroepiploic artery. Circulation 104:176, 2001.
220. Nunoo-Mensah J: An unexpected complication after harvesting of the radial artery for coronary artery bypass grafting. Ann Thorac Surg 66:929, 1998.
221. Ochsner JL, Moseley PW, Mills NL, Bower PJ: Long-term follow-up of internal mammary artery myocardial implantation. Ann Thorac Surg 23:118, 1977.
222. Ojha M, Leask RL, Johnston KW, et al: Histology and morphology of 59 internal thoracic artery grafts and their distal anastomoses. Ann Thorac Surg 70:1338, 2000.
223. O'Neill BJ: Clinical data: AVERT and QUO VADIS. Can J Cardiol 16(Suppl E):32E, 2000.
224. Ono M, Wolf RK, Angouras D, Schneeberger EW: Early experience of coronary artery bypass grafting with a new self-closing clip device. J Thorac Cardiovasc Surg 123:783, 2002.
225. Osswald BR, Blackstone EH, Tochtermann U, et al: Does the completeness of revascularization affect early survival after coronary artery bypass grafting in elderly patients? Eur J Cardiothorac Surg 20:120, 2001.
226. Ovrum E, Tangen G, Schiott C, Dragsund S: Rapid recovery protocol applied to 5,658 consecutive “on-pump” coronary bypass patients. Ann Thorac Surg 70:2008, 2000.
226a. Possati A, Goudino M, Prati F, et al: Long-term results of the radial artery used for myocardial revascularization. Circulation 108:1350, 2003.
227. Peterson LR, McKenzie CR, Ludbrook PA, et al: Value of saphenous vein graft markers during subsequent diagnostic cardiac catheterization. Ann Thorac Surg 68:2263, 1999.
228. Pfisterer ME, Kloter-Weber UC, Huber M, et al: Prevention of supraventricular tachyarrhythmias after open heart operation by low-dose sotalol: a prospective, double-blind, randomized, placebo-controlled study. Ann Thorac Surg 64:1113, 1997.

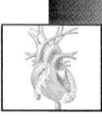

229. Quintilio C, Voci P, Bilotta F, et al: Risk factors of incomplete distribution of cardioplegic solution during coronary artery grafting. J Thorac Cardiovasc Surg 109:439, 1995.
230. Rand RP, Cochran RP, Aziz S, et al: Prospective trial of catheter irrigation and muscle flaps for sternal wound infection. Ann Thorac Surg 65:1046, 1998.
231. Rao V, Ivanov J, Weisel RD, et al: Predictors of low cardiac output syndrome after coronary artery bypass. J Thorac Cardiovasc Surg 112:38, 1996.
232. Rao V, Komeda M, Weisel RD, et al: Should the pericardium be closed routinely after heart operations? Ann Thorac Surg 67:484, 1999.
233. Reinecke H, Fetsch T, Roeder N, et al: Emergency coronary artery bypass grafting after failed coronary angioplasty: what has changed in a decade? Ann Thorac Surg 70:1997, 2000.
234. Ricci M, Salerno TA, Houck JP: Manubrium-sparing sternotomy and off-pump coronary artery bypass grafting in patients with tracheal stoma. Ann Thorac Surg 70:679, 2000.
235. Risk factors for deep sternal wound infection after sternotomy: a prospective, multicenter study. J Thorac Cardiovasc Surg 111:1200, 1996.
236. Roach GW, Kanchuger M, Mangano CM, et al: Adverse cerebral outcomes after coronary bypass surgery. Multicenter Study of Perioperative Ischemia Research Group and the Ischemia Research and Education Foundation Investigators. N Engl J Med 335:1857, 1996.
237. Rodriguez A, Bernardi V, Navia J, et al: Argentine Randomized Study: Coronary Angioplasty with Stenting versus Coronary Bypass Surgery in patients with Multiple-Vessel Disease (ERACI II): 30-day and one-year follow-up results. ERACI II Investigators. J Am Coll Cardiol 37:51, 2001.
238. Rodriguez A, Boullon F, Perez-Balino N, et al: Argentine randomized trial of percutaneous transluminal coronary angioplasty versus coronary artery bypass surgery in multivessel disease (ERACI): in-hospital results and 1-year follow-up. ERACI Group. J Am Coll Cardiol 22:1060, 1993.
239. Rodriguez RA, Giachino A, Hosking M, Nathan HJ: Transcranial Doppler characteristics of different embolic materials during in vivo testing. J Neuroimaging 12:259, 2002.
240. Rubens FD, Ruel M, Fremes SE: A new and simplified method for coronary and graft imaging during CABG. Heart Surg Forum 5:141, 2002.
241. Ruel MA, Rubens FD: Non-pharmacological strategies for blood conservation in cardiac surgery. Can J Anaesth 48:S13, 2001.
242. Ruel MA, Wang F, Bourke ME, et al: Is tranexamic acid safe in patients undergoing coronary endarterectomy? Ann Thorac Surg 71:1508, 2001.
243. Ruengsakulrach P, Sinclair R, Komeda M, et al: Comparative histopathology of radial artery versus internal thoracic artery and risk factors for development of intimal hyperplasia and atherosclerosis. Circulation 100:II139, 1999.
244. Sabik JF, Lytle BW, McCarthy PM, Cosgrove DM: Axillary artery: an alternative site of arterial cannulation for patients with extensive aortic and peripheral vascular disease. J Thorac Cardiovasc Surg 109:885, 1995.
245. Saginur R, Croteau D, Bergeron MG: Comparative efficacy of teicoplanin and cefazolin for cardiac operation prophylaxis in 3027 patients. The ESPRIT Group. J Thorac Cardiovasc Surg 120:1120, 2000.
246. Salasidis GC, Latter DA, Steinmetz OK, et al: Carotid artery duplex scanning in preoperative assessment for coronary artery revascularization: the association between peripheral vascular disease, carotid artery stenosis, and stroke. J Vasc Surg 21:154, 1995.
247. Sasajima T, Wu MH, Shi Q, et al: Effect of skeletonizing dissection on the internal thoracic artery. Ann Thorac Surg 65:1009, 1998.
248. Sauve JS, Thorpe KE, Sackett DL, et al: Can bruits distinguish high-grade from moderate symptomatic carotid stenosis? The North American Symptomatic Carotid Endarterectomy Trial. Ann Intern Med 120:633, 1994.
249. Schelbert HR: Measurements of myocardial metabolism in patients with ischemic heart disease. Am J Cardiol 82:61K, 1998.
250. Schwartz L, Kip KE, Frye RL, et al: Coronary bypass graft patency in patients with diabetes in the Bypass Angioplasty Revascularization Investigation (BARI). Circulation 106:2652, 2002.
251. Scott R, Blackstone EH, McCarthy PM, et al: Isolated bypass grafting of the left internal thoracic artery to the left anterior descending coronary artery: late consequences of incomplete revascularization. J Thorac Cardiovasc Surg 120:173, 2000.
252. Sedlis SP, Morrison DA, Lorin JD, et al: Percutaneous coronary intervention versus coronary bypass graft surgery for diabetic patients with unstable angina and risk factors for adverse outcomes with bypass: outcome of diabetic patients in the AWESOME randomized trial and registry. J Am Coll Cardiol 40:1555, 2002.
253. Selnes OA, Goldsborough MA, Borowicz LM Jr, et al: Determinants of cognitive change after coronary artery bypass surgery: a multifactorial problem. Ann Thorac Surg 67:1669, 1999.
254. Sergeant P, Blackstone E, Meyns B: Is return of angina after coronary artery bypass grafting immutable, can it be delayed, and is it important? J Thorac Cardiovasc Surg 116:440, 1998.
255. Serruys PW, Unger F, Sousa JE, et al: Comparison of coronary-artery bypass surgery and stenting for the treatment of multivessel disease. N Engl J Med 344:1117, 2001.
256. Seven-year outcome in the Bypass Angioplasty Revascularization Investigation (BARI) by treatment and diabetic status. J Am Coll Cardiol 35:1122, 2000.
257. Shapira OM, Alkon JD, Macron DS, et al: Nitroglycerin is preferable to diltiazem for prevention of coronary bypass conduit spasm. Ann Thorac Surg 70:883, 2000.
258. Shapira OM, Xu A, Vita JA, et al: Nitroglycerin is superior to diltiazem as a coronary bypass conduit vasodilator. J Thorac Cardiovasc Surg 117:906, 1999.
259. Shin H, Yozu R, Mitsumaru A, et al: Intraoperative assessment of coronary artery bypass graft: transit-time flowmetry versus angiography. Ann Thorac Surg 72:1562, 2001.
260. Simchen E, Galai N, Braun D, et al: Sociodemographic and clinical factors associated with low quality of life one year after coronary bypass operations: the Israeli coronary artery bypass study (ISCAB). J Thorac Cardiovasc Surg 121:909, 2001.
261. Sjoland H, Caidahl K, Wiklund I, et al: Impact of coronary artery bypass grafting on various aspects of quality of life. Eur J Cardiothorac Surg 12:612, 1997.
262. Sones FM, Shirey EK: Cine coronary arteriography. Mod Concepts Cardiovasc Dis 31:735, 1962.
263. Spence PA, Montgomery WD, Santamore WP: High flow demand on small arterial coronary bypass conduits promotes graft spasm. J Thorac Cardiovasc Surg 110:952, 1995.
264. Spiess BD, Ley C, Body SC, et al: Hematocrit value on intensive care unit entry influences the frequency of Q-wave myocardial infarction after coronary artery bypass grafting. The Institutions of the Multicenter Study of Perioperative Ischemia (McSPI) Research Group. J Thorac Cardiovasc Surg 116:460, 1998.
265. Stahle E, Tammelin A, Bergstrom R, et al: Sternal wound complications—incidence, microbiology and risk factors. Eur J Cardiothorac Surg 11:1146, 1997.
266. Starnes SL, Wolk SW, Lampman RM, et al: Noninvasive evaluation of hand circulation before radial artery harvest for

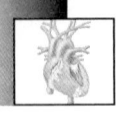

coronary artery bypass grafting. J Thorac Cardiovasc Surg 117:261, 1999.
267. Stoll C, Schelling G, Goetz AE, et al: Health-related quality of life and post-traumatic stress disorder in patients after cardiac surgery and intensive care treatment. J Thorac Cardiovasc Surg 120:505, 2000.
268. Stump DA, Rogers AT, Hammon JW, Newman SP: Cerebral emboli and cognitive outcome after cardiac surgery. J Cardiothorac Vasc Anesth 10:113, 1996.
269. Suda Y, Takeuchi Y, Ban T, et al: Twenty-two-year follow-up of saphenous vein grafts in pediatric Kawasaki disease. Ann Thorac Surg 70:1706, 2000.
270. Suematsu Y, Takamoto S, Ohtsuka T: Intraoperative echocardiographic imaging of coronary arteries and graft anastomoses during coronary artery bypass grafting without cardiopulmonary bypass. J Thorac Cardiovasc Surg 122:1147, 2001.
271. Suma H, Isomura T, Horii T, Sato T: Late angiographic result of using the right gastroepiploic artery as a graft. J Thorac Cardiovasc Surg 120:496, 2000.
272. Suzuki A, Kay EB, Hardy JD: Direct anastomosis of the bilateral internal mammary artery to the distal coronary artery, without a magnifier, for severe diffuse coronary atherosclerosis. Circulation 48:III190, 1973.
273. Sylivris S, Calafiore P, Matalanis G, et al: The intraoperative assessment of ascending aortic atheroma: epiaortic imaging is superior to both transesophageal echocardiography and direct palpation. J Cardiothorac Vasc Anesth 11:704, 1997.
274. Sylivris S, Levi C, Matalanis G, et al: Pattern and significance of cerebral microemboli during coronary artery bypass grafting. Ann Thorac Surg 66:1674, 1998.
275. Taggart DP, D'Amico R, Altman DG: Effect of arterial revascularisation on survival: a systematic review of studies comparing bilateral and single internal mammary arteries. Lancet 358:870, 2001.
276. Taggart DP, Browne SM, Halligan PW, Wade DT: Is cardiopulmonary bypass still the cause of cognitive dysfunction after cardiac operations? J Thorac Cardiovasc Surg 118:414, 1999.
277. Takach TJ, Beggs ML, Nykamp VJ, Reul GJ Jr: Concomitant cerebral and coronary subclavian steal. Ann Thorac Surg 63:853, 1997.
278. Takami Y, Ina H: Relation of intraoperative flow measurement with postoperative quantitative angiographic assessment of coronary artery bypass grafting. Ann Thorac Surg 72:1270, 2001.
279. Takami Y, Ina H: Effects of skeletonization on intraoperative flow and anastomosis diameter of internal thoracic arteries in coronary artery bypass grafting. Ann Thorac Surg 73:1441, 2002.
280. Tashiro T, Nakamura K, Sukehiro S, et al: Midterm results of free internal thoracic artery grafting for myocardial revascularization. Ann Thorac Surg 65:951, 1998.
281. Tewari P, Aggarwal SK: Combined left-sided recurrent laryngeal and phrenic nerve palsy after coronary artery operation. Ann Thorac Surg 61:1721, 1996.
282. Thatte HS, Khuri SF: The coronary artery bypass conduit: I. Intraoperative endothelial injury and its implication on graft patency. Ann Thorac Surg 72:S2245, 2001.
283. Tomasco B, Cappiello A, Fiorilli R, et al: Surgical revascularization for acute coronary insufficiency: analysis of risk factors for hospital mortality. Ann Thorac Surg 64:678, 1997.
284. Trehan N, Mishra M, Kasliwal RR, Mishra A: Surgical strategies in patients at high risk for stroke undergoing coronary artery bypass grafting. Ann Thorac Surg 70:1037, 2000.
285. Trick WE, Scheckler WE, Tokars JI, et al: Modifiable risk factors associated with deep sternal site infection after coronary artery bypass grafting. J Thorac Cardiovasc Surg 119:108, 2000.
286. Ura M, Sakata R, Nakayama Y, et al: Analysis by early angiography of right internal thoracic artery grafting via the transverse sinus: predictors of graft failure. Circulation 101:640, 2000.
287. Ura M, Sakata R, Nakayama Y, et al: Technical aspects and outcome of in situ right internal thoracic artery grafting to the major branches of the circumflex artery via the transverse sinus. Ann Thorac Surg 71:1485, 2001.
288. Uva MS, Braunberger E, Fisher M, et al: Does bilateral internal thoracic artery grafting increase surgical risk in diabetic patients? Ann Thorac Surg 66:2051, 1998.
289. Varnauskas E: Twelve-year follow-up of survival in the randomized European Coronary Surgery Study. N Engl J Med 319:332, 1988.
290. van Son JA, Falk V, Walther T, et al: Low-grade intimal hyperplasia in internal mammary and right gastroepiploic arteries as bypass grafts. Ann Thorac Surg 63:706, 1997.
291. Velez DA, Morris CD, Muraki S, et al: Brief pretreatment of radial artery conduits with phenoxybenzamine prevents vasoconstriction long term. Ann Thorac Surg 72:1977, 2001.
292. Vermes E, Mesguich M, Houel R, et al: Cardiac troponin I release after open heart surgery: a marker of myocardial protection? Ann Thorac Surg 70:2087, 2000.
293. Vineberg AM: Development of an anastomosis between the coronary vessels and a transplanted internal mammary artery. Can Med Assoc J 55:117, 1946.
294. Vural KM, Sener E, Tasdemir O: Long-term patency of sequential and individual saphenous vein coronary bypass grafts. Eur J Cardiothorac Surg 19:140, 2001.
295. Walpoth BH, Muller MF, Genyk I, et al: Evaluation of coronary bypass flow with color-Doppler and magnetic resonance imaging techniques: comparison with intraoperative flow measurements. Eur J Cardiothorac Surg 15:795, 1999.
296. Wareing TH, Davila-Roman VG, Daily BB, et al: Strategy for the reduction of stroke incidence in cardiac surgical patients. Ann Thorac Surg 55:1400, 1993.
297. Weintraub WS, Becker ER, Mauldin PD, et al: Costs of revascularization over eight years in the randomized and eligible patients in the Emory Angioplasty versus Surgery Trial (EAST). Am J Cardiol 86:747, 2000.
298. Wendler O, Hennen B, Markwirth T, et al: T grafts with the right internal thoracic artery to left internal thoracic artery versus the left internal thoracic artery and radial artery: flow dynamics in the internal thoracic artery main stem. J Thorac Cardiovasc Surg 118:841, 1999.
299. Wendler O, Tscholl D, Huang Q, Schafers HJ: Free flow capacity of skeletonized versus pedicled internal thoracic artery grafts in coronary artery bypass grafts. Eur J Cardiothorac Surg 15:247, 1999.
300. Whitlow PL, Dimas AP, Bashore TM, et al: Relationship of extent of revascularization with angina at one year in the Bypass Angioplasty Revascularization Investigation (BARI). J Am Coll Cardiol 34:1750, 1999.
301. Yoshikawa Y, Yagihara T, Kameda Y, et al: Result of surgical treatments in patients with coronary-arterial obstructive disease after Kawasaki disease. Eur J Cardiothorac Surg 17:515, 2000.
302. Yusuf S, Zucker D, Peduzzi P, et al: Effect of coronary artery bypass graft surgery on survival: overview of 10-year results from randomised trials by the Coronary Artery Bypass Graft Surgery Trialists Collaboration. Lancet 344:563, 1994.
303. Zerr KJ, Furnary AP, Grunkemeier GL, et al: Glucose control lowers the risk of wound infection in diabetics after open heart operations. Ann Thorac Surg 63:356, 1997.

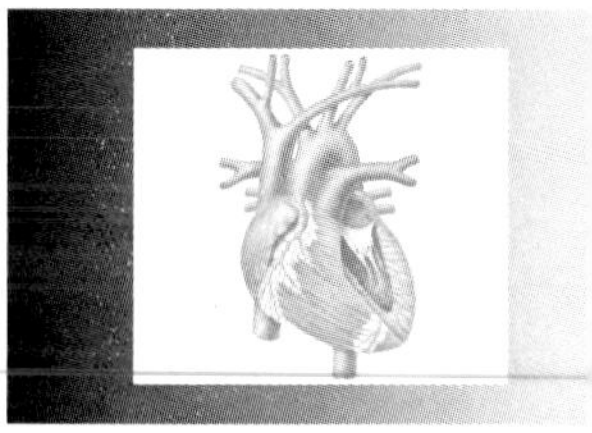

Alternative Approaches to Surgical Coronary Artery Bypass Grafting

CHAPTER 83

William E. Cohn and Audrey Rosinberg

INTRODUCTION

In 1967, Sabiston and colleagues reported the first clinically successful coronary artery bypass grafting (CABG). Other early pioneers included Favaloro, who is credited with popularizing the use of autogenous saphenous vein, and Kolesov, who performed the first mammary artery-to-coronary anastomosis. Over the several years that followed, centers around the world began performing the procedure in large numbers. Subsequent refinements in cardiopulmonary bypass (CPB), the introduction of cardioplegia, the growing acceptance of the left internal mammary graft, and the development of the intraaortic balloon pump resulted in continued improvements in outcome after CABG. By the early 1990s, over 350,000 procedures were being performed each year in the United States, with routine application in octogenarians, patients with severely impaired ventricular function, and patients with serious noncardiac morbidities.

As results continued to improve, and mortality and major morbidity rates in the 2% range became commonplace, many surgeons turned their efforts toward decreasing the invasiveness of CABG. Over the past several years, this effort has produced a number of variations of the traditional CABG intended to avoid CPB, minimize aortic manipulation, and minimize the trauma associated with surgical access. These variations include multivessel CABG without CPB, single-vessel CABG without CPB by way of a left minithoracotomy, videoscopic single-vessel CABG utilizing surgical robotics, and multivessel CABG by way of left minithoracotomy utilizing peripheral cannulation and CPB. Other new procedures include reoperative CABG through alternative incisions and grafting strategies and devices that minimize or eliminate aortic manipulation. This chapter describes these operations, discusses their relative merits, and summarizes current clinical results.

CARDIOPULMONARY BYPASS

Arguably, the development of the heart–lung machine by Gibbon and its early application by Kirklin were among the most important advances in the ultimate growth of CABG surgery. CPB, and ultimately the introduction of cardioplegia, provided a motionless, blood-free surgical field, which enabled the precision and reproducibility necessary for direct coronary anastomosis. Despite the obvious benefits of CPB, however, there is an increasing awareness of the potential deleterious effects. As the formed elements of the blood come in contact with the surfaces of the various components of the heart–lung machine, they are activated, resulting in a number of hematological and ultimately systemic changes. Typical sequelae include activation of complement, release of endotoxin, activation of leukocytes, increased expression of adhesion molecules, and release of inflammatory mediators, including cytokines, arachidonic acid metabolites, and free radicals to name but a few.[77] These sequelae occasionally manifest as coagulopathy, third-space fluid retention, and subtle end-organ dysfunction, including neurocognitive changes. The magnitude of this systemic inflammatory response (SIR) is generally modest, but can be quite severe, especially when the time on CPB is prolonged. Furthermore, it is well recognized that a small percentage of patients with preoperative end-organ dysfunction suffer significant morbidity when subjected to even a moderate degree of SIR.

Ongoing efforts have been directed at reducing the magnitude of the SIR associated with CPB. These efforts include decreasing the surface area and modifying the surface composition of the CPB circuit to minimize surface activation, minimizing hemodilution by decreasing the volume of crystalloid prime needed to institute CPB, avoiding the use of a cardiotomy sucker, and pretreating patients with various antiinflammatory medications, such as Trasylol.[43] Despite progress in these areas, performing CABG without CPB remains attractive.

MULTIVESSEL OFF-PUMP CORONARY ARTERY BYPASS

Off-pump coronary artery bypass grafting (OP-CAB) is as old as coronary surgery itself. Large case series dating back to the 1970s document its feasibility.[2,42,72] Nevertheless, OP-CAB only recently gained widespread acceptance and entered the mainstream of clinical practice, propelled by a greater awareness of the potential morbidity of cardiopulmonary bypass and aortic manipulation, and facilitated by improvements in surgical tools and techniques. OP-CAB is part of the procedural armamentarium of a growing proportion of surgeons worldwide and can be performed in virtually any patient requiring coronary revascularization.

The introduction of self-retaining coronary stabilizers and the development of techniques for their use are key factors that have led to resurgent interest in OP-CAB. When properly used, coronary stabilizers provide a relatively motionless and blood-free field, similar to that provided by CPB. The subsequent introduction of self-retaining cardiac positioning devices and the evolution of surgical techniques for rotating the heart enable precise anastomoses to be constructed on the inferior, posterior, and lateral walls of the beating heart while maintaining adequate hemodynamics without CPB.

Self-Retaining Coronary Stabilizers

A number of coronary artery stabilizers are available for clinical use. Current stabilizers can be categorized as compression, suction, or capture devices, depending on their design. Each type provides excellent immobility when used properly.

Compression-type stabilizers are generally two-pronged forks that are placed lightly on the epicardial surface such that the prongs are parallel to and flanking the coronary artery at the intended anastomotic site. The under surface of the prongs is designed to provide traction to avoid slippage. The fork is attached by way of an articulating arm to the retractor and can be locked tightly in position once the desired position has been achieved. Generally, the best stability occurs when only light downward force is used on the surface of the heart. Paradoxically, an increase in motion occurs when excessive downward force is applied. As such, the exposure techniques described later in this chapter should be used to present the target artery prior to positioning the stabilizer, rather than relying on the stabilizer to retract the heart. Compression-type stabilizers are advantageous in that they set up quickly and simply, and have an extremely low profile to allow unrestricted access to the coronary. For some aspects of the heart, however, slightly more downward pressure may be required with compression stabilizers to avoid slippage (Figure 83-1).

Suction-type stabilizers also are generally two-pronged forks attached to the retractor by means of an articulating arm. These stabilizers, however, are constructed with a series of ports on the undersurface of the prongs connected by sterile tubing to −100 to −300 mm Hg wall suction. The epicardium and epicardial fat flanking the vessel is sucked into these ports allowing the stabilizer to grip the surface of the heart. As such, less downward force is required at the anastomotic site. Suction stabilizers also set up quickly but require a regulated vacuum line. They have the added advantage of providing traction and countertraction of the fat surrounding the coronary, making them well suited for coronaries deep within the fat. Suction stabilizers tend to be slightly higher profile than compression types but, generally, access to the coronary is not problematic (Figure 83-2).

Capture-type stabilizers are usually fenestrated platforms that frame the intended anastomotic site. Silicone elastic tapes are passed deep to the coronary and locked to the platform under tension, pulling the epicardium up against the platform's undersurface (Figure 83-3A). Like suction, this

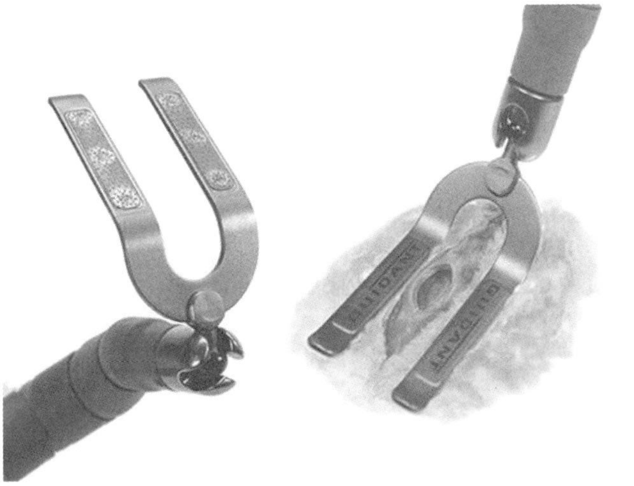

Figure 83–1 Compressive-type stabilizers are generally low profile, and have a textured bottom surface to improve their ability to grip the epicardium.

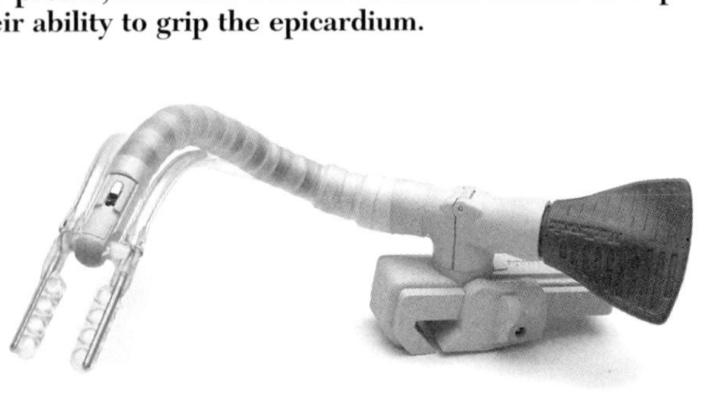

Figure 83–2 Vacuum-assisted stabilizers use a series of suction cups to grip the epicardium. Although slightly higher profile, they often require less downward force than compressive footplates.

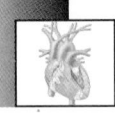

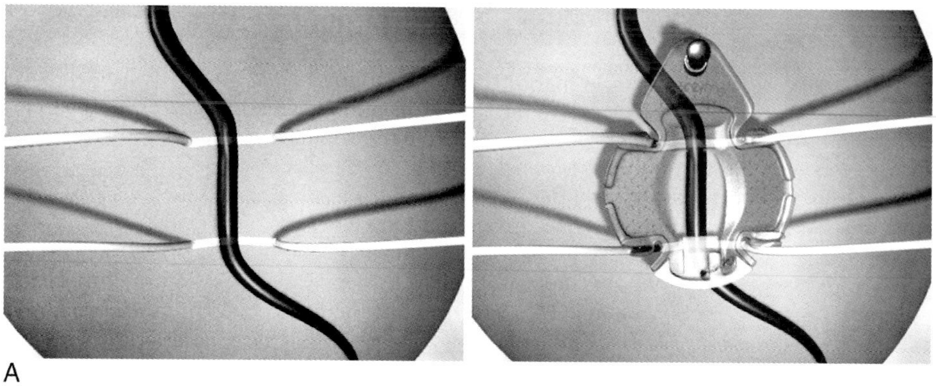

A

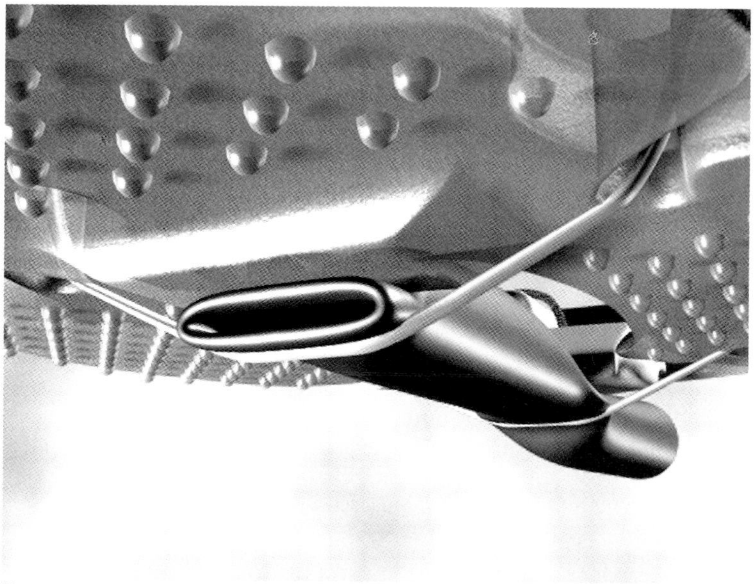

B

Figure 83–3 A, B, Capture-type stabilizers use silicone elastic tapes to ensure tight apposition of the textured surface of the footplate and the epicardial surface. This arrangement results in integrated coronary compression

effect reduces the demand for downward force to prevent slippage. Capture stabilizers, by virtue of their circumferential stabilization, provide superior anastomotic stability.[19] Additionally, the silicone elastic tapes compress the coronary against the platform's posterior aspect, providing integrated biplaner coronary occlusion (Figure 83-3B). Capture stabilizers arguably are more complex to position, however, and require proper spacing and alignment of the silicone elastic tapes to ensure adequate hemostasis. Furthermore, because of their larger size, they may not be well suited if tightly spaced sequential anastomoses are being constructed.

Maintaining Hemodynamic Stability during Multivessel OP-CAB

One of the greatest challenges in the early OP-CABs was maintaining hemodynamic stability while grafting coronaries on the lateral and posterolateral aspects of the heart. This challenge was greatest in patients with poor ventricular function and marginally compensated ischemia. Advances in surgical techniques including placement of deep pericardial retraction sutures, right vertical pericardiotomy and pleurotomy, and right hemisternal elevation, as well as the introduction of cardiac positioning devices and advances in anesthetic management, have largely eliminated this problem. To understand how these tools and techniques minimize the adverse effects of cardiac manipulation, it is important to understand the etiology of potential hemodynamic comprise when performing OP-CAB.

Mechanisms of Adverse Hemodynamic Effects

Left Ventricle

When a coronary stabilizer is positioned using excessive downward force, the stabilized aspect of the heart is constrained leading to diastolic dysfunction and decreased left ventricular end-diastolic volume (LVEDV), stroke volume, and cardiac output.[9] While volume loading and Trendelenburg positioning attenuate these effects by elevating left ventricular filling pressures, their recourse carries a risk of exacerbating intraoperative third space fluid sequestration and associated morbidity. Similarly, the use of short-acting α-adrenergic agents can effectively maintain perfusion pressure in this setting, but may be associated with an increased risk of perioperative mesenteric ischemia.[59] β-Adrenergic agents should similarly be avoided in the setting of yet-to-be-grafted coronary disease. There are also anecdotal reports of severe mitral regurgitation during exposure of the lateral wall, possibly related to deformation of subvalvular structures in combination with coronary insufficiency. Exposure techniques that minimize or eliminate left ventricular deformation are therefore desirable.

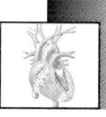

Right Ventricle

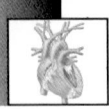

Exposure of the lateral wall of the left ventricle displaces the heart toward the right, resulting in the right ventricle being compressed against the pericardium and right side of the sternum. The relatively low pressure in the right ventricle makes it particularly vulnerable to deformation and reduction in right ventricular end-diastolic volume (RVEDV).[31,49] The decreased right ventricular stroke volume leads to poor left ventricular filling, and a drop in cardiac output. Volume loading and Trendelenburg positioning can compensate for this effect, as noted above, but not without potential risk. Right ventricular compromise is thought by many to be the dominant cause in many cases of hemodynamic instability that occur during exposure of the lateral wall. Various groups have proposed the use of right ventricular assist as palliation for right ventricular compromise during multivessel OP-CAB.[44,60] Clearly, however, exposure techniques that minimize right ventricular deformation are desirable.

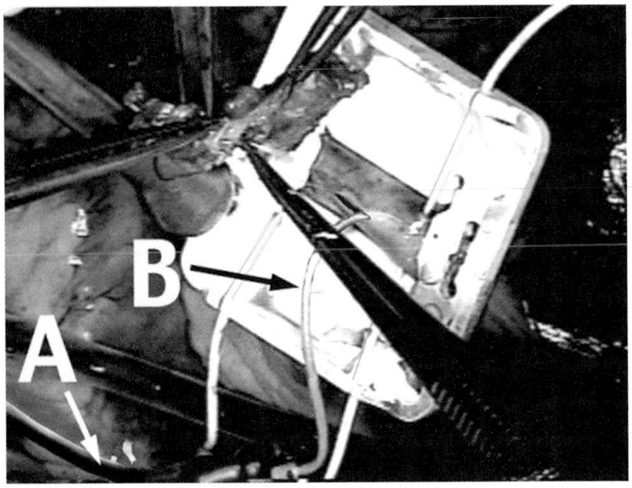

Figure 83–4 **A shunt connected to a 5 french cannula in the ascending aorta inserted into the coronary artery distal to the arteriotomy may be used to maintain brisk coronary flow while the graft is being constructed.**

Coronary Insufficiency

Intraoperative coronary insufficiency, secondary to decompensated coronary disease, transient coronary snaring during grafting, or poor perfusion pressure during heart manipulation, constitutes another mechanism that leads to hemodynamic instability. Communicating closely with the anesthesiologist, planning a revascularization strategy that minimizes myocardial ischemia, and using exposure techniques that maintain hemodynamic stability best prevent it. Although each patient should be managed on an individual basis, useful axioms exist. Patients with significant left main stenosis and marginally compensated ischemia may benefit from completion of the left internal mammary artery (LIMA)-to-left anterior descending (LAD) graft prior to manipulating the heart. Similarly, initial revascularization of occluded, collateralized coronary arteries should be carried out prior to transiently occluding those vessels that supply collaterals to them. The selective use of intracoronary shunts, aorta-coronary shunts, or assisted coronary perfusion devices[34] can be essential when grafting a moderately stenosed right coronary artery (RCA) proximal to the origin of the posterior descending branch (PDA), or a moderately stenosed LAD when grafting the proximal portion (Figure 83-4). The judicious use of an intraaortic balloon pump (IABP) can occasionally prove invaluable.[37]

Exposure Techniques

Depending on the size and shape of the patient's heart and the dimensions of the chest cavity, visualization of the proximal obtuse marginal and posterolateral branches of the circumflex system may be obstructed by the left hemisternum. Although intuitive attempts at improving exposure may involve applying additional rightward force to that aspect of the heart with the stabilizer, this maneuver frequently leads to hemodynamic compromise as well as paradoxically poor stabilization. Maximized access and stability at the anastomotic site with minimal compromise of cardiac performance are most readily achieved when the stabilizer is applied with little or no pressure: thus, coronary stabilizers should be used only to stabilize the anastomotic field rather than assist at retracting the heart. Exposure is best obtained with maneuvers such as the use of deep pericardial sutures, right pleurotomy and pericardiotomy, right hemisternal elevation, and apical suction devices, each of which is described below.

Deep Pericardial Sutures

One of the most important advances in exposure techniques for OP-CAB has been the use of deep pericardial sutures. First described by Lima,[45] these sutures, when placed under tension, create a ridge of pericardium that supports the base of the lateral left ventricle adjacent to the atrioventricular groove and allows the heart to be rotated rightward to assume an "apex-up" position (Figure 83-5). In this subluxed position, the apex of the heart points toward the ceiling and protrudes through the sternotomy incision, often above the plane of the sternal retractor. This generally allows for adequate exposure of the lateral and inferior aspects of the left ventricle prior to applying the coronary stabilizer.

Placement of deep pericardial sutures may vary between surgeons and according to the patient's anatomy. Generally, one or two 2-0 silk sutures are placed in the pericardium posterior to the left phrenic nerve immediately anterior to one or both left pulmonary veins, one deep in the oblique sinus behind the left atrium, and one to the left and posterior to the inferior vena cava (Figure 83-6). Care must be taken when placing these sutures to avoid injury to underlying structures such as the esophagus and lung.[79] The suture in the oblique sinus is particularly important to obtain good exposure of the lateral wall near the base of the heart. One commonly used technique consists of placing a single deep pericardial suture in this location, which is used to secure the midpoint of a 50-cm gauze strip deep in the oblique sinus. Subsequent traction on the two ends of the strip can then be adjusted to optimize exposure of different surfaces of the heart.

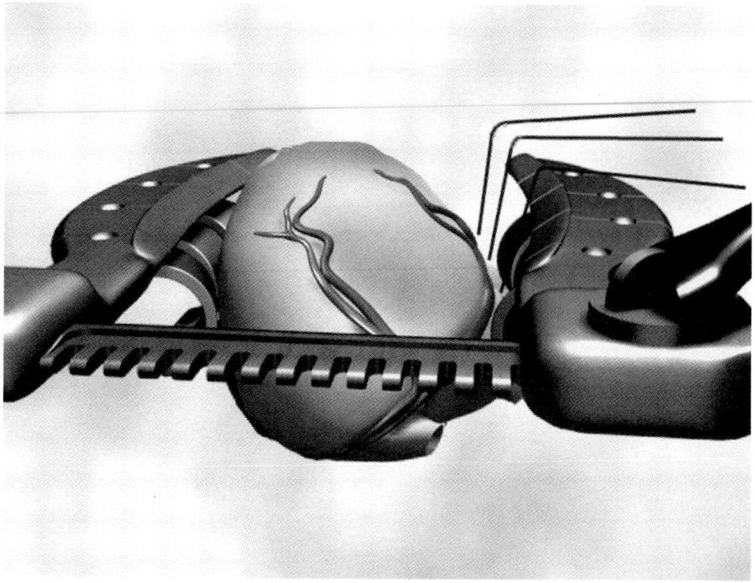

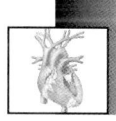

Figure 83–5 Deep pericardial sutures secured under tension deliver the heart into an "apex-up" position that provides adequate exposure of the lateral wall in many patients.

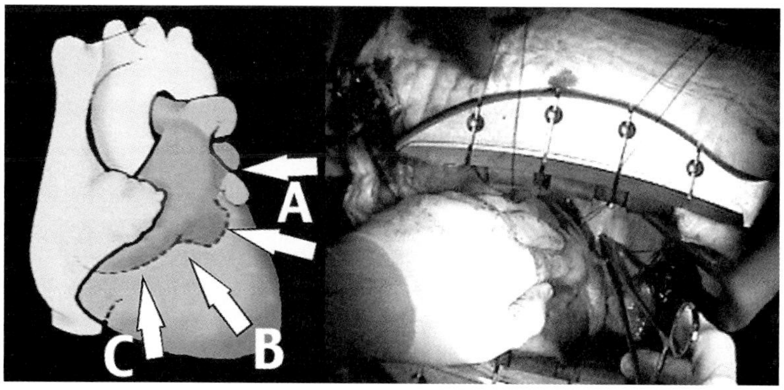

Figure 83–6 The diagram shows the approximate locations for the deep pericardial sutures. Most surgeons agree that the suture at "B" is of greatest importance for lateral wall exposure. The photo demonstrates operative exposure for placing the deep pericardial sutures, with the heart reflected up and to the right.

Regardless of the technique used, deep pericardial traction sutures generally allow for presentation of the lateral, inferior, and even posterior wall of the heart with little change in left ventricular geometry or left ventricular end-diastolic volume (LVEDV), providing adequate access for multivessel CABG while maintaining hemodynamic stability. In some patients, however, some or all of the additional maneuvers outlined below are necessary to effectively accomplish this aim.

Right Pleurotomy and Right Vertical Pericardiotomy

Right pleurotomy and right vertical pericardiotomy constitute helpful technical adjuncts for patients in whom lateral wall exposure is difficult. Human pericardium is quite flexible but very inelastic. This inelasticity accounts for the profound hemodynamic effects caused by acute tamponade despite a relatively small volume of intrapericardial fluid. As such, the posterior pericardium, right lateral pericardium, and diaphragmatic pericardium constitute a fixed-volume cusp or pocket. It is into this pocket that the right ventricle is compressed during extreme rightward rotation of the heart. In effect, pressure on the left ventricle results in right ventricular tamponade. Opening the right pleura widely and incising the pericardium vent the pocket, allowing the heart to herniate into the right pleural space while maintaining RVEDV.

Right lateral pericardiotomy can be performed with a right vertical incision extending from the cut edge of the initial anterior pericardiotomy, 2 cm cephalad and parallel to the diaphragm, down to the level of the inferior vena cava with care taken to avoid injury to the right phrenic nerve (Figure 83-7). The 2-cm rim of pericardium on the diaphragm facilitates closure of the pericardiotomy once grafting is complete. Caution should be exercised in measuring right-sided grafts as closure of the lateral pericardial incision may affect their lie. In some circumstances, one may also benefit from removing the right pericardiophrenic fat pad, which can be quite large, and decreasing tidal volume to provide additional room for the easily deformed right ventricle.

Some surgeons skilled in the OP-CAB procedure avoid right pleurotomy and lateral pericardiotomy on the contention that incising the lateral pericardium and entering an additional body cavity are inconsistent with the objective of decreased invasiveness. Although many cases can indeed be performed successfully without it, this maneuver in our opinion facilitates the reproducible performance of a precise anastomosis during multivessel OP-CAB. Furthermore, right pleurotomy does not leave a scar nor has it been associated with significant morbidity or additional length of stay after coronary surgery.

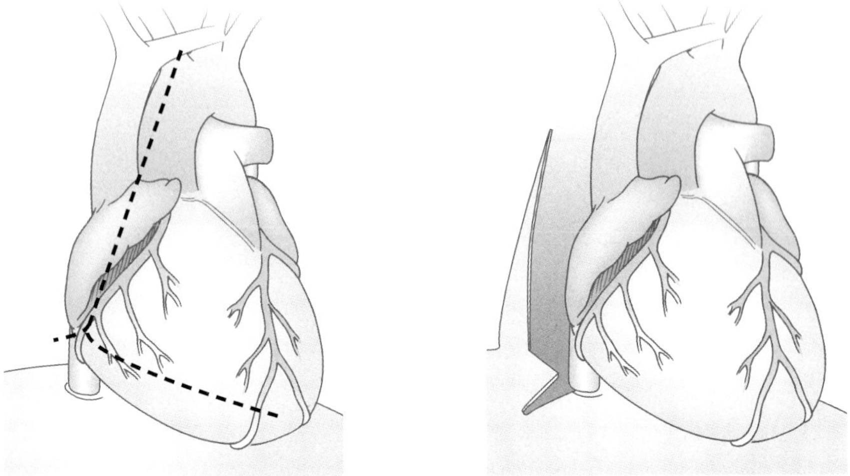

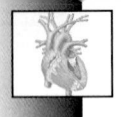

Figure 83–7 The right vertical pericardiotomy extends down the right side, parallel to the insertion of the pericardium into the diaphragm, toward the inferior vena cava. The right pleural space is opened widely as well.

Right Hemisternal Elevation

Asymmetrical right hemisternal elevation can further improve lateral wall exposure when used in conjunction with the techniques described above. Once the right pericardium and pleura are incised, the right half of the sternum and right blade of the retractor limit rightward displacement of the subluxed apex of the heart. By elevating these structures, the apex can clear the posterior aspect of the chest wall. This allows the entire heart to rotate into the right pleural space with little change in left and right ventricular geometry and end-diastolic volume (Figure 83-8). As a result of these maneuvers, the proximal obtuse marginal and posterolateral branches are brought toward the center of the operative field and into the surgeon's view.

Right hemisternal elevation is best accomplished if it is carried out as the sternotomy incision is being performed. By applying anterior traction on the right chest wall when the retractor is first spread, costal microfractures that inevitably form during sternal opening will predominantly occur in the right-sided ribs. The resulting increase in flexibility of the right chest wall will subsequently prevent the need for exaggerated tilting of the sternal retractor, which is often required to overcome the tendency of the left chest wall to rise after internal mammary artery harvest. The diaphragmatic insertion on the inferior aspect of the right hemisternum can also be released to facilitate right hemisternal elevation and create additional room for displacement of the apex of the heart into the right pleural space.

Apical Suction Devices

Recently, self-retaining apical suction retractors have been added to the operative armamentarium of OP-CAB surgeons. These tools are used to position the heart for exposure of its lateral and posterior surfaces with little impact on hemodynamics. These retractors generally consist of a suction cup mounted at the end of an articulating arm that can be locked in position relative to the retractor (Figure 83-9). The suction cup is placed at or near the apex of the heart and held in position by 300 mm Hg vacuum. Pulling the apex away from the base and pivoting the cardiac axis can achieve excellent exposure with little impact on left ventricular geometry and LVEDV. Although the use of these devices involves supplemental expenses in the conduct of OP-CAB, the easy affixation and their rapid setup make them an attractive adjunct for challenging patients. In many OP-CAB centers, apical suction retractors, in conjunction with right pleurotomy, vertical pericardiotomy, and sternal tilt, are used in the majority of cases (Figure 83-10).

Results after OP-CAB

The relative merit of OP-CAB, when compared to conventional CABG with CPB, remains unclear. Few topics in cardiac surgery have given rise to more debate. As a result, adoption of the OP-CAB technique has been sporadic. Current U.S. estimates (based on industry reports) suggest that between 18% and 25% of the 370,000 annual CABG

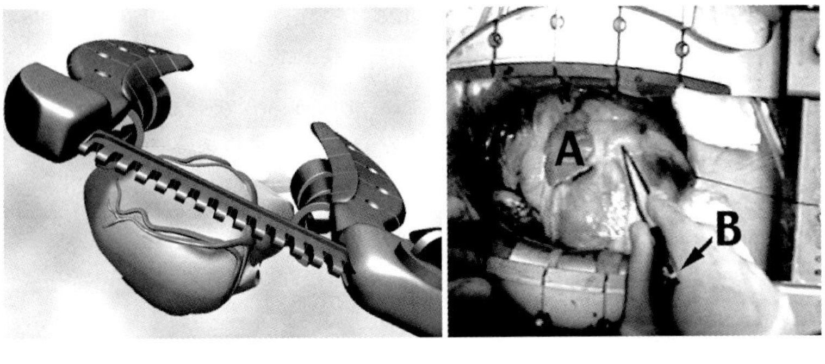

Figure 83–8 Tilting the right hemisternum, performing a vertical pericardiotomy, and opening the right pleura often allow one to position the apex of the heart in the right chest. Here the heart apex "A" is deep to the right hemisternum, and the left atrial appendage "B" is brought to the center of the operative field. This results in optimum exposure of the lateral wall, especially in patients with cardiomegaly.

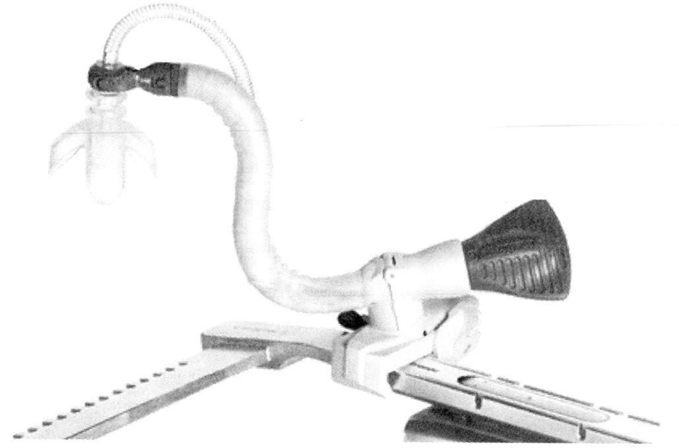

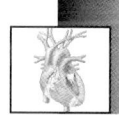

Figure 83–9 Apical suction devices allow one to rapidly position the heart without placement of deep pericardial sutures.

procedures are performed off pump. Interestingly, the small percentage of heart surgeons who perform predominantly OP-CAB perform the majority of these procedures, with the majority of surgeons performing fewer than 5% of their cases without CPB.

The well-documented low incidence of mortality and significant morbidity in the majority of both OP-CAB and conventional CABG patients compounds the difficulty in comparing these procedures.* As such, a large prospective randomized trial sufficient to show a statistical difference has not been performed to date. Several large retrospective, nonrandomized multicenter series have reported a lower incidence of death, stroke, IABP requirement, postoperative transfusion, time on ventilator, and length of stay for OP-CAB compared to contemporaneous conventional CABG at the same institutions† or to national database statistics.[15,55] The impact of selection bias, however, in determining operative technique for any given patient in these series may be a confounding variable. Similar results suggesting superiority of the OP-CAB procedure have been reported when propensity scores were used in an attempt to decrease the impact of selection bias.[47] Propensity scoring decreases dissimilarity

*References 3, 4, 11, 12, 15, 16, 35, 36, 46, 55–57.
†References 3, 11, 12, 16, 35, 36, 46, 56.

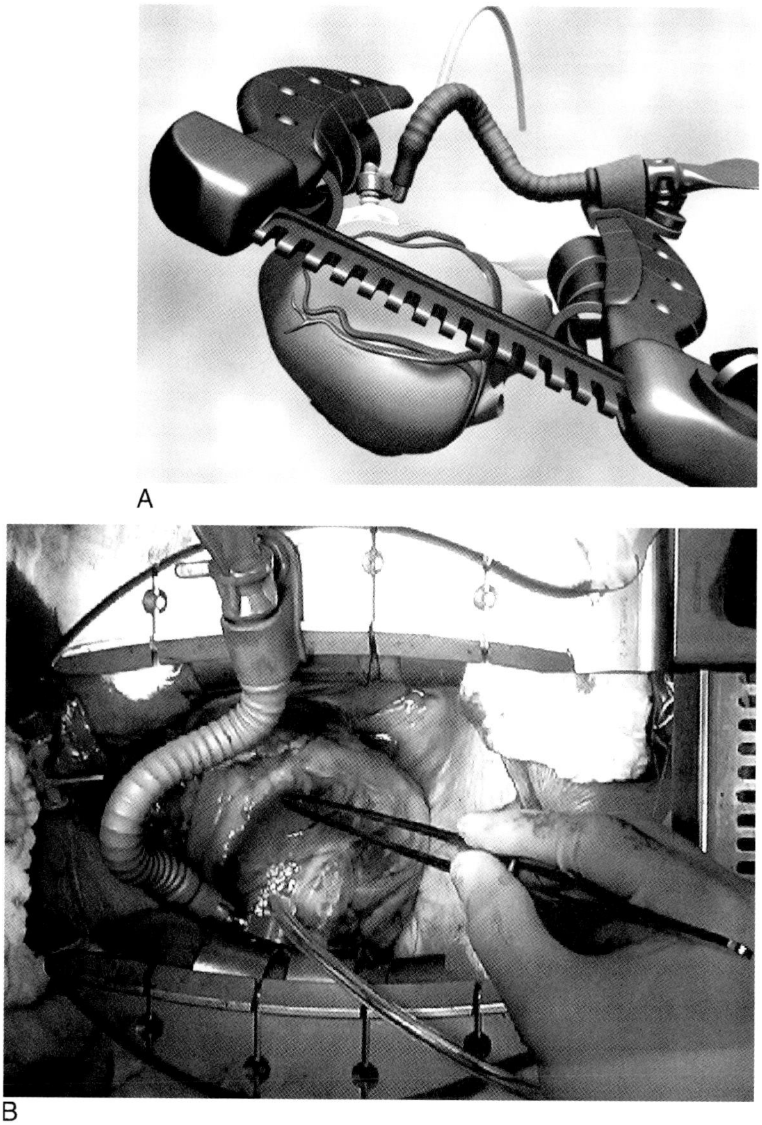

A

B

Figure 83–10 A, B, An apical suction device, when used in conjunction with right hemisternal elevation, vertical pericardiotomy, and right pleurotomy, provides optimal exposure of the high lateral wall.

between the two groups being compared with respect to major cardiac and noncardiac morbidities. The results, however, do not take into account intraoperative findings, such as small, calcified, diffusely atherosclerotic coronaries, intramyocardial or intraadipose coronaries, or other conditions that make revascularization technically more demanding, and at many centers, increase the likelihood of the procedure being performed with CPB. As such, technically difficult revascularizations are more prevalent in the conventional CABG group.

Although many of the reported advantages of OP-CAB can be debated, a decrease in postoperative coagulopathy and a reduced need for postoperative transfusion have been consistently found in essentially all OP-CAB series reported to date.* Reduced heparin requirements and preservation of platelet function in the absence of CPB are major factors. This finding has recently been confirmed in a prospective randomized study.[57]

Initial criticism aimed at OP-CAB centered on concerns with adequacy of revascularization and quality and reproducibility of the distal anastomosis. Indeed, early reports showed a small but significant decrease in the average number of grafts per patient when OP-CAB was performed compared to conventional CABG.[35,36] Subsequent evolution of tools and techniques for lateral and inferior wall exposure (vide supra), however, has allowed skilled OP-CAB surgeons to perform grafts to all aspects of the heart. More recent series report no difference in the average number of grafts constructed.[57] In addition, several well-documented series have demonstrated excellent graft patency.[54,56]

Although the debate continues, there is compelling evidence that OP-CAB is associated with decreased operative risk in some high-risk groups. This has been reported in several retrospective nonrandomized series,[3,63] as well as in series that looked specifically at the elderly, patients with reduced ejection fraction, and patients with renal failure.[4,40,64] There have been several reports documenting decreased risk associated with OP-CAB for reoperative patients as well.[5,65,73]

Reoperative OP-CAB can frequently be performed without dissecting out the ascending aorta or manipulating diseased grafts, making it is a very attractive approach. However, many surgeons consider the presence of heavily diseased but patent vein grafts a contraindication to OP-CAB because of the risk of graft embolization while the heart is being repositioned. A tailored left thoracotomy approach has been reported for reoperative grafting of the lateral wall in patients with patent LIMA-to-LAD grafts.[6,27] Through this exposure, a graft can readily be constructed from the descending thoracic aorta to lateral wall branches while avoiding the technical challenges associated with LIMA-graft mobilization. Long-term patency data for this type of graft are not available. Similarly, lower sternotomy and upper abdominal incisions have been described for constructing grafts to the inferior wall with the right gastroepiploic artery.[1,26]

Most surgeons agree that OP-CAB is ideally suited for revascularization of patients with significant atheroma or calcification of the ascending aorta. In this setting, free grafts are attached either to the side of the *in situ* LIMA as described initially by Tector et al[71] or to the innominate artery if disease free. Alternatively, free grafts can be attached to a disease-free area of the aorta with an automated anastomotic device,

*References 3, 4, 11, 12, 15, 16, 35, 36, 46, 55–57.

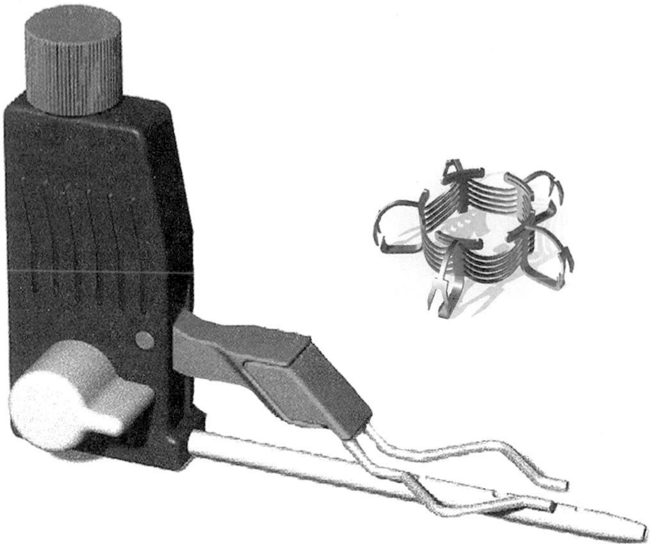

Figure 83–11 **Tools that facilitate construction of the proximal graft-to-aorta anastomosis without cross-clamp and automated anastomotic couplers may have an impact on the incidence of neurocognitive deficit after CABG.**

or with a clampless anastomotic facilitator that obviates the need for a partial-occluding clamp (Figure 83-11). Using a combination of palpation and epiaortic echo, an appropriate dime-sized area of relatively normal aorta can frequently be identified. OP-CAB allows these high-risk patients to undergo surgical revascularization with relative ease, while avoiding the certain hazards of cannulation and cross-clamping of the diseased aorta.

Neurocognitive Dysfunction after OP-CAB

Numerous published reports have demonstrated the new onset of subtle neurocognitive dysfunction (NCD) in some patients after CABG. Depending on the sensitivity of the tests used, the incidence has been reported to be between 5% and 60%. Specific deficits include short-term memory loss, reduced ability to perform simple calculations, and disturbances in personality and mood.[14,61,66] Many factors related to CPB, including SIR, alterations in cerebral blood flow, and microemboli, either from the CPB circuit or related to cannulation and cross-clamping, have been implicated.[22,66] Several groups have reported that OP-CAB is associated with significantly less SIR.[4,48,53] The magnitude of SIR, however, has not been shown to correlate with the severity of NCD in individual patients.[77] Furthermore, although a few studies have shown that OP-CAB is associated with a reduced incidence of NCD compared to conventional CABG with CPB,[22,80] other studies have shown no significant difference.[69,74] This failure of OP-CAB to favorably impact postoperative NCD has been largely attributed to the partial-occlusion aortic clamp and microemboli liberated during application and removal. Although OP-CAB obviates the need for placement of a perfusion catheter for CPB or a cross-clamp for cardiac arrest, the side-biting partial occlusion clamp, routinely used at many centers during construction of proximal anastomoses, arguably is equally traumatic. Avoidance of aortic manipulation, using composite grafts arising from the *in situ* LIMA and OP-CAB, has been shown to be an important factor in avoiding postoperative stroke.[13,39] A number of new devices recently introduced into clinical practice allow proximal anastomoses to be constructed off-pump without application of the partial-occlusion clamp (Figure 83-11). The impact these devices will have on NCD after OP-CAB has yet to be determined.

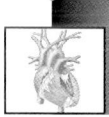

LIMITED ACCESS CORONARY ARTERY BYPASS

Additional efforts to minimize the invasiveness of CABG have focused on decreasing the trauma associated with surgical access. Although median sternotomy is relatively well tolerated, patients must refrain from heavy lifting for 2–3 months after surgery to allow union of the sternum. Although the incidence of wound complications is low, sternal wound infections generally require repeat operation, and can be life-threatening. Moreover, the musculoskeletal trauma associated with spreading the halves of the sternum is associated with a small degree of SIR that is synergistic with CPB in causing morbidity.[32,33] Avoiding sternotomy is therefore an attractive idea.

MIDCAB (MINIMALLY INVASIVE DIRECT CORONARY ARTERY BYPASS)

In 1995, Benetti et al introduced the MIDCAB procedure,[8] which was rapidly adopted by multiple centers in the United States and Europe.[28,67] The procedure is performed through a 7-cm anterior lateral thoracotomy, usually in the fifth intercostal space, and generally consists of a single-vessel off-pump bypass using the LIMA to bypass the LAD. Many early series documented satisfactory results with length of stay substantially shorter than for standard CABG and reduced requirement for transfusion.[7,20,28,67] Other reports suggested a reduced incidence of postoperative atrial fibrillation,[17] but this has been refuted.[37,70] Despite initial enthusiasm, MIDCAB is currently performed in large numbers in only a few U.S. centers. This decrease in utilization is due in part to the introduction and popularization of OP-CAB via median sternotomy. Technical hurdles intrinsic to MIDCAB also may have contributed.

Several early reports documented successful results with endoscopic LIMA harvest.[24,52] Many U.S. centers, however, chose to mobilize the LIMA using direct visualization through the thoracotomy to avoid the learning curve associated with videoscopic instrumentation and visualization. Direct harvest is often technically demanding and occasionally results in a LIMA graft of inadequate length. In addition, the vigorous chest wall retraction required for LIMA exposure results in significant early postoperative pain. Nevertheless, several U.S. centers skilled in MIDCAB continue to perform the procedure in large numbers and report excellent results.[50,68,76]

HYBRID MIDCAB APPROACH

Several recent reports have documented successful application of a hybrid strategy, combining a LIMA-to-LAD bypass (MIDCAB) with catheter-based interventions on the circumflex and right coronary arteries for the treatment of multivessel disease. In one multicenter series, videoscopic mobilization of the LIMA was performed with the aid of a voice-actuated robotic arm used to manipulate the scope[62] (Figure 83-12). In this series, the pericardium was opened using videoscopic techniques prior to performing the thoracotomy. In many patients this facilitated accurate placement of the chest wall incision, allowing the anastomosis between the LIMA and LAD to be

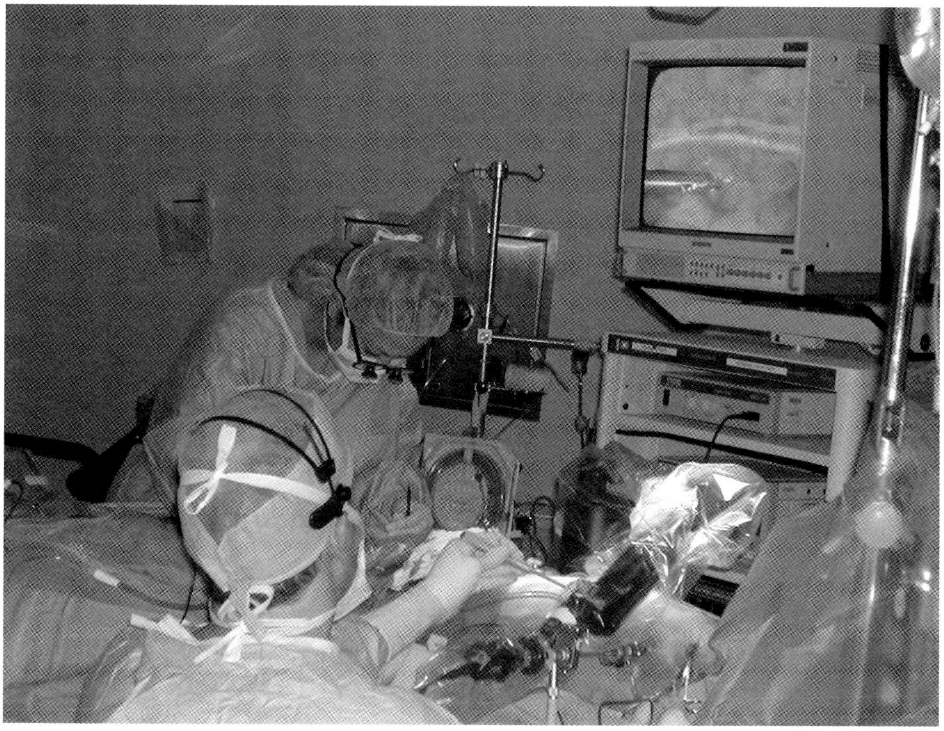

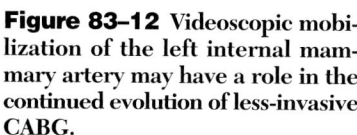

Figure 83–12 Videoscopic mobilization of the left internal mammary artery may have a role in the continued evolution of less-invasive CABG.

constructed without a rib spreader, using only soft tissue retractors and a specially designed bed-mounted stabilizer to expose the anastomotic site through the natural intercostal space[75] (Figure 83-13). Postoperative pain was reduced significantly with this approach. These reports have generated resurgent interest in the MIDCAB procedure at many centers.

COMPLETELY ENDOSCOPIC ROBOTIC-ASSISTED CABG

Several small series of completely closed-chest videoscopic LIMA-to-LAD procedures have been reported using surgical robots to mobilize the LIMA and to perform the sutured anastomosis, both with CPB[18,23,25] and without CPB.[10,18,51] The robots allow the surgeon to manipulate fully articulating videoscopic instruments by way of master–slave servos and microprocessor control. These instruments are designed to allow multiple degrees of freedom and can precisely emulate the surgeon's movements. An easy to use control environment, high-resolution displays that provide realistic three-dimensional steriopsis, and high magnification as well as tremor filtering and motion-scaling options offer the potential for superhuman precision. This precision compensates somewhat for absence of tactile feedback. Although extremely exciting, the routine use of surgical robotics in CABG surgery does not seem imminent. The robots themselves are quite expensive, and the learning curve for robotic totally endoscopic CABG (TECAB), especially if performed without CPB, is challenging. Surgeons skilled in the procedure can successfully perform only approximately one-in-three off-pump TECABs in carefully selected patients, resorting to a small MIDCAB incision to perform the anastomosis in the remainder. Future refinements in surgical robotic tools and techniques as well as refinements in automated distal anastomotic devices and other advances may have an impact in determining the ultimate utility of robotics in CABG procedures.

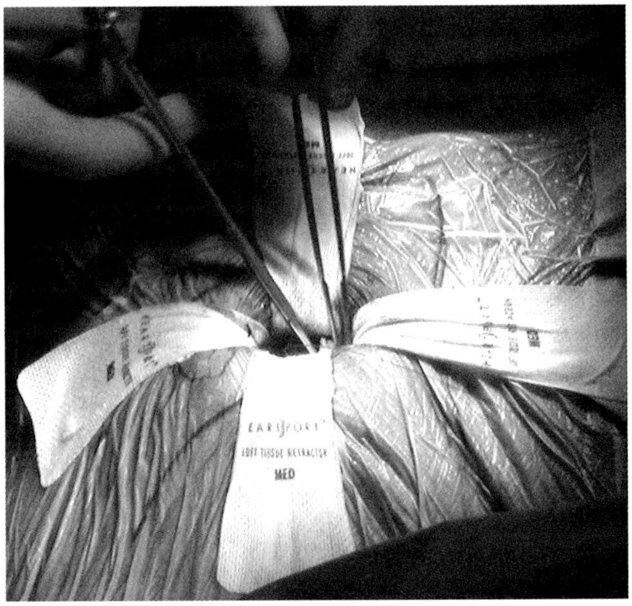

Figure 83–13 **In one type of less invasive bypass, accurate placement of the chest wall incision often allows the anastomosis between the LIMA and the LAD to be constructed through the natural interspace without placement of a rib spreader.**

PORT-ACCESS CABG

Heartport introduced port-access cardiac surgery in 1996 as a means of decreasing the trauma associated with surgical access. The strategy utilizes specialized catheters inserted into the femoral artery and vein that allow institution of cardiopulmonary bypass, balloon endoclamping of the ascending aorta, administration of antegrade cardioplegia, and venting of the ascending aorta. Additional catheters introduced percutaneously into the left jugular vein allow delivery of retrograde cardioplegia into the coronary sinus and venting of the pulmonary artery. A small chest incision can then be tailored for the desired procedure. Several series of multivessel CABG performed through small fifth intercostal space thoracotomies were published in the late 1990s using port access for institution of CPB with acceptable results,[29,30,58] but this procedure is no longer popular. Decreased enthusiasm is in part due to challenges associated with graft length and lie. Port access has remained an essential component of TECAB in several small series and remains an enabling technique in performing limited access mitral procedures and atrial septal defect repair. Advances in surgical robotics and automated distal anastomosis may have an impact on the ultimate role of port-access technology on the evolution of limited-access coronary artery bypass.

SUMMARY

Recent advances in surgical tools and techniques have given rise to a number of new options in the surgical management of coronary artery disease. Although additional data may be required before the relative merits of these options can be characterized, it is clear that this flexibility will allow the surgeon to tailor the operative approach to fit the patient. This becomes increasingly important given the increased prevalence of serious comorbidity and advanced age in patients referred for coronary bypass.

REFERENCES

1. Abraham R, Ricci M, Salerno T, et al: A minimally invasive approach for reoperative grafting of the right coronary artery. J Card Surg 17:289–291, 2002.
2. Ankeney JL: To use or not to use the pump oxygenator in coronary bypass operations. Ann Thorac Surg 19:108–109, 1975.
3. Arom KV, Flavin TF, Emery RW, et al: Safety and efficacy of off-pump coronary artery bypass grafting. Ann Thorac Surg 69:704–710, 2000.
4. Arom KV, Flavin TF, Emery RW, et al: Is low ejection fraction safe for off-pump coronary bypass operation? Ann Thorac Surg 70:1021–1025, 2000.
5. Ascione R, Lloyd CT, Underwood MJ, et al: Inflammatory response after coronary revascularization with or without cardiopulmonary bypass. Ann Thorac Surg 69:1198–1204, 2000.

6. Azoury FM, Gillinov AM, Lytle BW, et al: Off-pump reoperative coronary artery bypass grafting by thoracotomy: patient selection and operative technique. Ann Thorac Surg 71:1959–1963, 2001.
7. Bahit MC, Cabell CH, Dyke CK, et al: Highlights from the American College of Cardiology forty-ninth annual scientific sessions: March 18 to 21, 2001. Am Heart J 142:363–374, 2001.
8. Benetti FJ, Ballester C, Sani G, et al: Video assisted coronary bypass surgery. J Card Surg 10:620–625, 1995.
9. Biswas S, Clements F, Diodato L, et al: Changes in systolic and diastolic function during multivessel off-pump coronary bypass grafting. Eur J Cardiothorac Surg 20(5):913–917, 2001.
10. Boehm DH, Reichenspurner H, Detter C, et al: Clinical use of a computer-enhanced surgical robotic system for endoscopic coronary artery bypass grafting on the beating heart. Thorac Cardiovasc Surg 48:198–202, 2000.
11. Calafiore AM, Mauro MD, Contini M, et al: Myocardial revascularization with and without cardiopulmonary bypass in multivessel disease: impact of strategy on early outcome. Ann Thorac Surg 72:456–463, 2001.
12. Cartier R, Brann S, Dagenais F, et al: Systematic off-pump coronary artery revascularization in multivessel disease: experience of three hundred cases. J Thorac Cardiovasc Surg 199:221–229, 2000.
13. Chavanon O, Durand M, Hacini R, et al: Coronary artery bypass grafting with internal mammary artery and right gastroepiploic artery, with and without bypass. Ann Thorac Surg 73:499–504, 2002.
14. Clark RE, Brillman J, Davis DA, et al: Microemboli during coronary artery bypass grafting: genesis and effect on outcome. J Thorac Cardiovasc Surg 109:249–258, 1995.
15. Cleveland JC, Shroyer ALW, Chen AY, et al: Off-pump coronary artery bypass grafting decreases risk adjusted mortality and morbidity. Ann Thorac Surg 72:1282–1289, 2001.
16. Czerny M, Baumer H, Kilo J, Zuckerman A, et al: Complete revascularization in coronary artery bypass grafting with and without cardiopulmonary bypass. Ann Thorac Surg 71:165–169, 2001.
17. d'Amato TA, Savage EB, Wiechmann RJ, et al: Reduced incidence of atrial fibrillation with minimally invasive direct coronary artery bypass. Ann Thorac Surg 70:2013–2016, 2000.
18. Detter C, Boehm DH, Reichenspurner H, et al: Robotically-assisted coronary artery surgery with and without cardiopulmonary bypass—from first clinical use to endoscopic operation. Med Sci Monit 8:118–123, 2002.
19. Detter C, Deuse T, Christ F, et al: Comparison of two stabilizer concepts for off-pump coronary artery bypass grafting. Ann Thorac Surg 74:497–451, 2002.
20. Detter C, Reichenspurner H, Boehm DH, et al: Minimally invasive direct coronary artery bypass grafting (MIDCAB) and off-pump coronary artery bypass grafting (OPCAB): two techniques for beating heart surgery. Heart Surg Forum 5:157–162, 2002.
21. Detter C, Reichenspurner H, Boehm DH, et al: Single vessel revascularization with beating heart techniques—minithoracotomy or sternotomy? Eur J Cardiothorac Surg 19:464–470, 2001.
22. Diegeler A, Hiesch R, Schneider F, et al: Neuromonitoring and neurocognitive outcome in off-pump versus conventional coronary bypass operation. Ann Thorac Surg 69:1162–1166, 2000.
23. Dogan S, Aybek T, Andressen E, et al: Totally endoscopic coronary artery bypass grafting on cardiopulmonary bypass with robotically enhanced telemanipulation: report of 45 cases. J Thorac Cardiovasc Surg 123:1029–1030, 2002.
24. Duhaylongsod FG, Mayfield WR, Wolf RK: Thoracoscopic harvest of the internal thoracic artery: a multicenter experience in 218 cases. Ann Thorac Surg 66:1012–1017, 1998.
25. Falk V, Diegler A, Walther T, et al: Total endoscopic computer enhanced coronary artery bypass grafting. Eur J Cardiothorac Surg 17:38–45, 2000.
26. Fonger JD, Doty JR, Salazar JD, et al: Initial Experience with MIDCAB grafting using the gastroepiploic artery. Ann Thor Surg 68:431–436, 1999.
27. Fonger JD, Doty JR, Sussman MS, et al: Lateral MIDCAB grafting via limited posterior thoracotomy. Eur J Cardiothorac Surg 12:399–405, 1997.
28. Greenspun HG, Adourian UA, Fonger JD, et al: Minimally invasive direct coronary artery bypass (MIDCAB): surgical techniques and anesthetic considerations. J Cardiothorac Vasc Anesth 10:507–509, 1996.
29. Groh MA, Sutherland SE, Burton HG, et al: Port-access coronary artery bypass grafting: technique and comparative results. Ann Thorac Surg 68:1506–1508, 1999.
30. Grossi EA, Groh MA, Lefrk EA, et al: Results of a prospective multicenter study on port-access coronary bypass grafting. Ann Thorac Surg 68:1475–1477, 1999.
31. Grundeman PF, Borst C, Verlaan CW, et al: Exposure of circumflex branches in the tilted, beating porcine heart: echocardiographic evidence of right ventricular deformation and the effect of right or left heart bypass. J Thorac Cardiovasc Surg 118:316–323, 1999.
32. Gu JY, Mariani MA, Boonstra PW, et al: Complement activation in coronary artery bypass grafting patients without cardiopulmonary bypass: the role of tissue injury by surgical incision. Chest 116:892–898, 1999.
33. Gu JY, Mariani MA, van Oeveren W, et al: Reduction of the inflammatory response in patients undergoing minimally invasive coronary artery bypass grafting. Ann Thorac Surg 65:420–424, 1998.
34. Guyton RA, Thourani VH, Puskas JD, et al: Perfusion-assisted direct coronary artery bypass: selective graft perfusion in off-pump cases. Ann Thorac Surg 69(1): 171–175, 2000.
35. Hart JC, Spooner TH, Pym J, et al: A review of 1,582 consecutive octopus off-pump coronary bypass patients. Ann Thorac Surg 70:1017–1020, 2000.
36. Hernadez F, Cohn WE, Baribeau YR, et al: In-hospital outcomes of off-pump vs. on-pump coronary artery bypass procedures; a multicenter experience. Ann Thorac Surg 72(5):1528–1533, 2001.
37. Hravnak M, Hoffman LA, Saul MI, et al: Atrial fibrillation: prevalence after minimally invasive direct and standard coronary artery bypass. Ann Thorac Surg 71:1491–1495, 2001.
38. Kim KB, Lim C, Ahn H, et al: Intraaortic balloon pump therapy facilitates posterior vessel off-pump coronary artery bypass grafting in high-risk patients. Ann Thorac Surg 71(6):1964–1968, 2001.
39. Kobayashi J, Tagusari O, Bando K, et al: Total arterial off-pump coronary revascularization with only internal thoracic artery and composite radial artery grafts. Heart Surg Forum 6:30–37, 2002.
40. Koutlas TC, Elbeery JR, Williams JM, et al: Myocardial revascularization in the elderly using beating heart coronary artery bypass surgery. Ann Thorac Surg 69:1042–1047, 2000.
41. Kshettry VR, Flavin TF, Emery RW, et al: Does multivessel, off-pump coronary artery bypass reduce post-operative morbidity? Ann Thorac Surg 69:1725–1731, 2000.
42. Laborde F, Abdelmeguid I, Piwnica A: Aortocoronary bypass with extracorporeal circulation: why and when? Eur J Cardiothorac Surg 3:152–154, 1989.

43. Landis RC, Asimakopoulos G, Poullis M, et al: The antithrombotic and anti-inflammatory mechanisms of action of aprotinin. Ann Thorac Surg 72:2169–2175, 2001.
44. Lima LE, Jatene F, Buffolo E, et al: A multicenter initial clinical experience with right heart support and beating heart coronary surgery. Heart Surg Forum 4(1):60–64, 2001.
45. Lima R: Revascularizacion a o da artèria circunflexa sem auxilio da CEC. In XII encontro dos discipulos do dr. EJ Zerbini, Curitiba, 1995. Sessa ode videos. Curitiba, Parana, Sociedade dos discipulos do dr. EJ Zerbini Outtubro de 1995, 6.b.
46. Magee MJ, Dewey TM, Acuff T, et al: Influence of diabetes on mortality and morbitity: off-pump coronary artery bypass grafting versus coronary artery bypass grafting with cardiopulmonary bypass. Ann Thorac Surg 72:776–781, 2001.
47. Magee MJ, Jablonski, KA, Stamou SC, et al: Elimination of cardiopulmonary bypass improves early survival for multivessel coronary artery bypass patients. Ann Thorac Surg 73:1196–1202, 2002.
48. Matata BM, Sosnowski AW, Galinanes M: Off-pump bypass graft operation significantly reduces oxidative stress and inflammation. Ann Thorac Surg 69:785–791, 2000.
49. Mathison M, Edgerton JR, Horswell JL, et al: Analysis of hemodynamic changes during beating heart surgical procedures. Ann Thorac Surg 70:1355–1360; discussion 1360–1361, 2000.
50. Mehran R, Dangas G, Stamou SC, et al: One year clinical outcome after minimally invasive direct coronary artery bypass. Circulation 102:2799–2802, 2000.
51. Mohr FW, Falk V, Diegler A, et al: Computer-enhanced "robotic" cardiac surgery: experience in 148 patients. J Thorac Cardiovasc Surg 121:842–853, 2001.
52. Nataf P, Al-Attar N, Ramadan R, et al: Thoracoscopic IMA takedown. J Card Surg 15:278–282, 2000.
53. Okubo N, Hatori N, Ochi M, et al: Comparison of m-RNA expression for inflammatory mediators in leukocytes between on-pump and off-pump coronary artery bypass grafting. Ann Thorac Cardiovasc Surg 9:43–49, 2003.
54. Omeroglu SN, Kirali K, Guler M, et al: Midterm assessment of coronary artery bypass grafting without cardiopulmonary bypass. Ann Thorac Surg 70:844–849, 2000.
55. Plomondon ME, Cleveland JC, Ludwig ST: Off-pump coronary artery bypass is associated with improved risk adjusted outcomes. Ann Thorac Surg 72:114–119, 2001.
56. Puskas JD, Thourani VH, Marshall JJ, et al: Clinical outcomes, angiographic patency, and resource utilization in 200 consecutive off-pump coronary bypass patients. Ann Thorac Surg 71:1477–1484, 2001.
57. Puskas JD, Williams WH, Duke PG et al: Off-pump coronary artery bypass grafting provides complete revascularization with reduced myocardial injury, transfusion requirements, and length of stay: a prospective randomized comparison of 200 unselected patients undergoing off-pump versus conventional coronary artery bypass grafting. J Thorac Cardiovasc Surg 125:797–808, 2003.
58. Reichenspurner H, Guliemos V, Wunderlich J, et al: Port access coronary artery bypass grafting with the use of cardiopulmonary bypass and cardioplegic arrest. Ann Thorac Surg 65:413–419, 1998.
59. Reilly PM, Wilkins KB, Fuh KC, et al: The mesenteric hemodynamic response to circulatory shock: an overview. Shock 15(5):329–343, 2001.
60. Sharony R, Autschbach R, Porat E, et al: Right heart support during off-pump coronary artery bypass surgery—a multi-center study. Heart Surg Forum 5:13–16, 2002.
61. Sotaniemi KA, Mononen H, Hokkanen TE: Long term cerebral outcome after open heart surgery: a five year neuropsychological follow-up study. Stroke 17:410–416, 1986.
62. Stahl KD, Boyd WD, Vassiliades TA, et al: Hybrid coronary artery surgery and angioplasty in multivessel coronary artery disease. Ann Thorac Surg 74:1358–1362, 2002.
63. Stamou SC, Corso PJ: Coronary revascularization without cardiopulmonary bypass in high-risk patients: a route to the future. Ann Thorac Surg 71:1056–1061, 2001.
64. Stamou SC, Dangas G, Dullum MKC, et al: Beating heart surgery in octogenarians: perioperative outcome and comparison with younger age groups. Ann Thorac Surg 69:1140–1145, 2000.
65. Stamou SC, Pfister AJ, Dullum MK, et al: Late outcome of reoperative coronary revascularization on the beating heart. Heart Surg Forum 4:69–73, 2001.
66. Stump DA, Rogers AT, Hammon JW, et al: Cerebral emboli and cognitive outcome after cardiac surgery. J Cardiothorac Vasc Anesth 10:113–119, 1996.
67. Subramanian VA, McCabe JC, Geller CM: Minimally invasive direct coronary artery bypass grafting: two-year clinical experience. Ann Thorac Surg 64:1648–1655, 1997.
68. Subramanian VA, Patel NU: Current status of MIDCAB procedure. Curr Opin Cardiol 16:268–270, 2001.
69. Taggart DP, Browne SM, Halligan PW, et al: Is cardiopulmonary bypass still the cause of cognitive dysfunction after cardiac operations? J Thorac Cardiovasc Surg 118:414–420, 1999.
70. Cohn WE, Sirois CA, Johnson RG: Atrial fibrillation after minimally invasive coronary artery bypass grafting: a retrospective analysis. J Thorac Cardiovasc Surg 117:298–301, 1999
71. Tector AJ, Amundsen S, Schmahl TM, et al: Total revascularization with T grafts. Ann Thorac Surg 57:33–38, 1994.
72. Trapp WG, Bisarya R: Placement of coronary artery bypass graft without pump oxygenator. Ann Thorac Surg 19:1–9, 1975.
73. Trehan N, Mishra YK, Malhotra R, et al: Off-pump redo coronary artery bypass grafting. Ann Thorac Surg 70:1026–1029, 2000.
74. van Dijk D, Jansen EW, Hijman R, et al: Cognitive outcome after off-pump coronary artery bypass graft surgery: a randomized trial. JAMA 287:1405–1412, 2002.
75. Vassiliades TA: Atraumatic coronary artery bypass (ACAB): techniques and outcome. Heart Surg Forum 4:331–334, 2001.
76. Vassiliades TA, Rogers EW, Nielsen JL, et al: Minimally invasive direct coronary artery bypass grafting: intermediate term results. Ann Thorac Surg 70:1063–1065, 2000.
77. Wan S, LeClerc JL, Vincent JL: Inflammatory response to cardiopulmonary bypass: mechanisms involved and possible therapeutic strategies. Chest 112:676–692, 2000.
78. Westaby S, Saatvedt K, White S, et al: Is there a relationship between cognitive dysfunction and systemic inflammatory response after cardiopulmonary bypass? Ann Thorac Surg 71:667–672, 2001.
79. Yokoyama T, Baumgartner FJ, Gheissari A, et al: Off-pump versus on-pump coronary bypass in high risk subgroups. Ann Thorac Surg 70:1546–1550, 2000.
80. Zamvar V, Deglurkar I, Abdullah F, et al: Bleeding from the lung surface: a unique complication of off-pump CABG operation. Heart Surg Forum 4(2):172–173, 2001.
81. Zamvar V, Williams D, Hall J, et al: Assessment of neurocognitive impairment after off-pump techniques for coronary artery bypass graft surgery: prospective randomized controlled trial. BMJ 325:1268, 2002.

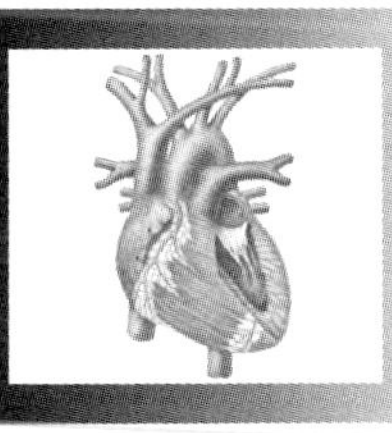

Bypass Conduit Options

Nabil A. Munfakh and Hendrick B. Barner

CHAPTER 84

INTRODUCTION

History

Coronary revascularization began in the 1960s with reports of successful coronary anastomosis by Kolesov.[60] Within a few years Favaloro and others demonstrated the feasibility of surgical revascularization of coronary obstruction in a large number of patients and the era of coronary artery bypass surgery began in earnest.[43] While these early pioneers of coronary surgery used the internal thoracic artery (ITA) and the saphenous vein, other conduits have been tried in an effort to improve outcome and extend the availability of the operation to patients in whom standard conduits are not available. In this chapter we review the various conduit options and discuss the rationale for using them.

Choice of Conduit

Conduit Factors

If patency were the only consideration, then the ITA would be the first choice and the second choice, but other considerations frequently prevail. Harvest time and whether the harvest can occur concomitantly or sequentially may be important. Ease of harvest and handling made the saphenous vein the conduit of choice in the early era and continues to be an important consideration in many situations. Experience of the surgeon is a factor because arterial conduits are more fragile and at risk for injury. The amount of conduit harvested is influenced by surgeon experience and also philosophy (complex grafting versus simple, i.e., one conduit for one distal anastomosis).

Patient Factors

Because the survival benefit of the ITA graft has not achieved significance before 8–10 years,[66,68] it can be argued that vein is an appropriate conduit for patients with reduced life expectancy whether related to age, poor left ventricular function, cancer, renal dialysis, pulmonary disease, or other comorbidities. On the other hand, the use of the left ITA for the left anterior descending artery has provided survival benefit immediately and at any age and this graft should be used with rare exceptions.[44,52,77] Patients with peripheral vascular disease and diabetes may be better served by not using the saphenous vein, so that it will be available for peripheral vascular reconstruction. Contraindications to use of the saphenous vein include varicose degeneration, superficial phlebitis, and deep vein occlusion in which the saphenous vein is an important collateral. Use of the *in situ* ITA may be compromised by prior chest wall irradiation, subclavian artery stenosis or occlusion, and ostial stenosis of the ITA, in which case a free ITA graft is possible.

VENOUS CONDUITS

Greater Saphenous Vein (GSV)

Anatomy and Histology

The GSV lies in the subcutaneous fat on the medial aspect of the leg from the saphenofemoral junction to the medial malleolus. Occasionally it is attached to the dermis or to the fascia. Short or long segments may be in duplicate. Below the knee, the vein is accompanied by the saphenous nerve, which should be preserved during harvest. The vein is usually larger proximally with a thicker, more fibrotic wall, while distally the vein is healthier, but may be small.

The vein wall is thicker than that of an arterial conduit, and the media is nourished by the vasa vasorum so that smooth muscle necrosis is usual after harvesting and it is replaced with fibrous tissue that converts the vein into a relatively rigid tube. This obviously restricts vasomotion after grafting. The endothelium of the vein is frequently damaged or lost (Figure 84-1), even with meticulous harvesting and preservation, but regenerates over weeks.[14]

Saphenous vein endothelial production of nitric oxide (NO) is inferior to that seen in arteries and decreases after grafting.[12,28,30,61,67] Because NO inhibits platelet adherence and aggregation, inhibits adherence of neutrophils, and directly or indirectly inhibits smooth muscle proliferation, it has been suggested that the state of the endothelium may promote atherosclerotic degeneration in vein grafts, while inhibiting it in arterial grafts.

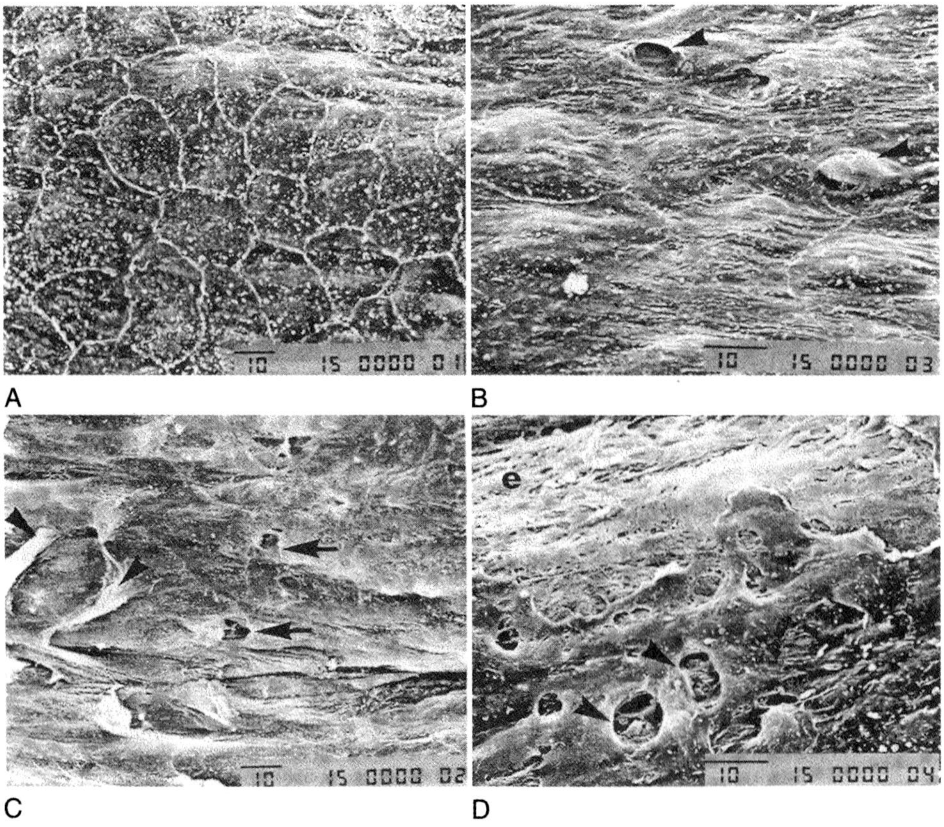

Figure 84–1 Scanning electron micrographs showing **(A)** well-preserved endothelial cells with prominent microvilli from saphenous vein stored in heparinized blood for 1 at 4° C. **B,** Minimal endothelial cell alterations are indicated by slight condensation of cell cytoplasm *(arrowheads)* after storage as in **A**. **C,** Separation of endothelial cells *(arrowheads)* and pitting *(arrows)* are noted after storage in **A** and **B**. In contrast to these is **D** in which vein stored in saline at room temperature manifests frank erosion (e) of endothelium with exposure of subendothelium and pitting *(arrowheads)* in the remaining endothelial cells.
(From Barner HB, Fisher VW: Endothelial preservation in human saphenous veins harvested for coronary grafting. J Thorac Cardiovasc Surg 100:148–149, 1990.)

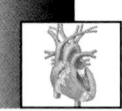

Harvesting Technique

An incision the length of the vein to be harvested is used by some, but we prefer multiple small incisions. Dissection should be as atraumatic as possible, forceps should handle only the adventitia of the vein, and stretch trauma minimized. Branches are controlled with clips or ligature. Endoscopic techniques have proven successful and require only two or three small incisions.[2,9,22,35] However, the learning curve of the endoscopic technique and cost of disposables have limited its use.

The vein is marked by placing a soft vascular bulldog clamp on the new distal end or by cannulating the new proximal end. The vein is distended with a physiological solution; we prefer heparinized blood with or without papaverine, at low pressure (no more than 150 mm Hg), to overcome harvest spasm, but avoid injury to endothelium. The commonest vein injury is branch avulsion, which is closed with 7-0 polypropylene to create a transverse suture line. Storage until use is in room temperature heparinized blood or physiological pH balanced salt solution. Incisions are closed after harvest with or without drains.

Grafting Strategies

Vein can be grafted to any target, but with the near ubiquitous use of the left ITA for the left anterior descending artery, the vein is restricted to other targets. Target size is important for vein graft flow with lower patency if the coronary is 1.5 mm or less.[72] Sequential vein grafting can overcome this disadvantage if the smaller coronary is grafted side to side with a larger coronary grafted distally. If a suitable vein is in short supply or to conserve vein, sequential grafting is also appropriate.

Table 84–1

Conduit Patency[a]

	Years postoperatively			
Conduit	*1*	*5*	*10*	*15*
Left ITA	99	95–98	85–95	88
Right ITA	98	95–98	80–85	65
RA	96	79		
RGA	95		63	
IEA		79		
GSV				
Current	80–95	73	55–75	32–40
Historic	80–85	75	45	

[a]Angiographic patency from 3, 13, 16, 29, 37, 38, 46, 103.
ITA, internal thoracic artery; RA, radial artery; RGA, right gastroepiploic artery; IEA, inferior epigastric artery; GSV, greater saphenous vein.

Clinical Results

Early randomized studies supported the use of bypass grafting with veins versus medical treatment for left main and two- or three-vessel coronary disease.[24] Because conduit patency correlates with survival and recurrence of ischemic events, there was and is great interest in angiographic follow-up. GSV closure in the first year approximates 12–20%[3,45] and is commonly related to low flow leading to layering of thrombus in the graft, which progresses to occlusion.[72] The golden period for vein grafts is from 1 to 5 years with a closure rate of 2–4%/year, which accelerates to 4–8%/year after the fifth year to give 10 year patency rates of 45–65%.[3,29,45,46] Sequential grafting improves patency particularly for side-to-side anastomoses.[29,37,59] Data from the current era reveal some improvement in vein graft patency to 72.5% at 7.5 years and 71% at 10 years[37,103] (Table 84-1). In one report all vein grafts were in addition to use of arterial conduits and directed to less important or remote coronary vessels.[37] These results reflect improved vein harvesting and preservation and frequent use of sequential grafting.[37]

Lesser Saphenous Vein (LSV)

Anatomy and Histology

The LSV lies posterior to the lateral malleolus and passes superiorly in the subcutaneous layer to the midpopliteal fossa where it perforates the fascia and joins the popliteal vein. Grossly and microscopically it is similar to the GSV.

Harvesting Technique

It can be harvested in the prone position (after bilateral GSV stripping) or supine by flexing the knee and rotating the hip internally or externally, or by flexing the hip and extending the knee, which requires a strong assistant. One or several incisions may be used.

Grafting Strategies

It is used exactly as the GSV.

Clinical Results

There are no long-term studies of the LSV and short-term observations report results similar to the GSV.[85,88]

Cephalic Vein

Anatomy and Histology

The vein extends from the subclavian vein to the subcutaneous tissue of the deltopectoral groove and passes along the lateral border of the biceps muscle through the antecubital fossa into the forearm where its anatomy is variable. The vein is small and its wall is much thinner than that of the GSV with little smooth muscle in the media.

Harvesting Technique

The vein is usually visible in the upper arm and a single incision is made over it and carried to near the antecubital fossa. If forearm vein is needed, a skin bridge is left over the fossa and a second incision is made in the forearm.

Grafting Strategies

It can be used similarly to the GSV, but if small it may be difficult to suture to the aorta and the thin wall could tear, so that use as a Y-graft from another vein graft would be preferable.

Clinical Results

Arm vein patency is significantly less than that of leg vein, so that it should be used only as a last resort.[97,113]

ARTERIAL CONDUITS

Left Internal Thoracic Artery

Anatomy and Histology

The left internal thoracic artery (ITA) arises from the left subclavian artery opposite the vertebral artery origin and passes through the thoracic inlet crossing dorsal to the subclavian vein with the phrenic nerve before passing deep to the endothoracic fascia just lateral to the sternal edge, which it follows to the sixth intercostal space. There it divides into the musculophrenic artery having a lateral course and the superior epigastric, which enters the rectus sheath.

The ITA is unique among the arterial conduits in that its muscular media has 6–12 elastic lamellae. The intima and subintima lie on the prominent internal elastic lamina, which has few and small fenestrations in contrast to other small arteries where more and larger fenestrations may allow entry of smooth muscle cells to the subintima and initiate plaque formation. The reduced smooth muscle mass results in less vigorous contraction compared to other muscular arteries when exposed to agonists. The internal elastic lamina in the ITA may limit the development of atherosclerosis.[96]

Harvesting Technique

After sternotomy the sternal leaf is elevated with a spreading type retractor or a table mounted pulling retractor. Historically brachial plexus trauma as well as rib fracture or costochondral separation was more common with the latter. The artery, with its larger medial vein, can usually be seen and palpated in its mid course just beyond the sternal edge after dissecting the mediastinal fat from the chest wall. Many prefer to open the pleura widely, but others prefer to leave the pleura intact when dissecting the conduit. It is common to harvest the left ITA with a 1- to 2-cm pedicle of endothoracic fascia, fatty areolar tissue, and two veins with all dissection using low current electrocautery. Others would clip all or some branches or use a combination of proximal clipping and distal cauterization. Skeletonization of the ITA is becoming popular because it provides a longer conduit and less compromise of sternal blood flow with improved healing.[31] Skeletonization implies dividing branches between clips to preserve distal branch structure and thereby collateral flow to the sternum.[36]

Grafting Strategies

Today nearly all patients should have the left ITA placed to the left anterior descending (LAD) coronary. If both ITAs are used the left ITA may be placed to the circumflex system and the right to the left anterior descending artery. Sequential grafting of the left ITA to one or more diagonal branches and occasionally to two sites on the LAD is practiced by many surgeons. Others are not comfortable with this strategy and believe that it has the potential to jeopardize distal ITA flow, which is usually the most important anastomosis. If directed to the circumflex system it is possible to perform sequential grafting to the ramus intermedius and the obtuse marginal branches and occasionally a more distal circumflex branch.

Clinical Results

Patency of the left ITA to the left anterior descending coronary is the gold standard for all conduits and all targets and approximates 99% at 1 year and 85–95% at 10 years.[3,8,38,103] Survival and freedom from ischemic events at 10 years were better in patients with two- or three-vessel disease when the left ITA was grafted to the left anterior descending artery versus saphenous vein, which was used for other targets in both groups.[60]

Right Internal Thoracic Artery

Anatomy and Histology

The right ITA has anatomy and histology similar to the left ITA.

Harvest Technique

Harvesting is no different from the left ITA except for the consideration that having a longer conduit is frequently helpful whether used *in situ* or as a free graft and therefore skeletonization is advantageous. Preservation of sternal blood flow to prevent sternal infection or poor healing is also a consideration since the left ITA is almost always harvested with the right ITA and bilateral ITA harvesting is associated with an increased incidence of sternal complications particularly in diabetics.

Grafting Strategies

The right ITA is somewhat limited compared to the left ITA in that it is further from two potential targets (left anterior descending and circumflex arteries) than the left ITA and the third target (posterior descending artery) may be too

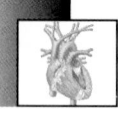

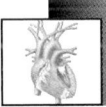

distant as well. Survival data support use of both ITAs for the left side of the heart.[68] The right ITA will usually reach the left anterior descending artery, but an anterior crossing position makes it vulnerable at reoperation. Routing it through the transverse sinus will minimize its exposure at reoperation and some would place it posterior to the superior vena cava as well.

Use as a free graft from the aorta has been common but there is a 10% or more loss of patency over time, which is improved if the anastomosis is made to a vein hood or to a pericardial patch.[16] Used as a Y-graft from another arterial conduit (usually the left ITA) may be optimal as it will reach any circumflex branch.[20] The extreme form of this strategy is the T-graft in which the right ITA is directed to the circumflex branches as well as branches of the right coronary artery.[105] This approach requires side-to-side grafting and perhaps crossing (diamond) anastomoses rather than parallel technique, which is easier and safer. It also raises the possibility of hypoperfusion due to technical imperfection or the single source of inflow for the entire heart.

Clinical Results

The right ITA has comparable patency to the left ITA when directed to the same targets (left anterior descending and obtuse marginal branches) whether placed anterior to the heart or through the transverse sinus. Patency is decreased when grafted to the distal circumflex branches or to branches of the right coronary artery as well as the right coronary artery itself.[16,19,38,103] When used as a Y-graft from the left ITA patency is unchanged.[20]

Survival data for the isolated right ITA or right ITA with associated vein grafts do not exist. Bilateral ITA grafting compared to left ITA for the left anterior descending coronary with a saphenous vein for all other targets is associated with improved survival and decreased reintervention (angioplasty and repeat coronary grafting) at 13 years with a smaller survival benefit in younger patients.[68]

Radial Artery

Anatomy and Histology

The radial artery begins with the ulnar artery at the brachial bifurcation in the antecubital fossa and has a relatively straight, superficial course to the wrist. It lies directly beneath the fascia in the distal third, beneath the brachioradialis muscle in the middle third, and several millimeters deep to the fascia proximally. It is accompanied by two venous comitantes and a small amount of fatty areolar tissue that constitute the "pedicle" for harvesting purposes. There are multiple small muscular branches on the dorsal surface. The lateral antibrachial cutaneous nerve lies deep in the subcutaneous tissue near but usually toward the radial side of the border of the brachioradialis muscle and may be damaged here. The other nerve at risk is the superficial radial nerve, which lies on the ulnar side of the radial artery and can be injured in the proximal or middle third if dissection strays from the artery. Distally the nerve passes deep and is not subject to injury. This nerve is sensory to the dorsum of the first metacarpal, the proximal phalanx of the thumb, and to the adjacent thenar eminence with 15–20% of patients having early dysfunction and 8% having chronic sensory disturbance after radial artery harvest.

The media is thicker than that of the other arterial conduits and devoid of elastic fibers. The wall of the artery is nourished from the lumen. Flow compromising atherosclerosis is rare and in 1–2% there is medial calcification (Mönckeberg's disease), usually associated with diabetes and/or renal failure and usually without intimal involvement. If extensive the conduit cannot be used but if mild to moderate we have used it.

Harvesting Technique

Determination of circulation to the hand is a prerequisite to radial artery harvest and we have used the Allen test for this, supplemented with a digital oximeter when palmar pigmentation prevented visual assessment of capillary refilling. The Allen test entails occlusion of both vessels at the wrist, having the patient make a tight fist for 15–30 s, opening the hand to a relaxed position, releasing the ulnar artery, and counting the seconds for capillary refilling of the palm with a cutoff of 12 s. Particular attention is paid to the thumb, which is the last digit to fill. In borderline situations repeat of the test will frequently reveal more rapid filling as collaterals dilate or are recruited. Some prefer Doppler study of the digital artery of the first ray but we have not found this necessary.

Incision begins and ends directly over the artery with a middle third ulnar curve to fit the brachioradialis muscle and avoid the lateral antibrachial cutaneous nerve. Depending on the length of the conduit required (maximum 20–24 cm in the male and 2 cm less in the female) a shorter incision is made. Some use one or two small incisions and an endoscopic technique.[33] We use low electrocautery for hemostasis to the level of the fascia but only for the fascia in the proximal third. The artery is mobilized as a pedicle using blunt and sharp dissection with division of branches between clips or with ultrasonic dissection and for branch division, which is our preferred method.[86] To safely harvest a maximal length we like to identify the brachial bifurcation. Occasionally the recurrent radial artery, which arises early, is a larger artery and can cause confusion. The brachial bifurcation may be low, which is a reason for always identifying the ulnar artery. In harvesting to the wrist crease a large branch or bifurcation may be seen and divided without impairing distal circulation. Median nerve injury has been reported and may relate to excessive use of electrocautery in controlling branches.

Grafting Strategies

Treatment of "harvest spasm" is mandatory for several reasons: the surgeon must know that the conduit is sound and does not have a harvest injury, the conduit must be able to contribute to myocardial blood flow perioperatively, and poor flow usually indicates persistent spasm or conduit injury and must be dealt with. We treat harvest spasm with intraluminal papaverine (2 mg/1 ml heparinized blood) usually followed by exposure to arterial pressure. Topical papaverine (3 mg/1 ml saline) can be sprayed on the pedicle or a sponge moistened with it can be placed on the pedicle. There has been wide interest in parenteral diltiazem perioperatively and orally thereafter, but we have not used it. Other calcium channel blockers (amlodipine, nifedipine, nicardipine) may be more effective[18] and nitroglycerin may be best.[18,90] Phenoxybenzamine is highly effective *in vitro*, but a parenteral preparation is not available in the United States.[101]

Because the radial artery is the longest arterial conduit it can reach any site in most hearts whether attached to the aorta or to another arterial conduit. When based on the aorta, we prefer an intermediary, which can be a vein hood or pericardial patch, to avoid the problem of a smaller hole and a thick-walled artery, which can become stenotic with healing. Some prefer to routinely attach it to an *in situ* internal thoracic artery, usually the left, in a "Y" or "T" configuration[4,20,32,54] (Figure 84-2). With use of the T-graft strategy side-to-side grafting with the ITA (30%) and the radial artery (90%) is routine. Many surgeons are not comfortable with these complex strategies, which require experience and expertise. Although crossing (diamond-shaped) anastomoses were anathema to arterial conduits, they are now employed when appropriate.

Clinical Results

Although the radial artery has been in use for more than a decade reported angiographic and clinical follow-up are only at 5–8 years whereas 10 years is minimum for demonstrating superiority to a venous conduit.[4,32,54] Survival and freedom from reintervention (the hardest end points) are comparable to other grafting strategies when used as an aortocoronary conduit, a Y-graft, or a T-graft.[4,20,32,54] One randomized study at 5 years compares the radial artery with the right ITA in younger patients and with the saphenous vein in older patients without survival or patency difference.[17]

RA patency to the left anterior descending coronary or proximal circumflex branches is comparable for either target and is also comparable to the ITA for these targets.[20] Radial artery patency from the aorta or from the left ITA is comparable.[54,69] Patency declines when the conduit is directed to the right coronary artery or distal circumflex branches, which is also true for the right and left ITA.[16,38,70] The radial artery is more sensitive to competitive coronary flow than is the ITA and should not be used for a coronary stenosis of less than 70–75% versus 50% for the ITA.[20,70]

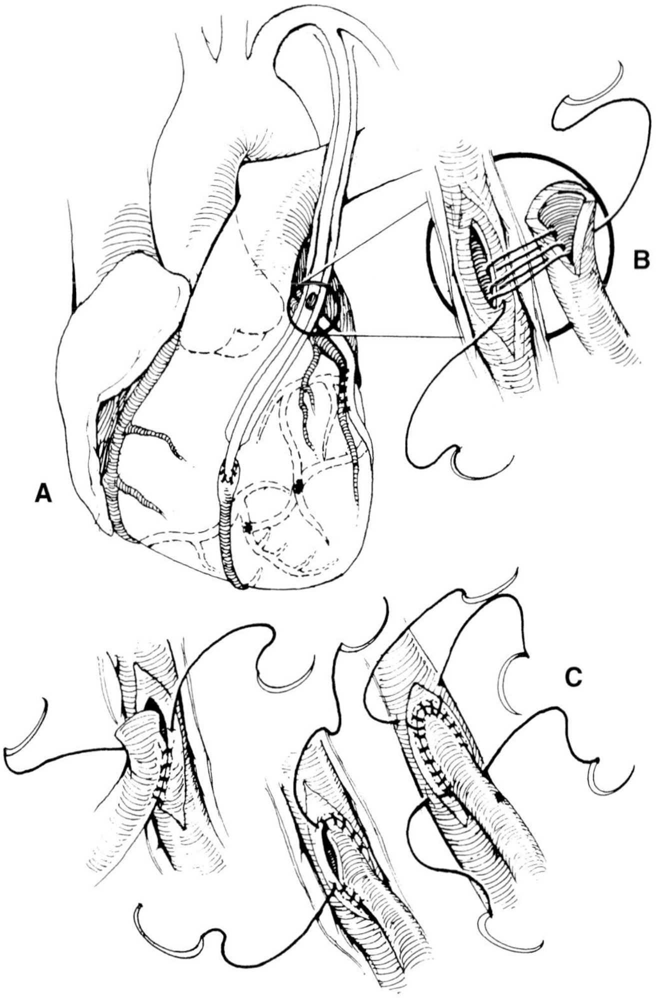

Figure 84–2 **A,** T-graft in which the radial artery has been anastomosed to the left internal thoracic artery (ITA) at the level of the left atrial appendage after incising the pericardium nearly to the phrenic nerve. The ITA is directed to the left anterior descending artery and the radial artery to the first obtuse marginal, the left posterolateral, and the right posterior descending arteries. **B,** End-to-side anastomosis performed to the pleural aspect of the ITA by rotating the pedicle 180 degrees and suspending it with two sutures. **C,** After completion of the anastomosis fine sutures are placed in a triangular configuration from the fascia of the ITA pedicle to the adventitia of the radial artery to reduce stress on the toe and heel of the anastomosis.
(From Barner HB: Conduit options for coronary artery bypass surgery. In Yang SC, Cameron DE, editors: Current Therapy in Thoracic and Cardiovascular Surgery. Harcourt Health Sciences [in press].)

Right Gastroepiploic Artery (RGA)

Anatomy and Histology

The RGA arises from the gastroduodenal artery and courses along the greater curvature of the stomach in the gastrocolic omentum. Because of its multiple branches it progressively decreases in size and at the short gastric branches usually becomes too small to be useful. It can vary significantly in size from patient to patient, and some have routinely assessed this with preoperative angiography. Similar to the RA, its media is essentially devoid of elastic fibers. It is smaller and with a thinner media than the RA.

Harvesting Technique

The median sternotomy incision is extended a short distance (4–8 cm) into the epigastrium and the stomach pulled up to expose the greater curvature where the gastroepiploic artery (GEA) is identified. Initially it was harvested as a bulky pedicle with mass ligatures or oversize clips, but most surgeons now use a skeletonizing technique. The thin walled branches are not amenable to electrocoagulation and are controlled with clips or ligatures. Dissection continues to the pylorus and distally to the short gastric branches depending on the size of the RGA, which should be at least 2.0 mm after dilating the conduit with intraluminal papaverine and blood for 10 min. This gives a usual length of 19 cm.[75]

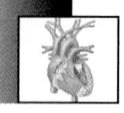

Grafting Technique

The mobilized GEA can be routed anterior or posterior to the stomach and anterior or posterior to the left lobe of the liver (Figure 84-3), and through or anterior (when directed to the left anterior descending artery) to the diaphragm.[104] An incision in the diaphragm could pinch the artery so that we make a cruciate incision or excise a small circle. The diaphragmatic opening should be 2.0 cm to the right of the anastomotic site so that the RGA can have a parallel approach to the target. It is tacked to the heart and diaphragm to maintain its position. The RGA can be used as a free graft from the aorta or another arterial conduit. Sequential grafting is appropriate when conduit size is optimal.[79]

Clinical Results

Early clinical patency was encouraging, but 10-year patency of 63% was the same as for SVG.[98] However, this series was operated before the significance of competitive coronary flow was fully appreciated and it is likely that this influenced patency.[99] Patency of the RGA is reduced with a coronary stenosis of less than 70–80% and also depends on conduit and coronary diameter and the location of the anastomosis.[79,106,107] A smaller conduit has been associated with subclinical ischemia. Early patency of free grafts has been excellent.[73] Intermediate patency has been excellent for sequential grafts in selected patients as well.[80] Abdominal complications have been rare with the most frequent being bleeding from the harvest bed or conduit.

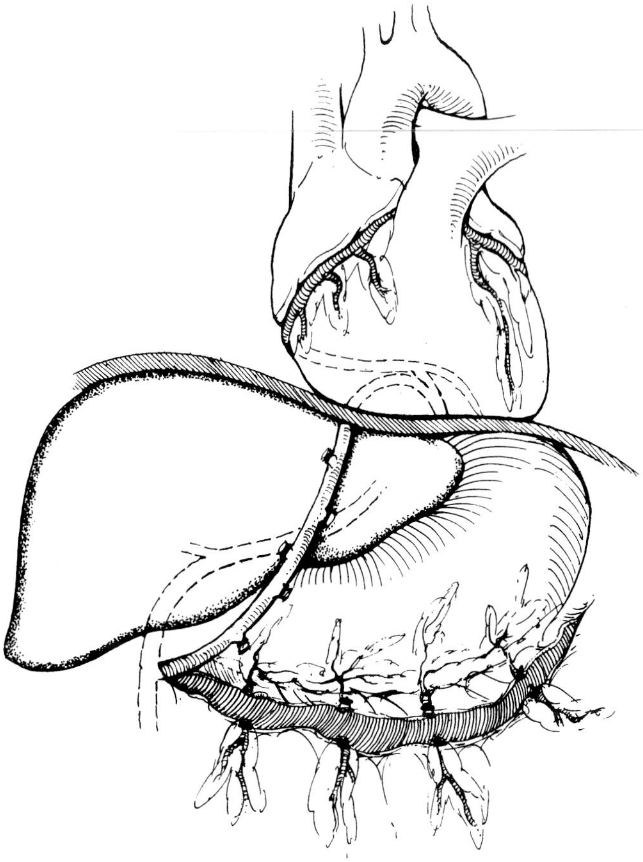

Figure 84–3 The right gastroepiploic artery has been skeletonized with clipping of branches and brought anterior to the stomach and left lobe of the liver to pass through the diaphragm well to the right of the posterior descending artery where an end-to-side anastomosis has been performed. The conduit pedicle is attached to the epicardium and to the diaphragm with fine suture to maintain its position. *(From Barner HB: Conduit options for coronary artery bypass surgery. In Yang SC, Cameron DE, editors: Current Therapy in Thoracic and Cardiovascular Surgery. Harcourt Health Sciences [in press].)*

Inferior Epigastric Artery (IEA)

Anatomy and Histology

The IEA arises from the external iliac artery under the inguinal ligament and ascends in a superoanterior course into the rectus sheath where it lies posterior to the muscle and may enter it at any time, which makes dissection extremely difficult. Its usable length varies greatly from 6–16 cm (mean 12 cm) because of bifurcation or an intramuscular course.[5]

The microanatomy is very similar to that of the RGA.[110] Medial calcification of the proximal 1–3 cm is seen and does not restrict flow but may preclude suturing.[5]

Harvesting Technique

A midline incision from umbilicus to symphysis allows medial entry into the rectus sheath and bilateral harvest. A near paramedian incision with lateral retraction provides less exposure to the proximal IEA than does a lateral rectus incision with medial muscle retraction. The artery is identified in the inferior sheath and mobilized with its vein and dissected proximally as near as possible to its origin and divided with knowledge that an anomalous obturator artery may rise from it near the external iliac artery. Distal dissection is continued to attain a desired length or until the IEA is not usable.

Grafting Strategy

After its introduction, it was used as a graft from the aorta.[6,13] Because of its inconsistent length and frequent difficulty in harvesting a long segment, it is best used as a short Y-graft from another arterial conduit.[21]

Clinical Results

Midterm patency when grafted from the aorta was 79%.[13] When used as a Y-graft, patency at a mean of 25.2 months was 100% (n = 25).[21] Rectus muscle necrosis has occurred without bothersome sequelae, but abdominal wall (skin and rectus muscle) necrosis requiring skin grafting occurred in 2 of 17 patients having bilateral ITA and IEA harvest.[6]

Other Arterial Conduits

Several other arteries have been used but in some instances by only one or two surgeons and in only a few patients. Two exceptions are the ulnar artery and lateral circumflex femoral artery. The splenic artery was used very early but dissection was difficult and splenectomy or pancreatitis were complications.[39] The inferior mesenteric artery was used in two patients.[92] The subscapular artery was used in three patients as a free graft via a left thoracotomy.[74] The thoracodorsal artery is a branch of the subscapular artery and has also been used as a free graft.[95] The left gastric artery can be brought through the diaphragm to the right coronary artery.[47,109]

Buxton used the ulnar artery in 21 patients when the Allen test was positive.[15] Dissection is difficult because the artery is deep within the forearm and near the median nerve proximally and the ulnar nerve distally with the possibility of trauma to these nerves.[15]

Of potential significance is the report of using the descending branch of the lateral femoral circumflex artery in 147 patients.[42] The artery is exposed in the anterolateral thigh between the rectus femoris and vastus lateralis muscles and harvested to an average length of 14.3 cm. Harvesting time averaged 18 min, and the proximal diameter was 2.5 cm with a distal diameter of 1.5 cm. It was used as a Y-graft from an *in situ* ITA graft to all potential targets but in 70% to a circumflex branch. Patency was 97.5% at 1 year (82 patients) and 93.7% at 3 years (48 patients).[42]

FACTORS INFLUENCING CONDUIT PATENCY

Arterial and venous grafts have different patencies related to their behavior and are considered separately.

Arterial Conduits

Arteries were designed for the arterial system, and, if handled carefully, their ultrastructure and physiological behavior are little altered by grafting to the coronary artery.[1,61] Failure is caused by intimal fracturing and thrombosis, profound spasm with secondary thrombosis, faulty anastomotic technique, severe coronary disease, and competitive coronary flow causing thrombosis. The degree of coronary stenosis causing competitive flow-induced thrombosis varies with the conduit (stenosis of less than 50–60% for the ITA and 70–80% for the other arterial conduits). In addition, the diameters of the coronary target and the conduit used to graft it influence conduit flow. The relative resistance to flow through the two systems (and the conduit is disadvantaged because of its greater length) determines which will prevail and supply most of the required flow to the myocardial bed. When graft forward flow is minimal or nonexistent, the ITA has the ability to remain patent (with to and fro flow) and with a reduced caliber (angiographic string sign) while the more muscular arterial conduits do not and frequently thrombose. This may be a consequence of the more muscular media, which when not continuously stimulated by flow-mediated endothelial release of NO closes the lumen. The vigor of measured stimulated contraction of arterial rings from the various conduits supports this notion,[27,53] but enhanced RA relaxation to NO may partially compensate.[91]

Venous Conduits

Vein grafts are not bothered with competitive flow because they are so much larger than coronary arteries. However, vein grafts close in the first year because of their large size, relatively sluggish flow, and intimal injury, which predisposes to thrombus formation. In addition, veins produce less prostacycline than arterial grafts[25] and have less NO-mediated relaxation,[67,91] which likely contributes to accelerated atherosclerosis in veins. Endothelial injury during harvesting, to which veins are particularly susceptible, can lead to early thrombosis or provide a nidus for the later formation of atheromas. Pathological or accelerated fibrous intimal hyperplasia caused some grafts to fail quickly in the 1970s and may have been caused by harvest injury.[11] Intimal hyperplasia is now considered a precursor to atherosclerosis, which closes grafts as early as the fifth year and progresses on.[11] Venous grafts have also shown accelerated atherosclerosis in hyperlipidemic states,[62] and this contributes to their poor long-term results when compared to arterial grafts. Vigorous reduction of risk factors, such as hyperlipidemia, can influence the progression of vein graft atherosclerosis.[10]

HYPOPERFUSION SYNDROME

Surgeons have learned that hypoperfusion of the heart after use of arterial conduits is more prevalent early in their experience and decreases over time.[23,49,108] Inadequate flow may be the result of untreated or inadequately treated spasm, irreversible spasm, intimal fracture or separation, and technical errors. Rarely it can be caused by none of the above but by inadequate flow capacity of the arterial conduit because of small size and/or greater need for flow. The decreasing incidence of hypoperfusion and the success of the T-graft (which places even greater flow demands on the ITA) suggest that arterial conduits are up to the task. There are data to indicate that subclinical hypoperfusion may be associated with arterial conduits.[56,80] This shortcoming is likely corrected over time (6 months in humans) because of remodeling of the conduit.[7,110,111] This physiological occurrence is based on the need for the endothelium to maintain sensed sheer stress in a narrow range (15–20 dyn-s/cm^2) by endothelial release of NO, which can increase (or decrease) vessel diameter by 10% acutely and by 50% chronically.

When hypoperfusion is of concern and the cause cannot be identified and corrected, a supplemental vein graft should be placed. In one specific instance (replacing a diseased but patent vein graft to the left anterior descending) we have been cautioned to use a vein graft or to leave the old vein graft if an arterial conduit is used.[78] Although we basically agree, we would commonly use the ITA (or another arterial conduit) in this setting and once cardiopulmonary bypass is discontinued and the patient is hemodynamically stable, occlude the vein graft temporarily. If stability persists, we would measure conduit flow, ligate the vein graft, and give protamine.

Although hypoperfusion may occur with vein grafts, it is usually easily recognizable (spasm or twist would be obvious and intimal fracture does not occur) and due to a technical error (failure to reverse the vein, faulty anastomosis) and is easily corrected.

ALTERNATIVE CONDUITS

Biological

Fresh GSV allografts were used prior to coronary grafting for femoral popliteal bypass with very poor patency at 1 year.

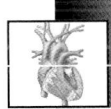

It was considered that cryopreservation might alter the antigenicity of the vein, but this proved ill-founded.[50,63,105] We have never found it necessary to use this conduit.

Bovine ITA treated with dialdehyde starch, sterilized with ethanol and propylene oxide and stored in deionized water and 1% propylene oxide solution, has had limited use as a bypass conduit with 15.8% (3 of 19) patency at 3–23 months and 14.3% (1 of 7) beyond 1 year.[34,76,98,100] We have not used this conduit.

Synthetic

Expanded polytetrafluoroethylene (PTFE) grafts have had limited success as a coronary conduit. Sapsford et al reported on 27 grafts in 16 patients with 27% patency on angiograms done at 12–29 months.[89] Chard et al reported 4 of 28 distal anastomoses patent at 45 months.[26]

A unique design placed a resistor in a 5-mm PTFE graft allowing a controlled arteriovenous fistula between the aorta and superior vena cava to increase graft flow yet allow arterial pressure in the graft proximal to the resistor. The graft is looped around the heart and multiple side-to-side anastomoses can be constructed.[40,41,112] However, success with this device has been poor and it is not currently available.

NEW STRATEGIES TO IMPROVE GRAFT PATENCY

Molecular studies of atherosclerosis and intimal hyperplasia have led to novel approaches to prevent graft occlusion. Intimal hyperplasia is the result of migration of smooth muscle cells from the media to the intima with subsequent proliferation of these cells. Endothelial cells, monocytes, macrophages, and platelets also play an important role in the complex mechanism of plaque formation. Intraoperative incubation of GSV with antisense DNA against c-*myc* confirmed significant vasculoprotective effects, reflected by the reduction in cell proliferation and decrease in several markers of injury.[71] Transfer of the endothelial-type nitric oxide synthase gene into the jugular vein has been done successfully in an animal model, and when these altered veins were grafted into the carotid circulation they demonstrated a significant reduction of graft neointima at 4 weeks postoperatively along with a reduction of proliferating cells and a decreased macrophage accumulation in the vein wall.[81] The nuclear transcriptional factor NFκB is important in the expression of genes for neutrophil and macrophage chemotactic factors, and for expression of adhesion molecules. Shintani et al reported on the successful transfection of aortocoronary saphenous vein grafts in dogs with a decoy to block this transcriptional factor and demonstrated a significant reduction in neointimal formation and proliferation of medial smooth muscle cells in grafts at 4 weeks postoperatively.[94] Whether these molecular approaches to inhibit graft stenosis will prove clinically useful is unknown at present.

Platelet inhibitors, heparin-like compounds, and angiotensin-converting enzyme inhibitors have all been shown experimentally to reduce intimal hyperplasia.[55,57,65,84,114] However, these efforts have not shown clinical effectiveness on graft patency with the exception of aspirin. Statins, which are widely used to reduce cholesterol, have recently been shown to inhibit neointima formation and inhibit smooth muscle proliferation in human saphenous vein segments *in situ*.[83]

Synthetic grafts fail in the coronary position because their surface is thrombogenic and their low flow rates allow significant fibrin deposition on the wall of the graft, which diminishes its lumen further and leads to further reduction in flow. Efforts at improving synthetic graft patency have been directed at lining the graft with an intact nonthrombogenic surface. Fibroblast growth factor, a potent stimulant of endothelial cells, has been used to treat PTFE to stimulate endothelial growth into these grafts.[51] Endothelial cell seeding of prosthetic grafts has been performed successfully in animals.[58,93] This technique requires harvesting autologous endothelial cells and growing them in culture to obtain sufficient cells to coat a graft. This technique has been used for peripheral vascular grafts in humans with some promising results.[82]

Therapeutic angiogenesis is another novel approach being tried in conjunction with coronary bypass procedures to improve myocardial revascularization. Angiogenesis holds the promise of improved myocardial perfusion by stimulating new vessel growth into the myocardium with the added benefit of improved graft runoff, which may improve patency. These techniques involve the administration of angiogenic proteins into the tissue directly or transfecting myocardial DNA with plasmid DNA for vascular endothelial growth factor.[48,64,87,101] These efforts have shown therapeutic benefit in improved angina scores in the early follow-up period of 6–12 months.

SUMMARY

As coronary bypass surgery has matured, it has become clear that arterial grafts are superior to vein conduit. The survival benefit of an ITA graft to the left anterior descending is clearly established as is the benefit of both ITAs directed to the left side. The use of multiple or only arterial conduits is associated with decreased need for reintervention. The benefit of arterial grafting is most clearly seen in the long term. Therefore, the surgeon must use appropriate judgment in deciding when an all-arterial revascularization is warranted as the operative time and complexity are clearly greater for multiple arterial grafts. Future advances in the therapeutic benefit of coronary bypass surgery clearly lie in the molecular realm of improved tissue perfusion with the induction of vascular neogenesis and with the prevention of vein graft atherosclerosis.

REFERENCES

1. Al-Bustami MH, Amrani M, Chester AH, et al: In vivo early and mid-term flow-mediated endothelial function of the radial artery used as a coronary bypass graft. J Am Coll Cardiol 39:573–577, 2002.
2. Allen KB, Griffith GL, Heimansohn, VA, et al: Endoscopic versus traditional saphenous vein harvesting: a prospective, randomized trial. Ann Thorac Surg 66:26–32, 1998.
3. Barner HB, Standeven JW, Reese J: Twelve year experience with internal mammary artery for coronary bypass. J Thorac Cardiovasc Surg 90:668–675, 1985.

4. Barner HB, Sundt TM III, Bailey M, et al: Intermediate term results of complete arterial revascularization in over 1000 patients using an internal thoracic artery/radial artery T-graft. Ann Surg 234:447–452, 2001.
5. Barner HB, Naumheim KS, Fiore AC: Use of the inferior epigastric artery as a free graft for myocardial revascularization. Ann Thorac Surg 52:429–436, 1991.
6. Barner HB, Naunheim KS, Peigh PS, et al: Inferior epigastric artery for myocardial revascularization. Eur J Cardio-Thorac Surg 7:478–481, 1993.
7. Barner HB: Remodeling of arterial conduits in coronary grafting. Ann Thorac Surg 73:1341–1345, 2002.
8. Berger PB, Alderman EL, Nadel A, et al: Frequency of early occlusion and stenosis in a left internal mammary artery graft to left anterior descending artery bypass graft after surgery through a median sternotomy on conventional bypass. Circulation 100:2353–2358, 1999.
9. Bitondo JM, Daggett WM, Torchiana DF, et al: Endoscopic versus open saphenous vein harvest: a comparison of postoperative wound complications. Ann Thorac Surg 73:523–528, 2002.
10. Blankenhorn DH, Nessin SA, Johnson RL: Beneficial effects of combined colestipol-niacin therapy on coronary atherosclerosis and coronary venous bypass grafts. JAMA 257:3233–3236, 1987.
11. Brody WR, Kosek, JC, Angell WW: Changes in vein grafts following aortocoronary bypass induced pressure and ischemia. J Thorac Cardiovasc Surg 64:846–851, 1972.
12. Broeders MAW, Doevendens PA, Maessen JG, et al: The human internal thoracic artery releases more nitric oxide in response to vascular endothelial growth factor than the human saphenous vein. J Thorac Cardiovasc Surg, 122:305–309, 2001.
13. Buche M, Schroeder E, Gurne O, et al: Coronary artery bypass grafting with the inferior epigastric artery. J Thorac Cardiovasc Surg 109:553–560, 1995.
14. Bush HL Jr, Jakubowski JA, Curl GR, et al: The natural history of endothelial structure and function in arterialized vein grafts. J Vasc Surg 3:204–215, 1986.
15. Buxton BF, Chan AT, Dixit AS, et al: Ulnar artery as a coronary bypass graft. Ann Thorac Surg 65:1020–1024, 1998.
16. Buxton BS, Ruengsakultach P, Fuller J, et al: The right internal thoracic artery graft—benefits of grafting the left coronary system and native vessels with a high grade stenosis. Eur J Cardio-Thorac Surg 18:255–261, 2000.
17. Buxton BS, Raman JS, Ruengsakulrach P, et al: Radial artery patency and clinical outcomes: five-year results of a randomized trial. J Thorac Cardiovasc Surg 125:1363–1371, 2003.
18. Cable DG, Caccitolo JA, Pearson PJ, et al: New approaches to prevention and treatment of radial artery graft vasospasm. Circulation 98:II-15–II-22, 1998.
19. Calafiore AM, Coutini M, Vitolla G, et al: Bilateral internal thoracic artery grafting: long-term clinical and angiographic results of in situ versus Y grafts. J Thorac Cardiovasc Surg 120:990–998, 2000.
20. Calafiore AM, Di Mauro M, D'Alessandro S, et al: Revascularization of the lateral wall: long-term angiographic and clinic results of radial artery versus right internal thoracic artery grafting. J Thorac Cardiovasc Surg 123:225–231, 2002.
21. Calafiore AM, di Giammarco G, Teodori G: Radial artery and inferior epigastric artery as composite grafts with internal mammary artery: improved midterm angiographic results. Ann Thorac Surg 60:517–524, 1995.
22. Carpino PA, Khabbaz KR, Bojar RM, et al: Clinical benefits of endoscopic vein harvesting in patients with risk factors for saphenectomy wound infections undergoing coronary artery bypass grafting. J Thorac Cardiovasc Surg 119:69–76, 2000.
23. Carrel T, Kujawski T, Zund G, et al: The internal mammary artery mal-perfusion syndrome: incidents, treatment, and angiographic verification. Eur J Cardio-Thorac Surg 9:190–197, 1995.
24. CASS Principal Investigators and their associates: Myocardial infarction and mortality in the coronary artery surgery (CASS) ramdomized trial. N Engl J Med 310:750–754, 1984.
25. Chaikhouni A, Crawford FA, Kochel, PJ, et al: Human internal mammary artery produces more prostacyclin than saphenous vein. J Thorac Cardiovasc Surg 92:88–91, 1986.
26. Chard RB, Johnson DC, Nunn GR, et al: Aorta-coronary bypass grafting with polytetrafluoroethylene conduits. J Thorac Cardiovasc Surg 94:132–134, 1987.
27. Chardigny C, Jebara VA, Acar C, et al: Vasoreactivity of the radial artery: comparison with the internal mammary and gastroepiploic arteries with implications for coronary artery surgery. Circulation 88(Pt. 2):115–127, 1993.
28. Chello M, Mastroroberto P, Perticone F, et al: Nitric oxide modulation of neutrophil-endothelium interaction: difference between arterial and venous coronary bypass grafts. J Ann Coll Cardio 31:823–826, 1998.
29. Christenson JT, Schmuziger M: Sequential venous bypass grafts: results 10 years later. Ann Thorac Surg 63:371–376, 1997.
30. Chua YL, Pearson PJ, Evora PRB, et al: Detection of intraluminal release of endothelium-derived relaxing factor from human saphenous veins. Circulation 88(Pt. 2):128–132, 1993.
31. Cohen AJ, Lockman J, Lorbergoyn M, et al: Assessment of sternal vascularity with single photon emission computed tomography after harvesting of the internal thoracic artery. J Thorac Cardiovasc Surg 118:496–502, 1999.
32. Cohen G, Tamariz MG, Sever JY, et al: The radial artery versus the saphenous vein graft in contemporary CABG: a case-matched study. Ann Thorac Surg 71:180–185, 2001.
33. Connolly MW, Tomillo LD, Stauder MJ, et al: Endoscopic radial artery harvesting: results of first 300 patients. Ann Thorac Surg 74:502–505, 2002.
34. Craig SR, Walker WS: The use of bovine internal mammary artery grafts in coronary artery surgery. Eur J Cardio-Thorac Surg 8:43–45, 1994.
35. Crouch JD, O'Hair DP, Keuler JP, et al: Open versus endoscopic saphenous vein harvesting: wound complications and vein quality. Ann Thorac Surg 68:1513–1516, 1999.
36. de Jesus RA, Acland RD: Anatomic study of the collateral blood supply of the sternum. Ann Thorac Surg 59:163–168, 1995.
37. Dion R, Glineur D, Derouck D, et al: Complementary saphenous grafting: long-term followup. J Thorac Cardiovasc Surg 122:296–304, 2001.
38. Dion R, Glineur D, Derouck D, et al: Long-term clinical and angiographic follow-up of sequential internal thoracic artery grafting. Eur J Cardio-Thorac Surg 17:407–417, 2000.
39. Edwards WS, Lewis CE, Blakeley WR, et al: Coronary artery bypass with internal mammary and splenic artery grafts. Ann Thorac Surg 15:35–40, 1973.
40. Emery RW, Joyce LV, Arom KV, et al: Operative considerations in implantation of the Perma-Flow graft. Ann Thorac Surg 58:1770–1773, 1994.
41. Emery RW, Mills NL, Teijeira FX, et al: North American experience with the Perma-Flow prosthetic coronary graft. Ann Thorac Surg 62:691–696, 1996.
42. Fabbrocini M, Fattouch K, Camporini G, et al: Descending branch of lateral femoral circumflex artery in arterial CABG: early and midterm results. Ann Thorac Surg 75:1836–1841, 2003.
43. Favaloro R: Saphenous vein autograft replacement of severe segmental coronary artery occlusion. Ann Thorac Surg 5:335–339, 1968.
44. Ferguson TB Jr, Coombs LP, Peterson ED: Internal thoracic artery grafting in the elderly patient undergoing coronary artery bypass grafting; room for process improvement? J Thorac Cardiovasc Surg 123:869–879, 2002.

45. Fitzgibbon GM, Leach AJ, Leon WJ, et al: Coronary bypass graft fate: angiographic study of 1179 vein grafts early, one year, and five years after operation. J Thorac Cardiovasc Surg 91:773–778, 1986.
46. Fitzgibbon GM, Leach AJ, Kafka HP, et al: Coronary bypass graft fate: long-term angiographic study. J Am Coll Cardiol 17:1075–1080, 1991.
47. Flege JB Jr: Left gastric to coronary artery bypass. Ann Thorac Surg 73:693, 2002.
48. Freedman SB, Isner JM: Therapeutic angiogenesis for coronary artery disease. Ann Intern Med 136:54–71, 2002.
49. Gaudino M, Trani C, Luciani N, et al: The internal mammary artery mal-perfusion syndrome: late angiographic verification. Thorac Surg 63:1257–1261, 1997.
50. Gelbfish J, Jacobowitz IJ, Rose DM, et al: Cryopreserved homologous saphenous vein. Early and late patency in coronary artery bypass surgical procedures. Ann Thorac Surg 42:70–73, 1980.
51. Greisler HP, Cziperle DJ, Kim DU, et al: Enhanced endothelialization of expanded PTFE grafts by fibroblast growth factor type I pretreatment. Surgery 112:244–255, 1992.
52. Grover FL, Johnson RR, Marshall G, et al: Impact of mammary grafts on coronary bypass operative mortality and morbidity. Ann Thorac Surg 57:559–569, 1994.
53. He G-W, Yang C-Q: Radial artery has higher receptor-mediated contractility but similar endothelial function compared with mammary artery. Ann Thorac Surg 63:1346–1352, 1997.
54. Iaco AL, Teodori G, Di Giammarco G, et al: Radial artery for myocardial revascularization: long-term clinical and angiographic results. Ann Thorac Surg 72:464–468, 2001.
55. Janiak P, Pillon A, Prost JF, et al: Role of angiotensin subtype 2 receptor in neointima formation after vascular injury. Hypertension 20:737–745, 1992.
56. Jegaden O, Bontemps L, de Gevigney G, et al: 2-D assessment by exercise thallium scintigraphy of myocardial revascularization using bilateral internal mammary and gastroepiploic arteries. Eur J Cardio-Thorac Surg 16: 131–134, 1999.
57. Kazi M, Lundmark K, Religa P, et al: Inhibition of rat smooth muscle cell adhesion and proliferation by non-anticoagulant heparins. J Cell Physiol 193:365–372, 2002.
58. Kent KC, Shindo S, Ikemoto T, et al: Species variation and the success of endothelial cell seeding. J Vasc Surg 92:271–276, 1989.
59. Kieser TM, Fitzgibbon GM, Keon WJ: Sequential coronary artery bypass grafts: long-term follow-up. J Thorac Cardiovasc Surg 91:767–772, 1986.
60. Kolesov VI: Mammary artery-coronary artery anastomosis as method of treatment for angina pectoris. J Thorac Cardiovasc Surg 54:535–544, 1967.
61. Kushwaha SS, Bustami M, Tadjkarimi, et al: Late endothelial function of free and pedicled internal mammary artery grafts. J Thorac Cardiovasc Surg 110:453–562, 1995.
62. Lardenoye JH, de Vries MR, Lowik CW, et al: Accelerated atherosclerosis and calcification in vein grafts: a study in APOE*3 Leiden transgenic mice. Circ Res 91:577–584, 2002.
63. Laub GW, Muralidharan S, Clancy R, et al: Cryopreserved allograft veins as alternative coronary artery bypass conduits: early phase results. Ann Thorac Surg 54:826–831, 1992.
64. Lee LY, Patel SR, Hackett NR, et al: Focal angiogene therapy using intramyocardial delivery of an adenovirus vector coding for vascular endothelial growth factor 121. Ann Thorac Surg 69:14–23, 2000.
65. Lindner V, Olson NE, Clowes AW, et al: Inhibition of smooth muscle cell proliferation in injured rat arteries. Interaction of heparin with basic fibroblast growth factor. J Clin Invest 90:2044–2049, 1992.
66. Loop FD, Lytle BW, Cosgrove DM, et al: Influence of the internal-mammary-artery graft on 10-year survival and other cardiac events. N Engl J Med 314:1–6, 1986.
67. Luscher TF, Diederich D, Siebenmann R, et al: Difference between endothelium-dependent relaxation in arterial and in venous coronary bypass grafts. N Engl J Med 319:462–467, 1988.
68. Lytle BW, Arnold JH, Loop FT, et al: Two internal thoracic artery grafts are better than one. J Thorac Cardiovasc Surg 117:855–872, 1999.
69. Maniar HS, Barner HB, Bailey M, et al: Radial artery patency: are aortocoronary conduits superior to composite grafting? Ann Thorac Surg 76:1498–1503, 2003.
70. Maniar HS, Sundt PM, Barner HB, et al: Effect of target stenosis and location on radial artery graft patency. J Thorac Cardiovasc Surg 123:45–52, 2002.
71. Mannion JD, Ormont ML, Shi Y, et al: Saphenous vein graft protection: effects of *c-MYC* antisense. J Thorac Cardiovasc Surg 115:152–156, 1998.
72. Marco JD, Barner HB, Kaiser GC, et al: Operative flow measurements in coronary bypass graft patency. J Thorac Cardiovasc Surg 71:545–549, 1976.
73. Matsurra A, Yasuura K, Yoshida K, et al: Transplantation of the en bloc vascular system for coronary revascularization. J Thorac Cardiovasc Surg 121:520–525, 2001.
74. Mills ML, Dupin CL, Everson CT, et al: Subscapular artery: an alternative conduit for coronary bypass. J Card Surg 8:66–71, 1993.
75. Mills NL, Hockmuth DR, Everson CT: Right gastroepiploic artery used for coronary artery bypass grafting: evaluation of flow characteristics and size. J Thorac Cardiovasc Surg 106:579–585, 1993.
76. Mitchell IM, Essop AR, Scott PJ, et al: Bovine internal mammary artery as a conduit for coronary revascularization: long-term results. Ann Thorac Surg 55:120–122, 1993.
77. Moon MR, Sundt TM, Pasque MK, et al: Influence of internal mammary artery grafting and completeness of revascularization on long-term outcome in octogenarians. Ann Thorac Surg 234:447–452, 2001.
78. Navia D, Cosgrove DM III, Lytle BW, et al: Is the internal thoracic artery the conduit of choice to replace a stenotic vein graft? Ann Thorac Surg 57:40–48, 1994.
79. Ochi M, Bessho R, Saji Y, et al: Sequential grafting of the right gastroepiploic artery in coronary artery bypass surgery. Ann Thorac Surg 71:1205–1209, 2001.
80. Ochi M, Hatori N, Fujii M, et al: Limited flow capacity of the right gastroepiploic artery graft: postoperative echocardiographic and angiographic evaluation. Ann Thorac Surg 71:1210–1214, 2001.
81. Ohta S, Komori K, Yonemitsu Y, et al: Intraluminal gene transfer of endothelial cell-nitric oxide synthase suppresses intimal hyperplasia of vein grafts in cholesterol-fed rabbit: a limited biological effect as a result of the loss of medial smooth muscle cells. Surgery 131:644–653, 2002.
82. Ortenwall P, Wadenvike H, Kutti J, et al: Endothelial cell seeding reduces thrombogenicity of Dacron grafts in humans. J Vasc Surg 11:403–410, 1990.
83. Porter KE, Naik J, Turner NA, et al: Simvastatin inhibits human saphenous vein neointima formation via inhibition of smooth muscle cell proliferation and migration. J Vasc Surg 36:150–157, 2002.
84. Powell JS, Muller RK, Baumgartner HR: Suppression of the vascular response to injury: the role of angiotensin-converting enzyme inhibitors. J Am Coll Cardiol 17(Suppl. B):137B–142B, 1991.
85. Raess DH, Mahomed Y, Brown JW, et al: Lesser saphenous vein as an alternative conduit of choice in coronary bypass operations. Ann Thorac Surg 41:334–336, 1986.

86. Ronan JW, Perry LA, Barner HB, et al: Radial artery harvest: comparison of ultrasonic dissection with standard technique. Ann Thorac Surg 69:113–114, 2000.
87. Rosengart TK, Lee LY, Patel SR, et al: Six-month assessment of a phase I trial of angiogenic gene therapy for the treatment of coronary artery disease using direct intramyocardial administration of an adenovirus vector expressing the VEGF 121 cDNA. Ann Surg 230:466–470, 1999.
88. Salerno TA, Charrette EJ: The short saphenous vein: an alternative to the long saphenous vein for aortocoronary bypass. Ann Thorac Surg 25:457–458, 1978.
89. Sapsford RN, Oakley GD, Talbot S: Early and late patency of expanded polytetrafluoroethylene vascular grafts in aortacoronary bypass. J Thorac Cardiovasc Surg 81:860–864, 1981.
90. Shapira OM, Xu A, Vita JA, et al: Nitroglycerin is superior to diltiazem as a coronary bypass conduit vasodilator. J Thorac Cardiovasc Surg 117:906–911, 1999.
91. Shapira OM, Xu A, Aldea GS, et al: Enhanced nitric oxide-mediated vascular relaxation in radial artery compared with internal mammary artery or saphenous vein. Circulation 100: II322–327, 1999.
92. Shatapathy P, Aggarwal BK, Punnen J: Inferior mesenteric artery as a free arterial conduit for myocardial revascularization. J Thorac Cardiovasc Surg 113:210–211, 1997.
93. Shepard AD, Eldrup-Jorgensen J, Keough EM, et al: Endothelial cell seeding of small caliber synthetic grafts in the baboon. Surgery 99:318–326, 1986.
94. Shintani T, Sawa Y, Takahashi T, et al: Intraoperative transfection of vein grafts with the NFκB decoy in a canine aortocoronary bypass model: a strategy to attenuate intimal hyperplasia. Ann Thorac Surg 74:1132–1137, 2002.
95. Simic O, Zambelli M, Zelic M, Dirjavec A: Thoracodorsal artery as a free graft for coronary artery bypass grafting. Eur J Cardio-Thorac Surg 16:94–96, 1999.
96. Sims FH, Chen X, Gavin JB: The importance of a substantial elastic lamina subjacent to the endothelium in limiting the progression of atherosclerotic changes. Histopathology 23:307–317, 1993.
97. Stoney WS, Alford WC, Burrus GR, et al: The fate of arm veins used for aortocoronary bypass grafts. J Thorac Cardiovasc Surg 84:522–526, 1984.
98. Suma H, Isomura T, Horii T, et al: Late angiographic result of using the right gastroepiploic artery as a graft. J Thorac Cardiovasc Surg 120:496–498, 2000.
99. Suma H: Personal communication, November 1, 2002.
100. Suma H, Wanibuchi Y, Takeuchi A: Bovine internal thoracic artery graft for myocardial revascularization: late results. Ann Thorac Surg 57:704–707, 1994.
101. Symes JF: Focal angiogenic therapy for myocardial ischemia. J Card Surg 15:283–290, 2000.
102. Taggart DP, Dipp N, Mussa S, et al: Phenoxybenzamine prevents spasm in radial artery conduits for coronary artery bypass grafting. J Thorac Cardiovasc Surg 120:815–817, 2000.
103. Tatoulis J, Buxton BF, Fuller JA: Patencies of 2127 arterial to coronary conduits over 15 years. Ann Thorac Surg 77:93–101, 2004.
104. Tavilla G, van Son JAM, Verhagen AF, et al: Retrogastric versus ante gastric routing and histology of the right gastroepiploic artery. Ann Thorac Surg 53:1057–1063, 1992.
105. Tector AJ, McDonald ML, Kress VC, et al: Purely internal thoracic artery grafts: outcomes. Ann Thorac Surg 72:450–455, 2001.
106. Tice DA, Urbino UR, Isom OW, et al: Coronary artery bypass with freeze-preserved saphenous vein allografts. J Thorac Cardiovasc Surg 71:378–380, 1976.
107. Uchida N, Kawaue Y: Flow competition of the right gastroepiploic artery graft in coronary revascularization. Ann Thorac Surg. 62:1342–1346, 1996.
108. Vajtai P, Ravichandran PS, Fessler CL, et al: Inadequate internal mammary artery graft as a cause of postoperative ischemia: incidence, diagnosis, and inaugement. Eur J Cardio-Thorac Surg 6:603–608, 1992.
109. Van Aaranhen EEHL, Schreur JH, Firouzi M, et al: The left gastric artery as an in situ conduit in coronary artery bypass grafting. Ann Thorac Surg 71:1013–1014, 2001.
110. Van Son JAM: Histology of the internal mammary artery versus the inferior epigastric artery. Ann Thorac Surg 53:1147–1149, 1992.
111. Wendler O, Hennen B, Markwirth T, et al: T-grafts with the right internal thoracic artery to left internal thoracic artery versus left internal thoracic artery and radial artery: flow dynamics in the internal thoracic artery mainstem. J Thorac Cardiovasc Surg 118:841–848, 1999.
112. Weyand M, Kerber S, Scmid C, et al: Coronary artery bypass with an expanded polytetrafluoroethylene graft. Ann Thorac Surg 67:1240–1244, 1999.
113. Wijnberg DS, Boeve WJ, Ebels P, et al: Patency of arm vein graft used in aorto-coronary bypass surgery. Eur J Cardio-Thorac Surg 4:510–513, 1990.
114. Yuda A, Takai S, Jin D, et al: Angiotensin II receptor antagonist L-158809, prevents intimal hyperplasia in dog grafted veins. Life Sci 68:41–48, 2000.

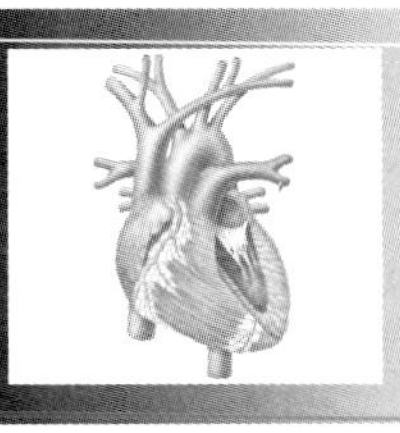

CHAPTER 85

Redo Coronary Artery Bypass Surgery

Bruce W. Lytle

Causes, Pathology, and Patient Population of Coronary Reoperations
Indications for Coronary Reoperations
Summary of Current Indications for Reoperation
Technical Aspects of Coronary Reoperations
Preoperative Assessment
Median Sternotomy, Conduit Preparation, and Cannulation
Stenotic Vein Grafts
Differently Invasive Strategies for Reoperative Coronary Surgery
The Results of Coronary Reoperations
Multiple Coronary Reoperations
Complementary End-Stage Revascularization Procedures
The Future of Coronary Reoperations

Reoperations present coronary artery surgeons with their greatest challenges. They involve multiple technical challenges including diffuse native coronary atherosclerosis, the presence of atherosclerotic vein grafts, and/or patent arterial grafts, lack of conduits for the construction of bypass grafts, and sternal reentry hazards. Patients undergoing reoperation for bypass grafting are different than those who undergo primary surgery. Their cardiac and noncardiac atherosclerosis is more advanced, they are more likely to have abnormal left ventricular function and noncardiac comorbidities, and the vascular pathologies that jeopardize myocardium are distinct and varied.

CAUSES, PATHOLOGY, AND PATIENT POPULATION OF CORONARY REOPERATIONS

The anatomical causes of the need for coronary reoperations include an ineffective or incomplete primary operation, the progression of coronary atherosclerosis in native coronary arteries, and bypass graft failure.[9,12,14] The relative contributions of these factors have changed with the evolution of bypass surgery and alternative treatments for coronary atherosclerosis. In the early years of bypass surgery technically inadequate primary operations were more frequent, leading to a substantial number of early (within 2–3 years of operation) reoperations. Today coronary surgeons are better microsurgical technicians, and early reoperations are less common. Also, primary operations for single- or double-vessel disease were common in the early years of bypass surgery and progression of native vessel atherosclerosis in ungrafted arteries was a common cause of reoperation. Now, most primary operations are performed for the treatment of triple-vessel disease, and when atherosclerotic progression occurs it usually involves distal disease in vessels previously grafted. When progression of native coronary atherosclerosis does contribute to the need for reoperation it is usually present in combination with bypass graft failure. The most important cause of reoperation is saphenous vein graft (SVG) failure based on pathological changes in SVGs: intimal fibroplasia and vein graft atherosclerosis (VGA).

The pathologies of vein grafts are important not only to understand the causes of reoperation but also to understand the natural history of postoperative patients treated conservatively and of the dangers associated with reoperations and percutaneous interventions for patients with previous bypass surgery.[1] Vein grafts examined within a month of operation often exhibit intimal disruption and mural thrombus, and when graft occlusion occurs at that time it is usually associated with thrombosis. Within 2–3 months a proliferative intimal fibroplasia may be identified in most SVGs. Intimal fibroplasia is concentric, diffuse, and cellular, changing with time into a more fibrous lesion. It may cause stenoses or occlusions but usually does not, and it is not friable. VGA is often recognized within a few years of operation and is characterized by lipid infiltration of areas of intimal fibroplasia. VGA is different than native vessel atherosclerosis in that fully developed VGA is diffuse, concentric, and superficial, mimicking the distribution of intimal fibroplasia. VGA is also extremely friable, and it is not encapsulated by an intima (Figure 85-1). Native vessel atherosclerosis, by comparison, is usually proximal, segmental, encapsulated, eccentric, and not friable. The unencapsulated, friable nature of VGA creates the risk of embolization during reoperation or interventional procedures. Mural thrombus is often associated with VGA and the presence of VGA stenoses predicts subsequent graft occlusion and clinical events.[15] VGA is present in most vein grafts examined more than 10 years after operation and produces stenoses and occlusions that increase in frequency with time. Late vein graft attrition leads to at least 30% of vein grafts being occluded by 10 postoperative years with another 30% exhibiting pathological changes angiographically.[5,13] There is now good evidence that treatment of postoperative patients with platelet inhibitors and statin type drugs decreases the rate of vein graft failure but even these antiatherosclerotic interventions have not eliminated VGA.[5,6]

Internal thoracic artery (ITA) grafts rarely develop atherosclerosis and patency rates of ITA grafts exceed those of vein grafts.[6,20] Patency rates of *in situ* left ITA (LITA) to left anterior descending (LAD) coronary artery grafts are more than 90% even 20 years after operation and there is unequivocal evidence that use of the LITA–LAD graft decreases the need for reoperation during the first 10 years after primary surgery when compared with the strategy of using only vein grafts.[8] Fewer long-term patency data are available regarding other types of ITA grafts, but evidence is accumulating that use of both ITAs as grafts at a primary operation provides incremental benefit over the use of only the LITA–LAD graft in terms of avoiding reoperation (Figure 85-2).[10]

For patients undergoing a primary bypass operation the likelihood of undergoing a reoperation will depend upon how long they live, the severity of their atherogenic diathesis, the details of the primary operation, the alternative therapies available, and physician and patient preference. Early studies showed that patient-related variables associated with a high rate of eventual reoperation included young age, normal left ventricular (LV) function, single- or double-vessel disease, and severe symptoms. Review of 4000 Cleveland Clinic Foundation patients who underwent primary operation during the 1971–1974 time frame showed that cumulatively, 10% of patients underwent reoperation by 10 and 25% of patients by 20 postoperative years.[4] Early in the bypass era there was concern that reoperations would overwhelm the surgical world. That has not happened for many reasons including a change in the population of patients undergoing primary operations to older patients with more extensive disease and shorter life expectancies, the use of ITA grafts, and the emergence of percutaneous treatments for graft and coronary artery stenoses. In the Society of Thoracic Surgeons' database the percentage of isolated coronary bypass operations that were reoperations ranged from 8.7% to 10.1% during the years 1998–2001.[23]

INDICATIONS FOR CORONARY REOPERATIONS

The randomized trials of bypass surgery vs. medical management that helped establish the indications for primary revascularization operations did not include patients undergoing reoperation, and because the vascular pathologies of reoperative candidates are different (particularly in regard to vein graft atherosclerosis), the same natural history of patients with native vessel atherosclerosis cannot be assumed to apply to patients postbypass surgery. No randomized trials exist comparing surgical treatment with the medical management of postoperative patients, but nonrandomized comparative studies have provided important information. First, early stenoses in vein grafts (<5 years

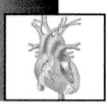

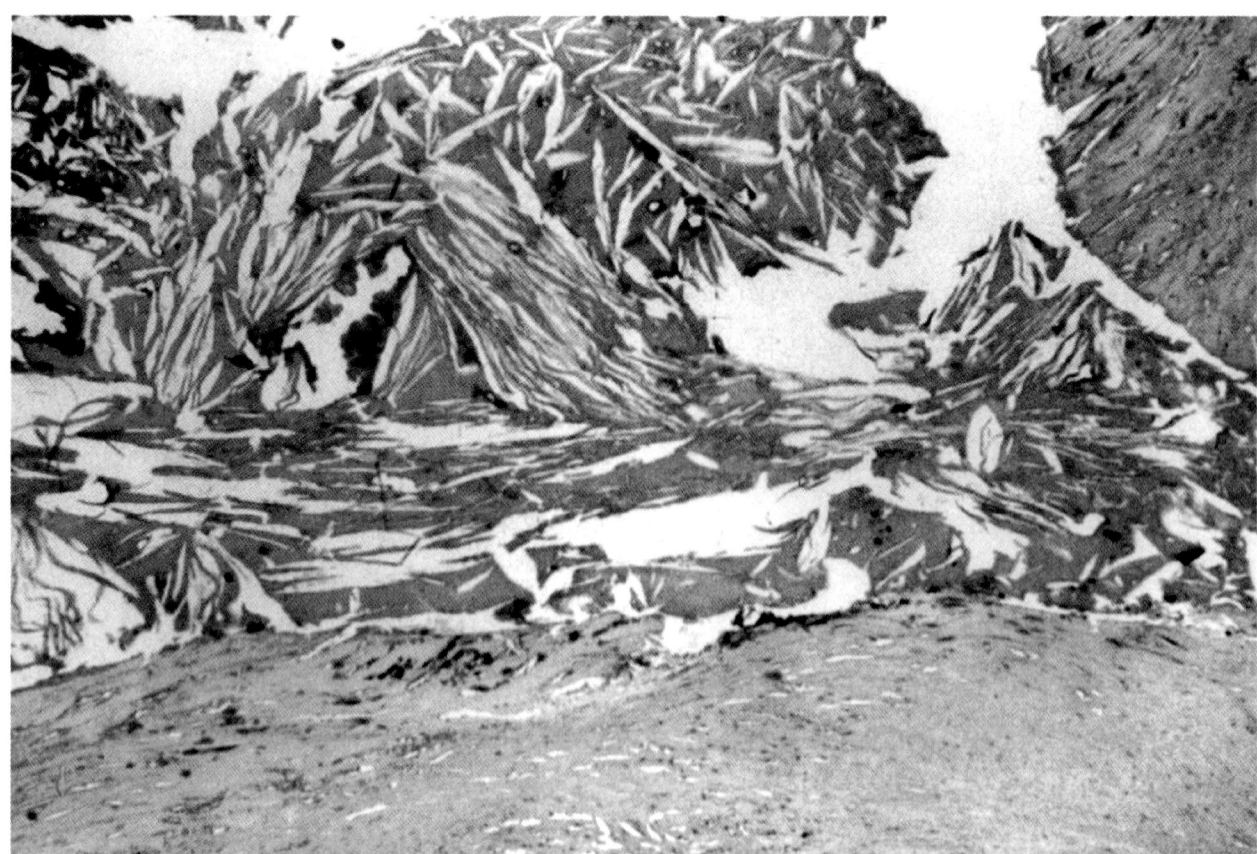

Figure 85–1 Vein graft atherosclerosis is a lesion that is unencapsulated and exceedingly friable, producing an unstable lesion that is prone to embolization.

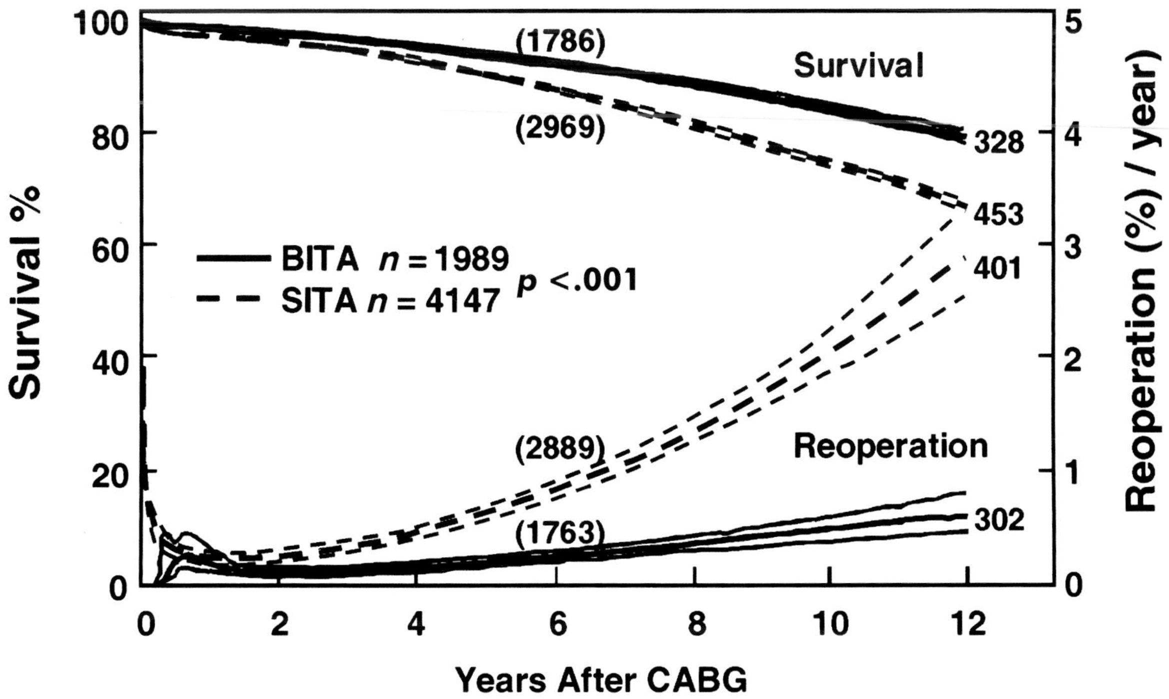

Figure 85–2 Comparison of survival and reoperation hazard function curves in propensity-matched patients receiving bilateral ITA (BITA) grafts and single ITA (SITA) grafts with or without additional vein grafts. BITA grafts result in lowering the rate of reoperation and in an improved survival rate.
(Reprinted with permission from Lytle BW, Blackstone EH, Loop FD, et al: Two internal thoracic artery grafts are better than one. J Thorac Cardiovasc Surg 117:855–872, 1999.)

after operation) do not predict unfavorable outcomes if patients are not highly symptomatic.[15] Second, patients with early stenoses in vein grafts who are highly symptomatic often exhibit marked improvement after reoperation.[16] Third, late (>5 years after operation) stenoses in vein grafts predict adverse outcomes when patients are managed medically, particularly if the stenotic vein graft subtends the LAD coronary artery (Figure 85-3).[15] Fourth, late stenoses in vein grafts appear to be consistently progressive. Fifth, reoperation can improve the survival rate of patients with late stenoses in vein grafts. This last observation is particularly true for patients with late stenoses in LAD vein grafts (Figure 85-3).[16] Sixth, patients with late stenosis in vein grafts who are highly symptomatic also experienced improved symptoms after reoperation.[16]

Functional studies may add to the accuracy of identifying patients likely to have unfavorable outcomes without reoperation.[7] Postoperative patients who demonstrate ischemia and an impaired exercise capacity are in more danger of death and cardiac events without reoperation than are those with more favorable stress tests.

SUMMARY OF CURRENT INDICATIONS FOR REOPERATION

Patients with atherosclerotic vein grafts appear to have a consistently progressive vascular pathology where stenoses continue to worsen and progress to occlusion in a relatively short period of time. Thus, significant stenoses in multiple vein grafts or vein grafts to the anterior descending coronary artery predict a bad outcome from the standpoint of survival without reoperation. Anatomical indications for reoperation are (1) atherosclerotic stenoses in vein grafts that supply the LAD, (2) stenoses in multiple vein grafts that supply large areas of myocardium, and (3) multivessel disease with a proximal LAD lesion with those lesions being native vessel stenoses, stenotic vein grafts, or a combination. Clinical indications for reoperation include significant angina caused by stenoses in vessels or grafts supplying viable myocardium subtended by graftable vessels and a positive functional test.

For some patients needing anatomical treatments, percutaneous treatments (PCT) can be useful and the degree to which PCT is effective is usually related to the specific vascular pathology being treated. Large stenotic native coronary arteries without long lesions or stenoses at major branching points may be stented safely and with low restenosis rates. However, many postoperative patients exhibit diffuse native vessel disease that is not particularly amenable to stenting.

To date the treatment of stenotic SVGs with percutaneous transluminal coronary angioplasty (PTCA) has been relatively ineffective, particularly over the long-term. PCT of early SVG stenoses caused by intimal fibroplasia is usually safe but restenosis rates have been high. The treatment of early anastomotic lesions is effective and restenosis rates have been lower in that setting. For patients with VGA, the procedure-related risks of interventional procedures have

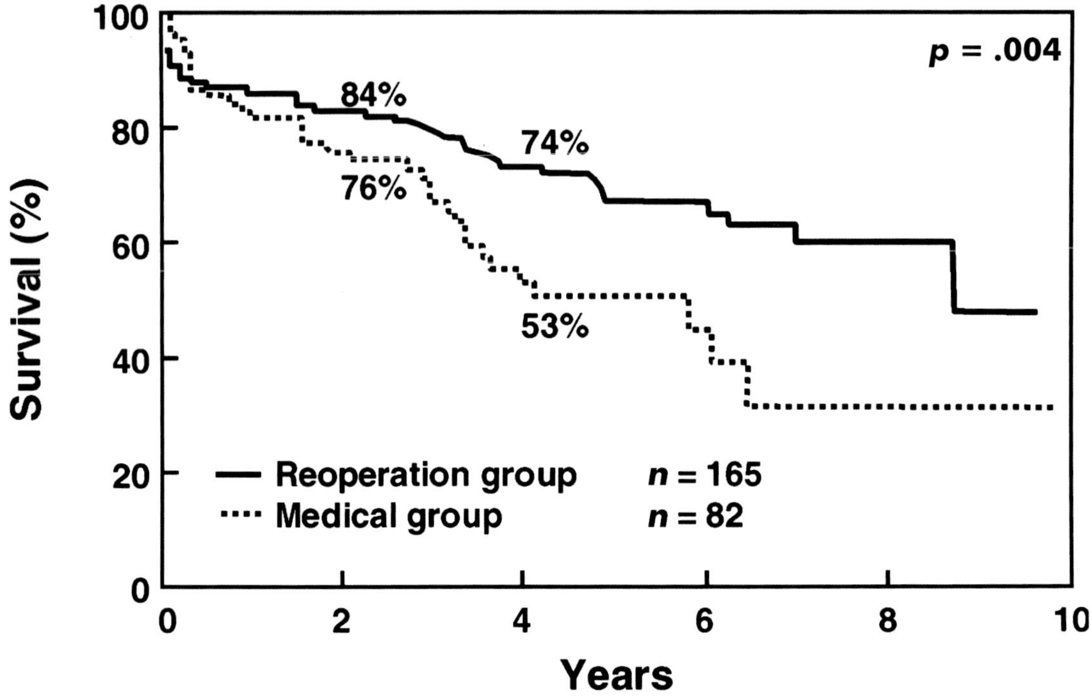

Number at	—	127	71	36	12	4
Risk	····	53	24	8	4	1

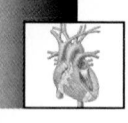

Figure 85–3 Comparison of late survival rates for patients with late stenoses >50% in vein grafts subtending the LAD coronary artery shows a distinct survival advantage for patients undergoing reoperation.
(Reprinted with permission from Lytle BW, Loop FD, Taylor PC, et al: The effect of coronary reoperation on the survival of patients with stenoses in saphenous vein bypass grafts to coronary arteries. J Thorac Cardiovasc Surg 105:605–614, 1993.)

been high, in large part because of atherosclerotic embolization, and long-term outcomes have been unfavorable, particularly when restenosis is defined as restenosis anywhere in the graft. The use of standard stents has been an improvement over balloon angioplasty alone, but not much of an improvement.[2] The impact of drug-coated stents on vein graft stenoses is not yet known.

Comparisons of surgical and percutaneous treatments for heterogeneous groups of patients with previous bypass surgery have shown roughly equivalent outcomes.[3,17] However, these analyses have not separated the patient subsets based on the vascular pathology needing to be treated, illustrating the difficulty of studying these very complex patient subsets. The relative use of reoperation and PCT for the anatomical treatment of patients with previous bypass surgery will depend upon multiple factors including the specific vascular pathology producing ischemia, the general health of the patient including specific contraindications to surgery, and the experience of the surgical and interventional teams.

TECHNICAL ASPECTS OF CORONARY REOPERATIONS

Reoperations are different and more difficult than primary operations. Potential technical problems during coronary reoperations are (1) sternal reentry, (2) aortic atherosclerosis, (3) atherosclerotic vein grafts, (4) patent arterial bypass grafts, (5) diffuse native coronary artery disease, (6) lack of bypass conduits, (7) locating coronary arteries, and (8) myocardial protection.

Perioperative myocardial infarction is the most common cause of in-hospital death following reoperation, and it is often anatomically based. There are many anatomical causes of myocardial infarction during reoperation including injury to bypass grafts, atherosclerotic embolization from vein grafts or from the aorta, myocardial devascularization following graft removal, hypoperfusion through new grafts, incomplete revascularization, early graft occlusion, air embolization, technical error, and failure to deliver cardioplegic solution. Myocardial protection during reoperation must not only provide a favorable metabolic environment but, more importantly, must be designed to avoid these anatomical causes of perioperative myocardial infarction.

PREOPERATIVE ASSESSMENT

Complete angiographic delineation of the native coronary and graft anatomy is important and may not be easy. If bypass grafts are not demonstrated by a preoperative coronary angiogram, it may be that those grafts are, in fact, not occluded but the angiographer failed to demonstrate their location. It is helpful to be able to examine old angiograms performed prior to previous operations to identify important coronary arteries and to help understand the operative notes, which are important to obtain if possible before embarking on a reoperation. Coronary arteries do not disappear and a large vessel that was present previously must be accounted for on the most recent angiogram.

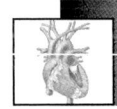

For a reoperation to have a high degree of success and achieve major improvement in the patient's clinical situation there must be some match-up between graftable coronary arteries and viable myocardium. Preoperative myocardial viability can be examined by thallium scanning, positron emission tomography, stress echocardiography, or magnetic resonance imaging.

It is important to know which bypass graft conduits are, or may be, available. Doppler studies can be used to establish ITA patency, but if the major goal of the operation is to use one or both ITAs to bypass important vessels, it is best to establish their patency by angiography. The same is true of the gastroepiploic artery if that is to be employed. Venous Doppler studies can be used to assess the presence of greater and lesser saphenous vein graft segments and arterial Doppler studies can assess radial artery status.

MEDIAN STERNOTOMY, CONDUIT PREPARATION, AND CANNULATION

A median sternotomy is used for most coronary reoperations (Figure 85-4). Situations associated with an increased risk of sternal reentry include right ventricular enlargement, a patent vein graft to the right coronary artery, an *in situ* right ITA (RITA) graft patent to a left coronary vessel, an *in situ* LITA graft that is directly beneath the sternum, aortic enlargement, multiple previous operations, and an injury during a previous sternal incision. In these situations arterial and venous access are obtained (Figure 85-4A and B) and radial artery and saphenous vein segments are prepared prior to the repeat sternotomy. In difficult situations cardiopulmonary bypass may be established prior to the sternotomy, but that is not our usual strategy. We commonly cut the sternal wires anteriorly but do not completely remove them and an oscillating saw is used to divide the anterior table of the sternum (Figure 85-4C). Once that is accomplished ventilation is stopped, the assistants elevate each side of the sternum with retractors, and the posterior table of the sternum is divided. Once the sternum is completely divided the wires that have been left in place posteriorly to protect underlying structures are removed. Other strategies to avoid or compensate for injury during repeat sternotomy include performing a small anterolateral right thoracotomy (Figure 85-4D), thoracoscopic lysis of substernal adhesions, and establishing peripheral cardiopulmonary bypass prior to the median sternotomy.

Once the sternum is opened, adhesions are lysed starting at the diaphragmatic level, extending the dissection into the thoracic cavities, and in a cranial direction. Working from the level of the diaphragm in the cranial direction is the safest approach to avoid graft injury. The innominate vein is freed from the sternum to prevent a stretch injury. The ITAs are then prepared. Scarring of the parietal pleura may make it difficult to obtain ITA length and the right ITA is often used as a free graft. If there is a patent left ITA graft in place that vessel is separated from the chest wall. Avoiding injury to a patent LITA graft is accomplished by being careful and is aided by the correct placement of the graft at the time of the previous operation. If the pericardium has been divided at a primary operation and the left ITA runs posterior to the lung, it is out of danger.

Reoperative candidates often have atherosclerosis of the ascending aorta and aortic arch, and intraoperative echocardiography is used to investigate this issue. Alternative arterial cannulation sites include the axillary artery and the femoral artery, but distal aortic and iliofemoral atherosclerosis often makes the axillary artery the preferred site.[21]

Manipulation of atherosclerotic vein grafts during the dissection of the heart may result in the embolization of debris into the distal coronary system and myocardial infarction. This is a major danger during reoperation that is not present during primary operations. If an atherosclerotic vein graft is present overlying the right atrium, graft manipulation can be lessened by cannulating the right atrium through the femoral vein (Figure 85-4B). When the right atrium is free of atherosclerotic grafts we employ a two-stage venous cannula through the right atrium into the inferior vena cava.

If a patent LITA graft is present, it is helpful to isolate that vessel such that it can be occluded with a clamp. When the location of a patent LITA graft is not obvious, the tissue between the aorta and the left lung is isolated by dissecting posteriorly on the medial aspect of the left lung and on the left lateral aspect of the aorta. The tissue contained between these two sites can be clamped with an atraumatic clamp, usually occluding the LITA graft.

Once we begin cardiopulmonary bypass a self-inflating balloon-tipped retrograde coronary sinus cardioplegia cannula is placed through the right atrium into the coronary sinus, the temperature is cooled to 34° C, the aorta is cross-clamped, and antegrade cardioplegia is given, followed by retrograde cardioplegia. Adequacy of delivery of retrograde cardioplegia is assessed by measuring the pressure in the coronary sinus, and noting the rate of cooling of the heart and the degree of distention of the cardiac veins. If retrograde delivery appears to be adequate, it is employed throughout the rest of the case. Dissection of the remainder of the left ventricle is accomplished once the heart has been arrested, a strategy that leads to an accurate dissection that is relatively atraumatic to the epicardium, decreases the amount of manipulation of atherosclerotic vein grafts, and aids in the identification and isolation of patent ITA grafts. An effective way to isolate a patent LITA–LAD graft is to dissect along the diaphragm to the left side of the apical portion of the LAD coronary artery and then continue the dissection proximally to the left of the patent LITA graft. The LITA graft will then be isolated in that strip of pericardium and can be identified and clamped. If retrograde cardioplegia delivery is adequate, a bulldog is placed over the patent LITA graft to prevent washout of cardioplegia. If severe scarring makes LITA control impossible, the graft is left open and the systemic temperature is decreased to 20° C to achieve cardiac arrest and myocardial protection.

Once the heart has been dissected out, the vessels to be grafted are identified. It is helpful to have a very clear idea of the previous bypass grafts that were performed as those grafts can be followed to identify the coronary vessels to be

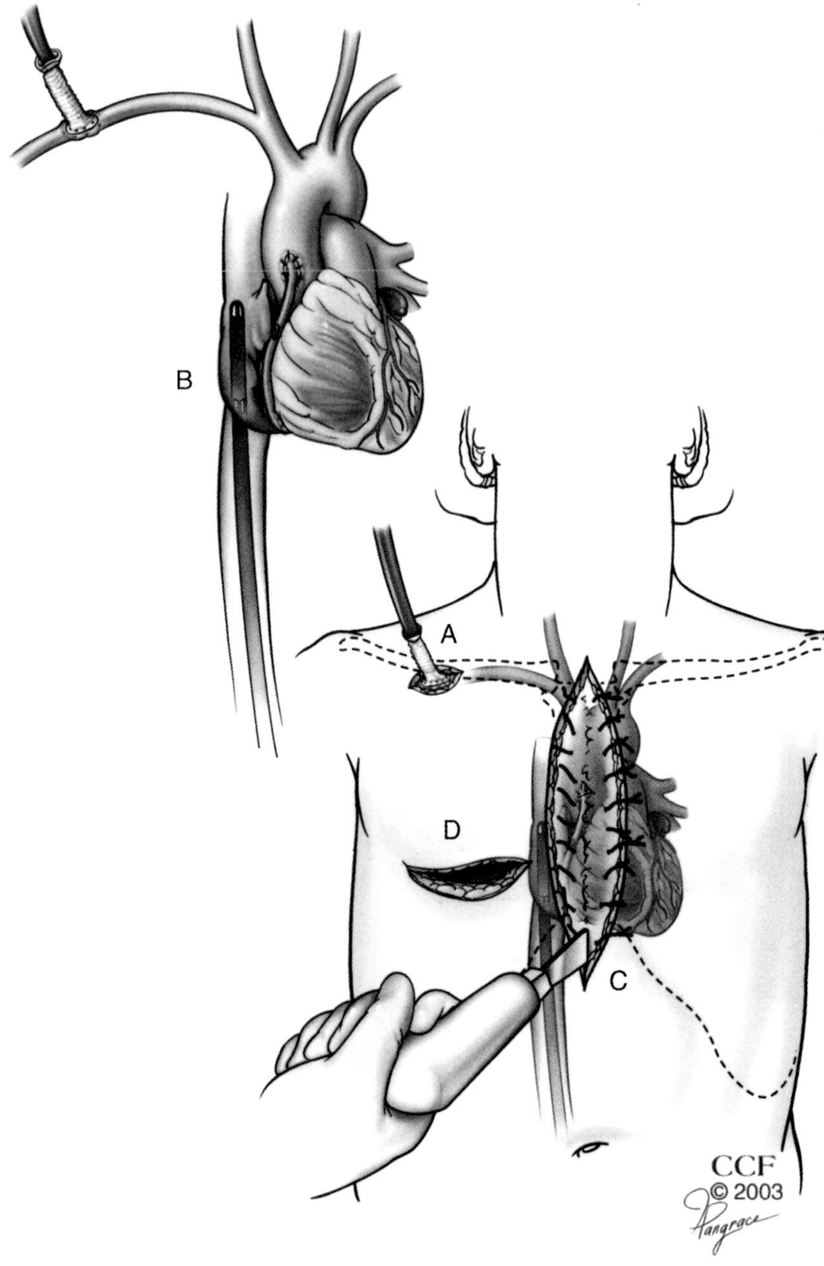

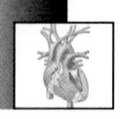

Figure 85–4 Strategies employed for safe sternal reentry during coronary reoperations include: **(A)** axillary artery cannulation for arterial access, **(B)** femoral venous cannulation to allow institution of cardiopulmonary bypass and avoid manipulation of an atherosclerotic SVG to the right coronary artery, **(C)** leaving the sternal wires intact posteriorly and using an oscillating saw to reopen the sternum, and **(D)** a small anterior right thoracotomy to allow safe separation of the right ventricle from the sternum.

grafted. It is common that the epicardial portions of the coronary arteries are heavily diseased and the intramyocardial portions may provide the best sites for anastomoses.

STENOTIC VEIN GRAFTS

The management of stenotic or patent but atherosclerotic vein grafts is a major issue during reoperations. In the early years of reoperative bypass surgery when most primary operations involved only one or two bypass grafts, our principle of management was to replace all vein grafts more than 5 years old regardless of their angiographic appearance in order to decrease the risk of atherosclerotic embolization at the time of reoperation and prevent premature SVG failure after it. For today's reoperative candidates that is often not possible because of the large number of grafts performed at previous operations and lack of bypass conduit availability. If patent or stenotic SVGs are removed at the time of reoperation it is necessary to replace them with conduits of equal size and effectiveness in order to avoid hypoperfusion. If a patent or stenotic vein graft is removed and replaced with a smaller arterial graft, hypoperfusion may result.[18] Thus, if a vein graft is stenotic it is best either to replace it with another vein graft or to leave the old vein graft in place and add an arterial graft to the coronary artery. A concern about the second strategy is that persistent flow through the old SVG might create competitive flow and produce an atretic arterial graft. If the vein graft has a greater than 50% stenosis, that usually does not occur.[25]

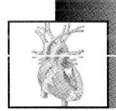

Arterial grafts can be effectively employed during most reoperations.[12] If not previously used, the LITA usually functions well as an *in situ* graft. The RITA is more difficult to use as an *in situ* graft at reoperation and in most instances is better used as a "free" graft. The use of the RITA as a free graft requires an inflow (proximal) anastomosis. The most common locations for a proximal arterial graft anastomosis are the aorta, a new LITA graft, or a previously constructed LITA graft. It is often the case that a previously constructed LITA graft has increased in size and is capable of providing inflow (Figure 85-5A).[24] Using this location as a site for a proximal RITA (or alternative arterial graft) anastomosis allows the length of the RITA that is available for grafting to be maximized (Figure 85-5B), and short segments of arterial grafts may be used to bridge distal LAD stenoses (Figure 85-5C). When constructing proximal anastomoses of arterial grafts to the aorta, we try to use the hood of either a new or an old vein graft as the anastomotic site, because a direct arterial graft anastomosis to the thickened reoperative aorta can be difficult (Figure 85-5D).

Because of the intramyocardial position of many coronary arteries, sequential ITA grafts may be difficult, and we more commonly employ composite "Y" type grafts that allow the individual limb of the graft to reach down into an intramyocardial area without kinking. SVG sequential grafts are more forgiving because of the large SVG size and are useful.

Alternative arterial bypass conduits such as the radial artery, the gastroepiploic artery, and the inferior epigastric artery also may have a role during reoperations. The radial artery is a large vessel that can be used as a single graft from the aorta to almost any coronary vessel and sometimes as a sequential graft based on its larger diameter (Figure 85-6). Early (<5 year) patency studies show a favorable patency rate for this graft. Until the radial artery is completely prepared, its use is uncertain because radial arterial line placement for monitoring during previous operations may have created intimal damage that may preclude use of at least part of the radial artery. The inferior epigastric artery is not a long vessel but may be helpful during reoperations as a composite graft, usually anastomosed to an ITA graft for inflow (see Figure 85-5C). The gastroepiploic artery used as an *in situ* graft can also be useful for grafting the posterior descending branch of the right coronary artery or the anterior descending coronary artery.

DIFFERENTLY INVASIVE STRATEGIES FOR REOPERATIVE CORONARY SURGERY

Although most reoperations are best performed through a median sternotomy because of the need to reach multiple regions of the heart, alternative reoperative strategies can provide an advantage in specific situations. Substantial proportions of primary operations are now being performed without the use of cardiopulmonary bypass and this "off-pump" approach is also appropriate for some reoperations. A disadvantage of reoperative off-pump surgery lies in the danger of manipulating patent but atherosclerotic vein grafts during dissection of the heart and causing embolization of atherosclerotic debris into coronary arteries. If all grafts are occluded, this is not a risk.

Target vessel revascularization strategies where limited areas are approached through alternative incisions and off-pump surgery is performed may be effective because the extensive epicardial dissection that may cause embolization is not needed. An increasingly common operation is to graft the circumflex coronary artery through a left thoracotomy with either a radial artery or SVG anastomosed to the descending thoracic aorta or subclavian artery and then to the circumflex artery, usually employing an off-pump strategy (Figure 85-7). This approach avoids the risk of damaging a patent LITA–LAD graft and avoids cardiopulmonary bypass. The disadvantages of this strategy are that intramyocardial circumflex vessels can be difficult to locate, the descending aorta may be atherosclerotic and a difficult site for a proximal anastomosis, and it makes use of the right ITA

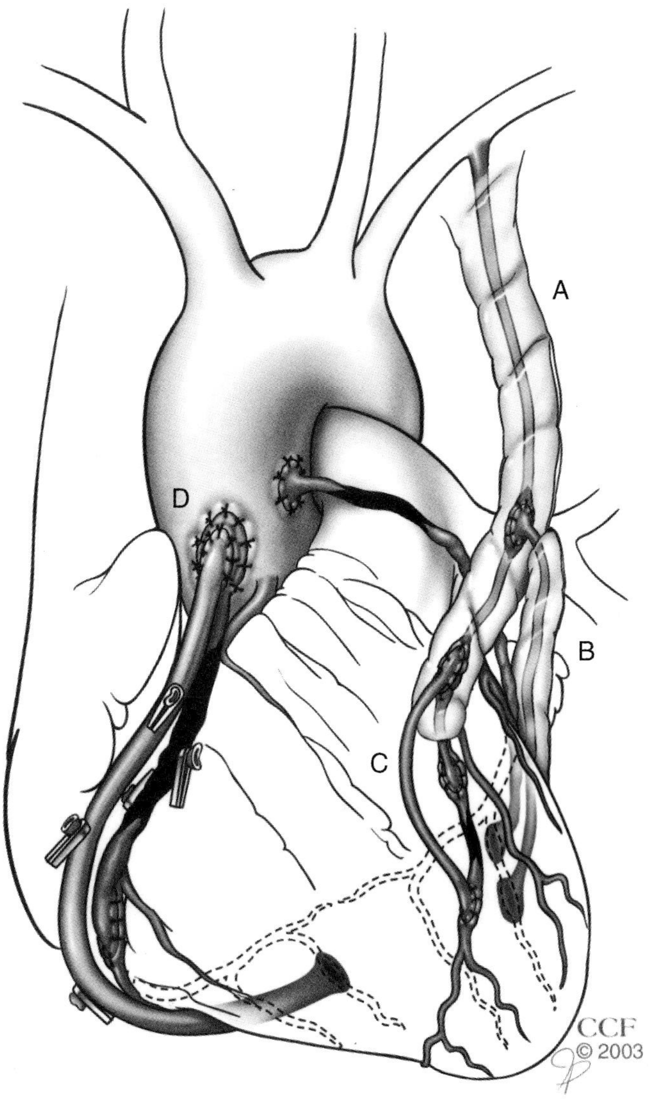

Figure 85–5 Multiple grafting strategies are often useful at reoperation. A new or previously placed left ITA graft (**A**) may be used as in-flow to maximize the length available for a free right ITA graft (**B**) or a small arterial graft segment (**C**) used to bridge a distal LAD stenosis. Often the hood of a previously placed vein graft (**D**) is the best location for a new arterial free graft or a vein graft.

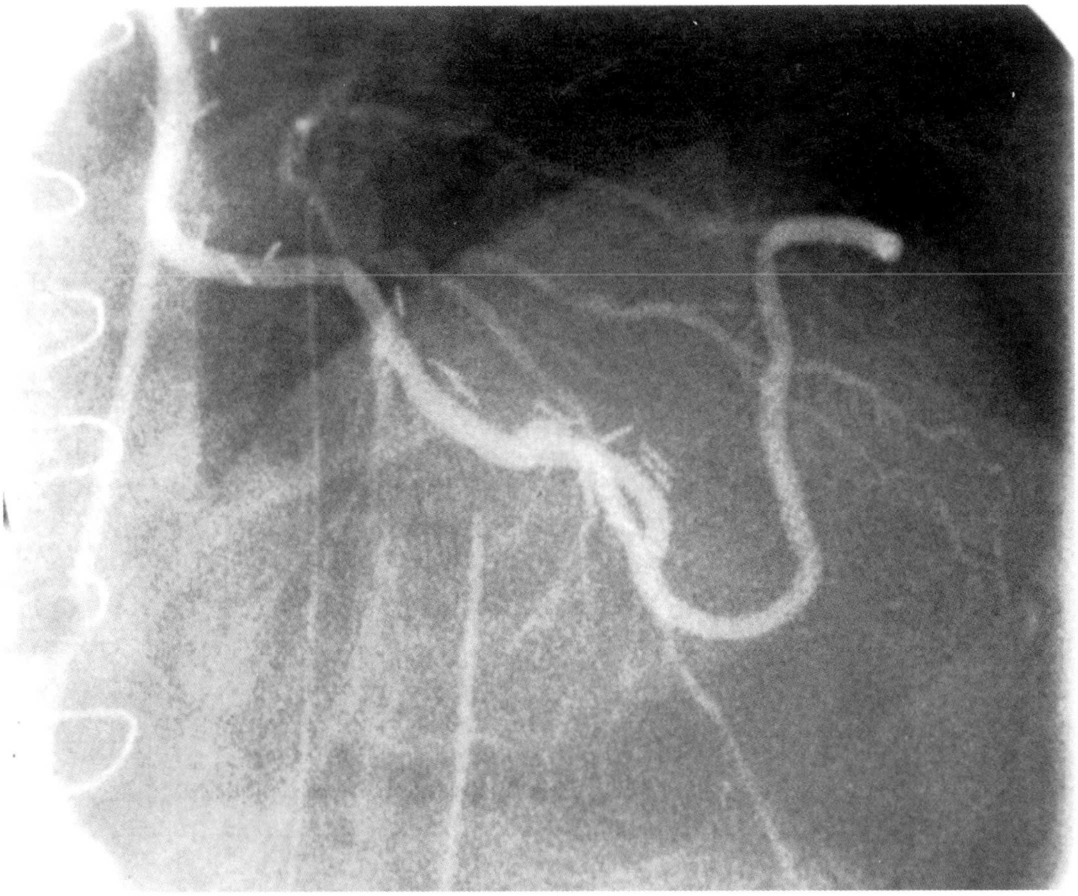

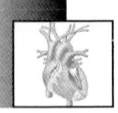

Figure 85–6 The radial artery, anastomosed to a previously constructed LITA–LAD graft, can be used to perform sequential grafting to multiple left-sided vessels.

difficult. In a situation where the LITA is patent to the LAD coronary artery and where there is a major circumflex branch available for grafting, it is usually our intent to use the right ITA to graft that circumflex vessel, thus maximizing long-term benefit.

The gastroepiploic artery may be used as an *in situ* graft to graft the posterior descending branch of the right coronary artery through the diaphragm with a small distal sternotomy or transdiaphragmatic approach or the anterior descending coronary artery through a distal sternotomy or small left thoracotomy. The left ITA may be used to graft the anterior descending coronary artery through a small left thoracotomy (MIDCAB) type approach and the right ITA may be used to graft the anterior descending artery as an *in situ* graft through a repeat median sternotomy. All of these strategies can be useful in specific situations where the goal is limited revascularization. However, most patients who are reoperative candidates need multiple grafts to multiple vessels.

THE RESULTS OF CORONARY REOPERATIONS

Coronary reoperations have been associated with increased risks when compared with primary operations. Data most reflective of widespread practice come from the Society of Thoracic Surgeons (STS) Database, and during the years 1998–2001 the mortality rate from reoperations ranged from 7.2% to 4.7%.[23] Centers with extensive experience with reoperations have noted improved survival rates with time and increasing experience. For example, at The Cleveland Clinic Foundation the in-hospital mortality rate of a first reoperation has been 3–4% from 1967 through 1991 and has been lowered to approximately 2% during the past decade.

Examination of clinical variables and their association with increased risk have shown that emergency operation is a very strong factor. There is not a standard definition of "emergency," but reported mortality rates for emergency coronary reoperations range from 13% to 40%. In the STS database for 1997 the mortality rates were 5.2% for elective reoperation, 7.4% for urgent reoperation, 13.5% for emergency reoperation, and 40.7% for "salvage" reoperation.[22] This incremental risk associated with emergency reoperation is greater than that seen for patients undergoing primary surgery. Advanced age has been associated with increased risk, but usually in association with other patient-related variables such as emergency operation, female gender, left ventricular dysfunction, renal failure, and left main stenosis.[27] Technical issues including the presence of patent ITA grafts and atherosclerotic vein grafts have been shown to increase the risk of reoperation in some series, although these factors can be overcome with experience. Perrault et al reviewed patients with atherosclerotic vein grafts and noted that the more atherosclerotic vein

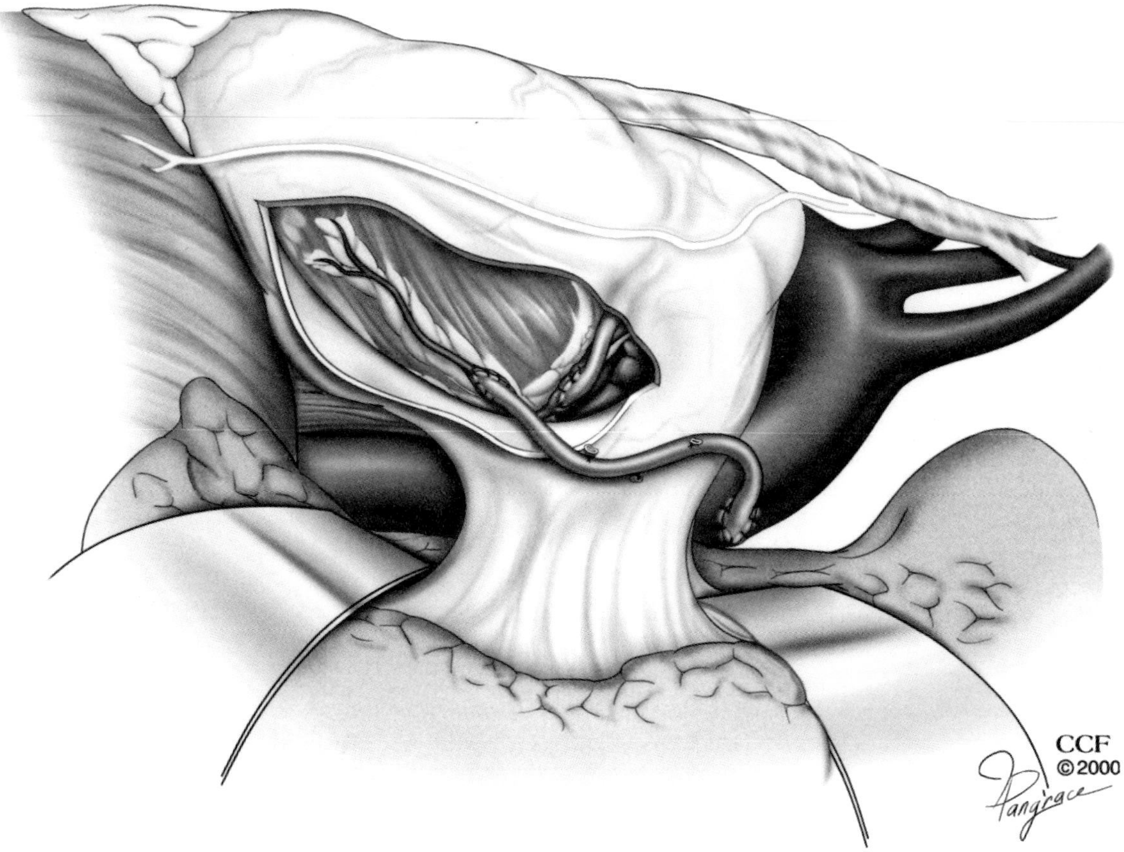

Figure 85–7 A left thoracotomy may be used for an off-pump anastomosis of a radial artery or vein graft to the circumflex coronary artery.

grafts were present the higher the mortality rate.[19] In some of our early experience we noted that an atherosclerotic vein graft to the LAD increased in-hospital risk but that effect was not strong, and in our most recent series we have found that atherosclerotic grafts do not increase mortality. This improvement in outcome appears to be based on the use of retrograde cardioplegia delivery and increased surgeon experience. The presence of a patent ITA graft has not increased risk in our series nor has the use of arterial grafts.[12]

Reoperations do not make patients as "perfect" as primary operations do. By the time patients undergo reoperation they have usually experienced significant progression of native vessel atherosclerosis, few undergo true "complete" revascularization, and the clinical results of reoperation reflect the imperfection of the anatomic correction.

Anginal symptoms are more common after reoperation than they are after a primary bypass operation. Follow-up of our series of reoperative patients at a mean interval of 72 months after operation showed that 64% of patients were classed as NYFC I, meaning that over a third had some symptoms.[14] However, only 10% of patients had class III or class IV symptoms. Long-term studies from Emory University have also noted at a 4-year follow-up that 41% of reoperative patients experienced some angina.[26] In addition, the late survival rates are not as good as those expected after a primary surgery. Weintraub and colleagues documented a 55% 10-year survival rate, and our most recent follow-up study found a survival of 69% for in-hospital intervals at the 10 postoperative year mark.[26] Left ventricular dysfunction, advanced age, and diabetes have been associated with decreased late survival rates, and as more reoperative candidates have those characteristics it would be surprising if the late survival after reoperation improved.

MULTIPLE CORONARY REOPERATIONS

Patients with more than one previous bypass operation present incremental problems. Lack of bypass conduits is common, and virtually all have very diffuse native vessel disease. Hospital risks have been increased for patients undergoing third or fourth procedures. In our early experience we noted an 8% mortality rate for third operations, although more recently the risks for patients less than 70 years of age have decreased to 1–2%. Likewise, the long-term survival rate is not quite as favorable, although in our most recent follow-up, 84% of patients with multiple previous operations were alive at 5 years and 66% at 10 years after operation.[11]

COMPLEMENTARY END-STAGE REVASCULARIZATION PROCEDURES

Substantial investigations have been directed toward indirect revascularization strategies that might apply to patients with coronary atherosclerosis so diffuse that neither bypass grafting nor PCT will result in complete or effective revascularization. Most patients judged candidates for these strategies have had previous bypass surgery.

Transmyocardial laser revascularization (TMLR) has been shown with randomized (although not blinded) trials to improve the symptom status of patients receiving only TMLR or TMLR in combination with bypass grafting. We rarely use TMLR in isolation but do use it in combination with bypass grafting during reoperation.

THE FUTURE OF CORONARY REOPERATIONS

A huge wave of patients needing coronary reoperations, once feared, has not materialized. However, recurrent ischemic syndromes after bypass surgery are common and are related to time. Despite advances in pharmacological and interventional therapies for coronary atherosclerosis, many patients still require reoperation and they present coronary surgeons with their most difficult challenges.

REFERENCES

1. Bourassa MG, Campeau L, Lesperance J: Changes in grafts and in coronary arteries after coronary bypass surgery. Cardiovasc Clin 21:83–100, 1991.
2. Brener SJ, Ellis SG, Apperson-Hansen C, et al: Comparison of stenting and balloon angioplasty for narrowings in aortocoronary saphenous vein conduits in place for more than five years. Am J Cardiol 79:13–18, 1997.
3. Cole JH, Jones EL, Craver JM, et al: Outcome of repeat revascularization in diabetic patients with prior coronary surgery. J Am Coll Cardiol 40:1968–1975, 2002.
4. Cosgrove DM, Loop FD, Lytle BW, et al: Predictors of reoperation after myocardial revascularization. J Thorac Cardiovasc Surg 92:811–821, 1986.
5. Fitzgibbon GM, Leach AJ, Kafka HP, et al: Coronary bypass graft fate: long-term angiographic study. J Am Coll Cardiol 17:1075–1080, 1991.
6. Gavaghan TP, Gebski V, Baron DW: Immediate postoperative aspirin improves vein graft patency early and late after coronary artery bypass graft surgery. A placebo-controlled, randomized study. Circulation 83:1526–1533, 1991.
7. Lauer MS, Lytle B, Pashkow F, et al: Prediction of death and myocardial infarction by screening exercise-thallium testing after coronary-artery-bypass grafting. Lancet 351:615–622, 1998.
8. Loop FD, Lytle BW, Cosgrove DM, et al: Influence of the internal mammary artery graft on 10-year survival and other cardiac events. N Engl J Med 314:1–6, 1986.
9. Loop FD, Lytle BW, Cosgrove DM, et al: Reoperation for coronary atherosclerosis: changing practice in 2509 consecutive patients. Ann Surg 212:378–386, 1990.
10. Lytle BW, Blackstone EH, Loop FD, et al: Two internal thoracic artery grafts are better than one. J Thorac Cardiovasc Surg 117:855–872, 1999.
11. Lytle BW, Cosgrove DM, Taylor PC, et al: Multiple coronary reoperations: early and late results. Circulation 80(4, Suppl. II):626, 1989.
12. Lytle BW, McElroy D, McCarthy PM, et al: The influence of arterial coronary bypass grafts on the mortality of coronary reoperations. J Thorac Cardiovasc Surg 107:675–683, 1994.
13. Lytle BW, Loop FD, Cosgrove DM, et al: Long-term (5 to 12 years) serial studies of internal mammary artery and saphenous vein coronary bypass grafts. J Thorac Cardiovasc Surg 89:248–258, 1985.
14. Lytle BW, Loop FD, Cosgrove DM, et al: Fifteen hundred coronary reoperations: results and determinants of early and late survival. J Thorac Cardiovasc Surg 93:847–859, 1987.
15. Lytle BW, Loop FD, Taylor PC, et al: Vein graft disease: the clinical impact of stenoses in saphenous vein bypass grafts to coronary arteries. J Thorac Cardiovasc Surg 103:831–840, 1992.
16. Lytle BW, Loop FD, Taylor PC, et al: The effect of coronary reoperation on the survival of patients with stenoses in saphenous vein to coronary bypass grafts. J Thorac Cardiovasc Surg 105:605–614, 1993.
17. Morrison DA, Sethi A, Sacks J, et al: Percutaneous coronary intervention versus repeat bypass surgery for patients with medically refractory myocardial ischemia (AWESOME Randomized Trial Registry Experience With Post-CABG Patients). J Am Coll Cardiol 40:1951–1954, 2002.
18. Navia D, Cosgrove DM, Lytle BW, et al: Is the internal thoracic artery the conduit of choice to replace a stenotic vein graft? Ann Thorac Surg 57:40–44, 1994.
19. Perrault L, Carrier M, Cartier R, et al: Morbidity and mortality of reoperation for coronary artery bypass grafting: significance of atheromatous vein grafts. Can J Cardiol 7:427–430, 1991.
20. The Post Coronary Artery-Bypass Graft Trial Investigators: The effect of aggressive lowering of low-density lipoprotein cholesterol levels and low-dose anti-coagulation on obstructive changes in saphenous-vein coronary artery bypass grafts. N Engl J Med 336:153–162, 1997.
21. Sabik JF, Lytle BW, McCarthy PM, et al: Axillary artery: an alternative site of arterial cannulation for patients with extensive aortic and peripheral vascular disease. J Thorac Cardiovasc Surg 109:885–891, 1995.
22. Society of Thoracic Surgeons National Database Committee, Durham, NC, 2003.
23. Society of Thoracic Surgeons National Database Annual Report 1997, Durham, NC.
24. Tector AJ, Kress DC, Amundsen SM, et al: Reoperation in patient with closed SVG and patent ITA-LAD graft: T-graft approach. Ann Thorac Surg 59:509–512, 1995.
25. Turner FE, Lytle BW, Navia D, et al: Coronary reoperations: results of adding an internal mammary artery graft to a stenotic vein graft. Ann Thorac Surg 58:1353–1355, 1994.
26. Weintraub WS, Jones EL, Craver JM, et al: In-hospital and long-term out come after reoperative coronary artery bypass graft surgery. Circulation 92(Suppl. II):II-50–II-57, 1995.
27. Yamamuro M, Lytle BW, Sapp SK, et al: Risk factors and outcomes after coronary reoperation in 739 elderly patients. Ann Thorac Surg 69:464–474, 2000.

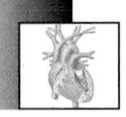

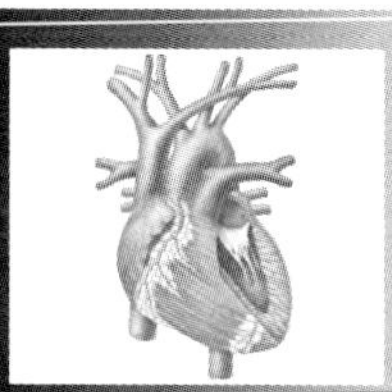

Ischemic Mitral Regurgitation

Lishan Aklog, Farzan Filsoufi, and David H. Adams

CHAPTER 86

INTRODUCTION

Although there has been increasing attention paid in the literature to ischemic mitral regurgitation (MR), its mechanisms, and its relatively poor prognosis, the management of this condition remains controversial. Before the assessment of various treatment strategies, it is important to precisely define ischemic MR and to understand its underlying mechanism.

Clinical Presentation

Ischemic MR has traditionally been characterized as acute or chronic, although this distinction is not very useful or precise. Some patients will develop acute MR during bouts of symptomatic or silent ischemia; this type will disappear with the resolution of the ischemia, and it has been referred to as *episodic transient ischemic MR*. Acute MR as a result of papillary muscle rupture after acute myocardial infarction (MI) is a relatively rare but dramatic condition; it most commonly occurs in patients without prior angina, with single-vessel coronary artery disease, and with an inferoposterior MI.

Acute postinfarction ischemic MR without papillary muscle rupture can be documented in many patients by physical examination (8–17%),[11,12,73] ventriculography (13–19%),[67–69] or echocardiography (38–74%).[7,11,12,72,106] Moderate to severe MR is present in up to 13% of these patients.[36,80] Although the MR will resolve over time in some patients, it will persist in others and lead to *chronic postinfarction ischemic MR*. In some patients, chronic ischemic MR will first appear up to 6 weeks (median, 7 days) after the MI as the infarcted left ventricle remodels. Risk factors for postinfarction ischemic MR include advanced age, female gender, prior acute MI, large infarct size, recurrent ischemia, multivessel coronary artery disease, and congestive heart failure.[13]

Definition

Carpentier's Functional Classification

Although several authors have proposed specific classification systems for ischemic MR, we believe that Carpentier's[20] functional classification of MR, which is based on leaflet motion, is as powerful for ischemic MR as it is for degenerative, rheumatic, and other etiologies. Carpentier type I dysfunction occurs despite normal leaflet motion, usually from pure annular dilatation or distortion resulting in poor leaflet coaptation. Type II dysfunction results from leaflet prolapse, when a portion of the free margin of one or both leaflets is not properly supported by the subvalvular apparatus and so rises above the plane of the annulus during systole, thereby preventing leaflet coaptation. Finally, type III dysfunction results from restricted leaflet motion. Here, the free margins of portions of one or both leaflets are pulled below the plane of the annulus into the left ventricle, thereby preventing them from rising up toward the plane of the annulus and coapting during systolic contraction. Restricted leaflet motion related to valvular or subvalvular pathology (usually rheumatic fibrosis) during systole and diastole is considered to be type IIIA dysfunction. Finally, in type III dysfunction the leaflet motion is restricted during systole and occurs when abnormal ventricular geometry or function leads to papillary muscle displacement, which pulls the otherwise normal leaflets down into the ventricle, away from each other, thus preventing proper coaptation of the leaflets. This usually results from prior MI or severe ventricular dilatation and dysfunction.

Ischemic MR can result from type I, II, or IIIB dysfunction. Pure annular dilation without apparent leaflet restriction can occur after basal infarctions, resulting in type I dysfunction. Acute papillary muscle rupture or chronic scarring and elongation can occur after papillary muscle infarctions, resulting in type II dysfunction. Type IIIB is the most common type of dysfunction seen in ischemic MR, and it results from papillary muscle displacement and tethering.

Type II Ischemic Mitral Regurgitation

From a surgeon's perspective, ischemic MR can be divided into two groups. Patients with type II dysfunction from papillary muscle rupture or elongation form one group. The indications for surgery and the ultimate management of these patients are not particularly controversial, and, assuming that valve replacement is not required for papillary muscle rupture, the principles of mitral valve repair are nearly identical to those used in other type II patients. Furthermore, the long-term prognosis is generally better than it is for those patients with type I or IIIB dysfunction.[39] The management of type II ischemic MR will be discussed separately at the end of this chapter.

Type I or IIIB Ischemic Mitral Regurgitation

The majority of ischemic MR patients have so-called functional ischemic MR from type I or IIIB dysfunction without any leaflet or subvalvular lesions. Although the term "functional MR" is commonly used to refer to MR without lesions of the mitral valve, its use should be discouraged, because it is an imprecise term and lacks the mechanistic and therapeutic correlates of the Carpentier functional classification.

Patients with type I or IIIB ischemic MR typically present with one of two clinical scenarios (Figure 86-1). The more common scenario is a patient with symptomatic multivessel coronary artery disease, with or without associated congestive heart failure symptoms, who is referred for surgical or percutaneous revascularization and who is noted to have mild to moderate MR on preoperative echocardiography or ventriculography. The other scenario is a patient with moderate to severe MR and primarily congestive heart failure symptoms who is referred for mitral valve surgery and who is noted to have multivessel coronary artery disease on preoperative catheterization.

We have proposed a set of criteria to use to define ischemic MR (Table 86-1).[6] Some of the clinical literature about ischemic MR is difficult to interpret because of imprecise definitions that lead to etiological and physiological heterogeneity within the patient population. We feel strongly that a relatively simple—but precise—definition of ischemic MR is critical to the presentation of a relatively homogenous group of patients for analysis.

Because many patients with nonischemic mitral valve disease have incidental coronary artery disease, we include only those with significant symptomatic multivessel coronary artery disease. We do not consider a documented clinical history of an MI mandatory for a patient to have ischemic MR. Although a prior MI is probably present in nearly all of these patients, it may be silent in many patients, especially in those with diabetes. Because acute transient ischemic MR is excluded, most patients without a documented clinical history of an MI will likely have experienced one or more subclinical events that will have led to the ischemic MR and, in many, to significant LV dysfunction. We do not insist on corroborating electrocardiographic or echocardiographic evidence of a

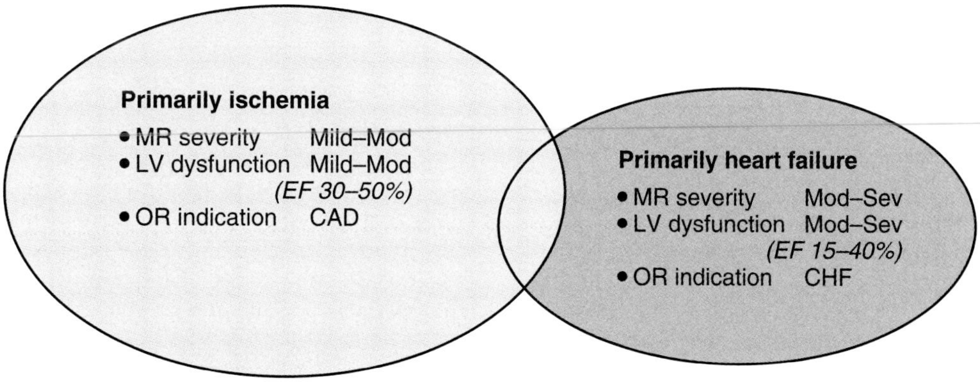

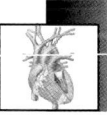

Figure 86–1 Schematic diagram illustrating the two most common—relatively distinct—clinical scenarios for patients presenting with ischemic mitral regurgitation. Most patients present with primarily ischemic symptoms and are noted on evaluation for coronary bypass surgery to have mild to moderate MR. A significant minority, however, primarily present with symptoms of congestive heart failure and are noted on evaluation for mitral valve surgery to have significant coronary artery disease; the latter tend to have worse left ventricular function. EF, Ejection fraction; OR, operative.

previously undocumented MI, because we did not think this would lead to a more clinically relevant group. It is possible that our definition would include a small number of patients with large areas of hibernating myocardium (without infarction) leading to papillary muscle displacement and type IIIB MR. We feel that it is appropriate to include these patients, because they share a common pathophysiological mechanism to those with true post-MI ischemic MR. It is also possible that some patients with MR soon after an acute MI will be included, despite the fact that they may have shown improvement in their MR (e.g., resolution of acute stunning, less volume overload) if they had been restudied later. We do not think that eliminating these patients by placing some arbitrary interval between the MI and documentation of MR is practical or helpful, because many patients will proceed to surgery within a few days of their MI, before repeat echocardiography can be performed.

In terms of the type of dysfunction, type I (annular dilatation with normal leaflet motion) or type IIIB (restricted leaflet motion during systole) dysfunction should be present without evidence of mitral stenosis, leaflet prolapse, or other leaflet pathology.

The MR grade should be at least mild or 2+ on semiquantitative assessment, preferably by transthoracic echocardiography performed while the patient is awake and not actively ischemic. General anesthesia and even the light sedation required for transesophageal echocardiography (TEE) can unload the ventricle and lead to underestimation of the degree of MR.[9,49] The unloading effects of an intraaortic balloon pump should also be taken into consideration, if one is present. During the past decade, state-of-the-art techniques for quantifying MR by echocardiography have emerged, and they are particularly useful for patients with ischemic MR. The preferred method is to calculate the regurgitant volume and the effective regurgitant orifice using the flow convergence proximal isovelocity surface area (PISA) method.[35,60] The Mayo group has suggested that the thresholds for significant MR should be lower (regurgitant volume >30; effective regurgitant orifice >20) in "functional" MR than in "organic" MR, given its impact on survival in this group.[74]

Table 86–1

Definition of Ischemic Mitral Regurgitation

1. Significant symptomatic multivessel coronary artery disease, with or without documented prior myocardial infarction
2. At least mild (grade 2+ out of 4+) mitral regurgitation a. Documented on preoperative echocardiogram or ventriculogram while patient is not actively ischemic b. No mitral stenosis
3. Type I or IIIb by Carpentier functional classification a. Annular dilatation with normal leaflet motion (Type I) *or* restricted leaflet motion during systole (Type IIIb) b. No leaflet prolapse (Type II), even if the etiology of prolapse is ischemic (e.g., papillary muscle rupture, elongated chordae from papillary muscle scarring) c. No other leaflet pathology

Ventriculography alone can be inadequate to assess MR, especially as hand injections with inadequate dye loads are frequently used to save time and minimize renal toxicity.[86]

PATHOPHYSIOLOGY

Normal mitral valve function involves a complex three-dimensional interaction between the leaflets, the annulus, the subvalvular apparatus, and the left ventricular wall. The mechanism by which myocardial ischemia and infarction perturb this carefully orchestrated process has been the focus of intensive laboratory investigation, most notably by groups at Stanford, the University of Pennsylvania, and Massachusetts General Hospital. These groups have carefully analyzed the geometric mechanisms of acute and chronic ischemic MR in several large animal models using biplane fluoroscopy, sonomicrometry, and two- and three-dimensional echocardiography.* Although these studies have several limitations (including the use of acute ischemia models, spatial resolution, and limited correlation between anatomical and physiological abnormalities), they provide significant insight into the pathophysiology of ischemic MR and potential treatment modalities.

The key pathophysiological components of type I and IIIB ischemic MR include annular changes (dilatation, distortion), subvalvular changes (papillary muscle displacement or tethering), and ventricular changes (dilatation with increased sphericity, wall motion abnormalities). Figure 86-2, A provides an overview of how these components interact to result in poor leaflet coaptation, which is the final common pathway for all types of MR.

Specific Geometric Abnormalities

Annular

Although annular dilatation is a common finding in clinical cases of chronic ischemic MR, the degree of dilatation can vary and does not necessarily correlate with the degree of MR. Some patients with significant ischemic MR have very little annular dilatation, and others with significant annular dilatation may not have much MR. The laboratory data support the notion that annular dilatation per se is not a

*References 30, 37, 40, 41, 44–47, 55, 56, 62, 66, 70, 71, 76, 77, 79, 81, 82, 98–102.

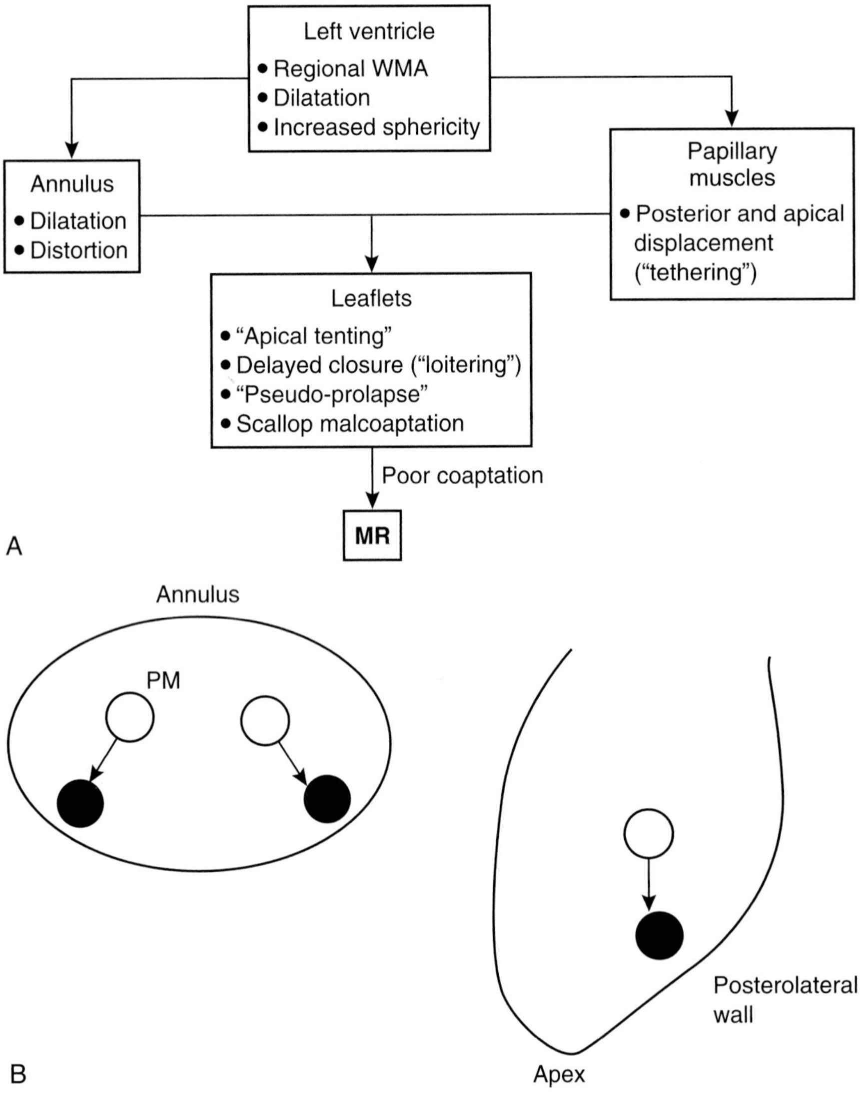

Figure 86–2 Schematic diagrams illustrating the pathophysiology of ischemic mitral regurgitation. A, The interaction between the left ventricle, the papillary muscles, the annulus, and the leaflets leading to poor leaflet coaptation as the final common pathway to mitral regurgitation. **B,** The geometry of papillary muscle displacement in ischemic mitral regurgitation; the tips are displaced posteriorly, apically, and away from each other. WMA, Wall motion abnormality.

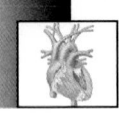

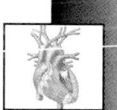

fundamental component of ischemic MR pathophysiology. Green and colleagues[48] showed that, in an acute sheep model, moderate degrees of annular dilatation do not necessarily lead to ischemic MR. Timek and others[98] recently noted that the mild degrees of annular dilatation that they observed during acute occlusion of the left anterior descending or distal left circumflex did not result in ischemic MR. This study and several others from the Stanford group noted the critical role of the septolateral (SL) dimension of the annulus in the pathophysiology of ischemic MR. The SL dimension is the anatomically correct term for what, in clinical practice, is commonly referred to as the anteroposterior (AP) dimension—the vertical or short axis of the annular ellipse that extends from the middle of the anterior annulus to the middle of the posterior annulus. The horizontal or long axis of the ellipse is referred to as the commissure-commissure (CC) dimension. These studies have shown that, in the sheep acute ischemia model, an increase in mitral annular area causes MR only to the extent that it increases the SL dimension. In fact, the CC dimension does not usually increase significantly with ischemia.[30,98–101] Furthermore, these researchers have shown that decreasing the SL dimension using a cinching device can abolish ischemic MR in sheep.[100,101] In severe cases of ischemic MR, the SL dimension can approach the CC dimension, which results in a circular annulus instead of the normal elliptical one.

Subvalvular

Papillary muscle displacement also plays a critical role in the pathophysiology of ischemic MR. It is important to distinguish this from papillary muscle dysfunction (or decreased papillary muscle shortening during systole), which has traditionally been implicated as a primary mechanism for ischemic MR. In fact, papillary muscle dysfunction does not cause ischemic MR. Timek and others[99] showed that the decreased shortening of one or both papillary muscles did not correlate with ischemic MR in the sheep. On the contrary, Messas and colleagues[76] demonstrated a paradoxical decrease in ischemic MR with papillary muscle dysfunction.

The primary alteration in papillary muscle geometry leading to ischemic MR is papillary muscle displacement or tethering. The pattern of displacement is actually fairly complex and cannot simply be described as apical tethering. The papillary muscle tips are displaced away from the midseptal (anterior) annulus (i.e., posterolaterally, apically, and away from each other) (Figure 86-2, *B*). The tethering distance has been shown to correlate with the severity of ischemic MR.[30,98,99] Experimental studies suggest that, although tethering of both papillary muscles is probably necessary to induce ischemic MR, displacement of the posteromedial papillary muscle usually predominates.

Left Ventricular

The initiating insult in ischemic MR is ventricular, specifically myocardial ischemia or infarction with remodeling that leads to regional annular and subvalvular distortion and ultimately poor leaflet coaptation. The independent contribution of global ventricular size and shape to the pathophysiology of ischemic MR is less clear. In an echocardiographic study of 102 patients, Kumanohoso and others[64] showed that, in comparison with those with anterior infarctions, patients with inferior infarctions had a higher incidence of ischemic MR despite less left ventricular dilatation and dysfunction; this was directly attributed to more severe posteromedial papillary muscle tethering in the inferior infarction group. Experimental data, however, have shown that regional left ventricular dysfunction does not lead to ischemic MR without some degree of left ventricular dilatation. It appears that the left ventricular sphericity is more important than the actual ventricular volumes or ejection fraction in the progression of ischemic MR.[105,108]

Leaflet Dysfunction

These changes in annular papillary muscle and left ventricular geometry interact to result in poor leaflet coaptation during systole, which is the final common pathway for ischemic MR. Specifically, an increase in the SL dimension leads to leaflet separation and delayed leaflet closure ("loitering") during systole.[41] Papillary muscle tethering leads to apical tenting of the leaflets (restriction of the motion of the free margins of the leaflets), which prevents them from rising to the plane of the annulus to coapt with one another; this has been well documented using quantitative echocardiographic methods in a clinical setting.[109] Tethering on the secondary chordae can result in an *effet de moete* deformation of the body of the leaflet, which further impairs coaptation (Figure 86-3). The contribution of the malcoaptation of the scallops of the posterior leaflet from papillary muscle tethering has been recently documented.[66,79]

A recent clinical study from the Cleveland Clinic used three-dimensional echocardiography to compare the mechanism of type IIIB MR as a result of ischemic versus dilated cardiomyopathy and reported very interesting findings.[65] Although the amount of apical tenting of the leaflets was significantly greater in the dilated cardiomyopathy patients, it was symmetrical along the line of coaptation. By contrast, in

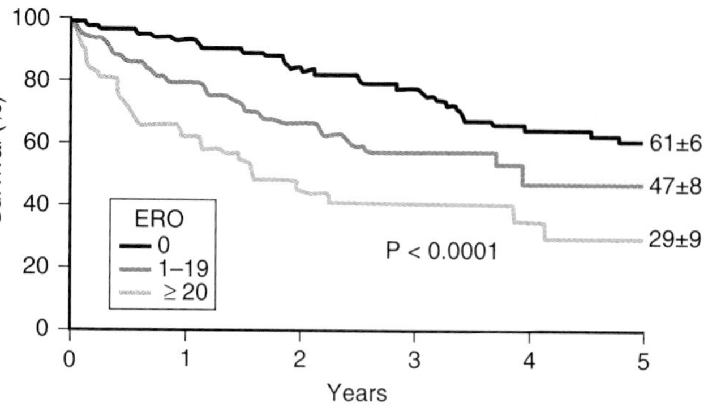

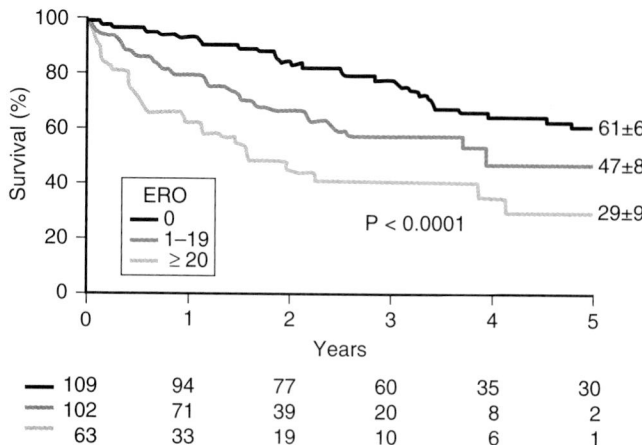

—	109	94	77	60	35	30
—	102	71	39	20	8	2
—	63	33	19	10	6	1

Figure 86–3 Survival curves documenting the significant relationship between the severity of mitral regurgitation and midterm survival after chronic myocardial infarction.[50] The severity of MR was assessed using quantitative techniques and expressed as an effective regurgitant orifice (given in mm^2). Even modest degrees of mitral regurgitation (<20) significantly reduced 3-year survival.

the ischemic cardiomyopathy patients, the tenting was asymmetrical, with less tenting of A2 and A3 as compared with A1. As a result, although there was less tenting in the ischemic group, there was paradoxically more MR, because the asymmetry led to A2 and A3 overriding P2 and P3 in a phenomenon that has been called "pseudoprolapse" (not true prolapse because neither leaflet margin rises above the plane of the annulus), which results in an eccentric, posteriorly directed MR jet. This explains why many dilated cardiomyopathy patients with severe bileaflet restriction have very little MR: the restricted leaflet edges are still able to coapt, even if the point of coaptation is well below the plane of the annulus.

SURGICAL DECISION MAKING

Surgical decision making in ischemic MR is complex and challenging, because the clinical literature is heterogeneous and often contradictory, which makes it difficult to synthesize and distill the information into concrete and practical clinical recommendations. There are multiple factors that must be considered, including the specific clinical scenario, the negative impact of ischemic MR on medium-term survival, the challenge of the intraoperative assessment of MR severity, the impact of coronary artery bypass grafting (CABG) alone on MR severity, the impact of CABG with or without mitral surgery on survival and late functional status, the additional operative risk of mitral valve surgery at the time and CABG, and the choice of valve repair versus replacement. We believe that the cumulative data about these various issues are coalescing into a set of principles that can guide modern surgical decision making for the treatment of this disease.

Decision Making in Specific Clinical Scenarios

Moderate to Severe Ischemic Mitral Regurgitation with Congestive Heart Failure

In this clinical scenario, the patient presents with moderate to severe MR, symptoms of congestive heart failure, or worsening left ventricular function and is referred primarily for mitral valve surgery. The preoperative coronary angiogram shows significant multivessel coronary artery disease that may or may not have been symptomatic. These patients usually have clear evidence of prior MI and at least moderate left ventricular dysfunction. They can be viewed as having MR as a result of ischemic cardiomyopathy, and if the ejection fraction is particularly low (<20%), the decision to operate in the absence of documented ischemia is similar to the one that needs to be made for patients with MR as a result of nonischemic cardiomyopathy. Surgical decision making in this clinical scenario is more straightforward. Patients with moderate to severe ischemic MR with symptoms of congestive heart failure and/or worsening left ventricular function should undergo combined mitral valve surgery and CABG as long as the expected operative morbidity and mortality are not prohibitive.

Mild to Moderate Ischemic Mitral Regurgitation at Coronary Artery Bypass Grafting

The more common clinical scenario is that of a patient with symptomatic multivessel coronary artery disease who is referred for CABG and who is noted to have mild to moderate MR on preoperative ventriculography or echocardiography. Although the patient may have shortness of breath as their angina equivalent or he or she may (sometimes in retrospect) have symptoms or signs of congestive heart failure, myocardial ischemia (acute coronary syndrome or chronic stable angina) usually dominates the clinical picture and is the primary indication for surgical intervention. Because the poor outcomes of percutaneous coronary intervention (PCI) in patients with ischemic MR are more widely appreciated,[34] this group may also include patients who would have otherwise undergone multivessel PCI for the coronary artery disease but who were noted to have MR and were thus referred for surgery.

Surgical decision making in this clinical scenario has been distinctly more controversial. Although most surgeons would agree that moderate to severe MR should be corrected at the time of CABG and that trace to mild MR can probably be left alone, the optimal management of mild to moderate ischemic MR remains controversial. Those favoring a conservative approach argue that the following are true:

1. Revascularizing ischemic areas will improve regional wall motion and correct the MR, which can then be assessed intraoperatively following grafting.[22]
2. Several studies suggest that performing CABG alone, even if some residual MR (RMR) persists, does not have an impact on long-term survival or functional status.[8,26]
3. Mitral valve surgery adds significantly to the operative risk of CABG, with most series reporting operative mortalities of >10%.[21,32,53,92,107]
4. Patients with ischemic MR tend to have relatively small left atria, thereby making mitral valve exposure and repair difficult for many surgeons.
5. Mitral valve replacement, if necessary, carries the added burden of long-term anticoagulation and the risk of reoperation.

Many surgeons, however, have advocated the more liberal use of mitral annuloplasty in patients with mild to moderate ischemic MR at the time of CABG, arguing the following:

1. Chronic ischemic MR is a dynamic condition that is very dependent on preload and afterload. The preoperative echocardiogram merely represents a brief snapshot of the severity of MR at the time of the study. The fact that many patients with "moderate" MR or less present with symptoms of congestive heart failure or enlarged left atria suggests that they probably have frequent episodes of more severe MR.
2. CABG alone will not correct moderate ischemic MR in many patients, especially those with scarring from myocardial infarction and those with annular and ventricular dilatation.
3. Significant residual MR can, according to several studies, result in late symptoms and decreased long-term survival.[3]
4. Mitral annuloplasty is nearly always technically feasible, and it alone will almost always correct moderate ischemic MR, thereby making mitral valve replacement almost never necessary.
5. The high operative mortality for combined mitral valve surgery and CABG reported in the literature is outdated and reflects a significant number of patients undergoing mitral valve replacement. Mitral valve repair can now be performed

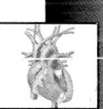

at the time of CABG, with an operative mortality as low as 3–4%.[1,15,38]

6. Leaving significant residual MR exposes the patient to the potential need for reoperative mitral valve surgery in the presence of patent grafts, which carries significant operative risk.

Impact of Ischemic Mitral Regurgitation on Survival

There is a growing body of evidence about the negative impact of even modest degrees of ischemic MR on medium-term survival in patients with coronary artery disease. The poor prognosis of patients with ischemic MR has been documented in a variety of clinical settings, with 3-year survival rates typically being in the 50–75%, range depending on the severity of MR and other patient characteristics.

After Myocardial Infarction

Several studies have documented the strong impact of MR on survival after acute MI.[22,23,64,85] In their analysis of a subgroup of 727 patients with acute MI from the survival and ventricular enlargement (SAVE) trial, Lamas and colleagues[67] found that even mild MR at the time of presentation was an independent predictor of mortality (relative risk, 2.0) and that this effect could not be attributed to differences in left ventricular function. Grigioni and others[50] found a direct correlation between survival and the severity of MR using quantitative echocardiography in patients at least 6 weeks after myocardial infarction (Figure 86-3).

After Percutaneous Coronary Intervention

Ellis and colleagues[34] reported a similar impact of MR on survival after PCI, especially in patients with left ventricular dysfunction. Three-year survival ranged from 46–76%; this was dependent on—as was the case with the post-MI patients above—the severity of MR (Figure 86-4). The authors suggested that PCI alone may be inadequate treatment for ischemic MR in these patients.

After Coronary Artery Bypass Grafting

The literature about the impact of preoperative MR in patients undergoing CABG has been mixed. Duarte and others[33] found that long-term survival in patients with moderate ischemic MR who underwent CABG alone was nearly identical to that of a control group without preoperative MR undergoing CABG during the same time period. Of note is that this group of patients differed significantly from those in recent studies of ischemic MR with regard to age and the incidence of left ventricular dysfunction and congestive heart failure.

Two large studies from the mid 1980s, however, suggested that preoperative MR is an independent risk factor for late death in patients undergoing CABG. Hickey and others[58] found that increasing MR severity had a progressively negative impact on survival, regardless of the treatment. Adler and colleagues[3] reported similar results in more than 2000 patients undergoing primary CABG. Uncorrected MR was an independent risk factor for late death, with a relative risk of 1.5 for each grade of MR. A recent study by Harris and colleagues[52] that compared CABG with and without mitral valve surgery in patients with 2–3+ MR showed 5-year survival rates of 60% and improved survival in Class III–IV patients who underwent concomitant mitral valve surgery (Figure 86-5).

Clinical Implications

Some have suggested that the MR, in any of these clinical scenarios, is merely a marker for severe underlying ischemic heart disease and not a direct cause of late death. The body of evidence supporting a direct impact of ischemic MR on late survival—although not definitive—is now quite strong. It is particularly compelling because, in many of the above studies, ischemic MR was also found to be a predictor of late mortality independent of the usual risk factors (e.g., age, ejection fraction, functional class), which argues against it simply being a confounding variable.

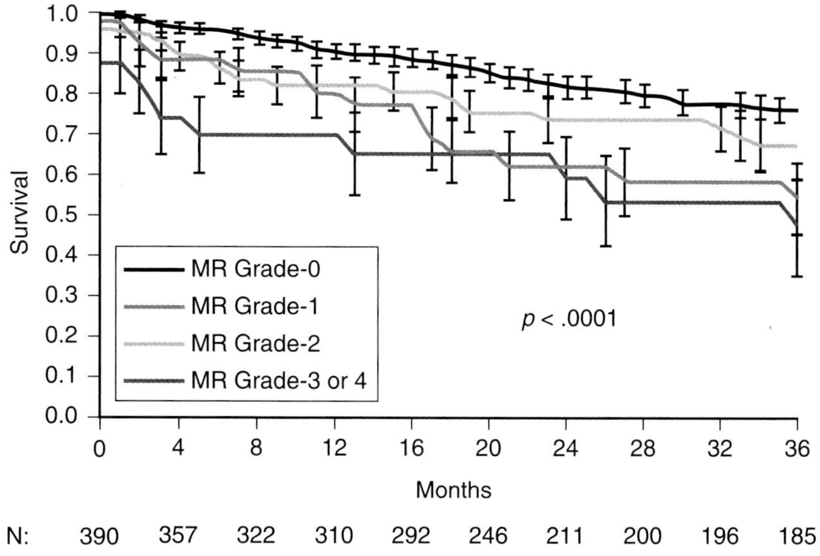

Figure 86–4 Survival curves documenting the significant relationship between the severity of mitral regurgitation and midterm survival in patients with ejection fractions of <40% who are undergoing percutaneous coronary intervention.[34] Three-year survival in patients with grade 2–4 mitral regurgitation was <60%, which suggests that percutaneous coronary intervention alone may not be adequate therapy for these patients.

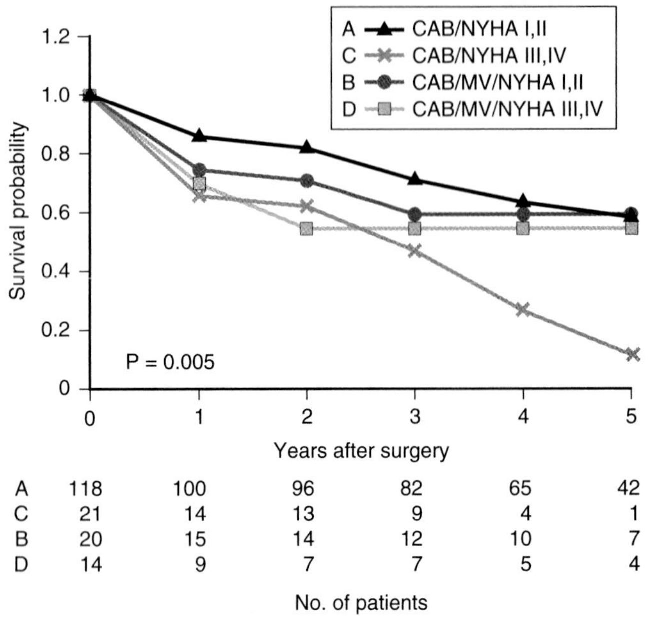

Figure 86–5 Survival curves documenting the impact of concomitant mitral valve surgery and functional (New York Heart Association) class on patients with ischemic mitral regurgitation undergoing coronary artery bypass surgery.[52] Patients within class III–IV undergoing concomitant mitral valve surgery had significantly better survival than those undergoing coronary artery bypass alone.

Although the strong impact of ischemic MR on survival supports intervening with the mitral valve in many patients with ischemic MR, the decision about whether to intervene in a specific patient can be complex and must take into account multiple factors, including the specific clinical presentation, the presence of comorbid conditions, and the expected operative morbidity and mortality. For purposes of surgical decision making, it is useful to separately consider the two most common clinical scenarios, which were noted earlier (see Figure 86-1).

Downgrading of Mitral Regurgitation by Intraoperative Transesophageal Echocardiography

The severity of MR is of paramount importance when deciding whether or not to intervene in ischemic MR at the time of CABG. As noted above, we feel that the MR severity should be based on a transthoracic echocardiogram performed in an awake patient who is not actively ischemic. The downgrading of MR by intraoperative TEE has now been well documented in the literature.

Our group showed that 90% of the patients with moderate (3+) MR who underwent intraoperative TEE had their MR downgraded to mild or less (0–2+). In nearly a third of these patients, there was no detectable MR on intraoperative TEE (Figure 86-6).[6] Bach and others[9] compared preoperative TEE in patients under intravenous conscious sedation with intraoperative TEE in patients under general anesthesia; they noted a significant decrease in the size of the regurgitant jet in patients with "functional" MR but not in those with flail leaflets. Grewal and colleagues[49] performed a similar study that was limited to patients with moderate or severe MR. Half of their patients were downgraded at least one grade, and this effect was again limited to those with "functional" MR.

The mechanism underlying this phenomenon is almost certainly the unloading effect of general anesthesia, which results in arterial and venous vasodilatation, which decrease afterload and preload, respectively. Although the effects of afterload on

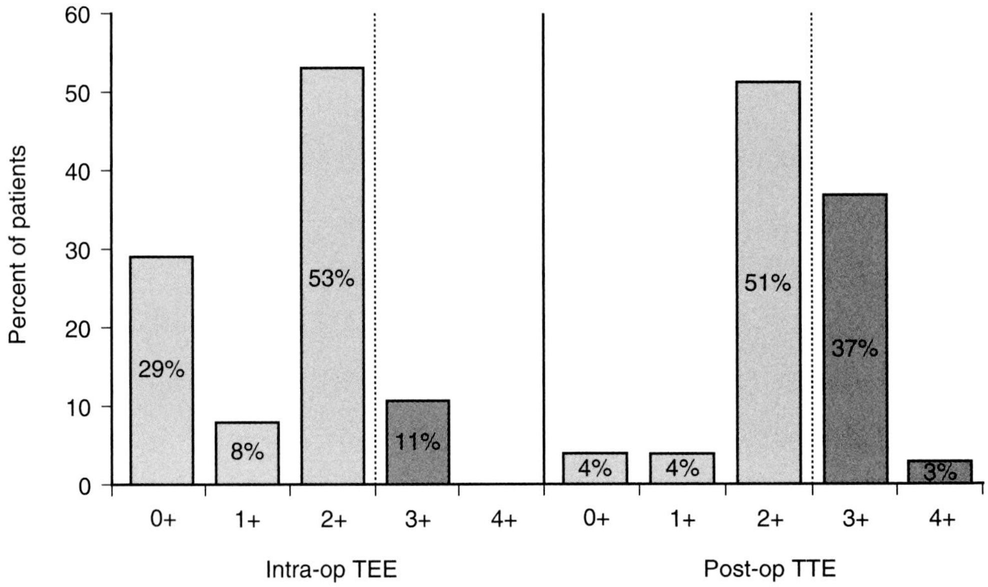

Figure 86–6 Bar graphs documenting the impact of coronary artery bypass grafting alone on patients with moderate (3+) ischemic mitral regurgitation (MR).[6] Nearly 90% of patients were downgraded to 2+ MR or less on intraoperative transesophageal echocardiography, which indicates that preoperative quantification of MR grade is critical. Although some patients had improvement in their MR grades with coronary artery bypass grafting alone, 40% were left with 3–4+ MR and only in <10% was the MR completely corrected (0–1+).

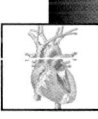

MR are generally well recognized, the effects of preload are underappreciated and may in fact be more important. Increased preload results in left atrial, left ventricular, and annular dilatation (which can increase leaflet separation) decrease leaflet coaptation and worsen MR severity. Grewal and others[49] documented that decreased end-diastolic and end-systolic volumes in patients under general anesthesia support the role of altered loading conditions in this phenomenon.

Although this finding supports careful, preoperative echocardiography in patients scheduled for CABG with suspected MR, it does not diminish the importance and utility of intraoperative TEE in this setting. On the contrary, TEE can provide important detailed anatomical information. In addition, intraoperative TEE with provocative testing to increase both preload and afterload may clarify the physiological importance of the MR and assist with intraoperative decision making if the preoperative assessment is equivocal or unavailable. However, two common practices should be strongly discouraged. Base the decision to intervene on: (1) a downgraded intraoperative TEE without provocative testing or (2) the MR severity on TEE following performance of the bypass grafts.

Coronary Artery Bypass Grafting Alone for Ischemic Mitral Regurgitation

Impact of Coronary Artery Bypass Grafting Alone on Severity of Mitral Regurgitation

A handful of studies have examined whether CABG alone corrects ischemic MR in a variety of settings (Table 86-2). Three support not intervening in mild to moderate ischemic MR. Balu and others,[10] in a report from 1982, presented preoperative and postoperative ventriculography data for a heterogeneous group of 12 patients with ischemic MR and suggested that CABG alone improves MR and functional status. This older study is limited by the small, heterogeneous patient population.

In a more recent report, Christenson and colleagues[22] reviewed 56 patients with severe left ventricular dysfunction (ejection fraction, ≤25%) and varying degrees of MR by preoperative echocardiography who underwent CABG alone. They observed that 93% of patients had no more than trace (0–1+) MR, and the remaining patients has mild (2+) MR on postoperative echocardiography. They conclude that "moderate co-existing MR seems to normalize after myocardial revascularization and should not be surgically corrected therefore at the primary operation."[22] This study, however, has several limitations that make it difficult to interpret and hence do not justify this broad recommendation. Most importantly, only 7 patients (13%) in this study had moderate (3+) preoperative MR, and more than 40% had trace (1+) MR. In addition, nearly 10% of these patients underwent concomitant left ventricular aneurysm repair, which can improve MR by decreasing ventricular dimensions; this may explain the unusually large increase in mean ejection fraction (18–44%) as compared with most reports about CABG in severe left ventricular dysfunction. The postoperative echocardiogram was performed anywhere from 3–36 months after surgery, thus making comparison of these results difficult. A similar study by Tolis and others[103] evaluated 49 patients with ejection fractions that were <30% and who had "mild-to-moderate" MR who underwent CABG alone. Mean MR grade decreased from 1.7 to 0.5, and the authors recommend CABG alone in this subgroup. These conclusions are limited by the fact that <10% of patients had 3+ MR and 40% had 1+ MR.

Three recent studies, however, have suggested that CABG alone does not completely correct ischemic MR. Czer and colleagues[28] used intraoperative TEE to compare 25 patients who underwent CABG alone with 24 patients who underwent suture annuloplasty. In the CABG alone group, there was no change in the annular diameter, leaflet-to-annulus ratio, or mean MR grade. This study was also limited by the fact that most patients had mild MR or less. In addition, the hazards of interpreting MR severity using TEE without controlling loading conditions have been described above. Ryden and others[93] reviewed 89 patients with 2+ MR undergoing CABG alone and reported that the MR was unchanged or worse in 38%.

A study from our group of patients at Brigham and Women's Hospital also concluded that CABG alone was not the optimal therapy for many patients with moderate ischemic MR.[6] One hundred and thirty-six patients with moderate ischemic MR underwent CABG alone. Among the 68 patients who underwent early postoperative transthoracic echocardiography (see Figure 86-5), 40% showed no improvement and were left with moderate or severe (3–4+) residual RMR. Approximately 50% of patients had some improvement and were left with mild (2+) RMR. Only a few remaining patients (<10%) had significant improvement, with no more than trace (0–1+) RMR.

Thus, current literature seems to suggest that, although CABG alone can decrease MR severity (especially in patients with mild ischemic MR and poor left ventricular function), it has an inconsistent and relatively weak impact on moderate ischemic MR, leaving many patients with 2+ or greater RMR.

Impact of Coronary Artery Bypass Grafting Alone on Late Outcomes

Although CABG alone may not correct ischemic MR, skeptics have argued that residual MR after CABG alone does not have an adverse impact on late functional status or survival. The Emory group[33] has addressed this in two reports about a cohort of 58 patients undergoing CABG alone for moderate MR between 1977 and 1983. In their most recent update,[33] 5- and 10-year actuarial survival was nearly identical to that of a control group without preoperative MR that underwent CABG during the same time period. The authors conclude that moderate ischemic MR should not be routinely corrected at the time of CABG.

Their patients differ from typical ischemic MR patients in most modern series. Specifically, they were relatively young (mean age, 63 years) with normal left ventricular function (mean ejection fraction, 53%) and little or no congestive heart failure (10% Class III or IV). These differences are important because, by their own analysis, evidence of congestive heart failure and age were independent predictors of late death. It is perhaps as important to note that nearly a quarter of their patients had nonischemic etiologies such as leaflet prolapse and rheumatic heart disease. Their univariate analysis shows a trend toward higher mortality in patients with

Table 86–2

Impact of Coronary Artery Bypass Grafting Alone on Mitral Regurgitation Severity

Author	*Year*	*n*	*Ejection fraction*	*Preoperative MR = 1+*	*Preoperative MR = 3+*	*Residual MR ≥ 2+*	*Concluded that CABG alone suffices*	*Comment*
Tolis[103]	2002	49	Mean, 22%	37%	10%	Mean, 0.5	Yes	
Aklog[6]	2001	68	Mean, 38%	0%	100%	90%	No	Only those with postoperative echocardiography (50%)
Czer[28]	1996	25		Mean, 1.7		Mean, 1.8	No	
Christensen[22]	1995	56	Mean, 18%	41%	13%	7%	Yes	10% had concomitant left ventricle aneurysm repair
Balu[10]	1982	12	34–75%	25%	25%	25%	Yes	MR assessed by ventriculogram

CABG, Coronary artery bypass grafting; MR, mitral regurgitation.

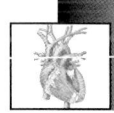

ischemic MR. Finally, they included both patients undergoing reoperation and those undergoing repair of left ventricular aneurysms. These differences raise the question of whether these long-term findings from a heterogeneous cohort of patients from the remote past can be applied to patients in the current era with a different preoperative profile.

Two other studies suggest that CABG alone does not have an impact on long-term survival in patients with moderate ischemic MR.[26,84] Both of these studies, however, were also limited by a heterogeneous patient population from the remote past with varying degrees of MR. One study compared patients with 2+ MR undergoing CABG alone with a case-matched control group without MR and showed no difference in 3-year survival or functional staus.[93]

Two large studies from the mid 1980s suggest that MR is an independent risk factor for late death in patients undergoing CABG. Hickey and others[58] from Duke University reviewed data from more than 2000 patients and found that increasing MR severity had a progressively negative impact on survival, regardless of the treatment. They recommended the more liberal application of concomitant mitral valve repair in moderate and severe MR. Adler and others[3] reported similar results in more than 2000 patients undergoing primary CABG. Uncorrected MR was an independent risk factor for late death, with a relative risk of 1.5 for each grade of MR.

There is limited information in the literature about the late functional status of patients undergoing CABG alone for moderate ischemic MR. The Emory study[33] reported a trend toward more class III and IV angina (29% vs. 6%) and congestive heart failure (14% vs. 6%) as compared with the case-matched controls. By contrast, Bolling and others[15] report that nearly all patients moved from class III–IV to class I–II after undergoing mitral valve repair at the time of CABG. These findings raise the possibility that, even if the significant rate of residual MR after CABG alone does not result in decreased long-term survival, it may adversely affect long-term functional status and quality of life. Concomitant mitral valve repair may therefore be justified (if it can be performed with relatively low operative risk) to improve long-term functional status. Bolling and others[16] and Chen and colleagues[21] have clearly demonstrated improved functional status after mitral valve repair in a broad group of patients with severe left ventricular function, many with an ischemic etiology. This may suggest that patients with left ventricular dysfunction may extract greater benefit from mitral valve repair at the time of CABG for moderate ischemic MR.

Impact of Coronary Artery Bypass Grafting with Mitral Valve Surgery on Late Outcomes

Multiple reports from the past 20 years suggest that late survival in patients with ischemic MR undergoing mitral valve surgery is suboptimal and significantly worse than it is in those with degenerative or rheumatic mitral valve disease.* Medium-term (3- to 5-year) survival in these studies ranged from 50–80%, depending on the risk profile. These poor outcomes are consistent with the overall poor prognosis of patients with ischemic MR in other contexts (e.g., medical therapy, angioplasty, CABG). Only a few studies have specifically compared the late outcomes of patients undergoing CABG alone with those undergoing concomitant mitral valve surgery. None of these were randomized or matched, and most are therefore limited by significant selection bias.[8,26,28,84]

Two recent studies have sought to directly compare outcomes of CABG alone with CABG/mitral valve surgery. Prifti and others[85] reviewed 99 patients with 2–3+ ischemic MR and ejection fractions of <30 who were split evenly between CABG alone and CABG/mitral valve surgery (nearly all repairs). Although the groups were comparable with regard to preoperative characteristics, concomitant mitral valve surgery led to improved ejection fraction, decreased left ventricular dimensions, and improved 3-year survival.

Harris et al[52] reviewed 196 patients with 2–3+ ischemic MR and an average ejection fraction of 39% (142 CABG alone; 44 concomitant mitral valve surgeries, mostly repairs). Those undergoing mitral valve surgery had somewhat more MR and a lot more Class III–IV congestive heart failure (41% vs. 15%). The operative mortality was much higher in this group (21% vs. 9%), but overall long-term survival was no different. In the subgroup of patients with class III–IV heart failure, however, concomitant mitral valve surgery provided a significant survival advantage (see Figure 86-6). An important secondary finding in this study was an approximately 50% incidence of 2+ or greater residual MR in patients undergoing mitral valve repair, a result that the authors acknowledge is suboptimal. The strong impact of RMR on survival, which we will discuss below, suggests that the survival benefit of concomitant mitral valve surgery would have been higher in the heart failure group—and may have been demonstrable in the overall group—if the residual MR rate had been as low as it was some other reports. In addition, concomitant mitral valve surgery would have faired much better if the operative mortality have been closer to the 4–10% reported in recent studies.

Overall, these data suggest that concomitant mitral valve surgery may improve late outcomes for patients with ischemic MR, especially for those with heart failure and if it can be performed with little additional operative risk and a low incidence of residual MR.

Residual Mitral Regurgitation After Coronary Artery Bypass Grafting/Mitral Valve Repair

Although concomitant mitral valve repair has become the preferred treatment for ischemic MR at the time of CABG, some surgeons remain skeptical that annuloplasty alone can adequately correct what is primarily a ventricular problem with secondary effects on the function of the valve. One of the reasons for this skepticism is the reports of residual MR after CABG/annuloplasty.

Incidence of Residual Mitral Regurgitation

Suture annuloplasty has been shown to have a significantly higher incidence of RMR in patients with ischemic MR. Hausmann and others[53] reported a 28% incidence of RMR of at least 2+ with this technique. Von Oppell and colleagues[107] had a 13% incidence of moderate RMR in a series in which most patients underwent suture annuloplasty. In a series of patients with 3–4+ ischemic MR, Czer and others[28] found

*References 21, 29, 52, 78, 87, 99, 104, 107.

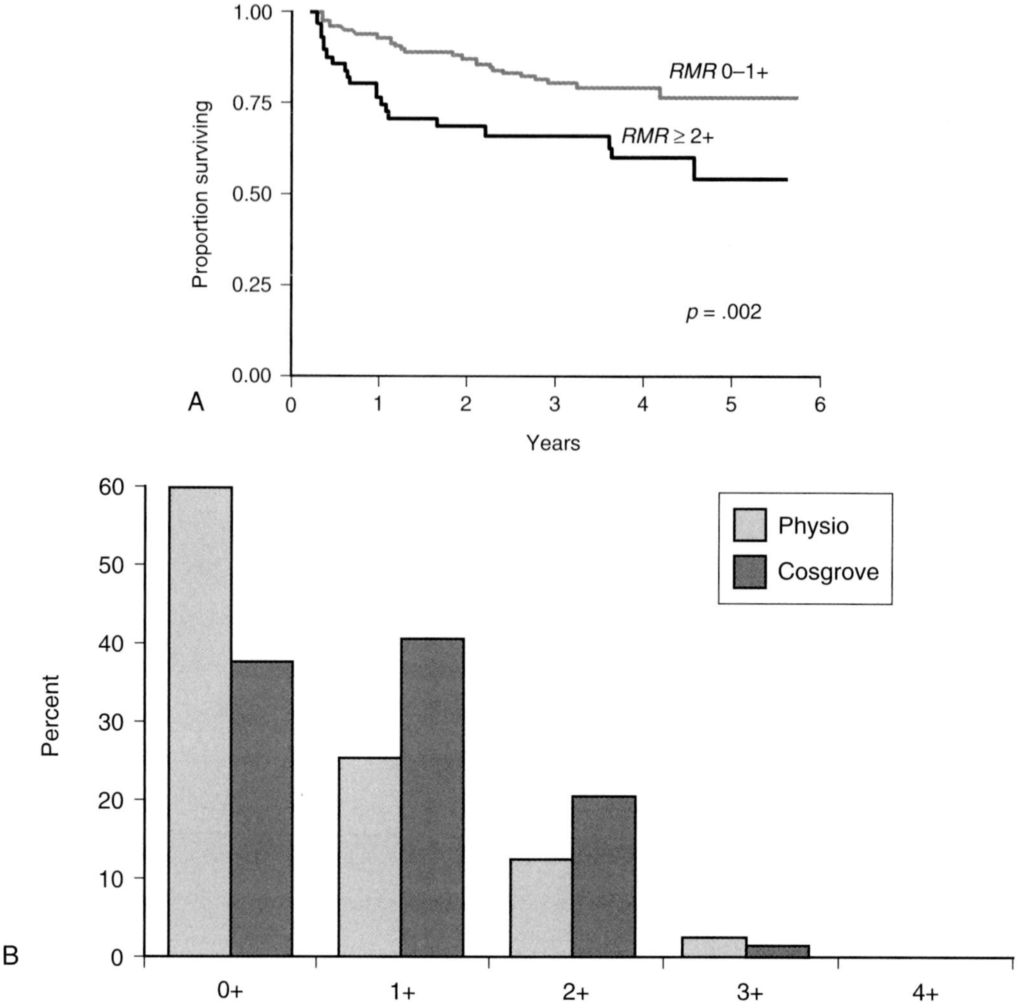

	0+	1+	2+	3+	4+
Physio	60%	26%	12%	2%	0%
Cosgrove	38%	40%	20%	1%	0%

Figure 86–7 Results from an analysis of the impact of residual mitral regurgitation (RMR) on survival after concomitant coronary artery bypass grafting and mitral valve annuloplasty for ischemic mitral regurgitation. A, RMR = 2+ had a significant impact on survival. **B,** Patients who received a complete semirigid remodeling annuloplasty ring (Carpentier-Edwards Physio, Edwards, Irvine, CA) had a significantly lower incidence of RMR than those who received a partial flexible posterior reduction annuloplasty band (Cosgrove-Edwards, Edwards, Irvine, CA).

that suture annuloplasty failed to decrease MR severity by 2 grades (i.e., RMR =2–3+) in 33% of patients.

The prosthetic ring/band annuloplasty has fared quite a bit better. We recently reported our experience with CABG/annuloplasty in patients with 3+ ischemic MR over a 7-year period and found a 12% incidence of RMR of at least 2+.[1] In the same report as above, Czer and colleagues[28] found that all but 1 patient (96%) who received a Carpentier ring had at least a 2-grade decrease in MR. Dion and others[32] were able to perform ring annuloplasty in all patients with ischemic MR resulting from annular dilatation or leaflet restriction, and they reported a 15% incidence of RMR. Bolling and colleagues[15] were able to perform annuloplasty alone in 46 out of 100 patients with severe MR undergoing CABG, with no RMR of at least 2+ in any patient. Finally, Tahta and others[97] reported that they had only 2 out of 100 patients with RMR of at least 2+ by intraoperative TEE after CABG/annuloplasty with a Duran (Medtronic, Minneapolis, MN) ring. The incidence of MR of at least 2+ increased to 29%, however, on follow-up TEE performed an average of 3 years postoperatively; this highlights the importance of distinguishing between residual and recurrent MR.

We recently reported about 288 patients (57% New York Heart Association Class III–IV; median ejection fraction, 35%) with Carpentier type I or IIIB ischemic MR (90% 3+ or 4+) who underwent CABG/annuloplasty (Figure 86-7). A complete remodeling with a semirigid ring (Carpentier-Edwards Physio, Edwards, Irvine, CA) was used in 92 patients, and a partial, restrictive, flexible band (Cosgrove-Edwards, Edwards, Irvine, CA) was used in 196 patients. RMR was assessed by echocardiography within 6 weeks of surgery. Nineteen percent of patients had residual RMR of at least 2+, whereas the remaining 81% had 0–1+ MR. Preoperative characteristics and 30-day mortality were

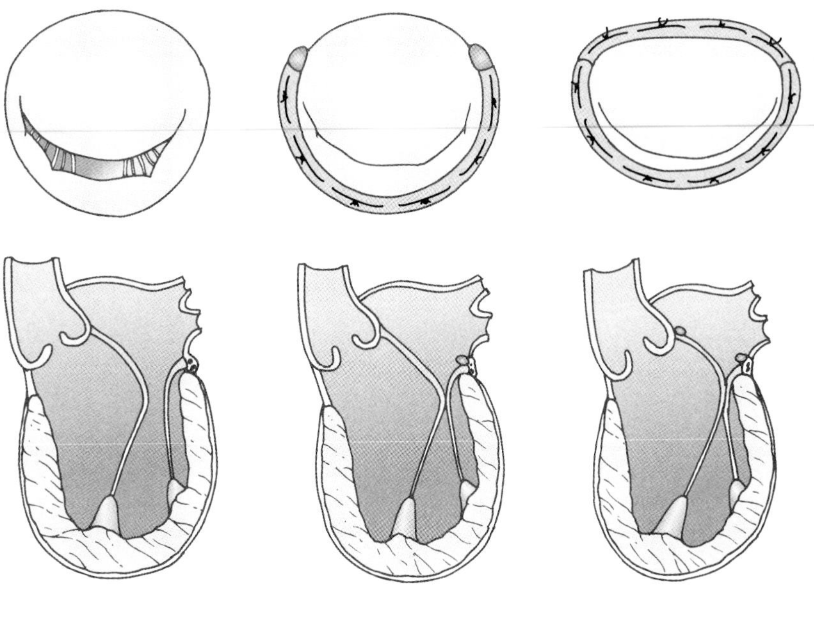

Figure 86–8 **Schematic diagrams demonstrating how a properly downsized remodeling annuloplasty ring *(far right)* predictably fixes the anteroposterior dimension, which should result in a larger surface of coaptation than a flexible partial reduction annuloplasty band *(middle)*.** The band will reliably reduce the posterior annulus to a specific size, but the degree to which it remodels the annulus and restores coaptation will depend on the relative degree of annular dilatation versus posterior leaflet restriction.

similar for these 2 groups. Complete resolution (RMR = 0+) was more likely with the Carpentier ring than the Cosgrove band (60% vs. 38%; $p = .001$). Carpentier ring patients had less RMR of at least 2+ (14% vs. 21%; $p = .10$). Univariable predictors of RMR of at least 2+ included preoperative 4+ MR and pulmonary hypertension; however, ventricular function was surprisingly not a predictor.

Possible Mechanisms of Residual Mitral Regurgitation

The mechanism of MR in these patients was impaired leaflet coaptation as a result of isolated annular dilatation (type I) and/or leaflet restriction (type IIIb). A flexible reduction annuloplasty device such as the Cosgrove-Edwards (Edwards, Irvine, CA) band or the Duran (Medtronic, Minneapolis, MN) ring seeks to improve leaflet coaptation by simply decreasing the annular circumference, which indirectly brings the leaflets together. A rigid or semirigid remodeling annuloplasty ring such as the Carpentier-Edwards Classic or Physio ring is designed to not only decrease the annular circumference but, in addition, to force the annulus back into its natural kidney shape. This should, in theory, decrease the SL dimension to a greater degree than would a flexible annuloplasty of the same size. This should, in turn, lead to a larger surface of coaptation and less RMR. The difference in reduction versus remodeling annuloplasty in patients with type IIIb MR is illustrated in Figure 86-9.

One possible explanation for RMR after CABG/annuloplasty is inadequate downsizing. Although important in type I patients, adequate downsizing is critical in type IIIb patients, especially those with left ventricular dilatation. In these patients, the AP dimension must be aggressively reduced to bring the restricted posterior leaflet close enough to the anterior leaflet to allow for adequate coaptation. Inadequate downsizing can lead to inadequate coaptation and RMR. We were not able to demonstrate inadequate downsizing; the distribution of ring/band sizes was not different between the groups. However, this does not rule out inadequate downsizing, because we suspect that the surgeon felt that he had adequately downsized if he placed a 26- or 28-mm ring, and he did not deliberately measure the annular dimensions and choose a ring 1–2 sizes smaller. We have recently begun to do the latter more systematically, and we have noticed a significant increase in patients receiving 24-mm rings. Other possible mechanisms for RMR include unsuspected mild prolapse and prominent clefts in patients with severe posterior leaflet restriction.

Impact of Residual Mitral Regurgitation on Survival

The more powerful finding of this study was that RMR had a significant impact on survival (see Figure 86-8, *A*). Three-year actuarial survival was lower in those with RMR of at least 2+ (65% vs. 80%). Univariable predictors of late mortality included RMR of at least 2+, age, New York Heart Association Class III–IV, cardiomyopathy, and renal failure. In the multivariable model, RMR of at least 2+ remained a strong independent predictor of late mortality (hazard ratio, 2.3; 95% confidence interval, 1.4–4.0).

The significant impact of even mild degrees of residual ischemic MR on survival should challenge surgeons to make every effort to minimize RMR after mitral annuloplasty. The literature does not, in our opinion, support a role for suture or pericardial annuloplasty in this disease. As mentioned above, the rates of RMR for these techniques are relatively high.[2,15,92,94] Grossi and others[107] showed a significant survival benefit (hazard ratio, 0.29) of ring annuloplasty over suture annuloplasty. Although we did not document a definite impact on survival, we found a lower incidence of RMR in patients who underwent a semirigid remodeling annuloplasty as compared with those who received a simple flexible reduction annuloplasty.

Additional Operative Risk of Mitral Valve Surgery in Ischemic Mitral Regurgitation

A critical piece of information that a surgeon contemplating concomitant mitral valve surgery for ischemic MR must consider is the additive operative risk of intervening on the mitral valve. A low operative risk would justify a more aggressive

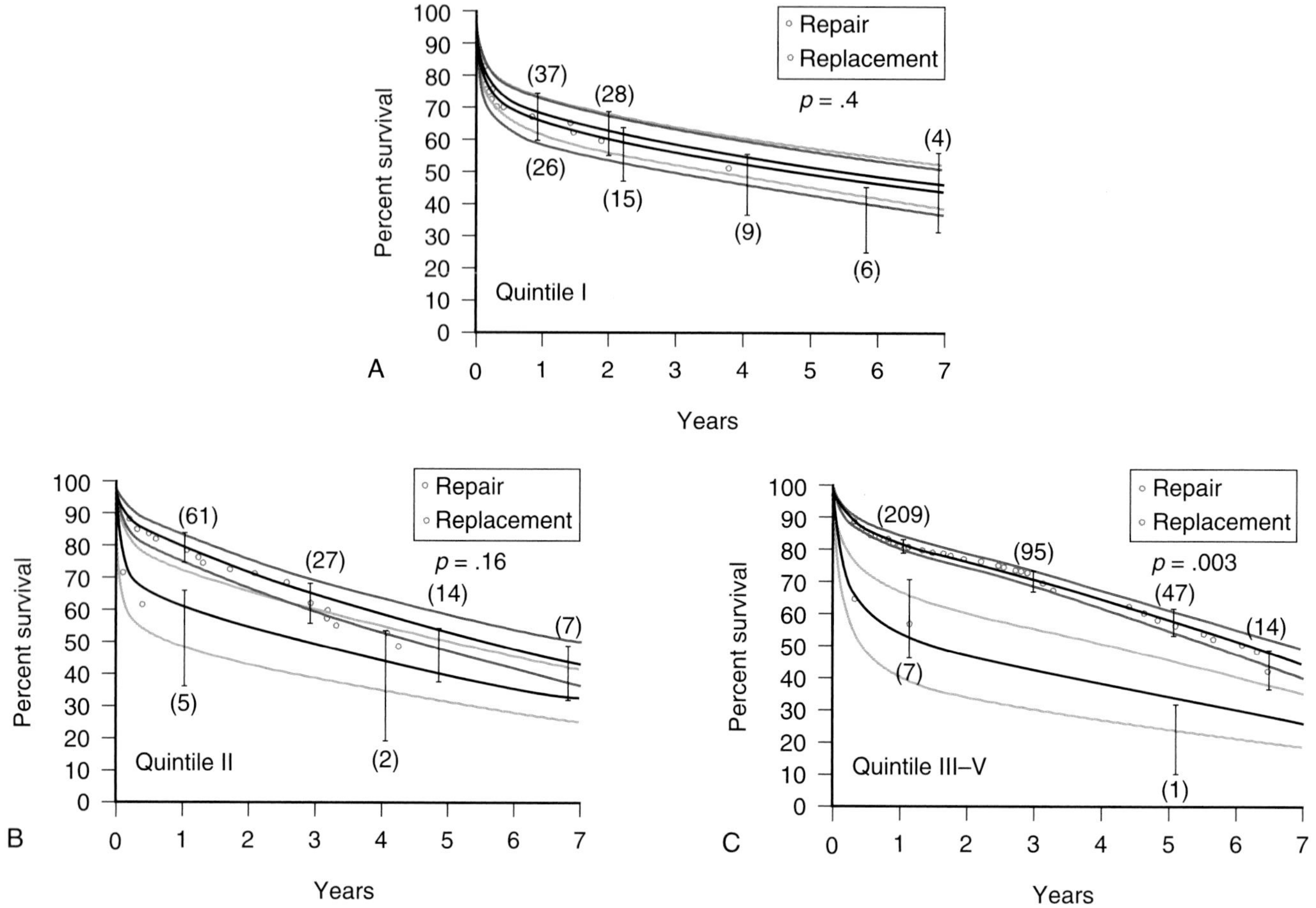

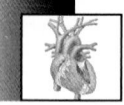

Figure 86–9 Survival curves documenting the impact of mitral valve repair versus replacement in patients with ischemic mitral regurgitation stratified by risk quintiles.[39] Most patients (quintiles III–V) saw a significant survival advantage from valve repair, whereas the highest-risk patients (quintile I) appeared to have similar survival with valve repair or replacement.

approach, given the likely benefit on late outcomes outlined above. A high incremental risk would justify a more conservative approach, although it depends on how high it is, because the benefit of mitral valve surgery may also be greatest in certain high-risk patients (e.g., Class III–IV heart failure).[52]

The operative risk for patients undergoing surgery for ischemic MR is clearly dependent on a number of preoperative factors, most notably age, left ventricular dysfunction, MR severity, and the usual cardiac surgical risk factors (e.g., age, urgency, comorbidities). Because there are no randomized or tightly controlled studies that compare CABG alone with CABG/mitral valve surgery and the patient characteristics vary widely among different clinical series, it is difficult to precisely quantify the additional operative risk of mitral valve surgery in a given patient with ischemic MR. Interpreting the clinical literature is also challenging, because uniform definitions of ischemic MR are not used. Many studies include patients with ruptured papillary muscles, chronic ischemic type II dysfunction, and even degenerative disease with incidental coronary artery disease. Nonetheless, there are enough clinical data (Table 86-3) to confirm certain apparent trends in the early outcomes of patients undergoing surgery for ischemic MR.

In most studies, the presence of ischemic MR does appear to increase the operative risk of CABG alone.* The 3–12% mortality rates seen in these studies are higher than those of most contemporary CABG series and than that of the 2002 Society of Thoracic Surgery database (2.5%, unadjusted).[20]

Concomitant mitral valve surgery/CABG has traditionally carried a much higher mortality rate than CABG alone or isolated mitral valve surgery; it is typically well over 10%. Several authors have demonstrated that the early and late outcomes of combined mitral valve and coronary bypass surgery depend strongly on the underlying etiology; in fact, they rely to the extent that they can be determined via retrospective analyses, with significantly worse outcome seen in patients with ischemic disease.[5,24,32,94] Although the reported operative mortality for mitral valve replacement at the time of CABG has remained relatively high,* the outcomes for mitral valve repair appear to be improving over time,† with most recent series reporting operative mortalities of well under 10%. For 2002, the Society of Thoracic Surgery database reported an 8% operative mortality rate for mitral valve repair/CABG (down from 12% in 1993) and an 11.5% mortality rate for mitral valve replacement/CABG (down from 17% in 1993). Our group recently reviewed early outcomes following CABG and mitral annuloplasty for moderate (3+) ischemic

*References 6, 8, 10, 22, 26, 84, 85, 88, 93, 103.

*References 18, 25, 26, 38, 43, 51, 53, 54, 61, 88, 92.

†References 1, 4, 14, 15, 25, 28, 32, 38, 39, 51, 53, 57, 61, 88, 95, 97, 107.

Table 86–3

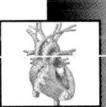

Operative Mortality for Ischemic Mitral Regurgitation Surgery

Coronary artery bypass grafting alone				*Coronary artery bypass grafting with valve repair*				*Coronary artery bypass grafting with valve replacement*			
Author	***Year***	***n***	***Mortality***	***Author***	***Year***	***n***	***Mortality***	***Author***	***Year***	***n***	***Mortality***
Tolis[103]	2002	49	2.9%	Szalay[95]	2003	91	6.6%	Bouchard[18]	2001	92	16%
Aklog[6]	2001	136	4.5%	Akar[4]	2002	102	8.8%	Grossi[51]	2001	71	20%
Ryden[93]	2001	89	12%	Tahta[97]	2002	100	12%	Gillinov[39]	2001	397	19%
Prifti[85]	2001	50	9%	Grossi[51]	2001	152	10%	Hausmann[53]	1999	197	14.2%
Czer[28]	1996	25	0%	Gillinov[39]	2001	397	6%	Cohn[25]	1995	56	8.9%
Christensen[22]	1995	56	3.6%	Bitran[14]	2001	25	0%	Ruvolo[92]	1995	67	13.4%
Rankin[89]	1989	129	11%	Adams[1]	2000	80	3.7%	He[54]	1991	36	11.1%
Arcidi[8]	1999	58	3.4%	Gangemi[38]	2000	16	6.3%	Rankin[89]	1989	42	45%
Connolly[26]	1986	85	11%	von Oppell[107]	2000	63	12.7%	Goor[43]	1988	40	12.5%
Pinson[84]	1984	83	4%	Hausmann[53]	1999	140	12.1%	Connolly[26]	1986	16	19%
				Bolling[15]	1996	100	4%	Kay[61]	1986	40	35%
				Czer[28]	1996	24	12.5%				
				Cohn[25]	1995	94	9.5%				
				Dion[32]	1995	37	14.6%				
				Hendren[57]	1991	84	9.2%				
				Rankin[89]	1989	40	18%				
				Kay[61]	1986	101	15%				

and found that operative mortality had decreased from 14% to 3.7% during the 1990s.[1] The latter was not dramatically different from the 2.9% mortality rate reported previously in an unmatched but contemporaneous group of patients undergoing CABG alone for moderate ischemic MR.[6]

So the critical question remains: What expected operative mortality should a surgeon incorporate into his or her decision-making process when considering whether to intervene on mild to moderate ischemic MR at the time of CABG? Although it obviously depends on the patient's

Table 86–4

Recommended Treatment of Ischemic Mitral Regurgitation at Coronary Bypass Surgery

Severe (4+) MR
- Mitral valve repair
  - Valve replacement for intraoperative failures (residual MR 2+ or greater)

Moderate (3+) MR
- Mitral valve repair, *unless*
  - additional operative morbidity and mortality would be prohibitive *or*
  - there is a strong indication for performing the CABG off-pump (e.g., heavily diseased ascending aorta)

Mild (2+) MR
- Mitral valve repair, *if*
  - additional operative morbidity and mortality would be low
  - signs and symptoms suggest periods of more severe MR (e.g., CHF, enlarged left atrium, atrial fibrillation)
  - there are appropriate anatomical findings on intraoperative TEE (e.g., poor surface of coaptation, tenting, annular dilatation)

MR, Mitral regurgitation; CABG, coronary artery bypass grafting; CHF, congestive heart failure; TEE, transesophageal echocardiography.

individual risk profile, we would argue that it should be about 3–5% for the typical patient in this clinical scenario at centers with broad experience with mitral annuloplasty for ischemic MR. One should remember that most of the series that report 6–12% mortality rates include patients with moderate to severe ischemic MR and congestive heart failure; these patients have higher operative risk, but the indication for mitral valve surgery remains strong for them.

Mitral Valve Repair Versus Replacement for Ischemic Mitral Regurgitation

Although mitral valve repair for ischemic MR carries the some of the same obvious benefits over replacement as it does for other etiologies (namely, avoiding the problems of long-term anticoagulation or bioprosthetic valve degeneration), the literature about the possible survival benefits of repair over replacement is less clear with regard to patients with ischemic disease than for those with degenerative, and, to a lesser extent, rheumatic disease.*

Two recent studies by Gillinov and colleagues[39] and Grossi and colleagues[51] have addressed this issue directly. They both applied sophisticated statistical techniques to analyze outcomes after repair or replacement in patients with all types (including type II) of ischemic MR. Gillinov and others found that, although the majority of patients benefited from valve repair (58% versus 36% 5-year survival), the highest-risk patients had similar survival with each procedure (Figure 86-9). The benefit of repair was diminished as certain characteristics appeared, such as lateral wall motion abnormalities and complex regurgitant jets. This suggested that, in some of these high-risk patients, a chordal-sparing valve replacement may be an acceptable alternative to repair. Grossi and others found better early survival (odds ratio, 0.43), complication-free late survival (odds ratio, 0.5), and a trend toward better overall survival and recommended valve reconstruction.

So, what role, if any, should valve replacement have in ischemic MR? Even if the benefit of repair is diminished in a small subgroup of patients, we are skeptical that a valve replacement will ultimately be superior to an appropriately downsized remodeling annuloplasty. Gillinov and others[39] used a remodeling annuloplasty in only a third of patients; the remainder received a partial restrictive band or pericardium. We have reported a significantly higher incidence of RMR with nonremodeling annuloplasties and a significant impact of RMR on late survival. Therefore, we feel that, in patients with ischemic MR, mitral valve replacement should be reserved for rare intraoperative failures, particularly in patients in whom the post-repair saline test or intraoperative transesophageal echocardiogram shows 2+ or greater RMR or a poor surface of coaptation.

Overall Recommendations for Ischemic Mitral Regurgitation During Coronary Artery Bypass Grafting

Although most surgeons agree that moderate to severe MR should be corrected at the time of CABG, there is still no consensus on the management of mild to moderate ischemic MR at the time of CABG. A preponderance of evidence seems to support a more liberal application of concomitant mitral valve surgery, which can be summarized in the following recommendations (Table 86-4):

1. All patients referred for CABG with suspected ischemic MR should undergo careful preoperative transthoracic echocardiography, preferably with quantitative assessment of MR severity while they are not actively ischemic. Those without complete preoperative assessment should undergo careful transesophageal echocardiographic assessment of their

*References 14, 18, 24, 25, 29, 53, 82, 83, 87, 89, 90, 94, 95, 96.

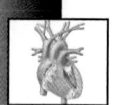

mitral valves to determine whether there is an anatomical substrate for type I or IIIB ischemic MR, and they should also receive provocative testing of the degree of MR if the TEE shows less MR than expected on the basis of the clinical picture.

2. Patients with severe ischemic MR should undergo concomitant mitral valve repair. Mitral valve replacement should be reserved for intraoperative failures (i.e., when an appropriately downsized remodeling annuloplasty does not correct the MR to 1+ or less).
3. Patients with moderate ischemic MR should undergo concomitant mitral valve repair unless preoperative factors suggest that the additional operative morbidity and mortality would be prohibitive (i.e., there is extensive mitral annular calcification or a strong indication for performing the CABG off pump [e.g., heavily diseased ascending aorta]).
4. Patients with mild ischemic MR should undergo concomitant mitral valve repair if none of the above risk factors are present and there are preoperative signs and symptoms that are suggestive of periods of more severe MR than have been documented (e.g., symptoms of congestive heart failure, enlarged left atrium, atrial fibrillation), especially if there is left ventricular dysfunction. In addition, anatomical findings present on intraoperative TEE should also be considered (e.g., minimal surface of coaptation, severe leaflet tenting coaptation depth, significant annular dilatation).

SURGICAL PRINCIPLES

Basic Principles

The basic principles of mitral valve repair for ischemic MR are not fundamentally different than those for degenerative disease. A successful outcome depends on the following:

1. careful review of the preoperative echocardiogram, with particular attention paid to the mechanism of MR, the direction of the MR jet(s), and specific anatomical abnormalities (e.g., calcification, thickening);
2. good visualization of the entire valve;
3. careful segmental valve analysis to confirm the mechanism of MR;
4. meticulous suture placement and ring sizing; and
5. consideration of adjunctive technique, if necessary.

Annuloplasty: Underlying Principles

The significant impact of even mild degrees of residual ischemic MR on survival should challenge surgeons to make every effort to minimize RMR after mitral annuloplasty. The literature does not, in our opinion, support a role for suture or pericardial annuloplasty in this disease. As mentioned above, the rates of RMR for these techniques are relatively high.[2,15,92,94] Grossi and others[107] showed a significant survival benefit (hazard ratio, 0.29) for ring annuloplasty over suture annuloplasty.

The laboratory evidence supporting a specific type of annuloplasty in general or specifically in ischemic MR is mixed.[14,26,30,51,91] Although the three-dimensional dynamic nature of mitral annulus and its contribution to ventricular function has been well documented, it is unclear what role this plays in pathological conditions such as ischemic MR. Some laboratory studies suggest that planar fixation of the annulus with a nonflexible ring impairs left ventricular function, whereas others dispute this.[17] In a recent study, we found a lower incidence of RMR in patients who underwent a semirigid remodeling annuloplasty as opposed to a simple flexible reduction annuloplasty (Figure 86-8B). In a recent editorial, Dr. Craig Miller emphasized the importance of correcting the SL dimension in ischemic MR, particularly in type IIIb dysfunction. He suggested that, at least in theory, this "may best be accomplished in patients with IMR by using stiffer rings...."[19]

Although we were able to document less RMR in patients undergoing a remodeling annuloplasty with a Carpentier ring, we do not have detailed echocardiographic data to provide a mechanism for this difference. We suspect, however, that it is most likely due to the importance of annular remodeling, specifically in the SL (or AP) dimension in patients with Carpentier type IIIb. As described earlier, a large body of data has been accumulated from several laboratories that describes the mechanisms that contribute to ischemic MR.[27,50,54,81] Several of these studies emphasize the importance of the SL dimension in ischemic MR.

A flexible reduction annuloplasty device such as the Cosgrove-Edwards band or the Duran ring seeks to improve leaflet coaptation by simply decreasing the annular circumference, which indirectly brings the leaflets together. A rigid or semirigid remodeling annuloplasty ring, such as the Carpentier-Edwards classic or physio ring, is not only designed to decrease the annular circumference but, in addition, to force the annulus back into its natural kidney shape. In accordance with its nature, it fixes the SL dimension to a specific value that based on the size of the anterior leaflet; this is less than what can be achieved by a flexible annuloplasty of the same size. This should, in turn, lead to a larger surface of coaptation and less RMR. A new remodeling annuloplasty ring designed specifically for the treatment of ischemic MR has recently been introduced into practice. The Carpentier-McCarthy-Adams IMR ETlogix (Edwards, Irvine, CA) ring is rigid; has a decreased AP diameter (i.e., is "automatically downsized"); is asymmetrical, with a narrower dimension at P2–P3; and has a slight dip at P2–P3 to accommodate the greater posterior leaflet restriction in this region.

As illustrated in Figure 86-9, a reduction annuloplasty will, to some degree, decrease the SL dimension, improve leaflet coaptation, and correct MR. The extent to which it accomplishes this, however, likely depends on the whether annular dilatation or posterior leaflet restriction is the dominant mechanism of MR. Even if the MR is mostly corrected with a nonremodeling annuloplasty in the short term, the long-term durability of the repair likely depends on the location and size of the surface of coaptation, which should be greater with a remodeling annuloplasty. Both Calafiore and others[32] and Yiu and others[108] have provided evidence that the coaptation depth or height (i.e., the distance between the annulus and the point at which coaptation begins) is important in patients with "functional"—but not specifically ischemic—MR.

The laboratory evidence supporting a specific type of annuloplasty in general or specifically in ischemic MR is mixed.[14,26,30,51,91] Although the three-dimensional dynamic nature of mitral annulus and its contribution to ventricular function has been well documented, it is unclear what role this plays in pathological conditions such as ischemic MR. Some laboratory studies suggest that planar fixation of the annulus with a non-flexible ring impairs left ventricular function, whereas others dispute this.[1,17,42]

Operative Techniques

Valve Exposure

The most common approach to patients with ischemic MR is a full sternotomy with cannulation of the ascending aorta and both vena cavae. After the completion of coronary bypass grafting, the mitral valve can be exposed either via the interatrial groove or transseptally. Patients with ischemic MR may have a small left atrial cavity, depending on the acuity of presentation. Despite this, however, excellent exposure of the valve can be obtained with a standard mitral valve retractor system if certain principles are followed. The interatrial approach is most commonly used and particular attention should be placed to the following: (1) complete dissection of the groove prior to atriotomy and (2) posterior extension of the inferior aspect of the atriotomy, with partial detachment of the right lower pulmonary vein. The transseptal approach may be useful in the setting of a small left atrium, concomitant tricuspid valve repair, or when an aortic prosthesis is present.

Valve Analysis

Before segmental valve analysis, it is often helpful to place an exposure suture in the posterior annulus at the junction between P1 and P2 to bring the valve apparatus anterior and lateral. Using 2 hooks, it is then possible to confirm the preoperative echocardiographic findings (i.e., posterior leaflet restriction [Carpentier Type IIIb dysfunction] due to posterior papillary muscle displacement) that most commonly affect P2 and P3. Associated annular dilatation is also commonly present.

Suture Placement

For implanting an annuloplasty ring, 2-0 braided sutures are the most commonly used. In general, sutures in the septal and lateral portions of the annulus should be placed using a backhand orientation, and sutures in the anterior and medial portions of the annulus are placed with a forehand orientation. Because of the potential increased tension in the setting of type IIIb dysfunction with associated annular dilatation, it is preferable to place the sutures very close together along the annulus, and suture crossover may be warranted. The full curve of the needle should be used to encourage deep, wide placement of individual sutures along the annulus. The anterior commissure is usually the most difficult area to expose, and it is usually approached last, after the placement of sutures along the septal, medial, and lateral portions of the annulus to place tension on prior sutures to expose this area of the annulus.

Sizing and Implantation

After sutures are placed about the annulus, standard ring sizers are used to select the appropriate ring. Placing gentle traction on marginal chords in the A-2 portion of the anterior leaflet with a hook allows the height and surface area of the anterior leaflet to be measured. An additional measurement to consider is the intercommissural distance.

Because leaflet restriction in ischemic MR results in less leaflet tissue available for coaptation, it is necessary to downsize the complete remodeling ring by 1 or 2 sizes to ensure an adequate surface of coaptation after annuloplasty. Systolic anterior motion will not occur, despite aggressive downsizing; this is because the restricted posterior leaflet cannot displace the anterior leaflet into the outflow tract. After a ring is selected (typically a size between 24 and 28 mm), the interrupted sutures are passed through it, with respect paid to the associated geometry of the annulus and the matching bite sizes on each. The individual sutures are then tied, thus securing the ring to the annulus.

After the downsized remodeling annuloplasty is completed, a saline test is used to confirm the line of coaptation along the margin of the leaflets. The typical appearance of a completed downsized remodeling annuloplasty is shown in Figure 86-10. Nearly the entire orifice is occupied by the anterior leaflet, thereby allowing the entire restricted posterior leaflet to contribute to coaptation.

Adjunctive Procedures

Although we suspect that the routine use of a remodeling annuloplasty and more aggressive downsizing will likely decrease the incidence of RMR after CABG/annuloplasty to well under 10%, it is possible that a small group of patients may exist in whom annuloplasty alone is insufficient to correct the MR. Adjunctive techniques may play a role here, but clinical experience is limited. Poor coaptation of the scallop of the posterior leaflet can occur with leaflet restriction; the clefts (P1P2 or P2P3) should be closed if this is suspected or a corresponding jet is noted on saline testing. Posterior leaflet extension, especially over the P3 scallop, has been used in patients with severe posterior leaflet restriction.[91] Kron and others[63] have treated ischemic MR with papillary muscle repositioning using a pledgeted suture attached to the annulus. The one series of edge-to-edge, Alfieri-type repair specifically in ischemic MR had an unacceptably high rate of early failure requiring reoperation,[75] as would have been predicted from laboratory data.[70] The risk of mitral stenosis is not insignificant if performed in the context of a downsized annuloplasty. Resection of secondary chordae,[31] ventricular plication,[96] and SL "cinching"[30] have been shown to have beneficial effects in animal models.

Mitral Valve Replacement

In selected patients, a chordal-sparing mitral valve replacement procedure should be considered if a downsized remodeling annuloplasty in combination with an adjunctive procedure does not correct the ischemic MR. A 2+ or greater RMR on the post-bypass TEE should prompt reexploration of the valve and consideration of valve replacement. The poor prognosis of patients with ischemic MR usually justifies the use of a bioprosthesis, even if the patient is in atrial fibrillation.

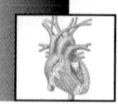

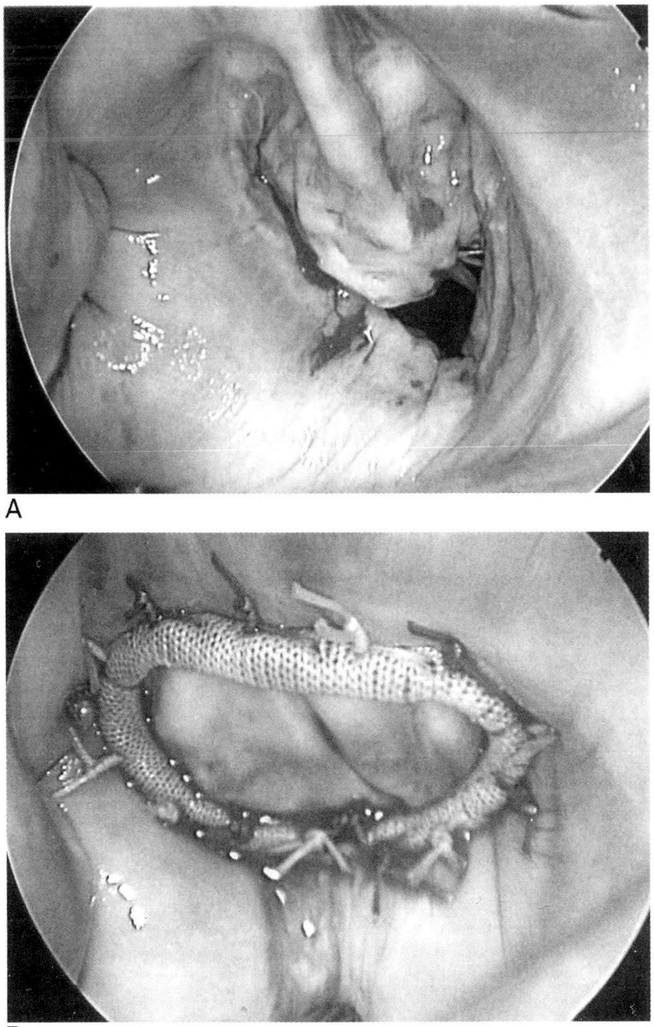

A

B

Figure 86–10 Intraoperative photographs of the mitral valve in a patient undergoing mitral annuloplasty for ischemic mitral regurgitation after myocardial infarction. A, The valve before repair showing several findings that are common to ischemic mitral regurgitation, including moderate annular dilatation, severe annular distortion (i.e., an increase in anteroposterior dimension with a loss of normal elliptical proportions), and posterior leaflet restriction that is greatest at the posteromedial aspect (P2–P3), with loss of leaflet coaptation in this region. **B,** The valve after successful downsized remodeling annuloplasty using a Carpentier-McCarthy-Adams IMR ETlogix (Edwards, Irvine, CA) ring. Note that the entire orifice area is taken up by the anterior leaflet, thereby allowing the entire restricted posterior leaflet to contribute to a large surface of coaptation.

TYPE II ISCHEMIC MITRAL REGURGITATION

Patients with ischemic MR secondary to Carpentier type II dysfunction form a subgroup with a clinical presentation and therapeutic approach that are distinct from the vast majority of patients with ischemic MR who have type I or IIIb dysfunction. In patients with type II Carpentier's functional classification, the leaflet motion of 1 or 2 leaflets is increased, thereby causing the free edge of the leaflet to override the plane of the mitral annulus during systole.[20a] In these patients, leaflet prolapse results from the rupture of 1 papillary muscle (partial or complete), from papillary muscle elongation, or, rarely, from isolated chordal rupture.

Papillary Muscle Rupture

Pathology and Pathophysiology

Papillary muscle rupture is a rare mechanical complication of myocardial infarction that carries a high mortality rate without early diagnosis and appropriate expeditious medical and surgical management; this complication occurs in 1–5% of patients who die after myocardial infarction.[108] Papillary muscle rupture can occur during the acute phase of myocardial infarction. However, most patients present within 2–7 days after myocardial infarction. The rupture involves the posteromedial papillary muscle (75%) more often than the anterolateral papillary muscle (25%). The vulnerability of posteromedial papillary muscle is explained by the fact that its vascular supply is dependent on 1 coronary artery (either the right coronary artery or the circumflex artery in right-or left-dominant systems, respectively).[35a] By contrast, the anterolateral papillary muscle is supplied by two major coronary arteries: the left anterior descending and the circumflex arteries. Complete papillary muscle rupture occurs in 30% of patients and results in bileaflet prolapse with severe MR. However, partial rupture of one papillary muscle involving one or more heads is more common. The myocardial infarction often involves a limited area of the myocardium, which may explain the fact that left ventricular function is relatively preserved in most patients.[97a]

Clinical Presentation and Differential Diagnosis

These patients often present with the sudden development of congestive heart failure and cardiogenic shock. The rapid clinical deterioration of a previously stable patient with a myocardial infarction should suggest the diagnosis of a mechanical complication of myocardial infarction. The sudden appearance of a systolic murmur and hemodynamic compromise may result from acute severe ischemic MR as a result of papillary muscle rupture or from ventricular septal rupture. Clinically it remains very difficult to distinguish between these two entities, despite differences in the characteristics of the murmurs; in ventricular septal rupture, the murmur is loud, prominent at the left sternal border, and associated with a thrill, whereas, in acute ischemic MR, it is softer, intense at the apex, and without a thrill. Another important condition in the differential diagnosis is extensive myocardial infarction with cardiogenic shock; this is associated with varying degrees of ischemic MR without papillary muscle rupture (type I or IIIb).

Rapid diagnostic evaluation is critical to establish the diagnosis and initiate treatment before the onset of complications of cardiogenic shock. Two-dimensional transthoracic echocardiography can document the MR and assess the left ventricular function, and it can usually visualize the ruptured papillary muscle head prolapsing into the left atrium. TEE may be necessary if the diagnosis of ruptured papillary muscle cannot be excluded in a patient with thermodynamically significant acute ischemic MR. Coronary angiography is necessary to document the extent of coronary artery disease.

Medical and Surgical Treatment

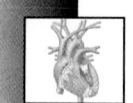

The principal goal of preoperative medical management is rapid hemodynamic stabilization, specifically for the preservation of cardiac output and arterial pressure to maintain peripheral organ perfusion and to preserve coronary blood flow; this usually requires the initiation of inotropic agents and the prompt insertion of an intraaortic balloon pump. This stabilization phase should occur while the operating room is being readied and should not delay the surgical management of these critically ill patients.

The goals of the surgical procedure are the correction of the MR and myocardial revascularization. Chordal-sparing mitral valve replacement remains the procedure of choice for most patients. Papillary muscle reimplantation can be attempted in selected patients, provided that necrosis of the supporting myocardial wall is limited and in the absence of an akinetic or dyskinetic wall. The nonprolapsed area of the valve serves as a reference point to determine the site and level of implantation of the papillary muscle remnant. At this site, a 5-mm-deep trench is created in the muscular wall. The papillary muscle remnant is trimmed to preserve only the fibrous cuff. The papillary muscle remnant is buried in the trench using interrupted 4/0 polypropylene sutures. The trench is then closed around the papillary muscle remnant using a figure-8 suture.

Papillary Muscle Elongation

Papillary muscle elongation results from the fibrotic transformation of the papillary muscle after myocardial infarction. The elongation of papillary muscle causes leaflet prolapse that results in MR. Most patients present with chronic ischemic MR and do not require emergency surgical treatment. Patients with severe MR should benefit from mitral surgery. In those with moderate MR, the latter should be corrected only if a coronary revascularization is undertaken. Mitral valve replacement with the preservation of subvalvular apparatus is the most common procedure.[17a,30a] However, mitral valve repair with papillary muscle shortening, as described by Carpentier, can be performed in selected patients.[20a] Papillary muscle shortening is performed by either burying the extra length of the papillary muscle into the trench created in the ventricle or by resecting the appropriate length of papillary muscle and suturing the fibrous cuff supporting the chords to the papillary muscle. Four to five circumferential simple sutures without pledgets should be used for this fixation. If the elongation involves only 1 papillary muscle head resulting in the prolapse of 1 segment of the valve (e.g., P3 segment prolapse), more conventional techniques of repair (e.g., resection of the prolapsed area combined with sliding valvuloplasty) can be performed safely.

REFERENCES

1. Adams DH, Chen RH, Byrne JG, et al: Improving outcomes in patients with moderate ischemic mitral regurgitation undergoing combined CABG and mitral annuloplasty. Circulation 102:II-462, 2000.
2. Adams DH, Filsoufi F, Aklog L: Surgical treatment of the ischemic mitral valve. J Heart Valve Dis 11(Suppl 1): S21–S25, 2002.
3. Adler DS, Goldman L, O'Neil A, et al: Long-term survival of more than 2,000 patients after coronary artery bypass grafting. Am J Cardiol 58:195–202, 1986.
4. Akar AR, Doukas G, Szafranek A, et al: Mitral valve repair and revascularization for ischemic mitral regurgitation: predictors of operative mortality and survival. J Heart Valve Dis 11:793–800; discussion 801, 2002.
5. Akins CW, Hilgenberg AD, Buckley MJ, et al: Mitral valve reconstruction versus replacement for degenerative or ischemic mitral regurgitation. Ann Thorac Surg 58:668–675; discussion 675–676, 1994.
6. Aklog L, Filsoufi F, Flores KQ, et al: Does coronary artery bypass grafting alone correct moderate ischemic mitral regurgitation? Circulation 104:168–175, 2001.
7. Alam M, Thorstrand C, Rosenhamer G: Mitral regurgitation following first-time acute myocardial infarction—early and late findings by Doppler echocardiography. Clin Cardiol 16:30–34, 1993.
8. Arcidi JM Jr, Hebeler RF, Craver JM, et al: Treatment of moderate mitral regurgitation and coronary disease by coronary bypass alone. J Thorac Cardiovasc Surg 95:951–959, 1988.
9. Bach DS, Deeb GM, Bolling SF: Accuracy of intraoperative transesophageal echocardiography for estimating the severity of functional mitral regurgitation. Am J Cardiol 76:508–512, 1995.
10. Balu V, Hershowitz S, Zaki Masud AR, et al: Mitral regurgitation in coronary artery disease. Chest 81:550–555, 1982.
11. Barzilai B, Davis VG, Stone PH, Jaffe AS: Prognostic significance of mitral regurgitation in acute myocardial infarction. The MILIS Study Group. Am J Cardiol 65:1169–1175, 1990.
12. Barzilai B, Gessler C Jr, Perez JE, et al: Significance of Doppler-detected mitral regurgitation in acute myocardial infarction. Am J Cardiol 61:220–223, 1988.
13. Birnbaum Y, Chamoun AJ, Conti VR, Uretsky BF: Mitral regurgitation following acute myocardial infarction. Coron Artery Dis 13:337–344, 2002.
14. Bitran D, Merin O, Klutstein MW, et al: Mitral valve repair in severe ischemic cardiomyopathy. J Card Surg 16:79–82, 2001.
15. Bolling SF, Deeb GM, Bach DS: Mitral valve reconstruction in elderly, ischemic patients. Chest 109:35–40, 1996.
16. Bolling SF, Deeb GM, Brunsting LA, Bach DS: Early outcome of mitral valve reconstruction in patients with end-stage cardiomyopathy. J Thorac Cardiovasc Surg 109:676–682; discussion 682–683, 1995.
17. Bolling SF, Pagani FD, Deeb GM, Bach DS: Intermediate-term outcome of mitral reconstruction in cardiomyopathy. J Thorac Cardiovasc Surg 115:381–386; discussion 387–388, 1998.

17a. Borger MA, Tau TM, Rao V: Reoperative mitral valve replacement: importance of preservation of the subvalvular apparatus. Ann Thorac Surg 74:1482–1487, 2002.

18. Bouchard D, Pellerin M, Carrier M, et al: Results following valve replacement for ischemic mitral regurgitation. Can J Cardiol 17:427–431, 2001.
19. Byrne JG, Aklog L, Adams DH: Assessment and management of functional or ischaemic mitral regurgitation. Lancet 355:1743–1744, 2000.
20. Carpentier A: Cardiac valve surgery—the "French correction." J Thorac Cardiovasc Surg 86:323–337, 1983.

20a. Carpentier A, Chauvaud S, Fabiani JN, et al: Reconstructive surgery of mitral valve incompetence: Ten-year appraisal. J Thorac Cardiovasc Surg. 79:338–348, 1980.

21. Chen FY, Adams DH, Aranki SF, et al: Mitral valve repair in cardiomyopathy. Circulation 98:II124–II127, 1998.
22. Christenson JT, Simonet F, Bloch A, et al: Should a mild to moderate ischemic mitral valve regurgitation in patients with poor left ventricular function be repaired or not? J Heart Valve Dis 4:484–488; discussion 488–489, 1995.
23. Christenson JT, Simonet F, Maurice J, et al: Mitral regurgitation in patients with coronary artery disease and low left ven-

tricular ejection fractions. How should it be treated? Tex Heart Inst J 22:243–249, 1995.
24. Cohn LH, Kowalker W, Bhatia S, et al: Comparative morbidity of mitral valve repair versus replacement for mitral regurgitation with and without coronary artery disease. 1988. Updated in 1995. Ann Thorac Surg 60:1452–1453, 1995.
25. Cohn LH, Rizzo RJ, Adams DH, et al: The effect of pathophysiology on the surgical treatment of ischemic mitral regurgitation: operative and late risks of repair versus replacement. Eur J Cardiothorac Surg 9:568–574, 1995.
26. Connolly MW, Gelbfish JS, Jacobowitz IJ, et al: Surgical results for mitral regurgitation from coronary artery disease. J Thorac Cardiovasc Surg 91:379–388, 1986.
27. Craver JM, Jones EL, Guyton RA: Short and long term outcome after mitral valve repair. Circulation 96:I-731, 1997.
28. Czer LS, Maurer G, Bolger AF, et al: Revascularization alone or combined with suture annuloplasty for ischemic mitral regurgitation. Evaluation by color Doppler echocardiography. Tex Heart Inst J 23:270–278, 1996.
29. Czer LS, Maurer G, Trento A, et al: Comparative efficacy of ring and suture annuloplasty for ischemic mitral regurgitation. Circulation 86:II46–II52, 1992.
30. Dagum P, Timek TA, Green GR, et al: Coordinate-free analysis of mitral valve dynamics in normal and ischemic hearts. Circulation 102:III62–III69, 2000.
30a. David TE, Uden DE, Strauss HD: The importance of the mitral apparatus in left ventricular function after correction of mitral regurgitation. Circulation 68:1176–1182, 1983.
31. Dion R. Ischemic mitral regurgitation: when and how should it be corrected? J Heart Valve Dis 2:536–543, 1993.
32. Dion R, Benetis R, Elias B, et al: Mitral valve procedures in ischemic regurgitation. J Heart Valve Dis 4(Suppl 2):S124–S129; discussion S129–S131, 1995.
33. Duarte IG, Shen Y, MacDonald MJ, et al: Treatment of moderate mitral regurgitation and coronary disease by coronary bypass alone: late results. Ann Thorac Surg 68:426–430, 1999.
34. Ellis SG, Whitlow PL, Raymond RE, Schneider JP: Impact of mitral regurgitation on long-term survival after percutaneous coronary intervention. Am J Cardiol 89:315–318, 2002.
35. Enriquez-Sarano M, Tribouilloy C: Quantitation of mitral regurgitation: rationale, approach, and interpretation in clinical practice. Heart 88:iv1–iv4, 2002.
35a. Estes EH Jr., Dalton FM, Entman ML, et al: The anatomy and blood supply of the papillary muscles of the left ventricle. Am Heart J 71:356–362, 1966.
36. Feinberg MS, Schwammenthal E, Shlizerman L, et al: Prognostic significance of mild mitral regurgitation by color Doppler echocardiography in acute myocardial infarction. Am J Cardiol 86:903–907, 2000.
37. Flachskampf FA, Chandra S, Gaddipatti A, et al: Analysis of shape and motion of the mitral annulus in subjects with and without cardiomyopathy by echocardiographic 3-dimensional reconstruction. J Am Soc Echocardiogr 13:277–287, 2000.
38. Gangemi JJ, Tribble CG, Ross SD, et al: Does the additive risk of mitral valve repair in patients with ischemic cardiomyopathy prohibit surgical intervention? Ann Surg 231:710–714, 2000.
39. Gillinov AM, Wierup PN, Blackstone EH, et al: Is repair preferable to replacement for ischemic mitral regurgitation? J Thorac Cardiovasc Surg 122:1125–1141, 2001.
40. Glasson JR, Komeda M, Daughters GT, et al: Early systolic mitral leaflet "loitering" during acute ischemic mitral regurgitation. J Thorac Cardiovasc Surg 116:193–205, 1998.
41. Glasson JR, Komeda M, Daughters GT 2nd, et al: Three-dimensional dynamics of the canine mitral annulus during ischemic mitral regurgitation. Ann Thorac Surg 62:1059–1067; discussion 1067–1068, 1996.
42. Gomez-Doblas JJ, Schor J, Vignola P, et al: Left ventricular geometry and operative mortality in patients undergoing mitral valve replacement. Clin Cardiol 24:717–722, 2001.
43. Goor DA, Mohr R, Lavee J: Preservation of the posterior leaflet during mechanical valve replacement for ischemic mitral regurgitation and complete myocardial revascularization. J Thorac Cardiovasc Surg 96:253–260, 1988.
44. Gorman JH 3rd, Jackson BM, Gorman RC, et al: Papillary muscle discoordination rather than increased annular area facilitates mitral regurgitation after acute posterior myocardial infarction. Circulation 96:II-124–II-127, 1997.
45. Gorman JH 3rd, Gorman RC, Jackson BM, et al: Distortions of the mitral valve in acute ischemic mitral regurgitation. Ann Thorac Surg 64:1026–1031, 1997.
46. Gorman JH 3rd, Gupta KB, Streicher JT, et al: Dynamic three-dimensional imaging of the mitral valve and left ventricle by rapid sonomicrometry array localization. J Thorac Cardiovasc Surg 112:712–726, 1996.
47. Gorman RC, McCaughan JS, Ratcliffe MB, et al: Pathogenesis of acute ischemic mitral regurgitation in three dimensions. J Thorac Cardiovasc Surg 109:684–693, 1995.
48. Green GR, Dagum P, Glasson JR, et al: Mitral annular dilatation and papillary muscle dislocation without mitral regurgitation in sheep. Circulation 100:II95–II102, 1999.
49. Grewal KS, Malkowski MJ, Piracha AR, et al: Effect of general anesthesia on the severity of mitral regurgitation by transesophageal echocardiography. Am J Cardiol 85:199–203, 2000.
50. Grigioni F, Enriquez-Sarano M, Zehr KJ, et al: Ischemic mitral regurgitation: long-term outcome and prognostic implications with quantitative Doppler assessment. Circulation 103:1759–1764, 2001.
51. Grossi EA, Goldberg JD, LaPietra A, et al: Ischemic mitral valve reconstruction and replacement: comparison of long-term survival and complications. J Thorac Cardiovasc Surg 122:1107–1124, 2001.
52. Harris KM, Sundt TM 3rd, Aeppli D, et al: Can late survival of patients with moderate ischemic mitral regurgitation be impacted by intervention on the valve? Ann Thorac Surg 74:1468–1475, 2002.
53. Hausmann H, Siniawski H, Hetzer R: Mitral valve reconstruction and replacement for ischemic mitral insufficiency: seven years' follow up. J Heart Valve Dis 8:536–542, 1999.
54. He GW, Hughes CF, McCaughan B, et al: Mitral valve replacement combined with coronary artery operation: determinants of early and late results. Ann Thorac Surg 51:916–922; discussion 923, 1991.
55. He S, Fontaine AA, Schwammenthal E, et al: Integrated mechanism for functional mitral regurgitation: leaflet restriction versus coapting force: in vitro studies. Circulation 96:1826–1834, 1997.
56. He S, Lemmon JD Jr, Weston MW, et al: Mitral valve compensation for annular dilatation: in vitro study into the mechanisms of functional mitral regurgitation with an adjustable annulus model. J Heart Valve Dis 8:294–302, 1999.
57. Hendren WG, Nemec JJ, Lytle BW, et al: Mitral valve repair for ischemic mitral insufficiency. Ann Thorac Surg 52:1246–1251; discussion 1251–1252, 1991.
58. Hickey MS, Smith LR, Muhlbaier LH, et al: Current prognosis of ischemic mitral regurgitation. Implications for future management. Circulation 78:I51–I59, 1998.
59. Hung J, Guerrero JL, Handschumacher MD, et al: Reverse ventricular remodeling reduces ischemic mitral regurgitation: echo-guided device application in the beating heart. Circulation 106:2594–2600, 2002.
60. Irvine T, Li XK, Sahn DJ, Kenny A: Assessment of mitral regurgitation. Heart 88:iv11–iv19, 2002.

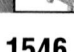

61. Kay GL, Kay JH, Zubiate P, et al: Mitral valve repair for mitral regurgitation secondary to coronary artery disease. Circulation 74:I88–I98, 1986.
62. Komeda M, Glasson JR, Bolger AF, et al: Geometric determinants of ischemic mitral regurgitation. Circulation 96:II-128–II-133, 1997.
63. Kron IL, Green GR, Cope JT: Surgical relocation of the posterior papillary muscle in chronic ischemic mitral regurgitation. Ann Thorac Surg 74:600–601, 2002.
64. Kumanohoso T, Otsuji Y, Yoshifuku S, et al: Mechanism of higher incidence of ischemic mitral regurgitation in patients with inferior myocardial infarction: quantitative analysis of left ventricular and mitral valve geometry in 103 patients with prior myocardial infarction. J Thorac Cardiovasc Surg 125:135–143, 2003.
65. Kwan J, Shiota T, Agler DA, et al: Geometric differences of the mitral apparatus between ischemic and dilated cardiomyopathy with significant mitral regurgitation: real-time three-dimensional echocardiography study. Circulation 107:1135–1140, 2003.
66. Lai DT, Tibayan FA, Myrmel T, et al: Mechanistic insights into posterior mitral leaflet interscallop malcoaptation during acute ischemic mitral regurgitation. Circulation 106:I40–I45, 2002.
67. Lamas GA, Mitchell GF, Flaker GC, et al: Clinical significance of mitral regurgitation after acute myocardial infarction. Survival and Ventricular Enlargement Investigators. Circulation 96:827–833, 1997.
68. Lehmann KG, Francis CK, Dodge HT: Mitral regurgitation in early myocardial infarction. Incidence, clinical detection, and prognostic implications. TIMI Study Group. Ann Intern Med 117:10–17, 1992.
69. Lehmann KG, Francis CK, Sheehan FH, Dodge HT: Effect of thrombolysis on acute mitral regurgitation during evolving myocardial infarction. Experience from the Thrombolysis in Myocardial Infarction (TIMI) Trial. J Am Coll Cardiol 22:714–719, 1993.
70. Levine RA, Hung J, Otsuji Y, et al: Mechanistic insights into functional mitral regurgitation. Curr Cardiol Rep 4:125–129, 2002.
71. Llaneras MR, Nance ML, Streicher JT, et al: Pathogenesis of ischemic mitral insufficiency. J Thorac Cardiovasc Surg 105:439–442; discussion 442–443, 1993.
72. Ma HH, Honma H, Munakata K, Hayakawa H: Mitral insufficiency as a complication of acute myocardial infarction and left ventricular remodeling. Jpn Circ J 61:912–920, 1997.
73. Maisel AS, Gilpin EA, Klein L, et al: The murmur of papillary muscle dysfunction in acute myocardial infarction: clinical features and prognostic implications. Am Heart J 112:705–711, 1986.
74. McCully RB, Enriquez-Sarano M, Tajik AJ, Seward JB: Overestimation of severity of ischemic/functional mitral regurgitation by color Doppler jet area. Am J Cardiol 74:790–793, 1994.
75. Menicanti L, Di Donato M, Frigiola A, et al: Ischemic mitral regurgitation: intraventricular papillary muscle imbrication without mitral ring during left ventricular restoration. J Thorac Cardiovasc Surg 123:1041–1050, 2002.
76. Messas E, Guerrero JL, Handschumacher MD, et al: Chordal cutting: a new therapeutic approach for ischemic mitral regurgitation. Circulation 104:1958–1963, 2001.
77. Messas E, Guerrero JL, Handschumacher MD, et al: Paradoxic decrease in ischemic mitral regurgitation with papillary muscle dysfunction: insights from three-dimensional and contrast echocardiography with strain rate measurement. Circulation 104:1952–1957, 2001.
78. Moainie SL, Guy TS, Gorman JH 3rd, et al: Infarct restraint attenuates remodeling and reduces chronic ischemic mitral regurgitation after postero-lateral infarction. Ann Thorac Surg 74:444–449; discussion 449, 2002.
79. Myrmel T, Lai DT, Lo S, et al: Ischemia-induced malcoaptation of scallops within the posterior mitral leaflet. J Heart Valve Dis 11:823–829, 2002.
80. Neskovic AN, Marinkovic J, Bojic M, Popovic AD: Early predictors of mitral regurgitation after acute myocardial infarction. Am J Cardiol 84:329–332[A8], 1999.
81. Otsuji Y, Handschumacher MD, Liel-Cohen N, et al: Mechanism of ischemic mitral regurgitation with segmental left ventricular dysfunction: three-dimensional echocardiographic studies in models of acute and chronic progressive regurgitation. J Am Coll Cardiol 37:641–648, 2001.
82. Otsuji Y, Kumanohoso T, Yoshifuku S, et al: Isolated annular dilation does not usually cause important functional mitral regurgitation: comparison between patients with lone atrial fibrillation and those with idiopathic or ischemic cardiomyopathy. J Am Coll Cardiol 39:1651–1656, 2002.
83. Oury JH, Cleveland JC, Duran CG, Angell WW: Ischemic mitral valve disease: classification and systemic approach to management. J Card Surg 9:262–273, 1994.
84. Pinson CW, Cobanoglu A, Metzdorff MT, et al: Late surgical results for ischemic mitral regurgitation. Role of wall motion score and severity of regurgitation. J Thorac Cardiovasc Surg 88:663–672, 1984.
85. Prifti E, Bonacchi M, Frati G, et al: Ischemic mitral valve regurgitation grade II-III: correction in patients with impaired left ventricular function undergoing simultaneous coronary revascularization. J Heart Valve Dis 10:754–762, 2001.
86. Pu M, Thomas JD, Vandervoort PM, et al: Comparison of quantitative and semiquantitative methods for assessing mitral regurgitation by transesophageal echocardiography. Am J Cardiol 87:66–70, 2001.
87. Rankin JS: Improving surgical strategies for ischemic mitral regurgitation. J Heart Valve Dis 2:533–535, 1993.
88. Rankin JS, Feneley MP, Hickey MS, et al: A clinical comparison of mitral valve repair versus valve replacement in ischemic mitral regurgitation. J Thorac Cardiovasc Surg 95:165–177, 1988.
89. Rankin JS, Livesey SA, Smith LR, et al: Trends in the surgical treatment of ischemic mitral regurgitation: effects of mitral valve repair on hospital mortality. Semin Thorac Cardiovasc Surg 1:149–163, 1989.
90. Rayhill SC, Castro LJ, Nizyporuk MA, et al: Rigid ring fixation of the mitral annulus does not impair left ventricular systolic function in the normal canine heart. Circulation 86:II26–II38, 1992.
91. Rendon F, Aramendi JI, Rodrigo D, et al: Patch enlargement of the posterior mitral leaflet in ischemic regurgitation. Asian Cardiovasc Thorac Ann 10:248–250, 2002.
92. Ruvolo G, Speziale G, Bianchini R, et al: Combined coronary bypass grafting and mitral valve surgery: Early and late results. Thorac Cardiovasc Surg 43:90–93, 1995.
93. Ryden T, Bech-Hanssen O, Brandrup-Wognsen G, et al: The importance of grade 2 ischemic mitral regurgitation in coronary artery bypass grafting. Eur J Cardiothorac Surg 20:276–281, 2001.
94. Seipelt RG, Schoendube FA, Vazquez-Jimenez JF, et al: Combined mitral valve and coronary artery surgery: ischemic versus non-ischemic mitral valve disease. Eur J Cardiothorac Surg 20:270–275, 2001.
95. Szalay ZA, Civelek A, Hohe S, et al: Mitral annuloplasty in patients with ischemic versus dilated cardiomyopathy. Eur J Cardiothorac Surg 23:567–572, 2003.
96. Szecsi J, Herijgers P, Sergeant P, et al: Mitral valve surgery combined with coronary bypass grafting: multivariate analysis of factors predicting early and late results. J Heart Valve Dis 3:236–242, 1994.
97. Tahta SA, Oury JH, Maxwell JM, et al: Outcome after mitral valve repair for functional ischemic mitral regurgitation. J Heart Valve Dis 11:11–18; discussion 18–19, 2002.

97a. Tavkoli R, Weber A, Vogt P, et al: Surgical management of acute valve regurgitation due to post-infarction papillary muscle rupture. J Heart Valve Dis 11:20–25, 2002.
98. Timek TA, Lai DT, Tibayan F, et al: Annular versus subvalvular approaches to acute ischemic mitral regurgitation. Circulation 106:127–132, 2002.
99. Timek TA, Lai DT, Tibayan F, et al: Ischemia in three left ventricular regions: Insights into the pathogenesis of acute ischemic mitral regurgitation. J Thorac Cardiovasc Surg 125:559–569, 2003.
100. Timek TA, Lai DT, Tibayan F, et al: Septal-lateral annular cinching abolishes acute ischemic mitral regurgitation. J Thorac Cardiovasc Surg 123:881–888, 2002.
101. Timek TA, Lai DT, Tibayan FA, et al: Septal-lateral annular cinching ('SLAC') reduces mitral annular size without perturbing normal annular dynamics. J Heart Valve Dis 11:2–9, 2002.
102. Timek TA, Nielsen SL, Green GR, et al: Influence of anterior mitral leaflet second-order chordae on leaflet dynamics and valve competence. Ann Thorac Surg 72:535–540; discussion 541, 2001.
103. Tolis GA Jr, Korkolis DP, Kopf GS, Elefteriades JA: Revascularization alone (without mitral valve repair) suffices in patients with advanced ischemic cardiomyopathy and mild-to-moderate mitral regurgitation. Ann Thorac Surg 74:1476–1480; discussion 1480–1481, 2002.
104. Umana JP, Salehizadeh B, DeRose JJ Jr, et al: "Bow-tie" mitral valve repair: an adjuvant technique for ischemic mitral regurgitation. Ann Thorac Surg 66:1640–1646, 1998.
105. Van Dantzig JM, Delemarre BJ, Koster RW, et al: Pathogenesis of mitral regurgitation in acute myocardial infarction: importance of changes in left ventricular shape and regional function. Am Heart J 131:865–871, 1996.
106. Vicente Vera T, Valdes Chavarri M, Garcia Alberola A, et al: [Mitral valve insufficiency in acute myocardial infarction. Assessment with pulsed and coded Doppler color]. Arch Inst Cardiol Mex 61:117–121, 1991.
107. von Oppell UO, Stemmet F, Brink J, et al: Ischemic mitral valve repair surgery. J Heart Valve Dis 9:64–73; discussion 73–74, 2000.
108. Wei JY, Hutchins GM, Bulkley BH; Papillary muscle rupture in fatal acute myocardial infarction: a potentially treatable form of cardiogenic shock. Ann Int Med 90:149–152, 1979.
109. Yiu SF, Enriquez-Sarano M, Tribouilloy C, et al: Determinants of the degree of functional mitral regurgitation in patients with systolic left ventricular dysfunction: a quantitative clinical study. Circulation 102:1400–1406, 2000.

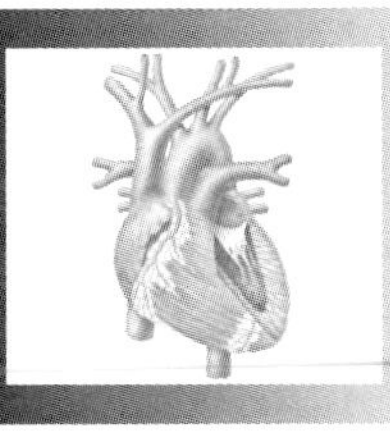

Postinfarction Ventricular Septal Defect

Abeel A. Mangi, Arvind K. Agnihotri, and David F. Torchiana

CHAPTER 87

INTRODUCTION

Disruption of the ventricular septum after myocardial infarction is an infrequent event. The resulting clinical syndrome can range from an asymptomatic murmur to an extensive left to right intracardiac shunt with resulting heart failure and shock. The first approaches to surgical management emphasized delayed repair allowing a period of time for fibrosis to occur so that tissue quality at the defect margins was more substantial.[19,29] Modern approaches recognize that potentially salvageable patients will deteriorate during this period of delay. As a result, early surgical intervention is now the accepted treatment.[15]

BACKGROUND

Historical Perspective

Postinfarction ventricular septal defect (VSD) was first recognized by Latham at autopsy in 1845.[51] The first antemortem diagnosis was made in 1923.[9] In 1956, Cooley accomplished the first successful surgical repair in a patient who had survived several weeks after septal perforation.[12] Most patients in the early era were brought to operation a month or longer after surviving acute infarction, in the belief that organization of the tissues surrounding the defect allowed a more secure closure.[19,29] Subsequently, improvements in myocardial protection, the design and refinement of surgical techniques, improved prosthetic materials, and the widespread use of cardiac ultrasound to permit the earlier diagnosis of VSD have all contributed to making earlier successful repair of this entity a possibility.[74]

Incidence and Demographics

Postinfarction VSD complicates 1–2% of myocardial infarctions, but accounts for 5% of deaths after myocardial infarction.[42,54] The incidence appears to be declining because of aggressive pharmacological and interventional management of acute myocardial infarction and better treatment of postinfarction hypertension.[16] Postinfarction VSDs occur more frequently in males (male to female ratio is 3:2) reflecting the higher incidence of coronary artery disease in the male population. The average age is 62 years (range 44–81 years). Septal rupture occurs most often after the first acute myocardial infarction.[67]

Etiology and Pathogenesis

Angiographic evaluation of patients with postinfarction VSD most often reveals a completely occluded culprit coronary artery.[12] Nearly two thirds of patients have single-vessel disease.[41] There is usually somewhat less extensive disease in other vessels and less collateralization.[58] Postinfarction VSDs are located most commonly (~60% of cases) in the anteroapical septum as a result of full-thickness anterior infarction secondary to occlusion of the left anterior descending artery. Twenty to 40% of patients with postinfarction VSD have rupture of the posterior septum because of inferoseptal infarction secondary to occlusion of a dominant right or a dominant circumflex coronary artery (Figure 87-1).[77] Simple rupture consisting of a direct through and through defect tends to be more common and is usually located anteriorly. Complex rupture with a more serpiginous tract is less common and is usually located inferiorly. Although most patients will develop a single VSD, 5–11% of patients may have multiple septal defects.

The myocardial infarction that sets the backdrop for a postinfarction VSD tends to be extensive and has been reported to involve 26% of the free wall on average when compared to only 15% in noncomplicated acute myocardial infarctions.[42] Postinfarction VSD usually develops 2–4 days after acute myocardial infarction but has been reported as soon as a few hours after acute myocardial infarction or up to 2 weeks later.[42,47,70] This time course correlates with histological findings that show extensive distribution of necrotic myocardium at this time, with relatively sparse onset of vasculogenesis, angiogenesis, or formation of fibrous connective tissue.[55,72] It has been hypothesized that "slippage" of myocytes during infarct expansion may allow blood to dissect through the necrotic myocardium from where it can enter the right ventricle (or the pericardial space in the setting of rupture of the free wall).[23,80] Similarly, autodigestion of necrotic myocardium may allow fissures to form through which blood can subsequently dissect.[6]

Pathophysiology

The primary determinant of outcome after postinfarction rupture of the ventricular septum is the development of heart failure (left, right, or biventricular), which is a function of both the size of the defect and the magnitude of the myocardial infarction. Left-sided heart failure tends to predominate in anterior VSDs, and right-sided failure predominates in posterior VSDs.[25,28,33] The extent of heart failure often cannot be explained solely by postinfarction failure of the ventricle.[64] With the opening of a defect in the ventricular septum, a proportion of each left ventricular ejection is diverted from the systemic circulation across the septum into the right ventricle, thereby compromising both forward systemic cardiac output and overloading the pulmonary circulation. The resulting cardiogenic shock can lead to end-organ malperfusion and organ failure, which may be irreversible and fatal. In addition, the normally compliant right ventricle may demonstrate severe diastolic failure after a prolonged left-to-right shunt. The resulting escalation in right ventricular diastolic pressures can ultimately result in flow reversal across the septum when right ventricular end-diastolic pressures exceed left ventricular end-diastolic pressures[4] and compound the situation further with systemic hypoxia.

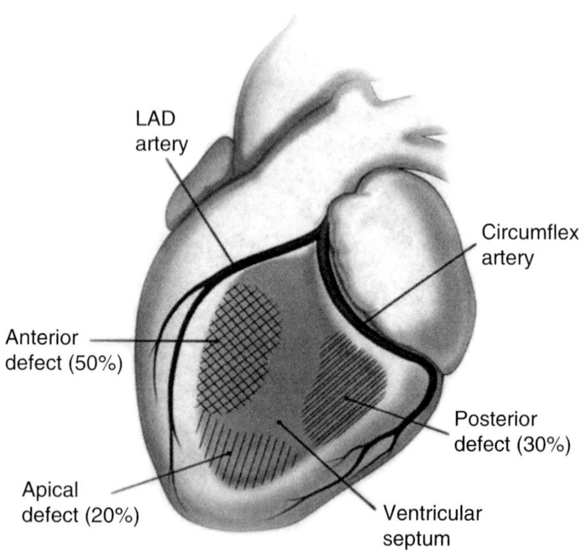

Figure 87–1 Schematic diagram depicting distribution of postinfarction VSDs.

Natural History

One quarter of patients with postinfarction VSD die within 24 h without surgical intervention. Half succumb to their illness within the first week, nearly two thirds die within 2 weeks, three quarters die within a month, and only 7% survive longer than 1 year.[7,61,67] These data have been confirmed in the recent SHOCK (SHould we emergently revascularize Occluded Coronaries in cardiogenic shocK) Multi-Center Trial in which subgroup analysis of patients suffering postinfarction VSD was performed. A total of 55 patients with postinfarction VSD were enrolled in the study a median of 16 h after infarction and went into shock 7.3 h thereafter. Of the 24 patients managed medically, only one survived (survival rate 4%). Thirty-one patients underwent operation to repair the VSD, of whom 21 underwent concomitant coronary artery bypass grafting. Of these, only six survived (survival rate 19%). The difference between the groups was statistically significant.[57]

The historic practice of waiting weeks after postinfarction rupture of the ventricular septum selected out patients with lesser pathology and a relatively mild hemodynamic insult.[17,28,45] It is clear that attempting to defer early operation in the hopes of maintaining hemodynamic stability deprives many patients of a chance of a successful outcome before irreversible end-organ damage supervenes.[8,39]

CLINICAL PRESENTATION, PREOPERATIVE MANAGEMENT, RISK STRATIFICATION

Presentation

Typically patients with postinfarction VSD will present several days after a myocardial infarction with a harsh new holosystolic murmur that may radiate to the axilla.[70] In more than half of patients this is associated with recurrent chest pain.[42] Clinical signs are generally those of right-sided heart failure, and pulmonary edema is rare. The electrocardiographic findings in these patients are the changes seen in antecedent anterior, septal, inferior, or posterior infarction. Up to one third of patients may develop transient atrioventricular conduction block that precedes rupture. Chest roentgenogram is generally nonspecific. Unfortunately, there is no reliable predictor of impending rupture.

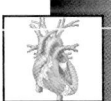

This clinical syndrome may resemble acute mitral regurgitation secondary to rupture of a papillary muscle. In fact, both entities may coexist, and sometimes can be distinguished only by imaging techniques. On physical examination, the murmur associated with postinfarction VSD is more prominent at the left lateral sternal border, is loud, and is associated with a thrill in over half of patients. Additionally, septal rupture is more commonly associated with anterior infarcts and conduction anomalies, whereas papillary muscle rupture is usually associated with posterior infarction and no conduction anomalies. If the patient is deemed salvageable, immediate placement of intraaortic balloon pump and early operation are the management strategy of choice.

Diagnosis

The classic technique for distinguishing between acute papillary muscle rupture and postinfarction VSD has been right heart catheterization, during which a greater than 9% step-up in the oxygen saturation between the right atrium and pulmonary artery is diagnostic of VSD in the appropriate clinical setting.[28] Additional findings such as elevated pulmonary-to-systemic flow ratios ($\dot{Q}_p/\dot{Q}_s$), which can range from 1.4:1 to 8:1, also verify the presence of the VSD and roughly correlate with size.[38] Neither of these techniques accurately localizes the defect. Color flow Doppler echocardiography can show the size and location of the defect, determine ventricular function, assess pulmonary artery and right ventricular pressures, and exclude concomitant mitral valve disease with sensitivity and specificity approaching 100%.[10,34,37,75]

Indications for Operation and Preoperative Management

As the natural history of untreated postinfarction VSD is dismal, the diagnosis of this entity suffices as an indication for operation in and of itself.[39] Patients in cardiogenic shock represent a surgical emergency. Occasionally, patients will be encountered who are already in established multisystem organ failure. This group of patients is unlikely to survive emergent repair and may benefit from a mechanical bridge (e.g., intraaortic balloon counterpulsation or ventricular assist device) for salvage prior to corrective operation. Patients who are in an intermediate status between shock and stable condition need to be operated on within 12–24 h after appropriate preoperative evaluations are completed. A small percentage of patients (<5%) who are completely stable with no clinical compromise can undergo repair on a semielective basis.

Preoperative management is directed toward maintaining hemodynamic stability and preventing end-organ damage. Specifically, therapy should be targeted toward reducing systemic vascular resistance (thereby reducing left to right shunting), maintaining cardiac output and peripheral perfusion, and maintaining or improving coronary blood flow. All three of these objectives can be accomplished by intraaortic balloon counterpulsation[36,59,68] as well as with directed pharmacological therapy.

Predictors of Risk

Patients with postinfarction VSD are a heterogeneous group in which both extremes of risk (that is, very low risk as well as very high risk) are possible. For the nonemergent, stable patients, excellent results can be achieved, probability of survival to discharge from the hospital is high, and long-term survival is comparable to that in common cardiac operations. On the other hand, patients in extremis tend to have dismal outcomes (Table 87-1).

In various studies, clinical variables have been used to identify the high-risk patient. In several studies, use of intraaortic balloon pump was correlated with increased early mortality,[2] presumably as a marker for disease severity. Other groups have demonstrated that posterior location of the septal rupture is associated with an increased operative mortality,[4,14,28,60] which may be due to a technically more difficult repair, to the increased risk of mitral regurgitation, and to right ventricular (RV) failure associated with an RV infarction. Proximal VSDs (closer to the atrioventricular

Table 87–1

Preoperative Predictors of Early and Late Death in Patients Undergoing Surgical Repair of Postinfarction VSD

Variable	*Predictor of early death*	*Predictor of late death*
Need for preoperative catecholamines	p = .001	p = NS
Emergent operation	p <.0001	p = NS
Anterior ventricular septal defect	p = .04	p = NS
Age > 65 years	p = .009	p = NS
Right heart failure	p = .01	p = .005
Elevation in blood urea nitrogen	p = .02	p = NS
Elevation of serum creatinine	p = NS	p <.05
Previous myocardial infarction	p = NS	p <.05
Presence of left main coronary disease	p = NS	p <.05

groove) have also been shown to strongly predict early mortality, presumably because they are associated with the largest infarctions.[13]

OPERATIVE MANAGEMENT

General Principles

Cardiopulmonary bypass is established with bicaval venous drainage and cannulation of the ascending aorta. The patient is cooled and cardiac standstill achieved with blood cardioplegia via the antegrade and retrograde routes. A variety of alternative strategies for myocardial protection are practiced at Massachusetts General Hospital (MGH), including continuous warm blood cardioplegia, fibrillatory arrest, and cold blood cardioplegia.[18,22,40,79] If myocardial revascularization is to be performed, this is done prior to opening the ventricle in order to optimize myocardial protection. The general principles of this operation include meticulous attention to myocardial protection, transinfarct approach to the VSD, thorough trimming of the left ventricular margins of the defect, conservative trimming of the right ventricular margin, close inspection of the papillary muscles and mitral apparatus, tension-free repair, placement of the patch on the endocardial surface, and buttressing the repair with Teflon felt to prevent sutures from cutting through the friable muscle.

Infarctectomy

Apical Amputation

The technique of apical amputation was first described by Daggett.[15] An incision is made through the infarcted apex of the left ventricle. Debridement of the necrotic myocardium back to healthy muscle results in amputation of the apex of the heart including the left ventricle, right ventricle, and septum. The remaining apical portions are then reapproximated to the apical septum using a row of interrupted mattress sutures of 0-Tevdek passed sequentially through a buttressing strip of Teflon felt, the left ventricular wall, a second strip of felt, the septum, a third strip of felt, the right ventricular wall, and a fourth strip of felt. After all these sutures have been tied, the closure is reinforced with an additional running suture.

Anterior Septal Rupture

These defects are approached through a left ventriculotomy through the infarct. If the defect is small, it can be closed by plication with primary closure.[71] Most defects are larger and require closure with a Dacron prosthetic patch after debridement of necrotic myocardium. This operation is performed by placing a series of pledgeted interrupted mattress sutures around the perimeter of the defect. Sutures are passed through the septum from right to left along the posterior rim and are passed from the epicardium to endocardium along the anterior rim. Once all the sutures are laid in, the patch is inserted and all sutures are pledgeted again and then tied. The edges of the ventriculotomy are then reapproximated in a double layer closure that is buttressed with Teflon felt or glutaraldehyde-preserved bovine pericardium (Figure 87-2).

Posterior/Inferior Septal Rupture

Posterior VSD poses the greatest technical challenge (Figure 87-3). Simple plication has an extremely high failure rate and is often complicated by reopening of the defect or by catastrophic disruption of the infarctectomy closure. Use of the following technique has been associated with improved operative results. After the establishment of cardiopulmonary bypass the left heart is vented via the right superior pulmonary vein. The heart is then delivered from the pericardial well as for bypass to the posterior descending coronary artery. The infarct may include both ventricles or may be limited to the left ventricle only. The left ventricle is opened in standard fashion and infarctectomy is performed. The mitral apparatus is inspected and mitral valve replacement is performed only in the setting of frank papillary muscle infarct. This is performed through a separate left atriotomy. The left ventricle needs to be aggressively debrided, but right ventricular debridement can be limited to only as much tissue as is needed to visualize the VSD. If the posterior septum has simply separated from the free wall, it can be reapproximated primarily in a double-layered buttressed closure. Larger defects require patch closure as described above. The only difference is that sutures are placed from the right side of the septum and from the epicardial side of the right ventricular free wall. The most important aspect of this operation is to perform a separate patch closure of the infarctectomy as primary closure of this large tissue defect with friable edges under tension is what has historically resulted in catastrophic disruption. We use a Hemashield Dacron graft for this purpose and pass sutures through the patch, which is seated on the epicardial surface of the heart and then through the margin of the infarctectomy, from the endocardium to epicardium. Use of an appropriately sized patch can result in restoration of normal ventricular geometry.

Infarct Exclusion with Endocardial Patch Repair

This technique emphasizes the importance of restoring normal ventricular geometry as an attempt to preserve or restore ventricular function.[3,22,40,71,78] The operative strategy is an extrapolation of Dor's technique of ventricular endoaneurysmorrhaphy[30] and involves intracavitary placement of an endocardial patch to exclude both the septal defect as well as the infarcted myocardium from the high-pressure zone of the ventricle, while maintaining ventricular geometry, which theoretically enhances ventricular function. Other theoretical benefits of this approach include avoiding resection of myocardium, which may further compromise ventricular function, and avoiding a suture line in friable muscle, which may diminish postoperative bleeding and disruption of the repair. David et al[25] have pioneered this technique, which involves exposing the interventricular septum via a left ventriculotomy through the infarcted anterior wall 1–2 cm from the left anterior descending coronary artery. Stay sutures are placed in the ventricular wall to aid in exposure of the septal defect. These authors have used a glutaraldehye-fixed bovine pericardial patch for the repair.

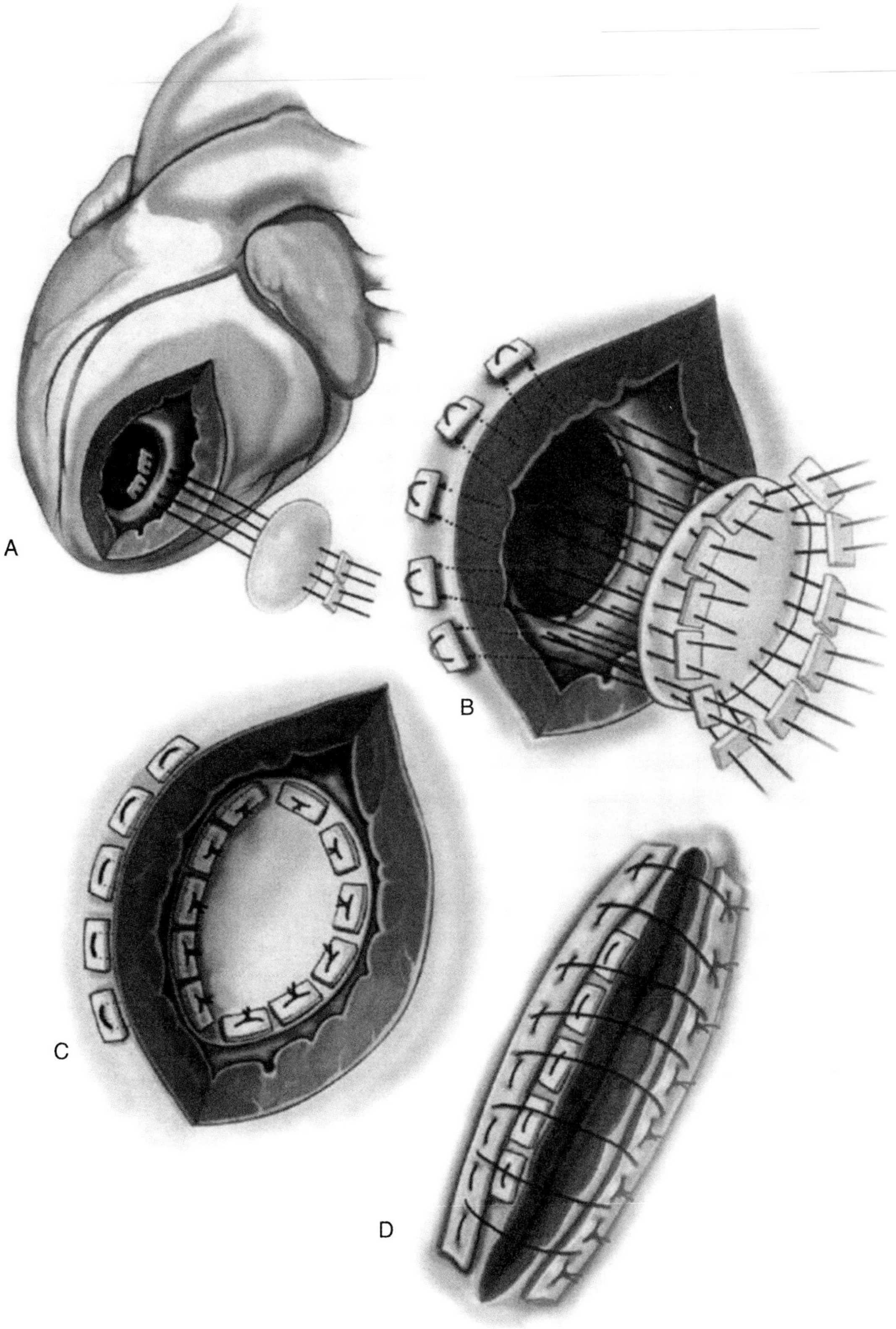

Figure 87–2 (A–D) Technique of repair of anterior postinfarction VSD by infarctectomy and patch repair.

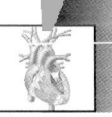

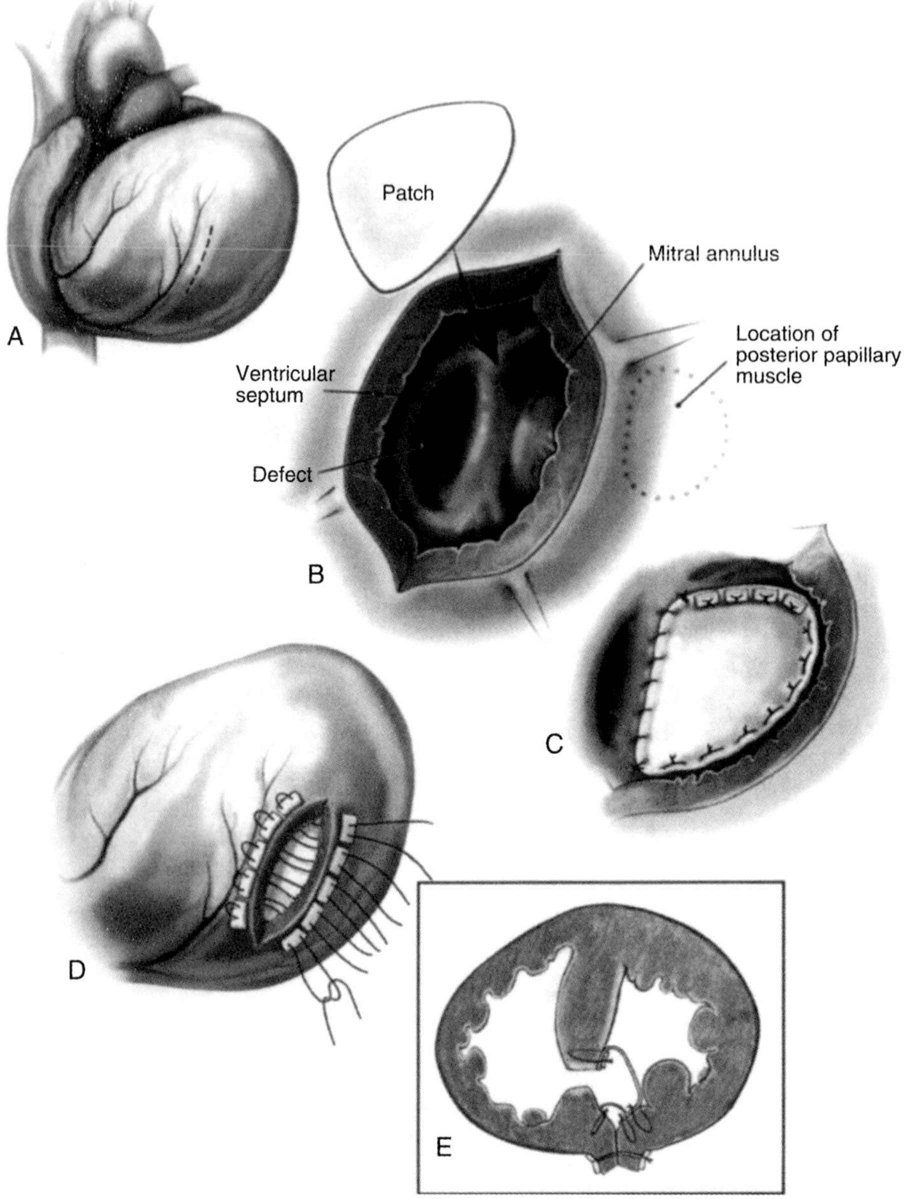

Figure 87–3 (A–E) Technique of repair of posterior postinfarction VSD by infarctectomy and patch repair.

This is tailored to the endocardial shape of the ventricular infarction (generally about 4 × 6 cm in size) and is then sutured to healthy muscle (on the endocardial surface) surrounding the septal defect with a continuous 3–0 polypropylene suture. The repair is then carried onto the noninfarcted endocardium of the anterolateral ventricular wall with stitches that are approximately 5–7 mm deep and 4–5 mm apart. The ventriculotomy is then closed over the patch in two layers and is buttressed with two strips of glutaraldehyde-fixed bovine pericardium. In case of a posterior septal defect, exposure is achieved via a posterior ventriculotomy with the heart elevated as for bypass grafting to the posterior descending artery. The repair commences with anchoring of the patch to the fibrous annulus of the mitral valve with a 3–0 continuous polypropylene suture starting at a point corresponding to the posteromedial papillary muscle and moving medially toward the septum until the noninfarcted endocardium is reached. The stitch is then transitioned onto the septal endocardium using the same technique as described above. In this area of the repair, the suture should be reinforced with interrupted, pledgeted sutures. The lateral edge of the patch is sutured to the posterior left ventricle along a line corresponding to the medial margin of the base of the posteromedial papillary muscle. These stitches again need to be full-thickness and buttressed with epicardial bovine pericardium or Teflon felt. Again, the ventriculotomy is closed in two layers of full-thickness sutures buttressed with bovine pericardium or Teflon felt.

Intraoperative Management

Coronary Artery Disease

The value of preoperative coronary artery angiography and coronary revascularization is controversial in this population.

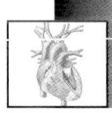

As many of these patients have multivessel coronary disease, bypassing significantly diseased vessels may increase both early and long-term survival when compared with patients not undergoing simultaneous bypass.* Our approach is to perform catheterization when the clinical scenario permits and to perform concomitant revascularization when indicated. The arguments against simultaneous revascularization are that it provides no additional benefit[44,56] and that it subjects patients to preoperative left heart catheterization, a time-consuming and potentially dangerous procedure. Other groups have proposed selective left heart catheterization and revascularization,[26,74] avoiding it in patients in whom a postinfarction VSD is thought to be the result of their first infarction, provided there is no history of angina and no electrocardiographic evidence of previous or ongoing ischemia in another territory.

Weaning from Cardiopulmonary Bypass

We have found routine intraoperative use of a transesophageal echocardiogram to be invaluable in assessing ventricular function, dimensions, residual shunt, and mitral regurgitation when weaning from bypass. For left heart dysfunction, we favor the use of intraaortic balloon counterpulsation and the use of a class of phosphodiesterase inhibitors such as milrinone in the postoperative setting. Strategies to ameliorate right heart failure aim to limit right ventricular afterload while maintaining systemic blood pressure. This can be achieved by right-sided administration of prostaglandin E1 (0.5–2.0 μg/min) with left-sided administration (via left atrial line) of norepinephrine.[21] Finally, inhaled nitric oxide (20–80 ppm) selectively dilates the pulmonary circuit and may be efficacious in ameliorating right heart failure.[65] Inability to separate from bypass is unusual if the repair has been successful. In the setting of inability to wean from cardiopulmonary bypass, institution of mechanical assist (left ventricular assist device, right ventricular assist device, or extracorporeal membrane oxygenation) may be considered.

Bleeding

Our group generally uses antifibrinolytic therapy with either aprotinin or ε-aminocaproic acid before commencing cardiopulmonary bypass in repair of postinfarction VSD. Other maneuvers to avoid postpump suture line bleeding include application of fibrin sealants to the proposed suture line prior to repair[69] or the use of biological glues following surgical repair.[32] As a last resort, Baldwin and Cooley[5] have employed placement of a left ventricular assist device solely as an adjunct to the repair of friable or damaged myocardium to decrease left ventricular distention, thereby controlling bleeding.

Delayed Repair

The occasional patient will present with evidence of severe end-organ dysfunction. As we have discussed above, the risk of repair may be prohibitive in these patients, and consideration should be given to delayed repair. Placement of a ventricular assist device for a defined period of time has the theoretical advantage of allowing reversal of end-organ dysfunction, allowing maturation of the infarct leading to firmer tissue that could make the closure less prone to technical failure, and permitting recovery of the stunned and energy-depleted myocardium. In our limited experience, this strategy has promise and merits further evaluation. Biventricular support is necessary if institution of left ventricular support results in right-to-left shunting.[49] An alternative in patients considered too sick to tolerate operation is placement of a temporary percutaneous closure device across the ventricular defect. Although, catheter-based approaches appear to be establishing a niche in the management of patients with recurrent or residual defects (the setting in which we have employed them),[8,43] it is unclear whether they have a role as primary therapy. In the acute setting, Landzberg and Lock[50] have reported that deployment of the CardioSEAL device failed in four out of seven patients. As device development continues to evolve, it may have a role as a bridge to definitive repair in the patient too unwell to tolerate operation.

*References 3, 17, 25, 28, 35, 48.

Principles of Postoperative Management

The postoperative care of these patients is similar to that of other patients undergoing extensive intracardiac operations. Early postoperative diuresis is important to decrease the arterial–alveolar gradient induced by the increased extravascular pulmonary fluid associated with cardiopulmonary bypass. A continuous furosemide drip may sometimes be needed. If the patient suffers from renal dysfunction, we favor early institution of continuous venovenous hemofiltration (CVVH). Intractable postoperative ventricular arrhythmias are treated with intravenous amiodarone.[66]

OUTCOMES

Operative Mortality

Operative mortality (death prior to discharge or within 30 days of operation) ranges from 30% to 50% (Table 87-1). Of note, David and colleagues[25] reported outstanding results with the infarct exclusion technique, having only a 19% early mortality. Regardless of technique, the most common cause of death following repair of a postinfarction VSD is low cardiac output (52%). Technical failures such as recurrent or residual VSD are the second most common causes of death (22%). Other causes of death include sepsis (17%), recurrent infarction (9%), cerebrovascular complications (4%), and intractable ventricular arrhythmias.

Long-Term Results

Most series report 5-year actuarial survival between 40% and 60% (Table 87-2). In the MGH experience, hospital survivors demonstrated 1-, 5-, and 10-year survivals of 91, 70, and 37%, respectively (Figure 87-4); 75% reported New York Heart Association class I functional status and 12.5% reported class II functional status.[16] These favorable results have also been reported by other groups. Gaudiani et al reported an 88% 5-year survival rate with 74% survivors in NYHA functional class I.[35] David et al reported a 66% 6-year survival,[25] and Davies et al reported a 5-year survival rate of 69%.[26]

Table 87–2

Summary of Recent Clinical Experience with Surgical Repair of Postinfarction VSD[a]

Institution	*City*	*Year*	*N*	*Hospital mortality*	*5-year survival*
Massachusetts General Hospital[1]	Boston	2002	114	37%	45%
University Hospital[63]	Zurich	2000	54	26%	52%[b]
Glenfield General Hospital[27]	Leicester	2000	117	37% (30 day)	46%
The Toronto Hospital[24]	Toronto	1998	52	19%	65%[b]
Southhampton General[20]	Southampton	1998	179	27%	49%
MidAmerica Heart Institute[46]	Kansas City	1997	76	41%	41%
Green Lane Hospital[31]	Auckland	1995	35	31% (30 day)	60%[b]
Hospital Cardiologique du Haut-Lévèque[28]	Bordeaux	1991	62	38%	44%
CHU Henri Mondor[53]	Créteil	1991	66	45%	44%

[a]Series with less than 25 patients and no 5-year follow-up were excluded from the table.
[b]Value estimated from published graphic or tabular data.

Recurrent Septal Defects

Ten percent to 25% of patients may develop a recurrent or residual VSD,[6] which may be due to reopening of a closed defect, the presence of an overlooked defect, or the development of a new defect in the early postoperative period. Small defects ($\dot{Q}_P:\dot{Q}_S < 2.0$) that occur as a result of peripatch leaks are usually asymptomatic and can be controlled with diuretic therapy. Larger defects ($\dot{Q}_P:\dot{Q}_S > 2.0$) or those causing symptoms or heart failure should be closed. These attempts may be made first in the catheterization laboratory.

SUMMARY

Although the prevalence of postinfarction VSDs had decreased with modern management of acute myocardial infarction, patients who do come to surgical attention are

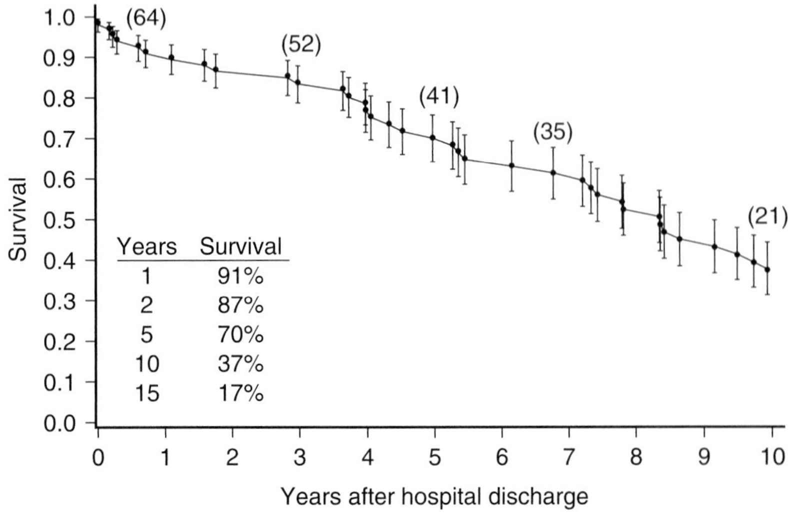

Figure 87–4 Survival after hospital discharge for repair of postinfarction VSD: the MGH experience.

older and sicker and have complex comorbidities. Surgery is complex and relatively infrequent and although the results are far better than no treatment at all, morbidity and mortality rates remain high. The use of predictive statistical models can assist us further in helping determine which patients should come to operation early, which patients would be better off temporized with the use of an assist device, and which patients should be turned down or treated percutaneously.

REFERENCES

1. Agnihotri AK, Madsen J, Daggett WM: Unpublished data from Massachusetts General Hospital experience.
2. Agnihotri AK, Daggett WM, Torchiana DF, et al: Surgical repair of postinfarction VSD: an analysis of risk. In preparation.
3. Alvarez JM, Brady PW, Ross DE: Technical improvements in the repair of acute postinfarction ventricular septal rupture. J Cardiac Surg 7:198, 1992.
4. Anderson DR, Adams S, Bhat A, Pepper JR: Postinfarction VSD: the importance of site of infarction and cardiogenic shock on outcome. Eur J Cardiothorac Surg 3:554, 1989.
5. Baldwin RT, Cooley DA: Mechanical support for intraventricular decompression in repair of left ventricular disruption. Ann Thorac Surg 54:176, 1992.
6. Beranek JT: Hyaline degeneration of the myocardium is implicated in the pathogenesis of postinarction heart rupture. Cor Notes 9:3, 1994.
7. Berger TJ, Blackstone EH, Kirklin JW: Postinfarction VSD. In Barratt-Boyes BG, Kirklin JW, editors: Cardiac Surgery. New York: Churchill Livingstone, 1993.
8. Blanche C, Khan SS, Matloff MJ, et al: Results of early repair of VSD after an acute myocardial infarction. J Thorac Cardiovasc Surg 104:961, 1992.
9. Brunn F: Diagnostik der erworbenen rupture der kammerscheidewand des herzens. Wien Arch Inn Med 53: 140, 1934.
10. Buckley MJ, Mudth ED, Daggett WM, et al: Surgical therapy for early complications of myocardial infarction. Surgery 70: 814, 1971.
11. Cooley DA: Postinfarction ventricular septal rupture. Sem Thorac Cardiovasc Surg 10(2):100, 1998.
12. Cooley DA, Belmonte BA, Zeis LB, Schnur S: Surgical repair of ruptured interventricular septum following acute myocardial infarction. Surgery 41:930, 1957.
13. Cox FF, Morshuis WJ, Plokker HWT, et al: Early mortality after surgical repair of post-infarction ventricular septal rupture: importance of rupture location. Ann Thorac Surg 61(6):1752–1757, 1996.
14. Cummings RG, Reimer KA, Catliff R, et al: Quantitative analysis of right and left ventricular infarction in the presence of postinfarction VSD. Circulation 77:33, 1988.
15. Daggett WM: Postinfarction VSD repair: retrospective thoughts and historical perspective. Ann Thorac Surg 50:1006, 1990.
16. Daggett WM, Buckley MJ, Akins CW, et al: Improved results of surgical management of postinfarction VSD. Ann Surg 196: 269, 1982.
17. Daggett WM, Guyton RA, Nundth ED, et al: Surgery for post-myocardial infarct VSDs. Ann Surg 186:260, 1977.
18. Daggett WM, Randolph JD, Jacobs ML, et al: The superiority of cold oxygenated dilute blood cardioplegia. Ann Thorac Surg 43:397, 1987.
19. Daicoff AR, Rhodes ML: Surgical repair of ventricular septal rupture and ventricular aneurysms. JAMA 203:457, 1968.
20. Dalrymple-Hay MJR, Monro JL, Livesey SA, Lamb RK: Postinfarction ventricular septal rupture: The Wessex Experience. Sem Thorac Cardiovasc Surg 10(2):111–116, 1998.
21. D'Ambra MN, LaRaia PJ, Philbin DM, et al: Prostaglandin E_1: A new therapy for refractory right heart failure and pulmonary hypertension after mitral valve replacement. J Thorac Cardiovasc Surg 89:567, 1985.
22. David TE: Surgical treatment of postinfarction ventricular septal rupture. Australasian J Card Thorac Surg 1:7, 1991.
23. David TE: Surgery for postinfarction VSDs. In David TE, editor: Mechanical Complications of Myocardial Infarction. Austin: R.G. Landes Company, 1993.
24. David TE, Armstrong S: Surgical repair of postinfarction VSD by infarct exclusion. Sem Thorac Cardiovasc Surg 10(2): 105–110, 1998.
25. David TE, Dale L, Sun Z: Postinfarction ventricular septal rupture: repair by endocardial patch with infarct exclusion. J Thorac Cardiovasc Surg 110:1315, 1995.
26. Davies RH, Dawkins KD, Skillington PD, et al: Late functional results after surgical closure of acquired VSD. J Thorac Cardiovasc Surg 106:592, 1992.
27. Deja MA, Szostek J, Widenka K, et al: Post infrarction VSD—can we do better? Eur J Cardiothorac Surg 18:194–201, 2000.
28. Deville C, Fontan F, Chevalier JM, et al: Surgery of postinfarction VSD: risk factors for hospital death and long-term results. Eur J Cardiothorac Surg 5:167, 1991.
29. Dobell ARC, Scott HJ, Cronin RFP, Reid EAS: Surgical closure of interventricular septal perforation complicating acute myocardial infarction. J Thorac Cardiovasc Surg 43:803, 1962.
30. Dor V, Saab M, Coste P, et al: Left ventricular aneurysm: a new surgical approach. Thorac Cardiovasc Surg 37:11, 1989.
31. Ellis CJ, Parkinson GF, Jaffe WM, et al: Good long-term outcome following surgical repair of post-infarction VSD. Aust NZ J Med 25:330–336, 1995.
32. Fabiani J-N, Jebara VA, Deloche A, et al: Use of surgical glue without replacement in the treatment of type A aortic dissection. Circulation 80:264, 1989.
33. Fanapazir L, Bray CL, Dark JF: Right ventricular dysfunction and surgical outcome in postinfarction VSD. Eur J Cardiothorac Surg 4:155, 1983.
34. Fortin DF, Sheikh KH, Kisslo J: The utility of echocardiography in the diagnostic strategy of postinfarction ventricular septal rupture: a comparison of two-dimensional versus Doppler color flow imaging. Am Heart J 121:25, 1991.
35. Gaudiani VA, Miller DC, Oyer PE, et al: Post-infarction VSD: an argument for early operation. Surgery 89:48, 1981.
36. Gold HK, Leinbach RC, Sanders CA, et al: Intra-aortic balloon pumping for VSD complicating acute myocardial infarction. Circulation 47:1191, 1973.
37. Harrison MR, MacPhail B, Gurley JC, et al: Usefulness of color Doppler flow imaging to distinguish VSD from acute mitral regurgitation complicating acute myocardial infarction. Am J Cardiol 64:697, 1989.
38. Heiffila J, Kareojosa M: Ruptured interventricular septum complicating acute myocardial infarction. Chest 66:675, 1974.
39. Heitmiller R, Jacobs ML, Daggett WM: Surgical management of postinfarction ventricular septal rupture. Ann Thorac Surg 41:683, 1986.
40. Hendren WG, O'Keefe DD, Geffin GA, et al: Maximal oxygenation of dilute blood cardioplegia solution. Ann Thorac Surg 58:1558, 1994.
41. Hill JD, Lary D, Keith WJ, Gerbode F: Acquired VSDs: evolution of an operation, surgical technique and results. J Thorac Cardiovasc Surg 70:440, 1975.
42. Hutchins GM: Rupture of the interventricular septum complicating myocardial infarction: pathologic analysis of 10 patients with clinically diagnosed perforation. Am Heart J 97:165, 1979.
43. Jones MT, Schofield PM, Dark JF: Surgical repair of acquired VSD: determinants of early and late outcome. J Thorac Cardiovasc Surg 93:680, 1987.

44. Kaplan MA, Harris CN, Kay JH, et al: Postinfarctional septal rupture: clinical approach and surgical results. Chest 69:734, 1976.
45. Kay HRL: In discussion of Daggett WM: surgical management of VSDs complicating myocardial infarction. World J Surg 2: 753, 1978.
46. Killen DA, Piehler JM, Borkon AM, et al: Early repair of postinfarction ventricular septal rupture. Ann Thorac Surg 63: 138–142, 1997.
47. Kitamura S, Mendez A, Kay JH: VSD following myocardial infarction: experience with repair through a left ventriculotomy and review of the literature. J Thorac Cardiovasc Surg 61:186, 1971.
48. Komeda M, Fremes SE, David TE: Surgical repair of the postinfarction VSD. Circulation 82(Suppl. 4):243, 1990.
49. Kshettry V, Salerno C, Bank A: Risk of left ventricular assist device as a bridge to heart transplant following postinfarction ventricular septal rupture. J Cardiac Surg 12:93–97, 1997.
50. Landzberg MJ, Lock JE: Transcatheter management of ventricular septal rupture after myocardial infarction. Sem Thorac Cardiovasc Surg 10:128–132, 1998.
51. Latham PM: Lectures on Subjects Connected with Clinical Medicine Comprising Diseases of the Heart. London: Longman Rees, 1845.
52. Lock JE, Block PC, McKay RG, et al: Transcatheter closure of VSDs. Circulation 78:361, 1988.
53. Loisance DY, Lordex JM, Deluze PH, et al: Acute postinfarction septal rupture: long-term results. Ann Thorac Surg 52:474–478, 1991.
54. Lundeberg S, Sodestrom J: Perforation of the interventricular septum in myocardial infarction: a study based on autopsy material. Acta Med Scand 172:413, 1962.
55. Mallory GK, White PD, Salcedo-Salgar J: The speed of healing of myocardial infarction: a study of the pathologic anatomy in seventy cases. Am Heart J 18:647, 1939.
56. Matsui K, Kay JH, Mendez M, et al: Ventricular septal rupture secondary to myocardial infarction: clinical approach and surgical results. JAMA 245:1537, 1981.
57. Menon V, Webb J, Hillis D, et al: Outcome and profile of ventricular septal rupture with cardiogenic shock after myocardial infarction: a report from the SHOCK registry. J Am Coll Cardiol 36:1010, 2000.
58. Miller S, Dinsmore RE, Greene RE, Daggett WM: Coronary, ventricular and pulmonary abnormalities associated with rupture of the interventricular septum complicating myocardial infarction. Am J Radiol 131:571, 1978.
59. Monatoya A: Ventricular septal rupture secondary to acute myocardial infarction. In Pifarre R, editor: Cardiac Surgery: Acute Myocardial Infarction and Its Complications. Philadelphia: Hanley and Belfus, 1992.
60. Moore CA, Nygaard TW, Kaiser DL, et al: Postinfarction ventricular septal rupture: the importance of location of infarction and right ventricular function in determining survival. Circulation 74:45, 1986.
61. Omayada A, Queen FB: Spontaneous rupture of the interventricular septum following acute myocardial infarction with some clinico-pathologic observations on survival in five cases. Personal communication.
62. Pae WE Jr, Pierce WS, Sapirstein JS: Intra-aortic balloon counterpulsation, ventricular assist pumping, and the artificial heart. In Baue AE, Geha AS, Hammond GL, et al, editors: Glenn's Thoracic and Cardiovascular Surgery. Stamford: Appleton & Lange, 1996.
63. Pretre R, Ye Q, Grünefelfder J, et al: Role of myocardial revascularization in postinfarction ventricular septal rupture. Ann Thorac Surg 69:51–55, 2000.
64. Radford MJ, Johnson RA, Daggett WM, et al: VSD following myocardial infarction: factors affecting survival. Clin Res 26:262A, 1978.
65. Rich GF, Murphy GD Jr, Roos CM, Johns RA: Inhaled nitric oxide: selective pulmonary vasodilatation in cardiac surgical patients. Anesthesiology 78:1028, 1993.
66. Saksena S, Rothbart ST, Shah Y: Clinical efficacy and electropharmacology of continuous intravenous amiodarone infusion and chronic oral amiodarone in refractory ventricular tachycardia. Am J Cardiol 54:347, 1984.
67. Sanders RJ, Kern WH, Blount SG: Perforation of the interventricular septum complicating myocardial infarction. Am Heart J 51:736, 1956.
68. Scanlon PJ, Monatoya A, Johnson SA: Urgent surgery for ventricular septal rupture complicating myocardial infarction. Circulation 72(Suppl. 2):185, 1985.
69. Seguin JR, Frapier JM, Colson P, Chaptal PA: Fibrin sealant for early repair of acquired VSD. J Thorac Cardiovasc Surg 104:748, 1992.
70. Selzer A, Gerbode F, Keith WJ: Clinical, hemodynamic and surgical considerations of rupture of the ventricular septum after myocardial infarction. Am Heart J 78:598, 1969.
71. Shumaker H: Suggestions concerning operative management of postinfarction VSDs. J Thorac Cardiovasc Surg 64:452, 1972.
72. Silver MD, Butany J, Chiasson DA: The pathology of myocardial infarction and its mechanical complications. In David TE, editor: Mechanical Complications of Myocardial Infarction. Austin: R.G. Landes Company, 1993.
73. Skehan JD, Carey C, Norrell MS, et al: Patterns of coronary artery disease in post-infarction ventricular septal rupture. Br Heart J 62:268, 1989.
74. Skillington PD, Davies RH, Luff AJ, et al: Surgical treatment for infarct-related VSDs. J Thorac Cardiovasc Surg 99:798, 1990.
75. Smyllie JH, Sutherland GR, Geuskens R, et al: Doppler color flow mapping in the diagnosis of ventricular septal rupture and acute mitral regurgitation after myocardial infarction. J Am Coll Cardiol 15:1455, 1990.
76. Sundt TM III, Kouchoukos NT, Saffitz JE, et al: Renal dysfunction and intravascular coagulation with aprotinin and hypothermic circulatory arrest. Ann Thorac Surg 55:1418, 1993.
77. Swithingbank JM: Perforation of the interventricular septum in myocardial infarction. Br Heart J 21:562, 1959.
78. Teoh KH, Christakis GT, Weisel RD, et al: Accelerated myocardial metabolic recovery with terminal warm blood cardioplegia. J Thorac Cardiovasc Surg 91:888, 1986.
79. Weisel RD: Myocardial protection during surgery for mechanical complications of myocardial infarction. In David TE, editor: Mechanical Complications of Myocardial Infarction. Austin: R.G. Landes Company, 1993.
80. Weisman HF, Healy B: Myocardial infarct expansion, infarct extension nad reinfarction: pathophysiologic concpts. Prog Cardiovasc Dis 30:73, 1987.

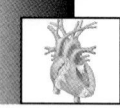

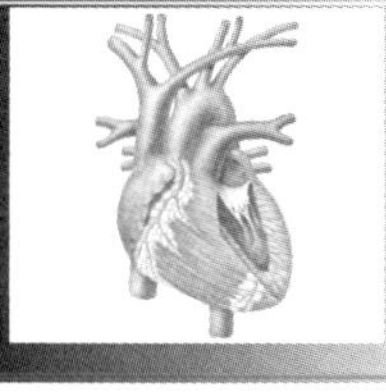

Therapeutic Angiogenesis

Marc Ruel and Frank W. Sellke

CHAPTER 88

INTRODUCTION

Coronary artery disease (CAD) persists as a leading cause of morbidity and mortality in the Western world. Despite increased awareness and better management of cardiovascular risk factors, CAD can involve the epicardial vasculature of some patients so diffusely that repeated attempts at catheter-based interventions and coronary artery bypass grafting (CABG) may be unsuccessful at alleviating ischemia and preventing acute coronary syndromes. This is most common in patients who have previously undergone CABG, in diabetics, in heart transplant recipients with cardiac allograft vasculopathy, and in patients of Indian descent or with a family history of early-onset CAD.[44,79–81,110,127] Overall, it is estimated that patients with myocardial ischemia who are not eligible for coronary bypass grafting on the basis of poor graftability have a 1-year myocardial infarction and mortality rate of 26% and 17%, respectively.[77] These patients constitute approximately 5% of patients who undergo coronary angiography at large referral centers, with many more having at least one myocardial territory found ungraftable at the time of CABG.[42,76] Although determination of ungraftability varies from one surgeon to another, technically accurate grafts with poor outflow have lower patency rates,[31] and failure to revascularize a single ischemic myocardial territory is associated with decreased survival and freedom from angina, regardless of the presence of a patent left internal thoracic artery bypass to the left anterior descending artery.[101]

Therapeutic angiogenesis aims at restoring perfusion to chronically ischemic myocardial territories by using growth factors without intervening on epicardial coronary arteries. Although this approach has received considerable scientific attention over the past decade, it has not yet been shown to provide clinical benefit and is therefore reserved for patients who have failed conventional therapies. Considering, however, that angiogenesis is a potent physiological process involved in growth and development of every animal and human, it is plausible that its use for therapeutic purposes, once its underlying mechanistic basis is better understood, could one day become a first-line modality for patients with CAD and other types of organ ischemia.

BACKGROUND

Vasculogenesis, Arteriogenesis, and Angiogenesis

At least three different processes may result in growth of new blood vessels: vasculogenesis, arteriogenesis, and true angiogenesis (Table 88-1).[90,113] *Vasculogenesis* occurs early in fetal development within new avascular tissue and consists of the differentiation of endothelial cells from angioblasts and endothelial progenitor cells, followed by their proliferation, coalescence, and recruitment of other cell types to complete the process of vascular formation *in situ*.[133] Although long considered to play no role in the response to chronic ischemia in adult tissues, vasculogenesis is now known to

Table 88–1

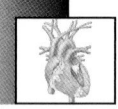

Biological Processes Leading to the Formation of New Blood Vessels

	Vasculogenesis	*Arteriogenesis*	*Angiogenesis*
Cell types involved	Endothelial stem cells	Endothelial cells; pericytes; smooth muscle cells; other	Endothelial cells
Primary stimulus	Development, also occurs in adult tissues	Not known (ischemia? inflammation?)	Inflammation, ischemia
End result	Fully formed vessels	Arterioles	Capillaries
Occurrence in adult tissues	Yes	Yes	Yes
Contribution to effective perfusion	Unclear	Major	Likely minimal
Growth factors involved	VEGF, Ang-1, Ang- 2	PDGF, Ang-1, Ang-2, FGFs(?)	FGFs, VEGFs

Modified with permission from Simons M, Bonow RO, Chronos NA, et al: Clinical trials in coronary angiogenesis: issues, problems, consensus: an expert panel summary. Circulation 102:E73, 2000.

Ang, angiopoietin; FGF, fibroblast growth factor; PDGF, platelet-derived growth factor; VEGF, vascular endothelial growth factor.

occur in adults, likely via recruitment of endothelial progenitor cells and other bone marrow–derived cells.

Arteriogenesis refers both to the process by which a postnatal vascular network remodels by maturation of preexisting collaterals in response to supply–demand imbalances ("angiogenic remodeling") and to the *de novo* formation by sprouting of mature blood vessels that contain pericytes and smooth muscle cells, which constitutes the actual goal of "therapeutic angiogenesis" modalities.

Angiogenesis refers in a strict sense to the sprouting into surrounding tissues of newly formed capillaries derived from preexisting vessels. Examples of this process are found in the border zone of a myocardial infarct or in granulation tissue during wound healing. These newly formed capillaries, however, lack a fully developed medial layer, have abnormal permeability, and cannot undergo vasomotor regulation. Thus the term "therapeutic *angiogenesis*" may constitute a misnomer, and the designative "therapeutic *arteriogenesis*" may better describe a process likely to result in the alleviation of ischemia; nevertheless, the former term is widely accepted and a distinction will not be taken further in the text.

Mechanisms of Angiogenesis

Vasodilation and increased capillary permeability from the sequestration of intercellular adhesion molecules such as vascular endothelial (VE)-cadherin and platelet endothelial cell adhesion molecule (PECAM)-1 are the initial steps in the physiological angiogenesis process (Figure 88-1). These events, mediated by the combined actions of nitric oxide (NO) and vascular endothelial growth factor (VEGF) on endothelial and smooth muscle cells, result in extravasation of plasma proteins, however limited by the negative feedback actions of angiopoietin-1 (Ang-1).[120] Subsequent detachment of smooth muscle cells and degradation of the surrounding perivascular matrix involve angiopoietin-2 (Ang-2) and metalloproteinases, which allow the migration of endothelial cells and liberation of endogenous growth factors such as fibroblast growth factor (FGF)-2 and VEGF from the matrix.

Proliferation of endothelial cells and their migration to distant sites are induced by several growth factors including VEGFs, FGFs (which recruit endothelial, mesenchymal, and inflammatory cells),[7] Ang-1 (chemotactic for endothelial cells and an inducer of sprouting),[115] and platelet-derived growth factors (PDGF; which recruit pericytes and smooth muscle cells around nascent vessel sprouts).[63] Endothelial cells then assemble into cords, form a lumen, and reexpress adhesion molecules such as VE-cadherin; these processes, mediated by VEGF, FGF-2, and Ang-1, may make endothelial cells resistant to apoptosis.[9,10,30] Cords and tubules can remain dormant or develop, branch, recruit periendothelial cells, and mature as functional vessels in order to meet local demands. The mechanisms responsible for these maturation processes are incompletely understood, but may involve PDGF-BB (smooth muscle chemotaxis),[63] Ang-1 (smooth muscle to endothelial cells interactions),[115] and FGF-2 (smooth muscle growth and vessel enlargement).[14] Table 88-2 outlines the role of substances involved in the angiogenic process.

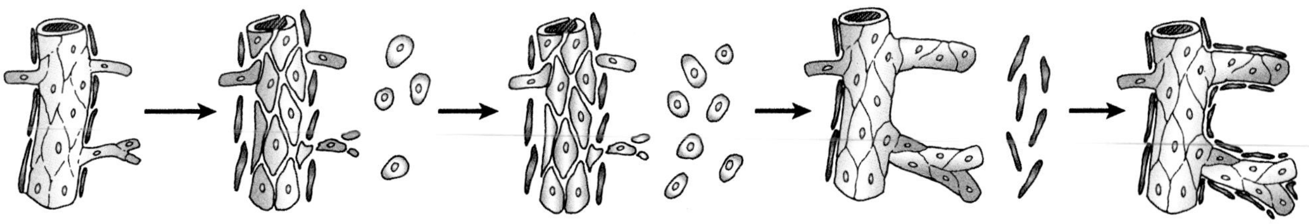

Figure 88–1 Mechanisms of angiogenesis.

Spontaneous Angiogenesis in Adult Tissues

The spontaneous occurrence of both arteriogenesis and angiogenesis has been demonstrated in animal models and humans under a variety of stresses including wound healing and inflammation,[24] peripheral vascular disease, chronic coronary insufficiency,[4,28,82] and acute myocardial ischemia.[4,38,46,59,121,131] For instance, serum levels of FGF-2 have been shown to be increased in patients with symptomatic CAD and normalize after successful revascularization.[43]

Basal or spontaneous angiogenesis may be enhanced by a number of commonly used substances. Nicotine, for instance, is proangiogenic and may worsen atherosclerotic plaques by promoting intimal proliferation.[36,83] Moderate ethanol concentrations and low-dose statins also have proangiogenic properties, and the use of statins has been associated with increased tissue perfusion in a hind limb ischemia model.[33,47] Adenosine and heparin appear to independently stimulate angiogenesis.[18,119] In a trial of IV adenosine and heparin administered daily for 10 days in patients with chronic stable angina, a 9% reduction in the extent and a 14% improvement in the severity of perfusion defects were noted on exercise thallium imaging in patients who received adenosine and heparin versus those who received placebo.[5]

Some commonly used medications have been shown to inhibit angiogenesis. These include captopril,[129] isosorbide

Table 88–2

Substances Involved in the Angiogenic Process

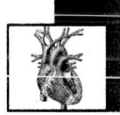

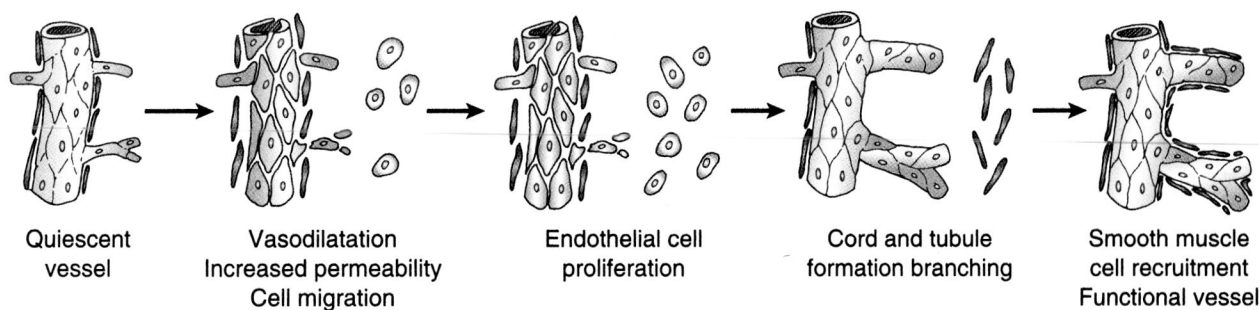

	Function
Nitric oxide	Vasodilatation; cofactor for VEGFs, FGFs, and other angiogens
Vascular endothelial growth factors	Vasodilatation; increased permeability; sequestration of VE-cadherin and PECAM-1; endothelial cell proliferation; formation of cords and lumens
Fibroblast growth factors	Endothelial cell proliferation; formation of cords and lumens; recruitment of inflammatory cells, pericytes, and smooth muscle cells; vessel maturation and enlargement (?)
Angiopoietin-1	Prevention of excessive vascular permeability; endothelial cell chemotaxis; formation of cords and lumens; vessel stabilization via smooth muscle to endothelial cell interactions
Angiopoietin-2	Vessel destabilization; detachment of smooth muscle cells; degradation of extracellular matrix (in conjunction with matrix metalloproteinases)
Platelet-derived growth factors	Chemotaxis/recruitment of pericytes and smooth muscle cells; branching of nascent rudimentary vessels
Cyclooxygenase-2	Vasodilatation; stimulation of angiogenesis

[a]Partial listing.
FGF, fibroblast growth factor; PECAM, platelet endothelial cell adhesion molecule; VE, vascular endothelial; VEGF, vascular endothelial growth factor.

dinitrate,[88] furosemide,[85] spironolactone,[72] as well as acetylsalicylic acid (ASA) and other antiinflammatory drugs whose antiangiogenic effects are related to inhibition of COX-2, the inducible isoform of cyclooxygenase.[72,73] Overall spontaneous angiogenic capacity has been shown to decrease with age in animals, correlated with decreases in myocyte PDGF production.[19]

Growth Factors and Delivery Strategies

Despite the complexity of the angiogenic process, therapeutic angiogenesis regimens have focused mainly on the administration of a single growth factor, with select isoforms of VEGF-A ($VEGF_{121}$, $VEGF_{165}$) and FGF (FGF-1, FGF-2, FGF-4) being most extensively studied. Delivery strategies may involve the actual angiogenic protein or the gene encoding for it; while proteins are administered directly, gene-based approaches usually employ naked plasmid DNA or a viral vector that encodes the gene to be incorporated by the host endothelial cells. Several routes of administration have been developed to deliver angiogenic substances to the ischemic myocardium in a single or repeated fashion; these include intravenous, intracoronary, left atrial, surgical perivascular, intrapericardial via a catheter placed under echo guidance, and catheter-based intramyocardial approaches guided by left ventricular electromapping. Table 88-3 outlines the relative advantages and disadvantages of protein versus gene-based approaches.

Gene Delivery Vectors

Gene-based approaches require vectors to incorporate an angiogenic gene into a target host cell and induce production of the encoded protein. Although naked plasmid DNA may be used for this purpose, its efficiency may be limited by the smaller fraction of plasmid DNA that actually enters the cell nucleus.[25,48] The use of adenoviruses is associated with higher transfection efficiency, and these viruses can be readily produced as replication-deficient mutants for gene transfer applications.[114] However, circulating antibodies to adenoviruses are common in the general population and may elicit an inflammatory response that could compromise the incorporation and expression of the gene.[29] Alternatives have been developed that include adeno-associated viruses, unique in their ability to transduce nondividing cells and allowing for a more prolonged transgene expression, and retroviral vectors.[48] Retroviruses differ from plasmid and adenoviral vectors in that their RNA is reverse transcribed to DNA and integrated into the host cell genome. Although this induces long-lasting expression of the incorporated gene, it also raises safety concerns with respect to potential overexpression.[113] In an attempt to increase the efficacy and safety of gene delivery vectors, research efforts also focus on the development of viral vectors allowing for up- or down-regulation of the gene of interest.

PRECLINICAL STUDIES

Ameroid Constrictor Model of Chronic Myocardial Ischemia

A large animal model of chronic myocardial ischemia is required for the preclinical evaluation of indirect revascularization modalities such as therapeutic angiogenesis. Because laboratory animals do not spontaneously develop CAD, coronary insufficiency must be experimentally created. Vessel embolization, surgical ligation, and thrombogenic copper coil implantation result in acute coronary occlusion and myocardial infarction; although a chronic ischemic area exists at the border of this infarct, it does not adequately model the ischemic myocardial territory of patients with severe angina.

A *collateral-dependent* (chronically ischemic) myocardial territory with minimal infarction can be created by surgical

Table 88–3

Protein versus Gene Therapy for Therapeutic Angiogenesis

	Protein therapy	*Gene therapy*
Duration of expression	+ (++ if sustained release)	++
Regulation of expression	+++	+
Dose–response	Unpredictable	Defined
Choice of delivery routes	+++	+++
Inflammatory reaction	+	+++
Potential for multiagent and repeated administration	++	+

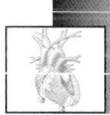

implantation and intermittent inflation of an external pneumatic coronary occluder[13,26] or by insertion of an ameroid constrictor around a major coronary artery, usually the proximal left circumflex.[105] The ameroid method results in progressive stenosis and occlusion of the encircled vessel over a period of 2–4 weeks. The constrictor consists of hygroscopic casein compressed into a cylindrical shape and enclosed within a stainless steel collar; when in contact with fluid, the casein expands in an inward direction because of the fixed metal ring and occludes the artery (Figure 88-2). Experimental protocols typically involve administration of growth factors 3–4 weeks after implantation of the ameroid, by which time it has closed and the myocardium been made ischemic.[94]

Pigs are an ideal model for the study of chronic myocardial ischemia because of their few native collateral vessels (unlike dogs, which have an interconnected coronary network) and their lack of propensity to normalize perfusion to the collateral-dependent myocardium. Even so, swine develop an endogenous angiogenic response to chronic myocardial ischemia that results in increased intercoronary collateral flow, and that mandates the use of ischemic controls in preclinical studies.[109,130] Compared to normal vessels, these collaterals have less medial smooth muscle, impaired endothelial-mediated vasodilatation, and altered endothelium-independent relaxation properties.[30,103]

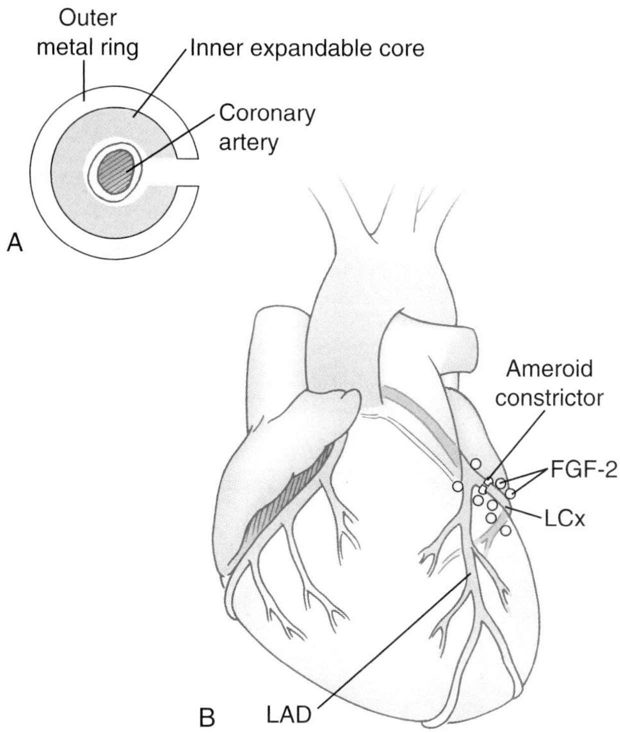

Figure 88–2 Ameroid constrictor model of chronic myocardial ischemia and sustained-release perivascular protein-based angiogenesis. A, Outward expansion of the inner casein core of the ameroid is prevented by the metal ring, resulting in progressive occlusion of the vessel. **B,** Ameroid inserted around the proximal left circumflex artery (LCx). Three weeks later, after complete closure of the ameroid, sustained-release FGF-2 beads are implanted around the occluded vessel and in the transition zone between the left anterior descending (LAD) and circumflex distributions.

Studies with Vascular Endothelial Growth Factor

Preclinical experience with VEGF has mainly involved its $VEGF_{165}$ and $VEGF_{121}$ isoforms, derived from alternative splicing of the VEGF-A gene. Both protein and gene-based approaches have been employed, and success reproducibly observed using either modality in limb ischemia models as well as in the setting of myocardial ischemia.* For instance, 2 μg of VEGF was administered perivascularly over 4 weeks in swine whose lateral myocardial territory was made ischemic by an ameroid occluder. Treated animals developed higher coronary flow and a 4-fold increase in capillary density of the collateral-dependent myocardium when compared with controls; furthermore, a decrease in the size of the ischemic zone was demonstrated on magnetic resonance imaging.[86]

The use of intracoronary, intrapericardial, or intravenous routes for the administration of VEGF has not always been as successful. In dog studies, a 28-day course of intracoronary VEGF injections was effective in increasing flow to the collateral-dependent territory above that of controls,[3] but a 7-day course did not produce any effect and actually exacerbated neointimal accumulation following endothelial injury.[54] In another study, injection of an adenoviral vector encoding for $VEGF_{165}$ through an indwelling pericardial catheter resulted in sustained pericardial transgene expression, but no increase in perfusion of the collateral-dependent territory could be demonstrated.[55] Finally, intravenous injection of $VEGF_{165}$ was found by Sato et al to be ineffective in a swine model.[97]

Studies with Fibroblast Growth Factor

Like VEGF, several isoforms of FGF exist, of which FGF-1 and FGF-2 have been most studied. Both FGFs are believed to induce angiogenesis as well as arteriogenesis by stimulating growth of a variety of cell types, including vascular smooth muscle cells and endothelial cells.[14]

FGF-1 is strongly expressed in ischemic myocardium and may play a role in the spontaneous formation of collaterals.[99] Its use to stimulate angiogenesis in large animals initially produced disappointing results likely because of the instability of wild-type FGF-1, which has a biological half-life of 15 min at 37° C.[84,123,125] After heparin binding and replacement of a single cysteine residue with a serine, which increased the half-life of FGF-1 1000-fold,[84] perivascular administration of its S^{117} mutant form was studied in a porcine ameroid model and resulted in improved collateral-dependent myocardial flow and left ventricular function.[66]

FGF-2 has been extensively studied in canine and porcine models of myocardial ischemia using multiple delivery strategies. Unger et al gave daily intracoronary bolus injections of 110 μg of FGF-2 in the distal circumflex artery of dogs for 28 consecutive days.[124] The transmural collateral flow in FGF-2-treated dogs significantly exceeded that of controls by the second week of treatment and was associated with an increase in vessel density. These investigators also conducted chronic studies with daily left atrial injections of FGF-2 for up to 13 weeks, in which the maximum effect attributable to the growth factor was temporally related to the presence of myocardial ischemia.[53] Chronic FGF-2

*References 34, 57, 68, 86, 97, 117, 118.

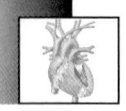

therapy was not associated with the occurrence of structural or vasoproliferative adverse effects for up to 6 months after treatment initiation.

Local perivascular administration of FGF-2 was studied in swine and led to increased perfusion of the collateral-dependent territory and a dose-dependent improvement in left ventricular ejection fraction both at rest and during pacing.[21,35,65] The protocol used 10 sustained-release heparin-alginate capsules, each containing 1 or 10 μg of FGF-2, implanted 3 weeks after ameroid placement around the occluded vessel and in the transition zone between the normal and collateral-dependent territories (Figure 88-2). Perivascular FGF-2 administration also normalized ischemia-induced impairments of endothelial-dependent vasodilatation.[106] In other studies, single-dose intrapericardial and intracoronary delivery of FGF-2 led to perfusion and contractility improvements; however, single-dose intravenous infusion was shown to be ineffective.[51,96]

The myocardial and tissue distribution of ^{125}I-labeled FGF-2 after intracoronary and intravenous administration was studied in swine with organ autoradiography.[50] The liver accounted for the majority of ^{125}I-labeled FGF-2 activity at 1 h after injection with either route; total cardiac specific activity at 1 h was 0.88% for intracoronary and 0.26% for intravenous administration and further decreased to 0.05% and 0.04% at 24 h, respectively (Figure 88-3A). In another study, the distribution of intravenous injections of FGF-2 was compared with that of perivascular sustained-release delivery.[20] The amount of FGF-2 deposited in arteries adjacent to sustained-release devices was 40 times that deposited in animals who received intravenous FGF-2 (Figure 88-3B). FGF-2 was also 5- to 30-fold more abundant in the kidney, liver, and spleen after intravenous injection than following perivascular release, indicating that perivascular delivery is more specific and effective than intravenous delivery at achieving local deposition of FGF-2.

Safety Profile

Although overexpression of VEGF in mice has been associated with the formation of angiomas and vascular tumors,[8,58] the occurrence of these adverse events or proliferative retinopathy has not been reported in large animal studies of growth factor therapy. Most studies were, however, of short-term duration and may have involved an insufficient number of animals to detect a rare occurrence of these events.

VEGF and FGF-2 are known to be associated with systemic hypotension that occurs in a dose-dependent fashion; in this regard, the doses of FGF-2 leading to hypotension are higher than for VEGF.[15,67] FGF-2 has also been associated with proliferative membranous nephropathy and proteinuria in mice, but this complication has not been observed in pre-

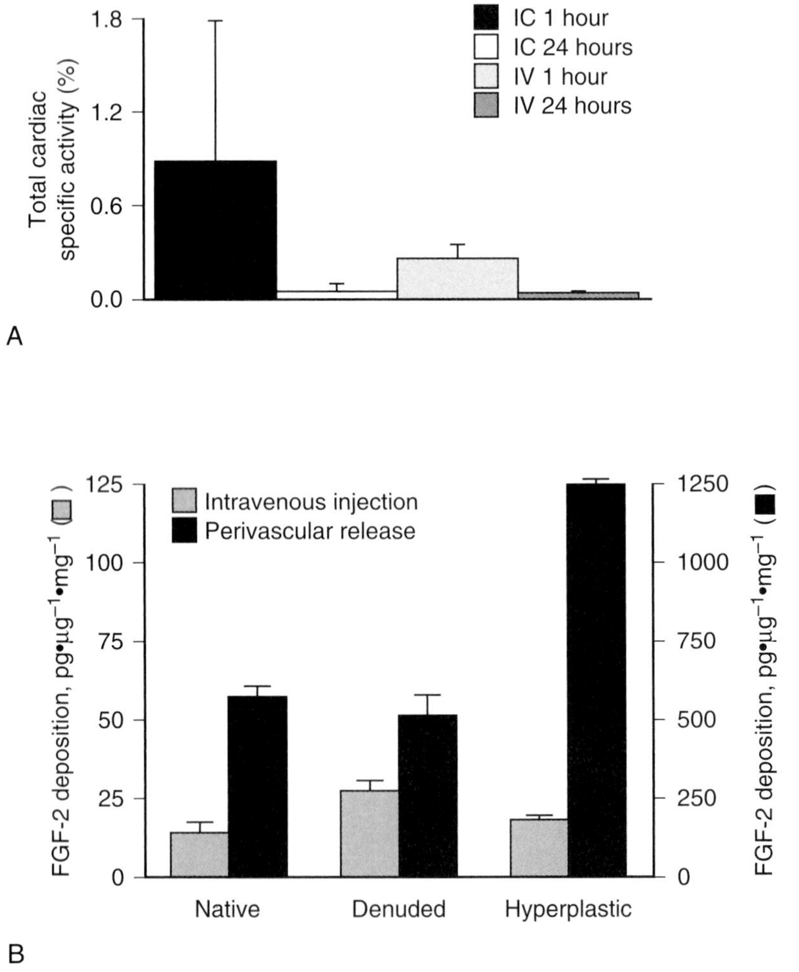

Figure 88–3 Tissue deposition after intravenous (IV), intracoronary (IC), and perivascular (using heparin- alginate sustained-released capsules) administration of FGF-2. A, Total cardiac specific activity after IC and IV injection of 25 μCi of ^{125}I-labeled FGF-2 in swine. Total specific cardiac activity with either method was less than 1% at 1 h and 0.1% at 24 h, with the liver accounting for most of the ^{125}I-labeled FGF-2 activity. **B,** Tissue deposition after a single intravenous injection versus perivascular administration of FGF-2 in intact carotid arteries ("native"), in arteries whose endothelium was denuded, and in arteries allowed to develop intimal hyperplasia 2 weeks after endothelial denudation. Deposition of FGF-2 was substantially lower with IV injection than with perivascular release for native arteries (factor of 40.0 less), denuded arteries (factor of 18.9 less), and hyperplastic arteries (factor of 67.1 less).

(**A** *from Laham RJ, Rezaee M, Post M, et al: Intracoronary and intravenous administration of basic fibroblast growth factor: Myocardial and tissue distribution. Drug Metab Dispos 27:821, 1999.* **B** *adapted from Edelman ER, Nugent MA, Karnovsky MJ: Perivascular and intravenous administration of basic fibroblast growth factor: Vascular and solid organ deposition. Proc Natl Acad Sci USA 90:1513, 1993.*)

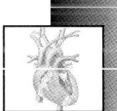

clinical or clinical studies.[23,95] Recently, VEGF has been linked with hypercoagulability; a relationship between serum VEGF and tissue factor levels was demonstrated in patients with atrial fibrillation and CAD.[11]

INDICATIONS AND SURGICAL TECHNIQUE

Indications for Angiogenic Therapy

Box 88-1 outlines the potential indications and contraindications to angiogenic therapy. The clinical effectiveness of therapeutic angiogenesis has not yet been proven. This modality should therefore be considered experimental and performed in the context of an approved clinical trial in consenting patients who have failed or are not amenable to conventional revascularization procedures.

Patients considered for therapeutic angiogenesis should have persistent, severe chronic stable angina imputed to at least one myocardial territory that cannot adequately or safely be revascularized with conventional methods.[92] The targeted myocardial territory should be ischemic and viable. Therapeutic angiogenesis should not be used to attempt emergency revascularization or salvage in the context of threatened proximal coronary occlusion.[113]

Absolute contraindications to therapeutic angiogenesis include a history of malignancy within the past 5 years, with the exception of basal or early-stage squamous skin cancers that are considered cured. Therapeutic angiogenesis should not be carried out in patients with proliferative retinopathy, vascular malformations, and low blood pressure. In addition, FGF-2 administration is contraindicated in patients with decreased creatinine clearance or proteinuria. Severely compromised left ventricular ejection fraction is a relative contraindication to angiogenic therapy, since delivery techniques involve procedural stress that could precipitate cardiac decompensation.

Box 88–1. Potential Indications and Contraindications to Angiogenic Therapy.

Potential indications	Contraindications
Chronic stable angina in the presence of ungraftable CAD in a major coronary distribution, with	Malignancy within past 5 years
Documentation of ischemia in the ungraftable territory	Vascular proliferative lesions
Evidence of ungraftability, such as previous failed attempts at PTCA and CABG	Diabetic retinopathy
Presence of viable myocardium in the ungraftable territory	Arteriovenous malformations
	Hemangiomas
	LVEF <30%
	Chronically low BP
	Impaired renal function (FGF-2)
	? Hypercoagulability (VEGF)

CAD, coronary artery disease; PTCA, percutaneous transluminal coronary angioplasty; CABG, coronary artery bypass grafting; LVEF, left ventricular ejection fraction; BP, blood pressure; FGF, fibroblast growth factor; VEGF, vascular endothelial growth factor.

Technique of Surgical Perivascular Implantation

The surgical perivascular implantation of angiogenic growth factors can be done in conjunction with CABG or as a sole therapy.[91,104] Both strategies may involve minimally invasive approaches in combination with multivessel off-pump CABG, ipsilateral or contralateral MIDCAB, or as sole therapy through a subxiphoid or small thoracotomy incision. In the future, implantation of angiogenic growth factors using a closed-chest videoscopic approach may constitute an ideal method of delivery.

Although a surgical approach can be used for the administration of virtually any type of angiogenic protein or gene vector, most of the experience has involved the perivascular delivery of FGF-2 protein using sustained-release beads at the time of CABG (Figure 88-4).[52,92,104] Controlled release of the FGF-2 derives from its avidity for heparin, which is bound to Sepharose beads and hardened into a capsule using a calcium chloride-alginate solution, without reduction in biological activity of the growth factor.[20,21,64] Once implanted, release of FGF-2 from the polymer occurs via first-order kinetics over a 4- to 5-week period; no inflammatory reaction results from placement of the polymer.

Perivascular implantation of FGF-2 using this delivery system in conjunction with CABG is performed through a median sternotomy. Attentive anesthetic management is crucial to minimize intraoperative cardiac ischemia. In this regard, particular attention should be given to the constant

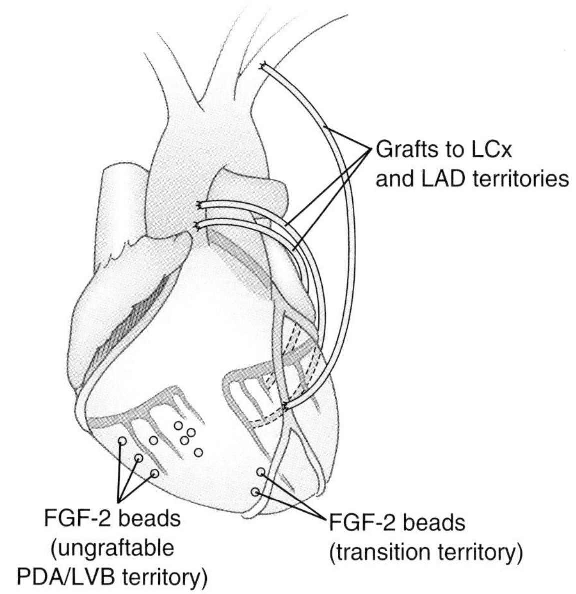

Figure 88–4 Implantation of sustained-release FGF-2 beads in the myocardial distribution of an ungraftable right coronary artery, in conjunction with CABG. LCx, left circumflex artery; LAD, left anterior descending (artery). PDA, posterior descending artery; LVB, left ventricular branches of the right coronary artery.
(Adapted with permission from Sellke FW, Laham RJ, Edelman ER, et al: Therapeutic angiogenesis with basic fibroblast growth factor: technique and early results. Ann Thorac Surg 65:1540, 1998.)

optimization of coronary perfusion pressure and ventricular afterload, oxygenation, and potassium and magnesium levels to prevent ventricular irritability. Monitoring of mixed venous oxygen saturation with a Swan–Ganz catheter and assessment of regional contractility and mitral valve function with transesophageal echocardiography (TEE) are desirable. After instituting cardiopulmonary bypass and cardioplegic arrest, distal coronary anastomoses to graftable coronaries are completed and nongraftability of the target territory is confirmed by direct inspection of the vessel. Multiple linear incisions are made in the epicardial fat surrounding the ungraftable vessel, and in the transition zone between the target territory and that supplied by a grafted or patent coronary artery, to enable the development of subepicardial collaterals between ischemic and normally perfused myocardium. Ten heparin-alginate beads, each containing 1 or 10 μg of human recombinant FGF-2, are inserted in the subepicardium and secured in place with a 6-0 polypropylene suture, with up to three beads placed in a single incision. As a quality control measure, two to six heparin-alginate beads from each batch are cultured aerobically and anaerobically to ensure sterility. Proximal anastomoses are then constructed, the patient is separated from cardiopulmonary bypass, and routine closure is performed. If intraoperative ischemia develops and leads to hemodynamic instability, an intraaortic balloon pump (IABP) is inserted. Postoperative pain should be managed attentively, and the use of a thoracic epidural catheter is advisable unless contraindicated by coagulopathy or heparin use.

CLINICAL STUDIES OF THERAPEUTIC ANGIOGENESIS

Protein Therapy

Surgical Perivascular Delivery

The safety of FGF-1 administration was demonstrated in a series of 20 patients conducted by Schumacher and colleagues, who injected 0.01 mg/kg of FGF-1 directly into the myocardium along a diffusely diseased left anterior descending (LAD) coronary artery to which the left internal thoracic artery (LITA) was also grafted.[87,100] Patients were followed up 12 weeks and 3 years later by selective injection of the LITA and quantitative evaluation of anterior myocardial collateralization with digital subtraction angiography. Although a local increase in collateral blush was observed along the LAD, nuclear imaging assessments of ischemia or functional parameters such as exercise capacity, Canadian Cardiovascular Society (CCS) angina class, or freedom from angina recurrence were not reported.

The safety and efficacy of perivascular FGF-2 administration were evaluated in a phase I, double-blind, randomized controlled trial that involved 24 patients concomitantly undergoing CABG.[52] In this study, patients in whom high-dose FGF-2 sustained-release capsules had been implanted in an ungraftable territory at the time of CABG had complete relief from angina and showed significant improvements in stress nuclear perfusion defect size at 3-month follow-up. These patients were subsequently followed at a mean of 32 months postoperatively with clinical assessment and nuclear imaging. Patients treated with either dose of FGF-2 experienced significantly more freedom from angina recurrence than controls (Figure 88-5).[92] Double-blinded nuclear imaging studies revealed that all but one patient in the control group had either persistence of a reversible perfusion defect or evidence of a new fixed defect in the ungraftable myocardial territory; this was, however, observed in only one of nine patients treated with FGF-2 (Figure 88-6). The remaining FGF-treated patients had disappearance of their ungraftable territory reversible perfusion defect and stability or decrease in the size of their fixed defect. FGF-treated patients also showed better late global left ventricular perfusion scores during pharmacological stress.[92] Although this study involved a small number of patients and may have been confounded by concomitant CABG, perivascular slow-release FGF-2 therapy appeared to result in persistent freedom from angina recurrence and sustained improvements in left ventricular perfusion.

Intravascular Delivery

Laham et al conducted a phase I, open-label dose-escalation trial evaluating the efficacy and safety of a single-bolus intracoronary administration of FGF-2 in 52 patients and showed that it may improve symptoms and myocardial perfusion.[49] These investigators then proceeded to a multicenter, randomized, double-blind, placebo-controlled trial of a single intracoronary infusion of FGF-2 at 0, 0.3, 3, or 30 μg/kg in 337 patients, the FGF Initiating RevaScularization Trial (FIRST).[112] Efficacy was evaluated at 90 and 180 days

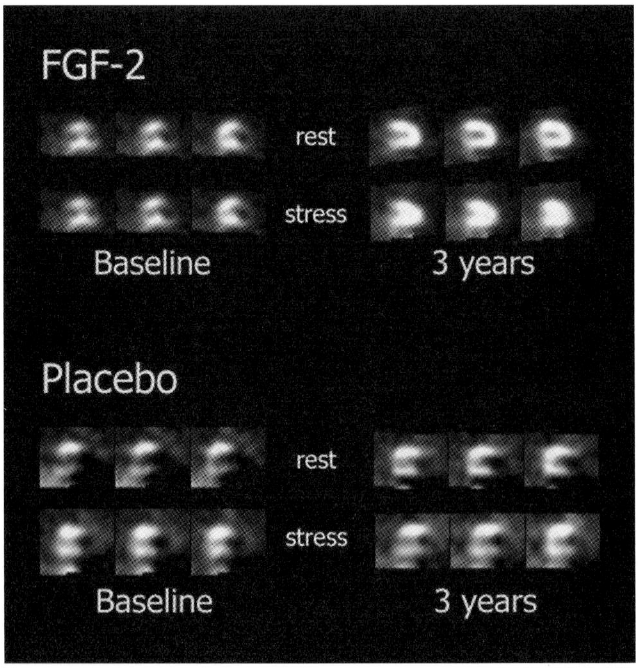

Figure 88–5 Baseline and 3 years' postoperative SPECT images of patients who received FGF-2 versus placebo beads implanted in an ungraftable inferoapical myocardial territory at the time of CABG. Horizontal long-axis views show complete resolution of the large inferoapical perfusion defect at rest and stress in the patient who received FGF-2, and no detectable change from baseline in the patient who received placebo. *(Reproduced with permission from Sellke FW, Ruel M: Vascular growth factors and angiogenesis in cardiac surgery. Ann Thorac Surg 75:S691–699, 2003.)*

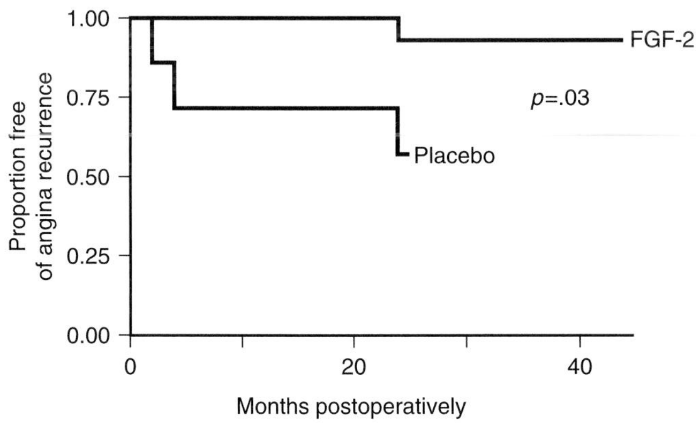

Figure 88–6 Freedom from angina in patients who underwent implantation of FGF-2 versus placebo in a major, nongraftable myocardial territory at the time of CABG.
(Reproduced with permission from Ruel M, Laham RJ, Parker JA, et al: Long-term effects of angiogenic therapy with FGF-2 protein. J Thorac Cardiovasc Surg 124:28–34, 2002.)

by exercise tolerance test, nuclear perfusion imaging, and angina questionnaire. Exercise tolerance was increased at 90 days in all groups but was not significantly different between placebo and FGF-treated groups. FGF-2 reduced angina symptoms, and these differences were more pronounced in highly symptomatic patients with baseline CCS angina class scores of III or IV. However, this benefit did not persist at 180 days because of continued improvement in the placebo group, and the trial was considered negative with respect to all main end points. Adverse events were similar across all groups, except for hypotension, which occurred more frequently in the 30 μg/kg FGF-2 group.

For peripheral vascular disease, FGF-2 was effective in increasing peak walking time at 90 days in a double-blind trial of 190 patients with moderate-to-severe intermittent claudication randomized to bilateral intraarterial lower limb infusions of placebo on days 1 and 30 (n = 63), FGF-2 (30 μg/kg) on day 1 and placebo on day 30 (single-dose, n = 66), or FGF-2 (30 μg/kg) on days 1 and 30 (double-dose, n = 61).[56] The improvement was, however, seen in the single-dose FGF-2 group only. Adverse event rates were not different among the three groups.

Intravenous and intracoronary administration of VEGF for myocardial ischemia was studied in a randomized, double-blind, phase II study: the Vascular Endothelial Growth Factor in Vascular Angina (VIVA) trial. This trial, like FIRST, was also negative with respect to symptom improvement, exercise time, and nuclear imaging end points.[37] It is possible that the effects of FGF-2 and VEGF in the FIRST and VIVA trials may have been compromised by the choice of intravascular delivery routes, which are nonspecific in their tissue distribution and carry the potential to worsen atherosclerosis.[61,75,83]

Gene Therapy

Surgical Perivascular Delivery

Rosengart et al examined the effects of direct administration of an adenoviral vector encoding for $VEGF_{121}$ as an adjunct to conventional CABG (in 15 patients) and as sole therapy (in 6 patients).[91] There was no control group and the main end points were related to safety. No systemic or cardiac-related adverse events related to vector administration were observed. All patients reported improvements in angina class, and postoperative nuclear imaging suggested increased contractility during stress conditions in the area of vector administration, but did not reveal an increase in myocardial perfusion.

Losordo et al initiated a small phase 1 trial to determine the safety and bioactivity of direct myocardial gene transfer (using naked plasmid DNA) of $VEGF_{165}$ as sole therapy in five patients with inoperable CAD and symptomatic myocardial ischemia.[70] The vector was administered by four 2.0-ml needle injections into the anterolateral left ventricular free wall through a small left anterolateral thoracotomy. The injections were not associated with side effects other than isolated premature ventricular complexes at the time of needle penetration. All patients had a significant reduction in angina as measured by nitroglycerin use, improved collateral scores on angiography, and reduced size of the ischemic defect on dobutamine nuclear imaging. These data were confirmed in a second open-label, uncontrolled phase 1 study from the same group in which 20 patients received either 125 or 250 μg of naked plasmid $VEGF_{121}$ injected directly into the myocardium via a minimally invasive thoracotomy.[116] Plasma VEGF concentrations increased at 14 days to a level 2-fold over pretreatment values and returned to baseline by 3 months. As in the previous study, patients reported decreased angina and reduced nitroglycerin use, and improvement was seen on radionuclide perfusion imaging.

Huwer et al used a protocol involving CABG and injection of plasmid DNA encoding for $VEGF_{165}$ and $VEGF_{167}$ at a dosage of 1000 μg each, directly into an area of myocardium not amenable to surgical revascularization. Overall results were marginal and an increase in nuclear perfusion in the region of gene application was observed in only 3 of 24 patients.[40]

Stewart et al recently reported the results of a phase 2, randomized, multicenter, 26-week study to assess the efficacy and safety of adenoviral $VEGF_{121}$ delivery via minimally invasive surgery versus maximum medical treatment in patients with severe angina and no other option for revascularization. Patients were randomized to receive $VEGF_{121}$ in 30 direct intramyocardial injections throughout the free wall of the left ventricle via minithoracotomy (32 patients), or continuation of optimal medical management (35 patients). Exercise treadmill time to 1-mm ST depression, time to angina, and total exercise duration were significantly improved in the VEGF group compared to the control group at 26 weeks. There were also significant improvements in CCS angina class and Seattle Angina Questionnaire scores at 12 and 26 weeks. Although the protocol was not blinded and improvements may have been due to a placebo effect or inflammation resulting from thoracotomy and vector administration, the study, in addition to suggesting efficacy, demonstrated no significant differences in adverse events between groups, no positive adenoviral cultures, and no significant changes in systemic VEGF levels.[114]

Catheter-Based Delivery

Vale et al conducted a pilot study of catheter-based myocardial gene transfer involving six patients with chronic myocardial ischemia who were randomized to receive 200 μg of naked plasmid VEGF-2 or placebo.[126] A steerable, deflectable 8F catheter incorporating a 27-gauge needle was advanced percutaneously and guided into the left ventricular myocardium by left ventricular electromechanical mapping. Despite the small number of patients, end points of angina frequency, nitroglycerin consumption, and stress myocardial perfusion on nuclear imaging revealed a trend in favor of the group transfected with VEGF-2 versus controls. These investigators proceeded to a trial involving 19 patients randomized to receive six injections of placebo or naked plasmid VEGF-2 in doses of 200, 800, or 2000 μg guided by left ventricular electromechanical mapping. Injections were safely performed and a significant improvement in CCS angina class was noted at 12 weeks in VEGF-treated versus placebo-treated patients, supporting the undertaking of a larger phase 2 trial.[69]

EFFICACY ISSUES

Delivery Routes and Duration of Effect

From the evidence currently available,[52,69,92] perivascular or intramyocardial administration of angiogenic factors constitutes the route of choice for angiogenic therapy, since it presents a more specific tissue distribution profile than intravascular techniques, does not result in rapid washout, is not limited by the endothelial barrier, and does not carry the potential of exacerbating intimal plaques. Protein administration also offers safety advantages over gene-based approaches[108] and may be delivered perivascularly using a sustained-delivery system without provoking an inflammatory response.[52,104,113] Although a surgical approach is required, this allows for the precise placement of beads within the ischemic territory as well as at the transition between normally perfused and collateral-dependent myocardium, promoting formation of subepicardial collaterals that may provide arterial inflow to the ischemic zone.

Duration of effect after single administration constitutes another pitfall of intravascular modalities. The pharmacokinetics and pharmacodynamics of a single FGF-2 dose administered by intracoronary or intravenous infusion were evaluated in 66 patients enrolled in the FIRST trial. Using either delivery route, the half-life of FGF-2 elimination was only 7.6 h and systemic exposure to FGF-2 was similar regardless of whether intracoronary or intravenous administration was used. Furthermore, Dor et al used a transgenic system for conditional switching of VEGF expression in mice, allowing for reversible induction of VEGF in the heart at any selected schedule.[16] These authors observed that VEGF caused chaotic connections with the existing network, formation of irregularly shaped sac-like vessels, and massive edema. Premature cessation of the VEGF stimulus led to regression of most acquired vessels, up to a critical transition time point beyond which remodeled new vessels persisted for months after withdrawing VEGF, conferring a long-term improvement in organ perfusion. The stimulation period that corresponds to this transition time point in humans is completely unknown, as is whether this course is growth factor specific or depends on patient-related factors.

Role of NO in Angiogenesis

There is interaction between the local availability of NO and the regulation of blood vessel growth mediated by the actions of VEGF and to a lesser extent FGF-2.[1,32,78,107] Diminished NO availability has been implicated in the inhibition of endothelial cell migration and capillary-like tube formation *in vitro*,[128] of basal and exogenous angiogenic responses in hypercholesterolemic rodents,[17,41] of basal angiogenesis in dogs,[74] and of the angiogenic response to exogenous FGF-2 in a hypercholesterolemic swine model of endothelial dysfunction (Figure 88–7). Given these data and the fact that therapeutic angiogenesis is not nearly as effective in patients with inoperable CAD as it has been in laboratory animals, the failure of effect observed in clinical trials may relate to a deficiency in the stimulated release of NO, whose production as well as that of other endothelium-derived substances is altered in end-stage CAD.[71,134] The current clinical indications for angiogenic therapy may therefore paradoxically target patients for whom the modality therapy is least likely to work, and it is plausible that the clinical efficacy of therapeutic angiogenesis may therefore benefit from concomitant modulation of the coronary microvascular endothelium in patients with end-stage CAD. Such research is ongoing and could bridge the missing link between successful animal models and disappointing clinical trials of angiogenic therapy.

Multiagent Therapy and Master-Switch Genes

Although the physiological events that result in angiogenesis are complex and incompletely understood, therapeutic angiogenic approaches so far have concentrated on the

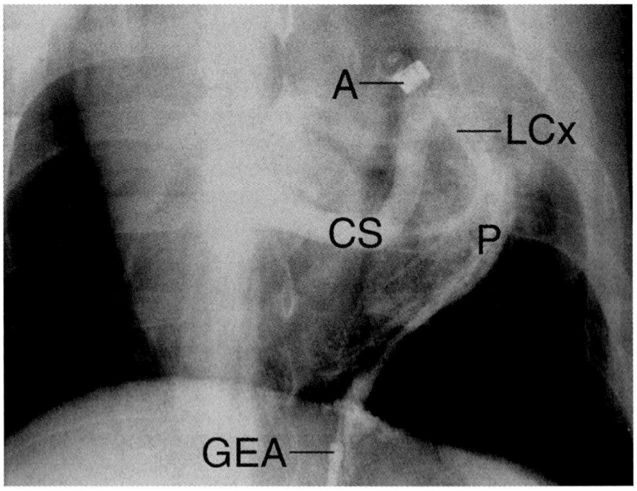

Figure 88–7 Gastroepiploic arteriogram (GEA) of a swine with chronic myocardial ischemia 7 weeks after apposition of a pedicled gastric submucosal patch. Patch contour (P), circumflex artery reconstitution (LCx), and occlusion at the ameroid constrictor (A) level, and drainage of contrast via the coronary sinus (CS) are seen. This model demonstrated that endogenous angiogenesis from an angiogenic organ could be stimulated to revascularize another without the need for growth factors.
(Reproduced with permission from Ruel M, Sellke FW, Bianchi C, et al: Myocardial revascularization using angiogenic properties of the gastric submucosa. Ann Thorac Surg 75: 1443–1449, 2003.)

administration of a single growth factor. Although this strategy was mandated by practicality and safety considerations as well as by the limited knowledge of potential interactions between growth factors, it is debatable whether single-agent approaches will ever result in clinically reproducible formation of long-lasting, functional vessels. Alternatively, the safety and efficacy of therapeutic approaches could also be increased by stimulating *endogenous* angiogenesis in response to ischemia or with combinations of exogenous growth factors. Experimental stimulation of endogenous angiogenesis without administration of exogenous growth factors was achieved by modulating the proangiogenic properties of the gastric submucosa in a swine model of chronic myocardial ischemia (Figure 88–8).[93]

Another alternative is the use of master-switch agents, which induce the basal cascades of angiogenesis-related genes, are up-regulated in the presence of ischemia, and mediate the endogenous angiogenic responses of animals and humans.[59,60,111] Hypoxia-induced factor (HIF)-1a is a prototype gene expressed in ischemic tissues that initiates the cascade of VEGF-dependent angiogenesis.[111] PR39, relaxin and sonic hedgehog are other master-switch agents with the propensity to induce the VEGF, FGF, and angiopoietin systems.[27,62,89,111,122] It is unknown whether the therapeutic use of these master-switch genes could lead to excessive, uncontrolled angiogenesis; their use should therefore be restricted until they are better understood and their tissue distribution reliably confined to a target tissue.

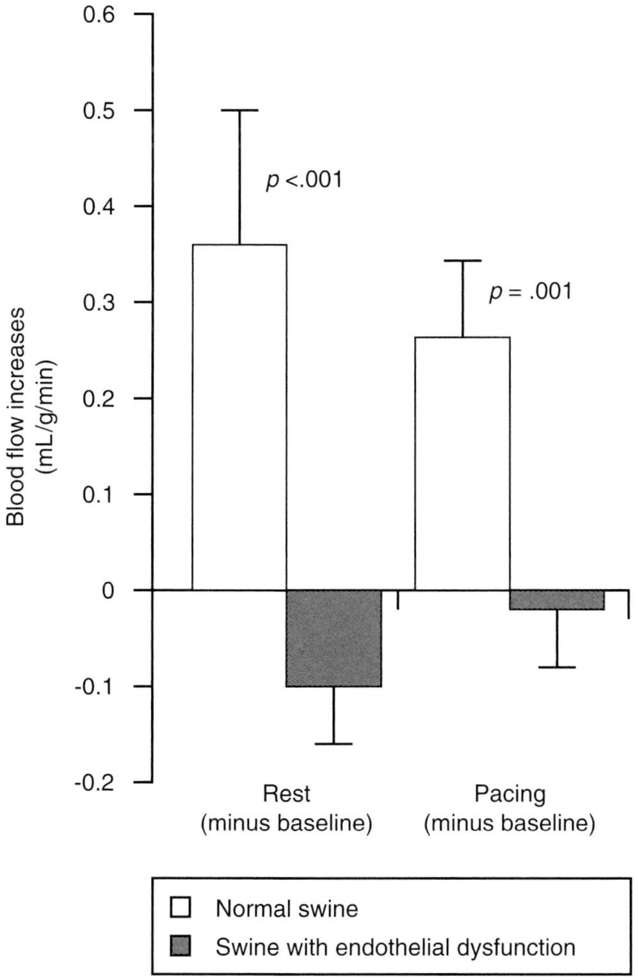

Figure 88–8 Lateral blood flow increases 4 weeks after perivascular FGF-2 therapy in normal swine and in swine with endothelial dysfunction secondary to chronic hypercholesterolemia. All swine had an ameroid constrictor placed around the circumflex coronary artery 7 weeks earlier. Only normal swine developed a functional angiogenic response; swine with endothelial dysfunction had no blood flow increase in response to FGF-2.

Combination of Therapeutic Angiogenesis with TMR

Experience in preclinical models of angiogenic therapy combined with transmyocardial laser revascularization (TMR) has been mixed, with some investigators reporting an increased inflammatory response from the addition of VEGF therapy to TMR in lieu of the enhanced angiogenic response that was anticipated.[22] Burkhoff and colleagues combined TMR and intramyocardial FGF-2 treatment directly into the channels in chronically ischemic dogs and found that this combination resulted in an increase in the density of large vessels (>50 μm), in keeping with the postulated arteriogenic effects of FGF-2 in ischemic tissues, but no augmentation of myocardial blood flow.[132] The combination of gene transfer vectors with TMR also produced mixed results, with one group showing that TMR enhanced the transfection efficiency of an expression plasmid encoding for VEGF at 6 weeks,[98] but another group reporting impaired transgene expression of an adenoviral vector gene and increased myocardial inflammation from combination of the two therapies.[39] No experience with combining angiogenic therapy with TMR in humans has yet been reported.

SUMMARY

Angiogenesis is a promising modality for the treatment of coronary disease. It is still experimental, reserved for selected patients with inoperable diffuse distal coronary disease, and likely more efficacious if performed with a perivascular/intramyocardial approach rather than with intravascular administration. Whether a sustained-release protein-, a gene-, or more recently a cell-based approach will prove safer and more effective than the others remains to be determined. With ongoing research efforts directed at overcoming the numerous limitations of current angiogenic regimens, it is plausible that stimulation of angiogenesis for therapeutic purposes will one day specifically recreate the natural process of vascularization that humans undergo during growth and development and become a major modality for the treatment of coronary artery disease.

REFERENCES

1. Arnal JF, Yamin J, Dockery S, Harrison DG: Regulation of endothelial nitric oxide synthase mRNA, protein, and activity during cell growth. Am J Physiol 267:C1381, 1994.
2. Asahara T, Masuda H, Takahashi T, et al: Bone marrow origin of endothelial progenitor cells responsible for postnatal vasculogenesis in physiological and pathological neovascularization. Circ Res 85:221, 1999.
3. Banai S, Jaklitsch MT, Shou M, et al: Angiogenic-induced enhancement of collateral blood flow to ischemic

myocardium by vascular endothelial growth factor in dogs. Circulation 89:2183, 1994.
4. Banai S, Shweiki D, Pinson A, et al: Upregulation of vascular endothelial growth factor expression induced by myocardial ischaemia: implications for coronary angiogenesis. Cardiovasc Res 28:1176, 1994.
5. Barron HV, Sciammarella MG, Lenihan K, et al: Effects of the repeated administration of adenosine and heparin on myocardial perfusion in patients with chronic stable angina pectoris. Am J Cardiol 85:1, 2000.
6. Bush MA, Samara E, Whitehouse MJ, et al: Pharmacokinetics and pharmacodynamics of recombinant FGF-2 in a phase I trial in coronary artery disease. J Clin Pharmacol 41:378, 2001.
7. Carmeliet P: Fibroblast growth factor-1 stimulates branching and survival of myocardial arteries: a goal for therapeutic angiogenesis? Circ Res 87:176, 2000.
8. Carmeliet P: VEGF gene therapy: stimulating angiogenesis or angioma-genesis? Nat Med 6:1102, 2000.
9. Carmeliet P, Collen D: Molecular basis of angiogenesis. Role of VEGF and VE-cadherin. Ann NY Acad Sci 902:249, 2000.
10. Chavakis E, Dimmeler S: Regulation of endothelial cell survival and apoptosis during angiogenesis. Arterioscler Thromb Vasc Biol 22:887, 2002.
11. Chung NA, Belgore F, Li-Saw-Hee FL, et al: Is the hypercoagulable state in atrial fibrillation mediated by vascular endothelial growth factor? Stroke 33:2187, 2002.
12. Chung NA, Lydakis C, Belgore F, et al: Angiogenesis in myocardial infarction. An acute or chronic process? Eur Heart J 23:1604, 2002.
13. Cohen MV, Yang XM, Liu Y, et al: A new animal model of controlled coronary artery occlusion in conscious rabbits. Cardiovasc Res 28:61, 1994.
14. Conway EM, Collen D, Carmeliet P: Molecular mechanisms of blood vessel growth. Cardiovasc Res 49:507, 2001.
15. Cuevas P, Garcia-Calvo M, Carceller F, et al: Correction of hypertension by normalization of endothelial levels of fibroblast growth factor and nitric oxide synthase in spontaneously hypertensive rats. Proc Natl Acad Sci USA 93:11996, 1996.
16. Dor Y, Djonov V, Abramovitch R, et al: Conditional switching of VEGF provides new insights into adult neovascularization and pro-angiogenic therapy. EMBO J 21:1939, 2002.
17. Duan J, Murohara T, Ikeda H, et al: Hypercholesterolemia inhibits angiogenesis in response to hindlimb ischemia: nitric oxide-dependent mechanism. Circulation 102:III370, 2000.
18. Dubey RK, Gillespie DG, Jackson EK: A(2B) adenosine receptors stimulate growth of porcine and rat arterial endothelial cells. Hypertension 39:530, 2002.
19. Edelberg JM, Lee SH, Kaur M, et al: Platelet-derived growth factor-AB limits the extent of myocardial infarction in a rat model: feasibility of restoring impaired angiogenic capacity in the aging heart. Circulation 105:608, 2002.
20. Edelman ER, Nugent MA, Karnovsky MJ: Perivascular and intravenous administration of basic fibroblast growth factor: vascular and solid organ deposition. Proc Natl Acad Sci USA 90:1513, 1993.
21. Edelman ER, Mathiowitz E, Langer R, Klagsbrun M: Controlled and modulated release of basic fibroblast growth factor. Biomaterials 12:619, 1991.
22. Fleischer KJ, Goldschmidt-Clermont PJ, Fonger JD, et al: One-month histologic response of transmyocardial laser channels with molecular intervention. Ann Thorac Surg 62:1051, 1996.
23. Floege J, Kriz W, Schulze M, et al: Basic fibroblast growth factor augments podocyte injury and induces glomerulosclerosis in rats with experimental membranous nephropathy. J Clin Invest 96:2809, 1995.
24. Folkman J, Shing Y: Angiogenesis. J Biol Chem 267:10931, 1992.
25. Freedman SB, Vale P, Kalka C, et al: Plasma vascular endothelial growth factor (VEGF) levels after intramuscular and intramyocardial gene transfer of VEGF-1 plasmid DNA. Hum Gene Ther 13:1595, 2002.
26. Fujita M, McKown DP, McKown MD, Franklin D: Changes in coronary flow following repeated brief coronary occlusion in the conscious dog. Heart Vessels 2:87, 1986.
27. Gavino ES, Furst DE: Recombinant relaxin: a review of pharmacology and potential therapeutic use. BioDrugs 15:609, 2001.
28. Gibson CM, Ryan K, Sparano A, et al: Angiographic methods to assess human coronary angiogenesis. Am Heart J 137:169, 1999.
29. Gilgenkrantz H, Duboc D, Juillard V, et al: Transient expression of genes transferred in vivo into heart using first-generation adenoviral vectors: role of the immune response. Hum Gene Ther 6:1265, 1995.
30. Goto F, Goto K, Weindel K, Folkman J: Synergistic effects of vascular endothelial growth factor and basic fibroblast growth factor on the proliferation and cord formation of bovine capillary endothelial cells within collagen gels. Lab Invest 69:508, 1993.
31. Graham MM, Chambers RJ, Davies RF: Angiographic quantification of diffuse coronary artery disease: reliability and prognostic value for bypass operations. J Thorac Cardiovasc Surg 118:618, 1999.
32. Granger HJ, Ziche M, Hawker JR Jr, et al: Molecular and cellular basis of myocardial angiogenesis. Cell Mol Biol Res 40:81, 1994.
33. Gu JW, Elam J, Sartin A, et al: Moderate levels of ethanol induce expression of vascular endothelial growth factor and stimulate angiogenesis. Am J Physiol Regul Integr Comp Physiol 281:R365, 2001.
34. Harada K, Friedman M, Lopez JJ, et al: Vascular endothelial growth factor administration in chronic myocardial ischemia. Am J Physiol 270:H1791, 1996.
35. Harada K, Grossman W, Friedman M, et al: Basic fibroblast growth factor improves myocardial function in chronically ischemic porcine hearts. J Clin Invest 94:623, 1994.
36. Heeschen C, Jang JJ, Weis M, et al: Nicotine stimulates angiogenesis and promotes tumor growth and atherosclerosis. Nat Med 7:833, 2001.
37. Henry TD, Abraham JA: Review of preclinical and clinical results with vascular endothelial growth factors for therapeutic angiogenesis. Curr Interv Cardiol Rep 2:228, 2000.
38. Hojo Y, Ikeda U, Zhu Y, et al: Expression of vascular endothelial growth factor in patients with acute myocardial infarction. J Am Coll Cardiol 35:968, 2000.
39. Hughes GC, Annex BH, Yin B, et al: Transmyocardial laser revascularization limits in vivo adenoviral-mediated gene transfer in porcine myocardium. Cardiovasc Res 44:81, 1999.
40. Huwer H, Welter C, Ozbek C, et al: Simultaneous surgical revascularization and angiogenic gene therapy in diffuse coronary artery disease. Eur J Cardiothorac Surg 20:1128, 2001.
41. Jang JJ, Ho HK, Kwan HH, et al: Angiogenesis is impaired by hypercholesterolemia: role of asymmetric dimethylarginine. Circulation 102:1414, 2000.
42. Jones EL, Craver JM, Guyton RA, et al: Importance of complete revascularization in performance of the coronary bypass operation. Am J Cardiol 51:7, 1983.
43. Katinioti AA, Tousoulis D, Economou E, et al: Basic fibroblast growth factor changes in response to coronary angioplasty in patients with stable angina. Int J Cardiol 84:195, 2002.
44. Kip KE, Faxon DP, Detre KM, et al: Coronary angioplasty in diabetic patients. The National Heart, Lung, and Blood Institute Percutaneous Transluminal Coronary Angioplasty Registry. Circulation 94:1818, 1996.
45. Klauber N, Browne F, Anand-Apte B, D'Amato RJ: New activity of spironolactone. Inhibition of angiogenesis in vitro and in vivo. Circulation 94:2566, 1996.

46. Kranz A, Rau C, Kochs M, Waltenberger J: Elevation of vascular endothelial growth factor-A serum levels following acute myocardial infarction. Evidence for its origin and functional significance. J Mol Cell Cardiol 32:65, 2000.
47. Kureishi Y, Luo Z, Shiojima I, et al: The HMG-CoA reductase inhibitor simvastatin activates the protein kinase Akt and promotes angiogenesis in normocholesterolemic animals. Nat Med 6:1004, 2000.
48. Laham RJ, Simons M, Sellke F: Gene transfer for angiogenesis in coronary artery disease. Annu Rev Med 52:485, 2001.
49. Laham RJ, Chronos NA, Pike M, et al: Intracoronary basic fibroblast growth factor (FGF-2) in patients with severe ischemic heart disease: results of a phase I open-label dose escalation study. J Am Coll Cardiol 36:2132, 2000.
50. Laham RJ, Rezaee M, Post M, et al: Intracoronary and intravenous administration of basic fibroblast growth factor: myocardial and tissue distribution. Drug Metab Dispos 27:821, 1999.
51. Laham RJ, Rezaee M, Post M, et al: Intrapericardial delivery of fibroblast growth factor-2 induces neovascularization in a porcine model of chronic myocardial ischemia. J Pharmacol Exp Ther 292:795, 2000.
52. Laham RJ, Sellke FW, Edelman ER, et al: Local perivascular delivery of basic fibroblast growth factor in patients undergoing coronary bypass surgery: results of a phase I randomized, double-blind, placebo-controlled trial. Circulation 100:1865, 1999.
53. Lazarous DF, Scheinowitz M, Shou M, et al: Effects of chronic systemic administration of basic fibroblast growth factor on collateral development in the canine heart. Circulation 91:145, 1995.
54. Lazarous DF, Shou M, Scheinowitz M, et al: Comparative effects of basic fibroblast growth factor and vascular endothelial growth factor on coronary collateral development and the arterial response to injury. Circulation 94:1074, 1996.
55. Lazarous DF, Shou M, Stiber JA, et al: Adenoviral-mediated gene transfer induces sustained pericardial VEGF expression in dogs: effect on myocardial angiogenesis. Cardiovasc Res 44:294, 1999.
56. Lederman RJ, Mendelsohn FO, Anderson RD, et al: Therapeutic angiogenesis with recombinant fibroblast growth factor-2 for intermittent claudication (the TRAFFIC study): a randomised trial. Lancet 359:2053, 2002.
57. Lee LY, Patel SR, Hackett NR, et al: Focal angiogen therapy using intramyocardial delivery of an adenovirus vector coding for vascular endothelial growth factor 121. Ann Thorac Surg 69:14, 2000.
58. Lee RJ, Springer ML, Blanco-Bose WE, et al: VEGF gene delivery to myocardium: deleterious effects of unregulated expression. Circulation 102:898, 2000.
59. Lee SH, Wolf PL, Escudero R, et al: Early expression of angiogenesis factors in acute myocardial ischemia and infarction. N Engl J Med 342:626, 2000.
60. Lee YM, Jeong CH, Koo SY, et al: Determination of hypoxic region by hypoxia marker in developing mouse embryos in vivo: a possible signal for vessel development. Dev Dyn 220:175, 2001.
61. Lemstrom KB, Krebs R, Nykanen AI, et al: Vascular endothelial growth factor enhances cardiac allograft arteriosclerosis. Circulation 105:2524, 2002.
62. Li J, Post M, Volk R, et al: PR39, a peptide regulator of angiogenesis. Nat Med 6:49, 2000. Published erratum appears in Nat Med 6(3):356, 2000.
63. Lindahl P, Bostrom H, Karlsson L, et al: Role of platelet-derived growth factors in angiogenesis and alveogenesis. Curr Top Pathol 93:27, 1999.
64. Lopez JJ, Edelman ER, Stamler A, et al: Local perivascular administration of basic fibroblast growth factor: drug delivery and toxicological evaluation. Drug Metab Dispos 24:922, 1996. Published erratum appears in Drug Metab Dispos 24(10):1166, 1996.
65. Lopez JJ, Edelman ER, Stamler A, et al: Basic fibroblast growth factor in a porcine model of chronic myocardial ischemia: a comparison of angiographic, echocardiographic and coronary flow parameters. J Pharmacol Exp Ther 282:385, 1997.
66. Lopez JJ, Edelman ER, Stamler A, et al: Angiogenic potential of perivascularly delivered aFGF in a porcine model of chronic myocardial ischemia. Am J Physiol 274:H930, 1998.
67. Lopez JJ, Laham RJ, Carrozza JP, et al: Hemodynamic effects of intracoronary VEGF delivery: evidence of tachyphylaxis and NO dependence of response. Am J Physiol 273:H1317, 1997.
68. Lopez JJ, Laham RJ, Stamler A, et al: VEGF administration in chronic myocardial ischemia in pigs. Cardiovasc Res 40:272, 1998.
69. Losordo DW, Vale PR, Hendel RC, et al: Phase 1/2 placebo-controlled, double-blind, dose-escalating trial of myocardial vascular endothelial growth factor 2 gene transfer by catheter delivery in patients with chronic myocardial ischemia. Circulation 105:2012, 2002.
70. Losordo DW, Vale PR, Symes JF, et al: Gene therapy for myocardial angiogenesis: initial clinical results with direct myocardial injection of phVEGF165 as sole therapy for myocardial ischemia. Circulation 98:2800, 1998.
71. Ludmer PL, Selwyn AP, Shook TL, et al: Paradoxical vasoconstriction induced by acetylcholine in atherosclerotic coronary arteries. N Engl J Med 315:1046, 1986.
72. Masferrer J: Approach to angiogenesis inhibition based on cyclooxygenase-2. Cancer J 7(Suppl. 3):S144, 2001.
73. Masferrer JL, Koki A, Seibert K: COX-2 inhibitors. A new class of antiangiogenic agents. Ann NY Acad Sci 889:84, 1999.
74. Matsunaga T, Weihrauch DW, Moniz MC, et al: Angiostatin inhibits coronary angiogenesis during impaired production of nitric oxide. Circulation 105:2185, 2002.
75. Mofidi R, Crotty TB, McCarthy P, et al: Association between plaque instability, angiogenesis and symptomatic carotid occlusive disease. Br J Surg 88:945, 2001.
76. Mukherjee D, Bhatt DL, Roe MT, et al: Direct myocardial revascularization and angiogenesis—how many patients might be eligible? Am J Cardiol 84:598, 1999.
77. Mukherjee D, Comella K, Bhatt DL, et al: Clinical outcome of a cohort of patients eligible for therapeutic angiogenesis or transmyocardial revascularization. Am Heart J 142:72, 2001.
78. Murohara T, Witzenbichler B, Spyridopoulos I, et al: Role of endothelial nitric oxide synthase in endothelial cell migration. Arterioscler Thromb Vasc Biol 19:1156, 1999.
79. Musci M, Loebe M, Wellnhofer E, et al: Coronary angioplasty, bypass surgery, and retransplantation in cardiac transplant patients with graft coronary disease. Thorac Cardiovasc Surg 46:268, 1998.
80. Musci M, Pasic M, Meyer R, et al: Coronary artery bypass grafting after orthotopic heart transplantation. Eur J Cardiothorac Surg 16:163, 1999.
81. Natali A, Vichi S, Landi P, et al: Coronary atherosclerosis in Type II diabetes: angiographic findings and clinical outcome. Diabetologia 43:632, 2000.
82. Nishigami K, Ando M, Hayasaki K: Effects of antecedent anginal episodes and coronary artery stenosis on left ventricular function during coronary occlusion. Am Heart J 130:244, 1995.
83. O'Brien ER, Garvin MR, Dev R, et al: Angiogenesis in human coronary atherosclerotic plaques. Am J Pathol 145:883, 1994.
84. Ortega S, Schaeffer MT, Soderman D, et al: Conversion of cysteine to serine residues alters the activity, stability, and

heparin dependence of acidic fibroblast growth factor. J Biol Chem 266:5842, 1991.
85. Panet R, Markus M, Atlan H: Bumetanide and furosemide inhibited vascular endothelial cell proliferation. J Cell Physiol 158:121, 1994.
86. Pearlman JD, Hibberd MG, Chuang ML, et al: Magnetic resonance mapping demonstrates benefits of VEGF-induced myocardial angiogenesis. Nat Med 1:1085, 1995.
87. Pecher P, Schumacher BA: Angiogenesis in ischemic human myocardium: clinical results after 3 years. Ann Thorac Surg 69:1414, 2000.
88. Pipili-Synetos E, Papageorgiou A, Sakkoula E, et al: Inhibition of angiogenesis, tumour growth and metastasis by the NO-releasing vasodilators, isosorbide mononitrate and dinitrate. Br J Pharmacol 116:1829, 1995.
89. Pola R, Ling LE, Silver M, et al: The morphogen Sonic hedgehog is an indirect angiogenic agent upregulating two families of angiogenic growth factors. Nat Med 7:706, 2001.
90. Risau W: Mechanisms of angiogenesis. Nature 386:671, 1997.
91. Rosengart TK, Lee LY, Patel SR, et al: Angiogenesis gene therapy: phase I assessment of direct intramyocardial administration of an adenovirus vector expressing VEGF121 cDNA to individuals with clinically significant severe coronary artery disease. Circulation 100:468, 1999.
92. Ruel M, Wu GF, Khan TA, et al: Inhibited angiogenic response to surgical FGF-2 protein therapy in a swine model of endothelial dysfunction. Circulation 108:II335–340, 2003.
93. Ruel M, Sellke FW, Bianchi C, et al: Endogenous myocardial angiogenesis and revascularization using a gastric submucosal patch. Ann Thorac Surg 75:1443–1449, 2003.
94. Ruel M, Laham RJ, Parker JA, et al: Long-term effects of surgical angiogenic therapy with fibroblast growth factor 2 protein. J Thorac Cardiovasc Surg 124:28, 2002.
95. Sasaki T, Jyo Y, Tanda N, et al: Changes in glomerular epithelial cells induced by FGF2 and FGF2 neutralizing antibody in puromycin aminonucleoside nephropathy. Kidney Int 51: 301, 1997.
96. Sato K, Laham RJ, Pearlman JD, et al: Efficacy of intracoronary versus intravenous FGF-2 in a pig model of chronic myocardial ischemia. Ann Thorac Surg 70:2113, 2000.
97. Sato K, Wu T, Laham RJ, et al: Efficacy of intracoronary or intravenous VEGF165 in a pig model of chronic myocardial ischemia. J Am Coll Cardiol 37:616, 2001.
98. Sayeed-Shah U, Mann MJ, Martin J, et al: Complete reversal of ischemic wall motion abnormalities by combined use of gene therapy with transmyocardial laser revascularization. J Thorac Cardiovasc Surg 116:763, 1998.
99. Schaper W, Ito WD: Molecular mechanisms of coronary collateral vessel growth. Circ Res 79:911, 1996.
100. Schumacher B, Pecher P, von Specht BU, Stegmann T: Induction of neoangiogenesis in ischemic myocardium by human growth factors: first clinical results of a new treatment of coronary heart disease. Circulation 97:645, 1998.
101. Scott R, Blackstone EH, McCarthy PM, et al: Isolated bypass grafting of the left internal thoracic artery to the left anterior descending coronary artery: late consequences of incomplete revascularization. J Thorac Cardiovasc Surg 120:173, 2000.
102. Sellke FW, Ruel M: Vascular growth factors and angiogenesis in cardiac surgery. Ann Thorac Surg 75:S691–699, 2003.
103. Sellke FW, Kagaya Y, Johnson RG, et al: Endothelial modulation of porcine coronary microcirculation perfused via immature collaterals. Am J Physiol 262:H1669, 1992.
104. Sellke FW, Laham RJ, Edelman ER, et al: Therapeutic angiogenesis with basic fibroblast growth factor: technique and early results. Ann Thorac Surg 65:1540, 1998.
105. Sellke FW, Li J, Stamler A, et al: Angiogenesis induced by acidic fibroblast growth factor as an alternative method of revascularization for chronic myocardial ischemia. Surgery 120:182, 1996.
106. Sellke FW, Wang SY, Friedman M, et al: Basic FGF enhances endothelium-dependent relaxation of the collateral-perfused coronary microcirculation. Am J Physiol 267:H1303, 1994.
107. Sellke FW, Wang SY, Stamler A, et al: Enhanced microvascular relaxations to VEGF and bFGF in chronically ischemic porcine myocardium. Am J Physiol 271:H713, 1996.
108. Shalala D: Protecting research subjects—what must be done. N Engl J Med 343:808, 2000.
109. Sharma HS, Wunsch M, Brand T, et al: Molecular biology of the coronary vascular and myocardial responses to ischemia. J Cardiovasc Pharmacol 20(Suppl. 1):S23, 1992.
110. Shaukat N, Lear J, Lowy A, et al: First myocardial infarction in patients of Indian subcontinent and European origin: comparison of risk factors, management, and long term outcome. BMJ 314:639, 1997.
111. Simons M: Therapeutic coronary angiogenesis: a fronte praecipitium a tergo lupi? Am J Physiol Heart Circ Physiol 280:H1923, 2001.
112. Simons M, Annex BH, Laham RJ, et al: Pharmacological treatment of coronary artery disease with recombinant fibroblast growth factor-2: double-blind, randomized, controlled clinical trial. Circulation 105:788, 2002.
113. Simons M, Bonow RO, Chronos NA, et al: Clinical trials in coronary angiogenesis: issues, problems, consensus: an expert panel summary. Circulation 102:E73, 2000.
114. Stewart DJ: A phase 2, randomized, multicenter, 26-week study to assess the efficacy and safety of BIOBYPASS (AdGVVEGF121.10) delivered through minimally invasive surgery versus maximum medical treatment in patients with severe angina, advanced coronary artery disease, and no options for revascularization. Circulation 106:2986, 2002.
115. Suri C, Jones PF, Patan S, et al: Requisite role of angiopoietin-1, a ligand for the TIE2 receptor, during embryonic angiogenesis. Cell 87:1171, 1996.
116. Symes JF, Losordo DW, Vale PR, et al: Gene therapy with vascular endothelial growth factor for inoperable coronary artery disease. Ann Thorac Surg 68:830, 1999.
117. Takeshita S, Weir L, Chen D, et al: Therapeutic angiogenesis following arterial gene transfer of vascular endothelial growth factor in a rabbit model of hindlimb ischemia. Biochem Biophys Res Commun 227:628, 1996.
118. Takeshita S, Zheng LP, Brogi E, et al: Therapeutic angiogenesis. A single intraarterial bolus of vascular endothelial growth factor augments revascularization in a rabbit ischemic hind limb model. J Clin Invest 93:662, 1994.
119. Tateno S, Terai M, Niwa K, et al: Alleviation of myocardial ischemia after Kawasaki disease by heparin and exercise therapy. Circulation 103:2591, 2001.
120. Thurston G, Suri C, Smith K, et al: Leakage-resistant blood vessels in mice transgenically overexpressing angiopoietin-1. Science 286:2511, 1999.
121. Tofukuji M, Metais C, Li J, et al: Myocardial VEGF expression after cardiopulmonary bypass and cardioplegia. Circulation 98:II242, 1998.
122. Unemori EN, Lewis M, Constant J, et al: Relaxin induces vascular endothelial growth factor expression and angiogenesis selectively at wound sites. Wound Repair Regen 8:361, 2000.
123. Unger EF, Banai S, Shou M, et al: A model to assess interventions to improve collateral blood flow: continuous administration of agents into the left coronary artery in dogs. Cardiovasc Res 27:785, 1993.
124. Unger EF, Banai S, Shou M, et al: Basic fibroblast growth factor enhances myocardial collateral flow in a canine model. Am J Physiol 266:H1588, 1994.

125. Unger EF, Shou M, Sheffield CD, et al: Extracardiac to coronary anastomoses support regional left ventricular function in dogs. Am J Physiol 264:H1567, 1993.
126. Vale PR, Losordo DW, Milliken CE, et al: Randomized, single-blind, placebo-controlled pilot study of catheter-based myocardial gene transfer for therapeutic angiogenesis using left ventricular electromechanical mapping in patients with chronic myocardial ischemia. Circulation 103:2138, 2001.
127. Varghese PJ, Arumugam SB, Cherian KM, et al: Atheromatous plaque reflects serum total cholesterol levels: a comparative morphologic study of endarterectomy coronary atherosclerotic plaques removed from patients from the southern part of India and Caucasians from Ottawa, Canada. Clin Cardiol 21:335, 1998.
128. Verma S, Wang CH, Li SH, et al: A self-fulfilling prophecy: C-reactive protein attenuates nitric oxide production and inhibits angiogenesis. Circulation 106:913, 2002.
129. Volpert OV, Ward WF, Lingen MW, et al: Captopril inhibits angiogenesis and slows the growth of experimental tumors in rats. J Clin Invest 98:671, 1996.
130. White FC, Carroll SM, Magnet A, Bloor CM: Coronary collateral development in swine after coronary artery occlusion. Circ Res 71:1490, 1992.
131. Xu X, Li J, Simons M, et al: Expression of vascular endothelial growth factor and its receptors is increased, but microvascular relaxation is impaired in patients after acute myocardial ischemia. J Thorac Cardiovasc Surg 121:735, 2001.
132. Yamamoto N, Kohmoto T, Roethy W, et al: Histologic evidence that basic fibroblast growth factor enhances the angiogenic effects of transmyocardial laser revascularization. Basic Res Cardiol 95:55, 2000.
133. Yancopoulos GD, Davis S, Gale NW, et al: Vascular-specific growth factors and blood vessel formation. Nature 407:242, 2000.
134. Zhang X, Zhao SP, Li XP, et al: Endothelium-dependent and -independent functions are impaired in patients with coronary heart disease. Atherosclerosis 149:19, 2000.

Transmyocardial Laser Revascularization

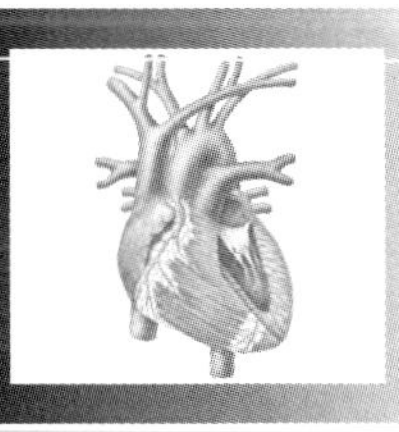

Keith A. Horvath

CHAPTER 89

INTRODUCTION

History

Before the advent of the conventional methods of myocardial revascularization (coronary artery bypass grafting [CABG] or percutaneous coronary interventions [PCI]), attempts were made to revascularize the heart by direct perfusion. An example of an operation designed to provide direct perfusion was Vinberg's method of implanting the internal mammary artery into the myocardium.[86] Additional attempts were based on Wearn's description of sinusoids that allowed blood to flow directly from the ventricle into the myocardium.[87] These arterioluminal connections provide perfusion in more primitive vertebrate hearts and clinically occur in children with pulmonary atresia, an intact ventricular septum, and proximal obstruction of the coronary arteries. Such attempts included myocardial acupuncture as performed by Sen and others[78] to establish direct perfusion and theoretically to recreate a coronary microcirculation similar to that of the reptilian heart. Additional methods of attempting to improve myocardial blood flow include Beck's creation of a form of superficial angiogenesis as a response to epicardial and pericardial inflammation.[7] combining the acupuncture, implantation, and inflammation techniques, Massimo and Boffi[63] as well as Borst and colleagues[88] used hollow tubes implanted in the myocardium to establish direct perfusion. Results from all of these procedures yielded limited success. The angina relief obtained was not longlasting, difficult to replicate, and, most importantly, eventually overshadowed by the ability to perform CABG. Since then, numerous patients have been successfully treated with conventional methods, such as CABG or PCI, but there are a significant and increasing number of patients who have exhausted the ability to undergo these procedures repeatedly, because of the diffuse nature of their coronary artery disease. As a result, they have chronic disabling angina that is often refractory to medical therapy. Transmyocardial laser revascularization (TMR) was developed to treat these patients. The mechanical trauma that resulted in poor long-term patency of myocardial acupuncture was overcome in theory by using a laser to create the channels. Although Mirhoseini et al[67,68] and Okada et al[72,73] pioneered the use of a laser to perform this type of revascularization in conjunction with coronary artery bypass grafting in the early 1980s, the use of a laser as sole therapy to establish its efficacy required advancements in the technology. The carbon dioxide (CO_2) laser used by Mirhoseini had a peak output of 80 W and therefore required a significant amount of time to complete a transmural channel. As a result, to optimally perform TMR, the heart had to be chilled and still. Increasing the output of the laser to 800 W allowed TMR to be performed on a beating heart. This breakthrough led to the widespread clinical application of TMR. Since then, over 10,000 patients have been treated with TMR around the world and results from individual institutions, multicenter studies, and prospective randomized control trials have been reported.*

Clinical Results

The early nonrandomized trials demonstrated that sole therapy TMR could be performed safely on patients with severe coronary artery disease who previously had no options. The significant angina relief seen in such patients led to prospective randomized studies to further demonstrate the efficacy of TMR. In these pivotal trials over 1000 patients were enrolled and randomized to receiving TMR or medical management for their severe angina.† The six trials employed a 1:1 randomization in which one half of the patients were treated with laser

*References 3, 5, 9, 13, 18, 21, 27, 34, 43, 53, 65, 77.

†References 1, 5, 9, 21, 43, 77.

and patients in the control group were continued on maximal medical therapy. All patients were followed up for 12 months.

METHODS

Patients

The entry criteria for these studies, and for sole therapy TMR in general, are as follows: patients had refractory angina that was not amenable to standard methods of revascularization as verified by a recent angiogram. They had evidence of reversible ischemia based on myocardial perfusion scanning, and their left ventricular ejection fractions were greater than 25%.

The typical profile of TMR patients is given in Table 89-1. Because the patients were equally randomized to the medical management group there were no significant demographic differences between the TMR and the control groups for any of these trials. Two different wavelengths of laser light were used. Three studies[5,9,43] employed a holmium:yttrium–aluminum–garnett (Ho:YAG) laser and three[1,21,77] used a carbon dioxide (CO_2) laser. The average patient age was 62 years and the majority were male (86%). Although there were significant differences in the baseline distribution of patients according to Canadian Cardiovascular Society (CCS) Angina Class, the majority of the patients were in angina class IV (61%). The ejection fractions for all of the patients were mildly diminished at 48 ± 10%. Many of the patients had suffered at least one previous myocardial infarction and had some prior revascularization, CABG, and/or PCI. Two of the trials[5,21] permitted a crossover from the medical management group to laser treatment for the presence of unstable angina that necessitated intravenous antianginal therapy for which they were unweanable over a period of at least 48 h. By definition, these crossover patients were less stable and significantly different than those who had been initially randomized to TMR or medical management alone.

Table 89–1

Baseline Characteristics of TMR Patients

Average age	62
Women	14%
CCS angina class III	39%
CCS angina class IV	61%
Ejection fraction (mean +/– SD)	48 +/– 10%
Previous MI	72%
Previous CABG	83%
Previous PTCA	37%
IDDM	32%

TMR, transmyocardial revascularization; CCS, Canadian Cardiovascular Society; MI, myocardial infarction; CABG, coronary artery bypass grafting; PTCA, percutaneous transluminal coronary angioplasty; IDDM, insulin-dependent diabetes mellitus.

Operative Technique

For sole therapy TMR, patients undergo a left anterior thoracotomy in the fifth intercostal space (Figure 89-1). The patient is placed in a supine position with the left side slightly elevated. Skin preparation includes at least one groin, particularly in patients with low ejection fractions or unstable angina who may require intraoperative placement of an intraaortic balloon pump. General anesthesia is established using a double-lumen endotracheal tube or a bronchial blocker to isolate the left lung. Although not mandatory, this facilitates the operation, particularly as most of the patients have pleural and mediastinal adhesions from previous bypass surgery. Additionally, a thoracic epidural catheter can be employed to provide postoperative pain control.

Once the ribs are spread by a retractor, the lung is deflated and the pericardium is opened to expose the epicardial surface of the heart (Figure 89-2). Care must be taken to avoid previous bypass grafts. The left anterior descending artery is identified and used as a landmark of the location of the septum. The inferior and posterior lateral portions of the heart can be reached through this incision with a combination of manual traction, placement of packing behind the heart, and, as illustrated, with the use of a right-angled laser handpiece. Channels are created starting near the base of the heart and then serially in a line approximately 1 cm apart toward the apex, starting inferiorly and working superiorly to the anterior surface of the heart. As there is some bleeding from the channels, commencement of the TMR inferiorly keeps the anterior area clear and expedites the procedure. The number of channels created depends on the size of the heart and on the size of the ischemic area. Myocardium that is thinned by scar, particularly when the scar is transmural, should be avoided as TMR will be of no benefit to these regions and bleeding from channels in these areas may be problematic.

The thoracotomy is then closed after the placement of a chest tube and, in the majority of the cases, the patient is extubated in the operating room.

The handpiece in Figure 89-2 is from a CO_2 laser and illustrates one of the differences between the two lasers employed for TMR. The CO_2 laser energy is delivered via hollow tubes and is reflected by mirrors to reach the epicardial surface. Channels of 1 mm are made with a 20–30 J pulse. The firing of the laser is synchronized to occur on the R wave of the ECG to avoid arrhythmias. The transmural channel is created by a signal pulse in 40 ms and can be confirmed by transesophageal echocardiography (TEE). The vaporization of blood by the laser energy as the laser beam enters the ventricle creates an obvious and characteristic acoustic effect as noted on TEE. The Ho:YAG laser achieves a similar 1-mm channel by manually advancing a fiber through the myocardium while the laser fires. Typical pulse energies are 2 J for

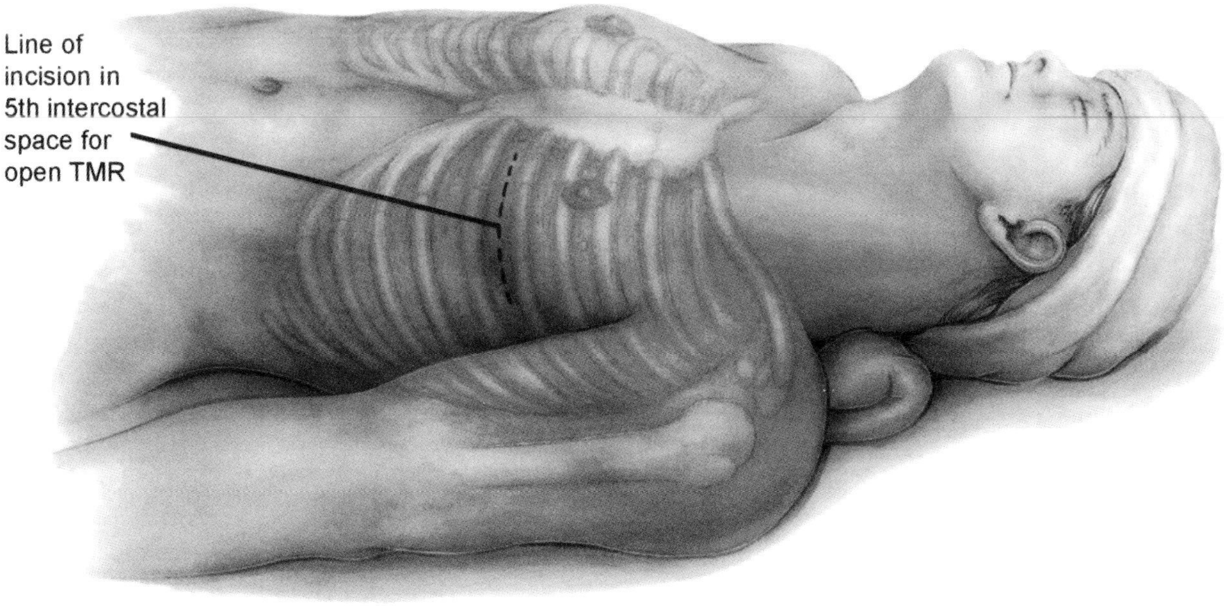

Figure 89–1 Sole therapy transmyocardial laser revascularization performed as an open surgical procedure is typically done through a left anterolateral thoracotomy in the fifth intercostal space. Exposure of the heart through this incision can typically be achieved without division of the ribs or costal cartilages.

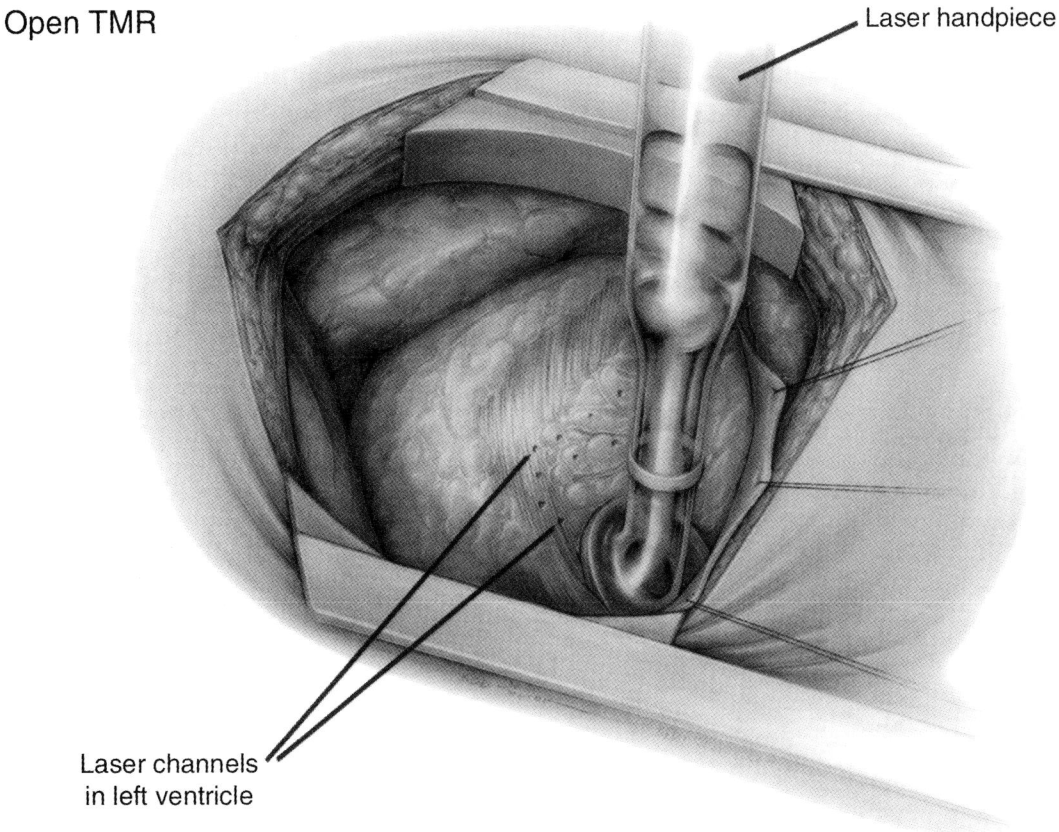

Figure 89–2 Channels are created in a distribution of one per square centimeter, starting inferiorly and then working superiorly to the anterior surface of the heart. The number of channels created depends on the size of the heart and on the size of the ischemic area.

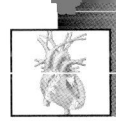

this laser with 20–30 pulses being required to traverse the myocardium. Detection of transmural penetration is primarily by tactile and auditory feedback.

End Points

The principal subjective end point for all of the trials was a change in angina symptoms. This was assessed by the investigator and/or a blinded independent observer. In addition to assigning an angina class, standardized questionnaires such as the Seattle Angina Questionnaire, the Short Form Questionnaire 36 (SF-36), and the Duke Activity Status Index were employed. These tests were used to detect changes in symptoms and quality of life. Objective measurements consisted of repeated exercise tolerance testing as well as repeat myocardial perfusion scans. Patients were reassessed at 3, 6, and 12 months postrandomization.

RESULTS

Mortality

Prior to the randomized studies, mortality rates in the 10–20%* range were reported for TMR patients. In the randomized trials, lower perioperative mortality rates were reported ranging from 1–5%.† One of the important lessons learned from these controlled trials that differ from the earlier studies was a decrease in the mortality when patients taken to the operating room were not unstable, specifically not taking IV heparin or nitroglycerin. When patients were allowed to recover from their most recent episode of unstable angina, and were able to be weaned from IV medications such that their operation could be performed 2 weeks later, the mortality dropped to 1%.[21] The 1-year survival for TMR patients was 85–95% and for medical management patients was 79–95%. Meta-analysis of the 1-year survival demonstrated no statistically significant difference between the patients treated with a laser and those who continued with their medical therapy.

Morbidity

Unlike mortality, the exact definition of various complications varied from one study protocol to the next, and therefore, morbidity data are difficult to pool. Nevertheless, the typical postoperative course had a lower incidence of myocardial infarction, heart failure, and arrhythmias than what has been documented in a similar cohort of patients, those who have reoperative CABG.†

Angina Class

The principal reason for performing TMR is to reduce the patient's anginal symptoms. This can be quantified by assessing the angina class preprocedure and postprocedure. Angina class assessment was performed by a blinded independent observer in all studies. This was done as the only angina assessment or as comparison with the investigators' assessments. Significant symptomatic improvement was seen in all studies for patients treated with the laser. Using a definition of success as a decrease of two or more angina classes, all of the studies demonstrated a significant success rate after TMR ranging from 25–76% (Table 89-2). Significantly fewer patients in the medical management group experienced symptomatic improvement and the success rate for these patients ranged from 0–32%. The seemingly broad range of success is due to differences between the baseline characteristics of the studies. It is more difficult to achieve a two angina class improvement if the baseline angina class is III. Studies that started with most patients in angina class III not surprisingly showed the lowest success rate. In contrast, the largest success rate for TMR was seen in the trial in which all of the patients were in class IV at enrollment. Of note, the medical management group in this study also showed the largest success rate.[5] This underscores some of the baseline differences between the studies.

Quality of Life and Myocardial Function

Quality-of-life indices as assessed by the Seattle Angina Questionnaire, the SF-36, and the Duke Activity Status Index demonstrated significant improvement for TMR-treated patients vs. medical management in every study. Global assessment of myocardial function by ejection fraction using echocardiography or radionuclide multigated acquisition scans showed no significant change in the overall ejection fraction for any of the patients, regardless of group assignment or study.

Hospital Admission

Another indicator of the efficacy of TMR was demonstrated in a reduction in hospital admissions for unstable angina or cardiac-related events postprocedure. A meta-analysis of the data provided indicates that the 1-year hospitalization rate of patients in the laser-treated group was statistically significantly less than for those treated medically. Medical man-

Table 89–2

One-Year Success Rate for Randomized Trials of TMR versus Medical Management (MM)[a]

Study	*Laser*	*MM (%)*	*TMR (%)*
Aaberge et al[1]	CO_2	0	39
Schofield et al[77]	CO_2	4	25
Burkhoff et al[9]	Ho:YAG	11	61
Frazier et al[21]	CO_2	13	72
Allen et al[4]	Ho:YAG	32	76

[a]Success rate = proportion of patients who experienced a decrease of two or more angina classes.

*References 13, 18, 27, 34, 37, 53, 65.
†References 1, 5, 9, 21, 43, 77.

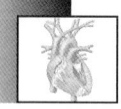

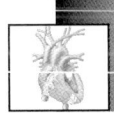

agement patients were admitted four times more frequently than TMR patients over the year of follow-up.[30]

Exercise Tolerance

Additional functional test assessment using exercise tolerance was also performed in three of the trials.[1,9,77] While the method of treadmill testing differed between the trials, the results demonstrate an improvement in exercise tolerance for TMR-treated patients. Two studies showed an average of 65–70 s improvement in the TMR group at 12 months compared to their baseline, while the medical management group had either an average of 5 s improvement or a 46 s decrease in exercise time over the same interval.[1,77] One additional trial demonstrated that the time to chest pain during exercise increased significantly and fewer patients were limited by chest pain in the TMR group, whereas the medical management group showed no improvement.[1]

Medical Treatment

All of the studies employed protocols that continued all of the patients on maximal medical therapy. For each study the frequencies and dosages of antianginal and cardiovascular drugs were similar between the two groups at baseline. TMR patients as a result of their symptomatic improvement had a reduction in their medication use over the year of follow-up. As many of these patients used a combination of short- and long-acting nitrates preoperatively, the trials demonstrated a significant decrease in the use of nitrates in TMR-treated patients while the medical management patients showed a slight increase in their nitrate usage. The overall medication use decreased or remained unchanged in 83% of the TMR patients and, conversely, the use of medications increased or remained unchanged in 86% of the medical management patients.[21]

Myocardial Perfusion

As previously stated, myocardial perfusion scans were obtained preoperatively to verify the extent and severity of reversible ischemia. The four largest randomized trials included follow-up scans as part of their study.[5,9,21,77] These results reflect over 800 of the patients randomized. The methodology of recording and analyzing these results differed in each study so it is difficult to pool the data. Nevertheless, review of the results demonstrated an improvement in perfusion for CO_2 TMR-treated patients. Fixed (scar) and reversible (ischemic defects) were tallied for both the TMR-treated patients and the medical management groups. A CO_2 study demonstrated a significant decrease in the number of reversible defects for both the TMR and the medical management patients.[77] This improvement in the reversible defects in the TMR group was seen without a significant increase in the fixed defects at the end of the study. However, the number of fixed defects in the medical management group had nearly doubled over the same interval. Similarly, there was a 20% improvement in the perfusion of previously ischemic areas in the CO_2 TMR group of another trial and in that same trial there was a 27% worsening of the perfusion of the ischemic areas in the medical management group at 12 months.[21] There was no difference in the number of fixed defects between the groups at 12 months, nor was there a significant change in the number of fixed defects for each patient compared with their baseline scans. The remaining two Ho:YAG studies that obtained follow-up scans showed no significant difference between the TMR and the medical management groups at 12 months and no significant improvement in perfusion in the TMR-treated patients over the same interval.[5,9]

Long-Term Results

Long-term results of Ho:YAG and CO_2 TMR also differ. As noted, after Ho:YAG TMR, significant short-term angina relief was demonstrated at 1 year, as the average angina class fell from 3.5 ± 0.5 at baseline to 1.8 ± 0.8 at 1 year ($p < 0.01$). However the average angina class at 3 years after Ho:YAG TMR significantly increased to 2.2 ± 0.7 ($p = 0.003$ vs. 1 year).[14,76] Additionally, at 3 years only 30% of the patients had a two class improvement in angina compared to their baseline and 70% had a one class improvement (Figure 89-3A). Long-term results with the CO_2 laser were markedly different. As reported, these results demonstrate a decrease in angina class from 3.7 ± 0.4 at baseline to 1.6 ± 1.0 at 5 years ($p = 0.0001$).[31] This was unchanged from the 1.5 ± 1.0 average angina class at 1 year of follow-up (p = ns vs. 5 years). Additionally, 68% of the patients at 5 years had a two or more angina class improvement and 17% had no angina with a length of follow-up out to 7 years (Figure 89-3B). As would be expected, the patient's quality of life improvements were also maintained long term. Additionally, one report of late clinical follow-up of another of the randomized control trials also demonstrated continued symptomatic improvement with CO_2 TMR.[2] This study is noteworthy in that the medical management arm of the original randomized trial was also followed long term. In this study with up to 5 years of follow-up, the average angina class for CO_2 TMR-treated patients decreased from 3.3 at baseline to 2.0 at follow-up. Over the same interval, the medical management group average angina class increased from 3.2 to 3.7. Only 3% of the medical management group showed a two class angina reduction at 5 plus years, whereas 24% of the TMR-treated patients maintained a two or greater class reduction in angina. Additionally, medical management patients were hospitalized twice as frequently for unstable angina as those treated with CO_2 TMR.

MECHANISMS

Understanding the mechanism of TMR starts with understanding the laser tissue interaction. Although numerous devices,[61,79] including ultrasound,[81] cryoablation,[46] radiofrequency,[15,91] heated needles,[32,89] as well as the aforementioned hollow and solid needles, have been used, none has engendered the same response that is seen with a laser. Additionally, numerous wavelengths of light have also been employed. These include xenon chloride (XeCl),[39,62] neodymium:YAG (ND:YAG),[90] erbium:YAG (Er:YAG),[25] and thulium–holmium–chromium:YAG lasers (THC:YAG).[42] All of these devices have been explored experimentally, but have not been pursued on a significant scale clinically. Only CO_2 and Ho:YAG are used for TMR. The result of any laser tissue interaction is dependent on both laser and tissue variables.[25,42,44] CO_2 has a wavelength of 10,600 nm, whereas

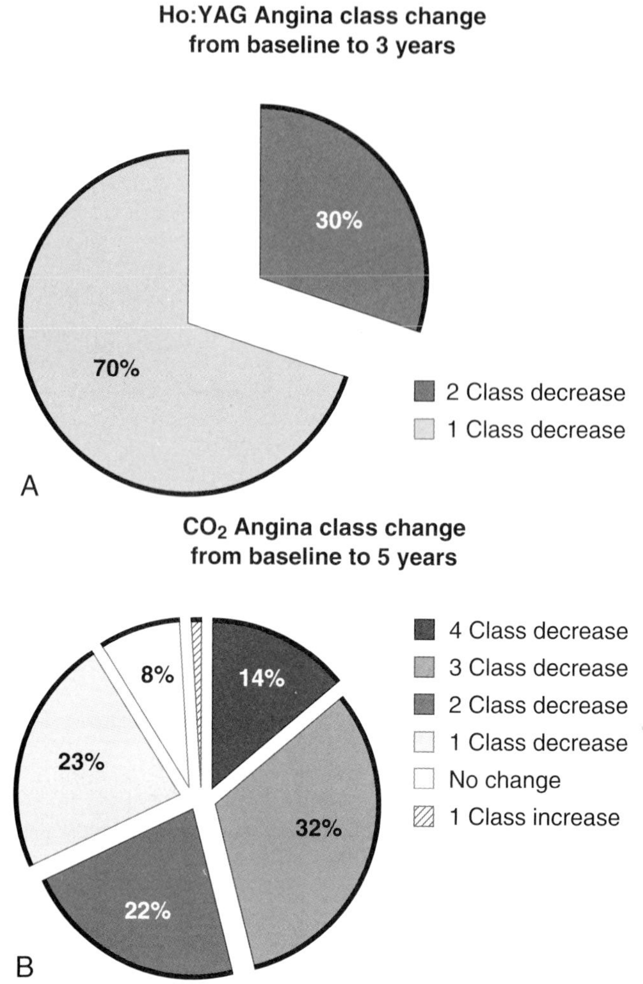

Figure 89–3 (**A**) Distribution of Ho:YAG TMR-treated patients by decrease in CCS angina class; baseline vs. 3 years. (**B**) Distribution of CO_2 TMR-treated patients by decrease in CCS angina class; baseline vs. 5 years.

Ho:YAG has a wavelength of 2120 nm. These infrared wavelengths are primarily absorbed in water and therefore rely on thermal energy to ablate tissue. One significant difference, however, is that the Ho:YAG laser is pulsed and the arrival of two successive pulses must be separated by time to allow for thermal dissipation, otherwise the accumulated heat will cause the tissue to explode under pressure. Such explosions create acoustic waves, which travel along the planes of lower resistance between muscle fibers and cause structural trauma as well as thermocoagulation.[45] The standard operating parameters for the Ho:YAG laser are pulse energies of 1–2 J and 6–8 W/pulse. The energy is delivered at a rate of 5 pulses/s through a flexible 1-mm optical fiber. It takes approximately 20 pulses to create a transmural channel. Despite the low energy level and short pulse duration, there are very high levels of peak power delivered to the tissue so that with each pulse there is an explosion (Figure 89-4). Additionally, the fiber is advanced manually through the myocardium, and it is therefore impossible to know whether the channel is being created by the kinetic energy delivered via the mechanical effects of the fiber or whether there has been enough time for thermal dissipation prior to the next pulse.

In contrast the CO_2 was used at an energy level of 20–30 J/pulse with a pulse duration of 25–40 ms. At this level, the laser photons do not cause explosive ablation and the extent of structural damage is limited. Additionally, a transmural channel can be created with a single pulse (Figure 89-4). Confirmation of this transmuralality is obtained by observing the vaporization of blood within the ventricle using TEE.

Finally the CO_2 laser is synchronized to fire on the R wave and with its short pulse duration arrhythmic complications are minimized. The Ho:YAG device is unsynchronized and due to the motion of the fiber through the myocardium over several cardiac cycles and is more prone to ventricular arrhythmias.

Patent Channels

As noted, the original concept of TMR was to create perfusion via channels connecting the ventricle with the myocardium. Clinical work demonstrated some evidence of long-term patency.[12,69] Additional experimental work showed some evidence of patency as well.[26,38,52,60] There are also significant reports from autopsy series and laboratories that indicate that the channels do not remain patent.[8,24,49,50,80] What evidence there is that channel patency may be a mechanism was only following CO_2 TMR (Figure 89–5). There has never been any evidence that Ho:YAG TMR channels stay patent.

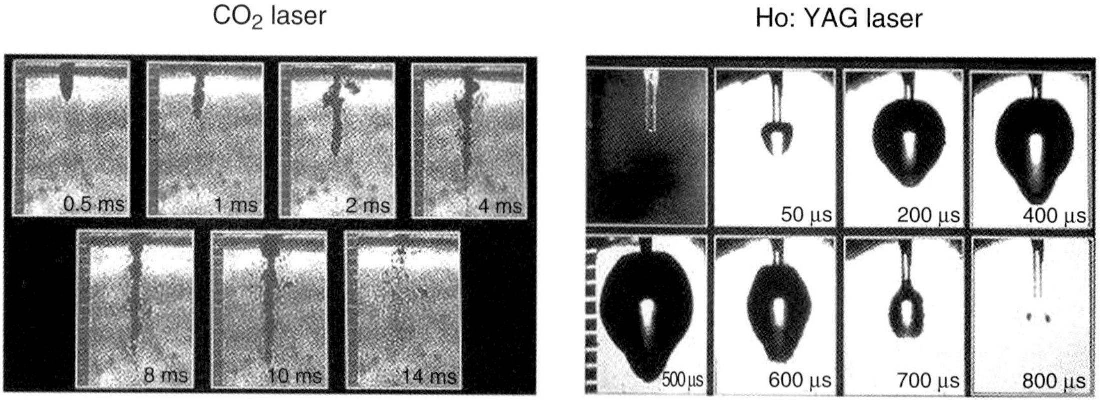

Figure 89–4 Sequential photography of the firing of a single pulse from a CO_2 laser and a Ho:YAG laser into water. The pulse duration and energy levels are the same as those being used clinically.

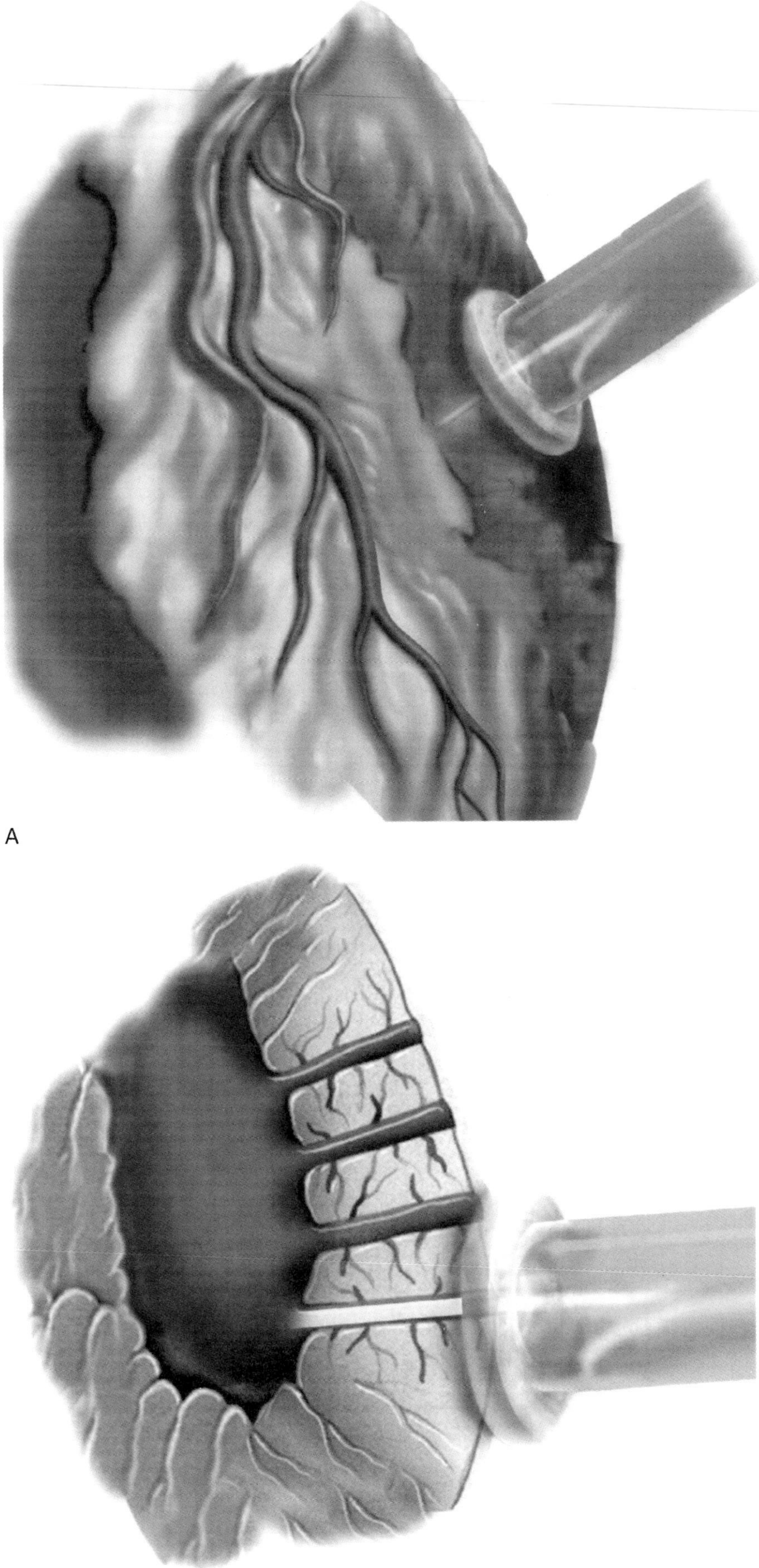

Figure 89–5 **A** and **B,** The CO_2 laser creates a transmural channel in a single 20-J pulse. Conceptually direct perfusion may occur via the channel. Evidence indicates the laser stimulates angiogenesis in and around the channel that leads to improved perfusion.

A

B

Denervation

In contrast to the open channel mechanism, damage to the sympathetic nerve fibers may explain the angina relief noted in clinical trials. The nervous system of the heart can function independently of inputs from extra cardiac neurons to regulate regional cardiac function by reflex action. This intrinsic system contains afferent neurons, sympathetic efferent, postganglionic neurons, and parasympathetic efferent postganglionic neurons. Because of this complex system, it is difficult to demonstrate true denervation. However, several experimental studies have demonstrated that denervation may indeed play a role in Ho:YAG TMR.[28,54,55] Experimental evidence to the contrary was obtained in a nonischemic animal model.[66] Regardless of the methodology employed in the laboratory, there is significant evidence of sympathetic denervation following positron emission tomography of Ho:YAG TMR-treated patients.[6] Although the studies were carefully carried out, it is difficult isolate the sympathetic afferent nerve fibers and the experiments were in the acute setting and address only the short-term effects.

Angiogenesis

The likely underlying mechanism for the clinical efficacy of TMR is the stimulation of angiogenesis. This mechanism fits the clinical picture of significant improvement in symptoms over time as well as a concomitant improvement in perfusion, as seen with the CO_2 laser. Numerous reports have demonstrated a histological increase in neovascularization as a result of TMR channels.* More molecular evidence of this angiogenic phenomenon was derived from work that demonstrated an upregulation of vascular endothelial growth factor (VEGF), messenger RNA, expression of fibroblast growth factor 2 (FGF-2), as well as matrix metalloproteinases following TMR.[33,58,74] Histologically, similar degrees of neovascularization have been noted after mechanical injury of various types. Needle injury has been demonstrated by immunohistochemistry to also stimulate growth factor expression and angiogenesis. The conclusion is that TMR-induced angiogenesis is a nonspecific response to injury.[10,11,61] Investigation of this using hot and cold needles, radiofrequency energy, and laser energy to perform TMR clearly demonstrates a spectrum of tissue response to the injury.[32] The results in a model of chronic myocardial ischemia to mimic the clinical scenario indicate that indeed neovascularization can occur after mechanical TMR, but if these new blood vessels grow in the midst of a scar, there will be little functional contribution from blood flow through these new vessels. The recovery of function with laser TMR was due to a minimization of scar formation and a maximization of angiogenesis.

This then becomes a critical question: if TMR induces angiogenesis, is there an ensuing improvement in function? Clinically, this has been demonstrated subjectively with quality of life assessments, but more importantly, it has been demonstrated objectively with multiple techniques, including dobutamine stress echocardiography,[16] positron emission tomography (PET),[22] and cardiac magnetic resonance imaging (MRI).[47,56] As further evidence of the angiogenic response, experimental data have mirrored the clinical perfusion results noted, with improvements in perfusion in porcine models of chronic ischemia where the ischemic zone was treated with CO_2 TMR.[36,40,51,60] This improved perfusion did lead to an improvement in myocardial function as well.

*References 8, 19, 41, 48, 50, 70, 82, 92, 93.

SUMMARY

Myocardial laser revascularization has been performed percutaneously,[57,71,89] thoracoscopically,[29] via thoracotomy,* and via sternotomy.[4,83,85] Aside from the percutaneous approach, any of the other surgical approaches have yielded similar symptomatic improvement. Several percutaneous trials have attempted to demonstrate a symptomatic improvement with the creation of 2–3 mm deep subendocardial divots achieved with a laser fiber fed via the peripheral artery into the left ventricle.[57,71,84] Even with the use of electromechanical mapping to verify the position of the fiber and the creation of the channel, the results from percutaneous myocardial revascularization (PMR) have been less favorable than those seen with TMR. A recent double-blinded randomized controlled trial showed no benefit to the laser-treated patients compared to the untreated control group.[57] As the patients were blinded to their treatment, the possibility of a significant placebo effect for PMR has been raised. Of note, the morbidity and mortality of PMR are reportedly similar to that seen with TMR. As a result, the United States Food and Drug Administration recently rendered PMR unapprovable. The failure of PMR to achieve the same clinical results seen with TMR may be due to several significant limitations. The first is the partial thickness treatment of the left ventricle. Even at the maximal estimated depth of 6 mm that has been reported with PMR, this is significantly less than the full thickness treatment of the myocardium that is achieved with an open TMR approach. Furthermore, there are typically fewer of these partial thickness channels created with PMR. The exact location of the channel and the establishment of a wide distribution of the channels from inside a moving ventricle are also problematic. Finally, the limitations of the Ho:YAG TMR are also applicable to PMR as that is the wavelength of light that has been employed.

Although the results of sole therapy TMR are encouraging and were necessary to confirm the efficacy of the procedure, the future of TMR is in combination therapy.[4,83,85] Perhaps prescient, Mirhoseini's description[67] of using TMR with CABG provides the likely clinical scenario for the future. As PCI techniques improve and evolve, the patients that undergo coronary artery bypass grafting will more likely than not have more diffuse disease and more occluded coronary arteries. As a result, some territories may be bypassable, but others may be better suited for TMR. A combination of both of these methods will provide a more complete revascularization. Early results with a randomized trial comparing CABG to CABG plus TMR indicated a mortality benefit to undergoing the combined procedure.[4] Unfortunately, the mortality rate for the CABG only patients in the study was high at 7.5% and may be the key contributing factor in the results. Additionally the patients were randomized based on

*References 1, 3, 5, 9, 21, 43, 77.

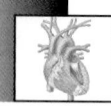

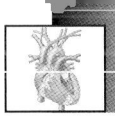

their angiograms and prior to investigation in the operating room. Nevertheless, these results indicate that the combined procedure is feasible, and, in fact, longer term outcomes of CABG plus TMR patients indicate that significant angina relief and low morbidity and mortality can be achieved in such high-risk patients.[83,85]

Other applications include the use of TMR in the treatment of cardiac transplant graft atherosclerosis. Although performed on a small number of patients, the results have indicated a benefit following TMR.[23,64] Finally, the combination of TMR plus other methods of angiogenesis may provide an even more robust response. Experimental work investigating these combinations has verified a synergistic effect with regard to histological evidence of significant angiogenesis and perhaps more importantly an improvement in myocardial function with a combination of TMR and gene therapy vs. either therapy alone.[17,20,35,59,75]

REFERENCES

1. Aaberge L, Nordstrand K, Dragsund M, et al: Transmyocardial revascularization with CO_2 laser in patients with refractory angina pectoris. Clinical results from the Norwegian randomized trial. J Am Coll Cardiol 35(5):1170–1177, 2000.
2. Aaberge L, Rootwelt K, Blomhoff S, et al: Continued symptomatic improvement three to five years after transmyocardial revascularization with CO_2 laser. J Am Coll Cardiol 39(10):1588–1593, 2002.
3. Agarwal R, Ajit M, Kurian VM, et al: Transmyocardial laser revascularization: early results and 1-year follow-up. Ann Thorac Surg 69(6):1993–1995, 2000.
4. Allen KB, Dowling RD, DelRossi AJ, et al: Transmyocardial laser revascularization combined with coronary artery bypass grafting; a multicenter, blinded, prospective, randomized, controlled trial. J Thorac Cardiovasc Surg 119:540–549, 2000.
5. Allen KB, Dowling RD, Fudge TL, et al: Comparison of transmyocardial revascularization with medical therapy in patients with refractory angina. N Engl J Med 341:1029–1036, 1999.
6. Al-Sheikh T, Allen KB, Straka SP, et al: Cardiac sympathetic denervation after transmyocardial laser revascularization. Circulation 100(2):135–140, 1999.
7. Beck CS: The development of a new blood supply to the heart by operation. Ann Surg 102:801–813, 1935.
8. Burkhoff D, Fisher PE, Apfelbaum M, et al: Histologic appearance of transmyocardial laser channels after 41/2 weeks. Ann Thorac Surg 61(5):1532–1535, 1996.
9. Burkhoff D, Schmidt S, Schulman SP, et al: Transmyocardial laser revascularization compared with continued medical therapy for treatment of refractory angina pectoris: a prospective randomized trial. Lancet 354:885–890, 1999.
10. Chu VF, Giaid A, Kuagn JQ, et al: Angiogenesis in transmyocardial revascularization: comparison of laser versus mechanical punctures. Ann Thorac Surg 68(2):301–307, 1999.
11. Chu V, Kuang J, McGinn A, et al: Angiogenic response induced by mechanical transmyocardial revascularization. J Thorac Cardiovasc Surg 118:849–856, 1999.
12. Cooley DA, Frazier OH, Kadipasaoglu KA, et al: Transmyocardial laser revascularization. Anatomic evidence of long-term channel patency. Tex Heart Inst J 21(3):220–224, 1994.
13. Cooley DA, Frazier OH, Kadipasaoglu KA, et al: Transmyocardial laser revascularization: clinical experience with twelve-month follow-up. J Thorac Cardiovasc Surg 111(4):791–797, 1996.
14. De Carlo M, Milano AD, Pratali S, et al: Symptomatic improvement after transmyocardial laser revascularization: how long does it last? Ann Thorac Surg 70(3):1130–1133, 2000.
15. Dietz U, Darius H, Eick O, et al: Transmyocardial revascularization using temperature controlled HF energy creates reproducible intramyocardial channels. Circulation 98:3770, 1998.
16. Donovan CL, Landolfo KP, Lowe JE, et al: Improvement in inducible ischemia during dobutamine stress echocardiography after transmyocardial laser revascularization in patients with refractory angina pectoris. J Am Coll Cardiol 15:281–285, 1997.
17. Doukas J, Ma CL, Craig D, et al: Therapeutic angiogenesis induced by FGF-2 gene delivery combined with laser transmyocardial revascularization. Circulation 102:1214, 2000.
18. Dowling RD, Petracek MR, Selinger SL, et al: Transmyocardial revascularization in patients with refractory, unstable angina. Circulation 98(Suppl. II):II73–II75, 1998.
19. Fisher PE, Khomoto T, DeRosa CM, et al: Histologic analysis of transmyocardial channels: comparison of CO_2 and holmium:YAG lasers. Ann Thorac Surg 64:466–472, 1997.
20. Fleischer KJ, Goldschmidt-Clermont PJ, Fonger JD, et al: One-month histologic response of transmyocardial laser channels with molecular intervention. Ann Thorac Surg 62:1051–1058, 1996.
21. Frazier OH, March RJ, Horvath KA: Transmyocardial revascularization with a carbon dioxide laser in patients with end-stage coronary artery disease. N Engl J Med 341:1021–1028, 1999.
22. Frazier OH, Cooley DA, Kadipasaoglu KA, et al: Myocardial revascularization with laser. Preliminary findings. Circulation 92(Suppl.):II58–II65, 1995.
23. Frazier OH, Kadipasaoglu KA, Radovancevic B, et al: Transmyocardial laser revascularization in allograft coronary artery disease. Ann Thorac Surg 65:1138–1141, 1998.
24. Gassler N, Wintzer HO, Stubbe HM, et al: Transmyocardial laser revascularization: histological features in human nonresponder myocardium. Circulation 95(2):371–375, 1997.
25. Genyk IA, Frenz M, Ott B, et al: Acute and chronic effects of transmyocardial laser revascularization in the nonischemic pig myocardium by using three laser systems. Lasers Surg Med 27:438–450, 2000.
26. Hardy RI, James FW, Millard RW, Kaplan S: Regional myocardial blood flow and cardiac mechanics in dog hearts with CO_2 laser-induced intramyocardial revascularization. Basic Res Cardiol 85(2):179–197, 1990.
27. Hattler BG, Griffith BP, Zenati MA, et al: Transmyocardial laser revascularization in the patient with unmanageable unstable angina. Ann Thorac Surg 68:1203–1209, 1999.
28. Hirsch GM, Thompson GW, Arora RC, et al: Transmyocardial laser revascularization does not denervate the canine heart. Ann Thorac Surg 68(2):460–468, 1999.
29. Horvath KA: Thoracoscopic transmyocardial laser revascularization. Ann Thorac Surg 65:1439–1441, 1998.
30. Horvath KA: Results of prospective randomized controlled trials of transmyocardial laser revascularization. Heart Surg Forum 5(1):33–40, 2002.
31. Horvath KA, Aranki SF, Cohn LH, et al: Sustained angina relief 5 years after transmyocardial laser revascularization with a CO_2 laser. Circulation 104(Suppl. I):I81–I84, 2001.
32. Horvath KA, Belkind N, Wu I, et al: Functional comparison of transmyocardial revascularization by mechanical and laser means. Ann Thorac Surg 72:1997–2002, 2001.
33. Horvath KA, Chiu E, Maun DC, et al: Up-regulation of VEGF mRNA and angiogenesis after transmyocardial laser revascularization. Ann Thorac Surg 68:825–829, 1999.
34. Horvath KA, Cohn LC, Cooley DA, et al: Transmyocardial laser revascularization: results of a multi-center trial using TLR

as sole therapy for end stage coronary artery disease. J Thorac Cardiovasc Surg 113:645–654, 1997.
35. Horvath KA, Doukas J, Lu CJ, et al: Myocardial functional recovery after FGF2 gene therapy as assessed by echocardiography and MRI. Ann Thorac Surg 74:481–487, 2002.
36. Horvath KA, Greene R, Belkind N, et al: Left ventricular functional improvement after transmyocardial laser revascularization. Ann Thorac Surg 66:721–725, 1998.
37. Horvath KA, Mannting F, Cummings N, et al: Transmyocardial laser revascularization: operative techniques and clinical results at two years. J Thorac Cardiovasc Surg 111(5):1047–1053, 1996.
38. Horvath KA, Smith WJ, Laurence RG, et al: Recovery and viability of an acute myocardial infarct after transmyocardial laser revascularization. J Am Coll Cardiol 25:258–263, 1995.
39. Hughes GC, Kypson AP, Annex BH, et al: Induction of angiogenesis after TMR: a comparison of holmium:YAG, CO_2, and excimer lasers. Ann Thorac Surg 70(2):504–509, 2000.
40. Hughes GC, Kypson AP, St Louis JD, et al: Improved perfusion and contractile reserve after transmyocardial laser revascularization in a model of hibernating myocardium. Ann Thorac Surg 67(6):1714–1720, 1999.
41. Hughes GC, Lowe JE, Kypson AP, et al: Neovascularization after transmyocardial laser revascularization in a model of chronic ischemia. Ann Thorac Surg 66:2029–2036, 1998.
42. Jeevanandam V, Auteri JS, Oz MC, et al: Myocardial revascularization by laser-induced channels. Surg Forum 41:225–227, 1990.
43. Jones JW, Schmidt SE, Richman BW, et al: Holmium:YAG laser transmyocardial revascularization relieves angina and improves functional status. Ann Thorac Surg 67:1596–1602, 1999.
44. Kadipasaoglu K, Frazier OH: Transmyocardial laser revascularization: effect of laser parameters of tissue ablation and cardiac perfusion. Sem Thorac Cardiovasc Surg 11:4–11, 1999.
45. Kadipasaoglu KA, Sartori M, Masai T, et al: Intraoperative arrhythmias and tissue damage during transmyocardial laser revascularization. Ann Thorac Surg 67(2):423–431, 1999.
46. Khairy P, Dubuc M, Gallo R: Cryoapplication induces neovascularization: a novel approach to percutaneous myocardial revascularization. J Am Coll Cardiol 35:5A–6A, 2000.
47. Kim RJ, Rafael A, Chen E, et al: Contrast-enhanced MRI predicts wall motion improvement after coronary revascularization. Circulation 100(Suppl.):I-797, 1999.
48. Kohmoto T, Fisher PE, DeRosa C, et al: Evidence of angiogenesis in regions treated with transmyocardial laser revascularization. Circulation 94:1294, 1996.
49. Kohmoto T, Fisher PE, Gu A, et al: Does blood flow through holmium:YAG transmyocardial laser channels? Ann Thorac Surg 61(3):861–868, 1996.
50. Kohmoto T, Fisher PE, Gu A, et al: Physiology, histology, and two week morphology of acute myocardial channels made with a CO_2 laser. Ann Thorac Surg 63:1275–1283, 1997.
51. Krabatsch T, Modersohn D, Konertz W, Hetzer R: Acute changes in functional and metabolic parameters following transmyocardial laser revascularization: an experimental study. Ann Thorac Cardiovasc Surg 6(6):383–388, 2000.
52. Krabatsch T, Schaper F, Leder C, et al: Histologic findings after transmyocardial laser revascularization. J Card Surg 11(5):326–331, 1996.
53. Krabatsch T, Tambeur L, Lieback E, et al: Transmyocardial laser revascularization in the treatment of end-stage coronary artery disease. Ann Thorac Cardiovasc Surg 4(2):64–71, 1998.
54. Kwong KF, Kanellopoulos GK, Nikols JC, Sundt TR III: Transmyocardial laser treatment denervates canine myocardium. J Thorac Cardiovasc Surg 114:883–890, 1997.
55. Kwong KF, Schuessler RB, Kanellopoulos GK, et al: Nontransmural laser treatment incompletely denervates canine myocardium. Circulation 98:1167–1171, 1998.
56. Laham RJ, Simons M, Pearlman JD, et al: Magnetic resonance imaging demonstrates improved regional systolic wall motion and thickening and myocardial perfusion of myocardial territories treated by laser myocardial revascularization. J Am Coll Cardiol 39:1–8, 2002.
57. Leon MB, Baim DS, Moses JW, et al: A randomized blinded clinical trial comparing percutaneous laser myocardial revascularization vs. placebo in patients with refractory coronary ischemia. Circulation 102:II–565, 2000.
58. Li W, Chiba Y, Kimura T, et al: Transmyocardial laser revascularization induced angiogenesis correlated with the expression of matrix metalloproteinase and platelet-derived endothelial cell growth factor. Eur J Cardiothorac Surg 19:156–163, 2001.
59. Lutter G, Dern P, Attmann T, et al: Combined use of transmyocardial laser revascularization with basic fibroblastic growth factor in chronically ischemic porcine hearts. Circulation 102:3693, 2000.
60. Lutter G, Martin J, Ameer K, et al: Microperfusion enhancement after TMLR in chronically ischemic porcine hearts. Cardiovasc Surg 9(3):281–291, 2001.
61. Malekan R, Reynolds C, Narula N, et al: Angiogenesis in transmyocardial laser revascularization: a nonspecific response to injury. Circulation 98(Suppl. II):II62–II66, 1998.
62. Martin JS, Sayeed-Shah U, Byrne JG, et al: Excimer versus carbon dioxide transmyocardial laser revascularization: effects on regional left ventricular function and perfusion. Ann Thorac Surg 69:1811–1816, 2000.
63. Massimo C, Boffi L: Myocardial revascularization by a new method of carrying blood directly from the left ventricular cavity into the coronary circulation. J Thorac Surg 34:257–264, 1957.
64. Mehra MR, Uber PA, Prasad AK, et al: Long-term outcome of cardiac allograft vasculopathy treated by transmyocardial laser revascularization early rewards, late losses. J Heart Lung Transplant 19:801–804, 2000.
65. Milano A, Pratali S, Tartarini G, et al: Early results of transmyocardial revascularization with a holmium laser. Ann Thorac Surg 65:700–704, 1998.
66. Minisi AJ, Topaz O, Quinn MS, et al: Cardiac nociceptive reflexes after transmyocardial laser revascularization: implications for the neural hypothesis of angina relief. J Thorac Cardiovasc Surg 122:712–719, 2001.
67. Mirhoseini M, Fisher JC, Cayton M: Myocardial revascularization by laser: a clinical report. Lasers Surg Med 3(3):241–245, 1983.
68. Mirhoseini M, Muckerheide M, Cayton MM: Transventricular revascularization by laser. Lasers Surg Med 2(2):187–198, 1982.
69. Mirhoseini M, Shelgikar S, Cayton M: Clinical and histological evaluation of laser myocardial revascularization. J Clin Laser Med Surg 8(3):73–77, 1990.
70. Mueller XM, Tevaearai HT, Chaubert P, et al: Does laser injury induce a different neovascularization pattern from mechanical or ischemic injuries? Heart 85:697–701, 2001.
71. Oesterle SN, Sanborn TA, Ali N, et al: Percutaneous transmyocardial laser revascularization for severe angina: PACIFIC randomized trial. Lancet 356:1705–1710, 2000.
72. Okada M, Ikuta H, Shimizu OK, et al: Alternative method of myocardial revascularization by laser: experimental and clinical study. Kobe J Med Sci 32:151–161, 1986.
73. Okada M, Shimizu K, Ikuta H, et al: A new method of myocardial revascularization by laser. Thorac Cardiovasc Surg 39(1):1–4, 1991.
74. Pelletier MP, Giaid A, Sivaraman S, et al: Angiogenesis and growth factor expression in a model of transmyocardial revascularization. Ann Thorac Surg 66:12–18, 1998.

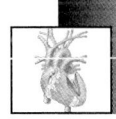

75. Sayeed-Shah U, Mann MJ, Martin J, et al: Complete reversal of ischemic wall motion abnormalities by combined use of gene therapy with transmyocardial laser revascularization. J Thorac Cardiovasc Surg 116:763–768, 1998.
76. Schneider J, Diegeler A, Krakor R, et al: Transmyocardial laser revascularization with the holmium:YAG laser: loss of symptomatic improvement after 2 years. Eur J Cardiothorac Surg 19(2):164–169, 2001.
77. Schofield PM, Sharples LD, Caine N, et al: Transmyocardial laser revascularization in patients with refractory angina: a randomized controlled trial. Lancet 353:519–524, 1999.
78. Sen P, Udwadia T, Kinare S, et al: Transmyocardial revascularization: a new approach to myocardial revascularization. J Thorac Cardiovasc Surg 50:181–189, 1965.
79. Shawl FA, Kaul U, Saadat V: Percutaneous myocardial revascularization using a myocardial channeling device: first human experience using the Angio Trax system. J Am Coll Cardiol 35:61A, 2000.
80. Sigel JE, Abramovitch CM, Lytle BW, et al: Transmyocardial laser revascularization: three sequential autopsy cases. J Thorac Cardiovasc Surg 115:1381–1385, 1998.
81. Smith NB, Hynynen K: The feasibility of using focused ultrasound for transmyocardial revascularization. Ultrasound Med Biol 24:1045–1054, 1998.
82. Spanier T, Smith CR, Burkhoff D: Angiogenesis. A possible mechanism underlying the clinical benefits of transmyocardial laser revascularization. J Clin Laser Med Surg 15:269–273, 1997.
83. Stamou SC, Boyce SW, Cooke RH, et al: One-year outcome after combined coronary artery bypass grafting and transmyocardial laser revascularization for refractory angina pectoris. Am J Cardiol 89:1365–1368, 2002.
84. Stone GW, Teirstein PS, Rubenstein R, et al: A prospective, multicenter, randomized trial of percutaneous transmyocardial laser revascularization in patients with nonrecanalizable chronic total occlusions. J Am Coll Cardiol 39:1581–1587, 2002.
85. Trehan N, Mishra Y, Mehta Y, et al: Transmyocardial laser as an adjunct to minimally invasive CABG for complete myocardial revascularization. Ann Thorac Surg 66:1113–1118, 1998.
86. Vinberg A: Clinical and experimental studies in the treatment of coronary artery insufficiency by internal mammary artery implant. J Int Coll Surg 22:503–518, 1954.
87. Wearn J, Mettier S, Klumpp T, et al: The nature of the vascular communications between the coronary arteries and the chambers of the heart. Am Heart J 9:143–164, 1933.
88. Walter P, Hundeshagen H, Borst HG: Treatment of acute myocardial infarction by transmural blood supply from the ventricular cavity. Eur Surg Res 3(2):130–138, 1971.
89. Whittaker P, Rakusan K, Kloner RA: Transmural channels can protect ischemic tissue. Assessment of long-term myocardial response to laser- and needle-made channels. Circulation 93:143–152, 1996.
90. Whittaker P, Spariosu K, Ho ZZ: Success of transmyocardial laser revascularization is determined by the amount and organization of scar tissue produced in response to initial injury: results of ultraviolet laser treatment. Lasers Surg Med 24:253–260, 1999.
91. Yamamoto N, Gu AG, Derosa CM, et al: Radio frequency transmyocardial revascularization enhances angiogenesis and causes myocardial denervation in a canine model. Lasers Surg Med 27:18–28, 2000.
92. Yamamoto N, Kohmoto T, Gu A, et al: Angiogenesis is enhanced in ischemic canine myocardium by transmyocardial laser revascularization. J Am Coll Cardiol 31(6):1426–1433, 1998.
93. Zlotnick AY, Ahmad RM, Reul RM: Neovascularization occurs at the site of closed laser channels after transmyocardial laser revascularization. Surg Forum 48:286–287, 1996.

Surgical Management of Heart Failure

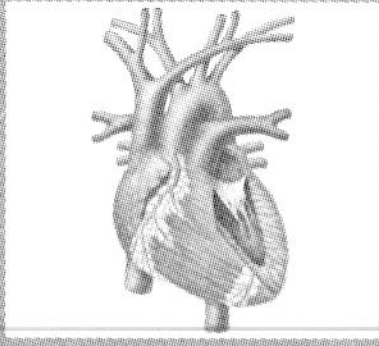

Pericardium and Constrictive Pericarditis

CHAPTER 90

Donald D. Glower

HISTORY

The earliest descriptions of the pericardium may date back to Hippocrates (460–377 B.C.).[36] Galen (129–210 A.D.) described the protective function of the pericardium and also reported a pericardial effusion in animals. Vesalius (1514–1564) carefully described the anatomy of the pericardium, and Rondelet (1507–1566) described pericarditis and pleuritis. Jean Riolan (1649) suggested treating pericarditis with trephination of the sternum, whereas a case of hemopericardium was reported by William Harvey (1649). The conditions of cardiac tamponade and constrictive pericarditis were described by Richard Lower (1669), John Mayow (1674), and Morgagni (1756). The pathophysiology of constrictive pericarditis was further clarified by Cheevers (1842).

Kussmaul (1873) noted the association between constrictive pericarditis and decreased intensity of the peripheral pulse (now termed *pulsus paradoxus*). Kussmaul also described inspiratory jugular venous distension, now termed *Kussmaul's sign* (versus normal inspiratory jugular venous collapse). Pick (1896) reported three patients with constrictive pericarditis and hepatic cirrhosis (a condition now known as Pick's cirrhosis)

The first successful pericardiotomy was performed by Romero in 1819, and the first pericardiocentesis was performed by Franz Schuh in 1840. Pericardial resection for constrictive pericarditis was proposed by Weill (1895) and Delorme (1898), with pericardiectomy ultimately performed by Rehn (1913) and Sauerbruch (1925). Early surgical treatment of constrictive pericarditis in the United States was reported by Beck (1930), Churchill (1936), and Blalock (1937). Radical pericardiectomy, including excision of thickened epicardium when necessary, was advocated by Holman (1955).

ANATOMY

The pericardium is a fibrous sac surrounding the heart and mediastinal great vessels. The outer wall of the pericardial sac consists of an outer fibrosa and an inner serosa.[37] Histologically the fibrosa is fibrocollagenous tissue with elastic fibers oriented along the lines of stress, and the pericardial serosa is composed of mesothelial cells with microvilli and an underlying basal lamina.[37]

This outer pericardial sac folds onto the heart and great vessels, where the epicardium and outer adventitial layer of the heart and great vessels constitute the visceral lining of the pericardial sac. Laterally the pericardium forms the medial walls of the pleural spaces. Inferiorly the pericardium is the superior surface of the central tendon of the diaphragm, and superiorly the pericardium blends with the deep cervical fascia. Anteriorly the pericardium is loosely joined to the xiphoid process and the sternal manubrium by ligamentous structures, and the anterior pericardium is otherwise separated from the posterior sternum by loose connective tissue and the thymus. Posteriorly and superiorly the pericardium envelops the great vessels, the venae cavae, and the pulmonary veins. The posterior pericardial space has two developmental recesses: the transverse sinus separating the great vessels from the pulmonary veins and the oblique sinus separating the left and right pulmonary veins (Figure 90-1).[37]

The arterial blood supply and venous drainage of the pericardium come from the pericardiophrenic branches of the internal mammary vessels bilaterally. The lymphatic drainage of the visceral pericardium is the tracheal and bronchial lymph chain, whereas the parietal pericardium shares lymphatic drainage with the sternum, diaphragm, and midmediastinum. The pericardium is innervated from the phrenic nerves, with some vagal innervation occurring via the esophageal plexus.[37]

The pericardium normally contains 15–35 ml of serous fluid. Pericardial fluid is a transudate containing less protein but more albumin than serum. Pericardial fluid therefore has a lower osmolality than does plasma.[37]

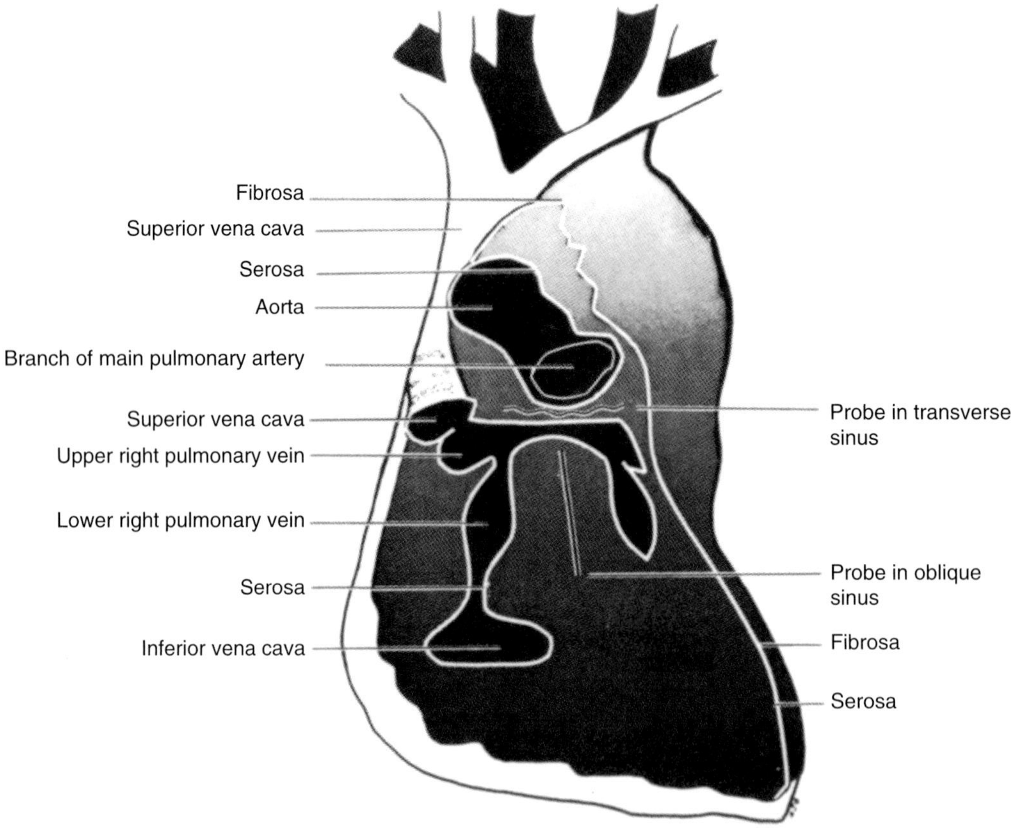

Figure 90–1 Anatomy of the posterior pericardial reflections. Note the transverse sinus and the oblique sinus.
(From Spodick DH: The Pericardium. New York: Marcel Dekker, Inc., 1997.)

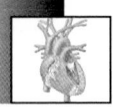

NORMAL PHYSIOLOGY

The pericardium and pericardial fluid minimize friction and energy loss during cardiac motion. On the other hand, the normal pericardium and its external attachments maintain cardiac position within the mediastinum in the presence of gravitational or other forces that could impair cardiac filling or function. The pericardium also serves as a barrier protecting the heart from inflammation or malignancy in adjacent structures.

The normal pericardium has mechanoreceptors connected to phrenic nerve and vagal nerve afferents, with stimulation lowering blood pressure, slowing heart rate, and contracting the spleen in dogs. Pericardial fluid contains prostacyclin, which can affect coronary artery vasomotor tone, and it has fibrinolytic properties that can lyse intrapericardial clot.

At rest, the normal pericardium probably has little restraining effect on cardiac systolic or diastolic function.[9] However, under conditions of acute cardiac dilation, the normal pericardium probably increases diastolic stiffness and limits diastolic filling of both left and right ventricles.[13,17] Under normal conditions, relatively little interaction between the left and right ventricles is mediated by the pericardium.[2,38]

Normal pericardial pressure at end-expiration is –2 mm Hg. Like pleural pressure, pericardial pressure decreases during inspiration and increases during expiration. As a result, inspiration normally decreases left ventricular stroke volume and decreases aortic blood pressure by <10 mm Hg. The mechanisms for these effects do not require an intact pericardium and are similar to the mechanisms of pulsus paradoxus (see later).

PATHOPHYSIOLOGY

Pericardial Effusion

Pericardial effusion (more than 50–100 ml) is the simple result of more fluid transuding into the pericardial space than is resorbed. Pericardial effusions requiring drainage typically contain 500–700 ml of fluid.[40] Eventually pericardial pressure rises high enough that resorption matches fluid production. Sustained increases in pericardial pressure over time cause the pericardial sac to stretch (as a result of material plasticity or creep), with slippage of pericardial collagen fibers and pericardial thinning. Causes of increased pericardial fluid production include inflammation or infection of the pericardium. Decreased pericardial fluid resorption can result from venous hypertension or lymphatic obstruction. If pericardial effusion increases pericardial pressure sufficiently, cardiac tamponade and pulsus paradoxus can result (see later).

Cardiac Tamponade

Cardiac tamponade has been defined as hemodynamically significant cardiac compression from accumulating pericardial contents that evoke and defeat compensatory mechanisms.[37] Cardiac tamponade can result from pericardial fluid, pus, blood, air, or tumor. In a normal pericardium, roughly 200 ml of acute pericardial fluid accumulation can produce tamponade, whereas larger volumes may be required in chronically enlarged pericardial sacs.

The initial effect of cardiac tamponade is decreased venous return to the right side of the heart resulting from a direct pressure effect and caused by effectively decreased right atrial and right ventricular diastolic compliance. Decreased right ventricular filling decreases stroke volume and thus cardiac output. Pulmonary venous return to the left side of the heart is decreased by increased left atrial pressure and by decreased right ventricular output. Central venous pressures of 14–30 mm Hg are typically associated with cardiac tamponade in euvolemic individuals, and lower venous pressures can occur with cardiac tamponade if hypovolemia also is present.

Left ventricular diastolic compliance and diastolic filling also are impaired by cardiac tamponade. Increased diastolic right ventricular pressure relative to left ventricular diastolic pressure can shift the interventricular septum leftward, thus decreasing preload of the interventricular septum and effectively decreasing left ventricular contractility. By combining these mechanisms, inspiration with cardiac tamponade can decrease systolic blood pressure by >10 mm Hg (pulsus paradoxus; see next section). Eventually arterial hypotension and increased intrapericardial pressure can decrease coronary perfusion sufficiently to decrease cardiac contractility as a result of global cardiac ischemia.

Diagnostic signs of cardiac tamponade are listed in Box 90-1.

Pulsus Paradoxus

Cardiac tamponade is associated with *pulsus paradoxus*, defined as a fall in systolic blood pressure of >10 mm Hg with inspiration. Pulsus paradoxus is thus an exaggeration of the normal inspiratory decrease in systolic blood pressure as a result of the same mechanisms (see Normal Physiology in the preceding). Although pulsus paradoxus is characteristic of cardiac tamponade, it also can be seen in chronic obstructive pulmonary disease, pulmonary embolism, obesity, right-sided heart failure, and ascites as a result of the same mechanisms.[2] Pulsus paradoxus may be absent in cardiac tamponade with severe left ventricular dysfunction, atrial

Box 90–1. Diagnostic Signs of Cardiac Tamponade.

Physical Examination

- Pulsus paradoxus

Pulmonary Artery Catheter Findings

- Central venous pressure >14 mm Hg
- Near-equalization of central venous pressure, pulmonary artery diastolic pressure, and capillary wedge pressures
- Decreased cardiac output

Echocardiography

- Right atrial compression
- Right ventricular diastolic collapse

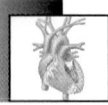

septal defect, severe aortic regurgitation, or positive pressure breathing.[37] Proposed mechanisms of pulsus paradoxus include the following:

1. Pooling of blood in the lungs during inspiration[10]
2. Increased right ventricular filling during inspiration caused by lower right ventricular pressure. In turn, right ventricular distension may shift the interventricular septum leftward, thus decreasing septal muscle preload and decreasing left ventricular stroke volume.[4]
3. Increased left ventricular afterload (aortic pressure minus pericardial pressure), which decreases left ventricular stroke work [29]

Constrictive Pericarditis

Constrictive pericarditis results when the volume of the pericardial sac itself is sufficiently reduced relative to cardiac volume so that cardiac filling is impaired. In constrictive pericarditis, pericardial fluid is generally absent or of normal volume. The wall of the pericardial sac is almost always thickened in constrictive pericarditis and may be 3–20 mm thick, versus 1–2-mm thickness for normal pericardium (Box 90-2).

Unlike cardiac tamponade, constrictive pericarditis impairs cardiac filling only in late diastole. Thus early diastolic filling of the right ventricle occurs briefly in constrictive pericarditis until the ventricle suddenly reaches the rigid constraint of the pericardium. The result is the pathopneumonic *"square root" sign* in the right and left ventricular diastolic filling pressure waveforms (Figure 90-2).

Similarly, in constrictive pericarditis, the central venous pressure tracing has a prominent *y* descent that corresponds to the initial dip of the "square root" sign of the right and left ventricular tracings. This *y* descent normally results from "diastolic collapse" of the normal venous pressure as rapid atrial filling occurs, and the *y* descent is exaggerated by constrictive pericarditis.

Box 90–2. Diagnostic Signs of Constrictive Pericarditis.

Physical examination

- Kussmaul's sign

Pulmonary artery catheter findings

- Central venous pressure >14 mm Hg
- Near-equalization of central venous pressure, pulmonary artery diastolic pressure, and capillary wedge pressures
- Decreased cardiac output
- "Square root" sign in right and left ventricular pressure tracings
- Prominent *y* descent in central venous pressure tracing

Echocardiography, computed tomography, or magnetic resonance imaging

- Pericardial thickening
- Right ventricular diastolic collapse
- Minimal pericardial fluid

Constrictive pericarditis also is associated with inspiratory jugular venous distension (*Kussmaul's sign*) (see Figure 90-2), which is less frequent in cardiac tamponade. Kussmaul's sign also can occur in right ventricular failure, restrictive cardiomyopathy, cor pulmonale, and acute pulmonary embolism.

Chronic elevation of venous pressures in constrictive pericarditis can result in hepatic congestion, cardiac cirrhosis, protein losing enteropathy, and nephrotic syndrome. Chronically, constrictive pericarditis alters the neurohormonal axis, with elevated levels of serum norepinephrine, renin, aldosterone, cortisol, growth hormone, and atrial natriuretic peptide.[1]

The differential diagnosis of constrictive pericarditis consists primarily of restrictive cardiomyopathy, which can occur simultaneously with constrictive pericarditis. Characteristic histology on myocardial biopsy, pulmonary capillary wedge pressure more than 5 mm Hg above central venous pressure, slower early diastolic filling, and impaired left ventricular systolic function all favor restrictive cardiomyopathy over constrictive pericarditis. Acute volume loading of 500 ml during right-sided heart catheterization accentuates the right-sided pressure findings of constrictive pericarditis and produces lesser changes in restrictive cardiomyopathy.

DIAGNOSIS

History and Symptoms

The presenting symptoms of pericardial disease can include fever, malaise, chest discomfort, shortness of breath, pedal edema, and abdominal distension. Medical history may reveal prior chest trauma, chest irradiation, or exposure to infectious agents such as tuberculosis.

Physical Examination

Physical examination of the patient with pericardial disease may reveal findings of fever, tachycardia, or tachypnea. The peripheral arterial pulse may paradoxically diminish during inspiration (*pulsus paradoxus*). Inspiratory jugular venous distension may be present (*Kussmaul's sign*). Chest examination may show dullness at the lung bases, muffled cardiac sounds, and a pericardial rub or pericardial knock. A prominent S_3 gallop may be present in constrictive pericarditis. Abdominal examination may demonstrate hepatomegaly or ascites, and pedal edema may be present. The extremities may be cool and constricted in tamponade.

Chest Radiograph

Chest radiograph may show cardiomegaly in pericardial effusion. Pericardial calcification can accompany constrictive pericarditis. Pleural effusion may be present in pericardial effusion, pericardial tamponade, and constrictive pericarditis. Chest radiograph also may demonstrate pneumopericardium or mediastinal mass as a result of pericardial cyst.

Electrocardiogram

Pericardial disease may be associated with atrial fibrillation, and the electrocardiogram (ECG) may show diminished

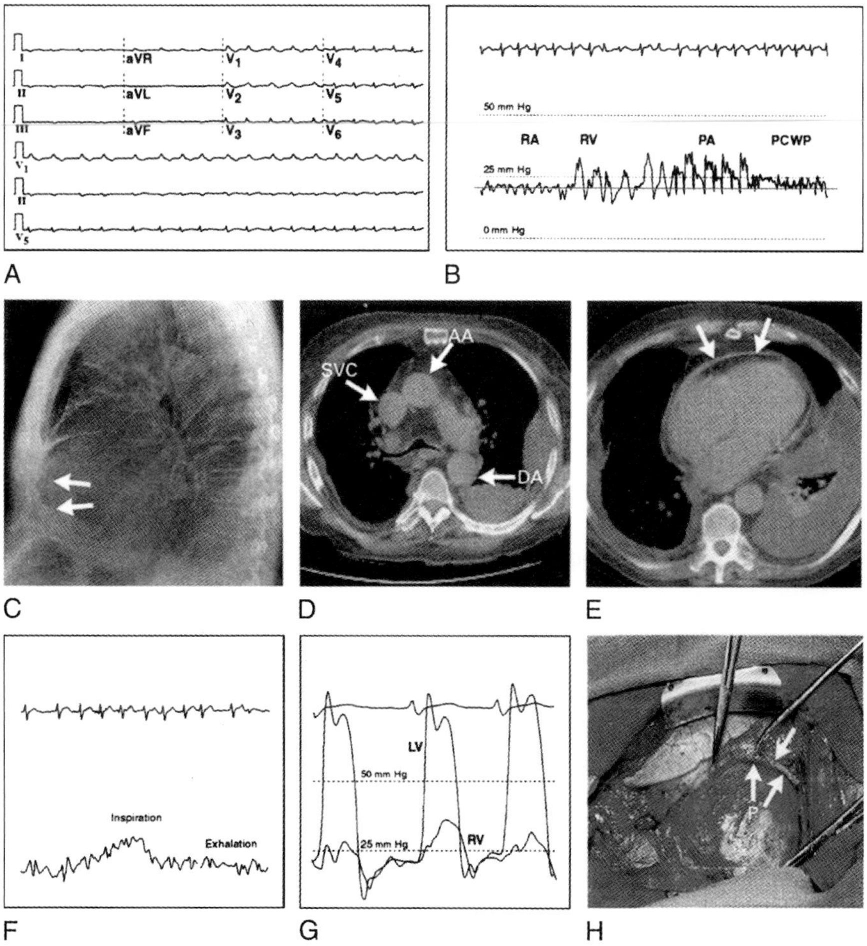

Figure 90–2 Images from a patient with constrictive pericarditis. (**A**) Electrocardiogram with low voltage. (**B**) Right-sided pressure tracings showing equalization of pressures in the right atrium (RA), right ventricle (RV), pulmonary artery (PA), and pulmonary capillary wedge pressure (PCWP). (**C**) Chest radiograph with pericardial calcification. (**D**) Computed tomography showing dilated superior vena cava (SVC) relative to ascending aorta (AA) and descending aorta (DA). (**E**) Computed tomography with thickened pericardium. (**F**) Inspiratory increase in right atrial pressure (Kussmaul's sign). (**G**) Simultaneous right and left ventricular pressure tracings with early diastolic pressure dip (characteristic "square root" sign). (**H**) Intraoperative findings of pericardial thickening (P).
(From Atwood JE, Osterberg L: Images in clinical medicine. Constrictive pericarditis. N Engl J Med 343:106, 2000.)

QRS voltage (see Figure 90-2). The four stages of ECG changes in acute pericarditis are as follows:

Stage I	ST elevation in all leads except AVR and V_1
Stage II	Normal ST segments but T wave flattening
Stage III	T wave inversion without Q waves or loss of R wave voltage
Stage IV	Normalization of T wave

Echocardiogram

Echocardiogram easily detects loculated or generalized pericardial effusion. Echocardiogram also can diagnose intrapericardial masses, pericardial cysts, pericardial calcification or thickening, or associated cardiac disease. The echocardiogram can be diagnostic of cardiac tamponade with findings of end-diastolic right atrial collapse, diastolic right ventricular collapse, and wide respiratory variation of blood flow velocity through cardiac valves (Figure 90-3).[5]

Computed Tomography

Computed tomography can demonstrate pericardial effusion, pericardial calcification and thickening, intrapericardial masses, and pericardial cysts (Figure 90-2). Relative to magnetic resonance imaging, computed tomography may be more sensitive in detecting calcification but has disadvantages of requiring intravenous contrast injection and more motion artifact.

Magnetic Resonance Imaging

Magnetic resonance imaging can demonstrate pericardial effusion, pericardial thickening, intrapericardial masses, pericardial cysts, and even intracardiac disease.[42] Compared with computed tomography, magnetic resonance imaging has the advantages of not requiring intravenous contrast injection and having less motion artifact. Magnetic resonance imaging may be less sensitive in detecting pericardial calcification than is computed tomography. Newer magnetic imaging techniques such as steady-state free-procession and spin tagging may provide better information than do older T_1- or T_2-weighted spin-echo techniques.[15,16]

Cardiac Catheterization

Cardiac fluoroscopy can demonstrate pericardial calcification or abnormally prominent swinging motion of the left ventricle over the cardiac cycle in pericardial effusion. Right-sided heart catheterization can be diagnostic of cardiac tamponade or pericardial constriction (see the preceding) (see Figure 90-2). Both tamponade and constriction

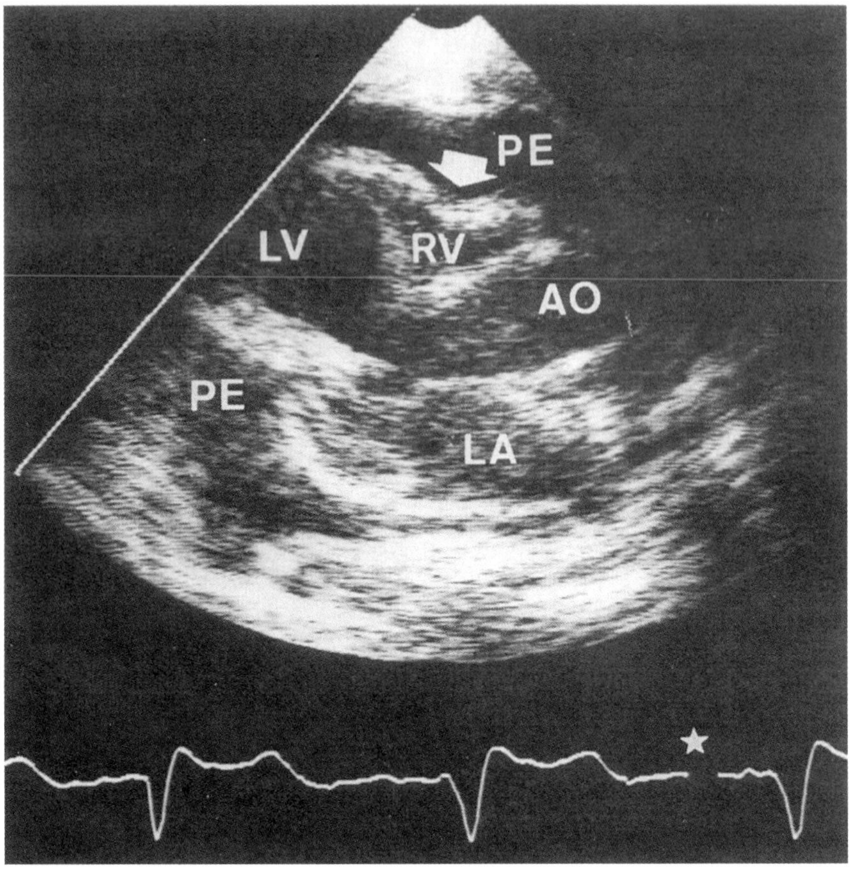

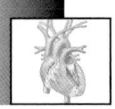

Figure 90–3 **Two-dimensional echocardiogram (parasternal long axis view) showing pericardial effusion (PE) and cardiac tamponade with collapse of the right ventricle (RV) at end-diastole (★).** AO, Aorta; LA, left atrium; LV, left ventricle. *(From Candell-Riera J: Tamponade and constriction: An appraisal of echocardiography and external pulse recordings. In Soler-Soler J, Permanyer-Miralda G, Sagrista-Sauleda J, editors: Pericardial Disease, pp. 17-45. Dordrecht, The Netherlands: Kluwer Academic Publishers, 1990.)*

show equalization and elevation of diastolic pressures in all four chambers of the heart. Physiological tamponade or constriction is unusual, with right atrial mean pressure under 14 mm Hg. Constriction may differentiated from tamponade or restrictive cardiomyopathy by the "square root" sign in the right and left ventricular tracings (see Figure 90-2), and the findings of cardiac constriction are accentuated by acute 500-ml volume challenge (see Constrictive Pericarditis in the preceding).

PERICARDIOCENTESIS

Pericardiocentesis is an effective means to rapidly treat cardiac tamponade and obtain pericardial fluid for diagnosis. Pericardiocentesis generally is performed with the patient in a supine position and using local anesthesia. A long pericardial needle is inserted to the patient's left of the xiphoid, inferior to the left costal margin (Figure 90-4). The needle is advanced toward the patient's left midscapula while maintaining aspiration on the needle. Cardiac puncture can be avoided by attaching an ECG to the needle. The needle is withdrawn if the ECG shows sudden negative deflection of the QRS complex, indicating contact with the myocardium. Alternatively, ultrasound or echocardiography may be used to guide the needle and avoid cardiac laceration.

Once the pericardial space is entered, the needle may be exchanged over a wire for a blunt pericardial catheter. The blunt pericardial catheter may be left in the pericardial space for several days to decrease the rate of recurrent effusion from 55% to 24%.[24] Pericardial fluid may be sent to the laboratory for blood cell count and differential, cytology (possibly including tumor markers), culture (including bacterial, fungus, and tuberculosis), and possibly biochemical examination (such as polymerase chain reaction [PCR] for tuberculosis, pH, specific gravity, lactic dehydrogenase, and protein content).[37]

Pericardiocentesis is rapid, requires little anesthesia, and is relatively safe. Complication rates vary from 5–50% and are increased in smaller effusion, when echo guidance is not used, and in the presence of coagulopathy.[24,35] The diagnostic yield from pericardiocentesis is limited to 20–30% because of an inability to obtain histological tissue, especially in malignant pericarditis.[6,25] Pericardiocentesis is less effective and diagnostic in hemopericardium with clot or in effusion with thick exudate. Although it is controversial, the optimal patients for pericardiocentesis are those with large anterior effusions and with either tamponade (therapeutic) or likely infectious or tuberculous etiology (diagnostic).[24] The rate of recurrent effusion and tamponade after successful pericardiocentesis is high, around 55%.[24]

Pericardial Biopsy

Pericardial biopsy can be performed percutaneously or surgically (see discussion of surgical procedures later in this chapter). Percutaneous pericardial biopsy is possible by dilating a pericardiocentesis needle tract to accept an intro-

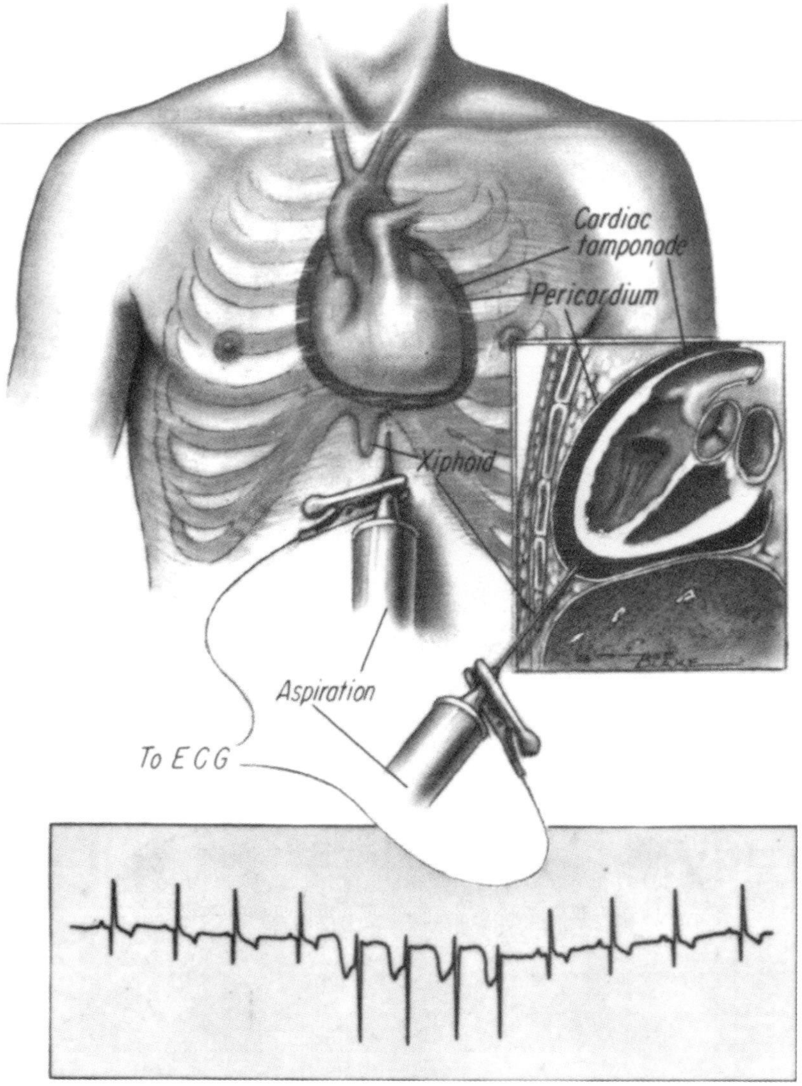

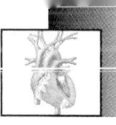

Figure 90–4 Technique of subxiphoid pericardiocentesis with electrocardiographic monitoring. Note negative QRS deflection indicating myocardial contact. ECG, Electrocardiogram.

ducer sheath. A bioptome can then be paced through the introducer using echocardiographic guidance to obtain pericardial biopsy.[39] The value and safety of percutaneous pericardial biopsy have not been established.

Combined with pericardiocentesis, histological examination (and possibly microbiological culture) of pericardial tissue can make the diagnosis of pericarditis and demonstrate the etiology of pericarditis in 30–50% of patients.[6,25] Pericardial tissue may be sent to the laboratory for hematoxylin–eosin and Gram stains and cultured for bacteria, fungus, and tuberculosis. Special stains may be used to detect certain forms of malignancy.

PERICARDIAL EFFUSION/NONCONSTRICTIVE PERICARDITIS

Diagnosis

The diagnosis of pericarditis requires the pathological demonstration of pericardial inflammation, scarring, or thickening. Thus certain diagnoses of pericarditis require pericardial biopsy, generally at operation for subxiphoid or transthoracic pericardial window. However, the diagnosis of pericarditis can be strongly supported by findings of pericardial effusion or pericardial thickening on echocardiography, computed tomography, or magnetic resonance imaging.

The diagnosis of pericardial effusion requires only an imaging study demonstrating more fluid than normal (>50–100 ml) in the pericardial space. Identifying the etiology of the pericarditis may require pericardiocentesis or pericardial biopsy.

Etiology and Treatment

A wide variety of etiologies exist for pericardial effusion and pericarditis (Table 90-1). Medical treatment for pericardial effusion varies with the etiology of the effusion as discussed later. Surgical treatment involves pericardiocentesis, subxiphoid pericardial window, or transpleural pericardial window. Pericardiocentesis and/or pericardial biopsy can be indicated to determine the etiology of the pericarditis and

Table 90–1

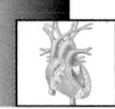

Etiologies of Pericarditis[6,21,26,32]

	Effusion	*Constriction*
Idiopathic	7–30%	50–70%
Malignant	20–50%	0
Tuberculous	5–10%	15%
Viral	5–15%	0
Bacterial	5–10%	0
Collagen-vascular	5–15%	1%
Uremic	10–15%	0
Radiation	5–15%	11%
Postoperative	5–25%	5–30%
Trauma	5%	1%

thus define the medical therapy. Pericardiocentesis also is indicated to acutely treat pericardial tamponade in a hemodynamically unstable patient and to achieve hemodynamic stability. Depending upon the etiology, single pericardiocentesis may only delay recurrent tamponade, necessitating more definitive treatment.[24]

Pericardial window is indicated in any patient with symptomatic pericardial effusion or in whom the etiology cannot otherwise be defined. Subxiphoid pericardial window can be performed using local anesthesia and therefore is preferable in patients who are hemodynamically unstable as a result of tamponade but in whom pericardiocentesis is deemed impractical or unsafe. Transpleural pericardial window is preferable in patients with good long-term prognosis but with significant likelihood of recurrent pericardial effusion.

Idiopathic Pericarditis

Idiopathic pericardial effusion is treated symptomatically. Symptoms of low-grade pain and fever can be treated with antiinflammatory agents such as indomethacin, ibuprofen, rofecoxib, or celecoxib. More severe or refractory symptoms almost always respond to a 2–3-week course of prednisone, beginning with 40 mg daily and tapering over the 2–3-week course. Other etiologies such as infection or uremia need to be excluded before treatment. Pericarditis can produce atrial fibrillation, which also may require treatment.

Chylopericardium

Chylopericardium can be idiopathic or follow thoracic surgery. Chylopericardium can be treated by pericardiocentesis or, if recurrent, by subxiphoid or transthoracic pericardial window with or without low thoracic duct ligation.[37]

Hemopericardium

Hemopericardium can result from trauma, recent mediastinal operation, coagulopathy, cardiac perforation caused by instrumentation, cardiac rupture, or aortic rupture. Acute hemopericardium resulting in cardiac tamponade requires emergent treatment (see Cardiac Tamponade section). In the absence of cardiac tamponade, the treatment of hemopericardium depends upon the underlying disease process. Hemopericardium caused by percutaneous cardiac puncture in the catheterization laboratory generally can be remedied by placing a pigtail catheter in the pericardial space, reversing anticoagulation, frequently aspirating the pigtail catheter, and watching for cessation of bleeding.

Hemopericardium caused by surgical diseases such as acute aortic dissection, cardiac or aortic rupture, or penetrating trauma is best treated by tube drainage of the pericardium *after* surgically correcting the source of bleeding. Hemopericardium caused by to blunt trauma or coagulopathy may require surgical drainage by either subxiphoid or transthoracic approach to prevent acute tamponade and late pericardial constriction.

Nonviral Infectious Pericarditis

The most common bacterial organisms causing pericarditis are *Staphylococcus*, *Streptococcus*, and gram-negative organisms in adults and *Haemophilus* or *Staphylococcus* in children. Bacterial pericarditis may occur from bacteremia or from contiguous spread from bacterial infection in the thoracic cavity. Symptoms of fever and chest pain are common. Diagnosis relies on culture or histological examination of pericardial fluid obtained by either pericardiocentesis or open pericardial drainage.

Bacterial pericarditis requires both appropriate antibiotic treatment and either acute or chronic pericardial drainage. Bacterial pericarditis may respond to one-time pericardial drainage with systemic antibiotic therapy for less virulent organisms such as *Streptococcus*. Pericardiectomy may be necessary if initial drainage fails, especially in organisms such as *Haemophilus*.[24]

Fungal or staphylococcal pericarditis responds better to more chronic drainage of the pericardium by the subxiphoid or transthoracic approaches.

Acute tuberculous pericarditis is best treated by intermittent pericardiocentesis as needed. Tube drainage of tuberculous pericarditis should be avoided to prevent chronic draining sinuses along the tube tract. Pericardiectomy or open pericardial drainage (preferably after 1 week of chemotherapy) may be necessary if initial drainage fails, and pericardial constriction can result in roughly one half of patients developing tuberculous pericarditis.[34]

Amebic or echinococcal pericarditis may require pericardiocentesis or tube drainage, depending upon the thickness and degree of loculation.

Viral Pericarditis

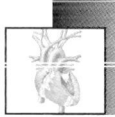

Several viruses, such as coxsackievirus, adenovirus, cytomegalovirus, human immunodeficiency virus (HIV), and herpes simplex virus, have been associated with pericarditis. Viral pericarditis often is a clinical diagnosis made with the assistance of viral serologies. Viral pericarditis often is accompanied by myocarditis, which can be documented on myocardial biopsy or indirectly suggested by acute deterioration of ventricular function. Viral pericarditis is usually self-limited, like idiopathic pericarditis. Pericardiocentesis or surgical pericardial drainage with biopsy is indicated as needed for diagnosis and/or symptoms.

Inflammatory Pericarditis

Connective tissue or inflammatory diseases such as rheumatoid arthritis and lupus can produce pericarditis in a minority of patients. The underlying condition should be treated if possible, and the pericardiocentesis or pericardial window is reserved for symptoms refractory to medical treatment or for the need to make a diagnosis.

Malignant Pericarditis

Malignant involvement of the pericardium generally is metastatic and occurs in roughly 10% of patients with noncardiac neoplasm. The most common tumors to involve the pericardium are lung (38%), breast (29%), lymphoma (7%), and others (26%).[14,32] Primary malignancy of the pericardium is rare and includes mesothelioma (50%), sarcoma, and malignant teratoma. Malignancy of the pericardium generally presents as cardiac tamponade as a result of malignant pericardial effusion. Pericardial constriction caused by malignancy is infrequent. Once pericardial effusion is demonstrated by an imaging study, the diagnosis of malignant pericardial effusion can be made by cytological examination of pericardial effusion in 20–30% of cases. Pericardial biopsy doubles the diagnostic yield of pericardiocentesis alone. The longevity of patients with malignant pericarditis is sufficiently low that subxiphoid drainage and transthoracic drainage have similar success rates. The median survival period for malignant pericardial effusion requiring surgical intervention is less than 6 months.[32] Rarely, good long-term results can be obtained by complete excision of localized primary tumors of the pericardium.

Radiation-Induced Pericarditis

Only a small fraction of patients receiving mediastinal irradiation develop clinically significant pericarditis. Early pericarditis developing within 1 month of initiating mediastinal irradiation generally is self-limited and needs only to be treated symptomatically, like idiopathic pericarditis. Treatment with pericardiocentesis or pericardial window should be reserved for significant refractory symptoms or concern about other etiologies. A small number of patients may develop constrictive pericarditis, usually 5–20 years after irradiation.

Postoperative Pericarditis

Only 10% of patients undergoing cardiac operation have clinically significant postoperative pericarditis, although all patients probably have some degree of pericarditis. Closure of the pericardium may increase the incidence of clinical pericarditis. Intraoperative use of bioabsorbable films may diminish pericardial scarring without the pericardial capsule formation associated with nonabsorbable pericardial substitute material.[28]

Symptoms typically appear 5–10 days after operation and are usually self-limited, resolving after 1–2 weeks. Treatment is similar to that of idiopathic pericarditis.

Uremic Pericarditis

Uremic pericarditis occurs in 20% of patients on hemodialysis and in 50% of patients with severe untreated renal disease. Patients may have chronic pericardial thickening, which classically can appear "shaggy." Other patients may have lesser pericardial thickening with significant pericardial effusions, which can cause cardiac tamponade.

Therapy for uremic pericarditis is focused on treating tamponade. No therapy has been shown to prevent or treat uremic pericardial tamponade short of pericardial drainage. Tamponade may respond to pericardiocentesis initially, but the incidence of recurrent tamponade in uremic pericardial effusion is highest with pericardiocentesis alone, better with subxiphoid pericardial window, and best with transthoracic pericardial window.[24]

CARDIAC TAMPONADE

Etiology

A common etiology of acute pericardial tamponade is hemopericardium after recent mediastinal operation or percutaneous cardiac instrumentation. Other causes of acute cardiac tamponade include pneumopericardium and hemopericardium caused by coagulopathy. Roughly one half of patients with chronic pericardial effusion have presenting symptoms of cardiac tamponade. Malignant effusion and uremic pericarditis are common causes of chronic cardiac tamponade (see Table 90-1).

Diagnosis

Cardiac tamponade can be diagnosed by right-sided heart catheterization or by echocardiography (see Box 90-1). At right-sided heart catheterization, cardiac output typically is reduced with elevation of central venous pressure of at least 14 mm Hg, and equalization of the central venous pressure, pulmonary artery diastolic pressure, and capillary wedge pressure. Echocardiography shows the pericardial space distended with fluid with right atrial compression and/or diastolic right ventricular collapse (see Figure 90-3).

Treatment

Cardiac tamponade resulting from hemopericardium within several days after a surgical procedure is almost always managed by returning to the operating room once coagulopathy is corrected. Back in the operating room, the hemopericardium should be evacuated (generally through the original surgical incision) and drains should be left in the pericardial space.

In the absence of a recent cardiac surgical procedure, patients with cardiac tamponade and hemodynamic compromise usually can be stabilized by emergent pericardiocentesis. Depending upon the etiology of the tamponade, a single pericardiocentesis may be all that is needed. Otherwise, a pigtail catheter may be left in the pericardium for up to 48 hours, or more definitive pericardial drainage by the subxiphoid or transpleural window may be desirable.

Subxiphoid pericardial window is ideal for many patients with tamponade in that local anesthesia can be used to avoid the hemodynamic embarrassment of general anesthesia in an unstable patient. Transpleural approaches are less suitable for the unstable patient because of intolerance of one-lung anesthesia or pleural insufflation of carbon dioxide. Patients for whom transpleural pericardial window has advantages should have initial pericardiocentesis to relieve tamponade before anesthetic induction for transpleural drainage.

CONSTRICTIVE PERICARDITIS

Etiology

The most common etiology of constrictive pericarditis in Western countries is idiopathic, with prior cardiac operation and mediastinal irradiation also being common (see Table 90-1). In earlier decades in the West and in developing countries today, tuberculosis is the leading cause of constrictive pericarditis. Pericardial closure at the time of routine cardiac operation can induce some degree of immediate pericardial constriction and decreased cardiac index[33] and probably increases the small but real incidence of late constrictive pericarditis. Although routine pericardial closure at the time of cardiac operation can decrease the risk of sternal reentry, some authors have therefore recommended avoiding pericardial closure in patients with ventricular dysfunction, risk of tamponade, or older age with low likelihood of reoperation.[33]

Diagnosis

The presence of pericardial thickening with minimal pericardial fluid on echocardiography, computed tomography, or magnetic resonance imaging supports the diagnosis, but is not sufficient to diagnose constriction (see Figure 90-2). Diagnosis of constrictive pericarditis requires demonstration of right-sided heart hemodynamics typical of constriction (see Figure 90-2). The findings at right-sided heart catheterization include decreased cardiac output, equalization of diastolic right-sided pressures, and characteristic "square root" sign with a steep *y* descent in right and left ventricular diastolic pressure tracings (see Box 90-2 and Figure 90-2). Detection of these findings can be augmented by 500 ml volume challenge at the time of right-sided heart catheterization.

Treatment

The treatment for pericardial constriction is pericardiectomy (see Pericardiectomy section). Patients should be referred before the onset of Class IV symptoms to minimize postoperative mortality and low cardiac output.[21] Rarely the underlying cause also may require treatment in some cases, such as tuberculous pericarditis. Long-term survival is not significantly different from that of the general population.[21]

PNEUMOPERICARDIUM

Pneumopericardium is a rare condition that most commonly results from severe chest trauma with associated lung injury or from spontaneous dissection of air from a ruptured bleb in neonates on positive pressure ventilation.[7] Symptoms are unusual, although tamponade occurs in 37% of patients. Treatment focuses on the underlying disease. Pericardiocentesis or pericardial tube drainage can be effective in those patients with tamponade. The mortality rate is high (58%) because of underlying disease.

PERICARDIAL CYSTS AND DIVERTICULA

Pericardial cysts and diverticula are thought to be congenital in origin and make up 10–20% of all mediastinal masses.[8,20] Pericardial cysts and diverticula have a fibrous wall lined with mesothelium, whereas bronchial cysts have bronchial epithelium. Pericardial cysts occur more often in men than in women. Most pericardial cysts and diverticula appear as asymptomatic masses on chest radiograph, whereas one third of patients have chest pain. Pericardial cysts are found at the right costophrenic angle in 77% of patients, at the left costophrenic angle in 22%, and in other areas (posterior mediastinum, hilar region, right paratracheal region, or aortic arch) in 8%.[18,20] Pericardial diverticula communicate with the pericardium and comprise 20% of combined pericardial cysts and diverticula.[18] Cysts or diverticula found to have low fluid density on computed tomography or magnetic resonance imaging need no further workup. Masses with density higher than transudate may need further workup to exclude other pericardial masses (Figure 90-5). Cysts or diverticula that need to be removed to exclude malignancy can be approached thoracoscopically or via thoracotomy. Even when malignancy is unlikely, some authors have recommended excision of most pericardial cysts to prevent complications of rupture, cardiac compression, or tracheal compression.[18]

PERICARDIAL TUMORS

Most pericardial tumors display malignant pericardial effusions as a result of malignant metastases from lung, breast, or lymphoma (see previous discussion on malignant pericardial effusion). Primary pericardial tumors include lipoma, hemangioma, lymphangioma, leiomyoma, neurofibroma, heterotopic thymus or thyroid, teratoma, mesothelioma, thymoma, liposarcoma, angiosarcoma, and synovial sarcoma. Half of all primary pericardial malignancies are mesotheliomas. The differential diagnosis includes pericardial cysts and pericardial diverticula (see the preceding), which often may be distinguished on computed tomography or magnetic resonance imaging.[41]

Once identified, primary pericardial tumors should be removed if possible. Depending upon location and size, median sternotomy, thoracotomy, or thoracoscopy may be used to approach primary pericardial tumors. Prognosis depends upon tumor type and extent. Lipomas, leiomyomas, and heterotopic tissue generally are resectable and have excellent prognosis. Mesotheliomas are almost always spread to contiguous structures in the pericardium, adjacent pleura, and occasionally mediastinal lymph nodes.

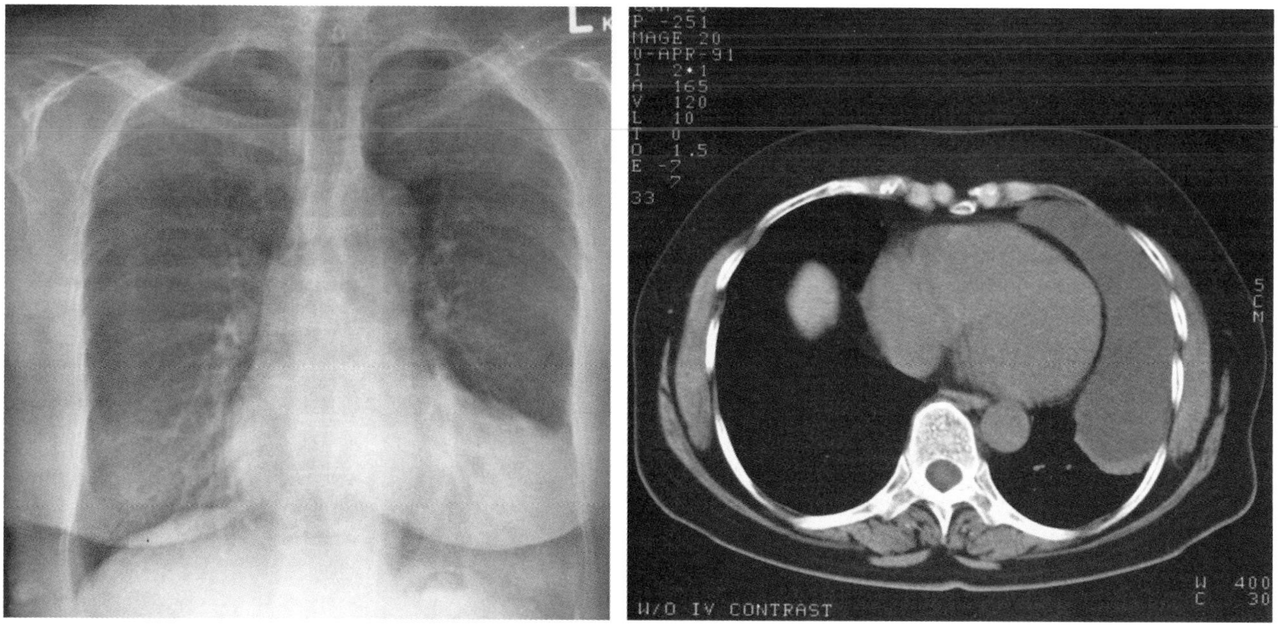

A B

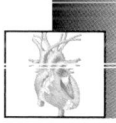

Figure 90–5 (**A**) Chest radiograph of a patients with a large left-sided pericardial cyst. (**B**) Computed tomographic scan of the same patients showing the pericardial cyst extending into the left hemithorax.

Mesotheliomas are rarely resectable, and no treatment has been shown to be effective. The survival rate with pericardial mesothelioma may be 40% at 6 months.[20]

PERICARDIAL DEFECTS

Congenital defects of the pericardium are rare, occurring in 1/10,000 autopsies with a 5:1 male:female predominance.[3] Roughly 30% of patients with pericardial defects have associated cardiac or pulmonary anomalies. The mean age at diagnosis is 20 years.[3] Complete absence of the pericardium is quite rare but generally is asymptomatic.

Partial pericardial defects occur most commonly on the left side[22] and can produce symptoms by compression of the left atrial appendage, allowing cardiac herniation, or even compressing coronary arteries. Partial pericardial defect may have some risk of death because of cardiac herniation or coronary compression. One third of patients are asymptomatic and are detected by abnormal chest radiograph. Symptoms of partial pericardial defect include sharp, fleeting chest pain that is often positional.[12] Other symptoms include dyspnea, sweating, syncope, and circulatory collapse.[3]

In complete or partial absence of the pericardium, chest radiograph is always abnormal, with rotation and leftward displacement of the heart placing the right-sided heart border over the spine. Computed tomography and magnetic resonance imaging similarly show displacement and rotation of the heart into the left side of the chest. Presence of a tongue of lung between the pulmonary artery and the aorta is pathognomonic for congenital absence of pericardium.[12]

Complete pericardial absence requires no treatment. Partial left pericardial defects not overlying the left ventricle may be observed if asymptomatic.[3] Patients with symptoms or partial pericardial defects overlying the left ventricle should be treated surgically to prevent cardiac herniation or compression. Surgical approaches include either sternotomy or thoracoscopy to perform pericardiectomy, repair the pericardial defect with a patch, or amputate the left atrial appendage.[3,22]

Pericardial rupture can occur as the result of blunt trauma and is associated with cardiac injury, cardiac rupture, and cardiac tamponade.[11] Pericardial rupture should be repaired to prevent cardiac herniation, but only after associated cardiac injuries are repaired. The mortality rate is over 50%.[19]

PERICARDIAL SURGICAL PROCEDURES

Subxiphoid Pericardial Window

For patients who require more extensive pericardial drainage than is possible through pericardiocentesis, the subxiphoid pericardial window is an excellent option that minimizes morbidity relative to other surgical alternatives. Subxiphoid pericardial window therefore is ideal for most patients hemodynamically compromised by cardiac tamponade. The subxiphoid pericardial window provides excellent drainage of the pericardial space, allows placement of large-bore pericardial tubes, and potentially drains the right pleural space. An additional advantage is that the subxiphoid pericardial window can be performed with either local or general anesthesia. Local anesthesia is preferable for patients who are hemodynamically compromised by pericardial tamponade.

After either anesthesia is established, a 6–12-cm incision is made in the midline from the cephalad end of the xiphoid to 1–2 cm inferior to the xiphoid (Figure 90-6). The linea alba is divided in a midline, and the xiphoid process is either removed or retracted. With sharp and blunt dissection continuing superiorly and to the patient's left, the pericardium is identified using upward retraction on the sternum and costal cartilages as necessary. Identification of the pericardium can be confirmed by needle aspiration of the pericardium to

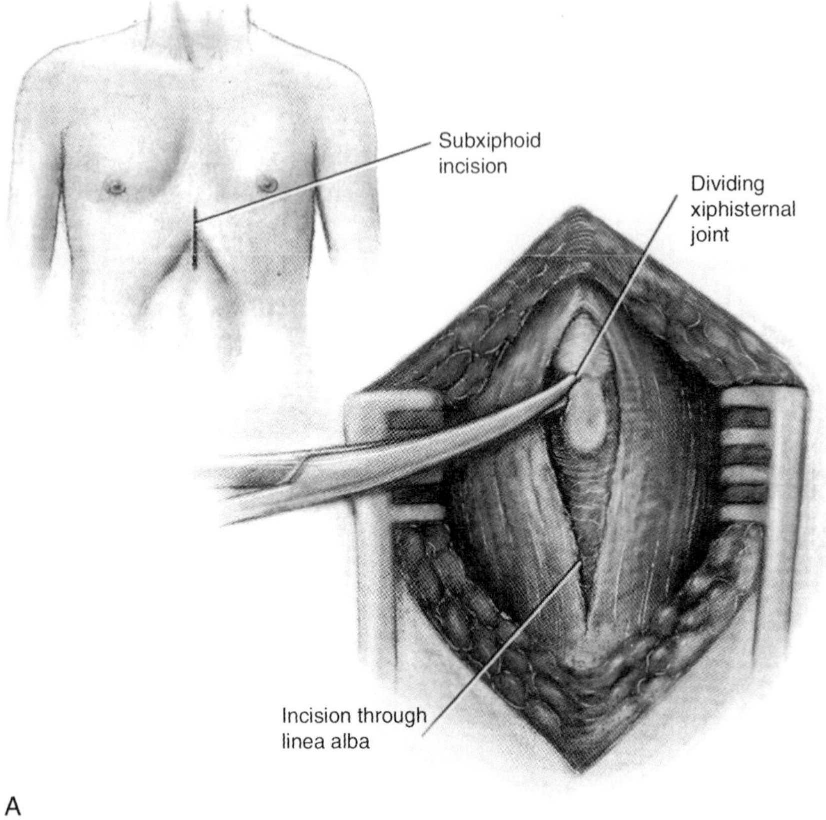

A

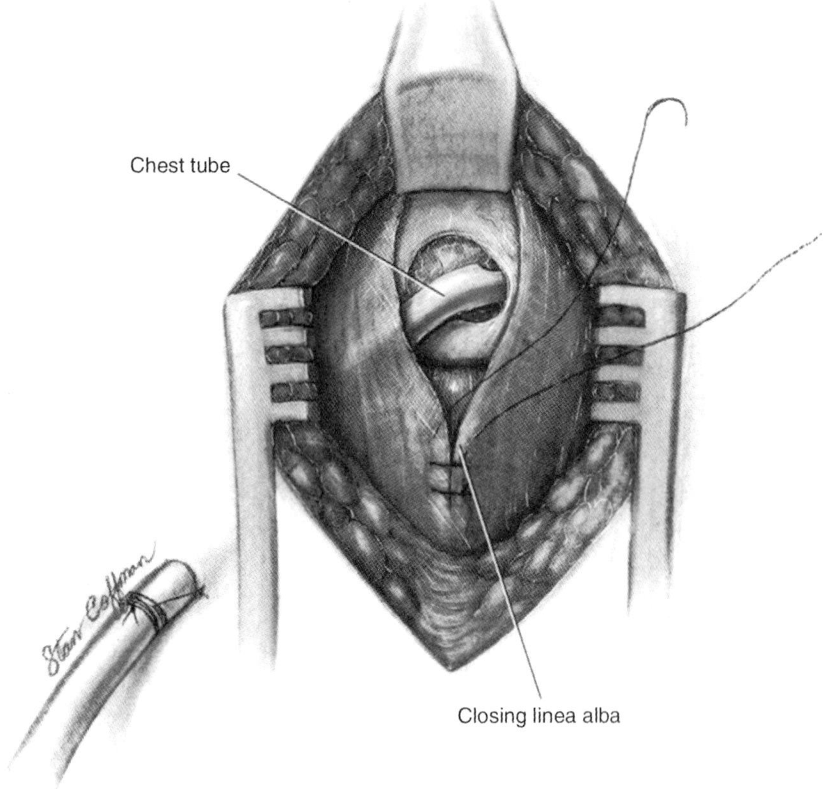

B

Figure 90–6 Technique of subxiphoid pericardial window. (**A**) A 7-cm subxiphoid incision is made, the linea alba opened, and the xiphoid process excised. (**B**) A 2 × 2 cm opening is made in the pericardium, and a tube drain is placed in the pericardial space. *(From Glower DD: Pericardial window. In Sabiston DC Jr., editor: Atlas of Cardiothoracic Surgery. Philadelphia: W.B. Saunders, 1995.)*

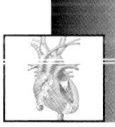

obtain fluid before incision into the pericardial space. Upon identifying the pericardium, a 4-cm-diameter piece of anterior pericardial is excised. The pericardium and pericardial fluid may be sent to the laboratory for histology and culture. Optionally, the pericardial window can be opened into the right pleural space to drain any right pleural effusion. An angled chest tube may then be placed on the diaphragm in the pericardial space, and an additional chest tube could be placed in the right pleural space. Chest tubes should be brought through the rectus muscle lateral to the incision. The linea alba and remaining incision are then closed.

The mortality rate directly related to subxiphoid pericardial window is 1% or less, and the survival rate is limited by the underlying disease (50–60% survival at 1 year).[32,40] The effectiveness in treating tamponade is nearly 100%, and the diagnostic yield is 40–80%.[23,25,40] Recurrent effusion or constriction can occur in 9–25% of patients[32,40] and may be more likely than after transthoracic pericardial resection and in patients with benign disease.[32]

Pericardioscopy

Pericardioscopy has been performed under general anesthesia using the same technique as subxiphoid pericardial window described in the preceding. Once the pericardial window has been created, a rigid mediastinoscope is introduced into the pericardial space. The pericardial space is inspected for gross diagnostic purposes, and endoscopically guided biopsies can be obtained. Pericardioscopy combined with pericardiocentesis and subxiphoid pericardial window has been reported to provide a specific diagnosis in 64% of cases, significantly greater than with pericardiocentesis or pericardial window alone.[25]

Transpleural Pericardial Window

A left thoracotomy generally is used to treat hemodynamically stable patients with pericardial effusion and with good long-term prognosis. Thoracotomy may be desired if simultaneous lung biopsy is needed, and chronic pericardial drainage may be more effective than subxiphoid approaches in nonmalignant pericarditis. Thoracotomy is relatively contraindicated in purulent pericarditis to avoid contamination of the pleural space.

A left thoracotomy (versus right thoracotomy) generally is preferred for open transpleural pericardial window because of the greater amount of pericardium accessible from the left side. The patient is placed supine with the left side elevated 30°. General anesthesia is standard, and left lung isolation is optional with either a double-lumen endotracheal tube or an endobronchial blocker. A 5–12 cm submammary incision is made, and the fifth or fourth intercostal space is entered. The lung is retracted laterally, and the internal mammary artery generally can be spared medially. The left anterior pericardium is opened anterior to the phrenic nerve, taking care not to injure the underlying heart and maintaining hemostasis on the pericardial edge with gentle electrocautery. Pericardium can be excised from 1–2 cm anterior to the phrenic nerve to the midsternal level. Pericardium posterior to the phrenic nerve also can be excised, although the indications for posterior pericardial resection are unclear. Because left thoracotomy generally is used in patients with good long-term prognosis, studies suggest that at least a 4 × 4 cm piece of pericardium should be excised to prevent recurrent pericardial effusion caused by adhesions.[32] A pleural drain is left in place, and the thoracotomy is closed in a standard fashion.

Transpleural pericardial window also may be performed using direct or video-assisted thoracoscopy in patients with pericardial effusion without hemodynamic compromise as a result of tamponade. Either right or left approaches may be used depending on where the greater pericardial pathology lies, but left thoracoscopy can have limited operating space because of the proximity of the distended pericardium to the chest wall. The patient is positioned in a lateral decubitus position (Figure 90-7). The trocar for the video thoracoscope initially is placed posteriorly, being careful to avoid pericardium, which might extend laterally. Two additional triangulated trocars are then placed for instrumentation. The pericardial window is then performed much as in the open transpleural approach in the preceding. An ultrasonic scalpel has been useful to achieve hemostasis on the pericardial edges without risk of ventricular arrhythmia caused by electrocautery.[27]

The mortality rate directly related to transthoracic pericardial window is 1% or less, although the operative mortality rate can be 19% for malignant disease and 5% for benign disease.[32] The effectiveness in treating tamponade is nearly 100%, and the diagnostic yield is 40–80%.[24,32] Recurrent effusion or constriction can occur in 5% of patients, versus 25% of patients with subxiphoid pericardial window.[32]

Transdiaphragmatic Pericardial Window

Transdiaphragmatic pericardial window can be performed using standard laparoscopic techniques or by resecting part of the diaphragm at the time of subxiphoid pericardial window. For the endoscopic approach, the camera is inserted supraumbilically with trocars in the right and left hypochondria. A 3–5-cm diameter opening in the diaphragm and pericardium is made to drain the pericardium into the peritoneal cavity.[31] As with thoracoscopic pericardial window, the ultrasonic scalpel has advantages over electrocautery of minimizing ventricular arrhythmias, smoke, and stimulation of the diaphragm.[30]

Pericardiectomy

Pericardiectomy usually is done through a median sternotomy, given the likelihood of pericardial adhesions that may be dense and the bilateral extent of the pericardium. Pericardiectomy is possible through bilateral thoracotomies, and left anterolateral thoracotomy has been used to achieve effective pericardiectomy.[21]

For sternotomy a midline incision is made from just inferior to the suprasternal notch to the inferior extent of the xiphoid process (Figure 90-8). The entire extent of the sternum is divided in the midline with a sternal saw, and the sternum is opened with a sternal retractor. A relatively thin area of anterior pericardium is incised, and a plane between the epicardium and the pericardium is established using sharp dissection. If possible, the pericardium is opened in the midline from the level of the diaphragm to the base of the great vessels. Tradition states that the left ventricle

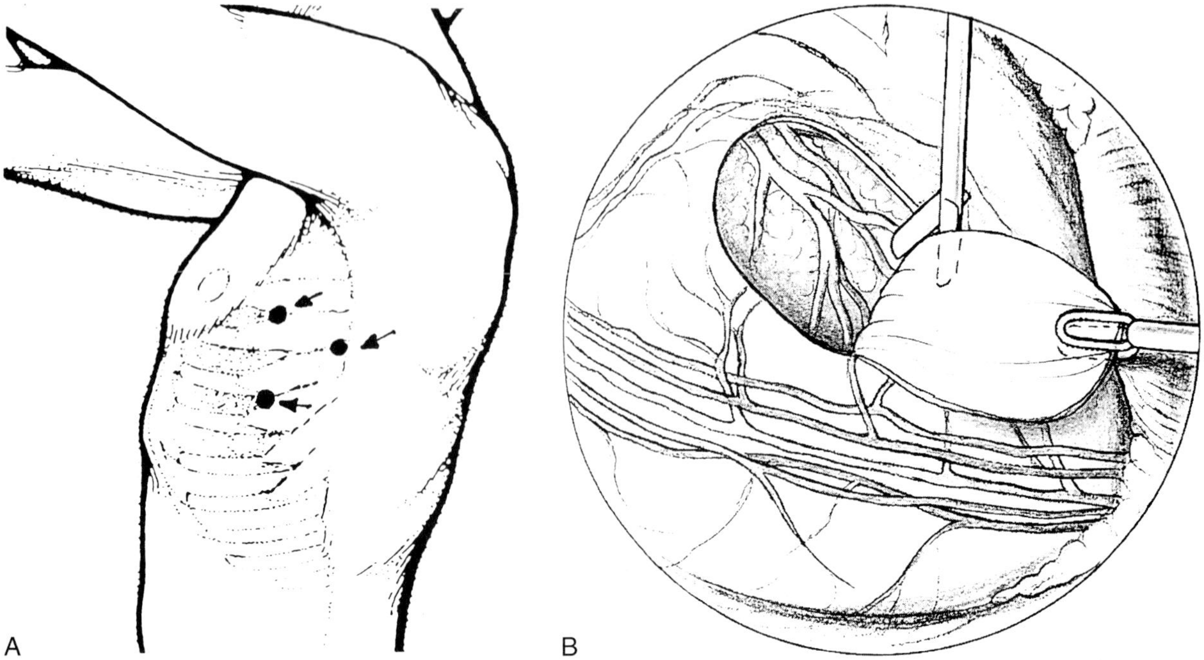

Figure 90–7 Thoracoscopic pericardial window with patient in the right lateral decubitus position. A, The three trocar sites are shown with the camera placed in the posterior port. **B,** Thoracoscopic view of the pericardial resection. *(From Inderbitzi R, Furrer M, Leupi F: Pericardial biopsy and fenestration. Eur Heart J 14:135–137, 1993)*

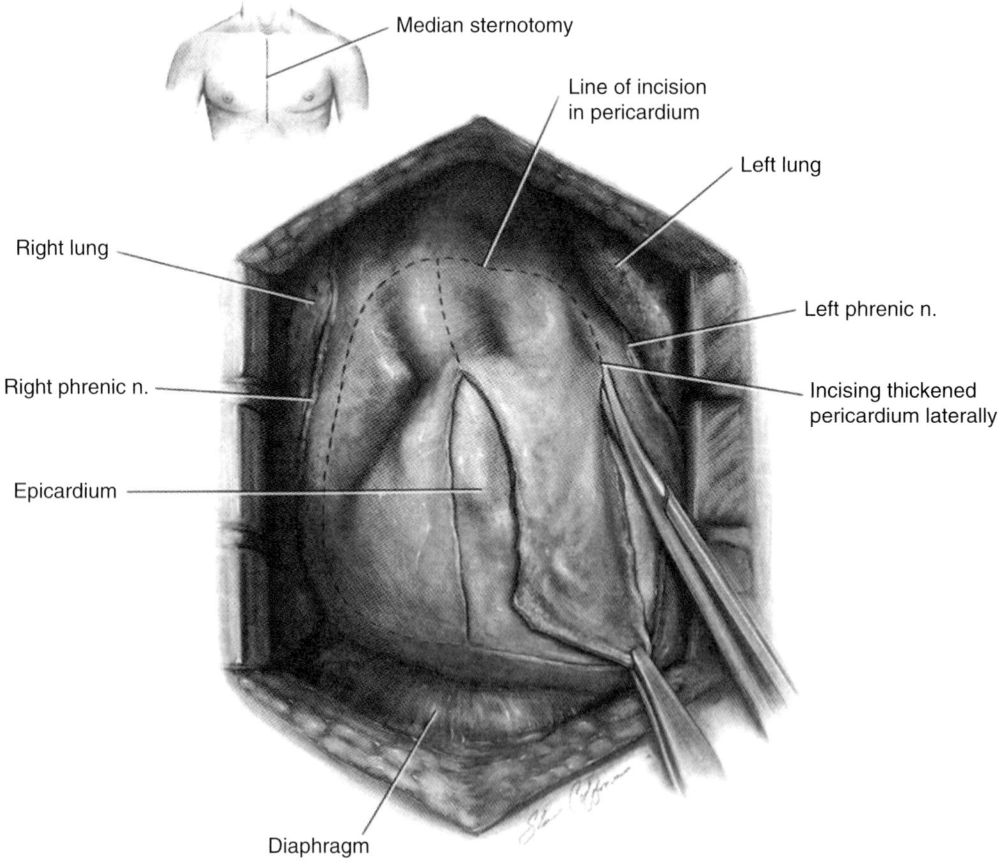

Figure 90–8 Technique of pericardiectomy. Median sternotomy is performed, and the pleural spaces are opened bilaterally. The anterior pericardium is excised from the diaphragm inferiorly to the great vessels superiorly and 1–2 cm anterior to the phrenic nerves bilaterally. As indicated, the diaphragmatic pericardium and the pericardium posterior to the phrenic nerves also may be excised. Unresectable, thickened epicardium may be scored.
(From Glower DD: Pericardiectomy for constrictive pericarditis. In Sabiston DC Jr., editor: Atlas of Cardiothoracic Surgery. Philadelphia: W.B. Saunders, 1995.)

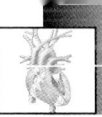

should be freed first to avoid right ventricular distension, although the frequency of this problem is unclear. The anterior pericardium is freed from 1–2 cm anterior to the right phrenic nerve to 1–2 cm anterior to the left phrenic nerve laterally, and from the anterior diaphragm inferiorly to the base of the great vessels superiorly. Occasionally dense epicardial scar may be impossible to remove without risk of cardiac injury. In that case the remaining epicardial scar may be carefully incised in a grid pattern of crossing lines 1–2 cm apart, although the effectiveness of this technique is unclear. Once freed from the epicardium, the pericardium can be excised using low electrocautery to achieve hemostasis. Care should be taken to avoid injury to the phrenic nerves, which may be difficult to identify.

Anterior pericardiectomy described in the preceding usually can be performed without cardiopulmonary bypass. Anterior pericardiectomy provides the majority of the hemodynamic benefit to be obtained in relieving constriction of the right ventricle. Pericardial scar between the inferior heart and the diaphragm may be excised to prevent inferior vena caval obstruction, but the benefits of resecting the diaphragmatic pericardium are unclear, given that the diaphragm itself cannot be resected. Resection of the atrial pericardium is felt by many to be less important than that of the ventricular pericardium,[21] making pericardiectomy via left thoracotomy practical in many cases. Finally, some authors have advocated excising pericardium posterior to the phrenic nerves bilaterally to decrease atrial constriction. Posterior pericardiectomy frequently requires cardiopulmonary bypass because of the cardiac manipulation necessary, and the necessary heparinization can result in significant blood loss in some cases of severe pericarditis. Once again, the necessity and advantages of posterior pericardiectomy remain unclear.

Pericardiectomy for constriction provides excellent symptomatic improvement, with 85% of late survivors being NYHA Class I and the remainder being Class II.[21] The operative mortality rate for pericardiectomy for constriction is 14%, primarily as a result of persistent low cardiac output in 70% of deaths.[21] The operative mortality rate varies with preoperative NYHA class, being 1% for Class I–II, 10% for Class III, and 46% for Class IV.[21]

REFERENCES

1. Anand IS, Ferrari R, Kalra GS, et al: Pathogenesis of edema in constrictive pericarditis. Circulation 83:1880–1887, 1991.
2. Baker AE, Dani R, Smith ER, et al: Quantitative assessment of independent contributions of pericardium and septum to direct ventricular interaction. Am J Physiol 275:H476–H483, 1998.
3. Bennett KR: Congenital foramen of the left pericardium. Ann Thorac Surg 70:993–998, 2000.
4. Brinker JA, Weiss JL, Lappe DL, et al: Leftward septal displacement during right ventricular loading in man. Circulation 61:626–633, 1980.
5. Candell-Riera J: Tamponade and constriction: An appraisal of echocardiography and external pulse recordings. In Soler-Soler J, Permanyer-Miralda G, Sagrista-Sauleda J, editors: Pericardial Disease, pp. 17–45. Dordrecht, The Netherlands: Kluwer Academic Publishers, 1990.
6. Corey GR, Campbell PT, Van Trigt P, et al: Etiology of large pericardial effusions. Am J Med 95:209–213, 1993.
7. Cummings RG, Wesley RLR, Adams DH, et al: Pneumopericardium resulting in cardiac tamponade. Ann Thorac Surg 37:511–518, 1984.
8. Davis RD Jr., Oldham HN Jr., Sabiston DC Jr.: Primary cysts and neoplasms of the mediastinum: Recent changes in clinical presentation, methods of diagnosis, management, and results. Ann Thorac Surg 44:229–237, 1987.
9. DeHert SG, tenBroecke PW, Rodrigus IE, et al: The effects of the pericardium on length-dependent regulation of left ventricular function in coronary artery surgery patients. J Cardiothorac Vasc Anesth 15:300–305. 2001.
10. Franklin DL, Van Critters RL, Rushmer RF: Balance between right and left ventricular output. Circ Res 10:17–25, 1962.
11. Galindo Gallego M, Lopez-Cambra MJ, Fernandez-Acenero MJ, et al: Traumatic rupture of the pericardium. Case report and literature review. J Cardiovasc Surg 37:187–191, 1996.
12. Gatzoulis MA, Munk MD, Merchant N, et al: Isolated congenital absence of the pericardium: Clinical presentation, diagnosis, and management. Ann Thorac Surg 69:1209–1215, 2000.
13. Glantz SA, Misbach GA, Moores WY, et al: The pericardium substantially affects the left ventricular diastolic pressure-volume relationship. Am J Physiol 42:433–441, 1978.
14. Hazelrigg SR, Mack MJ, Landreneau RJ, et al: Thoracoscopic pericardiectomy for effusive pericardial disease. Ann Thorac Surg 56:792–795, 1993.
15. Kojima S, Yamada N, Goto Y: Diagnosis of constrictive pericarditis by tagged cine magnetic resonance imaging. N Engl J Med 341:373–374, 1999.
16. Kovanlikaya A, Burke LP, Nelson MD, et al: Characterizing chronic pericarditis using steady-state free-precession cine MR imaging. Am J Roentgenol 179:475–476, 2002.
17. Krogmann ON, Traber J, Jakob M, et al: Determinants of left ventricular diastolic function during myocardial ischemia: Influence of myocardial structure and pericardial constraint. Coron Artery Dis 9:239–248, 1998.
18. Kutlay H, Yavuze, I, Han S, et al: Atypically located pericardial cysts. Ann Thorac Surg 72:2137–2139, 2001.
19. May AK, Patterson MA, Rue LW 3rd, et al: Combined blunt cardiac and pericardial rupture: Review of the literature and report of a new diagnostic algorithm. Am Surg 65:568–574, 1999.
20. McAllister HA Jr., Hall RJ, Cooley DA: Tumors of the heart and pericardium. Curr Prob Cardiol 24(2):57–116, 1999.
21. McCaughan BC, Schaff HV, Piehler JM, et al: Early and late results of pericardiectomy for constrictive pericarditis. J Thorac Cardiovasc Surg 89:340–350, 1985.
22. Miller DL, Katz NM, Kulkarni PK, et al: Right congenital pericardial defects. Am Heart J 126:1235–1238, 1993.
23. Moores DWO, Allen KB, Faber LP, et al: Subxiphoid pericardial drainage for pericardial tamponade. J Thorac Cardiovasc Surg 109:546–551, 1995.
24. Moores DWO, Dziuban SW Jr.: Pericardial drainage procedures. Chest Surg Clin N Am 5:359–373, 1995.
25. Nugue O, Millaire A, Porte H, et al: Pericardioscopy in the etiologic diagnosis of pericardial effusion in 141 consecutive patients. Circulation 94:1635–1641, 1996.
26. Oh KY, Shimizu M, Edwards WD, et al: Surgical pathology of the parietal pericardium: A study of 344 cases (1993–1999). Cardiovasc Pathol 10:157–168, 2001.
27. Ohtsuka T, Wolf RK, Wurnig P, et al: Thoracoscopic limited pericardial resection with an ultrasonic scalpel. Ann Thorac Surg 65:855–856, 1998.
28. Okuyama N., Wang CY, Rose EA, et al: Reduction of retrosternal and pericardial adhesions with rapidly resorbable polymer films. Ann Thorac Surg 68:913–918, 1999.

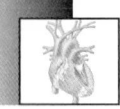

29. Olsen CO, Tyson GS, Maier GW, et al: Diminished stroke volume during inspiration: A reverse thoracic pump. Circulation 72:668–679, 1985.
30. Pataki N, Szelig L, Horvath OP, et al: Pericardial drainage using the transdiaphragmatic route: Refinement of the laparoscopic technique. Surg Endosc 16:1105, 2002.
31. Picardi EJ, Bedingfield J, Statz M, et al: Laparoscopic pericardial window. Surg Laparosc Endosc Percutan Tech 7:320–323, 1997.
32. Piehler JM, Pluth JR, Schaff HV, et al: Surgical management of effusive pericardial disease. J Thorac Cardiovasc Surg 90:506–516, 1985.
33. Rao V, Komeda M, Weisel RD, et al: Should the pericardium be closed routinely after heart operations? Ann Thorac Surg 67:484–488, 1999.
34. Sagrista-Sauleda J: Tuberculous pericarditis. In Soler-Soler J, Permanyer-Miralda G, Sagrista-Sauleda J, editors: Pericardial Disease, pp. 109–121. Dordrecht, The Netherlands: Kluwer Academic Publishers, 1990.
35. Selig MB: Percutaneous transcatheter pericardial interventions: Aspiration, biopsy, and pericardioplasty. Am Heart J 125: 269–271, 1993.
36. Spodick DH: Medical history of the pericardium. The hairy hearts of hoary heroes. Am J Cardiol 26:447–454, 1970.
37. Spodick DH: The Pericardium. New York: Marcel Dekker, Inc., 1997.
38. Sun Y, Beshara M, Lucariello RJ, et al: A comprehensive model for right-left heart interaction under the influence of pericardium and baroreflex. Am J Physiol 272:H1499–H1515, 1997.
39. Uthaman B, Endrys J, Abushaban L, et al: Percutaneous pericardial biopsy: technique, efficacy, safety, and value in the management of pericardial effusion in children and adolescents. Pediatr Cardiol 18:414–418, 1997.
40. Van Trigt P, Douglas J, Smith PK, et al: A prospective trial of subxiphoid pericardiotomy in the diagnosis and treatment of large pericardial effusion. Ann Surg 218:777–782, 1993.
41. Warren WH: Malignancies involving the pericardium. Semin Thorac Cardiovasc Surg 12:119–129, 2000.
42. White CS: MR evaluation of the pericardium and cardiac malignancies. Magn Reson Imaging Clin N Am 4:237–251, 1996.

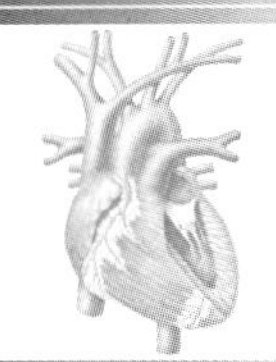

CHAPTER 91

Surgical Management of Hypertrophic Cardiomyopathy

William G. Williams, Ernest D. Wigle, Harry Rakowski, and Anthony C. Ralph-Edwards

INTRODUCTION

Hypertrophic cardiomyopathy (HCM) is a genetic disorder that affects 1 in 500 individuals in the general population (i.e., about one fourth of the prevalence of all forms of congenital heart disease).[13,14,21] HCM is inherited in an autosomal dominant pattern. Approximately 70% of cases are familial, and the rest are a result of spontaneous mutation. HCM is a heterogeneous disorder of sarcomere proteins, and to date 10 genes with as many as 34 discrete missense mutations have been identified. Mutations affecting β-myosin heavy chain, cardiac myosin-binding protein C, cardiac troponin T, troponin I, α-tropomyosin, regulatory myosin light chains, actin, and titin[13,15,21] have been characterized. In the future, when easily available genetic screening becomes available, better detection and outcome prediction may be possible. The troponin T and some β-myosin heavy chain mutations have been associated with a poor outcome.

Anatomically, HCM results in ventricular hypertrophy in the absence of an identifiable cause.[14,21,28,33] Hypertrophy is usually asymmetrical, and in 90% of patients it involves the interventricular septum. Most commonly the outlet septum (i.e., subaortic area) is the major focus of hypertrophy, but midventricular or apical septa may occur in isolation or concomitantly. Rarely (5%) the right ventricular outflow tract is stenosed. The extent of the hypertrophy varies tremendously and accounts for different manifestations of the disease.[14,16,21,28,33] Microscopically hypertrophied myocardium is associated with myocardial fiber disarray and fibrosis.

CLASSIFICATION OF HYPERTROPHIC CARDIOMYOPATHY

Based on hemodynamic data obtained via echocardiography or left ventricular catheterization, patients can be categorized as having either obstructive or nonobstructive forms of the disease (Box 91-1). The clinical manifestations of HCM vary depending on the extent and location of the hypertrophy and the resulting secondary hemodynamic effects.[31]

The obstruction may occur at rest, with provocation (latent), or intermittently (labile). The degree of obstruction varies directly with the inotropic state of the heart and inversely with the systemic vascular resistance and preload.

CLINICAL MANIFESTATIONS

The clinical presentation of HCM may be extremely varied. Common symptoms include dyspnea, fatigue, angina, palpitations, presyncope, syncope, and sudden death.

Dyspnea on exertion and fatigue are the most common symptoms in patients diagnosed with HCM. Dyspnea may be a result of poor left ventricular diastolic filling caused by either reduced compliance (secondary to hypertrophy) or impaired diastolic relaxation. In late stages of the disease, increasing left ventricular fibrosis may result in dilatation and further deterioration of compliance.

In patients with obstructive HCM, the associated mitral insufficiency related to systolic anterior motion of the anterior leaflet (SAM) increases left atrial pressure, resulting in limitation of exercise capacity, dyspnea, fatigue, and atrial arrhythmias.

Box 91–1. Classification of Hypertrophic Cardiomyopathy.

Nonobstructive HCM

- Abnormal diastolic function (impaired relaxation and impaired compliance)
- Normal or supernormal systolic function
- Impaired systolic (end-stage) systolic function (secondary to myocardial fibrosis)

Obstructive HCM

- Subaortic obstruction
- Midventricular obstruction
- Apical obstruction

Patients with extensive hypertrophy may develop angina as a result of inadequate endocardial perfusion. Concomitant coronary atherosclerosis may lead to regional ischemia, with the hypertrophied areas being at increased risk. In addition, 5% of patients with HCM have one or more intramyocardial coronary arteries, resulting in myocardial bridges that may compress the segment of coronary during systole. These myocardial bridges most often affect the left anterior descending artery. The systolic obliteration of the coronary lumen alters the diastolic flow pattern and has been linked to both angina and an increased risk of sudden death.[36,37]

Palpitations may be a result of supraventricular or ventricular arrhythmias. Atrial dilation occurs as a result of poor left ventricular diastolic function and mitral regurgitation. Patients with a left atrial diameter >50 mm are at increased risk of atrial fibrillation. The onset of supraventricular arrhythmia usually precipitates a marked increase in symptoms as a result of decreased cardiac output and hypotension, and often culminates in referral to the emergency department. The onset of atrial fibrillation also increases the risk of stroke. Ventricular arrhythmia may occur with HCM and is an ominous sign of increased risk of sudden death.[2–4,18,21,27] The mechanism of ventricular arrhythmia is not completely understood, but precipitating factors may relate to marginal endocardial perfusion, myocardial fibrosis, and, in some patients, an intramyocardial coronary artery.

Patients may suffer syncopal episodes as a result of vasovagal attacks or secondary to transient arrhythmia, including ventricular tachycardia or fibrillation. A history of sudden death is not uncommon among HCM patients and their relatives. Syncope is a major risk factor for sudden death. Increasing septal thickness also has been correlated with increased risk of sudden death.[25,29] Brief periods of ventricular tachycardia may not be associated with an increased risk of sudden death.[27]

HCM accounts for about one third of sudden deaths among young athletes.[21] The outcome of 16 patients with HCM who were resuscitated from ventricular tachycardia or fibrillation demonstrated that they were at increased risk for further malignant arrhythmia.[5]

Many patients are asymptomatic and may remain so.[9,14,16,21] The high prevalence of HCM in the general population (1 in 500) is further evidence that many individuals are asymptomatic. Symptoms in children are very uncommon, although they are not immune to sudden death.[36,37] Symptoms may first develop during adolescence, possibly as a result of accelerated development of myocardial hypertrophy. Most patients become symptomatic in their fourth or fifth decade. Because of the dynamic nature of the obstructive form of HCM, symptoms vary in intensity from day to day, depending on normal variation in endogenous inotropic state and peripheral vascular resistance.

PHYSIOLOGY OF OBSTRUCTIVE HYPERTROPHIC CARDIOMYOPATHY

Patients with asymmetrical septal hypertrophy develop left ventricular outlet obstruction, at the apex, at the midventricle, or most commonly in the subaortic area.[31–33]

In the most common variant of subaortic stenosis, the thickened septal wall protrudes into the left ventricular outlet just caudal to the aortic valve and opposite the mitral valve annulus and anterior mitral leaflet.[8] The thickened septum narrows the subaortic outlet. To compensate and maintain a normal cardiac output, the left ventricle contracts more vigorously to force blood through the diminishing diameter of the subaortic channel. Consequently, there is flow acceleration in the subaortic region, and a pressure gradient develops between the body of the left ventricle and the aorta. The left ventricle responds to this increased systolic pressure demand by generalized hypertrophy. Therefore a vicious circle ensues consisting of the hypertrophied septum obstructing the outlet, causing increased left ventricular work and subsequent hypertrophy that aggravates the outlet obstruction further.

The flow acceleration in the subaortic outlet affects the mitral valve and left atrium.[38] The anterior mitral valve leaflet is "lifted" toward the septum by the systolic venturi forces resulting from flow acceleration. Commonly the anterior leaflet moves toward the ventricular septum in midsystole, much as the airflow over an airplane wing lifts the airplane into the air.[39] The mitral valve leaflet displacement is referred to as systolic anterior motion, or SAM. Because of the leaflet displacement, normal coaptation of the mitral valve leaflets is prevented and regurgitation results. The mitral regurgitation as a result of SAM typically is posteriorly directed and occurs late in systole. The degree of regurgitation is proportional to the severity of the obstruction. Those factors that increase contractility, decrease peripheral resistance, or decrease preload increase the severity of SAM and the related mitral valve regurgitation.

It is important to recognize that the mitral regurgitation associated with subaortic obstruction occurs after SAM–septal contact and resolves when the outlet obstruction is relieved. Conversely, mitral regurgitation that occurs before SAM–septal contact is unrelated to the obstruction and persists after relief of the obstruction. Many patients experience regurgitation as a result of a combination of intrinsic valve anomalies (e.g., prolapse, myxomatous degeneration) and SAM.

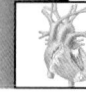

TREATMENT OF HYPERTROPHIC CARDIOMYOPATHY

Nonobstructive Hypertrophic Cardiomyopathy

Medical Treatment

Many patients remain asymptomatic or have mild symptoms and do not require treatment. They should, however, be assessed for the risk of sudden death. Because 50% of the siblings of patients may have the disease, it is important to screen all family members.

Patients who are symptomatic with nonobstructive HCM are managed medically with drugs that improve compliance, such as β-blockers to slow heart rate, or with calcium channel blockers to improve diastolic relaxation. Both agents improve left ventricular filling. The combination of β-blockers and verapamil should be avoided because it may increase the risk of sudden death.

Antiarrhythmic drugs may be indicated for patients at risk of atrial fibrillation or sudden death. Amiodarone is most commonly used, and its efficacy is supported by McKenna's data.[34,35]

However, a comparison of antiarrhythmic drugs versus automatic implantable cardioverter defibrillators (AICDs) for patients with HCM who had been resuscitated after episodes of near-fatal ventricular arrhythmia suggests that AICDs may be more effective than drugs.[19]

Anticoagulants should be considered for patients with chronic atrial fibrillation because they are at risk of stroke.

Implantable Defibrillators

Patients with HCM and a history of resuscitation from sudden death, documented ventricular tachycardia, or with a strong family history of sudden death should be considered for an implantable defibrillator.

In a multicenter study of 128 patients, Maron and associates[19] reported appropriate defibrillator discharge, and presumed salvage from what would have been sudden death, of 7% of patients per year. A similar proportion of patients had an inappropriate discharge, however.

We believe that patients resuscitated from sudden death should have coronary angiography to rule out a myocardial bridge. If myocardial bridge is present, they should undergo surgical unroofing of the coronary artery.[37]

Pacemaker Implantation for Hypertrophic Cardiomyopathy

Patients with the obstructive form of HCM (HOCM) may benefit from dual chamber (DDD) pacing, as first reported by McDonald et al.[23] The mechanism by which pacing may improve symptoms or lessen obstruction has been variously ascribed to asynchronous depolarization of the left and right ventricles causing paradoxical septal motion, a negative inotropic effect, decreased mitral valve SAM, increased end-systolic volume, or altered myocardial perfusion. The clinical benefit of pacing in HOCM is controversial. A recent prospective randomized double-blind crossover trial recommends that pacing not be used as primary therapy.[17] Pacing was associated with some symptomatic improvement and a modest reduction in outflow tract gradient of 40%, but objective exercise testing demonstrated no benefit, nor was there a change in left ventricular wall thickness on echocardiographic follow-up. The authors did concede that the elderly patient (>age 65 years) may benefit from DDD pacing.

Heart Transplantation

Between 5 and 10% of HCM patients may reach a terminal end-stage of dilated cardiomyopathy.[14,21,28,33] Thinning of the ventricular walls precedes this stage and leads to markedly dilated atrial and ventricular chambers. Therapy other than transplant is ineffective at this stage.

Myectomy for Patients with Hypertrophic Obstructive Cardiomyopathy

Patients who are symptomatic with the subaortic obstructive form of HCM will benefit from subaortic myectomy.[10,22,30,34,35] The indications for surgery include symptoms refractory to medical management, intolerance of medication, and some high-risk groups. Young patients with a thick septum (>24 mm) and those with a strong family history of sudden death should be considered for primary surgical treatment to improve prognosis. When genetic mapping becomes practical, it may help triage patients with high-risk genotypes toward primary surgical myectomy.

We do not consider that midventricular or apical obstruction is an indication for surgical myectomy, although the Mayo clinic group has reported success in a small group of patients with isolated midventricular obstruction.

Some patients have combined subaortic and midventricular obstruction, and they do benefit from myectomy that is extended toward the apex.

Preoperative Assessment

A careful clinical history and family history are important in assessing risk with and without surgery. Identification of concomitant disease is essential because additional cardiac lesions or other significant medical disorders alter the patient's risk.

The echocardiogram is invaluable in assessing both the extent and severity of the hypertrophy and in clarifying the function of the mitral valve.[7,38,39] Although this information should be available and reviewed before surgical consultation, a transesophageal echo assessment is essential in the operating room, both before and after the myectomy.[7]

In adult patients suitable for myectomy, the interventricular septum is greater than 17 mm and may be considerably thicker. The echo measurement is useful in gauging the depth of resection to be performed. The length of the hypertrophied septum is measured to determine what the length of the excision should be. Associated midventricular obstruction, which can be masked by the outlet stenosis, requires a longer resection to a level below the head of the papillary muscles.

The mitral valve regurgitation should be assessed by both echocardiography and contrast ventriculography for its quantity, direction, and timing (vide supra). Mitral regurgitation secondary to obstruction occurs after the SAM–septal contact and is characteristically posteriorly directed. Alterations in this pattern do exist and can resolve after successful myectomy, but significant regurgitation unrelated to obstruction may require concomitant mitral valve repair or replacement.

Because of the association of coronary artery myocardial bridges with HCM and the potential association with sudden death, every patient who is considered for surgery should have a selective coronary angiogram to document the presence or absence of both coronary artery disease and myocardial bridges.

Operative Technique of Myectomy

Myectomy is performed during cardiopulmonary bypass with single right atrial cannulation and venting of the left ventricle via the right superior pulmonary vein.

Myocardial hypothermia is used during bypass, but we avoid initiating cooling until after the myocardium has been arrested with blood cardioplegia at normal temperature. Once the normothermic cardioplegia arrests the heart, the cardioplegia is cooled and administration is continued until the myocardium reaches 15° C, generally requiring about 1500 ml of solution in total. Cooling the beating perfused heart may be dangerous because the hypertrophied heart may fibrillate and cardioplegic perfusion may not be distributed evenly. This situation can result in poor diastolic relaxation and difficulty with defibrillation after reperfusion. With warm induction cardioplegia, the heart usually recovers spontaneously during reperfusion, with or without a terminal dose of warm cardioplegia.

The septal resection is done through an oblique aortotomy that extends to, but not across, the sinotubular junction. Before the myectomy, the outflow tract and mitral and aortic valves should be carefully examined and the septal thickness and length of hypertrophy palpated to confirm the echo findings. Transmural palpation of the free left ventricular wall apical and distal to the septum provides a good guide as to what the septal thickness should be after resection.

The excision requires three incisions in the septum. It is illustrated in the accompanying diagram (Figure 91-1).

The initial septal subaortic incision is made with a #11 scalpel blade and starts 2 mm below the right cusp of the aortic valve, 2–3 mm to the right of its nadir. If this incision is started further to the right, it increases the risk of damaging the bundle of His, resulting in complete heart block. If the hypertrophy is unusually prominent on the right side of the outflow tract, the initial incision may be made further to the right but lower (10 mm from the aortic valve) in the septum and slanted to the left as it extends upward toward the aortic annulus. The depth of this initial incision depends on the estimate, by echo and palpation, of the septal thickness. The depth should leave a residual septal thickness of 5–8 mm, similar to the free left ventricular wall below the septum. The direction of the initial incision is toward the apex. For right-handed surgeons, the tendency is to direct the incision too far to the left of the apex. To avoid this, the surgeon can make the incision with the left hand. The length of the initial incision depends on the extent of the hypertrophy, but generally is 35–50 mm long in the adult patient. For patients with concomitant midventricular obstruction, the incision should extend at least to the level of the anteroseptal papillary muscle head. Transmural palpation of the incision is used to judge the adequacy of both its depth and length.

The second incision is made parallel to the first one and is 2 mm anterior to the left side of the mitral valve insertion. The septum is narrower here than on the right, so the second incision is not as long. Its depth is again determined by palpation, leaving a residual septal thickness of about 8 mm.

The third incision is made 2 mm below and parallel to the aortic annulus. It extends from the proximal extent of the first incision to the proximal extent of the second. The depth of this incision is only 2 mm because a deeper incision would become too shallow. Once the septum is exposed with this incision, it allows a second cut, also 2 mm deep, in a more anterior direction. A third 2-mm incision may be required to establish the depth of the resection, guided by transmural palpation and the depth of the first and second incisions. (The purpose of the superficial 2-mm-deep incisions is somewhat analogous to a series of short straight lines, each at an angle to one another, creating a curved line.) Once the appropriate depth of the third incision is established, the block of muscle to be excised is dissected distally toward the apex, confirming by repeated palpation that the direction and residual septal depth leave a residual septal thickness of 5–8 mm. Under the right–left commissure, the top of the resection is an acute angle as a result of the convergence of the annulus. As the dissection continues caudally, the resection located more distally under the commissure must be rounded to avoid perforating the septum below the pulmonary valve. On palpation of the residual septum, there should be no difference in thickness compared with the free left ventricular wall below the septum.

The cross-sectional area of the resected specimen should be approximately the area of the aortic valve. On average the resection measures 25 mm wide, 45 mm in length, and 15 mm in depth.

Before the aortic incision is closed, the mitral and aortic valves, including the mitral chordae, are inspected for inadvertent damage. The left ventricular cavity is irrigated to remove any loose pieces of muscle, and the bed of the resection is checked for muscle fragments.

Intraoperative Postmyectomy Transesophageal Echocardiography

Once off bypass, the adequacy of the myectomy is checked by transesophageal echo (TEE).[7,38,39] The outflow tract should be a normal diameter, and the mitral valve SAM should be absent, allowing the mitral valve to close in a normal plane of apposition. On Doppler interrogation, the mitral regurgitation should be considerably less or absent, and the left ventricular outflow gradient should be <10 mm Hg, with minimal or no increase in gradient after an induced extrasystole. It is not uncommon for some chordal SAM to persist. Color flow Doppler imaging should rule out a ventricular septal perforation, and usually identifies divided septal perforator arteries in the base of the resection.

Because the plane of the echo lies at a 30° angle to the plane of the myectomy, the medial wall of the resection appears on TEE as a prominent right-angled divot. Within a week of myectomy, this edge of the myectomy atrophies, thereby increasing the outlet diameter further.

Technique of Unroofing Coronary Artery Myocardial Bridge

An intramyocardial course of a coronary artery, usually the left anterior descending, may be associated with sudden

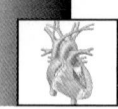

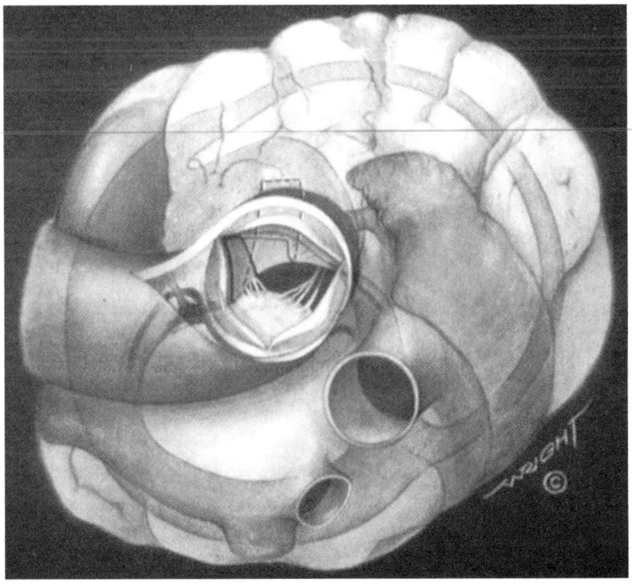

A

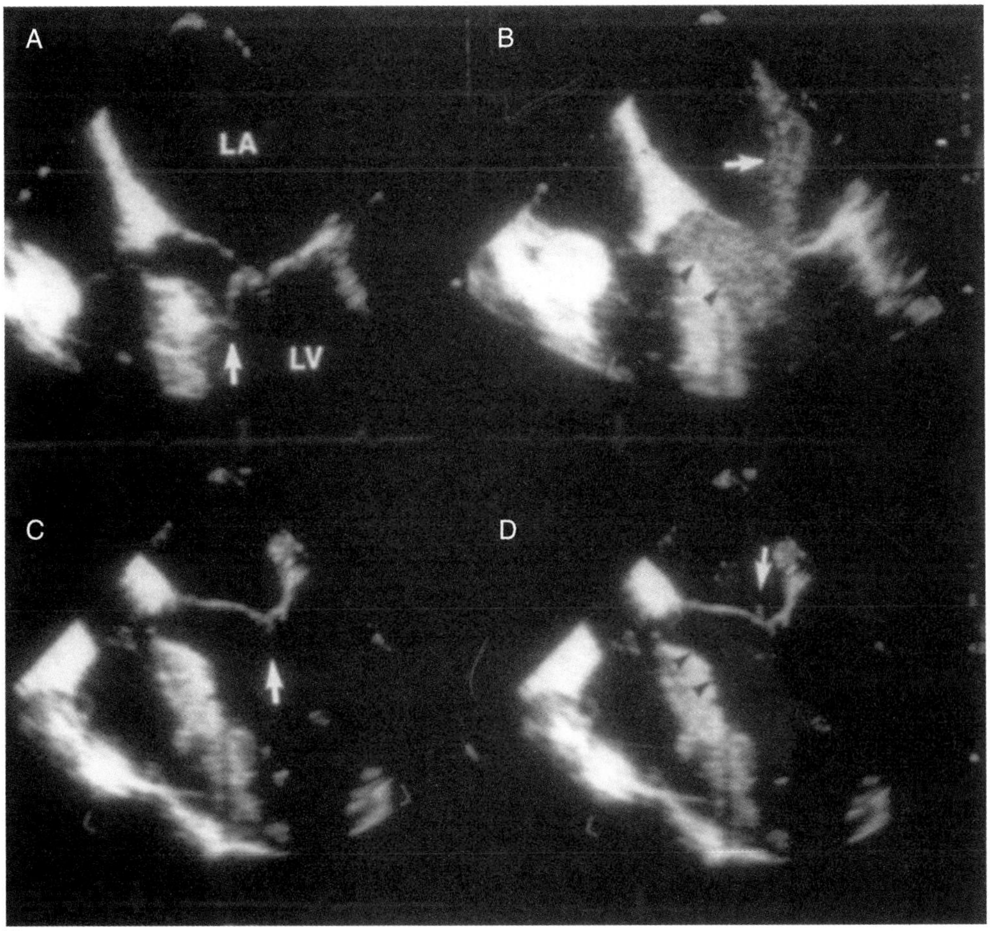

B

Figure 91–1 **A,** A surgeon's view of the heart from the patient's right side, looking toward the apex. The ascending aorta is shown open through an oblique aortotomy, exposing the trileaflet aortic valve. The protruding septum is seen in pink, narrowing the outflow tract opposite the mitral valve, shown in yellow. The stippled color indicates the thickness of the ventricular septum. The three incisions to complete the myectomy are labeled and described in the text. **B,** Panel A: The long-axis view of the left ventricular outflow tract by transesophageal echocardiography before myectomy. The thickened ventricular septum is evident, causing narrowing of the subaortic area. Panel B: The systolic anterior motion of the mitral valve has resulted in the SAM–septal contact *(arrow)*. Doppler imaging at that point in time shows turbulence into the left ventricular outflow tract and, at the same time, posteriorly directed mitral regurgitation. Panel C: Post-myectomy view of the enlarged left ventricular outlet showing the thinner outlet septum. Note that the plane of the mitral valve closure is normal. Panel D: Doppler imaging demonstrates resolution of the mitral regurgitation and normal flow across the subaortic outflow.

death, even in HCM patients without obstruction.[36,37] Systolic compression of the coronary artery may be impressive on cine angiography. Among our surgical patients with HOCM, 39 of 379 (10.2%) had a myocardial bridge. Whether the natural history of these patients results in an increased risk of death is unknown. However, for those who are having a myectomy, we attempt to unroof the coronary muscle bridge. The coronary artery distal to the tunnel is identified, and its superficial (anterior) surface is exposed by sharp dissection. The sharp dissection is then extended proximally along the plane of the artery until it reemerges onto the epicardial surface. The divided myocardium over the artery is usually 3–5 mm thick. Unfortunately, the course of the artery may be so deep that trabeculations of the right ventricular cavity are entered. In this situation, after the myocardial bridge has been divided, the opening into the

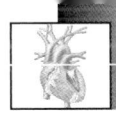

ventricle is repaired by pledgeted sutures placed deep into the coronary artery.

Postoperative Management

Patients who have had a myectomy are managed similarly to most patients with cardiac disease and benefit from an early extubation protocol.[1] Patients with HCM have increased myocardial contractility and require only an adequate preload. They seldom need inotropic support or afterload reduction, and both are contraindicated in patients with obstruction. Volume loading and atrial pacing should be used to manage low cardiac output, and hypotension may require a phenylephrine infusion to increase afterload. β-Agonists should be avoided if possible because these agents may induce arrhythmias or augment any existing residual subaortic gradient.

Postoperative atrioventricular (AV) block is common early after surgery, but permanent block is not common (4%). All patients should have temporary atrial and ventricular pacing wires, and all should be connected to backup ventricular demand pacing. It is not uncommon for patients who have had a myectomy to require temporary AV pacing for a few hours. Most patients resolve to sinus rhythm with a left bundle branch block, and therefore those with preoperative right bundle branch block are at high risk of developing postoperative complete AV block. Overall, about 4–5% of patients who have had a myectomy need permanent pacing.

Atrial arrhythmia, typically atrial fibrillation, is not uncommon a few days after myectomy, and we routinely prescribe sotalol the morning after myectomy and for 3 months after surgery to prevent or control atrial fibrillation.

Surgical Results of Myectomy

Since 1972 we have operated on 379 patients with HOCM. The median age at surgery is 44.2 years (range 0.2–76.4 years) (Figure 91-2). Thirty-nine were children (<18 years). Males predominated, 235 versus 144 (62% of the total).

Most patients were symptomatic before myectomy; the majority (59%) were New York Heart Association (NYHA) class III (Figure 91-3). Some younger children with high gradients and very thick septa were operated on in the absence of symptoms.

Lesions, in addition to HOCM, were present in 145 patients (38%) (Table 91-1).

A previous myectomy had been performed in 23 patients. Three of the previous operations were done by the author and 20 by other surgeons.

There were six early deaths (1.5%), and during a mean follow-up period of 6.1 years (median 4.9 years, range 0–26.5 years) there have been 36 late deaths. Survival is illustrated by the Kaplan–Meier method (Figure 91-4).

Survival at 10 years after myectomy is estimated to be 83% (±3%), and at 20 years, 68% (±8%) (Table 91-2).

Poorer preoperative NYHA class has some influence on early survival, but long-term survival is not different (Figure 91-5). The presence of associated pathology, especially coronary artery disease, by univariate analysis is associated with an increased risk of mortality (Figure 91-6). A myocardial bridge (n = 39) or surgical unroofing of a myocardial coronary artery bridge (n = 32) was not associated with early or late mortality. Permanent pacing, either before myectomy

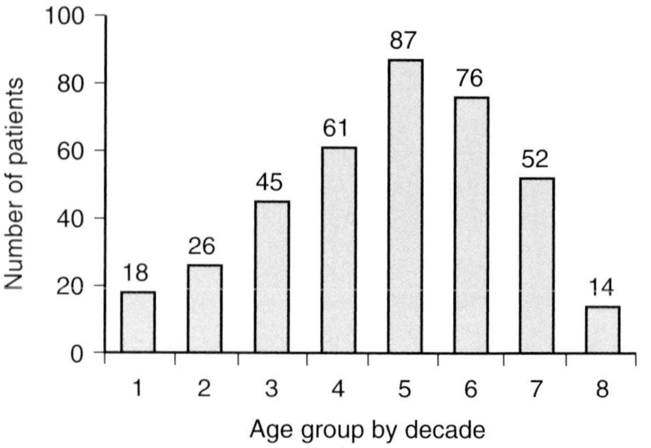

Figure 91–2 The histogram illustrates the age range at myectomy by decade. Median age is 44.2 years.

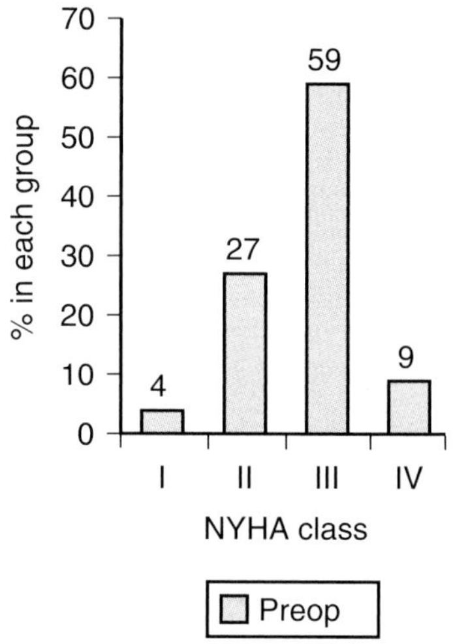

Figure 91–3 Preoperative New York Heart Association (NYHA) class.

Table 91–1

Major associated pathology	*N*	*% of total*
None	234	62%
Coronary artery	47	12%
Coronary myocardial bridge	39	10%
Mitral disease	29	8%
Midventricular stenosis	23	6%
Aortic disease	15	4%
RVOTO	8	2%

Some patients had more than one associated lesion; 28 patients had other miscellaneous lesions. RVOTO, right ventricular outflow tract

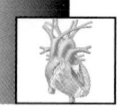

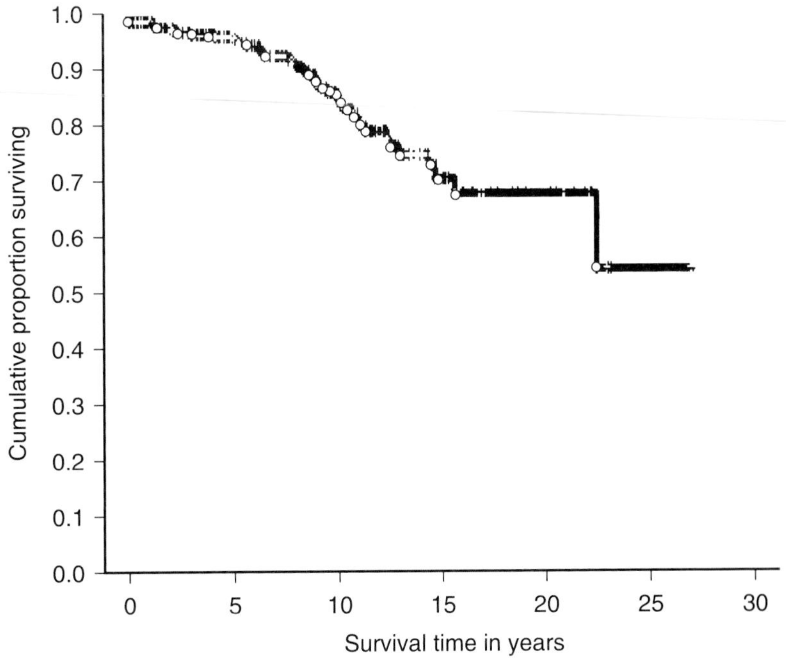

Figure 91–4 The Kaplan–Meier plot shows the survival after myectomy for 379 patients with obstructive hypertrophic cardiomyopathy. Survival at 5, 10, and 20 years is estimated to be 95%, 83%, and 68%, respectively.

Table 91–2

Univariate Risk Factors for Survival

Variables	*p*
Preoperative	
Age at myectomy: Children (39) vs. adults (339)	n.s.
Age by decade	n.s.
Male (234) vs. female (144)	n.s.
Associated pathology (144 vs. 235)	.01
Coronary artery disease (46 vs. 333)	<.001
Coronary myocardial bridge (39 vs. 340)	n.s.
Septal thickness	.017
Intraoperative	
Concomitant procedures (121 vs. 258)	.07
Coronary bypass (44 vs. 335)	<.001
Coronary unroofing (31 vs. 348)	n.s.
Aortic cross-clamp time (larger)	.05
Greater than median of 56-min pacemaker	n.s.

n.s., not statistically significant.

(n = 14) or after myectomy (n = 40), did not affect overall survival.

Early postoperative complications occurred in 20% of patients, the most important of which were strokes in six patients, one of whom had permanent severe long-term damage. Complete AV block requiring permanent pacing early after surgery occurred in 7% of the patients who had myectomy.

The hemodynamic changes that result from myectomy have been described previously.[7,38,39] Basically the myectomy enlarges the outlet to a normal diameter, thereby both relieving the outlet pressure gradient and normalizing the flow acceleration. This corrects the mitral valve SAM and allows the mitral leaflets to coapt normally, thereby relieving the mitral insufficiency. The intraoperative echo systolic pressure gradient among our patients decreased from 72 mmHg (±28) to 7 mmHg (±7), and the mitral regurgitation decreased from 58% moderate to severe before myectomy to 95% mild or less after myectomy.

Symptomatic improvement after myectomy is impressive, with 93% of patients becoming NYHA class I at the most recent follow up (Figure 91-7). Symptomatic improvement persists in most patients.

Reoperation has been required in only 11 patients, including four for recurrent (more likely persistent) outlet obstruction and one for midventricular obstruction. Three patients required a heart transplant, one required an aortic valve replacement after late endocarditis, one required a mitral valve replacement and atrial maze, and one other patient was reoperated on for an iatrogenic ventricular septal defect (VSD).

The median time to reoperation was 5.5 years (range 0–19 years). The probability of reoperation (n = 10) is illustrated by the Kaplan–Meier plot in Figure 91-8. Freedom from reoperation is 96% ± 1.5% at 10 years after myectomy. Recurrent subaortic stenosis was the indication for reoperation in only four patients. In one other patient, midventricular stenosis was the indication for reoperation. Three patients had a heart transplant, one had a mitral valve replacement and atrial maze, and the final patient was reoperated on for a VSD.

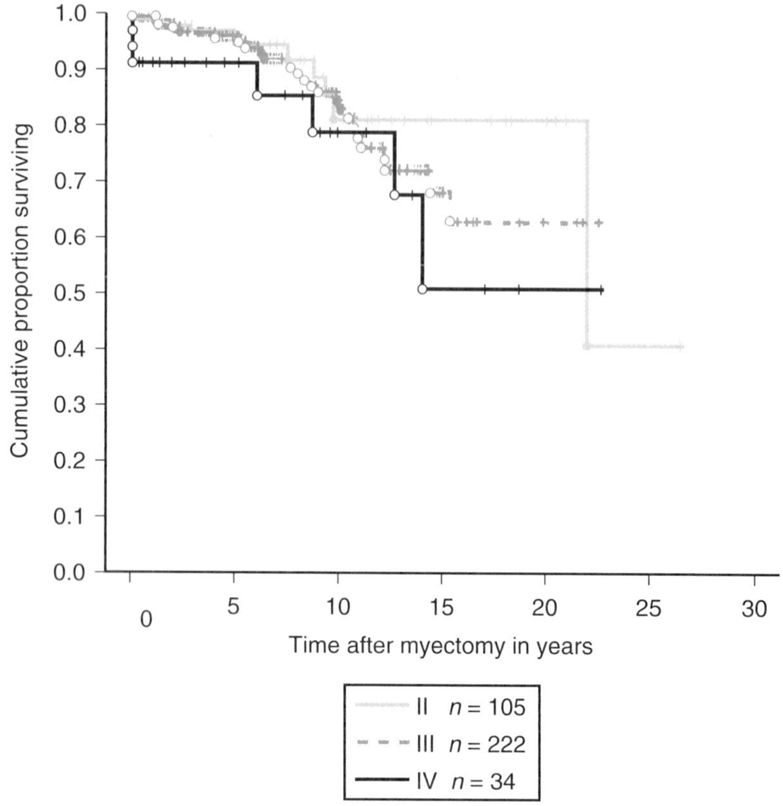

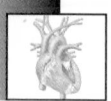

Figure 91–5 The early postmyectomy mortality rate is higher among patients with preoperative NYHA class IV symptoms. However, the overall mortality is not different. Not shown on the graph are 19 NYHA class I patients, among whom there are no deaths. Other univariate risk factors for mortality are shown in Table 91-2.

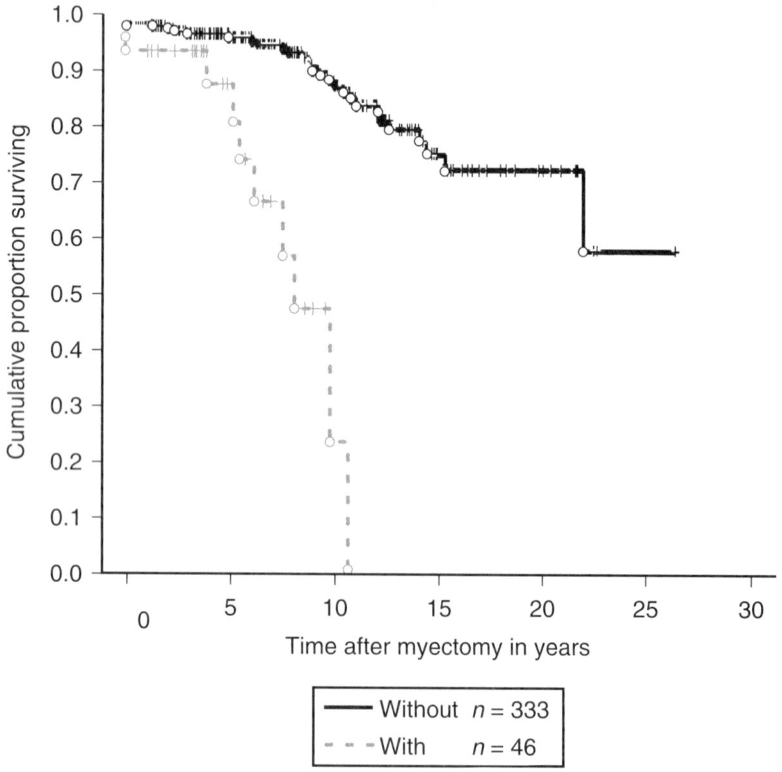

Figure 91–6 Coronary artery disease, present in 44 patients, was a significant predictor of increased prevalence of late death.

SUMMARY

HCM is a myocardial disease from a genetic mutation that results in myocardial hypertrophy in the absence of an obvious stimulus for that hypertrophy. Protein synthesis is altered in the subaortic region compared with elsewhere in the left ventricular wall.[11,12] HCM is not uncommon among the general population, occurring in perhaps 1 in 500 people. Manifestations of the disease are very diverse. The majority of patients are asymptomatic and have a normal life expectancy.

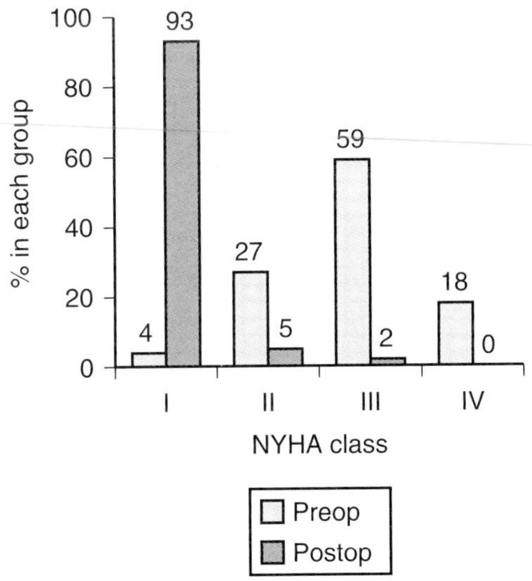

Figure 91–7 Symptomatic improvement of patients with the obstructive form of hypertrophic cardiomyopathy (HCM) after myectomy is impressive, with 93% becoming NYHA class I.

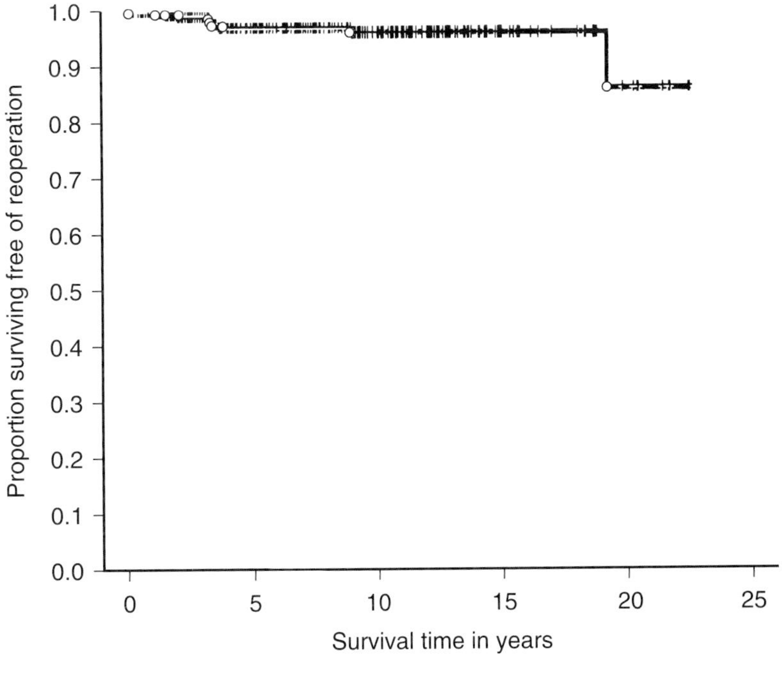

Figure 91–8 Only four patients required reoperation for subaortic obstruction, and one required reoperation for midventricular obstruction. The other six patients had reoperation for other reasons, including heart transplant (three patients), aortic valve replacement, mitral valve replacement, and ventricular septal defect (VSD).

However, symptoms from arrhythmias, altered diastolic function, or from apical, midventricular, or outlet obstruction, the latter usually associated with mitral valve regurgitation, may be severe and are associated with early death.

Surgical treatment is a useful therapeutic option for some patients with HCM. For those patients with HCM who are at high risk of sudden death, an implantable defibrillator should be considered. For the small number of patients with end-stage myocardial dysfunction, a heart transplant may be the only option.

Surgical myectomy for symptomatic patients with the obstructive form of HCM is a low-risk (1.5% mortality) procedure that improves symptoms in 93% of patients and may extend longevity. The results of surgical myectomy are a standard against which the recent advent of catheter alcohol-ablation of the blood supply to the septum should be compared.[20,26]

ACKNOWLEDGMENTS

The data included in this chapter are derived from the CVSDB,* the database of the division of cardiovascular surgery of the Hospital for Sick Children. The authors thank the data manager M. Gail Williams for her invaluable assistance.

*mgwillms@istar.ca

REFERENCES

1. Cregg N, Cheng DCH, Karski JM, et al: Morbidity outcome in patients with hypertrophic obstructive cardiomyopathy undergoing cardiac septal myectomy: Early-extubation anesthesia versus high-dose opioid anesthesia technique. J Cardiothorac Vasc Anesth 13:47–52, 1999.
2. Doevendans PA: Hypertrophic cardiomyopathy: Do we have the algorithm for life and death? Circulation 101:1224–1226, 2000.
3. Drory Y, Turetz Y, Hiss Y, et al: Sudden unexpected death in persons < 40 years of age. Am J Cardiol 68:1388–1392, 1991.
4. Elliott PM, Poloniecki J, Dickie S, et al: Sudden death in hypertrophic cardiomyopathy: Identification of high risk patient. J Am Coll Cardiol 36:2212–2218, 2000.
5. Elliott PM, Sharma S, Varnava A, et al: Survival after cardiac arrest or sustained ventricular tachycardia in patients with hypertrophic cardiomyopathy. J Am Coll Cardiol 33: 1596–1601, 1999.
6. Gilligan DM, Missouris CG, Boyd MJ, et al: Sudden death due to ventricular tachycardia during Amiodarone therapy in familial hypertrophic cardiomyopathy. Am J Cardiol 68: 971–973, 1991.
7. Grigg LE, Wigle ED, Williams WG, et al: Transesophageal echocardiography in obstructive hypertrophic cardiomyopathy: Clarification of pathophysiology and importance of intraoperative decision making. J Am Coll Cardiol 53:42–52, 1992.
8. Grigg LE, Wigle ED, Williams WG, et al: Transesophageal Doppler echocardiography in obstructive hypertrophic cardiomyopathy: Clarification of pathophysiology and importance in intraoperative decision making. J Am Coll Cardiol 20:53–54, 1992.
9. Hecht GM, Panza JA, Maron BJ: Clinical course of middle-aged asymptomatic patients with hypertrophic cardiomyopathy. Am J Cardiol 69:935–940, 1992.
10. Heric B, Lytle BW, Miller DP, et al: Surgical management of hypertrophic obstructive cardiomyopathy. Early and late results. J Thorac Cardiovasc Surg 110:195–208, 1995.
11. Li G, Li R-K, Mickle DAG, et al: Elevated insulin-like growth factor-1 and transforming growth factor-BI and their receptors in patients with idiopathic hypertrophic obstructive cardiomyopathy. Circulation 98:II144–150, 1998.
12. Li G, Borger MA, Williams WG, et al: Regional overexpression of IGF-1 and TGF-B1 in the myocardium of hypertrophic obstructive cardiomyopathy patients. J Thorac Cardiovasc Surg 123:89–95, 2002.
13. Maron BJ, Gardin JM, Flack JM, et al: Prevalence of hypertrophic cardiomyopathy in a general population of young adults: Echocardiographic analysis of 4111 subjects in the CARDIA study. Circulation 92:785–789, 1995.
14. Maron BJ: Hypertrophic cardiomyopathy. Lancet 350: 127–133, 1997.
15. Maron BJ, Moller JH, Seidman CE, et al: Impact of laboratory molecular diagnostic criteria for genetically transmitted cardiovascular diseases: Hypertrophic cardiomyopathy, long QT syndrome, and Marfan syndrome. Circulation 98:1460–1471, 1998.
16. Maron BJ, Casey SA, Poliac LC, et al: Clinical course of hypertrophic cardiomyopathy in a regional United States cohort. JAMA 281:650–655, 1999.
17. Maron BJ, Nishimura RA, McKenna WJ, et al: Assessment of permanent dual-chamber pacing as a treatment for drug-refractory symptomatic patients with obstructive hypertrophic cardiomyopathy. Circulation 99:2927–2933, 1999.
18. Maron BJ, Olivotto I, Spirito P, et al: Epidemiology of hypertrophic cardiomyopathy–related death. Circulation 102:858–864, 2000.
19. Maron BJ, Shen W-K, Link MS, et al: Efficacy of implantable cardioverter-defibrillators for the prevention of sudden death in patients with hypertrophic cardiomyopathy. N Engl J Med 342:365–373, 2000.
20. Maron BJ: Role of alcohol septal ablation in treatment of obstructive hypertrophic cardiomyopathy. Lancet 355: 425–426, 2000.
21. Maron BJ, Salberg L: Hypertrophic Cardiomyopathy: For Patients, Their Families, and Interested Physicians. New York: Futura Medical Publishing, 2001.
22. McCully RB, Nishimura RA, Tajik AJ, et al: Extent of clinical improvement after surgical treatment of hypertrophic obstructive cardiomyopathy. Circulation 99:2927–2933, 1999.
23. McDonald K, McWilliams E, O'Keefe B, et al: Functional assessment of patients treated with permanent dual chamber pacing as a primary treatment for hypertrophic cardiomyopathy. Eur Heart J 9:893–898, 1988.
24. McKenna WJ, Oakley CM, Krikler DM, et al: Improved survival with Amiodarone in patients with hypertrophic cardiomyopathy and ventricular tachycardia. Br Heart J 53:412–416, 1985.
25. McKenna WJ, Camm AJ: Sudden death in hypertrophic cardiomyopathy: Assessment of patients at high risk. Circulation 80:1489–1492, 1989.
26. Seggewiss H, Gleichman U, Faber L, et al: Percutaneous transluminal septal myocardial ablation in hypertrophic obstructive cardiomyopathy: Acute results and 3 month follow-up in 25 patients. J Am Coll Cardiol 31:252–258, 1998.
27. Spirito P, Rapezzi C, Autore C, et al: Prognosis of asymptomatic patients with hypertrophic cardiomyopathy and nonsustained ventricular tachycardia. Circulation 90:2743–2747, 1994.
28. Spirito P, Sideman CE, McKenna WJ, et al: The management of hypertrophic cardiomyopathy. N Engl J Med 336:775–785, 1997.
29. Spirito P, Bellone P, Harris KM, et al: Magnitude of left ventricular hypertrophy and risk of sudden death in hypertrophic cardiomyopathy. N Engl J Med 342:1778–1785, 2000.
30. Theodoro DA, Danielson GK, Feldt RH, et al: Hypertrophic obstructive cardiomyopathy in pediatric patients: Results of surgical treatment. J Thorac Cardiovasc Surg 112:1589–1599, 1996.
31. Wigle ED, Sasson Z, Henderson MA, et al: Hypertrophic cardiomyopathy. The importance of the site and extent of the hypertrophy. A review. Prog Cardiovasc Dis 28:1–83, 1985.
32. Wigle ED, Rakowski H: Hypertrophic cardiomyopathy: When do you diagnose midventricular obstruction versus apical cavity obliteration with a small nonobliterated area at the apex of the left ventricle? J Am Coll Cardiol 19:525–526, 1992.
33. Wigle ED, Rakowski H, Kimball BP, et al: Hypertrophic cardiomyopathy. Clinical spectrum and treatment. Circulation 92:1680–1692, 1995.
34. Williams WG, Wigle ED, Rakowski H, et al: Results of surgery for hypertrophic obstructive cardiomyopathy. Circulation 76:V104–V108, 1987.
35. Williams WG, Ralph-Edwards AC, Wigle ED: Surgical management of hypertrophic obstructive cardiomyopathy. Cardiol Rev 5:40–49, 1997.
36. Yetman A, Hamilton R, Benson L, et al: Factors associated with outcome in children with hypertrophic cardiomyopathy. Can J Cardiol 13:88C, 1997.
37. Yetman AT, McCrindle BW, MacDonald C, et al: Myocardial bridging in children with hypertrophic cardiomyopathy: A risk factor for sudden death. N Engl J Med 339:1201–1209, 1998.
38. Yu E, Chiam C, Siu S, et al: Left atrial structure and function post myectomy in patients with hypertrophic obstructive cardiomyopathy. Can J Cardiol 13:95C, 1997.
39. Yu EHC, Omran AS, Wigle D, et al: Mitral regurgitation in hypertrophic obstructive cardiomyopathy: Relationship to obstruction and relief with myectomy. J Am Coll Cardiol 36:2219–2225, 2000.

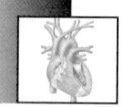

Left Ventricular Assist Devices

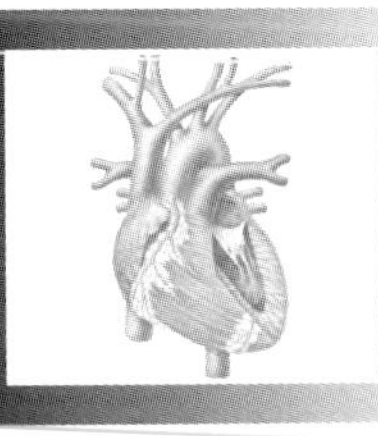

CHAPTER 92

Paul L. DiGiorgi, Eugene L. Kukuy, Yoshifumi Naka, and Mehmet C. Oz

INTRODUCTION

Left ventricular assist devices (LVADs) have become the standard of care for potential heart transplant patients with life-threatening heart failure refractory to medical and other surgical therapy. Significant advances in both the technology and clinical experience have taken place over the past 10 years. Indications for placement of VADs have broadened to include patients who were previously thought to be unsuitable for device insertion. The improving long-term success with device support has even led to the possibility of permanent support. Currently there is a wide array of devices, both available and in development. These range from univentricular percutaneous driveline-powered devices to fully implantable total artificial hearts. Both patient and device selection greatly impact outcome. This chapter provides a historical perspective, describes the indications for VAD placement, reviews current and future devices, and discusses intraoperative and postoperative management and complications.

HISTORICAL PERSPECTIVE

The first clinical implantation of an LVAD was reported by Hall and associates in 1963.[66] The intracorporeal device was anastomosed between the left atrium and descending aorta and consisted of an inner compressible blood chamber housed within an outer air chamber. With flow direction dictated by two ball valves and power provided by compressed air, the device could support the circulatory system in patients with postcardiotomy cardiac shock. In 1965 a subsequent paracorporeal version of the device was the first successful device used for cardiac shock after cardiotomy with subsequent explantation and discharge home.[34]

With the growing era of heart surgery and the need for adequate support devices, the Artificial Heart Program was formed in 1964. It became the Medical Devices Applications Branch of the National Heart and Lung Institute in 1970, gaining much support. The program's objectives included development of cardiac assist devices that could provide both short- and long-term circulatory assistance, including a permanent total artificial heart (TAH). In 1977 two requests for proposals (RFPs) were issued by the currently named National Heart, Lung, and Blood Institute (NHLBI). One was for the development of "Left Heart Assist Blood Pumps"[40]; the other was for "Development of Electrical Energy Converters to Power and Control Left Heart Assist Devices."[39] Another request was made in 1980 for the "Development of an Implantable Integrated Electrically Powered Left Heart Assist System"[38] to provide support for more than 2 years. The initial awardees included makers of the most commonly placed assist devices today: Abiomed, Baxter, ThermoCardioSystems, and Thoratec Labs.

The first successful bridge-to-transplant use of a TAH occurred in 1969,[23] whereas the first LVAD bridge to transplant occurred in 1978.[135] Although the patients survived to transplant, they succumbed to the then-common infectious complications of precyclosporine (Sandimmune; Sandoz Pharmaceutical Corporation, East Hanover, NJ) era panimmunosuppression. After cyclosporine use started, heart transplants increased and the potential need for bridging devices became increasingly apparent, given the scarcity of donor hearts and the resultant long wait times. As a result, the long-term support devices, developed through the NHLBI program, were approved for investigational use by the U.S. Food and Drug Administration (FDA) as a bridge to transplant. These included the Novacor LVAD (Baxter Healthcare Corp., Oakland, CA) and the HeartMate IP LVAD and VE LVAD (then Thermo Cardiosystems, Woburn, MA). The HeartMate IP LVAD was the first device approved for general clinical use in 1994. The cost and quality-of-life benefits of these assist devices were clearly realized with the ability to discharge LVAD patients to home and resume work awaiting heart transplant.[55]

In 1994 another RFP was issued for "Innovative Ventricular Assist Systems."[37] Resulting newer-generation VADs now include axial flow pumps and centrifugal pumps characterized by small sizes, quiet continuous flow, and total implantability. In addition, there is appreciation for the myocardial remodeling that takes place with LVAD unloading, providing potential insights into the selection of patients who will tolerate long-term LVAD explantation without transplant.[*] The growing long-term success of LVADs also has led to the serious consideration of LVADs as destination therapy for patients who are not transplant candidates.[158,160] The broad range of clinical options and device types available can create a therapeutic dilemma and mandates a careful review of pumps and their uses.

INDICATIONS

The traditional indication for VAD support was refractory cardiac failure in patients eligible for heart transplantation. Our patient population has expanded from patients with chronic heart failure to include a large proportion of patients with acute heart failure. Although some reports have shown better outcomes in stable patients awaiting heart transplant,[36,166] acceptable results have been obtained in the emergent patient population.[†] In addition, our own experience suggests similar survival rates between urgent and nonurgent LVAD placements.

There are now several clinical scenarios in which VADs are implanted. These include postcardiotomy cardiogenic shock (PCCS), acute myocardial infarction (AMI), acute decompensation of chronic heart failure, myocarditis, chronic heart failure in transplantation candidates, ventricular arrhythmias, and high-risk cardiac operations.

PCCS patients have shown significant survival benefits if identified early and appropriately treated.[69] Because most centers have the capability for short-term VAD support but not long-term VAD support and/or transplant, we created a network that rapidly identifies and transfers appropriate patients in our region. Initial evaluation optimizes short-term VAD support and transfers patients within 72 hours of decompensation. Long-term LVAD implantation, if necessary, is then performed within 5 days.

AMI patients suffer from cardiogenic shock about 6% of the time and have a mortality of almost 80%.[61,62] Even with early revascularization, 1-year survival remains less than 50%.[80] Many of these patients either suffer unrecoverable myocardial damage or lack suitable coronary anatomy for revascularization. Advanced mechanical support may be the only therapy available for these patients. Mechanical support can successfully bridge these patients to either recovery or transplant if necessary.[19,119]

Patients with long standing heart failure may decompensate acutely or over longer periods. These patients may not have been listed for transplant at the time of failure, although often they are followed at transplant centers. Acute decompensation can be triggered by several etiologies, including new ischemic injuries, arrhythmias, and infections. Patients already listed for heart transplant are the traditional group that has made up VAD populations. These patients tend to do well with VAD placement because rehabilitation can be optimized before transplant.[177]

LVAD implantation in acute myocarditis, particularly in young patients, most often is a bridge to recovery rather than transplantation. Unfortunately, it is difficult to determine which patients will benefit from short-term support or require long-term devices with subsequent transplantation.[84] Because recovery is more likely in this population, short-term VADs are more often placed with subsequent transition to long-term VADs if necessary.[21]

Patients with ventricular arrhythmias are unique in that, aside from the arrhythmia, their native cardiac function may not be significantly compromised. If pharmacological therapy and defibrillators have failed, VAD support may be warranted. VAD support has successfully been implemented in this scenario.[51,81,178]

Patients undergoing high-risk cardiac surgery may need mechanical ventricular support if the surgical procedure is not successful. We routinely arrange for LVAD backup for such cases. The patient is screened for transplant candidacy before surgery in case he or she needs LVAD support and heart transplant.

PATIENT SELECTION

The selection process for VAD implantation must reach a balance between highest-risk patients who have unacceptably high mortality rates and a too-conservative approach passing over patients who otherwise would have benefited from VAD support. Judicious use also is important because VAD implantation incurs significant social and financial investment.

According to the FDA, approval for transplant is required for VAD implantation, although this may be difficult in the setting of acute cardiac failure. The generally accepted hemodynamic criteria include systolic blood pressure less than 80 mmHg (or mean arterial blood pressure <65 mmHg), pulmonary capillary wedge pressure greater

---

*References 1, 43, 68, 74, 75, 96, 100, 111, 121, 125, 164, 186.

†References 21, 24, 69, 70, 109, 114.

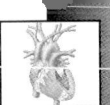

than 20 mmHg, systemic vascular resistance greater than 2100 dynes·sec/cm^5, urine output less than 20 ml/hour (adults) despite diuretics, and a cardiac output of less than 2 liters/min/m^2 despite maximal inotropic or intraaortic balloon pump support.[140] In addition, some centers are more specific about the use of inotropic agents, requiring at least two at specified doses.[179] In addition, several other factors must be taken into account. We use a system of cardiac and extracardiac factors when evaluating a patient for VAD placement, as summarized in Box 92-1.

Cardiac Factors

There are several cardiac factors that must be taken into account when considering VAD placement. Right heart failure (RHF) is one of the most important causes of perioperative mortality.[64,126] RHF complicating LVAD placement has been associated with low preoperative mean pulmonary arterial pressure and right ventricular stroke work index.[59] Hemodynamic indicators include left atrial pressures less than 10 mmHg, a cardiac index less than 1.8 liters/min/m^2, and a decreasing cardiac index developing in the setting of high pulmonary arterial and central venous pressures.[64] Pulmonary vascular resistance index and the transpulmonary gradient have been used to predict RHF in the post–heart transplant population.[22,103,174] However, these criteria were unable to distinguish survivors from nonsurvivors.[64] It should be remembered that normal preoperative pulmonary pressures do not necessarily indicate adequate right ventricular function. Although a patient may have a normal pulmonary vascular resistance in low cardiac output states, a fixed pulmonary vasculature can translate into pulmonary hypertension and RHF after instituting VAD support.

Although valve disease plays a role in patient selection for VAD implantation, most problems can be addressed at the time of surgery. Aortic insufficiency can cause shunting and loss of forward flow. The degree of aortic insufficiency may be underestimated in the preoperative setting. We therefore recommend intraoperative direct assessment with a left ventricular vent and believe that all regurgitant flow greater than 1.5 liters/min should be addressed. In patients who require long-term LVAD support as a bridge to transplant, our preferred strategy is to oversew an incompetent native aortic valve via the LVAD outflow aortotomy. In patients who have the potential for myocardial recovery and subsequent LVAD explant, the valve is repaired by resuspending the prolapsing cusp or by suturing it to the adjacent normal cusp, thereby creating a bicuspid valve. A mechanical valve should be oversewn with a patch to ensure that it will never open and reduce the incidence of thromboembolism. Mitral stenosis can compromise device inflow and may need to be corrected at the time of implant as well. Repair of other valve pathologies such as aortic stenosis and mitral regurgitation should be considered with regard to device weaning. If replacement is necessary, a tissue valve should be considered because of lower risk of thromboembolism and the avoidance of anticoagulation. Additionally, bubble studies should be performed and a patent foramen ovale repaired because hypoxia can result from right-to-left shunting after left-sided unloading from an LVAD. Tricuspid stenosis, although rare, should be treated because it reduces right atrial pressure and improves forward flow through the pulmonary circulation. Correction of tricuspid regurgitation, which is commonly found, has no benefit unless ascites is present. As left ventricular failure improves with device support, so will right ventricular failure and concomitant tricuspid regurgitation.

Preexisting coronary artery disease (CAD) is common in LVAD candidates. Adequate evaluation of CAD is important to maximize the benefits of VAD implantation. Right-sided bypasses may be necessary when implanting an LVAD to support right ventricular function. This is especially important for early postoperative right ventricular protection. In addition, ischemic complications such as angina and arrhythmias may still occur after VAD implantation and can be relieved by coronary bypass. Refractory, malignant arrhythmias themselves can be an indication for VAD implantation.[8,178] However, we usually do not perform left-sided bypasses for angina because angina after LVAD is uncommon. Unless ventricular recovery is likely, left-sided bypasses may not be warranted secondary to a relatively low-flow state after VAD implantation and the potential for early graft closure. However, there is a possibility that synchronized VAD support increases diastolic coronary flows by up to 97%.[185] If bypasses are performed, placement of the proximal anastomoses should take into account the LVAD outflow anastomosis site. We therefore recommend proximal bypass anastomoses on the lesser curvature of the aorta, providing ample room on the anterolateral aspect of the aorta to accommodate the LVAD outflow graft.

Box 92–1. Ventricular Assist Device Considerations.

1. Transplant candidate
2. Hemodynamic variables
   a. Cardiac index <2 liters/min/m^2
   b. Systolic blood pressure <80 mmHg
   c. Pulmonary capillary wedge pressure >20 mmHg
   d. On maximized medical therapy
3. Cardiac considerations
   a. Right ventricular function
   b. Valvular disease/prosthetic valves
   c. Ischemia/bypass grafts
   d. Arrhythmias
4. Noncardiac considerations
   a. Neurological function
   b. Infectious diseases
   c. Prothrombin time >16 seconds
   d. Urine output
   e. Blood urea nitrogen
   f. Bilirubin
   g. Pulmonary disease
   h. Body surface area <1.5 m^2

Modified from Williams M, Oz MC: Indications and patient selection for mechanical ventricular assistance. Ann Thorac Surg 71:S86–S91, 2001.

Noncardiac Factors

As more patients with postcardiotomy cardiogenic shock are evaluated for VAD implantation, neurological status has become an increasingly important and difficult assessment to make and remains an important determinant of mortality in transferred patients.[69] It is ethically permissible to discontinue support if patients are found to have unrecoverable neurological function. Ideally patients should have both thorough neurological evaluations and psychiatric evaluations to determine their ability to tolerate mechanical support.

Infection is the Achilles' heel of mechanical support. Infection is the most common complication of long-term VADs and accounts for substantial morbidity and even mortality among VAD patients.* The location of the infection can have a significant impact on outcome.[82] Patients ideally should have negative blood cultures at least 1 week before VAD implantation. This is especially true for patients with fungal infections because of the functional T-cell deficiency incurred by these patients.[4] Unfortunately, we have been unable to identify either fever or elevated white blood cell count as a risk factor for infection.[139] However, others have found elevated white blood cell count, although not fever, to be a risk factor for mortality.[144,179] As designs and treatments improve, VAD patients with infections do increasingly well after transplant.[171]

In our experience, renal failure has been the strongest predictor of mortality. We try to avoid placing devices in patients with serum creatinine levels greater than 5 mg/dl. Patients who have acute cardiac failure, however, may not show an elevated creatinine level until later. Blood urea nitrogen levels less than 20 mg/dl also have been associated with increased survival.[48] We have found urine output to be the best indicator of renal function. Urine output levels of less than 30 ml/h, despite diuretic use, have been an important indicator.[139] Although renal impairment is common in this population, recovery during the VAD support period is excellent.[57,58,64] Our recent reevaluation of risk factors showed a reduced significance of preoperative renal failure in survival after LVAD implantation.[153]

Hepatic function is an important factor in survival after use of a VAD. A prothrombin time of greater than 16 seconds is particularly ominous because patients require greater amounts of blood products. Increased transfusion requirements directly correlate with RHF. Coagulopathies should be treated aggressively with serine protease inhibitors (Aprotinin), vitamin K, and fresh-frozen plasma. Hepatic function, evidenced by bilirubin, has been proposed to be the best predictor of survival.[156] However, other studies have failed to associate bilirubin with survival.[48]

Reoperation can make VAD implantation more challenging technically, but its impact on mortality has varied in published reports.[48,139,156,179] We found reoperation to be a significant risk factor and use it as part of our screening scale to predict survival after implantation.

Other relative contraindications to VAD implantation include pulmonary failure exclusive of pulmonary edema and malignancy that precludes survival greater than 2 years. Presently, any condition excluding patients from transplant also excludes them as VAD candidates if this is known preoperatively.

Several studies have attempted to develop simple selection criteria for VAD implantation. These have been based on both unique clinical variables[179] and Acute Physiology and Chronic Health Evaluation II (APACHE II) scores.[64] In 1995 we published our own scoring scale as shown in Table 92-1.[139] Scores were based on the following seven relatively simple variables: (1) urine output, (2) central venous pressure, (3) mechanical ventilation, (4) prothrombin time, (5) reoperation, (6) white blood cell count, and (7) temperature. We found that scores greater than 5 correlated with increased mortality. Since then, based on increasing experience, we revised the scale and continued to use the score of 5 to predict increased mortality (Table 92-1). Using the new scale, a score greater than 5 corresponds with a 47% mortality versus 9% mortality for a score less than 5. The positive and negative predictive value of this scoring system is 79% and 70%, respectively.[153] However, it is important to remember that no scoring system serves as an absolute predictor for VAD candidacy or success. In addition, as both technology and patient selection evolve, these systems will become obsolete and new ones will need to be developed.

With appropriate selection of patients for VAD insertion, lives are saved, end-organ impairment is reduced, and transplantation risks are reduced. Ultimately the utilization of donor hearts will be maximized.

TYPES OF PUMPS

Extracorporeal

Centrifugal Pumps

Centrifugal devices have been the most commonly used pumps for postcardiotomy cardiac support.[142] Blood enters axially into the pump, is spun by the magnetically driven blades, and exits peripherally through the outlet port. Although they have been in clinical use for more than 20 years, initial enthusiasm diminished as a result of excessive hemolysis. Since then, many new designs have been

Table 92–1

Risk Factors for Poor Survival after Left Ventricular Assist Device Placement

Risk factor	*Score*
Mechanical ventilation	4
Reoperation	2
Previous LVAD	2
Central venous pressure >16 mm Hg	1
Prothrombin time >16 seconds	1

Modified from Rao V, Oz MC, Flannery MA, et al: Revised screening scale to predict survival after insertion of a left ventricular assist device. J Thorac Cardiovasc Surg 125:855–862, 2003.

*References 8, 72, 82, 171, 174, 177.

produced with improved hemodynamics.* Currently the two most commonly used pumps are the Biomedicus Bio-Pump (Medtronic, Inc., Minneapolis, MN) and the Sarns/3M Centrifugal System (Sarns/3M, Ann Arbor, MI). Centrifugal pumps are now considered by many to cause less hemolysis and blood element activation when compared with roller pumps.[118,128,199] None of the commonly used pumps have shown significant clinical advantages over another.[28]

Indications for centrifugal pump implantations are extracorporeal membrane oxygenation (ECMO), thoracic aortic surgery, postcardiotomy ventricular failure, bridge to a long-term ventricular assist device, and bridge to transplant. Besides thoracic aortic surgery, the major indication has been postcardiotomy ventricular failure.† Published outcomes have paralleled other short-term devices, with 56–68% of patients weaned and 21–44% of patients surviving to discharge.[85,88,104,132] Support duration is shorter than the other commonly used short-term device, the Abiomed BVS 5000, usually running less than 4 days. Popularity of centrifugal pumps primarily has been due to the lower price, ease of use, and greater availability they have historically enjoyed. However, this may change as more advanced systems such as the Abiomed BVS 5000 become commonplace and cost differences diminish.[26]

Major limitations have included seal disruption requiring close inspection,[29] mandatory anticoagulation, continued sedation with mechanical ventilation, and the inability to ambulate or rehabilitate patients while on the device. New generations of pumps, using magnetically coupled impellers, have nearly eliminated seal disruption. However, a full-time, bedside perfusionist is required to run each centrifugal pump system. Given these complications and limitations, especially in rehabilitation, extracorporeal centrifugal mechanical assist devices are mainly useful for short-term support in the patient with postcardiotomy ventricular failure and the bridge-to-transplant scenario.

The next generation of centrifugal pumps, however, now in bench and animal testing, is designed for long-term support with partial or total implantability (see later section on rotary pumps).‡

Abiomed BVS 5000

The Abiomed BVS 5000 (Abiomed Cardiovascular, Inc., Danvers, MA) is a short-term univentricular or biventricular support system composed of external pumps driven by a computer controlled drive console. The FDA first approved the product in 1992 for postcardiotomy support.[65] Since then, the indications for use have grown to include acute myocardial infarction, myocarditis, right ventricular support in conjunction with a long-term left ventricular support device, a bridge to recovery, and a bridge to transplant. As a result, the device has become one of the most commonly used means of short-term mechanical cardiac support.[87,192] It is the only device approved by the FDA for all patients with potentially reversible heart failure.

Advantages that have made the BVS system popular are the ease of insertion and simplicity in operation obviating the need for a full-time perfusionist. The system functions reliably for several days with average support duration between 5 and 9 days. This has been particularly helpful in community hospitals where there may be the need to transfer the patient to a transplant center for further treatment.[69,110] It has proven its effectiveness in the treatment of both acute myocarditis and postcardiotomy cardiogenic shock.[21,87,109,163] In addition, the cost may be closer to centrifugal pumps than previously expected.[26] For these reasons, the BVS system has become our standard for short-term bridging.

Disadvantages of this device include the requirement for continuous anticoagulation, limited mobility compared with implantable devices, and the requirement to remain in an intensive care unit (ICU). Flow rates are also limited compared with other devices. The maximum flow rate of 6 l/min may not be enough for septic or large patients. Although patients have been supported for as long as 90 days, the device is best suited for short-term use (<10 days).

Thoratec Device

The Thoratec ventricular assist device (Thoratec Laboratories Corp., Pleasanton, CA) consists of an externalized pneumatic pusher-plate pump positioned subcostally connected to a drive console. The drive is capable of univentricular or biventricular support with flows up to 7 l/min. The cannulas are tunneled exiting out the upper abdominal wall connected to the extracorporeal pump (Figure 92-1). The device was first used clinically in 1982 for postcar-

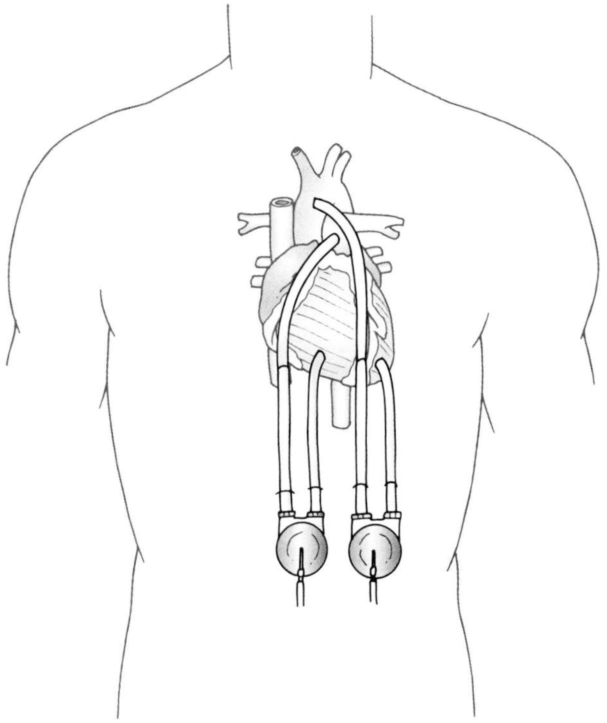

Figure 92–1 Thoratec ventricular assist device. Both the pumps and the drive console are external.
(Modified courtesy Thoratec Laboratories Corp., Pleasanton, CA.)

*References 14, 25, 27, 28, 30, 31, 105, 108, 124, 127, 136, 145, 181, 182, 189.
†References 28, 31, 85, 88, 131–133.
‡References 67, 130, 137, 165, 191, 193, 198.

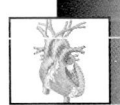

diotomy support[143] and in 1984 as a bridge to transplant.[77] It has received FDA approval as both a bridge to recovery and a bridge to transplant.

The main advantage of the Thoratec system is the ability to provide long-term biventricular support. This has become increasingly important with prolonged waiting periods for transplant. The Thoratec system is the only extracorporeal device that is used for long-term support. The paracorporeal position has some particular benefits as well. These include identification of clot and device exchange without invasive surgery. Survival to transplant has been good, up to 74% with support durations over 200 days.[47,50,52,93]

The major limitations of the Thoratec system are the limited mobility and rehabilitation potential as a result of a large drive console and the need for chronic anticoagulation. New, portable drive units will allow portability that should overcome the limitations of the original system.[49] In case of high output requirements, other devices may be desired because of flow limitations. The Novacor or HeartMate systems may be used in this case, in conjunction with the Thoratec system, providing right-sided support. Another alternative may be a TAH.

Even with limited portability and the need for chronic anticoagulation, the Thoratec VAD system provides a valuable adjunct to the cardiac assist device armamentarium because of its ability to provide long-term, biventricular support.

Adult Extracorporeal Membrane Oxygenation

ECMO provides mechanical cardiac support (univentricular or biventricular), as well as pulmonary support. Although neonatal use has been very successful, the adult experience has been mixed.

The main indications for ECMO are the need for mechanical assistance in the face of combined cardiovascular and pulmonary failure and pulmonary failure and pure respiratory failure. When it was initially used for postcardiotomy cardiogenic shock, survival was low (25%),[146] but with experience and improved circuits, survival increased to 40%.[175] ECMO benefits from potential peripheral cannulas insertion and versatility of small consoles. This has allowed potential implementation in areas outside of the operating room for both cardiac and pulmonary support.

Major limitations include requirement for sedation and possible paralysis, heparinization (except in cases of pure respiratory support), and the potential need for an intraaortic balloon pump to reduce afterload. A full-time perfusionist also is necessary to run the equipment. The duration of support is usually only 2–3 days, although it can last several days. Complications are common, including leg ischemia, renal failure, bleeding, and oxygenator failure, especially with venoarterial ECMO support.

Overall the successful use of ECMO in adults has been limited to select centers, and the epidemiological benefits remain minor.

Berlin Heart

The Berlin Heart (Mediport Kardiotechnik, Berlin, Germany) is a pneumatically driven paracorporeal support device capable of providing both univentricular and biventricular mechanical support. The system has been used in Europe since 1988. The blood pumps come in a variety of sizes, down to stroke volumes of about 10 ml, allowing for pediatric use.[73,86] Implantation is usually performed via a sternotomy with or without cardiopulmonary bypass and cardioplegic arrest.[99] The cannulas are brought out through the epigastrium to connect to the external blood pumps. Various drive consoles have been developed allowing patients to discharge to home while on ventricular support. The duration of implant lasts an average of 2 months and has lasted more than 500 days.

The Berlin Heart can provide biventricular or univentricular support. It has the advantage of pediatric applications and has proven its reliability and low rate of thromboembolic complications. Newer, portable consoles allow patients to be more mobile, with better rehabilitation and discharge to home.

Warfarin (Coumadin) is mandatory (international normalized ratio [INR] 2.5–3.5), along with aspirin and dipyridamole.[99] The pumps also require twice weekly inspection for thrombus formation. However, these high-maintenance requirements should provide reliable service for extended periods.

Intracorporeal

Intraaortic Balloon Pump

In use since the 1960s,[89] the intraaortic balloon pump (IABP) is the most commonly used cardiac assist device today. It is based on diastolic coronary blood flow augmentation and aortic counterpulsation. As a result, myocardial oxygen consumption is decreased by afterload reduction, whereas coronary blood flow is increased.[151] Percutaneous placement was developed by the 1980s, greatly increasing the use of the devices[16,176] by enabling placement by medical personnel other than surgeons outside of the operating room.

IABP is most commonly used in cardiogenic shock or ongoing myocardial infarction refractory to medical therapy. Preoperatively, IABP support is commonly used to stabilize patients with myocardial ischemia despite medical therapy before proceeding with revascularization. Survival differences have been shown with preoperative IABP placement, especially in patients with ejection fractions less than 25%[42] and less than 40%.[167] Intraoperatively it is used for patients failing weaning from cardiopulmonary bypass despite maximal medical therapy. Insertion of an IABP intraoperatively or postoperatively has been shown to be an independent predictor of death. Preoperative insertion has been associated with significantly increased survival.[187]

The IABP benefits from relatively rapid and easy insertion without necessarily requiring a surgical approach. The benefits of increased coronary perfusion, as well as reduced myocardial oxygen demand, are most realized in the ischemic heart, although other forms of cardiomyopathies also are benefited. It does not, however, provide the level of support of other assist devices. Anticoagulation with intravenous heparin is used to prevent thrombotic complications at both the insertion and balloon sites. Postoperative anticoagulation can be started with low-molecular-weight dextran and switched to heparin later. Vascular complications remain the most common source of morbidity, with rates varying

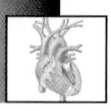

from 9–6%.[17,172] Most often this is related to the femoral artery, stressing the importance of common femoral artery insertion (rather than the superficial femoral artery). Given these complications, however, the IABP has become an important tool in supporting cardiac function without the need for significant surgical intervention.

Thoratec HeartMate

The HeartMate (Thoratec Laboratories Corp.) LVAD is an implantable, long-term, univentricular cardiac assist device (Figure 92-2). Based on work started in the mid-1960s, the first clinical implantation of the HeartMate took place in 1986. The HeartMate was the first mechanical circulatory support device to be approved by the FDA for bridging to transplant. Both a pneumatically driven (implantable pneumatic [IP]) and an electrically powered (vented electric [VE]) version exist. Most hospitals now have converted to the portable electric version, allowing discharge to home on support. Both systems function with a pusher-plate mechanism delivering up to 10 liters/min of flow. The driveline containing the electric cable and an air vent exits the skin to attach to the external drive console. Both inflow and outflow porcine valves are attached to the pump. The inflow cannula is attached to the left ventricular apex, and the outflow is via the ascending aorta. The blood-contacting portion of the pump incorporates titanium microspheres, and the flexible diaphragm is covered with textured polyurethane. This promotes the formation of a pseudointimal layer. This unique surface may be responsible for the low thromboembolic risk associated with the HeartMate despite the lack of anticoagulation.[33,159,173]

The main advantage of the HeartMate is the low thromboembolic rate (<5%) without anticoagulation.[112,173] Patients can be discharged home while awaiting transplant, where they can resume almost all their normal activities.

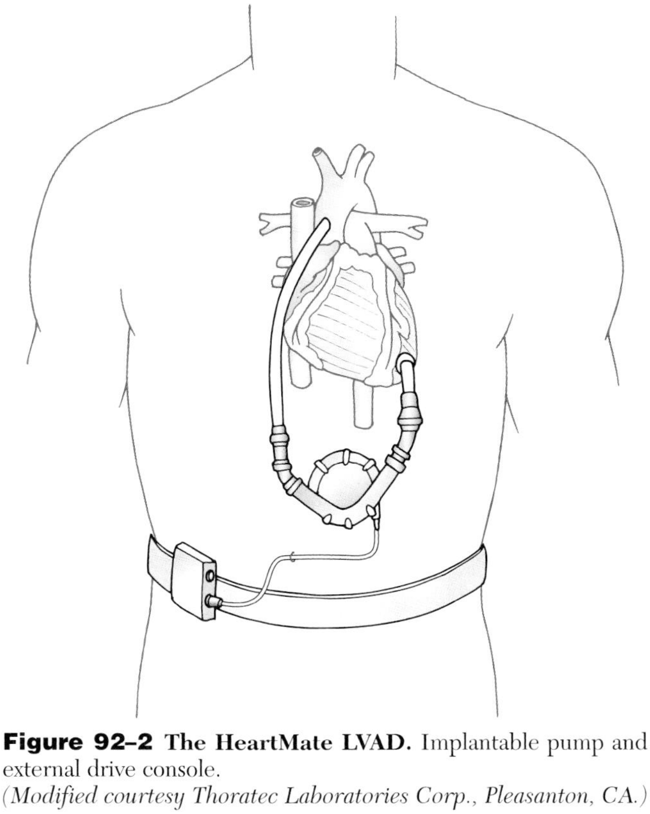

Figure 92–2 The HeartMate LVAD. Implantable pump and external drive console.
(Modified courtesy Thoratec Laboratories Corp., Pleasanton, CA.)

Patients must have a body surface area (BSA) of at least 1.5 m^2 to accommodate the abdominally placed pump. Proper screening of potential recipients is critical.[139] Early complications are related to technique. The major causes of perioperative mortality are hemorrhage and RHF. These have been reduced with the introduction of aprotinin (Bayer, Tarrytown, NY) and nitric oxide.[9,20,63,162,188] Flows of less than 3.0 liters/min (cardiac index <2.0) may predispose to clot formation inside the pump. If right-sided support was necessary, a different device would need to be placed. Device failure, requiring replacement, has been reported to occur in about 12% of patients.[112]

Although it belongs to only the first generation of relatively reliable mechanical cardiac assist devices, the HeartMate has enjoyed significant clinical success. As a result, the REMATCH (Randomized Evaluation of Mechanical Assistance for the Treatment of Congestive Heart Failure) study was undertaken using the device as an alternative, rather than as a bridge to transplantation.[160] One hundred twenty nine non–transplant candidates in New York Heart Association (NYHA) class IV heart failure were randomly assigned to receive either a HeartMate or an optimal medical therapy. There was a 48% reduction in the risk of death from any cause in the LVAD group compared with the medical therapy group. The 1- and 2-year survival rates were 52% versus 25% and 23% versus 8% for the LVAD and medical therapy groups, respectively.[158] These data, supporting mechanical therapy over medical therapy, may have profound effects on the treatment of end-stage heart failure in non–transplant candidates in the future.

Thoratec Intracorporeal VAD

Thoratec Intracorporeal VAD (Thoratec Laboratories Corp.) is an intracorporeal system that is the same size as the external Thoratec VAD but is housed in a titanium alloy casing and is implantable. The advantages of this system are its small size, reliability, implantable right ventricular support, and proven and extensively tested technology based on the currently used Thoratec system.[53,155] It is targeted toward patients who would benefit from long-term support and the benefits of an implanted device.

Novacor N1000PC

The Novacor N1000PC (World Heart Corporation, Ottawa, ON, Canada) is a wearable LVAD with an implantable pump and an externalized vent tube, controller, and batteries (Figure 92-3). Its dual pusher-plate design provides symmetrical movement, minimizing mechanical torque.[148,149] The pump is lined with a smooth polyurethane sac and has gelatin-sealed inflow and outflow grafts. The first successful bridge-to-transplant implantation took place in 1984, and the Novacor N1000PC received FDA approval for bridge to transplant in 1998. Inflow comes from the left ventricular apex, and outflow is through the ascending aorta with flows up to 10 liters/min. Patients can ambulate with little impairment after implantation. Many patients have been successfully discharged from the hospital to await transplant. It also has an excellent mechanical durability and reliability rate with few device failures.[95]

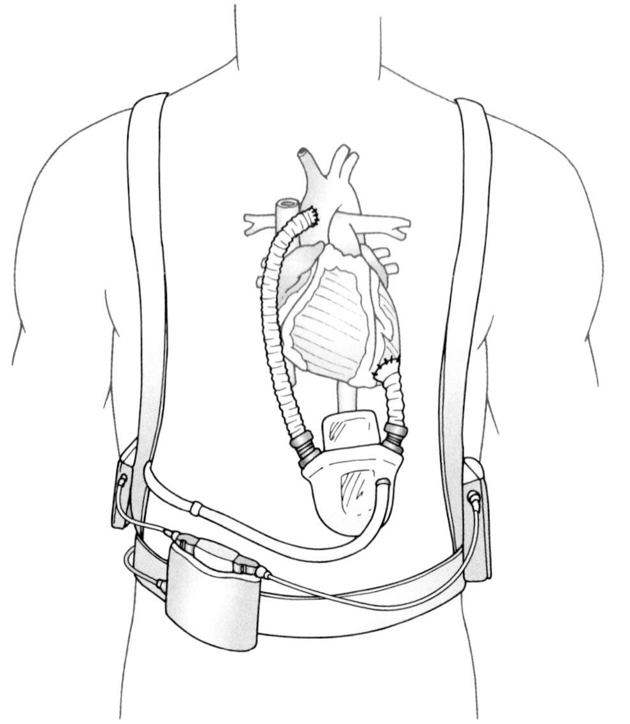

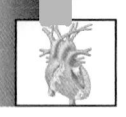

Figure 92–3 The Novacor N1000PC. Implantable pump and external drive console.
(Modified courtesy Baxter Healthcare Corporation, Berkeley, CA.)

Device-specific exclusion criteria include blood dyscrasias, presence of a prosthetic aortic valve, and a recipient BSA of less than 1.5 m.[152] As with most devices, preoperative multisystem organ failure is predictive of poor outcome as well.[94,139] Similarly, bleeding and RHF are the most significant perioperative complications. Anticoagulation must be maintained with warfarin (Coumadin) (INR 2–3) and aspirin. Despite anticoagulation, the embolic stroke rate associated with the Novacor device has been high (26%). However, recent inflow cannula–conduit modifications have dropped the embolic stroke rate to 12%.[152] Newer conduits using polytetrafluoroethylene (PTFE) may lower the embolic stroke rate further.

Novacor II

Novacor II (World Heart Corporation) is a concept heart created by a company with extensive LVAD experience. It is a totally implantable pump for definitive treatment of heart failure. Its unique dual-chamber, four-valve pump requires no volume compensator. The pusher plate is suspended and magnetically driven, thus providing for a system with few moving parts. The two chambers fill alternately, creating pulsatile flow.[157] The system also uses transcutaneous energy transfer technology to supply power. It is currently in preclinical testing.

LionHeart LVD-2000

The LionHeart LVD-2000 was designed with collaboration between Pennsylvania State University and Arrow International (Reading, PA). It is the first system designed specifically for destination therapy. It uses a transcutaneous energy transmission system (TETS) and an internal compliance chamber, allowing for complete implantation without percutaneous lines or connections. The pump consists of a titanium casing with an electric pusher-plate motor. Unidirectional blood flow is provided via two Delrin disk monostrut valves (27-mm inlet; 25-mm outlet). The inflow and outflow tracts are located in the ventricular apex and aorta, respectively. Maximum pump flow is 8 l/min with a stroke volume of 64 ml.[113] The controller is housed in a titanium casing that also contains rechargeable batteries. The control system is dependent on continual monitoring of end-diastolic volume; thus the patient's physiological demands control the filling volume of the pump.[113] The compliance chamber consists of a circular polymer sac and an attached subcutaneous port infusion system. This compliance chamber loses gas through the polymer and requires replenishment of gas once a month.[141] Recharging of the battery is accomplished through the TETS. The patient may be completely disconnected from the external power supply for a short period, relying on the internal backup batteries. The internal coil must be positioned under the skin so as to allow no more than 1 cm of tissue thickness between the coil and skin surface.[113,141]

The LionHeart system underwent initial studies in Europe using five centers, with 20 patients receiving the device. A U.S. clinical trial has begun with FDA approval for a phase I clinical human trial.[141]

HeartSaver LVAD

The HeartSaver LVAD (World Heart Corporation) is designed as a totally implantable, pulsatile LVAD system using TET coil for transcutaneous energy transfer. Similar to other LVADs, the inflow cannula is inserted into the apex of the left ventricle with outflow to the ascending aorta. The pump has an attached volume displacement chamber and is implanted into the left side of the chest as an entire unit. Preclinical work with the device is being done at the University of Ottawa Heart Institute, and numerous animal studies have shown promise.[71,122,123]

Rotary Pumps

Axial flow pumps represent one of the newest generations of assist devices. They can provide full cardiac support in a much smaller pump with fewer moving parts and less blood-contacting surface than pusher-plate devices. In addition to their small size, their design is notable for nonpulsatile flow. Several studies have demonstrated metabolic and neurohumoral changes in organ perfusion compared with pulsatile flow.* However, both clinical and long-term animal studies have failed to show significant differences in morbidity and mortality with axial flow pumps.† Clinically tested devices are the HeartMate II (Thoratec Laboratories Corp.), the DeBakey VAD (MicroMed Technology, Inc., Houston, TX), and the Jarvik 2000 (Jarvik Heart, Inc., New York, NY).

*References 2, 60, 76, 83, 98, 116, 134, 168–170, 183, 184, 194.
†References 32, 78, 79, 91, 102, 154, 161, 180, 190.

These devices weigh between 53 and 176 g and can generate flows in excess of 10 liters/min.

The Jarvik 2000 axial flow pump (Figure 92-4), the HeartMate II (Figure 92-5), and the DeBakey axial flow pump (Figure 92-6) all have similar features as mentioned in the preceding. Their small size allows better implantation into smaller patients than most pulsatile pumps. This also makes placement and explantation easier. With fewer moving parts there are fewer points of friction, therefore increasing their expected durability. Although there is controversy over long-term nonpulsatile flow, most patients maintain some native cardiac function and therefore continue to have pulsatile blood flow.

Unfortunately, if there is a device failure there are few options or backup mechanisms in place other than replacement. Additionally, because they lack valves, if device malfunction does occur the patient can develop the equivalent of wide-open aortic insufficiency. The DeBakey pump has already been successfully implanted in a small number of patients in Europe.[150,196] In addition, the HeartMate II and the Jarvik 2000 have been successfully implanted in humans.[195]

The latest in circulatory assist devices are centrifugal pumps being developed by several centers as the next generation of implantable assist devices. The HeartQuest System (MedQuest Products, Inc., Salt Lake City, UT) built on the Maglev (Magnetic Levitation) concept, allows for frictionless pumping, low thrombogenicity, minimal noise and vibration, and durability. These pumps have been tested in animals with promising results.[92] The VentrAssist (Micromedical Industries, Ltd., Chatswood, New South Wales, Australia) is another centrifugal pump currently undergoing animal testing. It has been implanted in animals without cardiopulmonary bypass. The centrifugal pump is hydrodynamically suspended, resulting in no wear, no hemolysis, and no need for anticoagulation.[197] Another centrifugal pump in development is the HeartMate III from the Thoratec Corporation. This pump is their third-generation pump, powered by a magnetically levitated centrifugal impeller. It is about one third the size of the HeartMate I pump and is about 3 times the volume of HeartMate II.[101,106] The Terumo "DuraHeartTM" LVAS (Terumo Cardiovascular Systems, Ann Arbor, Michigan) also incorporates a magnetically levitated impeller. The pump provides contact-free rotation of the impeller without wear and therefore is one of the most durable blood pumps. Many animal experiments have been conducted,

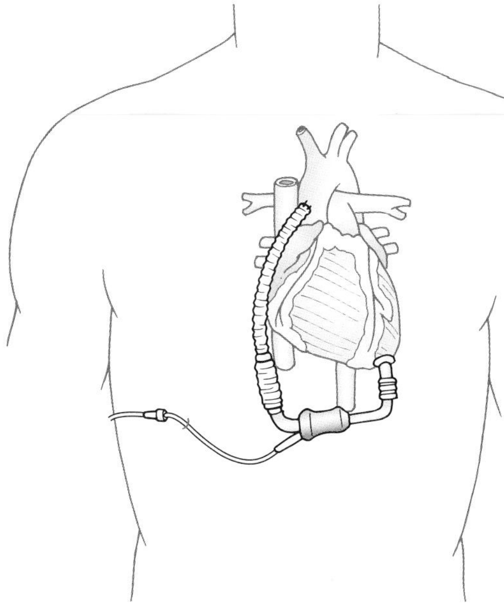

Figure 92–5 **HeartMate II.**
(Modified courtesy Thoratec Laboratories Corp., Pleasanton, CA.)

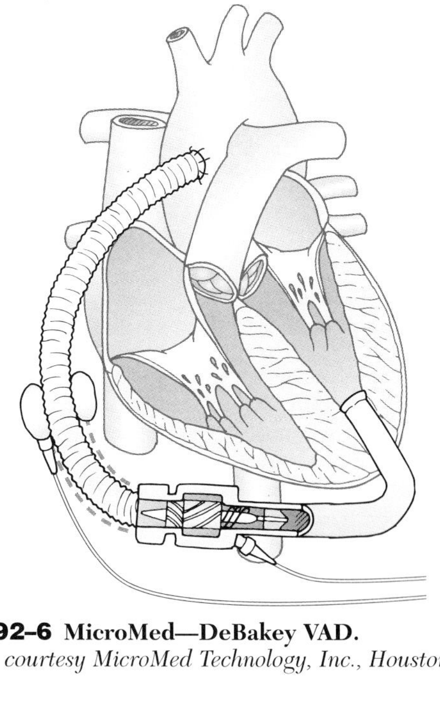

Figure 92–6 **MicroMed—DeBakey VAD.**
(Modified courtesy MicroMed Technology, Inc., Houston, TX.)

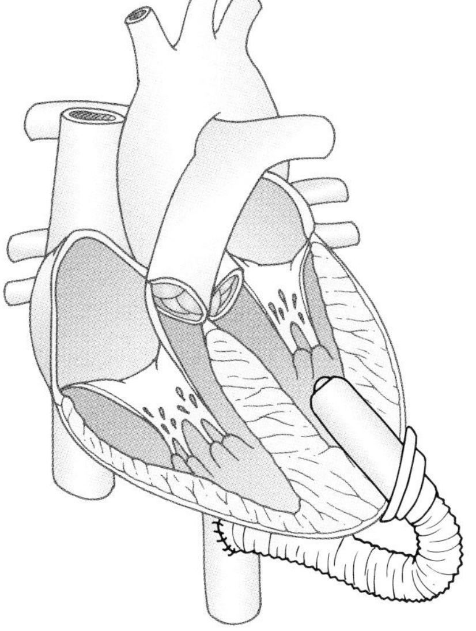

Figure 92–4 **Jarvik 2000.**
(Modified courtesy Texas Heart Institute, Houston, TX.)

with the longest thrombus-free operation being up to 864 days.[129,130] The first human clinical study began in 2002. The Kriton VAD (Kriton Medical, Inc., Miramar, FL) is also a small centrifugal pulsatile pump now used in long-term animal studies. The pump's displaced volume is 48 ml, and the pump is capable of pumping 15 liters/min in a pulsatile fashion. Because the pump's bearings also are magnetically suspended, the pump should last for years with minimal wear.[15]

Advantages of the new-generation centrifugal pumps include their smaller size, potential total implantability, and reliability as a result of few moving parts. The potential disadvantages of nonpulsatile flow remain to be seen with long-term support.

Cardiac Compression Devices

Epicardial compression devices support circulation by compressing the failing heart from its epicardial surface. The Anstadt cup was introduced in 1965 as a cardiac massage device used for cardiac arrest.[5] This early compression device held the heart in place with vacuum, but did not employ any means to synchronize with the cardiac cycle. Feasibility tests resulted in no device-related complications.[6] Newer devices consist of a cup or cuff with an internal inflatable diaphragm, an electrocardiogram sensor or trigger, and a compression driver console. The force generated by the compression device adds to the ventricular pressure generated by the native, contracting myocardium. Diastolic compliance is lessened, however, requiring higher filling pressures to obtain the same preload.[11,12]

Both Abiomed and Cardio Technologies, Inc. (CTI, Pine Brook, NJ) have compression devices under development. The CardioSupport System (CTI) is currently undergoing phase I trials in Europe. Early animal studies demonstrated successful support for up to 7 days.[147] The compression devices benefit from not having any blood–device interface, reducing the need for anticoagulation. The epicardial application should be relatively easier without the requirement for cardiopulmonary bypass. With variable compression strength, the devices are easily weaned as well. Potential problems include rhythm disturbances and myocardial injury that may result after prolonged use.[7]

DEVICE SELECTION

Device selection is invariably influenced by both availability and physician experience. Although much has been published on individual devices, few studies have compared assist devices at a single institution.[26,44] Currently there are two major indications for cardiac assist device support: bridge to recovery and bridge to transplant. Destination therapy, although probable, currently remains investigational.

There are currently five FDA-approved assist devices, in addition to the intraaortic balloon pump, for these indications: the Abiomed BVS 5000, the Thoratec device, the Novacor N1000PC, the Thoratec HeartMate Implantable Pneumatic, and the Thoratec HeartMate Vented Electric LVAD. In addition to the FDA devices, there are several other VADs in development and clinical use.

Important clinical issues when choosing a device include the expected duration of support, need for biventricular support, cost, device-related risks, patient characteristics, and United Network of Organ Sharing (UNOS) classification rules. Institutional standards of care, ranging from community practice to tertiary heart failure and transplant centers, also influence device selection.

Patients who may require mechanical circulatory support can be divided into the following three main categories. These different clinical scenarios and patient needs dictate the best type of device to use.

1. Profound shock: patients in acute, profound shock (e.g., postcardiotomy cardiac arrest, potentially with end-organ failure and RHF)
2. Decompensating congestive heart failure (CHF): more chronically ill patients who are transplant candidates
3. Non–transplant candidates: patients not at a transplant center and who have potentially recoverable myocardium

Patients in profound shock with end-organ dysfunction and RHF need early, excellent support to avoid permanent end-organ damage and increase their chances of survival. The preferred devices in such a scenario are the Abiomed BVS 5000, the Thoratec device, and the TAH (if available). These devices provide full biventricular support, reestablishing near-normal hemodynamics and allowing myocardial recovery.[65] Early implementation of biventricular support is critical in patients with severe biventricular failure.[21,109,163] While patients are on ventricular support, the potential for myocardial recovery and neurological status can be determined. If a prolonged support period is expected, a longer-term device should be implanted such as the Thoratec device or the TAH. Despite their severe cardiac failure, these patients can be successfully salvaged, with survival rates approaching that of the general cardiac transplantation population.[50,52]

Patients who suffer from more chronic CHF and who are transplant candidates may decompensate before receiving their transplant. In these patients the potential for long-term support must be considered. Hospital discharge and rehabilitation become important factors in choosing a device for this patient population.[41,94] Longer-term support with end-organ recovery and better rehabilitation is associated with better long-term survival.[13] Therefore the recommended devices are the implantable HeartMate and the Novacor LVAD. Treatment of RHF, if present, is mandatory. This can be done either medically or with a short-term VAD such as the Abiomed BVS 5000.

Non–transplant candidates may be patients at non–transplant centers or with recoverable cardiac function. Patients at non–transplant centers, who may benefit from a longer-term device and transplant workup, can be safely transferred once stabilized on short-term devices.[110] Many patients transferred on assist devices are successfully weaned without requiring a long-term implantable LVAD.[69,110] The preferred device for use in this setting is the Abiomed BVS 5000. A long-term device can be implanted later as required.

POSTOPERATIVE MANAGEMENT

Early Postoperative Management

There are several factors that we have found useful in the postoperative management of LVAD patients. Antibiotic prophylaxis is started preoperatively and continues for at least 3 days after implant. We treat RHF with milrinone and nitric oxide (NO).[9] In addition, we treat vasodilatory hypotension with intravenous arginine vasopressin (Parke-Davis, Morris Plains, NJ).[10] Aprotinin is continued in the postoperative period until hemorrhage has stopped. Ventricular arrhythmias are managed with appropriate pharmacological agents and cardioversion if necessary.

Late Postoperative Management

Late postoperative care focuses on rehabilitation and monitoring of the immunological changes[3] induced by the LVAD while awaiting heart transplantation. Patients with the vented electric Thoracic HeartMate LVAD are eligible for discharge to home while awaiting transplant.[18,41,117] Patients are followed up weekly in the LVAD clinic. Panel-reactive antibody levels are measured in Thoracic HeartMate LVAD patients biweekly.

LVAD Explant versus Transplant

Unless they are in a study, all LVAD patients are listed as heart transplant candidates. Long-term LVAD explantation is considered only if there is significant myocardial recovery evidenced by an exercise testing protocol. The profound ventricular unload provided by LVAD support can lead to reverse remodeling evident at a genetic, biochemical, and histological level.[56,97] LVAD flow is reduced to 2 l/min while patients exercise on a treadmill. Right heart catheterization and echocardiography are performed to determine the adequacy of ventricular function.[54] Although functional recovery allowing LVAD explantation has been reported,[120] our experience has shown only a small number of patients can be successfully weaned from their devices.[107]

Destination Therapy

Although they belong to only the first generation of relatively reliable mechanical cardiac assist devices, long-term LVADs (HeartMate and Novacor) have enjoyed significant clinical success. Improved long-term survival and quality of life has raised the question of destination therapy. As a result, the REMATCH study was undertaken using the device as an alternative, rather than as a bridge to transplant.[160] One hundred twenty-nine non–transplant candidates in NYHA class IV heart failure were randomly assigned to receive either a HeartMate device or an optimal medical therapy. There was a 48% reduction in the risk of death from any cause in the LVAD group compared with the medical therapy group. The 1- and 2-year survival rates were 52% versus 25% and 23% versus 8% for the LVAD and medical therapy groups, respectively.[158] These data, supporting mechanical therapy over medical therapy, may have profound effects on the treatment of end-stage heart failure in non–transplant candidates in the future.

COMPLICATIONS

There are six major complications that can occur after VAD implantation. Significant improvements have been made in reducing the morbidity of VAD support; however, challenges remain.

Postoperative bleeding frequently occurs after device placement. Normal postoperative bleeding is made excessive by preoperative heart failure leading to hepatic dysfunction, need for anticoagulation, coagulopathy caused by human–device interaction, extensive surgical dissection, and prolonged cardiopulmonary bypass time. Excessive perioperative bleeding occurs in 20–50% of patients. This rate, however, has decreased as the experience with the devices has grown.[45,115] Coagulation parameters, as well as complete blood cell count, must be monitored closely and products replaced as necessary. Death as a result of bleeding has been reported in up to 15% of patients.[35,115] Reexploration for bleeding also is common and at times can be planned. If excessive bleeding is noted at time of chest closure, the chest can be left open and packed and the patient taken to the ICU for resuscitation.

Infection is the most common complication of long-term VADs and accounts for substantial morbidity and even mortality among VAD patients.* There are some controversy and lack of definitions regarding what constitutes the various subgroups of device infection. LVAD infection can manifest as driveline, pocket, blood, and device endocarditis. The location of the infection can have a significant impact on outcome.[82] At times it can be difficult to decide if a pocket infection is present or exactly where the offending organism is harbored in an LVAD-supported patient with positive blood cultures and multiple catheters and intravenous lines. In addition to device infections, the patients are susceptible to the standard common infections seen in critically ill patients, such as pneumonia, line sepsis, and urinary tract infections. The reported infection rates in these patients is between 12% and 55%.[35,45,46,115] Pocket infections rates have been reported to be 11–24% for the HeartMate and Novacor systems, with the driveline infection rates even higher and in the range of 18–30% for the two devices.[45,115] There is much variability in these data because definitions for these infections have not been standardized and in many cases clinical presentation is ambiguous. Sepsis accounts for 21–25% of LVAD deaths and occurs in 11–26% of patients.[35,45,115,158] However, infection is not a contraindication to transplantation in this population, and transplantation can be accomplished successfully.[138]

Thromboembolism is a major concern in any patient with mechanical circulatory support because of the blood–device interface. The prevalence of embolism varies depending on the system used and varies from 7–47%, with the majority occurring in cerebral distribution in the 25% range.[45,115] The HeartMate device has the lowest thromboembolic rate, reported to be as low as 2–3%.[112,173] This is likely due to its uniquely textured blood–interface surface, which promotes a formation of neointima. This results in low levels of

*References 8, 72, 82, 171, 174, 177.

thrombus formation despite minimal anticoagulation with aspirin.[33,159,173] All other pumps require warfarin (Coumadin), as well as antiplatelet agents.

Mechanical failure is a complication on the decline. Constant modifications of pump design result in more reliable systems. The failure can occur in multiple places in the device itself or in the controller. The rate of failure is 10% or less, including the long-term studies with device duration longer than 1 year.[115,158] Device failure, however, does not always result in patient death. In many cases ample time or reserve is available to replace the device or the controller.

RHF is one of the most important causes of perioperative mortality.[64,126] In most cases the unloading and support of the left ventricle helps the right side. However, a rise in central venous pressure with a decrease in device flow and an empty left ventricle signals right ventricular failure. Inhaled nitric oxide significantly reduces right ventricular afterload, thereby increasing LVAD flows in patients with elevated pulmonary vascular resistance.[9,188] If this is inadequate, however, an RVAD should be implanted. The incidence of RHF is above 10%, with 20% of patients requiring prolonged inotropic support. RHF also is associated with high transfusion requirements, prolonged ICU admission, increased incidence of end-organ failure, and increased mortality.[90]

Multiple organ failure is another frequent complication in this population. Because of a significant amount of preoperative end-organ dysfunction and comorbid conditions, some of these patients do not fully recover despite restoration of cardiac output. Multiple organ failure is often the end result of a long cascade of complications, including sepsis, bleeding, and other events. Other times it may be the result of significant preoperative multiorgan dysfunction that worsens with added stress of surgery. Overall it accounts for 11–29% of VAD deaths.[115]

SUMMARY

LVADs are the standard of care for potential heart transplant patients with life-threatening heart failure refractory to medical therapy. Significant advances in both the technology and clinical experience have taken place over the past 10 years. Increasing technological advances, clinical experience, and broadening indications allow more patients to benefit from VAD support. Thus a critical niche can be filled while patients await heart transplant. For some patients, LVADs may even become an alternative to transplant. In turn, this results in more appropriate transplant candidates, increased survival, and better quality of life for patients who would otherwise not survive.

ACKNOWLEDGMENTS

Dr. Naka is the Herbert Irving Assistant Professor of Surgery at Columbia University.

Funding for VAD research has been provided by the Foundation for the Advancement of Cardiac Therapies (FACT).

REFERENCES

1. Altemose GT, Gritsus V, Jeevanandam V, et al: Altered myocardial phenotype after mechanical support in human beings with advanced cardiomyopathy. J Heart Lung Transplant 16:765–773, 1997.
2. Angell James JE, Daly M: Effects of graded pulsatile pressure on the reflex vasomotor responses elicited by changes of mean pressure in the perfused carotid sinus: Aortic arch regions of the dog. J Physiol 214:51–64, 1971.
3. Ankersmit H-J, Itescu S: Immunobiology of left ventricular assist devices. In Goldstein DJ, Oz MC, editors: Cardiac Assist Devices, pp. 193–211. Armonk, NY: Futura Publishing Company, Inc., 2000.
4. Ankersmit HJ, Tugulea S, Spanier T, et al: Activation-induced T-cell death and immune dysfunction after implantation of left-ventricular assist device. Lancet 354:550–555, 1999.
5. Anstadt GL, Blakemore WS, Baue AE: A new instrument for prolonged mechanical massage. Circulation 31(2 suppl):43, 1965 (abstract).
6. Anstadt MP, Bartlett RL, Malone JP, et al: Direct mechanical ventricular actuation for cardiac arrest in humans. A clinical feasibility trial. Chest 100:86–92, 1991.
7. Anstadt MP, Perez-Tamayo RA, Banit DM, et al: Myocardial tolerance to mechanical actuation is affected by biomaterial characteristics. ASAIO J 40:M329–M334, 1994.
8. Argenziano M, Catanese KA, Moazami N, et al: The influence of infection on survival and successful transplantation in patients with left ventricular assist devices. J Heart Lung Transplant 16:822–831, 1997.
9. Argenziano M, Choudhri AF, Moazami N, et al: Randomized, double-blind trial of inhaled nitric oxide in LVAD recipients with pulmonary hypertension. Ann Thorac Surg 65:340–345, 1998.
10. Argenziano M, Choudhri AF, Oz MC, et al: A prospective randomized trial of arginine vasopressin in the treatment of vasodilatory shock after left ventricular assist device placement. Circulation 96:II90, 1997.
11. Artrip JH, Yi GH, Levin HR, et al: Physiological and hemodynamic evaluation of nonuniform direct cardiac compression. Circulation 100:II236–II243, 1999.
12. Artrip JH, Yi GH, Shimizo J, et al: Maximizing hemodynamic effectiveness of biventricular assistance by direct cardiac compression studied in ex vivo and in vivo canine models of acute heart failure. J Thorac Cardiovasc Surg 120:379–386, 2000.
13. Ashton RC, Goldstein DJ, Rose EA, et al: Duration of left ventricular assist device support affects transplant survival. J Heart Lung Transplant 15:1151–1157, 1996.
14. Bianchi JJ, Swartz MT, Raithel SC, et al: Initial clinical experience with centrifugal pumps coated with the Carmeda process. ASAIO J 38:M143–M146, 1992.
15. Boyce SW, Crevensten G, Fine RB: An anatomically compatible, wearless, reliable, and nonthrombogenic centrifugal blood pump. Ann Thorac Surg 71:S190, 2001.
16. Bregman D, Nichols AB, Weiss MB, et al: Percutaneous intraaortic balloon insertion. Am J Cardiol 46:261–264, 1980.
17. Busch T, Sirbu H, Zenker D, et al: Vascular complications related to intraaortic balloon counterpulsation: An analysis of ten years experience. Thorac Cardiovasc Surg 45:55–59, 1997.
18. Catanese KA, Goldstein DJ, Williams DL, et al: Outpatient left ventricular assist device support: A destination rather than a bridge. Ann Thorac Surg 62:646–652, 1996.
19. Champsaur G, Ninet J, Vigneron M, et al: Use of the Abiomed BVS System 5000 as a bridge to cardiac transplantation. J Thorac Cardiovasc Surg 100:122–128, 1990.

20. Chang JC, Sawa Y, Ohtake S, et al: Hemodynamic effect of inhaled nitric oxide in dilated cardiomyopathy patients on LVAD support. ASAIO J 43:M418–M421, 1997.
21. Chen JM, Spanier TB, Gonzalez JJ, et al: Improved survival in patients with acute myocarditis using external pulsatile mechanical ventricular assistance. J Heart Lung Transplant 18:351–357, 1999.
22. Cloy MJ, Myers TJ, Stutts LA, et al: Hospital charges for conventional therapy versus left ventricular assist system therapy in heart transplant patients. ASAIO J 41:M535–M539, 1995.
23. Cooley DA, Liotta D, Hallman GL, et al: Orthotopic cardiac prosthesis for two-staged cardiac replacement. Am J Cardiol 24:723–730, 1969.
24. Copeland JG, Smith RG, Arabia FA, et al: The CardioWest total artificial heart as a bridge to transplantation. Semin Thorac Cardiovasc Surg 12:238–242, 2000.
25. Coselli JS, LeMaire SA, Ledesma DF, et al: Initial experience with the Nikkiso centrifugal pump during thoracoabdominal aortic aneurysm repair. J Vasc Surg 27:378–383, 1998.
26. Couper GS, Dekkers RJ, Adams DH: The logistics and cost-effectiveness of circulatory support: Advantages of the Abiomed BVS 5000. Ann Thorac Surg 68:646–649, 1999.
27. Curtis J, Wagner-Mann C, Mann F, et al: Subchronic use of the St. Jude centrifugal pump as a mechanical assist device in calves. Artif Organs 20:662–665, 1996.
28. Curtis JJ: Centrifugal mechanical assist for postcardiotomy ventricular failure. Semin Thorac Cardiovasc Surg 6:140–146, 1994.
29. Curtis JJ, Boley TM, Walls JT, et al: Frequency of seal disruption with the sarns centrifugal pump in postcardiotomy circulatory assist. Artif Organs 18:235–237, 1994.
30. Curtis JJ, Walls JT, Schmaltz RA, et al: Improving clinical outcome with centrifugal mechanical assist for postcardiotomy ventricular failure. Artif Organs 19:761–765, 1995.
31. Curtis JJ, Walls JT, Wagner-Mann CC, et al: Centrifugal pumps: Description of devices and surgical techniques. Ann Thorac Surg 68:666–671, 1999.
32. Dapper F, Neppl H, Wozniak G, et al: Effects of pulsatile and nonpulsatile perfusion mode during extracorporeal circulation: A comparative clinical study. Thorac Cardiovasc Surg 40:345–351, 1992.
33. Dasse KA, Frazier OH, Lesniak JM, et al: Clinical responses to ventricular assistance versus transplantation in a series of bridge to transplant patients. ASAIO J 38:M622–M626, 1992.
34. DeBakey ME: Left ventricular bypass pump for cardiac assistance. Clinical experience. Am J Cardiol 27:3–11, 1971.
35. Deng MC, Loebe M, El Banayosy A, et al: Mechanical circulatory support for advanced heart failure: Effect of patient selection on outcome. Circulation 103:231–237, 2001.
36. Deng MC, Weyand M, Hammel D, et al: Selection and outcome of ventricular assist device patients: The Muenster experience. J Heart Lung Transplant 17:817–825, 1998.
37. Department of Health and Human Services, National Institutes of Health, and the National Heart, Lung, and Blood Institute: Request for proposal. Innovative Ventricular Assist Systems. Bethesda, MD, 1994.
38. Department of Health and Human Services, National Institutes of Health, and the National Heart, Lung, and Blood Institute: Request for proposal. Development of an Implantable Integrated Electrically Powered Left Heart Assist System. Bethesda, Md, 1980.
39. Department of Health and Human Services, National Institutes of Health, and the National Heart, Lung, and Blood Institute: Request for proposal. Development of Electrical Energy Converters to Power and Control Left Heart Assist Devices. Bethesda, Md, 1977.
40. Department of Health and Human Services, National Institutes of Health, and the National Heart, Lung, and Blood Institute: Request for proposal. Left Heart Assist Blood Pumps. Bethesda, Md, 1977.
41. DeRose JJ, Umana JP, Argenziano M, et al: Implantable left ventricular assist devices provide an excellent outpatient bridge to transplantation and recovery. J Am Coll Cardiol 30:1773–1777, 1997.
42. Dietl CA, Berkheimer MD, Woods EL, et al: Efficacy and cost-effectiveness of preoperative IABP in patients with ejection fraction of 0.25 or less. Ann Thorac Surg 62:401–408, 1996.
43. Dipla K, Mattiello JA, Jeevanandam V, et al: Myocyte recovery after mechanical circulatory support in humans with end-stage heart failure. Circulation 97:2316–2322, 1998.
44. El Banayosy A, Arusoglu L, Kizner L, et al: Novacor left ventricular assist system versus HeartMate vented electric left ventricular assist system as a long-term mechanical circulatory support device in bridging patients: A prospective study. J Thorac Cardiovasc Surg 119:581–587, 2000.
45. El Banayosy A, Korfer R, Arusoglu L, et al: Device and patient management in a bridge-to-transplant setting. Ann Thorac Surg 71:S98–S102, 2001.
46. El Banayosy A, Minami K, Arusoglu L, et al: Long-term mechanical circulatory support. Thorac Cardiovasc Surg 45:127–130, 1997.
47. Farrar DJ: The Thoratec ventricular assist device: A paracorporeal pump for treating acute and chronic heart failure. Semin Thorac Cardiovasc Surg 12:243–250, 2000.
48. Farrar DJ: Preoperative predictors of survival in patients with Thoratec ventricular assist devices as a bridge to heart transplantation. Thoratec Ventricular Assist Device Principal Investigators. J Heart Lung Transplant 13:93–100, 1994.
49. Farrar DJ, Buck KE, Coulter JH, et al: Portable pneumatic biventricular driver for the Thoratec ventricular assist device. ASAIO J 43:M631–M634, 1997.
50. Farrar DJ, Hill JD: Univentricular and biventricular Thoratec VAD support as a bridge to transplantation. Ann Thorac Surg 55:276–282, 1993.
51. Farrar DJ, Hill JD, Gray LA, et al: Successful biventricular circulatory support as a bridge to cardiac transplantation during prolonged ventricular fibrillation and asystole. Circulation 80:III147–III151, 1989.
52. Farrar DJ, Hill JD, Pennington DG, et al: Preoperative and postoperative comparison of patients with univentricular and biventricular support with the Thoratec ventricular assist device as a bridge to cardiac transplantation. J Thorac Cardiovasc Surg 113:202–209, 1997.
53. Farrar DJ, Reichenbach SH, Rossi SA, et al: Development of an intracorporeal Thoratec ventricular assist device for univentricular or biventricular support. ASAIO J 46:351–353, 2000.
54. Foray A, Williams D, Reemtsma K, et al: Assessment of submaximal exercise capacity in patients with left ventricular assist devices. Circulation 94:II222–II226, 1996.
55. Frazier OH: The development of an implantable, portable, electrically powered left ventricular assist device. Semin Thorac Cardiovasc Surg 6:181–187, 1994.
56. Frazier OH, Benedict CR, Radovancevic B, et al: Improved left ventricular function after chronic left ventricular unloading. Ann Thorac Surg 62:675–681, 1996.
57. Frazier OH, Macris MP, Myers TJ, et al: Improved survival after extended bridge to cardiac transplantation. Ann Thorac Surg 57:1416–1422, 1994.
58. Friedel N, Viazis P, Schiessler A, et al: Recovery of end-organ failure during mechanical circulatory support. Eur J Cardiothorac Surg 6:519–522, 1992.
59. Fukamachi K, McCarthy PM, Smedira NG, et al: Preoperative risk factors for right ventricular failure after

implantable left ventricular assist device insertion. Ann Thorac Surg 68:2181–2184, 1999.
60. Gaer JA, Shaw AD, Wild R, et al: Effect of cardiopulmonary bypass on gastrointestinal perfusion and function. Ann Thorac Surg 57:371–375, 1994.
61. Goldberg RJ, Gore JM, Alpert JS, et al: Cardiogenic shock after acute myocardial infarction. Incidence and mortality from a community-wide perspective, 1975 to 1988. N Engl J Med 325:1117–1122, 1991.
62. Goldberg RJ, Gore JM, Thompson CA, et al: Recent magnitude of and temporal trends (1994–1997) in the incidence and hospital death rates of cardiogenic shock complicating acute myocardial infarction: The second National Registry of Myocardial Infarction. Am Heart J 141:65–72, 2001.
63. Goldstein DJ, Seldomridge JA, Chen JM, et al: Use of aprotinin in LVAD recipients reduces blood loss, blood use, and perioperative mortality. Ann Thorac Surg 59:1063–1067, 1995.
64. Gracin N, Johnson MR, Spokas D, et al: The use of APACHE II scores to select candidates for left ventricular assist device placement. Acute Physiology and Chronic Health Evaluation. J Heart Lung Transplant 17:1017–1023, 1998.
65. Guyton RA, Schonberger JP, Everts PA, et al: Postcardiotomy shock: Clinical evaluation of the BVS 5000 Biventricular Support System. Ann Thorac Surg 56:346–356, 1993.
66. Hall CW, Liotta D, Henly WS, et al: Development of artificial intrathoracic circulatory pumps. Am J Surg 108:685–692, 1964.
67. Hart RM, Filipenco VG, Kung RT: A magnetically suspended and hydrostatically stabilized centrifugal blood pump. Artif Organs 20:591–596, 1996.
68. Helman DN, Maybaum SW, Morales DL, et al: Recurrent remodeling after ventricular assistance: Is long-term myocardial recovery attainable? Ann Thorac Surg 70:1255–1258, 2000.
69. Helman DN, Morales DL, Edwards NM, et al: Left ventricular assist device bridge-to-transplant network improves survival after failed cardiotomy. Ann Thorac Surg 68:1187–1194, 1999.
70. Hendry PJ, Masters RG, Mussivand TV, et al: Circulatory support for cardiogenic shock due to acute myocardial infarction: A Canadian experience. Can J Cardiol 15:1090–1094, 1999.
71. Hendry PJ, Mussivand TV, Masters RG, et al: The HeartSaver left ventricular assist device: An update. Ann Thorac Surg 71:S166–S170, 2001.
72. Herrmann M, Weyand M, Greshake B, et al: Left ventricular assist device infection is associated with increased mortality but is not a contraindication to transplantation. Circulation 95:814–817, 1997.
73. Hetzer R, Loebe M, Potapov EV, et al: Circulatory support with pneumatic paracorporeal ventricular assist device in infants and children. Ann Thorac Surg 66:1498–1506, 1998.
74. Hetzer R, Muller J, Weng Y, et al: Cardiac recovery in dilated cardiomyopathy by unloading with a left ventricular assist device. Ann Thorac Surg 68:742–749, 1999.
75. Hetzer R, Muller JH, Weng YG, et al: Midterm follow-up of patients who underwent removal of a left ventricular assist device after cardiac recovery from end-stage dilated cardiomyopathy. J Thorac Cardiovasc Surg 120:843–855, 2000.
76. Hickey PR, Buckley MJ, Philbin DM: Pulsatile and nonpulsatile cardiopulmonary bypass: Review of a counterproductive controversy. Ann Thorac Surg 36:720–737, 1983.
77. Hill JD, Farrar DJ, Hershon JJ, et al: Use of a prosthetic ventricle as a bridge to cardiac transplantation for postinfarction cardiogenic shock. N Engl J Med 314:626–628, 1986.
78. Hindman BJ, Dexter F, Ryu KH, et al: Pulsatile versus nonpulsatile cardiopulmonary bypass. No difference in brain blood flow or metabolism at 27 degrees C. Anesthesiology 80:1137–1147, 1994.
79. Hindman BJ, Dexter F, Smith T, et al: Pulsatile versus nonpulsatile flow. No difference in cerebral blood flow or metabolism during normothermic cardiopulmonary bypass in rabbits. Anesthesiology 82:241–250, 1995.
80. Hochman JS, Sleeper LA, White HD, et al: One-year survival following early revascularization for cardiogenic shock. JAMA 285:190–192, 2001.
81. Holman WL, Roye GD, Bourge RC, et al: Circulatory support for myocardial infarction with ventricular arrhythmias. Ann Thorac Surg 59:1230–1231, 1995.
82. Holman WL, Skinner JL, Waites KB, et al: Infection during circulatory support with ventricular assist devices. Ann Thorac Surg 68:711–716, 1999.
83. Hornick P, Taylor K: Pulsatile and nonpulsatile perfusion: The continuing controversy. J Cardiothorac Vasc Anesth 11:310–315, 1997.
84. Houel R, Vermes E, Tixier DB, et al: Myocardial recovery after mechanical support for acute myocarditis: Is sustained recovery predictable? Ann Thorac Surg 68:2177–2180, 1999.
85. Hoy FB, Mueller DK, Geiss DM, et al: Bridge to recovery for postcardiotomy failure: Is there still a role for centrifugal pumps? Ann Thorac Surg 70:1259–1263, 2000.
86. Ishino K, Alexi-Meskishvili V, Hetzer R: Myocardial recovery through ECMO after repair of total anomalous pulmonary venous connection: The importance of left heart unloading. Eur J Cardiothorac Surg 11:585–587, 1997.
87. Jett GK: Abiomed BVS 5000: Experience and potential advantages. Ann Thorac Surg 61:301–304, 1996.
88. Joyce LD, Kiser JC, Eales F, et al: Experience with generally accepted centrifugal pumps: Personal and collective experience. Ann Thorac Surg 61:287–290, 1996.
89. Kantrowitz A, Tjonneland S, Freed PS, et al: Initial clinical experience with intraaortic balloon pumping in cardiogenic shock. JAMA 203:113–118, 1968.
90. Kavarana MN, Pessin-Minsley MS, Urtecho J, et al: Right ventricular dysfunction and organ failure in left ventricular assist device recipients: A continuing problem. Ann Thorac Surg 73:745–750, 2002.
91. Kawahito K, Damm G, Benkowski R, et al: Ex vivo phase 1 evaluation of the DeBakey/NASA axial flow ventricular assist device. Artif Organs 20:47–52, 1996.
92. Khanwilkar P: Oral presentation, ISHLT Third Fall Education Meeting. Mechanical Cardiac Support and Replacement II, November 9, 2001.
93. Korfer R, El Banayosy A, Arusoglu L, et al: Temporary pulsatile ventricular assist devices and biventricular assist devices. Ann Thorac Surg 68:678–683, 1999.
94. Kormos RL, Murali S, Dew MA, et al: Chronic mechanical circulatory support: Rehabilitation, low morbidity, and superior survival. Ann Thorac Surg 57:51–57, 1994.
95. Lee J, Miller PJ, Chen H, et al: Reliability model from the in vitro durability tests of a left ventricular assist system. ASAIO J 45:595–601, 1999.
96. Lee SH, Doliba N, Osbakken M, et al: Improvement of myocardial mitochondrial function after hemodynamic support with left ventricular assist devices in patients with heart failure. J Thorac Cardiovasc Surg 116:344–349, 1998.
97. Levin HR, Oz MC, Chen JM, et al: Reversal of chronic ventricular dilation in patients with end-stage cardiomyopathy by prolonged mechanical unloading. Circulation 91:2717–2720, 1995.
98. Levine FH, Philbin DM, Kono K, et al: Plasma vasopressin levels and urinary sodium excretion during cardiopulmonary bypass with and without pulsatile flow. Ann Thorac Surg 32:63–67, 1981.

99. Loebe M, Hennig E, Muller J, et al: Long-term mechanical circulatory support as a bridge to transplantation, for recovery from cardiomyopathy, and for permanent replacement. Eur J Cardiothorac Surg 11(suppl):S18–S24, 1997.
100. Loebe M, Muller J, Hetzer R: Ventricular assistance for recovery of cardiac failure. Curr Opin Cardiol 14:234–248, 1999.
101. Loree HM, Bourque K, Gernes DB, et al: The HeartMate III: Design and in vivo studies of a maglev centrifugal left ventricular assist device. Artif Organs 25:386–391, 2001.
102. Macha M, Litwak P, Yamazaki K, et al: Survival for up to six months in calves supported with an implantable axial flow ventricular assist device. ASAIO J 43:311–315, 1997.
103. Macris MP, Myers TJ, Jarvik R, et al: In vivo evaluation of an intraventricular electric axial flow pump for left ventricular assistance. ASAIO J 40:M719–M722, 1994.
104. Magovern GJ Jr: The biopump and postoperative circulatory support. Ann Thorac Surg 55:245–249, 1993.
105. Magovern GJ Jr, Christlieb IY, Kao RL, et al: Recovery of the failing canine heart with biventricular support in a previously fatal experimental model. J Thorac Cardiovasc Surg 94:656–663, 1987.
106. Maher TR, Butler KC, Poirier VL, et al: HeartMate left ventricular assist devices: A multigeneration of implanted blood pumps. Artif Organs 25:422–426, 2001.
107. Mancini DM, Beniaminovitz A, Levin H, et al: Low incidence of myocardial recovery after left ventricular assist device implantation in patients with chronic heart failure. Circulation 98:2383–2389, 1998.
108. Mann FA, Wagner-Mann CC, Curtis JJ, et al: A calf model for left ventricular centrifugal mechanical assist. Artif Organs 20:670–677, 1996.
109. Marelli D, Laks H, Amsel B, et al: Temporary mechanical support with the BVS 5000 assist device during treatment of acute myocarditis. J Card Surg 12:55–59, 1997.
110. McBride LR, Lowdermilk GA, Fiore AC, et al: Transfer of patients receiving advanced mechanical circulatory support. J Thorac Cardiovasc Surg 119:1015–1020, 2000.
111. McCarthy PM, Nakatani S, Vargo R, et al: Structural and left ventricular histologic changes after implantable LVAD insertion. Ann Thorac Surg 59:609–613, 1995.
112. McCarthy PM, Smedira NO, Vargo RL, et al: One hundred patients with the HeartMate left ventricular assist device: Evolving concepts and technology. J Thorac Cardiovasc Surg 115:904–912, 1998.
113. Mehta SM, Pae WE Jr, Rosenberg G, et al: The LionHeart LVD-2000: A completely implanted left ventricular assist device for chronic circulatory support. Ann Thorac Surg 71:S156–S161, 2001.
114. Minami K, El Banayosy A, Posival H, et al: Improvement of survival rate in patients with cardiogenic shock by using nonpulsatile and pulsatile ventricular assist device. Int J Artif Organs 15:715–721, 1992.
115. Minami K, El Banayosy A, Sezai A, et al: Morbidity and outcome after mechanical ventricular support using Thoratec, Novacor, and HeartMate for bridging to heart transplantation. Artif Organs 24:421–426, 2000.
116. Moores WY, Gago O, Morris JD, et al: Serum and urinary amylase levels following pulsatile and continuous cardiopulmonary bypass. J Thorac Cardiovasc Surg 74:73–76, 1977.
117. Morales DL, Catanese KA, Helman DN, et al: Six-year experience of caring for forty-four patients with a left ventricular assist device at home: Safe, economical, necessary. J Thorac Cardiovasc Surg 119:251–259, 2000.
118. Morgan IS, Codispoti M, Sanger K, et al: Superiority of centrifugal pump over roller pump in paediatric cardiac surgery: Prospective randomised trial. Eur J Cardiothorac Surg 13:526–532, 1998.
119. Mueller HS: Role of intra-aortic counterpulsation in cardiogenic shock and acute myocardial infarction. Cardiology 84:168–174, 1994.
120. Mueller J, Wallukat G, Weng Y, et al: Predictive factors for weaning from a cardiac assist device. An analysis of clinical, gene expression, and protein data. J Heart Lung Transplant 20:202, 2001.
121. Muller J, Wallukat G, Weng YG, et al: Weaning from mechanical cardiac support in patients with idiopathic dilated cardiomyopathy. Circulation 96:542–549, 1997.
122. Mussivand T, Henry PJ, Masters RG, et al: A totally implantable ventricular assist device. Results of in vivo studies. J Extra Corpor Technol 32:184–189, 2000.
123. Mussivand T, Hendry PJ, Masters RG, et al: Progress with the HeartSaver ventricular assist device. Ann Thorac Surg 68:785–789, 1999.
124. Naganuma S, Yambe T, Sonobe T, et al: Development of a novel centrifugal pump: Magnetic rotary pump. Artif Organs 21:746–750, 1997.
125. Nakatani S, McCarthy PM, Kottke-Marchant K, et al: Left ventricular echocardiographic and histologic changes: Impact of chronic unloading by an implantable ventricular assist device. J Am Coll Cardiol 27:894–901, 1996.
126. Nakatani S, Thomas JD, Savage RM, et al: Prediction of right ventricular dysfunction after left ventricular assist device implantation. Circulation 94:II216–II221, 1996.
127. Nakazawa T, Ohara Y, Benkowski R, et al: A pivot bearing-supported centrifugal pump for a long-term assist heart. Int J Artif Organs 20:222–228, 1997.
128. Nishinaka T, Nishida H, Endo M, et al: Less blood damage in the impeller centrifugal pump: A comparative study with the roller pump in open heart surgery. Artif Organs 20:707–710, 1996.
129. Nojiri C, Kijima T, Maekawa J, et al: Development status of Terumo implantable left ventricular assist system. Artif Organs 25:411–413, 2001.
130. Nojiri C, Kijima T, Maekawa J, et al: Recent progress in the development of Terumo implantable left ventricular assist system. ASAIO J 45:199–203, 1999.
131. Noon GP, Ball JW Jr, Papaconstantinou HT: Clinical experience with BioMedicus centrifugal ventricular support in 172 patients. Artif Organs 19:756–760, 1995.
132. Noon GP, Ball JW Jr, Short HD: BioMedicus centrifugal ventricular support for postcardiotomy cardiac failure: A review of 129 cases. Ann Thorac Surg 61:291–295, 1996.
133. Noon GP, Lafuente JA, Irwin S: Acute and temporary ventricular support with BioMedicus centrifugal pump. Ann Thorac Surg 68:650–654, 1999.
134. Noris M, Morigi M, Donadelli R, et al: Nitric oxide synthesis by cultured endothelial cells is modulated by flow conditions. Circ Res 76:536–543, 1995.
135. Norman JC, Brook MI, Cooley DA, et al: Total support of the circulation of a patient with post-cardiotomy stone-heart syndrome by a partial artificial heart (ALVAD) for 5 days followed by heart and kidney transplantation. Lancet 1:1125–1127, 1978.
136. Ohtsubo S, Naito K, Matsuura M, et al: Initial clinical experience with the Baylor-Nikkiso centrifugal pump. Artif Organs 19:769–773, 1995.
137. Ohtsuka G, Nakata K, Yoshikawa M, et al: Long-term in vivo left ventricular assist device study for 284 days with Gyro PI pump. Artif Organs 23:504–507, 1999.
138. Oz MC, Argenziano M, Catanese KA, et al: Bridge experience with long-term implantable left ventricular assist devices. Are they an alternative to transplantation? Circulation 95:1844–1852, 1997.
139. Oz MC, Goldstein DJ, Pepino P, et al: Screening scale predicts patients successfully receiving long-term implantable

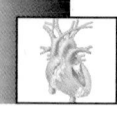

left ventricular assist devices. Circulation 92:II169–II173, 1995.
140. Oz MC, Rose EA, Levin HR: Selection criteria for placement of left ventricular assist devices. Am Heart J 129:173–177, 1995.
141. Pae WE Jr: Oral presentation, ISHLT Third Fall Education Meeting. Mechanical Cardiac Support and Replacement II, November 9, 2001.
142. Pae WE Jr, Miller CA, Matthews Y, et al: Ventricular assist devices for postcardiotomy cardiogenic shock. A combined registry experience. J Thorac Cardiovasc Surg 104:541–552, 1992.
143. Pennington DG, Bernhard WF, Golding LR, et al: Long-term follow-up of postcardiotomy patients with profound cardiogenic shock treated with ventricular assist devices. Circulation 72:II216–II226, 1985.
144. Pennington DG, McBride LR, Peigh PS, et al: Eight years' experience with bridging to cardiac transplantation. J Thorac Cardiovasc Surg 107:472–480, 1994.
145. Pennington DG, Merjavy JP, Swartz MT, et al: Clinical experience with a centrifugal pump ventricular assist device. Trans Am Soc Artif Intern Organs 28:93–99, 1982.
146. Pennock JL, Pierce WS, Wisman CB, et al: Survival and complications following ventricular assist pumping for cardiogenic shock. Ann Surg 198:469–478, 1983.
147. Perez-Tamayo RA, Anstadt MP, Cothran RL, et al: Prolonged total circulatory support using direct mechanical ventricular actuation. ASAIO J 41:M512–M517, 1995.
148. Portner PM, Oyer PE, Jassawalla JS, et al: An implantable permanent left ventricular assist system for man. Trans Am Soc Artif Intern Organs 24:99–103, 1978.
149. Portner PM, Oyer PE, Pennington DG, et al: Implantable electrical left ventricular assist system: Bridge to transplantation and the future. Ann Thorac Surg 47:142–150, 1989.
150. Potapov EV, Loebe M, Nasseri BA, et al: Pulsatile flow in patients with a novel nonpulsatile implantable ventricular assist device. Circulation 102:III183–III187, 2000.
151. Powell WJ, Daggett WM, Magro AE, et al: Effects of intra-aortic balloon counterpulsation on cardiac performance, oxygen consumption, and coronary blood flow in dogs. Circ Res 26:753–764, 1970.
152. Ramasamy N, Vargo RL, Kormos RL, et al: The Novacor left ventricular assist system. In Goldstein DJ, Oz MC, editors: Cardiac Assist Devices, pp. 323–340. Armonk, NY: Futura Publishing Company, Inc., 2000.
153. Rao V, Oz MC, Flannery MA, et al: Revised screening scale to predict survival after insertion of a left ventricular assist device. J Thorac Cardiovasc Surg 125:855–862, 2003.
154. Reddy RC, Goldstein AH, Pacella JJ, et al: End organ function with prolonged nonpulsatile circulatory support. ASAIO J 41:M547–M551, 1995.
155. Reichenbach SH, Farrar DJ, Hill JD: A versatile intracorporeal ventricular assist device based on the Thoratec VAD system. Ann Thorac Surg 71:S171–S175, 2001.
156. Reinhartz O, Farrar DJ, Hershon JH, et al: Importance of preoperative liver function as a predictor of survival in patients supported with Thoratec ventricular assist devices as a bridge to transplantation. J Thorac Cardiovasc Surg 116:633–640, 1998.
157. Robbins RC, Kown MH, Portner PM, et al: The totally implantable Novacor left ventricular assist system. Ann Thorac Surg 71:S162–S165, 2001.
158. Rose EA, Gelijns AC, Moskowitz AJ, et al: Long-term use of a left ventricular assist device for end-stage heart failure. N Engl J Med 345:1435–1443, 2001.
159. Rose EA, Levin HR, Oz MC, et al: Artificial circulatory support with textured interior surfaces. A counterintuitive approach to minimizing thromboembolism. Circulation 90:II87–II91, 1994.
160. Rose EA, Moskowitz AJ, Packer M, et al: The REMATCH trial: Rationale, design, and end points. Randomized Evaluation of Mechanical Assistance for the Treatment of Congestive Heart Failure. Ann Thorac Surg 67:723–730, 1999.
161. Sakaki M, Taenaka Y, Tatsumi E, et al: Influences of nonpulsatile pulmonary flow on pulmonary function. Evaluation in a chronic animal model. J Thorac Cardiovasc Surg 108:495–502, 1994.
162. Salamonsen RF, Kaye D, Esmore DS: Inhalation of nitric oxide provides selective pulmonary vasodilatation, aiding mechanical cardiac assist with Thoratec left ventricular assist device. Anaesth Intensive Care 22:209–210, 1994.
163. Samuels LE, Kaufman MS, Thomas MP, et al: Pharmacological criteria for ventricular assist device insertion following postcardiotomy shock: Experience with the Abiomed BVS system. J Card Surg 14:288–293, 1999.
164. Scheinin SA, Capek P, Radovancevic B, et al: The effect of prolonged left ventricular support on myocardial histopathology in patients with end-stage cardiomyopathy. ASAIO J 38:M271–M274, 1992.
165. Schima H, Schmallegger H, Huber L, et al: An implantable seal-less centrifugal pump with integrated double-disk motor. Artif Organs 19:639–643, 1995.
166. Schmid C, Deng M, Hammel D, et al: Emergency versus elective/urgent left ventricular assist device implantation. J Heart Lung Transplant 17:1024–1028, 1998.
167. Schmid C, Wilhelm M, Reimann A, et al: Use of an intraaortic balloon pump in patients with impaired left ventricular function. Scand Cardiovasc J 33:194–198, 1999.
168. Sezai A, Shiono M, Orime Y, et al: Major organ function under mechanical support: Comparative studies of pulsatile and nonpulsatile circulation. Artif Organs 23:280–285, 1999.
169. Sezai A, Shiono M, Orime Y, et al. Comparison studies of major organ microcirculations under pulsatile- and nonpulsatile-assisted circulations. Artif Organs 20:139–142, 1996.
170. Sezai A, Shiono M, Orime Y, et al: Renal circulation and cellular metabolism during left ventricular assisted circulation: Comparison study of pulsatile and nonpulsatile assists. Artif Organs 21:830–835, 1997.
171. Sinha P, Chen JM, Flannery M, et al: Infections during left ventricular assist device support do not affect posttransplant outcomes. Circulation 102:III194–III199, 2000.
172. Sirbu H, Busch T, Aleksic I, et al: Ischaemic complications with intra-aortic balloon counter-pulsation: Incidence and management. Cardiovasc Surg 8:66–71, 2000.
173. Slater JP, Rose EA, Levin HR, et al: Low thromboembolic risk without anticoagulation using advanced-design left ventricular assist devices. Ann Thorac Surg 62:1321–1327, 1996.
174. Springer WE, Wasler A, Radovancevic B, et al: Retrospective analysis of infection in patients undergoing support with left ventricular assist systems. ASAIO J 42:M763–M765, 1996.
175. Stolar CJ, Delosh T, Bartlett RH: Extracorporeal Life Support Organization 1993. ASAIO J 39:976–979, 1993.
176. Subramanian VA, Goldstein JE, Sos TA, et al: Preliminary clinical experience with percutaneous intraaortic balloon pumping. Circulation 62:I123–I129, 1980.
177. Sun BC, Catanese KA, Spanier TB, et al: 100 long-term implantable left ventricular assist devices: The Columbia Presbyterian interim experience. Ann Thorac Surg 68:688–694, 1999.
178. Swartz MT, Lowdermilk GA, McBride LR: Refractory ventricular tachycardia as an indication for ventricular assist device support. J Thorac Cardiovasc Surg 118:1119–1120, 1999.

179. Swartz MT, Votapka TV, McBride LR, et al: Risk stratification in patients bridged to cardiac transplantation. Ann Thorac Surg 58:1142–1145, 1994.
180. Taenaka Y, Tatsumi E, Sakaki M, et al: Peripheral circulation during nonpulsatile systemic perfusion in chronic awake animals. ASAIO Trans 37:M365–M366, 1991.
181. Taguchi S, Yozu R, Mori A, et al: A miniaturized centrifugal pump for assist circulation. Artif Organs 18:664–668, 1994.
182. Takami Y, Ohara Y, Otsuka G, et al: Preclinical evaluation of the Kyocera Gyro centrifugal blood pump for cardiopulmonary bypass. Perfusion 12:335–341, 1997.
183. Taylor KM, Wright GS, Bain WH, et al: Comparative studies of pulsatile and nonpulsatile flow during cardiopulmonary bypass. III. Response of anterior pituitary gland to thyrotropin-releasing hormone. J Thorac Cardiovasc Surg 75:579–584, 1978.
184. Taylor KM, Wright GS, Reid JM, et al: Comparative studies of pulsatile and nonpulsatile flow during cardiopulmonary bypass. II. The effects on adrenal secretion of cortisol. J Thorac Cardiovasc Surg 75:574–578, 1978.
185. Tedoriya T, Kawasuji M, Sakakibara N, et al: Coronary bypass flow during use of intraaortic balloon pumping and left ventricular assist device. Ann Thorac Surg 66:477–481, 1998.
186. Tomanek RJ, Cooper G: Morphological changes in the mechanically unloaded myocardial cell. Anat Rec 200: 271–280, 1981.
187. Torchiana DF, Hirsch G, Buckley MJ, et al: Intraaortic balloon pumping for cardiac support: Trends in practice and outcome, 1968 to 1995. J Thorac Cardiovasc Surg 113:758–764, 1997.
188. Wagner F, Dandel M, Gunther G, et al: Nitric oxide inhalation in the treatment of right ventricular dysfunction following left ventricular assist device implantation. Circulation 96(9 suppl):II-291–296, 1997.
189. Wagner-Mann C, Curtis J, Mann FA, et al: Subchronic centrifugal mechanical assist in an unheparinized calf model. Artif Organs 20:666–669, 1996.
190. Wakisaka Y, Taenaka Y, Chikanari K, et al: Long-term evaluation of a nonpulsatile mechanical circulatory support system. Artif Organs 21:639–644, 1997.
191. Wakisaka Y, Taenaka Y, Chikanari K, et al: Development of an implantable centrifugal blood pump for circulatory assist. ASAIO J 43:M608–M614, 1997.
192. Wassenberg PA: The Abiomed BVS 5000 biventricular support system. Perfusion 15:369–371, 2000.
193. Waters T, Allaire P, Tao G, et al: Motor feedback physiological control for a continuous flow ventricular assist device. Artif Organs 23:480–486, 1999.
194. Watkins WD, Peterson MB, Kong DL, et al: Thromboxane and prostacyclin changes during cardiopulmonary bypass with and without pulsatile flow. J Thorac Cardiovasc Surg 84:250–256, 1982.
195. Westaby S, Banning AP, Jarvik R, et al: First permanent implant of the Jarvik 2000 Heart. Lancet 356:900–903, 2000.
196. Wieselthaler GM, Schima H, Hiesmayr M, et al: First clinical experience with the DeBakey VAD continuous-axial-flow pump for bridge to transplantation. Circulation 101:356–359, 2000.
197. Woodard, J: Oral presentation, ISHLT Third Fall Education Meeting. Mechanical Cardiac Support and Replacement II, November 9, 2001.
198. Yamazaki K, Litwak P, Tagusari O, et al: An implantable centrifugal blood pump with a recirculating purge system (Cool-Seal system). Artif Organs 22:466–474, 1998.
199. Yoshikai M, Hamada M, Takarabe K, et al: Clinical use of centrifugal pumps and the roller pump in open heart surgery: A comparative evaluation. Artif Organs 20:704–706, 1996.

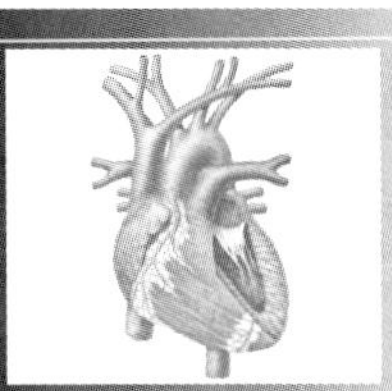

Total Artificial Heart

Robert D. Dowling

CHAPTER 93

HISTORY

The clinical use of cardiopulmonary bypass by Dr. Gibbon in 1953 was perhaps the most significant advance to usher in the current era of cardiac surgery. Four years later, Akutsu and Kolff[1] sustained the circulation of a dog for 90 minutes with two compact polyvinyl chloride pumps that were powered by an external air compressor. Unbeknownst to these investigators and the medical community, Demikhov had performed a similar experiment in 1937.[2,8] These pioneers were the first to struggle with many issues, including device compatibility, fit of the device in a narrow canine chest, problems related to device failure, and thrombus formation.

Initial survival in animals was extended from hours to days, and eventually to months. Pierce[15] reported the survival of a calf on an automatic device for just less than 1 year's time. The first clinical use of a total artificial heart was as a bridge to transplant in 1969 by Dr. Denton Cooley.[5] The Liotta artificial heart was placed in a patient who could not be weaned from cardiopulmonary bypass after resection of a ventricular aneurysm. The patient's circulation was supported for 39 hours, at which time a heart transplant was performed. Twelve years later, Cooley[4] described the second implantation of a pneumatic artificial heart. After 64 hours on support, the patient received a heart allograft. Unfortunately, neither of these patients survived. However, these early cases demonstrated that circulatory support with a pneumatic artificial heart was able to restore normal hemodynamics, preserve end-organ function, and allow for survival to transplantation.

The development of pneumatically powered devices continued at a number of laboratories, including Kolff's laboratory at the University of Utah. After extensive laboratory evaluation, clinical implants with this system were initiated. Initial trial design was to implant the Jarvik-7 device in patients who had failed all conventional methods of treatment, were felt to be at high risk of imminent death and were not considered to be transplant candidates.

On December 2, 1982, the Jarvik-7 was implanted in Dr. Barney Clark, who was suffering from end-stage heart failure. The Jarvik-7 device was pneumatically activated and required large percutaneous lines with the patient tethered to a large control console. Dr. Clark improved to the point where he was able to interact with his family, eat, and, ambulate for a few steps. He had multiple complications, including infections and stroke with resultant multisystem failure. The duration on support with the Jarvik-7 device was 112 days. After this implant, Dr. DeVries moved the clinical team to the Humana Heart Institute in Louisville, KY, where three additional implants were performed. One of the recipients, Bill Schroeder, survived over 600 days and achieved a place in history by being the first patient to be discharged from the hospital on a total artificial heart. The impact of the device on him and his family are described in a book authored by the patient's wife *(The Bill Schroeder Story)*.[3] Because of the cumbersome nature of the device and the patient's clinical course, he was never able to be transferred home, but did enjoy a significant period of time outside of a true hospital setting. There were significant infectious complications and stroke rate in this initial group of patients.

As the trial continued, it became clear to the medical community that the Jarvik-7 was not an acceptable device for destination therapy. In January 1990 the U.S. Food and Drug Administration (FDA) withdrew approval for clinical trials as destination therapy.[17] However, clinical trials with the Jarvik-7 heart as a bridge to transplant were initiated in 1985, with a number of successful case series reported. Subsequently, the Jarvik-7 system changed ownership and is currently known as the CardioWest Total Artificial Heart. This device has been in use since 1993, primarily by the group at the University of Arizona as a bridge to transplantation. With modern-day operative techniques and postoperative management strategies, this group has achieved very impressive results with this device, overcoming the earlier problems with infection and stroke.[6]

After the initiation of clinical trials of the Jarvik-7 heart, the National Heart, Lung, and Blood Institute initiated funding designed to stimulate development of a TAH with the potential of improving quality of life by allowing for patient discharge and improved ability to perform the activities of daily living. Initially, six centers were funded, with this number being decreased to two centers. The Penn State Total Electric Artificial Heart was developed in conjunction with the 3M Company, and the AbioCor Implantable

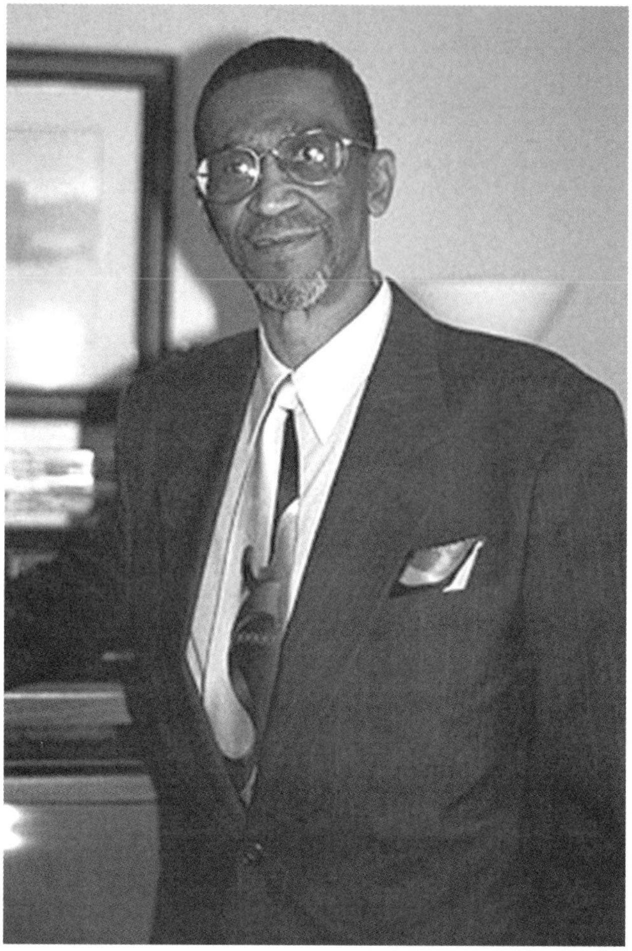

Figure 93–1 **Mr. Robert Tools, the first recipient of the AbioCor Implantable Replacement Heart, poses after recovering from the transplant operation.**

Replacement Heart (IRH) was developed by ABIOMED in conjunction with the Texas Heart Institute. Additional work done at the University of Louisville with the AbioCor IRH demonstrated consistent survival in a bovine model and complimented the preclinical work being done at the Texas Heart Institute under the direction of O.H. Frazier.[10,14]

Approval for a multicenter trial of the use of the AbioCor IRH was granted by the FDA in early 2001. On July 2, 2001, the device was implanted for the first time in Robert Tools, a decorated war veteran (Figure 93-1). This marked the first time that a totally implantable system had been used in a human to provide complete support of the circulation.

THE ABIOCOR IMPLANTABLE REPLACEMENT HEART

Device Description

The AbioCor IRH system is the first artificial heart system that does not require percutaneous lines or the need for percutaneous access.[11] This electrohydraulic system consists of both external and internal components. The four internal components are the thoracic unit, battery, controller, and transcutaneous energy transfer (TET) coil (Figure 93-2). The AbioCor thoracic unit (Figure 93-3) is placed in the chest in an orthotopic position after excision of the native ventricles. It consists of an energy converter and two pumping chambers that function as the left and right ventricles. The energy converter is situated between the chambers and contains a high-efficiency miniature centrifugal pump that operates unidirectionally to pressurize a low-viscosity hydraulic fluid. A two-position switching valve in the energy converter is used to alternate the direction of hydraulic flow between the left and right pumping chambers that results in alternate left and right systole. The rate of the switching valve determines the beat rate of the device and can be varied between 75 and 150 beats/min, resulting in a flow up to 8 liters/min. An atrial balance chamber is present and allows for adjustment of right-sided stroke volume to maintain right and left balance.[12,13] Essentially, a portion of hydraulic fluid is shunted into the balance chamber rather than to the right hydraulic pumping chamber. This decreases the volume ejected by the right side of the heart to compensate for bronchial blood flow. All blood-contacting surfaces of the AbioCor thoracic unit, including the trileaflet valves (24 mm internal diameter), are polyetherurethane (Angioflex), resulting in a smooth, continuous blood-contacting surface from the inflow cuffs to the outflow grafts.

The internal battery is lithium ion–based and is able to power the thoracic unit for brief (up to 20 minutes) periods. The internal controller drives the energy converter in the thoracic unit, monitors the implanted components, and transmits device performance data to a bedside console via radiofrequency (RF) telemetry. These RF transmissions convey information, including continuous real-time telemetry of hydraulic pressure waveforms, system-operating parameters, battery status, component temperature, and alarm information. The internal TET coil receives high-frequency power that is transmitted across the skin from the external TET coil. The internal TET system electronics converts this oscillating current to a direct current that is used to power the thoracic unit and recharge the internal battery.

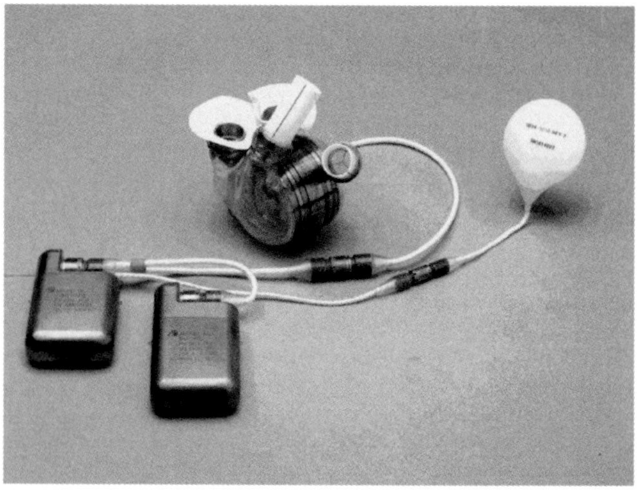

Figure 93–2 **The four internal components of the AbioCor Implantable Replacement Heart.** The AbioCor thoracic unit, the internal transcutaneous energy transfer (TET) coil, the internal battery, and the internal controller.

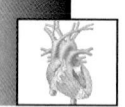

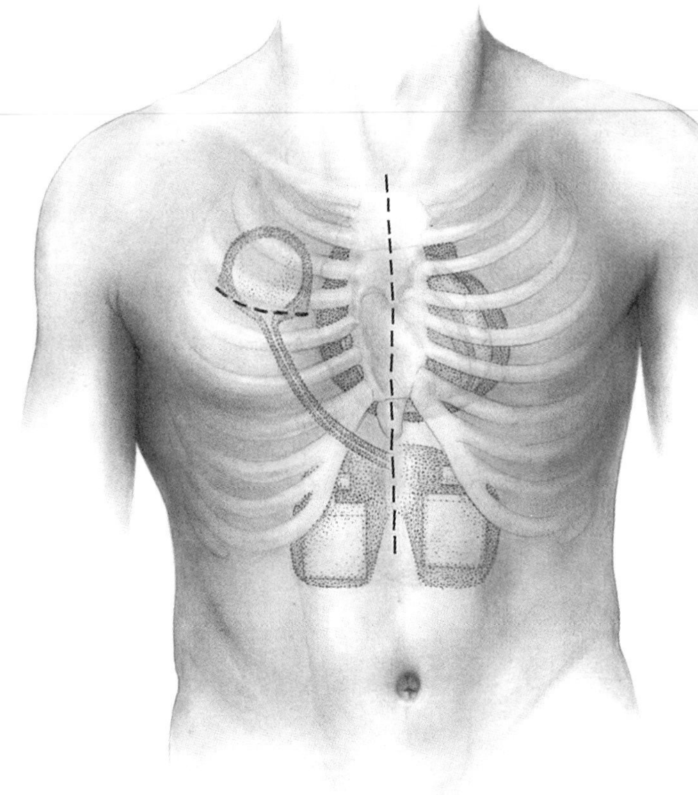

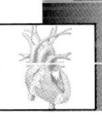

Figure 93–3 Diagrammatic presentation of the final position of internal components of the AbioCor device in the human body.

The four external components consist of an external TET coil, batteries, a TET module, and a bedside console. The external TET coil transfers energy across the skin to the internal TET coil. The external TET coil can be connected to either the bedside console or a portable TET module. When the patient is ambulatory, the external TET coil is connected to the portable TET module. The TET module delivers energy to the TET coil from external batteries and contains basic alarm systems that are activated if there is misalignment of the TET coils, low external battery voltage, or a general alarm indicating a potential problem with the system that is determined by reestablishing RF communication with the bedside console. The bedside console is used during implantation, during recovery, and when the patient is in his or her primary residence. The bedside console provides a display screen for control and monitoring of the implanted system via RF communication. The console can be remotely monitored when connected to a telephone jack via a laptop computer. The external batteries are lithium ion–based and are able to provide up to 1 hour of support per pound of battery. The external batteries can either be carried in a vest or a handbag, or attached to a nylon (Velcro) belt.

Operative Approach

The operative approach has been previously described.[9] At operation, an infraclavicular incision is made and the internal TET coil is placed anterior to the pectoral muscle fascia. A median sternotomy incision is then made, and the cable from the internal TET coil is passed to the lower part of the sternotomy incision. Figure 93-3 shows the location of the incisions and the position of the four internal components. The incision over the TET coil is then closed in layers. The TET coil is placed before heparinization to decrease the likelihood of a pocket wound hematoma. A sternal retractor is placed, and a pericardial cradle is created. Dissection for placement of the internal battery and controller is performed either in the preperitoneal space or deep to the rectus abdominus muscle. Standard bicaval cannulation is performed, cardiopulmonary bypass is initiated, and the aorta is cross-clamped. The right and left ventricles are excised just below the atrioventricular groove to allow for anastomosis of the atrial cuffs at the level of the annuli. The mitral and tricuspid valve leaflets are excised (Figure 93-4). The left atrial appendage is ligated, and the coronary sinus and patent foramen ovale (if present) are oversewn. The left atrial cuff of the device is trimmed to the appropriate diameter and sewn to the native left atrium at the level of the annulus using two layers of running 4-0 Prolene reinforced with felt strips. Leak testing is performed after the creation of each anastomosis to decrease the likelihood of suture line bleeding or air entrainment after placement of the device. Anastomosis of the right atrial cuff to the native right atrium is then performed in similar fashion, followed by leak testing (Figure 93-5). A cast model of the AbioCor thoracic unit is positioned in the chest to determine the appropriate length and orientation of the outflow grafts to the aorta and pulmonary artery. These outflow grafts are then sewn end-to-end to the great vessels with a running 4-0 Prolene suture. The aortic outflow graft is positioned anterior to the pulmonary artery graft. The AbioCor thoracic unit is then brought up to the operative field, and appropriate electrical connections are made (Figure 93-6).

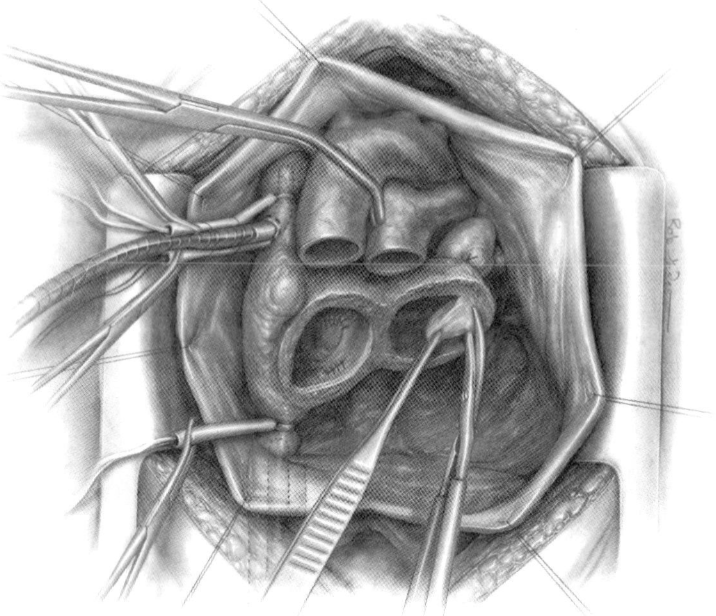

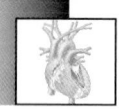

Figure 93–4 Cardiopulmonary bypass is initiated. The caval tapes are snared down. The aorta is cross-clamped. The ventricles are excised below the atrioventricular groove; mitral and tricuspid leaflets are excised. The left atrial appendage is ligated, and the coronary sinus is oversewn to prevent any venous bleeding from cut branches of draining veins.

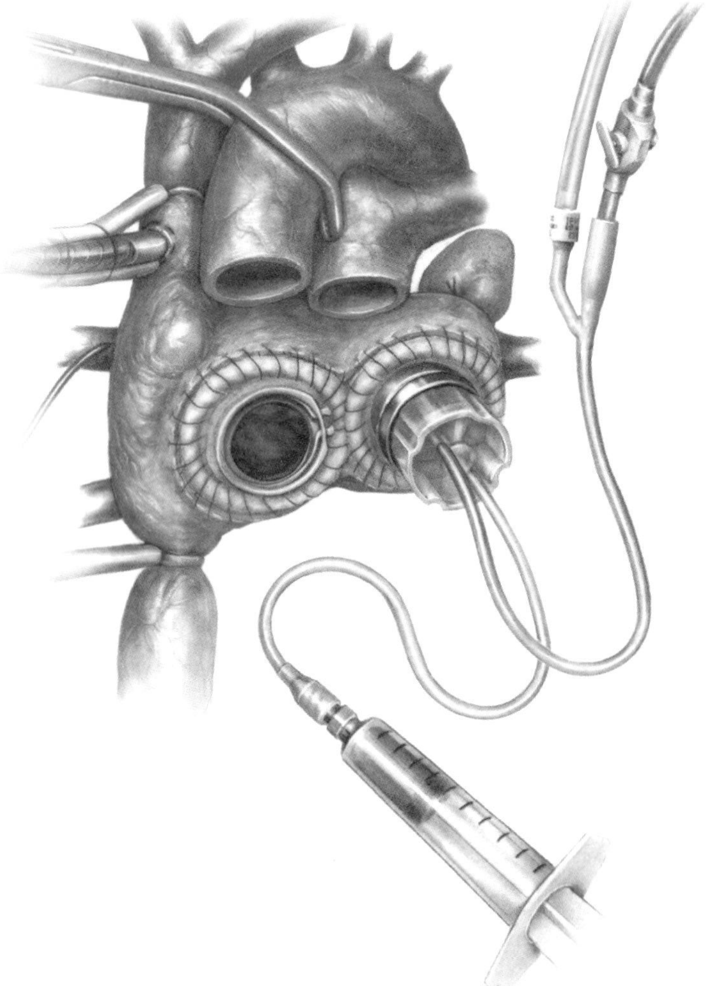

Figure 93–5 The atrial anastomosis is checked for leaks using an inflated Foley catheter to occlude the pulmonary veins while injecting saline into the left atrium. A similar procedure is then used to anastomose the right atrial cuff to the native right atrial remnant.

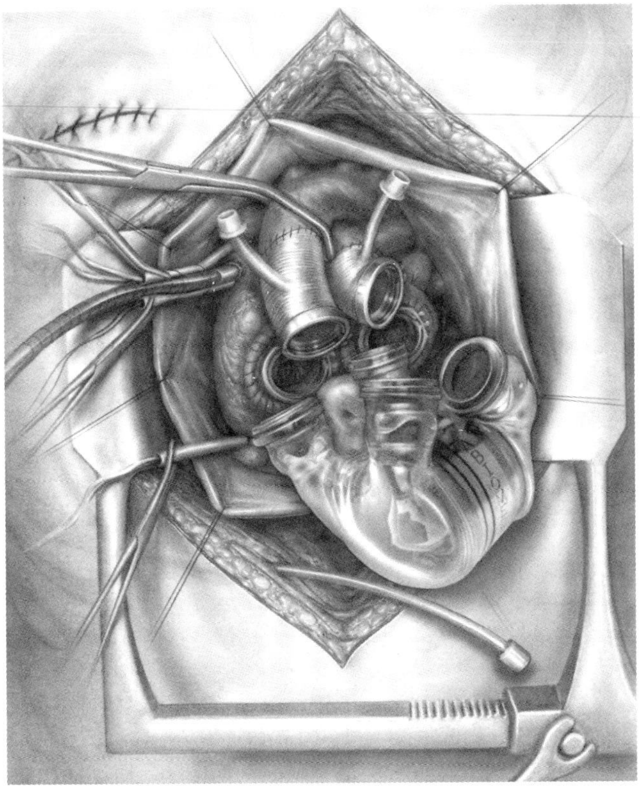

Figure 93–6 The AbioCor thoracic unit is brought up to the operative field.

The thoracic unit is placed in the pericardial space and attached to the left atrial cuff and outflow grafts via snap-lock connectors. The right ventricle of the thoracic unit is filled with saline, and the right atrial cuff is connected to the device. The caval tapes are released, and the device is completely de-aired by allowing blood and air to be ejected through the side ports arising from the outflow grafts. Once the right side of the heart has been de-aired, the side port of the pulmonary artery outflow graft is occluded. The left side of the heart is then de-aired through the side port on the aortic outflow graft. The device flow is increased up to 4–5 liters/min with the cross-clamp on and all the blood ejected through the side port of the left outflow graft and returned to the cardiopulmonary bypass circuit. Once the device is adequately de-aired, the cross-clamp is removed, the left side port is occluded, and the patient is weaned from cardiopulmonary bypass onto full device support (Figure 93-7). The left and right filling pressures are monitored and used to determine the beat rate and to adjust the balance chamber. Protamine is administered after demonstrating adequate hemodynamics. The sternal edges are approximated, and transesophageal echocardiography is performed to determine if there is impaired flow in the left pulmonary veins. Increased pulmonary vein flow velocity dictates the need to reposition the thoracic unit caudad and/or anterior. This is readily accomplished by placing sutures through the eyelets on the thoracic unit and around the left lower ribs. Proper hemostatis is ensured, followed by standard wound closure. A skilled anesthesia team that is familiar with the function of the device is essential.[16]

Clinical Trial

The clinical trial with the AbioCor IRH is designed as a destination therapy trial. Therefore patients selected for this initial clinical trial cannot be candidates for other types of operative therapies, including heart transplantation. As centers expand their criteria for acceptance into their transplant programs, this alone has significantly limited the number of potential candidates for destination therapy trials. Also, because of the nature of this clinical trial, it is felt that it would be appropriate to select patients with a high predicted mortality. A model (AbioScore) to predict 30-day survival in patients with end-stage heart failure was developed. It includes laboratory and clinical parameters such as age, serum sodium, serum creatinine, need for inotropes or intraaortic balloon pump, body mass index, left ventricular end-diastolic diameter, peak exercise oxygen consumption, presence of severe mitral regurgitation, and New York Heart Association (NYHA) class.

Patients considered as potential candidates for implantation of the AbioCor IRH must have a 30-day predicted mortality of greater than 70% based on this prognostic model or based on acute myocardial infarction (AMI) shock scores. Patients are excluded from the clinical trial if they have significant end-organ dysfunction that is not felt to be reversible, active infection, severe peripheral vascular disease, blood dyscrasia, or recent stroke or transient ischemic attack (TIA) as a result of atherosclerotic disease. All potential recipients undergo a complete psychosocial evaluation similar to that performed for potential transplant recipients. Great emphasis has been placed on selection of patients and their families who have a clear understanding of the clinical trial and will be able to endure a potentially long postoperative convalescence. Patients who meet all the appropriate criteria then undergo computed tomography of the chest. This is followed by AbioFit evaluation, which is a three-dimensional computerized image of the AbioCor thoracic unit superimposed on the imagery of the patient's mediastinal and chest wall structures. This computer simulation allows us to view the position of the AbioCor in the potential recipient's chest from every possible angle. This "virtual surgery" lets us determine if we can position the AbioCor thoracic unit in the chest without impinging on vital structures such as the left pulmonary veins and left lower lobe bronchus. Patients are excluded from the trial if the surgical team feels that this AbioFit evaluation suggests that the thoracic unit will not fit in the patient's chest.

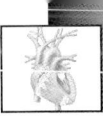

To date, 10 patients have been enrolled in the clinical trial at four centers. All implantable components have been well tolerated. There have been no patients with significant hemolysis or device-related infections. As anticipated in this most ill cohort of patients, there have been multiple morbidities. Three of the first five recipients had significant strokes. These patients were found at autopsy to have thrombus on the struts attached to the atrial cuffs that were placed to prevent potential inflow occlusion of the device by the mobile lateral walls of the left or right atrium. The blood pumps themselves were free of thrombus, as were the valves. As a result of this finding at autopsy, the atrial struts were removed from the atrial cuffs. Removal of the atrial struts does raise concern about the possibility of inflow obstruction of the device by the native atrial tissue. This has been addressed by redesigning the atrial cuffs to make them more conical and by the use of external atrial stenting, which is achieved by gluing a Teflon patch to the mobile part of the native atrial wall with Cryo Glue. This new design was initially demonstrated in the bovine model to prevent mobility of the atrial walls and has been successfully performed in the last four human recipients.

There have been many notable milestones in the initial phase of the clinical trial, including successful discharge of a patient to home for 11 months' time (Figure 93-8). Patient and family acceptance also has been high, primarily because of the quiet nature of the device and the absence of percutaneous lines. As noted earlier, the major adverse finding has been the development of thromboembolic events that appear to be related to thrombus formation on the atrial struts attached to the left atrial cuffs. As noted, these struts were removed after this discovery. The next series of patients will determine if removal of the atrial struts results in an acceptable level of thromboembolic events.

CARDIOWEST TOTAL ARTIFICIAL HEART

Device Description

The Jarvik-7 total artificial heart was originally developed in Dr. Willem Kolff's laboratory at the University of Utah. As noted earlier, in 1982, the initial clinical use of this device was as a destination therapy device. The Jarvik-7 total artificial heart changed ownership and became known as the CardioWest Total Artificial Heart. Further clinical trials were approved in 1993 after two modifications of the device. The CardioWest Total Artificial Heart is a pneumatic biventricular pulsatile pump that is implanted in the orthotopic position.[7] The two chambers are separate and after placement are simply attached to each other with a Velcro patch (Figure 93-9). After excision of the native ventricles, an atrial cuff that contains a quick connect is anastomosed to the native atrium at the level of the atrioventricular valve annulus. A 27-mm Medtronic-Hall inflow valve is present, leading to a spherical polyurethane chamber. One half of the chamber lining is immobile, whereas the other half is a four-layered diaphragm. The volume of the ventricular chamber is 72 ml, and the two ventricles and adjacent intraventricular space displace a total of 1500 ml. A steel reinforced pneumatic drive line exits from the ventricle. Pulses of air pressure from the console delivered via the drive line push the diaphragm, and thus the blood, through a 25-mm Medtronic-Hall valve into an outflow graft anastomosed to a great vessel. A negative pressure of 10–15 cm of water can be added to the device in diastole to improve ventricular filling at lower venous pressures. Cardiac outputs generally run in the range of 6–8 liters per minute.

Appropriate fitting criteria guidelines for placement for of the CardioWest Total Artificial Heart have been developed. Acceptable candidates must have a body surface area greater than or equal to 1.7 m^2, a cardiothoracic ratio of greater than 0.5, and a left ventricular diastolic dimension of greater than 66 mm. Additionally, potential recipients undergo a computed tomography of the chest and must be shown to have a combined ventricular volume of greater than 1500 ml and a distance from the sternum to the tenth thoracic vertebral body greater than 10 cm. The group at the University of Arizona considers the size of the device to be its major limitation and strictly follows the preceding size guidelines.

The use of transesophageal echocardiography has been of great value in ensuring a perfect position of the CardioWest Total Artificial Heart during chest closure. On occasion, right ventriculopexy to the anterior chest wall using umbilical tape or heavy suture attached to the body of the right ventricle is needed to allow for positioning of the device in the chest without compression of the pulmonary veins or the inferior vena cava.

Clinical Trials

Clinical results with the CardioWest Total Artificial Heart have markedly improved, likely as a result of better patient selection and better control of the coagulation system. Results of the international experience with the CardioWest Total Artificial Heart revealed that 70% of patients implanted survived to transplantation, with 91% of these transplanted patients being discharged to home.[2] More recently, Copeland compared the outcomes with the CardioWest device to the results obtained in his center with the Novacor Left Ventricular System and the Thoratec Ventricular System. Survival to transplantation was 75% for the CardioWest device, 87% for the Novacor device, and 38% for the Thoratec device.[14] A significant number of deaths in the left ventricular assist device (LVAD) groups were related to right ventricular failure, which is obviously eliminated by the use of a total artificial heart. With current anticoagulation management techniques, including the use of routine tests in addition to thromboelastography, the stroke rate with the CardioWest Total Artificial Heart has been dramatically decreased. The linearized stroke rates (events per patient/month) were 0.03 for the CardioWest device, 0.28 for the Novacor device, and 0.08 for the Thoratec device. The infection rate seen with the CardioWest device is similar to that seen with current-generation LVADs.

DEVICES UNDER DEVELOPMENT

In 2000, ABIOMED, Inc. purchased the Penn State electric total artificial heart. A hybrid design has been in development by ABIOMED combining the strengths of the AbioCor device with the strengths of the Penn State electric total artificial heart. This next-generation device is referred to as the AbioHeart. One major advantage of this new device is that it is significantly smaller (30% decrease in size) than current-generation devices. In addition, the compliance chamber has been removed from the thoracic unit, which also expedites fit in the human thorax.

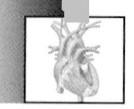

Additional advantages of the AbioHeart are likely to be improved membrane durability, decreased membrane trauma, and improved beat rate control. The inflow valves of the AbioHeart contain mechanical bileaflet valves, whereas the outflow valves consist of trileaflet valves that are fabricated from polyurethane. Initial preclinical trials with the device have been conducted at the University of Louisville. The first animal to receive this device survived for the proposed 30-day study period. There was excellent device func-

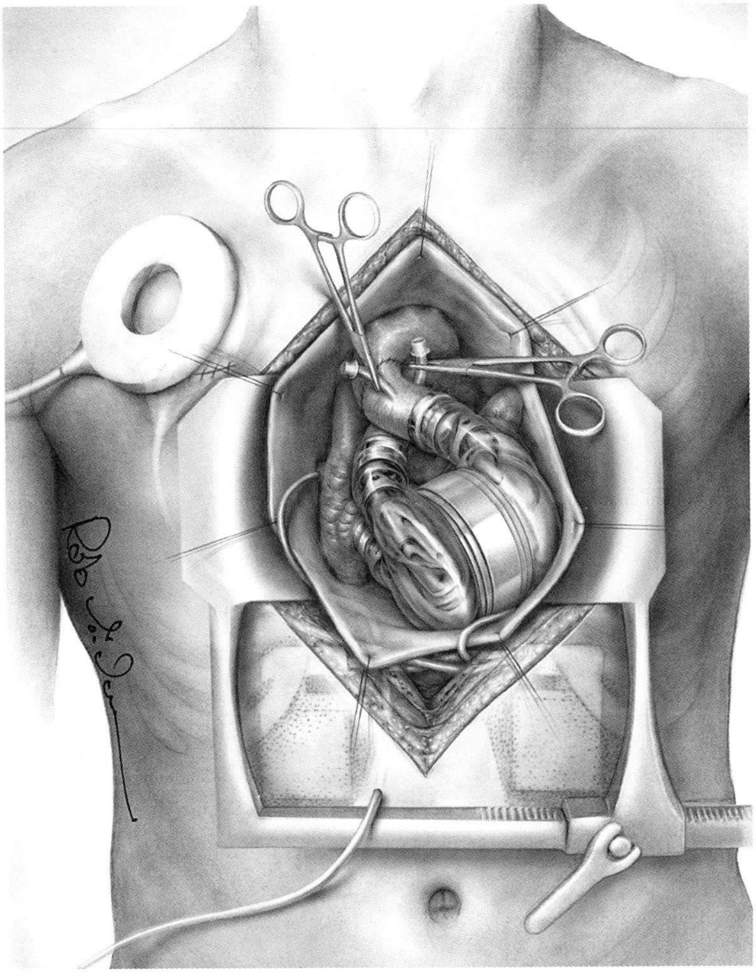

Figure 93–7 **The AbioCor Implantable Replacement Heart in its final position after complete deairing and occlusion of the side ports of the outflow grafts.**

tion without evidence of infection or hemolysis. The animal did recover to a full functional level of activity, including regular exercise on a treadmill. The second animal implanted with the device also demonstrated excellent device function. The animal was euthanized on the fourteenth postoperative day as a result of respiratory distress and was found to have a large hemothorax.

The MagScrew Total Artificial Heart has been a joint development between the Cleveland Clinic and Foster Miller Technologies. This device contains a MagScrew actuator, which is placed between alternating ejecting and passively filling ventricles.[18] The right and left pusher plates are guided in the actuator set but are not fixed to it. Therefore when the actuator drives the pusher plate of the front ventricle to eject, the other ventricle's motion is free of the actuator, so passive filling can occur in response to atrial filling pressures. Sophisticated control mechanisms that account for left-sided shunt flow and differences in vascular resistance between the pulmonary and systemic circulation have been developed. The ultimate configuration of the MagScrew Total Artificial Heart system is for a completely implantable system using TET, an internal battery, and control units.

Initial preclinical trials have been conducted at the Cleveland Clinic. The device was able to maintain physiological pressures with normal end-organ function. There was no evidence of hemolysis. The right and left atrial pres-

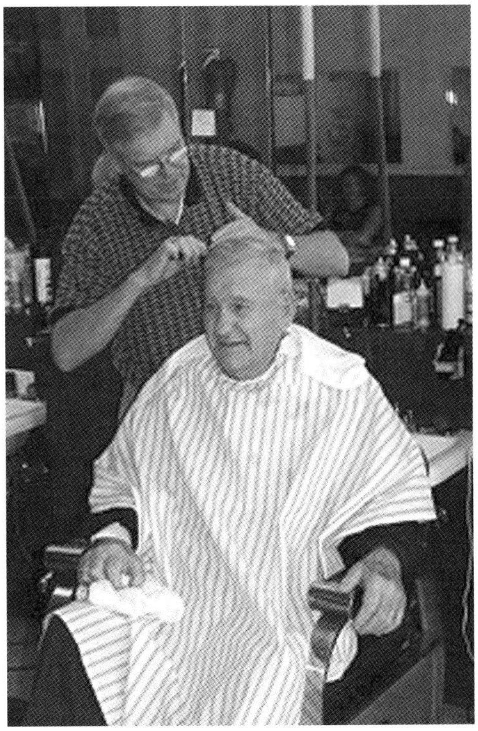

Figure 93–8 **Mr. Tom Christenson receiving a haircut at barber shop in Central City, KY, after discharge to home.**

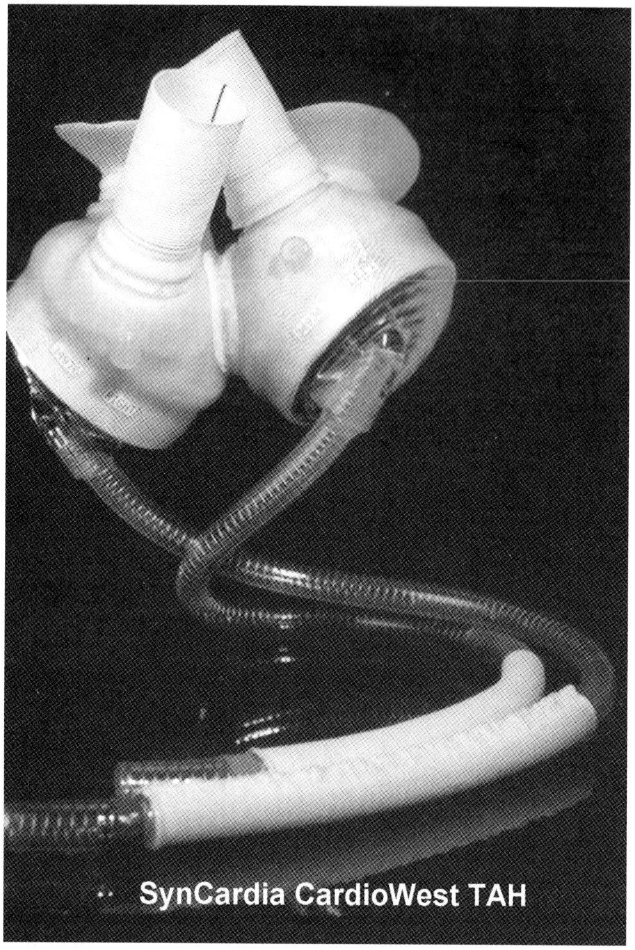

Figure 93-9 **CardioWest Total Artificial Heart showing the two separate chambers, outflow grafts, atrial cuffs, and drive lines.**

sures were well balanced, with the device demonstrating adequate preload sensitivity to changes in blood volume.

SUMMARY

The initial implant of a pneumatic total artificial heart in 1982 remains a landmark case. As the clinical trial progressed, it became clear that this particular device was not ready to be used as destination therapy, primarily because of the percutaneous drive lines and the need for a large console, which significantly limited the patient's mobility and therefore quality of life. The success of this clinical trial remains a matter of debate. However, it did clearly demonstrate that patients could have their entire circulation supported by an artificial device for prolonged periods. Indeed, the most recent experience with this device, now named the CardioWest Total Artificial Heart, has demonstrated that the major problems with the device, such as infection and stroke, were able to be addressed, with marked and dramatic improvement in patient outcomes in the bridge-to-transplant population. This clinical trial also highlighted the need for an electrically powered total artificial heart that could be totally implantable and allow for excellent patient mobility and transfer to home. Twenty years after Dr. Barney Clark received the first Jarvik-7 device, the AbioCor IRH was implanted in Robert Tools at the University of Louisville. This was the first clinical use of a totally implantable artificial heart. The initial clinical trial with this device is ongoing. Highlights of the trial include excellent device durability and discharge of a patient to home for 9 months' duration. The major downside of the clinical trial has been the high incidence of strokes, which has resulted in a design modification to the atrial cuffs. The next group of recipients of this device will help determine if these changes have a significant positive impact on decreasing the risk of stroke.

Preclinical trials with a number of other total artificial heart systems, including the AbioHeart and the MagScrew Total Artificial Heart, are underway with exciting preliminary data. We have entered an exciting era where experience with new-generation devices suggests that a clinically acceptable artificial heart as a permanent device is in the foreseeable future.

REFERENCES

1. Akutsu T, Kolff WJ: Permanent substitutes for valves and hearts. ASAIO Trans 4:230, 1958.
2. Arabia FA, Copeland JG, Smith RG, et al: International experience with the CardioWest total artificial heart as a bridge to heart transplantation. Eur J Cardiothorac Surg 11:S5–S10, 1997.
3. Barnette M: The Bill Schroeder Story, 1st ed., New York: Morrow, 1987.
4. Cooley DA: Staged cardiac transplantation: Report of three cases. Heart Trans 1:145, 1982.
5. Cooley DA, Liotta D, Hallman GL, et al: Orthotropic cardiac prosthesis for two-staged cardiac replacement. Am J Cardiol 24:723, 1969.
6. Copeland JG, Arabia FA, Smith RG, et al: Arizona experience with CardioWest Total Artificial Heart bridge to transplantation. Ann Thorac Surg 68:756–760, 1999.
7. Copeland J, Arabia F, Smith R, et al: Cardiac assist devices. In Goldstein DJ, Oz MC, editors: Intracorporeal Support: The CardioWest Total Artificial Heart, pp. 341–355, 2000.
8. Demikhov VP: Medquiz. In Haigh B, editor: Experimental Transplantation of Vital Organs, Moscow translation, pp. 212–213, 1960.
9. Dowling RD, Etoch SW, Gray LA Jr: Operative techniques for implantation of the AbioCor Total Artificial Heart. Oper Tech Thorac Cardiovasc Surg 7:139–151, 2002.
10. Dowling RD, Etoch SW, Stevens KA, et al: Current status of the AbioCor Implantable Replacement Heart. Ann Thorac Surg 71:S147–S149, 2001.
11. Dowling RD, Gray LA Jr, Etoch SW, et al: Initial experience with the AbioCor Implantable Replacement Heart system. JTCVS 2003 (in press).
12. Kung RT, Ochs BD, Singh PI: A unique left-right flow balance compensation scheme for an implantable total artificial heart. ASAIO J 35:468–470, 1989.
13. Kung RT, Yu LS, Ochs B, et al: An atrial hydraulic shunt in a total artificial heart. A balance mechanism for the bronchial shunt. ASAIO J 39:M213–M217, 1993.

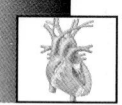

14. Parnis S, Yu LS, Ochs BD, et al: Chronic in vivo evaluation of an electrohydraulic total artificial heart. ASAIO J 40:M489–M493, 1994.
15. Pierce WS: The artificial heart—1986: Partial fulfillment of a promise. Trans Am Soc Artif Intern Organs 32:5, 1986.
16. Theilmeier KA, Pank JR, Dowling RD, et al: Anesthetic and perioperative considerations in patients undergoing placement of totally implantable replacement hearts. Semin Cardiothorac Vasc Anesth 5:335–344, 2001.
17. Statement on Jarvik Artificial Heart. Rockville, Md: FDA Press Office, January 11, 1990.
18. Weber S, Doi K, Massiello AL, et al: In vitro controllability of the MagScrew Total Artificial Heart. ASAIO J 48:606–611, 2002.

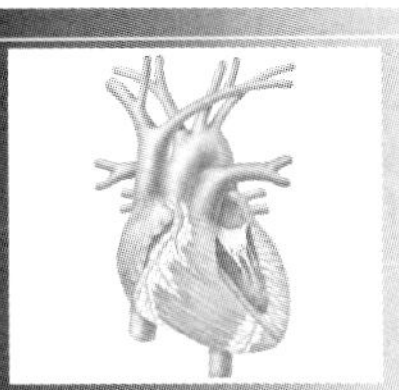

CHAPTER 94

Heart Transplantation

Leora B. Balsam and Robert C. Robbins

INTRODUCTION

The last 30 years have seen the evolution of heart transplantation from an experimental procedure to a mainstream therapeutic option for patients with end-stage heart failure. To date, over 60,000 heart transplants have been performed worldwide at more than 200 heart transplant centers.[40] Advances in surgical technique, immunosuppression, and infection prophylaxis have led to improved short-term and long-term results. The incidence of heart failure has been rising in the United States, and it is estimated that over 25,000 patients annually could benefit from cardiac transplantation.[22] Despite a growing need for this therapy, the number of transplant procedures performed worldwide remains stable, with donor organ supply being the primary limiting factor. Therefore in recent years, attempts have been made to expand the donor pool, as well as to develop alternative therapies, including improved medical treatment and mechanical assist devices.

This chapter reviews the current practice of heart transplantation. Emphasis is placed on selection and management of recipients, donor evaluation, operative technique, and postoperative management.

HISTORICAL BACKGROUND

Long before the success of clinical heart transplantation, experimental heart transplantation flourished in the laboratory. The earliest reports described heterotopic heart transplantation in animals, in which a second heart was anastomosed to vessels in the neck or abdomen. In 1905 Carrel and Guthrie[18] reported their findings that heterotopically transplanted hearts resume spontaneous contraction for several hours. The next several decades saw improved understanding of the physiology of heterotopically transplanted hearts, yet it was not until the late 1940s that transplantation of the heart into the thorax was reported. The pioneering work of Demikhov[27] included both heterotopic and orthotopic heart transplantation in the thorax. Amazingly, this work was performed before the advent of cardiopulmonary bypass. In the 1950s the use of hypothermia and mechanical pump oxygenators made orthotopic heart transplantation a potential reality. The technique of experimental orthotopic heart transplantation was refined by Lower and Shumway[53] at Stanford in the 1960s, and this team reported survival of up to 3 weeks in dogs after the procedure.[51] As advances were made in understanding the principles of tissue rejection, appropriate immunosuppressive regimens emerged. The Stanford group demonstrated long-term allograft survival in dogs when a combination of azathioprine and corticosteroids was administered after transplantation.[52]

In 1964 Hardy and associates[37] performed the first human heart transplant using a chimpanzee donor heart. The first human-to-human heart transplant was performed by Barnard in 1967 in Cape Town, South Africa.[9] The patient, a 57-year-old man with ischemic heart disease, died on the eighteenth postoperative day. Soon thereafter, Shumway and the Stanford group performed the first successful cardiac transplant in the United States.[79] Additional attempts at cardiac transplantation were made by leading cardiothoracic surgeons around the world without long-term success. Enthusiasm for the procedure waned as the problems of acute rejection and infection became more apparent, and only a handful of centers worldwide continued with programs of heart transplantation.

Over the next decade, the outcomes in transplantation improved as patient selection criteria were refined and postoperative care improved. Percutaneous endomyocardial biopsy, introduced by Caves and associates in 1973,[19] allowed for early diagnosis and treatment of acute rejection. Advances in immunosuppression, including the use of antithymocyte globulin, offered prophylaxis and treatment for acute rejection.[36] The introduction of cyclosporine in 1980 was particularly pivotal in the advancement of heart transplantation, and early studies in the United Kingdom by Calne and associates[17] and in the United States by the Stanford group demonstrated its efficacy.[63] Ultimately, combined immunosuppression regimens consisting of cyclosporine, azathioprine, and prednisone led to long-term patient survival.

This early success was followed by a dramatic increase in the number of cardiac transplant centers worldwide. The number of transplant procedures performed yearly grew rapidly in the late 1980s and reached its current plateau by the early 1990s.[40] Ongoing changes in surgical technique, organ preservation, and immunosuppression continue to yield better outcomes in the modern era of heart transplantation.

INDICATIONS AND EVALUATION FOR HEART TRANSPLANTATION

Recipient Selection

Over the years, selection criteria have emerged to identify patients who will benefit most from heart transplantation. The early reports of long-term survival after transplantation validated the effectiveness of transplantation as a treatment for end-stage heart failure, and since that time, the demand for transplantation has grown substantially. In the United States the heart transplant waiting list comprises over 4000 potential recipients, and the median waiting time to transplantation is 346 days.[85] The average waiting list mortality is 17% per year, and the mortality for patients in the highest medical urgency category is 45%.[90] Several trends in recipient selection have been notable, including a gradual relaxation of certain selection criteria, resulting in a larger pool of transplant candidates. Unfortunately, this increase in the number of potential recipients has not been matched by an increase in the donor organ supply. Despite liberalization of donor selection criteria and use of more marginal donor organs, the yearly donor organ pool remains stable at 2500 in the United States[85] and 3500 worldwide.[40] This disparity between the growing demand for organs and a limited donor pool has led to careful reevaluation of recipient selection criteria, as well as exploration of alternative medical and surgical therapies for heart failure. It is clear that organs must be allocated in the most rational and judicious manner possible.

Determining which patients with heart failure should be listed for transplantation involves careful review of the clinical history and a panel of laboratory and supplementary tests (Box 94-1). This process should be as objective as possible and is typically carried out by a team of physicians and nurses. Common indications include New York Heart Association (NYHA) class III or IV heart failure refractory

Box 94–1. Evaluation of Potential Cardiac Transplant Recipients.

Phase I: Assessment of Candidacy

General information

History and physical examination
CBC with differential and platelet count
Blood chemistry panel
Liver function tests
Renal function panel
Prothrombin and activated partial thromboplastin time
Urinalysis
Chest X-ray
Pulmonary function test

Assessment of cardiac function

Electrocardiography
Echocardiography
Radionuclide ventriculography[a]
Right-heart catheterization[a]
Left-heart catheterization[a]
Endomyocardial biopsy[a]
Peak exercise oxygen consumption (VO_2) testing

Screening tests

Stool guaiac × 3[a]
Mammography[a]
PSA screening[a]
Papanicolaou smear[a]
Bone densitometry[a]
Carotid duplex[a]

Infectious disease screening

HBsAg
HBV and HCV antibody
HIV serology
HTLV1 and HTLV2 serology
CMV IgM and IgG titers
Toxoplasma serology
EBV serology
RPR
PPD testing

Phase 2: Pretransplant Data

Blood type and antibody screening
HLA-DR typing
PRA screening
12-hour urine collection for creatinine clearance and total protein

[a]Performed if indicated by history, age, or physical examination.
CBC, Complete blood cell count; HBsAg, hepatitis B surface antigen; HTLV, human T-cell leukemia/lymphoma virus; Ig, immunoglobulin; EBV, Epstein-Barr virus; *RPR*, rapid plasma reagin; PPD, purified protein derivative.

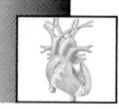

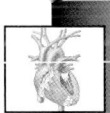

to maximal medical therapy, debilitating ischemia not amenable to interventional or surgical revascularization, and recurrent, symptomatic ventricular arrhythmias refractory to medical, implantable cardioverter defibrillator (ICD) and surgical treatment.[29] Patients with severe left ventricular dysfunction alone who remain symptom-free or are adequately managed with medical therapy should not be considered for transplantation.

For ambulatory patients, important techniques of risk-stratification have been developed to identify patients at low, moderate, or high risk of mortality while awaiting transplantation. Peak exercise oxygen consumption, or VO_2, is a measure that correlates well with waiting list mortality.[55] Patients with a peak VO_2 less than 14 ml/kg/min or less than 55% of the predicted peak VO_2 after reaching anaerobic threshold have moderate to high mortality risks and are likely to benefit from transplantation. Patients who achieve a peak VO_2 greater than 14 ml/kg/min have low mortality risks and will not benefit from transplantation. For all listed transplant candidates, peak VO_2 testing should be repeated at regular intervals and used to assess disease progression or improvement.[59] Patients whose VO_2 rises above 14 ml/kg/min should be removed from the active waiting list.

Aaronson and colleagues[2] at Columbia University have derived the Heart Failure Survival Score (HFSS) Index to risk-stratify ambulatory patients awaiting heart transplantation. This includes a noninvasive model, composed of seven parameters (diagnosis of ischemic cardiomyopathy, resting heart rate, left ventricular ejection fraction, mean blood pressure, peak VO_2, serum sodium, and presence of intraventricular conduction delay) and an invasive model, composed of eight parameters (diagnosis of ischemic cardiomyopathy, resting heart rate, left ventricular ejection fraction, mean blood pressure, peak VO_2, serum sodium, presence of intraventricular conduction delay, and mean pulmonary capillary wedge pressure). Both models can be used to identify a patient's pretransplant mortality risk. Deng et al[28] prospectively used the HFSS to assess the survival benefit associated with cardiac transplantation in all 889 adult patients listed for their first heart transplant in Germany in 1997. Using the HFSS, 12% were stratified into a high-risk group, 41% into a medium-risk group, and 47% into a low-risk group. The investigators found that only the high-risk group had reduced mortality risk at 1 year with transplantation. Limitations of this study include the short follow-up period and failure to assess alternate endpoints, including changes in quality of life and societal costs of treatment. Analysis of these endpoints and longer follow-up provide important information and may lead to modification of current recipient selection criteria.

Recent advances in medical therapy for heart failure have resulted in improved patient survival. In 2001 the COPERNICUS (Carvedilol Prospective Randomized Cumulative Survival) trial found that treatment of patients with severe heart failure with carvedilol reduced 1-year mortality to 11% compared with a placebo mortality of 19%.[64] Although no randomized trials of heart transplantation versus medical therapy have been performed, it is clear that in some cases, medical therapy yields an as good or better short-term outcome than transplantation. However, because the greatest mortality risk associated with transplantation occurs in the first year, long-term follow up is needed to compare late survival in medically treated cohorts with that in transplanted cohorts.

The most common diagnoses leading to heart transplantation in adults are idiopathic dilated cardiomyopathy and ischemic cardiomyopathy (Table 94-1). Approximately 90% of heart transplant patients carry these diagnoses. Of patients undergoing transplantation, 4% have valvular disease, 2% have congenital anomalies, and 2% undergo retransplantation. Survival after transplantation is related to underlying diagnosis. The 2002 Registry of the International Society for Heart and Lung Transplantation (ISHLT) lists diagnoses of congenital heart disease, ischemic cardiomyopathy, and other (diagnoses other than congenital, dilated cardiomyopathy or ischemic cardiomyopathy) as risk factors for 1-year mortality after heart transplantation. In addition, the diagnosis of ischemic cardiomyopathy is associated with an increased 5-year mortality.[40]

In the United Kingdom Aziz et al[6] performed a retrospective study of 220 heart transplant recipients and compared long-term survival of patients with underlying diagnoses of ischemic heart disease and dilated cardiomyopathy. At 5 years, survival was 96% in the dilated cardiomyopathy cohort and 47% in the ischemic heart disease cohort. At 10 years, survival was 92% in the dilated cardiomyopathy cohort and only 29% in the ischemic heart disease cohort. This provocative study suggests that the benefit of transplantation may be greater in patients with dilated cardiomyopathy. However, before changes are made in recipient selection criteria and organ allocation schemes, larger multicenter studies are needed.

Cardiac retransplantation is rare, with only 40–60 such procedures performed each year. It remains controversial, given the limited supply of donor organs. The most common indication is cardiac failure secondary to cardiac allograft

Table 94-1

Underlying Diagnoses of Adult Heart Transplant Recipients

Diagnosis	*Percentage of recipients (%)*
Ischemic cardiomyopathy	45
Dilated cardiomyopathy	45
Valvular disease	4
Congenital disease	2
Retransplantation	2
Miscellaneous	2

Data from Hertz MI, Taylor DO, Trulock EP, et al: The Registry of the International Society for Heart and Lung Transplantation: Nineteenth official report—2002. J Heart Lung Transplant 21:950, 2002.

vasculopathy (CAV). Survival outcomes are considerably worse than in primary transplantation, with a 1-year survival rate of 65%, a 2-year survival rate of 59%, and a 3-year survival rate of 55%. Srivastava et al[78] analyzed data from 514 retransplanted patients in the United Network for Organ Sharing (UNOS)/ISHLT database and found that survival was worst if the intertransplant interval was less than 6 months. In patients with an intertransplant interval longer than 2 years, 1-year survival was similar to primary transplantation. Therefore in carefully selected patients, there may be a role for retransplantation.

Absolute and relative contraindications to cardiac transplantation are listed in Box 94-2. Pulmonary hypertension, with a pulmonary vascular resistance greater than 3–4 Wood units despite maximal vasodilator therapy, is an absolute contraindication. In such cases, a newly transplanted heart is likely to suffer from acute right heart failure and the mortality risk to the patient is high. These patients may be candidates for combined heart and lung transplantation. Irreversible renal or hepatic dysfunction also is an absolute contraindication. In rare cases, multiorgan transplants have been performed, including combined heart and kidney transplants and combined heart and liver transplants. Active malignancy (excluding certain skin cancers) is an absolute contraindication. All potential recipients should undergo cancer screening with stool guaiac and chest X-ray. In addition, men should undergo prostate-specific antigen (PSA) screening and women should have mammography and a Papanicolaou (Pap) smear performed. Concomitant diseases, such as severe peripheral vascular disease or diabetes mellitus with secondary organ damage, are contraindications. In addition, certain primary diseases of the heart, such as amyloidosis, sarcoidosis, and giant cell myocarditis, may be contraindications because these diseases can recur in the transplanted heart. Relative contraindications to transplantation include age >65 years, obesity (>140% ideal body weight), osteoporosis, a history of substance abuse, a history of psychiatric disorder, a history of medical noncompliance, and lack of social support.[21,42]

Box 94–2. Recipient Contraindications to Heart Transplantation.

Absolute Contraindications

- Pulmonary hypertension (PVR >3–4 Wood units despite maximal therapy)
- Significant irreversible renal dysfunction (e.g., creatinine clearance <50 mg/ml/min)
- Significant irreversible hepatic dysfunction (e.g., bilirubin >3.0 mg/dl)
- Active malignancy
- Active infection
- Diabetes mellitus with secondary organ damage

Relative Contraindications

- Age >65
- Obesity
- Osteoporosis
- Active peptic ulcer disease
- Substance abuse
- Psychiatric disorder
- Noncompliance with medical care

Over time, the recipient age limit for heart transplantation has been increased. In its 2002 report, the ISHLT reported an increase in the proportion of recipients in the 50 to 64-year and the >65-year age ranges, and a concomitant decrease in the proportion of recipients in the 35 to 49-year age group. They identified age over 65 as a risk factor for increased 1- and 5-year mortality after transplantation.[40] However, single-center reports of good outcomes have been reported in carefully selected recipients up to age 75. Most centers attempt to risk-match recipients with appropriate donor organs, and knowledge of recipient age may influence this process. At the University of California, Los Angeles, an "alternative list" has been established for potential recipients over the age of 65, and donor organs that would not otherwise be used may be offered to these patients.[50]

In the end, the decision to list a patient for transplantation requires consideration of a multitude of medical, psychological, and social factors. Because transplantation requires a lifelong commitment on the part of both the patient and the transplant team, it is essential that the risks and benefits be carefully reviewed. Patients should be well apprised of these risks and must be willing to comply with lifelong immunosuppression, regular medical follow-up, and surveillance procedures.

Additional Tests Required for Listing

ABO blood typing is performed on all prospective recipients. In addition, prospective recipients should undergo screening for the presence of anti–human leukocyte antigen (HLA) antibodies. This is done by mixing the patient's sera with a panel of lymphocytes from random donors. A panel-reactive antibody (PRA) titer can be derived. In most centers a PRA greater than 10% prompts direct testing of a prospective recipient's sera against a prospective donor's lymphocytes.[14] This is referred to as a "cross-match." Most programs do follow-up PRA measurements every 4–6 months and after any sensitizing events (e.g., blood transfusion). Many programs offer therapy for sensitized patients, although the PRA threshold for treatment varies widely. Reported treatments include plasmapheresis, intravenous immunoglobulin, and immunosuppressive drugs such as cyclophosphamide and mycophenolate mofetil.[26,43,66,68,74] These may be used in combination, and various regimens have been described, including preoperative and intraoperative treatment.

HLA typing of the prospective recipient may be done before transplantation. However, prospective matching of recipient and donor HLA antigens is not routinely performed, because only a short period of donor heart ischemia (typically less than 6 hours) is tolerated.

RECIPIENT MANAGEMENT AFTER LISTING

Optimal medical management must be continued while the candidate awaits transplantation. The patient should be seen regularly by a cardiologist at the transplant center, usually every 3–4 months, and should be enrolled in a cardiac rehabilitation program. By optimizing patients' nutritional and physical condition before transplantation, the cardiologist minimizes the chances of postoperative complications.

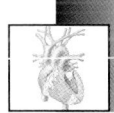

For patients with severe heart failure, oral medical therapy may be inadequate. In such cases patients may benefit from intravenous inotropes, including dobutamine, dopamine, and milrinone. Dobutamine, an β-1 adrenergic agonist, is most effective at doses less than 10 μg/kg/min. Dopamine, a sympathomimetic catecholamine, has both α- and β-agonist activity and should be used at doses less than 5 μg/kg/min; at higher doses, its arrhythmogenic and renal vasoconstrictive effects predominate. Milrinone, a phosphodiesterase inhibitor with inotropic and vasodilatory effects, is effective at doses of 0.5 μg/kg/min.

For heart failure refractory to all medical therapy, the use of mechanical assist devices may be necessary. Intraaortic balloon pump (IABP) counterpulsation, which reduces afterload and augments diastolic filling, may be beneficial in some cases. It is especially useful in patients with ischemic cardiomyopathy. These devices can be left in place for only a short period, usually several days, and are not effective if left ventricular ejection is severely compromised. There is a risk of infectious complications associated with IABP use, and 1-year mortality is increased in heart transplant recipients who have previously been supported with an IABP.[40] For patients with severe refractory ventricular failure, a left or right ventricular assist device (VAD) may be necessary. These devices divert blood from the ventricle and pump it back into the appropriate great vessel. The 2002 ISHLT Registry found a correlation between the use of a ventricular assist device and an increased 1-year mortality in heart transplant recipients.[40] The Cardiac Transplant Research Database (CTRD) group has reported that the relationship between ventricular assist device use and mortality depends on the length of time the device is left in place.[45] For patients who undergo transplantation within 30 days of device placement, the mortality is higher than for those who undergo transplantation after a longer period. It is likely that longer VAD placement allows for improved organ recovery and better patient rehabilitation, thereby resulting in a better outcome after transplantation.

With the development of improved mechanical assist devices, including fully implantable left ventricular assist devices (LVADs) and artificial hearts, it is likely that more patients with severe refractory heart failure will be bridged to transplantation with mechanical devices. The results of the REMATCH (Randomized Evaluation of Mechanical Assistance for the Treatment of Congestive Heart Failure) trial, which compared 1- and 2-year survival rates of patients with heart failure who were ineligible for transplantation treated with medical therapy versus LVAD placement, were encouraging.[70] Investigators found a 25% 1-year survival rate and an 8% 2-year survival rate in the medical therapy group, compared to a 52% 1-year survival rate and a 23% 2-year survival rate in the LVAD group.

A recent study by Aaronson and associates[1] at Columbia University retrospectively compared the use of LVADs and high-dose inotropes as bridges to transplantation in 104 patients. Survival to transplantation was 81% in the LVAD group, compared with 64% in the inotrope group. Moreover, survival after transplant was 95% at 3 years for the LVAD group but only 65% for the inotrope group. Although this preliminary study suggests that LVADs are superior to high-dose inotropes as a bridge to transplantation, larger prospective multicenter studies are needed to guide clinical practice.

In addition to use as a bridge to transplantation, it is likely that newer-generation LVADs may be used for long-term destination therapy. Although a large number of patients may benefit from this therapy, the cost is extremely high and will likely limit its scope.

ORGAN PROCUREMENT AND PRESERVATION

Donor Selection

The selection of donors for cardiac transplantation follows the list of guidelines outlined in Box 94-3. A primary screen is performed by specialists from organ procurement organizations, and information is collected regarding cause of death, body size, ABO blood type, serologies (including human immunodeficiency virus [HIV], hepatitis B virus [HBV], and hepatitis C virus [HCV]), and clinical course. A secondary screen is then performed by a transplant physician, including review of relevant history, baseline electrocardiogram (ECG), chest X-ray, laboratory data, and echocardiogram. A final screen is performed by the procuring surgeon, who directly inspects the organ.

Potential donors should meet requirements for brain death. Donors with a history of cardiac disease, including prior myocardial infarction and intractable ventricular arrhythmias, should be excluded.[38] In addition, donors with a history of severe chest trauma are excluded. Donor age of less than 55 is preferable, although on occasion older donors are considered. For all male donors over age 45 and female donors over age 50, cardiac catheterization with coronary angiography should be performed to rule out significant coronary artery disease.[90] Relative contraindications include positive hepatitis B or C serology, sepsis, history of cancer, prolonged hypotension or hypoxemia, and noncritical coronary artery disease.

In response to the donor organ shortage, there has been a trend toward liberalization of certain donor selection criteria. The Crystal City Guidelines, issued as a consensus

Box 94–3. Cardiac Donor Selection Criteria.

Age <55
No history of chest trauma or cardiac disease
No prolonged hypotension or hypoxemia
Meets hemodynamic criteria:
- MAP >60 mm Hg
- CVP 8–12 mm Hg
- Inotropic support <10 μg/kg/min dopamine or dobutamine

Normal ECG
Normal echocardiogram
Normal cardiac angiography[a]
Negative HBsAg, HCV, and HIV serologies

[a]Performed as indicated by donor age and history.
HBsAg, Hepatitis B surface antigen.

statement in 2002, describe strategies for maximizing the use of recovered donor hearts.[90] Expansion of the donor pool has been achieved by modification of criteria, including donor age, ischemic time, presence of mild left ventricular hypertrophy, mild valvular abnormality (or mild coronary artery disease), and use of hearts that have undergone arrest and resuscitation. Limited information is available regarding the long-term durability of organs derived from this expanded pool, although there is some evidence that certain donor factors, such as older age and prolonged ischemic time, may interact synergistically to increase recipient mortality risk.[25]

Donor Management

Aggressive hemodynamic and metabolic management of donors is essential and has been shown to result in higher organ retrieval rates. Patients suffering from acute brain injury are often hemodynamically unstable as a result of neurogenic shock, excessive fluid losses, and bradycardia. Meticulous fluid management is required, and intravascular volume replacement should be given to maintain a central venous pressure (CVP) between 5 and 10 mm Hg. Inotropic support should be weaned as much as possible. Blood transfusions are used sparingly to maintain a hematocrit level of 30%. If available, cytomegalovirus (CMV)-negative and leukocyte-filtered blood should be used. Diabetes insipidus is common in brain injury, and donors may require intravenous vasopressin to reduce excessive urine losses. Ventilator settings are adjusted to a FiO_2 of 40% or less, and positive end-expiratory pressure between 3 and 5 cm H_2O is used to prevent atelectasis.

A single echocardiogram may provide initial information about cardiac function, but may fail to predict long-term ventricular function. Echocardiographic dysfunction occurs in 10–37% of brain-dead patients, and the correlation between these abnormalities and actual pathological findings is often poor.[31] Placement of a pulmonary artery catheter is useful in assessing initial cardiac function, as well as response to therapy. Typical hemodynamic goals include a mean arterial pressure (MAP) >60 mm Hg, a CVP of 5–10 mm Hg, and a pulmonary capillary wedge pressure (PCWP) <12 mm Hg.

The Papworth group has reported an increase in organ retrieval of 30% by using an aggressive protocol for donor management.[81,88] This includes placement of a pulmonary artery catheter, donor management by a cardiac-trained anesthetist, and provision of hormonal therapy, including thyroxine, cortisol, antidiuretic hormone (ADH), and insulin. Using this protocol, the majority of donors originally deemed unacceptable by strict hemodynamic criteria are converted into acceptable donors.

The Crystal City Guidelines outline another management strategy for potential organ donors. The algorithm begins with conventional management (fluid resuscitation; correction of acidosis, hypoxemia, and anemia; weaning of inotropes) followed by an initial echocardiogram. If the left ventricular ejection fraction (LVEF) is greater than 45%, the heart is suitable for recovery. If the LVEF is less than 45%, hormonal resuscitation and hemodynamic management with a pulmonary artery catheter should be performed. The heart will be recovered only if appropriate hemodynamic parameters can be reached.[90]

Organ Allocation

Allocation schemes have been developed to facilitate organ distribution. In the United States organ allocation is governed by United Network for Organ Sharing (UNOS), and the current heart allocation algorithm takes into account medical urgency, time on the waiting list, and blood type.[69] The medical urgency categories include Status 1A, 1B, 2, and 7 and are defined in Table 94-2. In addition, the algorithm is modified by age, such that adolescent donor hearts are preferably allocated to pediatric recipients. Distribution occurs first locally and then regionally.

Donor and Recipient Matching

Prospective recipients and donors must be ABO blood type compatible. They should be size-matched, although differences up to 20% may be tolerated. For recipients whose pulmonary vascular resistance remains at the upper acceptable limit, a donor whose body size is at least equal to that of the recipient should be chosen to decrease the likelihood of acute right heart failure. In rare situations, small hearts may be heterotopically transplanted into larger recipients, but the outcomes in these cases are significantly worse than

Table 94–2

UNOS Medical Urgency Status Categories

Status level	*Category*
Status 1A	Patient is admitted to the listing transplant center hospital and has at least one of the following devices or therapies in place: 1. Mechanical circulatory support for acute hemodynamic decompensation that includes at least one of the following: Left and/or right ventricular device Total artificial heart IABP ECMO 2. Mechanical circulatory support with evidence of significant device-related complications 3. Mechanical ventilation 4. Continuous infusion of a single high-dose intravenous inotrope 5. Life expectancy <7 days
Status 1B	At least one of the following devices or therapies in place: 1. Left and/or right ventricular device 2. Continuous infusion of intravenous inotropes
Status 2	All other actively listed patients
Status 7	Patient is temporarily removed from active waiting list

IABP, Intraaortic ballon pump; ECMO, extracorporeal membrane oxygenation.

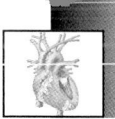

size-matched orthotopic heart transplantation.[16] In patients with an elevated PRA, a cross-match should be performed with the prospective donor. A positive cross-match portends a high likelihood of hyperacute rejection, and in such cases the donor organ cannot be accepted for that recipient.

Donor Operative Technique

Retrieval of the donor heart typically occurs as part of a multiorgan procurement. In many cases the cardiothoracic team will be working in conjunction with an abdominal team procuring the liver and/or kidneys. Communication between the two teams is essential. Slight modifications in the procurement procedure are necessary when either one or both lungs are also being procured.

A median sternotomy is performed, and the pericardium is opened longitudinally. The heart is carefully inspected for external signs of trauma, infarction, congenital anomalies, and overall right and left ventricular activity. The coronary arteries are palpated to rule out coronary artery disease. Significant abnormalities preclude use of the donor heart in transplantation. The ascending aorta is dissected from the pulmonary artery and encircled with umbilical tape. The superior vena cava (SVC) is mobilized to the level of the azygos vein and encircled with two heavy free ties. The inferior vena cava (IVC) is mobilized and surrounded with umbilical tape.

When the abdominal procurement team has completed their dissection, 30,000 units of heparin are administered to the donor. A cannula for infusion of cold cardioplegia is inserted into the ascending aorta. If the lungs are being procured, a pulmonoplegia line is inserted into the main pulmonary artery. Any central venous lines are withdrawn high into the SVC. The SVC is then doubly ligated and divided between the ligatures. The IVC is divided at the diaphragm. Sufficient length on the SVC and IVC will be needed for later bicaval anastomoses. Blood and perfusate from the liver will drain into the right pleural cavity, and suction should be available for its removal. The left side of the heart is decompressed by incising one of the pulmonary veins. Alternatively, if the lung also is being procured, the left side of the heart is decompressed by amputating the left atrial appendage. Once the heart has emptied, the aortic cross-clamp is placed and cold crystalloid cardioplegia (10 ml/kg) is rapidly infused into the aorta. Pulmonoplegia also is rapidly infused into the pulmonary artery if the lungs are being procured. While the plegic solutions are being delivered, the thoracic organs are topically cooled with several liters of ice-cold saline.

When the infusions are completed and the heart is cooled and arrested, the chest is emptied of the cold saline solution. The heart is rapidly excised by dividing the four pulmonary veins, the aorta (as high as possible), and the pulmonary artery (at its bifurcation or at the origin of its main right and left branches). If the lungs are procured, a small cuff of left atrial tissue may be retained with the pulmonary veins. Once removed from the donor, the heart is sterilely triple-bagged in cold 4° C saline or preservation solution and stored for transport.

Organ Preservation

Several strategies are used to improve cardiac preservation during organ retrieval and ischemic storage.[44] These include the use of hypothermia, cardioplegia, and preservation solutions. Hypothermia at 4–8° C markedly decelerates metabolism and is used during organ retrieval, storage, and transport. Cardioplegia is used to arrest electrical activity of the heart. Adequate decompression of the ventricles during organ retrieval limits injury to the heart during procurement. The heart may be stored in either cold saline or a variety of preservation solutions.[90] Most preservation solutions originally were designed for perfusion and storage of abdominal organs; experimental data in animals suggest that their use in cardiac transplantation may be advantageous, but little comparative clinical data are available. Preservation solutions may be delivered by continuous infusion during the storage period, but logistically this is difficult, and more often, organs are simply stored in bags containing the solution. Rarely, preservation solutions are used as alternatives to standard cardioplegia during organ procurement. Preservation solutions can be broadly categorized as "intracellular" and "extracellular" types, based on their differing ionic compositions. Intracellular solutions have a moderate to high potassium concentration and little calcium or sodium, whereas extracellular solutions have a high sodium concentration and a low to moderate concentration of potassium. In addition to electrolyte constituents, these solutions often contain impermeants and colloids to prevent the development of intracellular edema. Most contain glucose to prevent intracellular acidosis secondary to anaerobic metabolism. Many contain antioxidant additives to protect against reperfusion injury.

Cardiac preservation currently is limited to 4–6 hours of cold ischemic storage. Longer ischemic periods adversely affect recipient survival. Myocardial preservation is an active area of research, and progress in this area ultimately facilitates distant organ procurement and thereby increases the donor organ pool.

RECIPIENT OPERATIVE TECHNIQUE

Both orthotopic and heterotopic techniques for clinical heart transplantation are performed. Orthotopic transplantation is performed in the vast majority of cases, whereas heterotopic transplantation is reserved for cases in which the recipient has significant pulmonary hypertension or there is a marked size mismatch between recipient and donor (i.e., large recipient and small donor).

Several techniques of orthotopic heart transplantation have been described. For many years, the technique of Lower, Stofer, and Shumway, described in the 1960s, was the standard.[53] This technique, often referred to as the "biatrial technique" or the "standard technique," involves excision of the recipient heart at the midatrial level and sewing corresponding anastomoses between the donor and recipient left atrium, right atrium, aorta, and pulmonary artery. This technique allows for short operative times and avoids potential complications that result from individual vena caval and pulmonary vein anastomoses (in particular, stenosis and thrombosis). Disadvantages of the method include distortion of atrioventricular geometry, which can result in atrial enlargement, atrioventricular valve insufficiency, impaired atrial function and atrial thrombosis, and a propensity toward sinoatrial node dysfunction.[3,60] The proximity of the right atrial suture line to the sinoatrial node often resulted in necrosis of the sinoatrial node and postoperative dysfunction. Barnard[10] introduced an important modification of the technique in 1968; the incision in the donor heart's right atrium was extended from the opening of the IVC into the base of the right atrial appendage, rather than into the SVC, avoiding the region of the sinoatrial node.

The standard technique is still widely used at many transplant centers. However, newer "nonstandard" techniques, including the "bicaval" and "total" techniques, have been developed and offer the advantage of better preservation of atrial geometry.[11,30,73,76] In the bicaval technique, the native recipient's right atrium is excised and separate SVC and IVC anastomoses are made, in addition to left atrial, aortic, and pulmonary artery anastomoses. The total technique also uses separate SVC, IVC, aortic, and pulmonary artery anastomoses. However, rather than use a single left atrial anastomosis, the total technique describes separate right and left pulmonary vein anastomoses. The left atrial remnant is divided longitudinally, leaving left and right pulmonary vein cuffs, which are then anastomosed to the left and right pulmonary vein orifices in the donor heart's left atrium.

In a recent survey of 210 international transplant centers, 54% of centers reported that they used the bicaval technique most frequently.[4] Twenty-two percent reported using the standard technique most often, and 5% used the total technique most often. Reasons for converting to nonstandard techniques included concern over tricuspid valve dysfunction, right ventricular performance, and arrhythmias or heart block. Although several small studies have shown improved atrial function and decreased atrioventricular valvular insufficiency with the nonstandard techniques,[5,32,84] no large prospective randomized trials have been performed. A reported disadvantage of the bicaval and total techniques is the risk of SVC stenosis, particularly when there is a size mismatch between donor and recipient. A series from Stanford reported a 2.4% incidence of this complication.[82] The total technique may be associated with additional complications, including bleeding from inaccessible pulmonary vein suture lines and pulmonary vein stenosis.

Orthotopic Standard Technique

The recipient is positioned supine on the operating table. The chest is entered through a median sternotomy, and the pericardium is opened and reflected laterally. After heparinization, cardiopulmonary bypass (CPB) is initiated via cannulas in the ascending aorta, SVC, and IVC. Snares are placed around the SVC and IVC to affect total CPB. The patient is cooled to 28° C.

Once the donor heart has been brought to the operating room, excision of the recipient heart is performed. The aorta is cross-clamped just proximal to the aortic cannulation site. The right and left atrial walls, atrial septum, pulmonary artery, and aorta are divided. The division of the pulmonary artery and aorta should occur just above the semilunar valves (Figure 94-1A).

The donor heart is prepared for insertion into the recipient. The tissue between the orifices of the four pulmonary veins is excised, leaving a single large opening. The right atrium is opened, beginning from the lateral aspect of the IVC and extending into the base of the right atrial appendage. The heart is carefully examined for any valvular or congenital anomalies.

In the original description of the standard technique, anastomoses were performed in the following order: left atrium, right atrium, pulmonary artery, and aorta. In an attempt to achieve earlier reperfusion, some surgeons have altered the sequence of anastomoses. For example, the aortic anastomosis can be performed immediately after the left atrial or right atrial anastomoses and then the aortic cross-clamp can be removed. The original sequence of anastomoses is described as follows.

The anastomosis of the donor and recipient left atria is performed with a double-armed running 3-0 or 4-0 polypropylene suture. The first stitch is placed in the recipient left atrium at the level of the left superior pulmonary vein and at the base of the donor left atrial appendage. The suture line is continued around the superior and inferior borders of the left atrium and then tied along the interatrial septum. Once this suture line is complete, the left atrial appendage is cannulated with a line of cold saline to facilitate endocardial cooling. In addition, cold saline is continuously infused into the pericardial well to achieve topical cooling.

The two right atria are anastomosed with a double-armed running 4-0 or 5-0 polypropylene suture (Figure 94-1B). The fist stitch is placed though the midpoint of the donor septum, and the midpoint of the suture line along the atrial septum. The suture line is continued inferiorly first, and then the superior suture line is completed. The two ends of the suture are tied along the right atrial free wall. Once the right atrial anastomosis is completed, systemic rewarming is initiated.

The two pulmonary arteries are trimmed to an appropriate length and anastomosed with a running 4-0 polypropylene suture. The donor and recipient aortas also are trimmed and anastomosed with a running 4-0 polypropylene suture (Figure 94-1A).

The ascending aorta and pulmonary artery are cleared of air. The SVC and IVC snares are released, followed by the aortic cross-clamp. De-airing is continued as needed. Transesophageal echocardiography aids in de-airing the heart and assessing cardiac function. The line in the left atrial appendage is removed, and the hole is oversewn. Temporary atrial and ventricular wires are placed in the transplanted heart. The heart is then allowed to recover fully. Defibrillation may be necessary. After at least 30 minutes of reperfusion, the patient is gradually weaned from CPB and the cannulas are removed. Intravenous methylprednisolone (500 mg) is administered. Mediastinal drains are placed, as well as pleural chest tubes if the pleura has been opened. The chest is then closed in the standard fashion.

Orthotopic Bicaval Technique

In recent years the bicaval technique for orthotopic heart transplantation has become the preferred approach at most transplant centers. Several modifications distinguish it from the standard approach. First, the recipient SVC is cannulated just below the innominate vein junction and the IVC is cannulated at the diaphragm. Recipient cardiectomy is performed as a two-step procedure. In the first step, the heart is transected at the midatrial level, the aorta

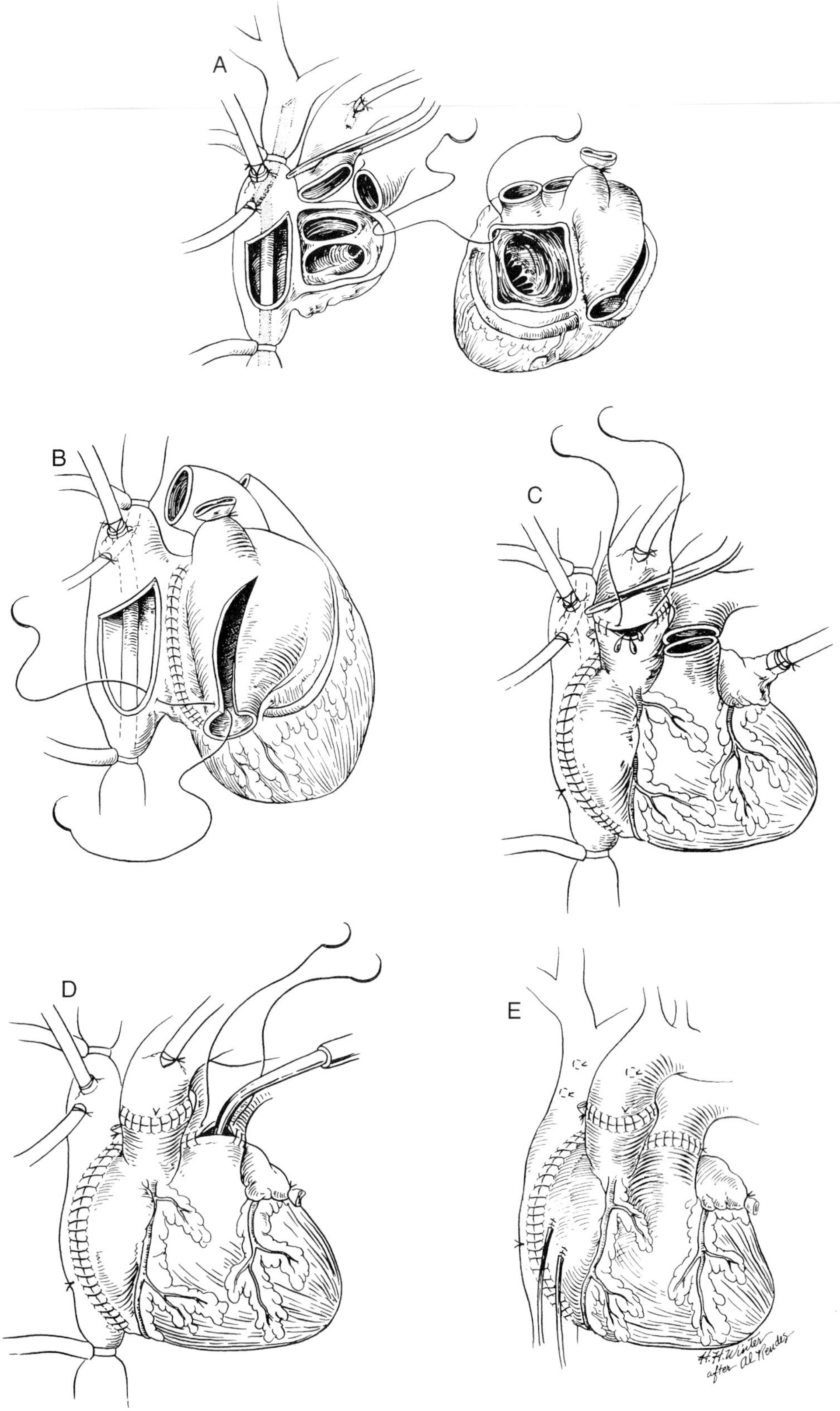

Figure 94–1 Biatrial or "standard" technique for orthotopic heart transplantation. A, Cannulation technique is similar to routine cardiac procedures with central cannulation. Tapes have been placed around the superior and inferior venae cavae, and the aorta has been cross-clamped to exclude the heart from the circulation. The recipient's heart has been excised at the atrioventricular groove. The superior vena cava (SVC) of the donor's heart has been ligated, and the left atrial anastomosis has been started. **B,** The left atrial anastomosis has been completed. The incision in the right atrium of the donor heart is curved away from the SVC and the adjacent sinoatrial node. The right atrial anastomosis is begun. **C,** The right atrial, pulmonary artery, and aortic anastomoses are completed. The aortic cross-clamp is removed, and the patient is weaned from cardiopulmonary bypass (CPB). When the heart is fully recovered, the bypass cannulas are removed.
(From Baumgartner WA, Reitz BA, Oyer PE, et al: Cardiac homotransplantations. Curr Probl Surg 16:1, 1979.)

and pulmonary artery are divided, and the heart is removed. In the second step, the posterior walls of both atria are removed; on the right side, the SVC and IVC are transected at their junction with the right atrium, and on the left side, the left atrium is trimmed, leaving a cuff of tissue around the pulmonary vein orifices (Figure 94-2A). The donor heart's left atrium is trimmed, leaving a single orifice where the pulmonary vein entry sites had been, and the right atrium remains intact. (Figure 94-2B). In the bicaval approach, the typical sequence of anastomoses is left atria, venae cavae, pulmonary arteries, and aortas. The left atrial, pulmonary artery, and aortic anastomoses

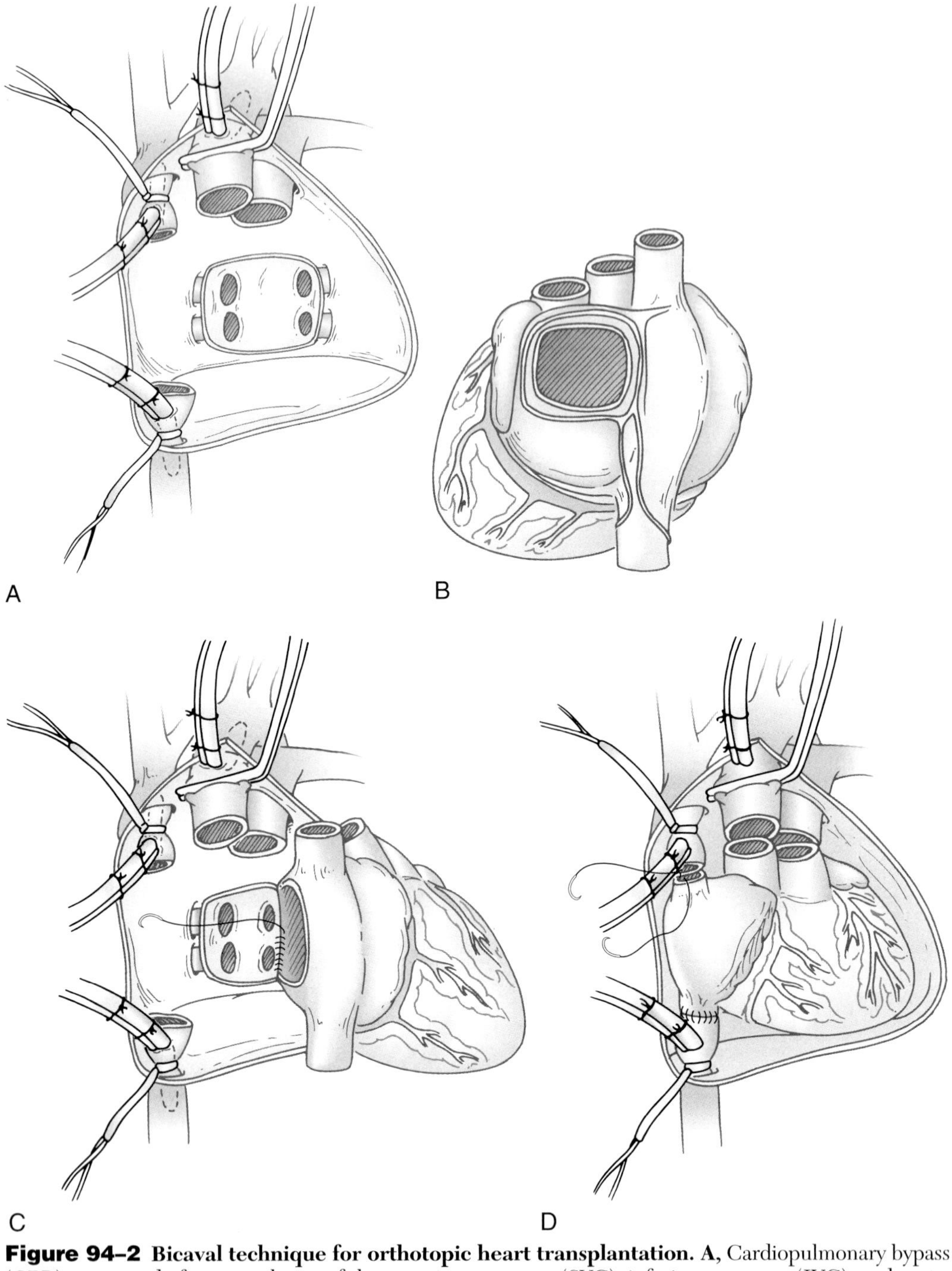

Figure 94–2 **Bicaval technique for orthotopic heart transplantation. A,** Cardiopulmonary bypass (CPB) is initiated after cannulation of the superior vena cava (SVC), inferior vena cava (IVC), and aorta. The aorta is cross-clamped, and native recipient cardiectomy is performed. A cuff of left atrial tissue is preserved around the four pulmonary vein orifices. **B,** The donor heart is prepared for transplantation. The left atrial tissue surrounding the four pulmonary vein orifices has been excised, leaving a single large orifice. **C,** The left atrial anastomosis is performed. **D,** The IVC anastomosis is completed, and the SVC anastomosis is performed. Once this is completed, the pulmonary artery and aortic anastomoses will be performed.

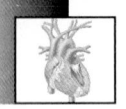

are performed as described earlier in the standard technique (Figure 94-2C). The SVC anastomosis is performed with a running 5-0 polypropylene suture and the IVC anastomosis with running 4-0 polypropylene suture (Figure 94-2D).

Orthotopic Total Technique

This technique is used at a small number of centers. It is similar to the bicaval approach, except that during recipient cardiectomy, the left atrial cuff surrounding the pulmonary vein orifices is divided longitudinally into separate right and

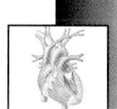

left pulmonary vein cuffs. Preparation of the donor heart requires separate excision of the right and left pulmonary veins, leaving two orifices on the donor heart's left atrium. Two left atrial anastomoses are fashioned, followed by the bicaval, pulmonary artery, and aortic anastomoses.

Heterotopic Technique

In this approach, the donor IVC and right pulmonary veins are ligated, followed by anastomosis of the donor and recipient left atria, SVC, aortas, and pulmonary arteries. SVC and aortic anastomoses are performed end-to-side, and a short length of graft is used to connect the pulmonary arteries (Figure 94-3). This heterotopic approach can be used when recipient pulmonary vascular resistance is markedly elevated, because in such cases acute right heart failure would likely develop after orthotopic transplantation. In addition, it has been used in cases of donor and recipient size mismatch when medical urgency for transplantation is high.[16] Improvements in mechanical assist devices and a growing experience in their use as a bridge to transplantation have made the indications for heterotopic heart transplantation less frequent.

RECIPIENT POSTOPERATIVE MANAGEMENT

Clinical Management in Early Postoperative Period

Upon completion of the transplant, the patient is taken to the intensive care unit. The patient remains mechanically ventilated with continuous monitoring of ECG, arterial blood pressure, and pulse oximetry. A central venous catheter and, in some cases, a pulmonary artery catheter, are used to assess hemodynamics. Temperature, urine output, and mediastinal drain output are monitored as well.

As with other patients undergoing cardiac surgery, dysrhythmias are frequent in the early postoperative period. Junctional rhythms are particularly common after orthotopic heart transplantation. Because cardiac output of the denervated transplanted heart is primarily rate dependent, the heart rate should be maintained between 90 and 110 beats per minute during the first few postoperative days.[61] Temporary pacing may be used to augment the heart rate. Less than 5% of patients have permanent sinus node dysfunction and require placement of a permanent transvenous pacemaker. The rate of sinus node dysfunction may be reduced when the bicaval technique is used.[32]

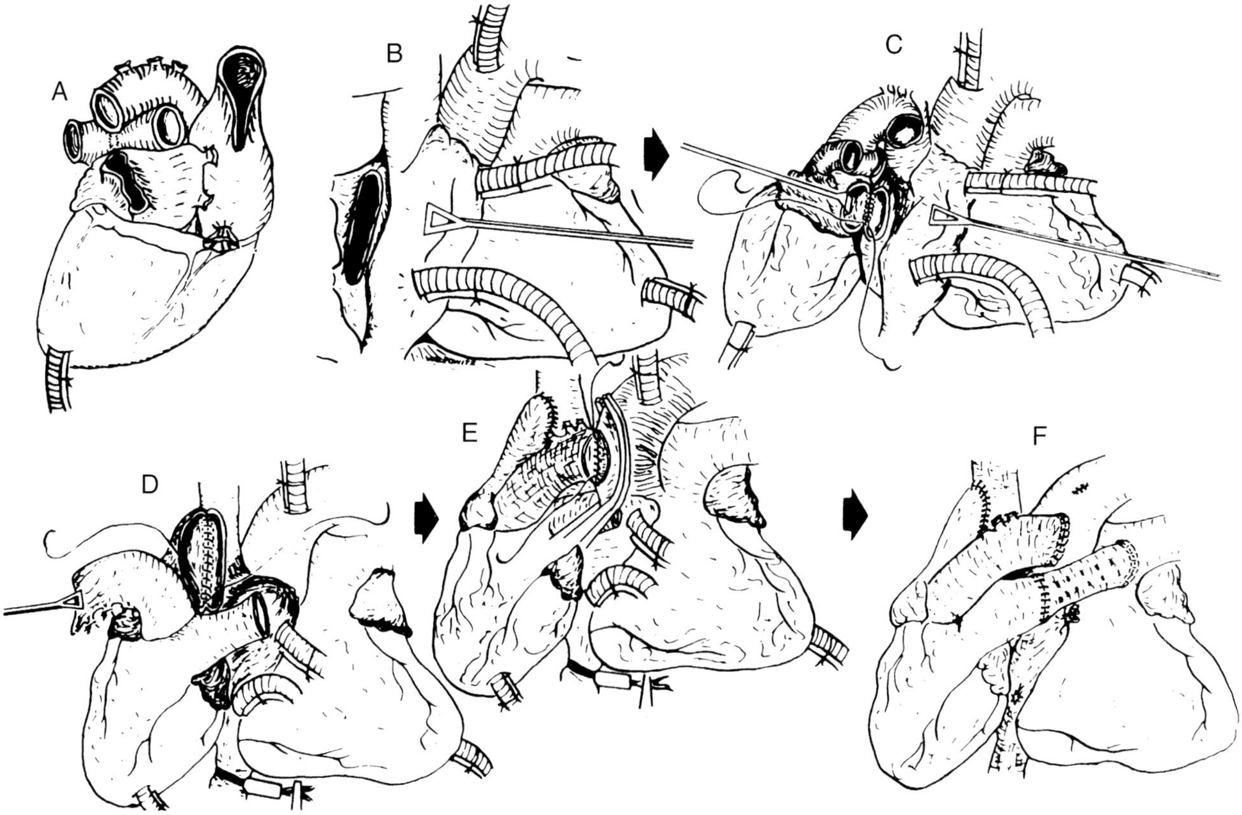

Figure 94–3 The heterotopic cardiac transplant. (**A**) Posterior view of the donor heart after preparation for anastomosis. (**B**) Left atriotomy. (**C**) Left atrial anastomosis. (**D**) Right atrial anastomosis. (**E**) Aortic anastomosis. (**F**) Completed anastomoses with a pulmonary-to-pulmonary arterial graft.
(A–E from Barnard CN, Wolpowitz A: Heterotopic versus orthotopic heart transplantation. Transplant Proc 11:309, 1979.)

In most cases, the postoperative course after transplantation is uncomplicated. The patient is extubated when alert and hemodynamically stable, typically within 24 hours of surgery. The patient is gradually weaned from inotropic support over the first few postoperative days. Invasive catheters are removed as soon as possible to reduce the risk of sepsis, and mediastinal drains are removed when drainage has fallen to less than 25 ml/h. Pacing wires are removed approximately 1 week after transplantation, provided that pacing is not required.

Early complications after transplantation include bleeding, depressed global myocardial performance, and right heart failure. Significant hemorrhage occurs in 3–4% of cases and may require surgical reexploration. The routine use of aprotinin and heparin-coated CPB circuits may decrease the incidence of bleeding. Depressed global myocardial performance is uncommon, but may occur in the setting of prolonged organ ischemia or inadequate preservation.[39] In such cases, aggressive hemodynamic and ventilatory management is necessary, and support from inotropic agents and vasopressors is needed. Hypovolemia, cardiac tamponade, sepsis, and bradycardia also may result in depressed myocardial performance and should be treated expeditiously if they are present. Right heart failure may occur after transplantation, particularly in recipients who have elevated preoperative pulmonary vascular resistance (PVR).[80] In such cases, the donor right ventricle is unable to work against the elevated PVR and begins to fail within hours after transplantation. Additional causes of right-sided heart dysfunction are technical failures, such as kinking or stenosis of the pulmonary artery anastomosis, which result in elevated pulmonary vascular resistance. Intraoperative transesophageal echocardiography should be performed routinely to assess right ventricular function. Treatment of right heart failure includes correction of any technical problems and medical treatment with inotropes and vasodilators. Refractory right heart failure may necessitate placement of a right ventricular assist device.

Maintenance Immunosuppression

In addition to careful monitoring of cardiac function during the immediate postoperative period, much focus is placed on institution of immunosuppression. In most cases, immunosuppression is initiated intraoperatively with intravenous methylprednisolone and continued postoperatively with a combination of intravenous and oral medications. Most centers have adopted multidrug immunosuppression regimens, employing triple drug combinations of a calcineurin inhibitor (cyclosporine or tacrolimus), an antiproliferative agent (azathioprine or mycophenolate mofetil), and corticosteroids. Immediately after transplantation, many of these medications can be administered intravenously, and once the patient is tolerating oral intake, they can be converted to oral immunosuppression. Because the risk of allograft rejection is highest in the first several months after transplantation, immunosuppression is most aggressive during this period. If patients remain free of rejection, immunosuppression gradually will be decreased over time. Typical immunosuppressive dosing regimens (early and late) are demonstrated in Box 94-4.

Box 94–4. Maintenance Immunosuppression for Heart Transplant Recipients.

Category 1: Calcineurin Inhibitor

Select one of the following:

A. Cyclosporine

3–10 mg/kg/day PO in divided doses twice daily
Adjust to maintain target serum trough level:
0–30 days after transplant: 150–200 ng/ml
>30 days after transplant: 50–150 ng/ml

B. Tacrolimus

0.10–0.15 mg/kg/day PO in divided doses twice daily
Adjust to maintain target trough level:
0–30 days after transplant: 10–20 ng/mg
31–90 days after transplant: 10–15 ng/ml
>90 days after transplant: 5–10 ng/ml

Category 2: Antiproliferative Agent

Select one of the following:

A. Mycophenolate mofetil

1000 mg PO bid

B. Sirolimus

1–2 mg PO qd
Adjust to maintain blood levels:
10–15 ng/ml (<30 days after transplant)
8–12 ng/ml (30–90 days after transplant)
8–10 ng/ml (>90 days after transplant)

C. Azathioprine

After transplant 2 mg/kg/day
Adjust to maintain WBC 4000–6000/mm^3

Category 3: Corticosteroid

Intraoperative methylprednisolone 500 mg IV
Immediate postoperative methylprednisolone 125 mg IV q8 × 3 doses
After transplant prednisone maintenance therapy and taper schedule

1–14 days after transplant:	1 mg/kg/day divided twice daily
15 days–6 weeks after transplant:	Taper to 0.5 mg/kg/day
6 weeks–3 months after transplant:	Taper to 0.2 mg/kg/day
4–6 months after transplant:	Taper to 0.1 mg/kg/day
>6 months after transplant:	Taper to 0.1 mg/kg qod and then discontinue as tolerated

PO, Per os (by mouth); bid, twice a day; qd, every day; WBC, white blood cell count; IV, intravenous.

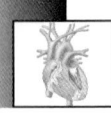

Multidrug immunosuppression targets multiple sites in the immune cascade, which lead to allograft rejection.[8] Calcineurin inhibitors block the activity of calcineurin, a calcium- and calmodulin-dependent phosphatase that is required for early T cell activation and interleukin-2 (IL-2) formation. Antiproliferative agents inhibit lymphocyte replication through a variety of mechanisms. Azathioprine inhibits the de novo and salvage pathways for purine biosynthesis. Mycophenolate mofetil (MMF) inhibits the de novo synthesis of guanine nucleotides. Because activated lymphocytes use the de novo pathway predominantly, MMF is thought to have greater selectivity than azathioprine. Corticosteroids inhibit lymphocyte proliferation by inhibiting macrophage production of cytokines, including IL-1 and IL-6.

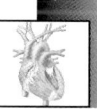

The drugs in these regimens act synergistically, allowing for dose reduction when used in combination. This helps minimize dose-dependent toxicity to the transplant recipient. Cyclosporine can cause nephrotoxicity, neurotoxicity, hypertension, hyperlipidemia, hirsutism, and gingival hyperplasia. Tacrolimus is also nephrotoxic and neurotoxic and has been associated with glucose intolerance and new-onset diabetes mellitus. Both cyclosporine and tacrolimus are metabolized by the liver and cause upregulation of the cytochrome p450 system. Azathioprine and MMF both cause dose-dependent bone marrow suppression. Finally, corticosteroids are associated with a myriad of side effects, including poor wound healing, development of cushingoid features, hypertension, diabetes mellitus, osteoporosis, and peptic ulcer disease.

Rapamycin, or sirolimus, is a new immunosuppressive agent that has been used successfully in renal and liver transplantation[47] and is now being used by some centers as a component of triple-therapy immunosuppression for heart transplantation. It inhibits mTOR (mammalian target of rapamycin), thereby blocking IL-2 signaling pathways.[8,33] Rapamycin also inhibits smooth muscle proliferation and has been used in drug-eluting coronary stents to inhibit neointimal hyperplasia. Experimental animal models show inhibition of cardiac allograft vasculopathy (CAV) with rapamycin treatment,[67] and it is hoped that rapamycin also will prevent CAV in clinical heart transplantation.

Few randomized prospective trials comparing immunosuppressive protocols in heart transplantation have been performed. As a consequence, practices vary widely from center to center. Moreover, most of the existing studies report only short-term findings. Taylor et al[83] performed a small prospective randomized multicenter study comparing the efficacy of tacrolimus-based immunosuppression to cyclosporine-based immunosuppression. At 1-year follow up, rejection rates were comparable in both groups, although the incidence of hypertension and hyperlipidemia was less in the tacrolimus group. A randomized multicenter trial comparing the triple drug regimens of cyclosporine/azathioprine/prednisone and cyclosporine/MMF/prednisone showed improved 1-year survival and greater freedom from rejection in the cyclosporine/MMF/prednisone group.[46] There was an increase in herpes simplex viral infection in the cyclosporine/MMF/prednisone group compared with that in the cyclosporine/azathioprine/prednisone group (21% versus 15%) but no difference in other infectious complications or malignancy.

Along with multidrug immunosuppression regimens, many centers employ cytolytic induction therapy to rapidly deplete lymphocytes in heart transplant recipients. This therapy occurs over a 3 to 10-day course, beginning immediately after transplantation. Several preparations of antilymphocyte antibodies are available, including antithymocyte globulin (ATG), OKT3, and IL-2 receptor antagonists.[8] ATG is a rabbit or equine polyclonal antibody preparation that results in rapid cytolytic depletion of T cells. Immunosuppression is profound and immediate. OKT3 is a mouse monoclonal antibody directed against the CD3 receptor of human T cells, which results in immediate destruction of T cells. IL-2 receptor antagonists, such as daclizumab and basiliximab, are humanized antibodies that effect the destruction of activated T cells expressing the IL-2 receptor on their cell surface.

Induction therapy has both advantages and disadvantages. Because immunosuppression is immediate, maintenance immunosuppression with other drugs can be delayed. In cases of hemodynamic instability or questionable renal function, this can be advantageous. Initial doses of ATG and OKT3 may be associated with a "cytokine release syndrome," which manifests with fever, chills, hypotension, and bronchospasm. Patients receiving these induction agents should be premedicated with acetaminophen, antihistamines, and corticosteroids and should be monitored closely. Because these preparations are raised in animals, patients may develop neutralizing antibodies, making prolonged and repeated courses impossible. Induction therapy with ATG and OKT3 may decrease the incidence of acute rejection in some cases, but in others, it simply delays the time of onset to rejection. Both are associated with a higher incidence of infectious complications and posttransplant lymphoproliferative disorder (PTLD).[8] The experience with IL-2 receptor blockade is more limited, but 1-year follow-up studies have shown a decrease in the frequency and severity of acute rejection and a decrease in development of CAV.[12,54] Long-term studies are needed to determine whether induction with IL-2 receptor antagonists provides a survival benefit or whether it affects the risk for infection or malignancy.

COMPLICATIONS

Hyperacute Rejection

Hyperacute rejection is a form of humorally mediated rejection. Preformed antibodies in the recipient recognize donor vascular endothelial antigens, resulting in activation of inflammatory and coagulation cascades. Graft vessels thrombose, and ultimately the organ will fail. ABO matching of donor and recipient has decreased the rate of hyperacute rejection. For recipients with an elevated PRA, prospective cross-matching of donor lymphocytes with recipient serum also has decreased the rate of hyperacute rejection.

Acute Rejection

The risk of acute rejection is highest during the first few months after transplantation, and then persists at a low constant level. Most heart transplant patients experience at least one episode of acute rejection, and there is a small mortality risk associated with each of these episodes. According to ISHLT data, acute rejection is the cause of death in approximately 1% of patients between 0 days and 3 years after transplantation.[40] More importantly, frequent and severe rejection episodes have been correlated with higher rates of CAV, which may lead to graft failure and patient death. In

1994 the CTRD group identified risk factors for recurrent rejection after heart transplantation.[48] In the first year after transplantation, these risk factors include shorter interval since previous rejection episode, young age, female gender, female donor, positive cytomegalovirus serology, prior infections, and OKT3 induction. After the first year, the dominant risk factors are a greater number of rejection episodes during the first year and the presence of prior cytomegalovirus infections.

The clinical presentation of acute rejection varies widely. Patients may be asymptomatic or may have presenting nonspecific clinical signs and symptoms, including fever, anorexia, leukocytosis, and mild hypotension. Rarely, acute rejection manifests with severe hypotension and circulatory collapse. Because clinical signs and symptoms lack a high degree of sensitivity or specificity in the diagnosis of acute rejection, the gold standard diagnostic test is a tissue biopsy. Percutaneous endomyocardial biopsy is performed as part of routine surveillance protocols after heart transplantation and also with the presence of a clinical suspicion of rejection. A bioptome is passed through a sheath in the right internal jugular vein and advanced though the tricuspid valve into the right ventricle, where tissue biopsies are taken. Pathologically, acute rejection can be a focal patchy process, so 4–6 biopsies should be taken to reduce sampling error.[15] A typical surveillance endomyocardial biopsy protocol includes weekly biopsies for the first 4 weeks after transplantation, biweekly biopsies for the next month, and then monthly biopsies through the sixth month after transplantation. If the patient is free from rejection at 6 months, the frequency of biopsies is reduced to every 3 months.

A standardized grading system for cardiac acute rejection was developed by the ISHLT Heart Rejection Study Group in 1989 and is illustrated in Table 94-3.[15] The system grades acute rejection with a score of 0 to 4, with 0 being no rejection and 4 being severe acute rejection.

Table 94–3

Cardiac Transplant Grading System for Acute Rejection

Grade	*Histological Appearance*
Grade 0	No rejection
Grade 1A	Focal infiltrate without necrosis
Grade 1B	Diffuse but sparse infiltrate without necrosis
Grade 2	Single focus with aggressive infiltration and/or focal myocyte damage
Grade 3A	Multifocal aggressive infiltrates and/or myocyte damage
Grade 3B	Diffuse inflammatory process with necrosis
Grade 4	Diffuse aggressive polymorphous ± infiltrate, ± edema, ± hemorrhage, ± vasculitis, with necrosis

Because of the cost, invasive nature, and potential for complications associated with endomyocardial biopsy, investigators currently are developing alternative noninvasive techniques to monitor cardiac allograft rejection.[58] Several emerging techniques are promising. These include allograft imaging techniques using magnetic resonance imaging (MRI),[56] wall motion analysis with tissue Doppler imaging,[24] electrical event monitoring with ventricular evoked response amplitude assessment,[7] identification of peripheral blood markers of rejection (e.g., P-selectin, prothrombin fragments, β-type natriuretic peptides, troponin),[57,75] imaging for necrosis with anti–myosin antibody-based scintigraphy,[41] and imaging for apoptosis with ^{99m}technetium-labeled Annexin V.[62]

Treatment of Acute Rejection

When a histological diagnosis of rejection is made, treatment consists of augmentation of immunosuppression. The degree of augmentation depends on the grade of rejection. A typical algorithm for the treatment of acute rejection is illustrated in Figure 94-4. In most cases, low-grade rejection (ISHLT grade 1A/B or 2) can be managed with adjustments in the patient's maintenance regimen. For higher-grade rejection, a pulse of high-dose intravenous corticosteroids is given. Endomyocardial biopsy is repeated after 7–14 days, and if rejection persists, patients may be treated with antilymphocyte antibody preparations or with conversion from one maintenance immunosuppressive drug to another. For example, tacrolimus may be used instead of cyclosporine, and sirolimus or MMF may be used instead of azathioprine. If rejection does not respond to this treatment, an additional pulse of steroids may be given. Acute rejection rarely is refractory to these measures. In such cases, total lymphoid irradiation,[71] plasmapheresis,[13] and conversion of azathioprine to cyclophosphamide or methotrexate have been used.[20]

Infection

An inherent complication of immunosuppression is increased risk for infection. Infection is associated with 18% of early deaths and nearly 40% of late deaths after heart transplantation.[35] The pathogens involved vary depending on the time after transplantation. Early infections occurring in the first month after transplantation are commonly caused by bacteria and manifest as pneumonia, urinary tract infections, wound infections, and line sepsis. Typical pathogens include *Pseudomonas aeruginosa, Staphylococcus aureus,* Enterobacteriaceae, and enterococci. The use of perioperative antibiotics and early removal of invasive catheters may prevent these infections. Late infections are typically caused by opportunistic viruses, protozoa, and fungi. They often occur after periods of augmented immunosuppression.

Cytomegalovirus (CMV) is the most common and clinically significant viral pathogen in heart transplant recipients.[72] It may cause a variety of syndromes and has been

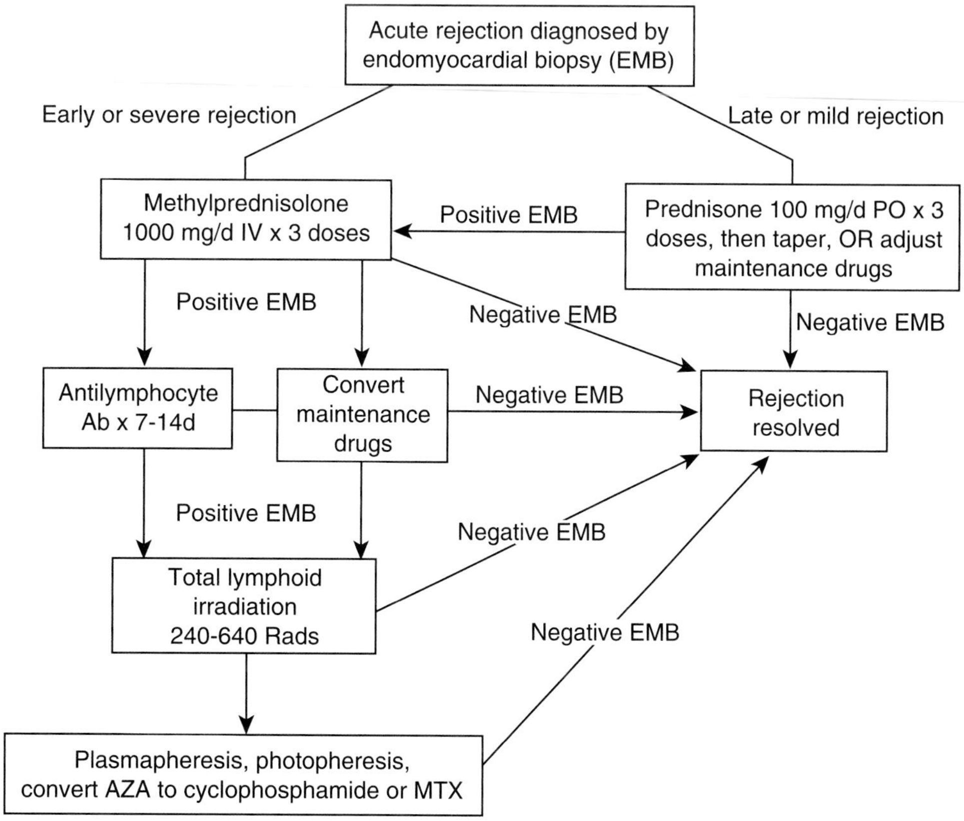

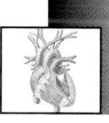

Figure 94–4 Treatment algorithm for acute rejection in heart transplant recipients. Ab, antibody; AZA, azathioprine; MTX, methotrexate.

implicated as a trigger for accelerated CAV. Heart transplant recipients are at high risk of CMV infection because their cell-mediated immunity, which is necessary to combat CMV, is impaired by conventional immunosuppressive drugs. CMV infection may present either as primary infection or as reactivation of a latent infection. It is most frequent at 1–4 months after transplantation. Primary CMV infection may develop in seronegative recipients receiving a heart from a CMV seropositive donor. In such cases, donor leukocytes or the allograft itself may harbor CMV and transmit it to the recipient. Reactivation of latent CMV may occur in seropositive recipients. The risk of CMV infection in different populations of cardiac transplant recipients is illustrated in Table 94-4. The seronegative recipient of a heart from a seropositive donor and those being treated for acute rejection with antilymphocyte antibody preparations are at highest risk.

Table 94–4

Risk of Cytomegalovirus (CMV) Disease in Different Populations of Cardiac Transplant Recipients

Donor CMV serotype	*Recipient CMV serotype*	*Antilymphocyte antibody therapy*	*Incidence of clinical disease (%)*
Positive	Negative	—	50–75
Positive or negative	Positive	—	10–15
Positive or negative	Positive	Induction	~25
Positive or negative	Positive	Antirejection	50–75
Negative	Negative	—	~0

From Rubin RH: Prevention and treatment of cytomegalovirus disease in heart transplant patients. J Heart Lung Transplant 19:731, 2000.

CMV infection may manifest as a mononucleosis-like syndrome or may be tissue invasive. The most common sites for tissue invasion are the lung, liver, and gastrointestinal tract. Less common sites include the retina and skin. Diagnosis is made by measurement of viral load with either quantitative polymerase chain reaction (PCR) or antigenemia assays; by direct culture of the virus from blood, urine, or tissue specimens; or by observation of characteristic histological changes (enlarged cells containing nuclear inclusion bodies). A combination of intravenous ganciclovir and hyperimmune globulin is used for treatment.[72]

Several populations of cardiac transplant patients benefit from prophylactic treatment against CMV infection. Serologically mismatched patients (seronegative recipient of heart from seropositive donor) are treated with a combination of ganciclovir and hyperimmune globulin for weeks to months after transplantation.[72,86] Often seropositive recipients also are treated with a course of ganciclovir to prevent reactivation infection. Finally, some groups have shown that administration of intravenous ganciclovir when antilymphocyte antibody therapy is used to treat rejection reduces the risk of CMV disease to baseline levels.

Protozoal pathogens after heart transplantation include *Pneumocystis carinii* and *Toxoplasma gondii.* Pulmonary infection with *P. carinii* can be prevented by routine postoperative prophylaxis with sulfa and trimethoprim or aerosolized pentamidine (for sulfa-allergic patients). Toxoplasmosis may occur in serologically mismatched patients (e.g., *T. gondii*-seronegative recipient of heart from *T. gondii*-seropositive donor), but may be prevented by prophylaxis with pyrimethamine.[35]

Invasive fungal infections are uncommon after cardiac transplantation, but when they occur, they cause significant morbidity and mortality. Fungal pathogens include *Candida albicans* and *Aspergillus.* Treatment consists of fluconazole, itraconazole, or amphotericin B.

Cardiac Allograft Vasculopathy

The long-term success of cardiac transplantation is limited by the development of CAV. CAV, also referred to as graft coronary artery disease, is an accelerated disease process that results in diffuse and heterogeneous narrowing of both large- and small-caliber vessels.[87] The predominant disease is fibrous neointimal hyperplasia, although atherosclerotic changes may be found as well. Significant CAV results in diminished coronary artery blood flow and may lead to arrhythmias, myocardial infarction, sudden death, or impaired left ventricular function with congestive heart failure. It is unusual for patients with severe CAV to have classic anginal symptoms, because the cardiac graft is denervated.

Analyzing data in the CRTD, Costanzo et al[23] reported that at 5 years, angiographically evident CAV was present in 42% of transplant patients. A total of 27% had mild disease, 8% had moderate disease, and 7% had severe disease. Risk factors for the development of CAV included older donor age, donor history of hypertension, donor male sex, recipient male sex, and recipient black race. The presence of severe disease was highly predictive of subsequent coronary artery disease–related events, including death and need for retransplantation. In 2002 the ISHLT Registry reported a 1-year posttransplant incidence of CAV of 8% and a 5-year posttransplant incidence of 33%.[40] In addition to advanced donor age and donor history of hypertension, recipient age less than 20 also was a risk factor. Aziz et al[6] stratified the incidence of CAV by underlying patient diagnosis and correlated a primary diagnosis of ischemic cardiomyopathy with an increased incidence of CAV.

The mechanistic etiology of CAV is poorly understood. It has been suggested that immunologically mediated damage to the coronary vascular endothelium is an important factor and that both alloantigen-dependent and alloantigen-independent processes are involved. The precise role of donor and recipient major histocompatibility complex (MHC) differences in this process has not been fully elucidated. Alloantigen-independent factors that have been implicated include graft ischemic time, oxidative stress resulting from ischemia and reperfusion, infection (particularly with CMV), and recipient metabolic characteristics such as hyperlipidemia and glucose intolerance.

Most transplant programs perform routine screening for CAV in heart transplant recipients. Yearly coronary angiography is recommended, although it lacks sensitivity and typically underestimates the presence of disease. Dobutamine stress echocardiography also may be used for routine screening.[77] Intracoronary ultrasound (ICUS), when available, is a more sensitive procedure that provides information about intimal area, lumen area, and plaque morphology.[34]

Treatment for CAV is limited. Because of the diffuse nature of the disease, patients rarely are candidates for coronary artery bypass grafting. Focal stenoses have been treated with angioplasty and stenting, but there is a high rate of restenosis. Ultimately, severe progressive disease may require retransplantation. Unfortunately, the overall survival rate after retransplantation is significantly worse than after primary transplantation. One-, 2- and 3-year survival rates are 65%, 59%, and 55%, respectively, compared with 84%, 80%, and 76% in primary transplantation.[40,78]

Because treatment options are limited, prevention of CAV is essential. Risk factor modification, including control of hyperlipidemia, hypertension, and hyperglycemia, may limit development of the disease. At-risk patients should receive routine prophylaxis against CMV. Experimental studies in animals have shown that modulation of the immune response by tolerance induction prevents CAV. Other techniques, including augmentation of endogenous nitric oxide activity and blockade of reperfusion injury, also prevent CAV. Application of these techniques to clinical transplantation may lead to improvement in long-term patient outcomes.

Neoplasm

The incidence of neoplasia is higher in transplant recipients than in the general population. This is undoubtedly a consequence of chronic immunosuppression. Moreover, because immunosuppressive regimens are particularly aggressive in thoracic organ transplantation, these patients develop malignancies more often than renal and liver transplant recipients.[49] The ISHLT reports that 29% of heart transplant recipients develop malignancies by the seventh year after transplantation.[40] Of these, the majority are skin

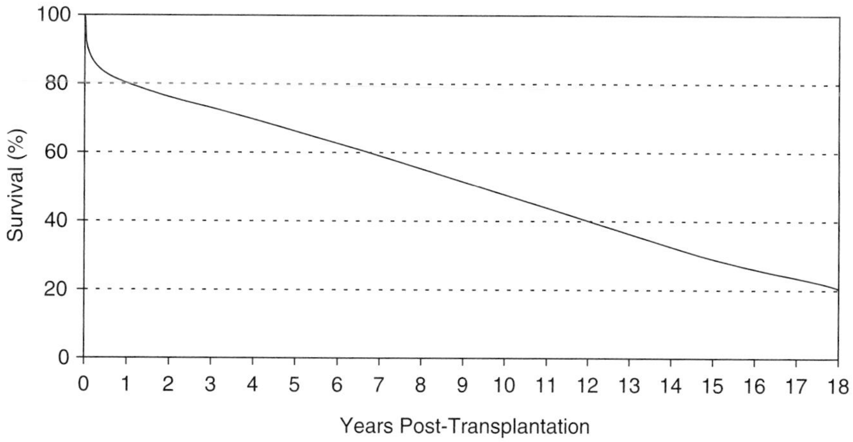

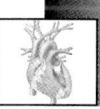

Figure 94–5 **Actuarial survival for heart transplants performed between 1982 and 2001.** Half-life = 9.3 years; conditional half-life = 11.8 years; *n* = 60,936.
(From Hertz MI, Taylor DO, Trulock EP, et al: The Registry of the International Society for Heart and Lung Transplantation: Nineteenth official report—2002. J Heart Lung Transplant 21:950, 2002.)

cancers (squamous cell carcinoma and basal cell carcinoma) and B-cell lymphoproliferative disorders. B-cell lymphoproliferative disorders cause the greatest degree of morbidity and mortality. They represent a spectrum of diseases, ranging from cellular hyperplasia to true lymphomas, and over 95% are associated with Epstein-Barr virus infection.[49] The mainstay of treatment for PTLD is reduction of immunosuppression and antiviral therapy, which yield a response rate of 30–40%. Chemotherapy, radiotherapy, and immunotherapy have been used successfully in some cases. Other malignancies that occur at higher frequency in the transplant population include Kaposi's sarcoma, carcinoma in situ of the cervix, and carcinoma of the vulva and anus. The incidence of solid organ tumors common in the general population (i.e., carcinoma of the lung, breast, colorectum, and prostate) is not higher in the transplant population.[65]

LONG-TERM RESULTS IN HEART TRANSPLANTATION

Analyzing data from 1982–2002, the ISHLT has published survival rates in heart transplant recipients. They have found 1-year, 5-year, 10-year, and 15-year survival rates of 80%, 66%, 47%, and 29%, respectively.[40] Patient half-life (i.e., time to 50% survival) is 9.3 years. These survival data are illustrated in Figure 94-5. Survival rates have been improving over time, and among patients transplanted in 1998–2001, the 1-year survival rate is 84%. The ISHLT lists the following as risk factors for 1-year mortality: mechanical assistance (e.g., extracorporeal membrane oxygenation [ECMO], IABP, VAD), previous transplant, underlying diagnosis of congenital heart disease or coronary artery disease, male recipient of female donor heart, PRA >25%, recipient bilirubin level >5 mg/dl, advanced donor and recipient age, donor history of coronary artery disease, and prolonged donor organ ischemia. Five-year mortality risk factors include CAV within the first year after transplant, rejection within the first year after transplant, retransplantation, and underlying diagnosis of coronary artery disease. The CTRD group also found that a combination of recipient and donor characteristics affect early and overall mortality.[89] Early mortality risk factors include younger recipient age, ventilator use, VAD use, previous sternotomy, elevated PVR, older donor age, female donor to male recipient, prolonged donor organ ischemia, and elevated donor inotropic support. Overall mortality risk factors include younger and older recipient age, recipient ventilator use, elevated recipient PVR, older donor age, female donor to male recipient, prolonged donor organ ischemia, and elevated donor inotropic support.

Approximately 40% of patients are hospitalized in the first year after transplant, often for treatment of rejection or infection. By the second year after transplant, only 20% are hospitalized. The vast majority report good functional status after transplantation, yet less than 40% of heart transplant recipients return to work after transplantation.

SUMMARY

The perseverance of early pioneers in heart transplantation has led to its current position as a mainstay of therapy for heart failure. For carefully selected patients, heart transplantation offers markedly improved survival and quality of life. Increasingly, however, the limitations of this procedure have become evident, and new strategies are developing to address these issues. In the years to come, limitations in donor organ availability, organ preservation, and immunosuppression will be important areas for growth and improvement. The development of donor specific tolerance is the Holy Grail of transplantation and ultimately could lead to longer graft survival, diminished need for immunosuppression, and fewer complications. Xenotransplantation is a major area of experimental research, and the recent development of transgenic pigs expressing human decay–accelerating factor (hDAF) has decreased the incidence of hyperacute rejection in nonhuman primates. Unfortunately, delayed xenograft rejection is a major obstacle limiting progress in this field. Finally, artificial hearts, mechanical assist devices, cell transplantation, and improved medical therapy should be explored as alternatives to transplantation in patients with heart failure.

REFERENCES

1. Aaronson KD, Eppinger MJ, Dyke DB, et al: Left ventricular assist device therapy improves utilization of donor hearts. J Am Coll Cardiol 39:1247–1254, 2002.

2. Aaronson KD, Schwartz JS, Chen TM, et al: Development and prospective validation of a clinical index to predict survival in ambulatory patients referred for cardiac transplant evaluation. Circulation 95:2660–2667, 1997.
3. Angermann CE, Spes CH, Tammen A, et al: Anatomic characteristics and valvular function of the transplanted heart: Transthoracic versus transesophageal echocardiographic findings. J Heart Transplant 9:331–338, 1990.
4. Aziz TM, Burgess MI, El Gamel A, et al: Orthotopic cardiac transplantation technique: A survey of current practice. Ann Thorac Surg 68:1242–1246, 1999.
5. Aziz T, Burgess M, Khafagy R, et al: Bicaval and standard techniques in orthotopic heart transplantation: Medium-term experience in cardiac performance and survival. J Thorac Cardiovasc Surg 118:115–122, 1999.
6. Aziz T, Burgess M, Rahman AN, et al: Cardiac transplantation for cardiomyopathy and ischemic heart disease: Differences in outcome up to 10 years. J Heart Lung Transplant 20:525–533, 2001.
7. Bainbridge AD, Cave M, Newell S, et al: The utility of pacemaker evoked T wave amplitude for the noninvasive diagnosis of cardiac allograft rejection. Pacing Clin Electrophysiol 22:942–946, 1999.
8. Baran DA, Galin ID, Gass AL: Current practices: Immunosuppression induction, maintenance, and rejection regimens in contemporary post-heart transplant patient treatment. Curr Opin Cardiol 17:165–170, 2002.
9. Barnard CN: The operation. A human cardiac transplant: an interim report of a successful operation performed at Groote Schuur Hospital, Cape Town. S Afr Med J 41:1271–1274, 1967.
10. Barnard CN: What we have learned about heart transplants. J Thorac Cardiovasc Surg 56:457–468, 1968.
11. Baumgartner WA, Traill TA, Cameron DE, et al: Unique aspects of heart and lung transplantation exhibited in the 'domino-donor' operation. JAMA 261:3121–3125, 1989.
12. Beniaminovitz A, Itescu S, Lietz K, et al: Prevention of rejection in cardiac transplantation by blockade of the interleukin-2 receptor with a monoclonal antibody. N Engl J Med 342:613–619, 2000.
13. Berglin E, Kjellstrom C, Mantovani V, et al: Plasmapheresis as a rescue therapy to resolve cardiac rejection with vasculitis and severe heart failure. A report of five cases. Transpl Int 8:382–387, 1995.
14. Betkowski AS, Graff R, Chen JJ, et al: Panel-reactive antibody screening practices prior to heart transplantation. J Heart Lung Transplant 21:644–650, 2002.
15. Billingham ME, Cary NR, Hammond ME, et al: A working formulation for the standardization of nomenclature in the diagnosis of heart and lung rejection: Heart Rejection Study Group. The International Society for Heart Transplantation. J Heart Transplant 9:587–593, 1990.
16. Bleasdale RA, Banner NR, Anyanwu AC, et al: Determinants of outcome after heterotopic heart transplantation. J Heart Lung Transplant 21:867–873, 2002.
17. Calne RY, White DJ, Rolles K, et al: Prolonged survival of pig orthotopic heart grafts treated with cyclosporin A. Lancet 1:1183–1185, 1978.
18. Carrel A, Guthrie C: The transplantation of veins and organs. Am Med 10:1101–1102, 1905.
19. Caves PK, Stinson EB, Graham AF, et al: Percutaneous transvenous endomyocardial biopsy. JAMA 225:288–291, 1973.
20. Chan GL, Weinstein SS, Vijayanagar RR: Treatment of recalcitrant cardiac allograft rejection with methotrexate. Cardiac Transplant Team. Clin Transplant 9:106–114, 1995.
21. Cimato TR, Jessup M: Recipient selection in cardiac transplantation: Contraindications and risk factors for mortality. J Heart Lung Transplant 21:1161–1173, 2002.
22. Costanzo MR, Augustine S, Bourge R, et al: Selection and treatment of candidates for heart transplantation. A statement for health professionals from the Committee on Heart Failure and Cardiac Transplantation of the Council on Clinical Cardiology, American Heart Association. Circulation 92:3593–3612, 1995.
23. Costanzo MR, Naftel DC, Pritzker MR, et al: Heart transplant coronary artery disease detected by coronary angiography: A multiinstitutional study of preoperative donor and recipient risk factors. Cardiac Transplant Research Database. J Heart Lung Transplant 17:744–753, 1998.
24. Dandel M, Hummel M, Muller J, et al: Reliability of tissue Doppler wall motion monitoring after heart transplantation for replacement of invasive routine screenings by optimally timed cardiac biopsies and catheterizations. Circulation 104: I184–I191, 2001.
25. Del Rizzo DF, Menkis AH, Pflugfelder PW, et al: The role of donor age and ischemic time on survival following orthotopic heart transplantation. J Heart Lung Transplant 18:310–319, 1999.
26. De Marco T, Damon LE, Colombe B, et al: Successful immunomodulation with intravenous gamma globulin and cyclophosphamide in an alloimmunized heart transplant recipient. J Heart Lung Transplant 16:360–365, 1997.
27. Demikhov VP: Experimental Transplantation of Vital Organs. New York: Consultants Bureau, 1962.
28. Deng MC, De Meester JM, Smits JM, et al: Effect of receiving a heart transplant: Analysis of a national cohort entered on to a waiting list, stratified by heart failure severity. Comparative Outcome and Clinical Profiles in Transplantation (COCPIT) Study Group. BMJ 321:540–545, 2000.
29. Deng MC, Smits JM, Packer M: Selecting patients for heart transplantation: Which patients are too well for transplant? Curr Opin Cardiol 17:137–144, 2002.
30. Dreyfus G, Jebara V, Mihaileanu S, et al: Total orthotopic heart transplantation: An alternative to the standard technique. Ann Thorac Surg 52:1181–1184, 1991.
31. Dujardin KS, McCully RB, Wijdicks EF, et al: Myocardial dysfunction associated with brain death: Clinical, echocardiographic, and pathologic features. J Heart Lung Transplant 20:350–357, 2001.30.
32. El Gamel A, Yonan NA, Grant S, et al: Orthotopic cardiac transplantation: A comparison of standard and bicaval Wythenshawe techniques. J Thorac Cardiovasc Surg 109:721–729, 1995.
33. Gambino A, Testolin L, Gerosa G, et al: New trends in heart transplantation. Transplant Proc 33:3536–3538, 2001.
34. Gao HZ, Hunt SA, Alderman EL, et al: Relation of donor age and preexisting coronary artery disease on angiography and intracoronary ultrasound to later development of accelerated allograft coronary artery disease. J Am Coll Cardiol 29:623–629, 1997.
35. Gentry LO: Cardiac transplantation and related infections. Semin Respir Infect 8:199–206, 1993.
36. Griepp RB, Stinson EB, Dong E Jr, et al: Use of antithymocyte globulin in human heart transplantation. Circulation 45:I147–I153, 1972.
37. Hardy J, Chavez CM, Kurrus F, et al: Heart transplantation in man: Developmental studies and report of a case. JAMA 188:1132–1140, 1964.
38. Harringer W, Haverich A: Heart and heart-lung transplantation: Standards and improvements. World J Surg 26:218–225, 2002.
39. Hauptman PJ, Aranki S, Mudge GH, Jr, et al: Early cardiac allograft failure after orthotopic heart transplantation. Am Heart J 127:179–186, 1994.
40. Hertz MI, Taylor DO, Trulock EP, et al: The Registry of the International Society for Heart and Lung Transplantation: Nineteenth official report—2002. J Heart Lung Transplant 21:950–970, 2002.

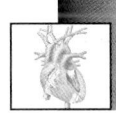

41. Hesse B, Mortensen SA, Folke M, et al: Ability of antimyosin scintigraphy monitoring to exclude acute rejection during the first year after heart transplantation. J Heart Lung Transplant 14:23–31, 1995.
42. Hunt SA: Who and when to consider for heart transplantation. Cardiol Rev 9:18–20, 2001.
43. Itescu S, Burke E, Lietz K, et al: Intravenous pulse administration of cyclophosphamide is an effective and safe treatment for sensitized cardiac allograft recipients. Circulation 105:1214–1219, 2002.
44. Jahania MS, Sanchez JA, Narayan P, et al: Heart preservation for transplantation: Principles and strategies. Ann Thorac Surg 68:1983–1987, 1999.
45. Jaski BE, Kim JC, Naftel DC, et al: Cardiac transplant outcome of patients supported on left ventricular assist device vs. intravenous inotropic therapy. J Heart Lung Transplant 20:449–456, 2001.
46. Kobashigawa J, Miller L, Renlund D, et al: A randomized active-controlled trial of mycophenolate mofetil in heart transplant recipients. Mycophenolate Mofetil Investigators. Transplantation 66:507–515, 1998.
47. Kreis H, Cisterne JM, Land W, et al: Sirolimus in association with mycophenolate mofetil induction for the prevention of acute graft rejection in renal allograft recipients. Transplantation 69:1252–1260, 2000.
48. Kubo SH, Naftel DC, Mills RM, Jr., et al: Risk factors for late recurrent rejection after heart transplantation: A multiinstitutional, multivariable analysis. Cardiac Transplant Research Database Group. J Heart Lung Transplant 14:409–418, 1995.
49. Kwok BW, Hunt SA: Neoplasia after heart transplantation. Cardiol Rev 8:256–259, 2000.
50. Laks H, Marelli D: The alternate recipient list for heart transplantation: A model for expansion of the donor pool. Adv Card Surg 11:233–244, 1999.
51. Lower RR, Shumway NE: Studies on orthotopic homotransplantation of the canine heart. Surg Forum 11:18–20, 1960.
52. Lower RR, Dong E, Shumway NE: Long-term survival of cardiac homografts. Surgery 58:110–119, 1965.
53. Lower RR, Stofer RC, Shumway NE: Homovital transplantation of the heart. J Thorac Cardiovasc Surg 41:196–204, 1961.
54. Mancini D, Beniaminovitz A, Edwards N, et al: Effect of Daclizumab induction therapy on the development of cardiac transplant vasculopathy. J Heart Lung Transplant 20:194, 2001.
55. Mancini DM, Eisen H, Kussmaul W, et al: Value of peak exercise oxygen consumption for optimal timing of cardiac transplantation in ambulatory patients with heart failure. Circulation 83:778–786, 1991.
56. Marie PY, Angioi M, Carteaux JP, et al: Detection and prediction of acute heart transplant rejection with the myocardial T2 determination provided by a black-blood magnetic resonance imaging sequence. J Am Coll Cardiol 37:825–831, 2001.
57. Masters RG, Davies RA, Veinot JP, et al: Discoordinate modulation of natriuretic peptides during acute cardiac allograft rejection in humans. Circulation 100:287–291, 1999.
58. Mehra MR, Uber PA, Uber WE, et al: Anything but a biopsy: Noninvasive monitoring for cardiac allograft rejection. Curr Opin Cardiol 17:131–136, 2002.
59. Miller LW: Listing criteria for cardiac transplantation: Results of an American Society of Transplant Physicians-National Institutes of Health conference. Transplantation 66:947–951, 1998.
60. Miniati DN, Robbins RC: Techniques in orthotopic cardiac transplantation: A review. Cardiol Rev 9:131–136, 2001.
61. Miniati DN, Robbins RC: Heart transplantation: A thirty-year perspective. Annu Rev Med 53:189–205, 2002.
62. Narula J, Acio ER, Narula N, et al: Annexin-V imaging for noninvasive detection of cardiac allograft rejection. Nat Med 7:1347–1352, 2001.
63. Oyer P, Stinson E, Jamieson S, et al: One year experience with Cyclosporin A in clinical heart transplantation. Heart Transplant 1:285–290, 1982.
64. Packer M, Coats AJ, Fowler MB, et al: Effect of carvedilol on survival in severe chronic heart failure. N Engl J Med 344:1651–1658, 2001.
65. Penn I: Incidence and treatment of neoplasia after transplantation. Transplantation 12:S328–S336, 1993.
66. Pisani BA, Mullen GM, Malinowska K, et al: Plasmapheresis with intravenous immunoglobulin G is effective in patients with elevated panel reactive antibody prior to cardiac transplantation. J Heart Lung Transplant 18:701–706, 1999.
67. Poston RS, Billingham M, Hoyt EG, et al: Rapamycin reverses chronic graft vascular disease in a novel cardiac allograft model. Circulation 100:67–74, 1999.
68. Ratkovec RM, Hammond EH, O'Connell JB, et al: Outcome of cardiac transplant recipients with a positive donor-specific crossmatch—preliminary results with plasmapheresis. Transplantation 54:651–655, 1992.
69. Renlund DG, Taylor DO, Kfoury AG, et al: New UNOS rules: Historical background and implications for transplantation management. United Network for Organ Sharing. J Heart Lung Transplant 18:1065–1070, 1999.
70. Rose EA, Gelijns AC, Moskowitz AJ, et al: Long-term mechanical left ventricular assistance for end-stage heart failure. N Engl J Med 345:1435–1443, 2001.
71. Ross HJ, Gullestad L, Pak J, et al: Methotrexate or total lymphoid radiation for treatment of persistent or recurrent allograft cellular rejection: A comparative study. J Heart Lung Transplant 16:179–189, 1997.
72. Rubin RH: Prevention and treatment of cytomegalovirus disease in heart transplant patients. J Heart Lung Transplant 19:731–735, 2000.
73. Sarsam MA, Campbell CS, Yonan NA, et al: An alternative surgical technique in orthotopic cardiac transplantation. J Card Surg 8:344–349, 1993.
74. Schmid C, Garritsen HS, Kelsch R, et al: Suppression of panel-reactive antibodies by treatment with mycophenolate mofetil. Thorac Cardiovasc Surg 46:161–162, 1998.
75. Segal JB, Kasper EK, Rohde C, et al: Coagulation markers predicting cardiac transplant rejection. Transplantation 72:233–237, 2001.
76. Sievers HH, Weyand M, Kraatz EG, et al: An alternative technique for orthotopic cardiac transplantation, with preservation of the normal anatomy of the right atrium. Thorac Cardiovasc Surg 39:70–72, 1991.
77. Spes CH, Klauss V, Mudra H, et al: Diagnostic and prognostic value of serial dobutamine stress echocardiography for noninvasive assessment of cardiac allograft vasculopathy: A comparison with coronary angiography and intravascular ultrasound. Circulation 100:509–515, 1999.
78. Srivastava R, Keck BM, Bennett LE, et al: The results of cardiac retransplantation: An analysis of the Joint International Society for Heart and Lung Transplantation/United Network for Organ Sharing Thoracic Registry. Transplantation 70:606–612, 2000.
79. Stinson EB, Dong E Jr, Schroeder JS, et al: Initial clinical experience with heart transplantation. Am J Cardiol 22:791–803, 1968.
80. Stobierska-Dzierzek B, Awad H, and Michler RE: The evolving management of acute right-sided heart failure in cardiac transplant recipients. J Am Coll Cardiol 38:923–931, 2001.
81. Stoica SC, Satchithananda DK, Charman S, et al: Swan-Ganz catheter assessment of donor hearts: Outcome of organs with

borderline hemodynamics. J Heart Lung Transplant 21:615-622, 2002.
82. Sze DY, Robbins RC, Semba CP, et al: Superior vena cava syndrome after heart transplantation: Percutaneous treatment of a complication of bicaval anastomoses. J Thorac Cardiovasc Surg 116:253–261, 1998.
83. Taylor DO, Barr ML, Radovancevic B, et al: A randomized, multicenter comparison of tacrolimus and cyclosporine immunosuppressive regimens in cardiac transplantation: Decreased hyperlipidemia and hypertension with tacrolimus. J Heart Lung Transplant 18:336–345, 1999.
84. Traversi E, Pozzoli M, Grande A, et al: The bicaval anastomosis technique for orthotopic heart transplantation yields better atrial function than the standard technique: An echocardiographic automatic boundary detection study. J Heart Lung Transplant 17:1065–1074, 1998.
85. 2001 Annual Report of the U.S. Scientific Registry of Transplant Recipients and the Organ Procurement and Transplantation Network. www.optn.org, 2002.
86. Valantine HA, Luikart H, Doyle R, et al: Impact of cytomegalovirus hyperimmune globulin on outcome after cardiothoracic transplantation: A comparative study of combined prophylaxis with CMV hyperimmune globulin plus ganciclovir versus ganciclovir alone. Transplantation 72:1647–1652, 2001.
87. Weis M, von Scheidt W: Cardiac allograft vasculopathy: A review. Circulation 96:2069–2077, 1997.
88. Wheeldon DR, Potter CD, Oduro A, et al: Transforming the "unacceptable" donor: Outcomes from the adoption of a standardized donor management technique. J Heart Lung Transplant 14:734–742, 1995.
89. Young JB, Naftel DC, Bourge RC, et al: Matching the heart donor and heart transplant recipient. Clues for successful expansion of the donor pool: A multivariable, multiinstitutional report. The Cardiac Transplant Research Database Group. J Heart Lung Transplant 13:353–364, 1994.
90. Zaroff JG, Rosengard BR, Armstrong WF, et al: Consensus conference report: maximizing use of organs recovered from the cadaver donor: Cardiac recommendations, March 28-29, 2001, Crystal City, Va. Circulation 106:836–841, 2002.

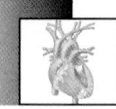

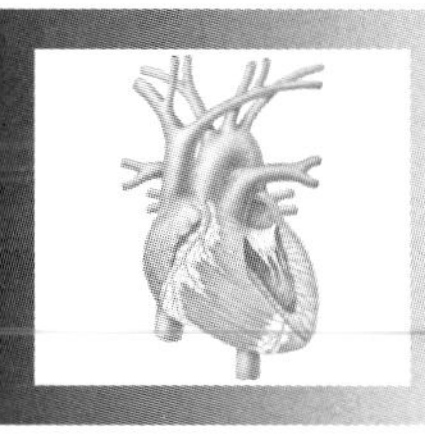

Heart–Lung Transplantation

Peter C. Kouretas and Bruce A. Reitz

CHAPTER 95

INTRODUCTION

The clinical realization of heart–lung transplantation evolved through much earlier experimental developments in the laboratory. Alexis Carrel[13] (Figure 95-1) and later Demikhov[22] and Marcus and associates[56] performed experiments that explored the possibility of heart–lung transplantation to replace diseased organs. When heart transplantation began in 1968, Cooley, Lillehei, and Barnard all performed human heart–lung transplants, with short survival. Progress in the laboratory translated to the clinical application of the first successful human heart–lung transplant performed at Stanford in 1981. Since these initial clinical transplants, the field of heart–lung transplantation and lung transplantation alone has undergone dramatic changes in all aspects, including indications, operative technique, and postoperative management. This chapter reviews the state of the art and current issues in the field of heart–lung transplantation.

INDICATIONS FOR HEART–LUNG TRANSPLANTATION

Recipient Diagnosis

Heart–lung transplantation initially was developed for patients with severe pulmonary vascular disease, such as individuals with primary pulmonary hypertension (PPH) and Eisenmenger's syndrome secondary to congenital heart disease. Indications have evolved to include any patient with end-stage cardiopulmonary disease, including individuals with septic lung disease associated with fairly normal heart function, as in the domino-donor procedure. The diagnostic profile of heart–lung transplant recipients reported to the Registry of the International Society for Heart and Lung Transplantation (ISHLT) through 2001 is depicted in Figure 95-2.[104]

Pulmonary hypertension secondary to congenital heart disease is the most frequent diagnosis, found in 32% of individuals who required heart–lung transplantation.[104] Cardiac lesions that may result in secondary pulmonary hypertension include atrial and ventricular septal defects, patent ductus arteriosus, truncus arteriosus, and other complex congenital anomalies, including univentricular heart with pulmonary atresia and hypoplastic left heart syndrome. Pulmonary hypertension secondary to congenital heart disease varies prognostically when compared with individuals with PPH. Despite comparable levels of pulmonary arterial pressures, individuals with Eisenmenger's syndrome have lower right atrial pressures, better cardiac index, and an overall better prognosis than patients with pulmonary hypertension without congenital heart disease.[38] Therefore hemodynamic variables are less reliable in this group than the presence of progressive symptoms as an indicator for transplantation (see later). Patients with significant hemodynamic derangements may be effectively managed with medical therapy and delay transplantation.

Secondary pulmonary hypertension with complex, irreparable cardiac defects must be treated with heart–lung transplantation. In a recent study there was a highly significant survival advantage for patients with Eisenmenger's syndrome caused by a ventricular septal defect (VSD) or multiple congenital anomalies who had a heart–lung transplant performed versus cardiac repair combined with lung transplantation.[112] In patients with simpler cardiac defects, one should consider repair of the cardiac defect combined with single or bilateral lung transplantation. Lung transplantation with intracardiac repair has evolved as a viable alternative to heart–lung transplantation for several reasons. First, right ventricular function improves after lung trans-

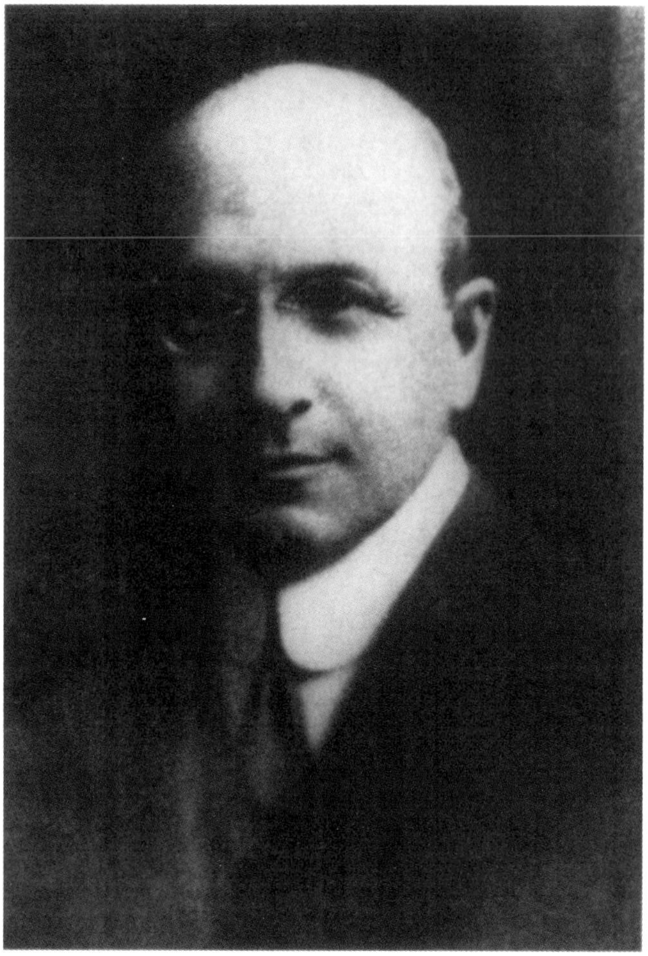

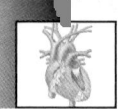

Figure 95–1 Alexis Carrel described the first heart–lung transplantation in a feline model in 1907. This experiment and numerous other observations predicted the eventual utility of the transplantation of organs. For these outstanding accomplishments, Carrel received the Nobel Prize in 1912.

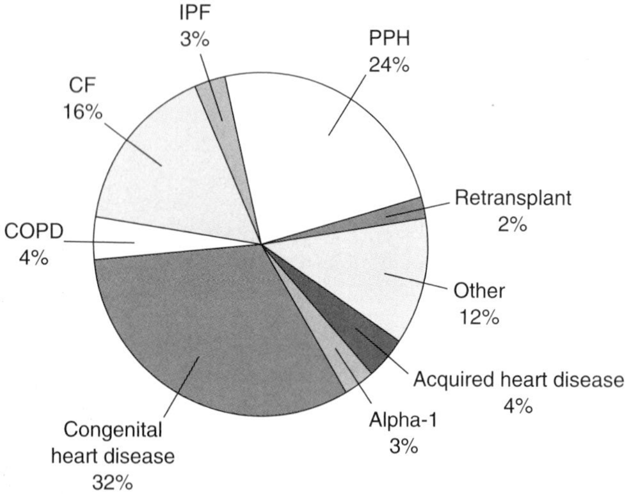

Figure 95–2 Indications for heart–lung transplantation. *(Modified from Trulock EP, Edwards LB, Taylor DO, et al: The Registry of the International Society of Heart and Lung Transplantation: Twentieth official adult lung and heart–lung transplant report—2003. J Heart Lung Transplant 22:625–635, 2003.)*

plantation secondary to normalization of pulmonary vascular resistance.[70] Also, there is an obvious organ donor shortage, as well as an avoidance of the denervation and graft coronary artery disease associated with cardiac transplantation.

PPH associated with irreversible right ventricular failure is the second most common indication for heart–lung transplantation, with 24% of recipients carrying this diagnosis.[104] In contrast to secondary pulmonary hypertension from congenital heart disease, abnormal hemodynamic parameters are closely related to increased mortality.[17] Therefore patients with PPH should be promptly referred to a transplant pulmonologist for initiation of intravenous (IV) pulmonary vasodilators. If severe right ventricular failure persists despite aggressive medical therapy, heart–lung transplantation may be indicated.

The role of heart–lung transplantation in the setting of PPH also has evolved over the last several years. Individuals with pulmonary vascular disease and improved right ventricular function after initiation of medical therapy also may be treated effectively with either single-lung transplantation (SLT) or double-lung transplantation (DLT). In the setting of PPH, DLT results in both greater hemodynamic improvements and shorter duration of postoperative mechanical ventilation than SLT.[8] It is the preferred operation in most transplant centers. Furthermore, comparable survival was noted after heart–lung transplantation and DLT in patients with PPH.[115] This has led to the recent trend in favor of DLT for PPH because of the potential for increased use of scarce donor organs. This trend has resulted in the decreased number of heart–lung transplants for PPH over the last 10 years. The subsets of patients who have fixed pulmonary vascular resistance not responsive to vasodilators and who have irreversible right-sided heart dysfunction are still candidates for heart–lung transplantation.

The remainder of heart–lung transplants are performed for a variety of disorders that result in end-stage pulmonary failure and irreversible cardiac failure. These include individuals with septic lung disease, such as cystic fibrosis and bronchiectasis, ischemic and restrictive cardiomyopathies with intercurrent end-stage lung disease, or acquired pulmonary vascular disease. Primary parenchymal lung disease, such as idiopathic pulmonary fibrosis, desquamative interstitial pneumonitis, and lymphangioleiomyomatosis, may present with severe right-sided heart failure and also may be a reason for heart–lung transplantation.

The introduction of the "domino" transplantation procedure renewed interest in heart–lung transplantation for septic lung disease. In this procedure the recipient of a heart–lung transplant served as a heart donor for a second recipient, thus maintaining donor organ allocation.[10,119] Recent studies have demonstrated equivalent survival in recipients of domino heart grafts compared with recipients of cadaveric heart grafts. However, this procedure is rarely performed, and bilateral lung transplant remains the procedure of choice for most septic or parenchymal lung disease.

The distribution of preoperative diagnoses treated with heart–lung transplantation at Stanford from 1981 to the present has been as follows: Eisenmenger's syndrome, 42%; PPH, 27%; cystic fibrosis, 14%; complex congenital heart disease, 10%; α-1 antitrypsin deficiency, 2%; cardiomyopathy with pulmonary hypertension, 2%; failure of SLT, 1%; congenital bronchiectasis, <1%; pulmonary lymphangioleiomyomatosis, <1%; and other diagnoses, 3%.[20]

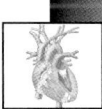

Recipient Selection Criteria

The selection of appropriate candidates for heart–lung transplantation is of paramount importance for success of the procedure. Any patient with end-stage cardiopulmonary disease with the capacity for full rehabilitation is a potential candidate for heart–lung transplantation. Suitable candidates should have a life expectancy of less than 1–2 years and generally have marked persistent functional disability with a New York Heart Association (NYHA) class designation of III or IV. Patients must otherwise be in good general health without other serious systemic illness. The occurrence of life-threatening complications, such as severe right-sided congestive heart failure with liver dysfunction, massive hemoptysis, or multiple syncopal episodes, suggests a poor prognosis and the need to list a patient as a candidate for heart–lung transplantation.

Recipients of heart–lung transplants generally are younger than heart transplant recipients, with an average age of 30 years versus 45 years, and are more likely to be female (54% versus only 19% female patients for heart transplant alone).[104] It must be determined that the patient and his or her family are emotionally prepared for transplantation. Each individual patient must be assessed for the presence of adequate emotional and psychosocial support to withstand the rigorous and intrusive medical regimen that he or she will be subjected to throughout his or her life. Heart–lung transplantation has become more common as a therapeutic option for complex congenital heart disease in infants and children.[59,94] These recipients also must be carefully evaluated, and they should have an extremely strong family support network in order to cope with the complex regimen and the frequent medical follow up.

The patient should be in the "window" for transplantation. The individual's disease process should be severe enough to warrant heart–lung transplantation, yet the patient must be well enough to survive the long wait until the transplantation occurs, as well as the surgical procedure itself.[57] The underlying disease determines the appropriate window. Survival with or without transplantation varies by disease process and by the patient's overall physical condition. Identification of a critical turning point in a patient's disease that signals an accelerated decline is the key to appropriate referral for transplantation. Pulmonary and cardiac clinical signs of this "transplantation window" include changes in the rate of decline in exercise capacity or pulmonary function, increasing frequency of infectious complications, increasing number and duration of hospitalizations, and increasing supplemental oxygen requirements. Other signs include increasing requirements for diuretics and increased hepatomegaly and bilirubin levels. Hyperbilirubinemia has been shown to be a marker for poor postoperative outcome in patients with pulmonary hypertension and right ventricular dysfunction. Patients with chronic bilirubin levels greater than 2.1 mg/dl who are undergoing heart–lung transplantation have been demonstrated to have significantly worse postoperative mortality of 58%.[47] The rate of perioperative complications, including coagulopathy, hepatic encephalopathy, poor wound healing, and impaired clearance of cyclosporine with resultant nephrotoxicity, also were significantly increased after heart–lung transplantation in such patients.[30]

Heart–lung transplantation should be undertaken before multisystem organ failure and severe malnutrition ensue. Many patients, while they await a suitable donor, become increasingly debilitated. Every opportunity to optimize their physical strength and nutritional status should be aggressively pursued.[89] Good physical performance before transplantation has been associated with improved postoperative recovery. Therefore patients should be referred for physical therapy early in an effort to improve their functional status and optimize their recovery potential.

In the past, most centers considered conditions associated with extensive adhesions, such as previous thoracotomy or sternotomy, septic lung disease, and previous chemical or surgical pleurodesis, an absolute contraindication to heart–lung transplantation. Historically these patients have an increase in morbidity and short-term mortality, primarily secondary to excessive blood loss and pulmonary issues associated with massive transfusions of blood products. The introduction of antifibrinolytic therapy (aprotinin) in thoracic organ transplantation has provided improved outcomes for this group of patients.[82] We now routinely accept patients with previous cardiac or thoracic surgery for heart–lung transplantation, and they represent a significant proportion of the current waiting list.

In patients selected for transplantation, routine pretransplant screening is performed for ABO blood group, the presence of preformed antibodies, human leukocyte antigen (HLA) and reaction of degeneration (DR) tissue types, and titers of antibodies against cytomegalovirus, herpes simplex virus, and toxoplasmosis. ABO compatibilities are strictly adhered to because isolated episodes of hyperacute rejection have been observed in transplants performed across ABO barriers. In addition to ABO compatibility, donor-recipient matching also is based on body size. In practice, matching donor and recipient height seems to be the most reproducible method for selecting the appropriate donor lung size. In general, the dimensions of the donor lungs should not be greater than 4 cm over those in the recipient. Other investigators have proposed that the simplest method of matching donor lung size to that of the recipient is to use their respective predicted total lung capacity (TLC) values.[69,101]

Once an appropriate donor–recipient match is made, the recipient is screened for preformed antibodies against a panel of 50 random donors. A percent reactive antibody (PRA) level greater than 25% prompts a prospective specific crossmatch between the donor and recipient. A positive crossmatch indicates the presence of antidonor circulating antibodies in the recipient, and the organ cannot be accepted for transplantation. Despite several retrospective studies that reveal improved graft survival with human leukocyte antigen (HLA) matching,[29,40,117] prospective HLA matching is not feasible given the short ischemic times that the heart–lung and lung blocks tolerate. Furthermore, in a recent multicenter study, HLA matching for lung transplantation did not have a large effect on clinical outcome, including the development of obliterative bronchiolitis.[73]

MANAGEMENT OF PATIENTS AWAITING TRANSPLANTATION

Given that the average waiting period for a heart–lung block is greater than 18 months, management of recipients after listing becomes a critical aspect of the preoperative plan. Routine medical care, including clinical surveillance, optimization of cardiopulmonary function, and management of disease-specific and age-specific issues, should be addressed during this time period. General considerations in the pretransplant period include appropriate surveillance protocols and screening for malignancies such as prostate, breast, and colon cancer. Other specific issues that should be addressed include appropriate prophylaxis for thromboembolism with warfarin,[24] and aggressive maximization of bone density because osteoporosis is an increasingly recognized clinical problem for patients on chronic steroids.[1] Optimization of nutrition and high-intensity pulmonary rehabilitation for awaiting patients should be implemented. Finally, psychosocial issues also need to be addressed during this time period, with referral for supportive counseling, support groups, and other training means to help each patient cope with the upcoming challenges.

Disease-specific issues in patients awaiting heart–lung transplantation also need to be addressed. These patients require optimum treatment of their heart failure with standard therapeutic measures such as sodium restriction, aggressive diuresis, and vasodilators. Afterload reduction with nitrates, hydralazine, and angiotensin-converting enzyme inhibitors prolong survival while awaiting transplantation.[14] In patients with PPH, supplemental oxygen is recommended to avoid hypoxic pulmonary vasoconstriction. Indications for outpatient oxygen therapy include an arterial partial pressure of oxygen ($Pa{O_2}$) of 55 mm Hg or less (or arterial oxygen saturation [$Sa{O_2}$] less than 88% on room air) at rest, during exertion, or while asleep.[66] The prognosis of PPH is determined by hemodynamic variables, with the following parameters associated with a poor outcome: increased mean pulmonary artery pressure (mPAP >85 mm Hg, median survival 12 months), increased mean right atrial pressure (RAP >20 mm Hg, median survival 1 month), and decreased cardiac index (CI <2.0 liters/min/m^2, median survival 17 months).[17] In addition to supplemental oxygen therapy, initiation of pulmonary vasodilator therapy improves the hemodynamics and survival while awaiting transplantation. Epoprostenol (Flolan) is a short-acting prostaglandin released normally by the endothelium that vasodilates the pulmonary vascular bed and inhibits platelet aggregation. Continuous infusion of epoprostenol has been demonstrated to significantly improve pulmonary hemodynamics, exercise capacity, and survival in patients with NYHA III and IV heart failure.[9,83] Patients may then be put on hold for transplant. Despite the improvement in pulmonary hemodynamics and survival, many patients' disease will progress, or they will develop tachyphylaxis. Therefore patients need to be followed closely and reactivated if any clinical deterioration is noted. Other interventions that may need to be considered in the setting of right ventricular failure in patients awaiting transplantation include creation of an interatrial shunt to decompress the pressure-overloaded ventricle.[44]

Patients with cystic fibrosis awaiting heart–lung transplantation have special needs. Pulmonary hygiene is of critical importance, given that more than 80% of patients are chronically colonized with *Pseudomonas aeruginosa*.[23] Pulmonary clearance techniques, institution of bronchodilators, and initiation of antibiotics in the setting of acute infection are lifelong requirements. Prophylactic antibiotics are not routinely given because of the development of multiresistant organisms.[75] Sinus disease and the predisposing risk of lower respiratory tract infections are risks in most patients with cystic fibrosis. Bilateral maxillary sinus antrostomies performed in the pretransplant period has resulted in fewer infectious complications in the posttransplant period.[53] In addition to infectious issues, other associated risk factors such as malnutrition secondary to malabsorption, pancreatic insufficiency, and diabetes mellitus need to be properly addressed.

SELECTION AND MANAGEMENT OF DONORS

The satisfactory criteria for heart–lung blocks are similar to those for hearts and lungs separately (Box 95-1). The lungs are the most delicate solid organ, with frequent parenchymal damage and neurogenic edema occurring after brain death, as well as the increased risk of aspiration. These factors result in only 10–20% of multiorgan donors with lungs suitable for donation. Preliminary donor evaluation includes a detailed history, review of electrocardiogram and echocardiogram, chest film, and arterial blood gas analysis. A donor age of less than 40 is preferred. However, potential donors aged 40 to 50 years may be considered at most transplant centers, provided they have normal cardiopulmonary functioning and a normal coronary arteriogram. Acceptance criteria also include no significant lung contusion or history of aspiration or sepsis. There should be no history of prior cardiac or pulmonary surgery. A donor chest film must be clear with no signs of pathology. An arterial blood gas analysis should reveal an arterial oxygen tension level greater than 350 mm Hg on a fractional inspired oxygen concentration ($FI{O_2}$) of 100%, and 100 mm Hg on an FIO_2 of 30%. Lung compliance is estimated by measuring peak inspiratory pressures, which should not exceed 30 cm H_2O. Tracheobronchial infection must be excluded with chest radiography, sputum Gram stain, and bronchoscopy. Finally, donor–recipient cardiopulmonary size matching must be established as outlined in the preceding.

Upon arrival at the donor hospital, the retrieval team assesses the chest film, recent arterial blood gas analyses, and hemodynamic parameters to confirm that there has been no deterioration in oxygenation or cardiac function. If possible, the bronchoscopic examination is repeated to ensure that there are no mucopurulent secretions suggestive of infection or aspiration, as in tracheobronchitis. Finally, visual and manual intraoperative assessment of the heart and lungs, confirming normal lung parenchyma with no palpable masses or evidence of contusion, is the final assessment.

Given the growing waiting lists and increased mortality before receiving a transplant, most centers have expanded their donor acceptance criteria with increased utilization of so-called marginal donors.[114] Thoracic trauma with a resultant pneumothorax is not a contraindication, provided there is not a continuous air leak. Furthermore, lungs that are mildly contused also can be used, provided there is not ongoing bleeding noted on bronchoscopy or major atelectasis. Prolonged intubation and ventilation greater than 70 hours, once thought to be a contraindication, also should be considered. As noted previously, older donors also are being considered, provided pulmonary functional parameters are normal and there is no significant coronary artery disease. Donors infected with hepatitis C virus are an evolv-

Box 95–1. Heart–Lung Donor Selection Criteria.

Age <40
Smoking history less than 20 pack years
Arterial Po_2 of 140 mm Hg on an FIo_2 of 40% or 350 mm Hg on an FIo_2 of 100%
Normal chest X-ray
Sputum free of bacteria, fungus, or significant numbers of white blood cells on Gram and fungal staining
Bronchoscopy showing absence of purulent secretions or signs of aspiration
Absence of thoracic trauma
HIV-negative status

ing area in cardiopulmonary transplantation. Hepatitis C–negative recipients have an increased risk of acquiring hepatitis, but the effect on patient survival remains unclear.[72] Absolute contraindications include severe coronary or structural heart disease, prolonged cardiac arrest, active malignancy (sometimes excluding primary brain cancers such as astrocytoma and skin cancers), positive smoking history of greater than 5 pack years, and positive human immunodeficiency virus (HIV) status.

Donor management after the declaration of brain death has evolved into a critical area where the opportunity exists for significantly improving the number and quality of potential donors. Aggressive management strategies implemented by organ procurement organizations (OPOs) make "unacceptable" lungs, defined as a Pao_2:FIo_2 ratio of less than 150, acceptable for transplant.[100] These "unacceptable" donors were treated with invasive monitoring, methylprednisolone, fluid restriction, inotropic agents, bronchoscopy, and diuresis. The resultant "acceptable" organs were successfully transplanted without compromise of either 30-day or 1-year graft survival.[100] The major goal in the initial management of these donors is the maintenance of hemodynamic stability and pulmonary function. Patients who have suffered an acute brain injury are usually hypovolemic, and appropriate fluid resuscitation is the initial step. Complicating factors include the development of diabetes insipidus, which should be treated with a vasopressin infusion (0.1–0.4 U/h).[39] Fluid administration is guided by the central venous pressure (CVP), keeping in mind that a CVP of greater than 8 mm Hg has been demonstrated to be an independent risk factor for the development of lung dysfunction.[71] Inotropic agents such as dopamine or phenylephrine are instituted to maintain perfusion pressure after intravascular volume has been repleted. The donor is not hyperventilated after brain death is declared, and a pH of 7.40 is the goal, thus avoiding pulmonary vasoconstriction. Positive end-expiratory pressure of 5 is maintained to prevent atelectasis, and higher levels are avoided, given the deleterious effect on cardiac output.

The pathophysiology of brain death and its deleterious effect on the cardiovascular system have been well described.[116] The resultant endocrine and metabolic derangements are a potential area of intervention in the marginal donor with hemodynamic instability. Hormonal therapy, including triiodothyronine (T_3), cortisol, insulin, and vasopressin, has been demonstrated to have beneficial effects on the hemodynamic profile of marginal donors.[65] Physiological resuscitation, guided by a better understanding of the pathophysiology of brain death, ultimately leads to increased number and quality of heart–lung donors.

HEART–LUNG PRESERVATION

The goal of optimum heart–lung preservation is to ameliorate the effect of ischemia–reperfusion (IR) injury on the allograft. In the initial heart–lung transplants, donor transportation to the transplant center with on-site procurement was considered essential because of a lack of confidence in lung preservation techniques. As with heart transplantation, better preservation techniques would expand the pool of available donors and would make donation more acceptable to referring hospitals and donors' families.

Minimization of IR injury ultimately results in optimization of allograft function in the posttransplantation period. "Nonspecific graft failure," which most likely represents IR injury, remains a significant cause of perioperative morbidity and possibly mortality.[18] Reperfusion injury may predispose to an increased risk of acute rejection secondary to the upregulation of histocompatibility class II antigens.[90] Understanding the pathophysiology of IR injury allows the implementation of strategies aimed at preserving function, minimizing injury, and prolonging allograft and patient survival.

The result of inadequate preservation is activation of the inflammatory cascade, resulting in pulmonary endothelial injury and increased capillary permeability. The resulting pulmonary interstitial and alveolar edema leads to diminished airway compliance, poor gas exchange, and increased pulmonary vascular resistance. Numerous recent studies have elucidated the role of the neutrophil and its interaction with the pulmonary endothelium in the pathogenesis of IR injury.[21,45,52] Reperfusion injury is caused in part by a complex interplay between leukocyte activation and subsequent release of inflammatory mediators and cytokines, with a final common pathway of pulmonary endothelial injury.

Since the early 1980s, various methods were developed to provide adequate preservation. These have varied from simple graft excision and cold storage to sophisticated auto perfusion with donor blood and a working heart–lung preparation. Today only the following two methods are actively employed: (1) perfusion with pulmonoplegia solutions and cold storage and (2) perfusion with cold donor blood, with both methods using pulmonary vasodilators. Pulmonary artery flush is the most widely adopted method of allograft preservation.[6] Pulmonary artery flush technique allows for rapid cooling of both lungs, with a significant improvement in allograft function noted after both the infusion rate (4 min) and total volume (60 ml/kg) were increased.[33] To counteract the reflex pulmonary vasoconstriction arising from preservation solutions, donors are pretreated with prostaglandins. These selective pulmonary vasodilators, alprostadil in North America and epoprostenol in Europe, improve the distribution of the pulmonary arterial flush and thus improve lung preservation. The role of retrograde flush through the left atrium also has been recently advanced, given the improved distribution of the flush in a porcine model.[110,111]

There are two types of crystalloid pulmonary artery flush solutions, intracellular and extracellular, both of which are designed to counteract the cellular swelling resulting from graft ischemia and hypothermia. The intracellular solutions, Euro-Collins (EC) and University of Wisconsin, are composed of electrolytes that mimic the intracellular environment. The extracellular solutions include the Wallwork solution, which uses donor blood, and low-potassium dextran (Perfadex). The most commonly used preservation solution is EC crystalloid solution, which has been modified with magnesium sulfate and 50% dextrose. A recent study has demonstrated that lung procurement with low-potassium dextran resulted in a significantly decreased incidence and severity of reperfusion injury with improved allograft function, as well as improved survival, when compared with EC.[63]

Recent investigations in the laboratory and clinic have demonstrated improvements in allograft preservation by modification of the pulmonary arterial flush solutions. The focus has been to intervene at the level of the leukocyte–endothelial interaction in an effort to preserve the function of the pulmonary endothelial cell. The impact of toxic inflammatory mediators elaborated by the leukocyte has been reduced by techniques such as leukocyte filtration,[51] introduction of monoclonal antibodies directed against antiintercellular adhesion molecules and selectins,[21,52,87] and vascular immunotargeting strategies.[45] Furthermore, treatments aimed at preserving pulmonary endothelial function by restoring endothelial-derived mediators such as nitric oxide and prostacyclin have been demonstrated to improve allograft pulmonary function.[41,64,86,105] Clearly these multiple avenues for the prevention of reperfusion injury in the pulmonary allograft illustrate that further changes in our current preservation scheme are forthcoming.

OPERATIVE TECHNIQUE FOR DONOR HEART–LUNG REMOVAL

In the early days of heart–lung transplantation, the donor was transported to the recipient hospital, and in an adjacent operating room, the recipient heart–lung block was excised simultaneously with donor organ preparation. Long-distance procurement is now the rule, given the improvements in donor selection, donor management, and preservation techniques. With numerous procurement teams working together, optimal communication is essential.

The donor operation is performed via a median sternotomy (Figure 95-3). The pericardium is opened vertically and laterally on the diaphragm and a pericardial cradle created. Both pleural spaces are then opened with inspection of both lungs and pleural spaces. In cases of trauma, cardiac and pulmonary contusions are immediately ruled out. The pulmonary ligaments are then divided inferiorly using electrocautery. The ascending aorta and aortic arch are dissected free and encircled with tapes. The superior and inferior venae cavae are then dissected free and also encircled with tapes. The azygos and innominate vein are ligated and divided which affords excellent exposure to the proximal trachea. The pericardium overlying the proximal trachea is incised vertically and encircled with a tape. Dissection of the distal trachea is kept to a minimum to avoid injury to the bronchial vessels at the carina.

The patient is administered 300 U/kg of IV heparin, and the aorta and pulmonary artery are cannulated. Approximately 15 minutes before applying the aortic cross-clamp, prostaglandin E_1 (PGE_1) is infused intravenously, initially at a rate of 20 ng/kg/min, and gradually increasing to a target rate of 100 ng/kg/min. During PGE_1 infusion, the mean arterial blood pressure should be maintained above 55 mm Hg. Inflow occlusion is accomplished by ligating the superior vena cava distally to avoid damage to the sinoatrial node. The inferior vena cava is clamped with a straight Potts clamp. The heart is allowed to empty, and the aortic cross-clamp is applied. Cold crystalloid cardioplegia (10 ml/kg) is administered via the aortic root. The inferior vena cava is incised, and the left atrial appendage is amputated immediately after initiating the pulmonoplegia, being mindful to ensure adequate venting and avoidance of cardiac distension. Pulmonoplegia with an EC solution at 4° C is rapidly infused through at a rate of 15 ml/kg/min for 4 minutes. During the administration of cold cardioplegia and pulmonary perfusate, copious amounts of cold topical saline are immediately poured over the heart and lungs. The lungs are ventilated with half-normal tidal volumes of room air while the dissection is completed, separating the heart–lung block from the posterior mediastinum from inferior to superior. The lungs are inflated to a three-fourths normal tidal volume, and the trachea is stapled with a TA-55 stapler and divided. The aorta is then divided, and the heart–lung block is removed, wrapped with sterile towels, and immersed in ice-cold saline at 4° C in preparation for transport (see Figure 95-3). Clinically we have used grafts preserved up to 6 hours with successful implantation and outcome.

OPERATIVE PROCEDURE

The operation to replace the heart and lungs is one of the most fascinating and challenging procedures for cardiothoracic surgeons. The anatomy that is seen and the areas of the thorax that are dissected are not commonly seen. Careful attention to details can simplify the procedure in even the most challenging patients.

Patients with PPH with end-stage right ventricular failure are usually the ideal candidates for heart–lung transplantation. These patients generally have not had previous cardiac or thoracic surgery or large mediastinal collaterals from cyanosis. On the other hand, patients with congenital heart disease and pulmonary atresia, or Eisenmenger's syndrome and cyanosis may have large mediastinal bronchial collaterals that require careful ligation. The most challenging aspect of the procedure is to remove the heart and lungs without injury to the phrenic, recurrent laryngeal, and vagus nerves. Careful attention to hemostasis is necessary before implantation of the graft, given that exposure of many of the areas of dissection is difficult.

The recipient procedure for heart–lung transplantation has evolved over the last decade, with two major changes often employed: the conversion from atrial cuff to bicaval anastomoses and the positioning of the pulmonary hila anterior to the phrenic nerve pedicle. The right atrial cuff anas-

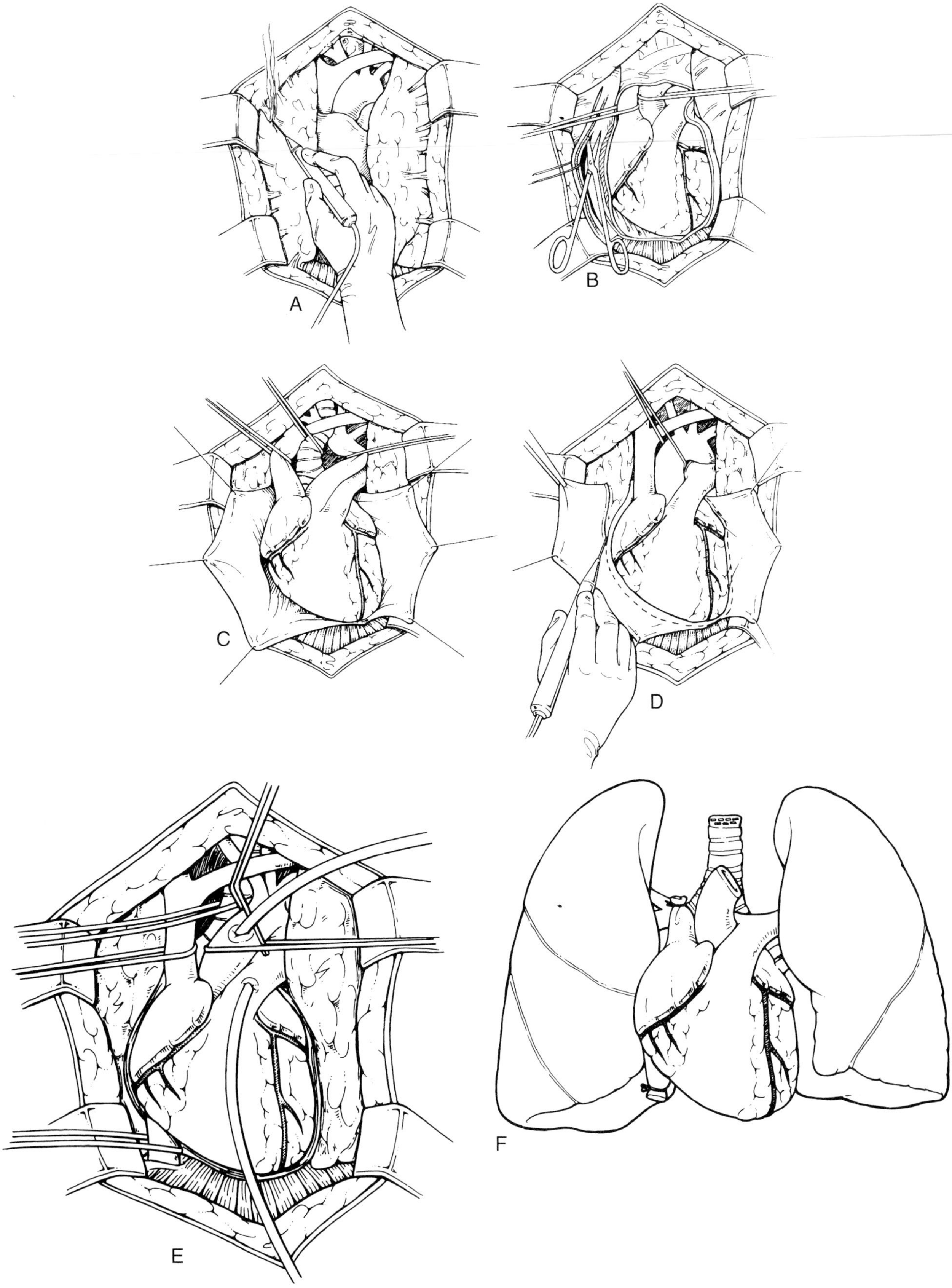

Figure 95–3 The donor operation. A, Through a median sternotomy, adhesions are lysed and the pulmonary ligaments are divided inferiorly. **B,** The pericardium is opened and cradled, followed by dissection of the ascending aorta, venae cavae, pulmonary artery, and trachea. **C,** Tapes are placed around the aorta, venae cavae, and trachea. **D,** The entire anterior pericardium is excised back to each hilum. **E,** Cardioplegia and pulmonoplegia are infused simultaneously into the aorta and main pulmonary artery after aortic cross-clamping. Application of topical cold Physiosol follows immediately. **F,** The venae cavae and aorta are divided, and the heart–lung block is dissected free from the esophagus and posterior hilar attachments. After the trachea is stapled and divided at the highest point possible, the entire heart–lung block is removed from the chest.
(From Yuh DD, Robbins RC, Reitz BA: Transplantation of the heart and lungs. In Edmunds LH, editor: Cardiac Surgery in the Adult, 1st ed., pp.1451–1475. New York: McGraw-Hill, Inc., 1997.)

tomosis initially was proposed in heart–lung transplantation to facilitate cannulation for cardiopulmonary bypass and eliminate the possibility of stenoses at the vena caval anastomoses. As in heart transplant alone, asynchronous contraction of both atrial cuffs is associated with increased incidence of atrioventricular valve regurgitation. Fewer postoperative arrhythmias also have been demonstrated as a clinical benefit.[60] Because the pulmonary hila are positioned anterior to the phrenic nerve pedicle, less posterior mediastinal dissection is required, resulting in decreased rates of phrenic and vagus nerve injury.[54] Another advantage to this technique is that it allows easier inspection of the posterior mediastinum for bleeding by rotation of the heart–lung block anteriorly and medially while still on cardiopulmonary bypass.

The patient is prepared for operation with the usual monitoring lines. After the induction of general anesthesia, the chest and both groins are prepared and draped in a sterile manner. A standard median sternotomy incision is made, and both pleural spaces are opened anteriorly (Figure 95-4). A portion of the pericardium is removed anteriorly, as well as much as 1.5 cm of the phrenic nerves. The ascending aorta and both venae cavae are dissected free and encircled with tapes. After fully heparinizing the recipient, the high ascending aorta and both venae cavae are cannulated separately, cardiopulmonary bypass instituted, and the patient cooled to 28° C. The aorta is cross-clamped, and a small amount of cardioplegia *may be* given to induce cardiac arrest.

The heart is excised first as in heart transplantation. Next, the lungs are removed sequentially. The right and left bronchi are skeletonized, and a stapling device (TA 30–4.8 mm) is used to occlude them. Cutting the bronchus distally allows the lung to be removed easily and avoids contamination from the open bronchus.

The native main pulmonary artery remnant is then removed. A portion of the pulmonary artery is left intact adjacent to the underside of the aorta in the region of the ligamentum arteriosum, which minimizes damage to the recurrent laryngeal nerve. The final step in the preparing the recipient is to open the pericardium at the superior part of the pericardial space just anterior to the right and left bronchi, allowing dissection back to the carina. The stapled ends of the right and left bronchi are grasped, and dissection is carried up to the level of the distal trachea. In this area it is important to stay directly on the bronchus, use electrocautery if possible, and avoid injury to the vagus nerve as it passes posterior to the bronchus and anterior to the esophagus. The vascular lymph nodes in this area may be very large, particularly in patients with cystic fibrosis. Bronchial vessels are individually identified and ligated or clipped. Patients with secondary pulmonary hypertension from congenital heart disease have large mediastinal bronchial collaterals that must be carefully ligated. Hemostasis is imperative in this area of dissection because exposure to this region is difficult after transplantation of the heart–lung block. The chest wall also is carefully inspected, and electrocautery or the argon beam coagulator is employed. After absolute hemostasis is ensured, the donor heart–lung graft is prepared for implantation.

The donor heart–lung block is removed from its sterile container and brought to the operative field in a basin with cold saline solution. The donor trachea is excised several rings above the carina, and the superior tracheal segment, with the clamp attached, is then removed from the field. The tracheobronchial tree is aspirated with a sucker that is later discarded. At the same time, a culture is taken directly from the trachea. The trachea is trimmed back so that only one complete cartilaginous ring is left just above the carina. A syringe full of normal saline is used to irrigate the bronchi and visualize them for retained secretions or any foreign body that might have been aspirated by the donor.

The heart–lung graft is then lowered into the chest with the lung hila anterior to the phrenic nerve pedicles (see Figure 95-4). A cold saline solution and gauze pads soaked in cold saline are placed over the lung and heart to maintain hypothermia during implantation. The recipient trachea is opened one cartilaginous ring above the carina, with all the adventitial peritracheal tissue that is adjacent to the superior tracheal segment left in place. Small bronchial vessels may require a Liga clip or suture; use of electrocautery at the cut edge of the trachea should be avoided. The tracheal anastomosis is performed with a running suture of 3-0 polypropylene, starting on the left side of the trachea and completing the posterior row from the inside. The same suture is continued anteriorly from outside the trachea. There should be a fairly close size match between donor and recipient, but any disparity generally can be accommodated by the flexible membranous part of the trachea. These bites usually go around at least one cartilaginous ring, and the donor trachea slightly invaginates the recipient trachea in most cases. When the tracheal anastomosis is complete, the chest is irrigated with several liters of ice-cold saline solution to cool the graft and to help remove any contamination from the trachea.

The recipient inferior vena cava is then anastomosed to the donor inferior vena cava using a running 4-0 polypropylene suture. At this point the patient is rewarmed toward 37° C, and the superior vena caval and aortic anastomoses are performed in an end-to-end fashion using a continuous 4-0 polypropylene suture (see Figure 95-4). After completion of the aortic anastomosis, the patient is placed in a slightly head-down position, the ascending aorta and pulmonary artery are aspirated for air, and the caval tapes and the aortic cross-clamp are removed. The tracheal tube is aspirated with sterile technique, and ventilation is resumed with room air. The left atrial opening at the appendage is repaired. When the patient's body temperature is almost normal and heart and lung function are satisfactory, cardiopulmonary bypass is discontinued and decannulation is performed routinely. The inspired concentration of oxygen is increased as required. Temporary pacing wires are applied to the donor right atrium and ventricle and brought out through the skin below the incision. Right-angled chest tubes are placed in the right and left pleural spaces, and a straight chest tube is placed in the mediastinum. Methylprednisolone (500 mg) is given to the recipient after heparin reversal with protamine sulfate.

The posterior mediastinum is then inspected for bleeding by carefully rotating the heart–lung block anteriorly and medially while the anesthesiologist uses hand ventilation. This maneuver is facilitated using the most recent modification, where the pulmonary hila are placed anterior to the phrenic nerves. Large amounts of warm saline solution at 37° C are used to irrigate both pleural spaces and the medi-

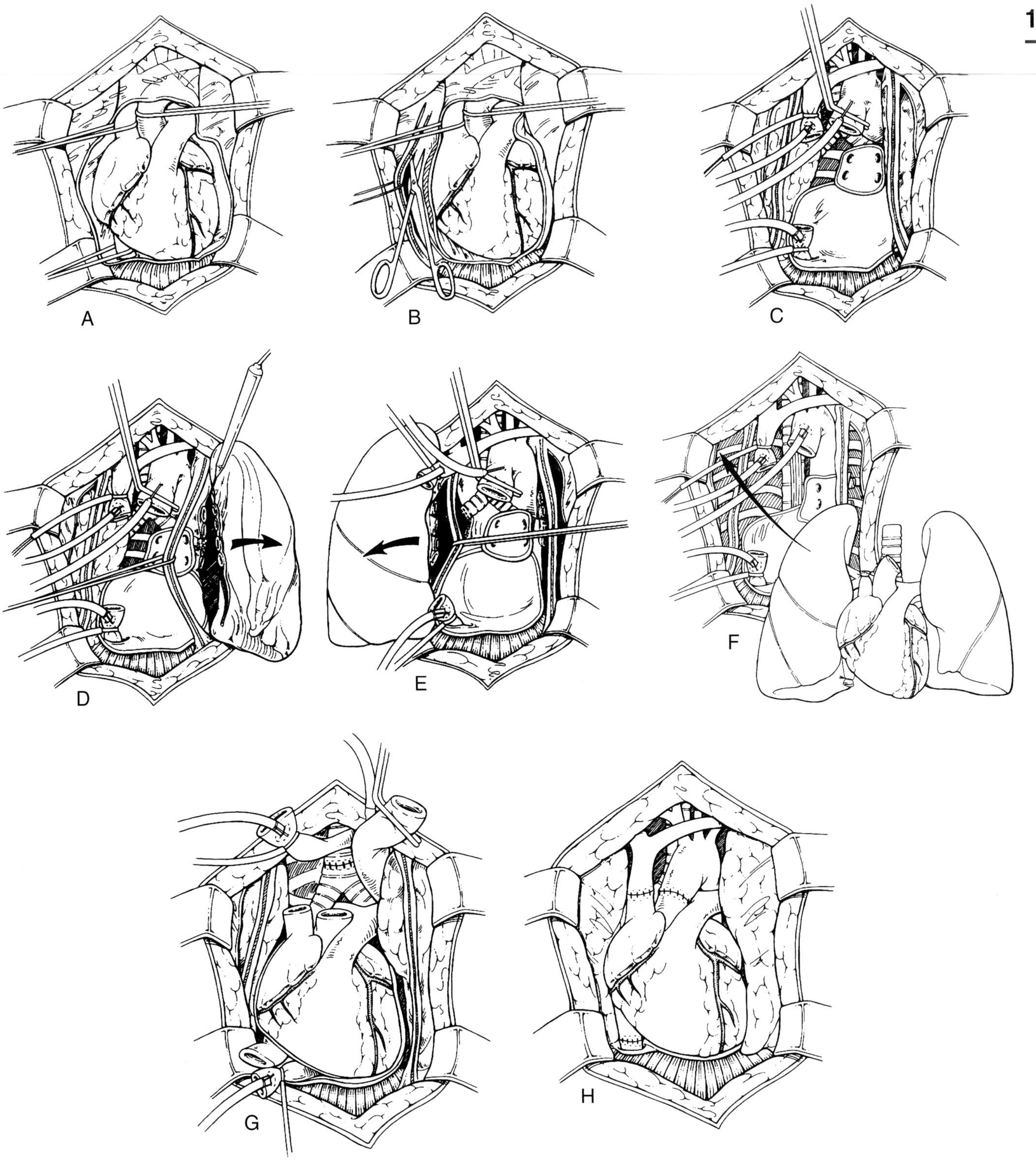

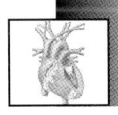

Figure 95–4 The recipient operation. A, Through a median sternotomy, the anterior pericardium is partially removed and the ascending aorta and both venae cavae are dissected and encircled with tapes. **B,** The right phrenic nerve is carefully separated from the right hilum. **C,** Cannulation for cardiopulmonary bypass consists of a cannula in the high ascending aorta and separate vena caval cannulas. Once on bypass, the native heart is excised in a manner similar to that for standard cardiac transplantation. **D–E,** Left and right pneumonectomies are performed by dividing the respective inferior pulmonary ligament, pulmonary artery and veins, and main stem bronchus. **F,** The heart–lung block is lowered into the chest, placing the hila anterior to each respective phrenic nerve pedicle. **G,** The tracheal anastomosis is performed with a continuous 3-0 polypropylene suture. **H,** The caval and aortic anastomoses are performed with a continuous 4-0 polypropylene suture.
(From Yuh DD, Robbins RC, Reitz BA: Transplantation of the heart and lungs. In Edmunds LH, editor: Cardiac Surgery in the Adult, 1st ed., pp.1451-1475. New York: McGraw-Hill, Inc., 1997.)

astinum. When hemostasis is satisfactory, the sternum is closed routinely with multiple stainless steel sternal wires.

POSTOPERATIVE MANAGEMENT

Intensive Care Unit

The immediate postoperative management of the patient undergoing heart–lung transplant is similar to that of any patient after cardiac surgery. Patients are allowed to awaken early in the postoperative course and are monitored closely for hemodynamic stability and bleeding. Endotracheal tube suctioning is performed when appropriate, and the patient is weaned from the ventilator in a routine manner. When the patient is alert and hemodynamically stable and blood gases and ventilatory mechanics are satisfactory, the patient is extubated. Strict attention is paid to fluid balance, and a vigorous diuresis is encouraged in most patients. As soon as possible, the patient is allowed to sit in a chair and begin ambulation. A physical therapist works with the patient to facilitate rapid rehabilitation.

There are several specific points that must be kept in mind when managing heart–lung transplant patients in the immediate postoperative period. Early graft dysfunction, manifested by progressive hypoxemia and hypercapnia, can be present in up to 10–15% of patients.[18] The proposed etiology is IR injury in the transplanted lung. This injury results in increased pulmonary capillary permeability, alveolar edema, impaired pulmonary compliance, and increased pulmonary vascular resistance with right ventricular dysfunction. Graft dysfunction can progress rapidly, and early treatment is essential. Initiation of pulmonary vasodilators such as alprostadil or inhaled nitric oxide (NO) may be necessary. Inhaled NO has been demonstrated to decrease the intrapulmonary shunt, optimizing ventilation–perfusion matching after lung transplantation.[3] In another study, inhaled NO administered in the setting of lung allograft dysfunction doubled the ratio of arterial oxygen tension to inspired oxygen fraction (PaO_2:FIO_2) within 1 hour of administration.[18] Furthermore, a significant reduction in airway complications, duration of mechanical ventilation, and mortality was noted.[18] In cases of persistent, severe pulmonary graft dysfunction refractory to all intervention, extracorporeal membrane oxygenation (ECMO) has been used successfully to stabilize gas exchange in several patients.[92]

Immunosuppression

The immunosuppression regimen for heart–lung transfer recipients includes induction therapy with polyclonal rabbit antithymocyte globulin (RATG) and maintenance therapy with cyclosporine, azathioprine, and prednisone. The protocol employed at Stanford University is depicted in Tables 95-1 and 95-2.

Induction therapy is used based on data showing the incidence of early acute rejection is decreased, as well as chronic rejection and obliterative bronchiolitis (OB).[26,78] Induction therapy is initiated with RATG 1.5 mg/kg IV on postoperative days (PODs) 1, 2, 3, 5, and 7 (see Table 95-1). If the patient is hemodynamically unstable or allograft func-

Table 95–1

Early Postoperative Immunosuppressive Regimen for Heart–Lung Transplant Recipients: Induction Therapy

Methylprednisolone	500 mg IV after engraftment 125 mg IV q8h for 3 doses
Rabbit antithymocyte globulin (RATG)	1.5 mg/kg IV on PODs 1, 2, 3, 5, and 7.
Premedication	Acetaminophen: 650 mg PO Diphenhydramine hydrochloride: 25–50 mg IV Hydrocortisone: 50–100 mg IV

PO, Per os (by mouth); IV, intravenous; POD, postoperative day.

Table 95–2

Early Postoperative Immunosuppressive Regimen for Heart–Lung Transplant Recipients: Maintenance Therapy

Cyclosporine	Start with 25 mg PO bid on POD 1, then titrate to 2–5 mg/kg/day in 2 divided doses to achieve target level, or use continuous IV infusion at one third the oral daily dose
Serum blood levels	
0–3 months	175–200 ng/ml
3–6 months	150–175 ng/ml
6–12 months	125–150 ng/ml
>12 months	125–150 ng/ml or less based on renal function, lymphoproliferative disorder, rejection history, drug interaction
Azathioprine	2 mg/kg/day PO or IV (start on POD 1 titrate to maintain white blood cell count >4000 mm³
Steroids	0.6 mg/kg/day in 2 divided doses beginning on POD 8 Wean to 0.2 mg/kg/day in 4–6 weeks

PO, per os (by mouth); bid, twice a day; IV, intravenous; POD, postoperative day.

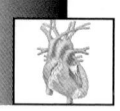

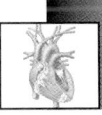

tion is compromised from reperfusion injury, RATG dosing is delayed for several days. From 1987 to 1993, induction therapy at Stanford University was switched from RATG to OKT3, the murine monoclonal antibody directed specifically against the T-cell (CD3) receptor. However, a greater incidence of acute pulmonary allograft rejection, postoperative infection, and OB was later demonstrated.[80] These findings resulted in a switch back to the polyclonal anti–T-cell antibody for induction therapy.

Methylprednisolone (500 mg IV) is administered intraoperatively and continued postoperatively at a dose of 125 mg IV every 8 hours for three doses. Maintenance prednisone is withheld for 1 week. Steroids are then restarted on POD 8 with a daily divided oral dose of prednisone 0.6 mg/kg, gradually tapered over the next 3–4 weeks to 0.1–0.2 mg/kg/day. The risk of airway complications after transplantation is not adversely affected by the use of postoperative steroids.[19]

In addition to steroids, maintenance immunosuppressive therapy includes azathioprine and cyclosporine. Azathioprine is initiated on POD 1 with a single evening dose of 2 mg/kg. The dose is titrated to maintain the leukocyte count greater than 4000 mm^3. Cyclosporine is also initiated on POD 1 and titrated slowly based on trough levels, with the goal of achieving therapeutic levels on the fifth postoperative day. This strategy avoids high serum levels and prevents the risk of nephrotoxicity. Patients who are unable to tolerate oral intake secondary to prolonged intubation or malabsorption are administered one third of the calculated total dose intravenously in a continuous manner.

Despite the fact that this immunosuppressive regimen has served heart–lung transplantation well, high rates of acute allograft rejection, infection, and chronic rejection, primarily manifested as OB, still exist. The quest for more efficacious and less toxic immunosuppressive regimens is a continual investigative challenge. Recent studies have suggested that conversion from cyclosporine to tacrolimus may prevent the progression of OB.[58] Mycophenolate mofetil has been demonstrated to have antiproliferative effects on T and B cells by inhibition of de novo purine biosynthesis with improved efficacy and reduced toxicity.[76] In addition, newer T-cell inhibitory agents such as sirolimus (rapamycin), which specifically block smooth cell proliferation, can potentially prevent both acute rejection and the manifestations of chronic rejection, also with less toxic side effects.[32,95]

COMPLICATIONS

Acute Rejection

The fine balance between adequate immunosuppression and the risk of infection and rejection remains one of the most difficult problems facing heart–lung transplantation, as with any lung transplant. The detection of acute rejection is rare in the first postoperative week, and the majority of episodes occur within the first year after transplantation. The diagnosis of acute rejection in the early posttransplant period is usually based on clinical parameters manifested by lung allograft dysfunction. Signs of acute rejection include dyspnea, low-grade fever, impaired oxygenation and ventilatory parameters, including a diminished forced expiratory volume in 1 second (FEV_1), and diffuse interstitial infiltrates on chest film (Figure 95-5).[37] Acute cellular rejection during the first month is associated with an infiltrate on chest radiograph in 75% of cases. After the first month, however, the chest film is normal or without change in 80% of patients.[61,74] The role of other modalities such as spirometry, computed tomography, and bronchoscopy with transbronchial biopsy (TBB) become increasingly important.

Given that acute allograft rejection in the early postoperative period is the single most significant risk factor for the development of subsequent OB, the role of surveillance modalities in detecting and treating early rejection become critical in the prevention of chronic rejection and the improvement in survival. Spirometric surveillance has been shown to be a reasonable screening tool for acute rejection. FEV_1 and forced expiratory flow rate 25–75% of vital capacity ($FEF_{25-75\%}$), were noted to be decreased during episodes of acute rejection, with $FEF_{25-75\%}$ being the best parameter to distinguish acute rejection from infection.[98] Given some lack of sensitivity and specificity of spirometric surveillance, however, TBB remains the gold standard for detection of rejection.

In heart–lung transplantation, the incidence of simultaneous rejection of both the heart and lung is rare,[99] and endomyocardial biopsy does not help diagnose acute lung rejection.[7] Furthermore, histological assessment by TBB is superior to cardiac biopsies because cardiac rejection is very rare without lung rejection, and thus the need for routine endomyocardial biopsies has been eliminated.[36] Surveillance bronchoscopy with TBB in heart–lung recipients is routinely performed at 2 and 4 weeks after transplantation and then at 2, 3, 6, and 12 months thereafter or as clinically indicated. At least five TBB specimens that have lung parenchyma are necessary for an adequate specimen.[121] Transbronchial biopsies performed in the setting of clinical symptoms were positive for rejection or infection in 72% of cases.[99] The yield for surveillance biopsies after 1 year in asymptomatic patients, however, is very low.[25] Late postoperative biopsies are therefore guided by clinical parameters, with any deterioration in pulmonary function leading to further evaluation.

A working formulation for the histological classification of pulmonary allograft rejection by The Lung Rejection Study Group of the ISHLT is presented in Table 95-3.[121] Rejection episodes occurring within the first 3 months, or those graded as moderate or severe (Figure 95-6), are treated with IV methylprednisolone at a dose of 1000 mg/day for 3 consecutive days, followed by an increased oral maintenance dose of 0.6 mg/kg/day, tapered to 0.2 mg/kg/day over 3–4 weeks. Both the chest radiograph and clinical symptoms usually improve rapidly after the initiation of pulse steroid therapy. In milder cases of rejection, or in those cases occurring after 3 months, treatment consists of increased oral prednisone, followed by a gradual taper over 3–4 weeks. Patients with steroid-resistant or persistent allograft rejection are treated with either monoclonal (OKT3) or polyclonal (RATG) antilymphocyte therapy. Other potential treatments in refractory and recurrent cases include switching to mycophenolate mofetil, rapamycin, or tacrolimus, as well as methotrexate, total lymphoid irradiation, or extracorporeal photochemotherapy.[4,12,81,109]

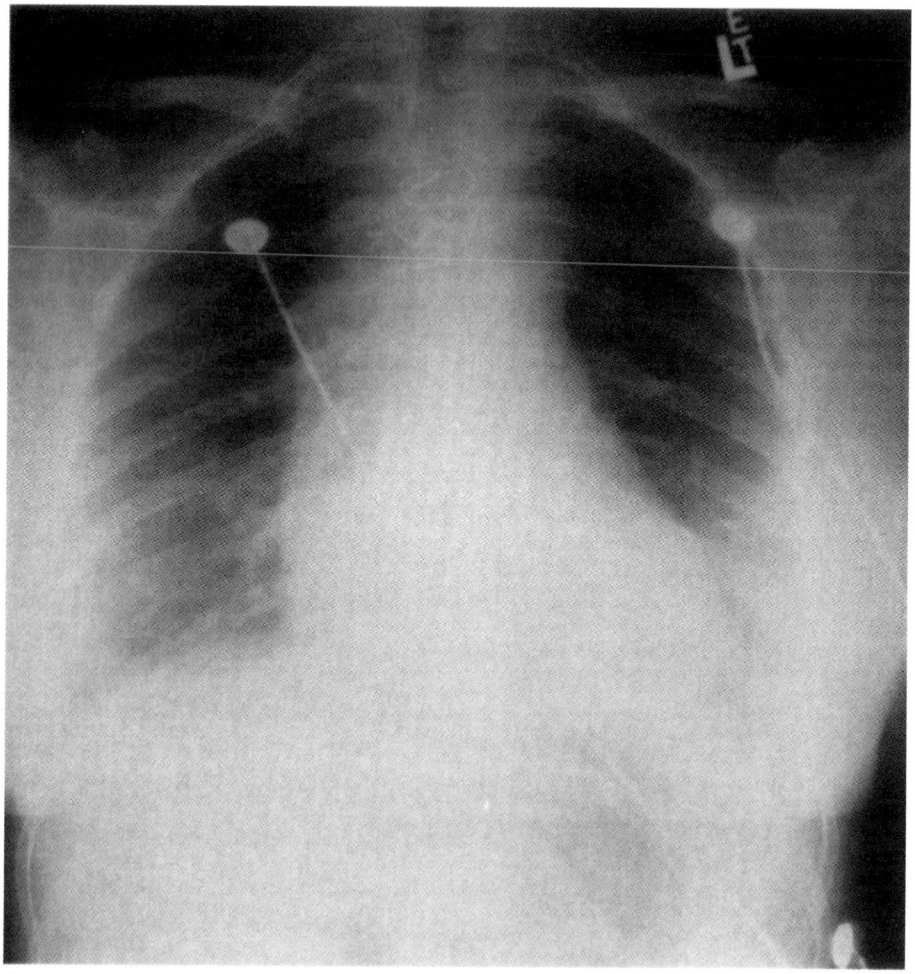

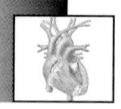

Figure 95–5 **Acute and resolving lung rejection. A,** Chest X-ray illustrates bilateral infiltrates characteristic of acute pulmonary rejection.

Infection

Infectious complications remain a significant cause of morbidity and mortality in heart–lung recipients. The spectrum of potential pathogens is extensive, yet some common patterns can be appreciated. Early postoperatively, bacterial infections are most prevalent, with the highest incidence noted in the first month after heart–lung transplantation.[46] Bacterial infections can manifest as pneumonia, mediastinitis, line sepsis, urinary tract infections, and skin infections. Gram-negative bacilli are the most common bacterial pathogens. Late after transplant, opportunistic pathogens such as viral, fungal, and protozoan species are more common.

Cytomegalovirus (CMV) is the most common viral pathogen in heart–lung transplants. CMV has been associated with pneumonitis in up to 50% of patients and is associated with an increased incidence of chronic rejection manifested as accelerated graft coronary artery disease and OB.[27,97] In addition to pneumonia, CMV infection can have presenting symptoms such as leukopenia and fever, gastroenteritis, hepatitis, and retinitis. CMV events occur within the first 12 months, with the majority becoming manifest within the first 3 months. Individuals at greatest risk of serious infections are seronegative recipients (R−) receiving a heart–lung block from a seropositive donor (D+), with an incidence of 90%. The incidence falls to 10% in recipients who are CMV-negative and receive a donor who is also negative. The diagnosis of CMV disease (symptomatic) or CMV infection (without symptoms) is established by several means: seroconversion from anti-CMV immunoglobulin M (IgM) negative to positive; a 4× rise in CMV immunoglobulin G (IgG) antibody titers; positive viral cultures from urine, blood, or dimercaprol (BAL); or CMV inclusion bodies on transbronchial biopsy.

Most transplant centers perform transplants across CMV serological barriers, implementing prophylactic measures in high-risk patients (D+R−). These patients receive prophylaxis with CMV γ-hyperimmunoglobulin (Cytogam) in addition to ganciclovir (DHPG).[118] This combination regimen resulted in a significant decrease in both CMV disease and CMV infection when compared with ganciclovir alone.[106] The protocol at Stanford University is to administer ganciclovir 5 mg/kg IV twice a day for 14 days, then 6 mg/kg once a day for 20 days. After DHPG, valcyte (valganciclovir) 900 mg is initiated for 6 weeks after transplant. Cytogam is given at a dose of 150 mg/kg IV within the first 72 hours after transplantation and then continued at a dose of 100 mg/kg at 2, 4, 6, and 8 weeks, followed by 50 mg/kg at weeks 12 and 16 after transplant.

Fungal organisms are the least frequent pathogens, yet these infections are associated with the greatest mortality. Fungal infections after lung, heart–lung, and heart trans-

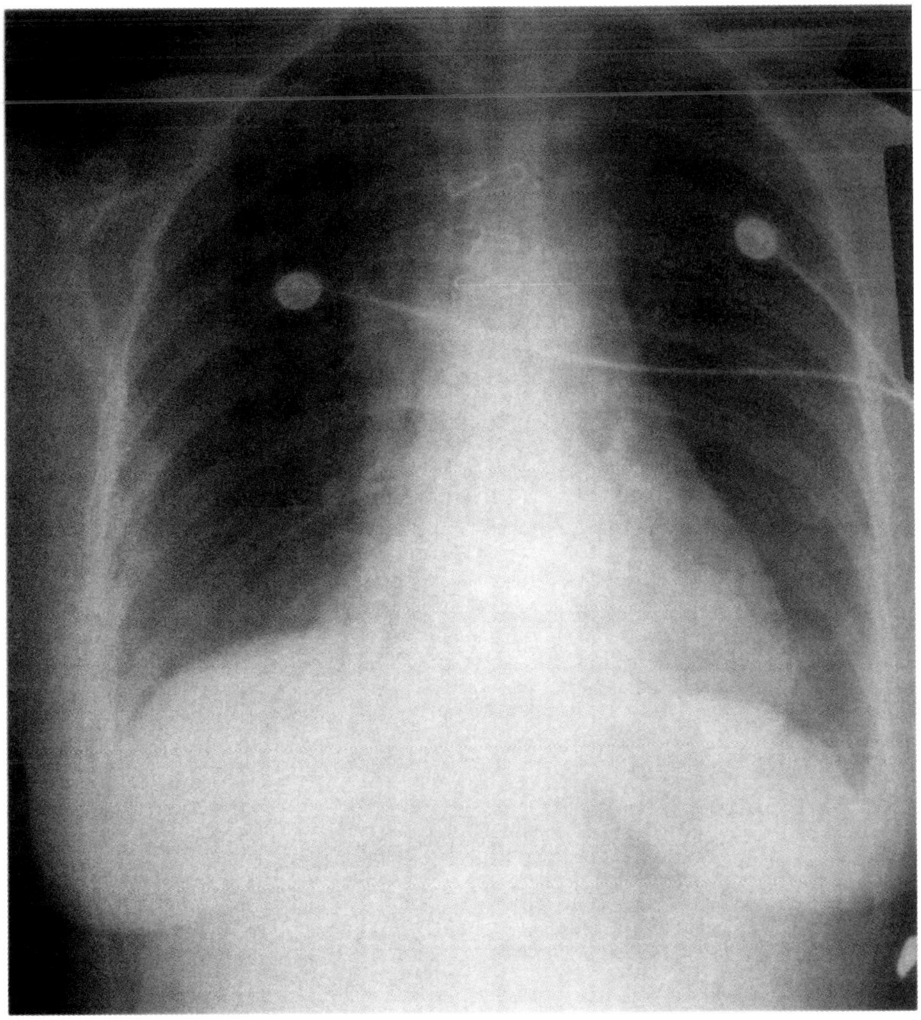
B

Figure 95–5 cont'd (**B**) Follow-up chest X-ray after pulsed methylprednisolone treatment of acute rejection demonstrating resolution of infiltrates. *(From Yuh DD, Robbins RC, Reitz BA: Transplantation of the Heart and Lungs. In Edmunds LH, editor: Cardiac Surgery in the Adult, 1st ed., pp.1451-1475. New York: McGraw-Hill, Inc., 1997.)*

plantation can be significantly lowered by prophylaxis with aerosolized amphotericin B.[77] Inhaled treatments with amphotericin B have been shown to decrease the rate of fungal infections at 3 months from 0.8 to 0.2, and the incidence fell twofold at 12 months when compared with a group that did not receive the inhaled treatment.[77] Bronchodilators are administered prophylactically before treatment to reduce bronchospasm. Fungal infections, diagnosed by sputum culture or computed tomography (CT) guided needle aspirate, are aggressively treated with IV amphotericin B administration.

Pneumocystis carinii pneumonia has been effectively prevented in heart–lung recipients since the initiation of prophylaxis with combination sulfamethoxazole and trimethoprim.[48] The dose of sulfamethoxazole and trimethoprim is 800 mg and 160 mg, respectively, twice daily, 3 days per week, adjusting the dose for renal insufficiency. If patients have a sulfur allergy or develop leukopenia, inhaled pentamidine (300 mg) is initiated once a month. *Toxoplasma gondii*–negative recipients receiving a seropositive donor are treated with a 6-week course of pyrimethamine 25 mg every day and leucovorin 10 mg every day. In addition, long-term prophylaxis typically includes clotrimazole (Mycelex Troches) for prevention of mucosal *Candida* infections.

Chronic Rejection—Obliterative Bronchiolitis

The main cause of long-term morbidity and mortality after heart–lung transplantation remains chronic rejection, primarily manifested as OB. The clinical diagnoses of bronchiolitis obliterans syndrome (BOS) and the pathological diagnoses of OB were defined in the working formulation by the ISHLT.[16] Bronchiolitis obliterans syndrome does not require histological diagnoses and is defined as a deterioration of graft function secondary to progressive airways disease. One must exclude other potential etiologies such as acute rejection and infection before diagnosing BOS. The clinical manifestations of BOS include a dry cough and progressive dyspnea. Interstitial pulmonary infiltrates are seen on chest film, and an obstructive pattern is seen on pulmonary function tests. Bronchiolitis obliterans syndrome can be staged, based on the deterioration of FEV_1 (Table 95-4).[16] OB, on the other hand, is a histological diagnoses based on the presence of eosinophilic fibrous scarring of the membranous and respiratory bronchioles with partial or complete obliteration of the lumen (Figure 95-7).[120]

The overall incidence of BOS/OB at 5 years after heart–lung transplantation, as reported by the ISHLT Registry, was approximately 48% (Figure 95-8).[104] Significant

Table 95–3

Working Formulation for Classification and Grading of Pulmonary Allograft Rejection

Grade	*Classification*	*Histological appearance (transbronchial biopsy)*
A	**Acute rejection**	
A0	Normal pulmonary parenchyma	Absence of an inflammatory infiltrate
A1	Minimal acute rejection	Rare, scattered perivascular and interstitial mononuclear cell infiltrates that are not obvious at low magnification
A2	Mild acute rejection	Larger, more frequent perivascular mononuclear cell infiltrates evident at low magnification; occasional neutrophils and eosinophils; alveolar septa free of lymphocytic infiltrate; concurrent lymphocytic bronchiolitis (B rejection) is often present
A3	Moderate acute rejection	Dense perivascular and interstitial mononuclear cell infiltrates that extend into the peribronchiolar alveolar septa
A4	Severe acute rejection	Diffuse perivascular, interstitial, and air-space mononuclear cell infiltrates; extend into alveolar septa; alveolar pneumocyte damage is prominent; hemorrhage, necrosis, necrotizing vasculitis also are evident
B	**Acute airway disease**	
B0	No air way inflammation	
B1	Minimal air way inflammation	Rare scattered mononuclear cells in the submucosa of the bronchi or bronchioles
B2	Mild air way inflammation	Circumferential mononuclear cells and occasional eosinophils within the submucosa of bronchi; no significant transepithelial migration of lymphocytes
B3	Moderate air way inflammation	Dense band-like infiltrate of mononuclear cells in the submucosa of bronchi; epithelial cell necrosis; marked lymphocyte transmigration through epithelium
B4	Severe air way inflammation	Dense band-like infiltrate of activated mononuclear cells in bronchi; dissociation of epithelium from basement membrane; epithelial ulceration and necrosis; fibrinopurulent exudates with neutrophils
BX	Ungradable because of sampling or infection	
C	**Chronic airway damage**	
C1	Active bronchiolitis obliterans	Intrabronchiolar and peribronchiolar submucosal mononuclear infiltrate; fibrosis; epithelial damage
C2	Inactive	Dense fibrous scarring without cellular infiltrates in the bronchioles
D	**Chronic vascular rejection**	Fibrointimal thickening of arteries and veins

From Yousem SA, Berry GJ, Cagle PT, et al: Revision of the 1990 working formulation for the classification of pulmonary allograft rejection: Lung Rejection Study Group. J Heart Lung Transplant 15:1–15, 1996.

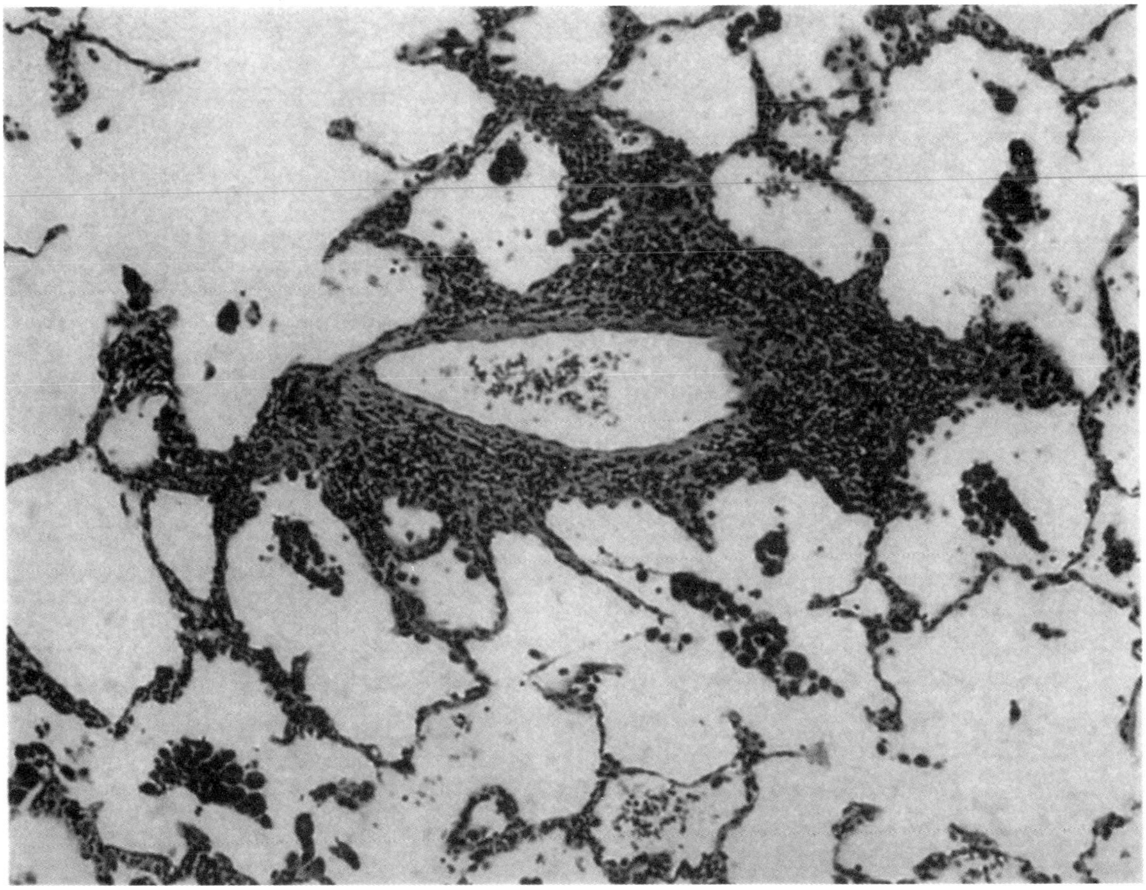

A

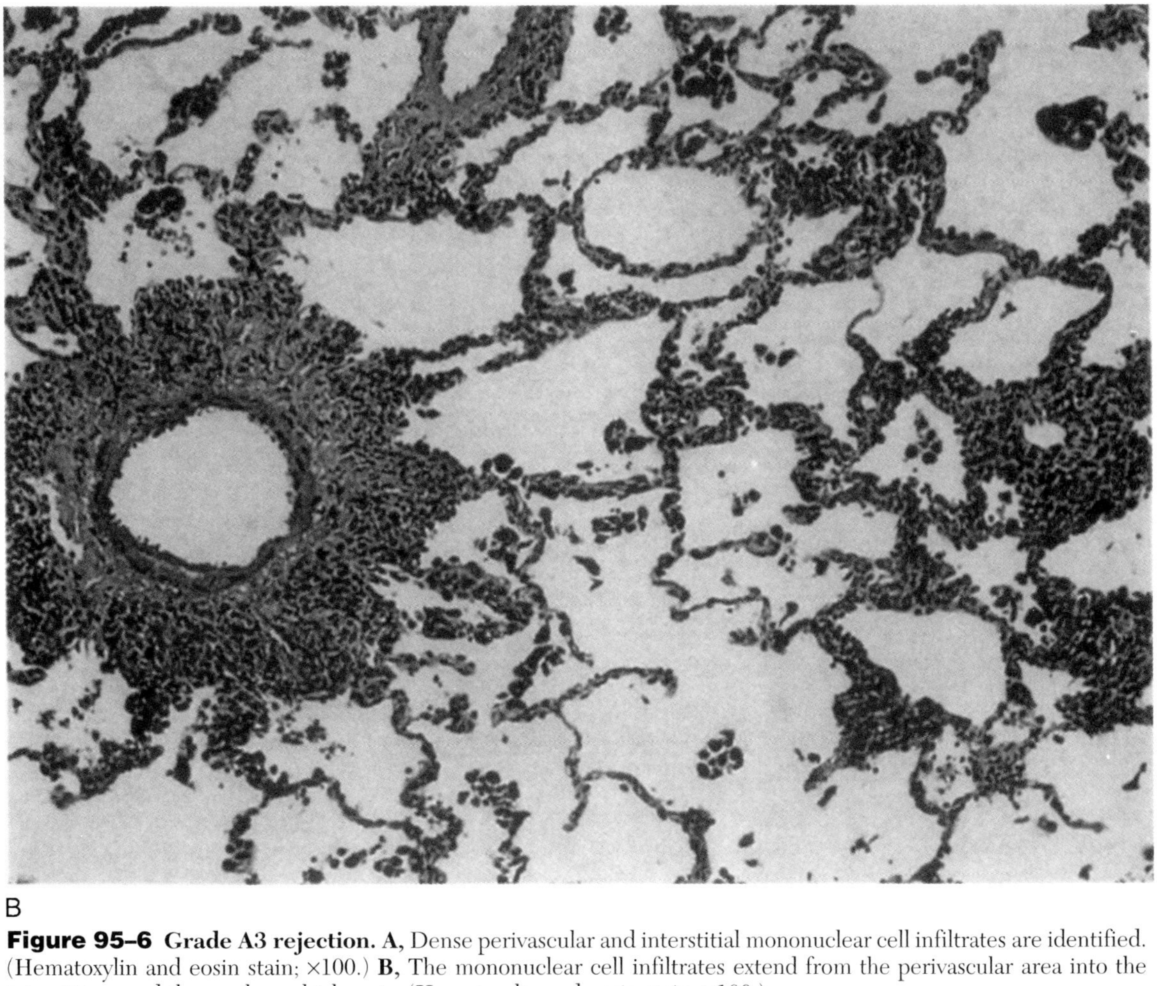

B

Figure 95–6 **Grade A3 rejection. A,** Dense perivascular and interstitial mononuclear cell infiltrates are identified. (Hematoxylin and eosin stain; ×100.) **B,** The mononuclear cell infiltrates extend from the perivascular area into the interstitium and the peribronchial septa. (Hematoxylin and eosin stain; ×100.)

risk factors associated with the development of OB include the frequency and severity of acute rejection, as well as the appearance of lymphocytic bronchiolitis on TBB.[26] Furthermore, organizing pneumonia, as well as CMV infection, significantly potentiates the effects of acute rejection.

A growing body of evidence supports the hypothesis that OB is an immunologically mediated process. In addition to its association with acute rejection, the disease is most commonly found in patients with the greatest degree of HLA mismatch.[30] Patients with OB have an increased number of mismatched major histocompatibility complex (MHC) class II antigens,[122] immunological mediators such as interleukin 2 (IL-2) and interleukin 6 (IL-6) in BAL fluid,[28] as well as a predominance of $CD8^+$ cytotoxic and suppressor cells on TBB.[62] CMV infection may have a stimulatory effect on the immune system that enhances the viral injury.[43] CMV prophylaxis with ganciclovir has been demonstrated to delay the onset of OB.[42] In addition to its immunological stimulus, CMV also has a direct stimulatory effect on the smooth muscle cells of the airways, as well as indirectly via the elaboration of growth factors and mitogenic mediators.[50] Better control of the immune response, prevention of acute rejection, and reducing CMV infection are the best therapy to prevent the incidence of BOS/OB.

For chronic surveillance, patients are provided with a portable spirometer so that expiratory flow can be checked frequently between clinic visits.[67,68] If there is any interval decrease or any signs of respiratory tract infection, the patient is instructed to contact the transplant center or primary care physician so that pulmonary function tests can be performed. Any subsequent alteration in $FEF_{25–75\%}$ prompts further evaluation with bronchoscopy and bronchoalveolar lavage, and transbronchial biopsy. After infection has been ruled out, augmentation of immunosuppression is the current mode of therapy. Cyclosporine and azathioprine doses are increased while monitoring renal function and leukocyte count. The prednisone dose also is increased to 1.0 mg/kg/day. In the event that there is acute rejection on the TBB, pulse-dose steroids are started (methylprednisolone 1 g IV for 3 days). In the setting of augmented immunosuppression, CMV prophylaxis with ganciclovir and fungal prophylaxis with inhaled amphotericin B are started.

Despite stabilization of pulmonary function with augmented immunosuppression, relapse rates are greater than 50% and mortality is significant.[79,108] The actuarial survival curves for heart–lung transplant patients are quite different for patients with BOS/OB and those patients without BOS/OB (Figure 95-9). Markedly better survival also was demonstrated in BOS stage 1 versus BOS stages 2 and 3.[79] The main cause of death is usually respiratory failure secondary to a superimposed pneumonia. Retransplantation often remains the only therapeutic option, although the results of retransplantation in patients who have developed end-stage OB are poor, with an actuarial survival rate of only 25% at 1 and 3 years after transplant.[2]

Chronic Rejection—Graft Coronary Artery Disease

Very few heart–lung recipients who survive the first year will die as a result of graft coronary artery disease.[85,107] There is a low incidence of cardiac allograft rejection.[7] The incidence of angiographically detectable coronary artery disease was only 11% at 5 years after a heart–lung transplant,[85] which is similar to the data from the ISHLT Registry (Figure 95-10).[104] This is in contrast to heart-only transplant recipients, in which as many as 50% of patients develop significant angiographic disease by 5 years and this is the major cause of mortality and retransplantation. A recent study using intracoronary ultrasound confirms the low incidence of transplant coronary artery disease in heart–lung recipients when compared with the heart-alone recipient group.[55] When the lung and heart are both transplanted, the lung is more immunologically active. This observation was confirmed in an animal model in which hearts transplanted in combination with lungs or spleen displayed an impressive reduction in myocardial rejection; this phenomenon is termed the "combi-effect."[113]

Table 95–4

Working Formulation for Bronchiolitis Obliterans Syndrome (BOS)

$0_{a\ or\ b}$	No significant abnormality: FEV_1 80% of baseline
$1_{a\ or\ b}$	Mild BOS: FEV_1 66–80% of baseline
$2_{a\ or\ b}$	Moderate BOS: FEV_1 51–65% of baseline
$3_{a\ or\ b}$	Severe BOS: FEV_1 50% of baseline

a, Without pathological evidence of obliterative bronchiolitis; *b*, with pathological evidence of obliterative bronchiolitis.

From Cooper JD, Billingham M, Egan T, et al: A working formulation for the standardization of nomenclature and for clinical staging of chronic dysfunction in lung allografts. J Heart Lung Transplant 12:713–716, 1993.

Complications of Immunosuppression

There are several side effects resulting from long-term immunosuppression. Cyclosporine causes nephrotoxicity, hypertension, hepatotoxicity, hirsutism, and gingival hyperplasia and is associated with an increased incidence of lymphoma. Azathioprine causes a generalized bone marrow depression manifested as leukopenia, thrombocytopenia, and anemia. Long-term use of steroids causes hypertension, diabetes, osteoporosis, and impaired wound healing. Induction therapy with either RATG or OKT3 can cause significant hemodynamic instability and respiratory compromise manifested as fever, hypotension, and bronchospasm. Patients are therefore premedicated with corticosteroids, acetaminophen, and antihistamines before administration.

One of the more troubling consequences of heart–lung transplantation is the development of posttransplant lymphoproliferative disorder (PTLD).[124] This is characterized by lymphadenopathy and often a diffuse lymphocytic infiltrate on TBB.[123] The treatment is immediate reduction in

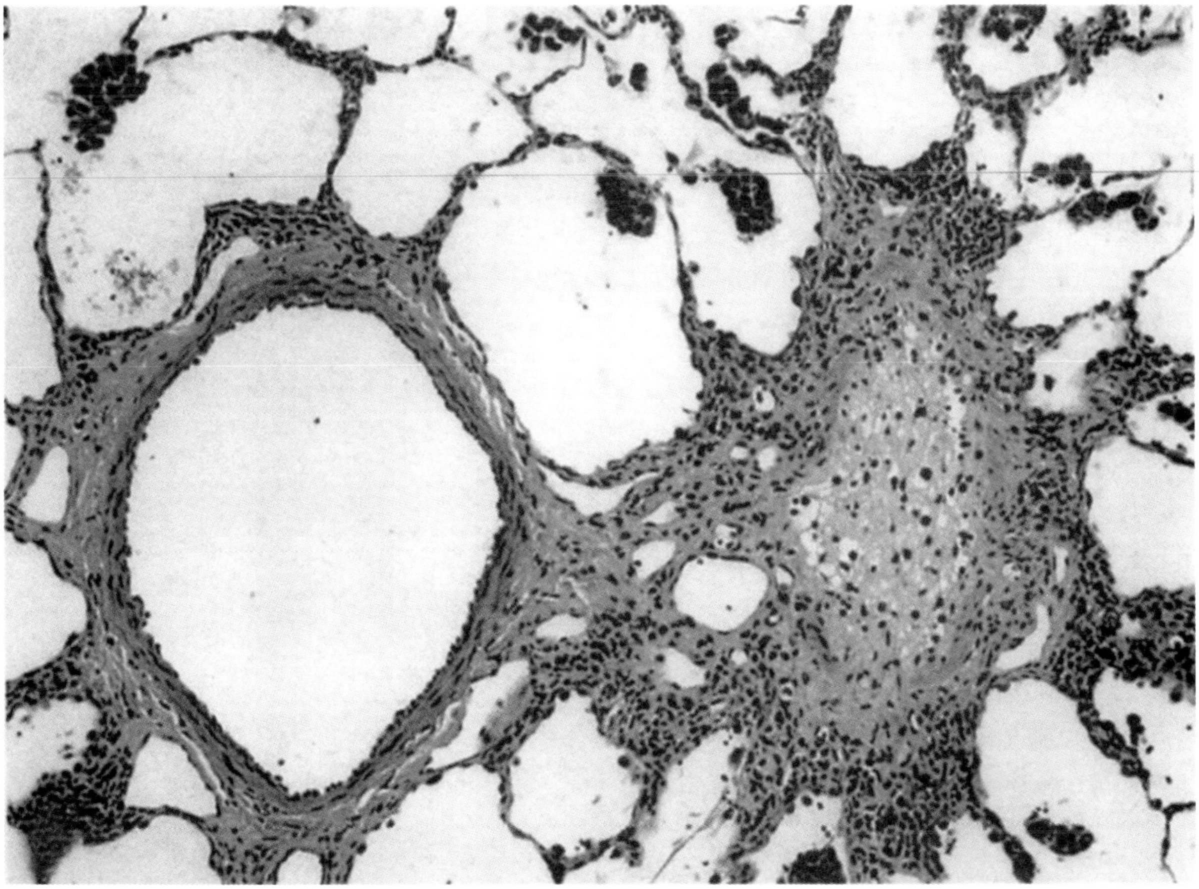

A

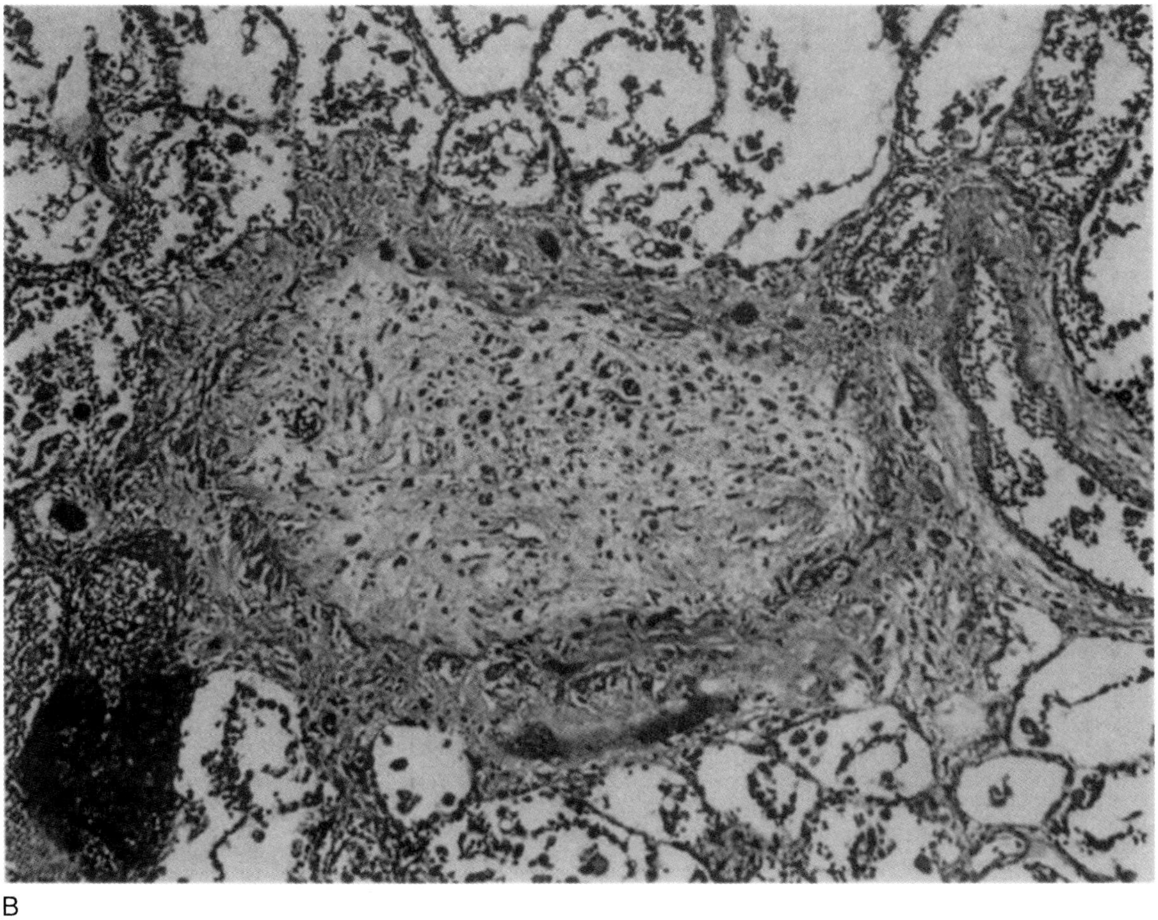

B

Figure 95–7 Active obliterative bronchiolitis (OB). OB is identified together with an intense chronic inflammatory cell infiltrate (grade Ca). Damage of the airway epithelium is evident. (**A,** Hematoxylin and eosin stain; ×100. **B,** Hematoxylin and eosin stain; ×100.)

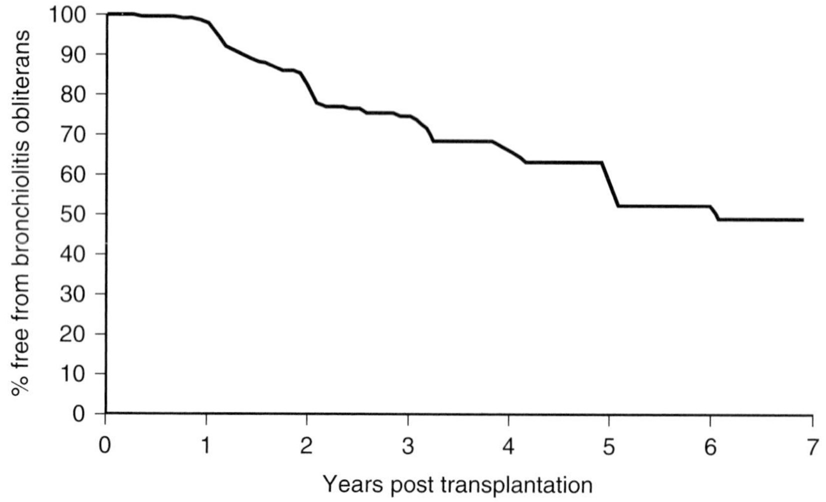

Figure 95–8 Freedom from obliterative bronchiolitis (OB) after heart–lung transplantation.
(Modified from Trulock EP, Edwards LB, Taylor DO, et al: The Registry of the International Society of Heart and Lung Transplantation: Twentieth official adult lung and heart–lung transplant report—2003. J Heart Lung Transplant 22:625–635, 2003.)

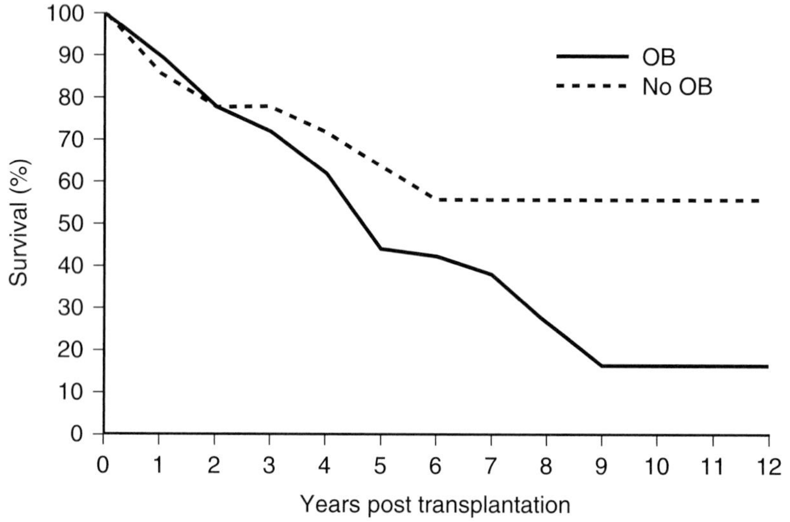

Figure 95–9 Survival rates with obliterative bronchiolitis (OB) after lung and heart–lung transplantation.
(Modified from Reichenspurner H, Girgis R, Robbins RC, et al: Stanford experience with obliterative bronchiolitis after lung and heart–lung transplantation. Ann Thorac Surg 62:1467, 1996.)

the intensity of the immunosuppression. The disease has essentially two forms: malignant and nonmalignant. Early onset of PTLD (less than 12 months after transplantation) is typically benign and resolves rapidly after reduced immunosuppression. Conversely, late PTLD is associated with a 70–80% mortality rate and typically resists a reduction in immunotherapy, as well as traditional chemotherapy.[5]

Additional Complications

Airway complications have become rare after heart–lung and lung transplantation secondary to improvements in surgical technique and postoperative management. The risk of a major airway complication after heart–lung transplantation is approximately half that of a single lung transplantation, with a reported incidence as low as 3.8%.[91] The incidence of airway complications is unrelated to steroid use in the preoperative or postoperative period.[19] Furthermore, no significant correlation could be identified with the ischemic interval, anastomotic wrapping, or date of first rejection episode.[15]

Abdominal complications after heart–lung transplantation remain a significant source of morbidity and mortality.[93] There is a high prevalence of symptomatic gastroparesis after heart–lung transplantation, probably as a result of vagotomy at the time of removal of the heart–lung block.[96] Gastroparesis with gastric distension can lead to gastroesophageal reflux with subsequent aspiration. Episodes of aspiration and the resultant inflammatory response can result in significant lung allograft dysfunction. Furthermore, whether this allograft injury predisposes the patient to an increased risk of BOS/OB remains to be determined.[11] Laparoscopic antireflux surgery also should be considered in patients with severe reflux disease after heart–lung transplantation, given the recent findings that pulmonary function and reflux symptoms were significantly improved.[49]

PHYSIOLOGY OF THE TRANSPLANTED LUNG

Standard measure of pulmonary function indicates that long-term function of the heart and lungs are well main-

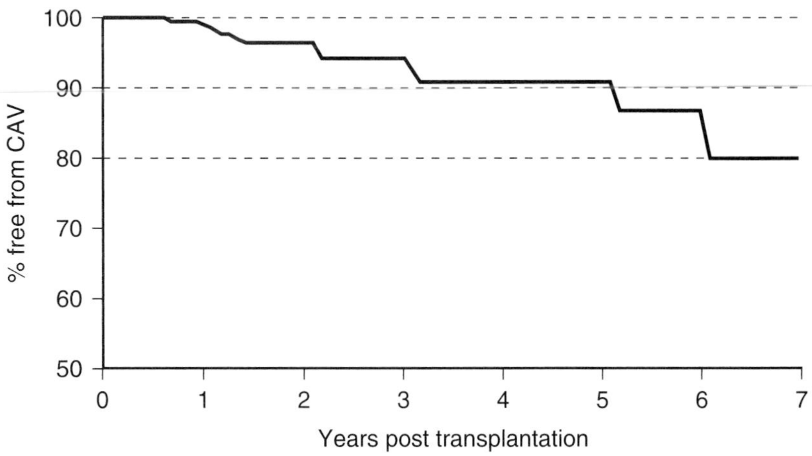

Figure 95–10 Freedom from accelerated graft coronary disease after heart–lung transplantation.
(Modified from Trulock EP, Edwards LB, Taylor DO, et al: The Registry of the International Society of Heart and Lung Transplantation: Twentieth official adult lung and heart–lung transplant report—2003. J Heart Lung Transplant 22:625–635, 2003.)

tained. Integrated cardiopulmonary function with exercise also is largely intact.[102,103] Some debate has centered around a bronchial hyperresponsiveness to a methacholine challenge.[34] There does appear to be decreased mucociliary clearance, which may be a contributing factor to the serious and repeated infections seen in heart–lung recipients.[35] In the absence of OB and severe recurrent infection, the function of the transplanted heart and lungs is conducive to an excellent quality of life.[102]

LATE RESULTS

A retrospective review of all 174 patients with end-stage cardiopulmonary disease who underwent heart–lung transplantation at Stanford University between 1981 and 2000 revealed that 40% of these patients were still alive, with a 5-year actuarial survival rate of 49% (Figure 95-11). This record compares closely with the worldwide experience with heart–lung transplantation, as reported by the ISHLT Registry (Figure 95-12).[104] A review of the last 10 years at Stanford from 1991–2002 reveals improved survival when compared with the previous decade (Figure 95-13).[20]

Causes of mortality after heart–lung transplantation differ over time after surgery. Early deaths, occurring less than 1 month after surgery, are most often due to infection (36% of overall deaths), hemorrhage (8–20%), acute respiratory disease syndrome (ARDS) (4%), and nonspecific graft failure (7–9%).[20,85] Acute rejection of the heart–lung graft is fairly uncommon, resulting in mortality in less than 2% of patients. Almost all rejection events in these patients occur within the first 3 months, with a linearized rejection rate twice as high for the lung (0.7 events/100 days) when compared with the heart (0.35 events/100 days). The most common cause of death after the immediate postoperative phase is OB. The overall prevalence of OB in patients surviving heart–lung transplantation longer than 3 months was 64%, with an overall mortality greater than 70% after 5 years of follow up.[79] Additional causes of late death include infection, malignancy, and coronary artery disease. The incidence and severity of transplant coronary artery disease is significantly less when compared with the heart transplantation population.[84] However, this complication remains an important cause of late death in heart–lung recipients.[85]

The long-term functional results after heart–lung transplantation are encouraging. Most recipients are able to

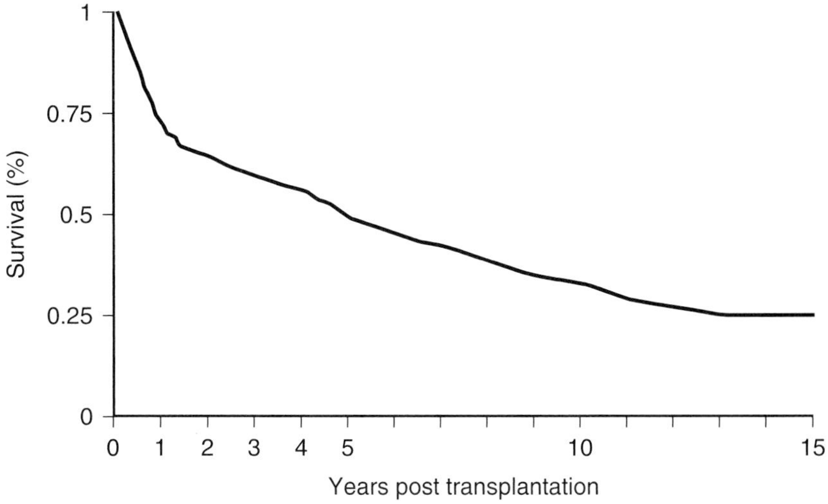

Figure 95–11 Actuarial survival of patients undergoing heart–lung transplantation at Stanford University, 1981–2000.

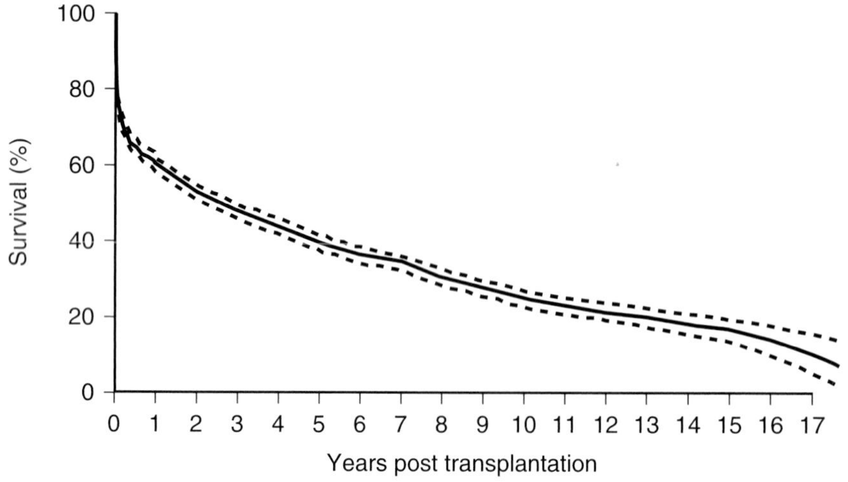

Figure 95–12 **Heart–lung transplantation actuarial survival based on data from the ISHLT Registry.** *(Modified from Trulock EP, Edwards LB, Taylor DO, et al: The Registry of the International Society of Heart and Lung Transplantation: Twentieth official adult lung and heart–lung transplant report—2003. J Heart Lung Transplant 22:625–635, 2003.)*

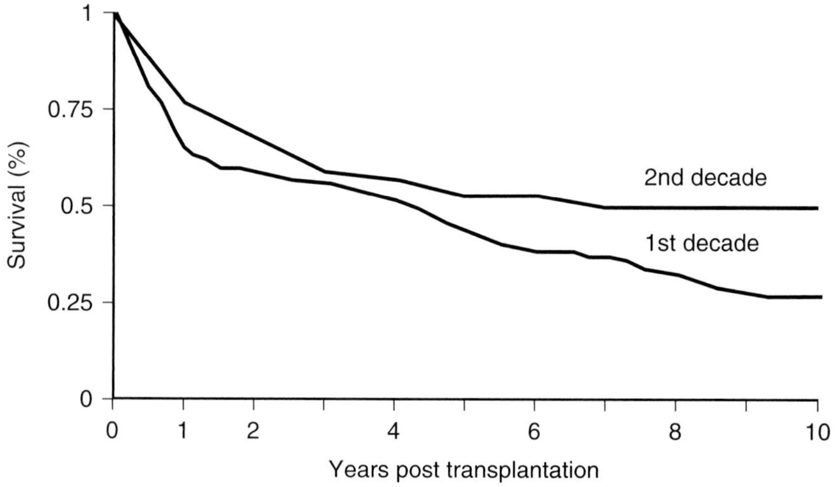

Figure 95–13 **Actuarial survival of patients undergoing heart–lung transplantation at Stanford University, comparison of the first decade (1981–1990) to the second decade (1991–2002).**

resume an active lifestyle without supplemental oxygen and demonstrate significant increases in exercise capacity after transplant.[88,103] Pulmonary function as measured by spirometry also is markedly improved after heart–lung transplantation.[103] Considering that heart–lung transplantation is performed in a subgroup of patients with a life expectancy of less than 2 years, despite maximal medical and nontransplant surgical therapy, the functional benefits of heart–lung transplantation become obvious.

FUTURE DEVELOPMENTS

Imperfections remain in the use of heart–lung transplantation for definitive treatment of end-stage cardiopulmonary disease. Significant improvements in selective immunosuppression and the development of precise immunotolerance are required before heart–lung transplantation can restore normal heart and lung function without significant long-term morbidity and mortality. The development of new immunosuppressive agents, the use of genetic engineering to formulate new humanized monoclonal antibodies, and the field of pharmacogenomics provide continued hope for an improved outlook for heart–lung transplant recipients. Novel approaches such as ex vivo gene therapy, the induction of immunotolerance, and xenotransplantation are promising areas of continual investigation.

REFERENCES

1. Adachi JD, Bensen WG, Brown J, et al: Intermittent etidronate therapy to prevent corticosteroid-induced osteoporosis. N Engl J Med 337:382–387, 1997.
2. Adams DH, Cochrane AD, Khaghani A, et al: Retransplantation in heart-lung recipients with obliterative bronchiolitis. J Thorac Cardiovasc Surg 107:450–459, 1994.
3. Adatia I, Lillehei C, Arnold JH, et al: Inhaled nitric oxide in the treatment of postoperative graft dysfunction after lung transplantation. Ann Thorac Surg 57:1311–1318, 1994.
4. Andreu G, Achkar A, Couetil JP, et al: Extracorporeal photochemotherapy treatment for acute lung rejection episode. J Heart Lung Transplant 14:793–796, 1995.

5. Armitage JM, Kormos RL, Stuart RS, et al: Posttransplant lymphoproliferative disease in thoracic organ transplant patients: Ten years of cyclosporine-based immunosuppression. J Heart Lung Transplant 10:877–886, 1991.
6. Baldwin JC, Frist WH, Starkey TD, et al: Distant graft procurement for combined heart and lung transplantation using pulmonary artery flush and simple topical hypothermia for graft preservation. Ann Thorac Surg 43:670–673, 1987.
7. Baldwin JC, Oyer PE, Stinson EB, et al: Comparison of cardiac rejection in heart and heart-lung transplantation. J Heart Transplant 6:352–356, 1987.
8. Bando K, Armitage JM, Paradis IL, et al: Indications for and results of single, bilateral, and heart-lung transplantation for pulmonary hypertension. J Thorac Cardiovasc Surg 108:1056–1065, 1994.
9. Barst RJ, Rubin LJ, Long WA, et al: A comparison of continuous intravenous epoprostenol (prostacyclin) with conventional therapy for primary pulmonary hypertension. The Primary Pulmonary Hypertension Study Group. N Engl J Med 334:296–302, 1996.
10. Baumgartner WA, Traill TA, Cameron DE, et al: Unique aspects of heart and lung transplantation exhibited in the 'domino-donor' operation. JAMA 261:3121–3125, 1989.
11. Berkowitz N, Schulman LL, McGregor C, et al: Gastroparesis after lung transplantation. Potential role in postoperative respiratory complications. Chest 108:1602–1607, 1995.
12. Cahill BC, O'Rourke MK, Strasburg KA, et al: Methotrexate for lung transplant recipients with steroid-resistant acute rejection. J Heart Lung Transplant 15:1130–1137, 1996.
13. Carrel A: The surgery of blood vessels. Johns Hopkins Hosp Bull 18:18, 1907.
14. Cohn JN, Archibald DG, Ziesche S, et al: Effect of vasodilator therapy on mortality in chronic congestive heart failure. Results of a Veterans Administration Cooperative Study. N Engl J Med 314:1547–1552, 1986.
15. Colquhoun IW, Gascoigne AD, Au J, et al: Airway complications after pulmonary transplantation. Ann Thorac Surg 57:141–145, 1994.
16. Cooper JD, Billingham M, Egan T, et al: A working formulation for the standardization of nomenclature and for clinical staging of chronic dysfunction in lung allografts. International Society for Heart and Lung Transplantation. J Heart Lung Transplant 12:713–716, 1993.
17. D'Alonzo GE, Barst RJ, Ayres SM, et al: Survival in patients with primary pulmonary hypertension. Results from a national prospective registry. Ann Intern Med 115:343–349, 1991.
18. Date H, Triantafillou AN, Trulock EP, et al: Inhaled nitric oxide reduces human lung allograft dysfunction. J Thorac Cardiovasc Surg 111:913–919, 1996.
19. Date H, Trulock EP, Arcidi JM, et al: Improved airway healing after lung transplantation. An analysis of 348 bronchial anastomoses. J Thorac Cardiovasc Surg 110:1424–1432, 1995.
20. Demers P, Robbins RC, Doyle R, et al: Twenty years of combined heart-lung transplantation at Stanford University. J Heart Lung Transplant 21:S77, 2003.
21. Demertzis S, Langer F, Graeter T, et al: Amelioration of lung reperfusion injury by L- and E-selectin blockade. Eur J Cardiothorac Surg 16:174–180, 1999.
22. Demikhov VP: Experimental Transplantation of Vital Organs, Vol. 1. New York: Consultant Bureau, 1962.
23. Fitzsimmons SC: The changing epidemiology of cystic fibrosis. J Pediatr 122:1–9, 1993.
24. Fuster V, Steele PM, Edwards WD, et al: Primary pulmonary hypertension: Natural history and the importance of thrombosis. Circulation 70:580–587, 1984.
25. Girgis RE, Reichenspurner H, Robbins RC, et al: The utility of annual surveillance bronchoscopy in heart-lung transplant recipients. Transplantation 60:1458–1461, 1995.
26. Girgis RE, Tu I, Berry GJ, et al: Risk factors for the development of obliterative bronchiolitis after lung transplantation. J Heart Lung Transplant 15:1200–1208, 1996.
27. Grattan MT, Moreno-Cabral CE, Starnes VA, et al: Cytomegalovirus infection is associated with cardiac allograft rejection and atherosclerosis. JAMA 261:3561–3566, 1989.
28. Griffith BP, Paradis IL, Zeevi A, et al: Immunologically mediated disease of the airways after pulmonary transplantation. Ann Surg 208:371–378, 1988.
29. Harjula AL, Baldwin JC, Glanville AR, et al: Human leukocyte antigen compatibility in heart-lung transplantation. J Heart Transplant 6:162–166, 1987.
30. Harjula AL, Baldwin JC, Oyer PE, et al: Recipient selection for heart-lung transplantation. Scand J Thorac Cardiovasc Surg 22:193–196, 1988.
31. Harjula A, Baldwin JC, Tazelaar HD, et al: Minimal lung pathology in long-term primate survivors of heart-lung transplantation. Transplantation 44:852–854, 1987.
32. Hausen B, Gummert J, Berry GJ, et al: Prevention of acute allograft rejection in nonhuman primate lung transplant recipients: Induction with chimeric anti-interleukin-2 receptor monoclonal antibody improves the tolerability and potentiates the immunosuppressive activity of a regimen using low doses of both microemulsion cyclosporine and 40-O-(2-hydroxyethyl)-rapamycin. Transplantation 69:488–496, 2000.
33. Haverich A, Aziz S, Scott WC, et al: Improved lung preservation using Euro-Collins solution for flush-perfusion. Thorac Cardiovasc Surg 34:368–376, 1986.
34. Herve P, Picard N, Le Roy LM, et al: Lack of bronchial hyperresponsiveness to methacholine and to isocapnic dry air hyperventilation in heart/lung and double-lung transplant recipients with normal lung histology. The Paris-Sud Lung Transplant Group. Am Rev Respir Dis 145:1503–1505, 1992.
35. Herve P, Silbert D, Cerrina J, et al: Impairment of bronchial mucociliary clearance in long-term survivors of heart/lung and double-lung transplantation. The Paris-Sud Lung Transplant Group. Chest 103:59–63, 1993.
36. Higenbottam T, Hutter JA, Stewart S, et al: Transbronchial biopsy has eliminated the need for endomyocardial biopsy in heart-lung recipients. J Heart Transplant 7:435–439, 1988.
37. Hoeper MM, Hamm M, Schafers HJ, et al: Evaluation of lung function during pulmonary rejection and infection in heart-lung transplant patients. Hannover Lung Transplant Group. Chest 102:864–870, 1992.
38. Hopkins WE, Ochoa LL, Richardson GW, et al: Comparison of the hemodynamics and survival of adults with severe primary pulmonary hypertension or Eisenmenger syndrome. J Heart Lung Transplant 15:100–105, 1996.
39. Iwai A, Sakano T, Uenishi M, et al: Effects of vasopressin and catecholamines on the maintenance of circulatory stability in brain-dead patients. Transplantation 48:613–617, 1989.
40. Iwaki Y, Yoshida Y, Griffith B: The HLA matching effect in lung transplantation. Transplantation 56:1528–1529, 1993.
41. Kawashima M, Bando T, Nakamura T, et al: Cytoprotective effects of nitroglycerin in ischemia-reperfusion-induced lung injury. Am J Respir Crit Care Med 161:935–943, 2000.
42. Keenan RJ, Lega ME, Dummer JS, et al: Cytomegalovirus serologic status and postoperative infection correlated with risk of developing chronic rejection after pulmonary transplantation. Transplantation 51:433–438, 1991.
43. Keller CA, Cagle PT, Brown RW, et al: Bronchiolitis obliterans in recipients of single, double, and heart-lung transplantation. Chest 107:973–980, 1995.
44. Kerstein D, Levy PS, Hsu DT, et al: Blade balloon atrial septostomy in patients with severe primary pulmonary hypertension. Circulation 91:2028–2035, 1995.

45. Kozower BD, Christofidou-Solomidou M, Sweitzer TD, et al: Immunotargeting of catalase to the pulmonary endothelium alleviates oxidative stress and reduces acute lung transplantation injury. Nat Biotechnol 21:392–398, 2003.
46. Kramer MR, Marshall SE, Starnes VA, et al: Infectious complications in heart-lung transplantation. Analysis of 200 episodes. Arch Intern Med 153:2010–2016, 1993.
47. Kramer MR, Marshall SE, Tiroke A, et al: Clinical significance of hyperbilirubinemia in patients with pulmonary hypertension undergoing heart-lung transplantation. J Heart Lung Transplant 10:317–321, 1991.
48. Kramer MR, Stoehr C, Lewiston NJ, et al: Trimethoprim-sulfamethoxazole prophylaxis for Pneumocystis carinii infections in heart-lung and lung transplantation—how effective and for how long? Transplantation 53:586–589, 1992.
49. Lau CL, Palmer SM, Howell DN, et al: Laparoscopic antireflux surgery in the lung transplant population. Surg Endosc 16:1674–1678, 2002.
50. Lemstrom KB, Bruning JH, Bruggeman CA, et al: Cytomegalovirus infection enhances smooth muscle cell proliferation and intimal thickening of rat aortic allografts. J Clin Invest 92:549–558, 1993.
51. Levine AJ, Parkes K, Rooney S, et al: Reduction of endothelial injury after hypothermic lung preservation by initial leukocyte-depleted reperfusion. J Thorac Cardiovasc Surg 120: 47–54, 2000.
52. Levine AJ, Parkes K, Rooney SJ, et al: The effect of adhesion molecule blockade on pulmonary reperfusion injury. Ann Thorac Surg 73:1101–1106, 2002.
53. Lewiston N, King V, Umetsu D, et al: Cystic fibrosis patients who have undergone heart-lung transplantation benefit from maxillary sinus antrostomy and repeated sinus lavage. Transplant Proc 23:1207–1208, 1991.
54. Lick SD, Copeland JG, Rosado LJ, et al: Simplified technique of heart-lung transplantation. Ann Thorac Surg 59:1592–1593, 1995.
55. Lim TT, Botas J, Ross H, et al: Are heart-lung transplant recipients protected from developing transplant coronary artery disease? A case-matched intracoronary ultrasound study. Circulation 94:1573–1577, 1996.
56. Marcus E, Wong SNT, Luisada AA: Homologous heart grafts: Transplantation of the heart in dogs. Surg Forum 2:212, 1951.
57. Marshall SE, Kramer MR, Lewiston NJ, et al: Selection and evaluation of recipients for heart-lung and lung transplantation. Chest 98:1488–1494, 1990.
58. Meiser BM, Uberfuhr P, Schulze C, et al: Tacrolimus (FK506) proves superior to OKT3 for treating episodes of persistent rejection following intrathoracic transplantation. Transplant Proc 29:605–606, 1997.
59. Michler RE, Rose EA: Pediatric heart and heart-lung transplantation. Ann Thorac Surg 52: 708–709, 1991.
60. Milano CA, Shah AS, Van Trigt P, et al: Evaluation of early postoperative results after bicaval versus standard cardiac transplantation and review of the literature. Am Heart J 140:717–721, 2000.
61. Millet B, Higenbottam TW, Flower CD, et al: The radiographic appearances of infection and acute rejection of the lung after heart-lung transplantation. Am Rev Respir Dis 140:62–67, 1989.
62. Milne DS, Gascoigne A, Wilkes J, et al: The immunohistopathology of obliterative bronchiolitis following lung transplantation. Transplantation 54:748–750, 1992.
63. Muller C, Furst H, Reichenspurner H, et al: Lung procurement by low-potassium dextran and the effect on preservation injury. Munich Lung Transplant Group. Transplantation 68:1139–1143, 1999.
64. Nawata S, Sugi K, Ueda K, et al: Prostacyclin analog OP2507 prevents pulmonary arterial and airway constriction during lung preservation and reperfusion. J Heart Lung Transplant 15:470–474, 1996.
65. Novitzky D: Donor management: State of the art. Transplant Proc 29:3773–3775, 1997.
66. O'Donohue WJ Jr: Home oxygen therapy. Clin Chest Med 18:535–545, 1997.
67. Otulana BA, Higenbottam T, Ferrari L, et al: The use of home spirometry in detecting acute lung rejection and infection following heart-lung transplantation. Chest 97:353–357, 1990.
68. Otulana BA, Higenbottam TW, Scott JP, et al: Pulmonary function monitoring allows diagnosis of rejection in heart-lung transplant recipients. Transplant Proc 21:2583–2584, 1989.
69. Ouwens JP, van der Mark TW, van der BW, et al: Size matching in lung transplantation using predicted total lung capacity. Eur Respir J 20:1419–1422, 2002.
70. Pasque MK, Trulock EP, Cooper JD, et al: Single lung transplantation for pulmonary hypertension. Single institution experience in 34 patients. Circulation 92:2252–2258, 1995.
71. Pennefather SH, Bullock RE, Dark JH: The effect of fluid therapy on alveolar arterial oxygen gradient in brain-dead organ donors. Transplantation 56:1418–1422, 1993.
72. Pereira BJ, Wright TL, Schmid CH, et al: A controlled study of hepatitis C transmission by organ transplantation. The New England Organ Bank Hepatitis C Study Group. Lancet 345:484–487, 1995.
73. Quantz MA, Bennett LE, Meyer DM, et al: Does human leukocyte antigen matching influence the outcome of lung transplantation? An analysis of 3,549 lung transplantations. J Heart Lung Transplant 19:473–479, 2000.
74. Rajagopalan N, Maurer J, Kesten S: Bronchodilator response at low lung volumes predicts bronchiolitis obliterans in lung transplant recipients. Chest 109:405–407, 1996.
75. Ramsey BW: Management of pulmonary disease in patients with cystic fibrosis. N Engl J Med 335:179–188, 1996.
76. Ransom JT: Mechanism of action of mycophenolate mofetil. Ther Drug Monit 17:681–684, 1995.
77. Reichenspurner H, Gamberg P, Nitschke M, et al: Significant reduction in the number of fungal infections after lung-, heart-lung, and heart transplantation using aerosolized amphotericin B prophylaxis. Transplant Proc 29:627–628, 1997.
78. Reichenspurner H, Girgis RE, Robbins RC, et al: Obliterative bronchiolitis after lung and heart-lung transplantation. Ann Thorac Surg 60:1845–1853, 1995.
79. Reichenspurner H, Girgis RE, Robbins RC, et al: Stanford experience with obliterative bronchiolitis after lung and heart-lung transplantation. Ann Thorac Surg 62:1467–1472, 1996.
80. Reichenspurner H, Robbins RC, Miller J, et al: RATG-induction therapy significantly reduces incidence of acute pulmonary rejection compared to OKT3 treatment. J Heart Lung Transplant 15:S103, 1996.
81. Ross HJ, Gullestad L, Pak J, et al: Methotrexate or total lymphoid radiation for treatment of persistent or recurrent allograft cellular rejection: A comparative study. J Heart Lung Transplant 16:179–189, 1997.
82. Royston D: Aprotinin therapy in heart and heart-lung transplantation. J Heart Lung Transplant 12:S19–S25, 1993.
83. Rubin LJ: Pathology and pathophysiology of primary pulmonary hypertension. Am J Cardiol 75:51A–54A, 1995.
84. Sarris GE, Moore KA, Schroeder JS, et al: Cardiac transplantation: The Stanford experience in the cyclosporine era. J Thorac Cardiovasc Surg 108:240–251, 1994.
85. Sarris GE, Smith JA, Shumway NE, et al: Long-term results of combined heart-lung transplantation: The Stanford experience. J Heart Lung Transplant 13:940–949, 1994.
86. Schmid RA, Hillinger S, Walter R, et al: The nitric oxide synthase cofactor tetrahydrobiopterin reduces allograft ischemia-

reperfusion injury after lung transplantation. J Thorac Cardiovasc Surg 118:726–732, 1999.
87. Schmid RA, Yamashita M, Boasquevisque CH, et al: Carbohydrate selectin inhibitor CY-1503 reduces neutrophil migration and reperfusion injury in canine pulmonary allografts. J Heart Lung Transplant 16:1054–1061, 1997.
88. Schwaiblmair M, Reichenspurner H, Muller C, et al: Cardiopulmonary exercise testing before and after lung and heart-lung transplantation. Am J Respir Crit Care Med 159: 1277–1283, 1999.
89. Schwebel C, Pin I, Barnoud D, et al: Prevalence and consequences of nutritional depletion in lung transplant candidates. Eur Respir J 16:1050–1055, 2000.
90. Shackleton CR, Ettinger SL, McLoughlin MG, et al: Effect of recovery from ischemic injury on class I and class II MHC antigen expression. Transplantation 49:641–644, 1990.
91. Shumway SJ, Hertz MI, Maynard R, et al: Airway complications after lung and heart-lung transplantation. Transplant Proc 25:1165–1166, 1993.
92. Slaughter MS, Nielsen K, Bolman RM III: Extracorporeal membrane oxygenation after lung or heart-lung transplantation. ASAIO J 39:M453–M456, 1993.
93. Smith PC, Slaughter MS, Petty MG, et al: Abdominal complications after lung transplantation. J Heart Lung Transplant 14:44–51, 1995.
94. Smyth RL, Scott JP, Whitehead B, et al: Heart-lung transplantation in children. Transplant Proc 22:1470–1471, 1990.
95. Snell GI, Levvey BJ, Chin W, et al: Sirolimus allows renal recovery in lung and heart transplant recipients with chronic renal impairment. J Heart Lung Transplant 21:540–546, 2002.
96. Sodhi SS, Guo JP, Maurer AH, et al: Gastroparesis after combined heart and lung transplantation. J Clin Gastroenterol 34:34–39, 2002.
97. Soghikian MV, Valentine VG, Berry GJ, et al: Impact of ganciclovir prophylaxis on heart-lung and lung transplant recipients. J Heart Lung Transplant 15:881–887, 1996.
98. Starnes VA, Theodore J, Oyer PE, et al: Evaluation of heart-lung transplant recipients with prospective, serial transbronchial biopsies and pulmonary function studies. J Thorac Cardiovasc Surg 98:683–690, 1989a.
99. Starnes VA, Theodore J, Oyer PE, et al: Pulmonary infiltrates after heart-lung transplantation: Evaluation by serial transbronchial biopsies. J Thorac Cardiovasc Surg 98:945–950, 1989b.
100. Straznicka M, Follette DM, Eisner MD, et al: Aggressive management of lung donors classified as unacceptable: Excellent recipient survival one year after transplantation. J Thorac Cardiovasc Surg 124: 250–258, 2002.
101. Tamm M, Higenbottam TW, Dennis CM, et al: Donor and recipient predicted lung volume and lung size after heart-lung transplantation. Am J Respir Crit Care Med 150: 403–407, 1994.
102. Theodore J, Marshall S, Kramer M, et al: The “natural history” of the transplanted lung: rates of pulmonary functional change in long-term survivors of heart-lung transplantation. Transplant Proc 23:1165–1166, 1991.
103. Theodore J, Morris AJ, Burke CM, et al: Cardiopulmonary function at maximum tolerable constant work rate exercise following human heart-lung transplantation. Chest 92:433–439, 1987.
104. Trulock EP, Edwards LB, Taylor DO, et al: The Registry of the International Society of Heart and Lung Transplantation: Twentieth official adult lung and heart-lung transplant report—2003. J Heart Lung Transplant 22:625–635, 2003.
105. Vainikka T, Heikkila L, Kukkonen S, et al: L-Arginine in lung graft preservation and reperfusion. J Heart Lung Transplant 20:559–567, 2001.
106. Valantine HA, Luikart H, Doyle R, et al: Impact of cytomegalovirus hyperimmune globulin on outcome after cardiothoracic transplantation: A comparative study of combined prophylaxis with CMV hyperimmune globulin plus ganciclovir versus ganciclovir alone. Transplantation 72: 1647–1652, 2001.
107. Valantine HA, Reichenspurner H, Girgis R, et al: CMV prophylaxis with CMV hyperimmune globulin and ganciclovir is more effective than ganciclovir alone. J Heart Lung Transplant 15:S57, 1996.
108. Valentine VG, Robbins RC, Berry GJ, et al: Actuarial survival of heart-lung and bilateral sequential lung transplant recipients with obliterative bronchiolitis. J Heart Lung Transplant 15:371–383, 1996.
109. Valentine VG, Robbins RC, Wehner JH, et al: Total lymphoid irradiation for refractory acute rejection in heart-lung and lung allografts. Chest 109:1184–1189, 1996.
110. Varela A, Montero C, Cordoba M, et al: Clinical experience with retrograde lung preservation. Transpl Int 9(1 suppl): S296–S298, 1996.
111. Varela A, Montero CG, Cordoba M, et al: Improved distribution of pulmonary flush solution to the tracheobronchial wall in pulmonary transplantation. Eur Surg Res 29:1–4, 1997.
112. Waddell TK, Bennett L, Kennedy R, et al: Heart-lung or lung transplantation for Eisenmenger syndrome. J Heart Lung Transplant 21:731–737, 2002.
113. Westra AL, Petersen AH, Prop J, et al: The combi-effect—reduced rejection of the heart by combined transplantation with the lung or spleen. Transplantation 52:952–955, 1991.
114. Wheeldon DR, Potter CD, Oduro A, et al: Transforming the “unacceptable” donor: Outcomes from the adoption of a standardized donor management technique. J Heart Lung Transplant 14:734–742, 1995.
115. Whyte RI, Robbins RC, Altinger J, et al: Heart-lung transplantation for primary pulmonary hypertension. Ann Thorac Surg 67:937–941, 1999.
116. Wijnen RM, van der Linden CJ: Donor treatment after pronouncement of brain death: A neglected intensive care problem. Transpl Int 4:186–190, 1991.
117. Wisser W, Wekerle T, Zlabinger G, et al: Influence of human leukocyte antigen matching on long-term outcome after lung transplantation. J Heart Lung Transplant 15:1209–1216, 1996.
118. Wreghitt TG, Hakim M, Gray JJ, et al: Cytomegalovirus infections in heart and heart and lung transplant recipients. J Clin Pathol 41:660–667, 1988.
119. Yacoub MH, Banner NR, Khaghani A, et al: Heart-lung transplantation for cystic fibrosis and subsequent domino heart transplantation. J Heart Transplant 9:459–466, 1990.
120. Yousem SA: Lymphocytic bronchitis/bronchiolitis in lung allograft recipients. Am J Surg Pathol 17:491–496, 1993.
121. Yousem SA, Berry GJ, Cagle PT, et al: Revision of the 1990 working formulation for the classification of pulmonary allograft rejection: Lung Rejection Study Group. J Heart Lung Transplant 15:1–15, 1996.
122. Yousem SA, Curley JM, Dauber J, et al: HLA-class II antigen expression in human heart-lung allografts. Transplantation 49:991–995, 1990.
123. Yousem SA, Dauber JA, Keenan R, et al: Does histologic acute rejection in lung allografts predict the development of bronchiolitis obliterans? Transplantation 52:306–309, 1991.
124. Yousem SA, Randhawa P, Locker J, et al: Posttransplant lymphoproliferative disorders in heart-lung transplant recipients: Primary presentation in the allograft. Hum Pathol 20:361–369, 1989.

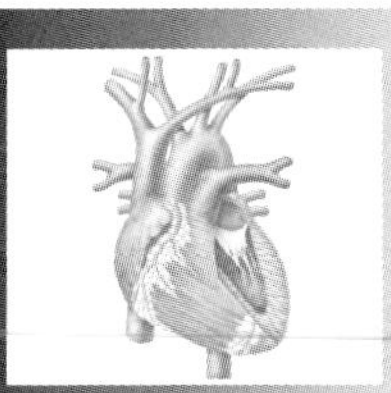

CHAPTER 96

Left Ventricular Reconstruction and the Surgical Treatment of the Failing Heart

Richard Lee, Katherine J. Hoercher, and Patrick M. McCarthy

INTRODUCTION

The application of nontransplant surgical therapies for heart failure is evolving. Cardiac surgery interventions have been performed for decades on patients with heart failure secondary to ischemic disease, valvular disease, and ventricular aneurysms. However, the perioperative morbidity and mortality of these interventions was significant, and their unpredictable outcomes limited the role of conventional surgery. This strategy has changed in the past decade. Today even the most severe left ventricular (LV) dysfunction is not in itself a contraindication to surgery. Carefully selected patients experience an improvement of their symptoms and, in many instances, may have an improved life expectancy.

Historically, patients with severe congestive heart failure were listed for heart transplantation. Although transplantation remains a very effective therapy for end-stage heart failure, it continues to be plagued by the limited number of donor organs and long-term morbidity.[152] Therefore it is no surprise that we currently seek to avoid or delay the need for cardiac transplantation whenever possible.

The implantation of left ventricular assist devices (LVADs) also has been proposed as a therapy for end-stage heart disease, either as an alternative to transplantation or as destination therapy. However, cost, infection, stroke, and mechanical failure remain significant barriers to this strategy in the current generation of devices as reported by both the REMATCH (Randomized Evaluation of Mechanical Assistance for the Treatment of Congestive Heart Failure) trial and our retrospective analysis of 244 device implants.[124,140]

Another confounding problem is the epidemiology of heart failure. In the past decade, although we have witnessed a decrease in death from coronary artery disease and stroke, we are seeing a significant increase in the incidence of heart failure with its tragic consequences.[151] In the United States alone, more than 5 million people suffer from congestive heart failure, with approximately 550,000 new cases diagnosed each year.[5] The aging population will only increase the magnitude of this problem.

Congestive heart failure (CHF) remains a terminal disease. After diagnosis, despite improvements in medical management, 5-year mortality is 60% for men and 45% for women.[102] In late-stage disease, (New York Heart Association [NYHA] class III and IV), even with maximal management, 1-year mortality is at least 20%; by 10 years, survivors are rare.[134,163]

In an effort to improve symptoms and survival in these patients, surgical interventions for patients with advanced heart failure are increasing and have resulted in a large paradigm shift in management.[97] Procedures and devices to arrest or reverse LV dilation and thus improve cardiac function are rapidly evolving. Advances in myocardial protection and perioperative management also have improved perioperative outcomes for a wide range of conventional surgery, such as coronary artery bypass grafting and valve surgery. In addition, mitral valve repair has become the procedure of choice for severe mitral regurgitation with LV dysfunction, allowing the preservation of the valvular–ventricular interaction and cardiac contractility. Also, low-gradient prostheses for aortic valve replacement allow patients with severe ventricular dysfunction to achieve maximal benefit after aortic valve replacement at a low risk. Also, with the application of novel techniques, surgical reconstruction of the dysfunctional left ventricle has made tremendous advances in recent years. This includes extending the reconstruction to include the LV septum, which had been neglected with conventional aneurysmectomy in the past.

Finally, LV reconstruction for dilated cardiomyopathy (the Batista procedure or partial left ventriculectomy) has been abandoned for the most part because of unacceptable perioperative mortality and morbidity, but the experience spawned a new generation of devices designed to change LV shape and reduce wall stress.

We have taken a "poly-surgery" approach to patients with severe LV dysfunction. That is, we apply a variety of surgical techniques that address all of the pathological aspects of heart failure. This chapter reviews the current and evolving surgical strategies for heart failure. We focus on ventricular reconstruction for both ischemic and nonischemic congestive heart failure and address the treatment of ischemia, valvular disease, and electrical dysfunction. It is also important to remember that the success of any surgical procedure for heart failure will yield the best results when combined with state-of-the-art pharmacological therapy, thereby producing a true synergistic benefit.

VENTRICULAR RECONSTRUCTION AND INTERVENTIONS FOR ISCHEMIC CARDIOMYOPATHY

Ventricular reconstruction is the active surgical attempt to restore the shape of the pathologically remodeled ventricle to one that is physiologically superior to the shape created in diseased states. In ischemic disease, remodeling usually occurs after a myocardial infarction, with residual akinetic or dyskinetic segments. Although the definitions are not universally standardized, dyskinetic segments are aneurysmal transmural scars, whereas akinetic segments are noncontributing segments of myocardium. Reconstruction, either alone or in conjunction with the correction of other cardiac disease, removes the diseased segment from the remaining functional segments of the left ventricle in an effort to improve cardiac function. At the Cleveland Clinic we frequently resect dyskinetic segments and may resect discrete near-transmural akinetic scars. We do not resect akinetic areas that have no scar.

The Past

The first surgical correction of a ventricular aneurysm occurred accidentally in 1937. Sauerbruch, thinking that he was operating on a mediastinal tumor, opened into the right ventricle and was forced to repair the false aneurysm.[145] Claude Beck was the first person to study this disease and attempt to correct the pathology. In 1944 Beck developed an animal model of LV aneurysm, attached strips of fascia lata to the aneurysm, and plicated the fascia lata as a means of repair.[16] He applied this technique to one patient, who died from an empyema 5 weeks postoperatively. The first successful surgical correction of an LV aneurysm did not occur until 1957. Through a left thoracotomy without cardiopulmonary bypass, Charles Bailey placed a large clamp on the base of the ventricular aneurysm, passed a horizontal mattress suture beneath it, and resected the aneurysm.[104] In 1958 Denton Cooley described the technique of open resection and simple closure on cardiopulmonary bypass.[47] This technique would become the standard of the profession for the next 30 years.

Although the technique remained unchanged, our understanding of LV aneurysm pathology and its role in CHF continued to evolve. The long-term survival in patients who were managed medically was disappointing. In 1953 Brushke and associates[32] reported a 5-year survival rate of 12% in patients with LV aneurysms who were medically managed. One year later, Schlichter and associates[147] reported the same 5-year survival rate of 12%, with the leading cause of death being CHF. This led to a more aggressive surgical approach by pioneers like Rene Favaloro. In 1968 Favaloro and colleagues[60] reported on a series of 130 patients who underwent resection for LV aneurysm with a hospital mortality of 13%. Follow up was obtained in 80 patients. There were 12 hospital deaths and 19 late deaths. Notably, however, of the 49 long-term survivors, 41 were free of symptoms.

The surgical resection of LV aneurysms slowly became applied; however, the results were not always predictable. In 1976 Lefemine and associates[101] reported on a series of 50 patients who underwent resection of aneurysm or akinetic segments with a hospital mortality of 22% and an additional late mortality of 20%. However, among survivors, 87% improved by at least one NYHA class. In 1979 Burton and associates[33] reported on a series of 169 patients who underwent resection of LV aneurysm with a hospital mortality of 18% and a 5-year survival rate of 60%. Of survivors, 90% were in NYHA class I or II.

Contemporary medical treatment of patients with ventricular aneurysms appeared to improve as well. In 1979 Proudfit and co-workers[137] reported a 5-year survival rate of 47% in 74 patients with LV aneurysms managed medically. In 1979 Grondin and associates[71] reported on a series of 40 patients with aneurysms who were medically managed. However, they divided the group into those with and without symptoms. After 10 years, survival was 90% in asymptomatic patients, but only 46% in patients who were symptomatic at the time of diagnosis. The causes of death were dominated by CHF, thromboembolism, and arrhythmias. Additional reports suggested that mortality was dependent on aneurysm size, with large aneurysms conferring a higher risk.[121] These reports of improved survival with medical management fostered a reluctance to apply surgery to the treatment of this disease. As recently as 1983 Cohen and co-workers[44] recommended that aneurysms be resected only after maximal medical management had failed. Indications in this group included heart failure, angina pectoris, recurrent thromboembolism refractory to anticoagulation, and refractory ventricular tachycardia.

In 1985 the traditional surgical technique of LV aneurysm was altered. Newer techniques described by

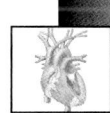

Jatene[86] and Dor et al[57] excluded the dysfunctional segment of the ventricular septum, as well as the free ventricular wall. After changing his technique, Jatene reduced his hospital mortality from 11.6% to 4.3%, and his late mortality from 12.6% to 3.5%. Dor applied his technique to areas of akinesia and dyskinesia. Although operative mortality was 12% in patients with large areas of akinesia, it was 0% in patients with small akinetic wall motion abnormalities.[58] In the subgroup of survivors with large akinetic areas, ejection fraction increased from 25% to 41%. Although other reports suggested an inferior outcome after reconstruction of akinetic segments as compared with dyskinetic segments, these surgeons used the traditional methods of aneurysm resection and linear closure.[48,109]

The research of the 1990s taught us that ventricular size and shape contribute to CHF and influence survival. Lee and associates[100] followed 382 patients with NYHA class III and IV heart failure referred for evaluation of cardiac transplantation. In patients with massively dilated left ventricles greater than 4 cm/m^2, the 2-year survival rate was 49%. In contrast, patients with left ventricles less than 4 cm/m^2 had a 75% 2-year survival rate.

Ventricular dilation also appears to effect survival after acute myocardial infarction. As part of the GUSTO (Global Utilization of Streptokinase and t-PA for Occluded Arteries) trial, Migrino and associates[117] evaluated end-systolic volume at 90–180 minutes into reperfusion during acute myocardial infarction. Patients with an end-systolic volume index greater than 40 ml/m^2 had a higher probability of mortality at 1 month and 1 year. In the SAVE (Survival and Ventricular Enlargement) trial, left ventricular size was a strong, independent risk factor for mortality after 2 years.[162]

Even after coronary artery bypass surgery, patients with large ventricles have a worse prognosis. Yamaguchi and co-workers[174] identified LV end-systolic volume index greater than 100 ml/m^2 as an independent risk factor for the development of CHF in ischemic cardiomyopathy. These reports helped cardiac surgeons focus on the importance of reconstruction of the left ventricle in ischemic cardiomyopathy.

The Present

At present, essentially four variations of left ventricular reconstruction are used that exclude the septum. These include a linear closure by Jatente (Figure 96-1), a modified linear closure by Mickleborough (Figure 96-2), a circular closure with a patch by Dor (Figure 96-3), and a double cerclage closure without a patch by McCarthy (Figure 96-4). All of these techniques involve an incision into the diseased anterior wall, an exclusion of the entire diseased segment, and a reduction in ventricular cavity size. In the majority of patients, reconstruction is done in the left anterior descending (LAD) distribution on the anterior portion of the left ventricle. However, reconstruction also has been performed on the posterior wall after circumflex or right coronary artery occlusion. Most of these patients undergo concomitant coronary artery bypass, and many also undergo mitral valve repair. Indications for the operation include patients with ischemic cardiomyopathy with worsening LV dysfunction, heart failure, angina pectoris, thromboembolism, or ventricular tachycardia. In other patients, severe coronary artery disease or mitral valve disease is the primary indication for surgical intervention, and the LV scar is reconstructed as a secondary procedure.

The RESTORE (Reconstructive Endoventricular Surgery, Returning Torsion Original Radius Elliptical Shape to the LV) Group recently reported on a series of 662 patients undergoing ventricular reconstruction for apical segments of akinesia and dyskinesia using the Dor technique.[9] Concomitant procedures included coronary artery bypass grafting (CABG) in 92%, mitral valve repair in 22%, and mitral valve replacement in 3%. Hospital mortality was 7.7%. In patients with only CABG and reconstruction, mortality was 4.9%. Postoperatively, ejection fraction increased from 30% to 40%, and LV end-systolic volume decreased from 96 ml/m^2 to 62 ml/m^2. At 3 years, survival was 89.4%. Survival was lower for patients with preoperative volumes greater than 80 ml/m^2. Freedom from hospital readmission for heart failure was 88.7%.

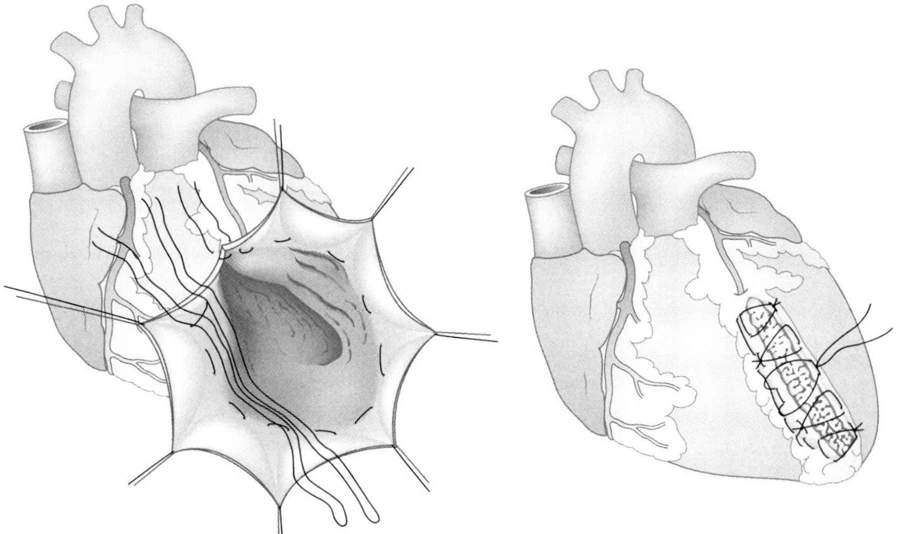

Figure 96–1 Dr. Adib Jatene of São Paulo, Brazil, introduced his technique of left ventricular (LV) reconstruction in the mid-1980s. This technique excluded the infarcted ventricular septum and achieved improved results as compared with traditional techniques of simple linear resection and closure.
(Reprinted with permission of Athanasuleas CL: Sem in Thor CV Surg 13:459–467, 2001.)

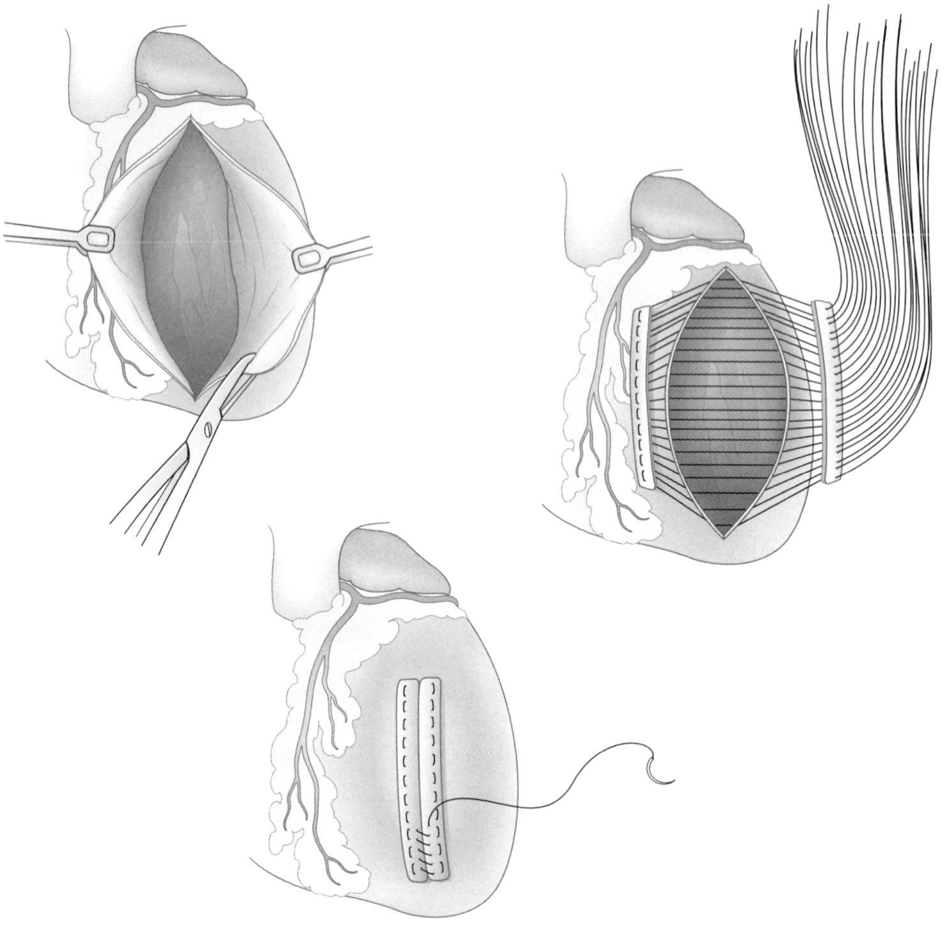

Figure 96–2 Dr. Lynda Mickleborough of Toronto, Canada, has great experience with a modified linear closure technique that excludes the septum utilizing a patch of bovine pericardium.
(Reprinted with permission. Ann Thor Surg 75:6–12, 2003.)

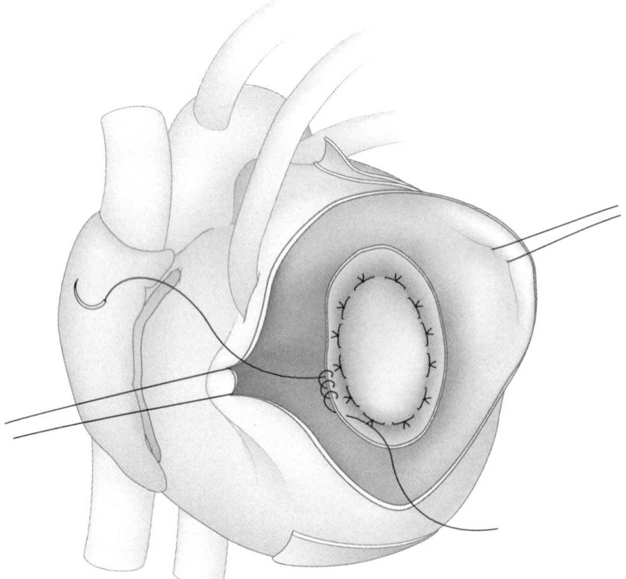

Figure 96–3 Dr. Vincent Dor of Nice, France, introduced his technique of left ventricular (LV) reconstruction in the mid-1980s, at the same time that Dr. Jatene introduced his technique. The Dor procedure incorporates a circular Fontan stitch and a patch to exclude the nonfunctional segment. Worldwide, this is the version of LV reconstruction that has been applied most frequently.
(Reprinted with permission. Semin Thorac Cardiovasc Surg 13:448–458, 2001.)

Mickleborough and co-workers[116] recently reported their results with a modified linear closure. One hundred and ninety-six patients with akinetic (57%) and dyskinetic (43%) segments underwent repair. Concomitant CABG was performed in 91% of patients. Preoperatively, 83% were in NYHA class III or IV. Hospital mortality was 2.6%. Actuarial survival rates at 1 and 5 years were 91% and 84%, respectively. Risk factors for a poor outcome at 5 years were 2+ or greater mitral regurgitation, CHF, and ventricular tachycardia. Among survivors, 80% were in NYHA class I or II.

At the Cleveland Clinic, LV reconstruction was performed in patients with a discrete left anterior descending scar, frequently with preoperative imaging consisting of magnetic resonance imaging (MRI) scan and/or three-dimensional (3D) echocardiography. Most patients had compensated heart failure or other indications for surgery such as severe coronary artery disease or mitral regurgitation. Currently, our technique of LV reconstruction is a double cerclage circular closure with no patch on the beating heart. One hundred and two consecutive patients undergoing this technique were reported, with a 1% hospital mortality.[35] A patch is used only in rare patients with a calcified aneurysm in whom the purse-string sutures may not create a neck, or in patients with a small LV cavity to avoid creating too small a cavity with a low stroke volume. Since January 1997, 224 patients (80% male, mean age 62

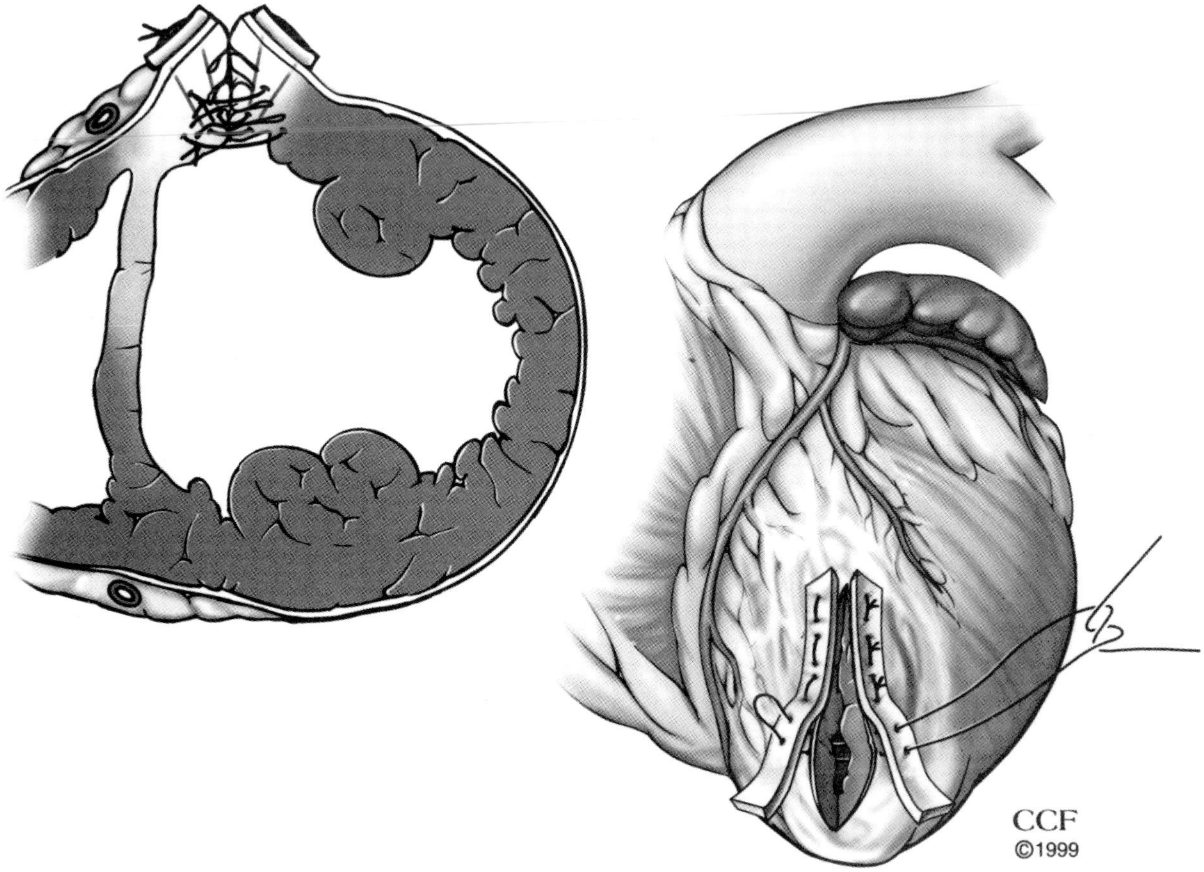

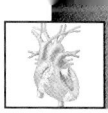

Figure 96–4 Dr. Patrick McCarthy of the Cleveland Clinic subsequently modified Dr. Dor's technique. This technique completely excludes the nonfunctional left ventricular (LV) segment with a Fontan stitch, but closes the ventricle in a manner that does not require any prosthetic material. This is our preferred technique of LV reconstruction. *(Reprinted with permission. Semin Thorac Cardiovasc Surg 14:137–142, 2002.)*

± 10 years) underwent LV reconstruction, 69% for dyskinetic and 31% for akinetic regions, as part of comprehensive surgical management of ischemic cardiomyopathy. Before surgery, 66% were in NYHA class III or IV. The mean preoperative ejection fraction was 26 ± 8.5%, and QRS duration was 121.8 ± 31.6 ms. Concomitant procedures included CABG in 85% of patients and mitral valve repair in 43%.

Overall survival at 30 days and 1, 2, and 3 years was 98%, 92%, 90%, and 86%, respectively. Freedom from readmission for heart failure at 1, 2, and 3 years was 80%, 70%, and 61%, respectively. Readmission was more common in older patients and those with a longer QRS duration, higher preoperative pulmonary artery diastolic pressures, postoperative pulmonary artery systolic pressures, and longer cardiopulmonary bypass times. Freedom from adverse events (e.g., transplant listing, return to NYHA class IV, LVAD, death) at 1, 2, and 3 years was 89%, 85%, and 83%, respectively. We did find that preoperative ventricular dysrhythmia was a powerful predictor of worse outcomes. Both adverse events ($p = .002$) and readmission ($p = .02$) were significantly higher in patients with a longer QRS duration. The presence of a preoperative implantable cardioverter defibrillator (ICD) also was associated with early mortality ($p = .001$). On the other hand, preoperative NYHA class, LV ejection fraction, preoperative ventricular volumes, prior cardiac surgery, and need for mitral valve repair were not risk factors for worse outcomes once the conduction disturbances were taken into account.

The Future

In the future, we need to define the appropriate candidates for LV reconstruction. With the advance in imaging technology, we should be better able to predict which patients will benefit from reconstruction and which will benefit from revascularization and valvular correction alone. In addition, the distinction between akinetic and dyskinetic segments must be clearly defined. Although there are several different methods of defining segment function, a simple, reproducible method has not yet been established. Finally, the effect of location of the aneurysm, the effect of a patch, and the indications for postoperative arrhythmia treatment need to be more completely understood.

On the horizon are the fields of gene and cellular transplantation. These modalities are in their infancy, but show encouraging early results.

GENE TRANSFER

Gene transfer involves the addition of genetic material into an already mature cardiac myocyte. Using the cell's own machinery, a target protein is produced to elicit a desired response. Already gene transfer has been used in animals to enhance myocardial perfusion[70,107] and improve cardiac performance.[53,83] However, several barriers to further application exist. These include a vehicle for gene transfer, mechanism of delivery, and choice of genetic material.

Unfortunately, the ideal vector for gene delivery does not exist. A vector should efficiently transfer a large piece of genetic material into a variety of selectable cell types without any adverse effects on either the target organ or the local cellular environment. At present, only a few vectors can achieve high levels of transgene expression. These include synthetic oligonucleotides, plasmids, adenoviral vectors, retroviral vectors, and lentivirus vectors. Each has advantages and disadvantages, but none are ideal. Future work should help produce a better vehicle.

The appropriate route of delivery is also still being determined. There has been success with direct myocardial injection, endocardial catheter-based techniques, pericardial gene delivery, and intravenous infusions.[13,64,73,159] More recently, autologous cells have been transfected and then injected into the myocardium.[175] This allows the injected cell to secrete the target protein. There are advantages and disadvantages to each of these routes. Moreover, different clinical situations may favor different modes of delivery. For example, concomitant cardiac surgery obviously lends itself to direct injection. Nonetheless, even the route of delivery is not yet firmly established.

Perhaps most importantly, the choice of gene or genes awaits identification. The four most promising targets include calcium homeostasis, β-adrenoreceptor signaling, adenylyl cyclase, and the V2 vasopressin receptor.

Both animal and human models suggest that a derangement in the sarcoplasmic Ca^{++} reuptake system after the completion of a contraction cycle is at least partly responsible for the decreased systolic force, prolonged relaxation, and elevated diastolic force in CHF.[7,74,75] An imbalance in expression of the sarcoplasmic calcium reuptake pump SERCA2a and its inhibitor phospholamban appears to be present in patients with CHF and is an obvious target for treatment.[77,88] Gene therapies directed toward calcium homeostasis have demonstrated early successes in isolated human myocytes and in vivo animal models of CHF.[52,83] This is perhaps the most promising target for gene therapy in heart failure to date.

Derangements in adrenergic signaling represent another potential target for gene therapy. Downregulation of β-adrenoreceptor, uncoupling from second messenger systems, and upregulation of β-adrenoreceptor kinase have all been demonstrated as significant components of heart failure.[30] In animal models, gene transfer–induced overexpression of β-adrenoreceptor and an inhibitor of β-adrenoreceptor kinase prevented the development of cardiomyopathy and improved contractility in a heart failure model.[149] Although patients receiving chronic β-agonist therapy have increased mortality, further investigation is needed to explore the β-adrenoreceptor as a potential therapeutic gene target.[125]

One mechanism for improved contractility after β-adrenoreceptor stimulation is an increase in cytosolic cyclic adenosine monophosphate (cAMP). Therefore the direct increase in cAMP has been another potential target. In fact, adenoviral-mediated cAMP increases have resulted in a sustained improvement in LV contractility.[99] However, similar to β-agonists, phosphodiesterase inhibitors have been shown to increase cardiac mortality and function.[110] Therefore a strategy that aims at increasing cAMP levels must be pursued with caution.

One potential target that may not be quite as obvious as the others is that of V2 vasopressin receptors (V2Rs), which promote the activation of adenyl cyclase. V2Rs are only physiologically expressed in the kidney and are not in the myocardium. However, gene transfer of the V2R into the myocardium and stimulation with desmopressin acetate (DDAVP) have been demonstrated to improve cardiac contractility.[172] Although the ideal gene has not yet been identified, an innovative approach such as this may help us find the appropriate gene or genes to help treat heart failure.

CELL TRANSPLANTATION

Once the myocardium is dead, it becomes a scar and can no longer contract. After myocardial infarction, even with reperfusion, a segment may have a significant area of myocardium that becomes a scar so that the segment, although viable, can no longer contribute to ventricular function. The segment is akinetic. The goal of cell transplantation is to repopulate areas of dead myocardium with a new pool of contractile cells to restore functioning in that segment of myocardium. The contribution of this target segment should improve overall cardiac function. Although there may be a role for cell transplantation in idiopathic cardiomyopathy, the majority of work to date has focused on ischemic disease.

Most studies have searched for the appropriate type of cell to repopulate the dead myocardium. The cells must be able to incorporate into the recipient myocardium. They must be able to survive, mature, and electromechanically couple with each other and the native myocardium. Both differentiated (fetal cardiac myocytes),[155] skeletal myoblasts,[85] fibroblasts,[144] smooth muscle cells,[103] and undifferentiated cells (stem cells)[126] have been used with varying degrees of success. This next section highlights some of the results.

Differentiated Cells

Both cardiac myocytes and skeletal myoblasts engraft and survive for at least several months in syngeneic myocardium.[95,157] However, only fetal myocytes have demonstrated the ability to develop intercalated disks.[155] Nonetheless, when fetal cardiac myocytes or skeletal myoblasts are transplanted 1 week after myocardial infarction, there is a similar functional improvement in LV function 1 month later.[148] Because of ethical issues and limited availability, fetal tissues have been virtually eliminated from clinical consideration. This, along with their accessibility and ease of handling, has made skeletal myoblasts the differentiated cell type of choice for cell transplantation.

Several limitations of differentiated cell transplantation may preclude the widespread application to the clinical setting. Although the transplantation of skeletal myoblasts increases the mass of contracting cells and improves ventricular performance, the greatest benefit occurs within days to weeks of myocardial infarction.[10] Unfortunately,

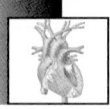

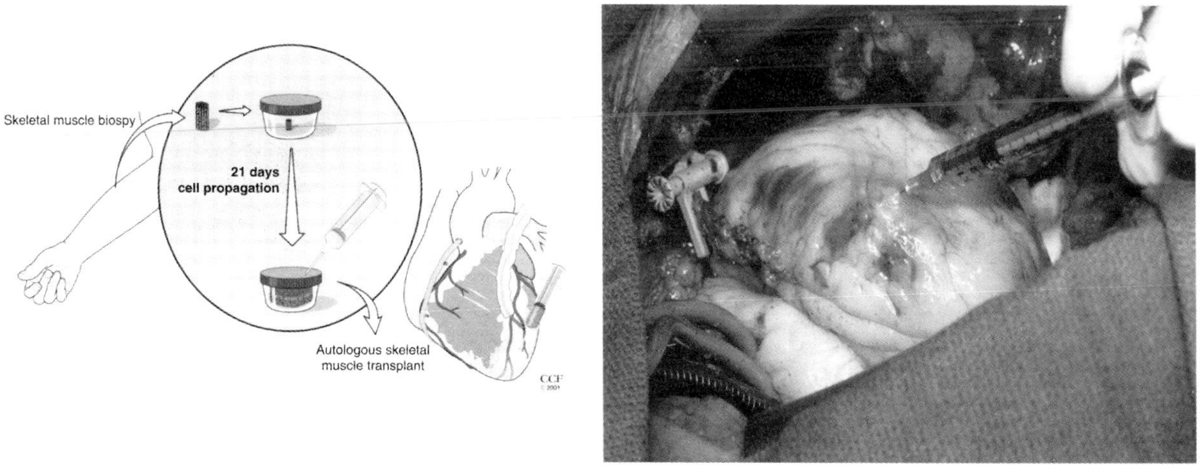

Figure 96–5 This figure illustrates the technique of skeletal myoblast transplantation. Skeletal muscle is harvested from an extremity; cells are then cultured for 3–4 weeks and then are directly injected into the ventricular myocardium.

harvesting and expanding these cells requires 3–4 weeks (Figure 96-5). Moreover, skeletal myoblast transplantation does not lead to the generation of blood vessels or cardiac myocytes.[123] To overcome these limitations, some attention has shifted to the transplantation of undifferentiated cells.

Undifferentiated Cells

Proliferating myocytes are present in human hearts after myocardial infarction.[17] Part of the normal physiological response to myocardial infarction involves mobilization of stem cells, "homing" of these cells into the damaged myocardium, and differentiation of at least some of these stem cells into cardiac myocytes.[17,84,153] Unfortunately, stem cell engraftment and differentiation into essential components of functional myocardium is an infrequent event.[84] However, if this natural repair mechanism can be potentiated or altered, significant myocardial regeneration may be achievable.

Mesenchymal stem cells can differentiate into cardiomyocytes,[108] and hematopoietic stem cells can differentiate into vascular structures.[164] Both have been studied for the treatment of acute myocardial infarction, and both have demonstrated an improvement in cardiac function in animal models.[94,168] This work in the laboratory has led to phase I trials in the clinical arena. Intracoronary injection of bone marrow–derived mononuclear cells within days after acute myocardial infarction appears to have improved LV contractility and perfusion.[160] Similar benefits have been demonstrated with direct myocardial injection. However, this treatment modality remains in its infancy and awaits further investigation (see Figure 96-5).

Significant achievements have been made in the areas of gene transfer and cell transplantation. However, numerous hurdles must be overcome before they become mainstream therapy for CHF. At present they mainly serve as important tools to understand the processes that cause CHF. Hopefully these tools will soon realize their potential and offer powerful weapons to combat this disease.

VENTRICULAR SURGERY FOR IDIOPATHIC CARDIOMYOPATHY

A common element in the progression and pathogenesis of heart failure is the development of LV remodeling, with subsequent deterioration in LV performance and increased morbidity and mortality.[111] In idiopathic cardiomyopathy, unlike ischemic cardiomyopathy, no discrete focal segment of diseased myocardium that can be excluded exists. Rather, the myocardium is globally diseased. Until recently, patients with idiopathic dilated cardiomyopathy and extreme ventricular dilatation were deemed inoperable and were referred for cardiac transplantation.[51] Surgical options to inhibit and reverse LV remodeling are at the forefront of the future of surgery for CHF.

Dynamic Cardiomyoplasty

Although originally intended as a method of providing mechanical support to the failing heart, dynamic cardiomyoplasty (DCMP) became the first widely used operation to inhibit ventricular remodeling. Carpentier and Chachques[38] performed the first successful surgery on a human in 1985. This breakthrough was accomplished by understanding that skeletal muscle could be transformed into a slow, fatigue-resistant muscle and by developing a pacing device that was capable of stimulating skeletal muscle in synchrony with cardiac contractions.[87]

This operation used the latissimus dorsi muscle as a wrap around the heart, using the implantation of the pacing device to condition the muscle into a fatigue-resistant pump.[2] Initially the procedure was designed to support the failing LV by augmenting systolic ejection and thus improve hemodynamics and symptoms of heart failure. However, it has been found that much of the benefit after DCMP appeared to be derived from the girdling effect of the wrap, which stabilized the remodeling process of the LV.[128]

In the past 15 years more than 800 patients have undergone DCMP. Reports from single centers have helped refine both patient experience and operative technique. Patients with NYHA class IV CHF experienced a prohibitively high operative mortality.[36,68] Importantly, evidence has shown that DCMP offers an improved functional status for many of the survivors, although in most instances, evidence for improvement of accompanying hemodynamic parameters was inconsistent.[87] Kass and colleagues[89] did demonstrate a leftward shift in end-systolic pressure volume relationships, as well as a reduction in LV volume at 12 months postoperatively in a small cohort of patients. However, these results are not consistently reproducible.

Despite the modest success of this procedure, it failed to gain widespread acceptance because of the high early mortality in those patients with advanced heart failure and a lack of demonstrated survival advantage over medical therapy. Results from a controlled randomized trial entitled Cardiomyoplasty-Skeletal Muscle Assist Randomized Trial (C-SMART) will be released in the near future. However, at present, the procedure is not routinely practiced, and the pacer is no longer commercially available.

Partial Left Ventriculectomy

In 1994 Randas Batista proposed the concept of ventricular volume reduction, or partial left ventriculectomy (PLV), as an alternative to cardiac transplantation.[14] The concept was based on Laplace's law and attempted to restore a normal diameter to the left ventricle by excising a portion of the lateral LV wall and thereby reducing the radius and the wall stress. The resected segment was the myocardium between the papillary muscles, or sometimes included papillary muscle transection and reimplantation. The procedure was most often performed with concomitant mitral valve repair or replacement.

From its inception, this procedure generated much controversy. Among the centers performing this operation, different surgical techniques were applied, postoperative outcomes were variable, and long-term survival and effects varied widely.

Follow-up of the earliest series of patients from Batista was inadequate, and hence any conclusions about the success of this surgery were impossible to ascertain. However, in 1997 researchers in Brazil and at Buffalo General Hospital reported on their combined experience of 120 patients undergoing partial left ventriculectomy.[15] Operative mortality was 22%, and survival at 2 years was 55%. Preoperatively, all patients were NYHA class IV and of the survivors, 57% were in NYHA class I and 33% were in NYHA class II.

In general, the outcomes after PLV at other centers generally were poor. However, varying patient selection and surgical techniques make comparison between centers difficult. Many of the earliest patients were not candidates for transplant and hence suffered a high mortality. Patients that would have been relisted for transplant or bridged with an LVAD at the Cleveland Clinic, for example, would have died at those centers. The procedure was thus abandoned at many centers. There was relatively little published information about these small series, with poor results, but it was obvious that the operation was not widely successful.

The most recent report from São Paulo, Brazil includes 37 patients with dilated cardiomyopathy with an operative mortality of 18.9% and actuarial survival rate of 56.7% at 24 months.[158] For the survivors, NYHA class improved from 3.5 ± 0.5 to 1.8 ± 0.9 ($p < .001$), and left ventricular ejection fraction (LVEF) increased from 17.1 ± 4.6% to 23 ± 8% ($p < .001$).

Other reports from England demonstrate a perioperative mortality of 22.5%, but only one late death in 14 patients.[6] This group included patients undergoing both idiopathic and ischemic cardiomyopathy. Results from Yugoslavia included 22 patients with three early deaths (13.6%) and four late deaths with a 1-year survival rate of 68 ± 10%.[67,135] Ejection fraction (EF) increased from 23.9 ± 6.8% to 40.7 ± 12.5% ($p < .001$) in survivors. Further study showed a decrease in LV circumferential end-systolic and end-diastolic stresses ($p = .0014$).

Between May 1996 and December 1998, 62 patients at the Cleveland Clinic underwent PLV for the treatment of advanced refractive heart failure. All but three in this group were candidates for cardiac transplantation and were either NYHA class III (39%) or NYHA class IV (61%). In general, this was an acutely ill population with a mean LVEF of 13.5%, peak oxygen consumption of 10.7 ml/kg/min, LV end-diastolic volume index of 330 ml/m^2, and 37% were inotrope dependent. Operative technique included excision of the lateral left ventricle between the papillary muscles with mitral valve repair, with papillary muscle reimplantation as needed.

In our initial publication from that series, we made several positive observations, including acute improvement in LV function, mitral regurgitation, and clinical functional class during early follow-up (mean period, 5 months). We also noted, however, the occurrence of unpredictable early failures and concluded that the operation should be approached with caution.[114]

A recent report of this operation as a surgical option for patients with advanced heart failure was recently performed to determine outcomes at 5 years. The primary end-points of this multivariable analysis were death, return to NYHA class IV, and relisting for transplantation. With a mean follow-up period of 3.3 ± 1.9 years, survival was 82%, 78%, and 52% at 1, 2, and 5 years, respectively. The risk of death (hazard function) consisted of two phases: an early phase that peaked at 4 months, followed by a constant hazard phase of 11% per year.[82] Event-free survival was 46%, 41%, and 23% at 1, 2, and 5 years, respectively. The observed 82% survival at 1 year, compared with the relatively poor event-free survival of 46% for the same time period, indicates the use of LVADs and transplantation in this population.

Although only young age was found to be a risk factor for failure in our early series, our more recent analysis demonstrated that increased pulmonary artery systolic pressure (>40 mm Hg) at evaluation was a powerful predictor of poor survival. Reduced maximum exercise oxygen consumption at baseline was associated with a rapid return to NYHA class IV heart failure. Furthermore, the higher the left atrial pressure, the lower was the event-free survival. With rare exceptions, late failure was not associated with redilation, drop in EF, or return of mitral regurgitation, even for patients undergoing papillary muscle resection.[63]

To date there remains a group of patients in our series who continue to benefit from PLV. The large number of early and late failures, however, continues to justify our decision to abandon the use of PLV as a surgical therapy for heart failure.

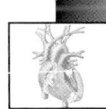

A number of reports have attempted to identify risk factors for heart failure. The Partial Left Ventriculectomy Second International Registry analyzed outcomes on 287 patients from 48 institutions in an effort to standardize inclusion and exclusion criteria and predict risk factors for heart failure after PLV.[90] Event-free survival (defined as freedom from death, LVAD, or listing for transplantation), was significantly reduced when PLV was performed as an emergent rather than as an elective procedure ($p < .001$). NYHA class IV preoperatively demonstrated an event-free survival of 39% at 2 years versus NYHA class less than IV, which was 59% ($p = .002$).

Mathematical modeling and finite element analysis predicted that PLV should improve systolic contractility, but was accompanied by decreased diastolic function, leading to overall depressed pump function.[56,139] Gorcsan et al[66] concluded that PLV, although resulting in improvements in EF and right ventricular (RV) ejection, was associated with accompanying LV stiffness. Additionally, the degree of improvement in LV function was associated with the degree of myocardial fibrosis present.

In summary, the PLV experience demonstrated that there are some patients with end-stage heart failure who respond to ventricular reconstruction with sustained benefit for years. However, the price to be paid for this surgical intervention generally was early heart failure and mortality. Failures remain unpredictable, and because of this, PLV should not be applied instead of cardiac transplantation. Much remains to be unraveled regarding the mystery of why PLV provides benefits to some patients and not to others.

ALTERNATIVE DEVICE THERAPIES

From lessons learned with dynamic cardiomyoplasty and PLV, two new devices have been developed to either prevent myocyte overstretch and provide passive LV constraint (Acorn CorCap, St. Paul, MN) or reshape the left ventricle without removing functioning myocardium (Myocor Myosplint, Maple Grove, MN).

The first such device is the Acorn CorCap, a meshlike polyester jacket that is surgically placed around the ventricles of the heart (Figure 96-6). Constructed from compliant woven mesh, it is designed to provide both flexibility and strength. The design of the mesh permits bidirectional compliance of the fabric, which allows it to conform easily to the heart, thus allowing the heart to return to a more normal ellipsoidal shape. CorCap placement often is performed with concomitant valve repair or coronary artery bypass.

Preclinical studies with CorCap have been reported from two different heart failure models. In an intracoronary microembolization canine heart failure model, Saavedra et al[141] have shown that long-term use of CorCap results in lowered end-diastolic and end-systolic volumes and shifted the end-systolic pressure volume relation to the left, compatible with reverse remodeling. In a canine heart failure model, Chaudhry et al[40] demonstrated an improvement in LV diastolic function and chamber sphericity, decreased wall stress, and no evidence of functional mitral regurgitation. In testing on the ovine heart failure model, Power and associates[136] reported similar findings of improved cardiac function, as evidenced by increased EF, fractional shortening, positive

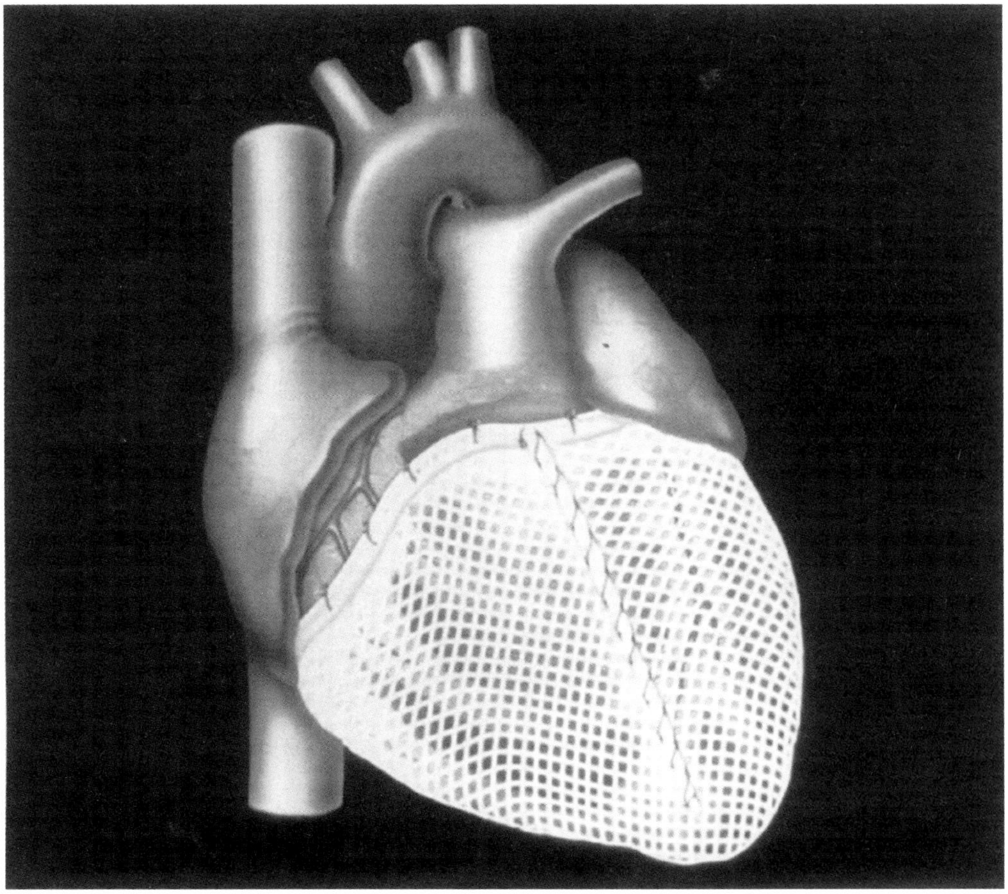

Figure 96–6 The Acorn CorCap is a meshlike polyester jacket that is surgically wrapped around a dilated left ventricle, often in conjunction with another cardiac procedure. Results of the randomized trial utilizing the device will soon be released.

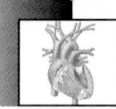

dP/dt, and negative dP/dt. In a study indicative of early reverse remodeling at the cellular level, Sabbah et al[142] found downregulation of a stretch-mediated p21 ras and sarcoplasmic reticulum adenosine triphosphatase (ATPase) after wrap placement in the canine model, suggesting that the CorCap can alter gene expression.

Recently the effect of CorCap on akinetic area development after acute myocardial infarction in an ovine model was investigated. After a baseline MRI study after creation of an anterior infarct in 10 sheep, the device was placed in five sheep, with the five remaining animals serving as controls. The terminal study done at 2 months after infarction revealed a significantly diminished area of akinesis in the CorCap group, with the relative area of akinesis following a similar pattern.[131]

Konertz et al[96] examined the safety and efficacy of the CorCap in a series of 27 patients suffering from cardiomyopathy with a mean NYHA class of 2.6 ± 0.1. Of these, 16 received concomitant cardiac surgery, principally mitral valve repair or replacement, and the remaining 11 patients received the CorCap only. In the device-only group, 5 of the 11 patients experienced adverse events, including two deaths during an average follow-up period of 12.2 ± 1.1 months, but none of the events were device related. Follow-up at 3 and 6 months reflected a significant improvement from pretreatment in EF (21% to 28% and 33%) and NYHA functional class (2.5 to 1.6 and 1.7), as well as a significant decrease in LV end-diastolic diameter (LVEDD) (74 mm to 68 mm and 65 mm) and LV end-systolic diameter (LVESD) (65 mm to 62 mm and 57 mm).

Raman et al[138] reported similar findings in a cohort of five patients undergoing CorCap placement with concomitant CABG. Midterm outcomes at 12 months follow-up demonstrated a significant decrease in LVEDD and LVESD, with an improvement in LVEF and NYHA functional class.

From these early safety and feasibility studies it appears that the CorCap device may be useful in preventing further cardiac dilation and may improve symptoms of heart failure without device-related morbidity or mortality. However, a randomized, prospective clinical trial of the Acorn CorCap is currently underway in Europe, the United States, and Australia to confirm these early observations.

Myocor Myosplint

The Myocor Myosplint was designed to change the geometry of the left ventricle, thereby decreasing wall stress and improving hemodynamics. The implant consists of two epicardial pads and a transventricular tension member. The two pads are located on the surface of the heart, with the load-bearing tension member passing through the ventricle connecting the pads and drawing the ventricular walls toward one another (Figure 96-7). Typically, three Myosplints are placed on the beating heart from the lateral left ventricle through the posterior intraventricular septum. The splints are then tightened to create a bilobular shape.

The Myosplint initially was studied in the canine heart failure model to assess outcomes at 1 month after

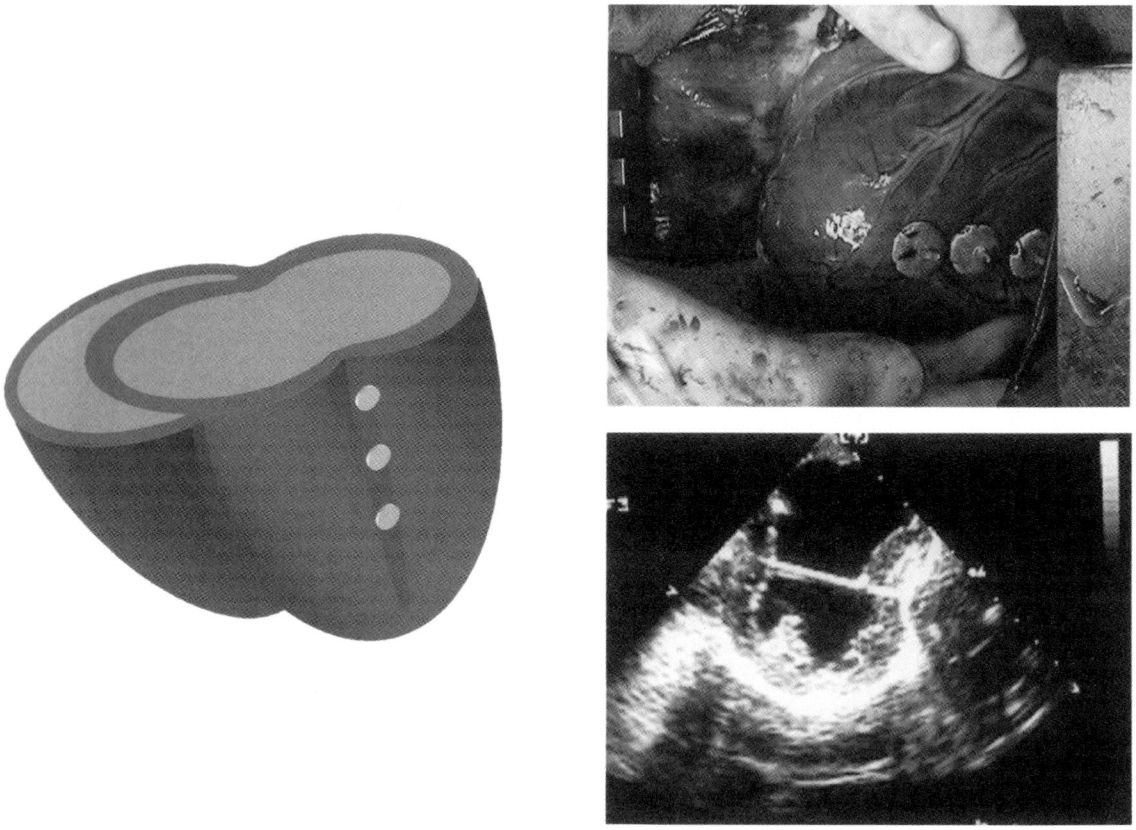

Figure 96–7 The Myosplint implants transventricular tension members to alter the geometry of the left ventricle into a bilobular shape. This reduces the tension on each of the individual ventricular segments and may promote reverse remodeling.

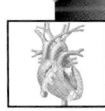

application. In this trial, heart failure was induced in 15 dogs over a period of 27 days. Of these, seven animals underwent sham surgery and eight animals received the Myosplint device. With the use of 3D echocardiographic calculations, LVEF significantly increased from 19% at baseline to 36% acutely and remained at 39% at 1 month after Myosplint implantation. Also, LV end-diastolic volume (LVEDV) and LV end-systolic volume (LVESV) significantly decreased and were sustained at 1 month after implantation. End-systolic wall stress (ESWS) significantly decreased by 39% acutely and by 31% at 1 month after implantation. Also, end-diastolic wall stress (EDWS) was significantly reduced by 30% acutely and by 41% at 1 month after implantation.[115]

Chronic human studies were first performed in seven patients with dilated cardiomyopathy and NYHA class III and IV. LVEDD in this group ranged from 72–102 mm. Mitral valve regurgitation was mild in three patients and moderate in four cases. Four patients underwent concomitant mitral valve repair at the time of Myosplint implant. At 3-month follow-up, one patient experienced worsening heart failure attributed to unrepaired and significant mitral regurgitation. The remaining six patients had improvement in symptoms of heart failure, with two of the patients being removed from the transplant waiting list. This early experience demonstrated that Myosplint implantation can be safely performed without significant adverse affects; however, these investigators noted that mitral valve repair should be done in any patient undergoing the Myosplint implant.[146]

The long-term effect of Myosplint therapy on cardiac function awaits results from a larger, randomized study. Currently the Myosplint is undergoing U.S. Food and Drug Administration (FDA) feasibility testing in the United States.

CORONARY ARTERY BYPASS SURGERY

Ischemic cardiomyopathy (ICM) currently represents the most common cause of CHF, ranging from 40–70% in different studies.[42,78] Ischemia, stunning, and hibernation are all viable myocardial states that are different from infarction. Ischemia is defined by adequate blood flow and intact function at rest with impaired flow reserve, and rapidly reversible function impairment with exercise. Myocardial stunning is ischemia with prolonged postischemic dysfunction. Hibernation describes myocardium that has impaired resting blood flow and function without response to exercise. All of these states frequently coexist in patients with ICM. However, their relative proportions are different and have tremendous importance for predicting improvement after CABG. Therefore preoperative assessment of the extent of myocardial viability has a tremendous impact on the decision to operate on patients with severe LV dysfunction. Providing more blood to scar tissue will not improve ventricular function.

At the Cleveland Clinic, MRI (when feasible) and positron emission tomography (PET) are the methods of choice in the preoperative assessment of myocardial viability. Newer MRI protocols assess the extent and distribution of scar and segmental perfusion and function relations, as well as associated aneurysm, LV thrombus, and mitral regurgitation. After a complete evaluation, we tend to offer surgery to patients with compensated CHF whom we believe will have improved ventricular function by increasing blood flow to ischemic, viable myocardium.

The evidence to operate on these patients comes from subsets of patients from earlier large randomized series. The Veteran's Affairs Cooperative Study of coronary bypass surgery demonstrated a survival advantage for patients with impaired ventricular function who underwent revascularization as compared with those who were medically managed.[78,167] In the Coronary Artery Surgery Study (CASS), patients with mild or moderately impaired ventricular function had an improved survival after CABG as compared with those who were medically treated.[127] Unfortunately, few patients with severe LV impairment were included. However, surgery also decreased the risk of sudden death in patients with a history of CHF. A second Veteran's Affairs (VA) trial in patients with unstable angina also demonstrated a survival advantage in patients with abnormal LV function who underwent bypass surgery.[150] The results of these studies have been further supported by data from the SOLVD (Studies of Left Ventricular Dysfunction) studies and other reports.[171] Patients taking angiotensin converting enzyme (ACE) inhibitors who had previously undergone revascularization have a lower mortality rate as compared with those who had not undergone bypass surgery.

Despite this information, surgeons were reluctant to operate on patients with poor ventricular function, because it usually translated into poor surgical outcomes. Fortunately, this has changed. The outcome after CABG in the setting of severe LV dysfunction has improved significantly over time. Table 96-1 reviews the largest series of CABG with severe LV dysfunction.[118] Perioperative mortality in more recent series has decreased and now approaches 2–8% at many institutions. Late survival, angina status, and NYHA class have improved in follow-up periods. In a series that assessed postoperative resting EF, EF improved in a majority of patients (Table 96-2).[97]

However, LV dysfunction remains a major marker of increased morbidity and mortality after CABG.[166] Patients with EF <20% are four times more likely to develop low cardiac output syndrome as compared with patients with normal EF. In the CABG Patch trial, patients with preoperative CHF had twofold greater perioperative mortality than those with normal ventricular function.[22] The impact of CHF on outcome after CABG also was noted in the SHOCK (Should We Revascularize Occluded Coronaries in Cardiovascular Shock) trial.[81] In this randomized trial of revascularization versus medical therapy for cardiogenic shock after myocardial infarction, patients who had CABG had 30-day and 1-year mortality of 47% and 53.3%, respectively. Although this is worse than the results of CABG in compensated CHF, patients in the medical therapy study arm had worse 30-day and 1-year mortality (56% and 66.4%, respectively).

Currently, coronary bypass surgery remains an important treatment for ICM with compensated CHF. Although these patients are at higher risk, morbidity and mortality have improved and have become acceptable. Future studies are needed to optimize imaging protocols for viability assessment and define the patients who will achieve the greatest benefit from revascularization.

Table 96–1

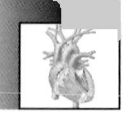

Results of CABG for Severe Left Ventricular Dysfunction

First author	*Number of patients*	*Years*	*Ejection fraction*	*Perioperative mortality (%)*	*Late mortality (%)*
Vlietstra	10	1966–72	<0.25	—	60 (2 yrs)
Manley	183	1968–71	mean 0.22	16	43 (5 yrs)
Yatteau	24	1968–72	<0.25	42	50 (2 yrs)
Oldham	11	1969–72	= 0.25	55	—
Zubiate	140	1969–75	<0.20	22	41.6 (6 yrs)
Faulkner	46	1969–75	mean 0.21	4	17 (2 yrs)
Mitchel	9	—	<0.20	0	11 (1 yr)
Fox	7	1971–74	<0.20	0	14
Jones	41	1973–77	<0.20	2.5	10 (1 yr)
Alderman	82	1975–79	= 0.25	8	37 (5 yrs)
Mochtar	62	1975–83	mean 0.25	4.8	30 (5 yrs)
Zubiate	93	1976–81	<0.20	5	50 (5 yrs)
Hochberg	51	1976–82	0.20–0.24	12	42 (3 yrs)
Hochberg	41	1976–82	<0.20	37	85 (3 yrs)
Sanchez	23	1982–89	mean 0.28	9	24 (2 yrs)
Kron	39	1983–88	<0.20	2.6	17 (3 yrs)
Blakeman	20	1984–88	mean 0.18	15	30 (1 yr)
Wong	22	1986–89	mean 0.25	9	23 (3 yrs)
Christakis	487	1982–90	<0.20	9.8	—
Hammermeister	251	1987–90	<0.20	9.2	—
Louie	22	1984–90	mean 0.23	13.6	28 (3 yrs)

Table 96–1

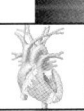

Results of CABG for Severe Left Ventricular Dysfunction—cont'd

First author	*Number of patients*	*Years*	*Ejection fraction*	*Perioperative mortality (%)*	*Late mortality (%)*
Milano	118	1981–91	<0.25	11	42 (5 yrs)
Shapira	74	1986–91	<0.30	—	13.5 (5 yrs)
Anderson	203	1983–92	mean 0.34	6	41 (5 yrs)
Hausmann	265	1986–92	mean 0.24	7.6	13 (3 yrs)
Kaul	210	1987–92	= 0.20	10	27 (5 yrs)
Mickleborough	79	1982–93	<0.20	3.8	32 (5 yrs)
Langenburg	96	1983–93	= 0.25	8.3	—
Elefteraides	135	1986–94	= 0.30	5.2	29 (4.5 yrs)
Iskandrian	269	1991–94	= 0.35	7.1	—
Kawachi	50	1982–95	= 0.30	8	26 (5 yrs)
Moshkovitz	75	1991–94	= 0.35	2.7	27 (4 yrs)
Trachiotis	156	1981–95	<0.25	3.8	35 (5 yrs)
Baumgartner	61	1990–96	<0.25	8	—
Cimochowski	111	1992–96	<0.35	1.8	—
Argenziano [CABG Patch]	454 no CHF 4 434 CHF	1993–96	= 0.35	3.5 no CHF 7.7 CHF	—
DeCarlo	80	1994–96	= 0.30	6.3	18 (2 yrs)
Luciani	116	1991–98	= 0.30	1.7	25 (5 yrs)

Reprinted from Kumpati GS, McCarthy PM, Hoercher KJ: Surgical treatments for heart failure. Cardiol Clin 19(4):669–681, 2002.

Table 96–2

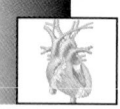

Improvement in Ejection Fraction (EF) after CABG for Severe Left Ventricular Dysfunction in Recent Series

First author	*Preoperative EF (mean+/–SD)*	*Postoperative EF (mean+/–SD)*	*Percentage of patients with EF increase (%)*	*Interval to postoperative EF*	*p*
Milano	0.21	0.27	N/A	N/A	< .005
Shapira	0.24	0.36	73 (>0.07)	5.8 mo	< .0001
Elefteraides	0.24	0.34	70 (= 0.05)	4.6 mo	< .0001
DeCarlo	0.27+/–0.04	0.38+/–0.08	N/A	N/A	< .001
Luciani	0.28+/–0.05	0.38+/–0.09	N/A	N/A	<0.001

Data from Kumpati GS, McCarthy PM, Hoercher KJ: Surgical treatments for heart failure. Cardiol Clin 19(4):669–681, 2002.
SD, Standard deviation; N/A, not applicable.

VALVULAR HEART DISEASE IN CONGESTIVE HEART FAILURE

Valvular disease itself is an important cause of CHF, but at times may be the effect of heart failure from another etiology. Once present, it continues to adversely affect patient survival and well-being and should be corrected. This section reviews the results of the surgical treatment of the aortic, mitral, and tricuspid valves and offers guidelines for the treatment of these high-risk patients.

The Aortic Valve

Clinicians commonly must make a judgment about the wisdom of operative intervention in patients with poor LV function in the following two types of aortic valve disease: (1) severe aortic stenosis with a low gradient and (2) severe aortic insufficiency with LV dilatation. This section addresses each of these clinical challenges.

Aortic Stenosis

Physiological changes from the increased afterload with aortic stenosis lead to a host of symptoms such as angina, dyspnea, syncope, and sudden death.[129] The guidelines for the management of patients with aortic valve disease generally are clear, but for patients with severe LV dysfunction the guidelines reflect conflicting evidence and the results of surgery have been difficult to predict.[26] Patients with severe aortic stenosis and low cardiac output may have only a modest transvalvular pressure gradient (i.e., <30 mm Hg). In these patients it may be difficult to determine the presence of severe aortic stenosis. In many cases of mild to moderate aortic stenosis, the valve does not open because of the underlying cardiomyopathy. Standard valve area formulas to calculate the severity of aortic stenosis are less accurate and may underestimate the valve area in low-flow states. Therefore these data should be interpreted with caution, and it is recommended that echocardiographic data be further validated with other diagnostic tests, which may include cardiac catheterization to determine the transvalvular gradient and dobutamine stress echo. In general, confirmation of severe aortic stenosis by at least two separate studies should provide assurance to the surgeon of the existence of true disease.[41]

Pereira, Asher, and others[130] reviewed the outcomes for three groups of patients with aortic stenosis at the Cleveland Clinic from 1990–1998. Group 1 included 68 patients who had aortic valve replacement (AVR) with aortic valve area (AVA) ≤0.75 cm^2, LVEF ≤35%, and mean gradient ≤30 mm Hg. Group 2 included 297 patients who had AVR with AVA ≤0.75 cm^2, LVEF ≤50%, and mean gradient ≤35 mm Hg. Finally, group 3 included 89 patients who did not receive AVR but who had AVA ≤0.75 cm^2, LVEF ≤35%, and mean gradient ≤30 mm Hg. A propensity analysis compared survival between a cohort of patients in group 1 (low gradient, AVR) versus group 3 (low gradient, no AVR).

Baseline characteristics in the surgical group with severe LV dysfunction were worse. However, the perioperative mortality was similar (5.9% among group 1 versus 4.0% in group 2). Many of the echocardiographic and cardiac catheterization data were worse for the low-gradient group 1 patients, and the surgery was more complex. With a multivariable analysis, the presence of elevated serum creatinine, older age, and moderate to severe RV dysfunction were the only significant predictors of mortality. In general, 1- and 4-year survival rates were good in both groups (Figure 96-8). One- and 4-year survival rates were 82% and 75%, respectively, for group 1 and 92% and 82% for group 2.

This information proved valuable by demonstrating that in the modern era, AVR can be performed in this patient population with operative mortality similar to patients with

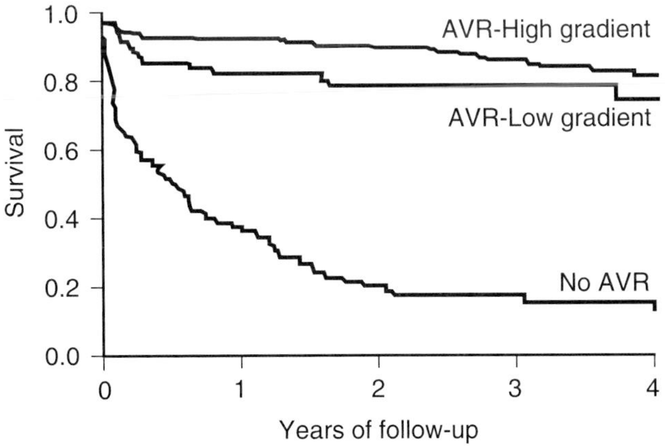

AVR-Highgrad	297	238	166	102	63
AVR-Lowgrad	68	47	32	25	21
No AVR	89	31	13	9	4

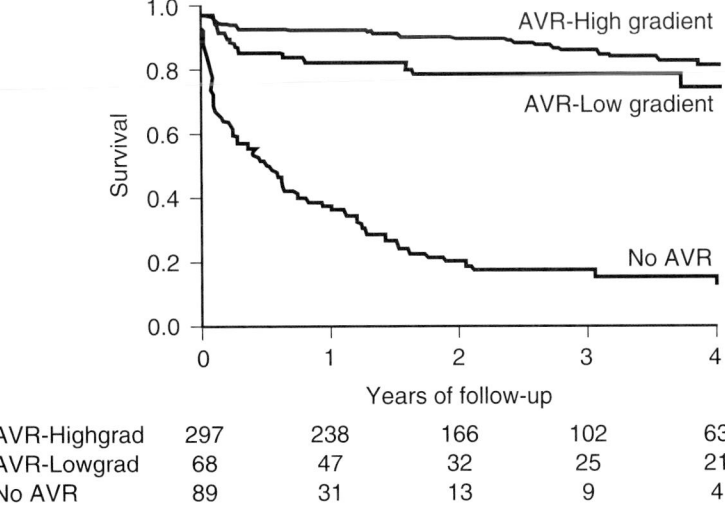

Figure 96–8 **Comparison of survival in patients with aortic valve stenosis after aortic valve replacement (AVR) (for high and low gradients) and medical management.**

better LV function. Conversely, the prognosis for patients who did not undergo AVR was dismal. As compared with the patients in group 1, the group 3 patients (severe LV, low gradient, no AVR) generally were older and had a higher percentage of NYHA class III or IV heart failure. Echocardiography also showed that the patients who did not have surgery had more mitral regurgitation and higher pulmonary artery systolic pressures, but similar aortic valve findings. Therefore a propensity-matched analysis was performed. Even in the propensity-matched group, survival was markedly diminished in the patients who had not undergone aortic valve surgery (see Figure 96-8). Furthermore, NYHA functional class improved in patients who underwent AVR.

Patients who have aortic stenosis with severe LV dysfunction and a low transvalvular gradient can undergo AVR at a slightly higher risk than patients with better ventricular function. However, late survival is much improved compared with the patients who did not undergo aortic valve surgery. Late improvement in NYHA functional class also is much better in patients who undergo aortic valve surgery.

Our results stand in contrast to previous reports, although the studies differed because of the exact patient population that was targeted for study.[24,31,45,154] Previous studies included patients before 1990 and therefore may have included patients with older prostheses with higher gradients, and poor myocardial protection. The literature on this subject generally consists of small patient series, and it is hard to draw firm conclusions. Nevertheless, if a physician faces a patient today with severe aortic stenosis and severe LV dysfunction, the diagnosis should be confirmed with studies such as dobutamine echocardiography, and then aortic valve surgery should be offered to these patients unless other medical conditions preclude this option.

Aortic Insufficiency

Patients who have symptomatic aortic insufficiency most often have dyspnea. Occasionally they have angina. Currently the indications for operative intervention include the following: (1) functional NYHA class III or IV symptoms with preserved LV function, (2) NYHA class II symptoms with progressive LV dilatation or angina, (3) asymptomatic patients with mild to moderate LV dysfunction, and (4) patients undergoing coronary artery bypass or other operations who have moderate to severe aortic insufficiency.[26] However, the guidelines for patients with severe LV dysfunction are less clear. Symptomatic patients with advanced LV dysfunction (EF <25%, and/or end-systolic dimension >60 mm) may have developed irreversible myocardial changes that are not improved by correction of the regurgitation.[116] Unfortunately, patients may not have presenting symptoms until advanced heart failure with severe LV dysfunction and ventricular dilatation is present.

In chronic aortic regurgitation, the left ventricle compensates by developing a large end-diastolic volume and eccentric cardiac hypertrophy.[62,72,129,133] A decrease in diastolic coronary flow from a profound reduction in diastolic perfusion pressure may even cause anginal symptoms.[130] The adaptive process leads to myocardial fibrosis. As aortic insufficiency continues, diastolic wall stress increases without a further increase in wall thickness, and myofibril slippage may develop. A vicious cycle ensues. Further increases in diastolic stress lead to further myocardial damage and fibrosis. It is difficult to determine the point at which the cycle becomes "irreversible," that is, the point when valve replacement does not improve cardiac function. The patients in this group present the greatest risk.[28]

Historically the natural history of patients with aortic regurgitation managed medically is dismal.[8] In the early days of cardiac surgery, operations in this group of patients were high risk.[29,43] However, several critical aspects of cardiac surgery have subsequently changed. At the time, cardioplegia was not common, the prostheses left high gradients, and perioperative care was less sophisticated. As practitioners' experience grew, the results improved.[27,61,93,169] However, the failures of that early experience left an unfavorable perception that continues today.

At the Cleveland Clinic, we reported outcomes in this high risk group of patients. We retrospectively examined 102 patients with chronic severe aortic insufficiency (AI) and LV dysfunction (EF ≤30%) who underwent isolated aortic valve surgery from 1972–1998.[113] Seven hundred and twenty-one patients with EF >30% who underwent isolated

AVR for AI served as controls. The severe LV group was older, had a higher NYHA class at baseline, and had more dilated ventricles.

Before 1980, 30-day operative mortality for patients with low EFs was high (24% versus 4%). From 1980–1990 there was some improvement, but operative mortality in the severe group remained high (14% versus 1%), as shown in Table 96-3. However, since 1990, hospital mortality was 0% for the severe LV group and 1% for the patients with better LV function. Furthermore, 5-year survival was markedly worse before 1980 for the patients with severe LV dysfunction, but it has not been significantly different since 1990. A substudy of patients with adequate early and late follow-up echocardiograms also documented favorable myocardial reverse remodeling (reduction in mass and volume, and increase in EF) over 2 years.[173]

We conclude from this experience that even with severe LV dysfunction, chronic aortic regurgitation should be treated with valve replacement in the modern era of cardiac surgery. Good early and late survival rates are expected, along with an improvement in ventricular function.

Aortic valve surgery for patients with the most advanced ventricular dysfunction can be performed with low risk. In the age of implantable LVADs, these operations can be carried out in centers that have LVAD capability as a "safety net" in case of early heart failure. However, this situation is rare. Today, with improved myocardial protection, better perioperative use of inotropes, and more advanced valve prostheses with low gradients, AVR can be safely performed for aortic insufficiency, even in patients with severe LV dysfunction.

Mitral Valve

A common complication of ischemic and nonischemic dilated cardiomyopathy is severe mitral regurgitation. In the setting of end-stage heart failure, as the left ventricle undergoes remodeling, the papillary muscles are displaced. The coaptation of the mitral valve leaflets is decreased, and a central jet of mitral regurgitation is produced with restricted posterior leaflet motion. This results in greater LV volume overload, increasing ventricular dilatation and dysfunction, and worsening mitral regurgitation. This is a vicious cycle in which ventricular dilatation begets mitral regurgitation and mitral regurgitation begets further dilatation.

Determination of the surgical candidacy of a symptomatic patient with mitral regurgitation and severe LV dysfunction has evolved over time. Mitral valve surgery in these patients was previously thought to be associated with a prohibitive operative mortality. Historically, physicians erroneously believed that the mitral regurgitation served as a pop-off mechanism to unload the diseased LV that had difficulty ejecting into the systemic aortic pressure.[92] They feared that a surgically replaced mitral valve would remove that pop-off mechanism and result in profound LV failure and perioperative death. This is in fact rare. A more thorough understanding of valvular–ventricular interaction with chordal preservation has improved postoperative ventricular function. In addition, the development of mitral valve repair techniques and improved myocardial protection have led to excellent surgical outcomes.

The resistance to correcting mitral valve pathology in patients with LV dysfunction was largely based on results produced by the use of traditional mitral valve replacement. This technique did not preserve the subvalvular apparatus.[50,105] Separating the valve from the ventricular wall caused further ventricular dilatation and decreased LV function. Subsequently, we have learned the importance of conserving the subvalvular apparatus in order to better preserve systolic function. This has allowed us to improve

Table 96–3

Thirty-Day Operative Mortality and Late Survival for Aortic Insufficiency Patients during Different Time Periods

Group	*n*	*30-day*	*1-yr (%)*	*5-yr (%)*	*10-yr (%)*	*15-yr (%)*
Severe LV <1980[a]	24	76	71	59	31	22
Control <1980[a]	181	96	90	80	66	54
Severe LV 1980–1990[b]	35	86	75	66	38	26
Control 1980–1990[b]	220	99	95	85	69	56
Severe LV >1990[c]	34	100	97	84	—	—
Control >1990[c]	270	99	96	88	—	—

Modified from McCarthy PM: Aortic valve surgery in patients with left ventricular dysfunction. Semin Thorac Cardiovasc Surg 14(2):137–143, 2002.

[a] $p < .0001$.

[b] $p < .0001$.

[c] $p = .3$.

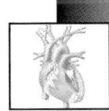

results in patients with severe LV dysfunction undergoing mitral valve surgery. We now have an increasing body of evidence that demonstrates a low operative mortality, good long-term survival, and an impressive freedom from readmissions for CHF.

Whether mitral valve repair or replacement is performed depends on the severity and etiology of the mitral valve disease and, in many cases, the skill and experience of the surgeon. In most instances, mitral valve repair has become the surgery of choice. The technique of mitral repair in patients who have LV dilatation and a central jet of mitral regurgitation reduces the mitral valve annulus using a small ring. The small ring (typically 26 mm) overcompensates for the LV dilatation and allows the leaflets to coapt again.[25,79]

Several groups have demonstrated good outcomes after mitral valve intervention in patients with severely diseased ventricles. Badhwar and Bolling[12] reported their results on 125 patients with 4+ mitral regurgitation who underwent mitral reconstruction. Mean EF was 14%, with a range from 8–24%. All underwent mitral valve repair with an undersized ring. There were five 30-day mortalities and 26 late deaths. The 1- and 2-year actuarial survival rates were 80% and 70%, respectively. Mean NYHA class improved from 3.2 to 1.8 after intervention. At 2 years, all patients demonstrated an improvement in cardiac output, EF, and end-diastolic volume (Table 96-4).

At the Cleveland Clinic, between 1990 and 1998, 44 patients with mitral regurgitation and a LVEF <35% underwent isolated mitral repair (n = 35) or replacement (n = 9). All patients had been hospitalized one to six times for management of heart failure (mean 2.3 ± 1.5) and were in NYHA class III or IV. The 1-, 2-, and 5-year survival rates were 89%, 86%, and 67%, respectively, with an improvement in NYHA class from 2.8 ± 0.8 preoperatively to 1.2 ± 0.5 at follow-up (Figure 96-9).[23]

Overall, the correction of mitral valve pathology in patients with severe LV function offers improvement of symptoms of CHF and good medium-term survival. In many instances, it provides an alternative to transplantation.

Tricuspid Valve

The most common form of tricuspid regurgitation is caused by annular dilatation from RV dilatation. The right-sided failure is usually the result of pulmonary hypertension from left-sided failure. Although this tricuspid regurgitation may improve with treatment of LV failure, longstanding tricuspid regurgitation may be permanent.[3] Here we address the implication of tricuspid regurgitation in the setting of CHF. The primary causes of tricuspid valve disease (rheumatic, traumatic, and infectious) are discussed in detail elsewhere.

The normal tricuspid valve does not always completely coapt in systole, and regurgitation may be found by echocardiography in 24–96% of normal individuals.[143,176] However, in pathological states, blood flows during systole into the right atrium, elevates right atrial pressure, and decreases cardiac output. When the mean right atrial pressure exceeds 10 mm Hg, peripheral edema usually results. As right

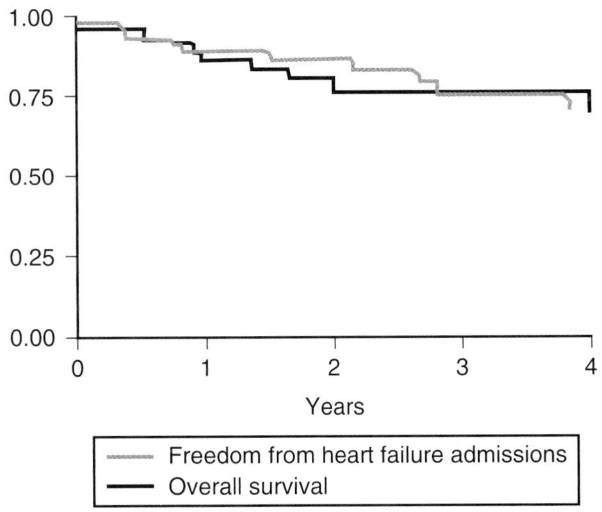

Figure 96–9 Survival and freedom from heart failure hospital admission after mitral valve repair.

Table 96–4

Comparison of Cardiac Function before and after Mitral Valve Repair in Patients with Severe Congestive Heart Failure

Echocardiographic parameter	*Preoperative (n = 125)*	*Postoperative (24 mo)*	*p*
End diastolic volume (ml)	281 ± 86	206 ± 88	< .001
Ejection fraction (%)	16 ± 5	26 ± 8	.008
Regurgitant fraction (%)	70 ± 12	13 ± 10	< .001
Cardiac output (liters/min)	3.1 ± 1.0	5.2 ± 0.8	.001
Sphericity index (D/liters)	0.82 ± 0.10	0.74 ± 0.07	.005

ventricular failure develops, symptoms of dyspnea and orthopnea develop. In the extreme form, hepatic dysfunction and ascites become clinical problems.

The decision to intervene on the tricuspid valve is usually determined by other cardiac pathology and is infrequently the primary indication for operative intervention. However, at the Cleveland Clinic we take an aggressive approach to tricuspid regurgitation and attempt repair in all patients undergoing cardiac surgery for concomitant disease with 2+ or greater regurgitation. In patients with CHF the valve is usually structurally normal and is amenable to repair rather than replacement. Repairs essentially come in three forms: the Kay technique, the De Vega technique, and ring annuloplasty. The Kay technique plicates the posterior leaflet and effectively converts the tricuspid into a bicuspid valve.[91] The De Vega technique narrows the annulus along the anterior and posterior leaflets with a purse-string suture.[55] The third technique fastens a ring along the anterior and posterior annuli.[37] A number of rings are commercially available. The two most widely practiced techniques are the De Vega technique and ring annuloplasty.

At the Cleveland Clinic we have recently reviewed different tricuspid valve annuloplasty techniques and established risk factors for failure of tricuspid valve repair in 790 patients from 1990–1999.[19] Four techniques were used: the Carpentier rigid ring, the Cosgrove flexible band, the De Vega procedure, and the customized Peri-Guard ring. One half of the patients had advanced CHF. Most (89%) had a concomitant mitral valve procedure. Severity of TR was stable across time with the Carpentier rigid ring, increased slowly with the Cosgrove flexible band, and increased more rapidly with both the De Vega procedure and the Peri-Guard ring. Risk factors for tricuspid valve repair failure included the following: higher preoperative tricuspid regurgitation grade, poor LV function, and repair type other than the Carpentier rigid ring annuloplasty. Tricuspid valve repair failure did not correlate with RV systolic pressure, ring size, preoperative NYHA functional class, or need for concomitant surgery.

Tricuspid valve annuloplasty did not consistently eliminate severe functional regurgitation, and across time tricuspid regurgitation increased in Peri-Guard and De Vega annuloplasties as opposed to ring techniques. Although a number of rings have been used, a newly designed ring, the MC3, incorporates the 3D structure of the ring into its repair and is currently our repair technique of choice. We hope that this technique will result in improved durability of tricuspid valve repair.

Other series have demonstrated that tricuspid valve repair can be performed in patients with heart failure with acceptable results. Kuwaki et al[98] reviewed their results with tricuspid repair in 260 patients. Ninety-seven percent of patients were in NYHA class III or IV. Hospital mortality was 8.9%. At 10 years, survival was 84%. Risk factors for late mortality were NYHA class IV and poor LVEF.

Repair of the tricuspid valve improves symptoms of CHF,[156] restores RV geometry, and increases EF (Figures 96-10 and 96-11).[122] Both the perioperative and long-term survival are encouraging after surgical treatment of tricuspid disease in this debilitated group of patients. Surgeons should take an aggressive approach to repair of the tricuspid valve as part of a strategy that corrects every significant anatomical problem in the diseased heart. In the surgical treatment of CHF, the tricuspid valve should not be forgotten.

ARRHYTHMIA SURGERY IN PATIENTS WITH HEART FAILURE

One of the evolving areas in the treatment of heart failure is that of arrhythmia surgery. Conduction abnormalities of the atrial and ventricular conduction systems are potential targets for therapies aimed at the improvement of cardiac function in CHF. Although these therapies have not been fully developed, substantial progress has already been made.

SURGICAL INTERVENTIONS FOR ATRIAL FIBRILLATION

The Cox-Maze Procedure

Atrial fibrillation (AF) is a common disease. It impacts more than 2 million people in the United States and is present in

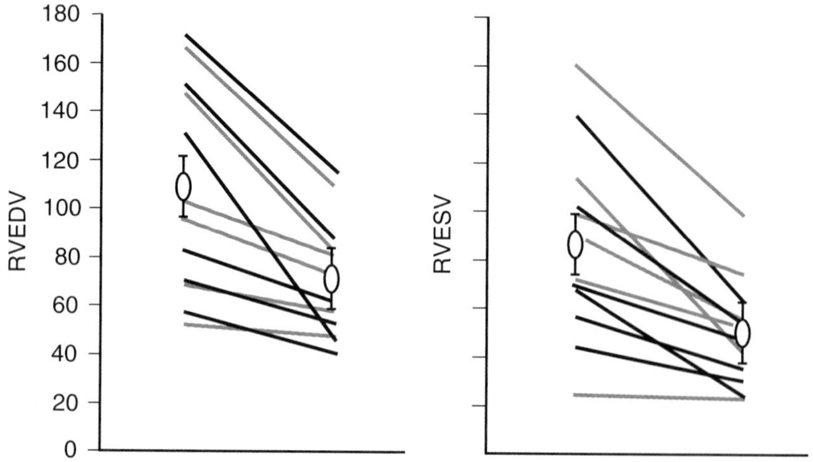

Figure 96–10 Reduction of end-diastolic and end-systolic right ventricular (RV) volumes after tricuspid valve repair.

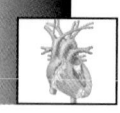

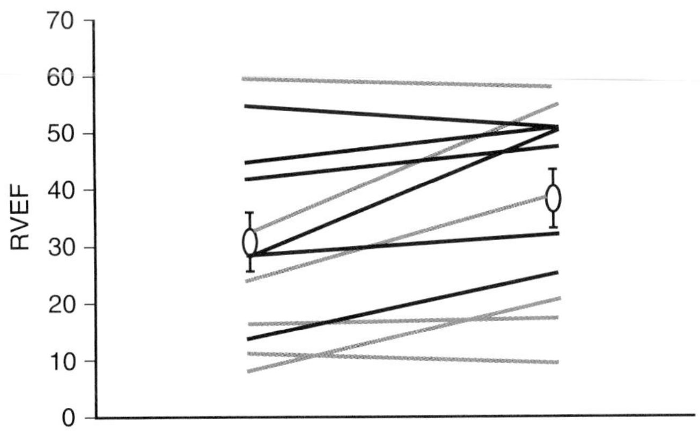

Figure 96–11 Improvement in right ventricular ejection fraction (RVEF) after tricuspid valve repair.

6% of Americans over the age of 65.[18] This leads to an impressive impact on the health care system. Each year, AF is responsible for 227,000 hospitalizations and 1.4 million outpatient visits. Permanent AF is responsible for a twofold increase in all-cause mortality and a fivefold increase in stroke. In addition, the loss of synchronous atrioventricular contraction may contribute to the symptoms of CHF.

Therapeutic options in the treatment of chronic AF remain limited. Rate control may be achieved by medical therapy. If this fails, patients may undergo radiofrequency ablation of the atrioventricular node and permanent pacemaker implantation. In patients with CHF, this strategy improves EF, exercise tolerance, and quality of life.[170] However, even with rate control, the loss of atrial transport function may further impair a patient who already has poor ventricular function. In addition, the patient still requires anticoagulation.

For the restoration of sinus rhythm and the improvement on the limitations of medical therapy, a number of surgical strategies have been employed. However, the gold standard remains the Maze III.[49] This procedure incorporates a series of linear incisions of both atria to establish lines of conduction block that prevent any potential reentrant circuits from occurring. This forces the heart into a regular rhythm. The procedure cures AF more than 90% of the time, with mortality less than 1%.[112] Unfortunately, the procedure is somewhat complex and requires the patient to spend a significant amount of time under cardiac arrest. Because of these reasons, surgeons have been slow to embrace the Maze as a routine procedure, especially in high-risk patients.

Two new developments may rapidly broaden the application of the Maze. First, we have a better understanding of the etiology of AF. In paroxysmal AF, the origin of the ectopic beats is the pulmonary veins in 94% of cases.[76] This suggests that the right-sided lesions may not be needed in this patient population. In addition, even in chronic AF, the left atrial lesions of the Maze may cure AF in 78% of patients.[161] This simplification may broaden the application of the Maze.

Second, numerous tissue ablation modalities are entering the clinical arena that dramatically reduce the time required to make a line of scar, and thus conduction block. These include unipolar radiofrequency, bipolar radiofrequency, cryothermy, and microwave techniques. These techniques not only decrease the time, but also markedly decrease the technical complexity of the Maze, as well as the potential for postoperative bleeding.

As the Maze becomes more widely applied, we will get a better understanding of the effect of rhythm restoration on heart failure. However, initial results are promising. Patients who have undergone isolated Maze procedures show reduced levels of heart failure markers such as brain natriuretic peptide and aldosterone 6 months after surgery.[4] More information will soon follow.

We expect a broader application of the Maze to yield an improvement in cardiac function and quality of life in patients with heart failure. As the technology evolves, we hope to eliminate AF and its detrimental effects on patients with CHF.

VENTRICULAR ELECTRICAL INTERVENTIONS

Biventricular Pacing

Approximately 30% of patients with CHF have a conduction delay affecting the onset of right or left ventricular systole.[59] This is apparent on the electrocardiogram, when the QRS interval is longer than 120 ms. This conduction delay alone may impair the coordination of cardiac contraction that would otherwise optimize cardiac ejection and total cardiac output. It may also contribute to mitral regurgitation. More importantly, the presence of a conduction delay is associated with an increased risk of death in patients with heart failure. Therefore strategies have evolved to "resynchronize" the ventricular electrical conduction system.

The first clinical improvement of CHF after the implantation of a dual-chamber pacemaker programmed to a short atrioventricular delay was reported by Hochleitner et al in 1990.[80] However, the subsequent decade led to various conflicting reports on the potential benefit of pacing in CHF.[106] Individual testing of patients appeared to be the only way to distinguish those who might benefit from atrioventricular resynchronization through a right-sided atrioventricular sequential pacing. However, the technique is cumbersome and invasive and does not always extrapolate to continued improvement. Therefore effort was shifted to LV-based biventricular pacing.

Several reports have suggested that the use of atrial-synchronized biventricular pacemakers may improve cardiac function and enhance the quality of life in patients with CHF. The Medtronic InSync and PATH-CHF (Pacing Therapies for Congestive Heart Failure) trials were prospective, uncontrolled trials that applied the use of biventricular pacing to patients with end-stage heart failure with a prolonged QRS duration.[11,69] The InSync trial demonstrated an improved NYHA classification and quality of life in patients after 1 year. The PATH-CHF trial demonstrated an improved 6-minute walk, quality of life, and EF after 1 year.

The MUSTIC (Multisite Stimulation in Cardiomyopathy) trial was a multicenter randomized case-controlled trial that demonstrated decreased hospitalization, improved 6-minute walk, and improved peak VO_2 max at 6 months after initiation of biventricular pacing.[39] Most recently, in a randomized, controlled study of 453 patients, the

MIRACLE (Multicenter InSync Randomized Clinical Evaluation) trial demonstrated an improvement in 6-minute walk, NYHA functional class, and EF, as well as a decrease in hospital readmission in patients undergoing cardiac resynchronization.[1]

Currently our cardiology colleagues incorporate biventricular pacing as part of the treatment of CHF in patients with prolonged QRS durations. The ideal candidates also have left bundle-branch block with a prolonged PR interval. As surgeons, we place permanent LV epicardial leads in all our patients with QRS durations >120 ms and LVEF <35% at the time of concomitant cardiac surgery. Although further investigations are underway, ventricular resynchronization appears to be an important tool in the multidisciplinary approach to heart failure that is being adopted by the cardiac surgeon.

IMPLANTABLE CARDIOVERTER DEFIBRILLATOR

Sudden cardiac death claims 300,000 lives in the United States each year.[65] In more than 80% of cases, sudden death is caused by the abrupt onset of ventricular tachycardia, which progresses to ventricular fibrillation.[54] Survival is determined by the time between onset and first defibrillation attempt.[132] Mirowski and co-workers[119] implanted the first implantable cardioverter defibrillator (ICD) at Johns Hopkins in 1980 to decrease the time to defibrillation and improve survival. By 1999, 50,000 devices had been implanted worldwide.

The results of two large prospective trials comparing ICDs to antiarrhythmic drug therapy in patients with life-threatening ventricular tachyarrhythmia have shown that the implantable defibrillator improves survival. At 3 years, the AVID (Antiarrhythmics Versus Implantable Defibrillator) trial demonstrated a 31% reduction in mortality, and the CIDS (Canadian Implantable Defibrillator Study) demonstrated a 20% reduction in mortality.[46,165] Although only the AVID trial demonstrated a statistical significant difference, there was a trend in survival reduction in the CIDS trial. Subsequently, ICD has become accepted as the treatment of choice in survivors of symptomatic sustained ventricular tachyarrhythmia.

Patients with heart failure constitute a large proportion of ICD recipients. Sudden cardiac death is responsible for approximately half of all cardiac deaths in patients with heart failure. However, as functional class deteriorates, the proportion of deaths that is sudden and unexpected decreases. Therefore a concern that an ICD will have little impact on overall survival in patients with heart failure has prompted investigation into the use of ICDs in this patient population.

Unsustained ventricular tachycardia in the setting of a previous myocardial infarction is associated with a 2-year mortality rate of approximately 20%.[21] The MADIT (Multicenter Automatic Defibrillator Implantation Trial) was designed to compare the effectiveness of prophylactic ICD implantation versus conventional medical therapy in patients with prior myocardial infarction, EF of 35% or less, unsustained ventricular tachycardia, and inducible, nonsuppressible ventricular tachycardia or ventricular fibrillation. The ICD group had a greater than 50% reduction in mortality (16% versus 39%).[120] The MUSTT (Multicenter Unsustained Tachycardia Trial) demonstrated an improved 5-year survival rate in patients with EFs less than 40% who received either an ICD or electrophysiology-guided drug therapy, with all the benefit coming from patients who received an ICD.[34] Although the CABG-Patch trial failed to demonstrate a survival benefit in patients with low EFs who received prophylactic ICD, electrophysiological testing was not performed, so not all the candidates may have been ideal recipients for the treatment.[22]

ICDs reduce mortality in patients with heart failure who have inducible ventricular arrhythmias. Several trials are underway to examine if ICDs improve survival in patients who do not have inducible ventricular arrhythmias. These include the Cardiomyopathy Trial (CAT), the Sudden Cardiac Death in Heart Failure Trial (SCD-HeFT), and MADIT II. These trials will help define the appropriate recipients of this therapy.

SUMMARY

CHF remains a terminal disease. Alternatives such as heart transplantation and ventricular assist devices are options for only a small percentage of people afflicted with this condition. As a result, thousands of people will die from this disease, and even more will have limited lives. We have chosen to take an aggressive approach to the treatment of CHF by fixing any abnormal anatomical or physiological characteristic of the diseased heart. We do not believe that any single parameter of cardiac function prohibits operative intervention. However, patient selection is paramount, because any intervention must improve cardiac function in order to improve the duration and quality of life in this high-risk group. In addition, this strategy should only be employed at a center that is prepared to offer all the resources that may be needed in the most challenging patients. Even more importantly, long-term medical management must be individually tailored to give these patients their best chance for a meaningful life.

REFERENCES

1. Abraham WT, Fisher WG, Smith AL, et al: Cardiac resynchronization in chronic heart failure. N Engl J Med 24:1845, 2002.
2. Acker MA: Dynamic cardiomyoplasty: At the crossroads. Ann Thorac Surg 68:750–755, 1999.
3. Ajayi AA, Adigun AQ, Ojofeitimi EO, et al: Anthropometric evaluation of cachexia in chronic congestive heart failure: The role of tricuspid regurgitation. Int J Card 71:79, 1999.
4. Albage A, Kenneback G, van der Linden J, et al: Improved neurohormonal markers of ventricular function after restoring sinus rhythm by the Maze procedure. Ann Thorac Surg 5:790, 2003.
5. American Heart Association: 2001 Heart and Stroke Statistical Update. Dallas: The Association, 2001.
6. Angelini GD, Pryn S, Mehta D, et al: Left-ventricular-volume reduction for end-stage heart failure. Lancet 350:489, 1997.
7. Arai M, Alpert NR, MacLennan DH, et al: Alterations in sarcoplasmic reticulum gene expression in human heart failure.

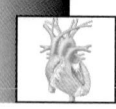

A possible mechanism for alterations in systolic and diastolic properties of the failing myocardium. Circ Res 72:463, 1993.
8. Aronow WS, Ahn C, Kronzon I, et al: Prognosis of patients with heart failure and unoperated severe aortic valvular regurgitation and relation to ejection fraction. Am J Cardiol 74:286–288, 1994.
9. Athanasuleas CL, Stanley AWH, Buckberg GD, et al: Surgical anterior ventricular endocardial restoration (SAVER) for dilated ischemic cardiomyopathy. Semin Thorac Cardiovasc Surg 13:448, 2001.
10. Atkins BZ, Hueman MT, Meuchel JM, et al: Myogenic cell transplantation improves in vivo regional performance in infarcted rabbit myocardium. J Heart Lung Transplant 18:1173, 1999.
11. Auricchio A, Stellbrink C, Sack S, et al: The Pacing Therapies for Congestive Heart Failure (PATH-CHF) study: Rationale, design and endpoints of a prospective randomized multicenter study. Am J Cardiol 83:130D, 1999.
12. Badhwar V, Bolling SF: Mitral valve surgery in the patient with left ventricular dysfunction. Semin Thorac Cardiovasc Surg 2002; 14:133–136, 2002.
13. Barr E, Carroll J, Kalynych AM, et al: Efficient catheter-mediated gene transfer into the heart using replication-defective adenovirus. Gene Ther 1:51, 1994.
14. Batista RJV, Santos JLV, Takeshita N, et al: Partial left ventriculectomy to improve left ventricular function in end-stage heart disease. J Card Surg 11:96–97, 1996.
15. Batista RJV, Verde J, Nery P, et al: Partial left ventriculectomy to treat end stage heart disease. Ann Thorac Surg 64:634–638, 1997.
16. Beck CS: Operation for aneurysm of the heart. Ann Surg 120:34, 1944.
17. Beltrami AP, Urbanek K, Kajsture J, et al: Evidence that human cardiac myocytes divide after myocardial infarction. N Engl J Med 344:1750, 2001.
18. Benjamin EJ, Wolf PA, D'Agostino RB, et al: Impact of atrial fibrillation on the risk of death: The Framingham Heart Study. Circulation 98:946, 1998.
19. McCarthy PM, Bhudia SK, Rajeswaran J, et al: Tricuspid valve repair: Durability and risk factors for failure. J Thorac Cardiovasc Surg 127:674–850, 2004.
20. Bhudia SK, McCarthy PM, Smedira NG, et al: Edge-to-edge (Alfieri) mitral repair: A versatile repair technique. Ann Thorac Surg 77:1598–1606, 2004.
21. Bigger JT, Fleiss JL, Kleiger R, et al: The relationships among ventricular arrhythmias, left ventricular dysfunction and mortality in the 2 years after myocardial infarction. Circulation 69:250, 1984.
22. Bigger JT, for the Coronary Artery Bypass Graft (CABG) Patch Trial Investigators: Prophylactic use of implanted cardiac defibrillators in patients at high risk for ventricular arrhythmias after coronary artery bypass graft surgery. N Engl J Med 337:1568, 1997.
23. Bishay ES, McCarthy PM, Cosgrove DM, et al: Mitral valve surgery in patients with severe left ventricular dysfunction. Eur J Cardiothorac Surg 17(3):213–221, 2000.
24. Blitz LR, Gorman M, Herrmann HC: Results of aortic valve replacement for aortic stenosis with relatively low transvalvular pressure gradients. Am J Cardiol 81:358–362, 1998.
25. Bolling S, Pagani FD, Deeb GM, et al: Intermediate-term outcome of mitral reconstruction in cardiomyopathy. J Thorac Cardiovasc Surg 115:381–388, 1998.
26. Bonow RO, Carabello B, de Leon A, et al: Guidelines for the management of patients with valvular disease: Executive summary. A report of the American College of Cardiology/American Heart Association Task Force on Practice Guidelines (Committee on Management of Patients with Valvular Disease). Circulation 98:1949–1984, 1998.
27. Bonow RO, Dodd JT, Maron BJ, et al: Long-term serial changes in left ventricular function and reversal of ventricular dilatation after valve replacement for chronic aortic regurgitation. Circulation 78:1108–1120, 1988.
28. Bonow RO, Nikas D, Elefteriades JA: Valve replacement for regurgitant lesions of the aortic or mitral valve in advanced left ventricular dysfunction. Cardiol Clin 13(1):73–83, 1995.
29. Bonow RO, Rosing DR, Maron BJ, et al: Reversal of left ventricular dysfunction after aortic valve replacement for chronic aortic regurgitation: Influence of duration of preoperative left ventricular dysfunction. Circulation 70(4):570–579, 1984.
30. Bristow MR, Ginsburg R, Minobe W, et al: Decreased catecholamine sensitivity and beta-adrenergic-receptor density in failing human hearts. N Engl J Med 307:205, 1982.
31. Brogan WC, Grayburn PA, Lange RA, et al: Prognosis after valve replacement in patients with severe aortic stenosis and a low transvalvular pressure gradient. J Am Coll Cardiol 21:1657–1660, 1993.
32. Bruschke AVG, Proudfit WF, Sones FM: Progress study of 490 consecutive non-surgical cases of coronary disease followed 5 to 9 years. II. Ventriculographic and other correlations. Circulation 47:1154, 1973.
33. Burton NA, Stinson EB, Oyer PE, et al: Left ventricular aneurysm: Preoperative risk factors and long-term operative results. J Thorac Cardiovasc Surg 77:65, 1979.
34. Buxton AE, Lee KL, Fisher JD, et al: A randomized study of the prevention of sudden death in patients with coronary artery disease. N Engl J Med 341:1882, 1999.
35. Caldeira C, McCarthy PM: A simple method of left ventricular reconstruction without patch for ischemic cardiomyopathy. Ann Thorac Surg 72:2148–2149, 2001.
36. Carpentier A, Chachques JC, Acar C, et al: Dynamic cardiomyoplasty at seven years. J Thorac Cardiovasc Surg 106:42–54, 1993.
37. Carpentier A, Deloche A, Hanania G, et al: Surgical management of acquired tricuspid valve disease. J Thorac Cardiovasc Surg 67:53, 1974.
38. Carpentier A, Chachques JC: Myocardial substitution with a simulated skeletal muscle: First successful clinical case. Lancet 1:1267, 1985.
39. Cazeau S, Leclercq C, Lavergne T, et al: Effects of multsite biventricular pacing in patients with heart failure and intraventricular conduction delay. N Engl J Med 344:873, 2001.
40. Chaudhry PA, Mishima T, Sharov VG, et al: Passive epicardial containment prevents ventricular remodeling in heart failure. Ann Thorac Surg 70:1275–1280, 2000.
41. Cheitlin MD, Alpert JS, Armstrong WF, et al: ACC/AHA guidelines for the clinical application of echocardiography: a report of the American College of Cardiology/American Heart Association Task Force on Practice Guidelines (Committee on Clinical Application of Echocardiography), developed in collaboration with the American Society of Echocardiography. Circulation 95:1686–1744, 1995.
42. Chen C, Gillam L, Chen L, et al: Temporal hierarchy in functional and ultrastructural recoveries between short-term and chronic hibernating myocardium after reperfusion. Circulation 92:I552, 1995 (abstract).
43. Clark DG, McAnulty JH, Rahimtoola S: Valve replacement in aortic insufficiency with left ventricular dysfunction. Circulation 61(2):411–421, 1980.
44. Cohen M, Packer M, Gorlin R: Indications for left ventricular aneurysmectomy. Circulation 67:717, 1983.
45. Connolly HM, Oh JK, Schaff HV, et al: Severe aortic stenosis with low transvalvular gradient and severe left ventricular dysfunction: Result of aortic valve replacement in 52 patients. Circulation 101:1940–1946, 2000.
46. Connolly SJ, Gent M, Roberts RS, et al: Canadian Implantable Defibrillator Study (CIDS): A randomized trial

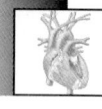

of the implantable cardioverter defibrillator against amiodarone. Circulation 101:1297, 2000.
47. Cooley DA, Collins HA, Morris GC, et al: Ventricular aneurysm after myocardial infarction. Surgical excision with the use of temporary cardiopulmonary bypass. JAMA 167:557, 1958.
48. Couper GS, Bunton RW, Birjiniuk V, et al: Relative risks of left ventricular aneurysmectomy in patients with akinetic scars versus true dyskinetic aneurysms. Circulation 82(suppl 5):IV248–256, 1990.
49. Cox JL, Jaquiss RD, Schuessler RB, et al: Modification of the Maze procedure for atrial flutter and atrial fibrillation. J Thorac Cardiovasc Surg 110:485, 1995.
50. David TE, Uden DE, Strauss HD: The importance of the mitral apparatus in left ventricular function after correction of mitral regurgitation. Circulation 68:II76–82, 1983.
51. Dec GW, Fuster V: Idiopathic dilated cardiomyopathy. N Engl J Med 331(23):1564–1575, 1994.
52. Del Monte F, Harding SE, Schmidt U, et al: Restoration of contractile function in isolated cardiomyocytes from failing human hearts by gene transfer of SERCA2a. Circulation 100:2308, 1999.
53. Del Monte F, Williams E, Lebeche D, et al: Improvement in survival and cardiac metabolism after gene transfer of sarcoplasmic reticulum Ca(2+)-ATPase in a rat model of heart failure. Circulation 104:1424–1429, 2001.
54. DeLuna AB, Coumel P, Leclercq JF: Ambulatory sudden death: Mechanisms of production of fatal arrhythmias on the basis of 157 cases. Am Heart J 117:151, 1989.
55. DeVega NF: La annulplastia selectiva: Reguable Y permanente. Rev Esp Cardiol 25:55, 1972.
56. Dickstein ML, Spotnitz HM, Rose EA, et al: Heart reduction surgery: An analysis of the impact on cardiac function. J Thorac Cardiovasc Surg 113:1032–1040, 1997.
57. Dor V, Kreitmann P, Jourdan J, et al: Interest of physiological closure (circumferential plasty on contractile areas) of left ventricle after resection and endocardiectomy for aneurysm or akinetic zone. Comparison with classical technique about a series of 209 left ventricular resections. J Cardiovasc Surg 26:73, 1985.
58. Dor V: Reconstructive left ventricular surgery for post-ischemic akinetic dilatation. Semin Thorac Cardiovasc Surg 9:139, 1997.
59. Farwell D, Patel NR, Hall A, et al: How many people with heart failure are appropriate for biventricular resynchronization? Eur Heart J 21:1246, 2000.
60. Favaloro RG, Effler DB, Groves LK, et al: Ventricular aneurysm-clinical experience. Ann Thorac Surg 6:227, 1968.
61. Fioretti P, Roelandt J, Bos RJ, et al: Echocardiography in chronic aortic insufficiency: Is valve replacement too late when left ventricular end-systolic dimension reaches 55 mm? Circulation 67(1):216–221, 1983.
62. Fischl ST, Gorlin R, Herman MV: Cardiac shape and function in aortic valve disease: Physiologic and clinical implications. Am J Cardiol 39:170–176, 1977.
63. Franco-Cereceda A, McCarthy PM, Blackstone EH, et al: Partial left ventriculectomy for dilated cardiomyopathy: Is this an alternative to transplantation? J Thorac Cardiovasc Surg 121:879–893, 2001.
64. Fromes Y, Salmon A, Wang X, et al: Gene delivery into the myocardium by intrapericardial injection. Gene Ther 6:683, 1999.
65. Gillum RF: Sudden coronary death in the United States. Circulation 79:756, 1989.
66. Gorcsan J 3rd, Feldman AM, Kormos RL, et al: Heterogenous immediate effects of partial left ventriculectomy on cardiac performance. Circulation 97:839–842, 1998.
67. Gradinac S, Miric M, Popvic Z, et al: Partial left ventriculectomy for idiopathic dilated cardiomyopathy: Early results and six-month follow-up. Ann Thorac Surg 66:1963–1968, 1998.
68. Grandjean PA, Austin L, Chan S, et al: Dynamic cardiomyoplasty: Clinical follow-up results. J Card Surg 6(suppl): 80–88, 1991.
69. Gras D, Mabo P, Tang T, et al: Multisite pacing as a supplemental treatment of congestive heart failure: Preliminary results of the Medtronic Inc. InSync Study. Pacing Clin Electrophysiol 21:2249, 1998.
70. Grines CL, Watkins MW, Helmer G, et al: Angiogenic Gene Therapy (AGENT) trial in patients with stable angina pectoris. Circulation 105:1291, 2002.
71. Grondin P, Kretz GK, Bical O, et al: Natural history of saccular aneurysms of the left ventricle. J Thorac Cardiovasc Surg 77:57, 1979.
72. Grossman W, Jones D, McLaurin P: Wall stress and patterns of hypertrophy in the human left ventricle. J Clin Invest 56:56–64, 1975.
73. Gunzman RJ, Lemarchand P, Crystal RG, et al: Efficient gene transfer into myocardium by direct injection of adenovirus vectors. Circ Res 73:1202, 1993.
74. Gwathmey JK, Copelas L, MacKinnonR, et al: Abnormal intracellular calcium handling in myocardium from patients with end-stage heart failure. Circ Res 61:70, 1987.
75. Gwathmey JK, Slawsky MT, Hajjar RJ, et al: Role of intracellular calcium handling in force-interval relationships of human ventricular myocardium. J Clin Invest 85:1599, 1990.
76. Haissaguerre M, Jais P, Shah DC, et al: Right and left atrial radiofrequency catheter therapy of paroxysmal atrial fibrillation. J Cardiovasc Electrophysiol 10:1575, 1999.
77. Hajjar RJ, Schmidt U, Kang JX, et al: Adenoviral gene transfer of phospholamban in isolated rat cardiomyocytes. Rescue effects by concomitant gene transfer of sarcoplasmic reticulum Ca(2+)-ATPase. Circ Res 81:145, 1997.
78. Hannan EL, Kilburn H Jr, O'Donnell JF, et al: Adult open heart surgery in New York State. An analysis of risk factors and hospital mortality rates. JAMA 264:2768–2774, 1990.
79. Hendren WG, Nemec JJ, Lytle BW, et al: Mitral valve repair for ischemic mitral insufficiency. Ann Thorac Surg 52:1246–1252, 1991.
80. Hochleitner M, Hortnagl H, Ng CK, et al: Usefulness of physiologic dual-chamber pacing in drug-resistant idiopathic dilated cardiomyopathy. Am J Cardiol 66:198–202, 1990.
81. Hochman JS, Sleeper LA, White HD, et al: One-year survival following early revascularization for cardiogenic shock. JAMA 285(2):190–192, 2001.
82. Hoercher KJ, Starling RC, McCarthy PM, et al: Partial left ventriculectomy: Lessons learned and future implications for surgical trials. Circulation 106:II418, 2002.
83. Hoshijima M, Ikeda Y, Iwanaga Y, et al: Chronic suppression of heart failure progression by a pseudophosphorylated mutant of phospholamban via in vivo cardiac rAAV gene delivery. Nat Med 8:864, 2002.
84. Jackson KA, Majka SM, Wang H, et al: Regeneration of ischemic cardiac muscle and vascular endothelium by adult stem cells. J Clin Invest 107:139, 2001.
85. Jain M, DerSimonian H, Brenner DA, et al: Cell therapy attenuates deleterious ventricular remodeling and improves cardiac performance after myocardial infarction. Circulation 103:1920, 2001.
86. Jatene AD: Left ventricular aneurysmectomy. J Thorac Cardiovasc Surg 89:321, 1985.
87. Jessup M: Dynamic cardiomyoplasty: Expectations and results. J Heart Lung Transplant 19(suppl 8S):S68–S72, 2000.
88. Kadambi VJ, Ponniah S, Harrer JM, et al: Cardiac-specific overexpression of phospholamban alters calcium kinetics and resultant cardiomyocyte mechanics in transgenic mice. J Clin Invest 97:533, 1996.
89. Kass DA, Baughman KL, Pak PH, et al: Reverse remodeling from cardiomyoplasty in human heart failure. External constraint versus active assist. Circulation 91:2314–2318, 1995.

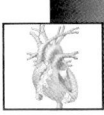

90. Kawaguchi AT, Suma H, Konertz W, et al: Partial left ventriculectomy: The 2nd International Registry report 2000. J Card Surg 16:10–23, 2001.
91. Kay JH, Maselli-Campagna G, Tsuji HK: Surgical treatment of tricuspid insufficiency. Ann Surg 163:53, 1965.
92. Kirklin JW: The replacement of cardiac valves. N Engl J Med 304(5):291–292, 1981.
93. Klodas E, Enriquez-Sarano M, Tajik AJ, et al: Aortic regurgitation complicated by extreme left ventricular dilation: Long-term outcome after surgical correction. J Am Coll Cardiol 27:670–677, 1996.
94. Kocher AA, Schuster MD, Szabolcs MJ, et al: Neovascularization of ischemic myocardium by human bone marrow derived angioblasts prevents cardiomyocyte apoptosis, reduces remodeling and improves cardiac function. Nat Med 7:430, 2001.
95. Koh GY, Soonpaa MH, Klug MG, et al: Stable fetal cardiomyocyte grafts in the hearts of dystrophic mice and dogs. J Clin Invest 96:2034, 1995.
96. Konertz WF, Shapland JE, Hotz H, et al: Passive containment and reverse remodeling by a novel textile cardiac support device. Circulation 104(12):I270–I275, 2001.
97. Kumpati GS, McCarthy PM, Hoercher KJ: Surgical treatments for heart failure. Cardiol Clin 19(4):669–681, 2001.
98. Kuwaki K, Morishita K, Tsukamoto M, et al: Tricuspid valve surgery for functional tricuspid valve regurgitation associated with left-sided valvular disease. Eur J Cardiothorac Surg 20:577, 2001.
99. Lai NC, Roth DM, Gao MH, et al: Intracoronary delivery of adenovirus encoding adenylyl cyclase VI increases left ventricular function and cAMP-generating capacity. Circulation 102:2396, 2000.
100. Lee TH, Hamilton MA, Stevenson LW, et al: Impact of left ventricular cavity size on survival in advanced heart failure. Am J Cardiol 72:672, 1993.
101. Lefemine AA, Govindarajan R, Ramaswamy K, et al: Left ventricular wall resection for aneurysm and akinesia due to coronary artery disease: Fifty consecutive patients. Ann Thorac Surg 23:461, 1977.
102. Levy D, Kenchaiah S, Larson MG, et al: Long term trends in the incidence and survival with heart failure. N Engl J Med 347:1397–1402, 2002.
103. Li RK, Jia ZQ, Weisel RD, et al: Smooth muscle cell transplantation into myocardial scar tissue improves heart function. J Mol Cell Cardiol 31:513, 1999.
104. Likoff W, Bailey CP: Ventriculoplasty: Excision of myocardial aneurysm. JAMA 167:557, 1958.
105. Lillehei CW, Levy MJ, Bonnabeau RC: Mitral valve replacement with preservation of papillary muscles and chordae tendineae. Circulation 94:2117–2123, 1996.
106. Linde C, Gadler F, Edner M, et al: Results of atrioventricular synchronous pacing with optimized delay in patients with severe congestive heart failure. Am J Cardiol 75:919–923, 1995.
107. Losordo DW, Vale PR, Hendel RC, et al: Phase ½ placebo-controlled, double-blind, dose-escalating trial of myocardial vascular endothelial growth factor 2 gene transfer by catheter delivery in patients with chronic myocardial ischemia. Circulation 105:2012–2018, 2002.
108. Makino S, Fukuda D, Miyoshi S, et al: Cardiomyocytes can be generated from marrow stromal cells. J Clin Invest 103:607, 1999.
109. Mangschau A: Akinetic versus dyskinetic left ventricular aneurysms diagnosed by gated scintigraphy: Difference in surgical outcome. Ann Thorac Surg 47:746, 1989.
110. Mann DL, Kent RL, Parsons B, et al: Adrenergic effects on the biology of the adult mammalian cardiocyte. Circulation 85:790, 1992.
111. Mann DL: Mechanisms and models in heart failure: A combinatorial approach. Circulation 100:999–1008, 1999.
112. McCarthy PM, Gillinov MA, Castle L, et al: The Cox-Maze procedure: The Cleveland Clinic experience. Semin Thorac Cardiovasc Surg 12:25, 2000.
113. McCarthy PM, Kumpati GS, Blackstone EH, et al: Aortic valve surgery for chronic aortic regurgitation with severe LV dysfunction: Time for a reevaluation? Circulation 104(suppl):II684, 2001.
114. McCarthy PM, Starling RC, Wong J, et al: Early results with partial left ventriculectomy. J Thorac Cardiovasc Surg 114:755–765, 1997.
115. McCarthy PM, Takagaki M, Ochiai Y, et al: Device-based change in left ventricular shape: A new concept for the treatment of dilated cardiomyopathy. J Thorac Cardiovasc Surg 122(3):482–490, 2001.
116. Mickleborough LL, Carson S, Ivanov J: Repair of dyskinetic or akinetic left ventricular aneurysm: Results obtained with a modified linear closure. J Thorac Cardiovasc Surg 121:675, 2001.
117. Migrino RQ, Young JB, Ellis SG, et al: End-systolic volume index at 90 to 180 minutes into reperfusion therapy for acute myocardial infarction is a strong predictor of early and late mortality. Circulation 96:116, 1997.
118. Milano CA, White WD, Smith LR, et al: Coronary artery bypass in patients with severely depressed ventricular function. Ann Thorac Surg 56:487–493, 1993.
119. Mirowski M, Reid PR, Power MM, et al: Termination of malignant ventricular arrhythmias with an implanted automatic defibrillator in human beings. N Engl J Med 303:322, 1980.
120. Moss AJ, Hall WJ, Cannom DS, et al: Improved survival with an implanted defibrillator in patients with coronary artery disease at high risk for ventricular arrhythmia. N Engl J Med 335:1933, 1996.
121. Mourdjinis A, Olsen E, Raphael MJ, et al: Clinical diagnosis and prognosis of ventricular aneurysms. Br Heart J 30:497, 1968.
122. Mukherjee D, Nader S, Olano A, et al: Improvement in right ventricular systolic function after surgical correction of isolated tricuspid regurgitation. J Am Soc Echocardiogr 13:650, 2000.
123. Murry CE, Wiseman RW, Schwartz SM, et al: Skeletal myoblast transplantation for repair of myocardial necrosis. J Clin Invest 98:2512, 1996.
124. Navia JL, McCarthy PM, Hoercher KJ, et al: Do left ventricular assist device (LVAD) bridge-to-transplantation outcomes predict the results of permanent LVAD implantation? Ann Thorac Surg 74(6):2051–2062, 2002.
125. O'Connor CM, Gattis WA, Uretsky BF, et al: Continuous intravenous dobutamine is associated with and increased risk of death in patients with advanced heart failure: Insights from the Flolan International Randomized Survival Trial (FIRST). Am Heart J 138:78, 1999.
126. Orlic D, Kajstura J, Chimenti S, et al: Bone marrow cells regenerate infarcted myocardium. Nature 410:701, 2001.
127. Passamani E, Davis KB, Gillespie MJ, et al: A randomized trial of coronary artery bypass surgery. Survival of patients with a low ejection fraction. N Engl J Med 312:1665–1671, 1985.
128. Patel HJ, Lankford EB, Polidori DJ, et al: Dynamic cardiomyoplasty: Its chronic effects on the failing heart. J Thorac Cardiovasc Surg 14:169–178, 1997.
129. Pathophysiology of Aortic Valve Disease in Cardiac Surgery in the Adult, pp. 835–858. L. Henry Edmunds, editor. New York: McGraw Hill, Inc., 1997.
130. Pereira JJ, Lauer MS, Bashir M, et al: Survival after aortic valve replacement for severe aortic stenosis with low transvalvular gradients and severe left ventricular dysfunction. J Am Coll Cardiol 39:1356–1363, 2002.
131. Pilla JJ, Blom AS, Brockman DJ, et al: Ventricular constraint using the acorn cardiac support device reduces myocardial

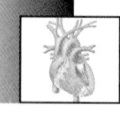

akinetic area in an ovine model of acute infarction. Circulation 106(12 suppl 1):I207–I211, 2002.
132. Pionkowski RS, Thompson BM, Gruchow HW, et al: Resuscitation time in ventricular fibrillation: A prognosis indication. Ann Emerg Med 12:733, 1983.
133. Pirwitz MJ, Lange RA, Willard JE, et al: Use of the left ventricular peak systolic pressure/end-systolic volume ration to predict symptomatic improvement with valve replacement in patients with aortic regurgitation and enlarged end-systolic volume. J Am Coll Cardiol 24:1672–1677, 1994.
134. Pitt B, Zannad F, Remme WJ, et al: The effect of spironolactone on morbidity and mortality in patients with severe heart failure. Randomized Aldactone Evaluation Study Investigators. N Engl J Med 341:689–700, 1999.
135. Popovic Z, Miric M, Gradinac S, et al: Effects of partial left ventriculectomy on left ventricular performance on patients with nonischemic dilated cardiomyopathy. J Am Coll Cardiol 32:1801–1808, 1998.
136. Power J, Raman J, Byrne M: Passive ventricular constraint is a trigger for a significant degree of reverse remodeling in an experimental model of degenerative heart failure and dilated cardiomyopathy. Circulation 102(suppl II):II502, 2000.
137. Proudfit WL, Bruschke AVG, Sones FM Jr: Natural history of obstructive coronary artery disease: Ten-year study of 601 nonsurgical cases. Prog Cardiovasc Dis 21:53, 1978.
138. Raman JS, Hata M, Storere JM, et al: The mid-term results of ventricular containment (ACORN WRAP) for end stage ischemic cardiomyopathy. Ann Thorac Cardiovasc Surg 7(5):278–281, 2001.
139. Ratcliffe MB, Jong J, Salahieh A, et al: The effect of ventricular volume reduction surgery in the dilated, poorly contractile left ventricle: A simple finite element analysis. J Thorac Cardiovasc Surg 116:566–577, 1998.
140. Rose EA, Gelijns AC, Moskowitz AJ, et al: Long term use of a left ventricular assist device for end stage heart failure. N Engl J Med 345(20):1432–1443, 2001.
141. Saavedra FW, Tunn R, Mishima T, et al: Reverse remodeling and enhanced adrenergic reserve from a passive external ventricular support in experimental dilated heart failure. Circulation 102(suppl II):II501, 2000.
142. Sabbah HN, Gupta RC, Sharov VG, et al: Prevention of progressive left ventricular dilation with the Acorn Cardiac Support Device (CSD) down regulates stretch-mediated P21ras, attenuates myocardial hypertrophy, and improves sarcoplasmic reticulum calcium cycling in dogs with heart failure. Circulation 102(suppl II):II683, 2000.
143. Sahn DJ, Maciel BC: Physiological valvular regurgitation: Doppler echocardiography and the potential for iatrogenic heart disease. Circulation 78:1075, 1988.
144. Sakai T, Li RK, Weisel RD, et al: Fetal cell transplantation: A comparison of three cell types. J Thorac Cardiovasc Surg 118:715, 1999.
145. Sauerbrunch F, O'Shaughnessy L: Thoracic Surgery, p. 235. Baltimore: William Wood & Co., 1937.
146. Schenk S, Reichenspurner H, Boehm DH, et al: Myosplint implant and shape–change procedure: Intra- and peri-operative safety and feasibility. J Heart Lung Transplant 21(6):680–686, 2002.
147. Schlichter J, Hellerstein HK, Katz LN: Aneurysm of the heart: A correlative study of 102 proved cases. Medicine 33:43, 1954.
148. Scorsin M, Hagege A, Vilquin JT, et al: Comparison of the effects of fetal cardiomyocyte and skeletal myoblast transplantation on postinfarction left ventricular function. J Thorac Cardiovasc Surg 119:1169, 2000.
149. Shah AS, Lilly RE, Kypson AP, et al: Intracoronary adenovirus-mediated deliver and overexpression of the beta(2)-adrenergic receptor in the heart: Prospects for molecular ventricular assistance. Circulation 101:408, 2000.
150. Sharma GV, Deupree RH, Khuri SF, et al: Coronary bypass surgery improves survival in high-risk unstable angina. Results of a Veterans Administration unstable angina cooperative study with an 8-year follow-up. Veterans Administration Unstable Angina Cooperative Study Group. Circulation 84:III260–III267, 1991.
151. Sharpe N, Doughty R: Epidemiology of heart failure and ventricular dysfunction. Lancet 352(suppl):3–7, 1998.
152. Sheehy E, Conrad SL, Brigham LE, et al: Estimating the number of potential donors in the United States. N Engl J Med 349(7):667–674, 2003.
153. Shintani S, Murohara T, Ikeda H, et al: Mobilization of endothelial progenitor cells in patients with acute myocardial infarction. Circulation 103:2776, 2001.
154. Smith N, McAnulty JH, Rahimtoola SH: Severe aortic stenosis with impaired left ventricular function and clinical heart failure: Results of valve replacement. Circulation 58:255–264, 1978.
155. Soonpaa MH, Koh GY, Klug MG, et al: Formation of nascent intercalated disks between grafted fetal cardiomyocytes and host myocardium. Science 263:98, 1994.
156. Staab ME, Nishimura RA, Dearani JA: Isolated tricuspid valve surgery for severe tricuspid regurgitation following prior left heart valve surgery. J Heart Valve Dis 8:567, 1999.
157. Stamm C, Westphal B, Kleine HD, et al: Autologous bone-marrow stem-cell transplantation for myocardial regeneration. Lancet 361:45, 2003.
158. Stolf NAG, Moreira LFP, Bocchi EA, et al: Determinants of midterm outcome of partial left ventriculectomy in dilated cardiomyopathy. Ann Thorac Surg 66:1585–1591, 1998.
159. Stratford-Perricaudet LD, Makeh I, Perricaudet M, et al: Widespread long-term gene transfer to mouse skeletal muscles and heart. J Clin Invest 90:626, 1992.
160. Strauer BE, Brehm M, Zeus T, et al: Repair of infarcted myocardium by autologous intracoronary mononuclear bone marrow cell transplantation in humans. Circulation 106:1913, 2002.
161. Sueda T, Nagata H, Shikata H, et al: Simple left atrial procedure for chronic atrial fibrillation associated with mitral valve disease. Ann Thorac Surg 62:1796, 1996.
162. Sutton MSJ, Pfeffer MA, Moye L, et al: Cardiovascular death and left ventricular remodeling two years after myocardial infarction. Circulation 96:3294, 1997.
163. Swedberg K, Kjekshus J, Snapinn S: Long-term survival in severe heart failure in patients treated with enalapril. Ten year follow-up of CONSENSUS I. Eur Heart J 20:136–139, 1999.
164. Takahasho T, Kalka C, Masuda H, et al: Ischemia and cytokine induced mobilization of bone marrow derived endothelial progenitor cells for neovascularization. Nat Med 5:434, 1999.
165. The Antiarrhythmics versus Implantable Defibrillators (AVID) Investigators: A comparison of antiarrhythmic-drug therapy with implantable defibrillators in patients resuscitated from near-fatal ventricular arrhythmias. N Engl J Med 337:1576, 1997.
166. The Multicenter Postinfarction Study Group: Risk stratification and survival after myocardial infarction. N Engl J Med 309:331–336, 1983.
167. The VA Cooperative Study Group: Eighteen-year follow-up in the Veterans Affairs Cooperative Study of Coronary Artery Bypass Surgery for Stable Angina. Circulation 86:121–130, 1992.
168. Tomita S, Li RK, Weisel RD, et al: Autologous transplantation of bone marrow cells improves damaged heart function. Circulation 100:II247, 1999.
169. Turina J, Milincic J, Seifert B, et al: Valve replacement in chronic aortic regurgitation: True predictors of survival after extended follow-up. Circulation 98:II100–II107, 1998.

170. Twidale N, Manada V, Nave K, et al: Predictors of outcome after radiofrequency catheter ablation of the atrioventricular node for atrial fibrillation and congestive heart failure. Am Heart J 136:647, 1998.
171. Veenhuyzen GD, Singh SN, McAreavey D, et al: Prior coronary artery bypass surgery and risk of death among patients with ischemic left ventricular dysfunction. Circulation 104:1489–1493, 2001.
172. Weig HJ, Laugwitz KL, Moretti A, et al: Enhanced cardiac contractility after gene transfer of the V2 vasopressin receptors in vivo by ultrasound-guided injection or transcoronary delivery. Circulation 101:1578, 2000.
173. Xu XF, Kumpati G, McCarthy PM, et al: Positive myocardial remodeling after surgical correction for isolated advanced aortic regurgitation complicated by severe left ventricular dysfunction. Circulation 104(17)(suppl):II494, 2001.
174. Yamaguchi A, Ino T, Adachi H, et al: Left ventricular volume predicts postoperative course in patients with ischemic cardiomyopathy. Ann Thorac Surg 65:434, 1998.
175. Yau TM, Fung K, Weisel RD, et al: Enhanced myocardial angiogenesis by gene transfer with transplanted cells. Circulation 104:I218, 2001.
176. Yoshida K, Yodhikawa J, Shakudo M: Color Doppler evaluation of valvular regurgitation in normals. Circulation 78:840, 1988.

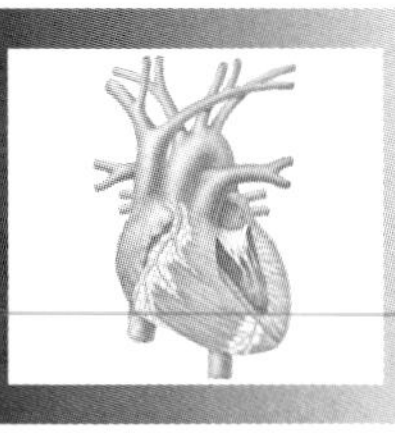

Cell Transplantation for Cardiovascular Disease

CHAPTER 97

Paul W. M. Fedak, Richard D. Weisel, and Ren-Ke Li

INTRODUCTION

Cardiac surgery has restored function in a variety of conditions that produce heart failure. Novel surgical interventions that may extend the surgical approaches for heart failure include robotics, mechanical assist devices, and ventricular remodeling procedures.[9] In addition to these advances, the future of cardiac surgery offers the promise of powerful new biological therapies to modify cardiovascular cells and tissues. Emerging cell-based therapies include cell transplantation for myocardial injury and the creation of bioengineered cardiovascular tissues to enhance the surgical repair of myocardial defects. These novel biological approaches may enhance the rapidly developing mechanical and surgical interventions for patients with cardiac disease by restoring and regenerating failing myocardium.

Historical Background

The ability to successfully isolate, purify, and expand mammalian cells in vitro offered the possibility of altering diseased tissues by way of cell transplantation. Cardiomyocytes have been isolated and cultured at various developmental stages from the hearts of many different species, including humans.[35,42] Cell transplantation for cardiac disease involves the isolation, expansion, and subsequent implantation of a population of cells into injured myocardium. In 1994 cardiomyocytes from transgenic fetal mice were first isolated, expanded in culture, and transplanted into syngenic mouse hearts.[78] The implanted cells survived the procedure and engrafted into the host myocardium. Nascent intercalated disks were observed connecting the engrafted fetal cardiomyocytes and the host myocardium. Importantly, cell engraftment did not compromise cardiac function or rhythm and chronic immune rejection was not encountered. Stable engraftment of transplanted cardiomyocytes was also observed in cardiomyopathic canine hearts without adverse effects, establishing the concept of cardiac cell transplantation in diseased hearts.[34] In 1996 our group provided the first evidence that cell transplantation improves cardiac function after myocardial injury.[39] Transplanted fetal cardiomyocytes formed a cardiac tissue that limited scar expansion and improved the systolic function of cryoinjured rat hearts. The field of cell transplantation for cardiovascular disease was now open for discovery. In 2000 cell transplantation was evaluated for possible clinical applicability and efficacy in a porcine model of myocardial infarction.[46] Use of autologous heart cells appeared to be clinically feasible, and their implantation after infarction improved regional perfusion and wall motion. In 2001 Menasche and colleagues[54] reported the first clinical use of cell transplantation for a patient with ischemic heart failure. By 2002 multicenter clinical trials were underway to evaluate cell transplantation for patients with ischemic cardiomyopathy. These preliminary clinical results are encouraging, and the future of cell transplantation for cardiovascular disease is promising.

SELECTION OF TISSUES AND DONOR CELLS FOR TRANSPLANTATION

Investigators have transplanted heart cells, skeletal muscle cells, bone marrow stem cells, smooth muscle cells, fibroblasts, and endothelial cells into injured hearts.[27,39,40,65,87] The cumulative experience with these diverse cells and tissues suggests that only specific cell types result in benefits after transplantation. However, the cells demonstrating beneficial effects are numerous and their phenotypes are sometimes quite dissimilar. In addition, these beneficial cells may mediate their effects through different pathways, and the success of cell therapy may thus depend on the particular type of myocardial injury being targeted. Accordingly, the selection of a particular type of tissue for cell isolation and expansion is critical to the overall success of cell transplantation in restoring and regenerating damaged myocardium. The ideal cells for transplantation should be isolated from tissues that are easy to harvest, grow rapidly in culture, and retain or modify their phenotype to complement the host tissue (Figure 97-1).

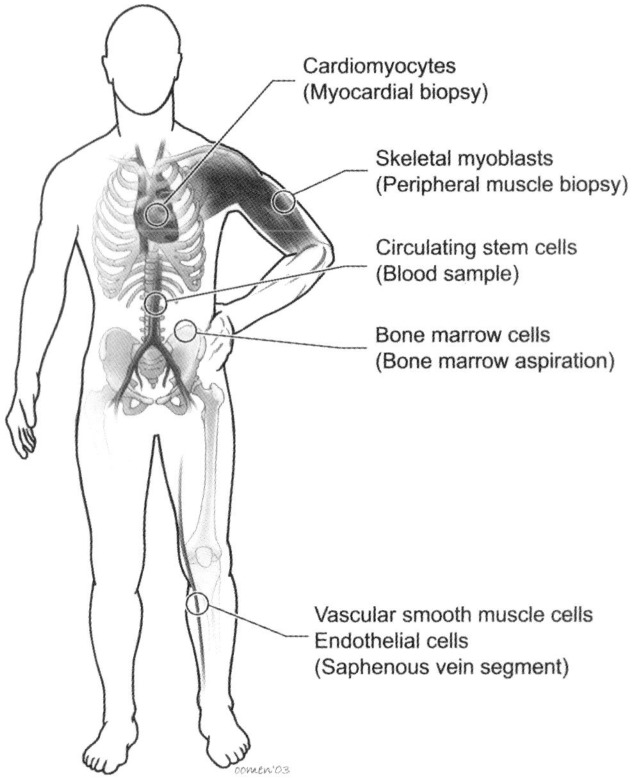

Figure 97–1 **Cell types and tissues used for cell transplantation into the heart.**

Heart Cells and Cardiomyocytes

When successfully isolated and cultured, fetal and neonatal cardiomyocytes retain organized sarcomeres and contract spontaneously and rhythmically while in vitro. The beating cells are connected by intercalated disks and form a cardiac-like tissue. Heart cells isolated and expanded from fetal myocardial tissue provided the critical proof of concept that cell transplantation to injured myocardium can provide functional benefits.[20,74,86] However, given the limited availability and ethical concerns surrounding fetal and neonatal tissues, the clinical application of cell transplantation has focused on using autologous cells from the diseased host. Accordingly, we and others entertained the prospect of using adult autologous heart cells for cell transplantation. There are important phenotypical differences between adult heart cells and fetal cardiomyocytes. Human heart cells from myocardial biopsies obtained from pediatric patients do not spontaneously contract in culture, but retain many biochemical and biological characteristics of human myocardium, such as contractile proteins. Adult heart cells have characteristics of both myofibroblasts and cardiomyocytes. These cells readily reproduce in culture and retain contractile elements, but do not spontaneously beat. In a porcine model of complete infarction, a small septal biopsy harvested noninvasively provided a source of healthy adult heart cells for transplantation that resulted in beneficial effects.[46] Heart cells extracted from the atrial appendage at routine cannulation sites for cardiac surgery resulted in similar benefits after transplantation into ischemic myocardium.[70] Despite the phenotypical changes associated with culturing adult heart cells and the limited capacity of differentiated cardiomyocytes to proliferate, repopulating damaged myocardium with healthy, contractile cardiomyocytes remains the ultimate goal of most cell transplantation therapies for cardiovascular disease. The transplantation of adult heart cells may repopulate the myocardium with cardiomyocytes in light of recent studies indicating that human hearts are capable of producing new cardiomyocytes.[2] Even though they have not been used clinically to date, autologous heart cells may provide an important benchmark with which all other cell types should be compared.

Skeletal Myoblasts

Skeletal myoblasts are endogenous skeletal muscle progenitor cells that serve to regenerate functional skeletal muscle tissue after injury. These cells are dormant in healthy skeletal tissues and proliferate and differentiate into mature skeletal muscle fibers when new tissue is necessary. Adult autologous skeletal myoblasts can be harvested from a small peripheral muscle biopsy, such as the arm or leg, and if successfully isolated from the donor tissue, they will grow rapidly in culture. Compared with both fetal and adult cardiomyocytes, skeletal myoblasts appear equally promising

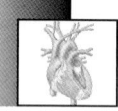

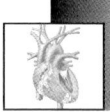

for cell transplantation into ischemic or infarcted hearts.* Scorsin et al,[75] with Menasche and colleagues, provided evidence in a rat coronary ligation model using fetal cells that skeletal myoblast transplantation improved postinfarction left ventricular (LV) function to a similar extent as cardiomyocytes. Transplanted skeletal myoblasts may not differentiate into cardiomyocytes after engraftment in the heart, but do modify their contractile phenotype after engraftment.[23,66] Skeletal myoblasts appear to be capable of contracting within the host tissue, allowing the potential to contribute to contractile force.[36] Given the unique qualities of these cells, autologous skeletal muscle cell transplantation was first to be employed in the clinical arena.[54]

Bone Marrow Cells

Bone marrow cells (BMCs) may offer unique advantages for cell transplantation in the heart. Adult autologous BMCs are readily harvested from a bone marrow aspiration, grow rapidly in culture, and retain or modify their phenotype to complement host tissues after implantation. In addition, quite uniquely, the bone marrow has a rich population of adult stem and progenitor cells (mesenchymal stem cells) that may be capable of forming varied tissues, including cardiac muscle (cardiomyocytes) and blood vessels (vascular smooth muscle cells and endothelial cells), the elements necessary for myocardial regeneration and revascularization.[59] With exposure to 5-azacytidine, bone marrow mesenchymal stem cells in culture differentiate into cells with cardiomyocyte-like characteristics and spontaneously beat.[50] After transplantation into a porcine myocardial infarct, we observed that BMCs in vivo also expressed muscle-specific markers and improved cardiac function.[84] Orlic and colleagues[60,61] regenerated the infarct area of mice with new muscle by transplanting a subpopulation of bone marrow stem cells. Accordingly, bone marrow is a promising alternative tissue source that may be capable of inducing both myogenesis and angiogenesis after cell transplantation. Not surprisingly, autologous BMCs, like skeletal myoblasts, also have been used clinically.[3,80,81]

Smooth Muscle Cells

Smooth muscle cells may offer some unique benefits over other cell types for clinical cell transplantation. First, smooth muscle cells can be readily harvested from easily accessible, small vascular segments (artery or vein). Second, smooth muscle cells expand rapidly and reliably in culture, even when harvested from adult tissues. Third, these muscle cells are capable of both hyperplasia and hypertrophy after engraftment in host myocardium, which may facilitate myocardial regeneration. Fourth, smooth muscle cells actively respond to external stresses and environmental stimuli, and in so doing, they may influence the remodeling process in the failing heart. Finally, vascular smooth muscle cells are capable of secreting angiogenic factors and extracellular matrix components, characteristics that may enhance cell engraftment and survival after implantation. Adult smooth muscle cells provide functional benefits after transplantation in experimental models of cardiac disease, similar to heart cells.[40,71] Smooth muscle cell transplantation has not been used clinically to date.

Endothelial Cells

Endothelial cells can be stimulated to proliferate, migrate, and create new vessels, given the right environmental cues. Implantation of adult endothelial cells can enhance new blood vessel formation in ischemic tissues.[32] Importantly, these data suggest that endothelial cells isolated from adults can be used for cell transplantation to relieve myocardial ischemia by angiogenesis. However, endothelial cell transplantation does not appear to augment global heart function despite significant angiogenesis. Compared with muscle cell transplantation, endothelial cells may not be capable of influencing chamber remodeling, preventing dilatation, and replacing lost contractile elements in the damaged heart. Endothelial cells alone may not be suitable to restore cardiac function in patients with extensive transmural myocardial infarctions. In contrast, if endothelial cells are implanted into ischemic myocardial tissue, the enhanced perfusion might recover hibernating muscle cell contractility and improve global heart function. Adult endothelial cells have not been used clinically to date.

Fibroblasts

Fibroblasts are a readily available and highly expansive cell type that is feasible for transplantation into the heart. Unfortunately, fibroblasts do not appear to improve contractile function despite successful engraftment.[26,71]

Circulating Stem Cells

Although it was once believed that a loss of myocardium is irreversible, studies now suggest that circulating stem cells are capable of homing to sites of myocardial injury to create new blood vessels and cardiomyocytes.[59] However, the quantity of progenitor cells capable of being recruited from the circulation is limited and, accordingly, innate myocardial repair is inadequate. Circulating stem cells can be isolated and expanded from the blood to enhance the repair of injured myocardial regions. Kawamoto and co-workers[28] evaluated the ability of circulating endothelial progenitor cells to contribute to myocardial angiogenesis. When ex vivo expanded human endothelial progenitor cells were injected intravenously into rats after myocardial infarction, the progenitor cells were recruited into the damaged myocardium, resulting in neovascularization and improved heart function.[28] Circulating stem cells have the potential to revolutionize the field of regenerative medicine, including cell transplantation for cardiovascular disease, although considerable challenges and numerous controversies remain to be addressed.

PROCEDURES, TECHNIQUES, AND COMPLICATIONS OF CELL TRANSPLANTATION

The conventional process of cell transplantation for cardiovascular disease involves a systematic approach to process donor cells in preparation for injection into the heart. The

*References 7, 12, 27, 51, 65, 75, 82.

optimal methods for cell processing are in evolution and may depend on such factors as the disease being targeted, the cell type being used, and the method of delivering the cells to the injured myocardium. A conventional sequence of events is outlined in Figure 97-2.

Cell Procurement and Processing for Transplantation

Cell Isolation and Purification

With sterile techniques, a tissue biopsy is obtained from the host. The tissue is minced, and the cells are released from interstitial matrix and adjacent cells using enzymatic digestion. Cells are then separated from residual tissue debris using centrifugation. Tissues are composed of a mix of cell types, and purification is critical to expand a specific line of cells. Purification of cells should be performed early during cell culturing and can be accomplished by techniques such as preplating, dilutional cloning, chemical selection, or a combination of these methods. Failure to purify a specific cell type often results in the overgrowth of fibroblasts in culture, a cell that is detrimental to cardiac function if injected into the heart in large proportions. Once the desired cells are isolated in solution, they are plated out on culture dishes in preparation for in vitro expansion.

Cell Expansion

Once isolated and plated, cells are maintained under strict culture conditions, allowing them to proliferate and expand in number. As the cells expand within the culture dishes, they must be subsequently passaged into new dishes as they reach confluence. This iterative process allows an adequate number of cells to be obtained for cell grafting and usually requires durations of 2–4 weeks, depending on the age of the donor tissue and the phenotype of the cells. It is important to note that passaging of cells in vitro may result in significant changes in cell characteristics and behaviors. Routine microscopy of the expanding cells is required to evaluate their health and phenotypes. Muscle cells (rectangular), endothelial cells (smaller and oval), and fibroblasts (spindle-shaped) can be readily distinguished in culture by light microscopy based on cell morphology alone. In some cases, cell expansion is not required and freshly isolated cells are injected into the heart.

Cell Storage

Once cells reach a desired number after expansion, they may be stored using cryopreservation. Storage of cells increases the feasibility of clinical autologous cell transplantation by allowing targeted cell therapy at predetermined intervals during the progression of cardiac disease. Cryopreserved cells can be reanimated in culture after storage, although the growth rate may be restricted. Our group previously established that cryopreservation of heart cells does not preclude successful transplantation in subcutaneous and myocardial scar tissue.[88] Our preliminary data also indicate that cryopreservation does not eliminate the ability of donor cells to restore cardiac structure and function in failing hearts. Improvements in cryopreservation techniques are still required to reduce injury and augment the rates of cell growth and survival after periods of storage.

Cell Modification and Preparation for Transplantation

In preparation for transplantation, cells are resuspended in culture medium at a desired concentration and volume for injection. For research experiments, the cells can be prelabeled with specific markers or genes for identification in vivo after engraftment.

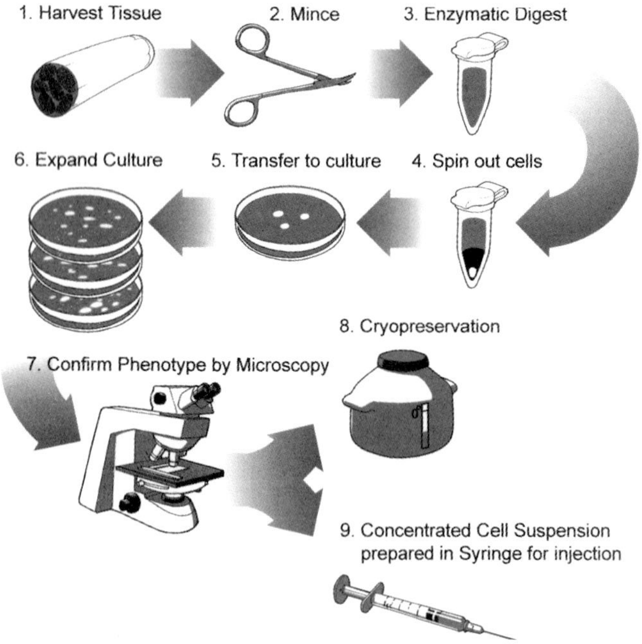

Figure 97–2 **A conventional method of cell procurement and processing for transplantation.**

Techniques of Cell Implantation

For use as an adjunct to cardiac surgery, direct epicardial delivery of donor cells by injection is perhaps most feasible and most reliable. The myocardium is entered at a 45° angle within the defect area on the beating or arrested heart, avoiding obvious epicardial vessels and deep injection into the lumen of the ventricle. Cell leakage can be minimized by suture closure of the needle tract after injection. Multiple injections of concentrated cell suspensions at minimal volumes are preferable to less frequent large volume injections. Noninvasive cell delivery has been successful with catheters in the coronary arterial system or by injection through the endocardium using a catheter advanced into the left ventricle.[14] In cases where abundant cells are required, prior seeding of the cells on a biodegradable mesh as a bioengineered muscle graft may facilitate cell transfer into the injured heart.

Complications

Acute Complications

The most frequent acute complications of cell transplantation include cell leakage and injury, inadequate

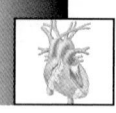

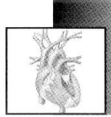

engraftment, embolization, and arrhythmias. With direct myocardial injection, some amount of cell leakage from the injection site in the dynamic beating heart is usually unavoidable. Careful injection techniques and suture closure of the injection site are recommended to avoid this important complication. Cell injury during delivery has been demonstrated as a result of the excessive shear forces associated with the injection process. An appropriate gauge needle and minimal tip length can minimize cell injury. Inadequate engraftment is a complex phenomenon that is not completely understood and is difficult to control. However, the benefits of cell transplantation may be seriously impaired if the cells do not maintain a stable engraftment after myocardial injection. Our preliminary data suggest that only about half of the cells that survive the injection process and are available for engraftment will ultimately survive and remain in the host tissue. Donor cells, air, fat, or other debris may embolize in the coronary system or systemic circulation if needle placement is not optimal. Emboli have the potential to cause serious consequences, but can be avoided by a careful and targeted technique of cell delivery. Acute arrhythmias have been encountered immediately after injection, resulting in heart block or asystole. These fatal complications are likely the result of coronary emboli, injection into the conduction system, severe ischemia from excessive injectant volume, or other causes. Serious acute arrhythmias are of concern, but are infrequent when an appropriate concentration and volume of cells and careful technique are employed.

Chronic Complications

The chronic complications associated with cell transplantation are less well understood, given the short follow-up involved in most experimental animal protocols and the limited application to date in humans. Cell transplantation may result in chronic complications such as cell rejection, cardiac arrhythmia, and cell proliferation. Donor cell survival after allogenic transplantation decreased with time from ongoing inflammation and cell rejection (lymphocytic infiltration) despite treatment with cyclosporine.[44] This also may occur to some extent after autologous cell transplantation. Stable autologous skeletal myoblast grafts have been observed in human cardiac scar tissue more than 1 year after transplantation.[23] Arrhythmia is a potential concern with cell grafting, and prophylactic implantable defibrillators have been employed in patients with severe ventricular dysfunction receiving cell transplantation.[52] In a clinical case series, 4 of 10 patients had arrhythmias. Other than ventricular arrhythmias, no serious complications have been associated with clinical cell transplantation to date.

CLINICAL APPLICATIONS OF CELL TRANSPLANTATION FOR CARDIOVASCULAR DISEASE

Cell transplantation can provide significant improvements in cardiac function after myocardial injury, making cardiac regeneration a promising therapeutic prospect for patients at risk of congestive heart failure. Proof-of-concept studies have been performed in several experimental animal models of human cardiovascular disease. In summary, transplanted cells survive in the failing myocardium, improve regional perfusion, increase wall thickness, and enhance wall motion, resulting in restored global cardiac function. In addition to these profound effects, cryoinjured mice demonstrated improved overall survival after cell transplantation with embryonic cardiomyocytes.[67] Whether these profound structural and functional benefits are sustainable over the long term is less well understood. Evidence suggests that the benefits are not transient, because cell transplantation improved cardiac function after myocardial infarction in rats up to 6 months after injection.[55] In addition, skeletal myoblasts remained stable and improved cardiac function in infarcted sheep for as long as 1 year after injection.[22] Clinical trials are currently underway, and the preliminary data are encouraging.

Coronary Artery Disease

Incomplete Infarction and Chronic Ischemia

The goals of cell transplantation in the setting of incomplete infarction and chronic ischemia are to improve regional perfusion, replace lost muscle mass, and prevent ongoing ischemia and infarct expansion. Endothelial cells and bone marrow cells are capable of stimulating angiogenesis and may be particularly suited for this clinical problem. We transplanted aortic endothelial cells into the myocardial scar tissue of adult rats.[32] The implanted cells enhanced blood vessel density as early as 1 week after injury. At 6 weeks, blood vessel density in the transplanted area was significantly greater than media-transplantation control animals. By labeling the donor cells with markers, we identified the transplanted cells in the endothelium of the newly forming blood vessels. Microsphere perfusion studies showed that the neovascularization increased regional blood flow after cell transplantation compared with controls. However, the increased angiogenesis did not result in an improvement in global heart function in this animal model. Although the adult endothelial cell transplantation stimulated angiogenesis, it cannot replace lost cardiomyocytes in the damaged heart and would not likely have significant benefits for patients with extensive, transmural myocardial infarctions with depressed cardiac function. In contrast, if the endothelial cells are implanted into ischemic myocardial tissue, the enhanced perfusion might permit recovery of contractile function of hibernating muscle cells and improve global heart function. Chekanov and colleagues[11] generated myocardial ischemia in sheep by placing an ameroid constrictor on the circumflex artery. Autologous endothelial cells isolated from jugular veins were implanted into the damaged area. Eight weeks after cell implantation, regional perfusion was significantly improved in the cell-transplanted group, but not in controls. Cardiac function in the cell-transplanted hearts was better than that in controls.

For patients with incomplete infarctions and chronic ischemia, BMCs may be the optimal cell type to increase perfusion and repopulate injured myocardium. Tomita and colleagues[83] implanted fresh isolated BMCs, cultured BMCs, and BMCs pretreated with 5-azacytidine into rat myocardial scar tissue induced by cryoinjury. Five weeks after transplantation, blood vessel density in the transplanted scar area in all cell groups was significantly greater than that in controls injected with the vehicle alone (culture medium). In some animals, transplanted cells were found as mature endothelial cells in the capillary wall of newly formed vessels. Thus BMCs are capable of transforming into useful endothelial cells in the formation of new vessels after transplantation. Use of untreated BMCs did not improve cardiac function in this study, perhaps a consequence of the model employed. In the cryoinjury model, no residual heart cells are available to provide clues to the engrafted marrow stromal cells to differentiate into muscle cells. In infarct models, residual cardiomyocytes in the damaged region may induce muscle differentiation and permit recovery of function. In a large animal model, Shake and colleagues[76] found that untreated marrow stromal cells did improve function after a myocardial infarction. We also found that marrow stromal cells improved cardiac function 4 weeks after occlusion of the left anterior descending coronary artery in pigs. Cultured BMCs pretreated with 5-azacytidine differentiated into cardiac-like muscle cells while in culture and also after engraftment in ventricular scar tissue, improving both regional perfusion and myocardial function.[84] Hamano and co-workers[24] determined that implanted autologous canine BMCs increased the blood vessel density in the transplant region almost twofold greater than in controls. In addition, Fuchs and colleagues[21] reported that freshly isolated BMCs from adult swine induced angiogenesis in ischemic myocardium after autologous transplantation.

BMCs have been used in humans with ongoing ischemia and muscle loss. Strauer and co-workers[81] transplanted autologous mononuclear BMCs in 10 patients with acute myocardial infarction by intracoronary injection during percutaneous transluminal angioplasty. After 3 months of follow up, myocardial regions of cell delivery demonstrated increased perfusion, viability, and wall motion compared with controls, suggesting improved myogenesis and angiogenesis after cell therapy. No adverse events were attributed to cell injection. In another early clinical report, Assmus and colleagues[3] examined BMC-derived progenitor cells, as well as circulating progenitor cells (CPCs) extracted from autologous blood samples. The use of CPCs would obviate the need for a bone marrow aspiration, facilitating clinical cell transplantation. Four months after acute myocardial infarction, intracoronary infusion of adult progenitor cells was associated with improved regional and global heart function, improved viability in the infarct area, and reduced LV end-systolic volumes. Interestingly, there was no difference in the ability of blood-derived versus bone marrow-derived progenitor cells to improve LV remodeling after myocardial infarction. Characterization of the progenitor cell phenotypes indicated that the CPCs were largely endothelial progenitor cells, whereas the bone marrow aspirate contained a population of hematopoietic, mesenchymal, and stromal stem cells. Therefore marrow stromal cells may be more likely to differentiate into muscle cells and improve heart function. The timing of cell delivery during acute myocardial infarction as opposed to chronic heart failure may confound early clinical reports. Specifically, donor cells were delivery to the injured region before significant scar formation and remodeling had occurred (within 5 days of coronary occlusion) in contrast to the majority of experimental animal studies. The differentiation of stem cells may have a "milieu-dependent" control mechanism such that "scar begets scar" and "muscle begets muscle." Early transplantation of progenitor cells before significant scar formation and LV remodeling may be desirable to optimize myogenesis and functional benefits. Unfortunately, early injection of cells may induce cell clearance by the inflammatory response to infarction, reducing cell survival and limiting the benefits of cell engraftment. We found that cells injected more than 7 days after cardiac injury resulted in better engraftment and better functional recovery after cell implantation.[45] Although the results with progenitor cell transplantation are encouraging, these preliminary trials using bone marrow and circulating progenitor cell transplantation in acute myocardial infarction to prevent heart failure were designed as phase I safety trials and, accordingly, efficacy must be interpreted with some caution because the treatment groups were compared with nonrandomized controls. The results of larger, randomized multicenter trials are eagerly anticipated.

Complete Infarction with Ventricular Dysfunction

The overriding goals of cell transplantation for complete infarction with ventricular dysfunction are to restore cardiac function and prevent the transition to congestive heart failure. Experimental animal models with regional ventricular dysfunction secondary to coronary ischemia, infarction, or localized cryoinjury indicate that diverse cell types when transplanted into the recipient myocardium can induce a profound biological phenomenon that restores contractile function and prevents or delays ventricular dilatation and maladaptive remodeling.[29,40,46,65,86]

What cell type is most appropriate for patients with complete infarction and ventricular dysfunction? BMC transplantation can stimulate angiogenesis and increase the capillary density, but global heart function may not be improved. For example, freshly isolated or cultured BMCs transplanted in rats after myocardial cryoinjury did not result in improved cardiac function.[83] Only bone marrow cells pretreated to form musclelike cells resulted in improved heart function after implantation into the myocardial scar tissue. In contrast, using a porcine model of chronic coronary occlusion, Shake and colleagues[76] locally injected BMCs into the injured heart. One month later, there was greater wall thickening in the area of cell transplantation and a corresponding improvement of heart function. These data suggest that angiogenesis induced by bone marrow transplantation may not improve heart function if the defect area is devoid of muscle (transmural scar). Both myogenesis and angiogenesis may be required to restore cardiac function in patients with transmural scar tissue. Accordingly, pretreated BMCs, subpopulations of adult bone marrow stem cells, or muscle cells themselves may be most appropriate for these patients. Fortunately, the majority of patients have persisting residual cardiomyocytes after infarction that may be sufficient to provide the clues to marrow stromal cells to differentiate into a muscle phenotype and improve function.

Muscle cell transplantation with heart cells, skeletal myoblasts, and smooth muscle cells successfully improved ventricular function after complete myocardial infarction. Preliminary evidence in patients also supports the use of muscle cell transplantation. Autologous human skeletal

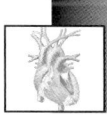

myoblasts expanded in culture from a thigh-muscle biopsy were directly injected into nonviable regions at the time of coronary artery bypass grafting or mechanical assist device insertion. Implanted autologous skeletal myoblasts formed viable grafts in failing human myocardium despite extensive fibrosis.[64] Patients with severe heart failure who received autologous skeletal myoblast transplants combined with coronary artery bypass grafting have reported improved symptoms and global heart function. Importantly, there was evidence of viability in the infarct region after clinical cell transplantation. These preliminary case series suggests that cell transplantation is a safe and potentially useful therapy for patients with heart disease, stimulating both myogenesis and angiogenesis. A randomized multicenter phase II trial led by Dr. Menasche in France is currently underway (MAGIC: Myoblast Autologous Grafting in Ischemic Cardiomyopathy). Other clinical trials using autologous skeletal myoblasts have confirmed the feasibility and safety of myoblast transplantation.[15] Similar clinical approaches at the time of coronary artery bypass grafting using subpopulations of adult bone marrow stem cells from autologous bone marrow aspirations have recently been reported.[80] Although these early clinical reports are not designed to evaluate efficacy, the preliminary data after midterm follow up is encouraging and supports the large body of animal studies indicating beneficial effects on remodeling, angiogenesis, and overall cardiac function.[53]

Complete Infarction with Ventricular Aneurysm

Cell-based therapies are designed to regenerate heart tissue and restore function after myocardial injury or loss. Because the engraftment process is limited after injection of cell suspensions, particularly in a large mature dyskinetic scar with poor perfusion and few remaining cardiomyocytes, patients with aneurysms and cardiac failure are unlikely to benefit from cell transplantation alone. Resection of the aneurysm and surgical remodeling of the ventricle to restore chamber size and shape may improve cardiac function. For surgical repair of LV aneurysms, ventricular restoration procedures such as the SAVER operation[4-6,18] may increase systolic function by normalizing LV chamber size and shape. A number of clinical studies using these emerging techniques have reported acceptable early and midterm results.[16,17,19] However, in the long term, chamber redilatation and decompensation is a concern with both modified and traditional aneurysm repairs.[19,57,77] Ventricular restoration procedures could be enhanced with use of an autologous muscle cell–seeded bioengineered graft in place of traditional, nonviable synthetic patch materials. Bioengineered muscle grafts may prevent recurrent dilatation and improve cardiac function after myocardial repair.

Fundamentally, cardiac tissue engineering involves seeding a biodegradable scaffold with muscle cells and allowing tissue formation in vitro before ultimately implanting the graft into the heart.[47] Ideally the seeded cells will grow into morphologically recognizable tissue before implantation and then integrate and remodel with the host tissue after implantation. Once implanted, the biodegradable scaffold will slowly dissolve and the seeded cells will retain their spatial architecture by synthesizing their own interstitial matrix scaffold. We seeded human pediatric heart cells on Gelfoam patches and subjected them to a mechanical stretch regimen to simulate the cardiac cycle of patch implantation into a beating heart.[1] Mechanical stretch resulted in the synthesis and formation of an organized, healthy matrix by the seeded cells, consistent with normal myocardium. These data and those of others suggest that heart cells retain the capacity to form cardiac-like tissue when provided with appropriate environmental cues, such as mechanical stretch.[1,10,30,31] Accordingly, we successfully created a contractile cardiac muscle graft using a Gelfoam scaffold and fetal cardiomyocytes.[41]

As mentioned previously, the interstitial matrix is a critical mediator of structural support and a key regulator of tissue architecture in vivo. The success of bioengineering heart muscle in vitro largely depends on the use of an appropriate matrix-like biomaterial capable of providing structural support, as well as the molecular cues necessary for tissue formation. We determined that specific biomaterials are capable of enhancing tissue formation while retaining structural support for a reasonable period.[62,63] Using these materials, we successfully replaced the right ventricular (RV) outflow tract in rats using a bioengineered smooth muscle graft.[62] Our studies and those of others indicate that bioengineered muscle grafts are capable of significant tissue formation and remodeling after implantation into the beating heart.[37,62,85] In contrast, nonbiodegradable patches such as Dacron (polyethylene terephthalate) and Gore-Tex (polytetrafluoroethylene [PTFE]) are nonviable, will not grow, have the potential for infection, and are incapable of significant remodeling and self-repair.

Although the optimal materials and environmental conditions for adequate tissue formation in the bioengineering of cardiac muscle grafts are largely unknown, some preliminary studies indicate that even our rudimentary constructs can improve the heart failure process. In a sheep model of a myocardial infarction, suturing a polypropylene mesh alone over the infarcted area prevented progressive LV expansion.[29] This technique maintained normal ventricular geometry and heart function for 8 weeks despite substantial tissue losses, suggesting that even noncontractile bioengineered muscle grafts may provide substantial benefits. Consequently, Leor and colleagues[37] showed that implantation of a bioengineered fetal rat cardiomyocyte graft onto the surface of a myocardial infarct attenuated ventricular dilatation. Our preliminary data in a rat of model of LV aneurysm from complete infarction confirm these intriguing findings. Eight weeks after implantation of a bioengineered smooth muscle graft, systolic function was improved by echocardiography and LV distensibility was reduced as compared with noncellular patch repairs. A complete resection of myocardial scar tissue and total replacement of the infarct area with bioengineered muscle grafts may avoid the long-term recurrent dilatation and decompensation complicating conventional therapies. Autologous bioengineered muscle grafts will likely replace synthetic materials for myocardial repair in the future.

Congestive Heart Failure

Nonischemic Dilated Cardiomyopathy

The heart failure epidemic is not restricted to patients with ischemic cardiomyopathy, and it appears that the benefits of cell transplant therapies may not be restricted to ischemia-based cardiac dysfunction. Cell transplantation has proved beneficial in animal models of nonischemic dilated cardiomyopathy (DCM).[58] Scorsin and co-workers[73] reported that cell transplantation improved heart function in mice with doxorubicin-induced DCM. Our group examined muscle cell transplantation in hamsters with an inherited form of DCM (delta-sarcoglycan gene deficiency), similar to some forms of human cardiomyopathy. Donor heart cells survived in the host myocardium after transplantation, prevented or delayed dilatation and wall thinning, and preserved heart function.[89] Because heart cells may be abnormal in these patients, we also transplanted autologous smooth muscle cells. The beneficial effects of smooth muscle cell transplantation on cardiac structure and function in DCM were similar to heart cell transplantation.[90] Thus muscle cell transplantation limited adverse LV remodeling and sustained LV function in DCM.

Cell transplantation also may improve the long-term benefits of LV remodeling surgery such as anterior ventricular endocardial restoration (SAVER) or mechanical cardiac restraint.[4-6] In a rat model, fetal cardiomyocyte transplantation combined with LV aneurysm repair prevented late LV dilatation and dysfunction.[72] Cell transplantation combined with LV remodeling surgery at the time of compensated LV dysfunction may prove to be the most effective approach to reverse LV dilatation, increase wall thickness, and prevent subsequent progression to heart failure in patients with DCM.

End-Stage Congestive Heart Failure

For patients with compensated ventricular dysfunction, targeted cell therapy at the onset of significant chamber dilatation and elevated wall stress may prevent decompensation, which would otherwise result in heart transplantation, ventricular device assistance, or death. Cell transplantation after the onset of cardiac decompensation may not be beneficial. The failing myocardium may be a poor host for donor cell engraftment because of severe wall stress, poor perfusion, and inflammatory infiltration. However, evidence for LV recovery (reverse remodeling) after left ventricular assist device (LVAD) assistance in decompensated DCM has been reported.[38,56] Thus after a period of hemodynamic unloading, cell transplantation may provide a stabilizing addition to the transient benefits offered by LVAD assistance and reverse remodeling. Clinical cell transplantation has been performed safely in LVAD-assisted failing hearts, but no data on possible benefits are yet available.[15,64]

MECHANISMS UNDERLYING THE BENEFITS OF CELL TRANSPLANTATION

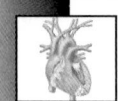

Active and Passive Mechanisms

The cellular and molecular mechanisms that mediate the functional benefits observed in the failing heart after cell transplantation are not clear. An active process whereby the engrafted cells replace lost contractile elements and contract synchronously with the host myocardium may occur. When we transplanted a cell suspension of cultured fetal and neonatal rat cardiomyocytes into the subcutaneous connective tissue of adult rat hind limbs, the injected cells formed spontaneously contractile cardiac-like muscle tissue.[43] These observations suggest that a similar process of active contraction could have occurred in myocardial scar tissue with injection of fetal heart cells. However, we also assessed the morphological and biochemical phenotypical changes that occurred in vitro with passaging of human pediatric and adult ventricular cardiomyocytes.[42] In contrast to fetal and neonatal heart cells, pediatric and adult human heart cells rapidly dedifferentiated in culture, lost their sarcomeres, and were rendered noncontractile. Additionally, adult cardiomyocytes were less expansive than the pediatric cells, which could be cultured for as long as 6 months. These cell culture data are not confirmatory, but they call into question the ability of adult heart cells to synchronously contract after cell transplantation into the beating heart. In addition, the number of cells that ultimately survive and engraft in the host myocardium after direct injection is significantly limited. Given this consistent observation of reduced cell survival after cell transplantation, active contraction of transplanted cells as the sole mediator of improved contractile function does not seem plausible. However, some suggest otherwise. Menasche and colleagues[52] recently demonstrated that skeletal myoblasts are capable of contraction after implantation into ischemic heart tissue. Others have shown that transplanted cells may have the potential for electromechanical coupling with host heart cells.[34,67,69,78] In these studies, however, functional improvements also could be explained by the ability of the engrafted cells to limit infarct expansion and improve angiogenesis. Although transplanted cells may indeed contract in host myocardium under specific conditions, it remains to be determined whether the active contraction of implanted cells is responsible for the improvements of systolic function observed after cell transplantation in failing hearts.

Matrix Remodeling

Although the functional characteristics of the cells themselves may be important, such as the ability to contract, it is possible that some of the beneficial effects of cell transplantation may be the result of a reorganization of the structural elements surrounding the engrafted cells. The interstitial or extracellular matrix (ECM) provides the structural framework for coordinated muscle cell contraction and also sequesters growth factors and cytokines that interact with local cell receptors to influence cellular behavior and survival. The myocardial matrix thus assembles a dynamic microenvironment in which molecular cues converge to maintain tissue architecture by regulating cell orientation, shape, growth (hypertrophy and proliferation), and survival (apoptosis).[25,48,49,68] Maladaptive remodeling of cardiac matrix impairs structural support for heart cells, leading to ventricular dilatation, increased wall stress, and both systolic and diastolic dysfunction.[8,33] Experimental and clinical studies indicate that the ECM is significantly degraded and remodeled in the failing heart,[79] and this process of matrix disruption has emerged as an important new target in the treatment of heart failure. Accordingly, therapeutic strategies that limit adverse matrix remodeling in failing myocardium, such as cell transplantation, may prevent ventricular dilatation and maintain the structural support necessary for effective cardiomyocyte contraction. In theory, because myocardial matrix disruption can decrease systolic performance without changing myocyte contractility,[8] engrafted cells could improve overall cardiac function without contributing to contractile function themselves simply by restoring deficient interstitial matrix components in the failing heart.

Cell Engraftment

How could cell transplantation influence the structural framework of the heart? The region of cell implantation must reorganize its structural components to accommodate and engraft the transplanted cells. Although the process of cellular engraftment is not well understood, it must involve the binding of implanted cells to host matrix elements. Without physical tethers to matrix elements, cells will not survive.[25,48,49,68] Thus in the process of engraftment, transplanted cells likely reorganize the degraded matrix of the host myocardium and secrete and incorporate new matrix elements within deficient areas (Figure 97-3). To maintain engraftment and their survival in host myocardium, implanted cells also may secrete bioactive peptides to stimulate angiogenesis (i.e., vascular endothelial growth factor [VEGF] and fibroblast growth factor [FGF]), as well as factors that influence cell hypertrophy, proliferation, and survival (Figure 97-4). These beneficial autocrine and paracrine mediators would influence adjacent heart cells, thereby restoring the balance of adverse bioactive mediators associated with heart failure. This cascade of events could prevent or delay adverse myocardial remodeling, even in the absence of donor cell contraction. As a consequence of cell engraftment, the restored myocardial matrix could improve the structural support for native heart cells, and in so doing, infarct expansion would be attenuated and regional function improved by a tethering effect to actively contracting host tissue.

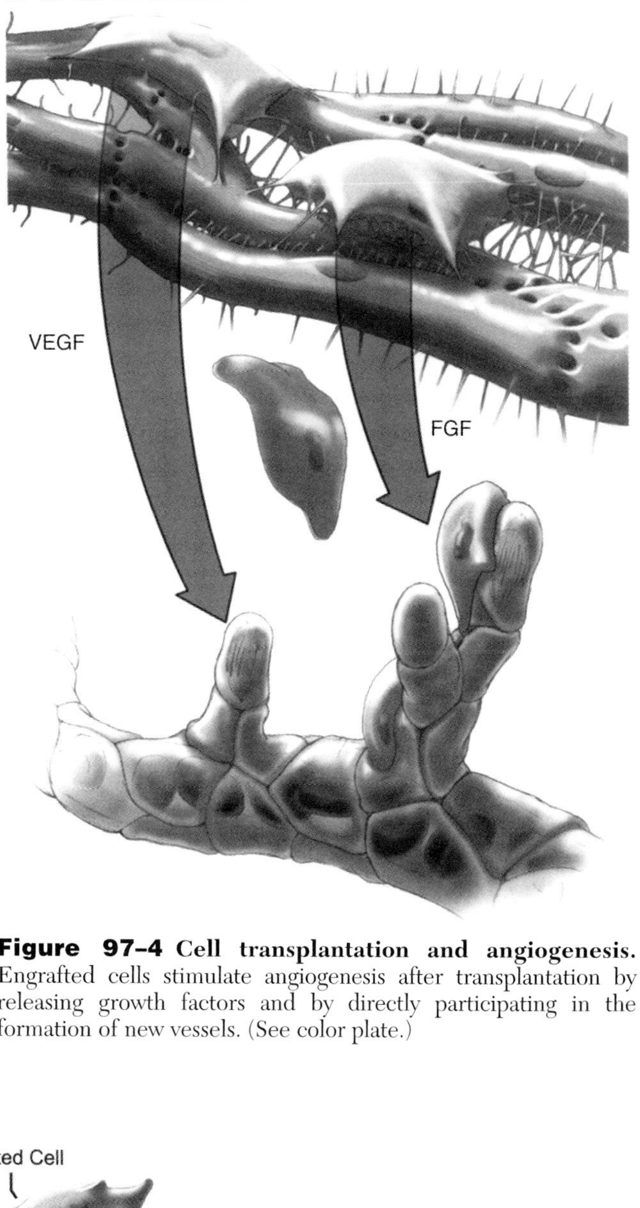

Figure 97–4 Cell transplantation and angiogenesis. Engrafted cells stimulate angiogenesis after transplantation by releasing growth factors and by directly participating in the formation of new vessels. (See color plate.)

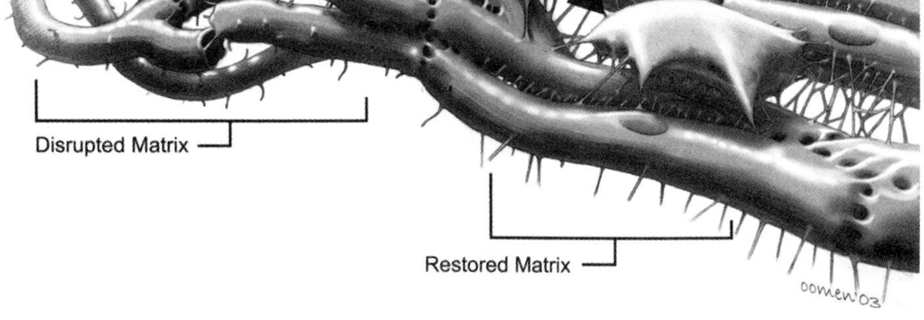

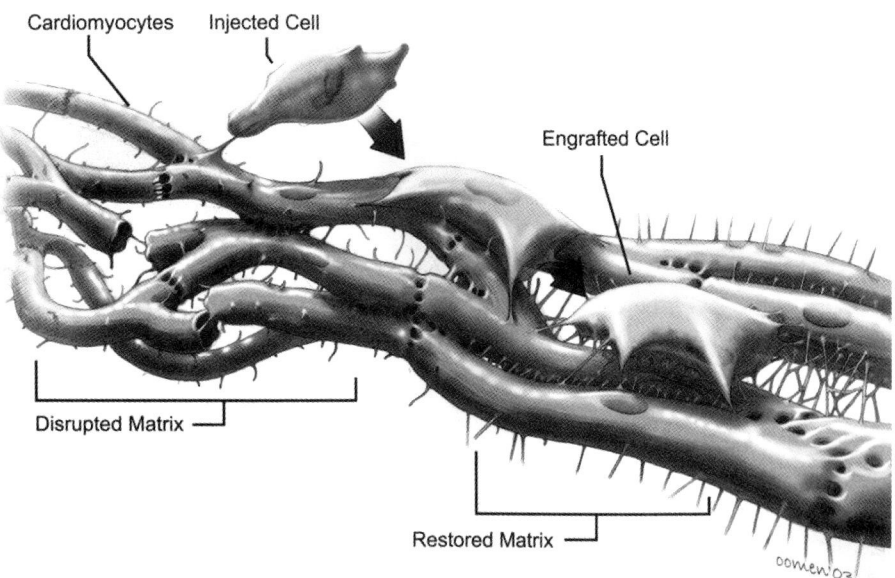

Figure 97–3 Cell engraftment in the failing heart. The interstitial matrix provides the structural support for cardiomyocytes, maintaining ventricular shape and function. The myocardial matrix is disrupted and degraded in the failing heart. The process of cell engraftment may replace and reorganize damaged structural elements after cell transplantation, preventing cardiac dilatation and restoring myocardial function in the failing heart. (See color plate.)

Angiogenesis

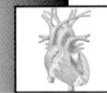

Transplanted cells stimulate angiogenesis by secreting bioactive growth factors (i.e., VEGF and FGF). In addition, the donor cells participate in the formation of new vessels by incorporating into the newly forming vessel wall (see Figure 97-4). Compared with gene or protein angiogenic therapies, not only does cell transplantation provide the signals for new vessels to grow into the ischemic region, but the donor cells provide the necessary cellular building blocks for new vessel formation in a region where cells are likely scarce. Angiogenesis in the absence of myogenesis may not influence overall heart function, but improving perfusion to the infarct region may itself modify the remodeling of both the injured region and the remaining myocardium. Increasing perfusion may salvage hibernating native cardiomyocytes and/or restore damaged cells. Increased perfusion also may aid in the restoration of injured matrix that in turn may facilitate donor cell incorporation, donor to host cell communications, and increased structural support and stability.

The cellular and molecular mechanisms that govern cell engraftment and subsequent improvements of cardiac function in the failing heart are likely multifactorial, complex, and far from understood. From the perspective that cardiac remodeling determines the clinical progression of heart failure and is emerging as a therapeutic target in heart failure of all etiologies,[13] the mechanisms underlying the benefits on remodeling with cell transplantation are an important area of future investigation.

SUMMARY

The restoration of cardiac function and regeneration of lost myocardium with cell transplantation and tissue engineering are promising new surgical tools for the growing number of patients at risk of heart failure. Autologous cell transplantation restores regional and global cardiac function after myocardial infarction or dilated cardiomyopathy by providing myogenesis, stimulating and participating in angiogenesis, and limiting maladaptive ventricular remodeling. Bioengineered muscle grafting offers the promise of myocardial regeneration by replacing irreversibly damaged myocardium with healthy autologous tissue to facilitate surgical remodeling of the failing heart.

REFERENCES

1. Akhyari P, Fedak PW, Weisel RD, et al: Mechanical stretch regimen enhances the formation of bioengineered autologous cardiac muscle grafts. Circulation 106:I137–I142, 2002.
2. Anversa P, Nadal-Ginard B: Myocyte renewal and ventricular remodelling. Nature 415:240–243, 2002.
3. Assmus B, Schachinger V, Teupe C, et al: Transplantation of progenitor cells and regeneration enhancement in acute myocardial infarction (TOPCARE-AMI). Circulation 106: 3009–3017, 2002.
4. Athanasuleas CL, Buckberg GD, Menicanti L, et al: Optimizing ventricular shape in anterior restoration. Semin Thorac Cardiovasc Surg 13:459–467, 2001.
5. Athanasuleas CL, Stanley AW Jr, Buckberg GD, et al: Surgical anterior ventricular endocardial restoration (SAVER) for dilated ischemic cardiomyopathy. Semin Thorac Cardiovasc Surg 13:448–458, 2001a.
6. Athanasuleas CL, Stanley AW Jr, Buckberg GD, et al: Surgical anterior ventricular endocardial restoration (SAVER) in the dilated remodeled ventricle after anterior myocardial infarction. RESTORE group. Reconstructive Endoventricular Surgery, returning Torsion Original Radius Elliptical Shape to the LV. J Am Coll Cardiol 37:1199–1209, 2001b.
7. Atkins BZ, Hueman MT, Meuchel JM, et al: Myogenic cell transplantation improves in vivo regional performance in infarcted rabbit myocardium. J Heart Lung Transplant 18: 1173–1180, 1999.
8. Baicu CF, Stroud JD, Livesay VA, et al: Changes in extracellular collagen matrix alter myocardial systolic performance. Am J Physiol Heart Circ Physiol 284:H122–H132, 2003.
9. Bolling SF, Smolens IA, Pagani FD: Surgical alternatives for heart failure. J Heart Lung Transplant 20:729–733, 2001.
10. Carrier RL, Papadaki M, Rupnick M, et al: Cardiac tissue engineering: cell seeding, cultivation parameters, and tissue construct characterization. Biotechnol Bioeng 64:580–589, 1999.
11. Chekanov V, Nikolaychik V, Tchekanov G, et al: Transplantation of autologous endothelial cells in a fibrin meshwork induces angiogenesis and improves myocardial function in an animal model of ischemic cardiomyopathy. Circulation 104:II260, 2001 (abstract).
12. Chiu RC: Cardiac cell transplantation: The autologous skeletal myoblast implantation for myocardial regeneration. Adv Card Surg 11:69–98, 1999.
13. Cohn JN, Ferrari R, Sharpe N: Cardiac remodeling—concepts and clinical implications: A consensus paper from an international forum on cardiac remodeling. Behalf of an International Forum on Cardiac Remodeling. J Am Coll Cardiol 35:569–582, 2000.
14. Dib N, Diethrich EB, Campbell A, et al: Endoventricular transplantation of allogenic skeletal myoblasts in a porcine model of myocardial infarction. J Endovasc Ther 9:313–319, 2002.
15. Dib N, McCarthy PM, Campbell A, et al: Safety and feasibility of autologous myoblast transplantation in patients with ischemic cardiomyopathy: Interim results from the United States experience. Circulation 106:II463, 2002 (abstract).
16. Di Donato M, Sabatier M, Dor V, et al: Akinetic versus dyskinetic postinfarction scar: Relation to surgical outcome in patients undergoing endoventricular circular patch plasty repair. J Am Coll Cardiol 29:1569–1575, 1997.
17. Di Donato M, Sabatier M, Dor V, et al: Effects of the Dor procedure on left ventricular dimension and shape and geometric correlates of mitral regurgitation one year after surgery. J Thorac Cardiovasc Surg 121:91–96, 2001.
18. Dor V, Saab M, Coste P, et al: Left ventricular aneurysm: A new surgical approach. Thorac Cardiovasc Surg 37:11–19, 1989.
19. Dor V, Sabatier M, Di Donato M, et al: Efficacy of endoventricular patch plasty in large postinfarction akinetic scar and severe left ventricular dysfunction: Comparison with a series of large dyskinetic scars. J Thorac Cardiovasc Surg 116:50–59, 1998.
20. Etzion S, Battler A, Barbash IM, et al: Influence of embryonic cardiomyocyte transplantation on the progression of heart failure in a rat model of extensive myocardial infarction. J Mol Cell Cardiol 33:1321–1330, 2001.
21. Fuchs S, Baffour R, Zhou YF, et al: Transendocardial delivery of autologous bone marrow enhances collateral perfusion and regional function in pigs with chronic experimental myocardial ischemia. J Am Coll Cardiol 37:1726–1732, 2001.

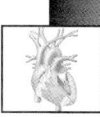

22. Ghostine S, Carrion C, Souza LC, et al: Long-term efficacy of myoblast transplantation on regional structure and function after myocardial infarction. Circulation 106:I131–I136, 2002.
23. Hagege AA, Carrion C, Menasche P, et al: Viability and differentiation of autologous skeletal myoblast grafts in ischemic cardiomyopathy. Lancet 361:491–492, 2003 (abstract).
24. Hamano K, Li TS, Kobayashi T, et al: Therapeutic angiogenesis induced by local autologous bone marrow cell implantation. Ann Thorac Surg 73:1210–1215, 2002.
25. Hornberger LK, Singhroy S, Cavalle-Garrido T, et al: Synthesis of extracellular matrix and adhesion through beta(1) integrins are critical for fetal ventricular myocyte proliferation. Circ Res 87:508–515, 2000.
26. Hutcheson KA, Atkins BZ, Hueman MT, et al: Comparison of benefits on myocardial performance of cellular cardiomyoplasty with skeletal myoblasts and fibroblasts. Cell Transplant 9:359–368, 2000.
27. Jain M, DerSimonian H, Brenner DA, et al: Cell therapy attenuates deleterious ventricular remodeling and improves cardiac performance after myocardial infarction. Circulation 103:1920–1927, 2001.
28. Kawamoto A, Gwon HC, Iwaguro H, et al: Therapeutic potential of ex vivo expanded endothelial progenitor cells for myocardial ischemia. Circulation 103:634–637, 2001.
29. Kelley ST, Malekan R, Gorman JH 3rd, et al: Restraining infarct expansion preserves left ventricular geometry and function after acute anteroapical infarction. Circulation 99: 135–142, 1999.
30. Kim BS, Nikolovski J, Bonadio J, et al: Cyclic mechanical strain regulates the development of engineered smooth muscle tissue. Nat Biotechnol 17:979–983, 1999.
31. Kim BS, Putnam AJ, Kulik TJ, et al: Optimizing seeding and culture methods to engineer smooth muscle tissue on biodegradable polymer matrices. Biotechnol Bioeng 57:46–54, 1998.
32. Kim EJ, Li RK, Weisel RD, et al: Angiogenesis by endothelial cell transplantation. J Thorac Cardiovasc Surg 122:963–971, 2001.
33. Kim HE, Dalal SS, Young E, et al: Disruption of the myocardial extracellular matrix leads to cardiac dysfunction. J Clin Invest 106:857–866, 2000.
34. Koh GY, Soonpaa MH, Klug MG, et al: Stable fetal cardiomyocyte grafts in the hearts of dystrophic mice and dogs. J Clin Invest 96:2034–2042, 1995.
35. Kohtz DS, Dische NR, Inagami T, et al: Growth and partial differentiation of presumptive human cardiac myoblasts in culture. J Cell Biol 108:1067–1078, 1989.
36. Leobon B, Garcin I, Vilquin JT, et al: Do engrafted skeletal myoblasts contract in infarcted myocardium? Circulation 106:II549, 2002 (abstract).
37. Leor J, Aboulafia-Etzion S, Dar A, et al: Bioengineered cardiac grafts: A new approach to repair the infarcted myocardium? Circulation 102:III56–III61, 2000.
38. Levin HR, Oz MC, Chen JM, et al: Reversal of chronic ventricular dilation in patients with end-stage cardiomyopathy by prolonged mechanical unloading. Circulation 91:2717–2720, 1995.
39. Li RK, Jia ZQ, Weisel RD, et al: Cardiomyocyte transplantation improves heart function. Ann Thorac Surg 62:654–660, 1996.
40. Li RK, Jia ZQ, Weisel RD, et al: Smooth muscle cell transplantation into myocardial scar tissue improves heart function. J Mol Cell Cardiol 31:513–522, 1999a.
41. Li RK, Jia ZQ, Weisel RD, et al: Survival and function of bioengineered cardiac grafts. Circulation 100:63–69, 1999b.
42. Li RK, Mickle DA, Weisel RD, et al: Human pediatric and adult ventricular cardiomyocytes in culture: Assessment of phenotypical changes with passaging. Cardiovasc Res 32: 362–373, 1996a.
43. Li RK, Mickle DA, Weisel RD, et al: In vivo survival and function of transplanted rat cardiomyocytes. Circ Res 78:283–288, 1996b.
44. Li RK, Mickle DA, Weisel RD, et al: Natural history of fetal rat cardiomyocytes transplanted into adult rat myocardial scar tissue. Circulation 96:II86, 1997.
45. Li RK, Mickle DA, Weisel RD, et al: Optimal time for cardiomyocyte transplantation to maximize myocardial function after left ventricular injury. Ann Thorac Surg 72:1957–1963, 2001.
46. Li RK, Weisel RD, Mickle DA, et al: Autologous porcine heart cell transplantation improved heart function after a myocardial infarction. J Thorac Cardiovasc Surg 119:62–68, 2000.
47. Li RK, Yau TM, Weisel RD, et al: Construction of a bioengineered cardiac graft. J Thorac Cardiovasc Surg 119: 368–375, 2000.
48. Lukashev ME, Werb Z: ECM signalling: Orchestrating cell behaviour and misbehaviour. Trends Cell Biol 8:437–441, 1998.
49. Lundgren E, Terracio L, Mardh S, et al: Extracellular matrix components influence the survival of adult cardiac myocytes in vitro. Exp Cell Res 158:371–381, 1985.
50. Makino S, Fukuda K, Miyoshi S, et al: Cardiomyocytes can be generated from marrow stromal cells in vitro. J Clin Invest 103:697–705, 1999.
51. Marelli D, Desrosiers C, el Alfy M, et al: Cell transplantation for myocardial repair: An experimental approach. Cell Transplant 1:383–390, 1992.
52. Menasche P: Myoblast transplantation: Feasibility, safety and efficacy. Ann Med 34:314–315, 2002.
53. Menasche P, Hagege A, Vilquin JT, et al: Transplantation of autologous skeletal myoblasts in patients with severe left ventricular function: A medium-term appraisal. Circulation 106:II463, 2002 (abstract).
54. Menasche P, Hagege AA, Scorsin M, et al: Myoblast transplantation for heart failure. Lancet 357:279–280, 2001.
55. Muller-Ehmsen J, Peterson KL, Kedes L, et al: Rebuilding a damaged heart: Long-term survival of transplanted neonatal rat cardiomyocytes after myocardial infarction and effect on cardiac function. Circulation 105:1720–1726, 2002.
56. Nakatani T, Sasako Y, Kobayashi J, et al: Recovery of cardiac function by long-term left ventricular support in patients with end-stage cardiomyopathy. ASAIO J 44:M516–M520, 1998.
57. Nishina T, Nishimura K, Yuasa S, et al: Initial effects of the left ventricular repair by plication may not last long in a rat ischemic cardiomyopathy model. Circulation 104:241–245, 2001.
58. Ohno N, Fedak PW, Weisel RD, et al: Cell transplantation in non-ischemic dilated cardiomyopathy. A novel biological approach for ventricular restoration. Jpn J Thorac Cardiovasc Surg 50:457–460, 2002.
59. Orlic D, Hill JM, Arai AE: Stem cells for myocardial regeneration. Circ Res 91:1092–1102, 2002.
60. Orlic D, Kajstura J, Chimenti S, et al: Transplanted adult bone marrow cells repair myocardial infarcts in mice. Ann N Y Acad Sci 938:221-230, 2001a.
61. Orlic D, Kajstura J, Chimenti S, et al: Bone marrow cells regenerate infarcted myocardium. Nature 410:701–705, 2001b.
62. Ozawa T, Mickle DA, Weisel RD, et al: Optimal biomaterial for creation of autologous cardiac grafts. Circulation 106:I176–I182, 2002a.
63. Ozawa T, Mickle DA, Weisel RD, et al: Histologic changes of nonbiodegradable and biodegradable biomaterials used to repair right ventricular heart defects in rats. J Thorac Cardiovasc Surg 124:1157–1164, 2002b.

64. Pagani F, DerSimonian H, Zawadzka A, et al: Autologous skeletal myoblasts transplanted in ischemia damaged myocardium in humans. Circulation 106:II463, 2002 (abstract).
65. Rajnoch C, Chachques JC, Berrebi A, et al: Cellular therapy reverses myocardial dysfunction. J Thorac Cardiovasc Surg 121:871–878, 2001.
66. Reinecke H, Poppa V, Murry CE: Skeletal muscle stem cells do not transdifferentiate into cardiomyocytes after cardiac grafting. J Mol Cell Cardiol 34:241–249, 2002.
67. Roell W, Lu ZJ, Bloch W, et al: Cellular cardiomyoplasty improves survival after myocardial injury. Circulation 105:2435–2441, 2002.
68. Ross RS, Borg TK: Integrins and the myocardium. Circ Res 88:1112–1119, 2001.
69. Ruhparwar A, Tebbenjohanns J, Niehaus M, et al: Transplanted fetal cardiomyocytes as cardiac pacemaker. Eur J Cardiothorac Surg 21:853–857, 2002.
70. Sakai T, Li RK, Weisel RD, et al: Autologous heart cell transplantation improves cardiac function after myocardial injury. Ann Thorac Surg 68:2074–2080, 1999a.
71. Sakai T, Li RK, Weisel RD, et al: Fetal cell transplantation: A comparison of three cell types. J Thorac Cardiovasc Surg 118:715–724, 1999b.
72. Sakakibara Y, Tambara K, Lu F, et al: Combined procedure of surgical repair and cell transplantation for left ventricular aneurysm: an experimental study. Circulation 106:I193–I197, 2002.
73. Scorsin M, Hagege AA, Dolizy I, et al: Can cellular transplantation improve function in doxorubicin-induced heart failure? Circulation 98:II151–II155, 1998.
74. Scorsin M, Hagege AA, Marotte F, et al: Does transplantation of cardiomyocytes improve function of infarcted myocardium? Circulation 96:II93, 1997.
75. Scorsin M, Hagege A, Vilquin JT, et al: Comparison of the effects of fetal cardiomyocyte and skeletal myoblast transplantation on postinfarction left ventricular function. J Thorac Cardiovasc Surg 119:1169–1175, 2000.
76. Shake JG, Gruber PJ, Baumgartner WA, et al: Mesenchymal stem cell implantation in a swine myocardial infarct model: Engraftment and functional effects. Ann Thorac Surg 73:1919–1925, 2002.
77. Sinatra R, Macrina F, Braccio M, et al: Left ventricular aneurysmectomy; comparison between two techniques; early and late results. Eur J Cardiothorac Surg 12:291–297, 1997.
78. Soonpaa MH, Koh GY, Klug MG, et al: Formation of nascent intercalated disks between grafted fetal cardiomyocytes and host myocardium. Science 264:98–101, 1994.
79. Spinale FG: Matrix metalloproteinases: Regulation and dysregulation in the failing heart. Circ Res 90:520–530, 2002.
80. Stamm C, Westphal B, Kleine HD, et al: Autologous bone-marrow stem-cell transplantation for myocardial regeneration. Lancet 361:45–46, 2003.
81. Strauer BE, Brehm M, Zeus T, et al: Repair of infarcted myocardium by autologous intracoronary mononuclear bone marrow cell transplantation in humans. Circulation 106:1913–1918, 2002.
82. Taylor DA, Atkins BZ, Hungspreugs P, et al: Regenerating functional myocardium: Improved performance after skeletal myoblast transplantation. Nat Med 4:929–933, 1998.
83. Tomita S, Li RK, Weisel RD, et al: Autologous transplantation of bone marrow cells improves damaged heart function. Circulation 100:II247–II256, 1999.
84. Tomita S, Mickle DA, Weisel RD, et al: Improved heart function with myogenesis and angiogenesis after autologous porcine bone marrow stromal cell transplantation. J Thorac Cardiovasc Surg 123:1132–1140, 2002.
85. Vacanti JP, Langer R: Tissue engineering: The design and fabrication of living replacement devices for surgical reconstruction and transplantation. Lancet 354: 32–34, 1999.
86. Watanabe E, Smith DM Jr, Delcarpio JB, et al: Cardiomyocyte transplantation in a porcine myocardial infarction model. Cell Transplant 7:239–246, 1998.
87. Weisel RD, Li RK, Mickle DA, et al: Cell transplantation comes of age. J Thorac Cardiovasc Surg 121:835–836, 2001.
88. Yokomuro H, Li RK, Mickle DA, et al: Transplantation of cryopreserved cardiomyocytes. J Thorac Cardiovasc Surg 121:98–107, 2001.
89. Yoo KJ, Li RK, Weisel RD, et al: Heart cell transplantation improves heart function in dilated cardiomyopathic hamsters. Circulation 102:III204–III209, 2000a.
90. Yoo KJ, Li RK, Weisel RD, et al: Autologous smooth muscle cell transplantation improved heart function in dilated cardiomyopathy. Ann Thorac Surg 70:859–865, 2000b.

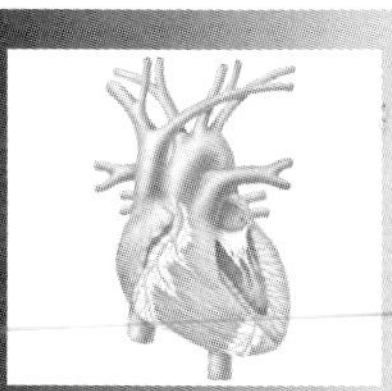

Surgery for Pulmonary Embolism

Patricia A. Thistlethwaite and Stuart W. Jamieson

CHAPTER 98

INTRODUCTION

Pulmonary thromboembolism is a significant cause of morbidity and mortality in the United States and worldwide. The estimated incidence of acute pulmonary embolism is approximately 630,000 per year in the United States based on clinical data[17] and is related to approximately 235,000 deaths per year based on autopsy data. Acute pulmonary embolism occurs half as often as acute myocardial infarction and is three times as common as cerebrovascular accident. It is the third most common cause of death (after heart disease and cancer).[28] Estimates of the incidence of acute pulmonary embolism, however, are generally thought to be low, because in 70–80% of patients in whom the primary cause of death was pulmonary embolism, the diagnosis was unsuspected premortem.[58,63]

Of patients who survive an acute pulmonary embolic event, approximately 2% will go on to develop chronic pulmonary hypertension.[11] Once pulmonary hypertension develops, the prognosis is poor, and this prognosis is worsened in the absence of intracardiac shunt. Patients with pulmonary hypertension caused by pulmonary emboli fall into a higher risk category than those with Eisenmenger's syndrome and encounter a higher mortality rate. In fact, once the mean pulmonary pressure in patients with thromboembolic disease exceeds 50 mm Hg, the 3-year mortality approaches 90%.[91] Therefore despite an improved understanding of pathogenesis, diagnosis, and management, pulmonary emboli and their long-term sequelae remain frequent and often fatal disorders.

Pulmonary embolism was first described by Laennec in 1819.[56] It was he who related the condition to deep venous thrombosis, and Virchow[114] later associated the three factors predisposing to venous thrombosis as stasis, hypercoagulability, and vessel wall injury. Virchow distinguished two types of thrombus in the pulmonary arteries of such patients: first, the embolus that arose as thrombus in a systemic vein and, second, the thrombus that occurs in situ within the pulmonary arteries distal to the occluding embolus as a result of the stagnant blood flow in that segment. To prove that pulmonary emboli arose from the peripheral venous circulation, Virchow inserted pieces of rubber or venous thrombi recovered from humans at autopsy into the jugular or femoral veins of dogs. When the animals were sacrificed, the foreign embolic material was found in the pulmonary arteries. Although pulmonary embolism can be caused by tumors, septic emboli, and foreign bodies, the overwhelming occurrence of pulmonary embolism is due to venous thromboembolism.[52]

ACUTE PULMONARY THROMBOEMBOLIC DISEASE

Clinical Points

The majority of pulmonary thromboembolic episodes are silent, and it is not until the amount of embolic material is substantial that the patient becomes symptomatic. After an acute, major thromboembolic episode, approximately 15–20% of patients die within 48 hours.[115] Most of the remaining patients resolve the emboli substantially by a variety of mechanisms. Therefore it is in the subgroup of patients who have a sudden fatal outcome (approximately 100,000 annually) that invasive therapy for acute pulmonary embolism might be considered.

Although the role of surgical therapy for the pulmonary hypertension resulting from chronic pulmonary emboli is now well established, the appropriate treatment for acute pulmonary embolism remains unclear. There are several reasons for this. Many patients die of massive pulmonary embolism in the terminal phases of another illness, which would make aggressive therapy inappropriate. For patients in whom invasive therapy is potentially indicated, there is substantial difficulty in defining which patients will respond to anticoagulation therapy for an acute massive pulmonary embolism in the limited amount of time available for both diagnosis and treatment before death occurs.

The hemodynamic response to a large, sudden pulmonary embolus relates to a variety of factors, most notably the size of the embolus, the degree of obstruction that it produced in the pulmonary vascular bed, and the underlying function of the lung that remains perfused. The degree of vascular obstruction is obviously related to the number of segmental arteries that are occluded, but also to prior pulmonary vascular capacitance. Thus the hemodynamic consequences of acute pulmonary embolism are also a reflection of factors such as the age of the patient and any possible previous thromboembolic events. The preexisting status of the right ventricle that governs the forward flow also is significant in determining the hemodynamic response to pulmonary embolism. Right ventricular function is affected by factors such as the degree of right ventricular hypertrophy or dilatation, tricuspid valve regurgitation, and the presence of coronary artery disease.

In addition to the mechanical factor of pulmonary artery obstruction, there are reflex and hormonal factors that can increase pulmonary vascular resistance (PVR) at the time of acute pulmonary embolism. Humoral factors, specifically serotonin, adenosine diphosphate (ADP), platelet-derived growth factor (PDGF), and thromboxane, are released from platelets attached to the thrombi,[36] whereas platelet-activating factor (PAF) and leukotrienes are secreted by neutrophils.[65] Anoxia and tissue ischemia downstream from emboli inhibit endothelium-derived relaxing factor (EDRF) production and enhance release of superoxide anions by activated neutrophils.[116] The combination of these humoral effects contributes to enhanced pulmonary vasoconstriction. Thus some patients with a relatively small embolus may have an exaggerated response to the degree of pulmonary vascular obstruction.

It has been demonstrated that in those patients without preexisting cardiac or pulmonary disease, an obstruction of less than 20% of the pulmonary vascular bed results in minimal hemodynamic consequences. It is only when the acute pulmonary obstruction exceeds 50–60% of the pulmonary vascular bed that cardiac and pulmonary compensatory mechanisms are overcome and cardiac output begins to fall.[76] Right ventricular failure occurs, which is accompanied by systemic hypotension as the amount of blood reaching the left ventricle decreases. The dilated right ventricle causes a shift of the ventricular septum to the left, further compromising left ventricular filling. Although patients with chronic pulmonary artery obstruction can have high pulmonary artery pressure levels that reflect the degree of obstruction, in acute pulmonary embolism the previously normal right ventricle cannot generate these pressures. Therefore in acute massive pulmonary embolism, pulmonary artery pressures may be normal, and a pulmonary artery mean pressure of 30–40 mm Hg may represent severe pulmonary hypertension.

Acute pulmonary embolism usually presents suddenly. Symptoms and signs vary with the extent of blockage, the magnitude of humoral response, and the preembolus reserve of the cardiac and pulmonary systems of the patient.[81] The clinical diagnosis is often missed or falsely made. Most pulmonary emboli occur without sufficient clinical findings to suggest the diagnosis, and in an autopsy series of proven emboli, only 16–38% of patients were diagnosed while still alive.[24] The acute disease is conveniently stratified into *minor, major* (submassive), or *massive* embolism on the basis of hemodynamic stability, arterial blood gases, and lung scan or angiographic assessment of the percentage of blocked pulmonary arteries.[34,41]

For patients with *minor pulmonary embolism,* physical examination may reveal tachycardia, rales, low-grade fever, and sometimes a pleural rub. Heart sounds and systemic blood pressure are often normal; sometimes the pulmonary second sound is increased. Less than one third of patients with acute pulmonary embolism have concurrent evidence of clinical deep venous thrombosis.[24] Room air arterial blood gases indicate a PaO_2 between 65–80 torr and a normal $PaCO_2$ around 35 torr.[34] Pulmonary angiograms typically show less than 30% occlusion of the pulmonary arterial vasculature.

Major pulmonary embolism is associated with dyspnea, tachypnea, dull chest pain, and some degree of cardiovascular changes manifested by tachycardia, mild to moderate hypotension, and elevation of central venous pressure.[34] Some patients may have syncope rather than dyspnea or chest pain. In contrast to massive pulmonary embolism, patients with major embolism (at least two lobar pulmonary arteries obstructed) are hemodynamically stable and have adequate cardiac output.[41] Room air blood gases reveal moderate hypoxia, with a PaO_2 between 50 and 60 torr, and mild hypocarbia, with a $PaCO_2$ ≤30 torr.[34] Echocardiograms may show right ventricular dilatation. Pulmonary angiograms indicate that 30–50% of the pulmonary vasculature is blocked; however, in patients with preexisting cardiopulmonary disorders, lesser degree of vascular obstruction may produce similar symptoms.

Massive pulmonary embolism is truly life-threatening and is defined as a pulmonary embolism that causes hemodynamic instability.[41] It is usually associated with occlusion of more than 50% of the pulmonary vasculature, but may occur with much smaller occlusions, particularly in patients with preexisting cardiac or pulmonary disease. The diagnosis is clinical, not anatomical. Patients develop acute dyspnea, tachypnea, tachycardia, and diaphoresis and may lose consciousness. Both hypotension and low cardiac output (<1.8 liters/min/m^2) are present. Cardiac arrest may occur. Neck veins are distended, central venous pressure is elevated, and a right ventricular impulse may be present. Room air blood gases show severe hypoxia (PaO_2 <50 torr), hypocarbia ($PaCO_2$ <30 torr), and acidosis.[34] Urine output falls, and peripheral pulses and perfusion are poor.

The clinical diagnosis of acute major or massive pulmonary embolism is unreliable and is incorrect in 70–80% of patients who have subsequent angiography.[29] The differentiation between major or massive pulmonary embolism and acute myocardial infarction, aortic dissection, septic shock, and other catastrophic states can be difficult and costly in time. Although plain chest X-ray, electrocardiogram, and insertion of a bedside Swan-Ganz catheter may add confirmatory information, they will not necessarily prove the diagnosis. Routine laboratory tests are usually normal.

The most common electrocardiographic abnormalities of acute pulmonary embolism are tachycardia and nonspecific

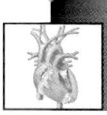

ST- and T-wave changes. The major value of the electrocardiogram is excluding a myocardial infarction. A minority of patients with massive embolism may show evidence of cor pulmonale, right axis deviation, or right bundle branch block.[24] Chest X-ray may show oligemia (Westermark's sign) or linear atelectasis (Fleischner lines), both of which are nonspecific findings. Ventilation–perfusion (V/Q) scans may provide confirmatory evidence, but these studies may be unreliable because pneumonia, atelectasis, previous pulmonary emboli, and other conditions may cause a mismatch in ventilation and perfusion that mimics positive results.[37]

In general, negative V/Q scans exclude the diagnosis of clinically significant pulmonary embolism. V/Q scans are usually interpreted as high, intermediate, or low probability of pulmonary embolism to emphasize the lack of specificity but high sensitivity of the test. Pulmonary angiograms provide the most definitive diagnosis for acute pulmonary embolism.[10] Using this technique, the diagnosis is established when there are filling defects or obstruction of pulmonary arterial branches, leading to irregular or absent contours or "streaming" of contrast material. Magnetic resonance imaging (MRI) is a better noninvasive method for the diagnosis of pulmonary emboli and provides specific information regarding flow within the pulmonary vasculature.[93] Unfortunately, this method is expensive, time consuming, and not widely available. Like angiography, it is generally not suitable for hemodynamically unstable patients. Transthoracic echocardiography (TTE) or transesophageal echocardiography (TEE) with color flow Doppler mapping can provide reliable information about the presence or absence of major thrombi obstructing the main pulmonary artery; however, these techniques are usually inadequate for visualization of the lobar vessels, where the embolic material is often localized. More than 80% of patients with clinically significant pulmonary embolism have abnormalities of right ventricular volume or contractility, often associated with acute tricuspid regurgitation.[15] In a subset of patients, abnormal flow patterns can be discerned in major pulmonary arteries during TEE.[87]

Prophylaxis

Although prophylactic measures should be considered and used for all patients undergoing major surgery or who have prolonged immobility, certain other patients also fall into a potentially high-risk group for pulmonary embolism. These include patients with previous embolism, malignancy, cardiac failure, obesity, or advanced age.[39] The prevalence of deep venous thrombosis of the thigh or pelvis, its strong association with pulmonary embolism, and the identification of the associated risk factors listed earlier provide the basis and rationale for prophylactic anticoagulation for the prevention of acute pulmonary embolism. Simple measures such as compression stockings probably should be prescribed more often and be used in most nonambulating patients in the hospital. Intermittent pneumatic compression devices are more cumbersome, but are also effective. These compression devices are available for the calf or the whole leg. They can provide a range of compression pressures, inflation and deflation duration, and sequential or nonsequential inflation, although a clear difference between these variations has not been demonstrated. Both compression stockings and pneumatic compression devices reduce the incidence of deep venous thrombosis after general surgery to approximately 40% of control patients.[3] Multiple studies have now shown that low-dose subcutaneous heparin or low-molecular-weight heparin given once a day reduces the incidence of deep venous thrombosis to approximately 35% and 18% of controls, respectively,[13,40] with a concomitant reduction in the incidence of pulmonary embolism. This reduction in thrombosis has not been associated with an excessive risk of bleeding.[13] Recent studies suggest that of patients who have deep venous thrombosis diagnosed in the hospital without pulmonary embolism, the probability of clinically diagnosed pulmonary embolism within the next 12 months is 1.7%.[85] If pulmonary embolism occurs, the probability of recurrent pulmonary embolism is 6.0%.[85] Six months of warfarin anticoagulation are recommended for patients who have deep venous thrombosis with or without pulmonary embolism as prophylaxis against recurrent disease.[96]

Supportive and Thrombolytic Therapy

The majority of patients who die of pulmonary embolism do so within 2 hours of the initial acute event, before the diagnosis can be firmly established, and before effective therapy can be instituted. Once the diagnosis is made, however, treatment will be either medical (supportive and thrombolytic therapy) or surgical (Figure 98-1).

Oxygen should be administered to alleviate hypoxic pulmonary vasoconstriction, and it is likely that a severely affected patient will require intubation and ventilatory support. Pharmacological agents, including cardiovascular pressors and vasoactive agents, may be instituted to stabilize the patient's hemodynamics. Once the circulation has been stabilized, both arterial and central venous catheters are placed to monitor cardiac output and pulmonary arterial oxygen saturation. There is debate as to whether pulmonary artery catheters, although obviously helpful in management, should be used in the setting of acute pulmonary embolism, because of the risk of dislodging further thromboembolic material. The electrocardiogram is monitored, a Foley catheter is inserted for accurate recording of urine output, and blood gas levels are obtained. Patients should be heparinized to prevent further propagation of thrombus at its origin and also in the pulmonary arterial tree. If there is no contraindication to anticoagulation, intravenous (IV) heparin is started with an initial bolus dose of 70 U/kg followed by 18–20 U/kg/h. Although heparin prevents propagation and formation of new thromboemboli, it rarely dissolves the existing clot. In most cases, the patient's intrinsic fibrinolytic system will lyse fresh thrombi over a period of days to weeks.[18] Heparin is monitored by measurement of activated partial thromboplastin times, which are maintained between 51–70 seconds (roughly twice that of controls) every 6–8 hours. The platelet count should be measured every 2–3 days to detect the presence of heparin-induced thrombocytopenia. Prothrombin times are also obtained at baseline to prepare for anticoagulation with warfarin later. For the early treatment of stable patients with acute pulmonary embolism, subcutaneous low-molecular-weight heparin (tinzaparin) given once daily has been shown to be as effective and safe as IV heparin with respect to recurrent thromboembolism, major bleeding, and death.[99]

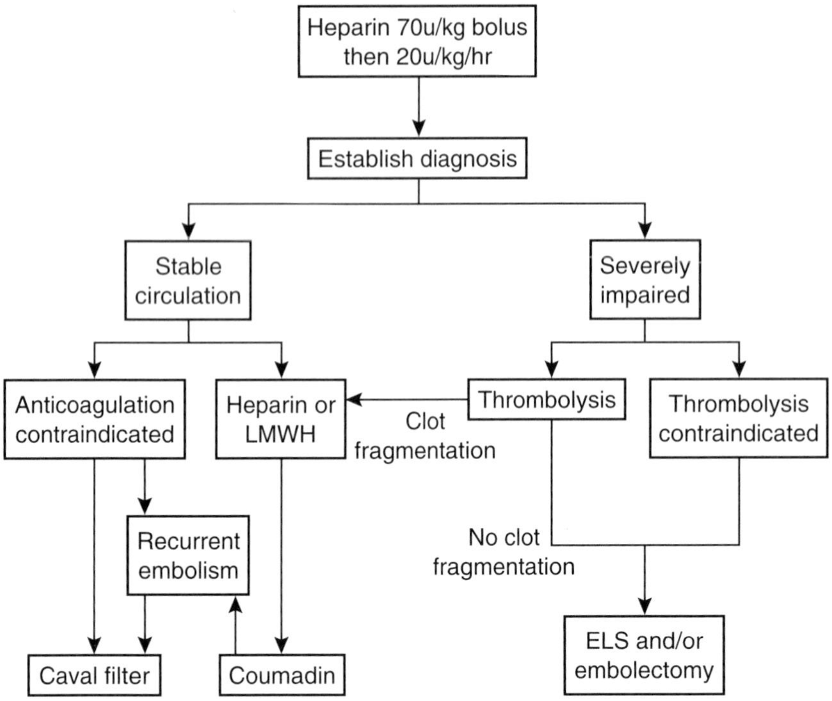

Figure 98–1 Acute pulmonary embolism treatment scheme. LMWH, low molecular weight heparin; ELS, extracorporeal life support.

The natural history of the clot in survivors of acute embolic events is fragmentation and progressive lysis. It therefore follows that the addition of streptokinase, urokinase, or recombinant tissue plasminogen activator improves survival by increasing the rate of lysis of fresh thrombi in the pulmonary arterial tree. Thromboembolytic agents dissolve thrombi by activating plasminogen to plasmin. Plasmin, when in proximity to a thrombus, degrades fibrin to soluble peptides. Circulating plasmin also degrades soluble fibrinogen and, to variable degrees, factors II, V, and VIII. In addition, increased concentrations of fibrin and fibrinogen degradation products contribute to coagulopathy by both inhibiting the conversion of fibrinogen to fibrin and interfering with fibrin polymerization. The thromboembolytic agents currently reported for the treatment of acute pulmonary embolism include streptokinase, urokinase, recombinant tissue plasminogen activator (rt-PA, alteplase), anisoylated plasminogen streptokinase activator complex (APSAC, anistreplase), and reteplase (Table 98-1).[89] Some new agents (so-called second generation thrombolytics) are variants of t-PA (tenecteplase, lanoteplase), staphylokinase, and saruplase, and are undergoing clinical testing.[90]

Although thrombolytic therapy has been shown to increase the rate of lysis of fresh pulmonary clots more than that of heparin alone,[25] there has been little difference measured in the amount of residual thrombus between the two treatments in early studies employing small cohorts of patients.[27,64,66] However, two recent trials comparing

Table 98–1

Thrombolytic Regimens for Massive Pulmonary Embolism

Drug	*Dose*	*Origin*
Alteplase (rt-PA)	10 mg as a bolus, followed by 90 mg in continuous infusion over 2 h	Recombinant DNA
Anistreplase (APSAC)	30 mg in 5 min	Recombinant DNA
Reteplase	Two bolus injections of 10 U, 30 min apart	Recombinant DNA
Streptokinase	250,000–500,000 U as a loading dose over 15 min, followed by 100,000/h for 24 h	Bacteria
Urokinase	4400 U/kg as a loading dose over 10 min, followed by 4400 U/kg/h for 12 h	Human urine

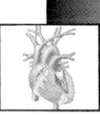

thrombolytic agents with IV heparin in acute pulmonary embolism have been large enough to detect a significant difference in the most important endpoint—mortality.[53,54] More recent experience suggests a trend toward better results with thrombolytic therapy because of a more rapid diminution in right ventricular afterload and dysfunction.[25] Compared with heparin therapy alone, thrombolytic agents carry a higher risk of bleeding problems, with up to 20% of patients experiencing a significant bleeding complication.[26,60] In general, thrombolytic therapy is contraindicated in patients with fresh surgical wounds, anemia, recent stroke, peptic ulcer, or bleeding dyscrasias.

In select incidences, mechanical removal of pulmonary thrombi has been reported with the use of a catheter device inserted under local anesthesia into the femoral or jugular vein.[30,79,95,109] Two types of catheters have been introduced into the pulmonary artery under fluoroscopy to remove embolic material. One such device consists of a small terminal cup attached to a flexible catheter.[30] Syringe suction is applied to the cup as a thrombus is engaged. The catheter and clot are removed en masse through the venotomy site, and this process may be repeated multiple times. A second reported device uses a rotational pigtail catheter system to mechanically fragment fresh pulmonary emboli under fluoroscopic visualization.[95] Successful catheter extraction of thrombus with clinically significant reduction in pulmonary arterial pressure varies between 61 and 84%, with the best results achieved for proximal, main pulmonary artery embolism.

Acute Pulmonary Embolectomy

Emergency pulmonary thromboembolectomy is indicated for suitable patients with life-threatening circulatory insufficiency, where the diagnosis of acute pulmonary embolism has been established. If a patient has been taken directly to the operating room without a definitive diagnosis, transesophageal or epicardial echocardiography and color Doppler mapping can confirm or refute the diagnosis in the operating room.[48,121] The primary difficulty with the broad application of operative embolectomy is that it is almost impossible to determine which patients will die without intervention. An emergency pulmonary embolectomy is most feasible (because of time) and most successful in patients who ultimately may not require it, which makes it difficult to establish the efficacy of this operation. Indications for acute surgical intervention include the following: (1) critical hemodynamic condition, with the patient deemed unlikely to survive, (2) definitive diagnosis of pulmonary embolism in the main or lobar pulmonary arteries with compromise of oxygen gas exchange, (3) unstable patients in whom thrombolytic or anticoagulation therapy is absolutely contraindicated, and (4) the presence of a large clot trapped within the right atrium or ventricle.

Acute pulmonary embolectomy was first described by Trendelenburg in 1908[111] using pulmonary artery and aortic occlusion, through a transthoracic approach. There were no surviving patients. Sharp[97] performed the first successful open embolectomy, using cardiopulmonary bypass.

For pulmonary embolectomy, a median sternotomy incision is used and cardiopulmonary bypass instituted. Tapes are placed around the superior and inferior venae cavae. The heart may be left beating, electrically fibrillated, or arrested with cold cardioplegic solution. Significant hypothermia is rarely needed because of the short duration of the operation. Two polypropylene sutures are placed in the mid–pulmonary artery for traction. A longitudinal incision is made between these sutures in the main pulmonary artery trunk 1–2 cm distal to the valve. If necessary, the incision may be extended directly into the left pulmonary artery. The emboli are extracted using forceps, suction, and balloon catheters. The right pulmonary artery also can be exposed and opened between the aorta and superior vena cava to allow better exposure in the distal segments, if necessary. A sterile pediatric bronchoscope may be used to visualize emboli in tertiary or quaternary pulmonary vessels, so that they may be cleared with balloon embolectomy or suction. After cleaning the pulmonary arterial tree lumina, the pleural spaces can be entered, and the lungs manually compressed to dislodge small distally lodged clots, which may then be suctioned out. The pulmonary arteriotomy is then closed with a 6-0 polypropylene suture. After restarting the heart, the patient is weaned from bypass, decannulated, and closed. The aim of this operation is to remove most of the embolic material, and no attempt is made to perform an endarterectomy.

As a corollary to this operation, some groups recommend either placement of an inferior vena caval filter or caval clipping before chest closure. Greenfield has recommended placement of an inferior vena caval filter under direct visualization before closing the chest.[32,101] Historically, some European surgeons clipped or plicated the intrapericardial vena cava at the end of the embolectomy to prevent migration of lower body clot into the pulmonary circulation; however, this procedure is associated with stasis in the venous system in the lower body and leg swelling.[104] In most centers that offer emergency pulmonary thromboembolectomy, no caval procedure is performed in the perioperative period and recurrent deep venous thrombosis or pulmonary embolism is treated by anticoagulation with warfarin for 6 months.[103] Percutaneously placed Greenfield filters are recommended only for patients with contraindications to anticoagulation or for patients with recurrent pulmonary embolism on therapeutic anticoagulation. The cone-shaped Greenfield filter is most widely used in the United States and is associated with a lifetime recurrent embolism rate of 5%, with a lifetime patency rate of 97%.[33,119]

Extracorporeal Life Support

The wider availability of long-term mechanical perfusion (termed extracorporeal life support [ELS]) using peripheral vessel cannulation to stabilize the circulation offers another approach to life-threatening pulmonary embolism. Most pulmonary emboli, even those that are massive, will dissolve with time. ELS can be instituted outside the operating room setting and can be implemented with rapidity in institutions where preparation for its emergency use has been made. With a trained team, needed equipment, and associated supplies readily available, ELS can be implemented within 15–30 minutes.[4] For hemodynamic support during the period of a life-threatening pulmonary embolism, venoarterial extracorporeal support can be instituted and maintained for a period up to several weeks, if necessary.[20,49]

This procedure begins with an IV heparin bolus of 1 mg/kg, followed by percutaneous or surgical cut-down of the femoral artery and femoral or internal jugular veins. If pulses are absent or weak, a larger incision is usually faster; however, because patients need heparin and have possibly received fibrinolytic drugs, a minimal wound is preferred. The tip of the venous catheter is advanced into the right atrium to obtain a flow rate of 2.5–4.0 liters/min using an emergency pump-oxygenator circuit primed with crystalloid.[117] The perfusion circuit consists of IV or arterial access tubes, a centrifugal pump, and a membrane oxygenator.[78] An electromagnetic flowmeter is placed on the arterial line, and an arterial filter is not applied. While the patient is on ELS, heparin is infused to maintain the activated clotting time between 150 and 180 seconds. In the initial hours after institution of ELS, activated clotting times are measured every 30 minutes, followed by every hour thereafter until decannulation. During the period of ELS support, thrombolytic drugs may be instilled directly into the pulmonary artery via a Swan-Ganz catheter to aid in clot lysis. ELS support may provide critical support to bridge an unstable patient to surgical embolectomy.[43]

Once oxygenation has been stabilized and PVR has normalized, the patient is decannulated and the cannulation sites surgically closed. ELS is usually discontinued in the operating room because vessels should be sutured closed because of the need for heparin and long-term anticoagulation.

Results of Acute Pulmonary Embolectomy

Mortality rates for emergency pulmonary thromboembolectomy vary widely, between 11 and 92% (Table 98-2).* It is difficult to compare these retrospective studies because of the difference in time in which the operations were performed, the preoperative hemodynamic state of the patient populations, and the variation in treatment plans. In general, greater surgical mortality was encountered if a patient had a preoperative cardiac arrest or required ELS support. For example, the mortality in patients who had suffered a cardiac arrest (45–75% perioperative mortality) is considerably worse than in those who have not, where mortality is

*References 1, 21, 22, 31, 35, 51, 68, 73, 94, 102, 105, 112, 113.

Table 98–2

Pulmonary Embolectomy Series: Comparative Mortality

Reference	*Time frame*	*No. of patients*	*Mortality (%)*	*Preoperative cardiac arrest (%)*
Mattox et al	1961–1981	39	56.4	56.4
Gray et al	1964–1986	71	30.0	35.2
Meyer et al	1968–1988	96	37.5	25.0
Stulz et al	1968–1994	50	46.0	38.7
Kieny et al	1970–1989	134	15.7	17.2
Tschirkov et al	1972–1976	24	29.2	16.7
Schmid et al	1975–1991	27	44.4	36.4
Doerge et al	1979–1998	41	29.3	34.1
Ullmann et al	1989–1997	40	35.0	47.5
Tayama et al	1990–2001	35	28.6	20.0
Aklog et al	1999–2001	29	10.3	3.4

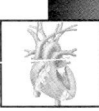

reported between 8 and 36%.[22,94] Consequently, although some groups report low mortality rates, this may be attributable to the selection of less ill patients as candidates for surgery. In patients in whom ELS is instituted during preoperative cardiac resuscitation, subsequent operative mortality ranges between 44 and 57%.[31,68] Thus the outcome depends largely on the preoperative condition of the patient. Primary causes of death include brain damage, cardiac failure, uncontrollable bleeding, and sepsis. Recurrent embolism after surgery is uncommon,[94,100] and approximately 80% of those who survive surgery maintain normal pulmonary artery pressures and exercise tolerance. In these patients, postoperative angiograms are normal or show obstruction in less than 10% of vessels. A minority of patients who have obstruction in more than 40% of pulmonary vessels after surgery also have significantly reduced pulmonary function and exercise tolerance.[100]

CHRONIC PULMONARY THROMBOEMBOLIC DISEASE

Incidence and Natural History

The natural history of pulmonary embolism is generally total embolic resolution, or resolution leaving minimal residua, with restoration of a normal hemodynamic status.[16] However, for unknown reasons, embolic resolution is incomplete in a small subset of patients. If the acute emboli are not lysed in 1–2 weeks, the embolic material becomes attached to the pulmonary arterial wall at the main pulmonary artery, lobar, segmental, or subsegmental levels.[86] With time, the initial embolic material progressively becomes converted into connective and elastic tissue. Often visualization of the pulmonary arteries by angioscopy a few weeks after unresolved pulmonary embolism reveals vessel narrowing at the site of embolic incorporation. In some patients, recanalization of some of the pulmonary arterial branches occurs, with the formation of fibrous tissue in the form of bands and webs.[19] By a mechanism that is poorly understood, this chronic obstructive disease may lead to a small vessel arteriolar vasculopathy characterized by excessive smooth muscle cell proliferation around small arterioles in the pulmonary circulation.[23] This small vessel vasculopathy is seen in the remaining open vessels, which are subjected to long exposure at high flow. Pulmonary hypertension results when the capacitance of the remaining open bed cannot absorb the cardiac output—because of either the degree of primary obstruction by embolus or the combination of a fixed obstructive lesion and secondary small vessel vasculopathy.

The incidence of pulmonary hypertension caused by chronic pulmonary embolism is even more difficult to determine than that of acute pulmonary embolism. There are more than 500,000 survivors of symptomatic episodes of acute pulmonary embolism per year.[9,75] The incidence of chronic thrombotic occlusion or stenosis in the population depends on which percentage of patients fails to resolve acute embolic material. One estimate is that chronic thromboembolic disease develops in only 0.5% of patients with a clinically recognized acute pulmonary embolism.[9] If these figures are correct and only patients with symptomatic acute pulmonary emboli are counted, approximately 2500 individuals would progress to chronic thromboembolic pulmonary hypertension in the United States each year. However, because many (if not most) patients diagnosed with chronic thromboembolic disease have no antecedent history of acute embolism, the true incidence of this disorder is probably much higher.

Regardless of the exact incidence, it is clear that acute embolism and its chronic relation, fixed chronic thromboembolic occlusive disease, are both much more common than is generally appreciated and are seriously underdiagnosed. In 1963 Houk and colleagues[42] reviewed the literature of 240 cases of chronic thromboembolic obstruction of major pulmonary arteries, but found that only six cases had been diagnosed correctly before death. Calculations extrapolated from mortality rates and the random incidence of major thrombotic occlusion found at autopsy supported the postulate that more than 100,000 people in the United States currently have pulmonary hypertension that could be relieved by operation. A recent autopsy analysis of 13,216 patients showed pulmonary thromboembolism in 5.5% of autopsies, and up to 31.3% in the elderly.[82]

It is unclear why acute emboli fail to resolve in a subset of patients who subsequently develop pulmonary hypertension. An identifiable hypercoagulable state is found in only a minority of patients. A lupus anticoagulant is present in 10–20% of patients with chronic thromboembolic pulmonary hypertension.[8,120] Inherited deficiencies of protein C, protein S, and antithrombin III, as a group, can be identified in up to 5% of this population.[14] Studies to identify abnormalities in the fibrinolytic pathway or within the pulmonary endothelium that would account for the incomplete thrombus dissolution have been unrevealing.[59,80,88]

Without surgical intervention, the survival of patients with chronic thromboembolic pulmonary hypertension is poor and is inversely related to the degree of pulmonary hypertension at the time of diagnosis. Riedel et al[91] found a 5-year survival rate of 30% among patients with a mean pulmonary artery pressure greater than 40 mm Hg at the time of diagnosis and 10% in those whose pressure exceeded 50 mm Hg. In another study a mean pulmonary artery pressure as low as 30 mm Hg was identified as a threshold for poor prognosis.[62]

Clinical Manifestations

Patients with chronic thromboembolic pulmonary hypertension usually have subtle or nonspecific presenting symptoms. The most common symptoms are progressive exertional dyspnea and exercise intolerance. These symptoms are a result of elevated dead space ventilation and a limitation in cardiac output from obstruction of the pulmonary vascular bed. As the disease progresses, additional symptoms such as edema, chest pain, lightheadedness, and syncope may develop. Early in the course of thromboembolic disease, physical findings may be limited to an accentuated P2, which may be easily overlooked during the physical examination. Nonspecific chest pains occur in approximately 50% of patients with more severe pulmonary hypertension. Hemoptysis can occur in all forms of pulmonary hypertension and probably results from abnormally dilated vessels distended by increased intravascular pressures. Peripheral edema, early satiety, and epigastric or right upper quadrant fullness or pain may develop as the right side of the heart fails and cor pulmonale develops.

Physical signs of pulmonary hypertension include a jugular venous pulse that is characterized by a large A wave. As the right side of the heart fails, the V wave becomes predominant. The right ventricle is usually palpable near the lower left sternal border, and pulmonary valve closure may be audible in the second intercostal space. Patients with advanced disease may be hypoxic and cyanotic. Clubbing is an uncommon finding. As the right side of the heart fails, a right atrial gallop may be auscultated and tricuspid insufficiency develops. Because of the large pressure gradient across the tricuspid valve in pulmonary hypertension, the murmur is high-pitched and may not exhibit respiratory variation. These findings differ from those usually observed in tricuspid valvular disease. A murmur of pulmonic regurgitation also may be detected, and a specific ausculatory finding is a flow murmur at the back—thought to result from stenosed pulmonary vessels.[7]

Diagnostic Evaluation of Chronic Thromboembolic Pulmonary Hypertension

Pulmonary vascular disease always must be considered in the differential diagnosis of unexplained dyspnea. The diagnostic evaluation serves three purposes: to establish the presence and severity of pulmonary hypertension; to determine its etiology; and, if thromboembolic disease is present, to determine whether it is surgically correctible.

Chest radiography is often unrevealing in the early stages of chronic thromboembolic pulmonary hypertension. As the disease progresses, several radiographic abnormalities may be found. These include peripheral lung opacities suggestive of scarring from previous infarction, cardiomegaly with dilation and hypertrophy of the right-sided chambers, and dilation of the central pulmonary arteries. Pulmonary function tests are often obtained in the evaluation of dyspnea and serve to exclude the presence of obstructive airways or parenchymal lung disease. There are no characteristic spirometric changes diagnostic of chronic thromboembolic pulmonary hypertension. Single-breath diffusing capacity for carbon monoxide (DLCO) may be moderately reduced, and it has been reported that 20% of patients have a mild to moderate restrictive defect caused by parenchymal scarring.[74] Arterial blood oxygen levels may be normal even in the setting of significant pulmonary hypertension. Most patients, however, experience a decline in Po_2 with exertion.[5]

Transthoracic echocardiography is the first study to provide objective evidence of the presence of pulmonary hypertension. An estimate of pulmonary artery pressure can be provided by Doppler evaluation of the tricuspid regurgitant envelope. Additional echocardiographic findings vary depending on the stage of the disease and include right ventricular enlargement, leftward displacement of the interventricular septum, and encroachment of the enlarged right ventricle on the left ventricular cavity with abnormal systolic and diastolic function of the left ventricle.[72] Contrast echocardiography may demonstrate a persistent foramen ovale, the result of high right atrial pressures opening the previously closed intraatrial communication.

Once the diagnosis of pulmonary hypertension has been established, distinguishing between major-vessel obstruction and small-vessel pulmonary vascular disease is the next critical step. Radioisotope V/Q lung scanning is the essential test for establishing the diagnosis of unresolved pulmonary thromboembolism. The V/Q scan typically demonstrates one or more mismatched segmental defects caused by obstructive thromboembolism. This is in contrast to the normal or "mottled" perfusion scan seen in patients with primary pulmonary hypertension or other small-vessel forms of pulmonary hypertension.[77]

It is important to note that during the process of reorganization, thromboemboli may recanalize or narrow the vessel lumen. Organized thrombi do not have the appearance of the intravascular filling defects seen with acute pulmonary emboli and appear as unusual filling defects, including fusiform or irregular narrowing, webs, bands, or completely thrombosed vessels that may resemble congenital absence of the vessel.[44] Organized material along a vascular wall of a recanalized vessel produces a scalloped or serrated luminal edge. A consequence of this partial recanalization is that the magnitude of the perfusion defects with chronic thromboembolic pulmonary hypertension frequently underestimates the actual degree of pulmonary vascular obstruction as determined by angiography or surgery.[92]

Cardiac catheterization provides essential information in the evaluation of patients with suspected thromboembolic pulmonary hypertension. Right ventricular catheterization allows for the quantification of the severity of pulmonary hypertension and assessment of cardiac function. Measurement of oxygen saturations in the vena cava, right ventricular chambers, and the pulmonary artery may document previously undetected left-to-right shunting. Coronary angiography and left-sided heart catheterization provide additional information about patients at risk for coronary artery or valvular disease and establish baseline measurements for cardiac output and left ventricular function. This information is crucial in the preoperative risk assessment of patients deemed candidates for pulmonary endarterectomy.

Pulmonary angiography is the gold standard for defining pulmonary vascular anatomy and is performed to identify whether chronic thromboembolic obstruction is present, to determine its location and surgical accessibility, and to rule out other diagnostic possibilities. Despite concerns regarding the safety of performing pulmonary angiography in patients with pulmonary hypertension, with careful monitoring, pulmonary angiography can be performed safely even in patients with severe pulmonary hypertension.[84] Biplane imaging is preferred, offering the advantage of lateral views that provide greater anatomical detail compared with the overlapped and obscured vessel images often seen with the anterior–posterior view. Maturation, organization, and recanalization of clot produces angiographic patterns of the following: (1) pouch defects, (2) webs or bands, (3) intimal irregularities, (4) abrupt narrowing of major vessels, and (5) obstruction of main, lobar, or segmental pulmonary vessels.[6]

In approximately 20% of cases the differential diagnosis between primary pulmonary hypertension and distal small-vessel pulmonary thromboembolic disease is hard to

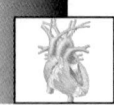

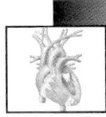

establish. In these patients, pulmonary angioscopy often may be helpful. The pulmonary angioscope is a diagnostic fiberoptic device that was developed to visualize the intima of central pulmonary arteries. It is inserted through a vascular sheath inserted in a central vein and passed through the right side of the heart into the pulmonary artery under fluoroscopic guidance. Inflation of a latex balloon affixed to the tip of the angioscope results in obstruction of blood flow in the artery and permits visualization of the arterial intima. The classic appearance of chronic pulmonary thromboembolic disease by angioscopy consists of intimal irregularity and scarring, with webbing of the vessel lumina.[83] The presence of embolic disease, occlusion of vessels, or the presence of gross thrombotic material also is diagnostic.

More recently, helical computed tomography (CT) scanning has been used to screen patients with suspected thromboembolic disease.[67,110] CT features of chronic thromboembolic pulmonary hypertension include evidence of organized thrombus lining the pulmonary vessels in an eccentric fashion, enlargement of the right ventricle and central pulmonary arteries, variation in size of segmental arteries (relatively smaller in the affected segments compared with uninvolved areas), and parenchymal changes compatible with pulmonary infarction.

Surgical Selection

Although previous attempts have been made, Allison et al[2] performed the first successful pulmonary thromboendarterectomy through a sternotomy using surface hypothermia in a patient with a 12-day history of pulmonary embolism, but only fresh clots were removed and an endarterectomy was not performed. Since then, there have been many occasional surgical reports of the surgical treatment of chronic pulmonary thromboembolism,[12,98] but by far the greatest surgical experience in pulmonary endarterectomy has been at the University of California, San Diego,[47] where over 1600 cases have been performed.

The three major reasons for considering a patient for pulmonary endarterectomy are hemodynamic, respiratory, and prophylactic. The hemodynamic goal is to prevent or ameliorate right ventricular compromise caused by pulmonary hypertension. The respiratory objective is to improve function by the removal of a large ventilated but unperfused physiological dead space. The prophylactic goals are to prevent progressive right ventricular dysfunction, retrograde extension of the clot, and the prevention of secondary vasculopathic changes in the remaining patent vessels. Pulmonary endarterectomy is considered in patients who are symptomatic and have evidence of hemodynamic or ventilatory impairment at rest or with exercise. Patients undergoing surgery usually exhibit a preoperative PVR greater than 300 dynes/sec/cm^{-5}, typically in the range of 800–1200 dynes/sec/cm^{-5}.[50] Although most patients have a pulmonary artery pressure that is less than systemic, the hypertrophy of the right ventricle that occurs over time makes pulmonary hypertension possible at suprasystemic levels. Therefore many patients have a level of PVR in excess of 1000 dynes/sec/cm^{-5} and suprasystemic pulmonary artery pressures. There is no upper limit of PVR level, pulmonary artery pressure, or degree of right ventricular dysfunction that excludes patients from operation. For those with milder pulmonary hypertension, the decision to operate is based on individual circumstances. Some patients elect to undergo surgery at this early stage of disease because of dissatisfaction with their exercise limitation or concerns about clinical deterioration in the future.

Those who choose not to pursue surgical intervention at early stages of the disease require close monitoring for progression of pulmonary hypertension. Because of the changes that can occur in the remaining patent (unaffected by clot or obstruction) pulmonary vascular bed subjected to the higher pressures and flow, pulmonary endarterectomy is usually offered to both symptomatic and asymptomatic patients whenever their angiograms demonstrate significant thromboembolic disease.[44]

Guiding Principles of the Operation

There are several guiding principles of the operation. It must be bilateral because, for pulmonary hypertension to be a major factor, both pulmonary arteries usually are substantially involved. The only reasonable approach to both pulmonary arteries is through a median sternotomy. Historically there were reports of unilateral operation, and occasionally this is still performed through a thoracotomy.[57] However, the unilateral approach ignores disease on the contralateral side, subjects the patient to hemodynamic jeopardy during the clamping of the pulmonary artery, and does not allow good visibility because of the continued presence of bronchial blood flow. In addition, collateral channels develop in chronic thromboembolic pulmonary hypertension not only through the bronchial arteries, but also from diaphragmatic, intercostal, and pleural vessels. The dissection of the lung in the pleural space via a median sternotomy, apart from bilateral access, avoids entry into the pleural cavities and allows for the ready institution of cardiopulmonary bypass.

Cardiopulmonary bypass is essential to ensure cardiovascular stability when the operation is performed and to cool the patient to allow circulatory arrest. Very good visibility is required, in a bloodless field, to define an adequate endarterectomy plane and then follow the pulmonary endarterectomy specimen deep into the subsegmental vessels. Because of the copious bronchial blood flow usually present in these cases, periods of circulatory arrest are necessary to ensure perfect visibility.[45] There have been sporadic reports of the performance of this operation without circulatory arrest.[38] However, it should be emphasized that although endarterectomy is possible without circulatory arrest, a complete endarterectomy is not. The circulatory arrest portions of the case are limited to the most distal portion of the endarterectomy process, deep in the subsegmental vasculature, and are usually limited to 20 minutes for each side with restoration of flow in between.

A true endarterectomy in the plane of the media must be accomplished. It is essential to appreciate that the removal of visible thrombus is largely incidental to this operation. Indeed, in most patients, no free thrombus is present; and on initial direct examination, the pulmonary vascular bed may appear normal. The early literature on this procedure indicates that thrombectomy often was performed without endarterectomy, and in these cases the pulmonary artery pressures did not improve, often resulting in death.

An inferior vena cava filter is always placed before surgery unless an obvious upper extremity or cardiac (e.g., intraventricular pacing wire, ventriculoatrial shunt) source is present. In the latter case, removal of any foreign material is undertaken, with alternative sites used, as with replacement of intravascular pacing leads with epicardial electrodes. Patients are treated with warfarin until the time of surgery, and this treatment is continued throughout the patient's life after surgery.

Pulmonary Endarterectomy—Surgical Technique

After a median sternotomy incision is made, the pericardium is incised longitudinally and attached to the wound edges. Typically the right side of the heart is enlarged, with a tense right atrium and a variable degree of tricuspid regurgitation. There is usually severe right ventricular hypertrophy, and, with critical degrees of obstruction, the patient's condition may become unstable with manipulation of the heart. Anticoagulation is achieved with the use of beef-lung heparin sodium (400 U/kg, IV) administered to prolong the activated clotting time beyond 400 seconds. Full cardiopulmonary bypass is instituted with high ascending aortic cannulation and two caval cannulas. These cannulas must be inserted into the superior and inferior venae cavae sufficiently to enable subsequent opening of the right atrium. The heart is emptied on bypass, and a temporary pulmonary artery vent is placed in the midline of the main pulmonary artery, 1 cm distal to the pulmonary valve. This marks the beginning of the left pulmonary arteriotomy.

After cardiopulmonary bypass is initiated, surface cooling with both a head jacket and a cooling blanket on the operating room table is begun. The blood is cooled with the pump oxygenator. During cooling, a 10° C gradient between arterial blood and bladder or rectal temperature is maintained.[118] Cooling generally takes 45 minutes to an hour. When ventricular fibrillation occurs, an additional vent is placed in the left atrium through the right superior pulmonary vein. This prevents the occurrence of atrial and ventricular distension resulting from the large amount of bronchial arterial blood flow that is common with these patients. It is most convenient for the primary surgeon to stand initially on the patient's left side. During the cooling period, some preliminary dissection can be performed, with full mobilization of the right pulmonary artery from the ascending aorta. All dissection of the pulmonary arteries takes place intrapericardially, and neither pleural cavity is entered. An incision is then made in the right pulmonary artery from beneath the ascending aorta under the superior vena cava and entering the lower lobe branch of the pulmonary artery just after the take-off of the middle lobe artery.

Any loose thrombus, if present, is removed. The endarterectomy cannot be performed in the presence of thrombus because it obscures the plane and prevents collapse of the endarterectomized specimen, hindering distal exposure. It is important to recognize that, first, an embolectomy without subsequent endarterectomy is ineffective and, second, in most patients with chronic thromboembolic hypertension, direct examination of the pulmonary vascular bed at operation generally shows no obvious embolic material. Therefore to the inexperienced or cursory glance, the pulmonary vascular bed may well appear normal even in patients with severe chronic embolic pulmonary hypertension. If the bronchial circulation is not excessive, the endarterectomy plane can be found during this early dissection. However, although a small amount of dissection can be performed before the initiation of circulatory arrest, it is unwise to proceed unless perfect visibility is obtained because the development of a correct plane is essential.

When the patient's temperature reaches 20° C, the aorta is cross-clamped and a single dose of cold cardioplegic solution is administered. Additional myocardial protection is obtained by the use of a cooling jacket wrapped around the heart. The entire procedure is now performed with a single aortic cross-clamp period with no further administration of cardioplegic solution. A modified cerebellar retractor is placed between the aorta and the superior vena cava. When back bleeding from bronchial collaterals obscures direct vision of the pulmonary vascular bed, thiopental is administered (500 mg–1g) until the electroencephalogram becomes isoelectric. Circulatory arrest is then initiated, and the patient undergoes exsanguination. It is rare that one 20-minute period for each side is exceeded. Although retrograde cerebral perfusion has been advocated for total circulatory arrest in other procedures, it is not helpful in this operation because it does not allow a completely bloodless field, and, with the short arrest times that can be achieved, it is not necessary.

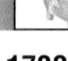

Any loose thrombotic debris encountered is removed. Then, a microtome knife is used to develop the endarterectomy plane posteriorly within the media of the vessel. Dissection in the correct plane is critical because if the plane is too deep, the pulmonary artery may perforate, with fatal results, and if the dissection plane is not deep enough, inadequate amounts of the partially resorbed thromboembolic material will be removed. Once the plane is correctly developed, a full-thickness layer is left in the region of the incision to ease subsequent repair. For the endarterectomy, gentle traction with forceps while sweeping the outer vessel wall layer away results in the progressive withdrawal of the endarterectomy specimen. The procedure is primarily performed with a long miniature sucker with a rounded tip.[44] As each lobar branch appears, it is grasped individually and the specimen is withdrawn until each segmental vessel branches again. Each of these subsegmental specimens is then extracted. Removal of each lobar and then segmental branch makes subsequent distal dissection easier. If a large mass of endarterectomized tissue begins to obscure visibility, it is excised. The entire specimen can thus be removed for a length of approximately 20 cm. The distalmost portion endarterectomy is performed with an eversion technique. Perforation at the level of the subsegmental vessels will become completely inaccessible later, so care must be taken to remain in the plane of the media for endarterectomy. Clear visualization in a completely bloodless field provided by circulatory arrest is therefore essential during development of the distal surgical plane. It is important that each subsegmental branch is followed and freed individually until it ends in a "tail," beyond which there is no further obstruction. Residual material should never be cut free; the entire specimen should "tail off" and come free spontaneously. Once the right-sided endarterectomy is completed, circulation is restarted and the arteriotomy is repaired with a continuous 6-0 polypropylene suture. The hemostatic nature of this closure is aided by the nature of the initial dissection, with the full thickness of the pulmonary artery being preserved immediately adjacent to the incision.

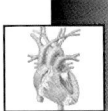

After completion of the repair of the right arteriotomy, the surgeon moves to the patient's right side. The pulmonary vent catheter is withdrawn, and an arteriotomy is made from the site of the pulmonary vent hole laterally to the pericardial reflection, avoiding entry into the left pleural space. Additional lateral dissection does not enhance intraluminal visibility, may endanger the left phrenic nerve, and makes subsequent repair of the left pulmonary artery more difficult. The left-sided dissection is virtually analogous in all respects to that accomplished on the right. The duration of circulatory arrest intervals during the performance of the left-sided dissection also is subject to the same restriction as the right. After the completion of the endarterectomy, cardiopulmonary bypass is reinstituted and warming is commenced. Methylprednisolone (500 mg IV) and mannitol (12.5 g IV) are administered, and during warming a 10° C temperature gradient is maintained between the perfusate and body temperature. If the systemic vascular resistance level is high, nitroprusside is administered to promote vasodilatation and warming. The rewarming period generally takes approximately 90 minutes, but varies according to the body mass of the patient.

When the pulmonary arteriotomy has been repaired, the pulmonary artery vent is replaced at the top of the incision. The right atrium is then opened and examined unless before cardiopulmonary bypass, a negative "bubble" test revealed no persistent foramen ovale on transesophageal echocardiography. Otherwise, any intraatrial communication (present in about 20% of patients) is closed at this point. Although tricuspid valve regurgitation is invariable in these patients and is often severe, tricuspid valve repair is not performed. Right ventricular remodeling occurs within a few days, with the return of tricuspid competence. If other cardiac procedures are required, such as coronary artery or mitral or aortic valve surgery, these are conveniently performed during the systemic rewarming period. Myocardial cooling is discontinued once all cardiac procedures have been concluded. The left atrial vent is removed, and the vent site is repaired. Air is evacuated from the heart, and the aortic cross-clamp is removed.

When the patient has rewarmed, cardiopulmonary bypass is discontinued. Dopamine hydrochloride is routinely administered at renal doses, and other inotropic agents and vasodilators are titrated as necessary to sustain acceptable hemodynamics. The cardiac output is generally high, with a low systemic vascular resistance. Temporary atrial and ventricular epicardial pacing wires are placed. Despite the duration of extracorporeal circulation, hemostasis is readily achieved, and the administration of platelets or coagulation factors is generally unnecessary. Wound closure is routine. A vigorous diuresis is usual for the next few hours, also the result of the previous systemic hypothermia. All patients are subjected to a maintained diuresis with the goal of reaching the patient's preoperative weight within 24 hours. Extubation is usually performed on the first postoperative day.

Thromboembolic Disease Classification and Prediction of Surgical Outcome

Recently four major types of pulmonary occlusive disease, based on anatomy and location of thrombus and vessel wall pathology, have been described.[72] This intraoperative classification of disease allows for the prediction of patient outcome after pulmonary endarterectomy.[108]

1. Type 1 disease (approximately 30% of cases of thromboembolic pulmonary hypertension; Figure 98-2): fresh thrombus in the main or lobar pulmonary arteries. In this situation, major vessel clot is present and visible on the opening of the pulmonary arteries. This clot usually reflects main or lobar pulmonary vessel wall disease, with stasis, and fresh propagation of clot into the major pulmonary vessels.
2. Type 2 disease (approximately 60% of cases; Figure 98-3): intimal thickening and fibrosis with or without organized thrombus proximal to segmental arteries. In these cases only thickened intima can be seen, occasionally with webs in the main or lobar arteries.
3. Type 3 disease (approximately 10% of cases; Figure 98-4): fibrosis, intimal webbing, and thickening with or without organized thrombus within distal segmental and subsegmental arteries only. This type of disease presents the most challenging surgical situation. No occlusion of vessels can be seen initially. The endarterectomy plane must be raised individually in each segmental and subsegmental branch. Type 3 disease is most often associated with presumed repetitive thrombi from indwelling catheters or ventriculoatrial shunts and sometimes represents "burned out" disease, where most of the embolic material has been reabsorbed.
4. Type 4 disease: microscopic distal arteriolar vasculopathy without visible thromboembolic disease. Type 4 disease does not represent classic chronic thromboembolic pulmonary hypertension and is inoperable. In this entity there is intrinsic small-vessel disease, although secondary thrombus may occur as a result of stasis. Small-vessel disease may be unrelated to thromboembolic events ("primary" pulmonary hypertension) or occur in relation to thromboembolic hypertension as a result of a high-flow or high-pressure state in previously unaffected vessels similar to the generation of Eisenmenger's syndrome.

It has been shown that patients with type 3 and 4 disease have more residual postoperative tricuspid regurgitation, higher postoperative pulmonary artery systolic pressures, and a higher postoperative PVR than those with type 1 or 2 disease.[108] Patients with distal thromboembolic disease (type 3–4) also had a higher perioperative mortality, required longer inotropic support, and had longer hospital stays compared with patients with type 1 or 2 thromboembolic disease. Thus the degree of improvement in pulmonary hypertension and tricuspid regurgitation after pulmonary endarterectomy is determined by the type and location of pulmonary thromboembolic disease.

Results of Pulmonary Endarterectomy

Although pulmonary endarterectomy is now performed at several major cardiovascular centers throughout the world, the majority of experience with this operation has been at

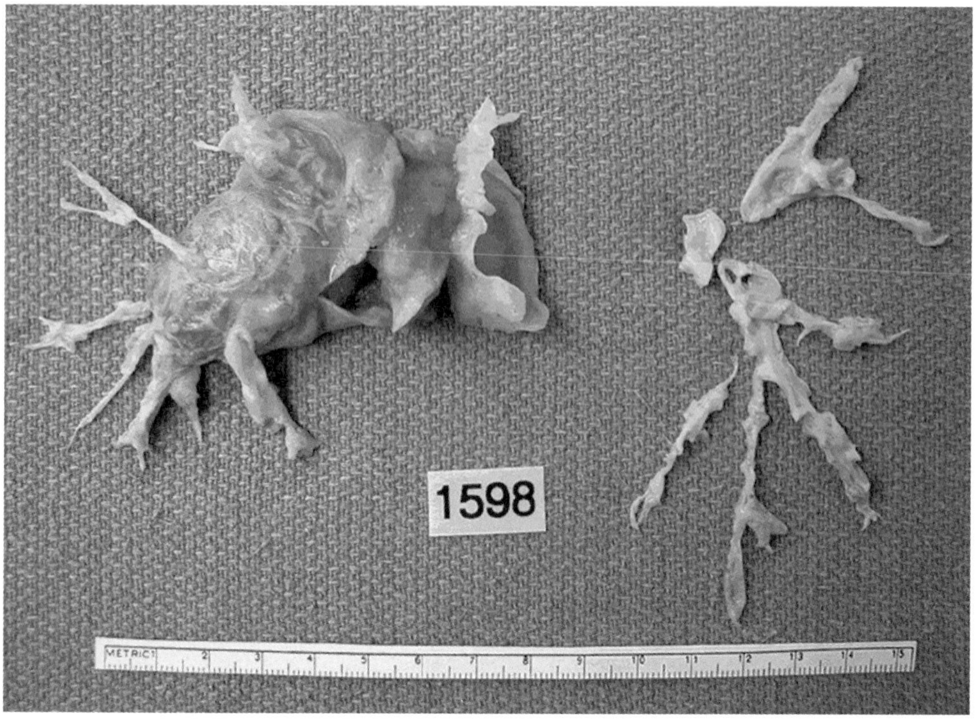

Figure 98–2 Surgical specimen removed from right and left pulmonary arteries. Evidence of fresh thrombus indicates type 1 disease. Note that removal of only the fresh material leaves a large amount of disease behind. The ruler measures 15 cm.

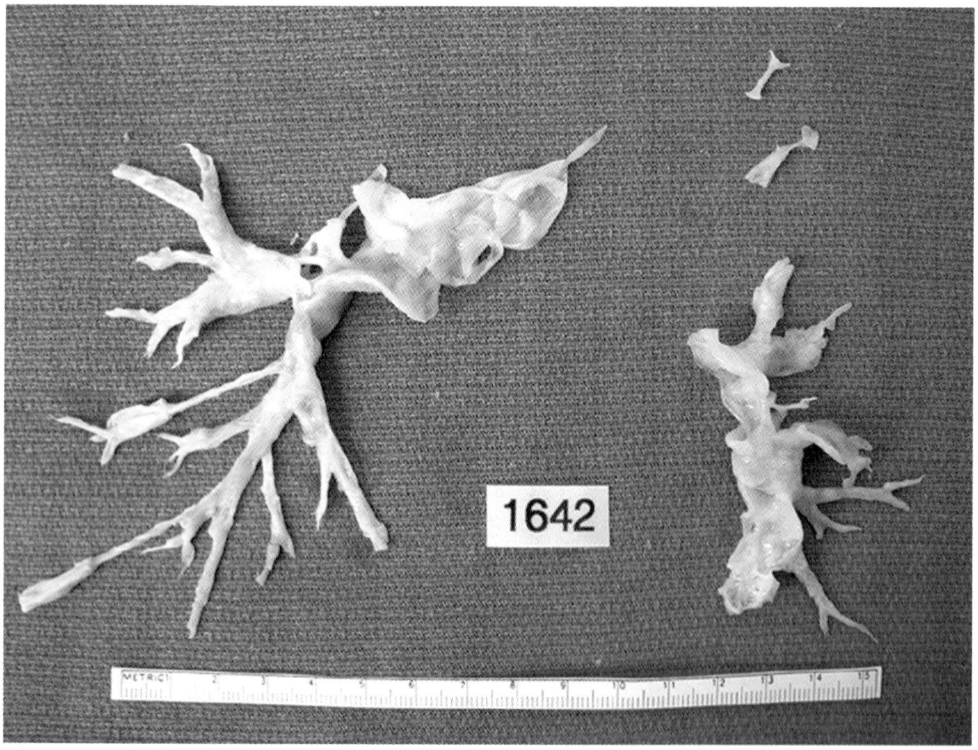

Figure 98–3 Surgical specimen removed from right and left pulmonary arteries indicating type 2 disease. Note the extent of dissection down to the tail end of each branch. The ruler measures 15 cm.

the University of California, San Diego (UCSD), where the technique of this operation was pioneered and refined. More than 1600 pulmonary endarterectomies have been performed at UCSD since 1970,[47] whereas the entire reported world literature on this operation (exclusive of UCSD) is approximately 300 cases. A total of 1400 cases have been completed at UCSD since 1990, when the surgical procedure was modified as described in this chapter. The mean patient age in the last 1300 patients at this one center was 52 years, with a range of 8–85 years. There was a slight male predominance, reflecting either disease predilection, surgical referral bias, or both. In nearly one third of cases, at least one additional cardiac procedure was performed at the time of operation. Most commonly, the adjunct procedure was closure of a persistent foramen ovale or atrial septal defect (26%) or coronary artery bypass grafting (8%).

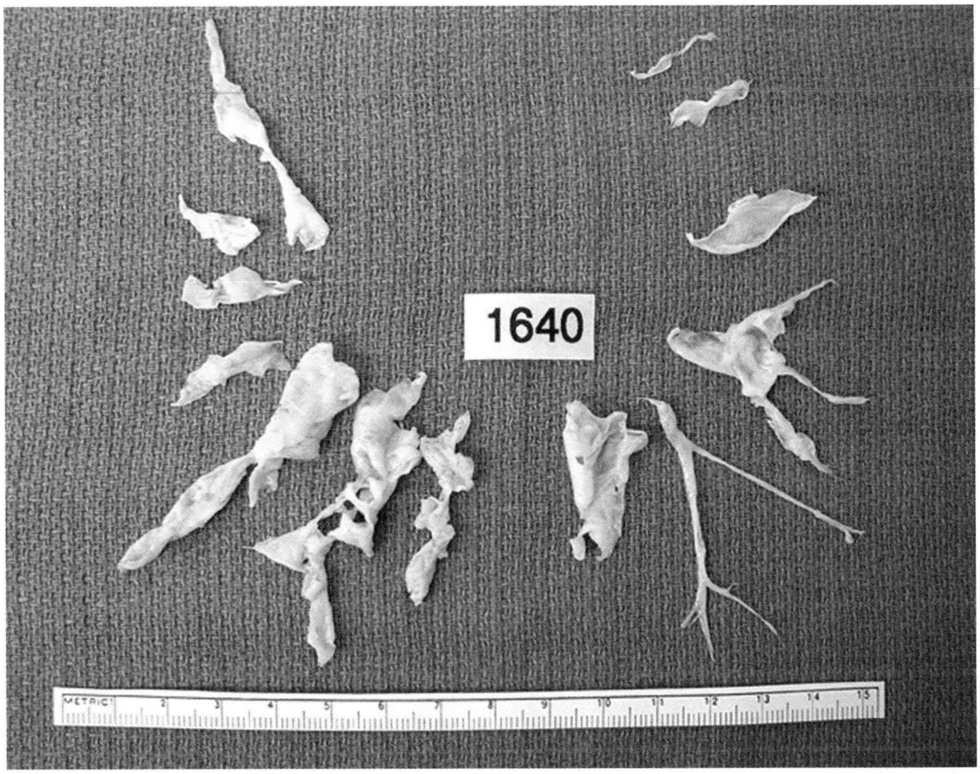

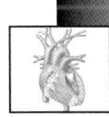

Figure 98–4 Surgical specimen removed from right and left pulmonary arteries. In this patient with type 3 disease, the dissection plane was raised at each segmental level. The ruler measures 15 cm.

With this operation, a reduction in pulmonary pressures and resistance to normal levels and corresponding improvement in pulmonary blood flow and cardiac output are generally immediate and sustained.[70] In general, these changes can be assumed to be permanent.[55,69] Table 98-3 lists the four largest published series of pulmonary endarterectomy results (all from UCSD) with respect to hemodynamic improvement.[46,47,107,108] Whereas before the operation, more than 50% of the patients were in New York Heart Association (NYHA) functional class III or IV in these studies, at 1 year after operation, 90% of patients were reclassified as NYHA functional class I or II. In addition, echocardiographic studies have demonstrated that, with the elimination of chronic pressure overload, right ventricular geometry rapidly reverts toward normal.[106] Right atrial and right ventricular hypertrophy and dilatation regress. Tricuspid valve function returns to normal within a few days as a result of restoration of tricuspid annular geometry after

Table 98–3

Postoperative Hemodynamic Parameters: Four Largest Series

Variable (mean)	*Jamieson et al 2003 n = 500*	*Thistlethwaite et al 2002 n = 202*	*Thistlethwaite et al 2001 n = 90*	*Jamieson et al 1993 n = 150*
Decrease in PAS (mm Hg)	29.0 ± 20.4	31.9 ± 18.9	34.7 ± 19.1	31.8
Decrease in PAD (mm Hg)	10.8 ± 10.5	13.1 ± 9.20	11.5 ± 8.70	ND
Decrease in PVR (dyne/sec/cm^{-5})	597.0 ± 404.2	547.2 ± 387.7	520.6 ± 285.7	637.5
Increase in CO (liters/min)	1.68 ± 1.64	1.62 ± 0.61	2.36 ± 1.68	1.8
Decrease in tricuspid regurgitant velocity (m/sec)	ND	1.37 ± 0.75	1.27 ± 0.87	ND

PAS, pulmonary artery systolic pressure; PAD, pulmonary artery diastolic pressure; PVR, pulmonary vascular resistance; CO, cardiac output; ND, not done.

the remodeling of the right ventricle; therefore tricuspid valve repair is not performed with this operation.[71]

Severe reperfusion injury is the single most frequent complication after pulmonary endarterectomy, occurring in up to 10% of patients.[61] Of patients with reperfusion injury, the majority resolve the problem with a short period of ventilatory support and aggressive diuresis. A minority of patients with severe lung reperfusion injury require long periods of ventilatory support, whereas extreme cases require venovenous extracorporeal support for oxygenation and blood carbon dioxide removal. Neurological complications from circulatory arrest have been eliminated mostly by shorter circulatory arrest periods and the use of a direct cooling jacket placed around the head. The head-wrap cooling jacket has been used in over 1000 cases of pulmonary endarterectomy at UCSD without complications[47] and provides even cooling to the surface of the cranium, particularly the posterior location. Perioperative confusion and stroke rates for pulmonary endarterectomy are similar to that seen with conventional open-heart surgery. In the UCSD series, reexploration for bleeding occurred at a rate of 2.5%, and 50% of patients required intraoperative or postoperative blood transfusion. Despite the length of this operation, wound infection occurred only in 1.8% of patients.

The largest risk factor for operation remains the severity of PVR and the ability to lower it to a normal range at operation. Those patients with high PVR with minimal vascular obstruction on angiogram (Type 4 small-vessel vasculopathy) have the worst prognosis, and surgery did not alleviate pulmonary hypertension in this population. Type 4 pulmonary hypertensive disease represents vascular obstruction at the arteriolar or capillary level ("primary pulmonary hypertension"). This small-vessel vasculopathy was not influenced by blind endarterectomy of the proximal pulmonary arterial tree. The majority of early deaths after this operation are in this subgroup, and future efforts are directed at more precisely determining who these patients are in the preoperative setting to avoid unnecessary operation.

In the UCSD experience, overall perioperative mortality was 9% for the entire cohort of patients, which encompasses a time span of 30 years. Most recently, surgical mortality for pulmonary endarterectomy approaches 4%. This reflects the learning curve for safely performing this operation and the refinements in surgical technique that enhance patient outcome.

A survey of surviving patients who underwent pulmonary endarterectomy between 1970 and 1995 in the UCSD series has formally evaluated long-term outcomes of this operation.[5] Questionnaires were mailed to 420 patients who had survived more than 1 year after the operation. Responses were obtained from 308 patients. Survival, functional status, quality of life, and the subsequent use of medical assistance were assessed. The survival rate after pulmonary endarterectomy was found to be 75% at 6 years or more. This survival rate exceeds single- or double-lung transplant survival rates for thromboembolic pulmonary hypertension. Ninety-three percent of the patients were found to be in NYHA class I or II, compared with approximately 95% of the patients being in NYHA class III or IV preoperatively. Of the working population, 62% of patients who were unemployed before the operation returned to work. Patients who had undergone pulmonary endarterectomy scored several quality-of-life components slightly lower than normal individuals, but significantly higher than the patients before pulmonary endarterectomy. Only 10% of patients used oxygen after surgery. In response to the question, "How do you feel about the quality of your life since your surgery?" 77% replied "much improved," and 20% replied "improved." These data appear to confirm that pulmonary endarterectomy offers substantial improvement in survival, function, and quality of life.

SUMMARY

Pulmonary hypertension caused by chronic pulmonary embolism is a condition that is underrecognized and carries a poor prognosis. Medical therapy for this condition is ineffective and only transiently improves symptoms. The only therapeutic alternative to pulmonary endarterectomy is lung transplantation. The advantages of pulmonary endarterectomy include a lower operative mortality, better long-term results with respect to survival and quality of life, and the avoidance of chronic immunosuppressive treatment and allograft rejection. Currently mortality rates for pulmonary endarterectomy are 4.4%, and the operation allows for sustained clinical benefit. These results make it the treatment of choice over transplantation for thromboembolic lung disease both in the short and long term.

Although pulmonary endarterectomy is technically demanding for the surgeon, requiring careful dissection of the pulmonary artery planes and the use of circulatory arrest, excellent results can be achieved. Improvements in operative technique developed over the last 4 decades allow pulmonary endarterectomy to be offered to patients with an acceptable mortality rate and anticipation of clinical improvement. With the increasing recognition of patients who have thromboembolic pulmonary hypertension and the realization that pulmonary endarterectomy is a safe and effective operation for this condition, it is anticipated that this will be an expanding area of surgical therapy in the future.

REFERENCES

1. Aklog L, Williams CS, Byrne JG, et al: Acute pulmonary embolectomy: A contemporary approach. Circulation 105:1416–1419, 2002.
2. Allison PR, Dunnill MS, Marshall R: Pulmonary embolism. Thorax 15:273–283, 1960.
3. Anderson FA Jr, Wheeler HB: Venous thromboembolism: Risk factors and prophylaxis. In Tapson VF, Fulkerson WJ, Saltzman HA, editors: Clinics in Chest Medicine: Venous Thromboembolism, Vol. 16, pp. 235–251. Philadelphia: W.B. Saunders, 1995.
4. Anderson HL 3rd, Delius RE, Sinard JM, et al: Early experience with adult extracorporeal membrane oxygenation in the modern era. Ann Thorac Surg 53:553–563, 1992.
5. Archibald CJ, Auger WR, Fedullo PF, et al: Long-term outcome after pulmonary thromboendarterectomy. Am J Respir Crit Care Med 160:523–528, 1999.
6. Auger WR, Fedullo PF, Moser KM, et al: Chronic major-vessel thromboembolic pulmonary artery obstruction: Appearance at angiography. Radiology 182:393–398, 1992.

7. Auger WR, Moser KM: Pulmonary flow murmurs: A distinctive physical sign found in chronic pulmonary thromboembolic disease. Clin Res 37:145A, 1989.
8. Auger WR, Permpikul P, Moser KM: Lupus anticoagulant, heparin use, and thrombocytopenia in patients with chronic thromboembolic pulmonary hypertension: A preliminary report. Am J Med 99:392–396, 1995.
9. Benotti JR, Ockene IS, Alpert JS, et al: The clinical profile of unresolved pulmonary embolism. Chest 84:669–678, 1983.
10. British Thoracic Society Standards of Care Committee Pulmonary Embolism Guideline Development Group: British Thoracic Society guidelines for the management of suspected acute pulmonary embolism. Thorax 58:470–483, 2003.
11. Carson JL, Kelley MA, Duff A, et al: The clinical course of pulmonary embolism. N Engl J Med 326:1240–1245, 1992.
12. Chitwood WR Jr, Sabiston DC Jr, Wechsler AS: Surgical treatment of chronic unresolved pulmonary embolism. Clin Chest Med 5:507–536, 1984.
13. Collins R, Scrimgeour A, Yusuf S, et al: Reduction in fatal pulmonary embolism and venous thrombosis by perioperative administration of subcutaneous heparin. Overview of results and randomized trials in general, orthopedic and urologic surgery. N Engl J Med 318:1162–1173, 1988.
14. Colorio CC, Martinuzzo ME, Forastiero RR, et al: Thrombophilic factors in chronic thromboembolic pulmonary hypertension. Blood Coagul Fibrinolysis. 12: 427–432, 2001.
15. Come PC: Echocardiographic evaluation of pulmonary embolism and its response to therapeutic interventions. Chest 101:151S–162S, 1992.
16. Daily PO, Dembitsky WP, Jamieson SW: The evolution and the current state of the art of pulmonary thromboendarterectomy. Semin Thorac Cardiovasc Surg 11:152–163, 1999.
17. Dalen JE, Alpert JS: Natural history of pulmonary embolism. Prog Cardiovasc Dis 17:259–270, 1975.
18. Dalen JE, Banas JS Jr, Brooks HL, et al: Resolution rate of pulmonary embolism in man. N Engl J Med 280:1194–1199, 1969.
19. Dartevelle P, Fadel E, Chapelier A, et al: Angioscopic video-assisted pulmonary endarterectomy for post-embolic pulmonary hypertension. Eur J Cardiothorac Surg 16:38–43, 1999.
20. Davies MJ, Arsiwala SS, Moore HM, et al: Extracorporeal membrane oxygenation for the treatment of massive pulmonary embolism. Ann Thorac Surg 60:1801–1803, 1995.
21. Del Campo C: Pulmonary embolectomy: A review. Can J Surg 28:111–113, 1985.
22. Doerge H, Schoendube FA, Voss M, et al: Surgical therapy of fulminant pulmonary embolism: Early and late results. Thorac Cardiovasc Surg 47:9–13, 1999.
23. Du L, Sullivan CC, Chu D, et al: Signaling molecules in nonfamilial pulmonary hypertension. N Engl J Med 348: 500–509, 2003.
24. Goldhaber SZ: Strategies for diagnosis. In Goldhaber SZ, editor: Pulmonary Embolism and Deep Vein Thrombosis, p. 79. Philadelphia: W.B. Saunders, 1985.
25. Goldhaber SZ: Thrombolytic therapy in venous thromboembolism: Clinical trials and current indications. In Tapson VF, Fulkerson WJ, Saltzman HA, editors: Clinics in Chest Medicine, Venous Thromboembolism, Vol. 16, pp. 307–320. Philadelphia: W.B. Saunders, 1995.
26. Goldhaber SZ: Modern treatment of pulmonary embolism. Eur Respir J Suppl 35:22s–27s, 2002.
27. Goldhaber SZ, Haire WD, Feldstein ML, et al: Alteplase versus heparin in acute pulmonary embolism: Randomized trial assessing right-ventricular function and pulmonary perfusion. Lancet 341:507–511, 1993.
28. Goldhaber SZ, Hennekens CH, Evans DA, et al: Factors associated with correct antemortem diagnosis of major pulmonary embolism. Am J Med 73:822–826, 1982.
29. Goodall RJ, Greenfield LJ: Clinical correlations in the diagnosis of pulmonary embolism. Ann Surg 191:219–223, 1980.
30. Gray HH, Miller GA, Paneth M: Pulmonary embolectomy: Its place in the management of pulmonary embolism. Lancet 1:1441–1445, 1988.
31. Gray HH, Morgan JM, Paneth M, et al: Pulmonary embolectomy for acute massive pulmonary embolism: An analysis of 71 cases. Br Heart J 60:196–200, 1988.
32. Greenfield LJ: Venous thrombosis and pulmonary thromboembolism. In Schwartz SI, editor: Principles of Surgery, 6th ed., pp. 989-1014. New York: McGraw-Hill, 1994.
33. Greenfield LJ, Proctor MC: Twenty-year clinical experience with the Greenfield filter. Cardiovasc Surg 3:199–205, 1995.
34. Greenfield LJ, Proctor MC, Williams DM, et al: Long-term experience with transvenous catheter pulmonary embolectomy. J Vasc Surg 18:450–458, 1993.
35. Gulba DC, Schmid C, Borst HG, et al: Medical compared with surgical treatment for massive pulmonary embolism. Lancet 343:576–577, 1994.
36. Gurewich V, Cohen ML, Thomas DP: Humoral factors in massive pulmonary embolism: An experimental study. Am Heart J 76:784–794, 1968.
37. Hagen PJ, Hartmann IJ, Hoekstra OS, et al: Comparison of observer variability and accuracy of different criteria for lung scan interpretation. J Nucl Med 44:739–744, 2003.
38. Hagl C, Khaladj N, Peters T, et al: Technical advances of pulmonary thromboendarterectomy for chronic thromboembolic pulmonary hypertension. Eur J Cardiothorac Surg 23:776–781, 2003.
39. Heit JA, Silverstein MD, Mohr DN, et al: The epidemiology of venous thromboembolism in the community. Thromb Haemost 86:452–463, 2001.
40. Hirsh J, Levine MN: Low molecular weight heparin. Blood 79:1–17, 1992.
41. Hoagland PM: Massive pulmonary embolism. In Goldhaber SZ, editor: Pulmonary Embolism and Deep Vein Thrombosis, p. 179. Philadelphia: W.B. Saunders, 1986.
42. Houk VN, Hufnagel CA, McClenathan JE, et al: Chronic thrombotic obstruction of major pulmonary arteries. Report of a case successfully treated by thromboendarterectomy, and a review of the literature. Am J Med 35:269–282, 1963.
43. Hsieh PC, Wang SS, Ko WJ, et al: Successful resuscitation of acute massive pulmonary embolism with extracorporeal membrane oxygenation and open embolectomy. Ann Thorac Surg 72:266–267, 2001.
44. Jamieson SW, Kapelanski DP: Pulmonary endarterectomy. Curr Probl Surg 37:165–252, 2000.
45. Jamieson SW, Nomura K: Indications for and the results of pulmonary thromboendarterectomy for thromboembolic pulmonary hypertension. Semin Vasc Surg 13:236–244, 2000.
46. Jamieson SW, Auger WR, Fedullo PF, et al: Experience and results with 150 pulmonary thromboendarterectomy operations over a 29-month period. J Thorac Cardiovasc Surg 106:116–127, 1993.
47. Jamieson SW, Sakakibara N, Manecke G, et al: Pulmonary endarterectomy: Experience and lessons learned in 1500 cases. Ann Thorac Surg 76:1457–1462.
48. Kasper W, Meinertz T, Henkel B, et al: Echocardiographic findings in patients with proved pulmonary embolism. Am Heart J 112:1284–1290, 1986.
49. Kawahito K, Murata S, Adachi H, et al: Resuscitation and circulatory support using extracorporeal membrane oxygenation for fulminant pulmonary embolism. Artif Organs 24:427–430, 2000.

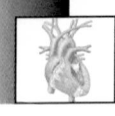

50. Kerr KM, Fedullo PF, Auger WR: Chronic thromboembolic pulmonary hypertension: When to suspect it, when to refer for surgery. Adv Pulm Hypertens 2:4–8, 2003.
51. Kieny R, Charpentier A, Kieny MT: What is the place of pulmonary embolectomy today? J Cardiovasc Surg 32:549–554, 1991.
52. Kniffin WD Jr, Baron JA, Barrett J, et al: The epidemiology of diagnosed pulmonary embolism and deep venous thrombosis in the elderly. Arch Intern Med 154:861–866, 1994.
53. Konstantinides S, Geibel A, Heusel G, et al: Heparin plus alteplase compared with heparin alone in patients with submassive pulmonary embolism. N Engl J Med 347:1143–1150, 2002.
54. Konstantinides S, Geibel A, Olschewski M, et al: Association between thrombolytic treatment and the prognosis of hemodynamically stable patients with major pulmonary embolism: Results of a multicenter registry. Circulation 96:882–888, 1997.
55. Kramm T, Mayer E, Dahm M, et al: Long-term results after thromboendarterectomy for chronic pulmonary embolism. Eur J Cardiothorac Surg 15:579–584, 1999.
56. Laennec RTH: Traite do l'auscultation mediate et des maladies des poumons et du Coeur. Paris: Brossen et Chaude, 1819.
57. Lambert V, Durand P, Devictor D, et al: Unilateral right pulmonary thromboendarterectomy for chronic embolism: A successful procedure in an infant. J Thorac Cardiovasc Surg 118:953–957, 1999.
58. Landefeld CS, Chren MM, Myers A, et al: Diagnostic yield of the autopsy in a university hospital and a community hospital. N Engl J Med. 318:1249–1254, 1988.
59. Lang IM, Marsh JJ, Olman MA, et al: Parallel analysis of tissue-type plasminogen activator and type 1 plasminogen activator inhibitor in plasma and endothelial cells derived from patients with chronic pulmonary thromboemboli. Circulation 90:706–712, 1994.
60. Levine MN: Thrombolytic therapy for venous thromboembolism: Complications and contraindications. In Tapson VF, Fulkerson WJ, Saltzman HA, editors: Clinics in Chest Medicine, Venous Thromboembolism, Vol. 16, pp. 321–328. Philadelphia: W.B. Saunders, 1995.
61. Levinson RM, Shure D, Moser KM: Reperfusion pulmonary edema after pulmonary artery thromboendarterectomy. Am Rev Respir Dis 134:1241–1245, 1986.
62. Lewczuk J, Piszko P, Jagas J, et al: Prognostic factors in medically treated patients with chronic pulmonary embolism. Chest 119:818–823, 2001.
63. Lindblad B, Eriksson A, Bergqvist D: Autopsy-verified pulmonary embolism in a surgical department: Analysis of the period from 1951 to 1988. Br J Surg 78:849–852, 1991.
64. Ly B, Arnesen H, Eie H, et al: A controlled clinical trial of streptokinase and heparin in the treatment of major pulmonary embolism. Acta Med Scand 203:465–470, 1978.
65. Malik AB, Johnson A: Role of humoral mediators in the pulmonary vascular response to pulmonary embolism. In Weir EK, Reeves JT, editors: Pulmonary Vascular Physiology and Pathophysiology, pp. 445-468. New York: Marcel Dekker, 1989.
66. Marder VJ, Sherry S: Thrombolytic therapy: Current status (2). N Engl J Med 318:1585–1595, 1988.
67. Matheus MC, Sandoval Zarate J, Criales Cortes JL, et al: Helical computerized tomography of the thorax in the diagnosis of unresolved chronic pulmonary thromboembolism. Arch Inst Cardiol Mex 70:456–467, 2000.
68. Mattox KL, Feldtman RW, Beall AC, et al: Pulmonary embolectomy for acute massive pulmonary embolism. Ann Surg 195:726–731, 1982.
69. Mayer E, Dahm M, Hake U, et al: Mid-term results of pulmonary thromboendarterectomy for chronic thromboembolic pulmonary hypertension. Ann Thorac Surg 61:1788–1792, 1996.
70. Menzel T, Kramm T, Mohr-Kahaly S, et al: Assessment of cardiac performance using Tei indices in patients undergoing pulmonary thromboendarterectomy. Ann Thorac Surg 73:762–766, 2002.
71. Menzel T, Kramm T, Wagner S, et al: Improvement of tricuspid regurgitation after pulmonary thromboendarterectomy. Ann Thorac Surg 73:756–761, 2002.
72. Menzel T, Wagner S, Kramm T, et al: Pathophysiology of impaired right and left ventricular function in chronic embolic pulmonary hypertension: Changes after pulmonary thromboendarterectomy. Chest 118:897–903, 2000.
73. Meyer G, Tamisier D, Sors H, et al: Pulmonary embolectomy: A 20-year experience at one center. Ann Thorac Surg 51:232–236, 1991.
74. Morris TA, Auger WR, Ysrael MZ, et al: Parenchymal scarring is associated with restrictive spirometric defects in patients with chronic thromboembolic pulmonary hypertension. Chest 110:399–403, 1996.
75. Moser KM, Auger WR, Fedullo PF: Chronic major-vessel thromboembolic pulmonary hypertension. Circulation 81:1735–1743, 1990.
76. Moser KM, Auger WR, Fedullo PF, et al: Chronic thromboembolic pulmonary hypertension: Clinical picture and surgical treatment. Eur Respir J 5:334–342, 1992.
77. Moser KM, Page GT, Ashburn WL, et al: Perfusion lung scans provide a guide to which patients with apparent primary pulmonary hypertension merit angiography. West J Med 148:167–170, 1988.
78. Newsome LR, Ponganis P, Reichman R, et al: Portable percutaneous cardiopulmonary bypass: Use in supported coronary angioplasty, aortic valvuloplasty, and cardiac arrest. J Cardiothor Vasc Anesth 6:328–331, 1992.
79. Obermaier R, Kroger JC, Benz S, et al: Successful catheter-guided local thrombolysis in acute pulmonary embolism in the early postoperative period after pancreatic head resection. Chirurg 73:945–949, 2002.
80. Olman MA, Marsh JJ, Lang IM, et al: Endogenous fibrinolytic system in chronic large-vessel thromboembolic pulmonary hypertension. Circulation 86:1241–1248, 1992.
81. Palevsky HI: The problems of the clinical and laboratory diagnosis of pulmonary embolism. Semin Nucl Med 21:276–280, 1991.
82. Panasiuk A, Dzieciol J, Nowak HF, et al: Pulmonary thromboembolism: Random analysis of autopsy material. Pneumonol Alergol Pol 61:171–176, 1993.
83. Pevec WC: Angioscopy in vascular surgery: The state of the art. Ann Vasc Surg 10:66–75, 1996.
84. Pitton MB, Duber C, Mayer E, et al: Hemodynamic effects on nonionic contrast bolus injection and oxygen inhalation during pulmonary angiography in patients with chronic major-vessel thromboembolic pulmonary hypertension. Circulation 94:2485–2491, 1996.
85. Poulsen SH, Noer I, Moller JE, et al: Clinical outcome of patients with suspected pulmonary embolism. A follow-up study of 588 consecutive patients. J Intern Med 250:137–143, 2001.
86. Presti B, Berthrong M, Sherwin RM: Chronic thrombosis of major pulmonary arteries. Hum Pathol 21:601–606, 1990.
87. Pruszczyk P, Torbicki A, Kuch-Wocial A, et al: Diagnostic value of transoesophageal echocardiography in suspected haemodynamically significant pulmonary embolism. Heart 85:628–634, 2001.
88. Rich S, Levitsky S, Brundage BH: Pulmonary hypertension from chronic pulmonary thromboembolism. Ann Intern Med 108:425–434, 1988.
89. Riedel M: Therapy for pulmonary thromboembolism. Part 1: Acute massive pulmonary embolism. Cor Vasa 38:93–102, 1996.

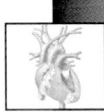

90. Riedel M: Acute pulmonary embolism 2: Treatment. Heart 85:351–360, 2001.
91. Riedel M, Stanek V, Widimsky J, et al: Long-term follow-up of patients with pulmonary thromboembolism. Late prognosis and evolution of hemodynamic and respiratory data. Chest 81:151–158, 1982.
92. Ryan KL, Fedullo PF, Davis GB, et al: Perfusion scan findings understate the severity of angiographic and hemodynamic compromise in chronic thromboembolic pulmonary hypertension. Chest 93:1180–1185, 1988.
93. Schiebler ML, Holland GA, Hatabu H, et al: Suspected pulmonary embolism: Prospective evaluation with pulmonary MR angiography. Radiology 189:125–131, 1993.
94. Schmid C, Zietlow S, Wagner TO, et al: Fulminant pulmonary embolism: Symptoms, diagnostics, operative technique, and results. Ann Thorac Surg 52:1102–1107, 1991.
95. Schmitz-Rode T, Janssens U, Duda SH, et al: Massive pulmonary embolism: Percutaneous emergency treatment by pigtail rotation catheter. J Am Coll Cardiol 36:375–380, 2000.
96. Schulman S, Rhedin AS, Lindmarker P, et al: A comparison of six weeks with six months of oral anticoagulant therapy after a first episode of venous thromboembolism. Duration of Anticoagulation Trial Study Group. N Engl J Med 332: 1661–1665, 1995.
97. Sharp EH: Pulmonary embolectomy: Successful removal of a massive pulmonary embolus with the support of cardiopulmonary bypass—a case report. Ann Surg 156:1–4, 1962.
98. Simonneau G, Azarian R, Brenot F, et al: Surgical management of unresolved pulmonary embolism. A personal series of 72 patients. Chest 107:52S–55S, 1995.
99. Simonneau G, Sors H, Charbonnier B, et al: A comparison of low-molecular-weight heparin with unfractionated heparin for acute pulmonary embolism. The THESEE Study Group. Tinzaparine ou Heparine Standard: Evaluations dans l'Embolie Pulmonaire. N Engl J Med 337: 663–669, 1997.
100. Soyer R, Brunet AP, Redonnet M, et al: Follow-up of surgically treated patients with massive pulmonary embolism: With reference to 12 operated patients. Thorac Cardiovasc Surg 30:103–108, 1982.
101. Stewart JR, Greenfield LJ: Transvenous vena caval filtration and pulmonary embolectomy. Surg Clin North Am 62: 411–430, 1982.
102. Stulz P, Schlapfer R, Feer R, et al: Decision making in the surgical treatment of massive pulmonary embolism. Eur J Cardiothorac Surg 8:188–193, 1994.
103. Tai NR, Atwal AS, Hamilton G: Modern management of pulmonary embolism. Br J Surg 86:853–868, 1999.
104. Tapson VF, Witty LA: Massive pulmonary embolism: Diagnostic and therapeutic strategies. In Tapson VF, Fulkerson WJ, Saltzman HA, editors: Clinics in Chest Medicine, Venous Thromboembolism, Vol. 16, pp. 329–340. Philadelphia: W.B. Saunders, 1995.
105. Tayama E, Ouchida M, Teshima H, et al: Treatment of acute massive/submassive pulmonary embolism. Circ J 66:479–483, 2002.
106. Thistlethwaite PA, Jamieson SW: Tricuspid valvular disease in the patient with chronic pulmonary thromboembolic disease. Curr Opin Cardiol 18:111–116, 2003.
107. Thistlethwaite PA, Auger WR, Madani MM, et al: Pulmonary thromboendarterectomy combined with other cardiac operations: Indications, surgical approach, and outcome. Ann Thorac Surg 72:13–19, 2001.
108. Thistlethwaite PA, Mo M, Madani MM, et al: Operative classification of thromboembolic disease determines outcome after pulmonary endarterectomy. J Thorac Cardiovasc Surg 124:1203–1211, 2002.
109. Timsit JF, Reynaud P, Meyer G, et al: Pulmonary embolectomy by catheter device in massive pulmonary embolism. Chest 100:655–658, 1991.
110. Touliopoulos P, Costello P: Helical (spiral) CT of the thorax. Radiol Clin North Am 33:843–861, 1995.
111. Trendelenburg F: Uber die operative behandlung der embolie der lungarterie. Arch Klin Chir 86:686–700, 1908.
112. Tschirkov A, Krause E, Elert O, et al: Surgical management of massive pulmonary embolism. J Thorac Cardiovasc Surg 75:730–733, 1978.
113. Ullmann M, Hemmer W, Hannekum A: The urgent pulmonary embolectomy: mechanical resuscitation in the operating theatre determines the outcome. Thorac Cardiovasc Surg 47:5–8, 1999.
114. Virchow R: Uber die verstopfung der lungenarterie. Reue Notizen auf Geb d Nature u Heilk 37:26, 1846.
115. Wakefield TW, Proctor MC: Current status of pulmonary embolism and venous thrombosis prophylaxis. Semin Vasc Surg 13:171–181, 2000.
116. Wei Z, Al-Mehdi AB, Fisher AB: Signaling pathway for nitric oxide generation with simulated ischemia in flow-adapted endothelial cells. Am J Physiol Heart Circ Physiol 281:H2226–H2232, 2001.
117. Wenger RK, Bavaria JE, Ratcliffe MB, et al: Flow dynamics of peripheral venous catheters during extracorporeal membrane oxygenation with a centrifugal pump. J Thorac Cardiovasc Surg 96:478–484, 1988.
118. Winkler MH, Rohrer CH, Ratty SC, et al: Perfusion techniques of profound hypothermia and circulatory arrest for pulmonary thromboendarterectomy. J Extracorporeal Technol 22:57–60, 1990.
119. Wittenberg G, Kueppers V, Tschammler A, et al: Long-term results of vena cava filters: Experiences with the LGM and the titanium Greenfield devices. Cardiovasc Intervent Radiol 21:225–229, 1998.
120. Wolf M, Boyer-Neumann C, Parent F, et al: Thrombotic risk factors in pulmonary hypertension. Eur Respir J 15:395–399, 2000.
121. Zlotnick AY, Lennon PF, Goldhaber SZ, et al: Intraoperative detection of pulmonary thromboemboli with epicardial echocardiography. Chest 115:1749–1751, 1999.

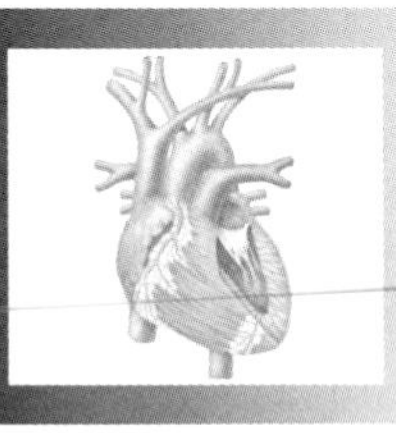

CHAPTER 99

Tumors of the Heart

John Liddicoat and A. Marc Gillinov

INTRODUCTION

With improved cardiac imaging and the development of cardiopulmonary artery bypass to enable intracardiac surgery, cardiac tumors have changed from a postmortem curiosity to a readily diagnosed and frequently treatable form of heart disease. Cardiac tumors can be located in the epicardium, myocardium, endocardium, or any combination of the three. In general, tumors that involve the parietal pericardium are not classified as cardiac tumors.

Tumors of the heart are classified as either primary or secondary. Primary tumors arise in the heart and are either benign or malignant. Secondary tumors are metastases from primary tumors arising elsewhere and hence are always malignant. Primary tumors are rare, with an autopsy incidence of less than 0.1%.[39] Secondary tumors are observed more commonly with a postmortem incidence of about 1%.[30] The prevalences of primary, benign neoplasms (Table 99-1); primary, malignant tumors (Table 99-2); and metastatic neoplasms (Table 99-3) were compiled by investigators at the Armed Forces of Pathology.[6,40]

Cardiac tumors have a variety of clinical features. Often symptoms are determined by the intracardiac location of the tumor. Intracavitary tumors can obstruct blood flow, causing signs and symptoms that mimic those of valvular heart disease. Intramyocardial tumors can trigger cardiac rhythm disturbances, including sudden death.[43] Intracavitary tumors can cause embolic events, resulting in symptoms related to the site of embolization. Cardiac tumors also can cause systemic symptoms mimicking collagen vascular disease, malignancy, or infective endocarditis.[43]

BENIGN PRIMARY CARDIAC TUMORS

Myxomas

Definition, Incidence, and Prevalence

Myxomas are the most common primary cardiac tumors. They are benign. Although myxomas have been reported in both genders and in all age groups, they are most often reported in women in the third to sixth decades of life. Myxomas usually occur sporadically, but at least 7% occur as a part of an autosomal dominant syndrome. In the latter situation the myxoma is a component of a larger syndrome referred to as the Carney complex.[7] In the Carney complex myxomas are associated with spotty pigmentation of the skin and endocrine hyperactivity. Myxomas that arise as a part of the Carney complex affect both sexes equally and at any age, arise as single or multiple lesions in all chambers of the heart, and tend to recur after surgical excision.[50]

Morphology

Arising from the endocardium, myxomas usually extend into a cardiac chamber. They are usually polypoid, pedunculated lesions with a smooth surface that is frequently covered with thrombus (Figure 99-1). The tumors range in size from 1–15 cm, but are most commonly about 5 cm in diameter with a weight of approximately 70 g.[24,27,32,37] Myxomas are thought to arise from pluripotent mesenchymal cells. Histologically, myxomas consist of a matrix of acid mucopolysaccharide (Figure 99-2).[38] The cells are polygonal or spindle-shaped and may form capillary-like channels that can communicate with arteries and veins located at the base of the tumor.[32]

Myxomas are most commonly found in the atria. Approximately 75% arise in the left atrium, and 15–20% arise in the right atrium.[32] Most left atrial myxomas are located on the border of the fossa ovalis, but they can originate from any place on the atrial wall. The remainder of myxomas are located in the ventricles. Myxomas arising from cardiac valves are rare.

Clinical Characteristics

Myxomas can display a variety of symptoms. In the sporadic form, the classic findings include emboli, congestive heart failure caused by obstruction of cardiac blood flow, and constitutional symptoms. These sequelae are related to the location, size, and mobility of the tumor.

Because most myxomas arise in the left atrium, systemic embolization is common, occurring in 30–50% of cases.[3,21,25] Left ventricular myxomas have an even higher propensity to embolize.[34] Right atrial myxomas rarely display clinical manifestations of emboli. Embolic material from myxomas can compromise blood flow to any organ, but the brain is most commonly affected. Myxoma should be included in

Table 99–1

Primary Benign Neoplasms of the Heart (1976–1993)

Tumor[a]	*Total*	*Surgical*	*Autopsy*	*Age ≤15 years at diagnosis*
Myxoma	114	102	12	4
Rhabdomyoma	20	6	14	20
Fibroma	20	18	2	13
Hemangioma	17	10	7	2
AV nodal	10	0	10	2
Granular-cell	4	0	4	0
Lipoma	2	2	0	0
Paraganglioma	2	2	0	0
Myocytic hamartoma	2	2	0	0
Histiocytoid cardiomyopathy	2	0	2	2
Fibrous histiocytoma	1	0	1	0
Epithelioid hemangioendothelioma	1	1	0	0
Bronchogenic cyst	1	1	0	0
Teratoma	1	0	1	1
Totals	100	146 (73%)	53 (27%)	45 (23%)

AV, atrioventricular.

From Roberts WC: Primary and secondary neoplasms of the heart. Am J Cardiol 80:671–682, 1997. Modified from Burke A, Virmani R: Tumors of the heart and great vessels. In Atlas of Tumor Pathology, 3rd series, Fascicle 16, p. 231. Washington, DC: Armed Forces Institute of Pathology, 1996.

[a]Excludes papillary fibroelastoma and lipomatous hypertrophy of the atrial septum.

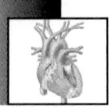

Table 99–2

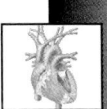

Primary Malignant Tumors of the Heart (1976–1993)

Tumor	*Total*	*Surgical*	*Autopsy*	*Age ≤15 years at diagnosis*
Sarcoma	137 (95%)	116	21	11 (8%)
Angiosarcoma	33	22	11	1
Unclassified	33	30	3	3
Fibrous histiocytoma	16	16	0	1
Osteosarcoma	13	13	0	0
Leiomyoma	12	11	1	1
Fibrous	9	9	0	1
Myxoma	8	8	0	1
Rhabdomyoma	6	2	4	3
Synovial	4	4	0	0
Lipoma	2	0	2	0
Schwannoma	1	1	0	0
Lymphoma	7	1	6	0
Totals	144 (100%)	117 (81%)	27 (19%)	11 (8%)

From Roberts WC: Primary and secondary neoplasms of the heart. Am J Cardiol 80:671–682, 1997. Modified from Burke A, Virmani R: Tumors of the heart and great vessels. In Atlas of Tumor Pathology, 3rd series, Fascicle 16, p. 231. Washington, DC: Armed Forces Institute of Pathology, 1996.

the differential diagnosis of any systemic embolic event, and any embolic material removed should undergo histological evaluation.

Myxomas also can display signs and symptoms related to cardiac obstruction. Typically the findings are related to the tumor's ability to impede the filling of the ventricles; in such instances, signs and symptoms may mimic those of mitral or tricuspid valve stenosis. Less commonly the tumors impede atrioventricular valve leaflet coaptation, causing regurgitation of the valve. Much less frequently, ventricular tumors obstruct the ventricular outflow and cause findings similar to those in aortic or pulmonic stenosis.

Constitutional symptoms include fever, malaise, rash, weight loss, and myalgia. Abnormal laboratory values, including elevated erythrocyte sedimentation rate, anemia, thrombocytopenia, and an elevated C-reactive protein, are common. These constitutional symptoms and laboratory findings are not related to tumor size or location.

Diagnosis

Echocardiography is the imaging modality of choice for diagnosis of myxomas. Tumor location and characteristics can be delineated by two-dimensional (2D) transthoracic echocardiography. Transesophageal echo may be used to further characterize the tumor.[35,36] The echocardiographic appearance of myxomas is usually distinctive, but other causes of intracardiac masses must be included in the differential diagnosis. In cases of diagnostic uncertainty, magnetic resonance imaging (MRI) and computed tomography (CT) may be helpful. Final diagnosis is confirmed by pathological examination.

Management

Surgical resection is the mainstay of treatment. The intracardiac mass is excised after establishing cardiopulmonary bypass and cardioplegic arrest. Bicaval cannulation is employed for venous return. Great care must be taken to minimize manipulation of the heart before cross-clamping the aorta to minimize the risk of tumor embolism. A variety of approaches are available for resection of left atrial tumors. Our preference is to approach them through a lateral, longitudinal incision in the left atrium. In cases where visualization is difficult, additional incisions in the right atrium and septum are employed.

The tumor is resected en bloc. Tumors that arise from a relatively well-defined pedicle can be excised without the need for full-thickness excision of a button of atrial wall. However, many surgeons prefer to excise a portion of the atrial wall, especially if the tumor arises from the interatrial septum or is relatively broad based. Tumors of the ventricle

Table 99–3

Metastatic Neoplasms of the Heart at Necropsy Order of Frequency of Cancers Encountered

Primary tumor	*Total autopsies*	*Metastases to heart*
Lung	1037	180 (17%)
Breast	685	70 (10%
Lymphoma	392	67 (17%)
Leukemia	202	66 (33%)
Esophagus	294	37 (13%)
Uterus	451	36 (8%)
Melanoma	69	32 (46%)
Stomach	603	28 (5%)
Sarcoma	159	24 (15%)
Oral cavity and tongue	235	22 (9%)
Colon and rectum	440	22 (5%)
Kidney	114	12 (11%)
Thyroid gland	97	9 (9%)
Larynx	100	9 (9%)
Germ cell	21	8 (28%)
Urinary bladder	128	8 (6%)
Liver and biliary tract	325	7 (2%)
Prostate gland	171	6 (4%)
Pancreas	185	6 (3%)
Ovary	188	2 (1%)
Nose (interior)	32	1 (3%)
Pharynx	67	1 (1%)
Miscellaneous	245	0
Total	6240	653 (10%)

From Roberts WC: Primary and secondary neoplasms of the heart. Am J Cardiol 80:671–682, 1997. Modified from Burke A, Virmani R (who combined studies of McAllister HA and Feoglio JJ Jr: Tumors of the cardiovascular system. In Atlas of Tumor Pathology, 2nd series, Fascicle 15, p. 111. Washington, DC: Armed Forces Institute of Pathology, 1978; and Mukai K, Shinkai T, Tominaga K, et al: The incidence of secondary tumors of the heart and pericardium: A 10-year study. Jpn N Clin Oncol 18:195, 1988).

may be resected without additional full-thickness excision of a portion of ventricular wall. Tumors arising from an atrioventricular valve usually can be resected without the need for valve replacement. Regardless of the site of origin, the atrioventricular valve in proximity to the tumor should be inspected for evidence of damage.

The results of surgical excision are good with a low risk of morbidity and mortality (0–3%).[16,28,46] Recurrence of atrial myxomas is infrequent. Sporadic myxomas recur in 1–3% of patients at an average of 2.5 years after surgery.[33] The risk of recurrence of familial myxomas ranges from 12–20%.[33,51] Therefore regular echocardiographic follow-up is recommended in the latter group. When myxomas recur, they should be resected.

Other Primary Benign Tumors

Rhabdomyoma

Rhabdomyoma is the most common cardiac tumor in children and the second most common benign cardiac tumor overall.[32] Most occur in children less than 1 year of age. Rhabdomyoma is a benign tumor composed of cardiac myocytes. About one half of patients with rhabdomyoma have tuberous sclerosis, and about one half of patients with tuberous sclerosis develop rhabdomyomas.[10] These tumors also occur sporadically or in conjunction with other rare congenital heart malformations.

Rhabdomyomas usually are found deep in the myocardium; they may extend into the cardiac chambers. They are of variable size, ranging from 1 mm to several centimeters. More than 90% of rhabdomyomas are multicentric. They invariably involve the ventricles. Most involve the left ventricle, and more than 80% involve the right

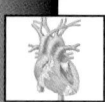

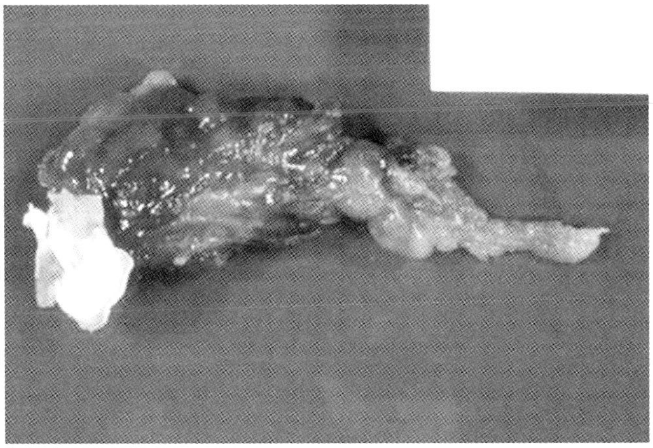

Figure 99-1 Pedunculated atrial myxoma with atrial tissue at base.

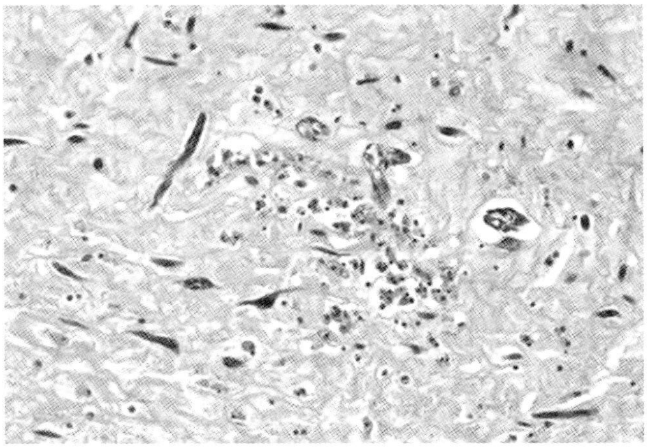

Figure 99-2 Hematoxylin and eosin (H & E) stain of myxoma. (See color plate.)

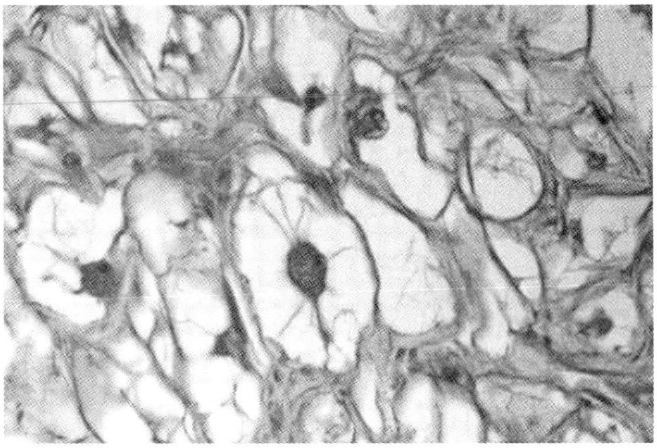

Figure 99-3 Rhabdomyoma spider cell. (See color plate.)

ventricle as well. Because of their morphological appearance and multicentric nature, rhabdomyomas are considered to be hamartomas rather than true tumors.[5] Pathologically they are distinguishable from the surrounding myocardium by their firm, gray, nodular characteristics.[8] Histological examination usually reveals classic "spider cells," which are glycogen-filled bodies with myofibrils extending radially from the nucleus to the periphery (Figure 99-3).[18,31] The specific cell type that gives rise to the tumor is still debated.[6,18]

Most children with rhabdomyomas display cardiac arrhythmias or obstructive symptoms in the first few days or weeks of life. Rhabdomyomas causing significant intracardiac obstruction to blood flow can result in death within 24 hours of birth; patients with less severe disease may be asymptomatic for years. The diagnosis is usually made by echocardiography. One of the curiosities of this tumor is the well-documented tendency for these tumors to regress.[1,2] Regression may be complete or partial. Smaller tumors in younger patients are most likely to regress.[8]

In most cases these tumors are not resected. Surgical resection is reserved for masses that cause significant cardiac obstruction.[12,19] Given the multicentricity of these lesions and their limited growth potential, the operative approach is conservative debulking, with the goal being relief of outflow obstruction with preservation of electrical conduction, and myocardial and valvular function. Occasionally, if a persistent, severe arrhythmia is present, preoperative endocardial mapping followed by tumor resection is performed.[15,23]

Fibroma

Cardiac fibromas are benign, rare tumors that occur predominantly in the pediatric age group. Like rhabdomyomas, fibromas are usually intramural tumors. However, unlike rhabdomyomas, they tend to present as solitary nodules rather than as multiple tumors. They are typically firm, gray nodules composed primarily of fibroblasts and collagen. They may contain calcific deposits.[17] The tumors are not encapsulated and may infiltrate the normal myocardium.[20] Cardiac fibromas average 5 cm in size.[20]

Typically children with cardiac fibromas have presenting symptoms of congestive heart failure, murmurs, or arrhythmias. Given the size of these tumors, an enlarged cardiac silhouette with an irregular border is often apparent on chest X-ray. The presence and location of the tumor can be confirmed by echocardiography. The infiltrative growth patterns of cardiac fibromas make them discernible from rhabdomyomas when imaged by MRI.

These tumors are bulky and have a predilection to grow. Spontaneous regression of this tumor has not been confirmed as it has for rhabdomyomas. Therefore complete surgical resection is indicated in most cases to prevent progressive heart failure.

Lipoma and Lipomatous Hypertrophy of the Interatrial Septum

Lipomas are encapsulated masses of adipose tissue that usually arise from the myocardium or pericardium.[32] Lipomas have also been reported on cardiac valves, where they simulate vegetations or myxomas.[13] They are usually small but can grow to be massive. Lipomas involving the pericardium may be mistaken for pericardial cysts and may be associated with pericardial effusions. Although most of these tumors are identified after death, they may be diagnosed by echocardiography and MRI. Most cardiac lipomas can be observed. However, lipomas causing obstructive symptoms or arrhythmias should be resected.

Lipomatous hypertrophy of the interatrial septum is a nonneoplastic condition of the heart. It is caused by fatty infiltration of the interatrial septum. It is a common, nonencapsulated lesion that occurs almost exclusively in obese people over 50 years of age.[44] These lesions can cause cardiac arrhythmias. The treatment of this condition is weight loss, not surgical resection.

Papillary Fibroelastoma

Papillary fibroelastomas are uncommon tumors of the heart. They are the most common tumors affecting cardiac valves.[14,41] They usually involve the valves of the left side of the heart.[11] Recently the second case of a pulmonary valve papillary fibroelastoma was reported.[42] In general these are tumors of adulthood. Although papillary fibroelastomas usually are asymptomatic, when symptoms occur, they are most frequently related to embolization. The tumors are identified by echocardiography. Surgical excision is advised, even in asymptomatic patients.[14,22,49]

Hemangioma

Cardiac hemangiomas are rare.[4] They can cause dyspnea and arrhythmias. They often are visualized as an abnormal blush on coronary angiography; resectability can be assessed by echocardiography, CT scan, and MRI. Surgical resection should be reserved for patients who are symptomatic. Surgical resection can resolve symptoms, even when complete excision is not possible. These tumors have been reported to resolve spontaneously.

MALIGNANT PRIMARY CARDIAC TUMORS

Angiosarcoma

Most malignant cardiac tumors are metastases from other malignancies.[37] Almost all primary malignant tumors of the heart are sarcomas[40]; angiosarcoma is the most common malignant primary cardiac tumor.[32] Angiosarcomas are usually solitary, large bulky masses that originate in the right atrium (Figure 99-4). They may extend into the right atrial cavity, causing valvular obstruction, right-sided heart failure, or hemorrhagic pericardial effusion with tamponade.[40] Most of these tumors metastasize, most commonly to the lung, liver, or brain.[48] Angiosarcomas are very aggressive, and survival after diagnosis ranges from 3–15 months.[4] Given their rapid growth and poor prognosis, surgical resection is rarely successful.

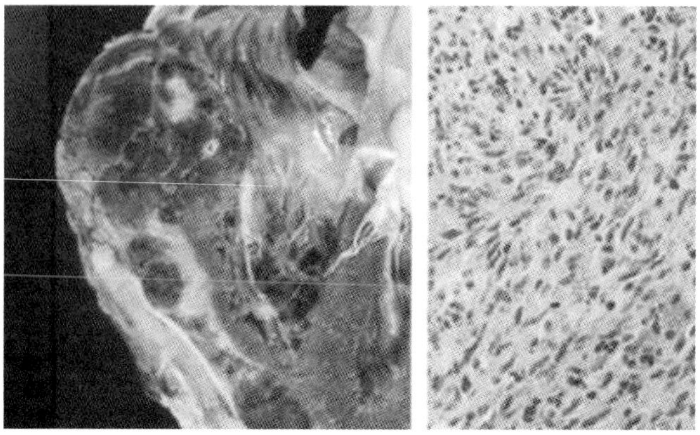

Figure 99–4 Angiosarcoma. (See color plate.)

Rhabdomyosarcoma

Rhabdomyosarcoma is the second most common cardiac sarcoma. Like angiosarcoma, it is more common in men.[26,29,44] Unlike angiosarcoma, rhabdomyosarcoma does not have a predilection for a particular cardiac chamber.[32] It may occur at multiple sites and extend into the pericardium. Patients may have cardiac obstructive or constitutional symptoms. Prognosis is poor, and surgical resection is usually ineffective.

Miscellaneous

Other uncommon primary cardiac malignancies include fibrosarcoma, liposarcoma, mesothelioma, lymphoma, leiomyosarcoma, and other rare sarcomas of varying cell types. These tumors may cause obstructive symptoms. Palliative surgery is sometimes indicated, but patients usually succumb to the malignancy. Primary lymphoma of the heart can be treated with radiotherapy and chemotherapy.[9,47]

SECONDARY CARDIAC TUMORS: METASTASES TO THE HEART

Metastatic tumors to the heart, or secondary tumors, are much more common than are primary cardiac tumors. Secondary tumors are usually carcinomas rather than sarcomas because of the relative frequency of these cancers.[40] Hematogenous spread is the most common mode of metastasis, but lymphatic spread and direct extension also occur. The pericardium is much more commonly involved than is the myocardium. Of patients with disseminated cancer, 10–20% develop cardiac involvement. However, only about 10% of these patients develop symptoms referable to cardiac metastases.[40] Symptoms occur most commonly in patients with pericardial metastases rather than intramural or intracavitary involvement. The symptoms associated with metastases are congestive heart failure and arrhythmias. Metastases to the heart should be suspected in patients with known neoplasms who develop congestive heart failure.

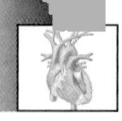

Carcinoma of the lung and breast may directly invade the parietal and visceral pericardium, causing myocardial restriction and pericardial effusion.[40] Melanoma commonly metastasizes to the myocardium, as does leukemia and lymphoma. The treatment of metastatic tumors depends on the tumor type and symptoms. Given the late stage at which cardiac metastases occur and the poor prognosis, few of these patients are candidates for cardiac surgical intervention. Lymphoma and leukemia may respond to chemotherapy or radiotherapy. Symptomatic malignant pericardial effusions may be drained by creation of a pericardial window.

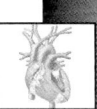

REFERENCES

1. Alakay AL, Ferry DA, Lin B, et al: Spontaneous regression of cardiac rhabdomyoma in tuberous sclerosis. Clin Pediatr 26:532, 1987.
2. Beghetti M, Gow RM, Haney I, et al: Pediatric primary benign cardiac tumors: A 15-year review. Am Heart J 134:1107, 1997.
3. Bortolotti V, Maraglino G, Rubino M, et al: Surgical excision of intracardiac myxomas: A 20-year follow-up. Ann Thorac Surg 49:449–453, 1990.
4. Brizzard C, Latremoville C, Jebara VA, et al: Cardiac hemangiomas. Ann Thorac Surg 36:484, 1993.
5. Bruni C, Prioleau PG, Ivey HH, et al: New fine structural features of cardiac rhabdomyoma: A case report. Cancer 46:2068, 1980.
6. Burke A, Virmani R: Tumors of the heart and great vessels. In Atlas of Tumor Pathology, 3rd series, Fascicle 16, p. 231. Washington, DC: Armed Forces Institute of Pathology, 1996.
7. Carney JA, Hruska LS, Beauchamp GD, et al: Dominant inheritance of the complex of myxomas, spotty pigmentation, and endocrine overactivity. Mayo Clin Proc 61:165–172, 1986.
8. Choi JY, Bae EJ, Noh CI, et al: Cardiac rhabdomyoma in childhood tuberous sclerosis. Cardiol Young 5:166, 1995.
9. Chou ST, Arkles LB, Gill GD: Primary lymphoma of the heart: A case report. Cancer 52:744, 1983.
10. Corno A, de Simone G, Catena G, et al: Cardiac rhabdomyoma: Surgical treatment in the neonate. J Thorac Cardiovasc Surg 87:725, 1984.
11. Darvishian F, Farmer P: Papillary fibroelastoma of the heart: Report of two cases and a review of the literature. Ann Clin Lab Sci 31:291, 2001.
12. DeLoma JG, Villagra F, DeLeon JP, et al: Rhabdomyoma of the heart: Surgical treatment. J Cardiovasc Surg 23:149, 1982.
13. Dollar AL, Wallace RB, Kent KM, et al: Mitral valve replacement for mitral lipoma associated with severe obesity. Am J Cardiol 64:1405, 1989.
14. Edwards FH, Hale D, Cohen A, et al: Primary cardiac valve tumors. Ann Thorac Surg 52:1127, 1991.
15. Engle MA, Ebert PA, Redo SF: Recurrent ventricular tachycardia due to resectable cardiac tumor: Report of two cases in two-year-olds in heart failure. Circulation 50:1052, 1974.
16. Fang BR, Vhiang CW, Hung JS, et al: Cardiac myxoma-clinical experience in 24 patients. Int J Cardiol 29:335–341, 1990.
17. Feldman PS, Meyer MW: Fibroelastic hamartoma (fibroma) of the heart. Cancer 30:314, 1976.
18. Fenoglio JJ, McAllister HA, Ferrans VJ: Cardiac rhabdomyoma: A clinicopathologic and electron microscopic study. Am J Cardiol 38:241, 1976.
19. Foster ED, Spooner EW, Farina MA, et al: Cardiac rhabdomyoma in the neonate: Surgical management. Ann Thorac Surg 37:249, 1984.
20. Freedom RM, Lee K-J, MacDonald C, et al: Selected aspects of cardiac tumors in infancy and childhood. Pediatr Cardiol 21:299, 2000.
21. Fyke FE, Seward JB, Miller FA, et al: Primary cardiac tumors: Experience with 30 consecutive patients since introduction of two-dimensional echocardiography. J Am Coll Cardiol 5:1465, 1985.
22. Gallo R, Kumar N, Prabhakar G, et al: Papillary fibroelastoma of mitral valve chordae. Ann Thorac Surg 55:1156, 1993.
23. Goldman S, Lortscher R, Pappas G: Surgical treatment of rhabdomyoma of the right atrium causing arrhythmias. J Thorac Cardiovasc Surg 89:802, 1985.
24. Goodwin JF: Diagnosis of the left atrial myxoma. Lancet 1:464–468, 1963.
25. Goodwin JF: The spectrum of cardiac tumors. Am J Cardiol 21:307, 1968.
26. Hajar R, Roberts WC, Folger GM Jr: Embryonal botryoid rhabdomyosarcoma of the mitral valve. Am J Cardiol 57:376, 1986.
27. Hall RJ, Cooley DA, McAllister HA, et al: Neoplastic heart disease. In Hurst JW, editor: The Heart, Arteries, and Veins, 7th ed., pp. 1382–1403. New York: McGraw-Hill, 1990.
28. Hanson EC, Gill CC, Razavi M, et al: The surgical treatment of atrial myxomas: Clinical experience and late results in 33 patients. J Thorac Cardiovasc Surg 89:298–303, 1985.
29. Hui KS, Green LK, Schmidt WA: Primary cardiac rhabdomyosarcoma: Definition of a rare entity. Am J Cardiovasc Pathol 2:19, 1988.
30. Lam KY, Dickens P, Chan ACL: Tumors of the heart. A 20-year experience with review of 12485 consecutive autopsies. Arch Pathol Med 117:1027–1031, 1993.
31. Landing BH, Farger S: Tumors of the cardiovascular system. In Atlas of Tumor Pathology, Sec. III, Fascicle 7. Washington, DC: U.S. War Department, 1956.
32. McAllister HA Jr, Fenoglio JJ Jr: Tumors of the cardiovascular system. In Atlas of Tumor Pathology, 2nd series, Fascicle 15, pp. 1-20. Washington, DC: Armed Forces Institute of Pathology, 1978.
33. McCarthy PM, Piehler JM, Schaff HV, et al: The significance of multiple, recurrent, "complex" cardiac myxomas. J Thorac Cardiovasc Surg 91:389, 1986.
34. Meller J, Teichholz LE, Pickard AD: Left ventricular myxoma: Echocardiographic diagnosis and review of the literature. Am J Med 63:816, 1977.
35. Mugge A, Daniel WG, Haverich A, et al: Diagnosis of noninfective cardiac mass lesions by two-dimensional echocardiography: Comparison of transthoracic and transesophageal approaches. Circulation 83:70–78, 1991.
36. Obeid AI, Marvasti M, Parker F, et al: Comparison of transthoracic and transesophageal echocardiography in the diagnosis of left atrial myxoma. Am J Cardiol 63:1006–1008, 1989.
37. Prichard RW: Tumors of the heart: Review of the subject and report of one hundred and fifty cases. Arch Pathol 51:98–128, 1951.
38. Reynen K: Cardiac myxomas. N Engl J Med 333(24): 1610–1617, 1995.
39. Reynen K: Frequency of primary tumors of the heart. Am J Cardiol 77:107, 1996.
40. Roberts WC: Primary and secondary neoplasms of the heart. Am J Cardiol 80:671–682, 1997.
41. Ryan PE, Obeid AI, Parker FB Jr: Primary cardiac valve tumors. J Heart Valve Dis 4:222, 1995.
42. Saad RS, Galvis CO, Bshara W, et al: Pulmonary valve papillary fibroelastoma: A case report and review of the literature. Arch Pathol Lab Med 125:933, 2001.
43. Shapiro LM: Cardiac tumours: Diagnosis and management. Heart 85(2):218–222, 2001.
44. Shirani J, Roberts WC: Clinical, electrocardiographic, and morphologic features of massive fatty deposits ("lipomatous hypertrophy") in the atrial septum. J Am Coll Cardiol 22:226, 1993.
45. Shrivastava S, Jacks JJ, White RS, et al: Diffuse rhabdomyatosis of the heart. Arch Pathol Lab Med 101:78, 1977.

46. St John Sutton MG, Mercier L-A, Giuliani ER, et al: Atrial myxomas: A review of clinical experience in 40 patients. Mayo Clin Proc 55:371–376, 1980.
47. Takagi M, Kugimiya T, Fukii T, et al: Extensive surgery for primary malignant lymphoma. J Thorac Cardiovasc Surg 33:570, 1992.
48. Thomas CR, Johnson GW, Stoddard MF, et al: Primary malignant cardiac tumors: Update 1992. Med Pediatr Oncol 20:519, 1992.
49. Topol EJ, Biern RO, Reitz BA: Cardiac papillary fibroelastoma and stroke: Echocardiographic diagnosis and guide to excision. Am J Med 80:129, 1986.
50. Vaughan CJ, Veugelers M, Basson CT: Tumors and the heart: Molecular genetic advances. Curr Op Cardiol 16:195–200, 2001.
51. Waller DA, Ettles DF, Saunders NR, et al: Recurrent cardiac myxoma: The surgical implications of two distinct groups of patients. Thorac Cardiovasc Surg 37:226–230, 1989.

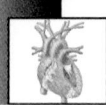

Congenital heart surgery

SECTION 3

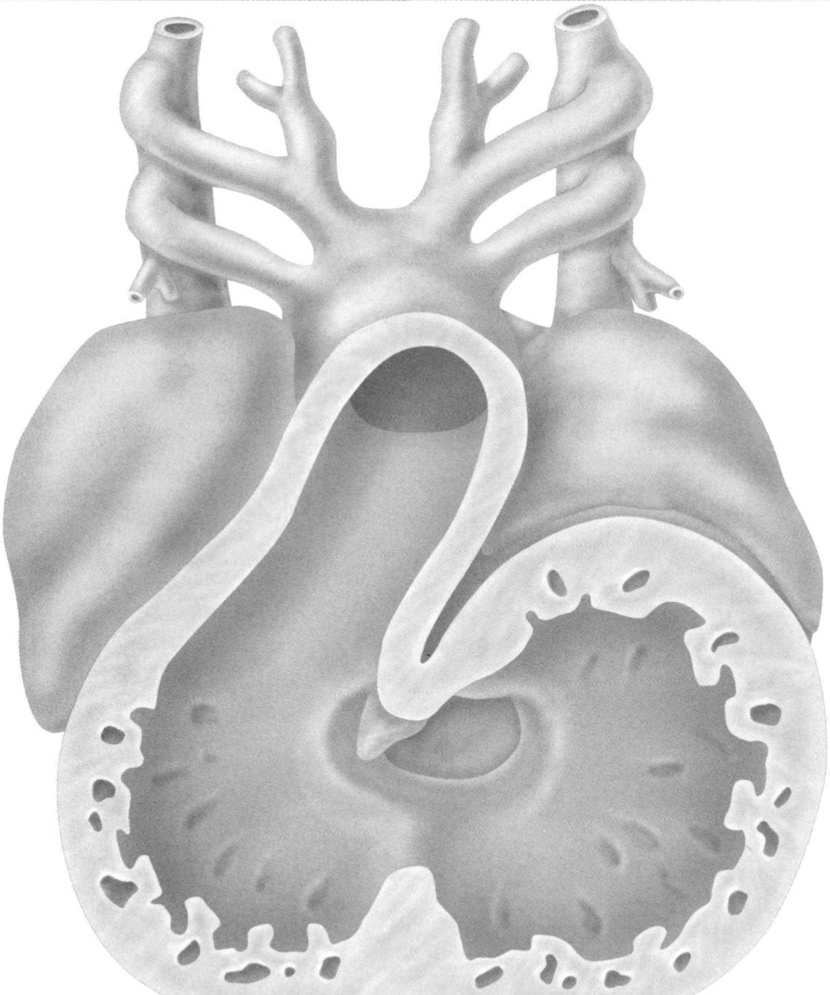

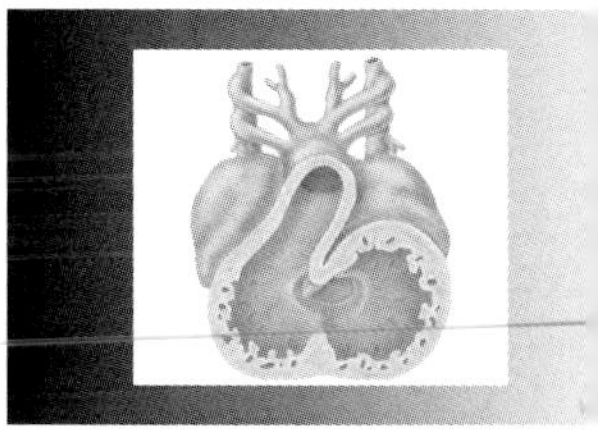

Cardiac Embryology and Genetics

Ivan P. Moskowitz and Amy L. Juraszek

CHAPTER 100

INTRODUCTION

The heart is the first functional organ to develop in the mammalian embryo. The developmental mechanisms responsible for cardiovascular morphogenesis have been the basis for study by classical embryologists for centuries and by molecular developmental biologists more recently. Major progress in our understanding of cardiac specification and morphogenesis has been obtained from the study of cardiovascular development in a number of invertebrate and vertebrate model systems, from *Drosophila* to mouse. The conservation of many aspects of heart development across phylogeny has provided the basis for our increased understanding of the underlying principles of cardiac development, and how congenital defects of the heart arise when development goes awry. Congenital heart malformations have long been recognized to be the result of developmental abnormalities affecting cardiac morphogenesis. Developmental defects can occur at any stage of heart development, resulting in phenotypes that vary widely, from severe morphological abnormalities resulting in early embryonic lethality to mild defects having little physiological impact. Given the rapid rate of information entering the field of cardiac embryology and the scope of this chapter, detailed genetic descriptions of specific morphogenetic events will not be discussed. Instead, illustrative examples are given to provide the reader with an understanding of current paradigms in the field. For the purposes of a cardiothoracic surgery textbook, greater detail is paid to developmental abnormalities of the heart that result in congenital heart defects in humans.

CARDIAC SPECIFICATION

Early in embryonic development, after gastrulation at approximately day 20 in human development, cells in the lateral mesoderm adopt a cardiogenic fate. The commitment of progenitor cells in the anterior left and right lateral plate mesoderm to the cardiogenic fate relies on inductive signals from the adjacent endoderm.[21,79,89] Specifically, the bone morphogenetic proteins (BMPs) expressed in the endoderm adjacent to the cardiogenic precursors play a role in cardiac induction and act with other signaling factors, including those from the fibroblast growth factor (FGF) family.[2,71,78,79] In vertebrates the heart-forming region is bounded by repressive signals in addition to inductive signals. Repressive signals include members of the *wnt* family of secreted molecules. Within the cardiogenic region, *wnt* antagonists oppose the repressive signals, allowing cells to commit to a cardiogenic fate.[57,76,96]

Several lines of evidence suggest that cardiogenic precursors within the lateral plate mesoderm contain prepatterned information regarding their ultimate positional identity and cell fate (Figure 100-1A). Lineage analysis has demonstrated that cells in the caudal cardiogenic mesoderm contribute to the atria, whereas cells in the rostral cardiogenic mesoderm contribute to the ventricles.[88] Explant experiments also demonstrate phenotypic differences between rostral and caudal precardiac mesoderm.[20,98] However, cell transplant experiments also demonstrate that rostral–caudal fates of cardiogenic precursors remain plastic and require instructive cues from outside the cardiogenic region.[31] Taken together, these results suggest that regional positional information is prepatterned within cardiogenic precursors before the development of the linear heart tube but that these positional identities appear not to be fixed until later. Several recent studies suggest that cell-type specification information, in addition to positional information, already resides within the field of cardiac progenitors. For example, precursors of both myocardial and endocardial cells can be found in the cardiogenic mesoderm, but no bipotential precursor has been identified.[13,94]

The definitive heart and associated vascular structures receive contributions not only from the precardiac mesoderm that forms the cardiac crescent, but also from

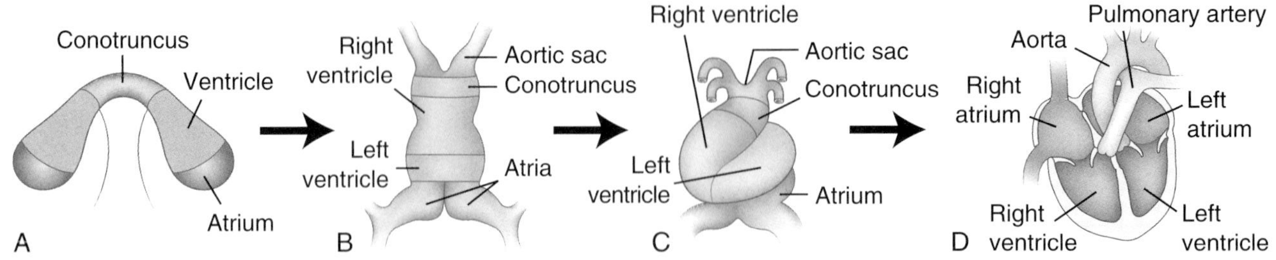

Figure 100–1 Model of cardiogenesis. **(A)** Cardiogenic precursors bilaterally positioned within the lateral plate mesoderm contain prepatterned information regarding their ultimate positional identity and cell fate, as modeled by color code. The convergence and fusion of the cardiac primordia form a linear heart tube **(B),** which undergoes rightward- or D-looping **(C).** **(D)** Rightward looping appropriately aligns the cardiac chambers for morphogenesis into the mature four-chambered structure. *(Modified from Moss and Adams, 6th ed., chapter 1, p. 4, figure 1.1.)*

two additional populations of cells. An "anterior heart-forming field" that lies adjacent to the crescent on its medial aspect has been identified and contributes to anterior structures of the outflow tract, as well as to the myocardial mass of the ventricles.[34,61,103] In addition, the neural crest, a population of multipotential migratory cells, contributes to the outflow tract of the heart and is specifically required for outflow tract septation.

Bilaterally symmetrical cardiogenic primordia are formed from the lateral fields of mesoderm in the early embryo. The convergence and fusion of the bilateral cardiac primordia form the primitive cardiac tube in the ventral midline (Figure 100-1B). The anterior margins of the cardiogenic mesoderm fuse first to form the cardiac crescent at approximately day 23 of human development.[19]

Fusion of the bilateral cardiac primordia then occurs in a rostral to caudal direction, with sequential addition of precardiac mesoderm at the caudal end of the developing heart tube.[20,67,74] The result is the formation of the primitive linear heart tube. The linear heart tube, already containing distinct myocardial and endocardial layers, initiates contractions at approximately 4 weeks of fetal development in humans. Morphological and molecular polarity along the heart tube (the anteroposterior axis) exists with distinct regions from anterior to posterior of the aortic sac, conotruncus, right ventricle, left ventricle, and atria (see Figure 100-1B).[12,33,70]

▸ BODY-PLAN LATERALITY AND CARDIAC LOOPING

The tubular heart undergoes a morphogenetic process of rightward looping in all vertebrates. During this process, the linear heart tube is converted into an S-shaped heart with a complex three-dimensional structure and asymmetry about the anterior–posterior, left–right, and dorsal–ventral axes (Figure 100-1C). Rightward looping is the visible start to the morphogenetic process that results in an asymmetrical, multichambered heart. The specificity of rightward looping is essential for the appropriate orientation of the developing cardiac chambers with one another, with the endocardial cushions that contribute to chamber septation, and with inflow and outflow vascular connections.

Rightward looping of the heart is the first visible indication of left–right asymmetry in the developing vertebrate body plan. The consistent directionality of this process suggests a highly conserved molecular control mechanism. Recent progress has been made in the molecular understanding of left–right patterning in the vertebrate embryo. This work demonstrates that significant molecular left–right differences are present in the embryo long before the visible morphogenetic event of rightward heart looping.

Early in embryonic development, during establishment of the lateral plate mesoderm, Hensen's node appears to control the genesis of left–right differences in gene expression despite its midline position. Beating cilia that project from the node undergo a counterclockwise vortexlike movement. Elegant studies in the mouse have demonstrated that the unidirectional beating of the cilia creates a leftward flow of fluid across Hensen's node. The unidirectional ciliary movement appears to be established by the inherent molecular chirality of the ciliary protein machinery and its molecular motor on the node.[64,65,93] The flow across the node may mediate the movement of secreted molecules across the node in a leftward direction. Such molecules could then function as left-sided determinants on the left side of the node. Alternatively, evenly distributed mechanosensory cilia may be specifically activated on the left side of the node by the fluid flow across the node (reviewed in Tabin and Vogan, 2003).[92] The resultant signal transduction downstream of the activated mechanosensory cilia in left-sided cells could then initiate a left-sided molecular cascade.

A molecular cascade for left–right determination has been identified, beginning with asymmetrical expression of the morphogen Sonic Hedgehog (Shh) on the left side of the node (Figure 100-2). Shh is able to induce left-sided perinodal expression of the left-sided determinant Nodal, a member of the transforming growth factor-β (TGF-β) signaling family.[46,66] The molecular ground state of laterality in fact appears to be "right-sidedness," with the expression of the Nodal normally repressed by BMP signaling. Shh induces the left-sided expression of Caronte, a secreted molecule, which overcomes BMP-mediated repression of Nodal in the lateral plate mesoderm.[72,108,110] Thus left-sided Shh results in the expression of Nodal locally and at a distance, and left-sided positional information is transferred to the left lateral plate mesoderm. One result of left-sided Nodal expression is the left-sided induction of Pitx2, a homeodomain-containing protein, throughout the left lateral plate mesoderm (see Figure 100-2). Pitx2 expression is maintained during subsequent organogenesis on the left side of the developing heart tube, gut,

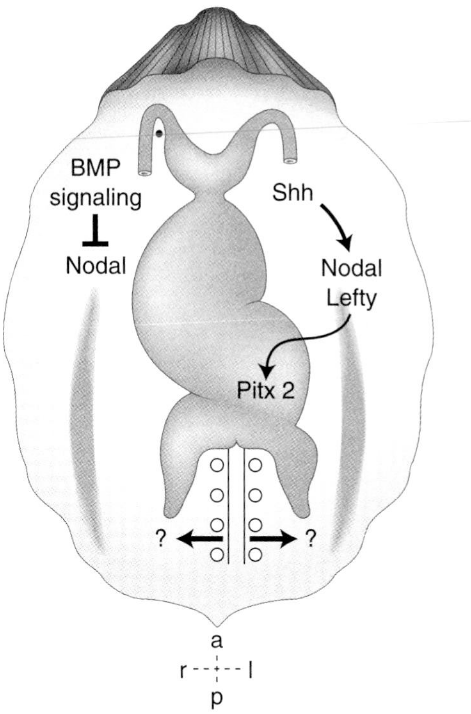

Figure 100–2 Molecular determination of the direction of cardiac looping. Summary of the molecular signaling pathways implicated in visceral left–right axis determination and right-handed cardiac looping.
(Modified from Moss and Adams, 6th ed., chapter 1, p. 9, figure 1.5.)

and lungs.* This cascade thereby transmits left-sided positional information from Hensen's node to the visceral organs.

Clinical Correlates of Abnormal Laterality: Heterotaxy Syndrome

The molecular hierarchy of left–right positional information establishes global left–right differences within the vertebrate body plan. Defects in the proper establishment of left–right differences of the visceral organs are generally known as heterotaxy syndrome (derived from the Greek, meaning "other arrangement"). Situs abnormalities can be grouped into distinct types of heterotaxy syndromes. Often the clinical phenotype reveals a predominance of one side. In simple terms, asplenia syndrome can be thought of as demonstrating a bilateral "right-sidedness" and polysplenia syndrome can be thought of as demonstrating bilateral "left-sidedness." The term *situs ambiguus* is used if the sidedness cannot be determined. Not surprisingly, mutations in the genes known to have a function in the normal establishment of left–right difference can result in heterotaxy syndrome, both in animal models and in human patients.[42]

Establishment of left–right asymmetry about Hensen's node has been demonstrated to require the *inversus viscerum (iv)* gene, encoding left–right dynein, the force-generating component in the cilia responsible for the vertical flow across the node. Mutation in *iv,* or other genes that contribute components to the functional ciliary motor, cause immotile cilia syndrome and a failure to generate the initial left–right asymmetry within Hensen's node.[90,91] Absence of asymmetry about the node results in randomized expression of left-sided determinants Nodal and Pitx2 in the lateral plate mesoderm.[10,68,75,91] The phenotypical result of the failure to generate the appropriate vector for laterality information is randomization of left- and right-sidedness within the visceral organs.

Mutations in single genes therefore can result in both polysplenia and asplenia syndromes, previously thought to be distinct entities and therefore having distinct etiologies. The finding that expression of left-sided determinants *Nodal* and *Pitx2* are randomized in these cases helps to explain the variability of defects seen in the heterotaxy syndromes. For example, *Pitx2* expression can be normal, presumably resulting in situs solitus, or reversed, presumably resulting in situs inversus (the left–right mirror image specification of the visceral organs).[14,55,59] However, it can also be bilateral, absent, or a range of relative left–right levels in between.[55] This range is similar to the wide range of situs abnormalities of the visceral organs observed in this model and in human patients with situs ambiguus. It also may help explain why previous efforts to categorize the specific morphology of heart defects in cases with asplenia and polysplenia have proven so difficult.[99]

The molecular hierarchy of left–right positional information establishes global left–right differences within the vertebrate body plan. The vertebrate heart has distinct left–right asymmetry, seen not only in its characteristic rightward-looping morphogenesis, but also in the resulting morphological, molecular, and physiological differences between its right and left sides. The process of rightward cardiac looping establishes the relative positions of the chambers of the developing heart and their vascular connections. The developing heart must therefore be able to interpret and act on asymmetrical left–right positional cues as they are established in the lateral mesoderm as a whole, as described in the preceding. The heart is therefore especially sensitive to alterations in the normal patterning of left–right differences. Cardiac malformations, especially routing abnormalities such as transposition of the great arteries (TGA) or double outlet right ventricle (DORV), are particularly common in heterotaxy cases. At this time, little is known about the molecules responsible for the specific transduction of left–right signaling information from the lateral plate mesoderm to the developing heart. However, recent work has identified some genes required for the generation of chamber-specific molecular differences within the developing heart.

CHAMBER SPECIFICATION AND THE CARDIOGENIC TRANSCRIPTIONAL PROGRAM

There is remarkable conservation of the early transcriptional hierarchy that specifies the cardiogenic fate between animal models as disparate as *Drosophila* and vertebrates. The *tinman* gene, encoding a homeodomain-containing transcription factor, is required for formation of the *Drosophila* dorsal vessel (the dorsal vessel in the fly is the analogue of the heart in vertebrates). Tinman directly activates transcription of several genes, including *pannier,* a GATA

*References 10, 25, 54, 68, 75, 80, 109.

transcription factor, and *Myocyte enhancer factor-2* (*Mef 2*), a MAD box containing transcription factor. MEF2 and Pannier then contribute to the downstream transcriptional activation of cardiomyocyte structural genes.[6,27,28,49]

Nkx2.5 is the vertebrate orthologue of the *Drosophila tinman* gene. *Nkx2.5* is expressed early in the cardiogenic mesoderm, in part a response to induction of the heart-forming region by BMPs from the endoderm.[41,48,53] Like Tinman in *Drosophila,* the NKX2-5 transcription factor plays a role in cardiogenic differentiation in vertebrates. NKX2-5 physically interacts with vertebrate GATA factors, and these transcription factors mutually activate each other's promoters. This establishes a positive molecular feedback loop that appears to strengthen the choice of "cardiomyocyte" fate. As in *Drosophila,* the GATA and MEF2 gene families have been demonstrated to play a role in the activation of a cardiomyocyte differentiation program throughout the myocardium. In vertebrates, three GATA family members, GATA-4, GATA-5, and GATA-6—demonstrate expression in cardiac lineages (reviewed in Reference 16). GATA factors are required for transcriptional control of several cardiac muscle structural genes. GATA family members act in cooperation with transcription factors from other families, including NKX2-5 and MEF2 to regulate the expression of target genes.[22,45,82] There are four MEF2 family members in vertebrates. As in *Drosophila,* these genes appear to directly activate structural genes of myocyte differentiation. For example, mice lacking the gene for one family member, *mef 2a,* die with cardiovascular abnormalities at the looping stage and fail to express a group of muscle-specific structural genes.[50,51]

NKX2-5 has roles in both cardiogenic differentiation and pattern formation of the vertebrate heart. The multifaceted nature of its action perhaps results from its promiscuous interactions with transcription factors of other classes. Aside from the GATA class of transcription factors, NKX2-5 is able to physically interact with the T-box transcription factor TBX-5. The *Tbx-5* gene is responsible for the human autosomal dominant disorder Holt–Oram syndrome. Cardiac manifestations of the loss of one copy of *Tbx-5* or *Nkx2-5* overlap and include atrial septal defects and conduction system abnormalities. NKX2-5 and TBX-5 have been shown to act synergistically on the promoters of genes with high levels of expression in the atria and the conduction system, including *atrial natriuretic factor* and *connexin 40*.[7,23]

Concomitant with the activation of a cardiomyocyte differentiation program is the development of regional differences between the chambers of the heart. As early as the tubular heart stage, the cardiac primordia demonstrate a segmental appearance. Morphologically, five primordial segments can be identified from posterior to anterior: sinus venosus/atrium, atrioventricular canal, left ventricle, right ventricle, and outflow tract (see Figure 100-1B). These morphologically distinct regions must be indicative of distinct transcriptional domains within the developing heart primordia. In fact, a growing number of transcription factors have been identified that demonstrate chamber-specific patterns of transcription.

The chamber-specific expression patterns of the Iroquois family member Irx4, a homeobox-encoding gene, suggested a role in ventricular versus atrial chamber specification. Irx4 is expressed specifically in the developing ventricular chambers of the heart and is excluded from the developing atria.[3] Irx4 has been demonstrated to play an important transcriptional role in the selection of ventricular fate. Loss of Irx4 function in the ventricles results in aberrant activation of atrial gene expression, whereas ectopic expression of Irx4 in atrial chambers results in the aberrant activation of ventricular gene expression. Further evidence for the separate genetic control of atrial and ventricular fate is demonstrated by the zebrafish mutants *lonely atrium* and *pandora,* in which the ventricular chamber fails to form but the atrial chamber appears morphologically intact.[11,87]

The β helix-loop-helix factors dHAND and eHAND have been demonstrated to play a role in determining molecular differences between the ventricles. The chamber-specific expression of the β helix-loop-helix factors dHAND and eHAND suggest that these genes may play a role in right versus left ventricular chamber specification. Although dHAND and eHAND are initially coexpressed throughout the precardiac mesoderm, dHAND expression becomes restricted to the right ventricular precursors during cardiac looping, whereas eHAND becomes restricted to left ventricular and conotruncal precursors.[84,85] Functional analysis of *dhand* has demonstrated a role in chamber formation and may provide a molecular candidate for a severe form of human congenital heart disease (CHD). Mice homozygous for a null *dhand* allele appear to lack a morphological right ventricle.[85] The phenotype of the heart in this animal model is similar to human right ventricular hypoplasia, establishing *dhand* as a candidate gene for this type of human CHD.

Irx4 and the *hand* genes suggest that the specification of chamber-specific modularity lies at least in part in the transcriptional localization of single genes. However, the notion that chamber identity as a whole is specified as a result of a small number of chamber-specific modules of gene expression is simplistic. The degree to which regulation of cardiac gene expression is a highly modular process has only begun to be understood. The analysis of the promoters of single cardiac-specific genes has demonstrated that a very large number of small promoter elements are required to recapitulate normal expression patterns (reviewed in Reference 16). The degree of modularity is so high that some elements drive expression in regions not previously thought to be molecularly distinct from their neighbors (reviewed in Reference 16). These findings suggest that complex combinatorial networks of transcription factors are required for the molecular regionalization of information within the developing heart.

SEPTATION OF THE ATRIA, VENTRICLES, ATRIOVENTRICULAR JUNCTION, AND OUTFLOW TRACT

Cardiac septation is a complex process that begins after looping morphogenesis has realigned the cardiac segments so that the right ventricle and left ventricle are located beside one another. Complete septation of the heart is not necessary for embryonic survival, which may in part explain the high incidence of septation defects seen in clinical cardiology practice. Four major components must develop to divide the heart into separate systemic and pulmonary circulations: (1) the atrial septum that separates the right and left atria, (2) the atrioventricular junction that contributes to atrial and ventricular septation, as well as to atrioventricular valve formation, (3) the ventricular septum that separates the right and left ventricles, and (4) the outflow tract or infundibular septum that separates the pulmonary from the aortic outflow tract.

Recent studies have resulted in a paradigm of atrial septal development newer than that presented by classical embryology studies.[35,43,105] The atrial septum includes septum secundum (secondary atrial septum), septum primum (primary atrial septum), and contributions from the atrioventricular cushions (Figure 100-3). Septum secundum is an infolding in the roof of the common primitive atrium. Septum primum develops from the dorsal wall of the atrium at 5 weeks gestation, grows toward the atrioventricular cushions as a crescentic muscular septum, and closes off the ostium primum (primary atrial communication) when it fuses with the atrioventricular cushions during the sixth week of fetal development. Septum primum carries a "cap" of distinct mesenchymal tissue along its leading edge that is critical for fusion of the primary atrial septum with the atrioventricular cushions.[105] As septum primum grows toward the atrioventricular cushions and divides the atria, it develops fenestrations that coalesce into the ostium secundum (secondary foramen) and allow for continued mixing of blood at the atrial level in the fetus.

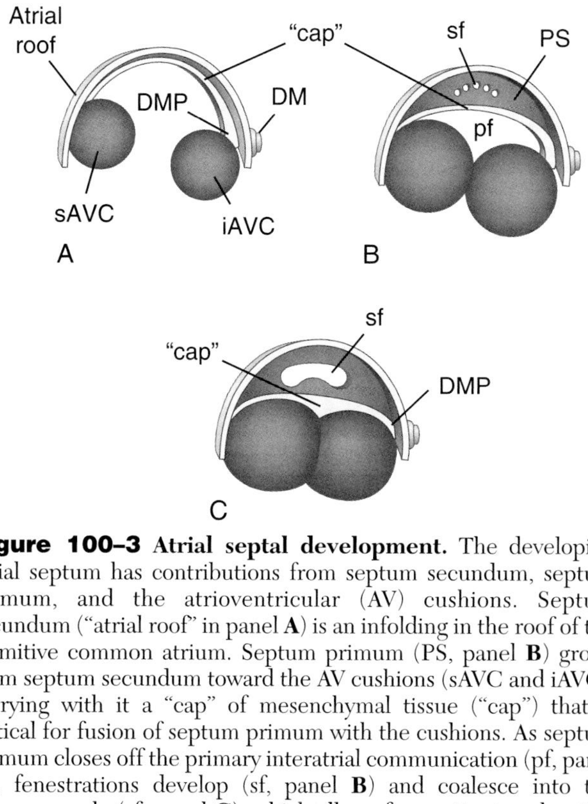

Figure 100–3 Atrial septal development. The developing atrial septum has contributions from septum secundum, septum primum, and the atrioventricular (AV) cushions. Septum secundum ("atrial roof" in panel **A**) is an infolding in the roof of the primitive common atrium. Septum primum (PS, panel **B**) grows from septum secundum toward the AV cushions (sAVC and iAVC), carrying with it a "cap" of mesenchymal tissue ("cap") that is critical for fusion of septum primum with the cushions. As septum primum closes off the primary interatrial communication (pf, panel **B**), fenestrations develop (sf, panel **B**) and coalesce into the foramen ovale (sf, panel **C**), which allows for continuing shunting of blood at the atrial level, which is necessary in the fetal circulation. DM, Dorsal mesocardium; DMP, dorsal mesenchymal protrusion.
(Modified from Wessels A, Anderson RH, Markwald RR, et al: Atrial development in the human heart: An immunohistochemical study with emphasis on the role of mesenchymal tissues. Anat Rec 259:288–300, 2000.)

Like the atrial septum, the ventricular septum is a complex structure including components derived from the atrioventricular cushions, the muscular ventricular septum, and the conal (infundibular) septum. In the early stages just after looping (31–35 days in the human), the muscular ventricular septum is a ridge of myocardium corresponding to the furrow of the primary fold on the outer curvature of the heart and separating the primitive left ventricle and primitive right ventricle.[44] In mammals the muscular septum develops from a ridge of infolded compact myocardium.[81] As the heart grows markedly in size along the outer curvature, the muscular septum grows concordantly with the ventricles.[12] The muscular septum fuses with the endocardial cushions of the atrioventricular junction and with the outflow tract to completely separate the right and left ventricles.

The atrioventricular junction (canal) segment of the developing heart initially connects the primitive atrium exclusively to the left ventricle (see Figure 100-1C). Complex remodeling must occur to allow for inflow from the atrium directly into both the right and left ventricles (see Figure 100-1D). In addition to establishing the right atrium to right ventricle continuity, the atrioventricular junction also gives rise to the endocardial cushions that will form the atrioventricular valves. (Endocardial cushions also form in the outflow tract and contribute to the semilunar valves and septation of the outflow tract.) The superior and inferior atrioventricular cushions fuse in the midline to form the atrioventricular septum, with resultant separation of the inflow into mitral (left side) and tricuspid (right side) components. The mesenchyme of the atrioventricular junction contributes to the portion of the atrial septum just proximal to the atrioventricular valves by fusing with the primary atrial septum. In addition, the atrioventricular septum mesenchyme forms the inlet portion of the ventricular septum (between the atrioventricular valves).

The growth and maturation of the endocardial cushions has been studied at the molecular level. Cardiac cushions begin as localized thickenings of the extracellular matrix between the endocardial and myocardial layers of the primitive heart tube, termed the cardiac jelly (Figure 100-4) (reviewed in ref. 24). The cushions begin as acellular structures that become populated by cells that have undergone an endothelial to mesenchymal transformation. JB3 is an antibody that recognizes fibrillin-2[73] and, in the heart, recognizes only the subset of cells ($JB3^+$) that have the potential to undergo the endothelial to mesenchymal transformation in the cushions (reviewed in ref. 62). The mesenchymal transformation is mediated by the myocardium of the atrioventricular junction via a number of molecules, including BMP-2, BMP-4, and neuregulin, an epidermal growth factor–like molecule, as well as the homeobox-containing transcription factor Msx-2.[1,24,86] ES proteins that form complexes with fibronectin also are present in the developing cushions and appear important for the regulation of the mesenchymal transformation (reviewed in refs. 24 and 62).

Contributions from the endocardial cushions and the cardiac neural crest are required for outflow tract septation (Figure 100-5). The endocardial cushions of the atrioventricular junction and the outflow tract are in physical continuity through the superior atrioventricular cushion, which extends along the inner curvature of the heart.[62] Extensive

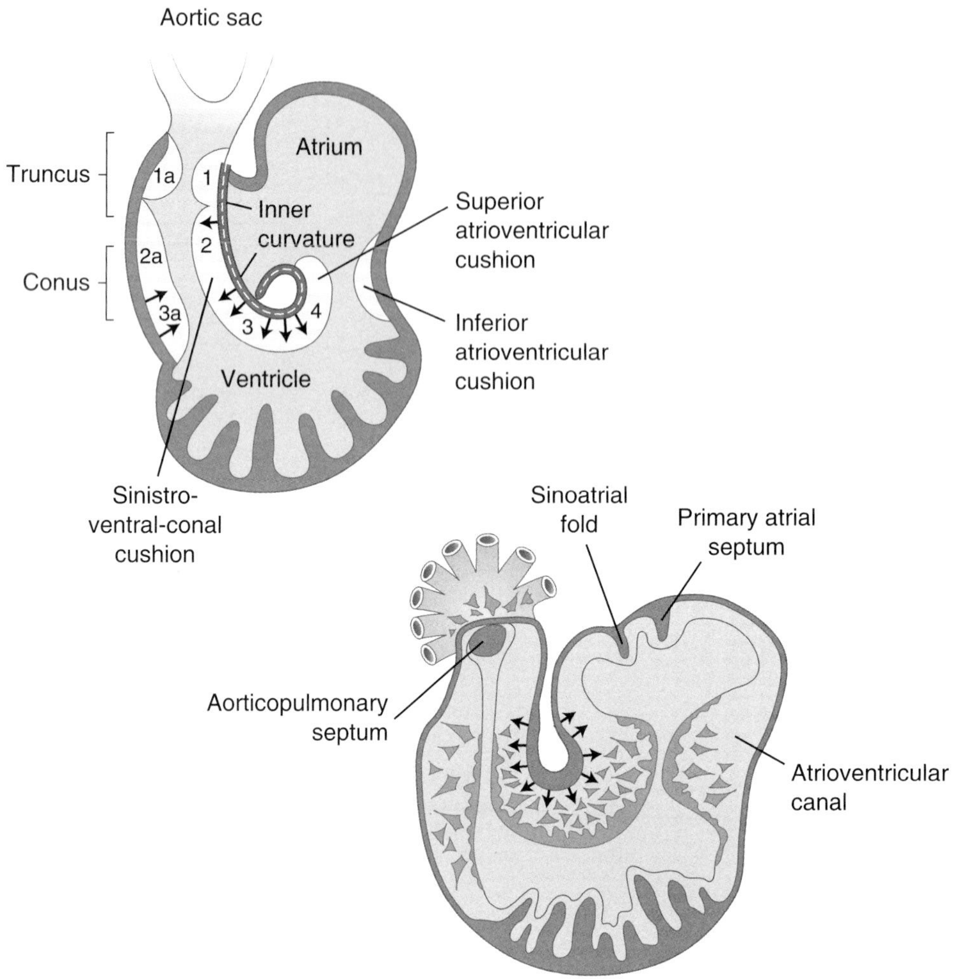

Figure 100–4 Cushion development. The endocardial cushions appear in the atrioventricular junction (atrioventricular canal) and in the outflow tract (conus and truncus) after looping of the heart tube. The superior AV cushion *(4)* is contiguous with the cushions of the outflow tract (*3, 3a, 2, 2a, 1,* and *1a*) along the inner curvature of the heart. Cushion tissue contributes to the formation of the valves and also to septation of the heart. The inner curvature undergoes significant remodeling and participates in myocardialization of the cushions *(arrows)*.
(Modified from Harvey RP, Rosenthal N, editors: Heart Development, p. 171. San Diego: Academic Press, 1999.)

remodeling of the inner curvature occurs to connect the right atrium to the right ventricle and the left ventricle to the aorta.[97] Septation of the outflow tract results from the development of two structures. Below the level of the semilunar valves, the conal septum (infundibular septum or muscular outflow tract septum) develops from myocardialization of the out flow tract cushions, a process that also involves contributions from the cardiac neural crest and the epicardium.[97] Above the level of the semilunar valves, the aorticopulmonary septum grows from the aortic sac toward the heart to separate the pulmonary from the aortic outflow tracts.

The three components of the ventricular septum (the inlet, muscular, and conal septae) must join together to completely separate the ventricles. The region of the membranous ventricular septum in the adult heart is the approximate location where these three components join. This finding suggests that a defect in the development of the inlet, muscular, or conal septae can result in a ventricular septal defect, suggesting a mechanistic rationale for the high frequency of defects at this anatomical location.

Clinical Correlates of Abnormal Chamber Septation

Common atrioventricular canal (also called endocardial cushion defect or atrioventricular septal defect) refers to a spectrum of lesions that have improper development of the atrioventricular junction as the underlying developmental abnormality. In such cases the atrioventricular junction has failed to undergo its normal septation and formation of separate atrioventricular valves, leaving a common atrioventricular valve providing inflow to both ventricles. The atrioventricular cushion contributions to atrial and ventricular septation also are abnormal, resulting in atrial septal defect of the ostium primum type and ventricular septal defect of the inlet (atrioventricular canal) type. This defect is reminiscent of the structure of the developing heart before atrioventricular junction septation by the developing endocardial cushions. Genes required for normal development of the atrioventricular endocardial cushions can result in common atrioventricular canal when mutated in a mouse model, as demonstrated by the ALK3 conditional receptor knockout.[30] Common atrioventricular canal therefore can be conceptualized as a developmental arrest, in which chamber septation fails to progress past the common atrioventricular junction.

Although complete common atrioventricular canal accounts for only 7.3% of all congenital malformations,[26] it is observed in approximately 40% of patients with trisomy 21 (Down syndrome).[100] These epidemiological data suggest that a gene important for the development of the atrioventricular junction resides on chromosome 21. To date, no single gene on chromosome 21 has been implicated in the genesis of common atrioventricular canal.[69]

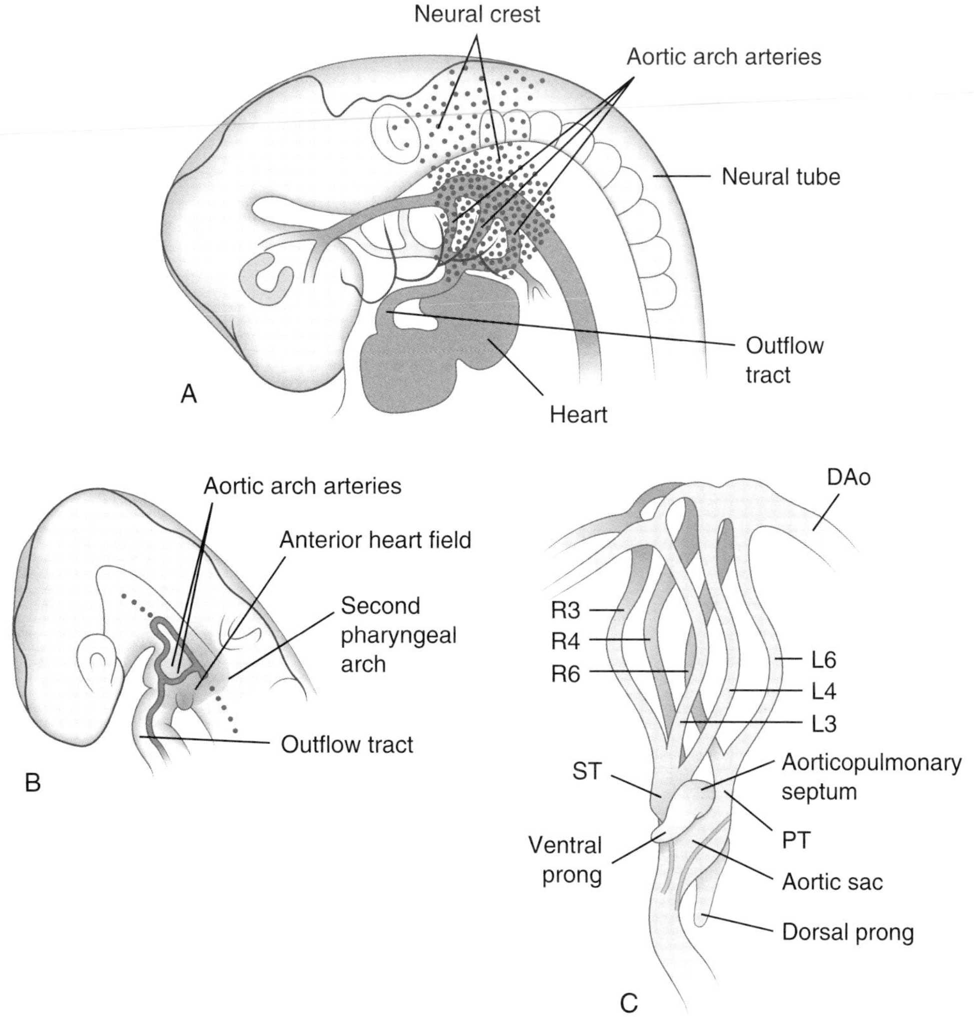

Figure 100–5 **Neural crest, anterior heart field, and outflow tract development. A,** The cardiac neural crest migrates into pharyngeal arches 3, 4, and 6, where it plays a crucial role in the patterning of the paired aortic arch arteries by preventing the regression of aortic arch arteries 3, 4, and 6, the precursors of the definitive great arteries. **B,** The anterior heart field is a recently described and separate migratory population of cells that originate near the second pharyngeal arch and contribute to cardiac outflow tract development. **C,** The neural crest cells condensing into two prongs that insert into the endocardial cushions of the developing outflow tract. The third aortic arch artery (L3 and R3) gives rise to the right and left carotid arteries. The left fourth arch artery (L4) becomes part of the definitive aortic arch, and the right fourth arch artery (R4) contributes to the proximal right subclavian artery. The left sixth aortic arch artery (L6) forms the ductus arteriosus. PT, pulmonary trunk; ST, systemic trunk.
(A and C are modified from Harvey RP, Rosenthal N, editors: Heart Development, pp. 180 and 182. San Diego: Academic Press, 1999. B is modified from Waldo KL, Kumiski DH, Wallis KT, et al: Conotruncal myocardium arises from a secondary heart field. Development 128:3179–3188, 2001.)

Isolated atrial septal defects are one of the most common congenital defects of the heart in humans. Secundum atrial septal defects result from a deficiency of septum primum in closing off the ostium secundum. Atrial septal defects also are frequently found in association with clinical syndromes. Secundum atrial septal defects are the most common structural defect resulting from the loss of one copy of the *Tbx-5* gene in Holt–Oram syndrome, an autosomal-dominant disorder.[4,47] Mutations in the *Nkx2-5* gene have been linked to autosomal-dominant secundum atrial septal defects,[5,77] and, more recently, mutations in the *GATA4* gene also have been linked to secundum atrial septal defects.[29] The finding that TBX-5, NKX2-5, and GATA4 all interact to regulate the expression of genes necessary for atrial septal development suggests that candidate genes for secundum atrial septal defects may lie downstream of these important transcription factors.

OUTFLOW TRACT DEVELOPMENT, THE ANTERIOR HEART FIELD, AND THE CARDIAC NEURAL CREST

Although the vertebrate heart develops primarily from the precardiac mesoderm (cardiac crescent), two other

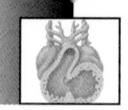

cell populations, the anterior heart field and the cardiac neural crest, are critical for normal outflow tract development.[34,36,61,103]

The existence of the anterior heart field was suspected 30 years ago, when Viragh and Challice[101] observed the transformation of epithelial to myocardial cells at the arterial pole of the developing mouse heart. De la Cruz and colleagues[17] utilized marking studies in living chick embryos to demonstrate that the distal outflow tract was a late addition to the developing heart. A series of recent studies show that a population of cells in the anterior mesoderm adjacent to the aortic sac (see Figure 100-5B), distinct from both the lateral cardiogenic mesoderm and the cardiac neural crest, contribute to the myocardium of the outflow tract in both avian[61,103] and murine models.[34] In the murine model, the anterior heart field contributions extend past the outflow tract and also contribute to the developing right ventricle to the level of the interventricular septum.[18,33] This finding may ultimately help explain observed gene expression differences between the right and left ventricles.

The cardiac outflow tract is initially a tubular structure connecting the primitive right ventricle to the aortic sac that must undergo septation to form the pulmonary artery and the aorta. In addition, the outflow tract must gain continuity with the primitive left ventricle. This occurs by a process termed "wedging," in which the subaortic conus is remodeled to allow the aortic valve to reach its normal adult position between the tricuspid and mitral valves. This process establishes fibrous continuity of the mitral and aortic valves (reviewed in ref. 37). The aorticopulmonary septum develops from the aortic sac mesenchyme and grows into the outflow tract, where it interacts with neural crest–derived cells in the endocardial cushions, ultimately dividing the outflow tract into the aorta and pulmonary artery (reviewed in ref. 104).

The cardiac outflow tract receives a large contribution of cells from the neural crest, a population of migratory pluripotent cells that arise adjacent to the developing neural tube. The cardiac neural crest is a subpopulation of the neural crest that originates from between the midotic placode to the third somite (see Figure 100-5A).[40] These cells migrate into the developing third, fourth, and sixth pharyngeal arches, where they interact with the third, fourth, and sixth aortic arch vessels, the progenitors of the definitive great arteries (aorta, carotid, and subclavian arteries, the main pulmonary artery, and ductus arteriosus). The aortic arch vessels develop as symmetrically paired structures, but undergo a highly specific and asymmetrical program of resorption, retaining the normal left aortic arch. The cardiac neural crest does not play a role in formation of the aortic arch vessels, but rather stabilizes the arch vessels and prevents their regression (see Figure 100-5C).[102] A subpopulation of the cardiac neural crest migrates further from the pharyngeal arches to the heart, where it forms the cardiac ganglia, participates in the septation of the outflow tract, and contributes to the formation of the semilunar valves.[39] The neural crest also interacts with the pharyngeal arch mesenchyme to form the thymus, thyroid, and parathyroid glands.

Animal models of neural crest defects have been useful in determining the etiology of some congenital heart malformations. Experimental ablation of the neural crest in avian embryos[38] demonstrated abnormal development of the heart and great arteries, as well as abnormalities of the glandular derivatives of the pharyngeal arches and pouches (thymus, thyroid, and parathyroid glands) (reviewed in ref. 36). Specifically, defects of the embryonic outflow tract were observed in embryos after neural crest ablation, including persistent truncus arteriosus, DORV, and tetralogy of Fallot. Ventricular septal defects of the infundibular septum also were common.[63] Interestingly, defects of the inflow portion of the heart occasionally were described as well, including double inlet left ventricle, straddling tricuspid valve, and tricuspid atresia, and they occurred in association with outflow defects.[63] Furthermore, abnormal aortic arch patterning occurred in virtually all embryos after neural crest ablation.[56,63,95] The arch abnormalities demonstrated great variability and included various types of interrupted aortic arch.

Murine models with cardiac phenotypes reminiscent of neural crest ablation include the Splotch mouse, bearing a mutation in the *Pax3* homeobox gene. Splotch homozygotes demonstrate persistent truncus arteriosus and aortic arch anomalies, as well as anomalies of the thymus, thyroid, and parathyroid glands. The homozygous mutation is lethal at embryonic day 14.[15] The Patch mutant mouse, bearing a deletion of a portion of chromosome 5, also demonstrates craniofacial, thymic, and outflow tract abnormalities, including arch patterning anomalies (reviewed in ref. 58). Initial efforts to understand this phenotype focused on the deletion of the gene for platelet-derived growth factor receptor (PDGFR). However, mice homozygous for a PDGFR-targeted null mutation do not consistently demonstrate cardiac anomalies, suggesting that other genes deleted in the Patch mutant must contribute to the cardiac phenotype.[83]

Retinoic acid, the active derivative of vitamin A, has been shown to play an important role in outflow tract development. Knockouts of the retinoic acid receptor in mice produce phenotypes reminiscent of neural crest ablation. There are two families of receptors, RAR and RXR, with each family containing three isoforms. Single-isoform knockouts produce no morphological defects; however, double mutants of RAR and RXR produce outflow tract defects (persistent truncus arteriosus, DORV, and arch anomalies), as well as craniofacial and thymic, thyroid, and parathyroid anomalies (reviewed in refs. 36 and 58). If vitamin A is administered, the cardiac phenotype may be rescued.[107] This suggests a role for retinoic acid signaling in neural crest migration and cardiac development.

Clinical Correlates of Abnormal Outflow Tract Development: DiGeorge Syndrome and 22q11 Deletion

DiGeorge syndrome is an autosomal dominant disorder whose phenotype includes cardiac defects of the outflow tract, in particular, interrupted aortic arch, persistent truncus arteriosus, tetralogy of Fallot, and aortic arch anomalies. The syndrome also includes parathyroid hypoplasia with resultant hypocalcemia, thymic hypoplasia with resultant T-cell deficit, cleft palate, and other craniofacial abnormalities. There are phenotypical similarities between DiGeorge, Takao (conotruncal anomaly face syndrome), and Shprintzen (velocardiofacial) syndromes, and in fact, the same molecular lesion is present in all three syndromes: deletion of 22q11. "CATCH22" or "CATCH phenotype" has been proposed as an acronym for the phenotype associated with these syndromes (*C*ardiac defects, *A*bnormal facies, *T*-cell deficit, *C*left palate, *H*ypocalcemia).[8,106] The phenotype demonstrates considerable variability between patients. 22q11 deletion is the most common deletion in humans, occurring in 1:4000 live births[9] with an average of 30 genes removed, although smaller and larger deletions are not infrequent (reviewed in ref. 18).

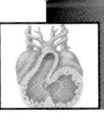

A vigorous search for candidate genes residing within the commonly deleted portion of human chromosome 22 has recently yielded some success in understanding the molecular underpinnings of the cardiac defects. Mouse models with deletions of the region of chromosome 16 syntenic to human chromosomal region 22q11 have been used to identify and test candidate genes (reviewed in ref. 58). Three independent groups have reported that haploinsufficiency of the T-box transcription factor gene *Tbx1* results in cardiac phenotypes consistent with DiGeorge syndrome.[32,52,60] However, not a single point mutation has been identified in any patient with DiGeorge syndrome; the phenotype in humans may require larger genetic alterations. The clinical variability seen among patients with DiGeorge syndrome has several possible sources, including variability in the size of the deletion, sensitivity to gene dosage from modifying genes (genetic background), or epigenetic factors. One study demonstrated that a targeted deletion of *Tbx1* in mice caused abnormal aortic arch patterning in 50% of embryos, implicating sensitivity to gene dosage in the variability of the DiGeorge phenotype.[60] When a larger deletion containing additional genes was studied, the mice showed parathyroid hypoplasia, thymic insufficiency, and a higher perinatal lethality, implicating deletion size. Another group demonstrated abnormal development of the fourth aortic arch in mice heterozygous for a *Tbx1* deletion.[52] Homozygous mutants were embryonic lethal with obliteration of the third, fourth, and sixth aortic arches.[52] In this model, *Tbx1*-haploinsufficient animals did not display thymic, parathyroid, or facial anomalies, again suggesting that a multiple gene deletion is required for the full clinical features of DiGeorge syndrome.[52]

ETIOLOGY OF CONGENITAL HEART DISEASE: THE RESULT OF A NATURAL SELECTION EXPERIMENT

The human circulatory system must provide nutrients and oxygen from distinct sources during embryonic, fetal, and neonatal development. Initially the developing embryo derives nutrition by passive diffusion from the maternal uterus after implantation. The development of the yolk sac circulation to transport nutrition from the yolk sac to the developing embryo is required during early embryonic development. The development of the fetal vascular system and heart are required to provide adequate circulation initially from the yolk sac and then from the placenta. Failure of circulatory development during these early stages results in early fetal lethality.

The dramatic transition from the fetal circulation to the adult circulation at birth clinically unmasks many congenital heart defects in the neonatal period. This transition involves the complete separation of pulmonary from the systemic circulation and requires the closure of the ductus arteriosus, functional closure of the foramen ovale, and the diversion of increased circulation to the low resistance vascular bed of the newly inflated lungs. Fetal circulation through the heart can be thought of as in-parallel, with oxygenated blood from the placenta traversing from the systemic venous return to the aorta via the foramen ovale to the left atrium (bypassing the right ventricle) and also via the ductus arteriosus into the descending aorta (bypassing the pulmonary vasculature). Postnatal circulation through the heart is in-series, with strict lines of flow from systemic venous return to the right side of the heart to the lungs to the left side of the heart to the aorta.

A survey of congenital heart defects suggests that most individual defects can be grouped into categories, each capable of supporting adequate in-parallel circulation but failing to establish proper in-series circulation. Unilateral blocks, such as valvar stenosis or atresia, are tolerated during fetal life because shunting across the foramen ovale and ductus arteriosus is able to bypass the obstruction. However, upon definitive separation into systemic and pulmonary circulations, unilateral blocks provide a serious obstacle to an in-series circulatory system. Septal defects or shunting lesions, such as atrial septal defects, ventricular septal defects, or patent ductus arteriosus, are tolerated during fetal life because the fetal circulation requires shunts at the atrial level and at the ductus arteriosus. It is the physiological results of the failure of these holes to close and establish an in-series circulation during the perinatal period that results in postnatal clinical presentation. Routing abnormalities such as TGA and double inlet or outlet abnormalities are also tolerated by a parallel circulatory system. Circulatory shunting across the foramen ovale and ductus arteriosus during fetal life causes these structural abnormalities to be phenotypically silent. Only upon definitive separation of the systemic and pulmonary circulatory routes do these abnormalities cause physiological deficits.

Thus the transition from fetal to neonatal circulation places unique demands on the developing circulatory system at birth. The result is a natural selection experiment, resulting in the clinical appearance of structural heart defects able to sustain fetal circulation yet unable to establish partitioned systemic and pulmonary circulations. The heart is the only organ to undergo such significant structural and physiological alterations within the perinatal temporal window. Congenital heart defects are the most common congenital defects to clinically present in the perinatal period because of the stringent structural alterations required of the heart during this critical time frame and the significant physiological impairment that results when these structural alterations fail.

This chapter demonstrates some of the remarkable progress that has been made in the molecular understanding of embryonic heart development and how specific structural defects of the heart arise when the activity of single genes is interrupted. The following decades will witness massive growth in our understanding of the molecular underpinning of heart development and their application to the diagnosis and treatment of congenital heart disease.

REFERENCES

1. Abdelwahid E, Rice D, Pelleniemi LJ: (2001). Overlapping and differential localization of Bmp-2, Bmp-4, Msx-2 and apoptosis in the endocardial cushion and adjacent tissues of the developing mouse heart. Cell Tissue Res 305:67–78, 2001.
2. Andree B, Duprez D, Vorbusch B, et al: BMP-2 induces ectopic expression of cardiac lineage markers and interferes with somite formation in chicken embryos. Mech Dev 70:119–131, 1998.
3. Bao ZZ, Bruneu BG, Seidman JG, et al: Regulation of chamber specific gene expression in the developing heart by Irx4. Science 283:1161–1164, 1999.
4. Basson CT, Bachinsky DR, Lin RC, et al: Mutations in human TBX5 [corrected] cause limb and cardiac malformation in Holt-Oram syndrome. Nat Genet 15(1):30–35, 1997.
5. Benson DW, Silberbach GM, Kavanaugh-McHugh A, et al: Mutations in the cardiac transcription factor NKX2.5 affect diverse cardiac developmental pathways. J Clin Invest 104(11):1567–1573, 1999.
6. Bour BA, O'Brien MA, Lockwood WL, et al: *Drosophila* MEF2, a transcription factor that is essential for myogenesis. Genes Dev 9:730–741, 1995.
7. Bruneau BG, Nemer G, Schmitt JP, et al: A murine model of the Holt-Oram syndrome defines roles of the T-box transcription factor Tbx5 in cardiogenesis and disease. Cell 106:709–721, 2001.
8. Burn J: Closing time for CATCH22. J Med Genet 36:737–738, 1999.
9. Burn J, Goodship J: Congenital heart disease. In Rimoin DL, Conner JM, Pyeritz RE, Emery AEH, editors: Emery and Rimoin's Principles and Practice of Medical Genetics, 3rd ed. London: Churchill-Livingstone, 1996.
10. Campione M, Steinbeisser H, Schweickert A, et al: The homeobox gene Pitx2: Mediator of asymmetric left-right signaling in vertebrate heart and gut looping. Development 126:1225–1234, 1999.
11. Chen CY, Schwartz RJ: Recruitment of the *tinman* homolog Nkx-2.5 by serum response factor activates cardiac alpha-actin gene transcription. Mol Cell Biol 16:6372–6384, 1996.
12. Christoffels VM, Habets PE, Franco D, et al: Chamber formation and morphogenesis in the developing human heart. Dev Biol 223:266–278, 2000.
13. Cohen-Gould L, Mikawa T: The fate diversity of mesodermal cells within the chicken heart field during early embryogenesis. Dev Biol 177:265–273, 1996.
14. Collignon J, Varlet I, Robertson EJ: Relationship between asymmetric nodal expression and the direction of embryonic turning. Nature 381:155–158, 1996.
15. Conway SJ, Henderson DJ, Copp AJ: Pax3 is required for cardiac neural crest migration in the mouse: Evidence from the splotch mutant. Development 124:505–514, 1997.
16. Cripps RM, Olson EN: Control of cardiac development by an evolutionarily conserved transcriptional network. Dev Biol 246:14–28, 2002.
17. De la Cruz MV, Gomez CS, Arteaga MM, et al: Experimental study of the development of the truncus and the conus in the chick embryo. J Anat 123:661–686, 1977.
18. Dees E, Baldwin HS: New frontiers in molecular pediatric cardiology. Curr Opin Pediatr 14:627–633, 2002.
19. DeHaan RL: Morphogenesis of the vertebrate heart. In DeHaan RL, Ursprung H, editors: Organogenesis, pp. 377–419. New York: Holt, Rinehart & Winston, 1965.
20. DeHaan RL: Regional organisation of prepacemaker cells in the cardiac primordia of the early chick embryo. J Embryol Ex Morphol 11:65–76, 1963.
21. DeHaan RL: In DeHaan RL, Ursprung H, editors: Organogenesis, pp. 377-420. New York: Holt, Rinehart & Winston, 1965.
22. Durocher D, Charron F, Warren R, et al: The cardiac transcription factors Nkx-2.5 and GATA-4 are mutual cofactors. EMBO J 16:5687–5696, 1997.
23. Durocher D, Chen CY, Ardati A, et al: The atrial natriuretic factor promoter is a downstream target for Nkx-2.5 in the myocardium. Mol Cell Biol 16:4648–4655, 1996.
24. Eisenberg LM, Markwald RR: Molecular regulation of atrioventricular valvuloseptal morphogenesis. Circ Res 77(1): 1–6, 1995.
25. Essner JJ, Branford WW, Zhang J, et al: Mesentoderm and left-right brain, heart and gut development are differentially regulated by Pitx2 isoforms. Development 127:1081–1093, 2000.
26. Ferencz C, Loffredo CA, Correa-Villasenor A, et al: Genetic and Environmental Risk Factors of Major Cardiovascular Malformations: The Baltimore-Washington Infant Study 1981-1989, pp.103–122. Armonk, NY: Futura Publishing Co., 1997.
27. Gajewski K, Kim Y, Lee YM, et al: D-Mef2 is a target for tinman activation during *Drosophila* heart development. EMBO J 16:515–522, 1997.
28. Gajewski K, Zhang Q, Choi CY, et al: Pannier is a transcriptional target and partner of Tinman during *Drosophila* cardiogenesis. Dev Biol 233:425–436, 2001.
29. Garg V, Kathiriya IS, Barnes R, et al: GATA4 mutations cause human congenital heart defects and reveal an interaction with TBX5. Nature 424(6947):443–447, 2003.
30. Gaussin V, Van de Putte T, Mishina Y, et al: Endocardial cushion and myocardial defects after cardiac myocyte-specific conditional deletion of the bone morphogenetic protein receptor ALK3. Proc Natl Acad Sci U S A 99(5):2878–2883, 2002.
31. Inagaki T, Garcia-Martinez V, Schoenwolf GC: Regulative ability of the prospective cardiogenic and vasculogenic area of the primitive streak during avian gastrulation. Dev Dyn 197:57–68, 1993.
32. Jerome LA, Papaioannou VE: DiGeorge syndrome phenotype in mice mutant for the T-box gene Tbx1. Nat Genet 27:286–291, 2001.
33. Kelly R, Buckingham M: The anterior heart-forming field: Voyage to the arterial pole of the heart. Trends Genet 18:210–216, 2002.
34. Kelly RG, Brown NA, Buckingham ME: The arterial pole of the mouse heart forms from Fgf10-expressing cells in pharyngeal mesoderm. Dev Cell 1:435–440, 2001.
35. Kim JS, Viragh S, Moorman AFM, et al: Development of the myocardium of the atrioventricular canal and vestibular spine in the human heart. Circ Res 88:395–402, 2001.
36. Kirby ML: Contribution of neural crest to heart and vessel morphology. In Harvey RP, Rosenthal N, editors: Heart Development. San Diego: Academic Press, 1999.
37. Kirby ML, Waldo KL: Neural crest and cardiovascular patterning. Circ Res 77(2):211–215, 1995.
38. Kirby ML, Gale TF, Stewart DE: Neural crest cells contribute to aorticopulmonary septation. Science 220: 1059–1061, 1983.
39. Kirby ML, Hunt P, Wallis K, et al: Abnormal patterning of the aortic arch arteries does not evoke cardiac malformations. Dev Dyn 208:34–47, 1997.
40. Kirby ML, Turnage KL Hays BM: Characterization of conotruncal malformations following ablation of "cardiac" neural crest. Anat Rec 213:87–93, 1985.
41. Koromuro I, Izumo S: Csx: A murine homeobox-containing gene specifically expressed in the developing heart. Proc Natl Acad Sci U S A 90:8145–8149, 1993.

42. Kosaki R, Gebbia M, Kosaki K, et al: Left-right axis malformations associated with mutations in ACVR2B, the gene for human activin receptor type IIB. Am J Med Genet 82:70–76, 1999.
43. Lamers WH, Moorman AFM: Cardiac septation: A late contribution of the embryonic primary myocardium to heart morphogenesis. Circ Res 91:93–103, 2002.
44. Lamers WH, Wessels A, Verbeek FJ, et al: New findings concerning ventricular septation in the human heart. Circulation 86:1194–1205, 1992.
45. Lee Y, Shioi T, Kasahara H, et al: The cardiac restricted homeobox protein Csx/Nkx2.5 physically associates with the zinc finger GATA4 and cooperatively activates atrial natriuretic factor gene expression. Mol Cell Biol 18:3120–3129, 1998.
46. Levin M, Johnson RL, Stern CD, et al: A molecular pathway determining left-right asymmetry in chick embryogenesis. Cell 82:803–814, 1995.
47. Li QY, Newbury-Ecob RA, Terrett JA, et al: Holt-Oram syndrome is caused by mutations in TBX5, a member of the Brachyury (T) gene family. Nat Genet 15(1):21–29, 1997.
48. Liberatore CM, Searcy-Schrick RD, Vincent EB, et al: Nkx-2.5 gene induction in mice is mediated by a Smad consensus regulatory region. Dev Biol 244:243–255, 2000.
49. Lilly B, Zhao B, Ranganayakulu G, et al: Requirement of the MADS domain transcription factor D-MEF2 for muscle formation in *Drosophila*. Science 267:688–693, 1995.
50. Lin Q, Lu J, Yanagisawa H, et al: Requirement of the MADS-box transcription factor MEF2C for vascular development. Development 125:4565–4574, 1998.
51. Lin Q, Schwarz J, Bucana C, et al: Control of mouse cardiac morphogenesis and myogenesis by transcription factor MEF2C. Science 276:1404–1407, 1997.
52. Lindsay EA, Vitelli F, Su H, et al: Tbx1 haploinsufficiency in the DiGeorge syndrome region causes aortic arch defects in mice. Nature 410:97–101, 2001.
53. Lints T, Parsons L, Hartley L, et al: Nkx-2.5: A novel murine homeobox gene expressed in early heart progenitor cells and their myogenic descendants. Development 119:419–431, 1993.
54. Logan M, Pagan-Westphal SM, Smith DM, et al: The transcription factor Pitx2 mediates situs-specific morphogenesis in response to left-right asymmetric signals. Cell 94:307–317, 1998.
55. Lowe LA, Supp DM., Sampath K, et al: Conserved left-right asymmetry of nodal expression and alterations in murine situs inversus. Nature 381:158–161, 1996.
56. Manner J, Seidl W, Steding G: Experimental study on the significance if abnormal cardiac looping for the development of cardiovascular abnormalities in neural crest ablated chick embryos. Anat Embryol 194:289–300, 1996.
57. Marvin MJ, Di Rocco G, Gardiner A, et al: Inhibition of Wnt activity induces heart formation from posterior mesoderm. Genes Dev 15:316–327, 2001.
58. Maschoff KL, Baldwin HS: Molecular determinants of neural crest migration. Am J Med Genet 97:280–288, 2000.
59. Meno C, Saijoh Y, Fujii H et al: Left-right asymmetric expression of the TGF beta-family member lefty in mouse embryos. Nature 381:151–155, 1996.
60. Merscher S, Funke B, Epstein JA, et al: Tbx1 is responsible for cardiovascular defects in velo-cardial-facial/DiGeorge syndrome. Cell 104:619–629, 2001.
61. Mjaatvedt CH, Nakaoka TH, Moreno-Rodriguez R, et al: The outflow tract of the heart is recruited from a novel heart-forming field. Dev Biol 238:97–109, 2001.
62. Mjaatvedt CH, Yamamura H, Wessels A, et al: Mechanisms of segmentation, septation, and remodeling of the tubular heart: Endocardial cushion fate and cardiac looping. In Harvey RP, Rosenthal N, editors: Heart Development. San Diego: Academic Press, 1999.
63. Nishibatake M, Kirby ML, Van Mierop LHS: Pathogenesis of persistent truncus arteriosus and dextroposed aorta in the chick embryo after neural crest ablation. Circulation 75:255–264, 1987.
64. Nonaka S, Tanaka Y, Okada Y, et al: Randomization of left right asymmetry due to loss of nodal cilia generating leftward flow of extra embryonic fluid in mice lacking KIF3B motor protein [published erratum appears in Cell 99(1):117, 1999]. Cell 95:829–837, 1998.
65. Okada Y, Nonaka S, Tanaka Y, et al: Abnormal nodal flow precedes situs inversus in iv and inv mice. Mol Cell 4:459–468, 1999.
66. Pagan-Westphal SM, Tabin CJ: The transfer of left-right positional information during chick embryogenesis. Cell 93:25–35, 1998.
67. Patten BM: Formation of the cardiac loop in the chick. Am J Anat 30:373–397, 1992.
68. Piedra ME, Icardo JM, Albajar M, et al: Pitx2 participates in the late phase of the pathway controlling left-right asymmetry. Cell 94:319–324, 1998.
69. Pierpont MEM, Markwald RR, Lin AE: Genetic aspects of atrioventricular septal defects. Am J Med Genet 97:289–296, 2000.
70. Redkar A, Montgomery M, Litvin J: Fate map of early avian cardiac progenitor cells. Development 128:2269–2279, 2001.
71. Reifers F, Walsh EC, Leger S, et al: Induction and differentiation of the zebrafish heart requires fibroblast growth factor 8 (fgf8/acerebellar). Development 127:225–235, 2000.
72. Rodriguez-Esteban C, Capdevila J, Economides AN, et al: The novel Cer-like protein Caronte mediates the establishment of embryonic left-right asymmetry [see Comments]. Nature 401:243–251, 1999.
73. Rongish BJ, Drake CJ, Argraves WS, et al: Identification of a developmental marker, the JB3-antigen, as fibrillin-2 and its de novo organization into embryonic microfibrous arrays. Dev Dyn 212:461–471, 1998.
74. Rosenquist GC, DeHaan RL: Migration of precardiac cells in the chick embryo: A radioautographic study. Carnegie Inst Wash Contrib Embryol 38:111–121, 1996.
75. Ryan AK, Blumberg B, Rodriguez-Esteban C, et al: Pitx2 determines left-right asymmetry of internal organs in vertebrates. Nature 394:545–551, 1998.
76. Schneider VA, Mercola M: Wnt antagonism initiates cardiogenesis in *Xenopus laevis*. Genes Dev 15:304–315, 2001.
77. Schott JJ, Benson DW, Basson CT, et al: Congenital heart disease caused by mutations in the transcription factor NKX2-5. Science 281(5373):108–111, 1998.
78. Schultheiss TM, Burch JB, Lassar AB: A role for bone morphogenetic proteins in the induction of cardiac myogenesis. Genes Dev 11:451–462, 1997.
79. Schultheiss TM, Xydas S, Lassar AB: Induction of avian cardiac myogenesis by anterior endoderm. Development 121:4203–4214, 1995.
80. Schweickert A, Campione M, Steinbeisser H, et al: Pitx2 isoforms: Involvement of Pitx2c or Pitx2b in vertebrate left-right asymmetry. Mech Dev 90:41–51, 2000.
81. Sedmera D, Pexieder T, Vuillemin M, et al: Developmental patterning of the myocardium. Anat Rec 258(4):319–337, 2000.
82. Sepulveda JL, Belaguli N, Nigam V, et al: GATA-4 and Nkx-2.5 coactivate Nkx-2 DNA binding targets: Role for regulating early cardiac gene expression. Mol Cell Biol 18: 3405–3415, 1998.
83. Soriano P: The PDGFα receptor is required for neural crest cell development and for normal patterning of the somites. Development 124:2691–2700, 1997.

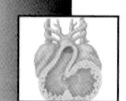

84. Srivastava D, Cserjesi P, Olson EN: A subclass of bHLH proteins required for cardiac morphogenesis. Science 270:1995–1999, 1995.
85. Srivastava D, Thomas T, Lin Q, et al: Regulation of cardiac mesodermal and neural crest development by the bHLH transcription factor, dHAND. Nat Genet 16:154–160, 1997.
86. Srivastava D, Baldwin HS: Molecular determinants of cardiac development. In Allen HD, Gutgesell HP, Clark EB, Driscoll DJ, editors: Moss and Adams' Heart Disease in Infants, Children, and Adolescents Including the Fetus and Young Adult. Philadelphia: Lippincott Williams & Wilkins, 2001.
87. Stainier DY, Fouquet B, Chen JN, et al: Mutations affecting the formation and function of the cardiovascular in the zebrafish embryo. Development 123:285–292, 1996.
88. Stalsberg H, DeHaan RL: The precardiac areas and formation of the tubular heart in the chick embryo. Dev Biol 19:128–159, 1969.
89. Sugi Y, Lough J: Anterior endoderm is a specific effector of terminal cardiac myocyte differentiation of cells from the embryonic heart forming region. Dev Dyn 200:155–162, 1994.
90. Supp DM, Brueckner M, Kuehn MR, et al: Targeted deletion of the ATP binding domain of left-right dynein confirms its role in specifying development of left right asymmetries. Development 126:5495–5504, 1999.
91. Supp DM, Witte DP, Potter SS, et al: Mutation of an axonemal dynein affects left-right asymmetry in inversus viscerum mice. Nature 389:963–966, 1997.
92. Tabin CJ, Vogan KJ: A two-cilia model for vertebrate left-right axis specification. Genes Dev 17:1–6, 2003.
93. Takeda S, Yonekawa Y, Tanaka Y, et al: Left-right asymmetry and kinesin superfamily protein KIF3A: New insights in determination of laterality and mesoderm induction by kif3a-/-mice analysis. J Cell Biol 145:825–836, 1999.
94. Tam PP, Parameswaran M, Kinder SJ, et al: The allocation of epiblast cells to the embryonic heart and other mesodermal lineages: The role of ingression and tissue movement during gastrulation. Development 124:1631–1642, 1997.
95. Tomita H, Connuck DM, Leatherbury L, Kirby ML: Relation of early hemodynamic changes to final cardiac phenotype and survival after neural crest ablation in chick embyos. Circulation 84:1289–1295, 1991.
96. Tzahor E, Lassar AB: Wnt signals from the neural tube block ectopic cardiogenesis. Genes Dev 15:255–260, 2001.
97. Van den Hoff MJB, Moorman AFM, Ruijter JM, et al: Myocardialization of the cardiac outflow tract. Dev Biol 212:477–490, 1999.
98. Van Mierop LHS: Location of pacemaker in chick embryo heart at the time of initiation of heartbeat. Am J Physiol 212:407–415, 1996.
99. Van Praagh S, Kakou-Guikahue M, Kim H-S, et al: Atrial situs in patients with visceral heterotaxy and congenital heart disease: Conclusions based on findings in 104 postmortem cases. Coeur 19:483–502, 1988.
100. Vaughan CJ, Basson CT: Molecular determinants of atrial and ventricular septal defects and patent ductus arteriosus. Am J Med Genet 97:304–309, 2000.
101. Viragh S, Challice CE: Origin and differentiation of cardiac muscle cells in the mouse. J Ultrastruct Res 42:1–24, 1973.
102. Waldo KL, Kumiski DH, Kirby ML: Cardiac neural crest is essential for the persistence rather than the formation of an arch artery. Dev Dyn 205(3):281–292, 1996.
103. Waldo KL, Kumiski DH, Wallis KT, et al: Conotruncal myocardium arises from a secondary heart field. Development 128:3179–3188, 2001.
104. Waller BR, McQuinn T, Phelps AL, et al: Conotruncal anomalies in the trisomy 16 mouse: An immunohistochemical analysis with emphasis on the involvement of the neural crest. Anat Rec 260:279–293, 2000.
105. Wessels A, Anderson RH, Markwald RR, et al: Atrial development in the human heart: An immunohistochemical study with emphasis on the role of mesenchymal tissues. Anat Rec 259(3):288–300, 2000.
106. Wilson DI, Burn J, Scambler P, et al: DiGeorge syndrome, part of CATCH22. J Med Genet 30:852–856, 1993.
107. Wilson JG, Roth JB, Warkany J: An analysis of the syndrome of malformations induced by vitamin A deficiency: Effects of restoration of vitamin A at various times during gestation. Am J Anat 92:189–217, 1953.
108. Yokouchi Y, Vogan KJ, Pearse RV 2nd, et al: Antagonistic signaling by Caronte, a novel Cerberus gene, establishes left-right asymmetric gene expression. Cell 98:573–583, 1999.
109. Yoshioka H, Meno C, Koshiba K, et al: Pitx2, a bicoid-type homeobox gene, is involved in a lefty signaling pathway in determination of left-right asymmetry. Cell 94:299–305, 1998.
110. Zhu L, Marvin MJ, Gardiner A, et al: Cerberus regulates left-right asymmetry of the embryonic head and heart. Curr Biol 9:931–938, 1999.

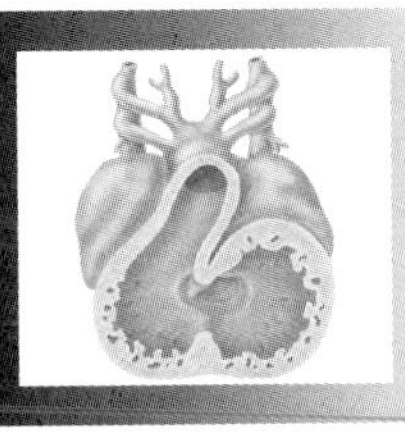

Segmental Anatomy

Richard Van Praagh

CHAPTER 101

INTRODUCTION

The cardiac segments are the anatomical and developmental "building blocks" out of which all human hearts, both normal and abnormal, are made.* The three main cardiac segments are the atria, the ventricles, and the great arteries (Figure 101-1).

The two connecting cardiac segments are the atrioventricular canal or junction and the infundibulum or conus arteriosus.

Segmental Sets or Combinations

How many types of human heart are there? Figure 101-1 provides a partial answer to this question. For each type of heart (see Figure 101-1), the atria, ventricles, and great arteries may be regarded as a set or combination: {atria, ventricles, great arteries}. Braces {} mean "the set of." The main cardiac segments are the members of the segmental set or combination.

Each segmental combination is recorded in venoarterial sequence, {atria, ventricles, great arteries}, because this is the natural or blood-flow order.

The two types of visceroatrial situs are shown in Figure 101-1. *Situs* means the pattern of anatomical organization. The situs of the viscera and the atria, which almost always are the same, may be *situs solitus,* that is, the usual, ordinary, or customary situs—hence the normal. Or the situs of the visceral and atria may be *situs inversus*—characterized by right–left reversal, but without anteroposterior or superoinferior change. Or the situs of the viscera and atria may be *situs ambiguus,* that is, the ambiguous or uncertain type of visceroatrial situs that may characterize the heterotaxy syndromes with asplenia or polysplenia that display anomalies of laterality.

In visceroatrial situs solitus, symbolized as {S,-,-} (see Figure 101-1, columns 1 and 2), the morphologically right atrium (RA) is right-sided (Figure 101-2), and the morphologically left atrium (LA) is left-sided (Figure 101-3).

*References 10, 14, 17, 3, 9, 4, 1, 7. References are arranged alphabetically at the end of the chapter but are cited in chronological, historical order in the text.

In visceroatrial situs inversus, symbolized as {I,-,-} (see Figure 101-1, columns 3 and 4), the mirror-image RA is left-sided and the mirror-image LA is right-sided.

In visceroatrial situs ambiguus, symbolized as {A,-,-} (not shown in Figure 101-1), the type of visceroatrial situs is not diagnosed. It should be understood that there are only two types of visceroatrial situs, solitus and inversus (see Figure 101-1). Undiagnosed visceroatrial situs (situs ambiguus) is not a specific third type of visceroatrial situs.

It also should be understood that the concepts of atrial isomerism and atrial appendage isomerism are considered to be erroneous.[16,20] Accurately speaking, atrial isomerism has never been documented (bilateral RA with bilateral inferior venae cavae, bilateral superior venae cavae, bilateral coronary sinus ostia, bilateral septa secunda, and bilateral broad triangular appendages; or bilateral LA with bilateral pulmonary veins, bilateral septa prima, and bilateral fingerlike appendages).

Two types of ventricular situs are shown in Figure 101-1: D-loop ventricles (see Figure 101-1, columns 1 and 4) and L-loop ventricles (see Figure 101-1, columns 2 and 3).

D-loop ventricles are solitus or noninverted ventricles that are associated with dextral or rightward looping of the straight heart tube, placing the morphologically right ventricle (RV) (Figure 101-4) to the right of the morphologically left ventricle (LV) (Figure 101-5).

L-loop ventricles are inverted or mirror-image ventricles that are associated with levo- or leftward looping of the straight heart tube, placing the mirror-image RV to the left of the mirror-image LV.

Chirality or Handedness[11]

The D-loop or solitus RV is right-handed (Figure 101-6). Figuratively speaking, the thumb of the right hand goes through the tricuspid valve. The fingers of the right hand go into the RV outflow tract. The palm of only the right hand faces the RV septal surface, and the dorsum of only the right hand faces the RV free wall surface.

The L-loop or inverted RV is left-handed (Figure 101-7). Figuratively speaking, the thumb of the left hand goes through the tricuspid valve. The fingers of the left hand go into the RV outflow tract. The palm of only the left hand faces the RV septal surface, and the dorsum of only the left hand faces the RV free wall surface.

Chirality is helpful because it defines ventricular situs (solitus or D-loop, versus inversus or L-loop), no matter what the ventricular spatial positions may be. The conventional definition of noninversion versus inversion is based on the sagittal plane, as in the definition of mirror-imagery: right–left reversal (relative to the sagittal plane), without

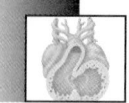

TYPES OF HUMAN HEART:
Segmental Sets and Alignments

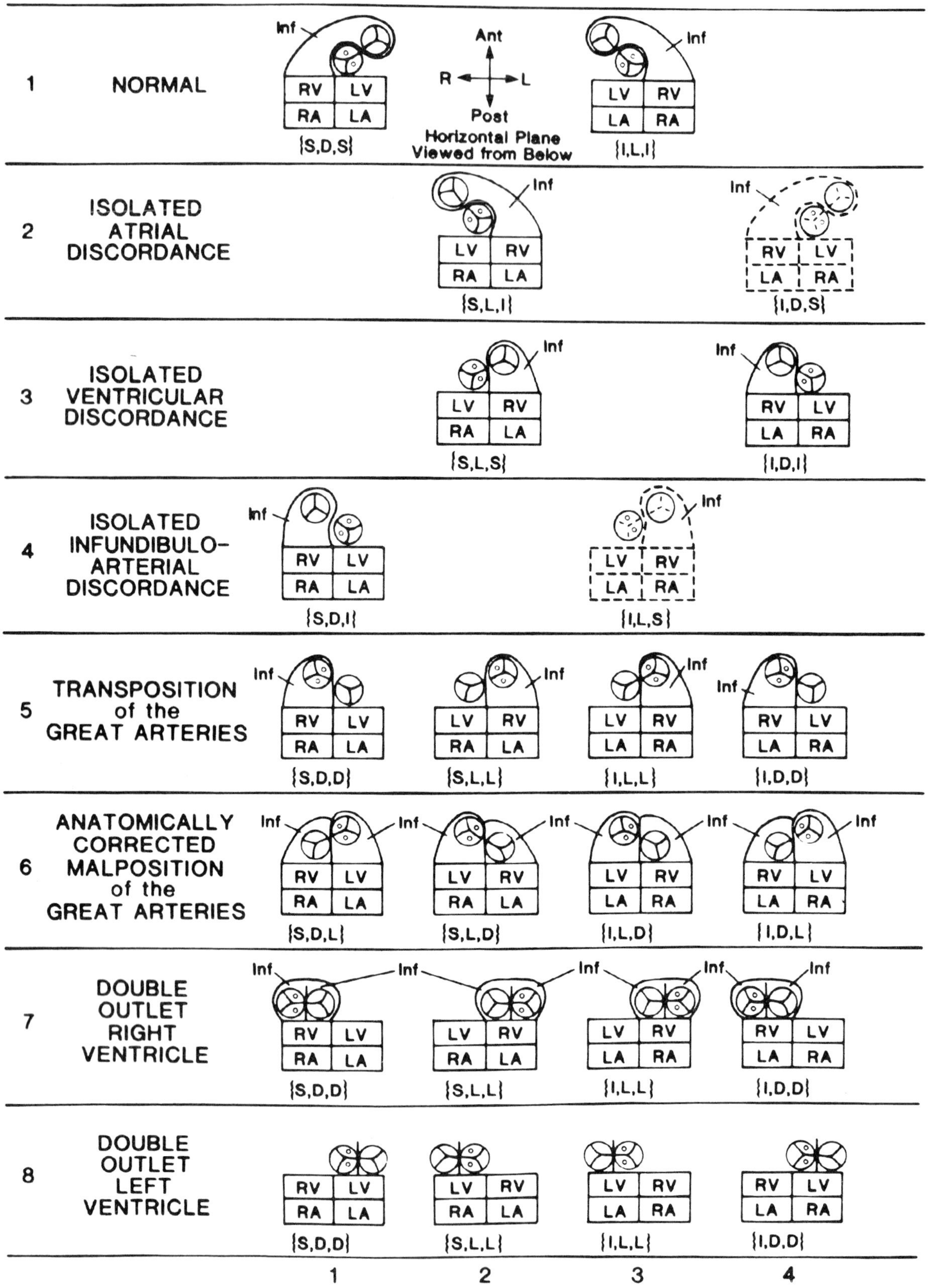

Figure 101–1 **Types of human heart, that is, segmental sets (combinations) and segmental alignments.** Heart diagrams are viewed from below, similar to subxiphoid two-dimensional echocardiograms. Cardiotypes depicted in broken lines had not been documented when this diagram was made. The aortic valve is indicated by coronary ostia. The pulmonary valve is indicated by the absence of coronary ostia. Braces {} mean "the set of." Segmental sets (combinations) are explained in the text. Ant, Anterior; Post, posterior; R, right; L, left; RA, morphologically right atrium; LA, morphologically left atrium; RV, morphologically right ventricle; LV, morphologically left ventricle; Inf, infundibulum.

(From Foran RB, Belcourt C, Nanton MA, et al: Isolated infundibuloarterial inversion {S,D,I}: A newly recognized form of congenital heart disease. Am Heart J 116:1337–1350, 1988.)

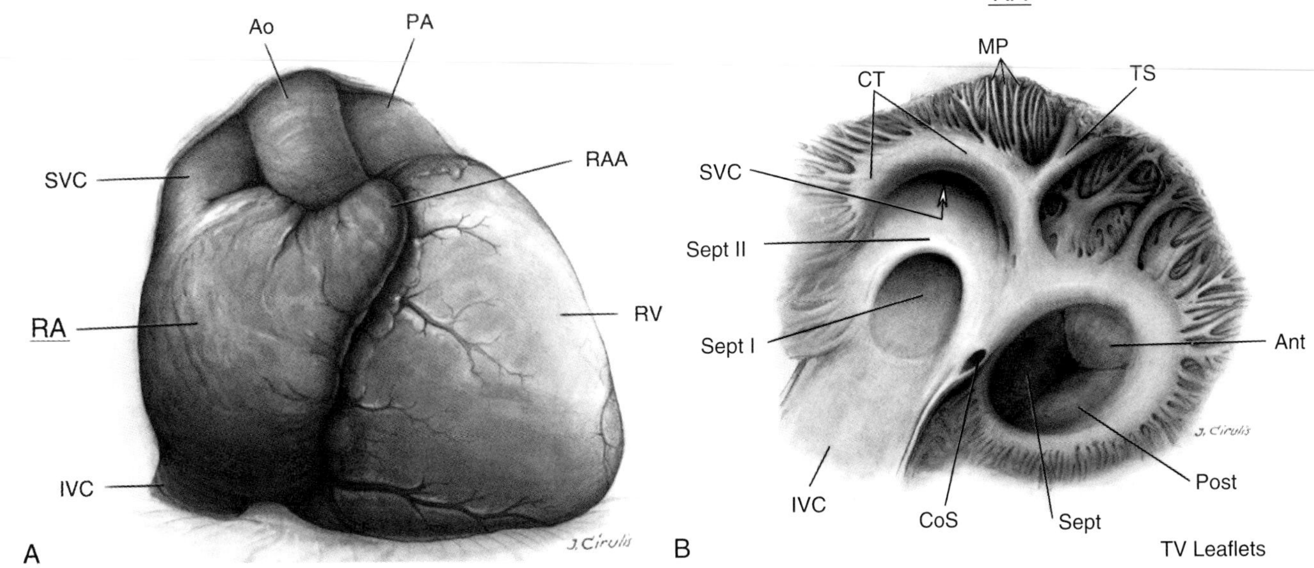

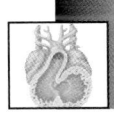

Figure 101–2 Morphologically right atrium (RA). (A) Exterior. **(B)** Interior. In **A,** note the large, broad, triangular right atrial appendage (RAA). The RA always receives the inferior vena cava (IVC) and normally receives the superior vena cava (SVC). *Ao,* Aorta; *PA,* pulmonary artery; *RV,* morphologically right ventricle. In **B,** note that the IVC is a highly reliable diagnostic marker of the RA, as is the ostium of the coronary sinus (CoS). The SVC is not a highly reliable diagnostic marker of the RA. The septal surface of the RA displays the superior limbic band of septum secundum (Sept II). Septum primum (Sept I) is the flap valve of the foramen ovale that opens into the left atrium prenatally. The crista terminalis (CT) or terminal crest lies lateral to the entry of the SVC. The CT internally corresponds to the sulcus terminalis or sinoatrial sulcus externally, where the sinoatrial node or pacemaker is located. Thus deep sutures into the CT should not be used in order to avoid the sick sinus syndrome. The musculi pectinati (MP) or pectinate muscles are prominent over the interior of the RAA. The tinea sagittalis (TS) or sagittal worm is also easily seen. Catheter tips can get lodged behind the TS, where an injudicious push can lead to perforation of the RA. The anterior (Ant), posterior (Post), and septal (Sept) leaflets of the tricuspid valve (TV) are seen from above. The membranous septum lies at the commissure between the Ant and Sept leaflets of the TV. The atrioventricular (AV) node and bundle of His unfortunately are invisible, so the surgeon must know where they are. Draw a mental line (not with a sucker, which may cause heart block) between the CoS ostium and the previously mentioned membranous septum (MS), beneath which the penetrating AV bundle passes to reach the ventricles. This CoS–MS line is where the AV node and the proximal unbranched AV bundle of His are located.
(From Van Praagh R, Vlad P: Dextrocardia, mesocardia, and levocardia. The segmental approach to diagnosis in congenital heart disease. In Keith JD, Rowe RD, Vlad P, editors: Heart Disease in Infancy and Childhood, 3rd ed., pp. 638–695. New York: Macmillan, 1978.)

superoinferior or anteroposterior change. Hence this conventional definition of inversion breaks down when the sagittal plane is not an appropriate frame of reference, as with superoinferior ventricles and crisscross atrioventricular (AV) relations in which the RV and the LV are both right-sided and left-sided. By contrast, chirality always applies accurately.

Chirality is a fundamental property of matter that also applies to the LV and to both atria. A solitus or D-loop LV is left-handed: only the palm of the left hand faces the LV septal surface. An inverted or L-loop LV is right-handed: only the palm of the right hand faces the inverted LV septal surface.

A solitus RA is right-handed: only the palm of the right hand faces the RA septal surface.

An inversus RA is left-handed: only the palm of the left hand faces the inverted RA septal surface. The solitus LA is left-handed: only the palm of the left hand faces the LA septal surface. The inversus LA is right-handed: only the palm of the right hand faces the inverted LA septal surface.

Thus the concept of handedness (chirality) applies to the RV (see Figures 101-6 and 101-7), but not only to the RV. Each type of ventricular situs (D-loop/L-loop) is both right-handed and left-handed.

D-loop ventricles may be symbolized as {-,D,-} (see Figure 101-1, columns 1 and 4). L-loop ventricles may be symbolized as {-,L,-} (see Figure 101-1, columns 2 and 3).

The two types of normal great arterial situs are solitus normally related great arteries (i.e., {-,-,S}) (see Figure 101-1, row 1, column 1), and inverted normally related great arteries (i.e.,{-,-,I}) (see Figure 101-1, row 1, column 3).

When the great arteries are abnormally related to each other, and abnormally aligned and connected relative to the underlying ventricular sinuses, the ventricular septum, and the atrioventricular valves, the semilunar interrelationships are described as follows.

When the aortic valve is right-sided (dextro- or D-) relative to the pulmonary valve, the semilunar interrelationship is symbolized as {-,-,D} (see Figure 101-1, columns 1 and 4). When the aortic valve is left-sided (levo- or L-) relative to the pulmonary valve, the semilunar interrelationship is symbolized as {-,-,L} (see Figure 101-1, columns 2 and 3).

When the aortic valve is directly anterior (antero- or A-) relative to the pulmonary valve, the semilunar interrelationship is symbolized as {-,-A} (not shown in Figure 101-1).

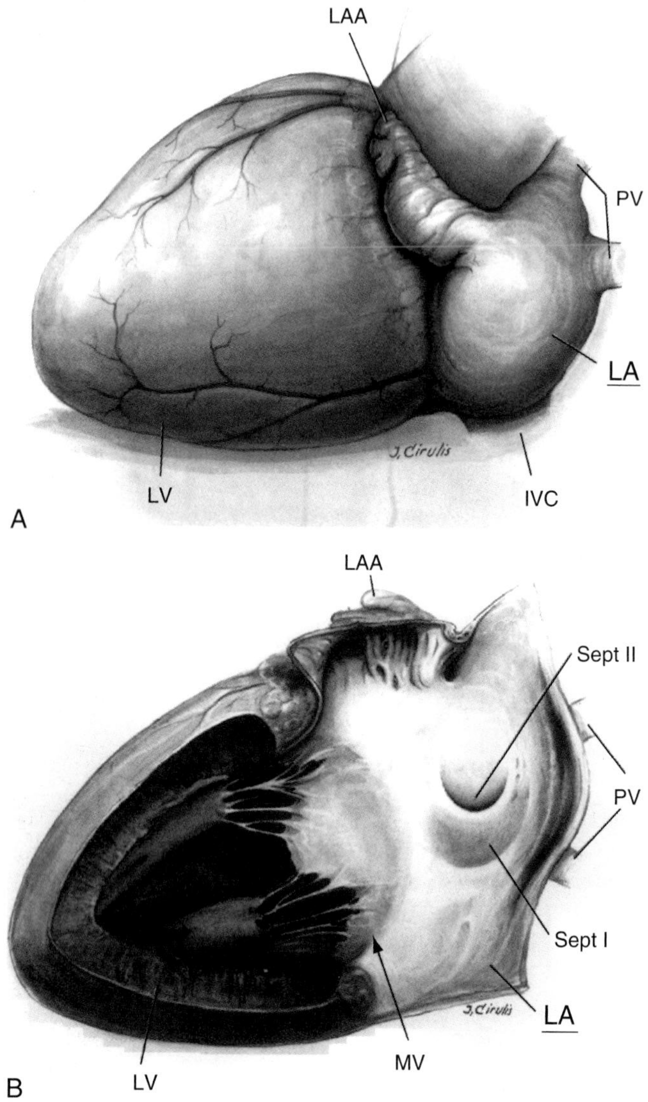

Figure 101–3 Morphologically left atrium (LA). **A,** Exterior. **B,** Interior. In **A,** note that the left atrial appendage (LAA) is long and thin, like a pointing finger. It is also relatively small and quite posterior. The pulmonary veins (PV) normally return to the LA, but abnormally do not return with totally anomalous pulmonary venous connection. The inferior vena cava (IVC) never connects directly with the LA, to our knowledge. LV, Morphologically left ventricle. In **B,** note that septum primum (Sept I) is easily seen on the septal surface of the LA, whereas septum secundum (Sept II) is partly covered by the more leftward Sept I. The pectinate muscles of the LA are largely confined within the small fingerlike LAA. MV, Mitral valve.

(From Van Praagh R, Vlad P: Dextrocardia, mesocardia, and levocardia. The segmental approach to diagnosis in congenital heart disease. In Keith JD, Rowe RD, Vlad P, editors: Heart Disease in Infancy and Childhood, 3rd ed., pp. 638–695. New York: Macmillan, 1978.)

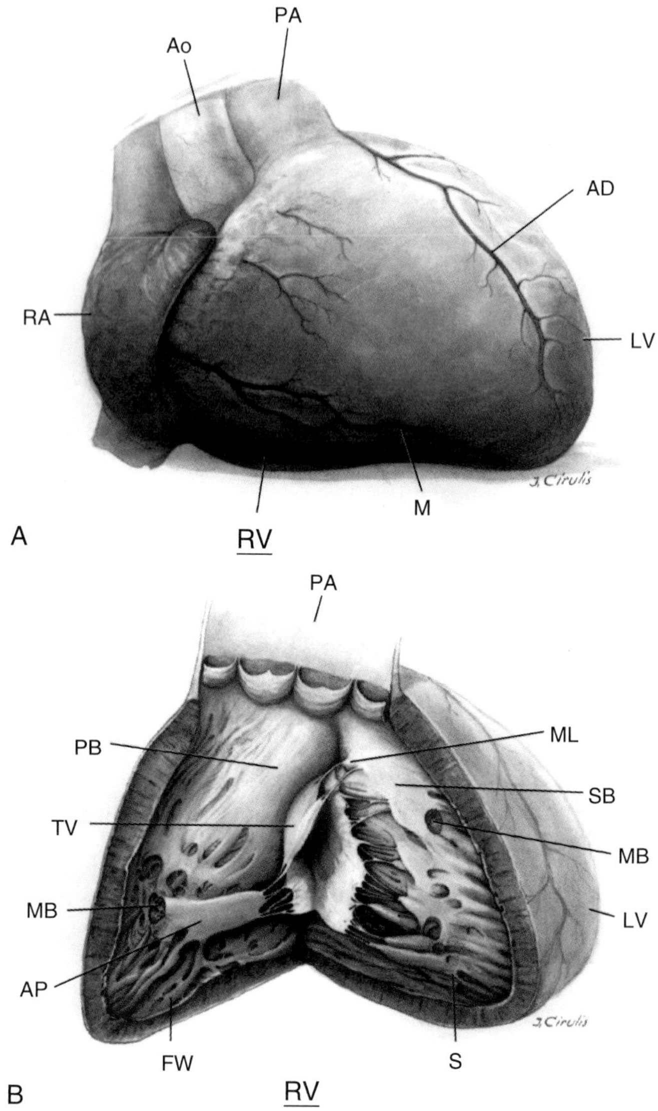

Figure 101–4 Morphologically right ventricle (RV). **A,** Exterior, drawing. **B,** Interior, drawing. **C,** Interior, photograph. In **A,** note that the exterior of the RV is triangular (as is the exterior of the right atrium [RA]). The anterior and diaphragmatic surfaces of the RV form an acute angle with each other of less than 90 degrees; hence this is called the acute margin of the heart, and the branch of the right coronary artery that runs along it is called the acute marginal branch (M). Two or more preventricular branches are also typical of the RV. The anterior descending (AD) branch of the left coronary artery indicates the location of the ventricular septum, to the left of which lies the left ventricle (LV). The ascending aorta (Ao) lies posterior and to the right of the main pulmonary artery (PA). In **B** and **C,** note that the conal septum (CS) and its parietal or free wall extension, the parietal band (PB), separate the pulmonary valve above from the tricuspid valve (TV) below. The septal band (SB) lies on the right ventricular septal surface anterosuperiorly. The SB gives off the moderator band (MB) that carries the right bundle branch of the AV conduction system from the septal band to the superior surface of the anterior papillary (AP) muscle of the RV, from whence the right bundle branch arborizes on the interior of the RV free wall as the Purkinje network. The muscle of Lancisi (ML), also known as the muscle of Luschka, or the medial papillary muscle anchors the anterior and septal leaflets of the tricuspid valve (TV) superiorly.

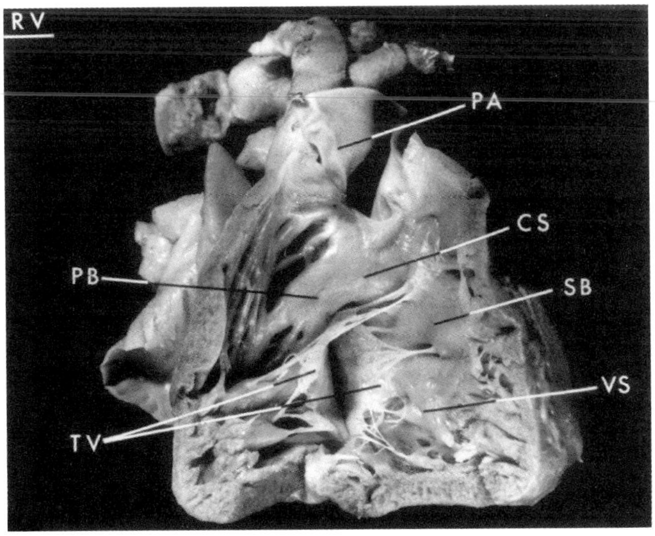

C

Figure 101–4 cont'd Immediately behind the ML lies the membranous septum, and immediately below the ML is where the right bundle branch of the conduction system emerges to run along the SB, close to its inferior margin. Often one can see the right bundle branch with the naked eye, and without special stains. Surgically this means that it is often possible to avoid transfixing the right bundle branch with surgical sutures during ventricular septal defect patch placement. Hence it is often possible surgically to avoid real right bundle branch block (as opposed to arborization block, which resembles right bundle branch block in the surface electrocardiogram, but not in the intracardiac electrocardiogram). Note that the TV attaches to the right ventricular septal surface via multiple chordae tendineas or tendinous chords; that is, the TV is "septophilic": It attaches to the surface of the ventricular septum (VS)—a diagnostic point that distinguishes the RV from the LV. Note also how coarse, few, and straight the RV trabeculations are—another distinguishing diagnostic feature of the RV. The RV sinus, body, or inflow tract—the main pumping portion—lies beneath the infundibulum, conus, or outflow tract. There is a ring of conal or infundibular muscle formed by the CS, PB, SB, and MB. This conal ring and the muscle above it form the conus or outflow tract. What the TV opens into, below the conal ring, is the RV sinus, body, or inflow tract. This main pumping portion of the RV is surprisingly small. From a functional standpoint, there is much "dead wood" in the RV: The conus is not a good pump. This understanding of the smallness of the main pumping portion of the RV strongly favors, when feasible, the arterial switch operation in the management of all kinds of transposition of the great arteries. *(From Van Praagh R, Vlad P: Dextrocardia, mesocardia, and levocardia. The segmental approach to diagnosis in congenital heart disease. In Keith JD, Rowe RD, Vlad P, editors: Heart Disease in Infancy and Childhood, 3rd ed., pp. 638–695. New York: Macmillan, 1978.)*

Segmental Alignments and Connections

The main cardiac segments (i.e., {atria, ventricles, great arteries}) can be aligned with each other in many different ways (see Figure 101-1). *Alignment* means what is aligned with what, or what opens into what (see Figure 101-1).

The main cardiac segments (i.e., {atria, ventricles, great arteries}) usually do not connect directly with each other (tissue-to-tissue) because of the interposition of the

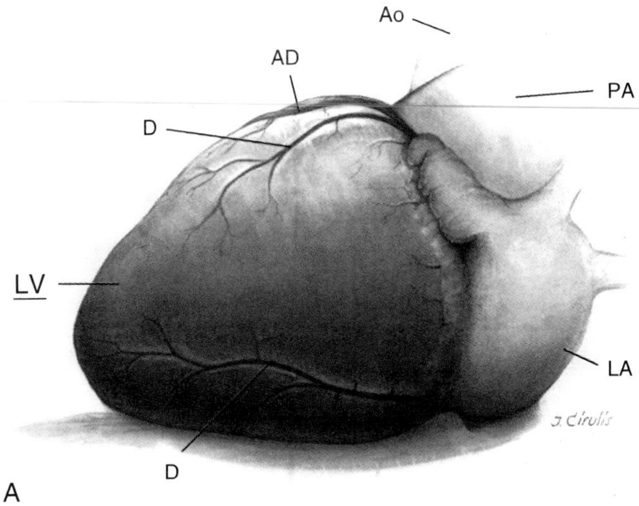

A

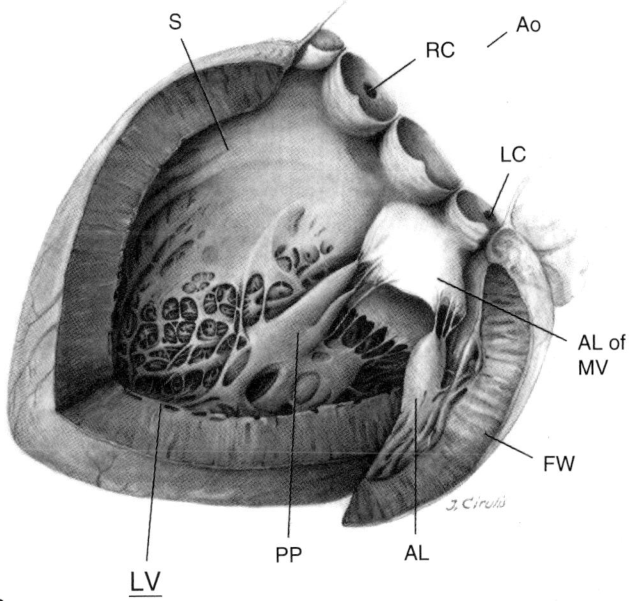

B

Figure 101–5 Morphologically left ventricle (LV). (**A**) Exterior, drawing. (**B**) Interior, drawing. (**C**) Interior, photograph. In **A**, note that the external shape of the LV is conical, like a bullet or a torpedo. The margin of the LV is described as obtuse (i.e., greater than 90 degrees). Hence the diagonal (D) branches of the left coronary arterial system are also known as obtuse marginal branches. The superior diagonal supplies the region of the superior or anterolateral papillary muscle group and the adjacent LV free wall. The inferior diagonal supplies the inferior or posteromedial papillary muscle group and the adjacent LV free wall. The anterior descending (AD) and the posterior descending (not seen) coronary arteries indicate the location of the ventricular septum. In **B** and **C,** the noncoronary (NC) and left coronary (LC) leaflets of the aortic valve are in direct fibrous continuity with the anterior leaflet (AL) of the mitral valve (MV), reflecting the normal absence of subaortic conal free wall myocardium. The anterosuperior portion of the left ventricular septal surface (S) is smooth or nontrabeculated. The inferior and apical portion of the left ventricular septal and free wall surfaces display a latticelike mesh of small, fine, oblique trabeculae carneae. The right coronary (RC) and left coronary (LC) ostia are seen emerging from their sinuses of valsalva. The noncoronary–left coronary commissure is normally located right above the middle of the anterior mitral leaflet.

(Continued)

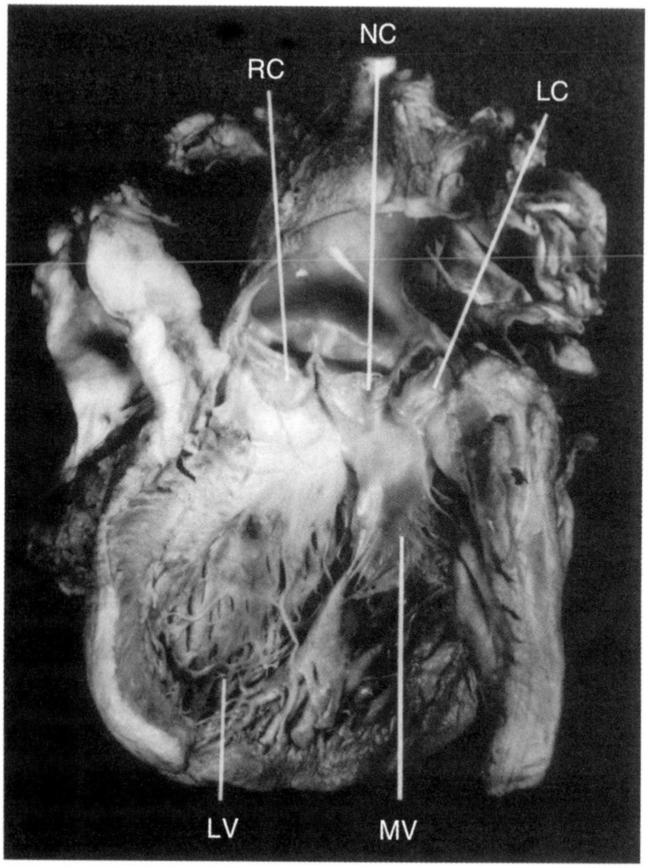

C

Figure 101–5 cont'd The noncoronary–right coronary commissure normally is located right above the membranous septum, which in turn is immediately above the left bundle of the atrioventricular conduction system. These landmarks beneath the aortic valve are highly relevant to surgical excision of discrete fibrous subaortic stenosis. The aortic commissures help indicate to the surgeon where various important and vulnerable structures are located. Often one can see both the anterior (superior) and the posterior (inferior) radiations of the left bundle branch of the conduction system, shown in **B**. Special stains are not needed. Because they are glycogen rich, the superior and inferior radiations often can be seen, yellow-white, arching across the smooth superior portion of the left ventricular septal surface. The superior radiation runs to the anterolateral (superior) papillary muscle group, and the inferior radiation courses to the posteromedial (inferior) papillary muscle group. The left ventricular papillary muscles are few, large, and arise from the left ventricular free wall—never normally from the left ventricular septal surface. Hence the papillary muscles of the LV have been described as "septophobic"—a point of diagnostic importance in distinguishing the LV from the right ventricle (RV).
(From Van Praagh R, Vlad P: Dextrocardia, mesocardia, and levocardia. The segmental approach to diagnosis in congenital heart disease. In Keith JD, Rowe RD, Vlad P, editors: Heart Disease in Infancy and Childhood, 3rd ed., pp. 638–695. New York: Macmillan, 1978.)

connecting segments (i.e., the atrioventricular [AV] junction and the conus arteriosus). *Connection* means what is connected with what, directly or tissue-to-tissue.

Thus the atria can be aligned with the ventricles in many different ways (see Figure 101-1), but the atria and the ventricles usually do not connect tissue-to-tissue—except at the bundle of His—because of the interposition of the tissues of the AV junction or canal. When the atria and the ventricles do connect directly, the result is AV bypass tracts with ventricular preexcitation, as in the Wolff-Parkinson-White syndrome. Normally the atria and the ventricles are electrically insulated from each other by the AV junction. Normally the atria and the ventricles are aligned, but the atria and the ventricles do not connect. Instead, the atria and the ventricles *are connected* (note the passive voice) by the AV junction.

Similarly, the ventricular sinuses (the pumping chambers) are aligned with the great arteries in many different ways (see Figure 101-1). However, the ventricular sinuses and the great arteries do not connect tissue-to-tissue because of the interposition of the conus arteriosus. Instead, the ventricular sinuses and the great arteries are connected (note the passive voice) in many different ways (see Figure 101-1) by the conal connector (Figure 101-8).

Thus intersegmental alignments and connections are different concepts. Both are important.

Segmental alignments may be *concordant*[173] (i.e., appropriate or normal), as when the RA opens into the RV or the LA opens into the LV, or the RV ejects into the pulmonary artery (PA) or the LV ejects into the aorta (Ao).

Segmental alignments may be *discordant*[17,3] (i.e., inappropriate or the opposite of normal), as when the RA opens into the LV or the LA opens into the RV, or the RV ejects into the Ao or the LV ejects into the PA.

AV alignments may be *concordant,* as when the segmental set is {S,D,-} (see Figure 101-1, column 1) or {I,L,-} (see Figure 101-1, column 3); *discordant,* as when the segmental combination is {S,L,-} (see Figure 101-1, column 2) or {I,D,-} (see Figure 101-1, column 4); *atretic,* as with tricuspid atresia or mitral atresia; *straddling,* as with straddling tricuspid valve or straddling mitral valve; *double-inlet,* as with double-inlet LV (with absent or markedly hypoplastic RV sinus) or double-inlet RV (with absent or markedly hypoplastic LV sinus); *common-inlet,* as with common AV canal and balanced RV and LV, common AV canal with common-inlet RV (when the LV is hypoplastic or absent), or common AV canal with common-inlet LV (when the RV sinus is hypoplastic or absent; or *double-outlet RA,*[6] when there is an RA-to-RV valve, an RA-to-LV valve, and an LA-to-LV (mitral) valve (three separate AV valves).

Ventriculoarterial (VA) alignments may be *concordant,* as with solitus normally related great arteries (i.e., {-,-,S}) (see Figure 101-1), with inverted normally related great arteries (i.e., {-,-,I}) (see Figure 101-1), or with anatomically corrected malposition of the great arteries (see Figure 101-1, row 6); *discordant,* as with transposition of the great arteries (TGA) (see Figure 101-1, row 5); or *double-outlet,* as with double-outlet right ventricle (DORV) (see Figure 101-1, row 7), double-outlet left ventricle (DOLV) (see Figure 101-1, row 8), or double-outlet infundibular outlet chamber (not shown in Figure 101-1).

The AV connections consist of the AV valves (leaflets and annuli) and the AV septum.

The VA connections consist of the conus arteriosus—septum and free wall(s) (see Figure 101-8). Development of the *subpulmonary conus,* with resorption of the subaortic conal free wall permitting aortic–mitral fibrous continuity, is associated with normally related great arteries (see Figure 101-8, subpulmonary conus).

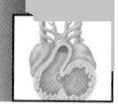

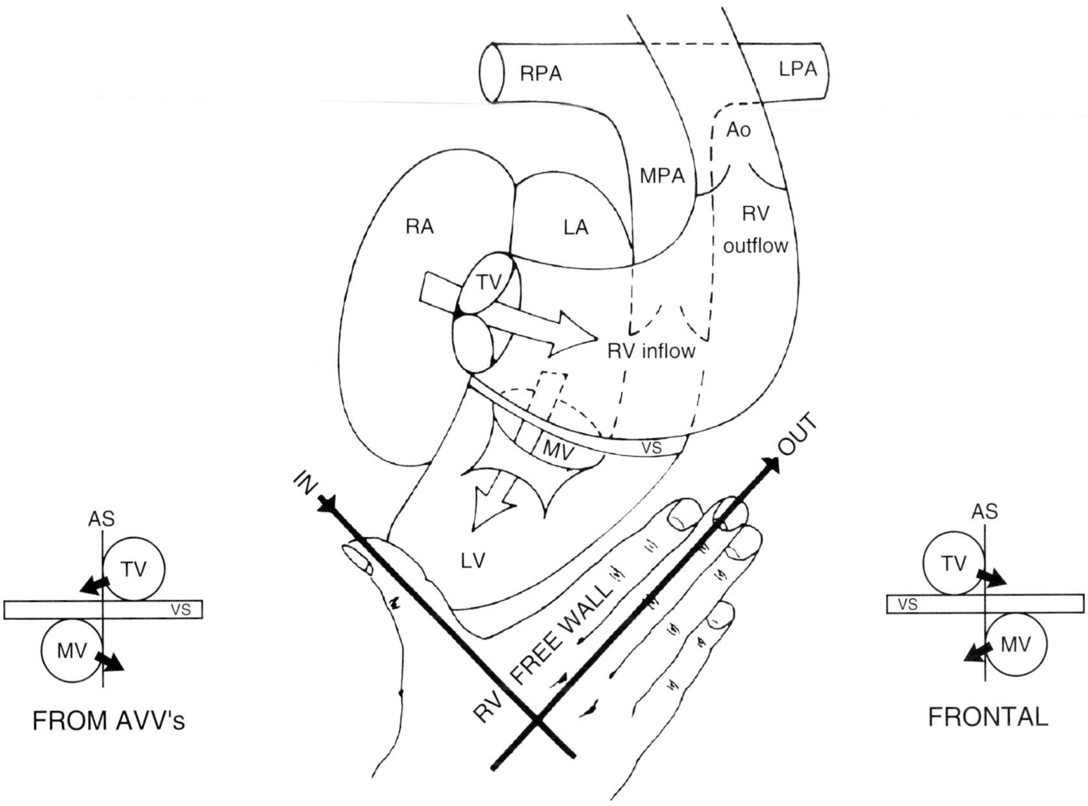

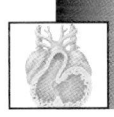

CRISSCROSS AV RELATIONS
TGA {S,D,L}

Figure 101–6 The D-loop right ventricle (RV) is right-handed. Figuratively speaking, the thumb of the right hand goes through the tricuspid valve (TV), indicating the RV inflow tract (IN). The fingers of the right hand go into the RV outflow tract (OUT). The palm of only the right hand faces the RV septal surface, and the dorsum of only the right hand is adjacent to the RV free wall surface. Handedness or chirality is helpful in making the diagnosis of the ventricular situs (D-loop versus L-loop) when the conventional definition of noninversion or inversion relative to the sagittal plane breaks down, as in this case of superoinferior ventricles with crisscross atrioventricular (AV) relations. Both ventricles are bilateral (right-sided and left-sided). Because D-loop RV is right-handed, some of our colleagues call D-loop ventricles right-hand topology. This is a case of physiologically uncorrected ("complete") transposition of the great arteries (TGA) {S,D,L} with AV concordance, ventriculoarterial (VA) discordance, superoinferior ventricles, and crisscross AV relations. Ao, Aorta; AS, atrial septum; AVVs, atrioventricular valves; LPA, left pulmonary artery; MPA, main pulmonary artery; MV, mitral valve; RPA, right pulmonary artery; VS, ventricular septum. Other abbreviations are the same as previously.
(From Van Praagh S, LaCorte M, Fellows KE, et al: Superoinferior ventricles, anatomic and angiocardiographic findings in 10 postmortem cases. In Van Praagh R, Takao A, editors: Etiology and Morphogenesis of Congenital Heart Disease, pp. 317–378. Mt. Kisco, NY: Futura Publishing Co., 1980.)

Development of the *subaortic conus,* with resorption of the subpulmonary conal free wall permitting pulmonary–mitral fibrous continuity, is associated with transposition of the great arteries (see Figure 101-8, subaortic conus).

Development of both the subaortic and the subpulmonary conus, without the resorption of subsemilunar conal free wall, results in a *bilateral conus,* with no semilunar–atrioventricular fibrous continuity. The bilateral conus is associated with DORV (see Figure 101-8, bilateral conus).

Absence or very marked deficiency of the subsemilunar conal myocardium rarely permits aortic–mitral and pulmonary–mitral fibrous continuity. *Absence or marked deficiency of the conus* may be associated with DOLV (see Figure 101-8, absent subsemilunar conus).

Thus the development of the conal connector between the ventricles and the great arteries is one of the most important morphological factors in determining the VA alignments.[13] The fact that the ventricular sinuses do not connect directly with the great arteries, but instead are connected via the conus arteriosus, is thus of great developmental significance.

SPECIFIC EXAMPLES AND SURGICAL RELEVANCE

The segmental anatomy of the heart is of great practical importance in congenital heart disease because it conveys the basic architectural "floor plan" of the heart (see Figure

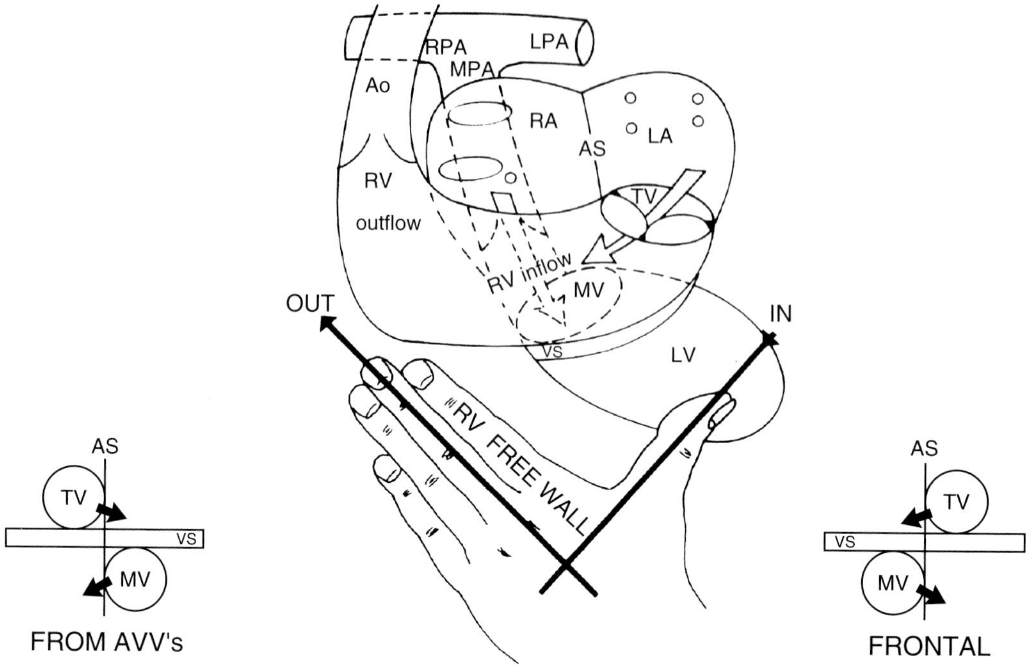

Figure 101–7 The L-loop right ventricle is left-handed. Figuratively speaking, the thumb of the left hand goes through the tricuspid valve (TV), representing the right ventricle (RV) inflow tract (IN). The fingers of the left hand go into the RV outflow tract (OUT). The palm of only the left hand faces the RV septal surface. The dorsum of only the left hand is adjacent to the RV free wall surface. Because L-loop RV is left-handed, some of our colleagues call L-loop ventricles left-hand topology. This is a case of congenital physiologically corrected TGA {S,L,D} with AV discordance and VA discordance, superoinferior ventricles, and crisscross AV relations. Some L-loop ventricles appear to be truly inverted, as with mirror-image dextrocardia in situs inversus totalis {I,L,I}. However, often L-loop ventricles, as with classical congenital physiologically corrected TGA {S,L,L}, or, as in this case—TGA {S,L,D}—may be only apparently inverted, that is, a solitus heart tube that has undergone L-looping (an L-malrotated solitus heart tube). L-loop formation has definitely occurred in both of the previous examples, but only one (i.e., {I,L,I}) may be truly inverted. This is why we prefer to talk about D-loop ventricles and L-loop ventricles (rather than noninverted and inverted ventricles, respectively). Thus when the ventricles are very malrotated, and consequently diagnostically potentially confusing, chirality is helpful. Abbreviations are the same as previously.
(From Van Praagh S, LaCorte M, Fellows KE, et al: Superoinferior ventricles, anatomic and angiocardiographic findings in 10 postmortem cases. In Van Praagh R, Takao A, editors: Etiology and Morphogenesis of Congenital Heart Disease, pp. 317–378. Mt. Kisco, NY: Futura Publishing Co., 1980.)

101-1). *In Figure 101-1, note that the vertical columns are organized in terms of the AV alignments:*

In column 1, all hearts have visceroatrial situs solitus and AV concordance (i.e., {S,D,-}).
In column 2, all hearts have visceroatrial situs solitus and AV discordance (i.e., {S,L,-}).
In column 3, all hearts have visceroatrial situs inversus and AV concordance (i.e., {I,L,-}).
In column 4, all hearts have visceroatrial situs inversus, and AV discordance (i.e., {I,D,-}).

In Figure 101-1, the horizontal rows are organized in terms of the ventriculoarterial alignments:

Rows 1 to 4 and 6 have VA concordance.
Row 5 has VA discordance (i.e., transposition of the great arteries).
Rows 7 and 8 have VA alignments with double-outlet: DORV (row 7) and DOLV (row 8).

The following are some specific examples of segmental anatomy and its surgical relevance.

1. The solitus normal heart is {S,D,S} (see Figure 101-1, row 1, column 1). There is AV and VA concordance.
2. The inverted normal heart is {I,L,I} (see Figure 101-1, row 1, column 3). There is AV and VA concordance.
3. Ventricular inversion with inverted normally related great arteries is {S,L,I} (see Figure 101-1, row 2, column 2). There is AV discordance with VA concordance. Intersegmental discordance at the AV junction means that the systemic and pulmonary circulations are physiologically uncorrected. Because the great arteries are normally related (i.e., inverted normally related), such patients need an atrial switch procedure (Senning or Mustard).
4. Isolated ventricular inversion is {S,L,S} (see Figure 101-1, row 3, column 2). There is AV discordance with VA concordance. Again, the presence of intersegmental discordance at the AV junction means that such patients have physiologically uncorrected, transposition-like circulations; hence an atrial switch operation is indicated. Isolated

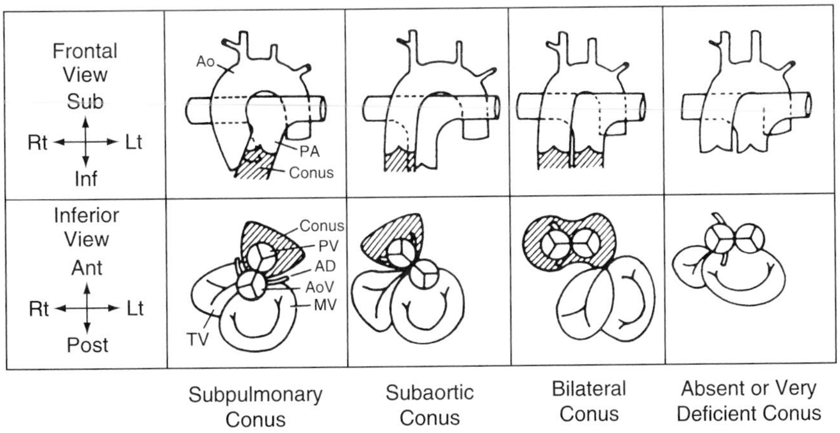

Figure 101–8 Anatomic types of subsemilunar infundibulum or conus arteriosus. The part of the conus that typically is involved in conotruncal malformations is the distal or subsemilunar part (i.e., the conal septum, the parietal band, and the subsemilunar free wall), not the proximal or apical septal band part of the conus. *The subpulmonary conus* is associated with normally related great arteries and, when underdeveloped, with tetralogy of Fallot. The subaortic conal free wall myocardium normally undergoes absorption, permitting aortic–mitral fibrous continuity. *The subaortic conus* typically is associated with transposition of the great arteries. Resorption of the subpulmonary conal free wall myocardium permits pulmonary–mitral fibrous continuity, both with typical D-TGA and typical L-TGA. When the distal or subsemilunar conus is bilateral (i.e., both subaortic and subpulmonary), neither the subaortic nor the subpulmonary conal free wall has undergone resorption (presumably apoptosis has failed to occur). Consequently, there is no semilunar–atrioventricular fibrous continuity. A *bilateral conus* is often associated with double-outlet right ventricle (DORV). Absence or marked deficiency of the subsemilunar conus rarely occurs. *Absence of the subsemilunar conal myocardium* can be associated with double-outlet left ventricle (DOLV), with aortic–mitral and pulmonary–mitral fibrous continuity. Thus the development of the conal connector between the ventricular sinuses below and the great arteries above is one of the most important morphogenetic factors that determine the definitive ventriculoarterial alignments. In view of its importance to diagnostic understanding and surgical management, it is suggested that the anatomic type of conus be included as a specific part of every diagnosis. AD, Anterior descending coronary artery; Ant, anterior; AoV, aortic valve; Inf, inferior; Lt, left; MV, mitral valve; PA, main pulmonary artery; Post, posterior; PV, pulmonary valve; Rt, right; Sup, superior; TV, tricuspid valve.
(Modified from Van Praagh R, Vlad P: Dextrocardia, mesocardia, and levocardia. The segmental approach to diagnosis in congenital heart disease. In Keith JD, Rowe RD, Vlad P, editors: Heart Disease in Infancy and Childhood, 3rd ed., pp. 638–695. New York: Macmillan, 1978.)

ventricular inversion {S,L,S} is the commonest type of AV discordance with VA concordance.[5]

5. Isolated ventricular noninversion is {I,D,I} (see Figure 101-1, row 3, column 4). Again, there is AV discordance with VA concordance, and hence an atrial switch procedure is desirable.
6. Isolated infundibuloarterial inversion is {S,D,I}[2] (see Figure 101-1, row 4, column 1). Because there is AV and VA concordance, there is no reason—based on the segmental anatomy—for the systemic and pulmonary circulations to be physiologically uncorrected. However, hearts with this rare segmental combination almost always also have inverted tetralogy of Fallot. It is the mirror-image tetralogy of Fallot type of pulmonary infundibular and valvular stenosis or atresia, with a subaortic ventricular septal defect, that requires surgical repair. Because the aortic valve lies to the left of the pulmonary valve, but the RV remains right-sided, this means that the right coronary artery runs across the stenotic pulmonary outflow tract—where the surgeon wants to make an incision to open up the obstructive subpulmonary infundibulum. Consequently, surgical repair of tetralogy of Fallot {S,D,I} may require a right ventricular-to-pulmonary artery conduit to "jump" the right coronary artery to avoid its transection. It is also sometimes possible, and preferable, to open up the pulmonary outflow tract by judicious myocardial resection,[8] thereby avoiding a free-standing conduit, which would have to be replaced every few years because of fibrotic obstruction of the conduit.
7. Typical complete transposition of the great arteries usually is TGA {S,D,D} (see Figure 101-1, row 5, column 1). There is AV concordance with VA discordance. Consequently, an arterial switch procedure usually is desirable to surgically correct the physiologically uncorrected systemic and pulmonary circulations. D-TGA (i.e., TGA with aortic valve to the right [Dextro or D] relative to the pulmonary valve) can have additional significant associated malformations, such as pulmonary stenosis or atresia with a ventricular septal defect. Hence, although segmental anatomy is important, it is not the whole story.

As now defined, all transpositions of the great arteries are *complete;* that is, both great arteries are placed completely across the ventricular septum and so rise above the anatomically inappropriate ventricle: Ao above RV, and PA above LV. Congenitally physiologically corrected TGA is also a complete TGA. *Partial* transpositions of the great arteries are now called either *DORV* (only the Ao is transposed above the RV, whereas the PA is not transposed above the LV), or *DOLV* (only the PA is transposed above the LV, but the Ao is not transposed above the RV).

8. Classical congenital physiologically corrected TGA typically is TGA {S,L,L} (see Figure 101-1, row 5, column 2). There is AV discordance and VA discordance. Two intersegmental discordances—at both the AV and VA junctions—physiologically cancel each other (as long as associated malformations such as pulmonary outflow tract stenosis or atresia with ventricular septal defect do not vitiate the potential physiological correction). These two intersegmental

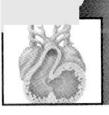

discordances potentially result in physiologically corrected destinations of the systemic venous blood stream, which flows to the transposed pulmonary artery, and of the pulmonary venous blood stream, which flows to the transposed aorta. So, two wrongs can make a right! However, they often do not—because of associated malformations.[15] Surgical management may involve repair of associated malformations only, or a double-switch procedure (atrial and arterial switch operations).

9. Physiologically uncorrected ("complete") TGA in situs inversus typically is TGA {I,L,L} (see Figure 101-1, row 5, column 3) with AV concordance and VA discordance.
10. Congenital physiologically corrected TGA in situs inversus typically is TGA {I,D,D} (see Figure 101-1, row 5, column 4) with AV and VA discordance.
11. The commonest form of anatomically corrected malposition of the great arteries is ACM {S,D,L} (see Figure 101-1, row 6, column 1) with AV and VA concordance.[12] In all forms of ACM, the ventricles have looped in one direction (to the right in this type), and the conotruncus (infundibulum and great arteries) have twisted in the opposite direction (to the left in this type). The result of these opposite twistings of the ventricular loop and the conotruncus is that, despite the presence of a serious malposition of the great arteries, each great artery nonetheless rises above the anatomically correct ventricle: Ao above LV and PA above RV. This is why these anomalies are called *anatomically corrected malpositions* of the great arteries.

It is noteworthy that ACM can be physiologically corrected, as in ACM {S,D,L}, or physiologically uncorrected, as in ACM {S,L,D} (see Figure 101-1, row 6, column 2) with AV discordance and VA concordance.

It is also noteworthy that VA concordance is not necessarily synonymous with normally related great arteries. In ACM, despite the presence of VA concordance, the VA alignments and connections are abnormal. The conus is either bilateral or subaortic.

12. The segmental anatomy of some of the anatomic types of DORV (see Figure 101-1, row 7) and DOLV (see Figure 101-1, row 8) are depicted, without associated malformations. In hearts with DORV[19] or DOLV,[18] the AV alignments are often concordant or discordant, depending on the AV segmental anatomy (see Figure 101-1). However, the VA alignments are never concordant or discordant, but double-outlet (RV or LV), by definition.

SUMMARY

An understanding of segmental anatomy is basic to the accurate diagnosis and successful surgical treatment of patients with complex congenital heart disease.

REFERENCES

1. Calcaterra G, Anderson RH, Lau KC, et al: Dextrocardia—value of segmental analysis in its categorization. Br Heart J 42: 497–507, 1979.
2. Foran RB, Belcourt C, Nanton MA, et al: Isolated infundibuloarterial inversion {S,D,I}: A newly recognized form of congenital heart disease. Am Heart J 116:1337–1350, 1988.
3. Kirklin JW, Pacifico AD, Bargeron LM, et al: Cardiac repair in anatomically corrected malposition of the great arteries. Circulation 48:153–159, 1973.
4. Otero Coto E, Quero Jimenez M: Aproximación segmentaria al diagnostico y clasificación de las cardiopatias congenitas. Fundamentos y utilidad. Rev Esp Cardiol 30:557–566, 1977.
5. Pasquini L, Sanders SP, Parness I, et al: Echocardiographic and anatomic findings in atrioventricular discordance with ventriculoarterial concordance. Am J Cardiol 62:1256–1262, 1988.
6. Pessotto R, Padalino M, Rubino M, et al: Straddling tricuspid valve as a sign of ventriculoatrial malalignment: A morphologic study of 19 postmortem cases. Am Heart J 138:1184–1195, 1999.
7. Rao PS: Systematic approach to differential diagnosis. Am Heart J 102:389–403, 1981.
8. Santini F, Jonas RA, Sanders SP, et al: Tetralogy of Fallot {S,D,I}: Successful repair without a conduit. Ann Thorac Surg 59:747–749, 1995.
9. Shinebourne EA, Macartney FJ, Anderson RH: Sequential chamber localization—logical approach to diagnosis in congenital heart disease. Br Heart J 38:327–339, 1976.
10. Van Praagh R: The segmental approach to diagnosis in congenital heart disease. In Bergsma D, editor: Birth Defects: Original Article Series, Vol. 8, pp. 4–23, 1972.
11. Van Praagh R, David I, Gordon D, et al: Ventricular diagnosis and designation. In Godman MJ, editor: Paediatric Cardiology, Vol. 4, pp. 153–168. London: World Congress, 1980. Edinburgh: Churchill Livingstone, 1981.
12. Van Praagh R, Durnin RE, Jockin H, et al: Anatomically corrected malposition of the great arteries {S,D,L}. Circulation 51:20–31, 1975.
13. Van Praagh R, Layton WM, Van Praagh S: The morphogenesis of normal and abnormal relationships between the great arteries and the ventricles: Pathologic and experimental data. In Van Praagh R, Takao A, editors: Etiology and Morphogenesis of Congenital Heart Disease, pp. 271–316. Mt Kisco, NY: Futura Publishing Co., 1980.
14. Van Praagh R, Ongley PA, Swan HJC: Anatomic types of single or common ventricle in man. Morphologic and geometric aspects of sixty autopsied cases. Am J Cardiol 13:367–386, 1964.
15. Van Praagh R, Papagiannis J, Grünenfelder J, et al: Pathologic anatomy of corrected transposition of the great arteries: Medical and surgical implications. Am Heart J 135:772–785, 1998.
16. Van Praagh R, Van Praagh S: Atrial isomerism in the heterotaxy syndromes with asplenia, or polysplenia, or normally formed spleen: An erroneous concept. Am J Cardiol 66:1504–1506, 1990.
17. Van Praagh R, Van Praagh S, Vlad P, et al: Anatomic types of congenital dextrocardia. Diagnostic and embryologic implications. Am J Cardiol 13:510–531, 1964.
18. Van Praagh R, Weinberg PM, Srebro J: Double-outlet left ventricle. In Adams FH, Emmanouilides GC, Riemenschneider TA, editors: Moss' Heart Disease in Infants, Children and Adolescents, 4th ed., pp. 461–485. Baltimore: Williams & Wilkins, 1989.
19. Van Praagh S, Davidoff A, Chin A, et al: Double-outlet right ventricle: Anatomic types and developmental implications based on a study of 101 autopsied cases. Coeur 13:389–439, 1982.
20. Van Praagh S, Santini F, Sanders SP: Cardiac malpositions with special emphasis on visceral heterotaxy (asplenia and polysplenia syndromes). In Fyler DC, editor: Nadas' Pediatric Cardiology, pp. 589–608. Philadelphia: Hanley & Belfus, Inc., 1992.

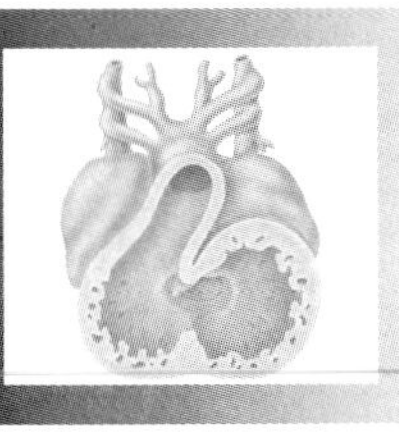

CHAPTER 102

Diagnostic Imaging: Echocardiography and Magnetic Resonance Imaging

Tal Geva

INTRODUCTION

Before the advent of cardiopulmonary bypass in the mid-1950s, little attention was given to the diagnosis of congenital heart disease (CHD), because no effective treatment was available. Physical examination, auscultation, electrocardiography, and radiography were the main diagnostic tools. Progress in open-heart techniques for repair of CHD required accurate and comprehensive delineation of cardiovascular anatomy and function. During the 1960s and 1970s, cardiac catheterization and angiography were the principal tools used for diagnosis of CHD. Echocardiography entered the arena in the late 1970s. The diagnostic capability of M-mode echocardiography proved insufficient in patients with CHD, but the rapid evolution of two-dimensional (2D) echocardiography during the following decade transformed the field. The technological advances in transducer design, image processing, and display, together with development and refinement of new imaging planes and examination techniques, allowed high-quality tomographic visualization of most cardiac defects.[35] The application of Doppler ultrasound to investigate blood flow allowed comprehensive hemodynamic assessment. By the mid-1980s, much of the necessary anatomical and hemodynamic information required for patient management could be obtained noninvasively, obviating the need for a diagnostic catheterization in many patients. During the 1990s, the field of pediatric cardiac imaging experienced accelerated progress in areas such as three-dimensional (3D) echocardiography and the application of magnetic resonance imaging (MRI) to CHD. At the same time, the proportion of cardiac catheterization procedures performed solely for diagnostic purposes has drastically declined. By the end of the 1990s, the majority of catheterization procedures in pediatric cardiology were therapeutic.

This chapter discusses the clinical application of the two main noninvasive diagnostic imaging modalities used for anatomical and physiological evaluation of preoperative and postoperative CHD—echocardiography and cardiovascular magnetic resonance (CMR) imaging.

ECHOCARDIOGRAPHY AND DOPPLER ULTRASOUND

Echocardiography is an ideal diagnostic tool in pediatric cardiology because of its noninvasive nature, relatively low cost, superb spatial and temporal resolutions, and ability to image cardiovascular anatomy and evaluate physiology in real time. In addition, modern cardiac ultrasound equipment is portable and adaptable to different environments such as the operating room, the intensive care unit, at the bedside, and in an outpatient office setting. In today's pediatric cardiology practice, echocardiography is the primary diagnostic modality used to evaluate anatomy and physiology preoperatively, intraoperatively, postoperatively, during follow-up of CHD, and prenatally.[35,111,116]

Description of Technique

For an echocardiographic image to be obtained, a burst of ultrasound energy is generated by a piezoelectric crystal and travels through the soft tissue at an average speed of approximately 1540 m/sec. When the propagating ultrasound wave encounters an interface between tissues with different acoustic properties, some of the energy is reflected back toward the transducer and some of the energy is refracted and continues to travel in the medium until it encounters the next interface. The returning ultrasound energy is then converted into an electrical energy that goes through a series of electronic processes, including amplification, filtering, postprocessing, and display.

M-Mode Echocardiography

A narrow beam of ultrasound energy is emitted toward the heart, and structures along the beam path reflect echoes back toward the transducer. A dot is displayed on the screen in a position corresponding to its distance from the transducer. This process is repeated rapidly to create an image. The distance from the transducer is displayed on the y-axis, and time is displayed on the x-axis (Figure 102-1). This provides an anatomically one-dimensional image of the heart that is characterized by excellent temporal and axial resolutions. In today's clinical pediatric echocardiography, M-mode is no longer used for anatomical imaging of the heart.[116] 2D-directed M-mode echocardiography is used primarily for evaluation of left ventricular dimensions and functions. In selected circumstances, when superior temporal resolution is required, 2D-directed M-mode echocardiography may be used to assess motion of specific structures such as native and prosthetic valve leaflets.

Two-Dimensional Echocardiography

With a rapid sweeping of an ultrasound beam through an arc, multiple "M-mode lines" are placed next to each other to construct a cross-sectional 2D image of the heart

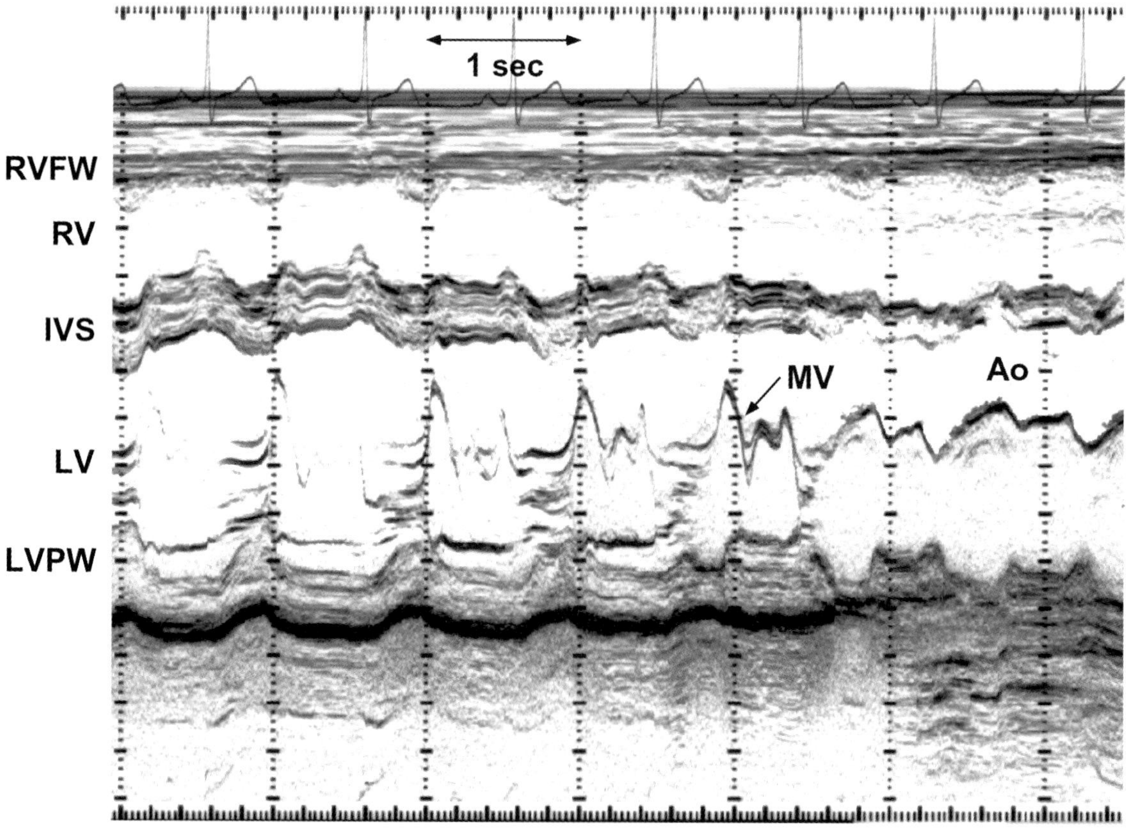

Figure 102–1 **M-mode tracing of the left ventricle and the aortic root.** Ao, Aortic root; IVS, interventricular septum; LV, left ventricle; LVFW, left ventricular free wall; MV, mitral valve; RV, right ventricle; RVFW, right ventricular free wall.

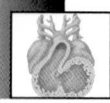

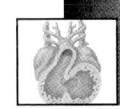

(Figure 102-2). This can be accomplished by rotating or rocking an ultrasonic crystal, as in mechanical transducers, or by electronically sweeping the sound beam through multiple piezoelectric crystals (transducer elements), as in phased array transducers. Recent advances in transducer technology and image processing permit very high frame rates (>200 Hz), a feature that greatly enhances temporal resolution.[96]

Three-Dimensional Echocardiography

Accurate spatial perception of an object depends on recognition of its three dimensions: length, width, and depth. Although an experienced examiner can mentally construct a 3D image of the heart from serial 2D tomographic images obtained by sweeping the transducer across the chest, 3D echocardiography offers enhanced perspective of cardiovascular structures and their interrelations. One approach for obtaining 3D echocardiographic images of the heart was based on computer reconstruction of contiguous 2D cross-sectional images. These efforts were hampered by difficulties in accurately registering the ultrasound image data in time and space and by long processing times. Advances in computer technology, development of gating techniques, improved software, and refinement of the user interface have resulted in shorter acquisition and reconstruction times and improved image quality.[24] The recent advent of real-time 3D echocardiography (RT-3DE) further enhances the potential of this technology to complement and perhaps eventually to replace 2D echocardiography in clinical practice. Using parallel image processing technique, RT-3DE sends and receives a pyramidal set of ultrasound energy from several thousand piezoelectric transducer elements to produce a 3D image (Figure 102-3).[24,113] Although the spatial and temporal resolutions of current RT-3DE technology are still limited, given the rapid evolution of the technology it is likely that image quality will continue to improve.

Doppler Echocardiography

The use of Doppler ultrasound to assess normal and abnormal hemodynamics has become an integral part of the echocardiographic examination.[35,111,116] The advent of 2D-directed Doppler interrogation has greatly enhanced the clinical application of this technique by allowing evaluation of flow characteristics in specific regions within the heart and great vessels. In today's echocardiography, spectral and color-coded Doppler flow mapping are used extensively to measure velocity and direction of blood flow (Figure 102-4). Calculations based on Doppler-derived measurements allow quantitative estimation of flow volume (such as cardiac output), pressure gradient across a stenotic region, cross-sectional flow area, and prediction of intracardiac pressures. Doppler echocardiography also provides qualitative and semiquantitative assessment of valve regurgitation, intracardiac and extracardiac shunts, as well as myocardial motion (tissue Doppler imaging). Detailed discussion of Doppler physics is beyond the scope of this text and can be found elsewhere.[25,35,111,129]

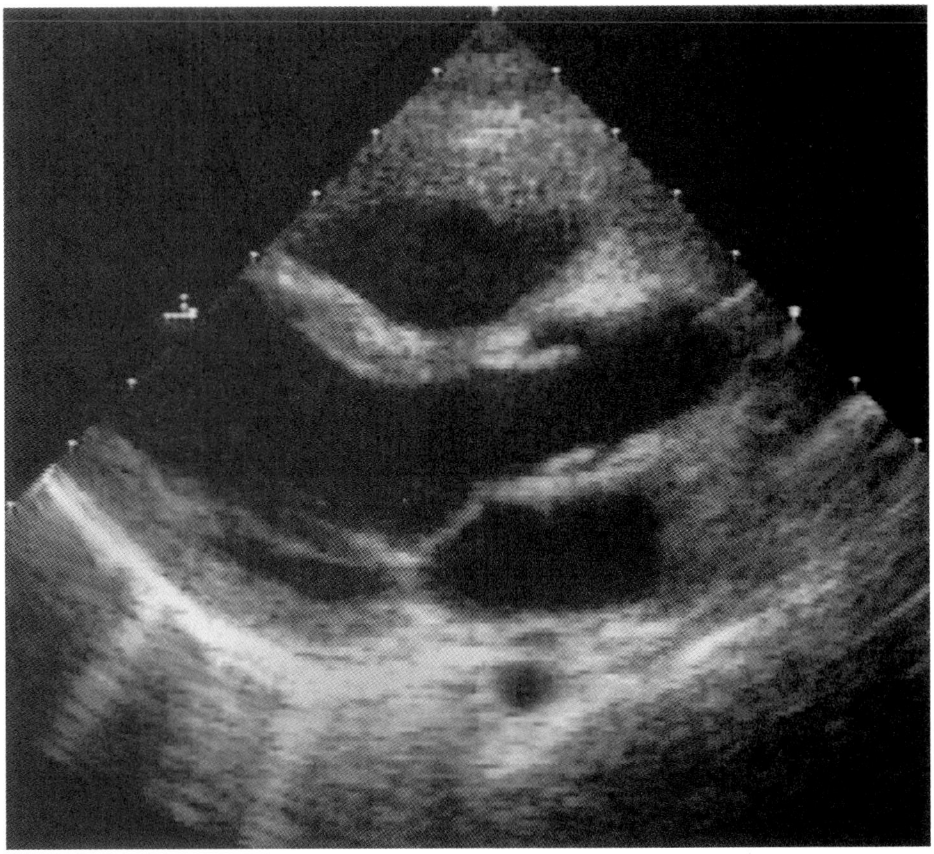

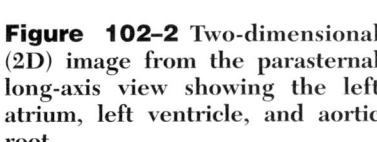

Figure 102-2 Two-dimensional (2D) image from the parasternal long-axis view showing the left atrium, left ventricle, and aortic root.

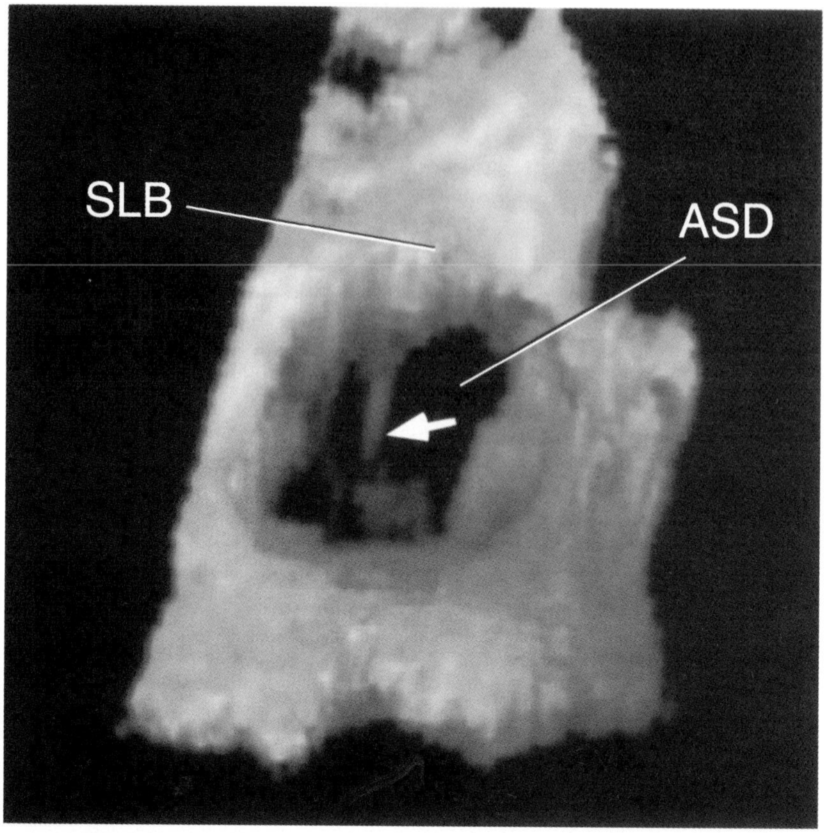

Figure 102–3 Three-dimensional (3D) echocardiographic imaging of a secundum atrial septal defect, viewed from the right atrial aspect. Note a remnant of septum primum *(arrow)* that traverses the defect. ASD, Atrial septal defect; SLB, superior limbic band of the fossa ovale.

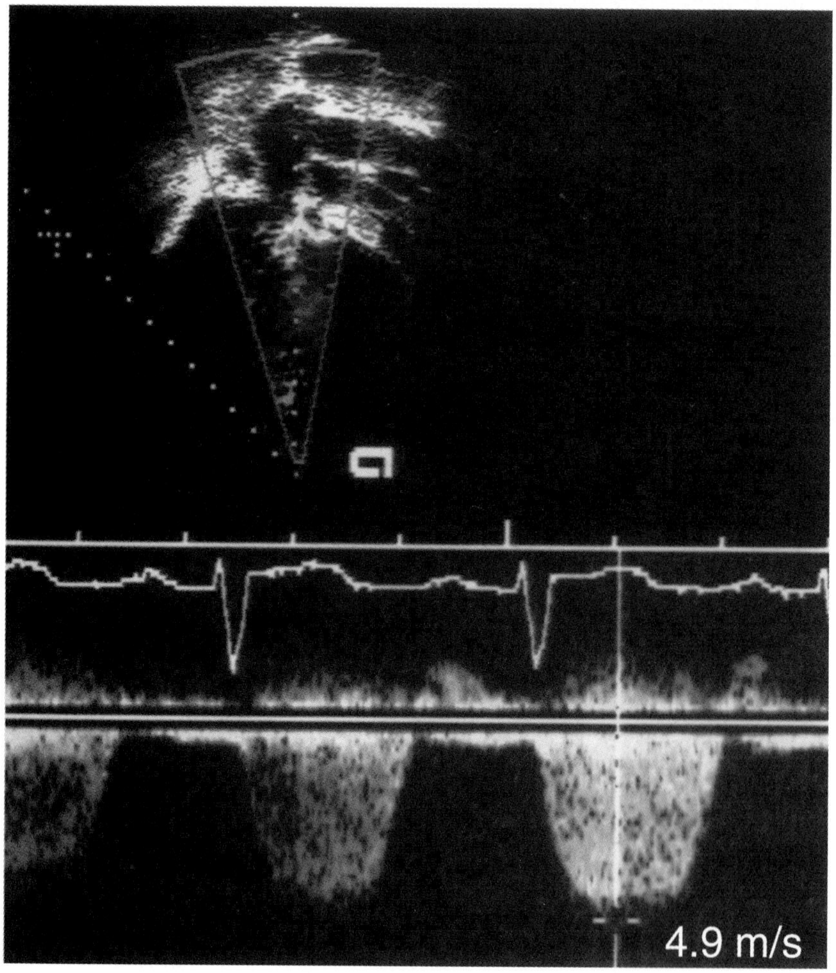

Figure 102–4 Doppler echocardiography. Visualization of a high-velocity jet by color Doppler aids in aligning the continuous wave Doppler cursor in a patient with {S,L,L} transposition of the great arteries with severe subpulmonary stenosis (predicted maximal instantaneous gradient ~96 mm Hg). (See color plate.)

Contrast Echocardiography

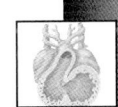

As early as the late 1960s, Gramiak et al[38] noted that intravascular injection of almost any solution resulted in a contrast effect detectable by echocardiography. Initially this technique was used to identify structures seen by M-mode echocardiography. Contrast echocardiography has been used to detect systemic[16] and pulmonary venous anomalies,[117] and for the detection of intracardiac and great artery level shunts.[2] In today's pediatric echocardiography, contrast studies are performed infrequently and are usually limited to detection of intracardiac shunts in patients with limited echocardiographic windows, patch or baffle leak after cardiac surgery, and in pulmonary arteriovenous malformations.[111,116]

Objectives of the Echocardiographic Examination

The objectives of the echocardiographic examination must be tailored to the individual patient. The initial evaluation should include a comprehensive survey of all anatomical elements of the central cardiovascular system. Subsequent examinations are often targeted to answer specific clinical questions. It is important, however, to repeat complete echocardiograms during follow up, even in patients who underwent a comprehensive initial examination, because of the dynamic nature of CHD. Examples include the late onset of discrete subaortic stenosis in patients with ventricular septal defect and/or coarctation of the aorta,[50] double-chambered right ventricle,[131] and supramitral stenosing ring.[70]

Examination Technique

Proper planning of the echocardiographic examination is important to ensure that all diagnostic information is obtained most efficiently. This is particularly relevant in sedated patients in whom the time available for data acquisition is limited. Ideally a complete segmental examination of cardiovascular anatomy and function should be performed in every new patient. This includes determination of visceral situs, heart position, atrial situs, systemic and pulmonary venous connections, ventricular situs, atrioventricular and ventriculoarterial alignments and connections, and coronary and great arterial anatomy. Assessment of ventricular function, intracardiac and vessel dimensions, and flow analysis across all valves, septa, chambers, and vessels are integral parts of the examination. In young children with suspected heart disease, the examination begins from the subxiphoid approach by determining the abdominal situs and then proceeding by scanning the heart and great vessels, employing a step-by-step segmental analysis (Figure 102-5A,B).[103] This approach is advantageous because it provides a wide-angle view of heart position and cardiovascular anatomy and function at an early

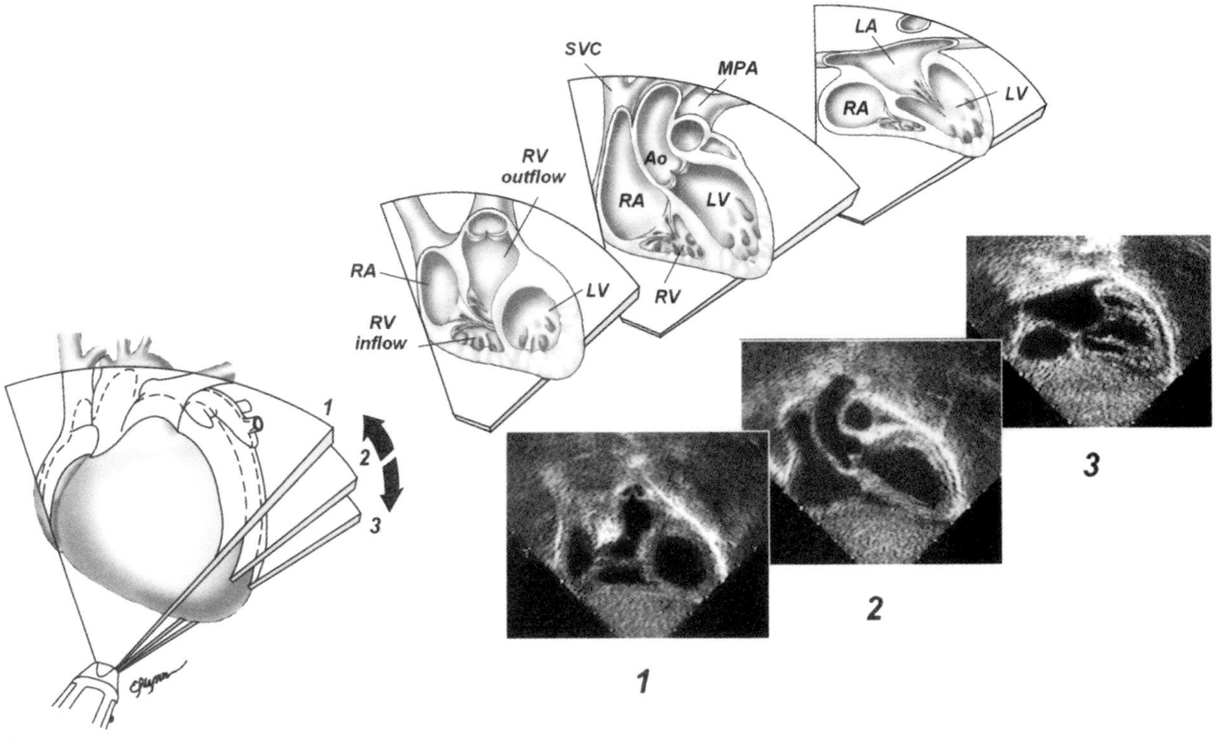

Figure 102–5 Standard 2-dimensional (2D) transthoracic imaging sweeps. A, Subxiphoid long-axis sweep. Slow gradual sweep starting at the level of the upper abdomen shows the connection of the inferior vena cava to the right atrium (RA). The left atrium (LA) is seen next. The connection of the pulmonary veins and the atrial septum can be demonstrated from this view. The left ventricle (LV) is seen along its long axis. Further superior angulation of the transducer depicts the left ventricular outflow tract, aortic valve, and ascending aorta (Ao). The superior vena cava (SVC) is seen to the right of the ascending aorta, and the main pulmonary artery (MPA) is seen to the left of the aorta. Further superior tilt of the transducer shows the right ventricular inflow and outflow (RV outflow) and the pulmonary valve. The sweep ends with anterior free wall of the right ventricle.

(Continued)

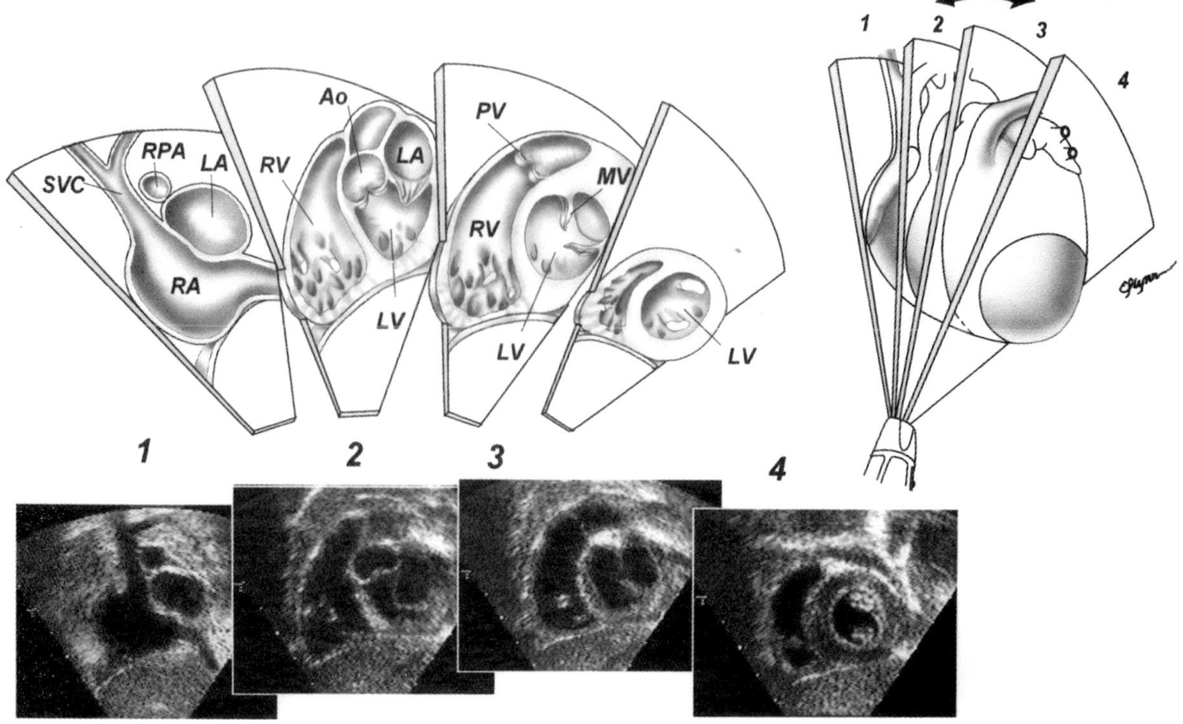

B

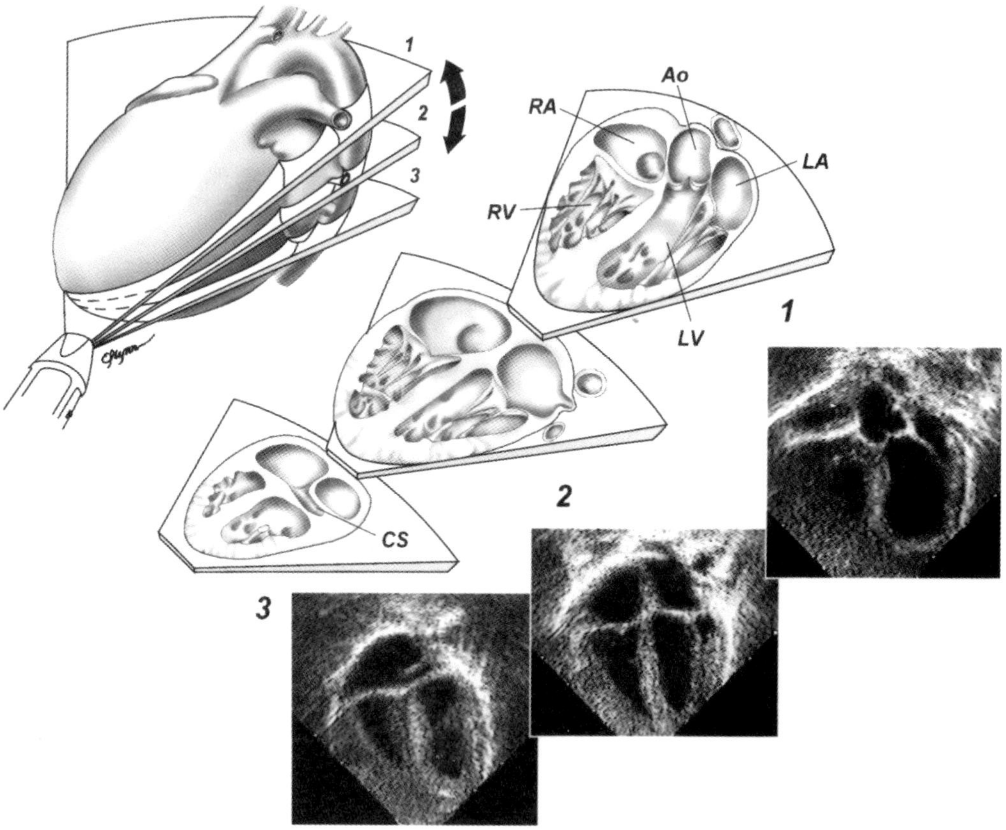

C

Figure 102–5 cont'd **B,** Subxiphoid short-axis sweep. From the subxiphoid long-axis view, the transducer is rotated clockwise ~90°. The sweep begins at the rightmost aspect of the heart and progresses from right to left through the cardiac apex. The superior vena cava (SVC) and inferior vena cava are seen entering the right atrium (RA). The right pulmonary artery (RPA) is seen in cross-section behind the SVC and above the left atrium (LA). The atrial septum is clearly seen in this plane. Sweeping the transducer leftward shows the base of the left ventricle (LV) and right ventricle (RV) and the atrioventricular (AV) valves. The aortic valve is seen in cross-section at this level. Further leftward tilt of the transducer depicts a cross-sectional view of the LV and mitral valve (MV), as well as the right ventricular outflow tract and pulmonary valve (PV). The sweep ends with imaging of the mid–muscular septum, the papillary muscles, and the apical portions of both ventricles. **C,** Apical four-chamber sweep. The transducer is positioned over the apex and angled to obtain a cross-sectional view of the atria and ventricles as shown in panel 2. The transducer is then angled posteriorly to image the posterior aspect of the heart (panel 3). In this plane, the coronary sinus (CS) can be viewed along the posterior left atrioventricular groove. Anterosuperior tilt of the transducer shows the left ventricular outflow tract and proximal ascending aorta (Ao).

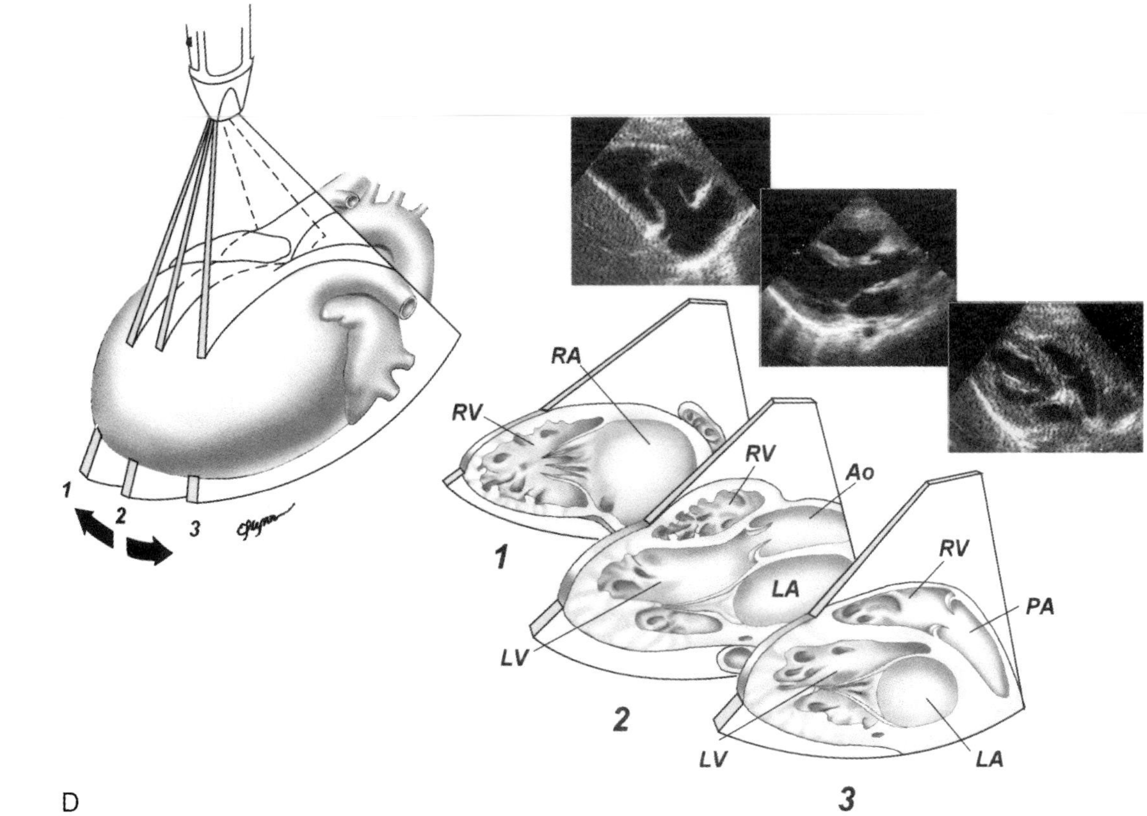

D

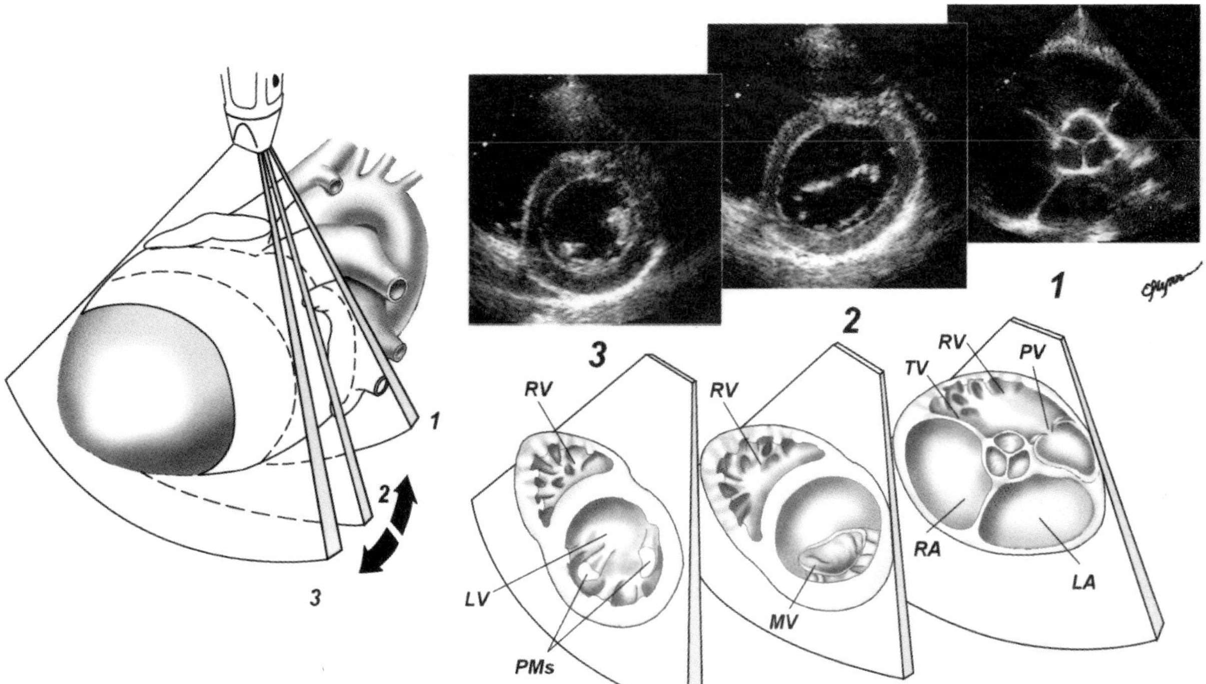

E

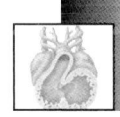

Figure 102–5 cont'd **D,** Parasternal long-axis sweep. The transducer is placed over the left precordium to the left of the sternum with the index mark toward the patient's right shoulder. A rightward and inferior tilt of the transducer towards the right hip shows the right atrium (RA), tricuspid valve, and right ventricular inflow (RV) (panel 1). The coronary sinus can be followed into the right atrium in this view. A leftward and superior tilt of the transducer toward the left shoulder depicts the right ventricular outflow tract (RV), pulmonary valve, and main pulmonary artery (PA) (panel 3). **E,** Parasternal short-axis sweep. From the parasternal long-axis view, the transducer (rd) is rotated clockwise ~90°. The sweep progresses from a plane that shows right and left atria (LA and RA), the atrial septum, the tricuspid valve (TV), right ventricle (RV), pulmonary valve (PV), and main pulmonary artery (panel 1) toward the apex. Panels 2 and 3 show cross-sectional views of the right ventricle (RV), left ventricle (LV), ventricular septum, mitral valve (MV), and papillary muscles (PMs) are obtained.

(Continued)

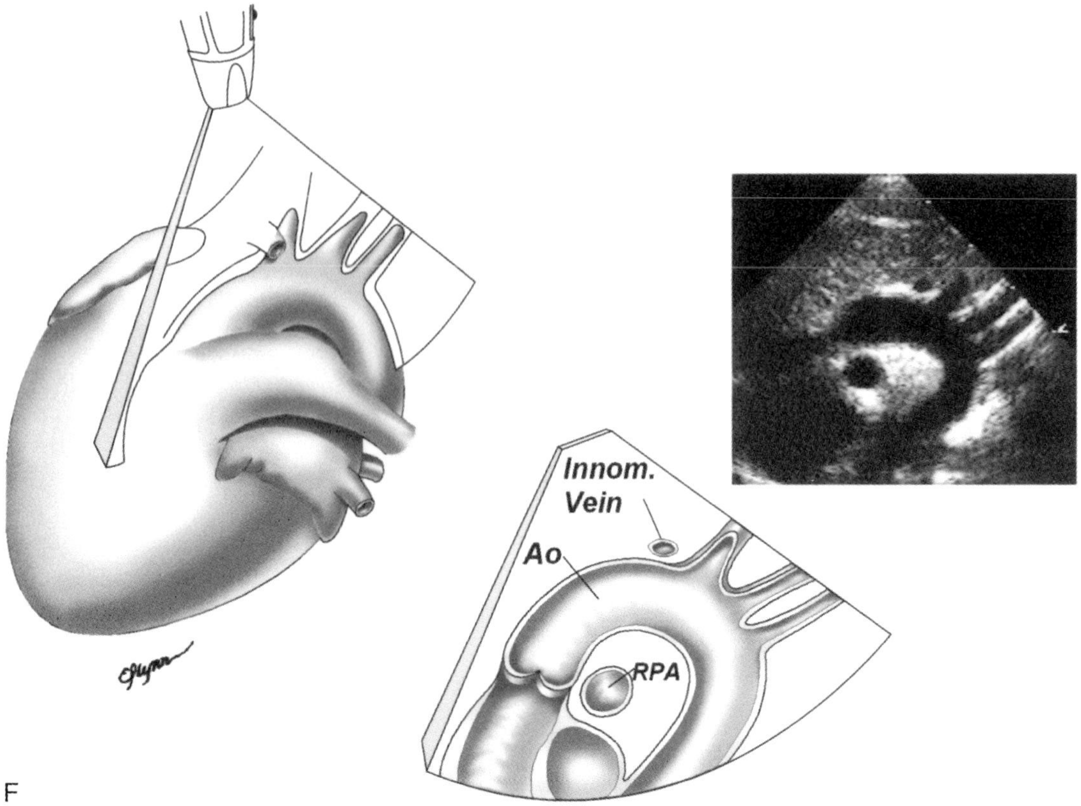

F

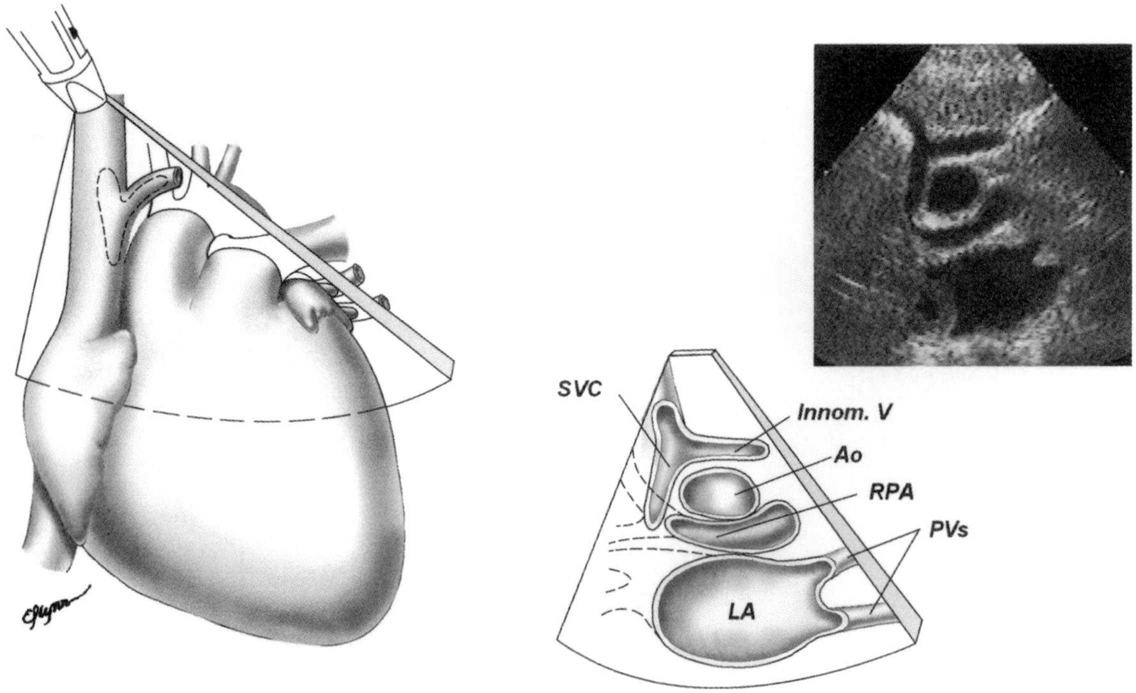

G

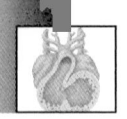

Figure 102–5 cont'd **F,** Aortic arch view from the suprasternal notch window. The innominate vein (Innom Vein) is seen anterior to the innominate artery. The right pulmonary artery (RPA) is seen in cross-section behind the ascending aorta. **G,** Suprasternal notch view in the transverse plane. The left innominate vein (Innom V) is seen draining into the superior vena cava (SVC). The distal ascending aorta (Ao) is seen superior to the right pulmonary artery (RPA), which is seen along its length above the left atrium (LA). Note the pulmonary veins entering the left atrium.

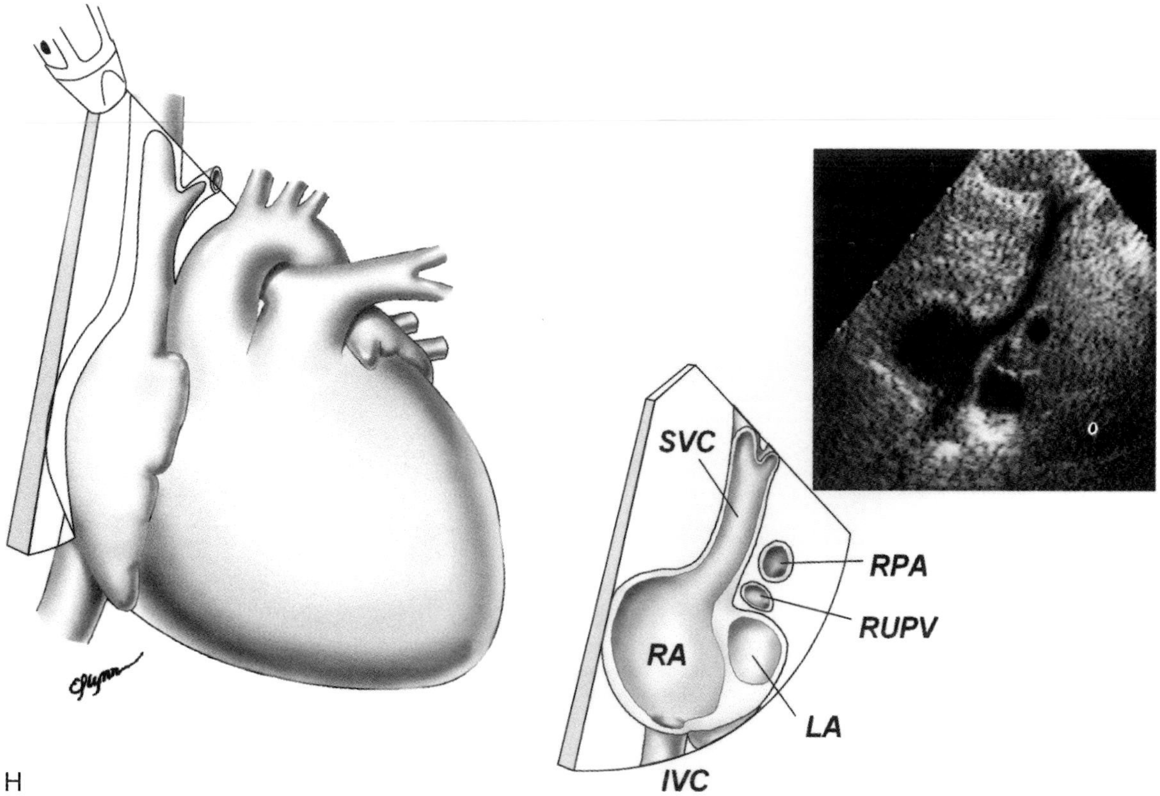

H

Figure 102–5 cont'd **H,** High right parasternal view in the sagittal plane view showing the superior vena cava (SVC) entering the right atrium (RA). This view allows demonstration of the sinus venosus septum.
(Reproduced with permission from Geva T: Echocardiography and Doppler ultrasound. In Garson A, Bricker JT, Fisher DJ, editors: The Science and Practice of Pediatric Cardiology, 2nd ed. Baltimore: Williams & Wilkins, pp. 789–843.)

stage in the examination. Subsequent 2D and Doppler analyses from the apical, parasternal, and suprasternal notch views supplement and confirm findings from the subxiphoid window (Figure 102-5C–G). The examination strategy should be tailored to the individual patient and modified according to the clinical situation as necessary. Although the standard views described in the preceding should be obtained in almost every patient, and represent the minimum acceptable examination, flexibility and improvisation are important to optimally utilize the full potential of echocardiography.

Anatomical Analysis

When an echocardiographic examination is performed and reviewed in a patient suspected of having CHD, a stepwise segmental approach to analysis of cardiac anatomy is taken. The fundamental principle of segmental analysis of CHD is to analyze each component of the heart separately according to its unique morphological features.[103] The heart is composed of five segments—three main segments and two connecting segments. The three main segments are the atria, the ventricles, and the great arteries. The atrioventricular canal, which includes the mitral and tricuspid valves and the atrioventricular septum, connects the atria with the ventricles. The infundibulum (or conus) connects the ventricles with the great arteries. When analyzing cardiac anatomy, each cardiac chamber must be identified individually according to its unique anatomical and morphological features and not according to its spatial position (right-sided or left-sided), valve of entry, or artery of exit. Throughout a systematic echocardiographic study, the examiner must go over a mental checklist of segments, their anatomical organization and position (situs), their connections and alignments with adjacent segments, and associated malformations. Using the aforementioned principles, any potential CHD can be accurately described in specific and precise terms. A detailed review of echocardiographic analysis of each cardiac segment can be found elsewhere.[103,111,116]

Special Echocardiographic Procedures

Transesophageal Echocardiography

Transesophageal echocardiography was first introduced in 1976 and appeared in pediatric use in 1989. The miniaturization of probes and development of multiplanar imaging have greatly increased its role as an adjunct to transthoracic imaging, during surgical repair of CHD (intraoperative transesophageal echocardiography), and to guide interventional catheterization procedures.

Indications and objectives

A transesophageal echocardiographic examination is usually performed to answer a limited set of clinical questions. It is advisable, however, to perform a comprehensive examination of the heart and blood vessels for additional unsuspected anatomical and/or hemodynamic anomalies

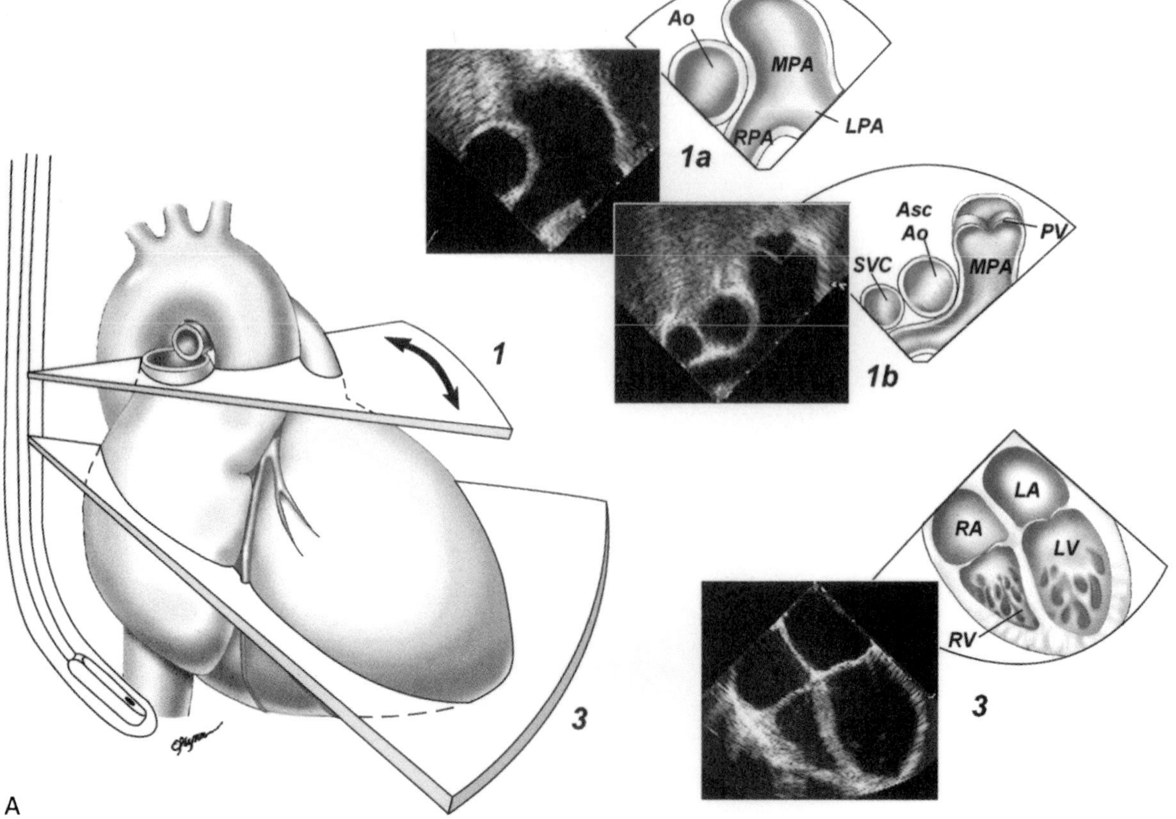

A

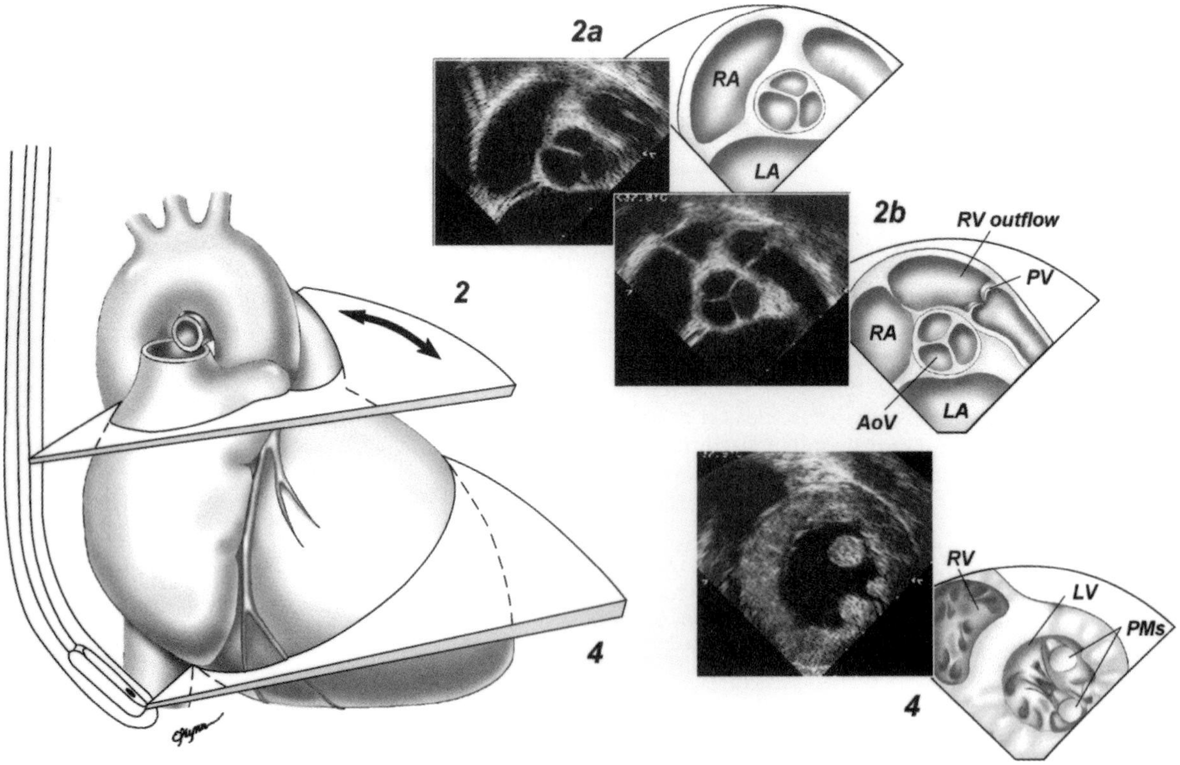

B

Figure 102–6 Transesophageal imaging. A, Transverse plane: Cross-sectional view at level 1a depicts the proximal ascending aorta (Ao), main pulmonary artery (MPA), and left and right pulmonary arteries (LPA and RPA, respectively). A rightward tilt of the transducer shows the RPA as it passes behind the superior vena cava (SVC) and ascending aorta (Asc Ao). For a four-chamber view (level 3), the transducer is advanced in the esophagus with slight retroflexion of the scope. **B,** Level 2 is parallel to the transthoracic parasternal short-axis view. In level 2a, the atrial septum is imaged by a slight rightward tilt of the transducer. In level 2b, the aortic valve (AoV) is seen in cross-section in the center of the image; the left atrium (LA), right atrium (RA), tricuspid valve, right ventricular outflow (RV outflow), pulmonary valve (PV), and the proximal main pulmonary artery are seen. With the transducer advanced into the lower esophagus and the scope anteflexed a cross-sectional view of the left ventricle (LV), mitral valve, and papillary muscles is obtained (level 4). Note that image orientation is the same as in transthoracic echocardiography.

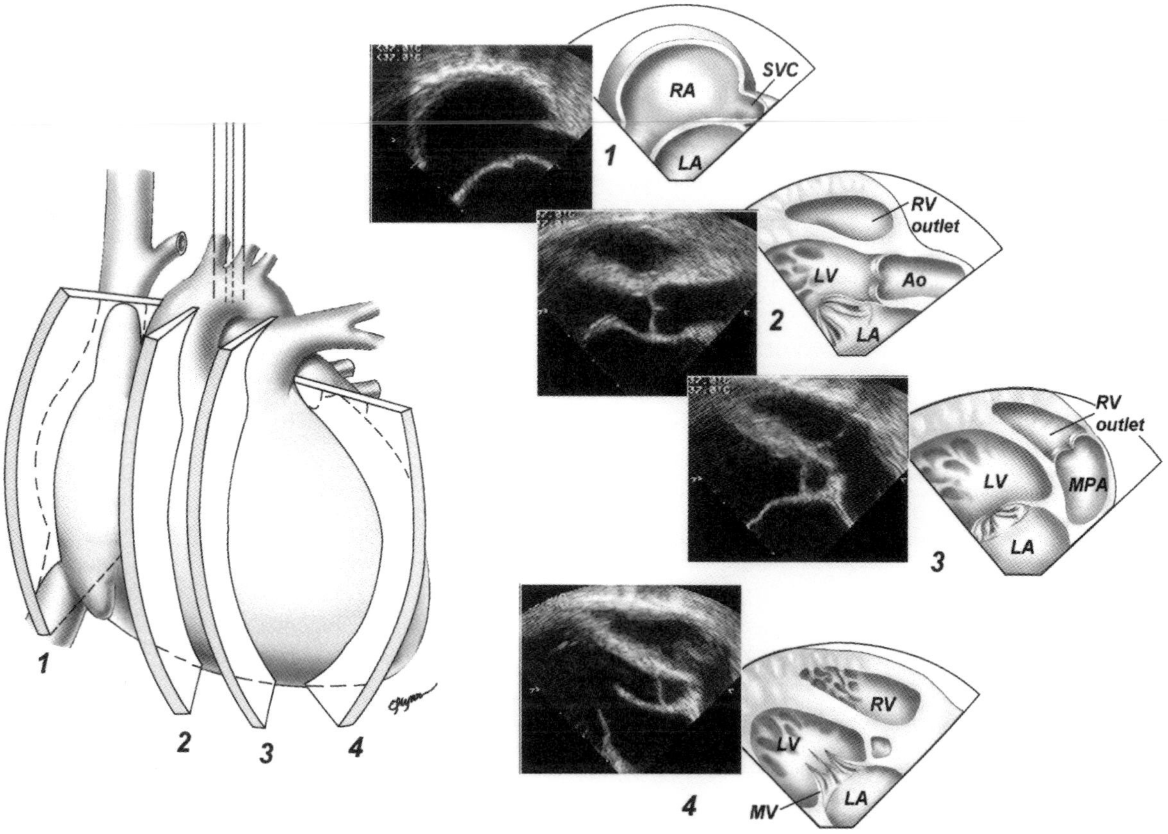

C

Figure 102–6 cont'd C, Vertical (longitudinal) plane: The sweep begins at a plane that crosses the superior vena cava (SVC), left atrium (LA), right atrium (RA), and atrial septum (level 1). Next, a leftward tilt of the transducer shows an image parallel to the transthoracic parasternal long-axis view of the left atrium (LA), mitral valve, left ventricle (LV), left ventricular outflow tract, and proximal aorta (Ao) (level 2). Further leftward tilt of the transducer (level 3) shows the right ventricular outflow tract (RV outlet), pulmonary valve, and main pulmonary artery (MPA). The sweep continues leftward to show the leftward aspects of the left atrium, mitral valve, and left ventricle (level 4). Further leftward tilt depicts the left atrial appendage and the left pulmonary veins (not shown). Note that image orientation is the same as in transthoracic echocardiography. *(Reproduced with permission from Geva T: Echcardiography and Doppler ultrasound. In Garson A, Bricker JT, Fisher DJ, editors: The Science and Practice of Pediatric Cardiology, 2nd ed. Baltimore: Williams & Wilkins, pp. 789–843.)*

(Figure 102-6). The availability of small biplane and multiplane probes designed for use in young infants weighing 3–3.5 kg or less has greatly enhanced the scope of transesophageal echocardiography in the pediatric age group.[34,62,120,121] Successful transesophageal echocardiographic examinations have been reported in patients weighing as little as 2.3 kg.[60,61] The role of transesophageal echocardiography in pediatric cardiology is continuously evolving. Although the transthoracic window is adequate in most situations, transesophageal echocardiography provides distinct advantages during cardiovascular surgery[34,61,69,72,120]; during video-assisted thoracoscopic procedures[65]; for guidance of interventional catheter procedures[59,128]; in the intensive care unit[34,71]; for detection of intracardiac thrombi and vegetations[26]; during assessment of prosthetic valves[21]; in selected patients on mechanical assist devices and extracorporeal membrane oxygenators[108]; and in selected patients with poor transthoracic windows, such as adults with CHD.[42]

Safety and complications

Although in expert hands transesophageal echocardiography is quite safe, complications have been reported, including oropharyngeal trauma and compression of airways and vascular structures.[30,104] Transesophageal echocardiography is contraindicated in patients with an unrepaired tracheoesophageal fistula, esophageal obstruction or stricture, perforated viscus, active gastrointestinal bleeding, in an unwilling or uncooperative patient who is inadequately sedated, or with an uncontrolled airway in a patient with respiratory or cardiac decompensation. Relative contraindications include cervical spine injury, immobility, or deformity; history of esophageal surgery; known esophageal varices or diverticulum; oropharyngeal deformities; and severe coagulopathy.[32,119]

Fetal Echocardiography

Examination of the fetal cardiovascular system in humans dates back to the late 1960s, when continuous wave Doppler was used to record fetal heart rate. Although Kleinman et al[53] had some success in detecting CHD in the fetus by M-mode echocardiography in the late 1970s, it was not until high-resolution 2D imaging became available in the mid-1980s that accurate delineation of cardiovascular anatomy became clinically routine. Today, prenatal detection of CHD can be reliably achieved by 17–20 weeks of gestation by transabdominal imaging. Using the transvaginal window, the heart and great vessels can be imaged as early as the late first trimester.[1]

Indications and Objectives

Although several studies have demonstrated a low detection rate of CHD by routine level I obstetric ultrasound,[12] cost–benefit considerations preclude universal fetal echocardiographic screening by expert pediatric echocardiographers. Alternatively, an approach based on targeting pregnancies that are at high risk for CHD is taken. Such an approach increases the yield of fetal echocardiography to approximately 30% when extracardiac anomalies are detected, to approximately 60% when level I scan detects possible CHD, and to nearly 100% when a second opinion is requested.[13,51] The indications for fetal echocardiography are summarized in Box 102-1.

Box 102–1. Indications for Fetal Echocardiography.

Fetal Risk Factors

- Extracardiac structural anomalies
- Chromosomal abnormalities
- Fetal dysrhythmias
  - Irregular rhythm
  - Tachyarrhythmia
  - Bradyarrhythmia
- Intrauterine growth retardation
- Nonimmune hydrops fetalis
- Suspected cardiac anomaly on level I scan
- Abnormal visceral situs

Maternal Risk Factors

- Congenital heart disease
- Exposure to teratogen (sample list only)
  - Lithium carbonate
  - Amphetamines
  - Alcohol
  - Anticonvulsants
  - Phenytoin
  - Trimethadione
  - Isotretinoin
- Maternal diabetes
- Phenylketonuria
- Maternal infection
  - Rubella
  - Toxoplasmosis
  - Coxsackie virus
  - Cytomegalovirus
  - Mumps virus

Familial Risk Factors

- Congenital heart disease
- Syndromes
  - Down
  - Marfan
  - Noonan
  - Tuberous sclerosis
  - Velocardiofacial

Modified from Kleinman C: Fetal echocardiography: Diagnosing congenital heart disease in the human fetus. In ACC Educational Highlights, pp. 10–14. Bethesda, MD: American College of Cardiology, 1996.

Description of Technique

Echocardiographic examination of the cardiovascular system in the fetus is based on the same principles of the segmental approach to diagnosis of CHD that are applied after birth. The main difference between examination of the fetus and the newborn is that the operator has no control over fetal position and, consequently, over the views obtained. Once fetal position is ascertained and the spatial coordinates are determined, the examination then continues according to the principles outlined in the previous sections. Given optimal acoustic windows and favorable fetal position, even the most complex cardiovascular anomalies can be detected (Figure 102-7). Defects that remain difficult to diagnose in utero include atrial septal defect, patent ductus arteriosus, small or moderate ventricular septal defect, coarctation of the aorta, and some valve and great vessel abnormalities.[8] The distinction between normal patency of the foramen ovale and an atrial septal defect is usually not possible in the fetus. Similarly, it is not possible to predict whether the normally patent ductus arteriosus will close after birth. In utero diagnosis of aortic coarctation may be difficult because the typical isthmic narrowing may not become apparent until after ductal closure.[8] However, the diagnosis may be suspected based on abnormal morphology of the transverse aortic arch (elongation and hypoplasia) and size discrepancy between the ventricles (right ventricle larger than left ventricle).[44]

Clinical Implications

Early prenatal diagnosis of major CHD allows parents to consider the option to terminate the pregnancy. It is also common to recommend amniocentesis to detect associated genetic abnormalities. When pregnancy continues, prenatal diagnosis of CHD allows proper planning for postnatal cardiac care. When intervention is anticipated immediately or shortly after birth (e.g., ductal-dependent anomalies or balloon atrial septostomy in transposition of the great arteries), delivery in a pediatric cardiac center is arranged. The currently available literature is conflicted on whether prenatal diagnosis of CHD leads to a significant reduction in mortality.[56,126] However, there is evidence that it can reduce morbidity in certain lesions.[56] Other advantages, such as psychological benefits to the parents, are also valuable.[114]

Fetal Arrhythmia

One of the major reasons for referral to fetal echocardiography is arrhythmia. Most commonly, irregular fetal heart rate is due to either conducted or blocked premature atrial contractions. These are usually benign and require follow-up only if they are frequent or associated with supraventricular tachycardia. Among the serious arrhythmias encountered in the fetus, supraventricular tachycardia and atrial flutter are the most common.[51] Premature ventricular contractions and ventricular tachycardia are rare in the fetus, but both have been reported.[51] Transplacental pharmacological therapy is indicated in fetuses with incessant tachyarrhythmia,

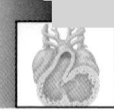

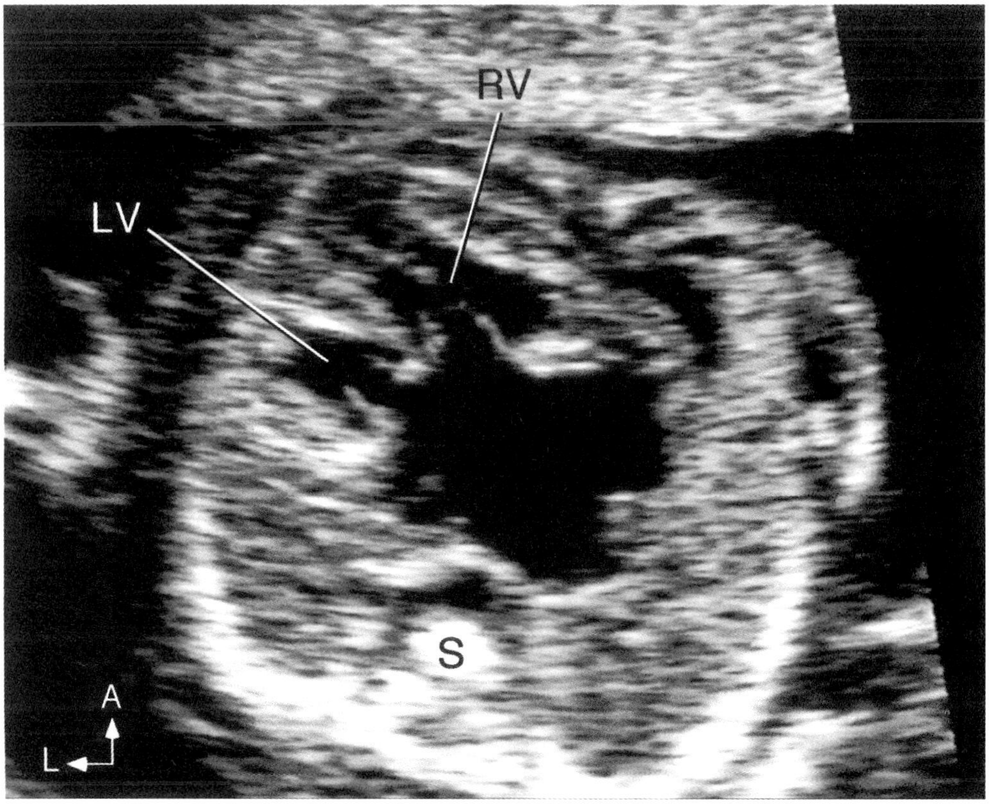

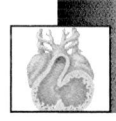

Figure 102–7 Fetal echocardiogram in a 24-week-old fetus with partial common atrioventricular (AV) canal as seen from a four-chamber view. The large deficiency of the atrial septum and apical displacement of the AV valve are clearly seen. A, Anterior; L, left; LV, left ventricle; RV, right ventricle; S, spine.

especially if signs of heart failure (e.g., enlargement of cardiac chambers, pericardial effusion, hydrops fetalis) are present. Complete heart block is the most common cause of prolonged bradycardia in the fetus.[52] The distinction between complete heart block and sinus bradycardia is important because the latter might indicate fetal distress. In fetuses with a structurally normal heart, maternal lupus erythematosus should be suspected. The most common structural CHDs associated with complete heart block are physiologically corrected transposition of the great arteries {S,L,L} and heterotaxy syndrome with polysplenia.

Fetal arrhythmias have been traditionally diagnosed by Doppler and M-mode echocardiography.[51] Both methods rely on simultaneous recording of signals from the atria and ventricles. Fetal position, however, may not always allow optimal alignment of the M-mode cursor or the Doppler beam. A newer method, tissue Doppler imaging with a high frame rate, provides a promising alternative to standard M-mode and Doppler echocardiography (Figure 102-8).[97]

Quantitative Analysis

Modern echocardiography allows accurate measurements of cardiovascular structures.[35,73,111,116] These measurements are helpful in deciding whether the size of a certain structure is within normal limits and in quantifying the degree of deviation from the expected norm.

Description of Technique

Measurements of linear dimensions (such as vessel diameter), cross-sectional areas (such as valve area), or volumetric dimensions (such as ventricular volume or mass) provide important quantitative information that can be used to assess the severity of disease process and to predict its course and prognosis. Because the pediatric age group encompasses a wide range of body sizes and because the heart and great vessels grow considerably from birth to adulthood, measured dimensions must be adjusted to allow meaningful comparisons between patients of different age and body size. For example, the mean value of the aortic valve annulus diameter is 0.74 cm in a 3.6-kg newborn (body surface area 0.24 m^2) and 1.95 cm in a 60-kg adolescent (body surface area 1.66 m^2). Indexing the aortic annulus diameter to body weight yields vastly different values (0.21 cm/kg in the newborn versus 0.032 cm/kg in the adolescent). Indexing the aortic valve diameter to the body surface area yields similarly unsatisfactory results (3.1 cm/m^2 in the newborn versus 1.17 cm/m^2 in the adolescent). Tanner[124] in 1949 and, more recently, Gutgesell and Rembold[41] noted that the growth of cardiac structures is not necessarily a linear function of the body surface area, the weight, the height, or the age. These findings are to be expected because the heart and great vessels grow much faster during the first 2–4 years of life compared with later childhood and adolescence. It was found that linear dimensions (such as diameters of valves and great vessels) should be indexed to the square root of the body surface area.[41,124] Returning to the previous example of the aortic valve diameter, indexing the valve diameter to the square root of the body surface area yields 0.74/0.49 = 1.51 cm/$m^{0.5}$ in the 3.6-kg newborn and 1.95/1.29 = 1.51 cm/$m^{0.5}$ in the 60-kg adolescent (Figure 102-9). Cross-sectional measurements (such as valve area) should be indexed to the body surface area.[41]

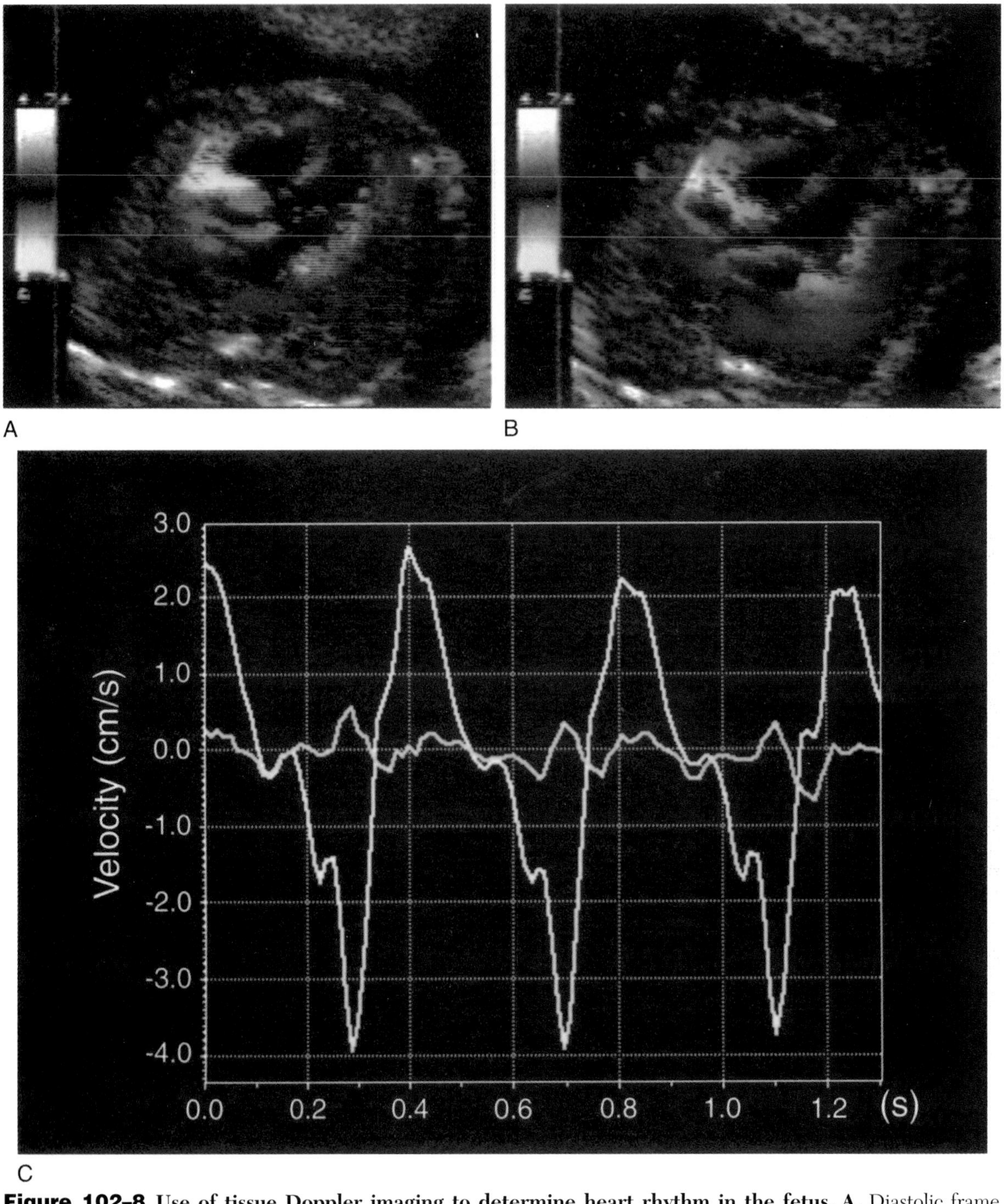

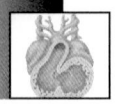

Figure 102–8 Use of tissue Doppler imaging to determine heart rhythm in the fetus. A, Diastolic frame showing left ventricular relaxation. **B,** Systolic frame showing ventricular contraction. **C,** Velocity–time curves of the left atrium *(green)* and left ventricle *(yellow)* showing the sequence of mechanical activation of the cardiac chambers in a fetus with normal atrioventricular (AV) conduction. The analysis is performed off-line using the digitally stored data. (See color plate for parts **A** and **B**.)

Left ventricular volume should be indexed to the body surface area raised to the power 1.28, and left ventricular mass should be indexed to the body surface area raised to the power 1.23 (SD Colan, unpublished data).

An alternative approach to comparing measurements between individuals is the use of Z scores.[35] The Z score is a statistical expression of the position of a data point relative to the regression line of a data set. The Z score is expressed as the number of standard deviations from the expected mean of a normal population. It is calculated as:

$$\text{Z value} = \frac{\text{Measured value} - \text{Mean value of normal population}}{\text{Standard deviation of normal population}}$$

Returning to the previous example of aortic valve diameter, the Z value of a 0.74-cm aortic valve diameter in a newborn

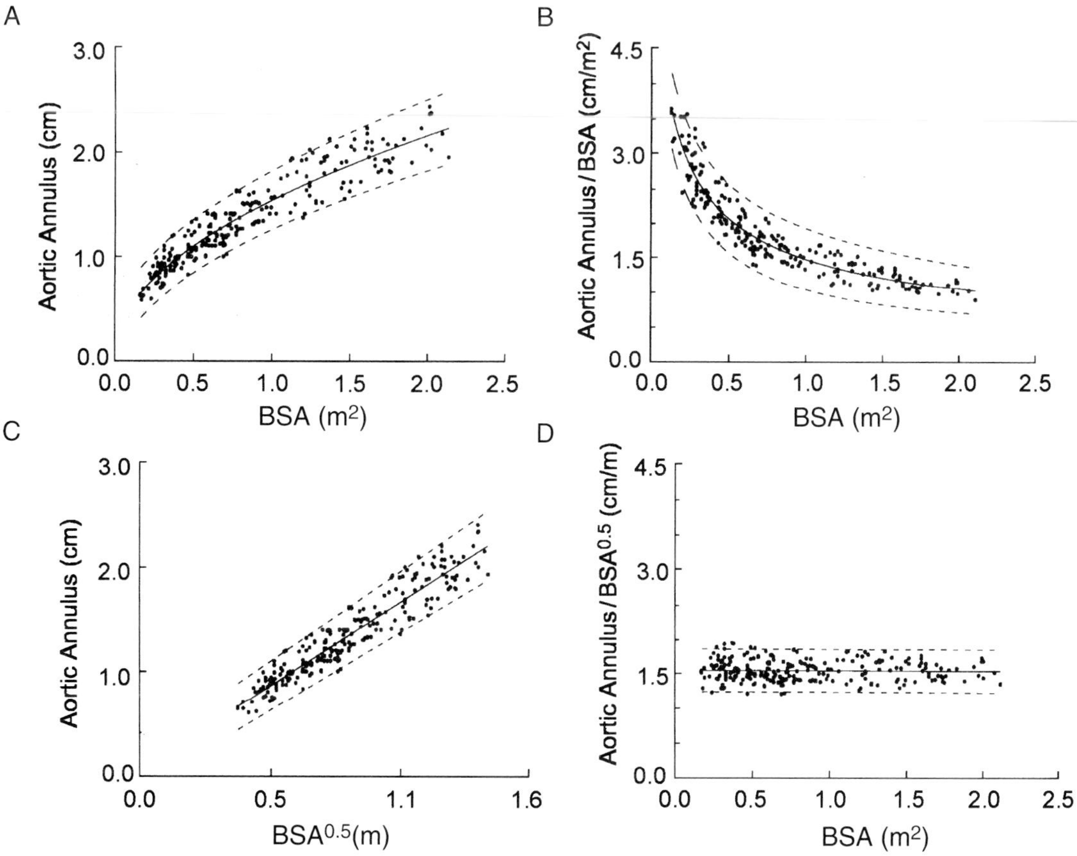

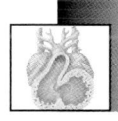

Figure 102–9 **Rationale for indexing linear measurements to the square root of body surface area (BSA). A,** Plot of aortic valve annulus diameter against body surface area showing a nonlinear curve. **B,** Plot of aortic valve annulus diameter indexed to body surface area against body surface area shows that the indexed diameter decreases exponentially as body surface area increases. **C,** Aortic valve annulus diameter plotted against the square root of body surface area showing a linear relationship. **D,** Plot of aortic valve diameter indexed to the square root of body surface area against body surface area showing that the indexed aortic valve diameter is the same in children and adults with widely varying body size.
(Reproduced with permission from Geva T: Echcardiography and Doppler ultrasound. In Garson A, Bricker JT, Fisher DJ, editors: The Science and Practice of Pediatric Cardiology, 2nd ed. Baltimore: Williams & Wilkins, pp. 789–843.)

with a body surface area of 0.24 m^2 is 0. That means that 0.74 cm is the mean value of aortic valve diameter in infants with that body size. In the adolescent with a body surface area of 1.66 m^2, the Z value of an aortic valve diameter of 1.95 cm is also 0. In other words, the same Z scores in the newborn and the adolescent indicate that both values are in the same position relative to the regression line of normal values and are comparable. An aortic valve diameter of 0.53 cm in the newborn would have a Z score of –2.0, which indicates that this value is two standard deviations below the expected mean. An aortic valve diameter of 0.96 cm in the same newborn would have a Z score of +2.0, which indicates that this value is two standard deviations above the mean. Thus expression of measurements as Z values allows comparison between patients, regardless of differences in body size.

Estimation of left ventricular volume is an important factor in determining the adequacy of chamber size in patients with left ventricular hypoplasia and in the evaluation of patients with volume overload. Numerous algorithms based on several geometric models have been developed for calculation of left ventricular volume. These have been reviewed in detail elsewhere.[35,111] The biplane Simpson's rule is considered among the most reliable methods for estimation of left ventricular volume. This method requires imaging of the left ventricle from two orthogonal views that share a common long axis: for example, the apical four- and two-chamber views (Figure 102-10A). Left ventricular volume is calculated according to:

$$V = \frac{\pi}{4} \times \sum_{i=1}^{N} a_i \times b_i \times \frac{L}{N}$$

where a_i = slice radius in the apical two-chamber view, b_i = slice radius in the apical four-chamber view, L = left ventricular length, N= number of slices, and V = volume.

Another method for estimation of left ventricular volume is the biplane area–length method, where $V = 5/6 \times \text{area} \times \text{length}$ (Fig 102-10B). Experience with assessment of left and right ventricular volumes by 3D reconstruction suggests that this technique is potentially more accurate than 2D echocardiographic techniques.[57] Left ventricular myocardial volume can be measured from the 2D echocardiogram by subtracting the endocardial volume from the epicardial volume. Left ventricular mass is calculated by multiplying the resultant myocardial volume by the density of muscle (1.055 g/ml). Because it is not influenced by acoustic windows and is independent of chamber geometry, MRI provides an excellent alternative to echocardiography in measuring chamber volume and mass and is considered the reference standard to which other techniques are compared (see subsequent section on MRI).

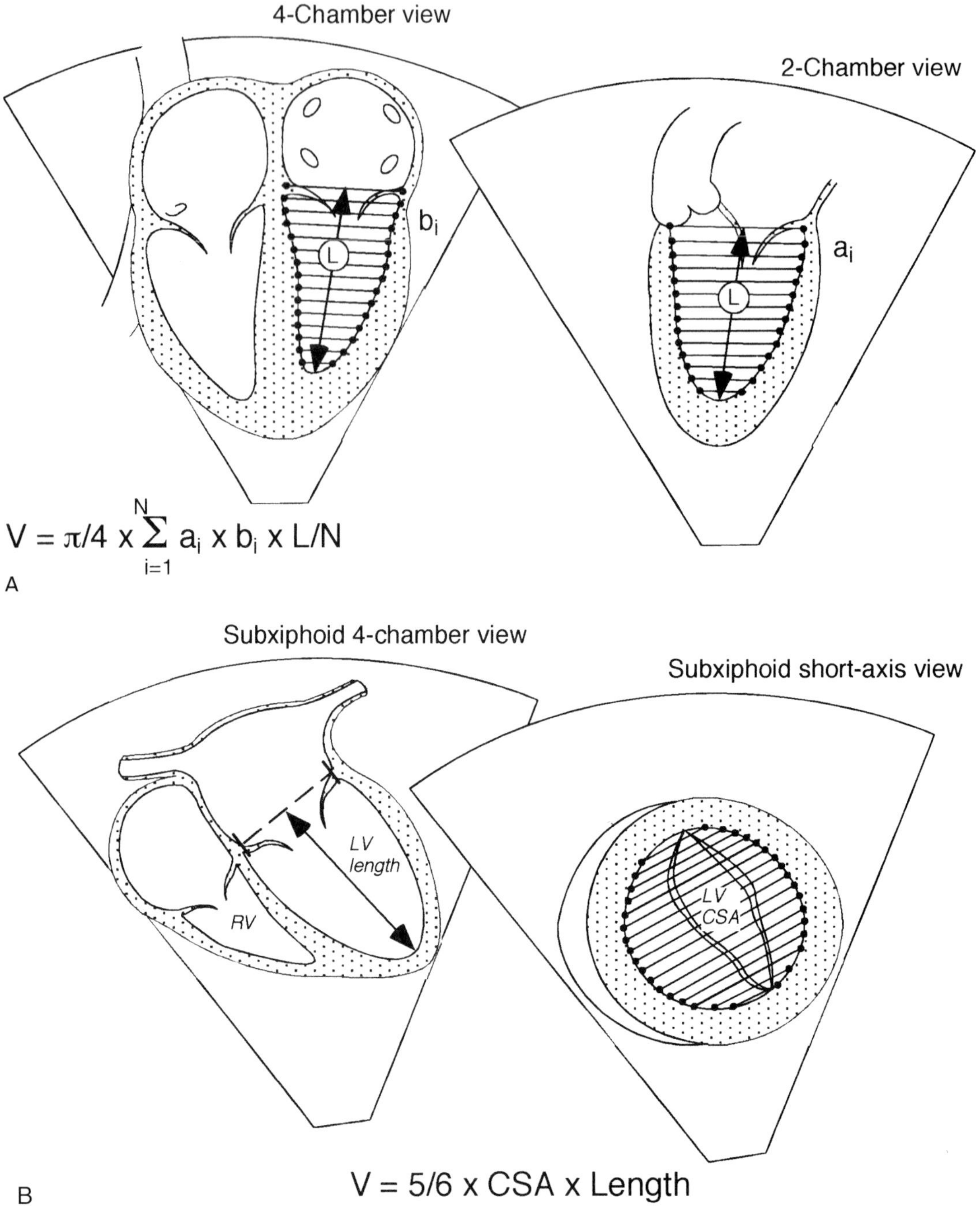

Figure 102–10 Methods for assessment of left ventricular volume by two-dimensional (2D) echocardiography. A, Biplane Simpson's rule for calculating left ventricular volume (see text for details). **B,** Area–length method for calculating left ventricular volume.
(Reproduced with permission from Geva T: Echcardiography and Doppler ultrasound. In Garson A, Bricker JT, Fisher DJ, editors: The Science and Practice of Pediatric Cardiology, 2nd ed. Baltimore: Williams & Wilkins, pp. 789–843.)

Ventricular Function

Left ventricular function can be assessed at several levels. The heart may be viewed as a pump designed to maintain adequate flow to vital organs.[17] This approach focuses on the external work performed by the heart, but it ignores the internal work and the functional state of the myocardium. The pump function of the heart can be assessed by measuring cardiac output and systemic and pulmonary venous blood pressures. It is known, however, that cardiac output and blood pressure can remain within the normal limits despite significant myocardial dysfunction.[17]

Ejection-phase indices of ventricular function, including shortening fraction, fractional area change, ejection fraction, velocity of circumferential fiber shortening (VCF), peak dP/dt, and systolic time intervals, measure global pump function.[17,35,111,116] Common to these indices is their dependence on loading conditions. These indices are unable to distinguish between the effect(s) of altered loading

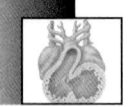

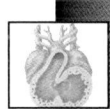

conditions and abnormalities in myocardial contractility. Hence abnormalities in preload and afterload can result in depressed shortening or ejection fractions, leading to the erroneous interpretation that myocardial contractility is depressed. Conversely, left ventricular myocardial contractility may be depressed even in the presence of normal shortening or ejection fractions. The advantage of most of these indices is their relative simplicity and ease of acquisition. Load-independent assessment of left ventricular systolic function requires a more sophisticated analysis. The interested reader is referred to the relevant chapters in this book and to other reviews of this topic.[17]

Doppler Evaluation of Pressure Gradients

Estimation of the pressure difference between adjacent compartments has been widely applied in clinical pediatric echocardiography (see Figure 102-4).[35,74,111,116] Among the most common uses is estimation of pressure drop across stenotic areas and prediction of pressure in cardiac chambers. For example, the systolic pressure in the right ventricle can be predicted from the peak pressure difference between it and the right atrium derived from the peak velocity of the tricuspid regurgitation jet. Right ventricular systolic pressure also can be assessed from knowledge of left ventricular pressure (by measurement of systemic blood pressure by sphygmomanometry) and the pressure drop across a ventricular septal defect. In principle, the pressure gradient across any two compartments connected by flow can be estimated by Doppler, provided that the limitations of the technique are taken into consideration and the sources of error in the application and interpretation of the technique are eliminated.

Calculation of Pressure Gradients

The Bernoulli equation relates pressure difference (ΔP) between two points separated by a distance (s) to the velocity at the two points (V_1 and V_2, respectively), the fluid density (for blood, ρ = 1060 kg/L), and the velocity-dependent viscous friction according to:

$$\Delta P = \overbrace{\frac{1}{2}\rho\left(V_2^2 - V_1^2\right)}^{\text{convective acceleration}} + \overbrace{\rho\int_1^2 \frac{d\vec{V}}{dt}\,d\vec{s}}^{\text{flow acceleration}} + \overbrace{R(\vec{V})}^{\text{viscous friction}}$$

For most clinical applications of the Bernoulli equation, the convective acceleration component of the formula is considered the most significant. After combining ρ for blood with conversion factors to mm Hg and velocity to m/sec, the coefficient calculates out to 3.98. In most clinical applications this factor is rounded to 4.0. The second term of the equation, flow acceleration, represents the pressure drop generated by flow acceleration. This phenomenon, however, is important only during a very brief period at the rapid acceleration phase when there is a lag between the velocity and the pressure curves. During that time period, the pressure gradient is not considered clinically important. The third term represents the force necessary to overcome viscous friction. When considering pressure drops across a discrete orifice, viscous friction becomes negligible. Hence for most clinical applications the formula is simplified based on the following assumptions: (1) the velocity proximal to the obstruction (V_1) is assumed to be negligible compared with the velocity just distal to the obstruction (V_2); (2) in most clinical situations peak flow acceleration occurs in early systole when the pressure gradient is irrelevant and can be ignored; and (3) viscous friction is assumed to be trivial. The Bernoulli equation can therefore be simplified: $\Delta P = 4(V_2)^2$. This formula has been shown to be valid in in-vitro flow models[127] and in a variety of clinical settings.[132] However, the assumptions that govern the use of the simplified Bernoulli equation may not always be correct. For example, in long-segment narrowing such as a Blalock–Taussig shunt, ignoring the viscous friction term of the Bernoulli equation may lead to significant underestimation of the pressure drop. The limitations and pitfalls that can potentially lead to errors in estimation of pressure gradients have been reviewed elsewhere.[35,111,115,116]

Safety and Complications

Because of the widespread use of echocardiography in the diagnosis and monitoring of children with suspected heart disease, safety of the technique is of prime importance. This is particularly relevant in fetal echocardiography, in which fetuses may be exposed to ultrasound energy early in gestation. To date, no reports on adverse effects from diagnostic ultrasound have been published. Physicians involved with diagnostic ultrasound must be aware that ultrasound is a form of mechanical energy that, under certain conditions, can cause biological damage to exposed tissue. This damage can result from conversion of mechanical energy to heat or from creation of gaseous microcavitations. Thus far, it appears that biological damage has been observed only in nonclinical laboratory conditions. The American Institute of Ultrasound in Medicine stated that "...no confirmed biologic effects on patients or instrument operator caused by exposure at intensities typical of present diagnostic ultrasound instruments have ever been reported. Although the possibility that such biologic effects may be identified in the future, current data indicate that the benefits to patients of the prudent use of diagnostic ultrasound outweigh the risks, if any, that may be present."[9]

MAGNETIC RESONANCE IMAGING

Cardiovascular magnetic resonance (CMR) imaging is a sophisticated noninvasive imaging modality that overcomes many of the limitations of echocardiography and cardiac catheterization. High-resolution static and dynamic images of the heart, blood vessels, and other thoracic structures are obtained regardless of body size and acoustic barriers. Moreover, CMR provides additional unique information that is not available by other imaging techniques. As a result of the rapid technological evolution in computer sciences, electronics, and engineering over the last decade, CMR has evolved from a technique that produced several static images in an hour-long examination to a modality capable of real-time imaging,[106,107] succinct dynamic 3D visualization of cardiovascular anatomy, and accurate quantification of blood flow[91] and myocardial function.[28] These capabilities have greatly expanded the role of CMR in preoperative and postoperative evaluation of infants, children, and adults with CHD.

MRI TECHNIQUES AND THEIR CLINICAL APPLICATIONS

In MRI, magnetic fields and RF energy are used to stimulate hydrogen nuclei in selected regions of the body to emit RF waves that are then used to construct images. As with other cardiovascular imaging modalities, a thorough understanding of the underlying imaging physics enhances the quality and interpretation of the diagnostic data. This section provides a practical introduction to cardiovascular MRI; a more detailed discussion can be found in other sources.[78,118]

For an image to be produced, the patient is first placed inside the scanner, which applies a static high-strength magnetic field. Most clinical scanners use static magnetic field strengths ranging from 0.5 tesla (T) to 3 T [1 tesla = 10,000 gauss (G); the strength of earth's magnetic field at its surface is approximately 0.5 G]. Higher magnetic field strengths are used mostly in research scanners. Once positioned within the scanner, a section of the patient's body is then excited using an RF pulse, and an echo is formed by means of a second RF pulse (spin echo) and/or gradient pulses (gradient echo). The signal from the echo is then processed by Fourier transformation, and the data are used to fill a line of matrix from which the image is generated.

Cardiac and Respiratory Gating

The heart, blood, and blood vessels are in relatively rapid motion compared with other body structures. Although the speed of MRI continues to improve, standard techniques are too slow to image the heart in real time with adequate spatial and temporal resolution for most applications. Rather, an image at a particular point during the cardiac cycle is built up from data acquired over multiple cardiac cycles. Consequently, synchronization with the cardiac cycle is required in order to "return" to the same point in the cycle and effectively freeze cardiac motion. Imaging may be synchronized or "gated" with a pulse oximetry trace (so-called peripheral gating) or, more optimally, with a high-quality electrocardiogram signal. Because images are constructed over multiple cardiac cycles, respiratory motion can degrade image quality. One approach to minimizing respiratory artifacts is to have the patient hold his or her breath during image acquisition. Although this solution is often quite effective, it cannot be used in patients who are too young or ill to cooperate. In such cases, respiratory motion compensation can be achieved by synchronizing image data acquisition to the respiratory cycle, as well as the cardiac cycle. Respiratory motion can be tracked by either a bellows device placed around the body or MRI navigator echoes that concurrently image the position of the diaphragm or heart. The principal limitation of respiratory gating is that it substantially prolongs scan times, because image data are only accepted during a portion of the respiratory cycle. A final strategy to minimize respiratory motion artifacts is to acquire multiple images at the same location and average them, thereby minimizing variations caused by respiration. As expected, the disadvantage of this approach is also increased scan time.

This discussion highlights the need for more rapid high-quality MRI techniques that obviate the need for cardiac gating and respiratory motion compensation. Recent advances in gradient coil performance and parallel acquisition methods have achieved this goal in the research environment and are becoming more widely available in the clinical arena.[4,66,90,106,107]

CMR examination is performed by repeatedly selecting a pulse sequence, prescribing an imaging location, and acquiring the image data to address specific clinical questions. The pulse sequence specifies how the magnetic field gradients and RF pulses are applied and read during image acquisition. Table 102-1 summarizes the features of some of the common CMR sequences used in clinical practice. In general, there are two major categories of pulse sequences: spin echo and gradient echo (Table 102-1). Spin echo sequences are characterized by applying an RF pulse that tips hydrogen protons by 90°, followed by a second 180° pulse, and are usually used to generate images in which flowing blood appears black. Gradient echo sequences apply RF pulses that are less than 90° (usually 15–60°), are faster than spin echo sequences, and are usually used to generate images in which flowing blood appears white. Adding preparatory pulses that alter tissue contrast can often modify a particular pulse sequence. In addition, there are numerous user-selectable imaging parameters that affect tissue contrast, image quality, and temporal and spatial resolution. The large choice of imaging techniques and parameters allow the operator to adjust image contrast for optimal anatomical definition and detection of abnormal tissue. They also provide the capability for sophisticated functional assessment. The following section reviews the more common cardiovascular MRI techniques with a focus on their clinical utility.

Anatomical Imaging and Tissue Characteristics

Spin echo pulse sequences are usually used to produce images in which flowing blood has low signal intensity and appears dark ("black blood" imaging). Other tissues appear as varying shades of gray. Although cardiac-gated spin echo sequences produce only one image per location and thus provide only static anatomical information, their advantages include high spatial resolution, excellent blood–myocardium contrast, and decreased artifact from metallic biomedical implants (e.g., sternal wires, stents, prosthetic valves). Spin echo sequences also are easily modified to alter tissue contrast and characterize abnormal structures. Their clinical uses include evaluation for arrhythmogenic right ventricular cardiomyopathy, cardiac tumors, constrictive pericardial disease, vessel wall abnormalities, and thoracic masses (Figure 102-11). Conventional spin echo sequences are hampered by relatively long scan times (several minutes, depending on heart rate and number of signal averages). More recently, fast spin echo sequences have been developed that allow one location to be imaged rapidly enough for the patient to hold his or her breath (10–15 seconds). A double inversion preparatory pulse is usually applied to suppress the blood signal,[15,22,112] and an additional inversion pulse may by applied to suppress the fat signal.

Table 102–1

Summary of MRI Techniques

Technique	*ECG triggering*	*Appearance of blood flow*	*Dynamic (cine[a]) vs. static[b]*	*Clinical application*
I. Spin Echo				
Standard spin echo	Yes	Dark	Static	Anatomy, tissue characterization
Fast spin echo with double inversion recovery	Yes	Dark	Static	Anatomy, tissue characterization, faster image acquisition relative to standard spin echo
II. Gradient Echo				
Segmented *k*-space fast gradient echo or steady-state free precession	Yes	Bright	Dynamic	Anatomy, ventricular function, blood flow imaging
Phase contrast	Yes	Bright	Dynamic	Flow quantification and characterization
Tagging	Yes	Bright	Dynamic	Analysis of myocardial mechanics and flow
Gadolinium-enhanced 3D MRA	No	Bright	Static	3D anatomical data set
MR fluoroscopy	No	Bright	Dynamic	Anatomy, function, guidance of interventional procedures
Delayed enhancement	Yes	Intermediate	Static	Myocardial viability

[a]Cine: Multiple images are obtained throughout the cardiac cycle in each anatomical location. The stacked images are then displayed on a computer screen in a cine-loop format.

[b]Static: A single image is obtained in each anatomical location.

Cine MRI

Cardiac-gated gradient echo sequences can be used to produce multiple images over the cardiac cycle in each anatomical location. These images can then be displayed in a cine loop format to demonstrate the motion of the heart and vasculature over the cardiac cycle. On such cine MR images, flowing blood produces a bright signal, and the myocardium and vessel wall are relatively dark ("bright-blood" imaging) (Figure 102-12). Using a segmented *k*-space technique, cine MRI scan times are reduced so that a single location can be imaged with good temporal and spatial resolutions in 5–15 seconds, thereby permitting breathhold scanning.[3] More recently, steady-state free precession cine MRI sequences have been developed that are even faster and have improved blood–myocardial contrast.[14,89]

Cine MRI is used to delineate cardiovascular anatomy and assess ventricular function. It is helpful for evaluating the systemic and pulmonary veins, atrial and ventricular septum, intracardiac baffles and pathways (e.g., after Fontan, Mustard, Senning, or Rastelli procedures), ventricular outflow tracts, ventricular–arterial conduits, pulmonary arteries, and the aorta. It is also useful in identifying stenotic and regurgitant jets, which appear as dark signal voids (see Figure 102-12). Myocardial tagging is a modification of cine MRI that allows for a sophisticated analysis of regional myocardial function (see section on ventricular function).[28,29,75,76]

MRI Assessment of Ventricular Function

The principal MRI sequence used for evaluation of ventricular function is gradient echo cine MRI. An electrocardiogram (ECG)-triggered segmented *k*-space fast (also termed "turbo") gradient recall echo sequence has been used extensively during the 1990s, and its accuracy and reproducibility in measuring left and right ventricular volumes, mass, and

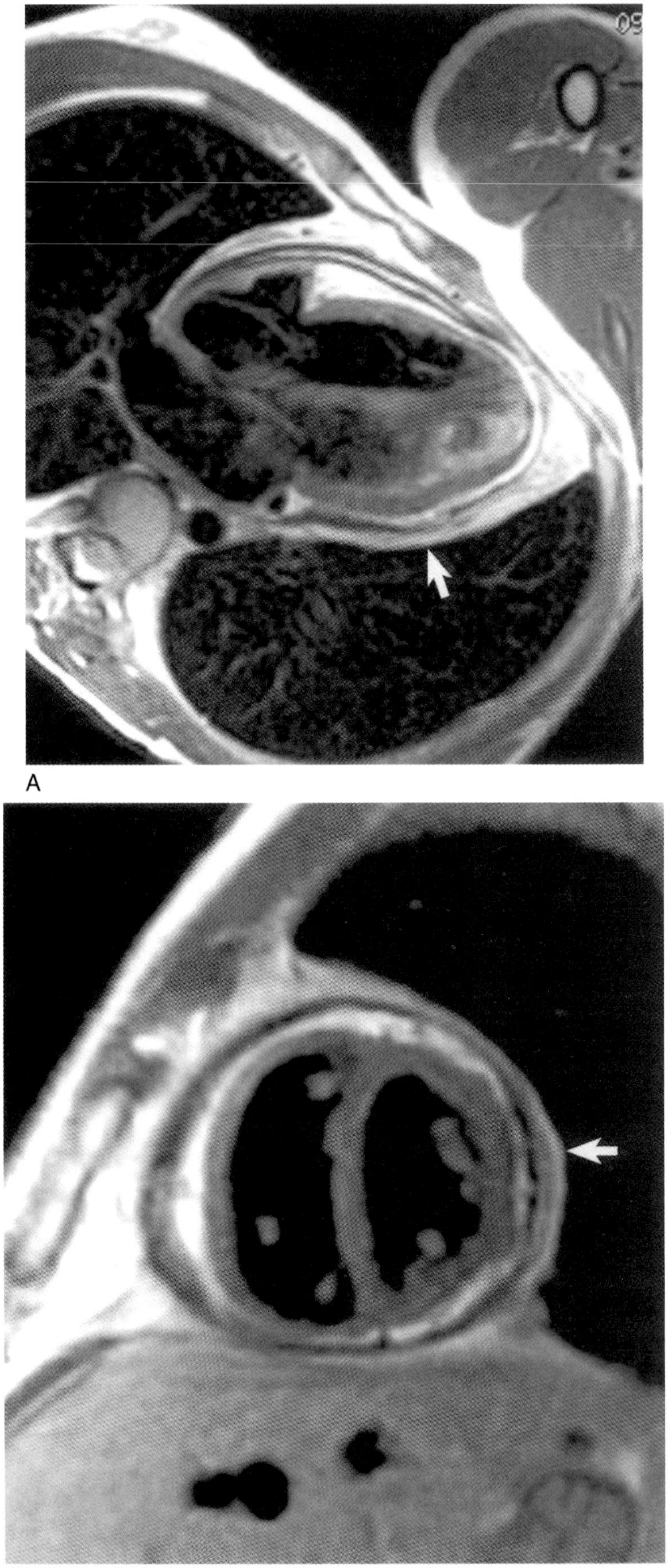

A

B

Figure 102–11 **Electrocardiogram (ECG)-triggered, breathhold, proton density–weighted, fast spin echo with double inversion recovery images showing a markedly thickened pericardium (*arrows*) in a 13-year-old girl with constrictive pericarditis. A,** Four-chamber plane. **B,** Short-axis plane.

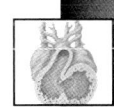

ejection fraction have been extensively validated.[39,63,85] A newer gradient echo imaging sequence, steady-state free precession, has been shown to provide a sharper contrast between the blood pool and the myocardium and to reduce motion-induced blurring during systole.[5,66,125]

Quantitative evaluation of ventricular function is achieved by obtaining a series of contiguous cine MRI slabs that cover the ventricles in short axis (Figure 102-13).[28,67,68,107] By the tracing of the blood–endocardium boundary, the slab's volume is calculated as the product of its cross-sectional area and thickness (which is prescribed by the operator). Ventricular volume is then determined by summation of the volumes of all slabs. The process can be repeated for each frame in the cardiac cycle to obtain a continuous time–volume loop or may be performed only on a diastolic and a systolic frame to calculate diastolic and systolic volumes. From these data one can calculate left and right ventricular ejection fractions and stroke volumes. Because the patient's heart rate at the time of image acquisition is known, one can calculate left and right ventricular output. Ventricular mass is calculated by tracing the epicardial borders, subtracting the endocardial volumes, and multiplying the resultant muscle volume by the specific gravity of the myocardium (1.05 g/mm^3). Most manufacturers of MRI scanners and some third-party companies offer software packages that automatically perform the previous calculations. Development of algorithms for automatic border detection have facilitated the application of these techniques, but further refinements are required to improve its accuracy.[31] Because of its accurate spatial and temporal registration of data, MRI measurements of chamber dimensions have become the accepted reference standard to which other methods are compared.[18,54] For example, Bellenger et al[7] measured left ventricular volumes in 64 patients with dilated cardiomyopathy.

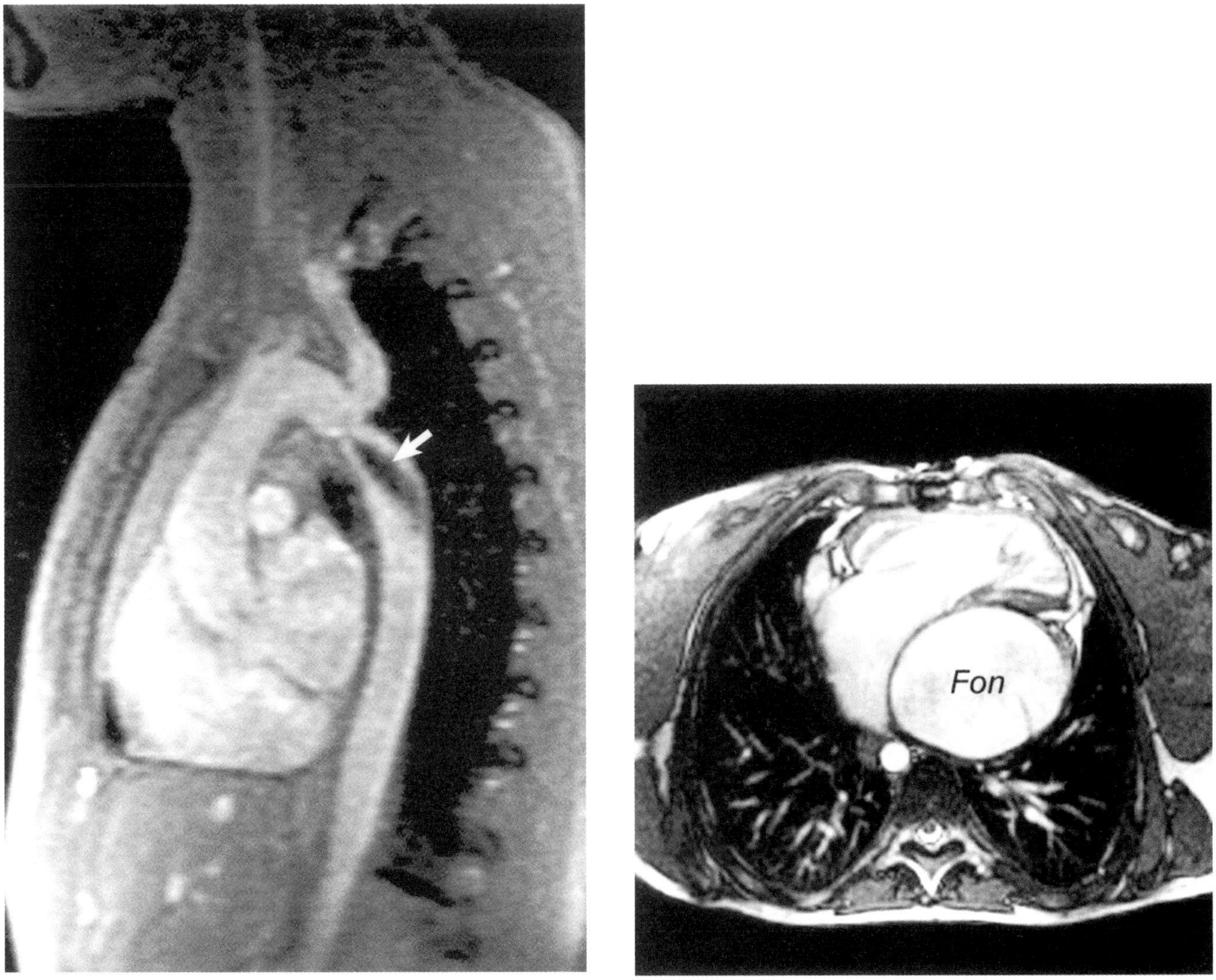

A B

Figure 102–12 Clinical applications of gradient echo cine magnetic resonance imaging (MRI). A, Electrocardiogram (ECG)-triggered, breathhold, segmented *k*-space, fast spoiled gradient echo multiphase sequence in a patient with severe coarctation of the aorta. The relatively long echo time allows for clear depiction of the dephasing jet in systole *(arrow)*, indicating high-velocity turbulent flow. **B,** Axial plane ECG-triggered, steady-state free precession multiphase sequence in a patient with heterotaxy syndrome and single ventricle who has had a Fontan operation. Note the left-sided Fontan pathway (Fon), as well as the clear depiction of intracardiac anatomy.

(Continued)

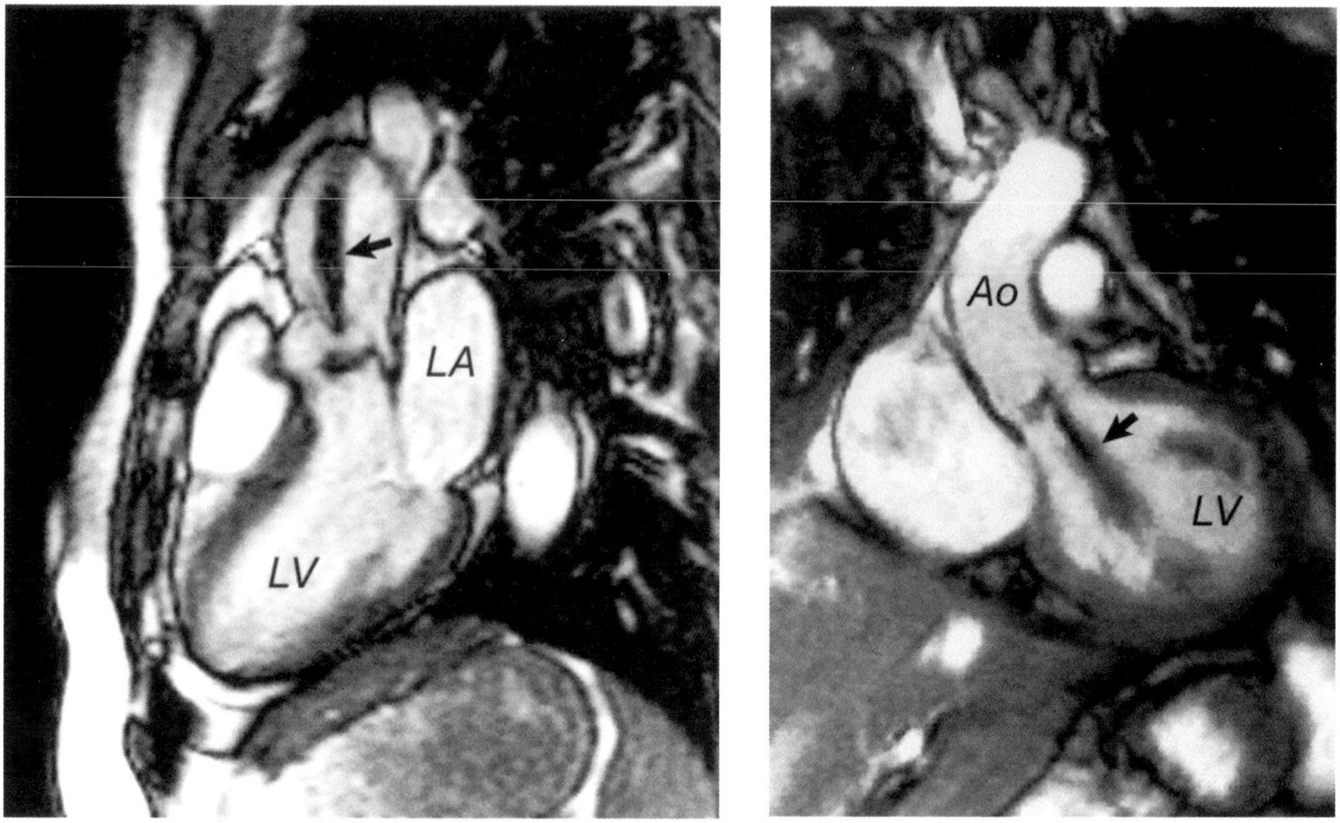

C D

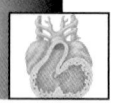

Figure 102–12 cont'd **C,** Systolic turbulent jet *(arrow)* in a patient with aortic valve stenosis. **D,** Diastolic turbulent jet *(arrow)* in a patient with aortic valve regurgitation. Ao, Aorta; LA, left atrium; LV, left ventricle.

They reported an intraobserver variability of 2.4 ± 2.5%, interobserver variability of 5.1 ± 3.7%, and interstudy variability (repeat MRI examinations) of 2.9 ± 1.2%. Normal MRI values of ventricular volume and mass in children, adolescents, and adults have been reported by Lorenz.[67]

Gradient echo cine MRI is also used to evaluate regional wall motion abnormalities and segmental wall thickening.[64] Dobutamine stress MRI has been reported to be a useful test in adults with coronary artery disease.[55,79,87] More recently, the use of an MRI-compatible supine cycle ergometer has been reported to allow assessment of ventricular function and valve regurgitation response to exercise.[99,100]

Another approach to MRI evaluation of ventricular function and myocardial mechanics is called myocardial tagging.[11] With a preparatory RF gradient echo pulse sequence such as spatial modulation of magnetization (SPAMM), the spin of the protons in selected parts of the image volume are flipped in such a way as to render them incapable of producing a signal. This results in stripes of signal void (dark stripes) across the image (Figure 102-14). Similarly, two sets of orthogonal stripes (tags) can be placed, producing a grid across the image. The grid or stripes are placed at the onset of the R wave and are followed by a gradient echo cine MRI sequence. As the myocardium moves during the cardiac cycle, the tags follow it and their rotation, translation, and deformation can be tracked, allowing for calculation of myocardial strain and strain rate.[10,27,49,80] This can be done during systole or diastole and in two or three dimensions. A recently described technique for the analysis of myocardial tagging data, harmonic phase imaging, greatly shortens the analysis time because it does not require manual tracing of the tags.[33]

Blood Flow Analysis

An ECG-gated, velocity-encoded cine MRI (VEC MRI) sequence, a type of gradient echo sequence, can be used to measure blood flow velocity and quantify blood flow rate.[77,86,91] The VEC MRI technique is based on the principle that the signal from hydrogen nuclei (such as those in blood) flowing through specially designed magnetic field gradients accumulates a predictable phase shift that is proportional to its velocity. Multiple phase images are constructed across the cardiac cycle in which the voxel intensity or brightness is proportion to blood velocity within that voxel. Flow quantification is performed by placing an imaging slab across a blood vessel or through the area at question within the heart (Figure 102-15A). The operator then determines whether flow velocity encoding is performed only perpendicular to the imaging plane (z axis) or in other directions as well (x and y axes). The data are then analyzed off-line using specialized software. A region of interest (ROI) is defined by the operator around the lumen of the relevant vessel, and the instantaneous mean velocity of each voxel is calculated (Figure 102-15,B–C). Flow rate is

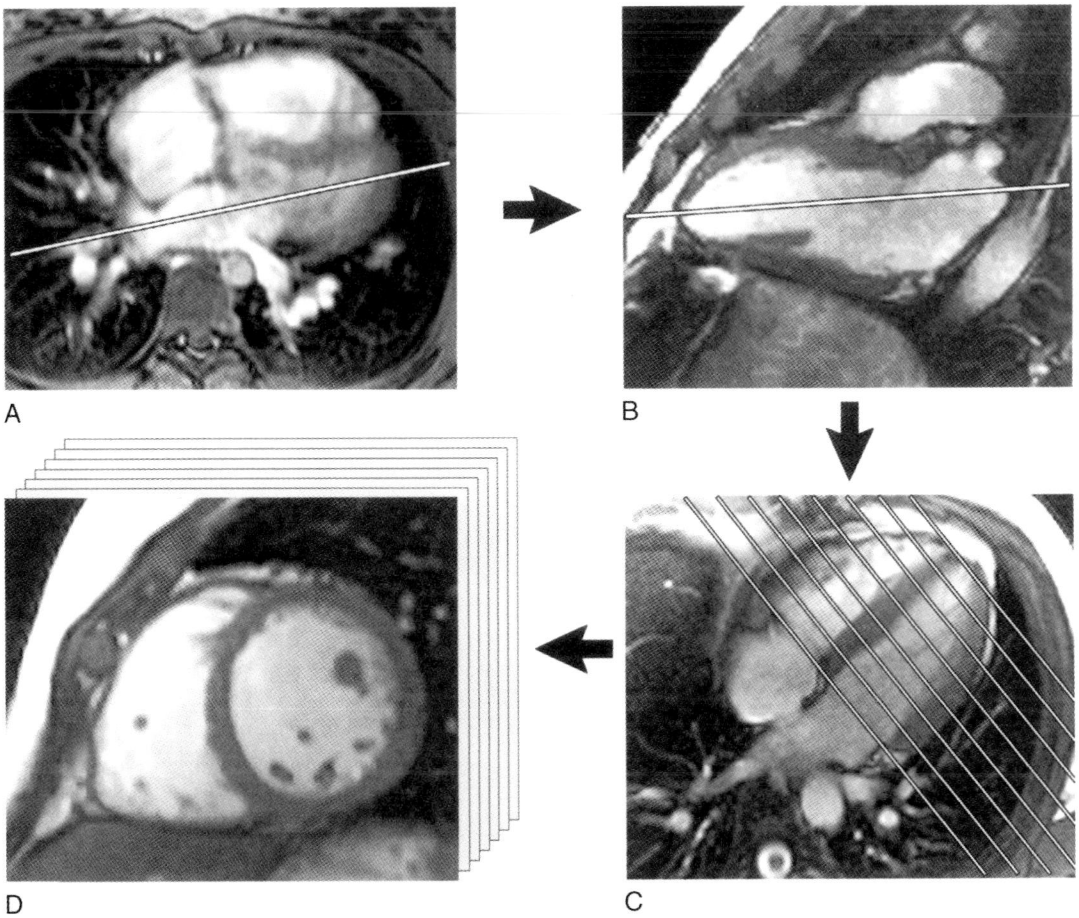

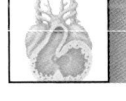

Figure 102–13 **Cine magnetic resonance imaging (MRI) technique for assessment of ventricular dimensions and function.** **A,** With a localizing image in the axial plane, an imaging plane is placed parallel to the left ventricular septal surface. **B,** Two-chamber plane. **C,** Four-chamber plane. **D,** Short-axis plane. For complete coverage of the ventricles, 12 contiguous imaging slabs are placed from the plane of the atrioventricular (AV) valves through the cardiac apex.

calculated as the product of the mean velocities within the ROI and its cross-sectional area. Integration of the instantaneous flow rates over the cardiac cycle yields the stroke volume (Figure 102-15D). This technique has been shown by in vitro and in vivo studies to be accurate and reproducible.[92] Cine phase contrast has been widely applied to measure systemic and pulmonary blood flow and their ratio, as well as flow in individual pulmonary arteries, across the mitral and tricuspid valves, across an atrial septal defect, in systemic and pulmonary veins, and in other individual blood vessels. This technique also allows accurate quantification of regurgitation volume and fraction across any cardiac valve.[95] An example of an important application of this technique in pediatric cardiology is the quantification of pulmonary regurgitation in patients who have undergone tetralogy of Fallot (TOF) repair (see Figure 102-15).[94] When flow encoding is performed in three spatial directions, multidimensional flow imaging and analysis can be accomplished by resolving the flow velocities and directions into flow vectors that can be viewed in cine-loop format (Figure 102-16). This technique allows unique imaging of blood flow in five dimensions (x, y, and z spatial dimensions, velocity, and time).[6] It also allows quantitative analysis of flow dynamics, including the ability to calculate the shear stress exerted by the flowing blood on the vessel wall.[83]

Contrast-Enhanced MR Angiography

Another approach for improving the contrast between vascular and nonvascular structures is to administer an exogenous intravenous contrast agent, typically a gadolinium chelate, that dramatically shortens the T_1 relaxation of blood, resulting in a bright signal on T_1-weighted sequences. This method of angiography is less prone to flow-related artifacts than other MR techniques and has a short acquisition time. Contrast-enhanced MR angiography (MRA) is usually performed without cardiac gating, using a 3D fast gradient echo acquisition lasting 15–30 seconds while the patient holds his or her breath.[81,93,122] The time delay between contrast administration and image acquisition determines the vascular territory illustrated, and several acquisitions can be performed. The entire procedure takes only a few minutes to perform and yields a high-contrast and high-resolution 3D data set depicting all or part of the thorax. The 3D data set can be navigated on dedicated workstations using a variety of image display techniques, including rapid construction of

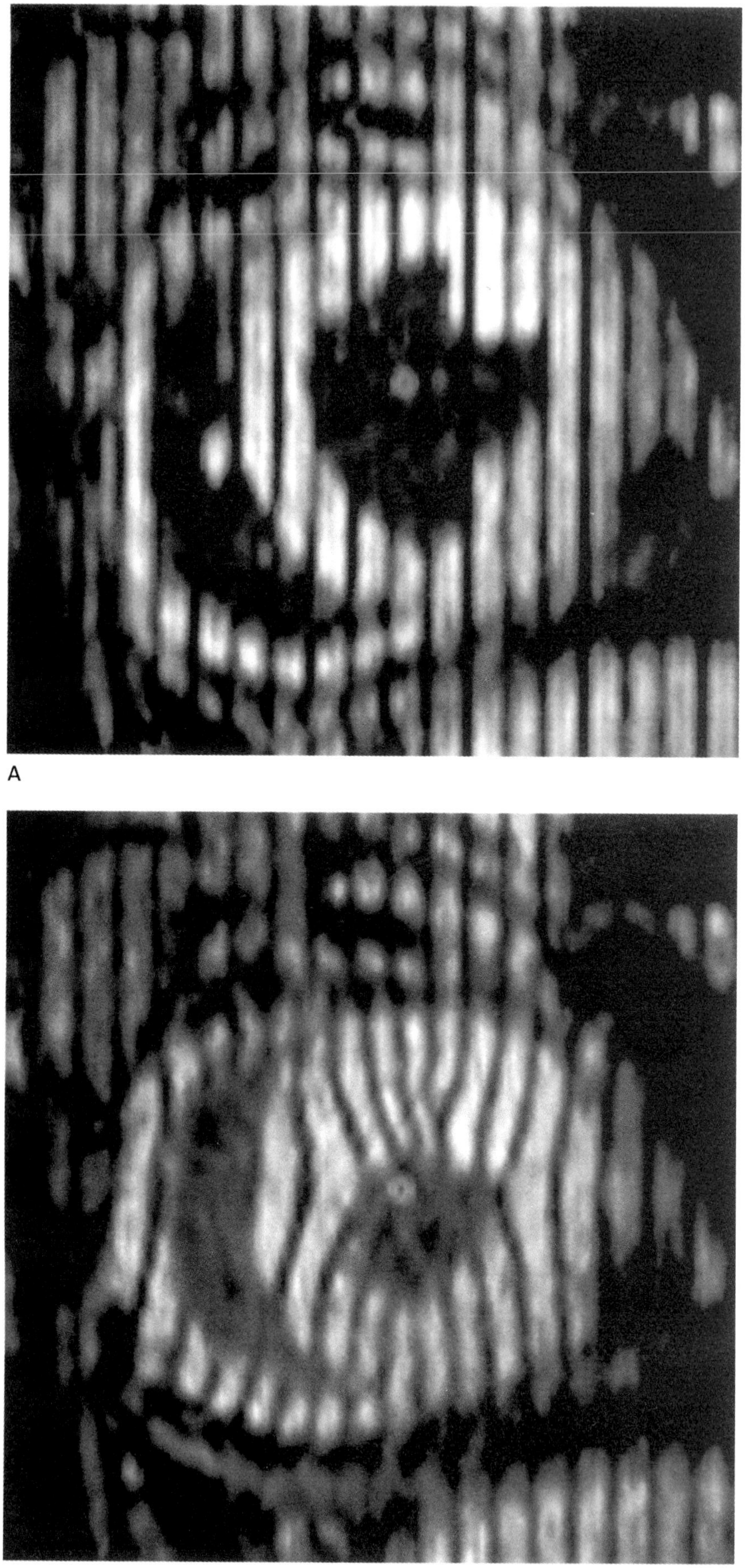

A

B

Figure 102–14 **Myocardial tagging.** **A,** Diastolic frame showing the undistorted tags before the onset of systole. **B,** Systolic frame showing distortion of the myocardial tags as a result of cardiac motion. Notice the undistorted tags on the chest wall and liver.

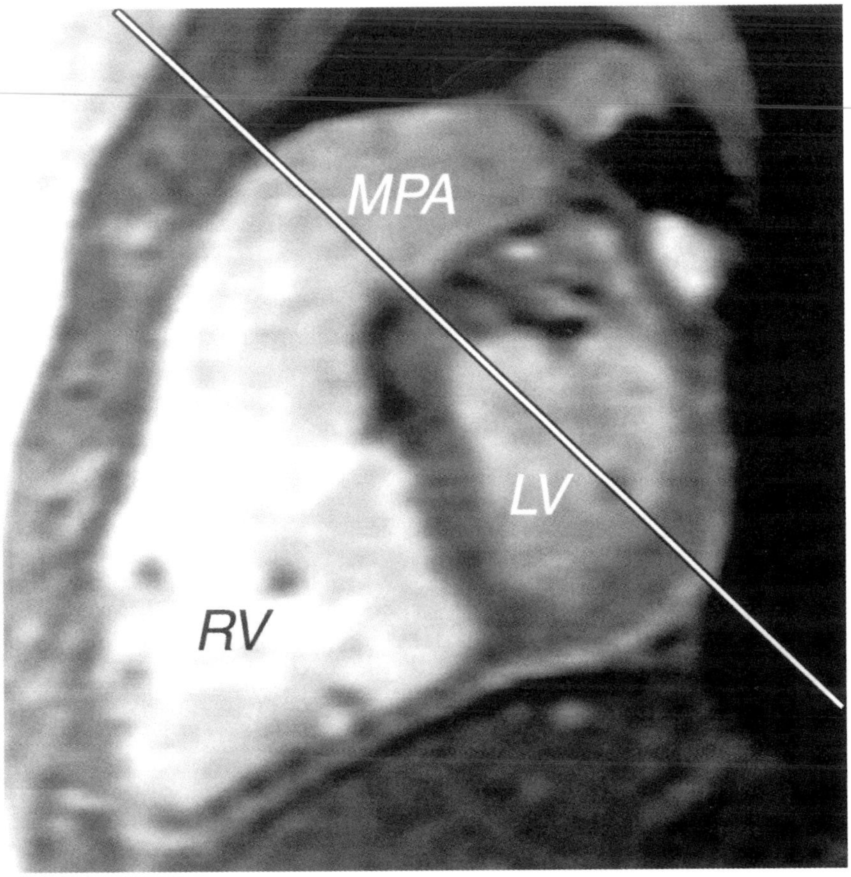

A

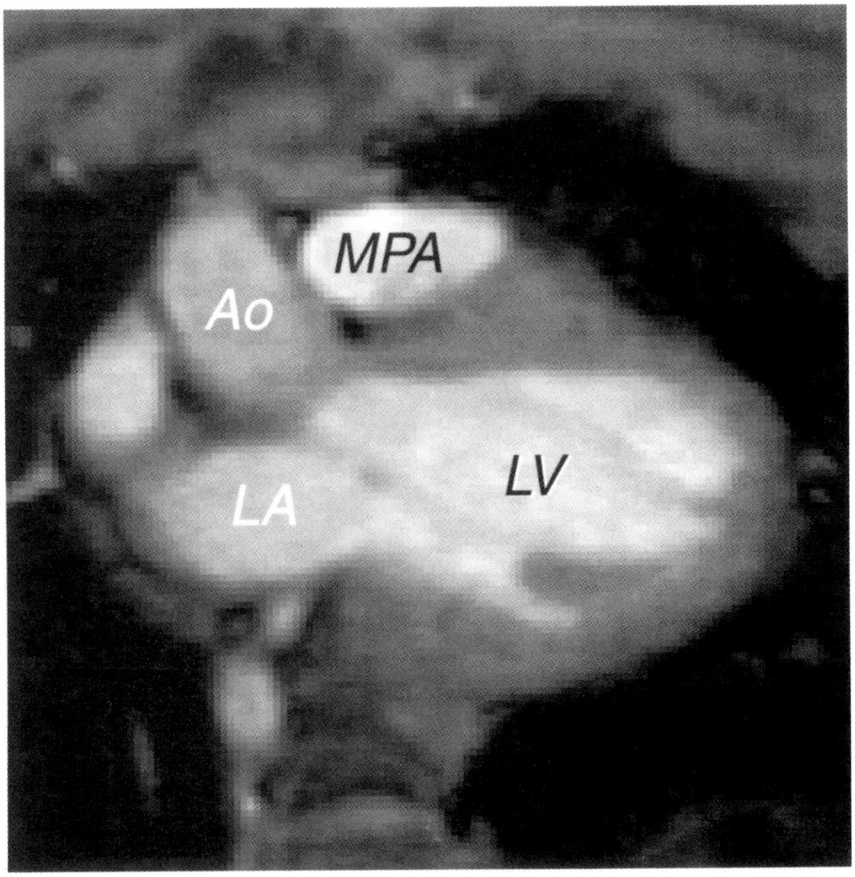

B

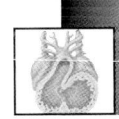

Figure 102–15 **Quantitative assessment of pulmonary regurgitation by velocity-encoded cine magnetic resonance imaging (MRI) in a 26-year-old patient with repaired tetralogy of Fallot. A,** An imaging plane is placed across the main pulmonary artery (MPA) (multiphase gradient echo cine MR). **B,** Magnitude image showing bright signal in the proximal main pulmonary artery (MPA).

(Continued)

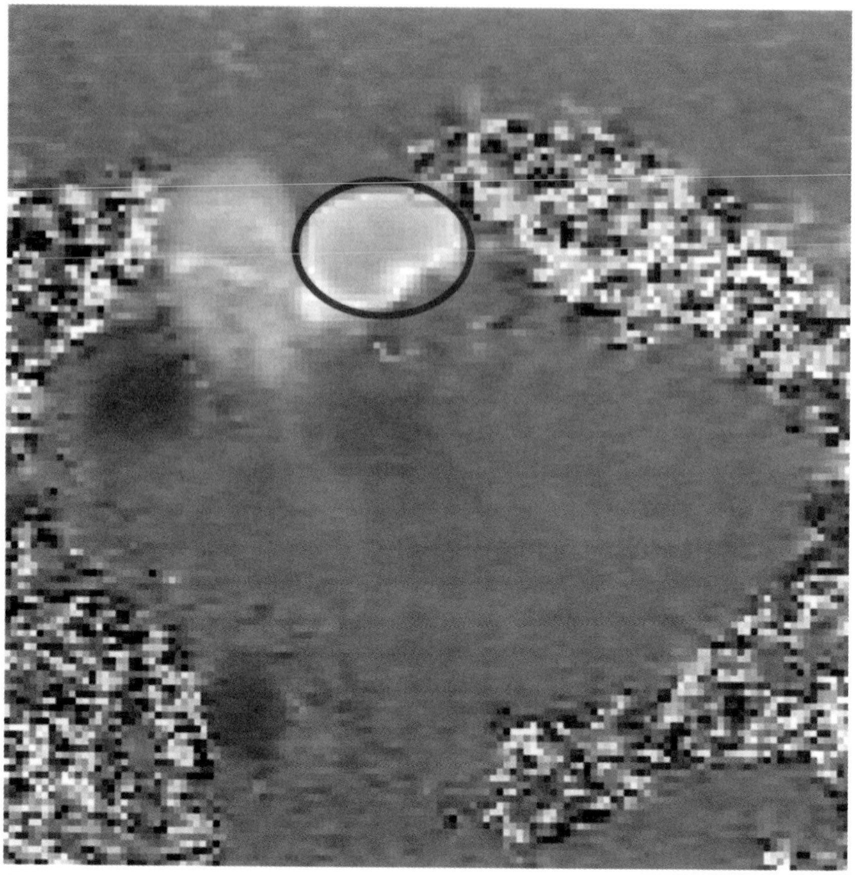

C

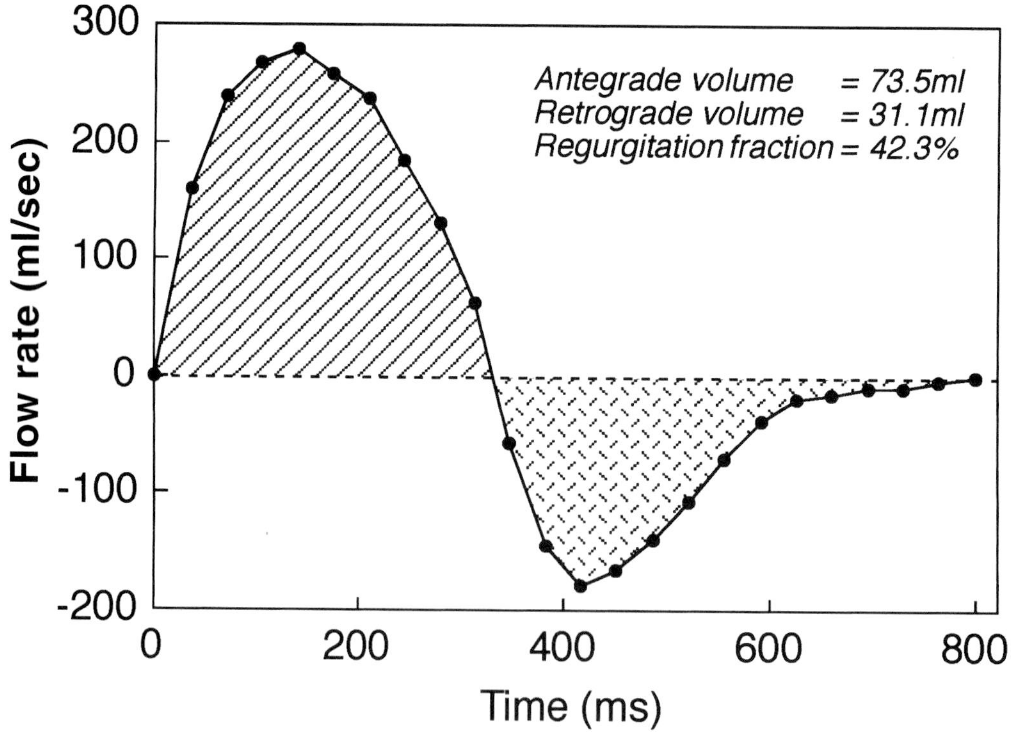

D

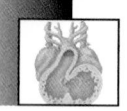

Figure 102–15 cont'd **C,** The corresponding phase image contains the velocity and directional data. Using a computer workstation, a region of interest *(oval)* is placed around the main pulmonary artery. **D,** The systolic flow-time integral *(area under the curve)* above the baseline yields the antegrade flow volume, and the diastolic flow-time integral below the baseline corresponds to the regurgitant flow volume. Regurgitation fraction is calculated as the ratio of retrograde (regurgitant volume) to antegrade volume.

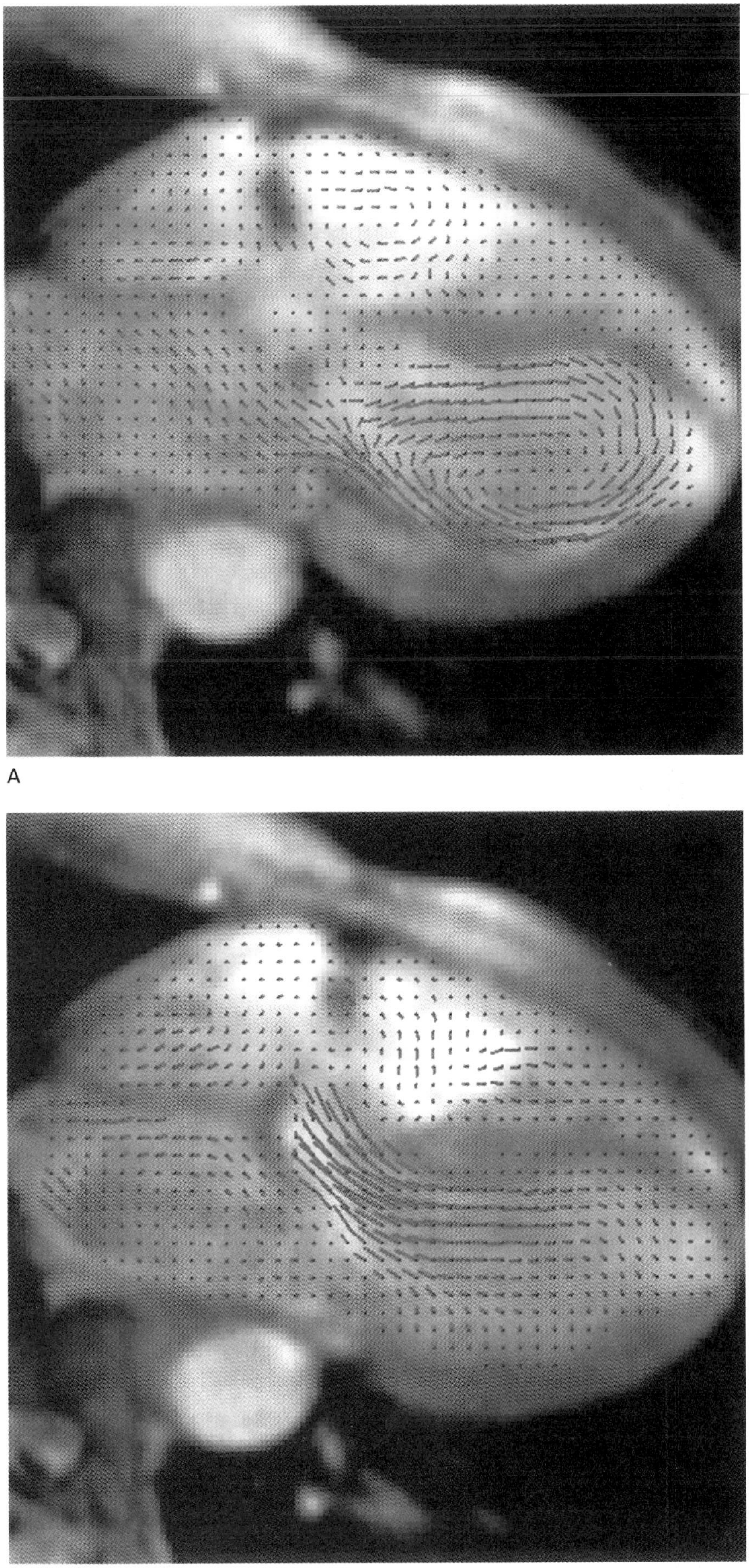

A

B

Figure 102–16 Three-dimensional (3D) flow vector map showing intracardiac diastolic (A) and systolic (B) flow pattern. The orientation of the vector corresponds to the instantaneous in-plane direction of blood flow, whereas the vector's length is proportional to instantaneous velocity. (See color plate.)

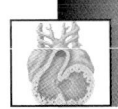

intuitive 3D models (Figure 102-17). Unlike cine MRI, conventional contrast-enhanced MRA is not time resolved. However, with continued improvements in imaging speed, cardiac-gated MRA will likely be possible in the near future. MRA is ideally suited to elucidate the anatomy of the aorta and its branches, pulmonary arteries, pulmonary veins, and systemic veins.[36,44,98] Although this technique is used mostly for imaging of extracardiac anatomy, we have found it useful in the evaluation of intraatrial systemic and pulmonary baffles (such as in Mustard or Senning operations and after Fontan procedures), as well as for imaging of the outflow tracts (such as in repaired TOF and the arterial switch operation). In addition, MRA clearly delineates the spatial relationships between vascular structures, the tracheobronchial tree, chest wall, spine, and other landmarks that may be useful for planning of interventional catheterization or surgical procedures.

Myocardial Ischemia and Viability

Although traditionally the diagnosis of myocardial ischemia has not been a focus of imaging in CHD, it clearly has relevance in patients who have congenital and acquired coronary abnormalities (e.g., anomalous origin of the left coronary artery, pulmonary atresia with intact ventricular septum, and Kawasaki disease). Moreover, myocardial ischemia is an important diagnostic challenge in postoperative and adult CHD. Several MRI techniques for imaging the coronary arteries with sufficient resolution to detect stenotic lesions are under evaluation, with some encouraging initial results.[19,20,123] However, the optimal approach and clinical utility of MR coronary angiography will likely remain in evolution for the next several years. MRI techniques are also available for assessment of regional left ventricular myocardial perfusion.[58,102] Typically, after a rapid intravenous gadolinium contrast injection, ultrafast, multislice imaging with an echo-planar pulse sequence is performed during a 20–30 second breathhold to image the first pass of contrast through the myocardium (Figure 102-18). The procedure can be repeated after administering a coronary vasodilator (e.g., adenosine or dipyridamole). Although offering superior spatial resolution compared with nuclear cardiology techniques without the use of ionizing radiation, the widespread application MR perfusion imaging has been limited by the need for time-intensive analysis and insufficient clinical validation. Alternatively, cine MRI can be used to detect focal wall motion abnormalities with pharmacological stress-induced ischemia. Initial studies have demonstrated that for dobutamine stress studies, MRI compares favorably with transthoracic echocardiography, primarily as

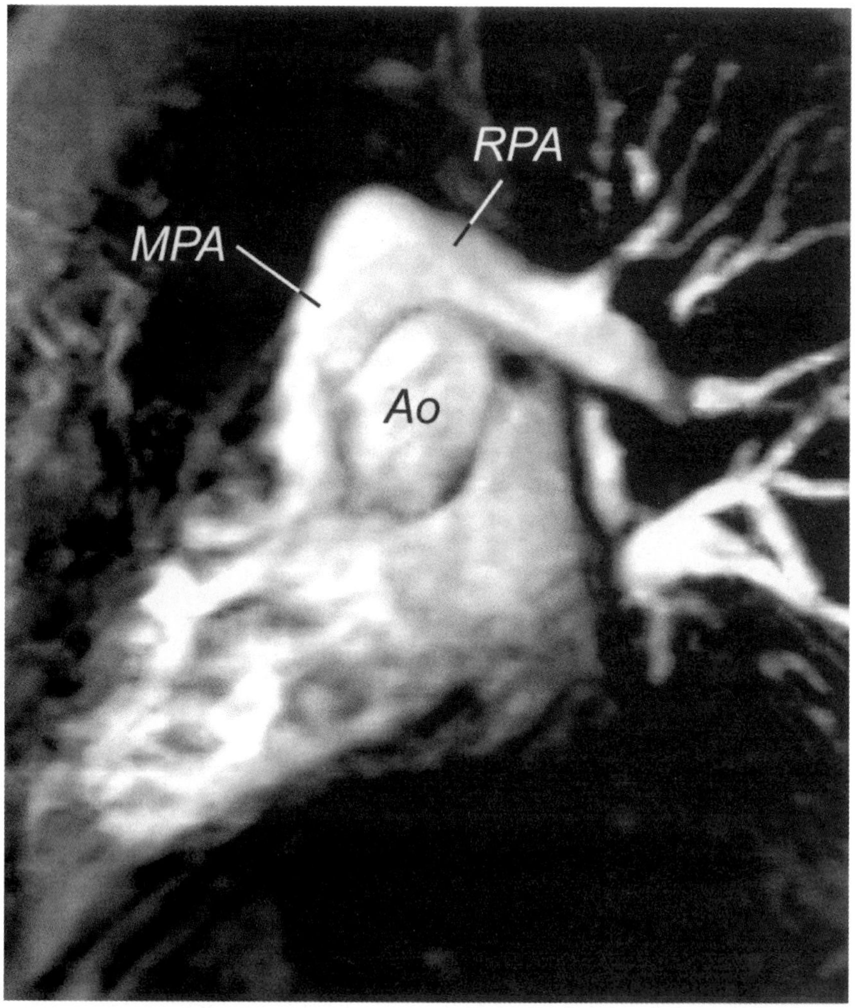

A

Figure 102–17 Gadolinium-enhanced three-dimensional (3D) magnetic resonance angiography (MRA) in a patient with D-loop transposition of the great arteries after an arterial switch operation. A, Subvolume Maximal Intensity Projection (MIP) image in an oblique sagittal plane showing the main (MPA) and right (RPA) pulmonary arteries.

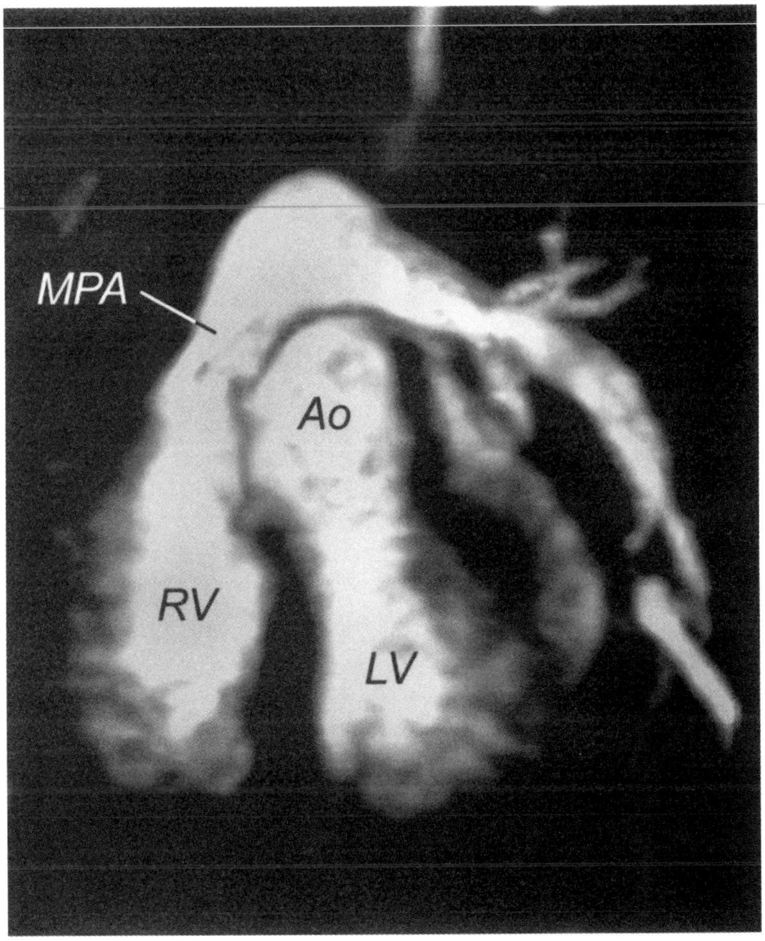

B

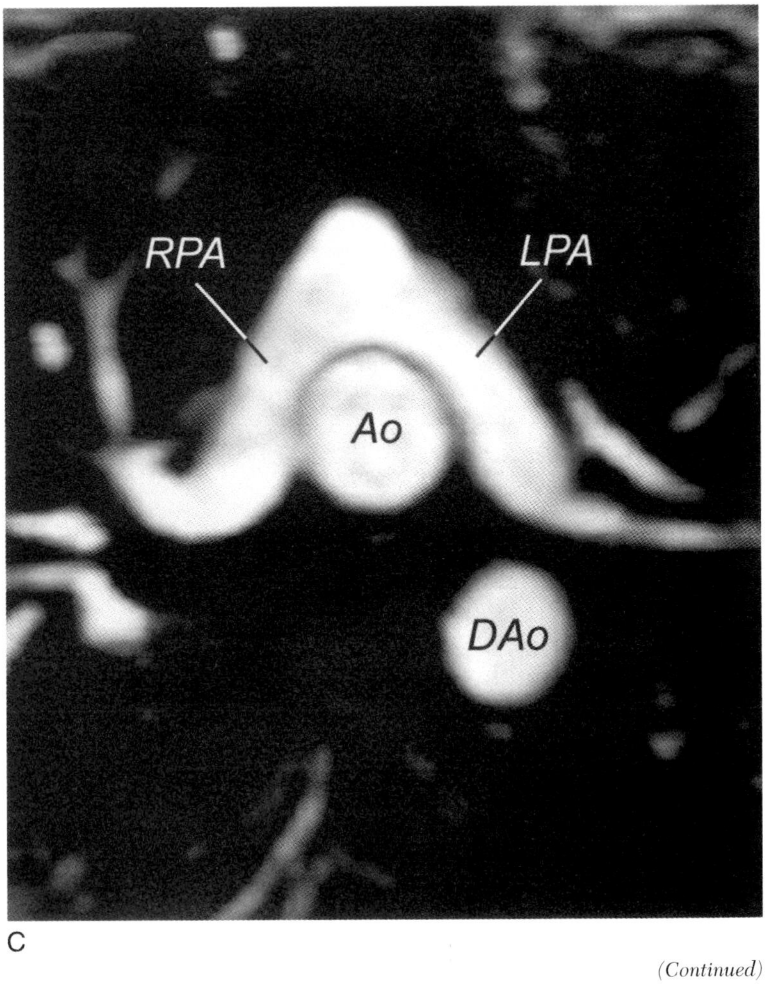

C

Figure 102–17 cont'd **B**, Leftward angulation of the imaging plane shows the left pulmonary artery. **C**, Axial plane MIP image demonstrates the left (LPA) and right (RPA) pulmonary arteries wrapped around the ascending aorta (Ao) (Lecompte maneuver).

(Continued)

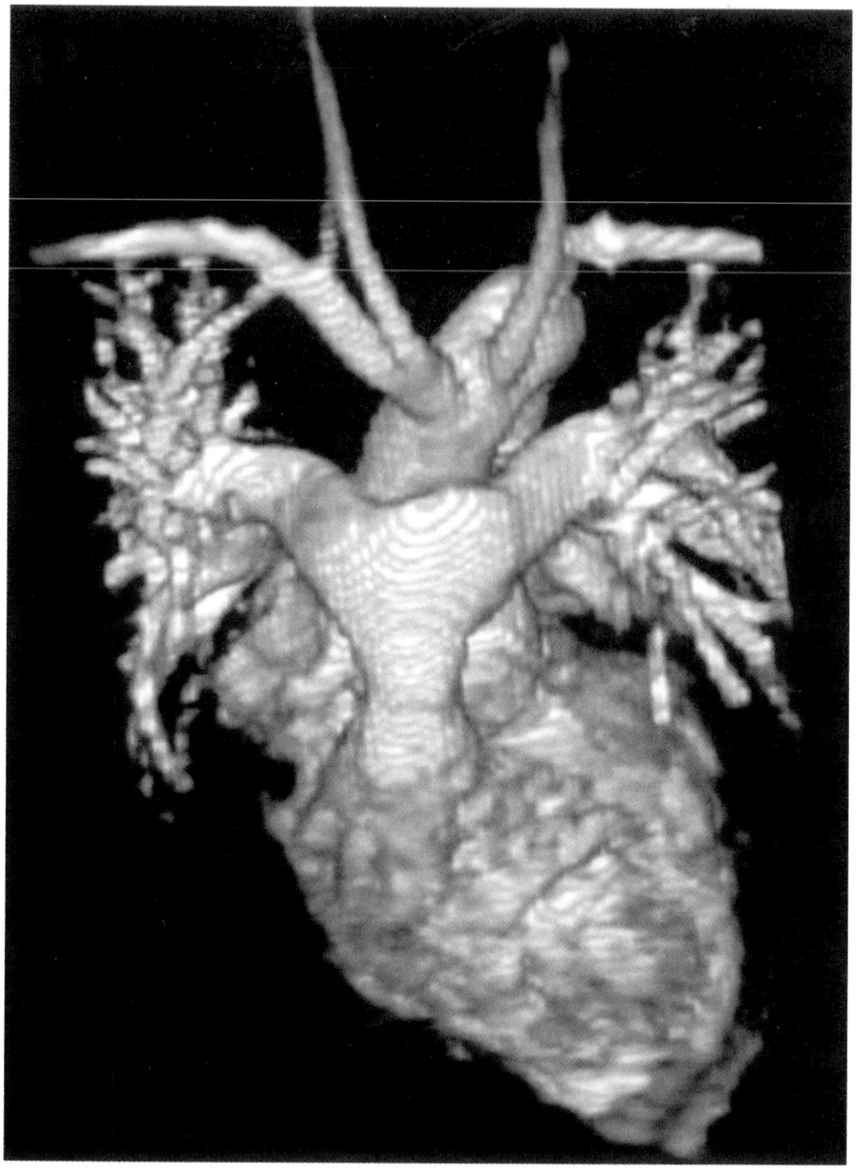

Figure 102–17 cont'd D, 3D volume reconstruction provides enhanced perception of the relationships between the great vessels. (See color plate.)

a result of its superior image quality.[46] Finally, there are a variety of MRI techniques that have been used to assess myocardial viability. In particular, there is growing evidence showing that hyperenhanced myocardial regions observed 10–15 minutes after the administration of gadolinium contrast agents (termed delayed myocardial enhancement) are indicative of irreversible myocardial injury (Figure 102-19).[47,84,88] Initial human studies assessing the utility of this technique in the diagnosis and management of myocardial ischemia are encouraging, and large-scale clinical trials are underway.[48]

Indications for CMR

The indications for CMR in patients with congenital and acquired pediatric heart disease are rapidly expanding. In general, the clinical reasons for a CMR examination may fall into one or more of the following three categories: (1) when transthoracic echocardiography is incapable of providing the required diagnostic information; (2) as an alternative to diagnostic cardiac catheterization with its associated discomfort, ionizing radiation exposure, contrast agent load, risks of morbidity and mortality, and high cost; and (3) for MRI's unique capabilities such as tissue imaging, myocardial tagging, and vessel-specific flow quantification.

General Considerations

Detailed preexamination planning is crucial given the wide array of imaging sequences available and the often complex nature of the clinical, anatomical, and functional issues in patients with CHD. The importance of a careful review of the patient's medical history, including details of all cardiovascular surgical procedures, interventional catheterizations, findings of previous diagnostic tests, and current clinical status, cannot be overemphasized. As is the case with echocardiography and cardiac catheterization, CMR examination of CHD is an interactive diagnostic procedure

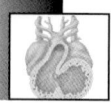

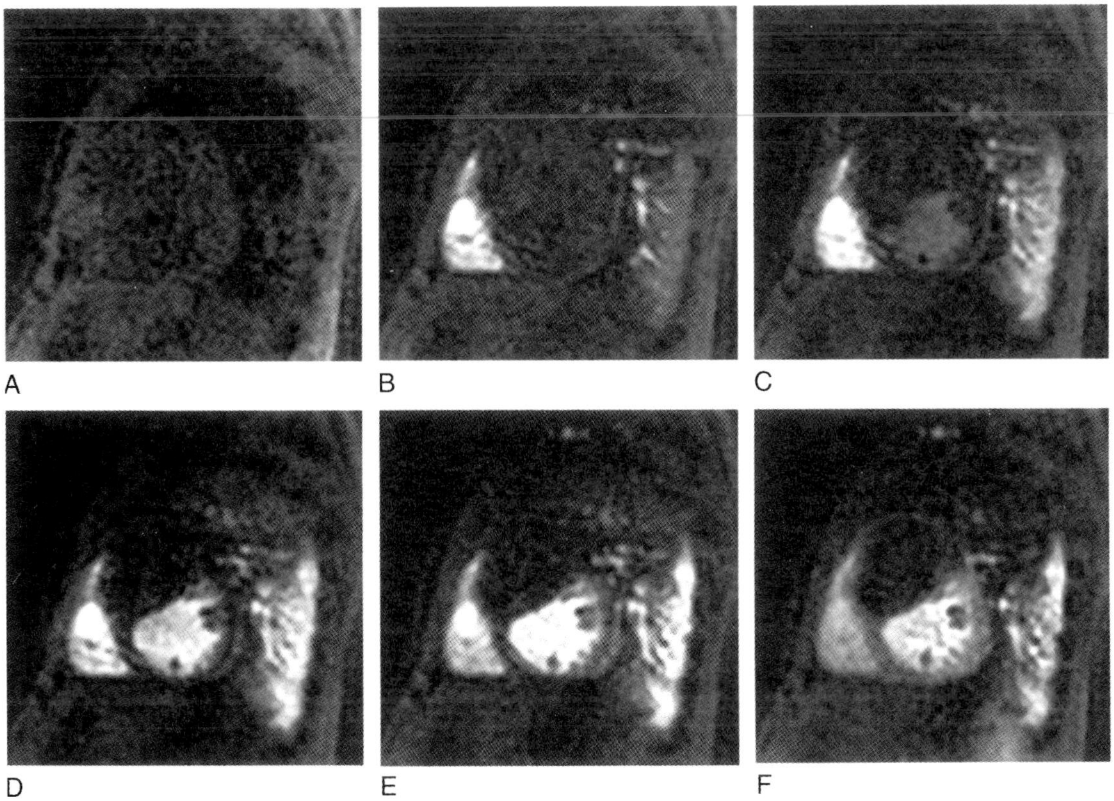

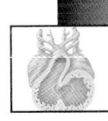

Figure 102–18 **First-pass myocardial perfusion scan in a patient with left ventricular fibroma. A,** At onset of scan there is no contrast in the heart. **B,** Arrival of contrast in the right ventricle. **C,** Arrival of contrast in the pulmonary veins and early enhancement of left ventricular cavity. **D,** Arrival of contrast in the left ventricular cavity (notice the unenhanced left ventricular myocardium). **E,** Arrival of contrast in the left ventricular myocardium (notice the hypoperfused tumor in the anterolateral aspect of the septum). **F,** Late myocardial enhancement with hypoperfused tumor.

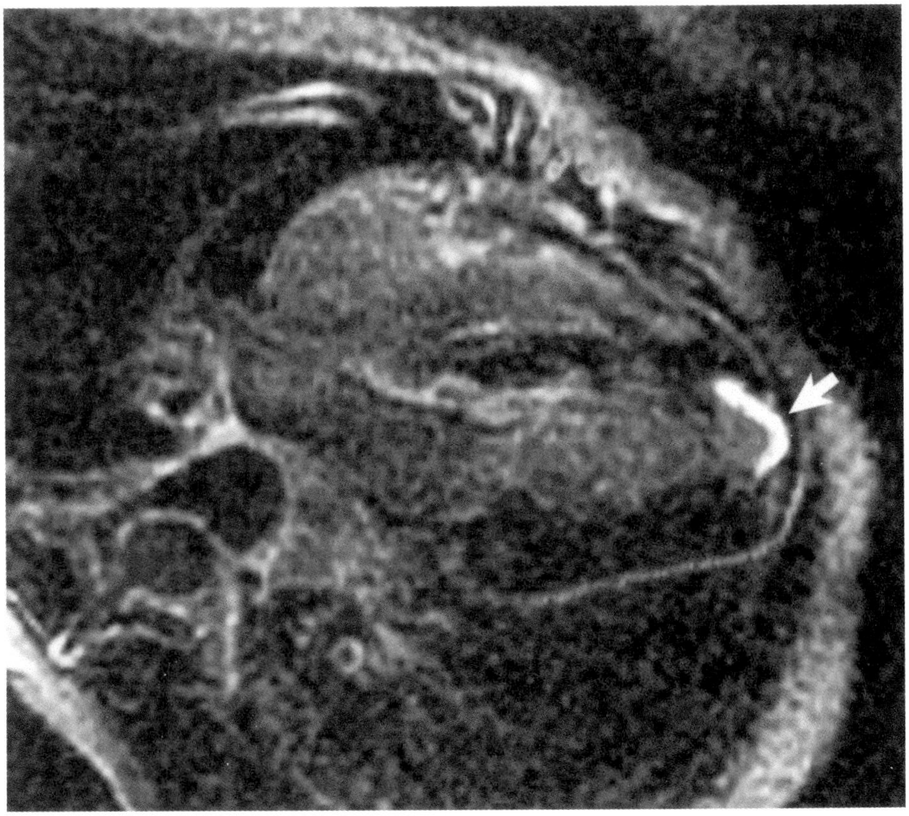

Figure 102–19 **Assessment of myocardial viability in an infant who underwent resection of myocardial tumor.** Nonviable myocardium produced bright signal (*arrow*) on post-gadolinium-delayed enhancement, inversion recovery T_1-weighted gradient echo sequence. Notice the dark signal from the viable left ventricular myocardium.

that requires on-line review and interpretation of the data by the supervising physician. The unpredictable nature of the anatomy and hemodynamics often require adjustment of the examination protocol; modification of imaging planes; adding, deleting, or changing sequences; and adjustment of imaging parameters. Reliance on standardized protocols and post-hoc reading alone in these patients might result in incomplete or even erroneous interpretation.

Sedation is often required in young patients who cannot cooperate with a CMR examination. Most patients younger than 5–6 years require sedation, and some patients between 6–10 years of age are capable of cooperation, whereas most children older than 10 years can undergo a CMR study without sedation provided their mental development is age-appropriate and they are not claustrophobic. Screening for sedation need is part of the scheduling process for CMR, and consultation with the referring cardiologist and parents is advised. Both conscious sedation and general anesthesia have been successfully used in CMR. In our experience, advantages of general anesthesia include a better safety profile (secured airways and close monitoring by a pediatric anesthesiologist); ability to suspend respiration, leading to improved image quality and a shorter examination time; and control over duration of sedation. Disadvantages of this approach include a higher cost and availability of skilled anesthesia personnel.

Safety and Complications

Standard clinical imaging scanners present no known hazards to biological materials. Three different magnetic fields are employed by such magnets: the relatively large static magnetic field, smaller but rapidly varying magnetic fields secondary to the magnetic field gradients, and RF pulses. Guidelines set by the FDA keep the strength of these fields well below levels that could cause significant biological effects. Animal studies evaluating the influence of static magnetic fields have not demonstrated significant biological effects for fields of up to 2 T.[130] Millions of patients have undergone MRI studies without any noticeable immediate or long-term sequelae. Pregnancy is presently a relative contraindication to MRI studies, although the magnetic field levels used in clinical imagers have no known effects on the embryo. Many women have undergone MRI imaging during all trimesters of pregnancy without reported ill effect on the mother, fetus, or resultant infant. When maternal and fetal health considerations require diagnostic studies, MRI imaging is preferable to methods that employ X-rays, such as computed tomography (CT) or angiography.

Implanted metallic objects are a subject of particular concern because they could potentially undergo undesirable torquing movements if the magnetic field were sufficiently strong and if they contained sufficient ferromagnetic material. Fortunately, surgical clips and sternotomy wires implanted in the chest and abdomen are typically only weakly ferromagnetic. Furthermore, these devices quickly become immobilized by surrounding fibrous tissue, and patients with these implants can be safely studied by MRI. The wires and clips, however, may cause image artifact. Similarly, patients with implanted intravascular coils, stents, and occluding devices can be imaged by MRI once the implants are believed to be immobile. Many centers choose to avoid exposing these patients to MRI for an arbitrarily chosen period after implantation (usually for several weeks), but such practice is not supported by conclusive published data. A decision to perform MRI examination shortly after cardiac surgery or implantation of a biomedical device must weigh the risk–benefit ratio for the individual patient.[109]

A number of devices are considered either a relative or absolute contraindication to MRI.[23,101,105,109,110] Presence of an intracranial, intraocular, or intracochlear metallic object is considered a contraindication to MRI. Prosthetic cardiac valves manufactured before 1964 may contain substantial ferromagnetic material, and most are considered a contraindication to MRI. The presence of a cardiac pacemaker is also considered a contraindication to MRI,[82] although some reports have suggested that scanning patients who have modern pacemakers may be possible.[37,43]

Because MRI scanners attract ferromagnetic objects, extreme caution should be employed in approaching magnets with objects containing iron or other ferromagnetic materials. Only especially designed MRI-compatible physiological monitoring equipment should be used in conjunction with MRI studies. There have been several reported cases of patient burns resulting from the use of MRI-incompatible pulse oximeters and electrocardiographic monitoring devices.

SUMMARY

Accurate diagnosis of CHD can be accomplished by the judicious use of a variety of modalities. Echocardiography has assumed a leading role as the primary diagnostic tool in pediatric cardiology because of its noninvasive nature and its ability to provide accurate comprehensive diagnostic information in real time, in a variety of clinical settings, and at a reasonable cost. CMR is rapidly becoming an important diagnostic tool in pediatric cardiology because of its ability to provide anatomical and functional information that cannot be obtained by echocardiography and, in some cases, by catheterization.

REFERENCES

1. Allan LD, Santos R, Pexieder T: Anatomical and echocardiographic correlates of normal cardiac morphology in the late first trimester fetus. Heart 77:68–72, 1997.
2. Allen HD, Sahn DJ, Goldberg SJ: New serial contrast technique for assessment of left to right shunting patent ductus arteriosus in the neonate. Am J Cardiol 41:288–294, 1978.
3. Atkinson DJ, Edelman RR: Cineangiography of the heart in a single breath hold with a segmented turboFLASH sequence. Radiology 178:357–360, 1991.
4. Baer FM, Crnac J, Schmidt M, et al: Magnetic resonance pharmacological stress for detecting coronary disease. Comparison with echocardiography. Herz 25:400–408, 2000.
5. Barkhausen J, Goyen M, Ruhm SG, et al: Assessment of ventricular function with single breath-hold real-time steady-state free precession cine MR imaging. AJR Am J Roentgenol 178:731–735, 2002.
6. Be'eri E, Maier SE, Landzberg MJ, et al: In vivo evaluation of Fontan pathway flow dynamics by multidimensional

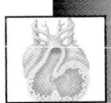

phase-velocity magnetic resonance imaging. Circulation 98:2873–2882, 1998.

7. Bellenger NG, Francis JM, Davies CL, et al: Establishment and performance of a magnetic resonance cardiac function clinic. J Cardiovasc Magn Reson 2:15–22, 2000.
8. Benacerraf BR, Pober BR, Sanders SP: Accuracy of fetal echocardiography. Radiology 165:847–849, 1987.
9. Bioeffects considerations for the safety of diagnostic ultrasound. American Institute of Ultrasound in Medicine. Bioeffects Committee. J Ultrasound Med 7:S1–S38, 1988.
10. Bogaert J, Rademakers FE: Regional nonuniformity of normal adult human left ventricle. Am J Physiol Heart Circ Physiol 280:H610–H620, 2001.
11. Bolster BD Jr, McVeigh ER, Zerhouni EA: Myocardial tagging in polar coordinates with use of striped tags. Radiology 177:769–772, 1990.
12. Buskens E, Grobbee DE, Frohn-Mulder IM, et al: Efficacy of routine fetal ultrasound screening for congenital heart disease in normal pregnancy. Circulation 94:67–72, 1996.
13. Buskens E, Stewart PA, Hess J, et al: Efficacy of fetal echocardiography and yield by risk category. Obstet Gynecol 87:423–428, 1996.
14. Carr JC, Simonetti O, Bundy J, et al: Cine MR angiography of the heart with segmented true fast imaging with steady-state precession. Radiology 219:828–834, 2001.
15. Chien D, Goldmann A, Edelman RR: High-speed black blood imaging of vessel stenosis in the presence of pulsatile flow. J Magn Reson Imaging 2:437–441, 1992.
16. Cohen BE, Winer HE, Kronzon I: Echocardiographic findings in patients with left superior vena cava and dilated coronary sinus. Am J Cardiol 44:158–161, 1979.
17. Colan SD: Assessment of ventricular and myocardial performance. In Fyler DC, editor: Nadas' Pediatric Cardiology, pp. 225–248. Philadelphia: Hanley & Belfus, 1992.
18. Danias PG, Chuang ML, Parker RA, et al: Relation between the number of image planes and the accuracy of three-dimensional echocardiography for measuring left ventricular volumes and ejection fraction. Am J Cardiol 82:1431–1434, A9, 1998.
19. Danias PG, Manning WJ: Coronary MR angiography: Current status. Herz 25:431–439, 2000.
20. Danias PG, Stuber M, Edelman RR, et al: Coronary MRA: A clinical experience in the United States. J Magn Reson Imaging 10:713–720, 1999.
21. Daniel WG, Mugge A, Grote J, et al: Comparison of transthoracic and transesophageal echocardiography for detection of abnormalities of prosthetic and bioprosthetic valves in the mitral and aortic positions. Am J Cardiol 71:210–215, 1993.
22. Edelman RR, Chien D, Kim D: Fast selective black blood MR imaging. Radiology 181:655–660, 1991.
23. Edwards MB, Taylor KM, Shellock FG: Prosthetic heart valves: Evaluation of magnetic field interactions, heating, and artifacts at 1.5 T. J Magn Reson Imaging 12:363–369, 2000.
24. Espinola-Zavaleta N, Munoz-Castellanos L, Attie F, et al: Anatomical three-dimensional echocardiographic correlation of bicuspid aortic valve. J Am Soc Echocardiogr 16:46–53, 2003.
25. Feigenbaum H: Echocardiography, 5th ed. Philadelphia: Lea & Febiger, 1994.
26. Feltes TF, Friedman RA: Transesophageal echocardiographic detection of atrial thrombi in patients with nonfibrillation atrial tachyarrhythmias and congenital heart disease. J Am Coll Cardiol 24:1365–1370, 1994.
27. Fischer SE, McKinnon GC, Scheidegger MB, et al: True myocardial motion tracking. Magn Reson Med 31:401–413, 1994.
28. Fogel MA: Assessment of cardiac function by magnetic resonance imaging. Pediatr Cardiol 21:59–69, 2000.
29. Fogel MA, Weinberg PM, Gupta KB, et al: Mechanics of the single left ventricle: A study in ventricular-ventricular interaction II. Circulation 98:330–338, 1998.
30. Frommelt PC, Stuth EA: Transesophageal echocardiographic in total anomalous pulmonary venous drainage: Hypotension caused by compression of the pulmonary venous confluence during probe passage. J Am Soc Echocardiogr 7:652–654, 1994.
31. Furber A, Balzer P, Cavaro-Menard C, et al: Experimental validation of an automated edge-detection method for a simultaneous determination of the endocardial and epicardial borders in short-axis cardiac MR images: Application in normal volunteers. J Magn Reson Imaging 8:1006–1014, 1998.
32. Fyfe DA, Ritter SB, Snider AR, et al: Guidelines for transesophageal echocardiography in children. J Am Soc Echocardiogr 5:640–644, 1992.
33. Garot J, Bluemke DA, Osman NF, et al: Fast determination of regional myocardial strain fields from tagged cardiac images using harmonic phase MRI. Circulation 101:981–988, 2000.
34. Gentles TL, Rosenfeld HM, Sanders SP, et al: Pediatric biplane transesophageal echocardiography: Preliminary experience. Am Heart J 128:1225–1233, 1994.
35. Geva T: Echocardiography and Doppler ultrasound. In Garson A, Bricker JT, Fisher DJ, et al, editors: The Science and Practice of Pediatric Cardiology, 2nd ed., Baltimore: Williams & Wilkins, 1997, pp. 789–843.
36. Geva T, Greil GF, Marshall AC, et al: Gadolinium-enhanced 3-dimensional magnetic resonance angiography of pulmonary blood supply in patients with complex pulmonary stenosis or atresia: Comparison with x-ray angiography. Circulation 106:473–478, 2002.
37. Gimbel JR, Johnson D, Levine PA, et al: Safe performance of magnetic resonance imaging on five patients with permanent cardiac pacemakers. Pacing Clin Electrophysiol 19:913–919, 1996.
38. Gramiak R, Shah PM, Kramer DH: Ultrasound cardiography: Contrast studies in anatomy and function. Radiology 92:939–948, 1969.
39. Graves MJ, Berry E, Eng AA, et al: A multicenter validation of an active contour-based left ventricular analysis technique. J Magn Reson Imaging 12:232–239, 2000.
40. Greil GF, Powell AJ, Gildein HP, et al: Gadolinium-enhanced three-dimensional magnetic resonance angiography of pulmonary and systemic venous anomalies. J Am Coll Cardiol 39:335–341, 2002.
41. Gutgesell HP, Rembold CM: Growth of the human heart relative to body surface area. Am J Cardiol 65:662–668, 1990.
42. Hirsch R, Kilner PJ, Connelly MS, et al: Diagnosis in adolescents and adults with congenital heart disease. Prospective assessment of individual and combined roles of magnetic resonance imaging and transesophageal echocardiography. Circulation 90:2937–2951, 1994.
43. Hofman MB, de Cock CC, van der Linden JC, et al: Transesophageal cardiac pacing during magnetic resonance imaging: Feasibility and safety considerations. Magn Reson Med 35:413–422, 1996.
44. Hornberger LK, Sahn DJ, Kleinman CS, et al: Antenatal diagnosis of coarctation of the aorta: A multicenter experience. J Am Coll Cardiol 23:417–423, 1994.
45. Jagannathan NR: Magnetic resonance imaging: Bioeffects and safety concerns. Indian J Biochem Biophys 36:341–347, 1999.
46. Keijer JT, van Rossum AC, van Eenige MJ, et al: Magnetic resonance imaging of regional myocardial perfusion in patients with single-vessel coronary artery disease: Quantitative comparison with (201)Thallium-SPECT and coronary angiography. J Magn Reson Imaging 11:607–615, 2000.

47. Kim RJ, Hillenbrand HB, Judd RM: Evaluation of myocardial viability by MRI. Herz 25:417–430, 2000.
48. Klein C, Nekolla SG, Bengel FM, et al: Assessment of myocardial viability with contrast-enhanced magnetic resonance imaging: Comparison with positron emission tomography. Circulation 105:162–167, 2002.
49. Klein SS, Graham TP Jr, Lorenz CH: Noninvasive delineation of normal right ventricular contractile motion with magnetic resonance imaging myocardial tagging. Ann Biomed Eng 26:756–763, 1998.
50. Kleinert S, Geva T: Echocardiographic morphometry and geometry of the left ventricular outflow tract in fixed subaortic stenosis. J Am Coll Cardiol 22:1501–1508, 1993.
51. Kleinman C: Fetal echocardiography: Diagnosing congenital heart disease in the human fetus. In ACC Educational Highlights, pp. 10–14. Bethesda, MD: American College of Cardiology, 1996.
52. Kleinman CS, Copel JA, Hobbins JC: Combined echocardiographic and Doppler assessment of fetal congenital atrioventricular block. Br J Obstet Gynaecol 94:967–974, 1987.
53. Kleinman CS, Hobbins JC, Jaffe CC, et al: Echocardiographic studies of the human fetus: Prenatal diagnosis of congenital heart disease and cardiac dysrhythmias. Pediatrics 65:1059–1067, 1980.
54. Kuhl HP, Bucker A, Franke A, et al: Transesophageal 3-dimensional echocardiography: in vivo determination of left ventricular mass in comparison with magnetic resonance imaging. J Am Soc Echocardiogr 13:205–215, 2000.
55. Kuijpers D, Ho KY, van Dijkman PR, et al: Dobutamine cardiovascular magnetic resonance for the detection of myocardial ischemia with the use of myocardial tagging. Circulation 107:1592–1597, 2003.
56. Kumar RK, Newburger JW, Gauvreau K, et al: Comparison of outcome when hypoplastic left heart syndrome and transposition of the great arteries are diagnosed prenatally versus when diagnosis of these two conditions is made only postnatally. Am J Cardiol 83:1649–1653, 1999.
57. Kuroda T, Kinter TM, Seward JB, et al: Accuracy of three-dimensional volume measurement using biplane transesophageal echocardiographic probe: In vitro experiment. J Am Soc Echocardiogr 4:475–484, 1991.
58. Laddis T, Manning WJ, Danias PG: Cardiac MRI for assessment of myocardial perfusion: Current status and future perspectives. J Nucl Cardiol 8:207–214, 2001.
59. Lai WW, al-Khatib Y, Klitzner TS, et al: Biplanar transesophageal echocardiographic direction of radiofrequency catheter ablation in children and adolescents with the Wolff-Parkinson-White syndrome. Am J Cardiol 71:872–874, 1993.
60. Lam J, Neirotti RA, Hardjowijono R, et al: Transesophageal echocardiography with the use of a four-millimeter probe. J Am Soc Echocardiogr 10:499–504, 1997.
61. Lam J, Neirotti RA, Lubbers WJ, et al: Usefulness of biplane transesophageal echocardiography in neonates, infants and children with congenital heart disease. Am J Cardiol 72:699–706, 1993.
62. Lam J, Neirotti RA, Nijveld A, et al: Transesophageal echocardiography in pediatric patients: Preliminary results. J Am Soc Echocardiogr 4:43–50, 1991.
63. Lamb HJ, Doornbos J, van der Velde EA, et al: Echo planar MRI of the heart on a standard system: Validation of measurements of left ventricular function and mass. J Comput Assist Tomogr 20:942–949, 1996.
64. Lamb HJ, Singleton RR, van der Geest RJ, et al: MR imaging of regional cardiac function: Low-pass filtering of wall thickness curves. Magn Reson Med 34:498–502, 1995.
65. Lavoie J, Burrows FA, Gentles TL, et al: Transoesophageal echocardiography detects residual ductal flow during video-assisted thoracoscopic patent ductus arteriosus interruption. Can J Anaesth 41:310–313, 1994.
66. Lee VS, Resnick D, Bundy JM, et al: Cardiac function: MR evaluation in one breath hold with real-time true fast imaging with steady-state precession. Radiology 222:835–842, 2002.
67. Lorenz CH: The range of normal values of cardiovascular structures in infants, children, and adolescents measured by magnetic resonance imaging. Pediatr Cardiol 21:37–46, 2000.
68. Lorenz CH, Walker ES, Morgan VL, et al: Normal human right and left ventricular mass, systolic function, and gender differences by cine magnetic resonance imaging. J Cardiovasc Magn Reson 1:7–21, 1999.
69. Ma MH, Hwang JJ, Lin JL, Shyu KG, et al: Detection of major aortopulmonary collateral arteries by transesophageal echocardiography in pulmonary atresia with ventricular septal defect. Am Heart J 126:1227–1229, 1993.
70. Manganas C, Iliopoulos J, Chard RB, et al: Reoperation and coarctation of the aorta: The need for lifelong surveillance. Ann Thorac Surg 72:1222–1224, 2001.
71. Marcus B, Wong PC, Wells WJ, et al: Transesophageal echocardiography in the postoperative child with an open sternum. Ann Thorac Surg 58:235–236, 1994.
72. Marx GR: Advances in cardiac imaging in congenital heart disease. Curr Opin Pediatr 7:580–586, 1995.
73. Marx GR, Geva T: MRI and echocardiography in children: How do they compare? Semin Roentgenol 33:281–292, 1998.
74. Maulik D, Nanda NC, Moodley S, et al: Application of Doppler echocardiography in the assessment of fetal cardiac disease. Am J Obstet Gynecol 151:951–957, 1985.
75. McVeigh E: Regional myocardial function. Cardiol Clin 16:189–206, 1998.
76. McVeigh ER, Atalar E: Cardiac tagging with breath-hold cine MRI. Magn Reson Med 28:318–327, 1992.
77. Mohiaddin RH, Gatehouse PD, Henien M, et al: Cine MR Fourier velocimetry of blood flow through cardiac valves: Comparison with Doppler echocardiography. J Magn Reson Imaging 7:657–663, 1997.
78. Mulkern RV, Chung T: From signal to image: Magnetic resonance imaging physics for cardiac magnetic resonance. Pediatr Cardiol 21:5–17, 2000.
79. Nagel E, Lehmkuhl HB, Bocksch W, et al: Noninvasive diagnosis of ischemia-induced wall motion abnormalities with the use of high-dose dobutamine stress MRI: Comparison with dobutamine stress echocardiography. Circulation 99:763–770, 1999.
80. Nagel E, Stuber M, Fleck E, et al: Myocardial tagging for the analysis left ventricular function. Magma 6:91–93, 1998.
81. Ohno Y, Kawamitsu H, Higashino T, et al: Time-resolved contrast-enhanced pulmonary MR angiography using sensitivity encoding (SENSE). J Magn Reson Imaging 17: 330–336, 2003.
82. Ordidge RJ, Shellock FG, Kanal E: A Y2000 update of current safety issues related to MRI. J Magn Reson Imaging 12:1, 2000.
83. Oshinski JN, Ku DN, Mukundan S Jr, et al: Determination of wall shear stress in the aorta with the use of MR phase velocity mapping. J Magn Reson Imaging 5:640–647, 1995.
84. Oshinski JN, Yang Z, Jones JR, et al: Imaging time after Gd-DTPA injection is critical in using delayed enhancement to determine infarct size accurately with magnetic resonance imaging. Circulation 104:2838–2842, 2001.
85. Pattynama PM, de Roos A, Van der Velde ET, et al: Magnetic resonance imaging analysis of left ventricular pressure-volume relations: Validation with the conductance method at rest and during dobutamine stress. Magn Reson Med 34:728–737, 1995.
86. Pelc NJ, Herfkens RJ, Shimakawa A, et al: Phase contrast cine magnetic resonance imaging. Magn Reson Q 7:229–254, 1991.

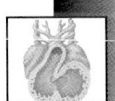

87. Pennell DJ, Underwood SR, Manzara CC, et al: Magnetic resonance imaging during dobutamine stress in coronary artery disease. Am J Cardiol 70:34–40, 1992.
88. Pereira RS, Prato FS, Wisenberg G, et al: The use of Gd-DTPA as a marker of myocardial viability in reperfused acute myocardial infarction. Int J Cardiovasc Imaging 17:395–404, 2001.
89. Plein S, Bloomer TN, Ridgway JP, et al: Steady-state free precession magnetic resonance imaging of the heart: Comparison with segmented k-space gradient-echo imaging. J Magn Reson Imaging 14:230–236, 2001.
90. Plein S, Smith WH, Ridgway JP, et al: Measurements of left ventricular dimensions using real-time acquisition in cardiac magnetic resonance imaging: Comparison with conventional gradient echo imaging. Magma 13:101–108, 2001.
91. Powell AJ, Geva T: Blood flow measurement by magnetic resonance imaging in congenital heart disease. Pediatr Cardiol 21:47–58, 2000.
92. Powell AJ, Maier SE, Chung T, et al: Phase-velocity cine magnetic resonance imaging measurement of pulsatile blood flow in children and young adults: In vitro and in vivo validation. Pediatr Cardiol 21:104–110, 2000.
93. Rajagopalan S, Prince M: Magnetic resonance angiographic techniques for the diagnosis of arterial disease. Cardiol Clin 20:501–512, v, 2002.
94. Rebergen SA, Chin JG, Ottenkamp J, van der Wall EE, et al: Pulmonary regurgitation in the late postoperative follow-up of tetralogy of Fallot. Volumetric quantitation by nuclear magnetic resonance velocity mapping. Circulation 88:2257–2266, 1993.
95. Reid SA, Walker PG, Fisher J, et al: The quantification of pulmonary valve haemodynamics using MRI. Int J Cardiovasc Imaging 18:217–225, 2002.
96. Rein AJ, Nadjari M, Bromiker R, et al: Detection of an obstructive membrane in the ductus arteriosus of a fetus using high frame rate echocardiography. Fetal Diagn Ther 13:250–252, 1998.
97. Rein AJ, O'Donnell C, Geva T, et al: Use of tissue velocity imaging in the diagnosis of fetal cardiac arrhythmias. Circulation 106:1827–1833, 2002.
98. Roche KJ, Krinsky G, Lee VS, et al: Interrupted aortic arch: Diagnosis with gadolinium-enhanced 3D MRA. J Comput Assist Tomogr 23:197–202, 1999.
99. Roest AA, Helbing WA, Kunz P, et al: Exercise MR imaging in the assessment of pulmonary regurgitation and biventricular function in patients after tetralogy of Fallot repair. Radiology 223:204–211, 2002.
100. Roest AA, Kunz P, Lamb HJ, et al: Biventricular response to supine physical exercise in young adults assessed with ultrafast magnetic resonance imaging. Am J Cardiol 87:601–605, 2001.
101. Rutledge JM, Vick GW 3rd, Mullins CE, et al: Safety of magnetic resonance imaging immediately following Palmaz stent implant: A report of three cases. Catheter Cardiovasc Interv 53:519–523, 2001.
102. Saeed M: New concepts in characterization of ischemically injured myocardium by MRI. Exp Biol Med 226:367-376, 2001.
103. Sanders S: Echocardiography and related techniques in the diagnosis of congenital heart disease. I. Veins, atria and interatrial septum. Echocardiography 1:185–217, 1984.
104. Savino JS, Hanson CW 3rd, Bigelow DC, et al: Oropharyngeal injury after transesophageal echocardiography. J Cardiothorac Vasc Anesth 8:76–78, 1994.
105. Sawyer-Glover AM, Shellock FG: Pre-MRI procedure screening: Recommendations and safety considerations for biomedical implants and devices. J Magn Reson Imaging 12:92–106, 2000.
106. Serfaty JM, Yang X, Aksit P, et al: Toward MRI-guided coronary catheterization: visualization of guiding catheters, guidewires, and anatomy in real time. J Magn Reson Imaging 12:590–594, 2000.
107. Setser RM, Fischer SE, Lorenz CH: Quantification of left ventricular function with magnetic resonance images acquired in real time. J Magn Reson Imaging 12:430–438, 2000.
108. Shanewise JS, Sadel SM: Intraoperative transesophageal echocardiography to assist the insertion and positioning of the intraaortic balloon pump. Anesth Analg 79:577–580, 1994.
109. Shellock FG: Metallic surgical instruments for interventional MRI procedures: Evaluation of MR safety. J Magn Reson Imaging 13:152–157, 2001.
110. Shellock FG, Shellock VJ: Cardiovascular catheters and accessories: Ex vivo testing of ferromagnetism, heating, and artifacts associated with MRI. J Magn Reson Imaging 8:1338–1342, 1998.
111. Silverman NH: Pediatric Echocardiography. Baltimore: Williams & Wilkins, 1993.
112. Simonetti OP, Finn JP, White RD, et al: "Black blood" T2-weighted inversion-recovery MR imaging of the heart. Radiology 199:49–57, 1996.
113. Sitges M, Jones M, Shiota T, et al: Real-time three-dimensional color Doppler evaluation of the flow convergence zone for quantification of mitral regurgitation: Validation experimental animal study and initial clinical experience. J Am Soc Echocardiogr 16:38–45, 2003.
114. Sklansky M, Tang A, Levy D, et al: Maternal psychological impact of fetal echocardiography. J Am Soc Echocardiogr 15:159–166, 2002.
115. Smith MD, Dawson PL, Elion JL, et al: Correlation of continuous wave Doppler velocities with cardiac catheterization gradients: An experimental model of aortic stenosis. J Am Coll Cardiol 6:1306–1314, 1985.
116. Snider AR, Serwer GA, Ritter SB: Echocardiography in Pediatric Heart Disease, 2nd ed. St. Louis: Mosby, 1997.
117. Snider AR, Silverman NH, Turley K, et al: Evaluation of infradiaphragmatic total anomalous pulmonary venous connection with two-dimensional echocardiography. Circulation 66:1129–1132, 1982.
118. Sodickson D: Clinical cardiovascular magnetic resonance imaging techniques. In Pennel D, editor: Cardiovascular Magnetic Resonance, New York: Churchill Livingstone, 2002, pp. 18–30.
119. Stevenson JG: Incidence of complications in pediatric transesophageal echocardiography: Experience in 1650 cases. J Am Soc Echocardiogr 12:527–532, 1999.
120. Stevenson JG: Role of intraoperative transesophageal echocardiography during repair of congenital cardiac defects. Acta Paediatr Suppl 410:23–33, 1995.
121. Stevenson JG, Sorensen GK, Gartman DM, et al: Transesophageal echocardiography during repair of congenital cardiac defects: Identification of residual problems necessitating reoperation. J Am Soc Echocardiogr 6:356–365, 1993.
122. Strecker R, Scheffler K, Klisch J, et al: Fast functional MRA using time-resolved projection MR angiography with correlation analysis. Magn Reson Med 43:303–309, 2000.
123. Stuber M, Botnar RM, Danias PG, et al: Contrast agent-enhanced, free-breathing, three-dimensional coronary magnetic resonance angiography. J Magn Reson Imaging 10:790–799, 1999.
124. Tanner J: Fallacy of per-weight and per-surface area standards, and their relation to spurious correlation. J App Physiol 2:1–15, 1949.
125. Thiele H, Paetsch I, Schnackenburg B, et al: Improved accuracy of quantitative assessment of left ventricular volume and ejection fraction by geometric models with

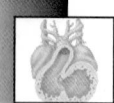

steady-state free precession. J Cardiovasc Magn Reson 4:327–339, 2002.
126. Tworetzky W, McElhinney DB, Reddy VM, et al: Improved surgical outcome after fetal diagnosis of hypoplastic left heart syndrome. Circulation 103:1269–1273, 2001.
127. Valdes-Cruz LM, Yoganathan AP, Tamura T, et al: Studies in vitro of the relationship between ultrasound and laser Doppler velocimetry and applicability to the simplified Bernoulli relationship. Circulation 73:300–308, 1986.
128. Van Der Velde ME, Perry SB: Transesophageal echocardiography during interventional catheterization in congenital heart disease. Echocardiography 14:513–528, 1997.
129. Weyman AE: Principles and Practice of Echocardiography, 2nd ed. Philadelphia: Lea & Febiger, 1993.
130. Wolff S, James TL, Young GB, et al: Magnetic resonance imaging: Absence of in vitro cytogenetic damage. Radiology 155:163–165, 1985.
131. Wong PC, Sanders SP, Jonas RA, et al: Pulmonary valve-moderator band distance and association with development of double-chambered right ventricle. Am J Cardiol 68: 1681–1686, 1991.
132. Yoganathan AP, Valdes-Cruz LM, Schmidt-Dohna J, et al: Continuous-wave Doppler velocities and gradients across fixed tunnel obstructions: Studies in vitro and in vivo. Circulation 76:657–666, 1987.

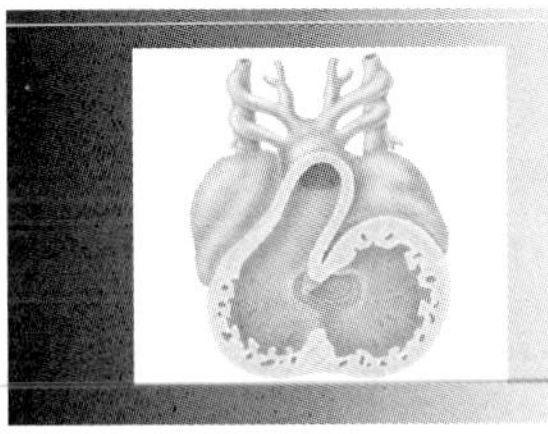

CHAPTER 103A

Cardiac Catheterization and Catheter-Based Interventions

Cardiac Catheterization

Peter Lang

INTRODUCTION

The role of cardiac catheterization in the study and care of children and adults with congenital heart disease has changed dramatically over the past six decades. The first cardiac catheterization performed on a patient with congenital heart disease took place in 1946. This catheterization was performed on an individual with an atrial septal defect (ASD) and confirmed preexisting notions of the pathophysiology of ASD that had been based on careful observations derived from physical examination and anatomical studies. Catheterizations performed over the next 10 years focused on physiological investigations. Relatively safe angiographic techniques propelled the development of surgery to treat children with congenital heart disease. During the first 20 years of surgery for congenital heart disease, advances in the understanding of the pathological anatomy, pathophysiology, and the consequences of surgical intervention could only develop because of the close interaction between the cardiac catheterization laboratory and the operating room. This relationship has become more complex during the past two decades. As the field of interventional catheterization has developed, it has ventured into the traditional domains of cardiac surgery. At the beginning of the 21st century, the treatment of many forms of complex congenital heart disease requires a coordinated interaction between cardiac catheterization and cardiac surgery. Indeed, the line between the two disciplines can often be difficult to distinguish. Cardiac surgeons and cardiologists who deal with congenital heart disease must be aware of the capabilities and limitations of their partners.

INDICATIONS

The advances in noninvasive imaging during the last 10 years have significantly decreased the need for anatomical assessment, which was the domain for many years of the angiographic component of cardiac catheterization. Angiography is still needed when there are poor echocardiographic "windows" or intervening bone or an air-filled lung. The development of magnetic resonance imaging (MRI) as a powerful diagnostic tool may further decrease the indications for anatomical definition by angiography. At this time, MRI of infants and young children often requires general anesthesia. The physician needs to consider the risks versus the benefits of the available diagnostic modalities.

In general, the use of angiography is indicated by the following:

1. When detailed anatomical definition of regions such as the branch pulmonary arteries beyond the hilum is needed.
2. When evaluation of the anatomy of complex ventricular septal defects (VSDs) is needed.
3. When there are inconsistencies between the findings on physical examination and/or noninvasive imaging and the clinical situation.

MRI has developed into the preferred imaging modality for defining abnormalities of the aortic arch, including obstructive lesions and vascular rings.

Hemodynamic assessment has become the primary indication for diagnostic catheterizations. Although physiological assessment can be made on estimates based on indirect echocardiographic observations, these assessments are less exact than those obtained at catheterization. This is particularly true of measurements of blood flow. Thus, determinations of pressure gradients and the resistance of vascular beds can be most accurately measured at catheterization. Often, these measurements are necessary for therapeutic decisions, compelling the use of cardiac catheterization to assist in critical recommendations to patients and families. Advances in MRI–derived flow measurements may further limit the need for invasive measurements. In preoperative patients, the surgeon's judgment of the adequacy or completeness of noninvasively acquired data may influence the decision to perform a catheterization. Thus, knowledge of the advantages and limitations of data gained by all available techniques is critical.

The first interventional (therapeutic) catheterization took place in Mexico City in 1954, when Dr. Rubio Alvarez and his colleagues were able to relieve obstruction of a severely stenotic pulmonary valve. Ten years later, Rashkind and

Miller opened the current era of interventional catheterization with the "creation of an atrial septal defect without thoracotomy". It was another decade and a half before Jean Kahn described her "new method for treating congenital pulmonary valve stenosis." The exploding field of interventional cardiac catheterization for the treatment of congenital cardiac defects has truly revolutionized the care of children since that time. Now, the lines between the disciplines of cardiology and cardiac surgery are truly blurred. Parents refer to the interventional cardiologists who close their child's ASDs as the physician who did the operation.

TECHNIQUES

There is no longer a "standard" cardiac catheterization. In years past, a physician could discuss performing a complete hemodynamic and angiographic evaluation for all children preparing to undergo palliative or corrective cardiac surgery. Those studies would involve admission to the hospital on the day prior to investigation. In many institutions, general anesthesia would be employed. Vascular access would be obtained, usually from the groin and large-bore catheters placed in the femoral vessels. A complete set of oxygen saturation data would be obtained through the right and left sides of the heart. Pressure measurements would be obtained from all heart chambers and great vessels. Oxygen consumption would be measured to allow for accurate determination of cardiac output, shunt flow, and vascular resistances. Angiography would then be performed, often in a rigid proscribed fashion, regardless of the underlying diagnosis. Right and left ventricular angiograms would be performed, as well as selective injections of great vessels. The child would remain in the hospital for another day for observation of vascular access sites, as well as the overall clinical status.

Using these protocols, an enormous amount of information was gathered that provided information regarding the natural history of congenital heart disease and uncovered previously unrecognized associations of malformations. An understanding of the variety of outcomes that may follow surgical intervention for most of the common congenital cardiac defects was developed. Such an approach has allowed full assessment of recent innovative surgical strategies such as the arterial switch operation for transposition of the great arteries. Despite these advantages of "complete" studies, catheterizations are currently performed in a focused fashion consistent with economic imperatives, current concepts of full disclosure of medical interventions, and a better understanding of the potential adverse outcomes of invasive procedures.

Cardiac catheterizations are now much more directed. The use of noninvasive diagnostic testing allows for shorter, focused examinations with concentration on specific areas of interest. A 2-year-old child who comes to the cardiac catheterization laboratory for occlusion of a patent ductus arteriosus should not need a left ventricular angiogram to rule out the presence of an associated VSD, since that information should be available from a prior echocardiogram. Similarly, the pulmonary artery pressure will have been estimated from the Doppler–derived pressure gradient between the aorta and the pulmonary artery. Thus, the physician will know in advance whether assessment of the pulmonary vascular bed is necessary. A complete hemodynamic and angiographic assessment need not be performed. Rather, a focused assessment of the ductus shape and size with rapid progression to occlusion will lead to a shorter, safer, and less expensive stay in the cardiac catheterization laboratory. Alternatively, if pulmonary artery hypertension is suspected on the basis of the noninvasive assessment, plans can be made for the administration of oxygen, nitric oxide, or other tests of pulmonary vascular reactivity, allowing for a planned procedure, rather than scrambling for equipment and personnel at the last minute.

PREMEDICATION AND SEDATION

There is wide institution variability in approaches to sedation for catheterization. Children with no major hemodynamic compromise can for the most part undergo a catheterization with conscious sedation. The use of intravenous morphine and/or midazolam works well for most children. Intramuscular injections of long-acting combinations of Demerol with phenothiazines have a long history of success and are generally effective, although injections can be traumatic. Adolescents and older children often do well with oral benzodiazepines prior to starting an intravenous line and instituting morphine and midazolam sedation. The benzodiazepines are helpful for relieving anxiety as well as the promotion of amnesia.

Children with hemodynamic compromise who are likely to be undergoing extensive procedures are most safely catheterized under general anesthesia. In past years, there had been a reluctance to initiate general anesthesia before obtaining "baseline" hemodynamic assessment. This remains true for individuals undergoing purely diagnostic studies or for those individuals in whom therapeutic interventions may depend on initial measurements. On the other hand, individuals with unstable hemodynamic situations (or situations that are liable to become unstable during the procedure) often come into the catheterization laboratory with prior noninvasive assessment of hemodynamics. The purpose of therapeutic intervention is often best served by a controlled procedure, under general anesthesia. In addition, individuals who require uncomfortable additional impositions, such as placement of a transesophageal echocardiographic probe for monitoring device closure of ASDs, are most humanely managed with general anesthesia. Consultation with members of the cardiac anesthesia team prior to cardiac catheterization in these situations serves not only the children but also the smooth performance of the cardiac catheterization.

Local anesthesia for percutaneous access in individuals undergoing cardiac catheterization with conscious sedation is generally obtained by using lidocaine. Close monitoring of patients during the entire progress of the catheterization procedure for changes in heart rate and blood pressure will allow maintenance of sedation and analgesia throughout the procedure. Skilled nursing personnel are critical to the endeavor, and the availability of anesthesiologists for consultation and assistance cannot be overestimated.

VASCULAR ACCESS

In a sense, vascular access is the most important part of a cardiac catheterization. It is the precursor to all that follows, and the manner it is achieved not only affects the catheterization at hand but also may limit the prospects for future procedures as well.

In some newborns, part or all of the study can be performed from the umbilical vessels. Umbilical arterial access is suitable for monitoring purposes. Simple catheter movements can often be performed, but complex manipulations are often limited by the tortuous course of the catheter. Similarly, umbilical venous access is preferred for simple monitoring and reaching easily accessible locations. For the performance of balloon atrial septostomy in infants with transposition of the great arteries, the direct course from the umbilical vein to the left atrium is ideal. The use of this technique spares the femoral vein from potential injury due to large catheters. On the other hand, complex manipulation through obstructed right heart structures is often time-consuming, frustrating, and unsuccessful.

The femoral approach is most commonly used in catheterizing individuals with congenital heart disease. The size of the femoral vessels allows for catheter entry. Control of the vessel after catheter removal is relatively easy and the procedure well-tolerated by individuals of all ages. Access from subclavian or jugular veins is often required due to anatomical constraints such as accessing the pulmonary vascular bed in children who have undergone superior vena cava to pulmonary artery anastomoses. Access from the subclavian or jugular veins is often required when multiple procedures using large-bore catheters have caused vascular compromise and loss of the femoral venous access. The internal jugular approach, while well tolerated and the access of choice for performing right heart biopsies, may be more difficult in young children in the absence of expert sedation.

The cardiologist and cardiac surgeon once again interact when planning vascular access. After surgery, the placement of femoral venous monitoring catheters in newborns may lead to thrombotic occlusion of these vessels and limit the ability for catheterizers to achieve planned goals in the future. Conversely, catheters in either the subclavian or jugular vein may lead to strictures and thrombotic complications that may drastically alter the ability to perform effective palliative and corrective surgeries involving the great veins of the upper thorax.

HEMODYNAMIC MEASUREMENTS

The use of noninvasive techniques such as echocardiography and MRI has greatly limited the need for hemodynamic assessment in the cardiac catheterization laboratory. It is the usual practice to make decisions regarding the need for cardiac surgery in children with most uncomplicated left-to-right shunts or obstructive lesions using noninvasive techniques. Still, there are instances when the direct measurement of pressure gradients in the cardiac catheterization laboratory is required. The assessment of pulmonary vascular resistance may be critical in determining whether an operation should be performed and when assessing the risks of such procedures.

Full discussion of all techniques used to assess hemodynamic parameters is beyond the scope of this chapter. However, certain principles need to be emphasized. First, when determining the severity of obstructive lesions, the general principle of Ohm's law, as it applies to hemodynamic variables, is critical. Pressure, or the pressure difference across a vascular bed, is proportional to flow and to resistance. Thus, if one is assessing the severity of a stenotic area one needs to know both the pressure difference (the gradient) and the flow (cardiac output). Simplistically, if a critically ill infant with aortic stenosis has a pressure gradient across the aortic valve of only 20 mm Hg with a cardiac output of 1 L/min/m^2, then that valve may be far more "obstructive" than in a situation with a child with a 50 mm Hg gradient across an aortic valve but a normal cardiac index of 5 L/min/m^2. It may be necessary to measure flow or cardiac output in the cardiac catheterization laboratory in order to fully understand the pressure gradient as estimated by a bedside echocardiogram.

Similar principles are applied when assessing the advisability of closing defects in older patients with intracardiac shunts and questionable pulmonary vascular beds. One might encounter a patient with a large VSD and systemic pressure in the pulmonary arteries with a pulmonary to systemic flow ratio of 3. All things being equal, once such a large VSD is closed, and the pulmonary flow reduced to one-third of its previous value, pulmonary artery pressure is likely to be reduced to one-third of its prior value. On the other hand, a similar patient with a pulmonary to systemic flow ratio of 1.5 is highly unlikely to achieve that outcome. Acute testing in the cardiac catheterization laboratory might be performed with agents such as oxygen or nitric oxide. If the pulmonary to systemic flow ratio is increased to 3, the physician might feel emboldened to perform the surgery, recognizing that similar treatment might be necessary after surgery to maintain pulmonary artery pressure at one-third systemic levels. If the overall clinical context leads the physician to believe that pulmonary vascular remodeling was likely, the use of cardiac catheterization with hemodynamic assessment under variable physiological conditions will have proved its value in aiding the clinical decision-making process.

Hemodynamic assessment can be critical, as in the above examples, but its place in modern practice of pediatric cardiology is under revision. Even in situations where assessment of pulmonary vascular resistance was deemed crucial to any decision-making process, such as evaluation of a patient for a Fontan procedure, is now under question. Children who have undergone bidirectional Glenn shunts and have thus "proved" that the pulmonary vascular bed can receive reasonable flow at low pressure may not need cardiac catheterization as an investigation before completing their Fontan operations. The success of treatment protocols based on noninvasive estimates of hemodynamic parameters will need to be compared with the more invasive investigations that have traditionally been employed.

ANGIOGRAPHY

Just as hemodynamic assessment in the cardiac catheterization laboratory has taken on a more limited role, angiography no longer remains the "gold standard" of imaging techniques. Physicians have long known that assessment of atrial anatomy is difficult using angiographic techniques and have relied on echocardiography for most of the assessment of venous and atrial anatomical detail. Those instances where angiography still held forth, such as the evaluation of complex venous drainage patterns in Heterotaxy syndrome, may now be easily visualized with MRI. Angiographic assessment of complex interventricular or intraventricular relationships can similarly be viewed by less invasive means. As the current era of catheterization comes to a close, angiography remains crucial to the evaluation of complex vascular patterns such as seen in the pulmonary vascular bed, the branching of the aortic arch, and the coronary arteries. As MRI and advanced computed tomography techniques develop further, it will be likely that the diagnostic approach will become noninvasive. When pathology amenable to interventional techniques is identified, angiography may be performed as a confirmatory diagnostic modality prior to intervention.

The aforementioned changes in the use of cardiac catheterization are not to be lamented. Reserving cardiac catheterization for situations that require focused measurement and intervention will increase the safety, decrease the cost, and improve the overall outcome of individuals with congenital heart disease.

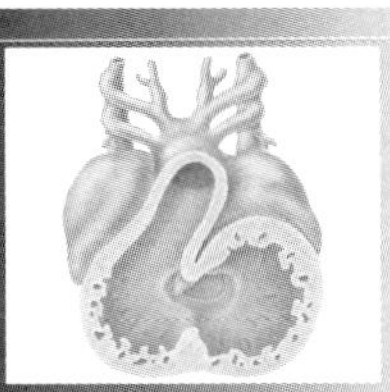

Cardiac Catheterization and Catheter-Based Interventions

Catheter-Based Interventions

CHAPTER 103B

Audrey C. Marshall

Introduction

INTRODUCTION

Interventional catheterization plays a larger role in the management of patients with congenital heart disease as catheter technology advances and training becomes more available. Simple congenital defects (e.g., isolated pulmonary or aortic valve stenosis, patent ductus arteriosus [PDA], atrial septal defect) are now routinely treated in the catheterization laboratory, without the need for surgery. For patients with more complex disease, interventional catheterization has been incorporated as part of a combined surgical/catheter approach to both repair and palliation. Although typical tetralogy of Fallot can be repaired with a single neonatal surgical procedure, variants such as tetralogy with multiple ventricular septal defects (VSDs) and tetralogy with pulmonary arterial hypoplasia pose significant problems for complete surgical repair. In these instances, catheter intervention (e.g., muscular VSD closure, pulmonary artery dilation) can be essential to adequate repair. Similarly, palliation of single-ventricle disease can be improved with the integration of transcatheter procedures. For patients who are undergoing the Fontan operation, surgical placement of a fenestration to augment cardiac output during the immediate postoperative period can be followed by elective transcatheter device closure. In these and many other settings, continued collaboration between the interventional cardiologist and the cardiac surgeon promises to improve the outcomes of children and adults with congenital heart disease.

Rashkind and Miller[61] reported the first balloon atrial septostomy in 1966; this provided a means of palliating the cyanotic infant with transposition of the great arteries. Currently, in the era of the neonatal arterial switch operation, septostomy in these patients allows for preoperative stabilization, and it remains life-saving in neonates who have inadequate mixing. Even among stable patients with evidence of adequate mixing who are maintained on a prostaglandin infusion, septostomy may be indicated to discontinue prostaglandins preoperatively, thereby attenuating hemodynamic lability and diminishing the need for mechanical ventilation and invasive monitoring.

There has been remarkably little change in the technique or equipment employed since the first description of septostomy. A balloon-tipped catheter introduced via the umbilical or femoral vein is positioned in the left atrium. Rapid acceleration of the inflated balloon across the septum into the right atrium results in the avulsion of septum primum from septum secundum, widely opening the foramen ovale and allowing for extensive mixing at the atrial level. Traditionally performed under fluoroscopic guidance in the catheterization laboratory, results have been equally satisfactory with echocardiographic guidance at the bedside in the intensive care unit (ICU), with only rare complications.[81]

Less frequently, creation of an atrial septal defect is indicated as a result of left atrial hypertension in neonates with hypoplastic left heart syndrome and an intact atrial septum. Left atrial hypertension may be evidenced by excessive cyanosis, a pulmonary venous obstructive pattern on chest radiography, or a restrictive atrial septum evident on Doppler interrogation. Although standard pull-through septostomy or blade septostomy can be effective for the short term, restenosis occurs in a significant proportion of patients.[54] Creation of an atrial defect using the transseptal puncture technique followed by static balloon dilation or stent placement allows for a larger, more durable opening of the atrial septum.[3]

Before the advent of balloon pulmonary valvotomy, a number of surgical approaches were developed that ranged from blind valvotomy to transarterial visualization with cardiopulmonary bypass. The disruption of commissural fusion achieved by passage of a dilator was easily replicated by the inflation of a dilating balloon mounted on a catheter shaft. Transcatheter balloon valvotomy is now the primary therapy for valvar pulmonary and aortic stenosis, with almost uniformly good results. With regard to semilunar valves, most patients will respond favorably to this simple mechanical enlargement of the valve orifice. By contrast, congenital mitral valve disease is often unresponsive to balloon dilation, and results are clearly related to the underlying valve morphology.

Since Kan and others[29] reported the first static balloon dilation of the pulmonary valve in 1982, this procedure has become widely accepted as the primary intervention of choice for valvar pulmonary stenosis. A number of dilating techniques have been applied with generally good results, and long-term follow-up information is available. Furthermore, techniques developed in older children have been successfully applied to the neonate with critical valvar pulmonary stenosis.[13,80]

In children with valvar pulmonary stenosis, the decision to intervene is based primarily on the Doppler-derived gradient by echocardiography. A gradient in excess of 50 mm

Hg should prompt referral for intervention. Symptoms with this degree of obstruction are rarely present.

An early series reported an average decrease in peak pulmonary valve gradient from 70–23 mm Hg after balloon dilation in a small group of patients.[42] These results were confirmed in a larger group by the work of the Valvuloplasty and Angioplasty of Congenital Anomalies (VACA) Registry Investigators, who cited a decrease from 71–28 mm Hg in 784 patients.[42,75] In this group, 89% of patients had a postprocedural gradient of <35 mm Hg. Some authors have reported disappointing results in the setting of dysmorphic valves.[75] In most patients who undergo successful balloon valvotomy, gradient relief is persistent (particularly when oversized balloons are used), with a balloon-to-annulus ratio of 1.2–1.4.[41,59]

Although the use of larger balloons in pulmonary valvotomy appears to improve immediate effect, experimental evidence of right ventricular outflow tract damage and the clinical observation of increased pulmonary insufficiency after oversized balloon dilation have supported a balloon-to-annulus ratio of 1.4 or less.[63] The long-term clinical relevance of resultant pulmonary insufficiency, which occurs in 10–40% of cases, remains undetermined.[50]

Pulmonary valvotomy is also effective in infants with critical pulmonary stenosis, and it may be pursued as a first step in the management of neonates with membranous pulmonary atresia and intact ventricular septum. These infants will present with cyanosis and possibly with congestive heart failure or low cardiac output. Echocardiographic evidence of suprasystemic right ventricular pressure serves as an additional indication for intervention. A highly stenotic valve can be safely crossed with a floppy-tipped wire, whereas an atretic valve—if thin and well formed—can be perforated with a standard straight wire or a radiofrequency wire.[66] After the valve is crossed, serial balloon dilations can achieve effective right ventricular decompression, potentially with less resultant pulmonary regurgitation than would be acquired surgically.[1] Major complications are uncommon (<1%), but they occur more frequently in neonates and infants than in older children.[13,75]

The first report of successful balloon dilation of an aortic valve appeared in 1984.[34] Aortic valve dilation presented a number of new concerns for the interventional cardiologist as compared with past experience with pulmonary valve dilation. Intrinsic differences in the compliance characteristics of the valve required a unique determination of optimal balloon-to-annulus ratio. Identification of the "ideal" balloon-to-annulus ratio at the aortic valve took on heightened importance because of the clear clinical implications of significant aortic regurgitation. Additionally, retrograde catheter courses (i.e., advancing the dilating catheter across the valve from the femoral artery) heightened the risk of vascular entry site injury and consequently imposed greater demand for low-profile equipment. Experience has shown a balloon-to-annulus ratio of 0.8–1.0 to be preferable to larger balloon-to-annulus ratios.[22] Although newer, lower-profile balloons have allowed the majority of procedures to be performed from the femoral artery, antegrade transvenous techniques have also been developed and employed successfully, with the potential for decreased morbidity related to femoral arterial injury.[39]

The procedure has been performed with good results in newborns, infants, and older children. Doppler-derived maximal instantaneous gradients in excess of 50 mm Hg are considered an indication for intervention in children and young adults. Aortic valve peak gradients fell from 77–30 mm Hg among patients in the largest reported series (n = 192).[64] Evaluation of the impact of the balloon-to-annulus ratio demonstrated no association between this ratio and a reduction in gradient, but higher balloon-to-annulus ratios were found to be associated with a greater incidence of increased aortic regurgitation.[71] This latter finding was contested by a later study that found no association when lower balloon-to-annulus ratios were used.[49] Major (life-threatening) complications occur in 5% of cases in the VACA registry, and femoral arterial thrombosis developed in 12%.[64]

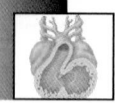

Freedom from reintervention was 75% at 4 years and 50% at 8 years after dilation of the aortic valve.[49] Many of these reinterventions consisted of repeat balloon dilation. Among patients who had previously undergone aortic valve dilation, redilation resulted in a 50% decrease in gradient.[68]

Aortic valvotomy has emerged as standard palliation for neonates with critical valvar aortic stenosis. These infants present with severe congestive heart failure and shock. Technically successful aortic valve dilation can be achieved in 73% of patients; survival was 88% over a follow-up period of 8 years, and freedom from reintervention was 64%.[16] In the smaller patients who underwent predominantly retrograde dilation, pulse loss in the catheterized extremity was universal, with 35% recovering a pulse after thrombolytic therapy. The advent of lower-profile balloons has allowed the procedure to be performed through sheaths as small as 3 or 4 Fr in the current era, which likely reduces the degree of arterial trauma.

Mitral valve dilation in patients with rheumatic mitral valve disease was first reported by Lock and others[37] in 1985. After the recognition of the significant surgical morbidity and mortality imposed by surgical management of congenital mitral stenosis in young children, Spevak and colleagues[74] attempted balloon angioplasty of the mitral valve in 9 patients, predominantly infants and toddlers. The procedure resulted in immediate gradient relief in 7 out of 9 patients with heterogeneous valve morphologies. The publication of 18 additional cases supported the short-term hemodynamic benefit of mitral valve dilation, with a 40% incidence of short-term symptomatic improvement. However, nearly 40% of patients developed at least moderate mitral regurgitation. Follow-up over a 2-year period showed only 70% survival at 2 years despite dilation, which was similar to the 55% predicted survival among similar patients undergoing surgery.[48]

The range of effective balloon-to-annulus ratios is greater in mitral valve disease than in semilunar valve disease, given the extreme heterogeneity of the mechanism of obstruction. In general, a conservative balloon is chosen first (1–3 mm smaller than the echocardiographic estimate of the annular diameter), and subsequent interventions are based on the appearance and effect of this first balloon. Moderate to severe regurgitation occurs after dilation in 22% of patients, and transient high-grade heart block occurs in a similar proportion.[48]

A variety of congenital and postoperative vascular obstructions—both venous and arterial—are responsive to balloon angioplasty. Although indications and results are varied, the principles of effective angioplasty are common, regardless of the dilation site. Effective angioplasty is achieved by creating a controlled tear in the vessel wall; ideally this is a partial tear through the media. The conditions under which this tear can be produced depend on the intrinsic compliance of the vessel wall and the severity of the obstruction. Mild stenoses and highly compliant lesions are particularly difficult to dilate effectively, but these can often be addressed effectively through the use of an endovascular stent. By contrast, severe noncompliant obstructions present significant risk of an uncontrolled transmural tear. The most common indications for balloon angioplasty in the treatment of congenital heart disease are coarctation of the aorta and pulmonary arterial stenosis.

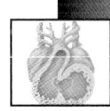

After pioneering work by Sos and others[73] and Lock and others[38] to test the feasibility of balloon dilation on postmortem or surgically excised specimens, Singer and colleagues[72] reported the first successful balloon dilation of recoarctation in a patient in 1982. Balloon dilation has since become the first line of therapy for treating recurrent coarctation after surgery. With regard to native coarctation, although the efficacy of balloon dilation as a primary intervention has been reported, advantages relative to primary surgical repair are debatable. Concern about relatively high restenosis rates and a 6% rate of late aneurysms have precluded the widespread acceptance of angioplasty as primary therapy for native coarctation.[76] In older children and adults, the success rates of the procedure—coupled with less-frequent occurrence of restenosis and relatively low risk—support balloon angioplasty as a reasonable first intervention.

Among infants who are less than 3 months old, authors have described favorable results of balloon dilation of native coarctation, which has reduced gradients of 48 mm Hg to 8 mm Hg.[33] However, in this same group, restenosis has been documented to occur in more than 50% of patients.[33,60] The high incidence of restenosis among infants after a successful initial dilation has been substantiated by other groups.[46] Therefore, in these younger patients, balloon dilation is pursued primarily as a palliative procedure. High rates of iliofemoral arterial complications, which were reported during the early experience with this infant population, have become of less concern as low-profile dilating balloon catheters have evolved.[8]

Results of angioplasty for recurrent, rather than native, coarctation have more strongly supported this therapy. Indications for dilation of coarctation in the older child or adult have traditionally included a gradient of more than 20 mm Hg or systemic hypertension. Kan and others[30] described the first 7 patients in 1983, and, in 1990, the VACA Registry results showed a reduction in gradient to less than 20 mm Hg in 78% of patients treated.[23] Immediate success did not appear to be related to the type of initial surgical procedure.[14,23] In 1991, Hijazi and others[24] argued that balloon dilations should be the treatment of choice for recurrent coarctation; this was based on an 88% success rate. However, these authors also noted that late aneurysm development could occur. The largest published experience suggests that one third of patients undergoing an acutely successful dilation of recurrent coarctation may require reintervention (based on follow-up of up to 12 years' duration).[78]

Coarctation was one of the first congenital lesions to be treated with the use of balloon-expandable endovascular stents.[51] Although the earliest series describes the use of aortic stents to treat severe coarctation, the procedure is increasingly used in patients with only mild obstruction. In cases of mild coarctation (<20 mm Hg), standard balloon angioplasty may be ineffective because of highly compliant low-grade obstruction. In these situations, stent placement can allow a well controlled enlargement of a mildly narrowed aorta. When gradients as low as 25 mm Hg were reduced to 5 mm Hg, there was an associated decrease in left ventricular end-diastolic pressure, which suggests an improvement in diastolic function.[40]

Proximal pulmonary arterial obstructions confined to the perihilar area can often be relieved surgically. However, more distal obstructions (often inaccessible to surgeons) are treated with balloon angioplasty. These obstructions can occur in association with congenital heart disease (most commonly tetralogy of Fallot variants) or along with arteriopathies such as Williams syndrome.

Indications for balloon dilation or stenting of pulmonary arteries include elevated right ventricular pressure (>½ systemic), diminished flow to the downstream lung as determined by angiography or lung perfusion scan, or hypertension in other segments of the lung as a result of flow diverted from the obstructed vessel. Postoperative anastomotic lesions generally respond well to standard balloon dilation, as do some congenital stenoses and hypoplasia; alternatively, pulmonary arterial obstruction resulting from vessel kinking or compression often requires stent placement to achieve relief.

Early during the pulmonary artery balloon dilation experience, low-pressure balloons were used, with successful dilations achieved in 38–59% of cases.[65,67,79] Results improved as high-pressure balloons came into use; these allowed for the relief of obstruction in up to 72% of vessels.[21] Despite the use of high-pressure balloons, a significant proportion of pulmonary arterial obstructions remain resistant to balloon angioplasty. The recent availability of cutting balloons has given rise to a new strategy in the treatment of resistant pulmonary arterial obstruction. The cutting balloon has been used to initiate controlled vascular injury at the site of resistant lesions; this initial tear can then be extended with standard angioplasty balloons.[62] By using small (<4 mm) cutting balloons on lesions that are resistant to high-pressure angioplasty, operators have achieved increased lumen diameter by more than 50% in 92% of vessels treated.[5]

Balloon angioplasty of pulmonary vessels is associated with a relatively high rate of complications, some of which are life-threatening. Vascular rupture and pulmonary edema have been reported after dilation attempts.[4] In patients with Williams syndrome, an 18% rate of postangioplasty aneurysm formation is higher than that described in other patient populations. Furthermore, the mortality rate (8%) is significantly higher in these patients than in those without arteriopathy.[20]

Balloon-expandable endovascular stents have been used successfully to relieve pulmonary arterial obstruction since the early 1980s. Stents have been used primarily in branch pulmonary artery stenoses in larger children because of the sizes of the stents available, the size of the delivery system, and the likelihood that surgical excision would eventually be necessary when the child outgrew the diameter of the stent. After experimental evidence that endovascular stents could be safely and effectively redilated, McMahon and others[44] reported about mechanisms of successful redilation in a large group of patients. The recent introduction of more-flexible, smaller, and lower-profile stenting systems has resulted in stents, being placed more frequently in compliant lesions of more distal vessels in smaller children.

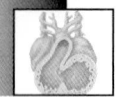

Homograft conduits, which are frequently employed in the surgical correction of conotruncal abnormalities, including tetralogy of Fallot and truncus arteriosus, often become obstructed as a result of contraction, kinking, neointimal "peel" accumulation, external compression, or simply patient growth. Standard balloon dilation of these obstructed conduits rarely provides definitive relief. By contrast, balloon-expandable stent placement can decrease the need for surgical reintervention.[26] Among 44 patients with right-ventricle-to-pulmonary-artery conduit obstruction who were treated with stent placement, acute results included a 50% decrease in conduit gradient and reduction of near-systemic right ventricular pressures to less than two-thirds systemic; freedom from reintervention after stent placement was 60% at 30 months.[57]

Pulmonary vein stenosis that occurs de novo or after repair of total anomalous pulmonary venous return remains a disease that is untreatable in the catheterization laboratory. On the basis of favorable results after balloon dilation angioplasty of other congenital lesions, Driscoll and colleagues[15] attempted pulmonary vein dilation in the early 1980s; early restenosis associated with clinical decline was observed. Similarly, when endovascular stents were applied to pulmonary venous obstruction nearly a decade later, progressive and intractable reobstruction was observed within months.[12,45] Stent modifications—such as the application of a physical barrier to intimal ingrowth (i.e., a covered stent) or drug-eluting properties—hold some promise, but results are as yet unreported.

Over the last 20 years, the variety of closure devices available to the interventional cardiologist has greatly increased. In 1989, the Rashkind PDA device was first placed in a patient. Currently the options for closure of PDA in the catheterization laboratory are numerous. Small PDAs are almost always amenable to coil occlusion, although the variety of coil sizes, configurations, and releasing mechanisms remains large. In addition, a number of intracardiac closure devices have been developed and marketed. Most of these devices were originally designed for the closure of atrial septal defects, and some have been adapted for use in other clinical settings, such as closure of the patent foramen ovale, VSD, and perivalvar leak. The underlying anatomy of the defect and the relationship of the defect to other cardiac structures dictates the qualities of the ideal closure device.

In 1967, Porstmann reported about the use of foam plugs to occlude PDA via a transcatheter approach.[56a] After this experience, a decade elapsed before the Rashkind PDA occluder was developed. Although it was more effective, the device continued to have a significant rate of residual flow in moderate-sized ductuses, and it never came to market. Ultimately, the Gianturco vascular occlusion coil was developed for occlusion of PDA and rapidly came into widespread use; now transcatheter closure is generally accepted as the first line of treatment for small PDAs (<3 mm). These vessels can be safely and effectively closed using a single coil that is chosen to provide a helical diameter that is twice the minimum ductus diameter.[36,47] Larger PDAs often require multiple coils, advanced coil delivery techniques, or alternative devices, with an attendant increase in rates of embolization and incomplete closure.[28,32,52]

Indications for PDA occlusion include hemodynamic considerations such as evidence of left ventricular volume load and right ventricular hypertension. In the case of small PDAs, the most common indication is to reduce the risk of bacterial endocarditis.

The duct can be traversed and closed from either the pulmonary arterial or the aortic approach; it is generally closed by leaving an occlusive device in the narrowest portion of the duct, but it can also be effectively closed by occluding the aortic ampulla.[25] Nearly half of small ducts can be closed using a single coil. Although some small ducts will require multiple coils, immediate complete closure rates in excess of 93% can be achieved.[25,53] The most common complication is distal coil embolization during placement, which occurs in 6% of procedures that are performed to close small ducti. When this occurs, the coil can be retrieved using transcatheter snaring techniques. Late embolizations and recanalization are extremely rare.

When the size of the duct exceeds 3 mm, it is likely to require multiple coils or another type of device. Owada and others[52] reported about the coil occlusion of PDAs that were 3.5 mm or larger; they had a 69% closure rate when using up to 4 coils. Patients who failed closure tended to be smaller, with greater shunts and a higher ratio of PDA diameter to aortic diameter.[52] These results of coil occlusion on large PDAs have led to the development of more sophisticated devices. One such device—the Amplatzer Ductal Occluder (AGA Medical, Golden Valley, MN)—has reportedly resulted in closure rates of 100% at 1-year follow-up for PDAs greater than 3.5 mm in diameter.[17]

Virtually all manner of native and prosthetic vascular communications have been occluded using an armamentarium of transcatheter closure devices. PDA remains the most common indication for coil occlusion in patients without associated heart disease. Among those with congenital heart defects, aortopulmonary collaterals account for the majority of interventions. Aortopulmonary collateral vessels, which are most commonly seen in variants of tetralogy of Fallot, can also be observed in almost every other form of cyanotic congenital heart disease. Indications for closure include volume load on the ventricle (particularly in single-ventricle circulations), the potential for competitive flow into the distal pulmonary arteries, and compromise of effective pulmonary blood flow. Closure of these vessels as a means of decreasing unwanted return into the field at the time of operation remains controversial.

Coil occlusion of aortopulmonary collaterals has been shown to result in complete closure in 72–76% of vessels in patients with congenital heart disease.[55,70] The technique used to close these vessels is simple, involving the use of coils that are 120–150% of the size of the diameter of the vessel. By contrast, closure of surgical aortopulmonary shunts is somewhat more challenging technically, and maneuvers have been described to improve success rates and diminish the risk of distal embolization of the coil.[9,55] Techniques have also been described for the closure of coronary fistulae and for venovenous collaterals and arteriovenous malformations.[2,19,27,56]

Transcatheter closure of secundum atrial septal defect has been shown to be feasible, safe, and effective, and it is becoming an increasingly available alternative to surgical closure. Furthermore, some data suggest that transcatheter closure of secundum defects may spare patients' cognitive function from possible deleterious effects of cardiopulmonary bypass, although this question remains debated.[77] Indications for closure include evidence of right ventricular volume load; less frequently, clinical heart failure or excessive cyanosis in the setting of additional right heart disease may lead to surgical or transcatheter closure.

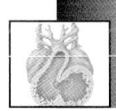

Although self-centering mechanisms (available with several of the currently available devices) aid in occlusive positioning of the device, some overlap of the device on the remnant of the atrial septum remains a requirement of closure. As a result, implanted devices may be significantly larger than the atrial defect. Furthermore, these devices are only appropriate when the defect is relatively far away from other cardiac structures, such as the superior vena cava or atrioventricular valves. Therefore, atrial septal defects of the sinus venosus or primum type are not currently treated in the catheterization laboratory.

The complication rate in a large series of patients treated with either the CardioSEAL device or the Amplatzer device was 8.6%.[11] Embolization or malposition of the device is the most common complication after device implantation.

Until recently, PFO was perceived as a largely benign anatomical variant. However, evidence of the association between PFO and cryptogenic stroke has been mounting, and the primary causative role of certain subtypes of PFO—particularly those associated with atrial septal aneurysm—has been hypothesized.[9a] Device closure of PFO for the prevention of recurrent paradoxical embolism was first reported in 1992.[7b] During the intervening 10 years, numerous additional indications for closure have been suggested, although recurrent cryptogenic stroke in the setting of a PFO with atrial septal aneurysm has emerged as the only unequivocal indication at this time.[6] Closure rates are expected to be 90–95%.

Surgery remains standard therapy for most types of VSD requiring closure. However, muscular defects (particularly at the apex or very anteriorly) or multiple defects (e.g., those seen in the "swiss cheese" septum) continue to pose a significant surgical challenge. The techniques for VSD device closure were developed to be used in conjunction with surgical approaches and in specific cases in which surgery was felt to be contraindicated. The earliest attempts at transcatheter closure of VSDs using a double-umbrella device were described by Lock in 1987.[7a,38a] Among 6 patients who were not considered candidates for operative closure, the authors described technical aspects of the procedure and feasibility. Bridges added to the experience with transcatheter VSD closure by reporting about a group of highly selected patients with muscular VSD occurring in association with complex heart lesions who underwent closure. It was suggested that preoperative transcatheter closure could simplify the subsequent surgical repair of relatively inaccessible lesions.

Postoperative defects have also been closed successfully with transcatheter devices, thereby obviating the need for reoperation. In fact, one subset of these residual defects—the "intramural" VSD seen in patients with conotruncal malformations after baffling of the left ventricle to a right ventricular aorta—is often detected only by angiography, and it is amenable to device closure without surgical revision of the patch.[58]

In contrast with closure of PDA or atrial septal defect, VSD closure is often associated with acute transient hemodynamic compromise during the implantation procedure. Hypotension (40%) and dysrhythmias (28.5%) constitute the most frequent adverse events that occur during VSD closure, and these warrant anticipatory involvement of the cardiac anesthesiologists.[35]

Until recently, more common types of VSD (e.g., paramembranous, conoventricular, inlet type) were not felt to be amenable to device closure. Membranous VSDs have been closed in a small group of selected patients with umbrella devices. Currently, U.S. trials of a device designed specifically for membranous defects are underway following encouraging initial reports.[25a] This device is characterized by an asymmetry of the closure discs, which minimize the override of the device on the left ventricular outflow tract septum and thereby minimizes the risk of aortic valve impairment.

In 1990, Bridges and colleagues[7] reported baffle fenestration as a modification of the Fontan procedure that could potentially decreasing surgical mortality and morbidity in high-risk patients. Eleven out of 20 patients had transcatheter closure of the fenestration during the early postoperative period, with a resultant increase in systemic saturations. If a fenestration is present, resting oxygen saturations of 90% or less and tolerance of test occlusion are indications for closure. For the nonfenestrated Fontan or for the patient whose fenestration has spontaneously closed prematurely, new defects can be created using catheter techniques, with a low incidence of complications.[31] When postoperative patients have high right atrial pressure, low output, and high systemic oxygen saturation in the absence of a baffle fenestration, the creation and dilation of a defect can result in significant hemodynamic improvement.

In large centers, between 55 and 75% of all catheterizations performed now involve intervention.[69] Because of their lesser degree of invasiveness, effective transcatheter interventions for congenital heart disease offer the potential for treatment at lower morbidity and cost. However, the indirect nature of these catheter procedures compromises their efficacy and also creates a unique set of potential complications. The overall rate of serious complications from interventional catheterization ranges from 4–6%.[10,18] Although relatively few of these complications (approximately 2%) will require emergent surgery, interventional procedures should not be undertaken unless surgical backup is available.[69] When complications requiring surgical intervention are encountered, vascular repair—either at the access site or at the site of intervention—is most common. Additional complications that may require surgery include valvar disruption, cardiac perforation, or foreign body or device malposition or embolization.[43] A collaborative relationship between the interventional cardiologist and the pediatric cardiac surgeon allows each to better understand the benefits and risks of the two different therapeutic modalities.

REFERENCES

1. Alwi M, Geetha K, Bilkis AA, et al: Pulmonary atresia with intact ventricular septum percutaneous radiofrequency-assisted valvotomy and balloon dilation versus surgical

valvotomy and Blalock Taussig shunt. J Am Coll Cardiol 35:468–476, 2000.

2. Armsby LR, Keane LF, Sherwood MW, et al: Management of coronary artery fistulae. Patient selection and results of transcatheter closure. J Am Coll Cardiol 39:1026–1032, 2002.
3. Atz AM, Feinstein JA, Jonas RA, et al: Preoperative management of pulmonary venous hypertension in hypoplastic left heart syndrome with restrictive atrial septal defect. Am J Cardiol 83:1224–1228, 1999.
4. Baker CM, McGowan FX Jr, Keane JF, Lock JE: Pulmonary artery trauma due to balloon dilation: recognition, avoidance and management. J Am Coll Cardiol 36:1684–1690, 2000.
5. Bergersen LJ, Perry SB, Lock JE: Effect of cutting balloon angioplasty on resistant pulmonary artery stenosis. Am J Cardiol 91:185–189, 2003.
6. Bridges ND, Hellenbrand W, Latson L, et al: Transcatheter closure of patent foramen ovale after presumed paradoxical embolism. Circulation 86:1902–1908, 1992.
7. Bridges ND, Lock JE, Castaneda AR: Baffle fenestration with subsequent transcatheter closure. Modification of the Fontan operation for patients at increased risk. Circulation 82:1681–1689, 1990.

7a. Bridges ND, Perry SB, Keane JF, et al: Preoperative transcatheter closure of congenital muscular ventricular septal defects. N Engl J Med 324:1312–1317, 1991.

7b. Bridges ND, Hellenbrand W, Latson L, et al: Transcatheter closure of patent foramen ovale after presumed paradoxical embolism. Circulation 86:1902–1908, 1992.

8. Burrows PE, Benson LN, Williams WG, et al: Iliofemoral arterial complications of balloon angioplasty for systemic obstructions in infants and children. Circulation 82:1697–1704, 1990.
9. Burrows PE, Edwards TC, Benson LN: Transcatheter occlusion of Blalock-Taussig shunts: technical options. J Vasc Interv Radiol 4:673–680, 1993.

9a. Cabanes L, Mas JL, Cohen A, et al: Atrial septal aneurysm and patent foramen ovale as risk factors for cryptogenic stroke in patients less than 55 years of age. Stroke 24: 1865–1873, 1992.

10. Cassidy SC, Schmidt KG, Van Hare GF, et al: Complications of pediatric cardiac catheterization: a 3-year study. J Am Coll Cardiol 19:1285–1293, 1992.
11. Chessa M, Carminati M, Butera G, et al: Early and late complications associated with transcatheter occlusion of secundum atrial septal defect. J Am Coll Cardiol 39:1061–1065, 2002.
12. Coles JG, Yemets I, Najm HK, et al: Experience with repair of congenital heart defects using adjunctive endovascular devices. J Thorac Cardiovasc Surg 110:1513–1519, 1995.
13. Colli AM, Perry SB, Lock JE, Keane JF: Balloon dilation of critical valvar pulmonary stenosis in the first month of life. Cathet Cardiovasc Diagn 34:23–28, 1995.
14. Cooper SG, Sullivan ID, Wren C: Treatment of recoarctation: balloon dilation angioplasty. J Am Coll Cardiol 14:413–419, 1989.
15. Driscoll DJ, Hesslein PS, Mullins CE: Congenital stenosis of individual pulmonary veins: clinical spectrum and unsuccessful treatment by transvenous balloon dilation. Am J Cardiol 49:1767–1772, 1982.
16. Egito ES, Moore P, O'Sullivan J, et al: Transvascular balloon dilation for neonatal critical aortic stenosis: early and midterm results. J Am Coll Cardiol 29:442–447, 1997.
17. Faella HJ, Hijazi ZM: Closure of the patent ductus arteriosus with the Amplatzer PDA device: immediate results of the international clinical trial. Catheter Cardiovasc Interv 51:50–54, 2000.
18. Fellows KE, Radtke W, Keane JF, Lock JE: Acute complications of catheter therapy for congenital heart disease. Am J Cardiol 60:679–683, 1987.
19. Fuhrman BP, Bass JL, Castaneda-Zuniga W, et al: Coil embolization of congenital thoracic vascular anomalies in infants and children. Circulation 70:285–289, 1984.
20. Geggel RL, Gauvreau K, Lock JE: Balloon dilation angioplasty of peripheral pulmonary stenosis associated with Williams syndrome. Circulation 103:2165–2170, 2001.
21. Gentles TL, Lock JE, Perry SB: High pressure balloon angioplasty for branch pulmonary artery stenosis: early experience. J Am Coll Cardiol 22:867–872, 1993.
22. Helgason H, Keane JF, Fellows KE, et al: Balloon dilation of the aortic valve: studies in normal lambs and in children with aortic stenosis. J Am Coll Cardiol 9:816–822, 1987.
23. Hellenbrand WE, Allen HD, Golinko RJ, et al: Balloon angioplasty for aortic recoarctation: results of Valvuloplasty and Angioplasty of Congenital Anomalies Registry. Am J Cardiol 65:793–797, 1990.
24. Hijazi ZM, Fahey JT, Kleinman CS, Hellenbrand WE: Balloon angioplasty for recurrent coarctation of aorta. Immediate and long-term results. Circulation 84:1150–1156, 1991.
25. Hijazi ZM, Geggel RL: Transcatheter closure of patent ductus arteriosus using coils. Am J Cardiol 79:1279–1280, 1997.

25a. Hijazi ZM, Hakim F, Hawcleh AA, et al: Catheter closure of perimembranous ventricular septal defects using the new Amplatzer membranous VSD occluder: initial clinical experience. Catheter Cardiovasc Interv 56:508–515, 2002.

26. Hosking MC, Benson LN, Nakanishi T, et al: Intravascular stent prosthesis for right ventricular outflow obstruction. J Am Coll Cardiol 20:373–380, 1992.
27. Hsu HS, Nykanen DG, Williams WG, et al: Right to left interatrial communications after the modified Fontan procedure: identification and management with transcatheter occlusion. Br Heart J 74:548–552, 1995.
28. Ing FF, Sommer RJ: The snare-assisted technique for transcatheter coil occlusion of moderate to large patent ductus arteriosus: immediate and intermediate results. J Am Coll Cardiol 33:1710–1718, 1999.
29. Kan JS, White RI, Mitchell SE, Gardner TJ: Percutaneous balloon valvuloplasty: a new method for treating congenital pulmonary valve stenosis. N Engl J Med 307: 540–542, 1982.
30. Kan JS, White RI, Mitchell SE, et al: Treatment of restenosis of coarctation by percutaneous transluminal angioplasty. Circulation 68:1087–1094, 1983.
31. Kreutzer J, Lock JE, Jonas RA, Keane JF: Transcatheter fenestration dilation and/or creation in postoperative Fontan patients. Am J Cardiol 79:228–232, 1997.
32. Kumar RK, Anil SR, Kannan BR, et al: Bioptome-assisted simultaneous delivery of multiple coils for occlusion of the large patent ductus arteriosus. Catheter Cardiovasc Interv 54:95–100, 2001.
33. Lababidi Z: Percutaneous balloon coarctation angioplasty: long-term results. J Interv Cardiol 5:57–62, 1992.
34. Lababidi Z, Wu JR, Walls JT: Percutaneous balloon aortic valvuloplasty: results in 23 patients. Am J Cardiol 53:194–197, 1984.
35. Laussen PC, Hansen DD, Perry SB, et al: Transcatheter closure of ventricular septal defects: hemodynamic instability and anesthetic management. Anesth Analg 80:1076–1082, 1995.
36. Lloyd TR, Fedderly R, Mendelsohn AM, et al: Transcatheter occlusion of patent ductus arteriosus with Gianturco coils. Circulation 88(4 Pt 1):1412–1420, 1993.
37. Lock JE, Khalilullah M, Shrivastava S, et al: Percutaneous catheter commissurotomy in rheumatic mitral stenosis. N Engl J Med 313:1515–1518, 1985.

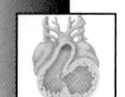

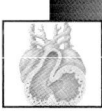

38. Lock JE, Niemi T, Burke BA, et al: Transcutaneous angioplasty of experimental aortic coarctation. Circulation 66:1280–1286, 1982.
38a. Lock JE, Bluck PC, McKay RG, et al: Transcatheter closure of ventricular septal defects. Circulation 78:361–368, 1988.
39. Magee AG, Nykanen D, McCrindle BW, et al: Balloon dilation of severe aortic stenosis in the neonate: comparison of anterograde and retrograde catheter approaches. J Am Coll Cardiol 30:1061–1066, 1997.
40. Marshall AC, Perry SB, Keane JF, Lock JE: Early results and medium-term follow-up of stent implantation for mild residual or recurrent aortic coarctation. Am Heart J 139:1054–1060, 2000.
41. McCrindle BW: Independent predictors of long-term results after balloon pulmonary valvuloplasty. Valvuloplasty and Angioplasty of Congenital Anomalies (VACA) Registry Investigators. Circulation 89:1751–1759, 1994.
42. McCrindle BW, Kan JS: Long-term results after balloon pulmonary valvuloplasty. Circulation 83:1915–1922, 1991.
43. McElhinney DB, Reddy VM, Moore P, et al: Surgical intervention for complications of transcatheter dilation procedures in congenital heart disease. Ann Thorac Surg 69:858–864, 2000.
44. McMahon CJ, El-Said HG, Grifka RG, et al: Redilation of endovascular stents in congenital heart disease: factors implicated in the development of restenosis and neointimal proliferation. J Am Coll Cardiol 38:521–526, 2001.
45. Mendelsohn AM, Bove EL, Lupinetti FM, et al: Intraoperative and percutaneous stenting of congenital pulmonary artery and vein stenosis. Circulation 88(5 Pt 2):II210–II217, 1993.
46. Mendelsohn AM, Lloyd TR, Crowley DC, et al: Late follow-up of balloon angioplasty in children with a native coarctation of the aorta. Am J Cardiol 74:696–700, 1994.
47. Moore JW, George L, Kirkpatrick SE, et al: Percutaneous closure of the small patent ductus arteriosus using occluding spring coils. J Am Coll Cardiol 23:759–765, 1994.
48. Moore P, Adatia I, Spevak PJ, et al: Severe congenital mitral stenosis in infants. Circulation 89:2099–2106, 1994.
49. Moore P, Egito E, Mowrey H, et al: Midterm results of balloon dilation of congenital aortic stenosis: predictors of success. J Am Coll Cardiol 27:1257–1263, 1996.
50. O'Connor BK, Beekman RH, Lindauer A, Rocchini A: Intermediate-term outcome after pulmonary balloon valvuloplasty: comparison with a matched surgical control group. J Am Coll Cardiol 20:169–173, 1992.
51. O'Laughlin MP, Perry SB, Lock JE, Mullins CE: Use of endovascular stents in congenital heart disease. Circulation 83:1923–1939, 1991.
52. Owada CY, Teitel DF, Moore P: Evaluation of Gianturco coils for closure of large (≥3.5 mm) patent ductus arteriosus. J Am Coll Cardiol 30:1856–1862, 1997.
53. Patel HT, Cao QL, Rhodes J, Hijazi ZM: Long-term outcome of transcatheter coil closure of small to large patent ductus arteriosus. Catheter Cardiovasc Interv 47:457–461, 1999.
54. Perry SB, Lang P, Keane JF, et al: Creation and maintenance of an adequate interatrial communication in left atrioventricular valve atresia or stenosis. Am J Cardiol 58:622–626, 1986.
55. Perry SB, Radkte W, Fellows KE, et al: Coil embolization to occlude aortopulmonary collateral vessels and shunts in patients with congenital heart disease. J Am Coll Cardiol 13:100–108, 1989.
56. Perry SB, van der Velde ME, Bridges ND, et al: Transcatheter closure of coronary artery fistulas. J Am Coll Cardiol 20:205–209, 1992.
56a. Porstmann W, Wierny L, Warnke H: Closure of persistent ducts arteriosus without thoracotomy. Ger Med Mon 12: 259–261, 1967.
57. Powell AJ, Lock JE, Keane JF, Perry SB: Prolongation of RV-PA conduit life span by percutaneous stent implantation. Intermediate-term results. Circulation 92:3282–3288, 1995.
58. Preminger TJ, Sanders SP, van der Velde ME, et al: 'Intramural' residual interventricular defects after repair of conotruncal malformations. Circulation 89:236–242, 1994.
59. Radtke W, Keane JF, Fellows KE, et al: Percutaneous balloon valvotomy of congenital pulmonary stenosis using oversized balloons. J Am Coll Cardiol 8:909–915, 1986.
60. Rao PS, Chopra PS, Koscik R, et al: Surgical versus balloon therapy for aortic coarctation in infants ≥3 months old. J Am Coll Cardiol 23:1479–1483, 1994.
61. Rashkind WJ, Miller WW: Creation of an atrial septal defect without thoracotomy. A palliative approach to complete transposition of the great arteries. JAMA 196:991–992, 1966.
62. Rhodes JF, Lane GK, Mesia CI, et al: Cutting balloon angioplasty for children with small-vessel pulmonary artery stenoses. Catheter Cardiovasc Interv 55:73–77, 2002.
63. Ring JC, Kulik TJ, Burke BA, Lock JE: Morphologic changes induced by dilation of the pulmonary valve anulus with overlarge balloons in normal newborn lambs. Am J Cardiol 55:210–214, 1985.
64. Rocchini AP, Beekman RH, Ben Shachar G, et al: Balloon aortic valvuloplasty: results of the Valvuloplasty and Angioplasty of Congenital Anomalies Registry. Am J Cardiol 65:784–789, 1990.
65. Rocchini AP, Kveselis D, Dick M, et al: Use of balloon angioplasty to treat peripheral pulmonary stenosis. Am J Cardiol 54:1069–1073, 1984.
66. Rosenthal E, Qureshi SA, Chen KC, et al: Radiofrequency-assisted balloon dilatation in patients with pulmonary valve atresia and an intact ventricular septum. Br Heart J 69:347–351, 1993.
67. Rothman A, Perry SB, Keane JF, Lock JE: Early results and follow-up of balloon angioplasty for branch pulmonary artery stenoses. J Am Coll Cardiol 15:1109–1117, 1990.
68. Satou GM, Perry SB, Lock JE, et al: Repeat balloon dilation of congenital valvar aortic stenosis: immediate results and midterm outcome. Catheter Cardiovasc Interv 47:47–51, 1999.
69. Schroeder VA, Shim D, Spicer RL, et al: Surgical emergencies during pediatric interventional catheterization. J Pediatr 140:570–575, 2002.
70. Sharma S, Kothari SS, Krishnakumar R, et al: Systemic-to-pulmonary artery collateral vessels and surgical shunts in patients with cyanotic congenital heart disease: perioperative treatment by transcatheter embolization. Am J Roentgenol 164:1505–1510, 1995.
71. Sholler GF, Keane JF, Perry SB, et al: Balloon dilation of congenital aortic valve stenosis. Results and influence of technical and morphological features on outcome. Circulation 78:351–360, 1988.
72. Singer MI, Rowen M, Dorsey TJ: Transluminal aortic balloon angioplasty for coarctation of the aorta in the newborn. Am Heart J 103:131–132, 1982.
73. Sos T, Sniderman KW, Retlek-Sos B, et al: Percutaneous transluminal dilatation of coarctation of the aorta post mortem. Lancet 2:970–971, 1979.
74. Spevak PJ, Bass JL, Ben-Shachar G, et al: Balloon angioplasty for congenital mitral stenosis. Am J Cardiol 66:472–476, 1990.
75. Stanger P, Cassidy SC, Girod DA, et al: Balloon pulmonary valvuloplasty: results of the Valvuloplasty and Angioplasty of Congenital Anomalies Registry. Am J Cardiol 65:775–783, 1990.

76. Tynan M, Finley JP, Fontes V, et al: Balloon angioplasty for the treatment of native coarctation: results of Valvuloplasty and Angioplasty of Congenital Anomalies Registry. Am J Cardiol 65:790–792, 1990.
77. Visconti KJ, Bichell DP, Jonas RA, et al: Developmental outcome after surgical versus interventional closure of secundum atrial septal defect in children. Circulation 100(19 Suppl):II145–II150, 1999.
78. Yetman AT, Nykanen D, McCrindle BW, et al: Balloon angioplasty of recurrent coarctation: a 12-year review. J Am Coll Cardiol 30:811–816, 1997.
79. Zeevi B, Berant M, Blieden LC: Midterm clinical impact versus procedural success of balloon angioplasty for pulmonary artery stenosis. Pediatr Cardiol 18:101–106, 1997.
80. Zeevi B, Berant M, Zalzstein E, Blieden LC: Balloon dilation of critical pulmonary stenosis in the first week of life. J Am Coll Cardiol 11:821–824, 1988.
81. Zellers TM, Dixon K, Moake L, et al: Bedside balloon atrial septostomy is safe, efficacious, and cost-effective compared with septostomy performed in the cardiac catheterization laboratory. Am J Cardiol 89:613–615, 2002.

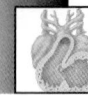

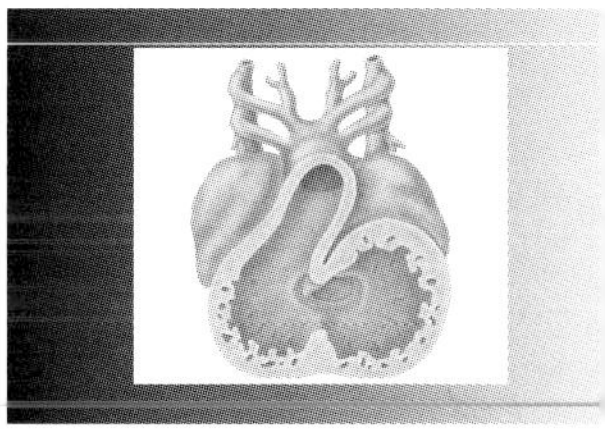

CHAPTER 104A

Surgical Approaches, Cardiopulmonary Bypass, and Mechanical Circulatory Support in Children

Surgical Approaches and Cardiopulmonary Bypass in Pediatric Cardiac Surgery

Pedro J. del Nido and Francis X. McGowan, Jr.

INTRODUCTION

Thoracic incisions traditionally used in adult cardiac and thoracic surgery have been used in children with varying success with respect to exposure, pain, and cosmetic result. There is a significant body of literature discussing various surgical approaches to intrathoracic structures for the treatment of congenital cardiac anomalies. Many reports focus on limiting the size of the incision to improve cosmetic results, and others focus on complications of some of these approaches, specifically in children.[31,146] The special considerations relevant to pediatric thoracic surgery relate to the lack of development and growth of soft tissue structures such as breast tissue, and bony structures such as ribs and vertebra. Thus incisions that fix growing bony structures, such as ribs in a posterior or lateral thoracotomy, may lead to scoliosis.[31] Anterior thoracic incisions also may injure structures that have not fully developed, such as breast tissue and pectoral muscles, resulting in chest wall deformities and sensory loss. Then again, the flexibility of the chest cage and ribs in young children permit the use of limited incisions with adequate exposure of relevant structures, whereas in adults this may not be possible without the risk of rib or sternal fracture or instability of the chest cage. Therefore in selecting the optimal approach to intrathoracic structures in children, consideration of all these factors is important to optimize exposure and for the safe conduct of the procedure, as well as to minimize pain and achieve a cosmetically acceptable result. Preoperative planning of the procedure is helpful, including determining which mediastinal structures need exposure for the surgical procedure and for cannulation for cardiopulmonary bypass. With the availability of thin-walled, wire-reinforced, small-diameter cannulas for use in children, cannulation for cardiopulmonary bypass often can be achieved with minimal extension of the thoracic incision beyond that needed for the repair itself. These approaches usually still provide sufficient exposure to use standard techniques for myocardial protection, such as use of cardioplegia and left ventricular venting.

Positioning of the child should be done in such a way that the surgeon and assistant have a direct view of the relevant anatomical structures and that also provides the anesthesiologist with access to the airway and major access lines. When a newborn or infant is placed supine on the table, it is important to remember that the head size is significantly larger in proportion to the chest, as compared with older children and adults. A shoulder roll should be used to elevate the shoulders and relieve some of the pressure from the occiput. Soft padding, including gel-filled plastic bags, should be placed under all pressure areas. Cooling blankets are used routinely in pediatric cardiac surgery; however, these require relatively direct patient contact to optimize heat transfer. More recently, perforated blankets filled with cold or heated air that is blown through have been used more frequently, with improved heat transfer properties compared with water-filled blankets. However, direct skin contact should be avoided with either method because of the risk of injury to the skin that can result in full-thickness skin loss, particularly in infants. For a lateral thoracotomy, an axillary roll is used to elevate the thorax and relieve pressure on the shoulder and potentially the brachial plexus. As with any thoracotomy incision, care must be taken not to extend the arm and shoulder under tension, even in infants, because this may cause injury to the brachial plexus.

For cosmetic purposes the skin incision can be placed below the actual entry site into the thorax, whether the incision is a sternotomy or a lateral intercostal approach. Care must be taken, however, to minimize creation of flaps, particularly in infants, because this often leads to breakdown of subcutaneous tissue with fat necrosis, resulting in wound separation. Excessive use of cautery, particularly in the subcutaneous fat in infants, is also another cause of fat necrosis and wound separation, often prolonging hospital stay and resulting in a poor cosmetic result.

THORACIC INCISIONS

Approaches to Extracardiac Structures in Infants and Children

Noncardiac thoracic surgery for the treatment of congenital cardiac defects or complications of cardiac surgery most often requires exposure to the posterior mediastinum. Exceptions include procedures for plication of the diaphragm or for unifocalization of aortopulmonary collaterals, which requires dissection of the hilum of the lung. A posterolateral incision extending from just anterior to the tip of the scapula to the midposterior scapula provides access, through the fourth, fifth, or sixth intercostal spaces (ICSs), to posterior mediastinal structures, as well as hilum of the lung, pericardium, and diaphragm (Figure 104A-1). If the upper half of the mediastinum needs exposure, an incision through the fourth ICS is optimal. For access to the hilum of the lung, the fifth ICS is optimal, and for access to the thoracic duct at the level of the diaphragm or to the central tendon of the diaphragm, a sixth ICS incision is optimal. The most common procedures where a thoracotomy is performed routinely are operations on the thoracic aorta or branches, such as surgery for repair of coarctation of the aorta or for ligation of patent ductus. Care should be taken to ensure that the appropriate interspace is entered, because exposure to the upper thorax can be very difficult in small children if the fifth or lower interspaces are entered. Although counting ribs (starting at the second rib, which has attachments of the anterior scalene) can be done, external landmarks also can be used. A useful landmark is the position of the areola when the arm is extended over the head. With the arm extended, the interspace below the position of the areola is usually the fourth ICS and can be used as a landmark to confirm identification of a particular interspace by other techniques. This method or identification of interspace is particularly useful in neonates and premature infants. Extensive division of the intercostal muscle is usually unnecessary in infants and small children because adequate exposure can be obtained by separating the ribs, which are more flexible in this age group, with less risk of fracture.

This same approach can be used for exposure of intrapericardial structures such as the pulmonary trunk for pulmonary artery banding and even for intracardiac procedures. Exposure to the inferior vena cava for cannulation through a posterolateral thoracotomy can be difficult, however, and may require division of one rib posteriorly. Closure of the thoracotomy incision, as in adults, should be done in layers, approximating the serratus muscle and fascia separate from the latissimus dorsi muscle and subcutaneous tissue. This approach minimizes distortion of the chest wall muscles and provides the best cosmetic results as well.

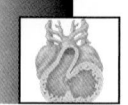

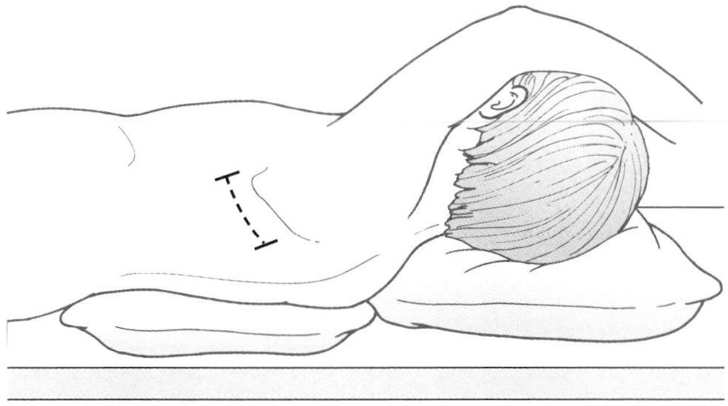

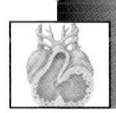

Figure 104A–1 Left posterolateral thoracotomy.

Other thoracotomy approaches, such as anterior thoracotomy for access to the pulmonary artery trunk or right atrium for closure of atrial septal defect, can be used but are associated with more incisional pain, frequently require at least partial detachment of the pectoralis muscle, and can cut across breast tissue in infants in whom identification of the breast mass is difficult. Although in postpubescent girls and adult women the incision for an anterolateral thoracotomy can be made in the inframammary position, often a flap is required to reach the fourth ICS, resulting in partial sensory loss in the skin over the flap and, in young women, is associated with asymmetrical growth of the breast tissue.[31] A transaxillary approach has been described for ligation of patent ductus and access to the transverse aortic arch and descending aorta. Either a transverse incision is made over the third interspace between the fold of the pectoralis muscle and scapula, or some have described a vertical incision from the axilla down to the fourth ICS. The third interspace is entered, which provides direct access to the distal aortic arch and arterial duct. However, exposure is limited, and extension of the incision, if more exposure is required, is difficult. In experienced hands, however, this approach is adequate for ductus ligation, even in small infants with a less visible incision.

Approaches to Cardiac Structures and Great Vessels

Full Sternotomy

The most commonly used incision for access to the heart and anterior mediastinal structures is a sternotomy. A vertical skin incision over the sternum itself, staying below the manubrium, permits full division of the sternum and provides an unobstructed view of all anterior mediastinal structures and direct access from branches of the aortic arch down to the inferior vena cava at the level of the diaphragm. This approach is necessary when the surgical procedure requires access to upper and lower mediastinal structures such as the aortic arch and right atrium, branch pulmonary arteries, and right ventricle. Examples include first-stage procedure for hypoplastic left heart syndrome, repair of truncus arteriosus, or pulmonary atresia with ventricular septal defect (VSD).

The incision in the pericardium is also vertical and, if placed directly over the cardiac structures that will be accessed, can facilitate exposure, particularly when transatrial procedures to access the ventricles are being performed. By opening the pericardium to the right of the midline and retracting the right side of the pericardium to the sternum, the ventricles fall away leftward, aiding exposure. Similarly, if exposure to the pulmonary trunk is required, such as in repair of tetralogy of Fallot, traction sutures on the left side of the pericardium can expose this area and facilitate repair. Sutures are used to suspend the pericardium and should also be used to rotate the heart to facilitate exposure. In cases in which the right atrium and venae cavae need exposure, suspension of the right-sided pericardial edge to the periosteum of the sternum often is required to visualize the lateral wall of the right atrium and inferior vena cava. If the left side of the pericardium is left unsuspended and incised along the edge of the diaphragm to the apex, the entire ventricular mass rotates away from the surgeon, facilitating exposure of the atrioventricular (AV) valves and interventricular septum to the level of the apex. A similar approach can be used to optimize exposure of the right ventricular (RV) outflow tract for surgery to correct tetralogy of Fallot. Here the pericardium at the level of the great vessels is suspended to the periosteum, leaving the pericardial edge at the diaphragm unsuspended, facilitating the view of the VSD through the ventriculotomy.

Limited Sternotomy Incisions

For many procedures a full sternotomy is not necessary to provide adequate access to all the relevant structures of the heart. Examples of the types of procedures in which a full sternotomy is unnecessary include any procedure in which the intracardiac repair is accomplished via a right atriotomy, such as repair of atrial septal defect, VSD, complete AV canal defect, transatrial repair of tetralogy of Fallot, and mitral valve repair. This is particularly true in infants and young children because of their pliable sternum and rib cage, which permits retraction with minimal force. For most procedures, the skin incision extends from the level of the areola (midthorax) down to the tip of the xiphoid process (Figure 104A-2). By detaching anterior diaphragm attachments to the cartilaginous segment of the rib cage anteriorly, access is gained to the anterior mediastinum. Before performing the partial sternotomy, blunt dissection is required to detach the pericardium and thymus from the sternum. A partial sternotomy can be performed either with a saw, or, in infants, heavy bandage scissors, which are sufficient for dividing the lower sternum. Once the partial sternotomy is completed, a narrow blade retractor such as an army–navy

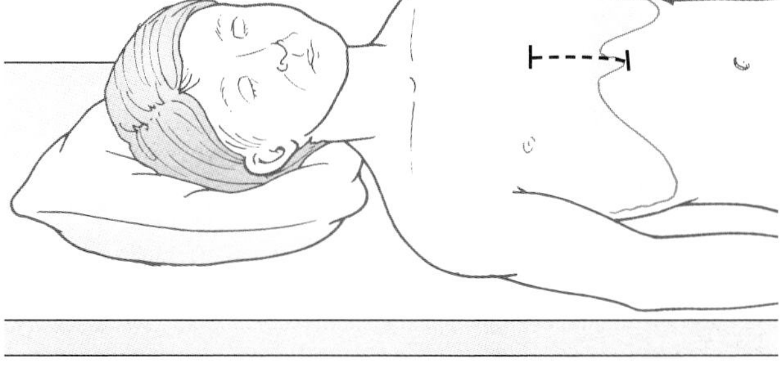

Figure 104A–2 Partial or limited sternotomy incision.

retractor is used to lift the sternum anteriorly and cephalad to provide exposure to the ascending aorta for cannulation. The retractor should not be placed on the skin and subcutaneous tissue because adequate exposure of the upper mediastinum will not be achieved and necrosis of the skin could occur from prolonged retraction. For the aorta to be exposed, however, caudal and anterior traction must be placed on the pericardium. This maneuver requires that thymus attachments to the pericardium be divided; otherwise there will be inadequate mobility of the pericardium and aorta. The pericardial incision must be made to the right of the midline, and the pericardium must be pinned to the right edge of the divided sternum to expose the right atrium and venae cavae.

For procedures in which the RV outflow tract or aortic root must be accessed, the partial sternotomy approach may still be used, but usually the skin and sternal incisions need to be extended superiorly by 1 or 2 cm. In this case traction sutures on the pericardium at the level of the pulmonary and aortic root suspend these structures into view, permitting adequate exposure.

Alternative Approaches to Cardiac Structures

Anterior or Anterolateral Thoracotomy

An anterior thoracotomy has been advocated for surgical repair of atrial septal defect and occasionally VSDs. The incision is made in the anterior fourth intercostal space, and in females great care must be taken to make the incision well below breast tissue. Dissection of the pericardial attachments to the sternum and thymus greatly facilitates exposure by permitting retraction of the pericardium down toward the diaphragm and bringing the ascending aorta closer into view. Direct cannulation of the ascending aorta is preferable to peripheral cannulation via femoral or axillary artery, because these vessels are small in children and stenosis at the cannulation site can result in claudication with exercise. In the past few years more flexible cannulas have become available in all sizes for pediatric use, and these have facilitated aortic cannulation. Some arterial cannula can be introduced over a guide wire, which makes insertion easier and safer. The cava can be cannulated directly, although the superior cava cannula is often best introduced via the right atrial appendage and directed retrograde into the superior vena cava (SVC). Aortic clamping to achieve cardiac arrest can be difficult with conventional arterial clamps because these were designed for application via a sternotomy. In small children a bulldog clamp is sufficient for aortic occlusion, and for larger children and teenagers, flexible clamps are now available. Cardioplegia can be delivered via a small flexible cannula inserted into the aortic root, or some have advocated transthoracic insertion of a needle into the aortic root.

Thoracoscopic Approach in Children

Because most cardiac procedures in children require cardiopulmonary bypass and intracardiac repair, port access for reconstruction has been applied almost exclusively to adult patients or, rarely, adult-sized adolescents. Thoracoscopic procedures in children have been, for the most part, confined to approaches to noncardiac structures or the pericardium. Examples include ligation of patent ductus, division of vascular rings, creation of a pericardial window, and, more recently, pacer lead insertion. Much of the instrumentation has been adapted from other surgical applications, and the thoracoscopic procedures have involved primarily dissection and ligation or division with little reconstruction or suturing.

Positioning and location of port incisions follows the same principles of thoracoscopy or thoracotomy in adults. For access to the distal transverse aortic arch and descending aorta, the patient should be in a full lateral decubitus position. For access to anterior mediastinal structures such as anterior pericardium or thymus, a partial decubitus position with the thorax tilted toward a supine position is optimal. Usually four incisions are required: two for the surgeon's instruments for the dissection, one for the scope and camera, and one for the assistant to introduce lung retractors or occasionally a grasper or suction. As with any thoracoscopic procedure, the central port is used for the camera, and the instrument ports are located at each side of the camera port, separated by sufficient distance to prevent the scope from interfering with instrument movement. In procedures in which a surgical robot is used to assist, the same port position is used, but the port for the lung retractor and suction is placed at the midaxillary line at the sixth or seventh intercostal space (Figure 104A-3).

For approach to anterior mediastinal structures, the same arrangement is used with respect to camera and instrument ports. In cases such as dissection of the right lobe of the thymus for thoracoscopic innominate artery suspension to relieve tracheal compression, the central port for the scope is placed at the anterior axillary line in the fourth ICS, and the two instrument ports are placed two or three interspaces to each side and 2–3 cm more anterior. A fourth port can be used for lung retraction and should be placed 1–2 intercostal spaces lower toward the diaphragm so as not to interfere with instrument motion. For the anterior pericardium the three ports are placed more inferiorly on the chest, using the fourth or fifth ICS for the scope and camera, and the instrument ports are placed 1–2 interspaces on either side.

CARDIOPULMONARY BYPASS IN CHILDREN

History

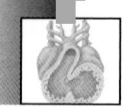

The use of extracorporeal circulatory techniques to repair congenital cardiac defects began in the 1950s, shortly after the initial development of the concept of cardiopulmonary bypass (CPB) and construction of a heart–lung machine. In 1953 Gibbon[61] repaired an atrial septal defect using the first heart–lung machine, which required 12–14 units of blood prime. At approximately the same time, Lillehei and colleagues[95] began using cross-circulation to repair a variety of defects in relatively young infants and children, including ventricular septal defects, atrioventricular canal, and tetralogy of Fallot, achieving a remarkable overall survival of greater than 60%. Shortly thereafter, Kirklin and others[86] developed a pump oxygenator derived from Gibbon's earlier efforts. This device required approximately half of the orig-

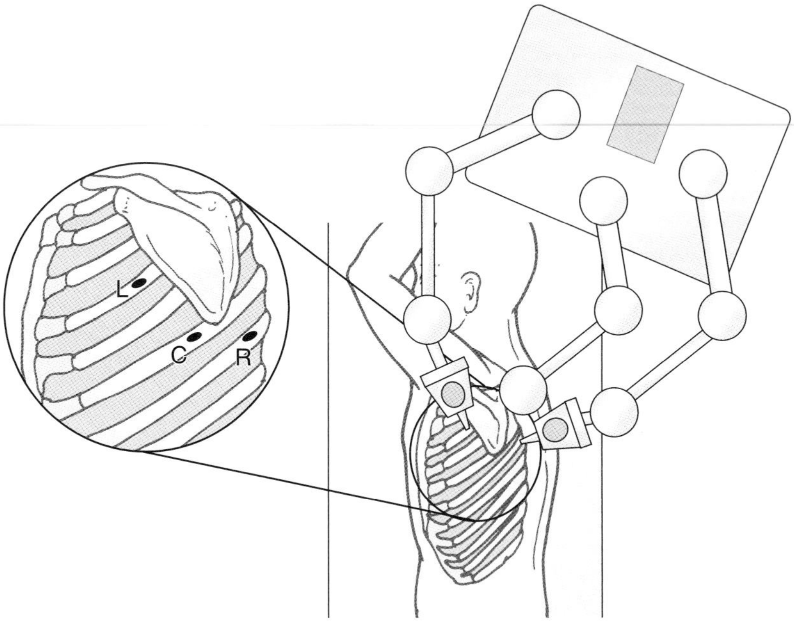

Figure 104A–3 Port position for robot-assisted thoracoscopic division of vascular ring. The scope and camera are introduced through the central Port (C) and instruments through the other two Ports for the left arm (L), and right arm (R).
(Modified from Mihaljevic T, Cannon JW, del Nido PJ: Robotically assisted division of a vascular ring in children. J Thorac Cardiovasc Surg 125:1163–1164, 2003.)

inal amount of fresh blood prime and extreme care to prevent severe foaming of blood, which was lethal; nonetheless, survival was 50%. These early reports prompted many subsequent investigations aimed at developing the scientific and technological knowledge needed to successfully undertake extracorporeal circulation in infants and children; in spite of these efforts, the morbidity and mortality of CPB remained high throughout the 1960s.

The next major advance occurred in the early 1970s, with the description of the use of deep hypothermic circulatory arrest in infants by Barratt-Boyes[11] and Castaneda.[26] These techniques relied primarily upon surface cooling, with exposure to the CPB circuit limited to a brief period of core cooling and rewarming, such that total CPB time was typically less than 20–30 min. Progressive and incremental advances in the design of circuit components and perfusion techniques for infants and small children occurred throughout the 1980s and into the early 1990s. As a result, the "toxicity" associated with the use of CPB in infants declined significantly, to the point where lengthy and complex repairs such as the arterial switch procedure for transposition of the great arteries and primary repair of tetralogy of Fallot currently can be undertaken in neonates and very young infants using CPB, with overall mortality less than 5%. Nonetheless, the morbidity associated with the use of CPB in infants and children is still widely held to be a major limitation to completely successful outcomes.

Key Differences between Pediatric and Adult Cardiopulmonary Bypass

There are many significant differences in circuit technology and the physiology of CPB in neonates, infants, and small children compared with adults. The surface area and volume of the CPB circuit relative to patient size and blood volume are much greater in neonates and infants. Arterial and venous cannulas are smaller, but more likely to deform or obstruct the aorta or venae cavae; their placement can be different and more variable than in adults, for example, separate superior and inferior vena caval cannulas or initial placement of the aortic cannula in the pulmonary artery (with retrograde systemic perfusion via the ductus arteriosus) during stage I repair of hypoplastic left heart syndrome. For hemodilution to be minimized, the size of various circuit components and tubing diameter are kept as small as possible. Nonetheless, hemodilution equivalent to 1–2 blood volumes from the circuit prime and cardioplegia is fairly common in neonates and small infants.

Deep hypothermic circulatory arrest, although used much less frequently than even a few years ago, is still employed much more often in children than in adults. Overall, pump flow rates can range from no flow (i.e., circulatory arrest) to more than 200 ml/min; mean arterial pressures can vary from 10–20 mm Hg during low-flow CPB to more than 50 mm Hg at full or high flow. Temperatures are typically lower in infant CPB (15–18° C core temperatures for deep hypothermia, 22–25° C for many other complex repairs), and different blood pH management strategies may be employed (e.g., alpha stat versus pH stat). In part because of these differences, the magnitude of neuroendocrine stress responses and systemic inflammatory responses to CPB, as well as their consequences, is generally believed to be more profound in neonates and infants than in adults.

Patient Factors

There are also numerous factors related to patient-specific variables and the diverse pathophysiology associated with congenital cardiac defects that further complicate CPB in this population. It is likely that neonates in general, and particularly those who are premature and/or weigh less than

1.8–2.0 kg, comprise a high-risk group as a result of immature organ function, as well as coexisting diseases such as sepsis, respiratory distress syndrome, or one or more other congenital anomalies.[172] The immature myocardium may be similarly prone to CPB-related dysfunction for several reasons, including its relatively deficient (compared with adult) contractile protein mass and organization of contractile proteins, the presence of fetal contractile protein isoforms, immature calcium cycling (which occurs primarily via the sarcolemmal membrane as opposed to the sarcoplasmic reticulum, which is less abundant and less well organized), and fewer mitochondria.

Various aspects of congenital heart disease can present additional complicating features. Hypertrophic and cyanotic hearts are more likely to be injured by ischemia and reperfusion and other consequences of congenital heart disease.[37,38,54,163] Aortopulmonary collaterals, which can be particularly significant in various cyanotic lesions, may promote pulmonary dysfunction as a result of high flow on CPB while compromising function of other organs as a result of "steal" from systemic perfusion; collaterals to the coronary circulation can washout cardioplegia and thereby hinder effective myocardial preservation. Pulmonary dysfunction after CPB may be more prevalent in infants with other routes of high pulmonary blood flow (e.g., truncus arteriosus, hypoplastic left heart syndrome, transposition of the great arteries) and in cyanotic infants.[1,172] Diffuse organ dysfunction is likely to be more common in patients who were severely cyanotic and hypoperfused at the time of delivery and/or the early neonatal period; most centers have found it beneficial in this situation to allow a period of stabilization of the circulation and recovery of organ function before undertaking CPB and cardiac surgery, using lesion-appropriate interventions such as prostaglandin E_1, inotropic support, ventilatory strategies to balance systemic and pulmonary blood flow, and even extracorporeal circulatory support (see later).

Differences in the Cardiopulmonary Bypass Circuit

A summary of the components of different-sized CPB circuits is shown in Table 104A-1.

Oxygenators

Oxygenator systems for infants and children must function over a wide range of pump flow rates (maximal flow rates range between 800–4000 ml/min and must be efficient over a range of flows equivalent up to 250 ml/kg), temperatures (10–38° C), hematocrits (15–40%), and line pressures (as a result of different-sized cannulas and tubing).

Virtually all current pediatric CPB applications use membrane-type oxygenators. There are essentially two types: microporous (hollow fiber or folded membrane) and nonporous membrane oxygenators. The major advantage of microporous-type membranes is their ability to effect gas exchange with a relatively modest membrane surface area, typically in the range of 0.3–1.5 m^2, depending on the specific oxygenator and configuration. Major disadvantages include some blood–gas contact at the start of CPB (until protein accumulation blocks the 0.05–0.25 μm pores) and protein leakage across the membrane, along with the potential for gas embolization if negative pressure develops on the blood side of the artificial membrane. Nonporous oxygenator membranes, typically of the folded sheet, silicone membrane variety, require a larger surface area to achieve gas exchange, but do not accumulate or leak protein as readily, and therefore are more often selected for longer-term circulatory support applications (e.g., extracorporeal membrane oxygenation [ECMO]).

To minimize hemodilution and the potential for fluid overload and edema, one needs to minimize priming volumes, which is defined as the volume of the membrane compartment plus the minimal amount required for the venous reservoir. Typical priming volumes of commercial

Table 104A–1

Sample Scheme for Infant and Pediatric Oxygenators[a]

Oxygenator	*Estimated total prime volume[b] (ml)*	*Membrane surface area (m^2)*	*Heat exchanger surface area (m^2)*	*Manufacturer's recommendation maximum flow rate (ml/min)*
Dideco Lilliput I (max 8 kg)	300–330	0.34	0.02	800
Dideco Lilliput II (max 20 kg)	425–575	0.64	0.02	2300
Cobe Optimini	790–1110	1	0.14	5000
Cobe Optima	1300–1420	1.9	0.14	8000

[a]Used under standard configuration.
[b]Assuming use of standard configuration, and usual tubing size and length for weight.

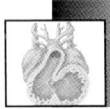

membrane oxygenators range from approximately 225–375 ml when used in the open configuration. The Dideco Lilliput hollow-fiber membrane oxygenator is an example of one with a smaller prime volume (~70 ml), but it is not available in an open system configuration.

Pumps

Most pediatric circuits use roller pumps. Pump flow rate is governed by the revolutions per minute (rpm) of the pump head, the degree of occlusion produced by the rollers, and the internal diameter of the tubing. A significant advantage is that pump flow is relatively independent of resistive and hydrostatic forces in the circuit. However, adequate flow is highly dependent on proper setting of roller head occlusion (which also affects the degree of blood trauma and hemolysis), as well as accurate knowledge of pump head rpm and tubing size. Failure to accurately account for any of these variables can lead to excessive or inadequate pump flow.

Tubing

Competing considerations govern selection of tubing size for infant and pediatric CPB (Table 104A-2). The internal diameter needs to be large enough to permit the required full flow rate (see later) without inordinately increasing circuit line pressures. On the other hand, the tubing should be as narrow and as short as practical to minimize priming volume. Some neonatal circuits use ¼-inch tubing on both the arterial and venous limbs, although most centers have further decreased the diameter of the arterial tubing to 3/16 inch; some use 3/16-inch tubing for both arterial and venous limbs (although vacuum-assisted venous drainage may be required in this instance).[172] The pump is usually situated as close to the surgical field as possible to reduce tubing length, which is a major contributor to overall circuit volume.

Table 104A–2

Infant and Pediatric CPB Tubing

Tubing diameter (in)	*Tubing volume (ml/ft)*	*Flow rate (ml/revolution)*
3/16	5.0	7.4
¼	9.7	13
3/8	21.7	27
½	38.6	45

Venous Drainage

As in adult circuits, venous blood usually flows from the patient to the venous reservoir of the CPB circuit by gravity. The level of blood in the venous reservoir serves as an important safety mechanism: It is a source of volume to increase arterial inflow and to assess the adequacy of venous return. If venous return and the level in the venous reservoir decline, causes such as unrecovered or lost blood in the surgical field, malpositioned venous cannulas, or excessive capillary leak can be identified, and interventions such as decreasing pump flow rate, adding volume, adjusting operating table height, or repositioning venous cannulas can be performed.

Many venous reservoirs are rigid and used in a configuration that is open to the atmosphere. Advantages include ease of removing entrained venous air, free flow of venous drainage (i.e., no air lockage or buildup of pressure in the reservoir), integration of the cardiotomy reservoir (as opposed to having a separate reservoir for cardiotomy suction), and the ability to accurately measure reservoir volume via calibration lines on the side of the chamber. This last feature is a useful aid to assess the patient's intravascular volume and therefore may facilitate weaning from CPB. Major disadvantages of open, rigid venous reservoirs include the presence of a blood–air interface, which may promote blood trauma and activation of the coagulation, fibrinolytic, and inflammatory cascades (see later) and the need for a larger priming volume.

A soft, collapsible venous reservoir bag that expands and contracts in relation to overall blood volume, venous return, and arterial inflow rate is being used with increasing frequency in infant CPB. Advantages include the absence of direct blood–air contact and the fact that air is not entrained if the venous reservoir becomes empty, which collapses the bag. A major disadvantage can be the inability to accurately measure venous reservoir volume and/or recognize subtle but important changes in venous return. Other relative disadvantages compared with rigid reservoirs include the need for a removal mechanism if air is entrained, the need for a separate cardiotomy suction reservoir, and the fact that venous drainage is significantly reduced if pressure builds up as a result of overfilling of the reservoir with blood volume or air.

Vacuum-assisted venous drainage has been used in pediatric patients.[132,172] Although it is not well studied in a controlled or prospective fashion at present, advantages may include the ability to reduce total circuit volume by using lower venous reservoir volume and 3/16-inch venous tubing, improving operating conditions to some extent by allowing use of smaller venous cannulas, and improving venous drainage through the small cannulas and tubing. Theoretically, the improvement of venous drainage could lead to reduced tissue and organ edema and congestion, improved organ function, and reduced inflammatory activation (e.g., via endotoxin release from congested, hypoperfused intestine). A major potential complication of vacuum-assisted venous drainage is venoarterial air embolism.[36]

Arterial Cannulas

Issues regarding cannula size are much more significant in infants and small children than in adults. Arterial cannulas for neonates and small infants must be of sufficient size to permit appropriate arterial inflow rates at reasonable line pressures, with minimal shearing or jetting of blood flow (which can damage the vessel intima, aortic valve, or blood elements), yet small enough to fit in small aortas without obstructing aortic flow (Table 104A-3). Small cannulas (i.e., 8 Fr) with a thin-walled, reinforced design that prevents cannula kinking and allows a larger luminal diameter for a given external diameter have become popular choices for infant bypass (Bio-Medicus, Minneapolis, MN). Care also needs to be taken not to kink or compress the infant's pliable aorta by the location and orientation of the aortic cannula and its tubing. As noted, the cannula itself can significantly obstruct flow in the vessel surrounding the cannula. Location of the tip can direct blood flow toward or away from specific vessels; for example, locating and directing the tip more distally toward the transverse arch may reduce flow through the right carotid artery and/or favor lower body perfusion at the expense of cerebral perfusion and optimal brain cooling.[82]

Certain congenital cardiac lesions require unique aortic cannulation sites. For example, the aortic cannula is typically placed more distally in the aorta for repairs that involve extensive proximal aortic surgery, such as the arterial switch procedure for transposition of the great vessels; this distal location may alter distribution of blood flow to the carotid vessels. Repair of interrupted aortic arch requires two arterial cannulas, one in each segment of the aorta (perfusing the head and lower body, respectively). The aortic cannula is placed in the pulmonary artery at the beginning of CPB for stage I repair of hypoplastic left heart syndrome because of the typically diminutive size of the ascending aorta in this lesion. The distal pulmonary arteries are occluded with tourniquets, and the aorta is perfused via the ductus arteriosus until the aortic reconstruction is completed, at which time the cannula is repositioned in the neoaorta.

Unlike adults, femoral arterial cannulation for CPB is not usually a viable option in infants and small children (weighing less than ~10–15 kg) because small vessel size precludes inserting an arterial cannula large enough to allow arterial inflow rates that are sufficient to completely meet metabolic needs (see later). In small infants (without recent sternotomy) the neck vessels are the preferred extrathoracic cannulation sites (see later). However, as a resuscitative measure in emergent situations (e.g., cardiopulmonary arrest in the cardiac catheterization laboratory, particularly where femoral vascular access is already in place), insertion of smaller perfusion cannulas in the femoral artery has often been lifesaving in terms of facilitating rapid establishment of extracorporeal support. Femoral access is performed occasionally for older children, either electively when there is concern that a cardiac chamber or vascular conduit lies immediately beneath the sternum, or emergently when one of these structures is entered inadvertently during the dissection.

Table 104A–3

Representative Pediatric Arterial Cannulas

Weight (kg)	*Standard arterial size (Fr)*	*Biomedicus pediatric Arterial size (Fr)*
<5	10	8
5–10	12	10
10–14	14	12
14–28	16	14
28–50	18	—

Venous Cannulas

Choice and location of venous cannulas also can be more complex and variable than is typically the case in adults and must take into account variations in venous anatomy and drainage, as well as the operative approach. Venous cannulas are available in a variety of sizes and have design features for particular indications (Table 104A-4). For example, thin-walled cannulas with multiple side holes enhance venous drainage; right-angled tips are frequently used in the SVC to improve alignment (and therefore drainage) and minimize impact on the surgical field; metal-tipped cannulas prevent kinking; and straight, short-tipped cannulas in the inferior vena cava (IVC) limit hepatic venous obstruction.

Overall, most repairs use separate SVC and IVC cannulas to achieve maximal collection of venous return and to minimize interference with the operative field. Common variations in venous anatomy that can complicate venous cannulation and must be taken into account include left or bilateral SVC, azygous or hemiazygous continuation of the IVC, and direct drainage of the hepatic veins into the atrium. A single atrial cannula is frequently used when deep hypothermic circulatory arrest is planned; in this instance, the venous cannula is removed after the patient is adequately cooled in order to have a clear operative field.

Regardless of location, it is important that the cannula is appropriately sited and that it causes as minimal obstruction to venous drainage as possible. Poor venous drainage may be difficult to detect and is more likely in patients with complicated venous anatomy. The consequences of impaired venous drainage and increased venous pressures are likely to be magnified during infant CPB because arterial perfusion pressure is frequently reduced. Obstruction of the SVC may promote cerebral edema and otherwise increases the risk of brain injury by decreasing cerebral blood flow (CBF) and hindering effective brain cooling. Many practitioners find monitoring of SVC pressure by a catheter placed in the internal jugular vein useful to detect possible SVC obstruction in this setting; the patient's head and face also should be inspected at regular intervals during CPB for the appearance of congestion or swelling. Monitoring CBF velocity using transcranial Doppler methodology might also be useful in this regard. IVC obstruction increases lower body venous pressures and potentially decreases hepatic, renal, and/or mesenteric perfusion; isolated hepatic vein obstruction also can occur. Consequences can include hepatic dysfunction, renal dysfunction, ascites, and perhaps increased inflammatory consequences as a result of mesenteric

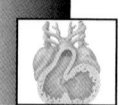

Table 104A–4

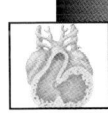

Representative Venous Cannulas for Pediatric CPB

		Metal tip right angle venous (Fr +)	
Weight (kg)	*Single venous (Fr)*[a]	*SVC*	*IVC*
<3.5	18	12	12
3.5–6	20	12	14
6–8	22	12	16
8–12	22	14	16
12–18	24	14	16–18
18–24	26	16	18–20
24–30	28	18–20	20
30–35	30	18–20	20
35–45	32	20	22
45–55	34	20–22	22–28

+, e.g., DLP.
[a]Bard, Terumo.

congestion.[55,72] Detection of IVC obstruction during CPB can be difficult and should be suspected whenever there is development of ascites, decreased urine output, or impaired venous return.

Filters

Almost all applications use 0.2-μm filters in the gas inflow lines to prevent bacterial or particulate contamination. Similarly, all crystalloid prime and cardioplegia solutions are passed through 0.2–μm filters before final addition to the CPB circuit. A 20- or 40-μm filter is used on the cardiotomy suction return line to remove macroaggregates and microaggregates and other debris from the blood returning from the surgical field. Exogenous blood is also filtered (typically through a 40-μm blood filter) before it is added to either the pump circuit or to cardioplegia. Specific removal of blood polymorphonuclear leukocytes using leukocyte-depleting filters placed in-line on the CPB circuit (which typically reduce circulating leukocyte counts in the patient by ~75%) is advocated by some centers as significant means to reduce reperfusion injury.[1,34]

Use of an arterial filter (40 μm) is somewhat more controversial. Many consider arterial filtering essential to limit the amount of microemboli and other debris from platelet and leukocyte microaggregates, traumatized blood elements, fat, and other sources, particularly because these might contribute to post-CPB neurological injury and damage to other organ systems. Some practitioners do not feel so strongly about these issues and omit arterial line filters, at least partly to reduce priming volume and hemodilution.[172]

Cardiopulmonary Bypass Prime

The priming volume of even the smallest neonatal and infant CPB circuits is usually equivalent to approximately 1.5–3 times the patient's blood volume. Thus dilution of red cells, clotting factors, and other plasma constituents is potentially of far greater magnitude than in adults. Physiological crystalloid solutions (e.g., Normosol) are the major component of CPB priming solutions in infants and children; colloidal primes are used infrequently. Significant additions to the infant CPB prime include packed red blood cells (or occasionally whole blood), as well as fresh frozen plasma or other colloids such as albumin.

Other agents that may be included in the pump prime include mannitol, steroids, heparin, and buffers (e.g., sodium bicarbonate or THAM [tris(hydroxymethyl)-aminomethane]). Mannitol is used primarily for its osmotic properties and is intended to reduce organ and cellular edema, as well as to promote diuresis and thereby contribute to renal protection. The osmotic diuresis may be particularly beneficial in some congenital cardiac operations in which a substantial amount of hemolysis from blood trauma caused by cardiotomy suction and high pump flow rates can occur. Stabilization of cellular membranes and various antioxidant properties, including radical scavenging, also have been attributed to mannitol. The significance of any of these effects is not proven in pediatric CPB. Steroids are used to reduce inflammatory effects of CPB (see later).

The use of albumin or other colloids to prime CPB circuits also is controversial.[16,126,170] There is evidence that reduced plasma protein concentrations and diminished plasma oncotic pressure can reduce lymphatic flow and increase capillary leak in the lung and other vascular beds.[23,101,145,149] Although fluid balance and weight gain were favorably influenced, a recent study that randomized pediatric CPB patients to crystalloid or colloid prime could not demonstrate significant differences in mortality or in length of mechanical ventilation, intensive care unit (ICU), or hospital stay.[145] These results are similar to those obtained in adults, in which albumin does prevent CPB-induced reductions in colloid oncotic pressure and lung water accumulation, but appears to have little effect on overall outcome or measures of pulmonary, myocardial, or renal function.

Hemodilution

As noted earlier, some centers have gone to substantial lengths to modify circuit design to reduce the degree of hemodilution associated with infant CPB and decrease the use of exogenous blood and other products. These modifications have included use of the smallest possible tubing, cannulas, and oxygenators; altered orientation of the CPB circuit to decrease tubing length; vacuum-assisted venous drainage to improve return through the small cannulas and tubing; and omission of arterial filters. Resultant priming volumes in the 180–250 ml range have been reported. Ultrafiltration techniques (see later) also are used to offset the hemodiluting effects of CPB and thereby reduce the requirement for donor blood and blood products. With the possible exception of ultrafiltration, there is no evidence that edema, the inflammatory response to CPB, or overall outcome is improved by these measures and, at present, it remains difficult to avoid the use of exogenous blood and/or blood products in patients weighing less than approximately 10 kg.

Both packed red cells and whole blood have been used to ensure age-, lesion-, and temperature-appropriate hematocrit levels during CPB. Packed red cells are readily available and are probably used by most centers to increase and maintain hematocrit levels during CPB. A major disadvantage of whole blood compared with packed red cells is the higher glucose load that accompanies whole blood; hyperglycemia may increase the risk of brain injury during cerebral ischemia. On the other hand, whole blood maintains plasma clotting factor concentrations more effectively, which can be significantly reduced by CPB in these patients (see later). Recently questions about the actual oxygen-carrying and delivery capacity of stored red blood cells have been raised.[162]

The optimal hematocrit level for neonatal and infant CPB remains controversial. Perhaps the most important consideration is the temperature and flow rate that are to be used (e.g., deep hypothermia, low-flow, or circulatory arrest). More profound degrees of hypothermia are used in pediatric patients to suppress metabolic demands and increase tolerance to periods of low flow (18–25° C) or absent flow (15–18° C). Although the oxygen-carrying capacity of hemoglobin increases at lower temperatures, its ability to donate oxygen to the tissues also is reduced. Moreover, the increase in blood viscosity that accompanies hypothermia is a significant impediment to microcirculatory flow and can lead to sludging and regional ischemia; the nonpulsatile flow patterns typical of most CPB applications may also decrease microcirculatory flow, particularly in the setting of increased viscosity. It also is important to note that the oxygen-carrying capacity of the non–red cell fluid component of blood (i.e., plasma) increases at decreasing temperatures asa result of the increased solubility of gas in the liquid phase that occurs as temperature declines; as a result, the net effect of hemodilution during hypothermia is to improve microvascular flow and oxygen delivery.

Despite these theoretical considerations, the optimal and maximal tolerable levels of hemodilution for a given degree of hypothermia are not established. Normovolemic hemodilution with hematocrit levels as low as 15% are believed to be well tolerated during normothermia in terms of cerebral and myocardial function as long as blood pressure, oxygenation, and cardiac output are maintained.[141,161] Long-standing practice at many centers has been to aim for hematocrit levels in the 18–22% range during deep hypothermic CPB and is based on the aforementioned improvements in blood rheology and overall oxygen-carrying capacity that accompany the combination of hemodilution and hypothermia. Animal studies and reports of children of the Jehovah's Witness faith undergoing hypothermic CPB suggest no detectable effect on overall outcome or cerebral or cardiovascular morbidity at hematocrit levels in the 10–18% range as long as low temperature, perfusion pressure, and flow rate are maintained.[71,76,141,164] Hematocrit levels of 10% or less in infants were associated with acidosis and other evidence of inadequate oxygen delivery.

More recent evidence has cast doubt on the safety of very low hematocrit levels during hypothermic CPB in infant patients. In experimental infant CPB models, higher hematocrit levels (in the 25–30% range) have been associated with enhanced preservation of brain high-energy phosphates, intracellular pH, tissue oxygenation, maintained capillary density and microvascular flow, reduced leukocyte activation, and reduced neurological injury.[45,46,78] A recent clinical study that randomized infants to either a low hematocrit level (mean hematocrit level 22% ± 3%) or high hematocrit level (28% ± 3%) strategy at the start of low-flow hypothermic CPB found lower postoperative cardiac index, higher serum lactate, and higher total body water levels in the low hematocrit group. At 1 year, overall neurological evaluations and Mental Development Index scores were similar in the two groups, but the low hematocrit group had significantly lower Psychomotor Development Index scores.[80] Our current practice is to aim to keep the hematocrit level between approximately 25 and 30% during all types of CPB. In addition to any direct effects, it is likely that the somewhat higher hematocrit level provides some degree of safety margin against other problems with perfusion, collaterals, and alterations in cerebral autoregulation and CBF.[65-67,76,85]

The optimal hematocrit level for weaning from CPB also is controversial. The overall goal is adequate systemic oxygen delivery. Based on the preceding, our current practice is to aim for hematocrit levels in the range of 25–30% during rewarming and for termination of CPB. These levels (and those perhaps even somewhat lower) are likely to be well tolerated by patients who have good myocardial function, minimal or no hemodynamic lesions, and a physiological repair with normal oxygen saturation at the conclusion of their surgery. Consideration should be given to increasing hematocrit level to improve oxygen-carrying capacity and oxygen delivery in patients with reduced myocardial function and/or palliative or staged operations that result in cyanosis. In these cases hematocrit levels of 40% or higher may be beneficial.

Pump Flow Rates during Pediatric Cardiopulmonary Bypass

Optimal pump flow rates for pediatric CPB are, as for adult CPB, based on considerations of adequate systemic oxygenation, oxygen delivery, and organ perfusion at normothermia as assessed by oxygen consumption and metabolic rate, mixed venous oxygen saturation, acid–base balance, and lactate production.[53] These are typically indexed to body weight. The higher metabolic rate of neonates and infants (approximately 1.5–2.5-fold greater than in adults) mandates proportionately higher flow rates during normothermic CPB (Table 104A-5).

Heparinization

The approach to anticoagulation during pediatric CPB is similar to that in adults. Heparin is administered in a dose of

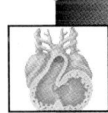

~4 mg/kg (400 U/kg) before initiation of bypass, either directly into the right atrium or into a central venous catheter; some centers include a portion of the total heparin dose in the CPB pump prime. Confirmation of heparin injection by blood aspiration, as well as the adequacy of heparin effect, should be performed before beginning CPB. The activated clotting time (ACT) is the primary method of monitoring the efficacy of heparin anticoagulation (and reversal) in infants and children. Typical guidelines require an ACT of >400 s before initiating CPB and maintaining ACTs between 400–600 s during CPB to prevent activation of blood coagulation pathways and clot formation. Inadequate concentrations of heparin are believed to be a major contributor to excessive activation of the coagulation and fibrinolytic systems.[28] Other methods of monitoring heparin effect, anticoagulation, and clotting parameters such as blood heparin concentration and thromboelastography are adjunctive at present, and are used mainly to assess residual heparin activity and diagnose and treat coagulopathies after termination of CPB.[112]

Although substantive data are scant, there is some general evidence that neonates and young infants are more sensitive to the effects of heparin administered for CPB and that the efficacy and duration of heparin-based anticoagulation is significantly more variable in neonates and young infants.[28,41,74,99,112] Potential mechanisms include the variable and generally lower levels of both procoagulant and anticoagulant factors present during the first few months of life and in some patients with congenital heart disease.[6,129,130,135] The degree of hypothermia, amount of hemodilution, and relative immaturity of drug metabolism also may contribute to increased and prolonged heparin effect in infants. Heparin resistance, on the other hand, is seen infrequently in infants, although sporadic examples resulting from recent heparin exposure or antithrombin III deficiency do occur. Heparin-induced thrombocytopenia and thrombosis appear to be less common in infants and children than in adult patients undergoing heart surgery, but the incidence may go up as the number of children who are repeatedly exposed in the operating room, catheterization laboratory, and other sites continues to increase.[127,154] At present there is only limited and anecdotal experience with the use of heparin alternatives such as hirudin and argatroban for anticoagulation during pediatric CPB.

Table 104A–5

Estimated Flow Rates for Normothermic Infant and Pediatric CPB

Body weight (kg)	*Flow range (ml/kg/min)*	*Usual "full flow" rate (ml/kg/min)*
<3	150–200	200
3–10	125–175	150
10–15	120–150	125
13–30	80–120	100

Heparin Reversal

Protamine sulfate is administered at the end of CPB to reverse the anticoagulant effects of heparin. As with heparin, there is little prospective, controlled information about the dosing of protamine in neonates and infants. Protamine dosing is usually based on body weight (3–4 mg/kg) or in a ratio to the heparin dose (mg:mg) of 1:1 or 1.3:1; in vitro titration to neutralize heparin in a patient sample also is employed by some. In general the target ACT after protamine administration is within ~10% of the pre-CPB baseline. The first two empirical methods usually result in relative protamine excess, which is intentional because of greater heparin sensitivity and duration in infants and other factors that may potentiate heparinization such as hemodilution, hypothermia, and delayed metabolic clearance. However, as for adults, there is evidence that empirical protamine dosing is associated with excess protamine administration and perhaps greater blood loss and transfusion requirements as compared with doses that directly measure blood heparin using titration or other methods.[74,99,102] Another argument against empiric dosing is that relatively small excesses of circulating protamine compared with heparin may have direct antiplatelet effects that can exacerbate bleeding after CPB.[68]

Typically the drug is administered slowly for a period of approximately 10 min. For unclear reasons, severe hypotensive, pulmonary vasoconstrictive, or anaphylactic/anaphylactoid reactions to protamine are uncommon in infants and children.[153] Of these, hypotension is most frequent, occurring in ~1.5% and 3% of protamine administrations. It is dose- and rate of administration–dependent, most likely caused by histamine release, usually fairly mild and transient, and responsive to volume replacement or calcium administration. Severe pulmonary vasoconstriction appears to be much less common in children than in adults, may be due to complement activation and/or pulmonary thromboxane release, and can be particularly problematic in patients with depressed contractile function.

Initiation of Pediatric Cardiopulmonary Bypass

CPB is initiated once the arterial and venous cannulas are correctly positioned and connected to the circuit, the absence of air in the arterial line (especially at the connection between cannula and circuit tubing) is confirmed, and adequate anticoagulation is established. Under most circumstances in neonates and infants, arterial inflow is slowly begun and then the venous line is unclamped. Rapid onset of bradycardia and loss of myocardial function can ensue when a cold prime is used. Therefore, when either normothermic or cold pump primes are used, full flow is usually reached fairly rapidly in neonates and infants to ensure adequate systemic perfusion and oxygen delivery. In situations in which it is important to keep the heart beating and potentially ejecting, electrolyte concentrations—specifically calcium and potassium—are usually normalized, along with the temperature of the prime solution, so as to maintain myocardial function and prevent myocardial distention during the initiation of bypass. Compromised venous drainage can also distend the heart and promote myocardial damage.

Large collateral vessels arising from the arterial tree (as can be seen in many forms of cyanotic heart disease, including tetralogy of Fallot and pulmonary atresia), patent ductus arteriosus, and surgical aortopulmonary shunts can promote run-off from the systemic circulation during CPB and thereby reduce perfusion pressure, effective organ (e.g., brain, heart, kidneys) blood flow, and cooling despite seemingly adequate total pump flow. Surgical control and effective occlusion of large aortopulmonary collateral vessels, surgical shunts, and the patent ductus arteriosus (PDA) is accomplished immediately before or shortly after commencing CPB. Significant aortopulmonary collateral vessels that are not important sources of pulmonary blood flow or contributors to arterial oxygenation can be coil-occluded in the cardiac catheterization laboratory before surgery, which also decreases the volume load on the systemic ventricle.

Monitoring during Pediatric Cardiopulmonary Bypass

Circuit Monitoring

Important CPB circuit variables include arterial line pressure, pump flow rate, oxygenator gases, and temperature. Arterial line pressure is measured via a pressure transducer placed in the arterial inflow limb. It can be substantially higher than patient arterial pressure because of the driving pressure required to achieve adequate flow through small-diameter infant arterial cannula and tubing, and typically is in the range of 225–260 mm Hg at mean arterial pressures of 40–60 mm Hg. Excessively high arterial line pressures (>300–400 mm Hg) can be due to tubing or cannula obstruction or cannula malposition and can result in circuit rupture. Many circuits also include a sensor on the oxygenator reservoir to detect critically low volume levels and one on the arterial line to detect air.

The flow output of roller pumps is governed by roller head rpm, occlusion pressure, and the internal tubing diameter. It is important to know that pump flow rate on roller pumps is not measured directly, but rather is calculated by the perfusionist (or electronics on the pump) based on these variables. Because the flow output of the pump is not measured directly, incorrectly measuring or inputting rpm, tubing size, or occlusion, as well as possible shunts within the circuit, can lead to potentially harmful perfusion errors (either increased or decreased). Unexpectedly low or high mean arterial pressure for the calculated flow rate may be the first clue to these possibilities. In the case of low flow in particular, abnormal biochemical variables will result if the condition is of sufficient magnitude and duration (see later).

Oxygenator gases can include oxygen, air, and carbon dioxide. Continuous in-line monitors of pH, PO_2, and PCO_2 values are used frequently. The gas "sweep speed" (flow rate) and oxygen concentration delivered to the oxygenator is controlled with a flowmeter or blender and measured with appropriate electrodes. Starting sweep speeds are usually at a ratio to pump flow rate of 1:1 for membrane oxygenators. However, the variability in pump flow rates, temperatures, and blood gas management strategies leads to wide variations in gas flow and composition in pediatric patients. Use of pH stat management can require altered gas sweep rates and the ability to add and precisely control carbon dioxide in the sweep gas.

Thermistors measure temperatures of the water bath and heat exchanger, along with arterial and venous blood temperatures. The temperature gradient between the patient and perfusate should not exceed 10° C; this may be especially important during rewarming to prevent formation of gaseous bubbles and emboli caused by decreased gas solubility as fluid temperature increases.

Patient Monitoring during Cardiopulmonary Bypass

Monitoring of mean arterial pressure is necessary during CPB. This is accomplished most often via catheters in either the radial or femoral arteries. Arterial catheter location occasionally can be governed by considerations such as prior surgical or shunt (e.g., Blalock–Taussig) sites and the current lesion and planned operation. Femoral arterial pressure monitoring (with or without concomitant radial arterial monitoring) is preferred by some for aortic reconstructions and for increased reliability when deep hypothermia is planned, particularly in small infants. Left atrial and central venous (SVC) or right atrial filling pressures also are measured routinely, depending on the surgery.

Nasopharyngeal, esophageal, and rectal temperatures are measured using appropriate thermistors. Nasopharyngeal or tympanic membrane temperatures are used most often and probably are the most accurate in terms of tracking brain temperature, although no extracranial site is truly reliable in this regard.[141] Rectal (or occasionally bladder) temperature is used to monitor core temperature. Esophageal temperature reflects aortic temperature and does not correlate well with core or brain temperatures.

Arterial and venous blood gases should be measured within 5–10 min after commencing and then at 15–30-min intervals for the remainder of CPB, and more frequently if there is evidence of compromised perfusion. In addition to pH, PO_2, and PCO_2 values, most analyzers are able to use the same samples to simultaneously measure hematocrit levels and serum electrolyte levels, including sodium, potassium, and ionized calcium. Many centers favor allowing or even promoting (for example, via the chelating effects of citrate in added blood products) reduced ionized calcium during CPB in an attempt to reduce the contribution of that cation to reperfusion injury. Ionized hypomagnesemia, another potential contributor to ischemia–reperfusion damage and dysrhythmias, has been found after pediatric CPB, although its clinical significance is uncertain at present.[109,123] Increasing blood lactate concentrations before and shortly after pediatric CPB have been suggested to correlate postoperative morbidity and mortality.[122]

The oxygen saturation of venous blood (SVO_2) is an important index of tissue perfusion, and it should be measured from venous blood samples at intervals as noted in the preceding discussion and also continuously via a calibrated in-line monitor on the venous line. Optimal and minimal acceptable values for SVO_2 during CPB, particularly as temperature and flow rate decrease, are not well defined. At normothermic or near-normothermic temperatures, SVO_2 can be interpreted in a fashion similar to non–CPB situations, and hence low values (~ <60–70%) should raise concern about inadequate tissue oxygen delivery (e.g.,

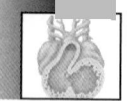

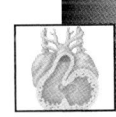

inadequate flow, low hemoglobin level) The development of shunting around major vascular beds that may occur as a consequence of CPB, in addition to any preexisting collateral vessels, may increase SVO_2 in an artifactual way; in other words, some degree of organ hypoperfusion may exist despite what appear to be acceptable SVO_2 values. At deeper levels of hypothermia, dissolved oxygen contributes an increasing proportion of total oxygen delivery, and the increased affinity of hemoglobin for oxygen impairs transfer from hemoglobin to tissue.[42] As a result, the interpretation of SVO_2 during deep hypothermia becomes more problematic, and it may be prudent to require substantially higher levels of SVO_2(~ >90%) when this measure is used to infer the adequacy of perfusion during deep hypothermic CPB.

Frequent monitoring of blood glucose level and efforts to maintain it in the normoglycemic range are important during CPB in neonates, infants, and children. The major cause of hypoglycemia appears to be limited hepatic glycogen stores and gluconeogenic capability, especially in neonates, and perhaps also in cyanotic and malnourished (e.g., congestive heart failure) infants and young children. Failure to provide exogenous glucose can result in severe hypoglycemia and neurological injury. The potential neurological consequences of hypoglycemia may be exacerbated by hypocarbia, which seems to lower the threshold for hypoglycemic neuronal damage, and by patient lesions (e.g., aortopulmonary collaterals) and bypass strategies that independently reduce cerebral autoregulation and/or CBF.[63,157,158]

Hyperglycemia also can be a frequent occurrence during pediatric CPB. Blood glucose level may increase as a result of increased supply from exogenous sources such as intravenous fluids and cardioplegia, as well as reduced glucose uptake, which is primarily due to increases in stress hormones such as cortisol, growth hormone, and catecholamines that counter the effects of insulin.[2] Additionally, deep hypothermia also can suppress glucose-stimulated insulin secretion during hypothermic CPB and for at least a few hours thereafter. It has become well accepted that hyperglycemia can potentiate cerebral ischemia–reperfusion injury under a variety of circumstances in both infants and children,[90,93,110] with a trend toward similar results in pediatric CPB patients, although these data are largely retrospective and uncontrolled.[63,165] Proposed mechanisms of hyperglycemic–ischemic brain injury include hyperosmolar cellular swelling from glucose loading and promotion of lactic acidosis and/or increased intracellular acidosis as a result of increased anaerobic glycolytic flux.

However, this issue remains controversial. Increased blood glucose concentration may be important for adequate brain glucose delivery when CBF and autoregulation are impaired. There was only a weak correlation between blood glucose with brain-specific creatine kinase isoenzyme (CK-BB) levels and no correlation with neurodevelopmental outcome in the Boston Circulatory Arrest study, and there was some evidence that post-CPB hyperglycemia was in fact protective, particularly against seizures, which are associated with worse neurodevelopmental outcomes.[20,143] Also, substantial data in a variety of non-CPB animal models indicate that preischemic hyperglycemia may protect immature brain from hypoxia, asphyxia, or hypoxia–ischemia.[24,70,173,174] One important caveat is that these studies were conducted almost exclusively in immature rat models in which circulation and ventilation were unsupported, and some of the protective effect of hyperglycemia may have been due to better maintenance of the circulation and/or ventilation in hyperglycemic animals (an effect that would be largely irrelevant during CPB).

Hypothermia

Hypothermia continues to be the mainstay for protection of the brain and other organs during CPB. Its major and most pervasive effect is to decrease metabolic rate and consequently metabolic demand for oxygen and other substrates. During ischemia, hypothermia slows consumption of high-energy phosphate compounds and also maintains them intracellularly, thereby facilitating recovery of adenosine triphosphate (ATP) and phosphocreatine during reperfusion. Hypothermia delays loss of ionic homeostasis during ischemia, particularly entry of sodium and calcium and resultant cellular edema, by energy-dependent, energy-independent, and membrane-stabilizing mechanisms.[84] Reduced amounts of free radical generation, inflammatory cytokine production, white cell activation, and leukocyte adhesion molecule synthesis have all been associated with hypothermia or hypothermic CPB. Hypothermia suppresses release of excitatory amino acid neurotransmitters during ischemia and reperfusion, which is likely to be an important cerebral protective mechanism, especially in neonatal and immature brain.[20,84]

Low-Flow Hypothermic Cardiopulmonary Bypass

The reductions in metabolic rate produced by hypothermia allow CPB flow rates to be reduced, thereby reducing the amount of blood returning to the heart and improving surgical conditions. Most centers use values of approximately 50 ml/kg/min or 0.70 l/min/m^2 for low-flow CPB. Studies in both adults and children have suggested the relative safety, particularly in terms of cerebral protection compared with deep hypothermic circulatory arrest, of this range of low-flow CPB in combination with hypothermia.[53,116,141,166,179]

Further reductions in pump flow to one fourth or less of normal rates may be used at deep levels of hypothermia (<18° C). However, there is no agreement on a "safe" degree of flow reduction for a given temperature in infants and children. Kern et al[85] have suggested that the critical pump flow rate in terms of the crucial juncture at which cerebral metabolism becomes flow dependent is between approximately 30–35 ml/kg/min at moderate hypothermia (26–29° C) and 5–30 ml/kg/min during deep hypothermia (18–22° C). The bulk of evidence suggests that cerebral autoregulation is markedly diminished or absent at temperatures below 20° C, and hence CBF becomes pressure passive at very low temperatures during CPB in infants.[67,141] Burrows and Bissonnette[21] have shown that a significant percentage of neonates and infants who undergo low-flow CPB (<22% of normal pump flow) have no detectable CBF as measured by transcranial Doppler and require higher perfusion pressures to reestablish CBF; similar results have been found by others at flow rates typical during profound (14–20° C nasopharyngeal temperature) hypothermic CPB, in which some infants lost CBF at flow rates as high as 25–35% of normal.[169] Thus it is possible that the result of low-flow CPB in at least some infants is the opposite of what

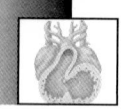

is intended in terms of using low flow to avoid deep hypothermic circulatory arrest; that is, low-flow hypothermic CPB may result in, rather than prevent, cerebral ischemia. The development of critical closing and opening pressures during may contribute to a no-reflow phenomenon and uneven brain cooling during low-flow CPB.[141] The notion of critical closing and opening pressures in the cerebral (and other vascular beds as well) also suggests that blood flow may be more dependent on arterial pressure than pump flow rate in these circumstances and that a minimum mean arterial pressure is necessary to maintain adequate flow to the brain and other organs.

Hypothermic protection of the brain during periods of low or absent flow depends on homogenous cooling of all brain regions. There is evidence that this may not occur, based on the temperature or oxygen saturation of jugular bulb venous blood, which indicates the likelihood of ongoing cerebral metabolic activity despite low tympanic or nasopharyngeal temperatures.[82,141] These data indicate that tympanic or nasopharyngeal temperatures may not identify subsets of patients with inadequately cooled brains. Risk factors for nonhomogenous and delayed brain cooling may include the position of the aortic cannula, vascular anomalies, aortopulmonary and other collaterals, blood gas or pH management strategy (see later), and the duration of cooling. For example, using alpha stat pH management, the duration of core cooling before a period of deep hypothermic circulatory arrest (DHCA) was the intraoperative variable most closely associated with postoperative cognitive outcome. Over cooling times between 11 and 18 min, increasing cooling time by 5 min increased development score by 26 points. It was speculated that shorter cooling times (~ <15 min) permitted ongoing metabolism in inhomogeneously cooled regions of the brain, making them susceptible to injury during the period of DHCA.[12] Also of interest, there was a trend for worse neurodevelopmental outcome (that did not reach not statistical significance) with cooling times longer than 20 min, perhaps as a result of the effects of prolonging exposure to the deleterious consequences of CPB, including microembolic events.

Deep Hypothermic Circulatory Arrest

DHCA has been used since the 1970s for the repair of congenital heart defects, primarily in neonates and small infants, and also occasionally in older children. Use of DHCA can decrease the length of time the patient is on CPB. This was an important advantage during the early congenital cardiac surgical experience, when limitations in CPB equipment and techniques put the neonate and small infant at increased risk. The impetus to minimize exposure to CPB has diminished as CPB methods for infants have improved. Continuous refinement of perfusion methods for neonates and infants has led to a reduction in DHCA use in many centers. Nonetheless, DHCA offers optimal surgical exposure in a small heart and chest by allowing removal of the perfusion cannulas, and its use (or similar alternatives such as DHCA alternated with periods of intermittent perfusion) is unavoidable for some lesions.

Both surface and core cooling are used before DHCA. Surface cooling is facilitated during the induction of anesthesia and surgical exposure and cannulation for CPB by lowering the room temperature as low as possible (<20° C), placing ice-filled bags around the head and neck, and positioning the patient on a cooling/warming blanket set to ~10° C. Using these methods, the usual rectal temperature at the time of initiating CPB is ~33° C (it is important to note that temperature-related dysrhythmias or ventricular fibrillation are rare in neonates and small infants at core temperatures >28–30° C). For most cases of DHCA, an ascending aortic arterial cannula (the pulmonary artery is cannulated initially for hypoplastic left heart syndrome) and single right atrial venous cannula are inserted. As noted, extremely rapid cooling (core temperature decreasing to 15–18° C in less than ~15 min) is usually avoided. The efficiency of different heat exchangers can vary widely, in part because of their surface areas relative to membrane surface area and flow rates (see Table 104A-1). Cooling is continued until both rectal and tympanic membrane temperatures are <18° C. Cardioplegia is administered, and CPB is then discontinued. Several pharmacological adjuncts are usually given as part of DHCA. Many include an α-blocker such as phentolamine or phenoxybenzamine in the pump prime to reduce vascular resistance, improve regional blood flow, and aid in homogeneous and effective cooling. High-dose methylprednisolone (30 mg/kg) is given for the reasons already discussed. Some administer sodium pentothal, 5–10 mg/kg, just before the start of DHCA to reduce cerebral electrical activity and metabolism; this is based in part on experience that up to 20–30% of neonatal brains will not be electrically silent despite tympanic and core temperatures ≤18° C. As discussed previously, a higher hematocrit level than used previously (~25–28% instead of 15–20%) is now favored by many based on evidence that it does not impair the hypothermic cerebral circulation and may be associated with improved myocardial function, less total body water accumulation, and perhaps improved performance on some neurodevelopmental tests at 1 year of age.[46,78] Finally, drainage of blood from the patient is promoted by several inflations of the lungs and manual compression of the abdomen. The venous cannula is then usually clamped and removed.

Before rewarming, initial steps are taken to remove air from the left ventricle, left atrium, and pulmonary veins. Cannulas are reinserted, and CPB is slowly resumed at 18° C.

There are different approaches to rewarming. In the oldest, rewarming begins immediately, maintaining a temperature differential between the warming circuit and patient venous blood of <10° C, and maximum water temperature is 42° C. Because concerns about cerebral injury after DHCA and information about the potential protective effects of hypothermia and harmful effects of even mild hyperthermia after a cerebral injury have increased, many centers currently undertake a period (~10–15 min) of 18° C perfusion on resumption of CPB after DHCA and try to limit both hyperthermic reperfusion (by keeping aortic perfusate temperatures lower) and post-CPB hyperthermia.[141,147,155,172] Before aortic cross-clamp removal, mannitol (0.25–0.5 g/kg) is frequently given. Ionized calcium, which had been allowed to decrease to ~0.4–0.8 mmol/L during cooling and early rewarming, is normalized once the heart has had a period of reperfusion and the core temperature has increased to ~30–32° C. It is probably important to keep both flow rate and mean arterial pressure at age-appropriate normal values because of the loss of cerebral autoregulation and consequent pressure-flow dependence of CBF after DHCA. Once calcium is normalized and the patient rewarmed to ~34° C, pulsatile ejection is stimulated by restricting venous return and ventilation begins; this is another opportunity to remove any residual intracardiac air. Observations of the heart, intracardiac filling pressures, arterial blood pressure, and other available information (e.g., contractility and filling on transesophageal echocardiography) are useful at this point to estimate the degree of inotropic support required when weaning from CPB. Typically, low doses of dopamine (~5–7.5 μg/kg/min) are all that is required.

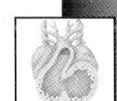

Management of Arterial Blood Gases during Pediatric Cardiopulmonary Bypass

Most centers adjust oxygen delivery to the CPB circuit such that arterial Po_2 values are in the range of approximately 400–600 torr. This hyperoxic approach is based on evidence that brain injury is greater during normoxic CPB compared with hyperoxic CPB.[128] Potential explanations for this effect include the fact that the brain mainly uses dissolved oxygen during deep hypothermic CPB, the amount of gas microemboli are decreased when nitrogen is omitted from the sweep gas, and oxygen microemboli are resorbed much faster than those containing nitrogen.[42,147] On the other hand, some centers favor significantly reducing Po_2 during CPB to reduce oxyradical production.[1,128] This mechanism may be especially important in cyanotic infants, in whom antioxidant reserves and scavenging enzyme systems may be downregulated.[1,35,128] The issue remains unresolved, and it is likely that the relative benefits of the two oxygenation strategies depend in part on the organ system in question. For example, reperfusing myocardium (especially cyanotic myocardium) at lower Po_2 may be beneficial for recovery of cardiac function, whereas it has recently been stated that the significance of hyperoxia-induced oxyradical injury to the brain is far less important than the deleterious effects of low perfusate Po_2, especially when CBF and cerebral autoregulation are impaired, as is the case with low flow deep hypothermic (or circulatory arrest) CPB.[147]

The optimal management strategy for pH and CO_2 during profound hypothermia, with or without DHCA, remains controversial. Both alpha stat and pH stat management strategies are used during pediatric CPB, and both have potential advantages and disadvantages. During hypothermia, the efficacy of the body's primary buffering systems (e.g., bicarbonate, phosphate) is markedly reduced and amino acids become the most important intracellular buffers as temperature falls; of these, the α-imidazole ring of histidine is the most effective proton acceptor (i.e., buffer). Water is less ionized (into H^+ and OH^-) as temperature falls and thus the pH of water (obviously the major fluid in the body) increases with falling temperature. The neutral point of water (i.e., the pH at which $[H^+] = [OH^-]$) also rises as temperature falls. This state (the pH where water is electrochemically neutral) is ~7.4 at 37° C and ~7.7–7.8 at profound hypothermic temperatures. Alpha stat management is based on preserving electrical neutrality at reduced temperatures and therefore the buffering capability of the α-imidazole ring of the amino acid histidine. Most enzyme, receptor, and metabolic systems function best at pH 7.4; several have been shown to function more efficiently at 20° C at pH ~7.7.[142,160] Blood from a normal patient cooled under alpha stat methods has a pH of ~7.4 and a CO_2 level of ~40 when the sample is warmed to 37° C in the blood gas analyzer. The alleged biochemical advantages of preserving electrochemical neutrality and intracellular buffering via alpha stat management include better preservation of metabolism and protein and enzyme function (by preserving intracellular pH [pH_i] and preventing abnormal charge accumulation on proteins), and slowing the diffusion of key charged intermediates such as adenosine diphosphate (ADP) and adenosine monophosphate (AMP) out of the cell, thereby promoting faster recovery of oxidative metabolism and high-energy phosphates when oxygen and substrate supply are restored.[160] Alpha stat management is likely to be associated with better preservation of cerebral autoregulation at mild to moderate hypothermic temperatures, lower CBF, and less brain swelling. These features may have a net beneficial effect in adults, in whom microemboli and cerebral edema appear to be major components of the insult compared with the higher brain blood flow and greater microemboli load associated with pH stat.[20,125] On the other hand, the alpha stat strategy causes a leftward shift in the oxyhemoglobin dissociation curve. In the setting of low flow, low perfusion pressures, and low temperatures, overall oxygen delivery under alpha stat management may be marginal to meet metabolic needs and CBF may be inadequate to evenly and effectively cool the brain.[17,20,77]

In contrast, pH stat uses a mathematical correction for the effects of temperature on pH and then adds CO_2 to the circuit to correct pH for the fall in temperature. pH stat therefore attempts to normalize the patient's pH (i.e., make it ~7.4) and Pco_2 at the hypothermic temperature; when this sample is analyzed at 37° C, it will be relatively acidotic (pH ~7.1–7.2) and hypercarbic (Pco_2 ~60–70 torr. The addition of CO_2 theoretically lowers pH_i and disrupts electrical neutrality. However, evidence suggests that pH stat may only minimally reduce pH_i.[7,167] The increase in CBF associated with pH stat, along with the rightward shift in the oxyhemoglobin dissociation curve, may favor even and effective brain cooling and oxygen delivery as long as perfusion pressure and flow are maintained. Hypercapnia decreases cerebral metabolic rate, energy use, glycolytic flux, and lactate production.[20,111,171,175] Hypercapnia and acidosis also may decrease excitatory amino acid neurotoxicity by inhibiting *N*-methyl-D-aspartate (NMDA) receptor function, glutamate release, and neuronal calcium fluxes.[20,133,171] Based on the work of Aoki and Swain and colleagues showing that cerebral pH_i becomes alkalotic during deep hypothermia even with pH stat management, it may be that the biochemical advantages of alpha stat are largely present during pH stat management and are supplemented by the effects of pH stat to increase CBF and oxygen availability because of its effect to rightward shift oxyhemoglobin dissociation.[8,166,167] These effects are likely to be paramount in the neonate and infant exposed to low flow or no flow because hypoxic and ischemic injury probably pose the greatest risk to the infant, in contrast to the adult with significant atherosclerosis and vascular disease managed at mild or moderate hypothermia, in whom minimizing microemboli and preserving autoregulation (and therefore favoring alpha stat management) may be the primary pathophysiological considerations. A small retrospective study using relatively brief cooling times (~ <15 min on average) suggested that pH stat might be preferable to alpha stat in terms of neurodevelopmental outcome when DHCA was used for Senning correction of arterial transposition.[79] In a larger, prospective, randomized single-center study, no consistent improvement or impairment could be related to pH management strategy during deep hypothermic CPB.[13] Overall, DHCA has been found to result in greater short-term (1 year of age) and long-term (8 years of age) functional neurological and neurodevelopmental deficits compared with low-flow CPB; interestingly, both pH strategies were associated with increased neurodevelopmental risk.[14]

Based on this information, many centers have begun to favor pH stat management for infant and pediatric CPB when deep hypothermia, low flow, or circulatory arrest are employed.[77-79,87,172] Patient factors also can influence this choice. The presence of cyanosis and aortopulmonary collaterals is considered by many to be an indication for pH stat management. CO_2 increases pulmonary vascular resistance, leading to improved systemic blood flow in these patients; cerebral perfusion is directly increased by CO_2 and also by the reduction in flow through the collaterals.[84,87,147]

Bleeding after Pediatric Cardiopulmonary Bypass

Bleeding is a significant problem after many cardiac surgical procedures in neonates, infants, and children. The cause in most cases is likely to be multifactorial. In addition to the difficulties surrounding heparinization and its antagonism by protamine discussed previously, there are numerous factors related to the patient, pathophysiology of the lesion, technical aspects of the operation, and the effects of CPB that can promote blood loss. Most of the procoagulant and anticoagulant blood factors are present in reduced concentration in neonates and infant; these concentrations approach adult values at varying rates over the first 6–12 months of life.[83,129,130,135] Infants therefore appear to be functionally balanced, albeit at a lower set-point, which enhances the effects of hemodilution by CPB. Reduced levels of both procoagulant and anticoagulant factors compared with age-matched controls have been found in many infants and children with congenital heart disease, particularly those with various forms of single ventricle physiology.[129-131] The etiology is unclear at present, as is whether these abnormalities are linked to any functional disturbances (either increased or decreased) in ability to clot.

Increased bleeding can occur in association with lesions that increase systemic venous pressures (e.g., Fontan physiology, Mustard or Senning atrial baffles, RV dysfunction) as a result of hepatic dysfunction, development of large venous collateral vessels, and high venous pressures. Hepatic dysfunction also can occur in lesions with significant systemic hypoperfusion (e.g., large left-to-right shunt, left-sided obstructive lesion such as critical coarctation). Cardiac lesions that generate large shear forces such as aortic stenosis and ventricular septal defects can promote the degradation of active von Willebrand factor multimers to less active and inactive monomers, leading to an acquired form of von Willebrand's disease. Prostaglandin E_1, used to maintain ductal patency preoperatively, can impair platelet function. Changes attributed to cyanosis that increase the risk of bleeding may include reduced platelet function, increased fibrinolysis, decreased total body amount of clotting factors (caused by polycythemia and hence decreased plasma volume), and the development of collateral vessels. Compared with most adult cardiac surgery, many congenital cardiac operations require extensive suture lines and reconstructions using tissue or prosthetic graft materials, often on high-pressure vessels (e.g., stage I operation for hypoplastic left heart syndrome, the arterial switch procedure). Reoperation also makes up a substantial part of pediatric cardiac surgery.

The effects of CPB on blood activation, coagulation, and fibrinolysis are arguably greater in neonates and infants because of the greater degree of hemodilution, deeper degrees of hypothermia, higher shear forces as a result of higher flow rates, more blood trauma and greater blood–air contact (higher flows, small tubing and cannulas, more cardiotomy suction), and proportionately greater degree of blood contact with the foreign surface. CPB reduces platelet number and causes platelet dysfunction by several mechanisms, including hypothermia, contact activation from the CPB circuit, activation via coagulation mechanisms, and cleavage of platelet adhesive receptors by fibrinolytic proteases that also are activated by CPB. Platelet number in neonates and small infants is approximately halved at the end of bypass surgery after protamine reversal, and platelet function is believed to be markedly impaired for the reasons outlined. Ongoing consumption of platelets and clotting factors caused by bleeding at complex and pressurized anastomotic sites can add to the problem.

Neonates who undergo CPB are likely to have normal platelet counts but reduced (compared with age-matched subjects, who, as already noted, have lower clotting factor levels compared with adult values) concentrations of factors II, VII, VIII, IX, and X. A subset of neonates may also have significantly lower fibrinogen levels at the outset, which can then be critically low at the end of bypass and be a major contributor to bleeding after bypass.[83] Other significant abnormalities at the end of CPB after protamine administration include further reductions and functionally low concentrations of factors V, VII, and VIII. Low platelet counts and fibrinogen concentrations after administration of protamine correlate with bleeding in neonates and small infants.[113]

Treatment of Bleeding after Cardiopulmonary Bypass

The treatment approach to bleeding after CPB in pediatric patients is based on the preceding considerations, driven by both the expected coagulation abnormalities and the presence of complex reconstructions and extensive vascular suture lines. Platelets are the initial therapy after adequate heparin reversal because of the documented deficiencies in platelet count and function. One to two units of platelets are typically administered to neonates and small infants to start, and up to 6–8 units in larger children. One rule of thumb is that each unit per 10 kg body weight increases platelet count by approximately 50,000/mm^3; the actual result in this setting is less, at least in part because of administration during ongoing bleeding and consumption. It also should be appreciated that platelets are supplied in fluid that is essentially plasma, so that a fair amount of clotting factors are supplied simultaneously. Cryoprecipitate is usually the next blood component administered after platelets and is chosen in part because it is a good source of fibrinogen in a relatively small volume. This sequence of platelets followed by cryoprecipitate has been shown to restore hemostasis in a majority of pediatric patients after CPB.[113] Fresh frozen plasma is usually reserved to replete measured factor deficiencies not amenable to cryoprecipitate, particularly because there is some evidence that it has little effect or may even be detrimental in most infants after CPB.[113] Some pediatric cardiac centers prefer to use fresh whole blood as the primary therapy after protamine reversal. When used within 48 h of collection, fresh whole blood contains active platelets and significant amounts of clotting factors and has been shown to reduce bleeding, transfusion requirements, and the use of other components in both neonates and adults.[100,117] A major limitation is difficulty obtaining reliable quantities within the 48-hour timeframe, in part because of required blood banking procedures and testing for infectious agents.

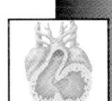

Although truly accelerated fibrinolysis is probably uncommon during pediatric CPB (and largely resolves after protamine administration),[112,113] it is likely that the activation of the fibrinolytic system that accompanies surgical trauma and bleeding, particularly in association with CPB-induced activation of coagulation and inflammatory cascades, has a significant role in consumption of clotting factors, generation of anticoagulant degradation products, and loss of adhesive receptors on platelets. For these reasons, antifibrinolytic agents such as ε-aminocaproic acid, tranexamic acid, and aprotinin have become increasingly popular. At present there is little controlled evidence that antifibrinolytic agents are beneficial in terms of blood loss, transfusion requirement, platelet dysfunction, and so on, in primary operations, although many centers use them for procedures such as arterial switch operations and stage I hypoplastic left heart reconstruction. There is substantial evidence in favor of their use for reoperation, particularly of the complex variety.[40,41,69,144] Theoretical concerns remain about potential deleterious prothrombotic consequences during low flow or deep hypothermic circulatory arrest and in tenuous anatomical or circulatory situations postoperatively (e.g., Fontan fenestration, coronary anastomoses, surgical shunts), although there are no direct reports of such and one retrospective study was unable to identify any role for these agents in similar problems.[25,69] Interestingly, meta-analyses of adult aprotinin studies indicate a protective effect against neurological injury, particularly stroke, that appears to be due at least in part to reduced patient reinfusion of shed blood.[124,159]

Organ Injury during Pediatric Cardiopulmonary Bypass

The damaging mechanisms of CPB include global (i.e., low flow or DHCA) and regional (e.g., heart, lung, gastrointestinal tract) periods of ischemia and reperfusion, activation of multiple limbs of the systemic inflammatory response, and intramyocardial and systemic air and particulate microemboli. During hypothermic CPB at full flow rates, the skeletal muscle functions as a large capacitance reservoir, and blood flow is shunted away from the vital organs to some extent. During low-flow hypothermic CPB, skeletal muscle vasculature constricts and flow to vital organs is preserved so that oxygen delivery is able to maintain oxygen consumption down to ~50% reduction in flow rate.[92] The presence of large collateral vessels, arterial obstructive lesions, cannula position, and other shunts from the systemic circulation may further compromise vital organ blood flow, as previously discussed.

Pulmonary Effects

The lungs are at significant risk for injury from CPB. This is likely to be due to hemodilution, inflammation, and ischemia and reperfusion effects.[18,150] Infants with current (e.g., infection, congestive heart failure, pulmonary overcirculation) or prior (e.g., respiratory distress syndrome, bronchopulmonary dysplasia) illness may be at greater risk. Manifestations of CPB-induced lung injury include loss of endothelium-dependent dilation and increased pulmonary vascular resistance, decreased compliance, decreased functional residual capacity, increased alveolar–arterial oxygen difference, leakage of fluid into the interstitial space, and reduced surfactant activity.[18,62,107,120,134] Hemodilution promotes fluid extravasation by reducing oncotic pressure. Activated complement, leukocytes, cytokines, and leukotrienes induce alveolar and capillary membrane damage, augment capillary leak, increase platelet and white blood cell plugging, and induce the release of additional mediators that further increase pulmonary vascular resistance and pulmonary parenchymal and vascular damage. Facilitating lung cooling by allowing a period of pulmonary blood flow on CPB during core cooling has been suggested as one means to reduce ischemic lung injury and its consequences.[27]

Renal Effects

As many as 3–7% of children have evidence of renal dysfunction after CPB.[136] Preoperative renal dysfunction or injury and low cardiac output after CPB may be the best predictors of renal dysfunction after CPB. Glomerular filtration rate and renal diluting and concentrating abilities are immature in neonates and very young infants. Low flow and reduced mean arterial pressure, nonpulsatile perfusion, and hypothermia lead to the production and release of hormones such as endothelin, catecholamines, antidiuretic hormone, atrial natriuretic factor, and rennin or angiotensin.[2,3,18,136] In addition to renal dysfunction, these factors may contribute to increased total body water, delayed fluid clearance after CPB, and related complications such as myocardial and pulmonary interstitial edema, delayed chest closure, and prolonged ventilatory support.

Brain Injury

Neurological injury continues to be one of the most problematic aspects of surgery for congenital heart disease. As overall operative mortality has declined in association with improved cardiac outcomes and life expectancy, quality-of-life issues have assumed greater importance. Prevention of neurological injury therefore has become increasingly important. Earlier retrospective series estimated the incidence of major neurological injuries after pediatric heart surgery to be between ~ 2 and 30%.[50,108,141] Although there appears to have been a progressive decline in major complications such as seizures, persistent choreoathetosis, and severe developmental delay (for reasons that are largely unknown), more subtle but significant cognitive and neurodevelopmental delays in IQ, language and motor skills, attention, learning skills, visual and spatial skills, and working memory recently have been found in children who underwent neonatal repair of arterial transposition, as well as in some single-ventricle patients and those who underwent complicated biventricular repairs; outcomes generally were worse in those who underwent DHCA.[14,15,51,52] Cognitive development also appears to be lower in school-age survivors of hypoplastic left heart syndrome and patients with Fontan physiology.[97,181] Risks for lower achievement included hypoplastic left heart syndrome, use of DHCA, and reoperation within 30 days.

It has become apparent that preoperative, intraoperative, and postoperative factors are involved.[96] The developing infant brain may be particularly susceptible to injury by hypoxia, ischemia–reperfusion, and the systemic inflammatory response because of its relatively fragile vasculature, high metabolic activity, and the fact that it is undergoing an intensive period of neuronal migration, axonal outgrowth, target finding and arborization, synaptogenesis, myelinization, astroglial development, and selective neuronal reduction (largely via apoptosis).[20] Most, if not all, of these processes are under the control of biochemical factors, neurotransmitters, and gene expression pathways that are likely to be affected by CPB and its consequences (e.g., cytokine and growth factor production, generation of oxyradical and nitroxyradical species, altered release and reuptake of excitotoxic amino acid neurotransmitters as a result of ischemia.).

A substantial number of children with congenital heart disease have genetic syndromes associated with developmental delay of various sorts, including Down syndrome and the CATCH-22 syndrome.[59] The latter is linked to microdeletions in the 22q11 region of chromosome 22, is associated with DiGeorge and velocardiofacial syndromes, manifests developmental delays in language and speech and mild hypotonia, and is present in 2–10% of children with congenital heart disease. It seems likely that other, as yet undefined genetic abnormalities result in both neurological problems and congenital heart disease. A sizable number of children with heart disease may have congenital brain malformations; more than 30% of infants with hypoplastic left heart syndrome have evidence of brain dysgenesis or other anomalies before surgery.[59,63,115] Low cardiac output, high venous pressures, thromboembolism, and chronic cyanosis are all likely to contribute to both gross and subtle neurocognitive lesions.[84,115,147]

Intraoperative causes of brain injury include abnormalities of cerebral autoregulation and cerebral perfusion, ischemia–reperfusion mechanisms, and emboli. Many of these factors have been discussed previously. The "safe" period of DHCA remains controversial and partly depends on how it is defined and under what conditions of flow, pH, temperature, cooling strategy, and patient population it is assessed. Using experimental energetic depletion or the cerebral metabolic rate for oxygen as the endpoint leads to estimates of 20–30 min or 40–65 min, respectively.[65,166] Clinical experience and some evidence suggests periods of DHCA as short as 20 min or as long as 45 min are possible before major complications such as seizures or choreoathetosis begin to increase in frequency.[20] Overall, the consensus has become that the risk of neurological injury and developmental abnormalities increase and IQ decreases in direct proportion to the duration of DHCA.*

This realization has led to evaluation of methods to avoid DHCA or reduce its duration, realizing that there are some anatomical circumstances where it cannot be avoided. The problems and potential for neurological dysfunction with low-flow hypothermic bypass have been discussed previously, and recent clinical outcome evidence supports the notion that this strategy is far from a perfect solution, although it is better than DHCA.[14,15,21,141,169] Intermittent resumption of hypothermic CPB to separate periods of DHCA and use of selective cerebral perfusion to avoid or reduce DHCA appear to be attractive options,[89,137-139] although they have yet to be subjected to widespread and thorough appraisals.[78]

The postbypass period also is receiving increased attention as a vulnerable period for neurological injury. As discussed, both low-flow deep hypothermic CPB and DHCA techniques can lead to compromises in CBF and metabolism. Therefore ensuring appropriate cardiac output, cerebral perfusion pressure, and oxygen delivery (i.e., appropriate hematocrit for the level of oxygen saturation and cardiac output) in the postoperative period are important. In addition to standard volume replacement and inotropic maneuvers, more novel strategies to support cardiac output in this setting include delayed sternal closure and ready use of ECMO.[47,106,172] Maintaining normothermic or even mildly hypothermic body temperatures in the first 24–48 h postoperatively also may be beneficial.[155]

The Stress Response to Cardiopulmonary Bypass

The stress response to CPB is characterized by the release of a large number and diverse group of neurohumoral substances, including catecholamines, endothelin, various prostaglandins, cortisol, and growth hormone. The concentrations measured in neonates and infants during and/or soon after CPB are some of the highest measured in humans and generally exceed those measured in adult CPB patients by fivefold to tenfold.[2,4] Stimuli include extensive and prolonged foreign surface contact, profound hypothermia, low flow, low perfusion pressure, and nonpulsatile perfusion. Clearance of many of these compounds by the liver, kidney, or lungs also may be delayed. Possible deleterious consequences include vasoconstriction and reduced organ perfusion, direct tissue injury, pulmonary hypertension, endothelial damage, and increased pulmonary vasoreactivity.

On the other hand, the release of many of these compounds and the overall response clearly has adaptive benefits. It is unclear what level, circumstances, or substances causes a net harmful response, to what extent acutely ill infants with congenital heart disease require some degree of stress response for hemodynamic stability, wound repair, and overall homeostasis, and to what degree the seemingly exaggerated response seen particularly in neonates and

---

*References 14, 44, 51, 52, 77, 180, 182.

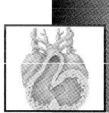

infants exposed to CPB is pathological and should be attenuated. Decreased stress response hormones and possibly improved morbidity and mortality have been associated with high-dose synthetic opioid administration to infants undergoing CPB and other stressful procedures.[4,5]

The Systemic Inflammatory Response to Cardiopulmonary Bypass

CPB causes a systemic inflammatory response via multiple mechanisms. These mechanisms include surgical trauma, blood contact with the CPB circuit, ischemia–reperfusion injury, and protamine administration.* These initiating events stimulate complex and interconnected cell- and humoral-based systems that include activation of the complement, coagulation, and fibrinolytic pathways; endotoxin release; cytokine production; endothelial activation and expression of leukocyte adhesion molecules; leukocyte and platelet activation; and production and release of oxyradicals, nitric oxide, prostanoids, eicosanoids, and proteolytic enzymes (e.g., myeloperoxidase and superoxide from activate neutrophils).

Complement activation occurs via both the alternate (stimulated by foreign surface contact, endotoxin, and kallikrein) and classical (protamine) pathways. Significant increases in activated complement fragments occur with initiation of bypass, and further still during rewarming, and these levels have correlated with renal, cardiac, and pulmonary dysfunction after CPB.[18,22,94,150,151] Various complement fragments cause white cell and platelet activation, white cell free radical production and degranulation, smooth muscle constriction, and capillary leak. Terminal complement fragments and the membrane attack complex can cause direct cell lysis.

Blood concentrations of bacterial endotoxin can increase because of its almost ubiquitous presence in sterile fluids and equipment, and also perhaps because of decreased intestinal perfusion, which also can augment reperfusion injury independent of endotoxin.[88,119] Endotoxin can directly injure endothelial cells and cause capillary leak, as well as stimulate the production of proinflammatory cytokines such as tumor necrosis factor (TNF), interleukin-1 (IL-1), interleukin-6 (IL-6), and interleukin-8 (IL-8). Cytokine production also can be stimulated by foreign surface contact, complement fragments, and other cytokines. Mechanisms of cytokine-induced tissue injury are multiple.

Cytokines such as IL-1 and TNF are directly toxic to endothelial and other cells; cause wasting, edema, and myocardial contractile dysfunction; and stimulate a number of cytotoxic and cytoprotective signaling mechanisms such as inducible (high-output and potentially cytotoxic) nitric oxide production, various proapoptotic and antiapoptotic pathways and proteins, enhanced oxyradical injury, and induction of cellular antioxidant enzymes. Levels of TNF and IL-1 are inconsistently increased by CPB in neonates and infants. Cytokine-induced nitric oxide (NO) production can result in profound hypotension (it is the major mechanism of vascular depression in septic shock), myocardial depression, and inhibition of cellular respiration and metabolism. IL-6 has been demonstrated in some studies to be a good predictor of clinical outcome and may be related to the extent of tissue injury.[18] IL-8 is a potent neutrophil chemoattractant and also causes leukocytosis and activation of neutrophil proteases and free radical enzymes. Increased IL-8 has been found in pediatric CPB in proportion to ischemic and total bypass times.[18,81,134,152] Some children have increased levels of some cytokines preoperatively; the cause(s) and significance of this finding are uncertain, but there is some evidence that neonates with a preoperative biochemical profile consistent with inflammation (e.g., increased plasma elastase and complement fragments) are more likely to manifest a capillary leak syndrome postoperatively.[152]

Neutrophil activation is believed to be an important mechanism of cellular injury during and after CPB. It is produced by a wide variety of stimuli, including foreign surface contact, endotoxin, cytokines, complement, platelet activating factor, and ischemia–reperfusion. Activated neutrophils express proadhesive molecules on their cell surface that are complementary to ones induced on endothelial and other cell membranes, marginate into the tissue, have increased lipoxygenase and myeloperoxidase activities (the source of superoxide and hypochlorous acid, respectively), and release neutrophil elastase. These products cause damage to lipids, proteins, and DNA. Elastase also causes endothelial damage, inactivates serine proteases in the coagulation pathway, and cleaves adhesive receptors from the platelet membrane.[20,176-178] Both myeloperoxidase and elastase, as well as evidence of neutrophil-mediated oxidant injury, have been detected after pediatric CPB.[1,18,91]

It recently has become apparent that CPB also induces a corresponding increase in antiinflammatory cytokines such as IL-10 and IL-1 receptor antagonist (IL-1ra). C-reactive protein (CRP), an acute phase protein that is a marker of inflammation and has antiinflammatory effects by decreasing neutrophil chemotaxis, also increases during and after pediatric CPB.* Transient immunosuppression mediated by these events and others such as loss of activated neutrophils and inhibition of cellular immune responses have also been found after pediatric CPB[165].

Overall there is substantial variability in the release pattern and plasma concentrations of cytokines in infants and children undergoing cardiac surgery compared with adults.[32,103,104,134,152] Although increased elements of the systemic inflammatory response generally are associated with increased risk of postoperative organ dysfunction and morbidity and mortality, better-designed studies with direct assays and endpoints are necessary to truly define any cause-and-effect relationship between systemic inflammatory response mediators and organ damage. It is also likely that the balance between proinflammatory and antiinflammatory stimuli and their diverse effects on a wide range of cellular types and functions must be taken into account.

Current Approaches to Limiting the Negative Consequences of Pediatric Cardiopulmonary Bypass

Many efforts and potential targets to decrease the negative impact of CPB in infants and children have been discussed

*References 9, 22, 32, 33, 60, 140, 150-152.

*References 18, 32, 33, 150, 152, 168.

 previously. These include modifications to reduce circuit area and volume, improve venous drainage, and define the optimal pH, hematocrit, temperature, flow rate, arterial pressure, and duration of CPB and/or DHCA.

Steroids

Administration of relatively high doses of steroids before pediatric CPB (either dexamethasone or methylprednisolone) may suppress the production of proinflammatory cytokines and improve organ function.[19,48,89,156] Because a major effect of steroid treatment is to alter gene expression and cellular activation, maximal effect may require administration some time before bypass (up to 8 h) and repeated dosing.[172] Improvements in body water accumulation, alveolar–arterial oxygen gradients, pulmonary artery pressure, and duration of mechanical ventilation and length of ICU stay have been observed.[19,48,172] Results from more extensive investigations in adults confirm beneficial alterations in the balance of proinflammatory to antiinflammatory mediators.[29] However, there were no significant effects on fluid balance and possibly detrimental effects on pulmonary function and glucose homeostasis (hyperglycemia). Furthermore, as with the stress response, it remains unclear whether broad-spectrum suppression of the systemic inflammatory response is beneficial. These differences may be due in part to the fact that steroids may be more likely to show a positive effect in neonates and infants, in whom the magnitude and consequences appear to be greater. On the other hand, it seems that caution is warranted until large, randomized, prospective, placebo-controlled studies with tightly regulated perioperative management are performed in pediatric patients.

Aprotinin

Aprotinin is another agent that has recently gained favor in terms of limiting the systemic inflammatory response to CPB in both infants and adults.[105,118,121,176] In addition to inhibiting fibrinolysis, it also has the ability to inhibit activation of the kallikrein and complement pathways, albeit at fairly high plasma concentrations. Inhibition of fibrinolytic proteases, in addition to reducing bleeding and helping maintain platelet function, also may decrease generation of fibrin degradation products, which also are proinflammatory. Oxygenation index and duration of mechanical ventilation also were improved by aprotinin in one recent study.[121] The incidence of anaphylactic reactions is reported to be between ~0.3 and 1.0% and is far more likely in conjunction with a reexposure. Although the risk of reexposure decreases significantly after approximately 6 months, it may be prudent to delay administration until surgical exposure and cannulation are complete in the setting of reoperative surgery and known (or potential) prior history of aprotinin treatment. At present there do not appear to be any other contraindications to aprotinin use in neonates and infants, although concern remains regarding the potential to favor clot formation, especially in low-flow or DHCA circumstances and certain surgical situations (e.g., low-flow pathways such as Glenn and Fontan connections, Fontan fenestrations, and coronary anastomoses).

Ultrafiltration

Both conventional and modified ultrafiltration are being used with increasing frequency during pediatric cardiac surgery. Potential beneficial mechanisms include hemoconcentration, removal of various inflammatory mediators and vasoactive compounds in the ultrafiltrate, and decreased total body water and tissue edema. Significant clinical improvements in tissue edema, post-CPB weight gain, hematocrit, blood pressure, global left ventricular function, lung compliance, oxygenation, and duration of mechanical ventilation have been reported, along with decreased postoperative bleeding, decreased postoperative transfusion and blood product requirements, and decreased pulmonary vascular resistance; one or more of these benefits have been observed in many, but not all, studies.* Less certain are the mechanisms responsible for these effects, because significant reductions in blood concentrations of inflammatory cytokines, complement fragments, and prostanoids have not been universally identified.[33,58,75] Although ultrafiltration techniques appear to be safe for infants and children, there is theoretical concern about removal of protective mediators and deleterious increases in viscosity and clotting factors (i.e., hypercoagulability). Future studies are needed to define the mechanisms of ultrafiltration effect and identify patients who are most likely to benefit.

REFERENCES

1. Allen BS: The clinical significance of the reoxygenation injury in pediatric heart surgery. Semin Thorac Cardiovasc Surg Pediatr Card Surg Annu 6:116–127, 2003.
2. Anand KJ, Hansen DD, Hickey PR: Hormonal-metabolic stress responses in neonates undergoing cardiac surgery. Anesthesiology 73:661–670, 1990.
3. Anand KJ, Hickey PR: Pain and its effects in the human neonate and fetus. N Engl J Med 317:1321–1329, 1987.
4. Anand KJ, Hickey PR: Halothane-morphine compared with high-dose sufentanil for anesthesia and postoperative analgesia in neonatal cardiac surgery. N Engl J Med 326:1–9, 1992.
5. Anand KJ, Sippell WG, Aynsley-Green A: Randomised trial of fentanyl anaesthesia in preterm babies undergoing surgery: effects on the stress response. Lancet 1:62–66, 1987.
6. Andrew M, Paes B, Milner R, et al: Development of the human coagulation system in the full-term infant. Blood 70:165–172, 1987.
7. Aoki M, Jonas RA, Nomura F, et al: Effects of aprotinin on acute recovery of cerebral metabolism in piglets after hypothermic circulatory arrest. Ann Thorac Surg 58:146–153, 1994.
8. Aoki M, Nomura F, Stromski ME, et al: Effects of pH on brain energetics after hypothermic circulatory arrest. Ann Thorac Surg 55:1093–1103, 1993.
9. Ashraf SS, Tian Y, Zacharrias S, et al: Effects of cardiopulmonary bypass on neonatal and paediatric inflammatory profiles. Eur J Cardiothorac Surg 12:862–868, 1997.
10. Bando K, Vijay P, Turrentine MW, et al: Dilutional and modified ultrafiltration reduces pulmonary hypertension after operations for congenital heart disease: A prospective ran-

*References 10, 30, 33, 49, 55, 57, 58, 73, 81, 98.

domized study. J Thorac Cardiovasc Surg 115:517–525; discussion 525–527, 1998.
11. Barratt-Boyes B: Complete correction of cardiovascular malformations in the first two years of life using profound hypothermia. In Barratt-Boyes BG, Neutze JM, Harris EA, editors: Heart Disease in Infancy, p. 35. Edinburgh: Churchill Livingstone, 1973.
12. Bellinger DC, Wernovsky G, Rappaport LA, et al: Cognitive development of children following early repair of transposition of the great arteries using deep hypothermic circulatory arrest. Pediatrics 87:701–707, 1991.
13. Bellinger DC, Wypij D, du Plessis AJ, et al: Developmental and neurologic effects of alpha-stat versus pH-stat strategies for deep hypothermic cardiopulmonary bypass in infants. J Thorac Cardiovasc Surg 121:374–383, 2001.
14. Bellinger DC, Wypij D, duDuplessis AJ, et al: Neurodevelopmental status at eight years in children with dextrotransposition of the great arteries: The Boston Circulatory Arrest Trial. J Thorac Cardiovasc Surg 126:1385–1396, 2003.
15. Bellinger DC, Wypij D, Kuban KC et al. Developmental and neurological status of children at 4 years of age after heart surgery with hypothermic circulatory arrest or low-flow cardiopulmonary bypass. Circulation 100:526–532, 1999.
16. Boks RH, van Herwerden LA, Takkenberg JJ, et al: Is the use of albumin in colloid prime solution of cardiopulmonary bypass circuit justified? Ann Thorac Surg 72:850–853, 2001.
17. Bove EL, West HL, Paskanik AM: Hypothermic cardiopulmonary bypass: A comparison between alpha and pH stat regulation in the dog. J Surg Res 42:66–73, 1987.
18. Brix-Christensen V: The systemic inflammatory response after cardiac surgery with cardiopulmonary bypass in children. Acta Anaesthesiol Scand 45:671–679, 2001.
19. Bronicki RA, Backer CL, Baden HP, et al: Dexamethasone reduces the inflammatory response to cardiopulmonary bypass in children. Ann Thorac Surg 69:1490–1495, 2000.
20. Burrows F, McGowan FX: Neurodevelopmental consequences of cardiac surgery for congenital heart disease. In Greeley W, editor: Perioperative management of the patient with congenital heart disease, p. 97. Baltimore: Williams & Wilkins, 1996.
21. Burrows FA, Bissonnette B: Cerebral blood flow velocity patterns during cardiac surgery utilizing profound hypothermia with low-flow cardiopulmonary bypass or circulatory arrest in neonates and infants. Can J Anaesth 40:298–307, 1993.
22. Butler J, Rocker GM, Westaby S: Inflammatory response to cardiopulmonary bypass. Ann Thorac Surg 55:552–559, 1993.
23. Byrick RJ, Kay C, Noble WH: Extravascular lung water accumulation in patients following coronary artery surgery. Can Anaesth Soc J 24:332–345, 1977.
24. Callahan DJ, Engle MJ, Volpe JJ: Hypoxic injury to developing glial cells: Protective effect of high glucose. Pediatr Res 27:186–190, 1990.
25. Casta A, Gruber EM, Laussen PC, et al: Parameters associated with perioperative baffle fenestration closure in the Fontan operation. J Cardiothorac Vasc Anesth 14:553–556, 2000.
26. Castaneda AR, Lamberti J, Sade RM, et al: Open-heart surgery during the first three months of life. J Thorac Cardiovasc Surg 68:719–731, 1974.
27. Chai PJ, Williamson JA, Lodge AJ, et al: Effects of ischemia on pulmonary dysfunction after cardiopulmonary bypass. Ann Thorac Surg 67:731–735, 1999.
28. Chan AK, Leaker M, Burrows FA, et al: Coagulation and fibrinolytic profile of paediatric patients undergoing cardiopulmonary bypass. Thromb Haemost 77:270–277, 1997.
29. Chaney MA: Corticosteroids and cardiopulmonary bypass: A review of clinical investigations. Chest 121:921–931, 2002.
30. Chaturvedi RR, Shore DF, White PA, et al: Modified ultrafiltration improves global left ventricular systolic function after open-heart surgery in infants and children. Eur J Cardiothorac Surg 15:742–746, 1999.
31. Cherup LL, Siewers RD, Futrell JW: Breast and pectoral muscle maldevelopment after anterolateral and posterolateral thoracotomies in children. Ann Thorac Surg 41:492–497, 1986.
32. Chew MS, Brandslund I, Brix-Christensen V, et al: Tissue injury and the inflammatory response to pediatric cardiac surgery with cardiopulmonary bypass: A descriptive study. Anesthesiology 94:745–753; discussion 5A, 2001.
33. Chew MS, Brix-Christensen V, Ravn HB, et al: Effect of modified ultrafiltration on the inflammatory response in paediatric open-heart surgery: A prospective, randomized study. Perfusion 17:327–333, 2002.
34. Chiba Y, Morioka K, Muraoka R, et al: Effects of depletion of leukocytes and platelets on cardiac dysfunction after cardiopulmonary bypass. Ann Thorac Surg 65:107-113; discussion 113–114, 1998.
35. Cowan DB, Weisel RD, Williams WG, Mickle DA: The regulation of glutathione peroxidase gene expression by oxygen tension in cultured human cardiomyocytes. J Mol Cell Cardiol 24:423–433, 1992.
36. Davila RM, Rawles T, Mack MJ: Venoarterial air embolus: A complication of vacuum-assisted venous drainage. Ann Thorac Surg 71:1369–1371, 2001.
37. del Nido PJ: Myocardial protection and cardiopulmonary bypass in neonates and infants. Ann Thorac Surg 64:878–879, 1997.
38. del Nido PJ, Mickle DA, Wilson GJ, et al: Inadequate myocardial protection with cold cardioplegic arrest during repair of tetralogy of Fallot. J Thorac Cardiovasc Surg 95:223–229, 1988.
39. D'Errico C, Shayevitz JR, Martindale SJ: Age-related differences in heparin sensitivity and heparin-protamine interactions in cardiac surgery patients. J Cardiothorac Vasc Anesth 10:451–457, 1996.
40. D'Errico CC, Munro HM, Bove EL: Pro: The routine use of aprotinin during pediatric cardiac surgery is a benefit. J Cardiothorac Vasc Anesth 13:782–784, 1999.
41. D'Errico CC, Shayevitz JR, Martindale SJ, et al: The efficacy and cost of aprotinin in children undergoing reoperative open heart surgery. Anesth Analg 83:1193–1199, 1996.
42. Dexter F, Kern FH, Hindman BJ, Greeley WJ: The brain uses mostly dissolved oxygen during profoundly hypothermic cardiopulmonary bypass. Ann Thorac Surg 63:1725–1729, 1997.
43. Dreyer WJ, Michael LH, Millman EE, et al: Neutrophil sequestration and pulmonary dysfunction in a canine model of open heart surgery with cardiopulmonary bypass. Evidence for a CD18-dependent mechanism. Circulation 92:2276–2283, 1995.
44. du Plessis AJ, Bellinger DC, Gauvreau K, et al: Neurologic outcome of choreoathetoid encephalopathy after cardiac surgery. Pediatr Neurol 27:9–17, 2002.
45. Duebener LF, Hagino I, Sakamoto T, et al: Effects of pH management during deep hypothermic bypass on cerebral microcirculation: Alpha-stat versus pH-stat. Circulation 106:I103–I108, 2002.
46. Duebener LF, Sakamoto T, Hatsuoka S, et al: Effects of hematocrit on cerebral microcirculation and tissue oxygenation during deep hypothermic bypass. Circulation 104:I260–I264, 2001.
47. Duncan BW, Hraska V, Jonas RA, et al: Mechanical circulatory support in children with cardiac disease. J Thorac Cardiovasc Surg 117:529–542, 1999.
48. El Azab SR, Rosseel PM, de Lange JJ, et al: Dexamethasone decreases the pro- to anti-inflammatory cytokine ratio during cardiac surgery. Br J Anaesth 88:496–501, 2002.

49. Elliott MJ: Ultrafiltration and modified ultrafiltration in pediatric open heart operations. Ann Thorac Surg 56:1518–1522, 1993.
50. Ferry PC: Neurologic sequelae of open-heart surgery in children. An 'irritating question.' Am J Dis Child 144:369–373, 1990.
51. Forbess JM, Visconti KJ, Bellinger DC, et al: Neurodevelopmental outcomes after biventricular repair of congenital heart defects. J Thorac Cardiovasc Surg 123:631–639, 2002.
52. Forbess JM, Visconti KJ, Hancock-Friesen C, et al: Neurodevelopmental outcome after congenital heart surgery: results from an institutional registry. Circulation 106:I95–I102, 2002.
53. Fox LS, Blackstone EH, Kirklin JW, et al: Relationship of whole body oxygen consumption to perfusion flow rate during hypothermic cardiopulmonary bypass. J Thorac Cardiovasc Surg 83:239–248, 1982.
54. Friehs I, del Nido PJ: Increased susceptibility of hypertrophied hearts to ischemic injury. Ann Thorac Surg 75:S678–S684, 2003.
55. Friesen RH, Campbell DN, Clarke DR, Tornabene MA: Modified ultrafiltration attenuates dilutional coagulopathy in pediatric open heart operations. Ann Thorac Surg 64:1787–1789, 1997.
56. Friesen RH, Thieme R: Changes in anterior fontanel pressure during cardiopulmonary bypass and hypothermic circulatory arrest in infants. Anesth Analg 66:94–96, 1987.
57. Gaynor JW: Use of ultrafiltration during and after cardiopulmonary bypass in children. J Thorac Cardiovasc Surg 122:209–211, 2001.
58. Gaynor JW: The effect of modified ultrafiltration on the postoperative course in patients with congenital heart disease. Semin Thorac Cardiovasc Surg Pediatr Card Surg Annu 6:128–139, 2003.
59. Gerdes M, Solot C, Wang PP, et al: Cognitive and behavior profile of preschool children with chromosome 22q11.2 deletion. Am J Med Genet 85:127–133, 1999.
60. Gessler P, Pfenninger J, Pfammatter JP, et al: Inflammatory response of neutrophil granulocytes and monocytes after cardiopulmonary bypass in pediatric cardiac surgery. Intensive Care Med 28:1786–1791, 2002.
61. Gibbon JH Jr: Application of a mechanical heart and lung apparatus to cardiac surgery. Minn Med 37:171–185; passim, 1954.
62. Gillinov AM, Redmond JM, Zehr KJ, et al: Inhibition of neutrophil adhesion during cardiopulmonary bypass. Ann Thorac Surg 57:126–133, 1994.
63. Glauser TA, Rorke LB, Weinberg PM, Clancy RR: Acquired neuropathologic lesions associated with the hypoplastic left heart syndrome. Pediatrics 85:991–1000, 1990.
64. Glauser TA, Rorke LB, Weinberg PM, Clancy RR: Congenital brain anomalies associated with the hypoplastic left heart syndrome. Pediatrics 85:984–990, 1990.
65. Greeley WJ, Kern FH, Ungerleider RM, et al: The effect of hypothermic cardiopulmonary bypass and total circulatory arrest on cerebral metabolism in neonates, infants, and children. J Thorac Cardiovasc Surg 101:783–794, 1991.
66. Greeley WJ, Ungerleider RM: Assessing the effect of cardiopulmonary bypass on the brain. Ann Thorac Surg 52:417–419, 1991.
67. Greeley WJ, Ungerleider RM, Kern FH, et al: Effects of cardiopulmonary bypass on cerebral blood flow in neonates, infants, and children. Circulation 80:I209–I215, 1989.
68. Griffin MJ, Rinder HM, Smith BR, et al: The effects of heparin, protamine, and heparin/protamine reversal on platelet function under conditions of arterial shear stress. Anesth Analg 93:20–27, 2001.
69. Gruber EM, Shukla AC, Reid RW, et al: Synthetic antifibrinolytics are not associated with an increased incidence of baffle fenestration closure after the modified Fontan procedure. J Cardiothorac Vasc Anesth 14:257–259, 2000.
70. Hattori H, Wasterlain CG: Posthypoxic glucose supplement reduces hypoxic-ischemic brain damage in the neonatal rat. Ann Neurol 28:122–128, 1990.
71. Henling CE, Carmichael MJ, Keats AS, Cooley DA: Cardiac operation for congenital heart disease in children of Jehovah's Witnesses. J Thorac Cardiovasc Surg 89:914–920, 1985.
72. Hickey PR, Andersen NP: Deep hypothermic circulatory arrest: A review of pathophysiology and clinical experience as a basis for anesthetic management. J Cardiothorac Anesth 1:137–155, 1987.
73. Hiramatsu T, Imai Y, Kurosawa H, et al: Effects of dilutional and modified ultrafiltration in plasma endothelin-1 and pulmonary vascular resistance after the Fontan procedure. Ann Thorac Surg 73:861–865, 2002.
74. Horkay F, Martin P, Rajah SM, Walker DR: Response to heparinization in adults and children undergoing cardiac operations. Ann Thorac Surg 53:822–826, 1992.
75. Huang H, Yao T, Wang W, et al: Continuous ultrafiltration attenuates the pulmonary injury that follows open heart surgery with cardiopulmonary bypass. Ann Thorac Surg 76:136–140, 2003.
76. Johnston WE, Jenkins LW, Lin CY, et al: Cerebral metabolic consequences of hypotensive challenges in hemodiluted pigs with and without cardiopulmonary bypass. Anesth Analg 81:911–918, 1995.
77. Jonas RA: Hypothermia, circulatory arrest, and the pediatric brain. J Cardiothorac Vasc Anesth 10:66–74, 1996.
78. Jonas RA: Deep hypothermic circulatory arrest: Current status and indications. Semin Thorac Cardiovasc Surg Pediatr Card Surg Annu 5:76–88, 2002.
79. Jonas RA, Bellinger DC, Rappaport LA, et al: Relation of pH strategy and developmental outcome after hypothermic circulatory arrest. J Thorac Cardiovasc Surg 106:362–368, 1993.
80. Jonas RA, Wypij D, Roth SJ, et al: The influence of hemodilution on outcome after hypothermic cardiopulmonary bypass: Results of a randomized trial in infants. J Thorac Cardiovasc Surg 126:1765–1774, 2003.
81. Journois D, Pouard P, Greeley WJ, et al: Hemofiltration during cardiopulmonary bypass in pediatric cardiac surgery. Effects on hemostasis, cytokines, and complement components. Anesthesiology 81:1181–1189; discussion 26A–27A, 1994.
82. Kern FH, Jonas RA, Mayer JE Jr, et al: Temperature monitoring during CPB in infants: does it predict efficient brain cooling? Ann Thorac Surg 54:749–754, 1992.
83. Kern FH, Morana NJ, Sears JJ, Hickey PR: Coagulation defects in neonates during cardiopulmonary bypass. Ann Thorac Surg 54:541–546, 1992.
84. Kern FH, Schulman S, Greeley WJ: Cardiopulmonary bypass: techniques and effects. In Greeley WJ, editor: Perioperative Management of the Patient with Congenital Heart Disease, pp. 67–120. Baltimore: Williams & Wilkins, 1996.
85. Kern FH, Ungerleider RM, Reves JG, et al: Effect of altering pump flow rate on cerebral blood flow and metabolism in infants and children. Ann Thorac Surg 56:1366–1372, 1993.
86. Kirklin JW: The middle 1950s and C. Walton Lillehei. J Thorac Cardiovasc Surg 98:822–824, 1989.
87. Kirshbom PM, Skaryak LA, DiBernardo LR, et al: Effects of aortopulmonary collaterals on cerebral cooling and cerebral metabolic recovery after circulatory arrest. Circulation 92:II490–II494, 1995.
88. Koike K, Moore EE, Moore FA, et al: Gut ischemia/reperfusion produces lung injury independent of endotoxin. Crit Care Med 22:1438–1444, 1994.

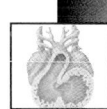

89. Langley SM, Chai PJ, Miller SE, et al: Intermittent perfusion protects the brain during deep hypothermic circulatory arrest. Ann Thorac Surg 68:4–12; discussion 12–13, 1999.
90. Lanier WL: Glucose management during cardiopulmonary bypass: Cardiovascular and neurologic implications. Anesth Analg 72:423–427, 1991.
91. Larson DF, Bowers M, Schechner HW: Neutrophil activation during cardiopulmonary bypass in paediatric and adult patients. Perfusion 11:21–27, 1996.
92. Lazenby W, Ko W, Zelano JA, et al: Effects of temperature and flow rate on regional blood flow and metabolism during cardiopulmonary bypass. Ann Thorac Surg 54:449–459, 1981.
93. LeBlanc MH, Huang M, Patel D, et al: Glucose given after hypoxic ischemia does not affect brain injury in piglets. Stroke 25:1443–1447; discussion 1448, 1994.
94. Li RK, Shaikh N, Weisel RD, et al: Oxyradical-induced antioxidant and lipid changes in cultured human cardiomyocytes. Am J Physiol 266:H2204–H2211, 1994.
95. Lillehei CW, Varco RL, Cohen M, et al: The first open-heart repairs of ventricular septal defect, atrioventricular communis, and tetralogy of Fallot using extracorporeal circulation by cross-circulation: A 30-year follow-up. Ann Thorac Surg 41:4–21, 1986.
96. Limperopoulos C, Majnemer A, Shevell MI, et al: Neurodevelopmental status of newborns and infants with congenital heart defects before and after open heart surgery. J Pediatr 137:638–645, 2000.
97. Mahle WT, Spray TL, Wernovsky G, et al: Survival after reconstructive surgery for hypoplastic left heart syndrome: A 15-year experience from a single institution. Circulation 102:III136–III141, 2000.
98. Maluf MA, Mangia C, Silva C, et al: Conventional and conventional plus modified ultrafiltration during cardiac surgery in high-risk congenital heart disease. J Cardiovasc Surg (Torino) 42:465–473, 2001.
99. Malviya S. Monitoring and management of anticoagulation in children requiring extracorporeal circulation. Semin Thromb Hemost 23:563–567, 1997.
100. Manno CS, Hedberg KW, Kim HC, et al: Comparison of the hemostatic effects of fresh whole blood, stored whole blood, and components after open heart surgery in children. Blood 77:930–936, 1991.
101. Marelli D, Paul A, Samson R, et al: Does the addition of albumin to the prime solution in cardiopulmonary bypass affect clinical outcome? A prospective randomized study. J Thorac Cardiovasc Surg 98:751–756, 1989.
102. Martindale SJ, Shayevitz JR, D'Errico C: The activated coagulation time: Suitability for monitoring heparin effect and neutralization during pediatric cardiac surgery. J Cardiothorac Vasc Anesth 10:458–463, 1996.
103. McBride WT, Armstrong MA, Crockard AD, et al: Cytokine balance and immunosuppressive changes at cardiac surgery: Contrasting response between patients and isolated CPB circuits. Br J Anaesth 75:724–733, 1995.
104. McBride WT, Booth JV: Human cytokine responses to cardiac operations: Prebypass factors. J Thorac Cardiovasc Surg 112:560–561, 1996.
105. McDonough J, Gruenwald C: The use of aprotinin in pediatric patients: A review. J Extra Corpor Technol 35:346–349, 2003.
106. McElhinney DB, Reddy VM, Parry AJ, et al: Management and outcomes of delayed sternal closure after cardiac surgery in neonates and infants. Crit Care Med 28:1180–1184, 2000.
107. McGowan FX Jr, Ikegami M, del Nido PJ, et al: Cardiopulmonary bypass significantly reduces surfactant activity in children. J Thorac Cardiovasc Surg 106:968–977, 1993.
108. Menache CC, du Plessis AJ, Wessel DL, et al: Current incidence of acute neurologic complications after open-heart operations in children. Ann Thorac Surg 73:1752–1758, 2002.
109. Mencia S, De Lucas N, Lopez-Herce J, et al: Magnesium metabolism after cardiac surgery in children. Pediatr Crit Care Med 3:158–162, 2002.
110. Michaud LJ, Rivara FP, Longstreth WT Jr, Grady MS: Elevated initial blood glucose levels and poor outcome following severe brain injuries in children. J Trauma 31:1356–1362, 1991.
111. Miller AL, Corddry DH: Brain carbohydrate metabolism in developing rats during hypercapnia. J Neurochem 36:1202–1210, 1981.
112. Miller BE, Guzzetta NA, Tosone SR, Levy JH: Rapid evaluation of coagulopathies after cardiopulmonary bypass in children using modified thromboelastography. Anesth Analg 90:1324–1330, 2000.
113. Miller BE, Mochizuki T, Levy JH, et al: Predicting and treating coagulopathies after cardiopulmonary bypass in children. Anesth Analg 85:1196–1202, 1997.
114. Miller BE, Tosone SR, Tam VK, et al: Hematologic and economic impact of aprotinin in reoperative pediatric cardiac operations. Ann Thorac Surg 66:535–540; discussion 541, 1998.
115. Miller G, Vogel H: Structural evidence of injury or malformation in the brains of children with congenital heart disease. Semin Pediatr Neurol 6:20–26, 1999.
116. Miyamoto K, Kawashima Y, Matsuda H, et al: Optimal perfusion flow rate for the brain during deep hypothermic cardiopulmonary bypass at 20 degrees C. An experimental study. J Thorac Cardiovasc Surg 92:1065–1070, 1986.
117. Mohr R, Martinowitz U, Lavee J, et al: The hemostatic effect of transfusing fresh whole blood versus platelet concentrates after cardiac operations. J Thorac Cardiovasc Surg 96:530–534, 1988.
118. Mojcik CF, Levy JH: Aprotinin and the systemic inflammatory response after cardiopulmonary bypass. Ann Thorac Surg 71:745–754, 2001.
119. Moore EE, Moore FA, Franciose RJ, et al: The postischemic gut serves as a priming bed for circulating neutrophils that provoke multiple organ failure. J Trauma 37:881–887, 1994.
120. Morita K, Ihnken K, Buckberg GD, et al: Pulmonary vasoconstriction due to impaired nitric oxide production after cardiopulmonary bypass. Ann Thorac Surg 61:1775–1780, 1996.
121. Mossinger H, Dietrich W, Braun SL, et al: High-dose aprotinin reduces activation of hemostasis, allogeneic blood requirement, and duration of postoperative ventilation in pediatric cardiac surgery. Ann Thorac Surg 75:430–437, 2003.
122. Munoz R, Laussen PC, Palacio G, et al: Changes in whole blood lactate levels during cardiopulmonary bypass for surgery for congenital cardiac disease: An early indicator of morbidity and mortality. J Thorac Cardiovasc Surg 119:155–162, 2000.
123. Munoz R, Laussen PC, Palacio G, et al: Whole blood ionized magnesium: Age-related differences in normal values and clinical implications of ionized hypomagnesemia in patients undergoing surgery for congenital cardiac disease. J Thorac Cardiovasc Surg 119:891–898, 2000.
124. Murkin JM: Attenuation of neurologic injury during cardiac surgery. Ann Thorac Surg 72:S1838–S1844, 2001.
125. Murkin JM, Farrar JK, Tweed WA, et al: Cerebral autoregulation and flow/metabolism coupling during cardiopulmonary bypass: The influence of $Paco_2$. Anesth Analg 66:825–832, 1987.
126. Myers G: A comparative review of crystalloid, albumin, pentastarch, and hetastarch as perfusate for cardiopulmonary bypass. J Extra-Corporeal Technol 29:30–35, 1997.

127. Newall F, Barnes C, Ignjatovic V, Monagle P: Heparin-induced thrombocytopenia in children. J Paediatr Child Health 39:289–292, 2003.
128. Nollert G, Nagashima M, Bucerius J, et al: Oxygenation strategy and neurologic damage after deep hypothermic circulatory arrest. II. Hypoxic versus free radical injury. J Thorac Cardiovasc Surg 117:1172–1179, 1999.
129. Odegard KC, McGowan FX Jr, DiNardo JA, et al: Coagulation abnormalities in patients with single-ventricle physiology precede the Fontan procedure. J Thorac Cardiovasc Surg 123:459–465, 2002.
130. Odegard KC, McGowan FX Jr, Zurakowski D, et al: Coagulation factor abnormalities in patients with single-ventricle physiology immediately prior to the Fontan procedure. Ann Thorac Surg 73:1770–1777, 2002.
131. Odegard KC, McGowan FX Jr, Zurakowski D, et al: Procoagulant and anticoagulant factor abnormalities following the Fontan procedure: Increased factor VIII may predispose to thrombosis. J Thorac Cardiovasc Surg 125:1260–1267, 2003.
132. Ojito JW, Hannan RL, Miyaji K, et al: Assisted venous drainage cardiopulmonary bypass in congenital heart surgery. Ann Thorac Surg 71:1267–1271; discussion 1271–1272, 2001.
133. Ou-Yang Y, Kristian T, Mellergard P, Siesjo BK: The influence of pH on glutamate- and depolarization-induced increases of intracellular calcium concentration in cortical neurons in primary culture. Brain Res 646:65–72, 1994.
134. Ozawa T, Yoshihara K, Koyama N, et al: Clinical efficacy of heparin-bonded bypass circuits related to cytokine responses in children. Ann Thorac Surg 69:584–590, 2000.
135. Peters M, ten Cate JW, Jansen E, Breederveld C: Coagulation and fibrinolytic factors in the first week of life in healthy infants. J Pediatr 106:292–295, 1985.
136. Picca S, Principato F, Mazzera E, et al: Risks of acute renal failure after cardiopulmonary bypass surgery in children: A retrospective 10-year case-control study. Nephrol Dial Transplant 10:630–636, 1995.
137. Pigula FA, Gandhi SK, Siewers RD, et al: Regional low-flow perfusion provides somatic circulatory support during neonatal aortic arch surgery. Ann Thorac Surg 72:401–406; discussion 406–407, 2001.
138. Pigula FA: Arch reconstruction without circulatory arrest: Scientific basis for continued use and application to patients with arch anomalies. Semin Thorac Cardiovasc Surg Pediatr Card Surg Annu 5:104–115, 2002.
139. Pigula FA: Competing perfusion strategies: Effect on microvascular oxygen tension. J Thorac Cardiovasc Surg 125:456, 2003.
140. Plotz FB, van Oeveren W, Bartlett RH, Wildevuur CR: Blood activation during neonatal extracorporeal life support. J Thorac Cardiovasc Surg 105:823–832, 1993.
141. Pua HL, Bissonnette B: Cerebral physiology in paediatric cardiopulmonary bypass. Can J Anaesth 45:960–978, 1998.
142. Rahn H, Reeves RB, Howell BJ: Hydrogen ion regulation, temperature, and evolution. Am Rev Respir Dis 112:165–172, 1975.
143. Rappaport LA, Wypij D, Bellinger DC, et al: Relation of seizures after cardiac surgery in early infancy to neurodevelopmental outcome. Boston Circulatory Arrest Study Group. Circulation 97:773–779, 1998.
144. Reid RW, Zimmerman AA, Laussen PC, et al: The efficacy of tranexamic acid versus placebo in decreasing blood loss in pediatric patients undergoing repeat cardiac surgery. Anesth Analg 84:990–996, 1997.
145. Riegger LQ, Voepel-Lewis T, Kulik TJ, et al: Albumin versus crystalloid prime solution for cardiopulmonary bypass in young children. Crit Care Med 30:2649–2654, 2002.
146. Rosengart TK, Stark JF: Repair of atrial septal defect through a right thoracotomy. Ann Thorac Surg 55:1138–1140, 1993.
147. Scallan MJ: Brain injury in children with congenital heart disease. Paediatr Anaesth 13:284–293, 2003.
148. Schulze-Neick I, Penny DJ, Rigby ML, et al: L-arginine and substance P reverse the pulmonary endothelial dysfunction caused by congenital heart surgery. Circulation 100:749–755, 1999.
149. Schupbach P, Pappova E, Schilt W, et al: Perfusate oncotic pressure during cardiopulmonary bypass. Optimum level as determined by metabolic acidosis, tissue edema, and renal function. Vox Sang 35:332–344, 1978.
150. Seghaye MC, Duchateau J, Grabitz RG, et al: Complement activation during cardiopulmonary bypass in infants and children. Relation to postoperative multiple system organ failure. J Thorac Cardiovasc Surg 106:978–987, 1993.
151. Seghaye MC, Duchateau J, Grabitz RG, et al: Complement, leukocytes, and leukocyte elastase in full-term neonates undergoing cardiac operation. J Thorac Cardiovasc Surg 108:29–36, 1994.
152. Seghaye MC, Grabitz RG, Duchateau J, et al: Inflammatory reaction and capillary leak syndrome related to cardiopulmonary bypass in neonates undergoing cardiac operations. J Thorac Cardiovasc Surg 112:687–697, 1996.
153. Seifert HA, Jobes DR, Ten Have T, et al: Adverse events after protamine administration following cardiopulmonary bypass in infants and children. Anesth Analg 97:383–389, table of contents, 2003.
154. Severin T, Zieger B, Sutor AH: Anticoagulation with recombinant hirudin and danaparoid sodium in pediatric patients. Semin Thromb Hemost 28:447–454, 2002.
155. Shum-Tim D, Nagashima M, Shinoka T, et al: Postischemic hyperthermia exacerbates neurologic injury after deep hypothermic circulatory arrest. J Thorac Cardiovasc Surg 116:780–792, 1998.
156. Shum-Tim D, Tchervenkov CI, Jamal AM, et al: Systemic steroid pretreatment improves cerebral protection after circulatory arrest. Ann Thorac Surg 72:1465–1471; discussion 1471–1472, 2001.
157. Sieber F, Derrer SA, Saudek CD, Traystman RJ: Effect of hypoglycemia on cerebral metabolism and carbon dioxide responsivity. Am J Physiol 156:H697–H706, 1989.
158. Siesjo BK, Ingvar M, Pelligrino D: Regional differences in vascular autoregulation in the rat brain in severe insulin-induced hypoglycemia. J Cereb Blood Flow Metab 3:478–485, 1983.
159. Smith PK, Datta SK, Muhlbaier LH, et al: Cost analysis of aprotinin for coronary artery bypass patients: Analysis of the randomized trials. Ann Thorac Surg 77:635–642; discussion 642–643, 2004.
160. Somero G, White FN: Enzymatic consequences under alpha stat regulation. In Rahn H, Prakash O, editors: Acid-Base Regulation and Body Temperature, pp. 55–80. Boston: Nijhoff, 1985.
161. Spahn DR, Smith LR, Veronee CD, et al: Acute isovolemic hemodilution and blood transfusion. Effects on regional function and metabolism in myocardium with compromised coronary blood flow. J Thorac Cardiovasc Surg 105:694–704, 1993.
162. Spiess BD: Blood transfusion for cardiopulmonary bypass: The need to answer a basic question. J Cardiothorac Vasc Anesth 16:535–538, 2002.
163. Stamm C, Friehs I, Cowan DB, et al: Inhibition of tumor necrosis factor-alpha improves postischemic recovery of hypertrophied hearts. Circulation 104:I350–I355, 2001.
164. Stein JI, Gombotz H, Rigler B, et al: Open heart surgery in children of Jehovah's Witnesses: Extreme hemodilution on cardiopulmonary bypass. Pediatr Cardiol 12:170–174, 1991.
165. Steward DJ, Da Silva CA, Flegel T: Elevated blood glucose levels may increase the danger of neurological deficit following profoundly hypothermic cardiac arrest. Anesthesiology 68:653, 1988.

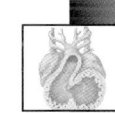

166. Swain JA, McDonald TJ Jr, Griffith PK, et al: Low-flow hypothermic cardiopulmonary bypass protects the brain. J Thorac Cardiovasc Surg 102:76–83; discussion 83–84, 1991.
167. Swain JA, McDonald TJ Jr, Robbins RC, Balaban RS: Relationship of cerebral and myocardial intracellular pH to blood pH during hypothermia. Am J Physiol 260:H1640–H1644, 1991.
168. Tarnok A, Schneider P: Pediatric cardiac surgery with cardiopulmonary bypass: Pathways contributing to transient systemic immune suppression. Shock 16(suppl 1):24–32, 2001.
169. Taylor RH, Burrows FA, Bissonnette B: Cerebral pressure-flow velocity relationship during hypothermic cardiopulmonary bypass in neonates and infants. Anesth Analg 74:636–642, 1992.
170. Tigchelaar I, Gallandat Huet RC, Korsten J, et al: Hemostatic effects of three colloid plasma substitutes for priming solution in cardiopulmonary bypass. Eur J Cardiothorac Surg 11:626–632, 1997.
171. Tombaugh GC, Sapolsky RM: Evolving concepts about the role of acidosis in ischemic neuropathology. J Neurochem 61:793–803, 1993.
172. Ungerleider RM, Shen I: Optimizing response of the neonate and infant to cardiopulmonary bypass. Semin Thorac Cardiovasc Surg Pediatr Card Surg Annu 6:140–146, 2003.
173. Vannucci RC: Experimental biology of cerebral hypoxia-ischemia: Relation to perinatal brain damage. Pediatr Res 27:317–326, 1990.
174. Vannucci RC, Mujsce DJ: Effect of glucose on perinatal hypoxic-ischemic brain damage. Biol Neonate 62:215–224, 1992.
175. Vannucci RC, Towfighi J, Heitjan DF, Brucklacher RM: Carbon dioxide protects the perinatal brain from hypoxic-ischemic damage: An experimental study in the immature rat. Pediatrics 95:868–874, 1995.
176. Wachtfogel YT, Kucich U, Hack CE, et al: Aprotinin inhibits the contact, neutrophil, and platelet activation systems during simulated extracorporeal perfusion. J Thorac Cardiovasc Surg 106:1–9; discussion 9–10, 1993.
177. Wachtfogel YT, Kucich U, James HL, et al: Human plasma kallikrein releases neutrophil elastase during blood coagulation. J Clin Invest 72:1672–1677, 1983.
178. Wachtfogel YT, Pixley RA, Kucich U, et al: Purified plasma factor XIIa aggregates human neutrophils and causes degranulation. Blood 67:1731–1737, 1986.
179. Watanabe T, Orita H, Kobayashi M, Washio M: Brain tissue pH, oxygen tension, and carbon dioxide tension in profoundly hypothermic cardiopulmonary bypass. Comparative study of circulatory arrest, nonpulsatile low-flow perfusion, and pulsatile low-flow perfusion. J Thorac Cardiovasc Surg 97:396–401, 1989.
180. Wells FC, Coghill S, Caplan HL, Lincoln C: Duration of circulatory arrest does influence the psychological development of children after cardiac operation in early life. J Thorac Cardiovasc Surg 86:823–831, 1983.
181. Wernovsky G, Stiles KM, Gauvreau K, et al: Cognitive development after the Fontan operation. Circulation 102:883–889, 2000.
182. Wypij D, Newburger JW, Rappaport LA, et al: The effect of duration of deep hypothermic circulatory arrest in infant heart surgery on late neurodevelopment: The Boston Circulatory Arrest Trial. J Thorac Cardiovasc Surg 126:1397–1403, 2003.

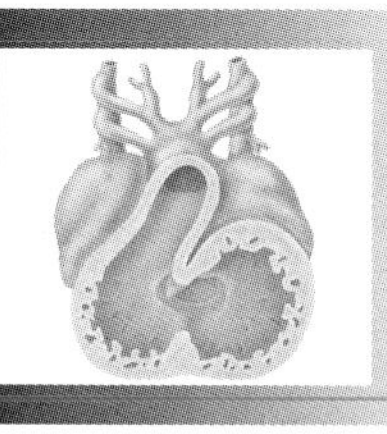

CHAPTER 104B

Surgical Approaches, Cardiopulmonary Bypass, and Mechanical Circulatory Support in Children

Mechanical Circulatory Support

Peter C. Laussen and Stephen J. Roth

INTRODUCTION

Mechanical support of the circulation for infants and children has an important role in providing short-term circulatory support during reversible myocardial failure, as a means of cardiopulmonary support before and after cardiac surgery, and also as a potential bridge to cardiac transplantation. Modalities of support include extracorporeal membrane oxygenation (ECMO), intraaortic balloon pump (IABP) counterpulsation, and ventricular assist devices (VADs). Although a variety of assist devices are available for adult-sized patients, the need for miniaturization has delayed their application in children; ECMO is therefore the most common form of mechanical circulatory support for pediatric patients. ECMO was first introduced as an important method of respiratory support in pediatric patients with severe lung disease, and institutions with an established ECMO program have been able to effectively transition this methodology to provide biventricular support and oxygenation in pediatric patients with a failing circulation.[19,43,83] There are no established guidelines for the indications and management of cardiac ECMO support, and there is considerable interinstitutional variability with respect to utility and outcomes, depending on experience and philosophy. VADs offer the potential for both short- and longer-term support of circulation in patients who do not have concurrent pulmonary parenchymal or vascular disease, and there is increasing interest in developing this form of support as an effective longer-term bridge to transplantation.

EXTRACORPOREAL MEMBRANE OXYGENATION

Overview of Utility

The use of ECMO to support children with impaired gas exchange as a result of acute respiratory failure has become an accepted and successful therapy, particularly in neonates with a variety of parenchymal and vascular lung diseases (e.g., meconium aspiration, respiratory distress syndrome, diaphragmatic hernia, persistent hypertension of the newborn).[83] The positive effect of ECMO on outcome in these patients depends mainly on the early diagnosis of severe pulmonary failure, the prompt institution of ECMO, and the reversible nature of the pulmonary dysfunction. However, the advent of other therapies such as high-frequency oscillatory ventilation, surfactant therapy, permissive hypercapnia, and inhaled nitric oxide has led to a reduction in the need for ECMO in neonates.[24,42,80] According to the cumulative data reported by the Extracorporeal Life Support Organization (ELSO) Registry, 77% of all neonates who have been placed on ECMO for respiratory support have survived to discharge from hospital.[24] The outcome for older patients is considerably lower, with the reported cumulative survival for pediatric and adult patients placed on ECMO for respiratory support being approximately 50%.

In contrast to respiratory ECMO, over the past decade there has been a steady increase in the number of patients and institutions using ECMO to support a failing circula-

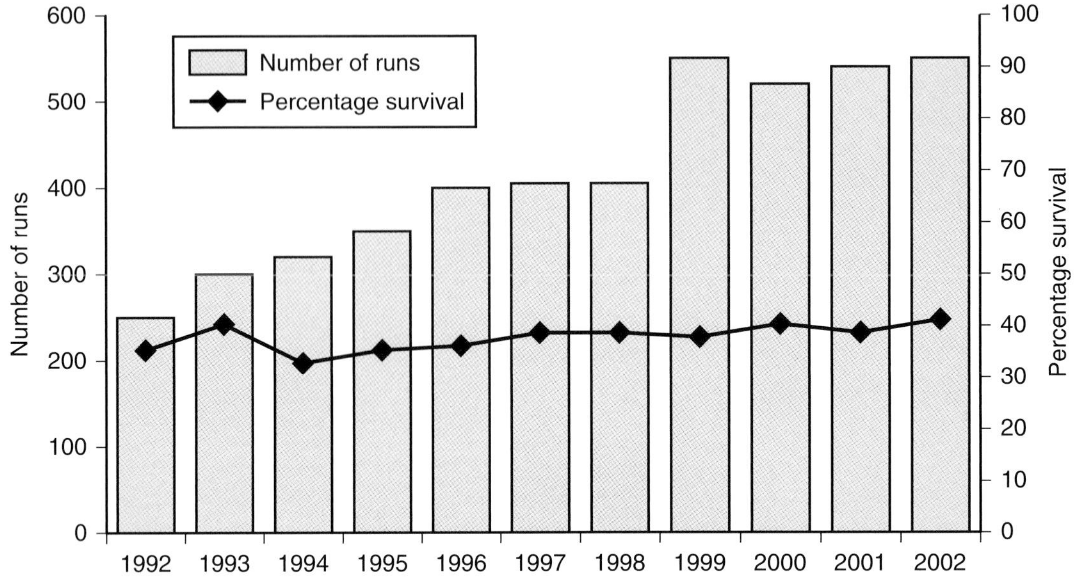

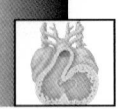

Figure 104B–1 **Number of cardiac extracorporeal membrane oxygenation (ECMO) runs and survival for all patients receiving cardiac ECMO support reported to the Extracorporeal Life Support Organization (ELSO) Registry over the past 10 years.**

tion, mostly after congenital cardiac surgery or as a bridge to transplantation.* Another more controversial indication for cardiac ECMO has been its rapid deployment during resuscitation from cardiac arrest.† Despite the increased enthusiasm for ECMO support of the circulation, the survival to discharge as reported by ELSO (38% neonates and 39% pediatric patients, Figure 104B-1) has not increased over the past decade and has lagged behind considerably compared with the experience with respiratory ECMO (Table 104B-1).[24]

*References 1, 6, 14, 20, 24, 38, 44–46, 49, 63, 65, 72.

†References 1, 14, 16, 20, 23, 36.

Table 104B–1

Neonatal Respiratory and Cardiac ECMO: Differences in Survival Reported by the ELSO Registry for Specific Diagnostic Groups

Diagnosis	*Survived (%)*
Meconium aspiration syndrome	94
Primary pulmonary hypertension	79
Sepsis	75
Air leak syndrome	70
Congenital diaphragmatic hernia	53
Cardiac disease	37

Extracorporeal Life Support Organization (ELSO): International Summary, July 2003.

The majority of cardiac patients are placed on ECMO after surgery. Adverse outcomes after cardiac ECMO are primarily related to irreversible underlying cardiac disease and to the presence of significant end-organ injury. Recovery from severe myocardial dysfunction while on mechanical support will occur, provided the myocardium has sustained a transient and reversible injury. ECMO facilitates ventricular recovery by reducing myocardial wall tension, increasing coronary perfusion pressure, and maintaining systemic perfusion with oxygenated blood. In infants, in whom myocardial failure is frequently biventricular and is associated with respiratory insufficiency or pulmonary hypertension, ECMO is the preferred means of mechanical support. In contrast to the concept of "resting the lungs" for patients who are placed on ECMO for respiratory failure and lung injury, it is important that the heart regain contractile function and conduction as soon as possible to maintain a workload and avoid involution of the myocardial mass. This requires frequent evaluation, often with echocardiography, and it is critical that overdistension of the heart be avoided. It also is important to appreciate the differences between the ECMO circuit and management compared with routine cardiopulmonary bypass (CPB) used during cardiac surgery. The ECMO circuit is a "closed" circuit and has limited ability to handle any air in the venous limb of the circuit, and careful de-airing of both the arterial and venous cannulas is essential when connecting to the ECMO circuit.

The average duration for cardiac ECMO runs reported to ELSO over the past 15 years has increased slightly from approximately 4–5 days to 5–7 days; the longest reported run has been 62 days.[24] These data highlight the fact that ECMO should be viewed only as a relatively short-term support of the circulation, and beyond 7 days the chances of successful decannulation and survival decrease substantially. These data also support the need to develop longer-term mechanical support devices, particularly as a bridge to transplantation. The significant time limitation associated with cardiac ECMO means that ideally, only patients with known reversible cardiac disease should be considered candidates for cardiac ECMO, but this is often not possible when a rapid decision needs to be made to place a patient on ECMO because of cardiac arrest or severe low cardiac output state.

In general, institutions with an efficient and well-established ECMO service are more likely to use this form of support for the failing circulation, and surgeon bias, case type, surgical techniques, and CPB management are additional confounding factors that make comparisons among institutions difficult.[77] Although it could be argued that ECMO should be readily available in any center undertaking complex congenital cardiac surgery, establishing a structured and coordinated team approach to cannulation is key for any ECMO service.[20] In our experience at Children's Hospital Boston, the introduction of a dedicated cardiac ECMO program and development of a rapid response system for use during active resuscitation has contributed to an increase in the survival to discharge for ECMO circulatory support from 45% in 1995 to 59% in 2002 irrespective of diagnosis or indication for cardiac support.[23]

Indications

According to the ELSO Registry outcomes based on broad diagnostic categories, patients placed on ECMO because of complications related to fulminant myocarditis have the highest survival (Table 104B-2), although this lags behind the successful outcomes achieved with ECMO for respiratory support in neonates. The survival from cardiac ECMO to discharge from hospital according to cardiac surgery procedure is shown in Table 104B-3. The heterogeneity of procedures for which ECMO has been used is well demonstrated, but the survival rate is poor across all groups and there is no specific cardiac procedure or diagnostic group for which ECMO is a proven therapy.

Rather than trying to determine indications for cardiac ECMO according to specific diagnosis or procedure, the indications can be examined within five broad categories: preoperative resuscitation; inability to wean from cardiopulmonary bypass; postcardiotomy; cardiomyopathy, myocarditis, and bridge to transplantation; and after-in-hospital cardiac arrest and CPR.

Table 104B–2

International Summary of ELSO Registry through July 2003: Survival for Cardiac ECMO Runs Based on Broad Diagnostic Categories

Diagnosis	*Survived (%)*
Congenital cardiac defect	38
Cardiac arrest	26
Cardiogenic shock	42
Cardiomyopathy	49
Myocarditis	58

Table 104B–3

ELSO Registry July 2003 International Summary: Selected Cardiac Runs by Procedure

Procedure	*Total Reported Cardiac ECMO (%)*	*Survived (%)*
Anomalous venous return repair	2.5	42
Aortic outflow repair	1.3	33
Arterial switch	4.8	38
ASD repair	0.3	29
AV canal repair	1.5	42
Bidirectional Glenn shunt	0.5	31
Fontan procedures	2.3	25
Heart transplant	5.7	45
Mitral valve repair	1.9	41
Rastelli repair	0.9	36
Stage 1 palliation (Norwood)	5.1	29
Systemic to pulmonary artery shunts	2.1	37
Tetralogy repair	3.5	45
VSD repair	2.1	36

ELSO, Extracorporeal Life Support Organization; ECMO, extracorporeal membrane oxygenation; ASD, atrial septal defect; AV, atrioventricular; VSD, ventricular septal defect.

Preoperative Resuscitation

ECMO may be beneficial for critically ill patients before cardiac surgery, enabling preoperative stabilization, optimization, and prevention of end-organ dysfunction before repair. These patients represent a small group, they are usually are newborns, and indications include severely low cardiac output states (e.g., critical aortic stenosis), pulmonary hypertension (e.g., obstructed total anomalous pulmonary venous drainage), or severe hypoxemia (e.g., transposition of the great arteries and pulmonary hypertension).[31,33,77]

Inability to Wean from Cardiopulmonary Bypass

The reported survival of patients placed on ECMO because they were unable to wean directly from CPB in the operating room (i.e., without any period of stability off CBP) is poor.[1,6,49,77] Aside from issues such as primary myocardial dysfunction, pulmonary hypertension, severe hypoxemia, and refractory dysrhythmias, unrecognized residual or irreparable defects are major factors in determining successful outcome in this circumstance.[6] These defects must be searched for in the operating room, preferably in combination with echocardiography and the careful measurement of oxygen saturations and intracardiac pressures. Ideally, only children with potentially reversible myocardial injury who cannot be weaned from CBP should be considered candidates for ECMO, although this may be extremely difficult to determine in the operating room immediately after cardiac surgery. Considerations include preoperative condition, intraoperative course, and likelihood of being a transplant candidate.

Severe hemorrhage is a major problem in the transition from the CPB circuit to the ECMO circuit. Although a lower activated clotting time (ACT) (160–180 seconds) can be used, often small doses of protamine are necessary to assist with the initial control of bleeding. We usually administer 1 mg/kg increments of protamine until a target ACT of 180 seconds is achieved. Infusions of antifibrinolytic drugs such as aprotinin (bolus 30,000 IU/kg, infusion 10,000 IU/kg/h), tranexamic acid (bolus 100 mg/kg, infusion 10 mg/kg/h), or ε aminocaproic acid (bolus 100 mg/kg, infusion 30 mg/kg/h) should be considered. Exploration of the chest may be necessary, particularly if the bleeding persists at >10 ml/kg/h and problems with ECMO flow are encountered because of decreased venous cannula drainage from a tamponade-like effect. The large transfusion requirement may place considerable burden on the supply of donor blood products. As an alternative, it is possible to connect a chest tube to cell saver tubing to enable blood to be collected in the cell saver reservoir and subsequently spun for retransfusion.

When a patient is placed on ECMO in the operating room, it is important that discussions with the patient's family be clear and direct. Recovery of myocardial function should be expected within 2–3 days,[22] and if this is not evident, either listing for cardiac transplantation if appropriate or withdrawal from support must be considered.

Postcardiotomy

ECMO is an effective therapeutic option for infants and children who have had a period of relative stability after successful termination of CBP, and where significant residual cardiac defects are excluded. Myocardial or respiratory failure causing a low cardiac output state, hypoxemia, or pulmonary hypertension and cardiac arrest are the major indications in this group. This is a large group of patients, and reported survival rates are as high as 60–70%, provided ECMO is instituted rapidly and effectively.*

Cardiomyopathy, Myocarditis, and Bridge to Transplantation

Patients who have acute fulminant myocarditis can be managed successfully with ECMO.[21,24] Although some of these patients may be candidates for VADs, even though their disease is usually biventricular, ECMO is often preferable. Patients with fulminant myocarditis may arrive at the hospital undergoing full cardiac arrest, but more commonly are in shock from an extremely low cardiac output state or have hemodynamically significant dysrhythmias, including ventricular tachycardia or heart block. The heart is usually distended and is contracting very poorly. Prompt institution of ECMO may allow sufficient resuscitation and stabilization to prevent end-organ injury and enable the myocardium to rest while awaiting potential recovery. After instituting ECMO, the heart must be fully decompressed and urgent left atrial vent placement may be necessary.[7] The heart may not begin to eject for the first 24–36 hours after starting ECMO, although recovery of electrical activity within the first few hours should be expected. If recovery of ventricular ejection is not evident within 2–3 days, ECMO can be continued either as a bridge to heart transplantation or as a bridge to alternate longer-term support with a VAD if feasible.†

ECMO should be viewed as a short-term bridge to transplantation because of the limited donor availability and the time-related risks for complications, such as infection, bleeding, end-organ impairment, problems secondary to immobilization, and difficulties in maintaining adequate nutrition.[18,67] In our experience at Children's Hospital Boston, the median time spent on ECMO awaiting heart transplantation is currently 140 hours (range 26–556 hours), but only 50% of our listed patients have been effectively bridged. In a small number of older and larger children, ECMO has been used to initially resuscitate the circulation and end-organs, and if a donor heart has not become available by day 6 or 7 of ECMO, we have successfully transitioned from ECMO to longer-term VAD.

ECMO also has been used to effectively support the failing heart after transplantation. This may be necessary immediately after transplantation because of graft failure, usually in the setting of pulmonary hypertension and acute right ventricle failure of the donor heart. ECMO also is effective to support the heart during periods of acute rejection.[26] The inflammation and myocardial edema are similar to that seen with fulminant myocarditis and lead to a similar spectrum of clinical features. ECMO allows the transplanted heart to decompress with decreased wall tension while antirejection therapy is increased. In our experience, survival to discharge for this indication is currently 64%, and the median duration of ECMO support has been 4 days.

*References 1, 6, 14, 49, 66, 77.

†References 13, 15, 18, 22, 25, 26, 35, 45, 51, 74.

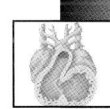

After-in-Hospital Cardiac Arrest and CPR

Survival and outcome of in-hospital resuscitation in pediatric patients after a cardiac arrest continues to be extremely poor.* Even within a highly monitored and resource-intensive area such as a pediatric intensive care unit, the survival rate after cardiac arrest has only been reported to be between 9–31%. The duration of cardiac arrest and resuscitation also is an important determinant of subsequent outcome, and a number of reports have noted a critical threshold of approximately 15 minutes.[61,70] However, there are reports of successful use of ECMO to support children after prolonged periods of cardiac arrest that have been unresponsive to closed or open cardiac massage and all other usual interventions.[1,16,23] Again, it is important to emphasize that the underlying lesion, in conjunction with the effectiveness of cardiopulmonary resuscitation (CPR) while instituting ECMO, are the major determinants of outcome when mechanical support is used in this setting. Although the exact place of ECMO in the CPR algorithm remains ill defined, patients with a witnessed arrest and rapid institution of effective CPR, and who have no apparent recovery of cardiac function within 10–15 minutes of initiating resuscitation and no contraindications, may be suitable candidates for ECMO.

*References 61, 70, 73, 76, 81, 82.

Determining the relative contraindications to ECMO support during active resuscitation attempts can be difficult (Table 104B-4). Preferably, discussions regarding the use of ECMO in certain patients should be undertaken before an event occurs, although clearly this is not always possible. In our experience we have been able to successfully use our rapid response ECMO system during CPR in patients with acquired and structural heart disease, and in patients with two or single ventricle defects. In the latter group, neonates who have a sudden, reversible event, such as acute thrombosis and obstruction to a systemic-to-pulmonary artery shunt after a Norwood procedure, have been readily resuscitated with ECMO. On the other hand, patients with cavopulmonary corrections (i.e., Fontan or bidirectional Glenn anastomosis) have been difficult to resuscitate using ECMO, in part because of limitations with cannulation, and inability to maintain adequate systemic oxygen delivery and avoid cerebral venous hypertension during CPR with chest compressions. Although we have used ECMO in the resuscitation of patients with pulmonary hypertension and those with systemic outflow obstruction, the severe limitation to cardiac output and oxygenations during CPR in these patients has meant that their overall outcomes on ECMO have been poor because of the development of severe end-organ injury.

Despite a small number of series reporting their successes using ECMO during active resuscitation and chest compressions,[1,16,23,32,36] in contrast, the ELSO Registry reports only a 26% survival to discharge for patents placed

Table 104B–4

ECMO Support during Active Cardiopulmonary Resuscitation

	Resuscitation Event	*Considerations*
Indications	• Witnessed and monitored event (e.g., tamponade, arrhythmia, systemic to pulmonary artery shunt obstruction) • Immediate and effective BLS and CPR • No response to ALS in 10 min • Acceptable cardiac transplant candidate (e.g., fulminant myocarditis)	• In-hospital: ICU, OR, catheterization laboratory • Effective ECMO system and resources • Primed circuit (vacuumed or crystalloid) • Equipment and personnel immediately available
Contraindications		
Absolute	• Non–witnessed or monitored event • Known comorbidities that preclude listing of transplantation	• Out-of-hospital arrest • Other congenital or chromosomal abnormalities • Sepsis • CNS injury • Renal failure
Relative	• Effective ECMO support system not established • Known comorbidities that preclude effective CPR (e.g., pulmonary hypertension, systemic outflow tract obstruction, semilunar or AV valve insufficiency, hypertrophic cardiomyopathy, cavopulmonary connection)	• Circuit not immediately available • Equipment and personnel not trained or in-house

ECMO, Extracorporeal membrane oxygenation; ICU, intensive care unit; OR, operating room; BLS, basic life support; CPR, cardiopulmonary resuscitation; ALS, advanced life support.

on ECMO in this circumstance.[24] To avoid significant delays a "rapid response" ECMO system has been established at some institutions.[23,36] The success of a rapid response system depends on a multidisciplinary approach, with equipment being immediately available, and the personnel with assigned roles being in-house, including cardiac surgery and intensive care fellows, respiratory and ECMO specialists, and trained nursing staff. At Children's Hospital, Boston, a vacuum and carbon dioxide (CO_2)-primed circuit using a roller pump and a 0.8- to 1.5-m^2 membrane oxygenator is available at all times and is suitable for children weighing up to approximately 15 kg. Even in older children this circuit initially provides sufficient flow for resuscitation, stabilization, and hopefully prevention of end-organ damage, until a larger oxygenator can be spliced into the circuit. Generally, however, for older children and adults, a new circuit with a hollow-fiber membrane is used, which takes little time to de-air and can be established within 15 min; once stable on ECMO, the hollow-fiber membrane can be exchanged for a conventional membrane for longer-term support as necessary. An alternative rapid response system has been described, which uses a heparin-coated circuit, centrifugal pump, and hollow-fiber membrane with a priming volume of only 250 ml and a priming time of only 5 min.

In postoperative cardiac patients, atrial and aortic cannulation via a reopened sternotomy is usually the access mode of choice. In other patients, experienced practitioners can rapidly gain access via the neck vessels. During resuscitation the circuit is primed with crystalloid supplemented with 5% albumin. We do not wait for donor blood to be crossmatched to complete a blood prime of the circuit because of the inevitable delay. We prefer to reestablish organ perfusion as soon as possible, and once ECMO is satisfactorily established, blood products can be added or the priming crystalloid removed via hemofiltration. To assist with neurological protection, where possible we maintain mild hypothermia (34–35° C) for the first 12h after placing a patient on ECMO during active resuscitation. Using the rapid response system, we can be ready to place a patient on ECMO within 15 min, and the main limitation then becomes problems associated with cannulation. We have deployed the rapid response system during active resuscitation in more than 90 children since 1996 and have been able to achieve an improved survival to discharge of 58% in this group of patients.

CIRCUIT AND CANNULA MANAGEMENT

The ECMO system circuit includes a reservoir, membrane oxygenator, and heat exchanger. The ECMO and cannula guidelines used at Children's Hospital Boston, are shown in Tables 104B-5 and 104B-6. The circuit volume can range from approximately 350 ml (in neonates) to 2–3 liters (adult). Before cannulation, heparin is administered and the ACT is usually maintained between 180 and 200 by continuous heparin infusion. Occasionally, ACTs are maintained at somewhat lower levels in the presence of significant bleeding. At times, large doses of drugs such as heparin, fentanyl, or midazolam may be necessary because of binding to the circuit and oxygenator or dilution by bleeding. Perfusion flow rates in infants and small children typically range from 100–150 ml/kg/min during full circulatory support. Blood products are administered to keep the hematocrit level typically between 35–45%, and the platelet count is greater than 100,000/mm^3.

Arteriovenous cannulation is usually employed for cardiac ECMO, although venovenous bypass can be used in patients who require ventilatory support only. In the immediate postoperative period, mediastinal cannulation, using single right atrial and ascending aortic cannulas, is often preferable because cannulation can be rapidly achieved, along with left atrial decompression if necessary. For the risk of infection to be reduced further, if possible, the skin is closed over the cannulas and the chest, or a surgical scialastic membrane is used instead. Alternatively, the internal jugular vein and carotid artery can be used, with the potential advantage of less bleeding, a more stable cannula position, and, by avoiding an open sternum, a possible reduction in the risk of infection. If neck cannulation is used, the carotid artery can be either ligated or repaired; despite concerns about uneven cerebral blood flow, ligation seems to be surprisingly well tolerated clinically, whereas reconstruction requires long-term follow up because of the increased risk of stenosis at the anastomotic site.[12,41] The femoral vessels in infants and very young children may not accommodate cannulas of sufficient size to permit complete circulatory support. However, these sites have been used occasionally to provide resuscitation and stabilization in acute emergency situations (e.g., in the cardiac catheterization laboratory) or when femoral access has already been established.

Children with complex structural cardiac defects may have associated abnormalities with systemic venous damage (e.g., heterotaxy syndromes) or have undergone previous cardiac catheterization or interventions that may have caused occlusion of femoral vessels. Therefore it is essential that the venous and arterial anatomy be well known and documented to prevent inappropriate cannulation attempts.

The daily management of a patient on ECMO or other forms of extracorporeal life support requires a meticulous assessment of cardiorespiratory function, end-organ perfusion and injury, evolving complications such as bleeding or sepsis, and the mechanics of the ECMO circuit.[79] If a patient fails to wean from ECMO or there is a delay in anticipated recovery of myocardial function, the possibility of a residual surgical problem must always be considered. This is usually difficult to diagnose by echocardiography alone, and cardiac catheterization (i.e., diagnostic or interventional) should be considered.

Assessing the adequacy of flow and systemic perfusion soon after initiation of ECMO is of paramount importance. Inadequate flow states and/or persistent hypotension despite perceived adequate flow require immediate analysis and intervention (Table 104B-7). Venous cannula malposition or inadequate size limits venous drainage if a roller pump is used, thereby contributing to circuit chatter and bladder collapse. This should be addressed immediately, and the venous cannula should be repositioned, an additional venous cannula placed, or the existing cannula upsized. When ECMO flow appears inadequate to meet the needs of the patient and limited venous drainage restricts additional flow, interpretation of arterial and atrial pressures may aid the formulation of a differential diagnosis. For example, if the atrial pressure is low and venous drainage is inadequate, this may represent

Table 104B–5

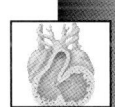

ECMO Circuit Guidelines: Children's Hospital Boston

Weight (kg)	*2–15*	*16–20*	*21–35*	*36–60*	*>60*	*Stat (>15 kg)*
Circuit	Neonatal	Pediatric	Pediatric	Adult	Adult	Stat
Membrane (m^2)	0.8–1.5	2.5	3.5	4.5	4.5	Optima
Prime						
5% albumin (ml)	50	100	100	100	100	100
Packed red blood cells (l/ml)	500	1000	1000	1500	1500	1000
Fresh-frozen plasma (l/ml)	200	400	400	500	500	400
Cryoprecipitate (U)	2	3	3	4	4	3
Platelets (U)	2	4	4	6	6	6
Medications						
Heparin (U)	500	500	500	800	800	500
THAM (ml)	100	200	300	300	300	200
Calcium gluconate (mg)	1500	3000	3000	4000	4000	3000
Flows						
Minimum (ml/min)	100	200	250	300	600	0.5
Maximum (l/min)	1.8	4.5	5.5	6.5	6.5 (ea)	8.0
Sweep gas range (l/min)	1–4.5	2–8	2–11	2–13	2–13	0.5–20
Membrane volume (ml)	174	455	575	665	1330	260
Circuit volume (ml)	580	1500	1600	2500	3200	1000

PRBC, Packed red blood cells; FFP, fresh-frozen plasma; THAM, tris-hydroxymethyl aminomethane; Normosol, isotonic crystalloid solution (sodium 140 mEq/l, chloride 90 mEq/l, potassium 5 mEq/l, magnesium 3 mEq/l).

hypovolemia from ongoing or unrecognized bleeding. Conversely, high atrial pressures with inadequate venous drainage may represent tamponade physiology that requires surgical exploration in a postoperative patient, or may reflect left ventricle overdistension from inadequate decompression or aortic valve regurgitation. Elevated postmembrane pressures may reflect malposition of the arterial cannula or a cannula that is too small and needs to be revised. Elevated premembrane pressures (i.e., >350 mm Hg) at normal flows without change in postmembrane pressure, or evidence of blood-to-gas leak, constitute membrane oxygenator dysfunction and may dictate oxygenator replacement. Extensive thrombus or consumptive coagulopathy with hypofibrinogenemia and thrombocytopenia constitutes other indications for circuit replacement.

Echocardiography, especially transesophageal (and occasionally cardiac catheterization), is used to assess cardiac structure and contractile function and to detect residual lesions and the need for left atrial decompression.[7,53] Venting the left atrium may be necessary to lower the left atrial pressure and decrease left ventricular wall stress, thereby minimizing ongoing myocardial injury. Adequate decompression can be assessed early by echocardiography and signs of pulmonary edema. Strategies to assist with decompressing the ventricle include placing a vent in the left atrium either by direct placement through an open chest or by a transcatheter approach in the catheterization laboratory[7] and augmenting ventricular ejection with inotropic agents.

Once ECMO is successfully established, inotropic support is usually reduced, and vasodilators may be required to improve systemic perfusion and enable appropriate flow rates. F_{IO_2} and ventilatory support also are decreased to a low respiratory rate (5–10 breaths/min), low peak inspiratory pressures (20–25 cm H_2O), and low levels of positive end-expiratory pressure (PEEP) to preserve lung volume and limit inactivation of alveolar surfactant.

Considerations regarding cannulation and flow rates once on ECMO may be specific to the underlying cardiac defect or surgical repair. For example, the management of an aortopulmonary shunt is critical in patients with single ventricle physiology. Systemic and pulmonary flow should be balanced by either partially clipping the shunt or using high ECMO flows. On ECMO, circuit flows up to 200 ml/kg/min or more are usually necessary to maintain adequate systemic perfusion while accounting for run-off into the pulmonary circulation through the shunt. Although partial temporary narrowing of the shunt may be advisable in some circumstances, it is unwise to completely occlude the only source of pulmonary blood flow to the pulmonary endothelium. It is possible to bypass the membrane oxy-

Table 104B–6

ECMO Cannula Size According to Patient Weight

Weight (kg)	*Venous (Fr)*	*Arterial (Fr)*
2–4	8–14	8–10
5–15	15–19	12–15
16–20	19–21	15–17
21–35	21–23	17–19
35–60	23	19–21
60+	23	21

genator in patients following the Norwood procedure with a modified Blalock–Taussig shunt without lung disease if higher flows are maintained and the shunt is patent.[37] This maneuver simplifies the circuit and may permit less use of heparin. ECMO thus effectively becomes a VAD.

Problems related to cannula placement and adequacy of venous drainage may be particularly evident in patients with complex venous anatomy, such as heterotaxy syndrome, and in patients with a cavopulmonary connection. The site of cannulation is affected by vessel patency, and the underlying physiology might influence the number of venous cannulas used. For example, patients with a superior cavopulmonary anastomosis (bidirectional Glenn shunt [BDG]) as the primary source of pulmonary blood flow frequently require separate venous drainage of the superior vena cava (SVC) and inferior vena cava (IVC), unless there is congenital interruption of the infrahepatic IVC with drainage of lower body blood to the azygos vein. In the latter case a single venous cannula in the SVC might be sufficient. On the other hand, placement of a cannula in the SVC may be detrimental in patients with BDG physiology because of the potential for reduced cerebral venous drainage and therefore decreased cerebral perfusion. This is also a concern for patients with Fontan physiology; although it may be possible to achieve adequate drainage with a venous cannula placed in the Fontan baffle, an additional SVC catheter is often necessary to achieve the desired or necessary flow rates on ECMO.[8]

Weaning from Extracorporeal Membrane Oxygenation

The strategies for weaning from cardiac ECMO are often quite different from those used to wean patients who are on ECMO for respiratory support. For patients with structurally normal hearts who require ECMO support for respiratory illness, the ability to wean is dependent on resolution of the primary pulmonary process, often with little need for support of the myocardium beyond moderate inotropic support, fluid and electrolyte management, and nutritional support. Once lung compliance and gas exchange have normalized, improvement of the lungs on chest radiograph is apparent, and a stable circulation with sufficient negative fluid balance has been achieved, the patient is sedated, paralyzed, and fully ventilated and the ECMO circuit is clamped.

When considering weaning from ECMO used for circulatory support, a thorough understanding of the underlying cardiac physiology and cardiorespiratory interactions and an appreciation for the expected range of oxygen saturation levels is important. Because of the increased risk of complications and mortality in patients with cardiac disease when the duration of mechanical circulatory support extends beyond 7 days, consideration as to when and how to wean cardiac patients from ECMO should begin once circulatory stability has been established. The disease process and circumstances resulting in hemodynamic failure or cardiac arrest may influence the expected duration of mechanical support. For example, patients who fail to separate from CPB after cardiac surgery as a result of severe pulmonary hypertension usually respond to a period of 24–48 hours on ECMO with inhaled nitric oxide (NO) therapy and inotropic support of the right side of the heart. Similarly, patients who have a low cardiac output state or suffer cardiac arrest after

Table 104B–7

Causes of Inadequate ECMO Flow and Perfusion

	Cannula	*Anatomical*	*Physiological*
Inadequate venous drainage	Too small Malpositioned Air occlusion	Heterotaxy syndromes Vessel occlusion/stenosis	Hypovolemia Tamponade Nonvented, distended ventricle
Inadequate systemic perfusion	Too small (high postmembrane pressure) Malpositioned Occlusion	Aortic valve regurgitation Vessel stenosis	Systemic vasoconstriction or vasodilation

cardiac surgery may have residual defects that allow rapid weaning and decannulation soon after reoperation. The likelihood of recovery of ventricular function should be decided within the first 48–72 hours so that cardiac transplantation status can be ascertained. ECMO instituted for catheter intervention or arrhythmia ablation procedures may be discontinued within hours of patient cannulation.[10] In contrast, patients with severe cardiomyopathies or those awaiting heart transplantation may require mechanical assistance for a much longer period. Patients with severe bronchiolitis as a result of respiratory syncytial virus complicating repair of congenital heart disease on CPB typically require 2–3 weeks of ECMO support for respiratory failure.

Patients requiring cardiovascular support with ECMO are partially weaned within the first 48 hours in order to assess myocardial function by echocardiography and hemodynamic evaluation. An acceptable PaO_2 obtained while the ECMO circuit is clamped varies substantially according to the underlying anatomy and pathophysiology. If transthoracic cannulation was used and problems with bleeding were encountered during the ECMO run, the mediastinum may require exploration before or during the weaning process. If only a short period of reconditioning of the myocardium is anticipated, the patient is frequently sedated and paralyzed, dopamine infusion is increased to 5–10 μg/kg/min, intravascular volume status is optimized, and ventilator settings are adjusted according to lung compliance and expected arterial O_2 saturation. ECMO flow is decreased by 25–50% over a period of time until the circuit is clamped. Volume is infused to achieve appropriate preload. Echocardiographic assessment of ventricular systolic function, valvular function, systemic and pulmonary outflow obstruction, and location and direction of intracardiac shunts is useful before weaning, as well as if there is a change in hemodynamics after the circuit has been clamped. Arterial blood gases, serum lactate levels, and systemic and mixed venous oxygen saturation levels are important guides to the stability of the circulation, ventilation, and adequacy of perfusion after the circuit has been clamped. Decannulation from ECMO is undertaken once the patient has maintained a stable circulation and acceptable gas exchange for a period of up to 4 hours.

VENTRICULAR ASSIST DEVICES

The experience with VADs in infants and children remains relatively small, mainly because of technical limitations and the smaller number of suitable pediatric patients who would benefit from univentricular support.[20,29,64] In adults, VAD support is useful as a bridge to transplantation and allows for recovery of end-organ function, elimination of edema, and improvement in nutrition, and it provides rehabilitation of critically ill patients. An important component of these benefits is the ability of the device to allow for ambulation, which cannot be accomplished currently with ECMO and centrifugal VADs. The main problem in adapting the VADs used for adult patients are size limitations and flow requirements; the risk for thromboembolic complications increases with lower flow.

As with ECMO, the selection of appropriate candidates is crucial and surgical problems or residual defects should be excluded where possible. Whereas ECMO can be instituted by peripheral cannulation of neck or femoral vessels, VADs require direct cannulation of the heart through a sternotomy. For this reason the VAD experience in infants and small children has been primarily in postcardiotomy patients.[20] The reported survival rates with VADs are similar to those achieved with cardiac ECMO,[22,29,38,75] and left ventricular support devices (LVADs), right ventricular support devices (RVADs), or dual-support VADs (Bi-VADs) can successfully support the circulation, depending on the circumstances. The majority of reported pediatric patients have received LVADs, which have been particularly beneficial in patients with an ischemic myocardium secondary to an anomalous origin of left coronary artery from the pulmonary artery and for "retraining" of the poorly prepared left ventricle after an arterial switch procedure.[17,39,54]

There are a number of advantages of the VAD circuit when compared with ECMO. They are relatively simple in design, take less time to prime, and require little technical assistance once established. Bleeding complications and requirement for blood products and platelet transfusions generally are less in patients on VADs compared with those on ECMO.[38,41] Requirement for heparinization and maintaining a prolonged ACT is proportionately less. Because of the lower complication rate, a VAD may be more suitable for long-term support as a bridge to transplantation.[20,38]

Another possible advantage of VADs is superior left ventricular drainage and unloading, a prerequisite for myocardial rest and potential recovery.[20,41,52] However, although increased ventricular wall stress during ECMO has been demonstrated experimentally, if the left atrium is adequately vented, equivalent ventricular decompression is provided when compared with a VAD. Whenever a patient is placed on a VAD, the response of the unsupported ventricle must be closely monitored. Ideally the reduction in left atrial pressure during LVAD support, associated with adequate decompression of the left ventricle, reduces pulmonary venous pressures and improves right ventricular function. Unfortunately, based on adult data, right ventricular failure can still develop in up to 25% of patients especially in LVAD-supported patients with ischemic myocardium, preexisting anatomical defects, or after prolonged bypass procedures.[62,68,69]

A variety of systems have been modified for use in pediatric patients and may be classified as pulsatile or nonpulsatile devices.

Nonpulsatile Devices

Primarily because of technical limitations with pulsatile pumps, most VADs for small children are nonpulsatile systems, either roller pumps or a centrifugal pump such as the Bio-Medicus circuit (Medtronic, Bio-Medicus, Minneapolis, MN). The centrifugal pump, in which blood is entrained by creating a vortex using spinning cones, is very sensitive to changes in preload and systemic resistance. This proves to be useful in adapting inotropic support or afterload reduction in preparation of weaning. Furthermore, the pump is designed to create constant flow rather than pressure, thereby reducing the risk of accidental line disruption. The Bio-Medicus centrifugal pump can be used in infants and older children, and because gravity is not needed to achieve venous drainage, the pump housing can be placed close to the patient and is readily portable.

Impeller-type pumps such as the intraventricular axial flow pump are under evaluation. Electromechanically coupled, the inlet flow is achieved by apical ventricular cannulation with outlet cannulation of the ascending or descending aorta. Hemolysis is a concern with axial flow and roller pumps, and this possible complication needs to be monitored closely.[57]

Pulsatile Devices

Pulsatile devices used in adult patients have been modified or developed for use in older children (usual surface area >1.2 m^2 to achieve a flow rate of at least 2 l/min). Successful use of the Heartmate VAD (Thermocardiosystems, Woburn, MA) has been reported in adolescents with body surface areas ranging from 1.4–2.2 m^2.[28] The implantation of the Thoratec VAD (Thoratec Laboratories Corp., Berkeley, CA) has been reported in children as young as 11 years of age,[48] and in our experience at Children's Hospital Boston, the smallest patient who has undergone implantation of this device has a body surface area of 1.35 m^2.

The MEDOS HIA VAD (MEDOS Medizintechnik AG, Stolberg, Germany) and Berlin Heart VAD (Berlin Heart AG, Berlin, Germany) are paracorporeal pneumatic devices that are currently being evaluated and offer the potential for longer-term support in infants and small children.[4,34,47,71] Produced in various sizes, which can deliver low stroke volumes, a measured amount of compressed air delivered through a pneumatic line compresses the ventricular chamber or bladder, thereby enforcing ejection of blood. Diastolic pump filling is achieved by either gravity or gentle suction. Because of the high resistance of the small-bore cannulas, positive pressures of up to 350 mm Hg and negative suction of 100 mm Hg at pumping rates of up to 180 beats/min may be necessary, increasing the power requirements for the driving unit considerably, compared with adult devices. Polyurethane trileaflet valves with low transvalvular pressure gradients and rapid closure, as well as the use of heparin-coated systems, may reduce the thromboembolic risk, one of the major problems associated with VADs.

INTRAAORTIC BALLOON COUNTER PULSATION

Intraaortic balloon counter pulsation (IABP) is commonly used for the treatment of myocardial failure in adults, especially in the postoperative period. When used in infants and children, however, results have been disappointing, with survival rates of less than 50%.[2,60,78] Many factors contribute to the reduced efficacy in children. Heart failure in pediatric patients is often due to either right ventricular or biventricular dysfunction, conditions in which the IABP is not effective. Placement of an IABP in the pulmonary artery has been reported, but is usually problematic, in part because of the small balloon size required and the increased compliance of the pulmonary artery.[56,58] The relatively rapid heart rate of infants and small children and the variable delay between aortic valve closure and the appearance of the arterial tracing on the oscilloscope make effective timing of inflation and deflation more difficult. At heart rates greater than 160 beats/min, the IABP is often reduced to a 1:2 or even 1:4 pumping frequency to facilitate cycle timing, at the same time decreasing the effectiveness to 50–80%.[9,59] The aorta is typically more distensible in both infants and children, and therefore both coronary flow augmentation during diastole (balloon inflation) and afterload reduction during systole (balloon deflation) are likely to be less. In addition, the effect of diastolic augmentation on normal coronaries, prevailing in the pediatric population, has been questioned.[3,11] Severe cyanotic heart disease in children can be accompanied by extensive aortopulmonary collateral vessels, which permit shunting of blood into the pulmonary circulation during balloon inflation, thus reducing augmentation of coronary blood flow.

The smallest balloon system available for children is 2.5 ml, which can be used for neonates as small as 2 kg. In general, for children weighing less than 30 kg, a balloon volume of 0.5 ml/kg is recommended. For balloon inflation, helium is preferred over CO_2, allowing a faster pneumatic response because of its low density. Interestingly, the incidence of vascular complications, such as bleeding, emboli, or limb ischemia, correlates well with the adult population, where it is reported in about 10–20%. Other potential complications are infection, renal dysfunction, mesenteric occlusion or embolism, and cerebrovascular accidents.[5,50]

Over the past years, numerous technical improvements have been made to enhance efficacy in the pediatric population. These include modified pumping consoles and small-sized catheters, improved tracking at higher heart rates, more rapid inflation and deflation, and the use of M-mode echocardiography for cycle timing.[55] Further studies are necessary to evaluate the importance of IABP support for pediatric patients.

LONGER-TERM OUTCOME FROM MECHANICAL SUPPORT

Formal, prospective evaluation of the longer-term outcomes of children receiving mechanical support of the circulation has not been undertaken. Despite the successful deployment of mechanical support to enable cardiac recovery and discharge from hospital, longer-term cardiac function and the functional status of patients should be determined. Besides cardiac status, end-organ injury and residual deficits need to be evaluated, particularly neurological outcomes.[32] The ELSO Registry data indicate a combined neurological complication rate of 26% in all patients receiving cardiac ECMO, with seizures being the most common neurological event (9.5%). In a recent retrospective report of the outcome, infants supported with ECMO after cardiotomy (median follow up 55 months), only 50% of survivors were determined to have no motor or cognitive deficit of any sort.[27] As the technology and indications for mechanical support of the circulation in children continue to evolve and advance, simultaneous outcome studies will be essential.

REFERENCES

1. Aharon AS, Drinkwater DC, Churchwell KB, et al: Extracorporeal membrane oxygenation in children after repair of congenital cardiac lesions. Ann Thorac Surg 72:2095–2102, 2001.

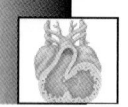

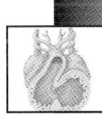

2. Akomea-Agyin C, Kejriwal NK, Franks R, et al: Intraaortic balloon pumping children. Ann Thorac Surg 67:1415–1420, 1999.
3. Amsterdam EA, Awan NA, Lee G, et al: Intra-aortic balloon counterpulsation: Rationale, application and results. Cardiovasc Clin 11(3):79–96, 1981.
4. Asfour B, Weyard M, Kececioglu D, et al: A novel paracorporeal mechanical assist device for newborns and infants allows bridging to transplantation. Transplant Proc 29(8):3330–3332, 1997.
5. Beckman CB, Geha AS, Hammond GL, et al: Results and complications of intraaortic balloon counterpulsation. Ann Thorac Surg 24(6):550–559, 1977.
6. Black MD, Coles JG, Williams WG, et al: Determinants of success in pediatric cardiac patients undergoing extracorporeal membrane oxygenation. Ann Thorac Surg 60(1):133–138, 1995.
7. Booth KL, Roth SJ, Perry SB, et al: Cardiac catheterization of patients supported by extracorporeal membrane oxygenation. J Am Coll Cardiol 40:1681–1686, 2002.
8. Booth KL, Roth SJ, Thiagarajan RR, et al: ECMO support of Fontan and bidirectional Glenn circulation. Ann Thorac Surg (in press).
9. Cadwell CA, Quaal SJ: Intra-aortic balloon counterpulsation timing [see comments]. Am J Crit Care 5(4):254–261; quiz 262–263, 1996.
10. Charmichael TB, Walsh EP, Roth SJ: Anticipatory use of venoarterial extracorporeal membrane oxygenation for a high-risk interventional cardiac procedure. Resp Care 47: 1002–1006, 2003.
11. Chatterjee S, Rosensweig J: Evaluation of intra-aortic balloon counterpulsation. J Thorac Cardiovasc Surg 61(3):405–410, 1971.
12. Cheung PY, Vickar DB, Hallgren RA, et al: Carotid artery reconstruction in neonates receiving extracorporeal membrane oxygenation: A 4-year follow-up study. Western Canadian ECMO Follow-Up Group. J Pediatr Surg 32(4): 560–564, 1997.
13. Dalton HJ, Siewers RD, Fuhrman BP, et al: Extracorporeal membrane oxygenation for cardiac rescue in children with severe myocardial dysfunction. Crit Care Med 21(7): 1020–1028, 1993.
14. del Nido PJ: Extracorporeal membrane oxygenation for cardiac support in children. Ann Thorac Surg 61:336–339, 1996.
15. del Nido PJ, Armitage JM, Fricker FJ, et al: Extracorporeal membrane oxygenation support as a bridge to pediatric heart transplantation. Circulation 90(5 pt 2):II66–II69, 1994.
16. del Nido PJ, Dalton HJ, Thompson AE, Siewers RD, et al: Extracorporeal membrane oxygenator rescue in children during cardiac arrest after cardiac surgery. Circulation 86(suppl 5):II300–II304, 1992.
17. del Nido PJ, Duncan BW, Mayer JE Jr, et al: Left ventricular assist device improves survival in children with left ventricular dysfunction after repair of anomalous origin of the left coronary artery from the pulmonary artery. Ann Thorac Surg 67(1):169–172, 1999.
18. Delius RE: As originally published in 1990: Prolonged extracorporeal life support of pediatric and adolescent cardiac transplant patients. Updated in 1998. Ann Thorac Surg 65(3): 877–878, 1998.
19. Duncan BW, editor: Mechanical Support for Cardiac and Respiratory Failure in Pediatric Patients. New York: Marcel Dekker, 2001.
20. Duncan BW: Mechanical circulatory support for infants and children with cardiac disease. Ann Thorac Surg 73:1670–1677, 2002.
21. Duncan BW, Bohn DJ, Atz AM, et al: Mechanical circulatory support for the treatment of children with acute fulminant myocarditis. J Thorac Cardiovasc Surg 122:440–448, 2001.
22. Duncan BW, Hraska V, Jonas RA, et al: Mechanical circulatory support in children with cardiac disease. J Thorac Cardiovasc Surg 117(3):529–542, 1999.
23. Duncan BW, Ibrahim AE, Hraska V, et al: Use of rapid-deployment extracorporeal membrane oxygenation for the resuscitation of pediatric patients with heart disease after cardiac arrest. J Thorac Cardiovas Surg 116(2):305–311, 1998.
24. Extracorporeal Life Support Organization: ECLS Registry Report: International Summary, pp. 1–15. Ann Arbor: Extracorporeal Life Support Organization, 2003.
25. Gajarski RJ, Mosca RS, Ohye RG, et al: Use of extracorporeal life support as a bridge to pediatric cardiac transplantation. J Heart Lung Transplant 22:28–34, 2003.
26. Galantowicz ME, Stolar CJ: Extracorporeal membrane oxygenation for perioperative support in pediatric heart transplantation. J Thorac Cardiovasc Surg 102(1):148–151; discussion 151–152, 1991.
27. Hamrick SEG, Gremmels DB, Keet CA, et al: Neurodevelopmental outcome of infants supported with extracorporeal membrane oxygenation after cardiac surgery. Pediatrics 111:e671–e675, 2003.
28. Helman DN, Addonizio LJ, Morales DLS, et al: Implantable left ventricular assist devices can successfully bridge adolescent patients to transplant. J Heart Lung Transplant 19: 121–126, 2000.
29. Hetzer R, Loebe M, Potapov EV, et al: Circulatory support with pneumatic paracorporeal ventricular assist device in infants and children. Ann Thorac Surg 66(5):1498–1506, 1998.
30. Hetzer, R., Muller J, Weng Y, et al: Cardiac recovery in dilated cardiomyopathy by unloading with a left ventricular assist device. Ann Thorac Surg 68(2):742–749, 1999.
31. Hunkeler NM, Center CE, Donze A, Spray TL, et al: Extracorporeal life support in cyanotic congenital heart disease before cardiovascular operation. Am J Cardiol 69(8): 790–793, 1992.
32. Ibrahim AE, Duncan BW, Blume ED, Jonas RA: Long-term follow-up of pediatric cardiac patients requiring mechanical circulatory support. Ann Thorac Surg 69:186–192, 2000.
33. Ishino K, Alexi-Meskishvili V, Hetzer R: Preoperative extracorporeal membrane oxygenation in newborns with total anomalous pulmonary venous connection. Cardiovasc Surg 7(4):473–475, 1999.
34. Ishino K, Loebe M, Uhlemann F, et al: Circulatory support with paracorporeal pneumatic ventricular assist device (VAD) in infants and children. Eur J Cardiothrac Surg 11:965–972, 1997.
35. Ishino K, Weng Y, Alexi-Meskishvili V, et al: Extracorporeal membrane oxygenation as a bridge to cardiac transplantation in children. Artif Organs 20(6):728–732, 1996.
36. Jacobs JP, Ojito JW, McConaghey TW, et al: Rapid cardiopulmonary support for children with complex congenital heart disease. Ann Thorac Surg 70:742–750, 2000.
37. Jaggers JJ, Forbess JM, Shah AS, et al: Extracorporeal membrane oxygenation for infant postcardiotomy support: Significance of shunt management. Ann Thorac Surg 69:1476–1483, 2000.
38. Karl TR: Extracorporeal circulatory support in infants and children. Semin Thorac Cardiovasc Surg 6(3):154–160, 1994.
39. Karl TR, Horton SB, Mee RB: Left heart assist for ischemic postoperative ventricular dysfunction in an infant with anomalous left coronary artery. J Card Surg 4(4):352–354, 1989.
40. Karl TR, Iyer KS, Sano S, et al: Infant ECMO cannulation technique allowing preservation of carotid and jugular vessels. Ann Thorac Surg 50(3):488–489, 1990.
41. Karl TR, Sano S, Horton S, Mee RB: Centrifugal pump left heart assist in pediatric cardiac operations. Indication, technique, and results. J Thorac Cardiovasc Surg 102(4): 624–630, 1991.

42. Kennaugh JM, Kinsella JP, Abman SH, et al: Impact of new treatments for neonatal pulmonary hypertension on extracorporeal membrane oxygenation use and outcome. J Perinatol 17(5):366–369, 1997.
43. Kern F, et al: Extracorporeal circulation and circulatory assist devices in the pediatric patient. In Lake C, editor: Pediatric Cardiac Anesthesia, pp. 219–257. Stamford, Conn: Appleton & Lange, 1998.
44. Khan A, Gazzaniga AB: Mechanical circulatory assistance in paediatric patients with cardiac failure. Cardiovasc Surg 4(1): 43–49, 1996.
45. Kirshbom PM, Bridges ND, Myung RJ, et al: Use of extracorporeal membrane oxygenation in pediatric thoracic organ transplantation. J Thorac Cardiovasc Surg 123:130–136, 2002.
46. Klein MD, Shaheen KW, Wittlesby GC, et al: Extracorporeal membrane oxygenation for the circulatory support of children after repair of congenital heart disease. J Thorac Cardiovasc Surg 100(4):498–505, 1990.
47. Konertz W, Hotz H, Schneider M, et al: Clinical experience with the MEDOS HIA-VAD system in infants and children: A preliminary report. Ann Thorac Surg 63(4):1138–1144, 1997.
48. Korfer R, El-Banayosy A, Arusoghi L, et al: Single-center experience with the Thoratec ventricular assist device. J Thorac Cardiovasc Surg 119:596–600, 2000.
49. Kulik TJ, Moler FW, Palmisaro JM, et al: Outcome-associated factors in pediatric patients treated with extracorporeal membrane oxygenator after cardiac surgery. Circulation 94(suppl 9):II63–II68, 1996.
50. Lazar JM, Ziady GM, Dermmer SJ, et al: Outcome and complications of prolonged intraaortic balloon counterpulsation in cardiac patients. Am J Cardiol 69(9):955–958, 1992.
51. Levi D, Marelli D, Plunkett M, et al: Use of assist devices and ECMO to bridge pediatric patients with cardiomyopathy to transplantation. J Heart Lung Transplant 21:760–770, 2002.
52. Loebe M, Muller J, Hetzer R: Ventricular assistance for recovery of cardiac failure Curr Opin Cardiol 14(3):234–248, 1999.
53. Marcus B, Alkinson JB, Wong PC, et al: Successful use of transesophageal echocardiography during extracorporeal membrane oxygenation in infants after cardiac operations. J Thorac Cardiovasc Surg 109(5):846–848, 1995.
54. Mee RB, Harada Y: Retraining of the left ventricle with a left ventricular assist device (Bio-Medicus) after the arterial switch operation. J Thorac Cardiovasc Surg 101(1):171–173, 1991 (letter).
55. Minich LL, Tani LY, McGough EC, et al: A novel approach to pediatric intraaortic balloon pump timing using M-mode echocardiography. Am J Cardiol 80(3):367–369, 1997.
56. Moran JM, Opravil M, Gorman AJ, et al: Pulmonary artery balloon counterpulsation for right ventricular failure: II. Clinical experience. Ann Thorac Surg 38(3):254–259, 1984.
57. Oku T, Harasaki H, Smith W, Nose Y: Hemolysis. A comparative study of four nonpulsatile pumps. ASAIO Trans 34(3):500–504, 1988.
58. Opravil M, Gorman AJ, Krejcie TC, et al: Pulmonary artery balloon counterpulsation for right ventricular failure: I. Experimental results. Ann Thorac Surg 38(3):242–253, 1984.
59. Pantalos GM, Minich LL, Tani LY, et al: Estimation of timing errors for the intraaortic balloon pump use in pediatric patients. ASAIO J 45(3):166–171, 1999.
60. Park JK, Hsu DT, Gersony WM: Intraaortic balloon pump management of refractory congestive heart failure in children. Pediatr Cardiol 14(1):19–22, 1993.
61. Parra DA, Totapally BR, Zahn E, et al: Outcome of cardiopulmonary resuscitation in a pediatric cardiac intensive care unit. Crit Care Med 28:3296–3300, 2000.
62. Pavie A, Leger P: Physiology of univentricular versus biventricular support. Ann Thorac Surg 61(1):347–349; discussion 357–358, 1996.
63. Pennington DG, Swartz, MT: Circulatory support in infants and children. Ann Thorac Surg 55(1):233–237, 1993.
64. Pennington DG, Swartz MT, Lohmann P, McBride LR: Cardiac assist devices. Surg Clin North Am 78(5):691–704, vii, 1998.
65. Raithel SC, Pennington DG, Boegner E, et al: Extracorporeal membrane oxygenation in children after cardiac surgery. Circulation 86(suppl 5):II305–II310, 1992.
66. Rogers AJ, Trento A, Siewers RD, et al: Extracorporeal membrane oxygenation for postcardiotomy cardiogenic shock in children. Ann Thorac Surg 47(6):903–906, 1989.
67. Sable CA, Shaddy RE, Suddaty EC, et al: Impact of prolonged waiting times of neonates awaiting heart transplantation. J Perinatol 17(6):481–488, 1997.
68. Santamore WP, Austin EH, 3rd, Gray LA Jr: Overcoming right ventricular failure with left ventricular assist devices. J Heart Lung Transplant 16(11):1122–1128, 1997.
69. Santamore WP, Gray LA Jr: Left ventricular contributions to right ventricular systolic function during LVAD support. Ann Thorac Surg 61(1):350–356, 1996.
70. Schindler MB, Bohn D, Cox PN, et al: Outcome of out-of-hospital cardiac or respiratory arrest in children. N Engl J Med 335:1473–1479, 1996.
71. Shum-Tim D, Duncan BW, Hraska V, et al: Evaluation of a pulsatile pediatric ventricular assist device in an acute right heart failure model. Ann Thorac Surg 64(5):1374–1380, 1997.
72. Sidiropoulos A, Hotz H, Konertz W: Pediatric circulatory support. J Heart Lung Transplant 17(12):1172–1176, 1998.
73. Slomin AD, Patel KM, Ruttimann UE, Pollack MM: Cardiopulmonary resuscitation in pediatric intensive care units. Crit Care Med 25:1951–1955, 1997.
74. Thiagarajan RR, Roth SJ, Margossian S, et al: Extracorporeal membrane oxygenation as a bridge to cardiac transplantation in a patient with cardiomyopathy and hemophilia A. Int Care Med 29:985–988, 2003.
75. Thuys CA, Mullaly RJ, Horton SB, et al: Centrifugal ventricular assist in children under 6 kg. Eur J Cardiothorac Surg 13(2):130–134, 1998.
76. Von Seggern K, Egar M, Fuhrman BP: Cardiopulmonary resuscitation in a pediatric ICU. Crit Care Med 14(4): 275–277, 1986.
77. Walters HL 3rd, Hakimi M, Rice MD, et al: Pediatric cardiac surgical ECMO: Multivariate analysis of risk factors for hospital death. Ann Thorac Surg 60(2):329–336; discussion 336–337, 1995.
78. Webster H, Veasy LG: Intra-aortic balloon pumping in children. Heart Lung 14(6):548–555, 1985.
79. Wessel DL, Almodovar MC, Laussen PC: Intensive care management of cardiac patients on extracorporeal membrane oxygenation. In Duncan BW, editor: Mechanical Support for Cardiac and Respiratory Failure, pp. 75–111. New York: Marcel Dekker, 2000.
80. Wilson JM, Bower LK, Thompson JE, et al: ECMO in evolution: The impact of changing patient demographics and alternative therapies on ECMO. J Pediatr Surg 31(8): 1116–1122; discussion 1122–1123, 1996.
81. Zaritsky A: Cardiopulmonary resuscitation in children. Clin Chest Med 8(4):561–571, 1987.
82. Zaritsky A: Outcome following cardiopulmonary resuscitation in the pediatric intensive care unit. Crit Care Med 25:1937, 1997.
83. Zwischenberger JB, Bartlett RH, editors: ECMO. Extracorporeal Cardiopulmonary Support in Critical Care. Ann Arbor: Extracorporeal Life Support Organization, 1995.

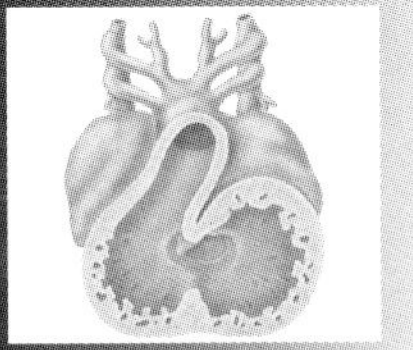

Pediatric Anesthesia and Critical Care

Kirsten C. Odegard and Peter C. Laussen

CHAPTER 105

INTRODUCTION

The management of congenital heart disease has progressed significantly over the past three decades. Most congenital heart lesions are now amenable to either anatomical or physiological repair early in infancy. Advances in diagnostic and interventional cardiology, the evolution of surgical techniques and conduct of cardiopulmonary bypass, and refinements in postoperative management have all contributed to a substantial decrease in morbidity and mortality associated with congenital heart disease (CHD). The approach to repairing CHD as early as possible, preferably in the neonatal period, has had significant implications for the anesthetic care of these critically ill infants during cardiac surgery. For this challenge to be met, a clear understanding of neonatal respiratory and cardiac physiology, neonatal responses to anesthesia and surgery, and the pathophysiology of complex congenital heart defects is necessary.

PATHOPHYSIOLOGY

Care of the critically ill neonate requires an appreciation of the special structural and functional features of immature organs. The neonate appears to respond more quickly and extremely to physiologically stressful circumstances; this may be expressed in terms of rapid changes in, for example, pH, lactic acid, glucose, and temperature.[5]

The physiology of the preterm and full-term neonate is characterized by a high metabolic rate and oxygen (O_2) demand (twofold to threefold increase compared with adults), which may be compromised at times of stress because of limited cardiac and respiratory reserve. The myocardium in the neonate is immature, with only 30% of the myocardial mass comprising contractile tissue, compared with 60% in mature myocardium. In addition, neonates have a lower velocity of shortening, a diminished length–tension relationship, and a reduced ability to respond to afterload stress.[9,20] Because the compliance of the myocardium is reduced, the stroke volume is relatively fixed and cardiac output is heart rate–dependent; therefore the Frank–Starling relationship is functional only within a narrow range of left ventricular end-diastolic pressure. The cytoplasmic reticulum and T-tubular system are underdeveloped, and the neonatal heart is dependent on the transsarcolemmal flux of extracellular calcium both to initiate and sustain contraction.

Cardiorespiratory interactions are important in neonates and infants. In simple terms, ventricular interdependence refers to a relative increase in ventricular end-diastolic volume and pressure causing a shift of the ventricular septum and diminished diastolic compliance of the opposing ventricle.[13] This effect is particularly prominent in the immature myocardium. Therefore a volume load from an intracardiac shunt or valve regurgitation, and a pressure load from ventricular outflow obstruction or increased vascular resistance, may lead to biventricular dysfunction. For example, in neonates with tetralogy of Fallot and severe outflow obstruction, hypertrophy of the ventricular septum may contribute to diastolic dysfunction of the left ventricle and an increase in end-diastolic pressure. This does not improve immediately after repair in the neonate, because it takes some weeks to months for the myocardium to remodel. Therefore an elevated left atrial pressure is not an unexpected finding after neonatal tetralogy repair. This circumstance may be further exacerbated if there is a persistent volume load to the left ventricle after surgery, such as from residual ventricle septal defects (VSDs).

The mechanical disadvantage of an increased chest wall compliance and reliance on the diaphragm as the main muscle of respiration limits ventilatory capacity in the neonate. The diaphragm and intercostal muscles have fewer type I muscle fibers (i.e., slow-contracting, high-oxidative fibers for sustained activity), and this contributes to early fatigue when the work of breathing is increased. In the newborn only 25% of fibers in the diaphragm are type I, reaching a mature proportion of 55% by 8–9 months of age.[11,37] Diaphragmatic function may be significantly compromised by raised intraabdominal pressure, such as from gastric distension, hepatic congestion, and ascites.

The tidal volume of full-term neonates is between 6 and 8 ml/kg, and, because of the previous mechanical limitations, minute ventilation is dependent on respiratory rate. The resting respiratory rate of the newborn infant is between 30 and 40 breaths per minute, which provides the optimal alveolar ventilation to overcome the work of breathing and match the compliance and resistance of the respiratory system. When the work of breathing increases, as with parenchymal lung disease, airway obstruction, cardiac failure, or increased pulmonary blood flow, a larger proportion of total energy expenditure is required to maintain adequate ventilation. Infants therefore fatigue readily and fail to thrive.

The neonate has a reduced functional residual capacity (FRC) secondary to increased chest wall compliance (FRC being determined by the balance between chest wall and lung compliance). Closing capacity also is increased in newborns, with airway closure occurring during normal tidal ventilation.[44] Oxygen reserve is therefore reduced, and, in conjunction with the increased basal metabolic rate and oxygen consumption 2–3 times that of adult levels, neonates and infants are at risk for hypoxemia. However, atelectasis and hypoxemia do not occur in the healthy neonate because FRC is maintained by dynamic factors, including tachypnea, breath stacking (early inspiration), expiratory breaking (expiratory flow interrupted before zero flow occurs), and laryngeal breaking (auto positive end-expiratory pressure [PEEP]).

Organ immaturity of the liver and kidney may be associated with reduced protein synthesis and glomerular filtration, such that drug metabolism is altered and synthetic function is reduced. These problems may be compounded by the normal increased total body water of the neonate compared with the older patient, along with the propensity of the neonatal capillary system to leak fluid out of the intravascular space.[45] This is especially pronounced in the neonatal lung, in which the pulmonary vascular bed is almost fully recruited at rest and the lymphatic recruitment required to handle increased mean capillary pressures associated with increases in pulmonary blood flow may be unavailable.[19]

The caloric requirement for neonates, especially preterm neonates, is high (100–150 kcal/kg/24 h) because of metabolic demand. The task of supplying nutrition for growth becomes even more difficult when necessary limits are placed on the total amount of fluid that may be administrated either parentally or by the enteral route. Hyperosmolar feedings have been associated with an increased risk of necrotizing enterocolitis (NEC) in the preterm neonate or to the neonate born at term who has decreased splanchnic blood flow of any cause (e.g., left-sided obstructive lesions).[62]

PHYSIOLOGICAL APPROACH TO CONGENITAL HEART DISEASE

Specific classification of congenital heart defects is difficult because of the complex nature of many lesions. Identification and classification on the basis of physiology provide an organized framework for the intraoperative anesthetic management and postoperative care of children with complex CHD.

MIXING

Intraatrial mixing of pulmonary and systemic venous return is essential for maintenance of cardiac output in defects with right or left atrioventricular valve atresia (e.g., tricuspid atresia or hypoplastic left heart syndrome [HLHS]) and those with an anatomically parallel pulmonary and systemic circulation, such as D-transposition of the great vessels (D-TGA). If complete mixing occurs, the systemic arterial oxygen saturation (Sao_2) should be approximately 85% in room air, although this may be highly variable, depending on the amount of pulmonary blood flow. Inadequate mixing across a restrictive atrial septal defect (ASD) can cause significant desaturation secondary to reduced pulmonary blood flow or pulmonary edema from pulmonary venous hypertension. The septal defect can be enlarged either by catheter balloon septostomy or balloon dilation, or surgically by atrial septectomy.

SIMPLE SHUNTS

Shunts causing an increase in pulmonary blood flow may be simple or complex, occurring between the ventricles, atria, or great arteries and are described by the relative amount of pulmonary (Qp) to systemic (Qs) blood flow (Qp/Qs). Patients may be acyanotic or cyanotic, have one or two ventricles, or have a single outflow trunk, yet have a significant increase in Qp/Qs and be at risk for congestive heart failure (CHF) and pulmonary hypertension (Table 105-1).

In patients with large left-to-right shunts and low pulmonary vascular resistance, a substantial increase in pulmonary blood flow can occur. If the increase in pulmonary blood flow and pressure continues, structural changes occur within the pulmonary vasculature, until eventually pulmonary vascular resistance (PVR) becomes persistently elevated.[33,52] The time course for developing pulmonary vascular obstructive disease (PVOD) depends on the amount of shunting, but changes may be evident by 4–6 months of age in some lesions. The progression is more rapid when both the volume and pressure load to the pulmonary circulation are increased, such as with a large VSD. As PVR decreases in the first few months after birth, and the hematocrit falls to its lowest physiological value, the increased left-to-right shunt, and therefore volume load on the systemic ventricle, can lead to congestive cardiac failure and failure to thrive.

The end-diastolic volume is increased in patients with an increased Qp/Qs ratio, but the time course over which irreversible ventricular dysfunction develops is variable.

Table 105–1

Simple Shunts: Defects or Surgical Procedures Contributing to an Increased Qp/Qs

Type of shunt	*Acyanotic*	*Cyanotic*
Two ventricles	ASD VSD CAVC DORV	D-TGA/VSD PA/VSD
Single ventricle		TA+/–TGA HLHS DORV/MA Norwood procedure BT shunt
Aortopulmonary connection	PDA Truncus arteriosus A-P window	PA/MAPCA

Qp, Pulmonary blood flow; Qs, systemic blood flow; ASD, atrial septal defect; VSD, ventricular septal defect; CAVC, complete atrioventricular canal; DORV, double-outlet right ventricle; D-TGA, D-transposition of the great arteries; PA, pulmonary atresia; TA, tricuspid atresia; MA, mitral atresia; HLHS, hypoplastic left heart syndrome; BT, Blalock–Taussig; PDA, patent ductus arteriosus; MAPCA, multiple aortopulmonary collateral arteries; A-P, aortopulmonary.

Generally if surgical intervention to correct the volume overload is undertaken within the first 2 years of life, residual dysfunction is uncommon.[25]

The volume load on the systemic ventricle and increased end-diastolic pressure contributes to increased lung water and pulmonary edema by increasing pulmonary venous and lymphatic pressures. Compliance of the lung is therefore decreased, and airway resistance is increased secondary to small airway compression by distended vessels.[8,34,40] Lungs may feel stiff on hand ventilation and deflate slowly. Besides cardiomegaly on chest radiograph, the lung fields are usually hyperinflated. Ventilation–perfusion mismatch contributes to an increased alveolar-to-systemic arterial O_2 ($A\text{–}aO_2$) gradient and dead space ventilation.[42] Minute ventilation is therefore increased, primarily by an increase in respiratory rate. Pulmonary artery and left atrial enlargement may compress main stem bronchi, causing lobar collapse. Symptoms and signs of CHF to note in neonates and infants are shown in Box 105-1.

Manipulating PVR is an important means of limiting pulmonary blood flow and pressure. During anesthesia PVR can be maintained or increased by using a low FIO_2 and altering ventilation to achieve a normal pH and $PaCO_2$.[55] Care must be taken on induction of anesthesia because patients may have a diminished contractile reserve. Preload, contractility, and heart rate must be maintained; afterload reduction is often well tolerated and reduces pulmonary flow and myocardial work.

Box 105–1. Symptoms and Signs of Cardiac Failure in a Neonate and Infant.

Poor growth

Poor feeding
Diaphoresis

Increased work of breathing

Tachypnea
Grunting
Flaring of ala nasi
Chest wall retraction

Decreased cardiac output

Tachycardia
Gallop rhythm
Cardiomegaly
Poor extremity perfusion
Hepatomegaly

COMPLEX SHUNTS

In complex shunts there is either presence of additional pulmonary or systemic outflow obstruction; the Qp/Qs is determined by the size of the orifice, the outflow gradient, and resistance across the pulmonary or systemic vascular bed. The obstruction may be fixed, as with valvular stenosis, or dynamic as in forms of tetralogy of Fallot (TOF).

OUTFLOW OBSTRUCTION

Severe outflow obstruction in the newborn may be associated with ventricular hypertrophy and vessel hypoplasia distal to the level of obstruction. The increased pressure load may cause ventricular failure, with mixing or shunting at the atrial and/or ventricular level necessary to maintain cardiac output if there is complete outflow obstruction. Maintenance of preload, afterload, and normal sinus rhythm is important to prevent a fall in cardiac output or coronary hypoperfusion. Because the time course to develop significant ventricular dysfunction is longer in patients with a chronic pressure load compared with a chronic volume load, symptoms of CHF are uncommon unless the obstruction is severe and prolonged.

PULMONARY HYPERTENSION

Pulmonary hypertension may be idiopathic or secondary to increased pulmonary artery flow and pressure or pulmonary venous obstruction. Factors that increase PVR and pulmonary pressures include light anesthesia with a poorly attenuated stress response, hypoxemia, hypoventilation with a fall in functional residual capacity and respiratory acidosis, metabolic acidosis, hypothermia, prolonged bypass with associated inflammatory response and capillary leak, and protamine and blood product administration, such as platelets (Box 105-2).

Box 105–2. Causes of Abnormally Elevated Pulmonary Artery Pressure and Pulmonary Hypertension.

Left-to-right shunt lesion (e.g., large VSD or PDA)
Pulmonary arteriolar smooth muscle hypertrophy (e.g., pulmonary vascular obstructive disease)
Increased pulmonary venous pressure
Mechanical obstruction of the pulmonary circulation:
- Anatomical defects (e.g., pulmonary vein or branch pulmonary artery stenosis)
- Pulmonary embolus

Raised intrathoracic pressure
Lung hyperinflation
Lung hypoinflation and hypoplasia
Decreased alveolar oxygen tension
Acidemia (respiratory or metabolic)
Inflammatory response to cardiopulmonary bypass
Drugs: protamine
Hyperviscosity (from polycythemia)
Blood product administration (e.g., platelets)
Artifactual (e.g., monitoring problems, catheter malpositions)

PDA, Patent ductus arteriosus.

After repair of defects with large left-to-right shunts, pulmonary artery pressures (PAPs) may remain elevated immediately after bypass as the pulmonary arteries remain initially "reactive" to factors that increase PVR. Factors on bypass contributing to this include compression and atelectasis of the lung and pulmonary edema from inadequate venting of the left atrium or from the humoral and cellular response to bypass. Attenuation of the stress response with deep anesthesia using high-dose narcotics[31] prevents increases in PVR. A high inspired oxygen concentration and hyperventilation to induce a respiratory alkalosis reduces PVR, and boluses of bicarbonate may be necessary to maintain a metabolic alkalosis.[17,46,57] Ideally the pH should be approximately 7.45–7.50, and the arterial CO_2 should be 30–35 mm Hg. Remember, a strategy of hyperventilation to induce a respiratory alkalosis and lower PVR may have an adverse effect on central nervous system (CNS) recovery by lowering cerebral blood flow. The pattern of ventilation and maintenance of lung volumes is important; atelectasis and decreases in lung compliance may cause a significant rise in PVR and pulmonary pressures. Changes in ventilation must be made cautiously and frequently reassessed.

Several intravenous (IV) vasodilators, including the nitric oxide (NO) donors nitroprusside and glycerol trinitrate, the phosphodiesterase (PDE) inhibitors amrinone and milrinone, the eicosanoids prostaglandins E_1 and I_2, tolazoline, and isoproterenol, have been used to treat postoperative patients with elevated PVR.[28] The chief limitation with these pharmacological agents is that their vasodilatory effects are not specific to the pulmonary vasculature, so that vasodilation of the systemic vasculature and systemic hypotension may accompany reduction of pulmonary hypertension.

Inhaled NO selectively dilates smooth muscle cells in small pulmonary vessels and lowers PVR.[49] The selective effect of inhaled NO on the pulmonary vasculature is due to rapid uptake and inactivation by hemoglobin as NO diffuses from alveoli to the lumen of lung capillaries. The usefulness of inhaled NO for CHD patients with pulmonary hypertension has been documented in several populations.[7] After surgery NO has been shown to reduce PAP and PVR in patients with pulmonary venous obstruction such as total anomalous pulmonary venous connection (TAPVC) and mitral stenosis, to a lesser extent in patients with a large preexisting left-to-right shunt and those with cavopulmonary connections (Fontan physiology),[24] and in patients with pulmonary hypertensive crises related to cardiopulmonary bypass (CPB). NO also has improved both pulmonary hypertension and impaired gas exchange in patients who have undergone lung transplantation. Patients with a variety of other pulmonary vascular or parenchymal diseases, including persistent pulmonary hypertension of the newborn,[26,53] primary pulmonary hypertension, acute respiratory distress syndrome,[21] and acute chest syndrome in sickle cell disease[6] also have shown significant improvements in oxygenation from treatment with inhaled NO.

The role of newer pulmonary vasodilating drugs such as the PDE type V inhibitor sildenafil (Viagra) and endothelin-I–blocking drugs such as bosentan is under investigation. The utility of these drugs in CHD is yet to be established.

PREOPERATIVE EVALUATION

Patients with complex defects require frequent evaluation and often repeat cardiac operations as a staged approach to surgical repair. Previous anesthetic, bypass, or surgical problems should be noted. In general, providing continuity of care in these patients, such as a dedicated cardiac anesthesia service, is useful to ensure consistent management practices and allows for a longer-term relationship and confidence with patients and families.

Failure to thrive is an important indicator of cardiopulmonary compromise. Symptoms as described in Box 105-1 should be noted. Murmurs and extra heart sounds may be difficult to interpret if tachycardic, but a palpable thrill usually indicates a significant murmur. In older children, failure to thrive, lethargy, and poor exercise tolerance are significant symptoms. Orthopnea, syncope, and palpitations also may be described. Recurrent respiratory infections and wheezing are common in patients with left-to-right shunts. Four-limb blood pressures should be compared, and room air baseline peripheral arterial saturations should be noted, along with potential airway problems. The chest X-ray should be analyzed for cardiomegaly, pulmonary congestion, airway compression, and atelectasis. Echocardiographic assessment and cardiac catheterization results provide valuable information about anatomical structure, myocardial function, intracardiac pressures, shunting, and gradients across obstructions. They should be interpreted in conjunction with the cardiologist and surgeon. Patients with cardiac failure are often stabilized on digoxin, diuretics, and oral vasodilators such as captopril. Preoperative digoxin levels and hypokalemia must be checked.

The consequences of chronic hypoxemia also need special consideration. Polycythemia increases oxygen-carrying capacity, but when the hematocrit level rises above 65%, the increased blood viscosity causes stasis and potential thrombosis and exacerbates tissue hypoxia. Dehydration must be avoided and IV maintenance fluids commenced while fasting preoperatively. Bleeding disturbances are common in cyanotic patients[38] and may be due to thrombocytopenia, defective platelet aggregation, or clotting factor abnormalities.

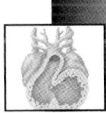

MONITORING

The monitoring used for any specific patient should depend on the child's condition and the magnitude of the planned procedure. For elective patients, noninvasive monitoring is placed before induction of anesthesia, including electrocardiogram (ECG), pulse oximetry, capnography, and a noninvasive blood pressure cuff.

ECG monitoring is essential because significant rhythm disturbances may occur before and after bypass, particularly with VSD and outflow tract surgery. Myocardial ischemia occurs in pediatric patients because of anatomical and shunt-related problems, rather than coronary occlusive disease. Anomalous coronary arteries are associated with a number of complex defects such as transposition of the great vessels and pulmonary atresia. Ischemia also occurs when coronary perfusion pressure falls, such as in HLHS, truncus arteriosus, and critical aortic stenosis. Ventricular fibrillation may occur in these settings,[30] particularly on induction of anesthesia. Ischemia after bypass may result from air embolism or complications related to surgery, such as coronary reimplantation or coronary compression from conduits.

Pulse oximetry is an important monitor before and after bypass because peripheral arterial saturation levels provide an indicator of pulmonary blood flow. The anesthesiologist needs to know the patient's baseline, prebypass peripheral O_2 saturation (Spo_2), and anticipated level after surgery. Causes for lower than expected Spo_2 in patients with single ventricle physiology include pulmonary venous desaturation and intrapulmonary shunt, reduced pulmonary blood flow, or low cardiac output. For patients who have undergone a two-ventricle repair, a lower than expected Spo_2 is usually secondary to intrapulmonary shunting because of either parenchymal lung disease such as atelectasis or edema, or restrictive pulmonary defects such as pleural effusion or pneumothorax. After neonatal right ventricular outflow tract repair, such as TOF or truncus arteriosus, a small atrial communication is an advantage, providing a right-to-left atrial shunt. Although these patients may be cyanosed immediately after surgery, as the compliance of the right ventricle (RV) improves, the right-to-left shunt decreases and the Spo_2 rises.

Once anesthetized, a direct arterial line is placed percutaneously or via a cutdown. The site of the arterial line placement needs careful consideration. For example, patients undergoing placement of a modified Blalock–Taussig shunt from the subclavian or innominate artery should have the radial arterial line placed in the opposite extremity. Similarly, a right radial arterial line is necessary when repair of coarctation of the aorta is proposed. The arch anatomy and possible aberrant arterial vessels are additional considerations when planning arterial access. Aortic root pressure monitoring may be necessary immediately after bypass if the peripheral arterial pressure is damped from hypothermia or low output state. Caution is necessary when flushing arterial catheters in neonates and infants because retrograde flow into the carotid arteries is possible.[14]

Some centers routinely employ central venous pressure monitoring for all cardiovascular surgery. Percutaneous central venous access enables titration of volume replacement and administration of vasoactive infusions before CPB, and during CPB it may provide a measure of the adequacy of cerebral venous drainage. In neonates and infants, central venous lines should be used with caution because of the risk of superior vena cava thrombosis, which can have significant sequelae if collateral veins are poorly developed. Transthoracic right and left atrial lines can be inserted by the surgeon for hemodynamic pressure monitoring and drug infusions after bypass.[23] They have a low complication rate, may be left in situ for a longer period during postoperative recovery, and are easily removed in the intensive care unit (ICU). Swan–Ganz catheters are rarely used in pediatric cardiac surgery because of anatomical limitations. Direct pulmonary artery catheters are inserted by the surgeon to measure pulmonary saturations, detect residual outflow tract gradients, and for thermodilution measurement of cardiac output.

It is important to know the anatomy of central venous drainage before attempting percutaneous cannulation. Heterotaxy syndrome and possible vein occlusions after previous catheterization are considerations, and, if in doubt, ultrasound evaluation of the position and size of a central vein before cannulation is useful.

Cerebral protection is a concern during bypass for congenital heart surgery, particularly because deep hypothermic arrest or low flow bypass is commonly used. Tympanic or nasopharyngeal temperature monitoring is used to assess the adequacy of cerebral cooling and rewarming. Continuous electroencephalogram (EEG) monitoring,[56] transcranial Doppler,[32] and frontal lobe infrared spectroscopy or cerebral oximetry can be used to evaluate cerebral blood flow velocity and perfusion, and O_2 delivery and extraction.

INTRAOPERATIVE ECHOCARDIOGRAPHY

Intraoperative transesophageal echocardiography (TEE) has gained an established role in intraoperative monitoring of patients undergoing repair of CHD.[35,47,61] The development of smaller probes has allowed transesophageal monitoring to replace epicardial echocardiographic imaging in neonates, and such monitoring is now routinely performed. Placement of a transesophageal probe after the induction of anesthesia in the operating room (OR) enables reevaluation of the anatomy before surgical intervention but, more importantly, the adequacy of surgical repair can be evaluated as soon as the patient is weaned from CPB. Interference of the probe with the airway and the effect on unstable hemodynamics before and after CPB must be carefully evaluated to avoid complications of this monitoring.

INDUCTION OF ANESTHESIA

Because of the potential for rapid and dramatic hemodynamic changes in young patients with CHD, especially infants, complete preparation of anesthetic and monitoring equipment and required drugs is essential. Adequate assistance should be immediately available during the induction of anesthesia in case problems develop.

The choice of induction technique is influenced by the response to premedications, the parent–child–anesthesiologist relationship, and the anesthetic management plan. In older patients who have minimal compromise of their cardiac reserve, the choice of induction techniques is large. Inhalation, IV, or intramuscular induction of anesthesia can be accomplished, provided individual pathophysiological limitations are understood. Cooperative children with an adequate cardiac reserve and difficult IV access or a morbid fear of needles can have anesthesia induced cautiously with inhaled anesthetics, even if the patients are cyanotic. An inhalation induction with sevoflurane is suitable for most infants and children, provided they have stable ventricular function and adequate hemodynamic reserve. This emphasizes the importance of preoperative evaluation when planning the induction technique. Inhalational induction can be used safely in patients with cyanotic heart disease, although uptake may be slower because of the right-to-left shunt.[60] Saturations generally increase, provided cardiac output is maintained and airway obstruction avoided.

An intravenous induction should be used for all patients with severely limited hemodynamic reserve, particularly those with severe ventricular failure or pulmonary hypertension. In situations where hemodynamic instability during induction is likely, starting an inotropic agent such as dobutamine or dopamine before induction should be considered. Although the stress of placing an IV may be considerable for some patients, particularly those with difficult IV access after previous procedures, this is preferable to the potential myocardial depression during an inhalation induction with sevoflurane or halothane.

Fentanyl 15–25 µg/kg, in combination with pancuronium 0.2 mg/kg, provides hemodynamic stability and prompt airway control and attenuates the stress-induced increase in PVR associated with intubation. Ketamine 1–3 mg/kg IV is safe and reliable, providing hemodynamic stability and minimal increases in PVR. It is particularly useful in patients with severe CHF and ventricular outflow tract obstructions. Atropine 20 µg/kg or glycopyrrolate 10 µg/kg are traditionally given concurrently because of increased secretions. If IV access is difficult and stressful in infants, a combination of ketamine 4 mg/kg, glycopyrrolate 10 µg/kg, and suxamethonium 2 mg/kg intramuscularly allows prompt induction and airway control.

Etomidate is an anesthetic induction agent with minimal cardiovascular and respiratory depression. An intravenous dose of 0.2–0.3 mg/kg induces rapid loss of consciousness with duration of action of 3–5 minutes. Etomidate may be used as an alternative to the synthetic opioids for induction of anesthesia in patients with limited myocardial reserve.

Barbiturates and propofol can be used in patients with normal ventricular function. Titrated doses are suitable for short procedures such as cardioversion or TEE. Midazolam 0.1–0.2 mg/kg also is a useful adjunct during a narcotic induction, but may cause hypotension in patients dependent on a high sympathetic drive.

MAINTENANCE OF ANESTHESIA

Anesthesia maintenance techniques depend on the patient's preoperative cardiorespiratory status and pathophysiology of the underlying cardiac defect, the surgical procedure, the conduct of CPB, potential postoperative surgical problems, and the anticipated postoperative management. Once induction of anesthesia and control of the airway are accomplished and monitoring is adequate, anesthesia can be maintained with inhaled anesthetics or additional intravenous drugs as dictated by the response of each patient, intraoperative events, and postoperative plans.

Stress responses to pain and other noxious stimuli are profound in even the youngest neonates, regardless of postconceptual age.[3,5] These hormonal and metabolic stress responses can be deleterious,[4] particularly in patients with marginal hemodynamic reserve. High-dose narcotic techniques provide excellent hemodynamic stability and are commonly used to maintain anesthesia, with the choice of agent and dose dependent on the planned procedure, duration of bypass, and the anticipated postoperative management. Patients with good cardiac function undergoing relatively short bypass procedures, such as ASD closure, can be extubated in the OR or soon after surgery. Fentanyl 10–20 µg/kg in combination with isoflurane or sevoflurane is suitable before bypass. During CPB, awareness is a potential problem. Methods to prevent this vary between anesthesiologists, but isoflurane 1% can be continued on the bypass machine or intermittently doses of midazolam might be given. After bypass, inhalational agents are titrated as required according to hemodynamic responses.

STRESS RESPONSE

In general terms the "stress response" is a systemic reaction to injury, with hemodynamic, endocrinological, and immunological effects (Box 105-3). Stress and adverse postoperative outcome have been linked closely in critically ill newborns and infants. This is not surprising given their precarious balance of limited metabolic reserve and increased resting metabolic rate. Metabolic derangements such as altered glucose homeostasis, metabolic acidosis, salt and water retention, and a catabolic state contributing to protein breakdown and lipolysis are commonly seen after major stress in sick neonates and infants.[58] This complex of maladaptive processes may be associated with prolonged mechanical ventilation courses and ICU stay, as well as increased morbidity and mortality.

The neuroendocrine stress response is activated by afferent neuronal impulses from the site of injury, traveling via sensory nerves through the dorsal root of the spinal cord to the medulla and hypothalamus. Anesthesia can therefore have a substantial modulating effect on the neuroendocrine pathways of the stress response by virtue of providing analgesia and loss of consciousness.

It is important to distinguish between suppression of the endocrine response and attenuation of hemodynamic responses to stress. Because of their direct effects on the myocardium and vascular tone, anesthetic agents can readily suppress the hemodynamic side effects of the endocrine stress response. The same is true when inotropic and vasoactive agents are administered during anesthesia. However, the postoperative consequences of the endocrine stress response, particularly fluid retention and increased catabolism, remain unabated. Relying on hemodynamic

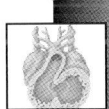

Box 105–3. Systemic Response to Injury.

Autonomic nervous system activation

Catechol release
Hypertension, tachycardia, vasoconstriction

Endocrine response

Anterior pituitary:	↑ ACTH, GH
Posterior pituitary:	↑ Vasopressin
Adrenal cortex:	↑ Cortisol, aldosterone
Pancreas:	↑ Glucagon, insulin resistance
Thyroid:	↓/→ $T_{4/3}$

Metabolic response

Protein catabolism
Lipolysis
Glycogenolysis/gluconeogenesis
Hyperglycemia
Salt and water retention

Immunological response

Cytokine production
Acute phase reaction
Granulocytosis

ACTH, Adrenocorticotrophic hormone; GH, growth hormone.

variables to assess the level of "stress" is therefore often inaccurate. Metabolic indices such as hyperglycemia and hyperlactatemia also are indirect markers of "stress," particularly because they are influenced by other factors such as fluid administration and cardiac output.

The effect of surgical stress has been particularly evaluated in neonates and infants undergoing cardiac surgery.[2,4,66] A conclusion from these studies supported the notion that reducing the stress response with large-dose opioid anesthesia, and extending this into the immediate postoperative period, was important to reduce the morbidity and mortality associated with congenital heart surgery in neonates.

However, these studies were performed over a decade ago, and during the intervening period, there have been substantial changes in the perioperative management of children with heart disease, as well as the management of CPB in general. Along with these changes, outcomes have improved considerably. In the early experience of bypass in neonates and infants, the use of high-dose opioid anesthesia to modulate the stress response was perceived to be one of the few clinical strategies available that was associated with the demonstrable improvement in morbidity and mortality.[2] More recently, it has been demonstrated that opioids do not in fact modify the endocrine or metabolic stress response initiated by CPB; despite this, mortality and morbidity continue to remain low.

Whereas the neonate may be more labile to changes in intravascular pressures, pulmonary vascular resistance, and cardiac output than older children, in fact the neonate is quite capable of coping with the acute phase of surgical stress. It is less common nowadays to see neonates in the immediate postbypass period with extensive peripheral edema or anasarca and, along with that, impaired ventricular function, reactive pulmonary hypertension, and substantial alterations in lung compliance and airway resistance. An example of this is the incidence of postoperative pulmonary hypertensive events. Pulmonary hypertensive crises were more common a decade or more ago in infants who had been exposed to weeks or months of high pulmonary pressure and flow, such as truncus arteriosis, complete atrioventricular canal defects, and transposition of the great arteries with VSDs. High-dose opioids were an important component of management for patients at risk for pulmonary hypertensive crises; however, this occurs much less frequently nowadays, when patients are operated upon at an earlier age and are therefore less likely to have significant or irreversible changes in the pulmonary vascular bed. Therefore changes in surgical practice, and in particular the timing of surgery, have meant that the longer-term pathophysiological consequences of various defects are less apparent than what they were 10–20 years ago. A strategy of high-dose opioid anesthesia to blunt the stress response may therefore be a less critical determinant of outcome.

This does not mean that high-dose synthetic opioids are not necessary for neonatal cardiac surgery. Synthetic opioids are potent analgesics and provide hemodynamic stability because of their lack of negative inotropic or vasoactive properties. Because of the limited physiological reserve, the pathophysiology of underlying cardiac defects, and the clinical consequences of the systemic inflammatory response to bypass in the neonates, using an anesthetic technique that has minimal hemodynamic side effects is clearly desirable.

The main aim is to provide an anesthetic that maintains hemodynamic stability and allows the anesthesia team to concentrate on all other aspects of the surgery, bypass, and post-CPB care. Sudden changes in hemodynamics before and after bypass may develop secondary to myocardial dysfunction, residual anatomical lesions, loss of sinus rhythm, changes in preload state, variable pulmonary vascular resistance, and alterations in mechanical ventilation, to mention a few; using a high-dose opioid anesthesia technique allows the anesthesiologist to focus on an evolving hemodynamic picture without the distraction of side effects from anesthetic drugs.

DISCONTINUATION OF CARDIOPULMONARY BYPASS

The effects of prolonged CPB relate in part to the interactions of blood components with the extracorporeal circuit, causing a systemic inflammatory response. This is magnified in children because of the large bypass circuit surface area and priming volume relative to patient blood volume. The clinical consequences include increased interstitial fluid and generalized capillary leak, and potential multiorgan dysfunction. Total lung water is increased with an associated decrease in lung compliance and increase in A–aO_2 gradient. Myocardial edema results in impaired ventricular systolic and diastolic function. A secondary fall in cardiac output by 20–30% is common in neonates in the first 6–12 hours after surgery, contributing to decreased renal function and oliguria.[63] Sternal closure may need to be delayed because of mediastinal edema and associated cardiorespiratory compromise when closure is attempted. Ascites, hepatic ingestion, and bowel edema may affect mechanical ventilation, cause a prolonged ileus, and delay feeding. A coagulopathy after CPB may contribute to delayed hemostasis.

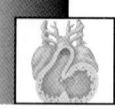

When weaning from CPB, an organized approach must be taken to prepare for termination of CPB so that a smooth transition is ensured. There should be communication between the surgeon and the anesthesiologist regarding anticipated difficulties in terminating CPB. Blood volume is assessed by direct visualization of the heart and monitoring right or left atrial filling pressures. When filling pressures are adequate, the patient fully warmed, acid–base status normalized, heart rate adequate, and sinus rhythm achieved, the drainage from the venous cannula is retarded, flow is reduced gradually, and the patient weaned from CPB. The need for vasopressor and inotropic support during weaning from bypass is determined by close observation of the heart during the rewarming phase.

Optimal ventricular filling pressures are estimated using filling pressures from preoperative catheterization data, the appearance of the heart, and infusion of small increments of volume while watching filling and systemic arterial pressures. The direct measurement of oxygen saturations from chambers of the heart enables calculations of a residual intracardiac shunt immediately after surgery, and direct pressure measurements across systemic and pulmonary outflow tracts enables detection of significant residual obstruction. TEE can be used to evaluate ventricular function, as well as assess surgical repair.

After discontinuing bypass, and despite full rewarming on bypass, rebound mild hypothermia often develops in neonates and infants. Active measures to decrease radiant and evaporative losses are necessary because of the increased metabolic stress, pulmonary vasoreactivity, coagulopathy, and potential for dysrhythmias associated with hypothermia. However, hyperthermia must also be actively avoided because of the associated increased metabolic rate and potential for ongoing neurological injury, particularly when myocardial function may be depressed and cerebral autoregulation impaired.[59]

Hemostasis may be difficult to obtain if bypass has been prolonged and if there are extensive, high-pressure (often concealed) suture lines. Prompt management and meticulous control of surgical bleeding is essential to prevent the complications associated with a massive transfusion. Besides hemodilution of coagulation factors and platelets, complex surgery with long bypass times increases endothelial injury and exposure to the nonendothelialized surface of the pump circuit, thereby stimulating the intrinsic pathway and platelet activation and aggregation.

POSTOPERATIVE MANAGEMENT

The optimal postoperative management of patients with CHD requires a multidisciplinary approach. A thorough understanding of the precise anatomical diagnosis, pathophysiology, and details of the surgical and CPB technique is necessary. For most patients, postoperative recovery is uncomplicated, and in general, when the patient's clinical progress or postoperative cardiorespiratory function does not follow the expected course, myocardial function must be evaluated and possible residual defects investigated, either with echocardiography and/or cardiac catheterization.

SEDATION AND ANALGESIA

The assessment of adequate analgesia in children can be difficult, particularly when they are paralyzed and ventilated. Primarily, autonomic signs such as hypertension, tachycardia, pupillary size, and diaphoresis are used. If unparalyzed, children will grimace and withdraw from a painful stimulus, and if breathing spontaneously, changes in respiratory pattern such as tachypnea, grunting, and splinting of the chest wall may be evident.

However, changes in autonomic signs do not only reflect pain. Other causes include awareness as patients emerge from anesthesia and sedation, fever, hypoxemia, hypercapnea, changes in vasoactive drug infusions, and seizures. If not diagnosed correctly, patients may receive additional opioid or benzodiazepine doses when hypertensive and tachycardic, which only contributes to tolerance and possible withdrawal symptoms later.

SEDATIVES

Chloral hydrate is commonly used to sedate children before medical procedures and imaging studies.[15] It can be administered orally or rectally in a dose ranging from 50–80 mg/kg (maximum dose 1 g), with an onset of action within 15–30 minutes with a duration of action between 2–4 hours. Chloral hydrate should be used to promote intermittent sedation in the ICU and not be prescribed as a repetitive scheduled medication.[1] Administered intermittently, it can be used to supplement benzodiazepines and opioids, may assist sedation during drug withdrawal, and is useful as a nocturnal hypnotic when trying to establish normal sleep cycles.

Benzodiazepines are the most commonly used sedatives in the ICU because of their anxiolytic, hypnotic, and amnestic properties. Although they provide excellent conscious sedation, they may cause dose-dependent respiratory depression and result in significant hypotension in patients with limited hemodynamic reserve. After chronic administration, tolerance and withdrawal symptoms are common.

Opioid analgesics are the mainstay of pain management in the ICU. They also can provide sedation for mechanically ventilated patients, as well as blunt hemodynamic responses to procedures such as endotracheal tube suctioning. Intermittent dosing of opioids can provide effective analgesia and sedation after surgery, although periods of oversedation and undermedication can occur because of peaks and troughs in drug levels. A continuous infusion is therefore advantageous.

Intermittent morphine doses of 0.05–0.1 mg/kg IV or as a continuous infusion at 50–100 μg/kg/hr provides excellent postoperative analgesia for most patients. The sedative property of morphine is an advantage over the synthetic opioids; however, histamine release can cause systemic vasodilation and an increase in pulmonary artery pressure.

The synthetic opioids, fentanyl, sufentanil, and alfentanil, have a shorter duration of action than morphine and do not cause histamine release, therefore producing less vasodilation and hypotension. Fentanyl is commonly prescribed after cardiac surgery. It blocks the stress response in a dose-related fashion while maintaining both systemic and pulmonary hemodynamic stability.[31,29] Chest wall rigidity is an idiosyncratic and dose-related reaction that can occur with a rapid bolus in newborns and older children. A continuous infusion of fentanyl 5–10 μg/kg/hr provides analgesia after surgery, although it often needs to be combined with a benzodiazepine to maintain sedation. Large variability between children in fentanyl clearance exists, making titration of an infusion difficult. The experience with extracorporeal membrane oxygenation (ECMO) indicates that tolerance and dependence to a fentanyl infusion develops rapidly and significant increases in infusion rate may be required.

The development of tolerance is dose- and time-related, and is a particular problem after cardiac surgery in patients who received a high-dose opioid technique to maintain anesthesia. Physical dependence with withdrawal symptoms such as dysphoria, fussiness, crying, agitation, tachypnea, tachycardia, diaphoresis, and feeding intolerance may be seen in children and can be managed by gradually tapering the opioid dose or administering a longer-acting opioid such as methadone. Methadone has a similar potency to morphine with the advantage of a prolonged elimination half-life between 18 and 24 hours. It can be administered intravenously and is absorbed well orally.

Alternate methods of opioid delivery that are often effective after cardiac surgery include patient-controlled analgesia (PCA) and epidural opioids, as either a bolus or continuous infusion. Patients receiving epidural opioids must be closely monitored for potential respiratory depression, and side effects include pruritus, nausea, vomiting, and urinary retention.

ASSESSMENT OF CARDIAC OUTPUT

A complete evaluation of cardiac output (CO) should be the initial focus of management in the ICU after cardiac surgery. Low CO is associated with longer duration of mechanical ventilatory support, ICU stay, and hospital stay, all of which can increase the risk of morbidity and/or mortality. Data from physical examination, routine laboratory testing, and bedside hemodynamic monitoring are all considered during the initial assessment.

Postoperative patients with low CO can display a variety of abnormalities on physical examination or of bedside monitoring and laboratory values. These manifestations of low CO are listed in Table 105-2. The mechanism(s) underlying low CO in a specific patient can be related to a number of factors. These include residual or unrecognized anatomical cardiovascular defects, the type of surgical procedure (e.g., RV dysfunction after right ventriculotomy), surgical complications (e.g., compromised coronary artery perfusion), dysrhythmia (supraventricular or ventricular) or loss of atrioventricular conduction, low preload (ongoing bleeding), high afterload (e.g., systemic vasoconstriction related to CPB), metabolic derangement (e.g., hypocalcemia, hypomagnesemia) and pulmonary hypertension (primarily affects RV function).

In neonates and infants an approximate 30% fall in CO within 9–12 hours after surgery can be anticipated even when the surgical repair is excellent. This pattern has been documented best for neonates with transposition of the great arteries (D-TGA),[63] but also occurs in neonates undergoing complete repair of TOF or truncus arteriosus. Pharmacological support of the myocardium may be necessary and anticipated to mitigate the effects of decreased cardiac index (CI) in these patients, including increase in

Table 105–2

Manifestations of Low Cardiac Output after Cardiac Surgery

Examination	
	Core hyperthermia Tachycardia or bradycardia Hypotension (for age and weight) Narrow pulse pressure Decreased peripheral perfusion: Hepatomegaly Ascites Oliguria
Monitoring	
Arterial waveform	Blunted or dampened upstroke Narrow pulse pressure
RAP or CVP, LAP (decreased)	Low intravascular fluid status Inadequate preload
RAP or CVP, LAP (increased)	Poor ventricular function Residual volume load Residual outflow tract obstruction Ischemia Loss of NSR Atrioventricular valve regurgitation/stenosis Tamponade
Laboratory and Radiographic	
Svo_2	Decreased with an increased AV O_2 difference (>25–30%)
Acid–base balance	Metabolic acidosis with increased anion gap Increased arterial lactate Elevated BUN and Cr Increased liver transaminases
Chest radiography	Cardiac enlargement Pulmonary edema Pleural effusion

RAP, Right atrial pressure; CVP, central venous pressure; LAP; left atrial pressure; NSR, normal sinus rhythm; Svo_2, systemic venous oxygen saturation; AV, arteriovenous; BUN, blood urea nitrogen; Cr, creatinine.

inotropic support with dopamine or additional drugs such as milrinone to lower afterload.

Strategies for treating the patient with low CO should focus on one or a combination of the factors contributing to CO, such as contractility, preload, afterload, and heart rate. Because decreased myocardial contractility occurs frequently after reparative or palliative surgery with CPB, pharmacological enhancement of contractility is commonly used in the ICU. Before treatment with an inotrope is initiated, the volume status, serum ionized Ca^{++} level, and cardiac rhythm should be evaluated. Dopamine is usually the initial treatment of hypotension, and it increases contractility by elevating intracellular Ca^{++} from direct binding to myocyte β_1-adrenoceptors and by increasing norepinephrine levels. At a dose >5 μg/kg/min, dopamine should be infused through a central venous catheter to avoid superficial tissue damage should extravasation occur. The dose is titrated to achieve the desired systemic blood pressure, although some patients, especially older children and adults, may develop an undesirable dose-dependent tachycardia. Dobutamine may be less effective than dopamine as a single agent in the treatment of moderate hypotension because it reduces systemic vascular resistance (SVR).[41]

If a patient does not respond adequately to dopamine at 10–15 μg/kg/min and has severe hypotension (>30% decrease in mean arterial blood pressure for age), treatment with epinephrine should be considered. Epinephrine can be added to dopamine at a starting dose of 0.05–0.1 μg/kg/min, with subsequent titration of the infusion to achieve the target systemic blood pressure. At high doses (i.e., ≥0.5 μg/kg/min), epinephrine can produce significant renal and peripheral vasoconstriction plus significant tachycardia, and those who require persistent doses of epinephrine >0.3–0.5 μg/kg/min should be evaluated for the possibility of mechanical circulatory support. Norepinephrine at doses of 0.01–0.2 μg/kg/min can be considered in patients with severe hypotension and low SVR (e.g., "warm" or "distributive" shock), inadequate coronary artery perfusion, or inadequate pulmonary blood flow with a systemic-to-pulmonary artery shunt. A combination of low-dose epinephrine (e.g., <0.1 μg/kg/min) or dopamine with an IV afterload reducing agent such as nitroprusside or milrinone frequently is beneficial to support patients with significant ventricular dysfunction accompanied by elevated afterload. Epinephrine is preferred to the equally potent inotrope norepinephrine because it generally is well tolerated in pediatric patients and causes less dramatic vasoconstriction.

If the rhythm cannot be determined with certainty from a surface 12- or 15-lead ECG, temporary epicardial atrial pacing wires, if present, can be used with the limb leads to generate an atrial ECG.[50] Temporary epicardial atrial and/or ventricular pacing wires are routinely placed in most patients to allow mechanical pacing if sinus node dysfunction or heart block occurs in the early postoperative period. Because atrial wires are applied directly to the atrial epicardium, the electrical signal generated by atrial depolarization is significantly larger and thus easy to distinguish compared with the P wave on a surface ECG. Sinus tachycardia, which is common and often secondary to medications (e.g., sympathomimetics), pain and anxiety, or diminished ventricular function, must be distinguished from a supraventricular, ventricular, or junctional tachycardia. Heart block can diminish CO by producing either bradycardia or loss of atrioventricular synchrony or both. Complete heart block may be transient in approximately one third of cases, but if it persists beyond postoperative day 9–10, it is unlikely to resolve, and a permanent pacemaker is indicated.

Elevated afterload in both the pulmonary and systemic circulations frequently follows surgery with CPB.[64] An increase in systemic afterload from elevated SVR may significantly increase myocardial work and reduce end-organ perfusion. Treatment of elevated SVR includes recognizing and improving conditions that exacerbate vasoconstriction (e.g., pain and hypothermia) and administering a vasodilating agent such as a PDE inhibitor (e.g., amrinone or milrinone) or an NO donor (e.g., nitroprusside).[10,39]

FLUID MANAGEMENT

Fluid management in the immediate postoperative period is critical, because of the inflammatory response to CPB and significant increase in total body water that often occurs. Capillary leak and interstitial fluid accumulation are continuous after surgery in neonates and infants, often necessitating ongoing volume replacement. A fall in CO and increased antidiuretic hormone secretion contribute to delayed water clearance and potential prerenal dysfunction. During bypass, optimizing the circuit prime hematocrit and oncotic pressure, attenuating the inflammatory response with steroids and protease inhibitors such as aprotinin, and the use of modified ultrafiltration techniques may help limit interstitial fluid accumulation.[12,16,18] During the first 24 hours after surgery, maintenance fluids should be restricted to 50% of full maintenance, and volume replacement titrated to appropriate filling pressures and hemodynamic response.

Oliguria is common in the first 24 hours after complex surgery and CPB. CO should be enhanced with volume replacement and vasoactive drug infusions, if necessary, before diuretics can be effective. In addition, low-dose dopamine (3 μg/kg/min) has the advantage of redistributing renal blood flow to promote diuresis. Fenoldopam mesylate, a selective dopamine (DA_1) receptor agonist that causes smooth muscle relaxation, leading to both renal and splanchnic vasodilation, has been used to provide renal protection during periods of ischemia and hypoxia, such as during hypothermic CPB.[27] At a dose of 0.1–0.5 μg/kg/min it also may have a role in postoperative ICU management to enhance renal perfusion by decreasing renal vascular resistance.

Furosemide 1–2 mg/kg IV every 8 hours is a commonly prescribed loop diuretic that is excreted into the renal tubular system before producing diuresis; low CO therefore reduces its efficacy. Bolus dosing may result in a significant diuresis over a short period, thereby causing changes in intravascular volume and possibly hypotension. A continuous infusion of 0.2–0.3 mg/kg/hr after an initial bolus of 1 mg/kg IV often provides a consistent and sustained diuresis without sudden fluid shifts. Chlorothiazide 10 mg/kg IV or orally (PO) every 12 hours also is an effective diuretic, particularly when used in conjunction with loop diuretics.

Peritoneal dialysis, hemodialysis, and continuous venovenous hemofiltration (CVVH) provide alternate renal replacement therapy in patients with persistent oliguria and renal failure.[22,48] Besides enabling water and solute clearance, nutritional support can be increased. A peritoneal dialysis catheter can be placed into the peritoneal cavity at the completion of surgery or later in the ICU. Indications in the ICU include the need for renal support, to reduce intraabdominal pressure from ascites that may be compromising mechanical ventilation, and to improve fluid management to allow administration of parenteral nutrition. Drainage may be significant in the immediate postoperative period as third-space fluid losses continue, and replacement with albumin and/or fresh frozen plasma may be necessary to treat hypovolemia and hypoproteinemia. For enhancement of fluid excretion if oliguria persists, low-volume peritoneal dialysis may be effective, although a persistent communication between the peritoneum, mediastinum, and/or pleural cavities after surgery limits the effectiveness of peritoneal dialysis and is a relative contraindication.

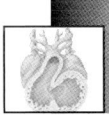

PULMONARY FUNCTION AND MECHANICAL VENTILATION

Altered respiratory mechanics and positive pressure ventilation may have a significant influence on hemodynamics after congenital heart surgery. Although changes in alveolar O_2 (PaO_2), $PaCO_2$, and pH significantly affect PVR, the mean airway pressure and changes in lung volume during positive pressure ventilation also affect PVR, preload, and ventricular afterload. Therefore the approach to mechanical ventilation should not only be directed at achieving a desired gas exchange, but also directed at the potential cardiorespiratory interactions of positive pressure ventilation. This is particularly critical during weaning.

Altered lung mechanics and ventilation–perfusion abnormalities are common problems in the immediate postoperative period.[36,43] Besides preoperative problems secondary to increased Qp/Qs, additional considerations include the surgical incision and lung retraction, increased lung water after CPB, possible pulmonary reperfusion injury, surfactant depletion, and restrictive defects from atelectasis and pleural effusions. In general, neonates and infants, with their limited physiological reserve, should not be weaned from mechanical ventilation until hemodynamically stable, and factors contributing to an increase in intrapulmonary shunt and altered respiratory mechanics have improved.

An increase in mean intrathoracic pressure during positive pressure ventilation decreases preload to both pulmonary and systemic ventricles, but has opposite effects on afterload to each ventricle (i.e., decreases afterload to systemic ventricle, but increases afterload on the pulmonary ventricle).[51,54] Changes in lung volume have a major effect on PVR, which is lowest at FRC, whereas both hypoinflation and hyperinflation may result in a significant increase in PVR.[65] An increase in PVR increases the afterload or wall stress on the RV, compromising RV function and contributing to decreased left ventricular (LV) compliance secondary to interventricular septal shift. In addition to low CO, signs of RV dysfunction, including tricuspid regurgitation, hepatomegaly, ascites, and pleural effusions, may be observed. An increase in mean intrathoracic pressure increases the afterload on the RV from direct compression of extraalveolar and alveolar pulmonary vessels. Patients with normal RV compliance, and without residual volume load or pressure load on the ventricle after surgery, usually show little change in RV function from the alteration in preload and afterload that occurs with positive pressure ventilation. However, these effects can be magnified in patients with restrictive RV physiology or poor diastolic function after congenital heart surgery, particularly neonates who have required a right ventriculotomy for repair of TOF, pulmonary atresia, or truncus arteriosus, and patients with concentric RV hypertrophy.

The systemic arteries are under higher pressure and are not exposed to radial traction effects during inflation or deflation of the lungs. Therefore changes in lung volume affect LV preload, but the effect on afterload is dependent on changes in intrathoracic pressure alone rather than changes in lung volume. Wall stress is directly proportional to the transmural LV pressure (i.e., the difference between the intracavity LV pressure and surrounding intrathoracic pressure). An increase in intrathoracic pressure, as occurs during positive pressure ventilation, therefore reduces the transmural gradient and wall stress on the LV. This is one explanation for the beneficial effect of positive pressure ventilation and PEEP in patients with LV failure. In addition, patients with LV dysfunction may have impaired pulmonary mechanics secondary to increased lung water, decreased lung compliance, and increased airway resistance. The work of breathing is increased, and neonates and infants in particular can fatigue early because of limited respiratory reserve. A significant proportion of total body oxygen consumption is directed at the increased work of breathing in neonates and infants with LV dysfunction, contributing to poor feeding and failure to thrive. Therefore positive pressure ventilation has an additional benefit in patients with significant volume overload and systemic ventricular dysfunction by reducing the work of breathing and oxygen demand.

Weaning from positive pressure ventilation may be difficult in patients with persistent systemic ventricular dysfunction. During spontaneous respiration the transmural pressure across the systemic ventricle is increased, and this sudden increase in wall stress may contribute to pulmonary edema and low CO state. Therefore it is often beneficial to continue vasoactive support during weaning and extubation if there is concern for ventricular dysfunction.

WEANING FROM MECHANICAL VENTILATION

Although most patients who have had no complications with repair or CPB will wean without difficulty after congenital cardiac surgery, some patients with borderline cardiac function and residual volume overload may require prolonged mechanical ventilation and a slower weaning process. Weaning is a dynamic process, and continued reevalauation is necessary.

The method of weaning varies between patients. Most patients can be weaned using either a volume- or pressure-limited mode by simply decreasing the intermittent mandatory ventilation (IMV) rate. Guided by physical examination, hemodynamic criteria, respiratory pattern, and arterial blood gas measurements, the mechanical ventilator rate is gradually reduced. Patients with limited hemodynamic and respiratory reserve may demonstrate tachypnea, diaphoresis, and shallow tidal volumes as they struggle to breathe spontaneously against the resistance of the endotracheal tube. The addition of pressure- or flow-triggered pressure support of 10–15 cm H_2O above PEEP is often beneficial in reducing the work of breathing.

Numerous factors that contribute to the inability to wean from mechanical ventilation after congenital heart surgery are shown in Box 105-4. In general, however, residual cardiac defects after surgery causing either a volume or pressure load must be excluded by echocardiography or cardiac catheterization if a patient fails to wean from ventilation as expected.

INDICATIONS FOR EARLY TRACHEAL EXTUBATION

The heterogeneous nature of congenital cardiac defects and wide age range makes it difficult to establish rigid protocols for cardiovascular and respiratory management after surgery. Each patient must be viewed individually and managed according to preoperative condition and stability, surgeon preference, any surgical or CPB-related complications, and postoperative cardiorespiratory status (Table 105-3). In keeping with the strategy of early surgical intervention and repair to promote improved longer-term growth and development, and with less emphasis on complete suppression of the stress response in the immediate postoperative period, it is possible to expeditiously move patients through the ICU in a safe yet efficient fashion.

Patients undergoing selected non-CPB or closed cardiac surgery and thoracic procedures are usually suitable for early tracheal extubation. This includes infants and older children undergoing procedures such as patent ductus arteriosus and vascular ring ligation. Infants and older children undergoing repair of coarctation of the aorta may benefit from early extubation to avoid the hypertension and tachycardia that often accompanies a slow wean from mechanical ventilation in the ICU after surgery. The risk of rebound hypertension and need to protect high-pressure surgical suture lines often dictates early blood pressure control with vasodilating and β-blocking drugs. In addition, mild to moderate hypothermia is often deliberately induced during surgery in an effort to optimize spinal cord protection while the aorta is cross-clamped, and tracheal extubation should be delayed until patients are normothermic.

In our experience, neonates and infants who require surgical modification to pulmonary blood flow, either from placement of a pulmonary artery band or creation of a systemic-to-pulmonary artery shunt, are not suitable for early extubation management protocols; we routinely continue mechanical ventilation and deep sedation for at least the first postoperative night until cardiorespiratory stability is attained.

Children undergoing relatively short bypass procedures using mild to moderate hypothermia, such as ASD repair, small VSD closure, and right ventricle-to-pulmonary artery conduit replacement, are often suitable for weaning and extubation either in the OR or early after ICU admission.

Box 105–4. Factors Contributing to the Inability to Wean from Mechanical Ventilation after Congenital Heart Surgery.

Residual cardiac defects

Volume load
Pressure load
Ventricular dysfunction
Dysrhythmias

Pulmonary restrictive defects

Pulmonary edema
Pleural effusion
Atelectasis
Ascites
Chest wall edema
Phrenic nerve injury

Airway

Edema/subglottic stenosis
Retained secretions
Vocal cord injury
Extrinsic compression
Bronchomalacia

Metabolic

Inadequate nutrition
Diuretic therapy (contraction alkalosis)

Sepsis

Table 105–3

Considerations for Planned Early Extubation after Congenital Heart Surgery

Patient factors	Limited cardiorespiratory reserve Pathophysiology of specific congenital heart defects Timing of surgery and preoperative management
Anesthetic factors	Premedication Drug distribution and maintenance of anesthesia on CPB Postoperative analgesia requirements
Surgical factors	Extent and complexity of surgery Residual defects Risks for bleeding and protection of suture lines
Conduct of CPB	Degree of hypothermia Level of hemodilution Myocardial protection Modulation of the inflammatory response and reperfusion injury
Postoperative management	Myocardial reserve Cardiorespiratory interactions Neurological recovery Analgesia management

CPB, Cardiopulmonary bypass.

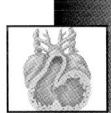

These patients generally have a stable preoperative clinical status, demonstrate few complications related to CPB, and have an uncomplicated postoperative course.

Infants who are in stable clinical condition before surgery and who are undergoing a complete repair using moderate to deep hypothermia on CPB, such as those undergoing closure of a large VSD, complete atrioventricular canal defect, or TOF, are often suitable for early extubation in the first 6–12 hours after surgery, provided they have stable cardiac output, stable gas exchange, and no surgical complications such as bleeding. Nevertheless, if there has been a large volume load on the ventricle before surgery or a labile pulmonary vascular resistance secondary to increased pulmonary blood flow, cautious management should be guided by hemodynamic and respiratory function as patients begin to emerge from sedation.

Infants and older children undergoing some types of LV outflow tract repair, including subaortic stenosis repair with the Konno operation or subaortic membrane resection, and aortic valvuloplasty or replacement, usually have well-preserved and often hyperdynamic ventricular systolic function. Hypertension and tachycardia frequently are a management concern in these patients in the immediate postoperative period. Not only does this increase the risk for disruption of suture lines, but the increased myocardial work may contribute to ischemia and increase the likelihood for ventricular tachyarrhythmias. This is especially a concern during emergence from anesthesia and sedation. Provided ventricular function is stable, hemostasis has been secured, and there are no concerns for ventricular tachyarrhythmias, it is often preferable for these patients to be extubated early after surgery (6–12 hours), rather than undergoing a more prolonged weaning process.

After creation of a cavopulmonary connection, when a bidirectional Glenn (BDG) shunt or a modified Fontan procedure, patients usually benefit from early tracheal extubation. Effective pulmonary blood flow is enhanced during spontaneous ventilation because of the lower mean intrathoracic pressure, but despite this goal, these patients should only be weaned once hemodynamic stability has been achieved. After a BDG procedure, it is usually possible to extubate the trachea within 12 hours of surgery.

After the modified Fontan procedure, patients also can typically be weaned and extubated within 12 hours of surgery. In the current surgical era of almost routine fenestration of the right atrial baffle, the arterial oxygen saturation should be in the 80–90% range after surgery, and, provided the patient is well perfused, has a transpulmonary gradient of 5–10 mm Hg, and does not have an acidosis or persistent large volume requirement, transfer from the ICU within 2–3 days of surgery can be accomplished.

The response to surgery and bypass can vary considerably among neonates and is often unpredictable. At Children's Hospital Boston, neonates undergoing two-ventricle repairs are usually managed with sedation and/or paralysis in the immediate postoperative period until hemodynamic and respiratory stability has been attained, although there are clear differences, depending on diagnosis and procedure. For example, after procedures such as an uncomplicated arterial switch operation for D-TGA, or repair of an interrupted aortic arch with VSD closure, many neonates are sufficiently stable to begin to wean from mechanical ventilation and be extubated by the first or second postoperative day.

On the other hand, neonates who have undergone a right ventriculotomy, such as after neonatal repair of TOF or truncus arteriosus, commonly demonstrate restrictive RV physiology in the immediate postoperative period. A low CO state with increased right-sided filling pressure may be evident, and continuing sedation and paralysis are often necessary for the first 48–72 hours until diastolic function improves.

Neonates undergoing a Norwood-type procedure for HLHS or other forms of single ventricle with aortic arch obstruction can pose considerable management problems in the immediate postoperative period. This is one group of patients in whom sedation and paralysis should be continued initially after surgery to minimize the stress response and any imbalance between oxygen supply and demand until a stable circulation and gas exchange have been achieved. Inotrope and vasoactive support is usually required, often combined with afterload reduction to reduce myocardial work and improve systemic perfusion. Volume replacement to maintain preload is essential, and monitoring mixed venous O_2 saturation as an indicator of CO is beneficial.

INTENSIVE CARE UNIT DISCHARGE

The cost of intensive care medicine is high. As the mortality and morbidity associated with congenital cardiac surgery

Box 105–5. Criteria for Intensive Care Unit Discharge.

Cardiovascular

- Stable blood pressure and systemic perfusion without requiring intravenous vasoactive support
- Invasive intravascular monitoring not indicated
- Stable cardiac rhythm (usually sinus) and no need for external pacing using temporary wires

Respiratory

- Adequate ventilation rate and pattern, no signs of airway obstruction, and effective cough
- Appropriate oxygenation (according to physiology after surgery)
- Restrictive pulmonary defects that would limit ventilation or oxygenation, including atelectasis, pneumothorax (after chest tube removal), or pleural effusion
- Neurological status adequate to protect airway

Fluid and metabolism

- Afebrile
- Advancing on caloric requirements with stable glucose levels
- Even fluid balance with stable diuretic management
- Stable electrolyte balance with appropriate supplementation

Appropriate nursing intensity

- Minimal chest physical therapy or bronchodilator treatments
- Established nutrition plan (enteral or parenteral)
- Controlled analgesic or sedation requirements
- Appropriate nursing staff numbers according to the intensity of care

have declined, length of ICU stay, total hospital stay, and cost-effectiveness have become important outcome variables. The timing of discharge from the ICU is therefore an important management decision. For the majority of patients who have a stable hemodynamic and respiratory status, the decision to transfer out of the ICU is not difficult. The function of all organ systems should be assessed and considered in this decision, although the focus is on cardiovascular and respiratory function. In addition to poor CO and residual anatomical lesions, there are a variety of noncardiac problems that can complicate recovery and prolong ICU stay (Box 105-5). It is important to emphasize that this decision should be multidisciplinary, with particular attention paid to nursing availability and experience, and availability of adequate monitoring.

REFERENCES

1. American Academy of Pediatrics CoD: Guidelines for monitoring and management of pediatric patients during and after sedation for diagnostic and therapeutic procedures. Pediatrics 89:1110–1115, 1992.
2. Anand KJ, Hansen DD, Hickey PR: Hormonal-metabolic stress responses in neonates undergoing cardiac surgery. Anesthesiology 73:661–670, 1990.
3. Anand KJ, Hickey PR: Pain and its effects in the human neonate and fetus. N Engl J Med 317:1321–1329, 1987.
4. Anand KJ, Hickey PR: Halothane-morphine compared with high-dose sufentanil for anesthesia and postoperative analgesia in neonatal cardiac surgery. N Engl J Med 326:1–9, 1992.
5. Anand KJ, Sippell WG, Aynsley-Green A: Randomised trial of fentanyl anaesthesia in preterm babies undergoing surgery: Effects on the stress response. Lancet 1:62–66, 1987.
6. Atz AM, Wessel DL: Inhaled nitric oxide in sickle cell disease with acute chest syndrome. Anesthesiology 87:988–990, 1997.
7. Atz AM, Wessel DL: Inhaled nitric oxide in the neonate with cardiac disease. Semin Perinatol 21:441–455, 1997.
8. Bancalari E, Jesse MJ, Gelband H, Garcia O: Lung mechanics in congenital heart disease with increased and decreased pulmonary blood flow. J Pediatr 90:192–195, 1977.
9. Baum VC, Palmisano BW: The immature heart and anesthesia. Anesthesiology 87:1529–1548, 1997.
10. Benzing G 3rd, Helmsworth JA, Schreiber JT, Kaplan S: Nitroprusside and epinephrine for treatment of low output in children after open-heart surgery. Ann Thorac Surg 27:523–528, 1979.
11. Berman W: The hemodynamics of shunts in congenital heart disease. In Johansen K, Burggren WW, editors: Cardiovascular shunts: Phylogenetic, Ontogenetic, and Clinical Aspects, pp. 399–410. New York: Raven Press, 1978.
12. Booker PD: Intra-aortic balloon pumping in young children. Paediatr Anaesth 7:501–507, 1997.
13. Bove AA, Santamore WP: Ventricular interdependence. Prog Cardiovasc Dis 23:365–388, 1981.
14. Butt WW, Gow R, Whyte H, et al: Complications resulting from use of arterial catheters: Retrograde flow and rapid elevation in blood pressure. Pediatrics 76:250–254, 1985.
15. Cote CJ: Sedation for the pediatric patient. A review. Pediatr Clin North Am 41:31–58, 1994.
16. Davies MJ, Nguyen K, Gaynor JW, Elliott MJ: Modified ultrafiltration improves left ventricular systolic function in infants after cardiopulmonary bypass. J Thorac Cardiovasc Surg 115:361–369; discussion 369–370, 1998.
17. Drummond WH, Gregory GA, Heymann MA, Phibbs RA: The independent effects of hyperventilation, tolazoline, and dopamine on infants with persistent pulmonary hypertension. J Pediatr 98:603–611, 1981.
18. Elliott MJ: Ultrafiltration and modified ultrafiltration in pediatric open heart operations. Ann Thorac Surg 56:1518–1522, 1993.
19. Feltes TF, Hansen TN: Effects of an aorticopulmonary shunt on lung fluid balance in the young lamb. Pediatr Res 26:94–97, 1989.
20. Friedman WF: The intrinsic physiologic properties of the developing heart. Prog Cardiovasc Dis 15:87–111, 1972.
21. Gerlach H, Rossaint R, Pappert D, Falke KJ: Time-course and dose-response of nitric oxide inhalation for systemic oxygenation and pulmonary hypertension in patients with adult respiratory distress syndrome. Eur J Clin Invest 23:499–502, 1993.
22. Giuffre RM, Tam KH, Williams WW, Freedom RM: Acute renal failure complicating pediatric cardiac surgery: A comparison of survivors and nonsurvivors following acute peritoneal dialysis. Pediatr Cardiol 13:208–213, 1992.
23. Gold JP, Jonas RA, Lang P, et al: Transthoracic intracardiac monitoring lines in pediatric surgical patients: A ten-year experience. Ann Thorac Surg 42:185–191, 1986.
24. Goldman AP, Delius RE, Deanfield JE, et al: Pharmacological control of pulmonary blood flow with inhaled nitric oxide after the fenestrated Fontan operation. Circulation 94:II44–II48, 1996.
25. Graham TP Jr: Ventricular performance in congenital heart disease. Circulation 84:2259–2274, 1991.
26. Group TNINOS: Inhaled nitric oxide in full-term and nearly full-term infants with hypoxic respiratory failure. N Engl J Med 336:597–604, 1997.
27. Halpenny M, Lakshmi S, O'Donnell A, et al: Fenoldopam: Renal and splanchnic effects in patients undergoing coronary artery bypass grafting. Anaesthesia 56:953–960, 2001.
28. Heymann MA: Control of the pulmonary circulation in the perinatal period. J Dev Physiol 6:281–290, 1984.
29. Hickey PR, Hansen DD: High-dose fentanyl reduces intraoperative ventricular fibrillation in neonates with hypoplastic left heart syndrome. J Clin Anesth 3:295–300, 1991.
30. Hickey PR, Hansen DD, Wessel DL, et al: Blunting of stress responses in the pulmonary circulation of infants by fentanyl. Anesth Analg 64:1137–1142, 1985.
31. Hickey PR, Hansen DD, Wessel DL, et al: Pulmonary and systemic hemodynamic responses to fentanyl in infants. Anesth Analg 64:483–486, 1985.
32. Hillier SC, Burrows FA, Bissonnette B, Taylor RH: Cerebral hemodynamics in neonates and infants undergoing cardiopulmonary bypass and profound hypothermic circulatory arrest: assessment by transcranial Doppler sonography. Anesth Analg 72:723–728, 1991.
33. Hoffman JI, Rudolph AM, Heymann MA: Pulmonary vascular disease with congenital heart lesions: Pathologic features and causes. Circulation 64:873–877, 1981.
34. Howlett G: Lung mechanics in normal infants and infants with congenital heart disease. Arch Dis Child 47:707–715, 1972.
35. Hsu YH, Santulli T Jr, Wong AL, et al: Impact of intraoperative echocardiography on surgical management of congenital heart disease. Am J Cardiol 67:1279–1283, 1991.
36. Jenkins J, Lynn A, Edmonds J, Barker G: Effects of mechanical ventilation on cardiopulmonary function in children after open-heart surgery. Crit Care Med 13:77–80, 1985.
37. Keens TG, Bryan AC, Levison H, Ianuzzo CD: Developmental pattern of muscle fiber types in human ventilatory muscles. J Appl Physiol 44:909–913, 1978.
38. Kontras SB, Sirak HD, Newton WA Jr: Hematologic abnormalities in children with congenital heart disease. JAMA 195:611–615, 1966.
39. Lawless ST, Zaritsky A, Miles M: The acute pharmacokinetics and pharmacodynamics of amrinone in pediatric patients. J Clin Pharmacol 31:800–813, 1991.

40. Lees MH, Way RC, Ross BB: Ventilation and respiratory gas transfer of infants with increased pulmonary blood flow. Pediatrics 40:259–271, 1967.
41. Leier CV, Heban PT, Huss P, et al: Comparative systemic and regional hemodynamic effects of dopamine and dobutamine in patients with cardiomyopathic heart failure. Circulation 58:466–475, 1978.
42. Levin AR, Ho E, Auld PA: Alveolar-arterial oxygen gradients in infants and children with left-to-right shunts. J Pediatr 83:979–987, 1973.
43. Lister G, Talner N: Management of Respiratory Failure of Cardiac Origin. New York: Churchill Livingstone, 1981.
44. Mansell A, Bryan C, Levison H: Airway closure in children. J Appl Physiol 33:711–714, 1972.
45. Mills AN, Haworth SG: Greater permeability of the neonatal lung. Postnatal changes in surface charge and biochemistry of porcine pulmonary capillary endothelium. J Thorac Cardiovasc Surg 101:909–916, 1991.
46. Morray JP, Lynn AM, Mansfield PB: Effect of pH and PCO_2 on pulmonary and systemic hemodynamics after surgery in children with congenital heart disease and pulmonary hypertension. J Pediatr 113:474–479, 1988.
47. Muhiudeen IA, Roberson DA, Silverman NH, et al: Intraoperative echocardiography for evaluation of congenital heart defects in infants and children. Anesthesiology 76:165–172, 1992.
48. Paret G, Cohen AJ, Bohn DJ, et al: Continuous arteriovenous hemofiltration after cardiac operations in infants and children. J Thorac Cardiovasc Surg 104:1225–1230, 1992.
49. Pepke-Zaba J, Higenbottam TW, Dinh-Xuan AT, et al: Inhaled nitric oxide as a cause of selective pulmonary vasodilatation in pulmonary hypertension. Lancet 338:1173–1174, 1991.
50. Perry J, Walsh EP: Diagnosis and Management of Cardiac Arrhythmias. Baltimore: Williams & Wilkins, 1998.
51. Pinsky MR, Summer WR, Wise RA, et al: Augmentation of cardiac function by elevation of intrathoracic pressure. J Appl Physiol 54:950–955, 1983.
52. Rabinovitch M, Haworth SG, Castaneda AR, et al: Lung biopsy in congenital heart disease: A morphometric approach to pulmonary vascular disease. Circulation 58:1107–22, 1978.
53. Roberts JD Jr, Fineman JR, Morin FC 3rd, et al: Inhaled nitric oxide and persistent pulmonary hypertension of the newborn. The Inhaled Nitric Oxide Study Group. N Engl J Med 336:605–610, 1997.
54. Robotham JL, Lixfeld W, Holland L, et al: The effects of positive end-expiratory pressure on right and left ventricular performance. Am Rev Respir Dis 121:677–683, 1980.
55. Rudolph AM, Yuan S: Response of the pulmonary vasculature to hypoxia and H^+ ion concentration changes. J Clin Invest 45:399–411, 1966.
56. Rung GW, Wickey GS, Myers JL, et al: Thiopental as an adjunct to hypothermia for EEG suppression in infants before circulatory arrest. J Cardiothorac Vasc Anesth 5:337–342, 1991.
57. Schreiber MD, Heymann MA, Soifer SJ: Increased arterial pH, not decreased $PaCO_2$, attenuates hypoxia-induced pulmonary vasoconstriction in newborn lambs. Pediatr Res 20:113–117, 1986.
58. Shew SB, Jaksic T: The metabolic needs of critically ill children and neonates. Semin Pediatr Surg 8:131–139, 1999.
59. Shum-Tim D, Nagashima M, Shinoka T, et al: Postischemic hyperthermia exacerbates neurologic injury after deep hypothermic circulatory arrest. J Thorac Cardiovasc Surg 116:780–792, 1998.
60. Tanner GE, Angers DG, Barash PG, et al: Effect of left-to-right, mixed left-to-right, and right-to-left shunts on inhalational anesthetic induction in children: A computer model. Anesth Analg 64:101–107, 1985.
61. Weintraub R, Shiota T, Elkadi T, et al: Transesophageal echocardiography in infants and children with congenital heart disease. Circulation 86:711–722, 1992.
62. Wernovsky G, Rubenstein SD, Spray TL: Cardiac surgery in the low-birth weight neonate. New approaches. Clin Perinatol 28:249–264, 2001.
63. Wernovsky G, Wypij D, Jonas RA, et al: Postoperative course and hemodynamic profile after the arterial switch operation in neonates and infants. A comparison of low-flow cardiopulmonary bypass and circulatory arrest. Circulation 92: 2226–2235, 1995.
64. Wessel DL: Hemodynamic responses to perioperative pain and stress in infants. Crit Care Med 21:S361–S362, 1993.
65. West JB: Respiratory Physiology: The Essentials. Baltimore: Williams & Wilkins, 1974.
66. Wood M, Shand DG, Wood AJ: The sympathetic response to profound hypothermia and circulatory arrest in infants. Can Anaesth Soc J 27:125–131, 1980.

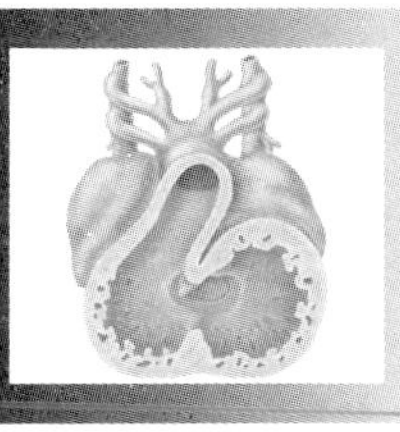

Congenital Tracheal Disease

Carl Lewis Backer, Constantine Mavroudis, and Lauren D. Holinger

CHAPTER 106

INTRODUCTION

The two most common congenital tracheal anomalies in infants and children are tracheomalacia and tracheal stenosis. Congenital tracheal stenosis is most commonly caused by complete cartilage tracheal rings and is the most common indication for surgical intervention.[11] The normal trachea has an anterior arch-shaped cartilage and a posterior membranous trachea. In children with complete tracheal rings the cartilage ring is circumferential and the membranous trachea is absent (Figure 106-1). In contrast, tracheomalacia is associated with a broad membranous trachea. This results in "floppiness," resulting in tracheal narrowing, particularly during expiration. The word "tracheomalacia" is derived from the Greek word *malakia,* meaning softness. The circumference of the trachea is normal, but the structure is less rigid. Tracheomalacia is a chronic condition that infrequently requires surgical intervention. Patients with tracheal stenosis often have associated anomalies, most commonly pulmonary artery sling and congenital cardiac anomalies.[8] Pulmonary artery sling is present in one third of patients with congenital tracheal stenosis. Major intracardiac anomalies are present in 25% of the patients with congenital tracheal stenosis.

Significant historical milestones in pediatric tracheal surgery are shown in Table 106-1. The classification of tracheal stenosis was first proposed by Drs. Cantrell and Guild from the University of Washington, Seattle in 1964.[13] They classified these patients into the following three morphological types: (1) funnel-like stenosis, (2) segmental stenosis, and (3) generalized hypoplasia. They also noted the frequent association of a tracheal right upper lobe bronchus that is present in 20% of these patients (Figure 106-2). In the Congenital Heart Surgery Nomenclature and Database Project, we classified congenital tracheal stenosis as congenital-complete tracheal rings, postintubation, traumatic, or congenital web.[4] Localized stenosis is defined as less than 50% of the tracheal length, and long-segment stenosis as greater than 50% of the tracheal length.[4] In a series of landmark publications in the 1960s, Dr. Hermes Grillo from Massachusetts General Hospital defined the surgical approach to the trachea and tracheal release procedures for resection.[21] He and others helped define the blood supply of the trachea.[41] The first successful operation for congenital stenosis of the trachea was reported by Dr. Kimura from Kobe Children's Hospital in Kobe, Japan, in 1982.[31] He used a costal cartilage graft to augment the tracheal lumen of a 12-month-old infant with tracheal stenosis secondary to complete tracheal rings (cartilage tracheoplasty). The use of pericardium to augment the tracheal lumen was first performed by Dr. Farouk Idriss from Children's Memorial Hospital in 1982.[27] The operation was facilitated by the use of cardiopulmonary bypass for respiratory support during the procedure. Slide tracheoplasty was first reported by Victor Tsang from Brompton Hospital in London, England, in 1989.[42] Its use in the United States has been championed by Dr. Grillo and his associates.[22] Claus Herberhold and Martin Elliott from Great Ormond Street, London, England, performed the first successful use of a tracheal homograft to augment the lumen of a patient with a failed prior intervention for tracheal stenosis from congenital tracheal rings in 1994.[17] We reported the use of a free tracheal autograft for infants with congenital tracheal stenosis in 1998; the first operation was performed in 1996.[6] Pulmonary artery sling repair was first performed by Dr. Willis J. Potts at Children's Memorial Hospital in 1953.[39] The left pulmonary artery was divided at its origin from the right pulmonary artery and reanastomosed anterior to the trachea.

CLINICAL PRESENTATION AND DIAGNOSTIC TECHNIQUES

The diagnosis of congenital tracheal stenosis should be suspected in any infant who has stridor (noisy breathing), respiratory distress, apnea, cyanosis, wheezing, retractions, or

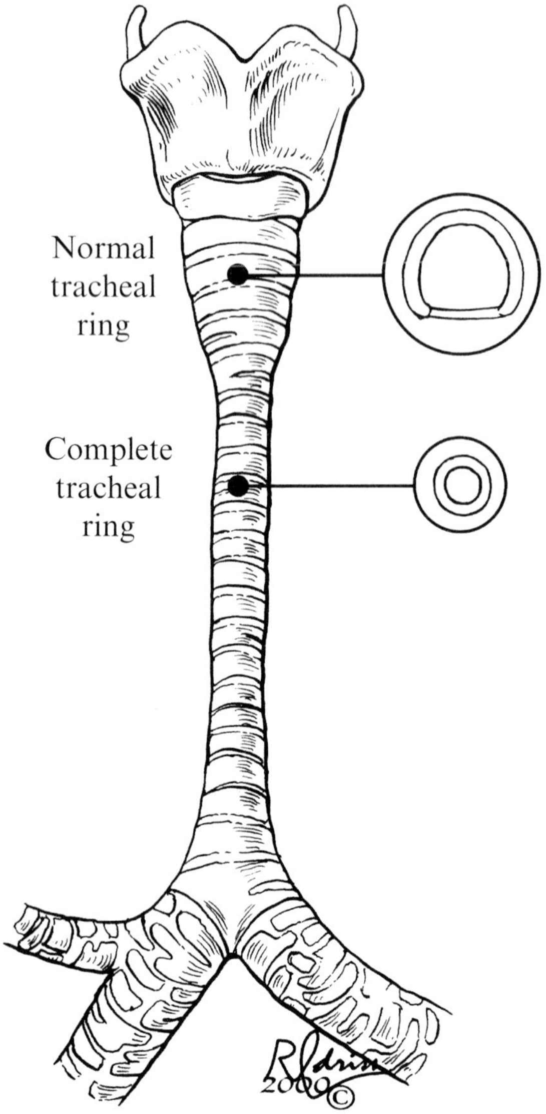

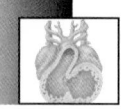

Figure 106–1 **Complete tracheal rings.** This is an illustration of the trachea of an infant with long-segment tracheal stenosis secondary to complete tracheal rings. There are three normal tracheal rings immediately below the cricoid. The upper cutaway shows a normal tracheal ring with the anterior cartilage and flat posterior membranous trachea. This is followed by 18 complete tracheal rings that progress almost to the carina. These complete tracheal rings are illustrated in the lower cutaway—there is a complete cartilage ring with a substantially reduced tracheal lumen. The tracheal lumen in some of these infants is as small as 1.5–2 mm.

Table 106–1

Notable Historical Events in Pediatric Tracheal Surgery

Year	*Event*	*Surgeon*
1953	Pulmonary artery sling repair	Potts
1964	Tracheal stenosis classification	Cantrell
1969	Tracheal resection limitations	Grillo
1980	Cartilage tracheoplasty	Kimura
1982	Pericardial tracheoplasty, cardiopulmonary bypass	Idriss
1989	Slide tracheoplasty	Goldstraw
1994	Tracheal homograft	Elliott
1996	Tracheal autograft	Backer

respiratory failure requiring intubation. A common clinical presentation is as a "difficult intubation." The child presents when being anesthetized and intubated for a surgical procedure. At that time the endotracheal tube selected for the patient's size fails to pass into a normal location within the trachea, because of the tracheal stenosis. These patients should be evaluated with a chest radiograph, computed tomography (CT) scan and/or magnetic resonance imaging (MRI), bronchoscopy, and echocardiography. The chest radiograph often demonstrates the diminutive nature of the tracheal lumen. It reveals lung agenesis or hypoplasia. CT scan or MRI shows the tracheal lumen in cross section and provides the length of the tracheal stenosis. A tracheal right upper lobe can be identified if present. Three-dimensional (3D) reconstruction generates a remarkable graphic representation of the tracheal pathology (Figure 106-3).[35]

Our experience has been that CT is most useful because it requires less sedation and there is less movement artifact than with MRI. A pulmonary artery sling (if present) is demonstrated if the CT scan is performed with contrast. A pulmonary artery sling also can be seen with MRI. For the sick neonate who is transferred with a critically positioned endotracheal tube and congenital tracheal stenosis, transthoracic echocardiography has been our diagnostic procedure of choice to demonstrate a pulmonary artery sling.[2] In addition, echocardiography should be performed on all of these infants because of the 25% incidence of congenital heart disease found in patients with congenital tracheal stenosis.[8] The single most important diagnostic procedure in all patients is rigid bronchoscopy. This can be performed as a separate procedure before the planned tracheal operation or at the time of the tracheal procedure. Often the congenital tracheal stenosis is so severe that even the smallest-diameter bronchoscope will not pass through the stenosis. In this situation a fine telescope (outer diameter 1.8 mm) may be passed through the stenosis without the bronchoscope. In some severe cases distal visualization of the trachea is unable to be obtained by bronchoscopy for fear of occluding the tracheal lumen. In the past we occasionally used contrast tracheobronchography, but with the excellent images generated by CT scan, we and others feel that the risks of contrast tracheograms outweigh the benefits (Box 106-1).[37]

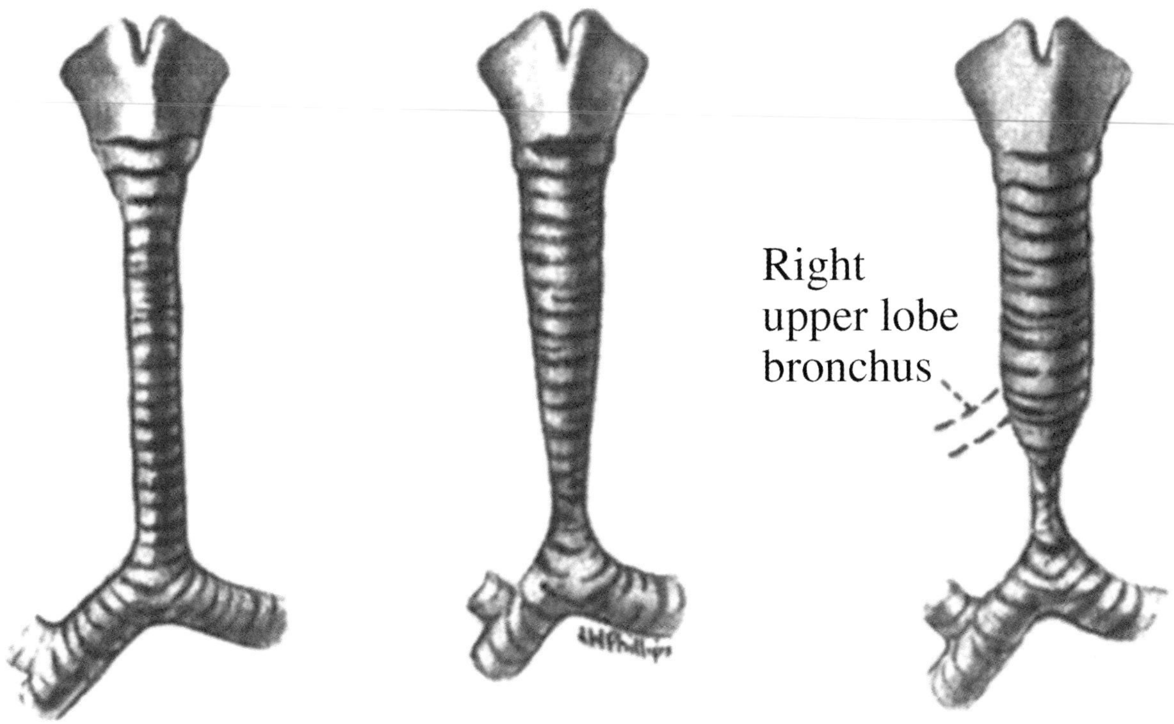

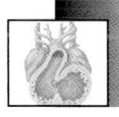

Figure 106–2 **Diagram of the three morphological variants of congenital stenosis of the trachea.** *Left*, Generalized hypoplasia; *center*, funnel-like stenosis; *right*, segmental stenosis. The occurrence of an anomalous right upper lobe bronchus (tracheal right upper lobe), as in the case presented, is most common in the segmental form.
(From Cantrell JR, Guild HC: Congenital stenosis of the trachea. Am J Surg 108:297, 1964.)

SURGICAL TECHNIQUES

Cartilage Tracheoplasty

The first successful report of a surgical procedure for long-segment congenital tracheal stenosis was a cartilage tracheoplasty performed by Kimura and associates[31] from Kobe Children's Hospital in Japan. They operated on a 12-month-old female infant referred with recurrent respiratory distress since birth. By bronchoscopy the entire trachea was seen to be stenotic. The left bronchus was of normal caliber, and the right lung was completely aplastic. Through a median sternotomy incision the left bronchus was incised and cannulated for ventilation. A longitudinal incision was made through the entire length of the anterior wall of the trachea. Two separate pieces of costal cartilage were used to fill the defect in the anterior wall of the trachea. The grafts were attached to the tracheal edges with interrupted 5-0 Dexon sutures. This patient required prolonged intubation and ventilation, but was successfully extubated 2 months postoperatively.

We feel that the surgical technique of cartilage tracheoplasty for the infant with long-segment congenital tracheal stenosis is best performed with the use of cardiopulmonary bypass. The approach is through a median sternotomy in which the midline incision is extended onto the neck, or (preferably) a collar incision is used for further exposure of the trachea in the neck. The cartilage graft can be harvested via the median sternotomy incision as shown in Figure 106-4. Median sternotomy is performed while preliminary preparation of the cartilage graft is being done. The trachea is dissected and exposed on its anterior surface. The patient is heparinized and cannulated for cardiopulmonary bypass via the right atrium and ascending aorta. Extracorporeal circulation is initiated with cooling to 32° C, so the heart remains beating in normal sinus rhythm. Ventilation is stopped. A scalpel is then used to open the anterior wall of the stenotic trachea through the extent of the stenosis (Figure 106-5). Although we previously used bronchoscopic guidance for the assessment of the degree of stenosis, in most cases it is possible to perform this by visualizing the trachea through the tracheal incision with the use of headlight illumination. The segment of costal cartilage is then tailored to a size and shape suitable for the anterior opening of the trachea. Care is taken to preserve the perichondrium. The perichondrium is placed on the luminal surface, and the graft is secured with interrupted absorbable monofilament suture (PDS) (Figure 106-6). Intraluminal suture exposure is avoided, and the graft is seated on the tracheotomy rather than being allowed to prolapse into the lumen. After completion of the graft suture line, the anesthesiologist inflates the lungs with air and the suture line is confirmed to be airtight, with additional sutures placed as necessary. Bronchoscopy is performed to confirm the tracheal lumen adequacy and clear retained secretions. The endotracheal tube is repositioned in the midportion of the cartilage graft. The patient is ventilated and weaned from cardiopulmonary bypass. The tracheal suture line is sealed with Tissel glue. Hemoclips are placed in the soft tissue adjacent to the trachea to mark the location of the cartilage graft. Sternotomy is closed in the standard fashion. Patients are maintained on heavy sedation and with muscle relaxation to minimize motion of the endotracheal tube in the airway. One week after the proce-

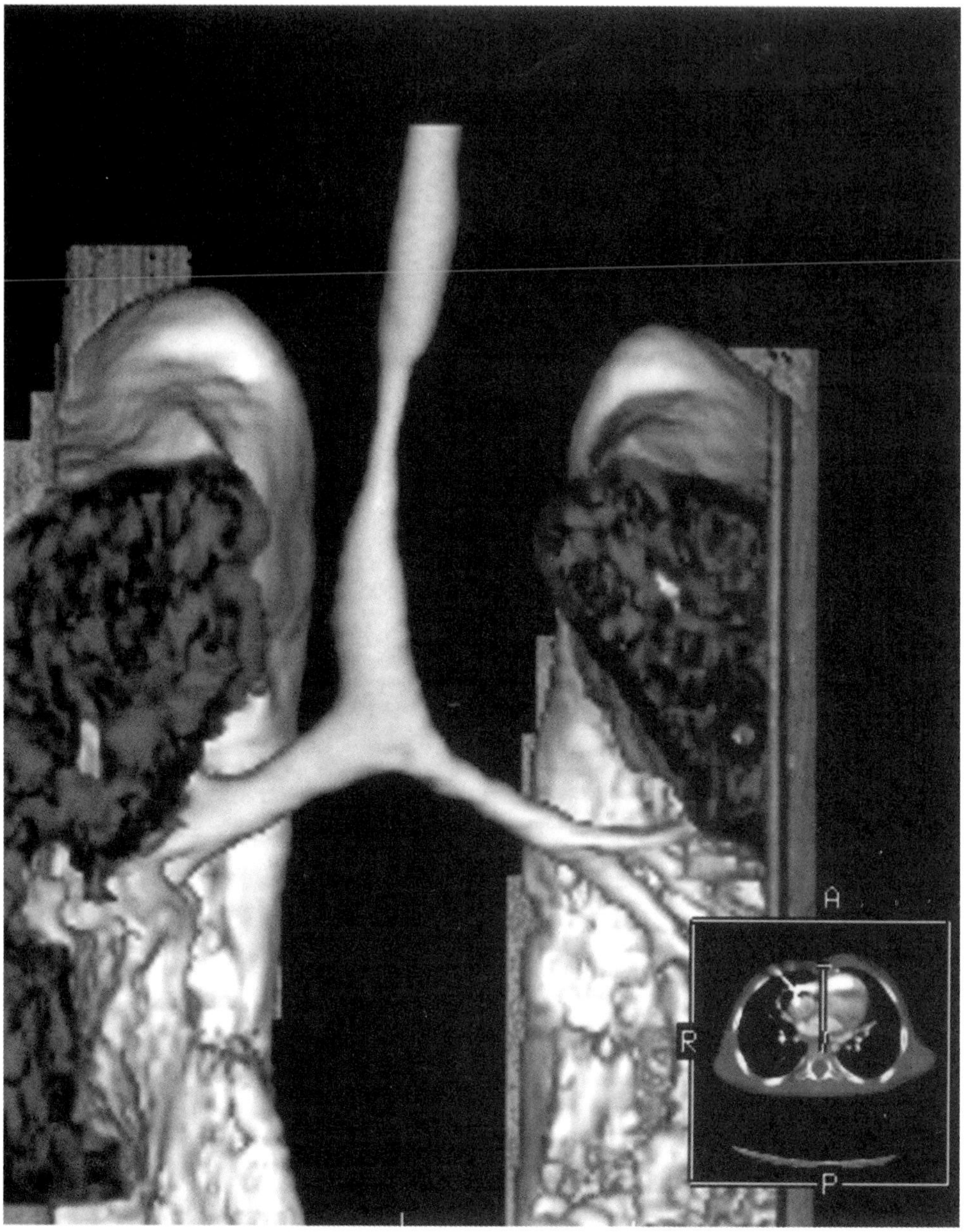

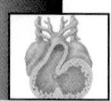

Figure 106–3 Computed tomography (CT) with three-dimensional (3D) reconstruction reveals a significant tracheal stenosis in the midportion of this child's trachea. The pathology at the time of surgery was essentially identical to the pathology indicated by the CT scan. This child underwent a successful tracheal autograft.

Box 106–1. Diagnostic Techniques for Infants with Complete Tracheal Rings.

- Chest radiograph
- Computed tomography (CT) with contrast, including three-dimensional (3D) reconstruction
- Rigid bronchoscopy
- Echocardiography (rule out pulmonary artery sling, congenital cardiac anomalies)

dure, the patient is reexamined with rigid bronchoscopy. If necessary, granulation tissue is removed and secretions are suctioned. If the airway appears to be stable and adequately healed, the patient is weaned from the ventilator over the next several days and extubated. Follow-up bronchoscopies are performed as necessary until the trachea is cleared of granulation tissue.

The long-term follow-up of these infants is that the graft becomes incorporated into the tracheal structure and grows with the patient. In addition, reepithelialization of the graft site with ciliated columnar epithelium occurs.[38] In our series of patients we have used the cartilage tracheoplasty exclusively for reoperations after failed pericardial tracheoplasty.[5] The results of this procedure are shown in Table 106-2.[5,19,30,34,43]

Pericardial Tracheoplasty

Pericardial tracheoplasty was first performed by Dr. Farouk Idriss in 1982 at Children's Memorial Hospital.[27] This procedure also marked the first use of cardiopulmonary bypass for a patient undergoing an operation for complete tracheal rings. Idriss reported on five infants with long-segment tracheal stenosis, all operated on through a median sternotomy with extracorporeal circulation that had a pericardial patch inserted to augment the tracheal lumen. There were no

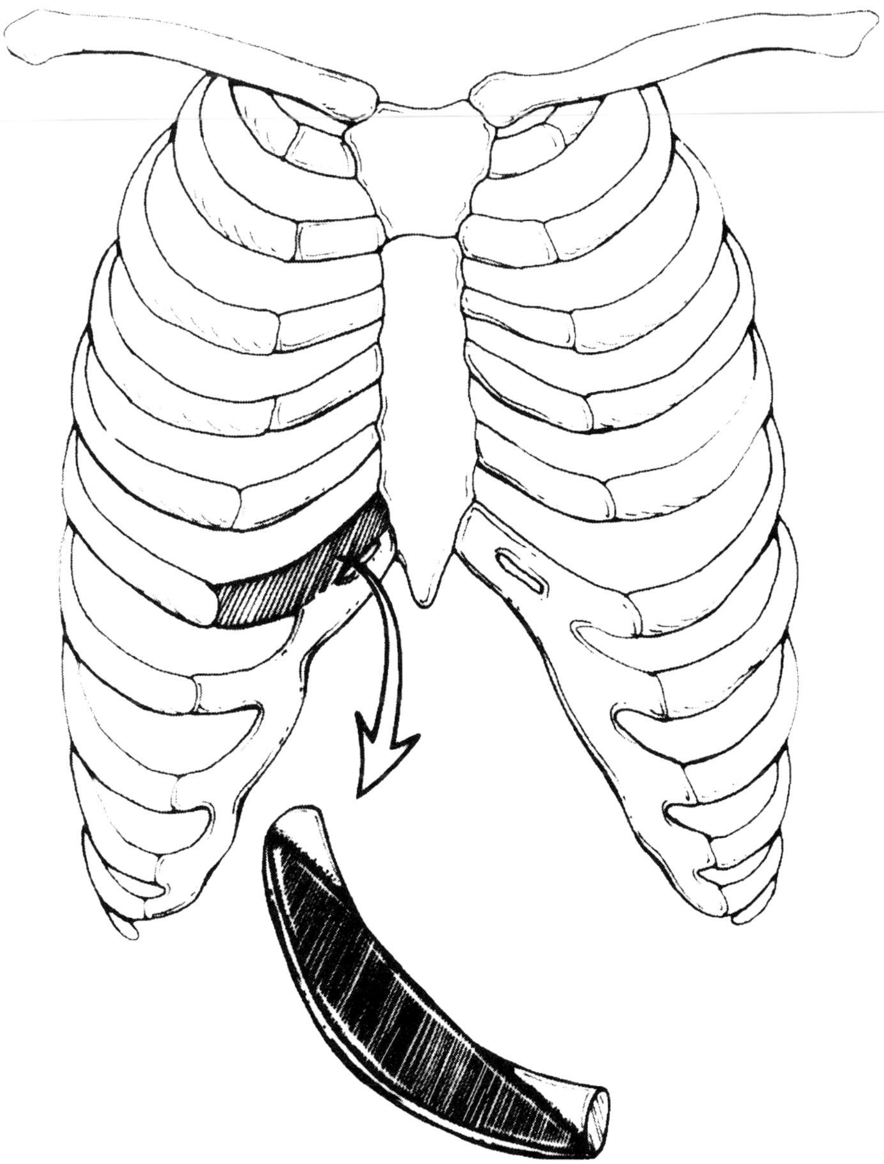

Figure 106–4 Before the median sternotomy, a segment of cartilage is harvested from the sixth or seventh rib. The cartilage is then tailored to correspond to the subsequent tracheal opening.
(From Jaquiss RD, Lusk RP, Spray TL, Huddleston CB: Repair of long-segment tracheal stenosis in infancy. J Thorac Cardiovasc Surg 110:1504–1512, 1995.)

deaths or infections. This technique was the procedure of choice at Children's Memorial Hospital for the next 15 years. The approach in all of these patients was through a median sternotomy with the use of cardiopulmonary bypass for respiratory support.

The innominate artery and vein are dissected free and encircled with vessel loops. These may then be retracted superiorly or inferiorly to address the various components of the trachea. The aorta is mobilized from its pericardial attachments and retracted with a small pledgetted suture to the left. The anterior surface of the trachea is freed from pericardial attachments so that it may be completely visualized from cricoid to carina if necessary. Initially we assessed the area of stenosis with intraoperative rigid bronchoscopy. A 25-gauge needle was passed through the anterior surface of the trachea to identify bronchoscopically the site of maximal stenosis. More recently we have, based on the 3D CT scan reconstruction, identified preoperatively the area of stenosis to be addressed and then opened this anteriorly with a No. 11 blade. If the surgeon opens the trachea slowly and visualizes the posterior tracheal wall, the area of complete tracheal rings can be incised successfully without carrying the incision too far. Once the full extent of the tracheal stenosis has been opened, a suitably shaped pericardial patch is fashioned. This patch frequently is quite long (4–6 cm in length) and may need to extend from the diaphragmatic surface to the brachiocephalic vessels. The width of the patch is usually 2–3 cm, which is clearly wider than the tracheal opening. However, there is some shrinking of the patch over time after patch placement, and this can be managed by inserting a larger patch than the tracheal opening might suggest. We do not place the patch in glutaraldehyde, but simply keep it in a sponge soaked in saline during the dissection and opening of the trachea. The patch is anchored in place using interrupted Vicryl (Polyglactin 910; Ethicon, Inc., Somerville, NJ) or PDS sutures (Figure 106-7). The suturing begins in the area of the carina, which is the most critical location. With the suturing begun here once the lower portion of the patch is in place, less blood and fluid tend to accumulate in the tracheal lumen because this is the most inferior point of the dissection. After the patch is in place, rigid bronchoscopy is repeated to assess the tracheal lumen and suction free blood and secretions. The endotracheal tube is replaced and is positioned so that the tip of the tube is below

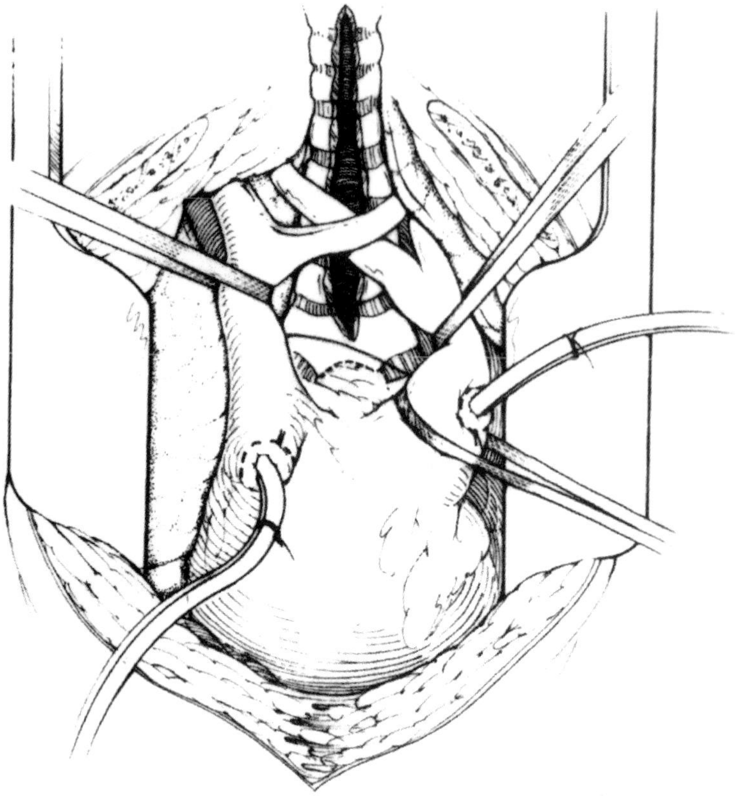

Figure 106–5 Exposure of the trachea through a sternotomy is demonstrated, including the relative positions of bypass cannulas and retraction of the great vessels for optimum exposure. Tracheal incision has been performed to the carina.
(From Jaquiss RD, Lusk RP, Spray TL, Huddleston CB: Repair of long-segment tracheal stenosis in infancy. J Thorac Cardiovasc Surg 110:1504–1512, 1995.)

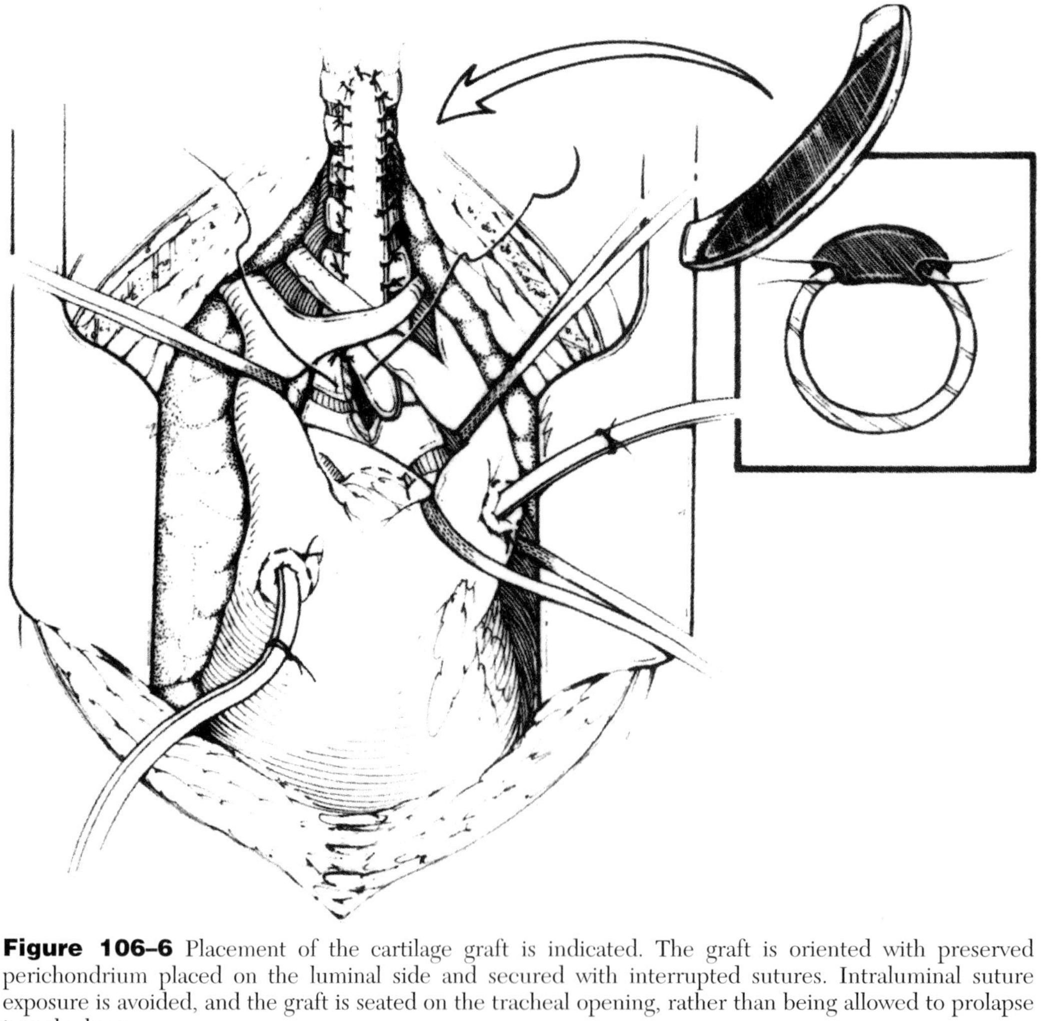

Figure 106–6 Placement of the cartilage graft is indicated. The graft is oriented with preserved perichondrium placed on the luminal side and secured with interrupted sutures. Intraluminal suture exposure is avoided, and the graft is seated on the tracheal opening, rather than being allowed to prolapse into the lumen.
(From Jaquiss RD, Lusk RP, Spray TL, Huddleston CB: Repair of long-segment tracheal stenosis in infancy. J Thorac Cardiovasc Surg 110:1504–1512, 1995.)

Table 106–2

Results of Cartilage Tracheoplasty

Surgeon	*Year*	*Patients*	*Mortality*
Lobe[34]	1987	4	1 (25%)
Tsugawa[43]	1988	5	1 (25%)
Backer[5]	1997	4	1 (25%)
Kamata[30]	1997	11	5 (45%)
Huddleston[19]	2002	10	1 (10%)
Total		34	9 (25%)

the lowest point of the tracheal patch. The endotracheal tube acts as a stent for the pericardial patch. If the patch goes all the way to the carina, the endotracheal tube is positioned at an appropriate point just above the carina so that it does not irritate the carina. The patient is ventilated, and the anesthesiologist inflates the lungs to a pressure of 35 or 40 cm of water to test the patch for air leaks. Any leaks are controlled with additional sutures. The patient is then ventilated and weaned from cardiopulmonary bypass. The heparin is reversed with protamine. The edges of the patch are sealed with a very fine spray of Tissell glue (Baxter Health Care Corp., Glenlake, CA). The extent of the pericardial patch is marked with small hemoclips placed in the soft tissues of the adjacent mediastinum at the superior and inferior portions of the pericardial patch. For the prevention of patch tracheomalacia, fine monofilament Prolene sutures are used to take partial-thickness bites of the pericardium and fix it to the posterior wall of the ascending aorta and the innominate artery. This acts as a suspending device, holding the patch open. These patients are kept on muscle relaxants and heavily sedated for 1 week. Repeat bronchoscopy is performed. If there is an adequate repair with a good tracheal lumen and minimal granulation tissue, the patient is then weaned from the ventilator and extubated in 5–7 days. Many of these patients, however, have patch tracheomalacia, necessitating a prolonged period of intubation for 1 or 2 more weeks after the first successful bronchoscopy. Repeat bronchoscopies are performed as needed to clear granulation tissue and retained secretions. Over several months' time the patch becomes reepithelialized with pseudostratified columnar epithelium.[14]

The results of pericardial patch tracheoplasty at several different centers are illustrated in Table 106-3.[3,5,10,10a] Our impression with the pericardial tracheoplasty was that we had a low operative mortality (7%) but a fairly prolonged hospitalization with a mean hospital stay of slightly over 2 months. In addition, these patients required frequent bronchoscopic examinations for resection of granulation tissue, which tended to occur chiefly at the carinal area where there was a critical junction of the pericardial patch, the carina, and the irritation from the distal end of the endotra-

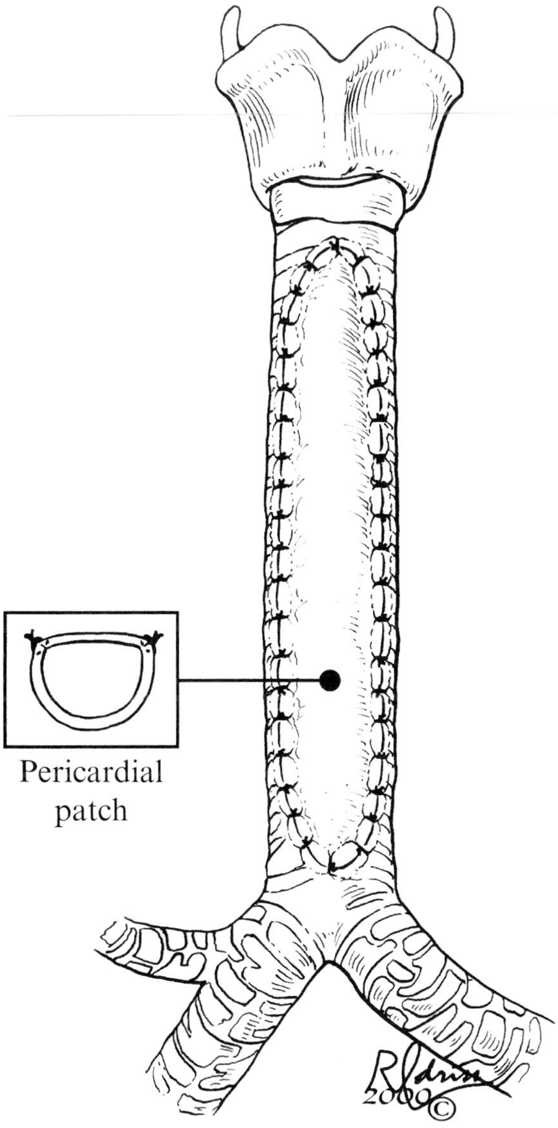

Figure 106–7 Illustration of a completed pericardial patch tracheoplasty. The pericardium is anchored with interrupted Vicryl sutures. In cross-selection *(inset)*, the tracheal lumen is shown now to be normal in size.
(From Backer CL, Mavroudis C, Gerber ME, et al: Tracheal surgery in children: An 18-year review of four techniques. Eur J Cardiothorac Surg 19:777–784, 2001.)

Table 106–3

Results of Pericardial Tracheoplasty

Surgeon	*Year*	*Patients*	*Mortality*
Bailey[3]	1994	13	6 (47%)
Backer[5]	1997	28	5 (18%)
Brown[10,10a]	2002	20	3 (15%)
Total		61	14 (23%)

cheal tube. In addition, a significant percentage of these patients required a repeat procedure in the form of either a tracheotomy to stent the patch (n = 3), Palmaz intraluminal expandable wire stent (n = 3), or reoperation with either a repeat pericardial patch (n = 2) or a cartilage graft (n = 4) tracheoplasty.[5] It was because of these chronic problems with the pericardial tracheoplasty that we turned to the tracheal autograft technique in 1996.

Tracheal Autograft Technique

The principle of the tracheal autograft technique is to shorten the trachea and use the excised piece of trachea as an anterior patch (autograft). Our first group of patients was reported in 1998 and consisted of six infants whose mean age was 4.9 months and mean weight was 5.4 kg.[6] All patients were operated on through a median sternotomy with cardiopulmonary bypass. Four patients had simultaneous pulmonary artery sling repair, and two patients required intracardiac repair of a congenital heart defect. The trachea was incised anteriorly through the area of stenosis, the midportion of the stenotic trachea was excised, and an end-to-end anastomosis was carried out posteriorly. The excised tracheal segment (mean length 1.8 cm) was used as a free autograft patch. In 4 of those first 6 patients the autograft was augmented in the upper trachea with pericardium. All patients survived and were extubated and discharged at a mean of 13 and 23 days, respectively. Since that initial successful experience, the tracheal autograft has become our procedure of choice for infants with long-segment tracheal stenosis.[9]

The operation is performed through a median sternotomy approach. If the tracheal stenosis extends up to the cricoid, a collar incision is made in the neck as a "T" from the median sternotomy incision. This incision tends to heal better than a midline extension of the median sternotomy onto the neck. The strap muscles are divided in the midline. The thymus is partially excised, preserving only the cervical heads. The innominate artery and vein are dissected free. Dissection of the trachea is performed anteriorly to identify externally the site of the stenosis. Unlike the pericardial tracheoplasty, some dissection must be performed circumferentially and posteriorly to facilitate the removal of the midportion of the trachea for the autograft. Attention must be paid to the lateral blood supply of the tracheal wall and a decision made regarding which vessels can be preserved for an adequate blood supply to the eventual anastomosis. In most cases the carinal attachments are freed, as are the pericardial attachments of the right and left main stem bronchi. After cardiopulmonary bypass has been initiated and the aorta retracted to the left, the trachea is opened in the midline through the extent of the tracheal stenosis. This is done in most cases now without the use of bronchoscopic guidance. The midportion of the tracheal stenosis (typically 6–8 complete tracheal rings with a mean length of 1.8 cm) is then excised. The posterior trachea is brought together with interrupted 6.0 PDS (Ethicon, Inc.) sutures (Figure 106-8). This leaves an anterior opening that is then augmented with

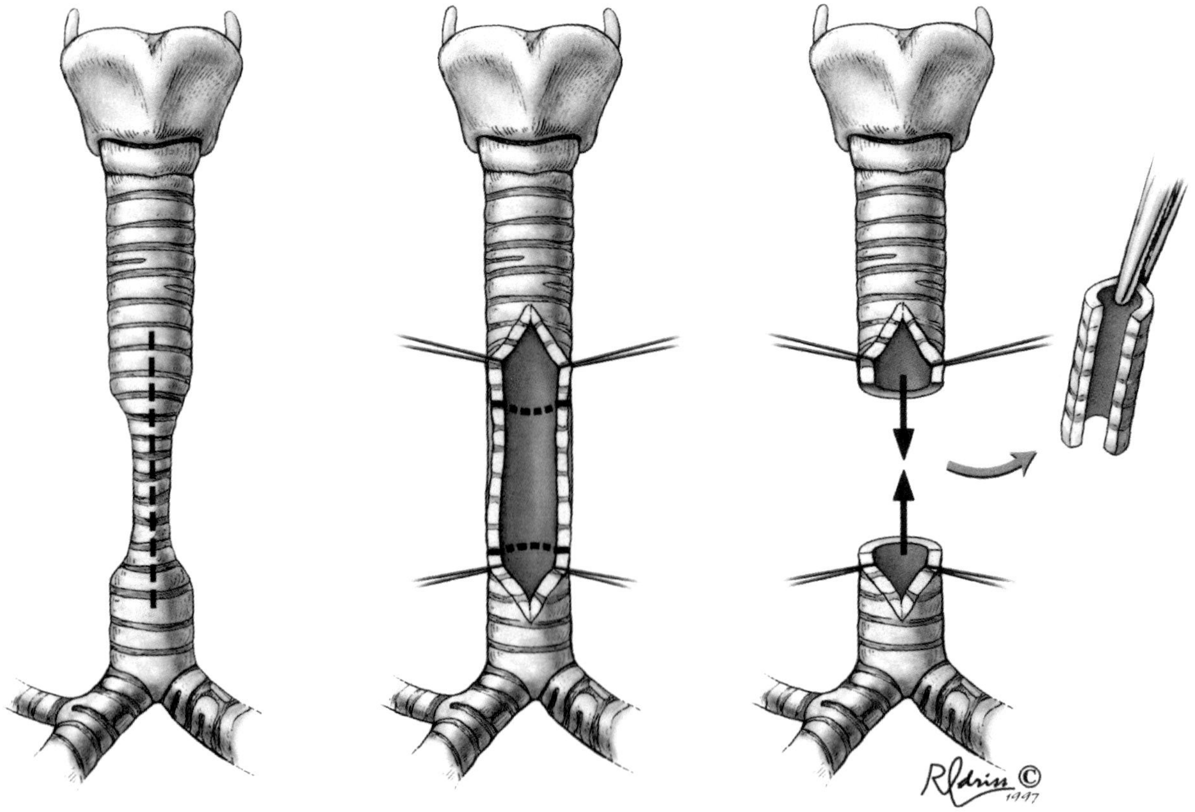

Figure 106–8 Tracheal autograft. An anterior longitudinal incision is performed through the complete extent of the tracheal rings *(left)*. The midportion of the trachea is excised to be used as the tracheal autograft *(center)*. The two remaining orifices of the trachea are reapproximated posteriorly *(right)*.
(From Backer CL, Mavroudis C, Dunham ME, et al: Repair of congenital tracheal stenosis with a free tracheal autograft. J Thorac Cardiovasc Surg 113:869–874, 1998.)

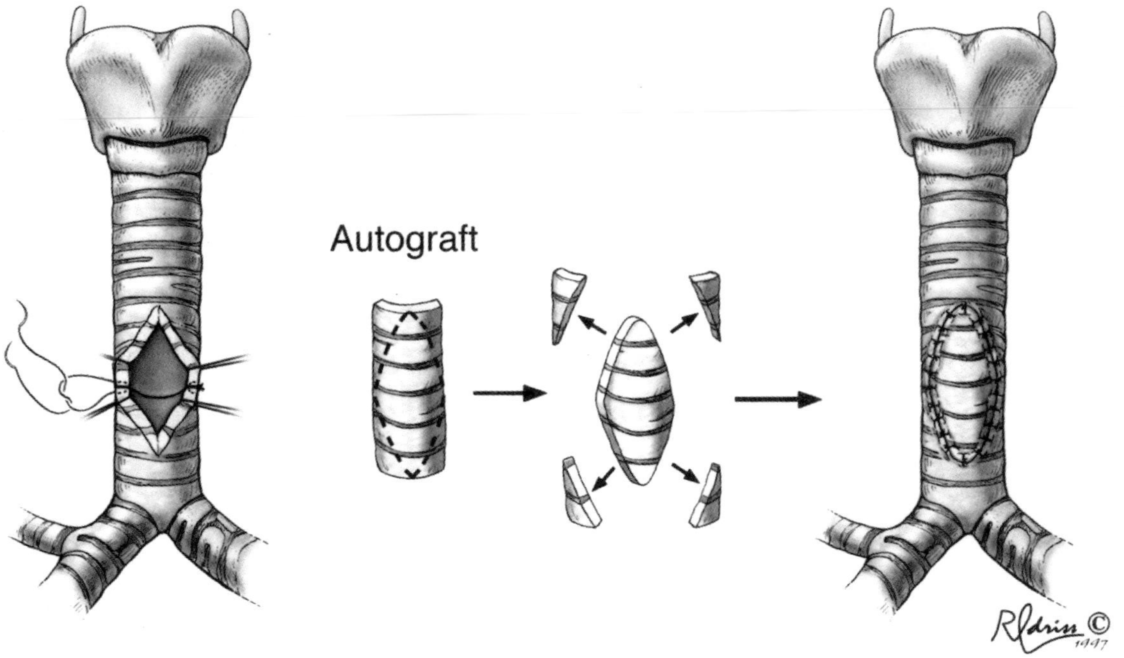

Figure 106–9 **Tracheal autograft.** The posterior tracheal anastomosis is performed with interrupted 6-0 PDS sutures *(left)*. The autograft is prepared by trimming the corners of the autograft *(center)*. The autograft is sutured in place to cover the remaining opening in the anterior trachea *(right)*.
(From Backer CL, Mavroudis C, Dunham ME, et al: Repair of congenital tracheal stenosis with a free tracheal autograft. J Thorac Cardiovasc Surg 113:869–874, 1998.)

the autograft. The corners of the autograft are trimmed so that the autograft fits into the anastomosis. The autograft does not shrink like pericardium and therefore does not need to be oversized. The autograft is sutured in place with multiple interrupted 6-0 PDS sutures (Figure 106-9). If the autograft is not long enough to completely augment the anterior tracheal lumen, the superior portion of the tracheal opening that is remaining after autograft insertion is patched with pericardium (Figure 106-10). This patch tends to be relatively short (1.5–2 cm in length) and, because of the additional support, has less chance for patch tracheomalacia. The placement of the endotracheal tube depends on the anatomy. If the autograft completes the procedure, the tube may be positioned either above the autograft or through the area of the autograft if it is in a superior location. For patients in whom pericardium is used for augmentation, the tube is usually positioned in the midportion of the autograft. The soft tissues of the mediastinum adjacent to the autograft are marked with hemoclips superiorly and inferiorly to identify the superior and inferior borders and the junction of the pericardium with the autograft. After the patients have been ventilated and assessed for air leaks, they are weaned from cardiopulmonary bypass. The autograft is sealed with Tissell glue, and the autograft suture line is sometimes compressed by the innominate artery. In this case a cervical strap muscle is mobilized and brought in as an interposition between the innominate artery and the tracheal autograft. We have now performed the tracheal autograft technique in 19 patients with one early death for an early mortality of 5% and two late deaths for a late mortality of 11%. The early death occurred in a patient who also had simultaneous repair of tetralogy of Fallot with an anomalous left coronary artery that required extracorporeal membrane oxygenation (ECMO) support for low cardiac output postoperatively. The child expired of myocardial infarction and necrotizing pneumonia with a patent trachea.

Of the two late deaths, one occurred 18 months postoperatively when the trachea was perforated during bronchoscopy elsewhere. The other death occurred 4 months postoperatively from a trachea-to-carotid fistula in a child with an absent right lung and anomalous brachiocephalic vessels. Our series is currently the only published series using this technique.[6,8,9] We have had personal communication, however, with several other surgeons who have successfully used this technique.

Tracheal Resection

In the article by Cantrell and Guild published in 1964 that reported the three morphological varieties of congenital tracheal stenosis, the authors also reported a successful case of tracheal resection of segmental stenosis in a child.[13] This was a 7-year-old child who had a tracheal right upper lobe and a bridging bronchus to the carina. The bridging bronchus was stenotic. The bridging bronchus was excised, and the carina was brought up to the main trachea. An anastomosis was performed with interrupted sutures of braided stainless steel. The child survived the operation and was asymptomatic on follow up. Tracheal stenosis amenable to tracheal resection with end-to-end anastomosis was originally thought to be feasible for stenosis involving up to 50% of the total tracheal length. However, recent evidence from Massachusetts General Hospital has indicated that resections of more than 30% of the trachea have a substantial failure rate.[44] This has been our impression also and is interestingly corroborated by our tracheal autograft series, where the average autograft length excised was 6–8 tracheal rings (33% of the trachea). Our current recommendation is

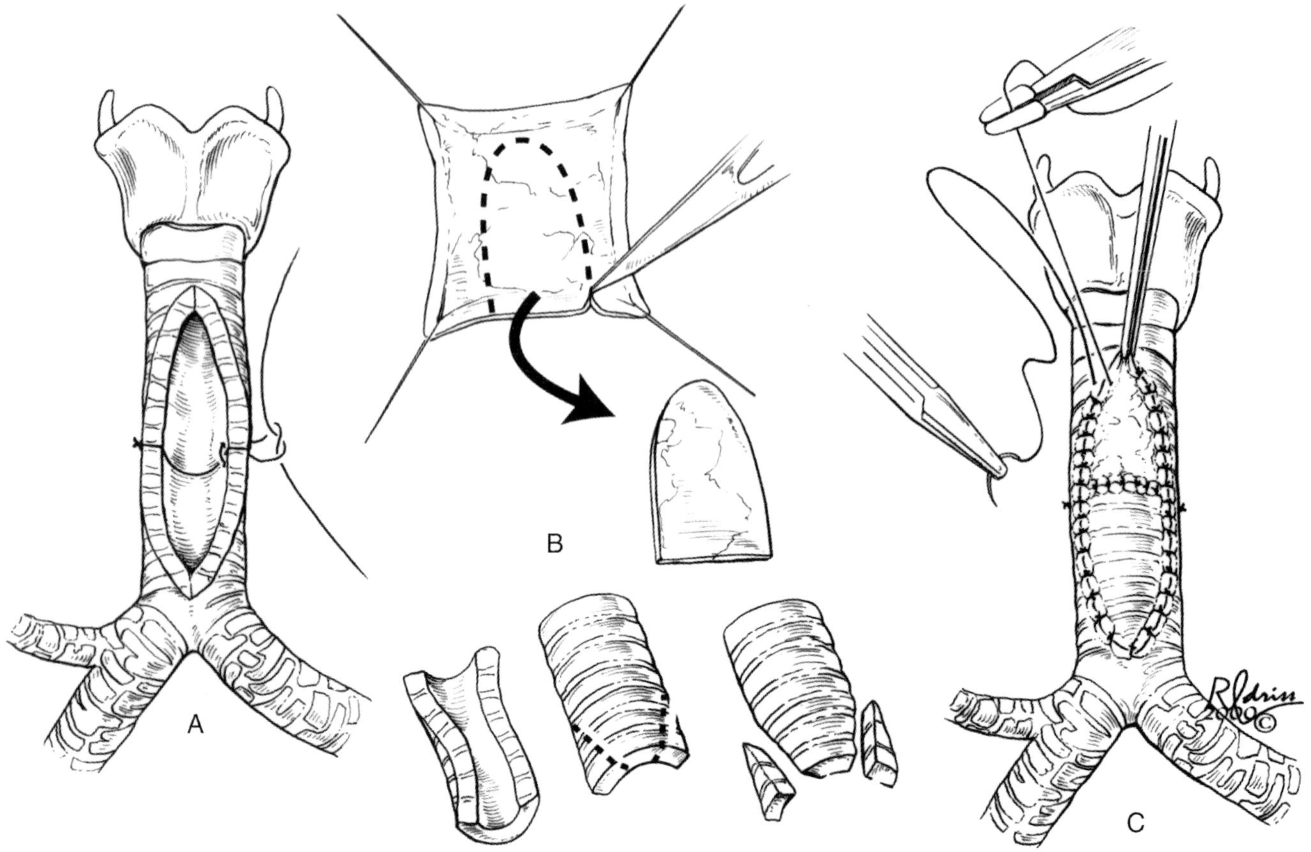

Figure 106–10 **Composite tracheal autograft. A,** The posterior anastomosis is performed. **B,** The autograft is trimmed, cutting only the inferior corners of the autograft. A portion of pericardium is harvested and tailored. **C,** The autograft is sutured in place anteriorly adjacent to the carina. The pericardial patch is inserted superiorly to complete the repair.
(From Backer CL, Mavroudis C, Gerber ME, et al: Tracheal surgery in children: An 18-year review of four techniques. Eur J Cardiothorac Surg 19:777–784, 2001.)

that tracheal resection should be performed only if the stenosis is less than one third of the total tracheal length. This is usually 6–8 complete tracheal rings.

We have performed all of the tracheal resections in our series through a median sternotomy approach with the use of cardiopulmonary bypass. The dissection is similar to that of the tracheal autograft. If the focal area of stenosis cannot be identified externally, intraoperative bronchoscopy with the use of the illuminated tip of the bronchoscope for guidance can demonstrate the area of the complete tracheal rings. The technique of passing a fine needle through the anterior trachea also is useful for some patients. The technique that we currently employ is to incise the trachea through the length of the stenosis in a longitudinal fashion. This incision is exactly the same as that performed for the tracheal autograft technique. The incision is extended proximally and distally until the extent of the complete tracheal rings has been encompassed. If this length is less than 30% of the trachea (6–8 complete tracheal rings), the segment is then simply excised. The two ends are brought together, and the anastomosis is performed with interrupted PDS sutures (Figure 106-11). Before the anterior sutures are tied, the trachea is suctioned free of secretions and blood with a fine plastic suction catheter. However, if the length of the stenosis is too long for a successful end-to-end anastomosis, the operation can be easily converted to the tracheal autograft technique. Results of tracheal resection in infants and children are shown in Table 106-4.[9,15,25,44] The overall mortality in over 70 patients was 8%. The median age in our tracheal resection patients at Children's Memorial Hospital was 4 months, and the mean number of excised tracheal rings was 5. Mean hospital stay was 14 days. The one death (out of 12 patients) occurred 2.5 months postoperatively in a child with biliary atresia awaiting a liver transplant.

Slide Tracheoplasty

Slide tracheoplasty was first reported by Victor Tsang and Peter Goldstraw from Brompton Hospital, London, England, in 1989.[42] They operated on two patients with complete tracheal rings; one survived and one died. The slide tracheoplasty has been reported as being performed either through a cervical collar incision or through a median sternotomy approach. The procedure has been performed with and without cardiopulmonary bypass. The midportion of the tracheal stenosis is transected (Figure 106-12). The two tracheal halves are then opened longitudinally, one anteriorly and one posteriorly (different surgeons have reported placing these openings either inferiorly or superiorly). The illustrations show an anterior tracheotomy inferiorly and a posterior tracheotomy superiorly (Figure 106-13).

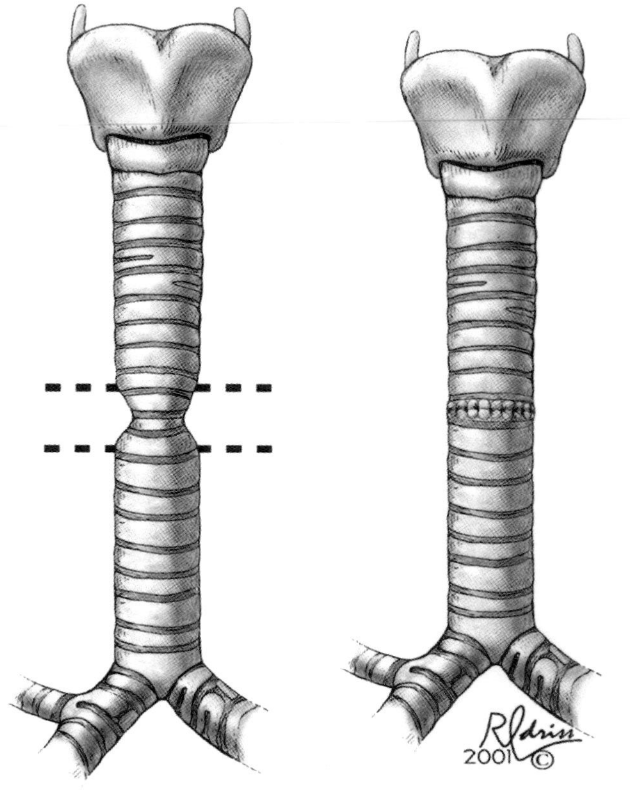

Figure 106–11 **Tracheal resection.** The localized segment of tracheal stenosis is excised. The trachea is extensively mobilized, specifically in the right and left main stem bronchi and carina. This allows the trachea to be brought together without tension for an end-to-end anastomosis using interrupted PDS sutures.
(From Backer CL, Mavroudis C, Holinger LD: Repair of congenital tracheal stenosis. Semin Thorac Cardiovasc Surg Pediatr Card Surg Annu 6:33–50, 2003.)

The two openings are then "slid" together and approximated with interrupted absorbable sutures for the anastomosis (Figure 106-14). The end result is a trachea that is half the original length with four times the internal luminal diameter (Figure 106-15). The configuration of the anastomosis is

Table 106–4

Results of Tracheal Resection

Surgeon	*Year*	*Patients*	*Mortality*
Ziemer[25]	1997	8	1 (12%)
Jonas[15]	1999	6	1 (16%)
Grillo[44]	2002	46	2 (4%)
Backer[9]	2002	12	1 (8%)
Total		72	5 (7%)

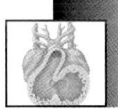

shown in the small inset. The results of the slide tracheoplasty are reported in Table 106-5.* The overall mortality was 12% in 33 patients.

We have used the slide tracheoplasty in three patients with excellent results in one patient and marginal results in the other two.[16] One patient developed significant granulation tissue and a "figure of 8" configuration to the trachea. This has been reported by other surgeons. The granulation tissue required multiple bronchoscopic procedures for removal, and the "figure of 8" configuration led to placement of airway stents. The patient eventually expired of sepsis. The second patient also had frequent bronchoscopic procedures for granulation tissue, developed recurrent stenosis and tracheomalacia, and required a tracheostomy and placement of stents. In contrast, the results reported by Dr. Grillo and also Manning and associates[23,40] have been quite good and are encouraging for the application of this technique.

Homograft Tracheoplasty

The homograft tracheoplasty technique was first performed in adults by Claus Herberhold of Germany. Herberhold

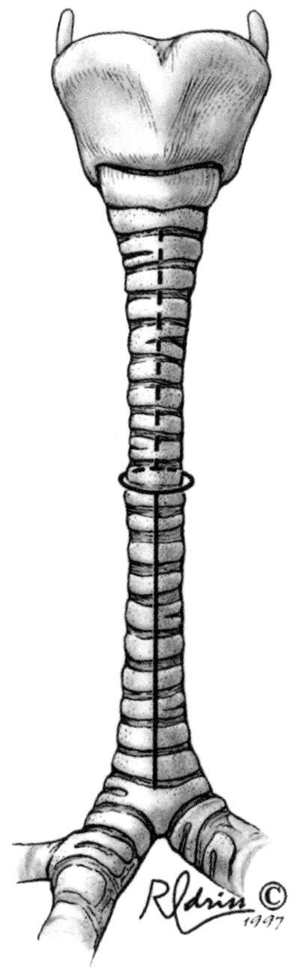

Figure 106–12 **Slide tracheoplasty.** The trachea is transected at the midpoint of the long-segment congenital tracheal stenosis. The superior position of the trachea is incised posteriorly, and the inferior aspect of the trachea is incised anteriorly.
(From Dayan SH, Dunham ME, Backer CL: Slide tracheoplasty in the management of congenital tracheal stenosis. Ann Otol Rhinol Laryngol 106:914–919, 1997.)

*References 1, 16, 23, 33, 36, 40, 42.

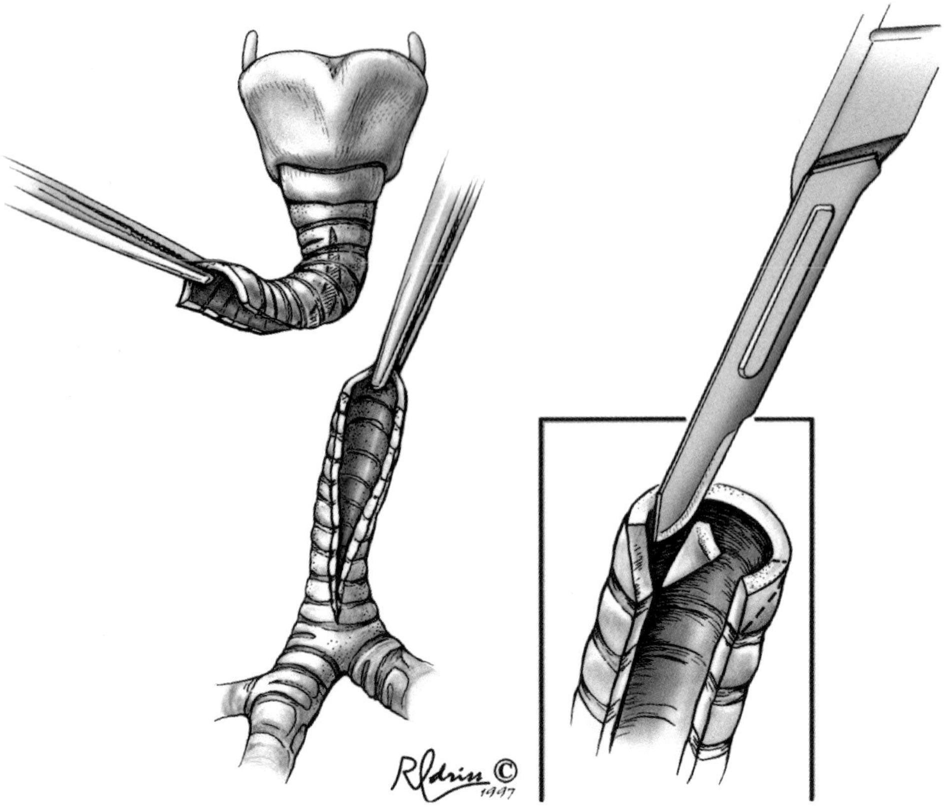

Figure 106–13 Slide tracheoplasty. The upper trachea has been opened posteriorly, and the lower trachea has been opened anteriorly. The corners of the transected trachea are trimmed so that the leading edge will fit into the V-portion of the other component. *(From Dayan SH, Dunham ME, Backer CL: Slide tracheoplasty in the management of congenital tracheal stenosis. Ann Otol Rhinol Laryngol 106:914–919, 1997.)*

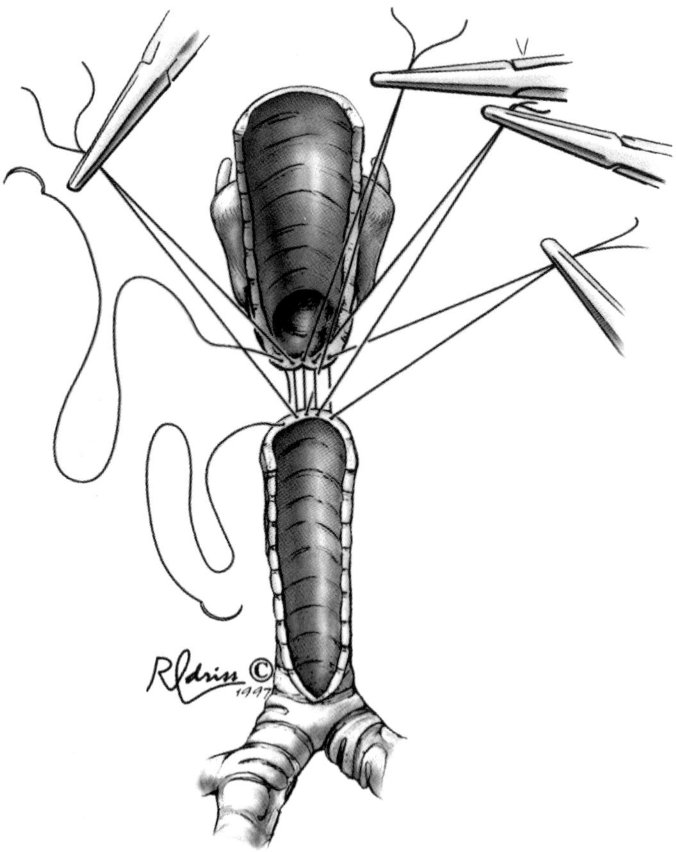

Figure 106–14 Slide tracheoplasty. This illustrates the beginning of the long anastomotic suture line that is performed with an interrupted 6-0 PDS suture while the patient is on cardiopulmonary bypass. *(From Dayan SH, Dunham ME, Backer CL: Slide tracheoplasty in the management of congenital tracheal stenosis. Ann Otol Rhinol Laryngol 106:914–919, 1997.)*

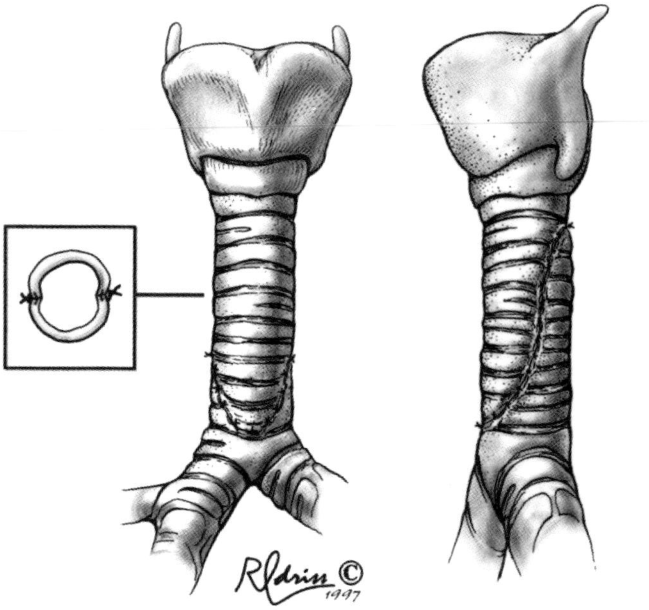

Figure 106–15 **Anterior (*left*) and lateral views (*right*) of the anastomosed trachea.** The tracheal length has been reduced by almost half, and the internal luminal diameter has been increased by four times. The cross-sectional appearance of the trachea is shown in the inset.
(*From Dayan SH, Dunham ME, Backer CL: Slide tracheoplasty in the management of congenital tracheal stenosis. Ann Otol Rhinol Laryngol 106:914–919, 1997.*)

Table 106–5

Results of Slide Tracheoplasty

Surgeon	*Year*	*Patients*	*Mortality*
Tsang[42]	1989	2	1 (50%)
Lang[33]	1999	2	0
Harrison[1]	2000	3	0
Matute[36]	2001	4	0
Backer[9]	2002	3	1 (33%)
Grillo[23]	2002	8	0
Manning[40]	2003	11	2 (18%)
Total		33	4 (12%)

and Elliott first applied the technique to a child in 1994.[17] Jacobs and Elliott reported the largest series of patients undergoing this procedure.[28] Most of these patients were infants who had a prior failed operation for complete tracheal rings. Cadaveric trachea is harvested, fixed in formalin, washed in thimerosal, and stored in acetone. The operation is performed through a median sternotomy with the use of cardiopulmonary bypass. The stenosed tracheal segment is opened to widely patent segments proximally and distally. The anterior cartilage is partially excised, and the posterior tracheal muscle or tracheal wall remains. A temporary silicone rubber intraluminal stent is placed, and absorbable sutures secure the homograft (that is trimmed appropriately) in position. Regular postoperative bronchoscopic treatments clear granulation tissue. The stent is removed endoscopically after endothelialization occurs over the homograft. In Jacobs et al's initial report there were 24 patients, most of whom were reoperations.[28] There were four deaths, for an overall mortality of 17%. Jacobs et al[29] recently reported the North American experience with the homograft, and there were six patients with one early death. This continues to be used as an alternative for the patient who has failed a previous primary procedure.

Pulmonary Artery Sling

A pulmonary artery sling is found in one third of patients who have tracheal stenosis.[8] The left pulmonary artery originates anomalously from the right pulmonary artery and courses posterior to the trachea on the way to the left lung. This compresses the right main bronchus and distal trachea (Figure 106-16). The first pulmonary artery sling repair was reported by Willis J. Potts from Children's Memorial Hospital.[39] Potts operated on a 5-month-old child who had severe right bronchial compression without a known diagnosis. He approached the patient through a right thoracotomy. He made the intraoperative diagnosis of a pulmonary artery sling with origin of the left pulmonary artery from the right pulmonary artery. Potts considered several surgical alternatives, including a pneumonectomy. He stated, "A pneumonectomy might be done but the possibility of this extreme course of action was only given brief consideration because of the defeatist attitude it elicited in the face of an unusual situation." Potts clamped and divided the left pulmonary artery and transposed it anterior to the tracheobronchial tree. He then reanastomosed the pulmonary artery. The patient survived the operation, but in a report nearly 25 years later was found to have an occluded left pulmonary artery.[12]

Historically the next series of patients who underwent pulmonary artery sling repair were operated on through a left thoracotomy.[32] This allowed better exposure for the anastomosis. However, many of these patients continued to have significant problems with left pulmonary artery stenosis and/or occlusion. Starting in 1985 we began using the median sternotomy approach and cardiopulmonary bypass for all of these patients.[7] The left pulmonary artery is divided and transposed anterior to the trachea. However, instead of being reanastomosed at its original site from the right pulmonary artery, we implanted it into the main pulmonary artery at a site selected to approximate the normal origin of the left pulmonary artery (Figure 106-17). Our

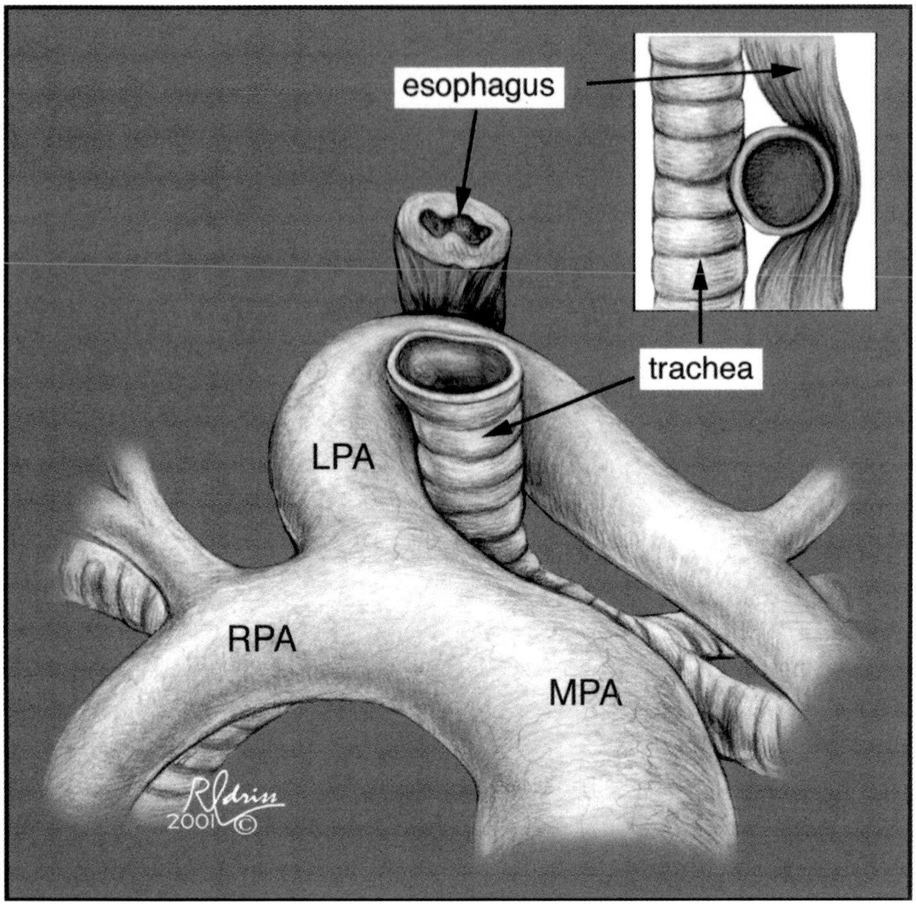

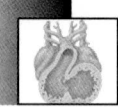

Figure 106–16 Pulmonary artery sling. The left pulmonary artery originates from the right pulmonary artery and acts as a "sling" pulling on and compressing the distal trachea and right main bronchus. The inset shows anterior compression of the esophagus by the anomalous left pulmonary artery on the lateral view. *LPA,* Left pulmonary artery; *MPA,* main pulmonary artery; *RPA,* right pulmonary artery.
(From Mavroudis C, Backer CL: Vascular rings and pulmonary artery sling. In Mavroudis C, Backer CL, editors: Pediatric Cardiac Surgery, 3rd ed. Philadelphia: Mosby, 2003.)

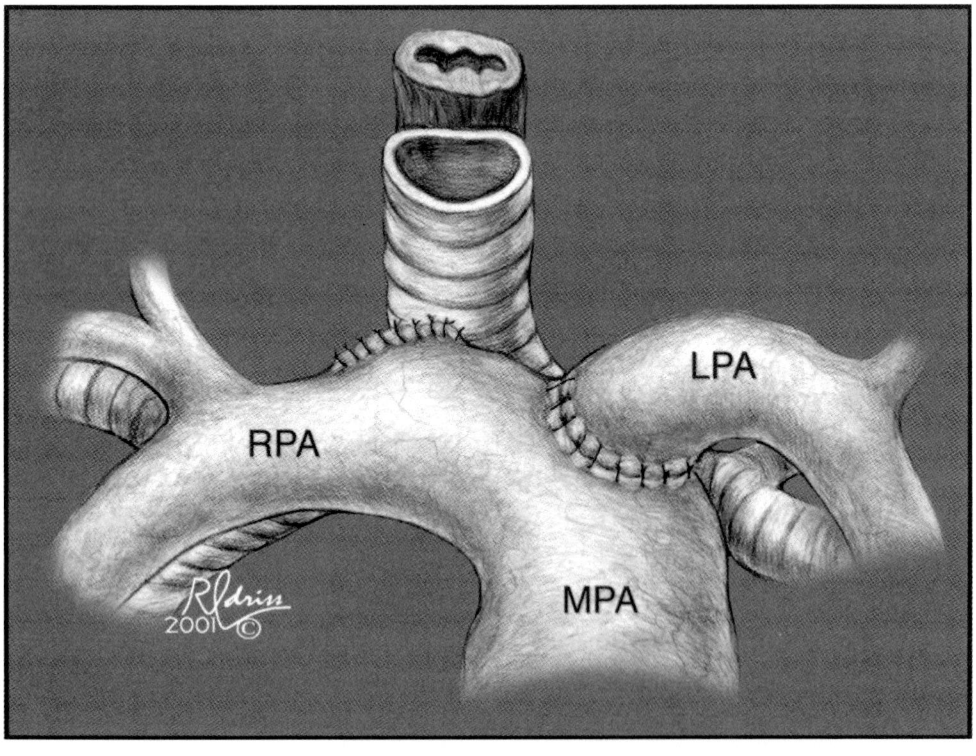

Figure 106–17 Pulmonary artery sling repair. The right pulmonary artery origin of the left pulmonary artery has been oversewn with interrupted sutures (to prevent right pulmonary artery stenosis). The left pulmonary artery has been anastomosed to an opening created in the main pulmonary artery, again with interrupted sutures. The left pulmonary artery is now anterior to the trachea.

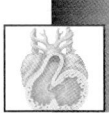

current series of patients undergoing pulmonary artery sling now numbers 33 patients. Twenty-two of these patients have had associated tracheal stenosis secondary to complete tracheal rings (66%). There have been no early deaths. There have been four late deaths, all related to complications from complete tracheal rings. Two of these deaths occurred before 1985. All patients repaired with cardiopulmonary bypass (25) have a patent left pulmonary artery, and the mean blood flow to the left pulmonary artery by nuclear scan is 36%.[7]

Tracheomalacia

Tracheomalacia can be a difficult entity to deal with in the infant and young child. Tracheomalacia can be classified as primary or secondary. Secondary causes include tracheoesophageal fistula and external compression from vascular structures (i.e., the innominate artery), cardiac structures, congenital cysts, and neoplasms. Tracheomalacia accounts for almost half of all congenital tracheal anomalies that present with stridor.[26] Symptoms depend on the location, length, and severity of the pathology. Intrathoracic tracheomalacia typically produces expiratory stridor or wheezing, which mimics asthma. Symptoms also may include a harsh barking cough, hyperextension of the neck, recurrent respiratory infections, and, when associated with compression by an anomalous innominate artery, reflex apnea.

Lateral chest X-ray (CXR) shows narrowing of the trachea during expiration. The diagnosis is confirmed at bronchoscopy if spontaneous respiration is maintained during bronchoscopy—the wide posterior membranous trachea is observed to collapse anteriorly during expiration. These dynamics are not observed when the child is paralyzed and ventilated with positive pressure. CT scan with contrast medium is carried out after bronchoscopy to define the nature of underlying suspected extrinsic compression.

Most patients with mild to moderate tracheomalacia eventually grow out of the tracheomalacia and do not require surgical intervention. However, a small number of patients who have severe tracheomalacia require intubation, ventilation, and usually very high positive end-expiratory pressure (PEEP) to keep the airway open and allow adequate ventilation of the patient. For these severe cases of tracheomalacia there are several surgical alternatives.

The first option is tracheostomy. This may obviate the need for positive pressure ventilation because the tracheostomy tube holds open the trachea. With associated bronchomalacia, PEEP may be necessary. There has been increasing experience with discharging these patients on home ventilation. Many children's hospitals have separate services for these patients who become chronically ventilator dependent for a variety of reasons. As the trachea matures and the cartilage gains more strength, these patients eventually can be weaned from their ventilators.

A second alternative is to bronchoscopically place a balloon expandable wire stent (Figure 106-18). We have reported our experience with the use of Palmaz (Johnson & Johnson International Systems Co., Warren, NJ) stents in infants, and most of these have been placed for tracheomalacia and bronchomalacia.[20] The most common indications in our series were after pericardial tracheoplasty or for patients with tetralogy of Fallot and absent pulmonary valve who have severe compression of the tracheobronchial tree from enlarged pulmonary arteries. These stents were quite effective in selected patients, but several patients had complications with significant granulation tissue formation. Filler and colleagues[18] from Toronto also have reported their results with these stents. In our current practice these stents usually are used as a measure of last resort in infants who have not responded to tracheostomy and positive pressure ventilation.

A surgical procedure for infants with tracheomalacia was reported by Hagl and associates[24] from Heidelberg, Germany. This operation is performed through either a thoracotomy or a median sternotomy approach. External stabilization of the severely dysplastic distal trachea (n = 6) or left main bronchus (n = 2) was achieved by suspending the malacic segment within an oversized and longitudinally opened ring-reinforced polytetrafluoroethylene prosthesis. Multiple pledgetted sutures were placed extramucosally to the dysplastic tracheal wall and the dyskinetic pars membranacea, as well as to the polytetrafluoroethylene prosthesis in a radial orientation. Guided by simultaneous video-assisted bronchoscopy, reexpansion of the collapsed segments was achieved by gentle traction on the sutures while tying (Figure 106-19). They reported excellent results in 6 of 7 patients.

Postintubation Stenosis

The largest series of pediatric patients undergoing tracheal surgery for a postintubation stenosis was recently reported from Massachusetts General Hospital.[44] Dr. Wright and colleagues reported 72 patients evaluated for postintubation stenosis over a nearly 25-year period. Of these patients, 31 were treated with tracheal resection and 17 were treated with laryngotracheal resection. Postintubation tracheal stenosis typically occurs from a stricture caused by scarring at the site of compression of the tracheal mucosa by the balloon from the endotracheal tube. Historically, balloons used in the past were low volume and high pressure. Since converting to high-volume, low-pressure balloons, the incidence of postintubation stenosis has diminished significantly. Evaluation of postintubation stenosis is chiefly with bronchoscopy. The larynx should undergo a detailed examination to identify commonly associated superglottic (arytenoid scarring and fixation), glottic (vocal cord paralysis or granulomas), or proximal subglottic pathology. These commonly associated problems may require attention before the tracheal stenosis is repaired. The technical details of the tracheal resection for these patients are similar to that of resection for patients with congenital stenosis secondary to complete tracheal rings.

Tracheal Web

Web-like diaphragms most often occur at the subcricoid level. These webs typically do not involve a significant length of the trachea. Tracheal webs are evaluated in a similar fashion to other patients with tracheal stenosis, and bronchoscopy continues to be the primary diagnostic tool. Tracheal webs have been removed or excised bronchoscopically with biopsy

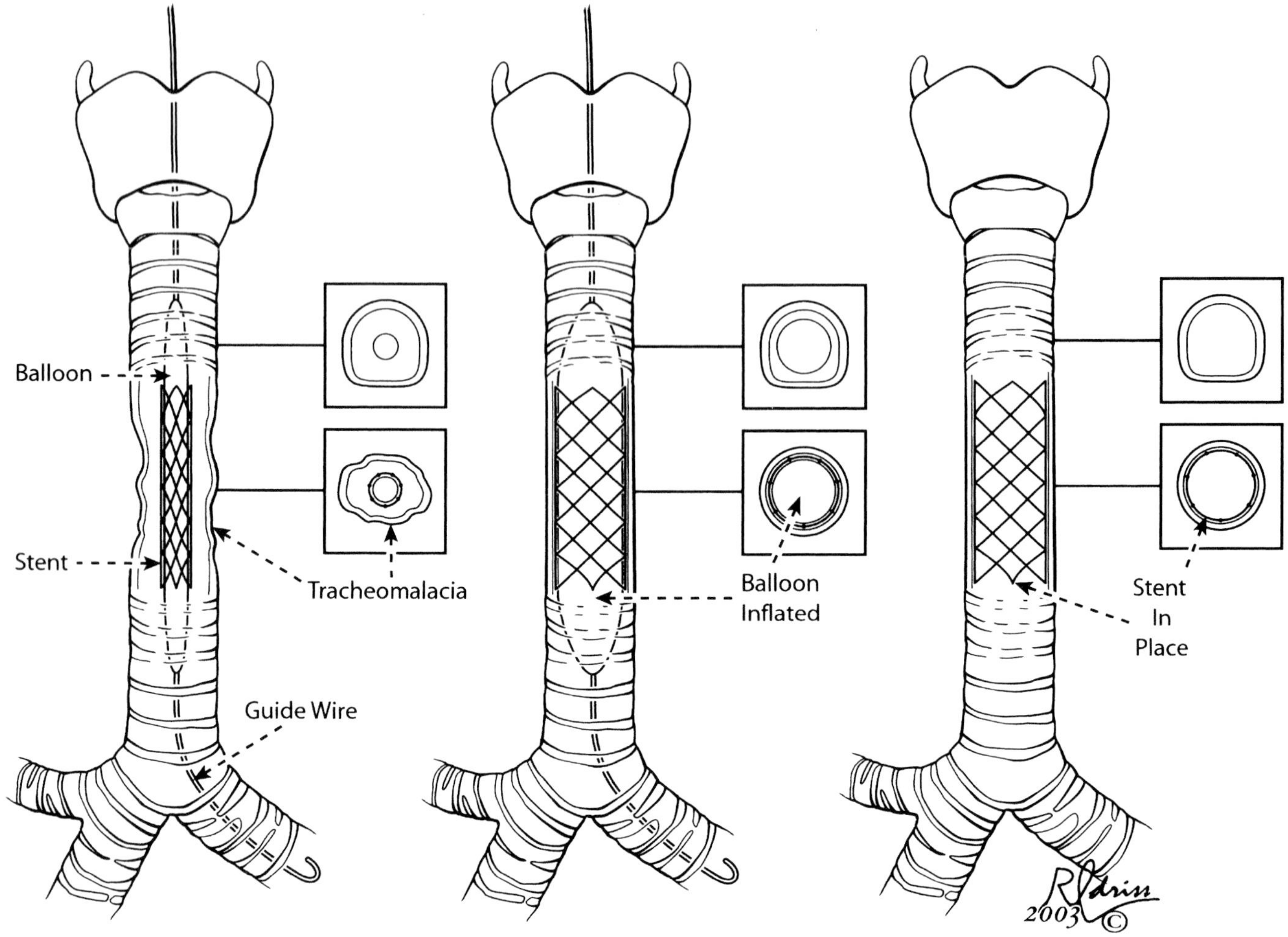

Figure 106–18 **Palmaz stent insertion in a child with severe tracheomalacia. A,** The Palmaz stent (mounted on a balloon-tipped catheter) has been positioned in the mid trachea. Positioning of the stent is with both fluoroscopy and bronchoscopy. **B,** The balloon is inflated, compressing the stent against the tracheal wall. **C,** The balloon catheter has been removed, and the stent is now in place. The tracheal lumen is held open by the stent.

forceps and occasionally with the use of an insulating cauterizing electrode. Laser therapy also may be successful. If this should fail, a tracheostomy done below the web may be a temporary solution, allowing the patient to grow and have a definitive resection later in life. In most cases these webs are cared for by the pediatric otolaryngologist, with only occasional need for tracheal resection by the thoracic surgeon.

SUMMARY

The most common indication for a surgical procedure on an infant or small child's trachea is tracheal stenosis secondary to complete tracheal rings. These infants present a significant challenge in their clinical management, requiring close cooperation between the pediatric cardiothoracic surgeons and the otolaryngologists. We recommend tracheal resection for short segments (6–8 tracheal rings, one third of the trachea) and a tracheal autograft for long-segment stenosis. We use a median sternotomy approach and cardiopulmonary bypass for all patients. If the patient has an associated pulmonary artery sling or intracardiac anomaly, that lesion should be repaired simultaneously. Bronchoscopic expertise is absolutely required to make the diagnosis, and for postoperative airway management. Other centers are achieving excellent results with cartilage, slide, and pericardial tracheoplasty. Each institution must arrive at its own best practice. The outlook for these patients has evolved significantly from the mid-1970s, when most of these patients died, to the current era, where the mortality for complete tracheal rings is now approximately 15%. The postoperative management of these patients is complex and requires extreme attention to detail and vigilance with regard to airway management.

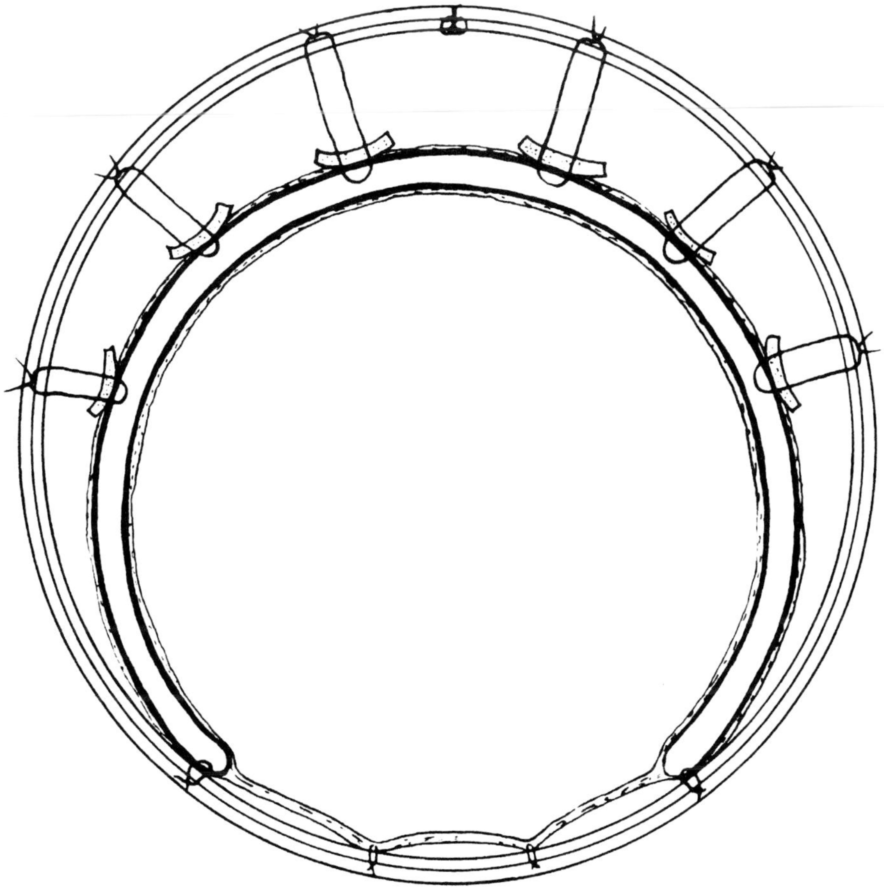

Figure 106–19 **Schematic cross-sectional view of tracheal external stabilization with "onlay" fixation of the flaccid pars membranacea and free suspension of the malacic cartilaginous portions within an oversized polytetrafluoroethylene prosthesis.**
(From Hagl S, Jakob H, Sebening C, et al: External stabilization of long-segment tracheobronchomalacia guided by intraoperative bronchoscopy. Ann Thorac Surg 64:1412–1421, 1997.)

REFERENCES

1. Acosta AC, Albanese CT, Farmer DL, et al: Tracheal stenosis: The long and the short of it. J Pediatr Surg 35:1612–1616, 2000.
2. Alboliras ET, Backer CL, Holinger LD, et al: Pulmonary artery sling: Diagnostic and management strategy. Pediatrics 98:530, 1996 (abstract).
3. Andrews TM, Cotton RT, Bailey WW, et al: Tracheoplasty for congenital complete tracheal rings. Arch Otolaryngol Head Neck Surg 120:1363–1369, 1994.
4. Backer CL, Mavroudis C: Congenital Heart Surgery Nomenclature and Database Project: Vascular rings, tracheal stenosis, pectus excavatum. Ann Thorac Surg 69:S308–S318, 2000.
5. Backer CL, Mavroudis C, Dunham ME, Holinger LD: Reoperation after pericardial patch tracheoplasty. J Pediatr Surg 32:1108–1112, 1997.
6. Backer CL, Mavroudis C, Dunham ME, Holinger LD: Repair of congenital tracheal stenosis with a free tracheal autograft. J Thorac Cardiovasc Surg 115:869–874, 1998.
7. Backer CL, Mavroudis C, Dunham ME, Holinger LD: Pulmonary artery sling: Results with median sternotomy, cardiopulmonary bypass, and reimplantation. Ann Thorac Surg 67:1738–1744, 1999.
8. Backer CL, Mavroudis C, Gerber ME, Holinger LD: Tracheal surgery in children: An 18-year review of four techniques. Eur J Cardiothorac Surg 19:777–784, 2001.
9. Backer CL, Mavroudis C, Holinger LD: Repair of congenital tracheal stenosis. Semin Thorac Cardiovasc Surg Pediatr Card Surg Annu 5:173–186, 2002.
10. Bando K, Turrentine MW, Sun K, et al: Anterior pericardial tracheoplasty for congenital tracheal stenosis: Intermediate to long-term outcomes. Ann Thorac Surg 62:981–989, 1996.

10a. Brown JW: Personal communication, November 2002.

11. Benjamin B, Pitkin J, Cohen D: Congenital tracheal stenosis. Ann Otol Rhinol Laryngol 90:364–371, 1981.
12. Campbell CD, Wernly JA, Koltip PC, et al: Aberrant left pulmonary artery (pulmonary artery sling): Successful repair and 24 year follow-up report. Am J Cardiol 45:316–320, 1980.
13. Cantrell JR, Guild HC: Congenital stenosis of the trachea. Am J Surg 108:297–305, 1964.
14. Cheng ATL, Backer CL, Holinger LD, et al: Histopathologic changes after pericardial patch tracheoplasty. Arch Otolaryngol Head Neck Surg 123:1069–1072, 1997.
15. Cotter CS, Jones DT, Nuss RC, Jonas R: Management of distal tracheal stenosis. Arch Otolaryngol Head Neck Surg 25: 325–328, 1999.
16. Dayan SH, Dunham ME, Backer CL, et al: Slide tracheoplasty in the management of congenital tracheal stenosis. Ann Otol Rhinol Laryngol 106:914–919, 1997.
17. Elliott MJ, Haw MP, Jacobs JP, et al: Tracheal reconstruction in children using cadaveric homograft trachea. Eur J Cardiothorac Surg 10:707–712, 1996.
18. Filler RM, Forte V, Fraga JC, Matute J: The use of expandable metallic airway stents for tracheobronchial obstruction in children. J Pediatr Surg 30:1050–1056, 1995.
19. Forsen JW Jr, Lusk BP, Hudddleston CB: Costal cartilage tracheoplasty for congenital long-segment tracheal stenosis. Arch Otolaryngol Head Neck Surg 128:1165–1171, 2002.
20. Furman RH, Backer CL, Dunham ME, et al: The use of balloon-expandable metallic stents in the treatment of

pediatric tracheomalacia and bronchomalacia. Arch Otolaryngol Head Neck Surg 125:203–207, 1999.
21. Grillo HC: Surgical approaches to the trachea. Surg Gynecol Obstet 129:347–352, 1969.
22. Grillo HC: Slide tracheoplasty for long-segment congenital tracheal stenosis. Ann Thorac Surg 58:613-621, 1994.
23. Grillo HC, Wright CD, Vlahakes GJ, MacGillivray TE: Management of congenital tracheal stenosis by means of slide tracheoplasty or resection and reconstruction, with long-term follow-up of growth after slide tracheoplasty. J Thorac Cardiovasc Surg 123:145–152, 2002.
24. Hagl S, Jakob H, Sebening C, et al: External stabilization of long-segment tracheobronchomalacia guided by intraoperative bronchoscopy. Ann Thorac Surg 64:1412–1421, 1997.
25. Heinemann MK, Ziemer G, Sieverding L, et al: Long-segment tracheal resection in infancy utilizing extracorporeal circulation. In Imai Y, Momma K, editors: Proceedings of the Second World Congress of Pediatric Cardiology and Cardiac Surgery, pp. 711-713. New York: Futura Publishing Co., 1998.
26. Holinger LD, Green CG, Benjamin B, Sharp JK: Tracheobronchial tree. In Holinger LD, Lusk RP, Green CG, editors: Pediatric Laryngology and Bronchoesophagology. Philadelphia: Lippincott-Raven, 1997.
27. Idriss FS, DeLeon SY, Ilbawi MN, et al: Tracheoplasty with pericardial patch for extensive tracheal stenosis in infants and children. J Thorac Cardiovasc Surg 88:527–536, 1984.
28. Jacobs JP, Elliott MJ, Haw MP, et al: Pediatric tracheal homograft reconstruction: A novel approach to complex tracheal stenoses in children. J Thorac Cardiovasc Surg 112:1549–1558, 1996.
29. Jacobs JP, Quintessenza JA, Andrews T, et al: Tracheal allograft reconstruction: The total North American and worldwide pediatric experiences. Ann Thorac Surg 68:1043–1051, 1999.
30. Kamata S, Usui N, Ishikawa S, et al: Experience in tracheobronchial reconstruction with a costal cartilage graft for congenital tracheal stenosis. J Pediatr Surg 32:54–57, 1997.
31. Kimura K, Mukohara N, Tsugawa C, et al: Tracheoplasty for congenital stenosis of the entire trachea. J Pediatr Surg 17:869–871, 1982.
32. Koopot R, Nikaidoh H, Idriss FS: Surgical management of anomalous left pulmonary artery causing tracheobronchial obstruction. Pulmonary artery sling. J Thorac Cardiovasc Surg 69:239–246, 1975.
33. Lang FJ, Hurni M, Monnier P: Long-segment congenital tracheal stenosis: Treatment by slide-tracheoplasty. J Pediatr Surg 34:1216–1222, 1999.
34. Lobe TE, Hayden CK, Nicolas D, Richardson CJ: Successful management of congenital tracheal stenosis in infancy. J Pediatr Surg 22:1137–1142, 1987.
35. Manson D, Babyn P, Filler R, Holowka S: Three-dimensional imaging of the pediatric trachea in congenital tracheal stenosis. Pediatr Radiol 24:175–179, 1994.
36. Matute JA, Romero R, Garcia-Casillas MA, et al: Surgical approach to funnel-shaped congenital tracheal stenosis. J Pediatr Surg 36:320–323, 2001.
37. Nicotra JJ, Mahboubi S, Kramer SS: Three-dimensional imaging of the pediatric airway. Int J Pediatr Otorhinolaryngol 41:299–305, 1997.
38. Oue T, Kamata S, Usui N, et al: Histopathologic changes after tracheobronchial reconstruction with costal cartilage graft for congenital tracheal stenosis. J Pediatr Surg 36:329–333, 2001.
39. Potts WJ, Holinger PH, Rosenblum AH: Anomalous left pulmonary artery causing obstruction to right main bronchus. Report of a case. JAMA 155:1409–1411, 1954.
40. Rutter MJ, Cotton RT, Azizkhan RG, Manning PB: Slide tracheoplasty for the management of complete tracheal rings. J Pediatr Surg 38:928–934, 2003.
41. Salassa JR, Pearson BW, Payne WS: Gross and microscopical blood supply of the trachea. Ann Thorac Surg 24:100–107, 1977.
42. Tsang V, Murday A, Gillbe C, Goldstraw P: Slide tracheoplasty for congenital funnel-shaped tracheal stenosis. Ann Thorac Surg 48:632–635, 1989.
43. Tsugawa C, Kimura K, Muraji T, et al: Congenital stenosis involving a long segment of the trachea: Further experience in reconstructive surgery. J Pediatr Surg 23:471–475, 1988.
44. Wright CD, Graham BB, Grillo HC, et al: Pediatric tracheal surgery. Ann Thorac Surg 74:308–314, 2002.

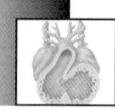

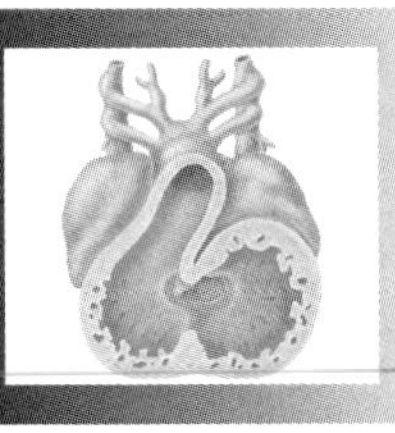

Patent Ductus Arteriosus and Vascular Rings

Redmond P. Burke

CHAPTER 107

PATENT DUCTUS ARTERIOSUS

As time went on there was an urge to attack several blood vessel anomalies which had been seen previously at autopsies during my training two years before. The first consideration had to do with possibly attacking a ductus arteriosus that had remained patent. How could one be closed off surgically? It had never been accomplished anywhere before. Possible surgical approaches to a ductus were practiced on humans in the autopsy room and on animals. After deciding clearly on the best approach, there seemingly would be no difficulty or risk in ligating a patent ductus. Our first operation for such a procedure was performed on a seven-year-old girl on August 26, 1938. The postoperative course was uneventful and without worry. The next morning she was up and out of bed and around the ward. She was discharged in ten days. Our patent ductus operations were always done through a left antero-lateral approach through the third intercostal space.

Eleven children were operated upon satisfactorily for ductus closure by ligation. The twelfth was a fourteen-year-old girl also treated by ligation. She was well at the time of hospital discharge. Two weeks after that, there was a party for her at her home. While dancing with friends, she suddenly collapsed on the floor and was instantly dead! The family permitted an autopsy examination, which showed that the ductus ligature had cut through, permitting massive hemorrhage. I never again ligated a ductus. All subsequent patients were handled by careful local dissection placing double clamps on the ductus, then cutting the ductus in half and meticulously closing each end by suturing. This became the standard technique, giving completely satisfactory results. It was used with total satisfaction up through the last ductus operation I performed, which was number 1,610, in March 1972.[100]

—Robert E. Gross

History

The development of medical therapy for patent ductus arteriosus (PDA) encompasses a half century of medical pioneering and technological innovation, and epitomizes the surgeon's quest to reduce therapeutic trauma. Innovative approaches have been developed to achieve both closure and persistent patency, to achieve different therapeutic goals in congenital heart therapy. Galen first described the ductus arteriosus, and Harvey demonstrated its function in fetal circulation. The first successful surgical ligation of PDA, which was also the first successful operation for congenital heart disease, was performed by Dr Robert Gross at Children's Hospital Boston in 1938, when he was 33 years old.[56] Powell and Decancz reported surgical ligation in premature infants in 1963. Porstmann et al[111] described a series of transcatheter device closures in 1971. Prostaglandins were used to open the ductus arteriosus to palliate patients with congenital heart defects in the early 1970s.[106] Friedman and associates[47] reported PDA closure in premature newborns with indomethacin in 1976. Laborde et al[78] described video-assisted thoracoscopic surgery (VATS) PDA closure in 1993, the same year that Rothman and Tong[115] described the first coil occlusion of a PDA. A gene locus associated with PDA was identified by Mani et al in 2002.[90]

Genomics

In the United States PDA appears in approximately 1 of 2500 births, with a 2:1 predilection for females. A genetic basis for persistently patent ductus arteriosus has been described by analysis of genetic linkage. In Iran PDA accounted for a higher fraction of congenital heart disease (15%) than in the United States (2–7%) and had a high level of parental consanguinity (63%). Recurrence of PDA among siblings was 5%. A genome-wide analysis of linkage in 21 unrelated consanguineous PDA cases demonstrated linkage of PDA to a 3-centimorgan interval of chromosome 12q24, with linkage in 53% of kindreds. These findings suggest a recessive component to PDA and implicate a single locus, PDA1. PDA has been found in association with fetal hydantoin, warfarin, and rubella syndromes, Down syndrome, and trisomy 13.

Anatomy

The ductus arteriosus derives from the sixth aortic arch, connecting the main or proximal left pulmonary artery to the descending aorta. Ductal shape, length, and diameter are variable, which may influence the efficacy of various therapeutic approaches. The duct is usually cone shaped, broader at the aortic end, and may present as a bilateral, right-sided, or missing structure. The ductus serves as an alternate pathway for right ventricular cardiac output away from the dormant pulmonary circulation in utero, and ductal closure marks the transition from fetal to adult circulation. Anatomical relationships include the left recurrent laryngeal nerve, controlling the left vocal cord, which separates from the vagus nerve anterior to the aorta and courses around the PDA from anterior to posterior before entering the tracheoesophageal groove. This nerve is a useful anatomical landmark and must be protected during PDA ligation. Occasionally the ductus arises from the arch proximal to the left subclavian artery, and the recurrent nerve is found passing under the arch instead of under the ductus. Such variations in ductal anatomy, and surgical confusion, have been associated with spectacular misadventures—including ligation of the left pulmonary artery and the aorta.

Pathophysiology and Indications for Surgery: Premature, Full Term, Adult

Premature

Persistently patent ductus arteriosus may follow several pathophysiological trajectories in premature newborns. Survival of extremely premature infants (<27 weeks of gestational age) has steadily improved over the past two decades. Unexplained metabolic acidosis and respiratory deterioration on day 3 or 4 in a ventilated premature neonate may be the first sign of a PDA. The incidence of PDA increases with decreasing birth weight: from 7% in very low birth weight premature newborns (VLBW, less than 1500 g) to 42% in extremely low birth weight infants (ELBW, less than 1000 g).[43,128] PDA produces significant left-to-right shunt with an increase in left ventricular output and decreased pulmonary compliance. Ductal closure is impeded by immature or insufficient smooth muscle and insensitivity to increased oxygen tension. Ductal patency depends on circulating prostaglandins acting on specific receptors within the ductus. There is a coordinated regulation of fetal and maternal prostaglandins at the time of birth that affect ductal closure. This regulation may be altered by the increasing use of selective cyclooxygenase inhibitors for the management of preterm labor.[114] Other circulating vasodilators, which cannot be cleared from the circulation by immature lungs, may contribute to ductal persistence. Maternal residence at high altitude increases the incidence of PDA. Systemic effects result from diastolic steal and retrograde diastolic blood flow away from the splanchnic and renal circulations. Ductal closure may be associated with pulmonary artery branch stenosis, creating a murmur; however, this usually resolves by a corrected age of 3 months.[5] In extremely premature newborns the presence of a PDA plays a major role in the development of chronic lung disease (CLD). Efforts to prevent CLD in ELBW infants should include early closure of the PDA.[11]

Randomized controlled trials of therapeutic PDA closure in premature newborns have fallen into the following three groups: (1) prophylactic treatment in the first 24 hours, (2) presymptomatic treatment on ultrasound evidence of a PDA or the first clinical signs, and (3) treatment when the PDA becomes hemodynamically significant. These approaches do not differ significantly in the incidence of mortality, bronchopulmonary dysplasia, necrotizing enterocolitis (NEC), or retinopathy of prematurity. Prophylactic treatment with indomethacin may reduce the incidence of intraventricular hemorrhage. Clinical decisions on the treatment of the ductus are individualized and based on gestational age, respiratory condition, and the magnitude of the ductal shunt.[73]

Surgeons must be able to safely ligate persistent PDA in extremely small patients with complex multisystem dysfunction, including hyaline membrane disease, NEC, bronchopulmonary dysplasia, pulmonary hemorrhage,[72] intracranial hemorrhage, adrenal insufficiency,[136] renal dysfunction, and sepsis. Studies of primary medical versus primary surgical therapy for premature newborns with PDA support primary medical therapy, including fluid restriction, diuretics, and nonsteroidal antiinflammatory medications. Medical treatment is associated with more renal dysfunction than is primary surgery, whereas the rates of NEC and intracranial hemorrhage are similar. In extremely premature infants, use of indomethacin during the first 48 hours of life has been associated with a reduced need for PDA ligation, but an increased risk of NEC with intestinal perforation.[48] Vasoconstriction induced by bolus injection of indomethacin reduces organ perfusion secondary to decreased cerebral, renal, and mesenteric blood flow.[29] Ibuprofen recently has been shown to have fewer gastrointestinal side effects when used for neonatal duct closure[2] and may be indicated for patients with renal dysfunction.[32] Premature neonates failing medical therapy should undergo surgical ligation to avoid the complications of persistent left-to-right shunting.

Full Term

In full-term newborns the ductus usually closes within the first 10 hours of life by physical examination, and within 2 days by echocardiography.[51] Complex maternal and fetal prostaglandin interactions regulate ductal closure.[114] Anatomical studies show that smooth muscle constriction in response to increased oxygen tension, and breakdown of the internal elastic membrane, allow contact and coalescence of the mucoid-filled ductal media.[62] Persistent ductal flow allows left-to-right shunting with left ventricular volume overload and pulmonary overcirculation, leading to congestive heart failure, failure to thrive, and pulmonary hypertension. The time course of onset of pulmonary hypertension for untreated PDA is unpredictable and multifactorial. PDA may alter local vascular immune response mechanisms, creating a nidus for bacterial endocarditis.[35] PDA turbulence sufficient to produce a murmur is commonly thought to be capable of producing a jet lesion and increasing the risk of endocarditis, justifying closure. There is no consensus on the need to close the silent ductus identified by echocardiography, which may not produce cardiopulmonary dysfunction, but may still be a risk for infection.[110]

Adult

Natural history studies from the 1960s suggest that 40% of patients with untreated PDA would die by age 45.[26] Adult patients may have undiagnosed PDA and suspected Eisenmenger's syndrome. Diagnostic catheterization to measure pulmonary resistance changes to oxygen and nitric oxide are indicated to determine operability in patients with longstanding PDA and suspected pulmonary hypertension.

PDA aneurysm has been described as an underdiagnosed problem, and potential complications include rupture, erosion, infection, and thromboembolism.[89] Ductal aneurysm may appear spontaneously, after PDA surgery, or after transcatheter occlusion.[91] Neonatal ductal aneurysm can be diagnosed echocardiographically. Asymptomatic neonatal ductal aneurysms usually resolve spontaneously by thrombosis and should be managed expectantly with surgical closure if the aneurysm persists beyond a few days.[129] Prompt surgical treatment is recommended for all spontaneous ductal aneurysms in patients older than 2 months of age and in all patients with postoperative ductal aneurysm. Ductal aneurysm in older patients may present with hoarseness related to traction on the recurrent nerve, producing vocal cord paralysis,[102] or it may obstruct the left main stem bronchus.[116] Calcification and infection of ductal aneurysm in adults are common. For surgical resection or aneurysmorrhaphy, cardiopulmonary bypass support is recommended.

Diagnosis

Physical examination and echocardiography form the foundation for PDA diagnosis. A characteristic systolic machinery murmur radiating from the pulmonic area to the midclavicle is highly suggestive, and confirmation with transthoracic echocardiography is routine. The left atrial-to-aortic diameter ratio is a reliable predictor of significant PDA shunt in premature newborns with pulmonary disease.[80] Diagnostic catheterization for PDA has largely given way to interventional catheterization for device closure after echocardiographic diagnosis.

Therapeutic Options for Patent Ductus Arteriosus

The advent of transcatheter device closure has altered the treatment algorithm for PDA. In institutions with active interventional cardiology, transcatheter device closure is routinely and effectively used for infants, children, and adults with PDA.[109] Primary surgical closure is usually reserved for premature newborns and patients with large ducts who have failed attempted device closure. Vascular access for device closure is traumatic in premature newborns, and the use of multiple or large devices for large ducts has produced left pulmonary artery stenosis and aortic obstruction by device protrusion. Surgical support may be required to manage device complications,[66,109] ideally in collaboration with the interventional cardiologist. Embolized or failed devices may be snared and pulled to the femoral insertion point, where the surgeon may retrieve the device by cutdown. Transaortic or transatrial retrieval on cardiopulmonary bypass may be necessary to retrieve larger devices that have embolized or are obstructing the left pulmonary artery or aorta. Conversely, the interventional cardiologist may support the surgeon if a small residual leak is detected after attempted surgical ligation, because these residual defects are readily closed by transcatheter device.

Early controversies in PDA surgical technique involved the ideal method of closure, with advocates of various forms of suture ligation (double or triple), clip ligation (single or double), and division. No technique has prevented a low incidence of recanalization, although division would seem to best minimize this risk. Several thoracotomy approaches have been described for PDA ligation or division, including anterolateral thoracotomy, posterolateral thoracotomy with a transpleural or retropleural approach, and axillary thoracotomy. Surgical approaches continue to evolve in an effort to reduce incisional trauma.

Thoracotomy

PDA traditionally is approached via a left thoracotomy under general anesthesia, with adequate intravenous access for rapid volume infusion in the event of bleeding. Intraoperative transesophageal echocardiography is often used in patients weighing more than 2 kg to confirm closure. Patients are placed in a right lateral decubitus position, and a subscapular or axillary muscle sparing incision is made to allow entry through the third or fourth intercostal space. The left upper lobe is retracted medially, with a malleable retractor fixed to the rib spreader. Overretraction may produce bradycardia from vagus nerve traction, or arrhythmia from contact with the heart. The left lower lobe is retracted inferiorly with a second malleable retractor. The parietal pleura overlying the duct is opened vertically, creating a medial flap that can be suspended with stay sutures. The vagus and recurrent nerves are usually visible and can be left undisturbed as the upper and lower angles of the PDA are dissected (Figure 107-1). The upper angle typically is more challenging because the duct is often firmly attached to the undersurface of the aortic arch by a vascular tissue plane. Blunt dissection in this plane can be bloody, particularly in

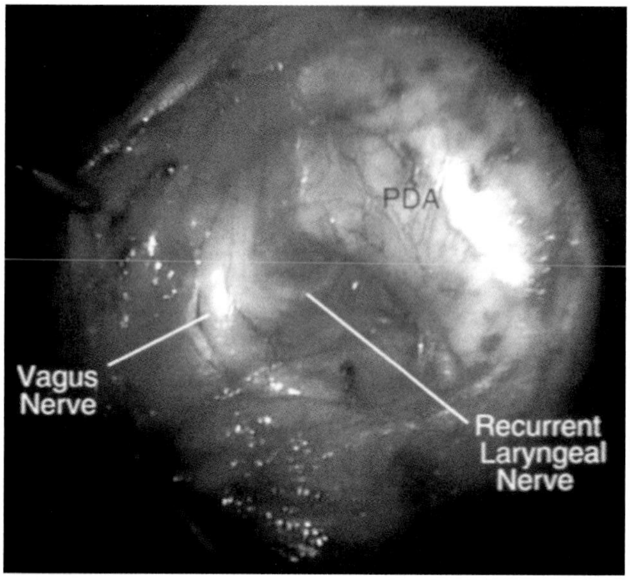

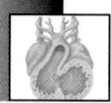

Figure 107–1 **Intraoperative image of patent ductus arteriosus (PDA) and the proximity of vagus and recurrent laryngeal nerves.**

premature neonates with platelet dysfunction from recent indomethacin therapy or sepsis. Cautery dissection must be precise to avoid damaging the ductus and nerves. Once the upper and lower angles are developed, a vascular clip can be applied, or the duct can be dissected circumferentially and encircled with sutures proximally and distally. When direct dissection around a large duct is not progressing or feels dangerous, a subtraction dissection can be performed. The aorta is dissected above and below the duct and rotated medially to expose the posterior ductal wall, allowing double passage of a suture for ligation. Small adventitial bites are used to maintain enough suture separation to allow safe division. For short, wide ducts, Potts-type nonslipping vascular clamps may be placed to allow duct division and running suture closure of the stumps, flush with the aorta and pulmonary artery. Ductal laceration and bleeding requires prompt control of the proximal and distal aorta, cooling and volume resuscitation by anesthesia, and transpericardial exposure to control the main pulmonary artery. Once proximal and distal control is achieved, repair is straightforward.

Surgeons may be asked to deal with residual PDA flow, infection, hemolysis, or aneurysm formation after device closure. It is technically possible to ligate a ductus that has a transcatheter device in its lumen without lacerating the duct wall.[28] More often, proximal and distal clamping of the pulmonary artery and aorta, above and below the PDA, are needed to allow transection of the duct, device removal, and oversewing of the stumps.

Results of large surgical series demonstrate that open PDA ligation or division has been a reliable, effective, safe procedure for decades. Potential complications include pneumothorax, hemothorax, chylothorax, residual leak, recurrent nerve injury,[44] chest wall trauma, left pulmonary artery injury,[110] and aortic injury. The incidence and risk of recanalization after surgical closure are unclear. Surgical series report very low incidence of this complication, whereas an echocardiographic study of recanalization suggests a high incidence (20%) of residual ductal flow after surgical ligation in one center.[124] Coil closure of a small residual leak after surgical ligation of a large duct is safe and effective.

Video-Assisted Thoracoscopic Surgery

The chest wall morbidity of thoracotomy includes scoliosis,[67,120,138] pain syndromes,[36] breast deformity,[27] and scapular deformity. To reduce this trauma, video-assisted thoracoscopy has been used increasingly for PDA ligation. In 1993 Laborde et al[78] described a video-assisted approach to PDA using three thoracostomies. A four-port approach allowing two-handed dissection was developed at Children's Hospital Boston.[25] This approach has been adopted by many,* but not all, congenital heart centers. The technique is not intuitive and there is a learning curve affecting the duration of operations. The risk of catastrophic bleeding appears greater than with an open approach, although this danger has not been demonstrated in reported series.

Instrumentation for video-assisted repair of congenital heart defects must accommodate a wide range of thoracic and ductal sizes and shapes. Instruments for precise dissection, cautery, retraction, suturing, and clip application have been developed. Endoscopic trocars and instruments are used to transverse the pediatric intercostal space, which varies from 2 mm in the premature newborn to 6 mm in the adolescent child. A 4-mm diameter, 30 degree face angle, three-chip endoscopic imaging system provides 4 × magnification with excellent illumination. Digital capture systems allow intraoperative images to be saved for future reference. A mechanical arm stabilizes the endoscope, freeing the assistant for retraction. Voice-activated mechanical arms are available.

Positioning and anesthetic management are similar to that for PDA surgery by thoracotomy (Figure 107-2). Isolated lung ventilation is not necessary; however, surgery is facilitated by having the anesthesiologist watch the endoscopic image to calibrate the ventilation to facilitate the procedure. The four-trocar VATS technique consists of a series of small (4–12 mm) incisions on the left-sided chest wall for patients with a left aortic arch. Three incisions are in the line of a standard posterolateral thoracotomy, and the fourth is in the axilla. The first assistant stands on the patient's right, managing lung retraction with a fan-shaped expandable retractor, or with two cotton-tipped applicators (for premature newborns). Retractors are advanced and manipulated under direct endoscopic vision to avoid lung injury. The surgeon stands on the patient's left, using a grasper in the left hand through the axillary port and the cautery in the right hand through the most posterior port. A low table position improves the surgeon's ability to maneuver endoscopic instruments. Port locations are marked with a surgical pen, and incisions are made. Blunt dissection and entry into the pleural space with a curved hemostat allows placement of smooth trocars. During trocar insertion, care is taken to avoid pushing the parietal pleura away from the chest wall. This creates a pleural tent, which obscures the endoscopic operative field. Strict hemostasis is imperative to maintain a clear endoscopic image. Lens fogging is common and resolves as the endoscope temperature stabilizes. Pediatric trocars allow atraumatic insertion of a 2.7-

*References 20, 30, 37, 38, 108, 132, 139.

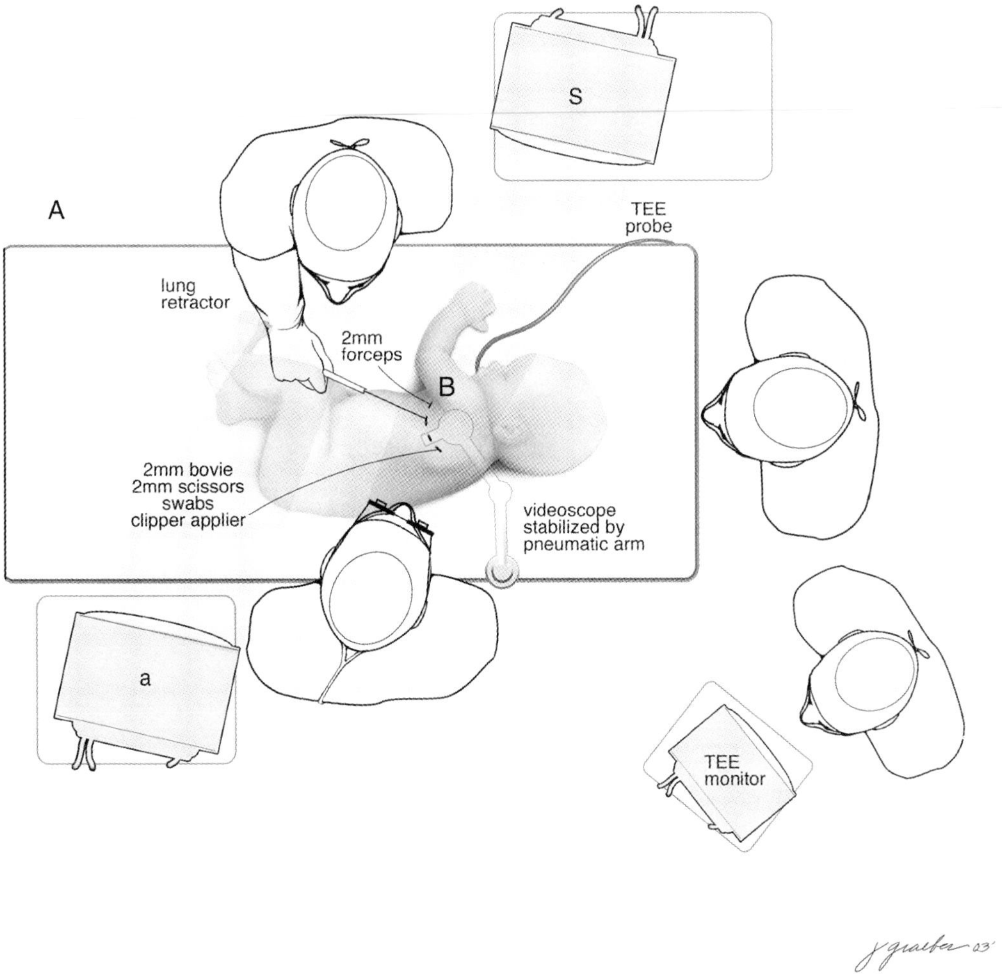

Figure 107–2 Operating room setup for video-assisted thoracoscopic ligation of patent ductus arteriosus (PDA). A, Operating room setup: Monitors are aligned for the surgeon (S) and assistant (a). **B,** Thoracostomy parts.

mm grasper, an expanding fan-shaped lung retractor, and a 4-mm 30° angled endoscope. The larger posterior port admits an L-shaped cautery dissector and the clip appliers, which can accommodate small, medium, or large vascular clips. Elevating the parietal pleura over the duct with a grasper allows the upper and lower duct angles to be dissected, as in an open procedure. Complete back wall dissection usually is not necessary and may increase the risk of bleeding from ductal injury. The crossing hemiazygos vein can be divided between clips when needed for exposure. The vagus and recurrent laryngeal nerves are easily seen, but are not specifically dissected. It is possible to use a neural probe to identify the recurrent nerve.[105] A mechanical arm holds the videoscope in position, providing a stable camera image. Effective PDA closure can be achieved with a single clip, double clips,[38] or endoscopic ligation.[70] When clips are used, care is taken to ensure proper clip position before closure to avoid pinching the ductal wall with the distal ends of the clip, which could leave a residual lumen or tear the duct wall (Figure 107-3). Rapid conversion to thoracotomy is possible to control bleeding. Cauterizing the pleural edges may prevent chylous leak. Intraoperative transesophageal echocardiography (TEE) is useful to confirm ductal closure.[81] Once the lung is reexpanded, the thoracostomy tube is removed in the operating room. Patients are extubated in the operating room and transferred to the ward, where they rapidly resume a regular diet. Recovery usually is complete by the evening of surgery, and patients generally do not require narcotics for pain management.[84]

Laborde et al[79] have reported a series of 332 patients ranging from 1.2–65 kg, undergoing VATS PDA interruption without mortality and with very low residual flow rates (six patients required second procedures for residual flow, five were successful, and one persists). Complete closure rates have reached 100%.[14,103] Complications have been minimal, with recurrent nerve injury rates ranging from zero[50] to 1.8%.[79] Catastrophic bleeding has not been reported.

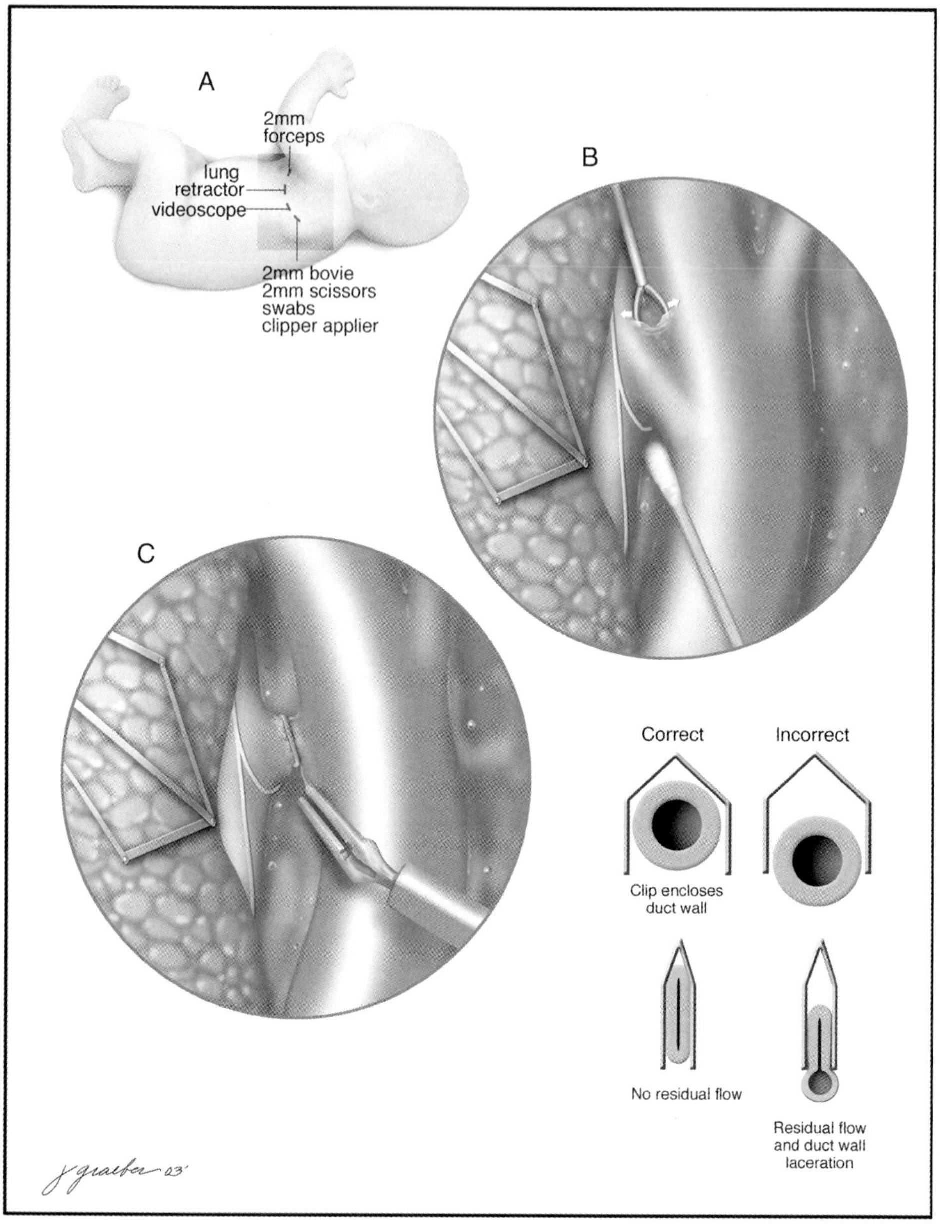

Figure 107–3 Video-assisted dissection technique for ligation of patent ductus arteriosus (PDA).

Median Sternotomy

Median sternotomy has been reserved for patients with wide, short, and/or calcified PDAs where there is potential need for cardiopulmonary bypass support. These defects can be repaired with a transpulmonary artery approach during bypass with temporary occlusion of the branch pulmonary arteries to protect the pulmonary circulation. Adults with PDA are difficult to close with VATS—the aorta is rigid and the dissection is more difficult. Given the morbidity of these incisions, most patients, particularly adults, are referred for primary transcatheter device closure of PDA.[131]

Ductal ligation or division as a secondary procedure during open heart surgery is performed frequently. The takeoffs of the right and left pulmonary arteries must be clearly identified, and the recurrent nerve swept away, before ligation. In several ductal-dependent lesions, such as pulmonary atresia with intact ventricular septum, the ductus may be tortuous and friable and should be avoided until preparations for cardiopulmonary bypass are complete.

Robotics

PDA ligation with robotic assistance has been described.[82] Two general systems are available—robotically controlled endoscopes (which can be voice activated) and robotically controlled instrument manipulators. Current systems are physically large and expensive. There are several limitations to robotic surgery with available technology. Robotic systems have no effective force or tactile feedback, preventing the surgeon from sensing or calibrating the force being applied to tissues. Current systems have widely spaced operating arms, designed for surgery on adult patients, and instruments generally require 7-mm ports, restricting their

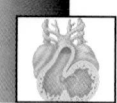

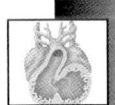

applicability in the pediatric thorax. Robotic surgery must be performed entirely with visual cues, and endoscopic depth perception and resolution do not yet match direct visualization with operative loupes. Depth perception is limited, except with very large two-chip endoscopes (10 mm), which do not fit through the infant intercostal space without unacceptable trauma. Engineering constraints create a time lag between the surgeon's hands and the instrument tips, which affects operative precision. Instrument changes are time consuming, and robotic cardiac procedures have taken considerably longer than either open or VATS techniques.

Therapeutic Approach in Premature Newborns

Primary medical therapy for premature newborns is successful in 60% of patients. Fluid restriction and diuretics are combined with indomethacin therapy to achieve ductal closure. Premature newborns generally are not candidates for transcatheter device closure, because vascular trauma and thermal instability are difficult to control in the catheterization laboratory.

Open surgical ligation or clipping is the mainstay of surgical therapy for premature newborns with PDA. Reducing surgical trauma is particularly important in these patients. Surgery generally is performed in the neonatal intensive care unit to minimize the risk of hypothermia. Operative mortality rates are low[21] and do not appear to be influenced by birth weight, age at operation, degree of preexisting pulmonary disease, or prior use of indomethacin.[134] In series of VLBW premature newborns, surgery-related mortality of 3% and overall mortality of 10% have been reported.[104] Potential surgical morbidity includes tension pneumothorax (which can be fatal[76]), bleeding, chylothorax, phrenic nerve injury, wound infection, and residual flow. Complications such as pneumothorax, pleural effusion, recurrent nerve injury, and phrenic nerve injury have been described. Phrenic nerve injury and diaphragm paralysis may produce significant pulmonary morbidity.[68]

VATS has been applied to premature newborns as small as 570 g, with 100% closure rates,[61] and without recurrent or phrenic nerve injury, chylothorax, pneumothorax, or bleeding. VATS for premature newborns has been performed both in the neonatal intensive care unit setting and in the operating room, with operative times averaging 1 hour.[23] Thermal instability is a constant concern in premature newborns undergoing surgical closure of patent ductus, and careful attention to maintaining overhead and bed warming, avoiding cold irrigation, and monitoring temperature during procedures is critical. Interestingly, it does not appear that resting energy expenditure is increased in extremely premature newborns before or after PDA ligation.[50] Heat generation from VATS endoscopes has been reported to have the potential to increase patient temperature during surgery on premature newborns.[122,127] Despite anatomical simplicity, the therapeutic options for PDA have evolved into a relatively complex algorithm, combining surgical, medical, and transcatheter technologies.

VASCULAR RING AND PULMONARY ARTERY SLING

In June 1945 our attention was drawn to a teenage boy who had difficulty in swallowing and also had rather noisy respiratory sounds in the chest. Roentgenographic studies quickly and clearly showed a pulsating vessel behind the esophagus, pressing upon it. Also, there was a pulsation on the anterior surface of the trachea. These facts could very clearly be substantiated by roentgen studies with a swallow of barium, and also by injecting a little radiopaque material down the trachea. At surgical exploration, there was an amazing finding of a "double aortic arch," the first part of the ascending aorta splitting, with half going up and across behind the esophagus and the other limb going up in front of the trachea, both branches meeting on the left side to form the descending aorta. The anterior arch was of much larger size than the rear one. It was not at all difficult to divide the posterior arch and suture closed each end thereof. This completely freed the esophagus from its compression. The anterior arch, being the larger of the two, was intentionally saved. Severance of the posterior arch had relieved tension on the anterior limb and allowed it to swing free from the trachea. It was all a surprise, and a very happy outcome.[100]

—Robert E. Gross

History

Vascular ring comprises a set of unusual anatomical anomalies of the aorta and arch vessels producing tracheal and esophageal compression. Bayford[12] described the "obstructed deglutition" produced by an aberrant subclavian artery as a prank of nature, giving rise to the term "dysphagia lusoria." Glaevecke and Doehle[53] described pulmonary artery sling in 1897. Gross[55] performed the first successful division of a vascular ring in 1945, 7 years after he first ligated a patent ductus. Edwards[41] outlined the embryological development of the aortic arch and its variations in 1948. Potts and associates[112] repaired a pulmonary artery sling in 1954. The first VATS vascular ring division was performed in 1993 at Children's Hospital Boston,[22] the same institution where Gross had performed the first open surgical division 48 years earlier.

Genomics

Vascular rings comprise 1 or 2% of congenital heart disease. Genetic factors determining aortic arch development and its perturbations are now being elucidated. The internal organs of all vertebrates are asymmetrically organized across the left–right axis. The development of this asymmetry is controlled by a molecular pathway that includes the signaling molecule Nodal and the transcription factor Pitx2, proteins encoded by genes that are predominantly expressed on the left side of all vertebrate embryos studied to date.[19] At the genome level, cardiac neural crest cells are known to play multiple roles during development of the inflow and outflow tract of the heart and the aortic arch. In 2002 Liu et al[87] showed that the Pitx2 gene contributes to aortic arch development, suggesting that a major function of the Pitx2-mediated left–right asymmetry pathway is to pattern the aortic arches. The homeobox gene, Lbx1, specifies a subpopulation of cardiac neural crest necessary for normal heart development.[117] Acute ethanol toxicity during the time of neural crest cell migration produces vascular rings in animal models.[33]

Cardiovascular anomalies are present in 75–80% of patients with a chromosome 22q11 deletion and include various vascular rings.[93,94,99] Because of the possible association between right aortic arch and band 22q11 deletion, a fluorescence in situ hybridization (FISH) test may be of value. Routine screening for cardiovascular anomalies, including echocardiography and other imaging studies to identify the laterality and branching pattern of the aortic arch, is indicated in patients diagnosed with 22q11 deletion beyond 6 months of age and is particularly critical for patients with respiratory or feeding disorders who may have a vascular ring.[96] Patients with congenital laryngeal web[95] or hypoparathyroidism[74] also should have genetic screening for chromosome 22q11 deletion syndrome and may have associated vascular ring formation. Twenty percent of patients with double aortic arch may have associated cardiac malformations, including tetralogy of Fallot,[133] D-transposition of the great arteries,[77,126,135] ventricular septal defect,[34] and atrioventricular canal.[121] A unique vascular ring has been reported in association with situs inversus totalis and corrected transposition of the great arteries.[45]

Anatomy

Vascular ring anatomy is commonly described by referring to the embryological development of the six pairs of pharyngeal arch arteries that develop in conjunction with the branchial pouches (Figure 107-4). These symmetrical arches appear in sequence and follow a pattern of segmental regression, producing the usual configuration of arch anatomy with a leftward descending thoracic aorta. Regression usually occurs in the distal sixth arch and the right-sided dorsal aorta, leaving the left fourth arch to become the aortic arch and the right fourth arch to become the innominate artery. The distal left sixth arch becomes the ductus arteriosus, and the proximal sixth arches form the proximal branch pulmonary arteries. Vascular rings and compressive vascular anatomy develop when this process of development is altered, with resulting complete or partial encirclement or compression of the trachea and esophagus. The pulmonary arteries are formed when lung buds from the splanchnic plexus fuse with the sixth aortic arches bilaterally. Aberrant migration of the left pulmonary artery behind the trachea results in the pulmonary artery ring–sling complex.

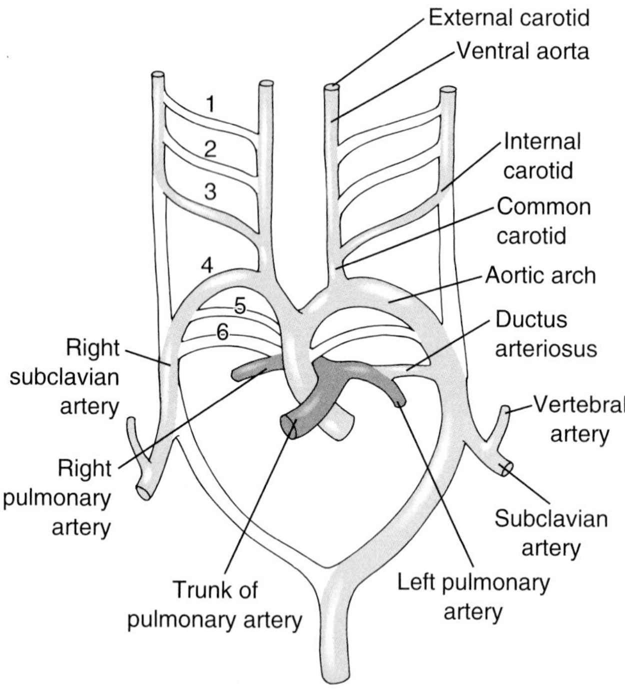

Figure 107-4 Aortic arch development. *(Modified from Gray H: Anatomy of the Human, 1918.)*

Clinical Presentation and Diagnostic Techniques for Vascular Rings

Vascular rings encircle the trachea and esophagus, usually causing compression of both structures. Findings on presentation are diverse and may include a harsh cry, inspiratory stridor, dysphagia, chronic cough, bronchopneumonia, poor growth, failure to thrive, difficulty feeding, respiratory distress, wheezing, cyanosis, and hyperinflation of the lungs. The extent of respiratory impairment depends on the severity of compression, which can vary considerably. Less commonly, patients may suffer primarily from swallowing problems related to esophageal compression. These typically manifest as vomiting and feeding intolerance in infants and younger children and as dysphagia later in life. Swallowing dysfunction may contribute to respiratory symptoms when a food bolus compresses the membranous trachea. Respiratory compromise generally is more problematic in younger patients, whereas dysphagia presents at an older age as children shift to solid foods. Children may have esophageal foreign bodies stuck at the level of the ring.[31] Adult patients may display a wide range of respiratory and gastrointestinal symptoms and associated pathophysiology.[54,65,71]

Although it is now possible to diagnose right and double fetal aortic arch using prenatal ultrasound,[1] the diagnosis is frequently missed. It is common for patients with vascular ring to be misdiagnosed with "asthma,"[49,86,101] or "reflux,"[113] and patients with vascular ring often go undiagnosed for over a year after the onset of symptoms.[75] Tracheal compression by a vascular ring causes upper airway obstruction with noisy breathing heard during inspiration and expiration, which can be distinguished from asthma, where the noise is heard mainly at the end of expiration. Airway compression by the vascular ring can produce a characteristic "seal-barking" cough. A high index of suspicion for vascular ring in patients with respiratory symptoms can be lifesaving. Fatal aortoesophageal fistula has been described in several cases of undiagnosed tight vascular rings, which were created iatrogenically by nasogastric tubes.[4,98,107] Parents may report noisy breathing since birth or may not be aware of obvious noises. There may be a history of obstructive sleep apnea. Physical examination findings include low-pitched inspiratory and expiratory gargling sounds, inspiratory stridor, and expiratory wheezes. Neck flexion may increase respiratory symptoms, with improvement on neck extension.

Chest radiography is not particularly useful in the diagnosis of vascular ring, except as a screening tool identifying a right aortic arch in patients with respiratory symptoms. The barium esophagram remains an effective minimally invasive technique to complete the diagnosis.[123] The patterns of posterior and lateral impressions on the esophagus are characteristic of the common forms of vascular ring (Figure 107-5). Transthoracic echocardiography (TTE) is effective in diagnosing vascular rings, particularly when associated cardiac abnormalities are suspected.[85] (TEE is usually avoided in the presence of esophageal obstruction. Computed tomography (CT) and magnetic resonance imaging (MRI) are accurate noninvasive imaging modalities for diagnosing and visualizing vascular ring anatomy [58,69,88]; however, they may require sedation, complicating management in infants with potential airway obstruction. Generating three-dimensional reconstructions of arch anatomy may facilitate operative planning.[60] MRI studies have shown that symptomatic patients with vascular rings have significantly altered tracheal geometry compared with asymptomatic patients.[46] Patients with associated tracheal disease and patients who have had previous vascular ring surgery may benefit from MRI reconstructions, because more complex operative procedures, including tracheoplasty, may be necessary.[119] MRI also has been useful for delineating unusual anatomical variants producing true vascular rings[118] or ring-type symptoms.[59]

Bronchoscopy is performed routinely, but is not necessary, to confirm tracheal compression before surgery and relief of compression after repair. Pulmonary function may be useful[130]; however, these studies are not performed routinely. In some older patients, pulmonary function studies may be useful to document improvement after repair. Pulmonary function studies before and after vascular ring division suggest persistent airway abnormalities despite anatomical correction.[17,92]

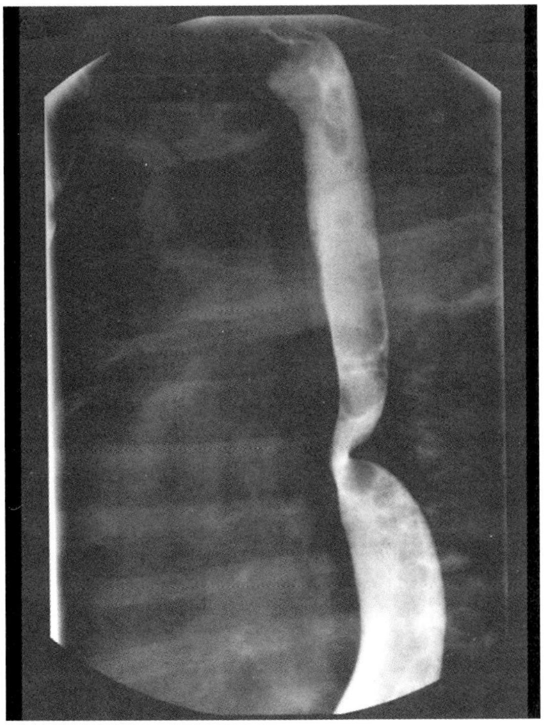

Figure 107–5 Barium esophagram. The lateral view shows esophageal constriction from a double aortic arch with an atretic left arch in a 9-month-old girl with inspiratory stridor.

Management

Tracheoesophageal compression syndromes present in four general pathoanatomical classes, each having unique manifestations and surgical approaches. These general classes and their nomenclature recently have been organized to facilitate database management and risk stratification.[6] The four ring types include double aortic arch, right aortic arch with left ligamentum, innominate compression, and pulmonary artery sling. Surgery is indicated in symptomatic patients. Reports of medical management demonstrate persistent symptoms in most patients, making this approach difficult to justify. Justification for surgery in asymptomatic patients diagnosed incidentally is less clear, and these patients may be managed expectantly. Traditional surgery for double aortic arch and the right aortic arch rings is performed through a left thoracotomy. A right thoracotomy is used to approach a left-sided aortic arch with a right-sided ligamentum.

Double Aortic Arch

Double aortic arch represents a persistence of both right and left fourth embryonic branchial arches joining the aortic portion of the truncoaortic sac to their respective dorsal aorta. The ascending aorta bifurcates anterior to the trachea, encircling the trachea and esophagus. The innominate artery does not form. The right arch is dominant in 80% of patients, the left in 15%, and they are rarely equal. The larger right arch usually crosses posterior to the esophagus and joins with the left arch in the posterior mediastinum to form the descending aorta. The distal left arch is often atretic, and the distal right arch is rarely so.

Double aortic arch is rarely associated with congenital heart disease, but when present, tetralogy of Fallot and transposition of the great vessels are most common. Clinical manifestations are related to the nature of malformation and tightness of the ring. If both arches are widely patent, the rings are tight and patients develop stridor in the first weeks of life. Rings with one hypoplastic or atretic arch are usually less tight. These patients may have presenting symptoms at 3–6 months of age. Double aortic arch rarely presents in adulthood. Most patients develop symptoms by 1 year of age, often in the first month of life, and rarely after 6 months. Stridor, a nonproductive cough, or a hoarse cry may be noted soon after birth. Solid foods are not handled well, and vomiting may precede or follow choking. Children with double aortic arch are often small and poorly developed and hold their head in hyperextension. Infants feed poorly as a result of respiratory distress and may have life-threatening episodes of apnea and cyanosis. Repeated severe respiratory infections may occur.

Physical examination may be within normal limits, but coughing, dyspnea, drooling, or dysphagia may be seen. Cardiac examination is most often normal. Lung examination may or may not show evidence of pneumonia. Radiographs may show no significant abnormalities. Tracheal deformities sometimes can be detected or at least suspected from the shadow of the air column in the trachea without contrast. Both arches may be seen on either side of the trachea in the anteroposterior projection. There also may be evidence of hyperinflation of either or both lungs as a result of obstruction of the lower trachea and main stem bronchi. An esophagram may not only establish the diagnosis, but also identify the structures making up the constricting ring. In double aortic arch the right arch indentation on an anterior esophagram is usually wider and more superior than that of the left arch. Computerized imaging (CT and/or MRI) is often obtained to confirm spatial relationships between the vessels, trachea, and esophagus.

With a dominant right arch the surgical approach to double aortic arch is via a left thoracotomy under general anesthesia, with or without single lung ventilation. The parietal pleural overlying the left subclavian artery is opened, and the dissection is carried from the left subclavian artery down onto the arch elements. The atretic segment of the arch is usually the most distal or posterior portion. Division is performed at the atretic segment, or at the descending aortic insertion of the most diminutive segment (Figure 107-6). With a dominant left arch an approach via median sternotomy or left thoracotomy is possible. The distal right arch is divided at its insertion into the descending aorta.

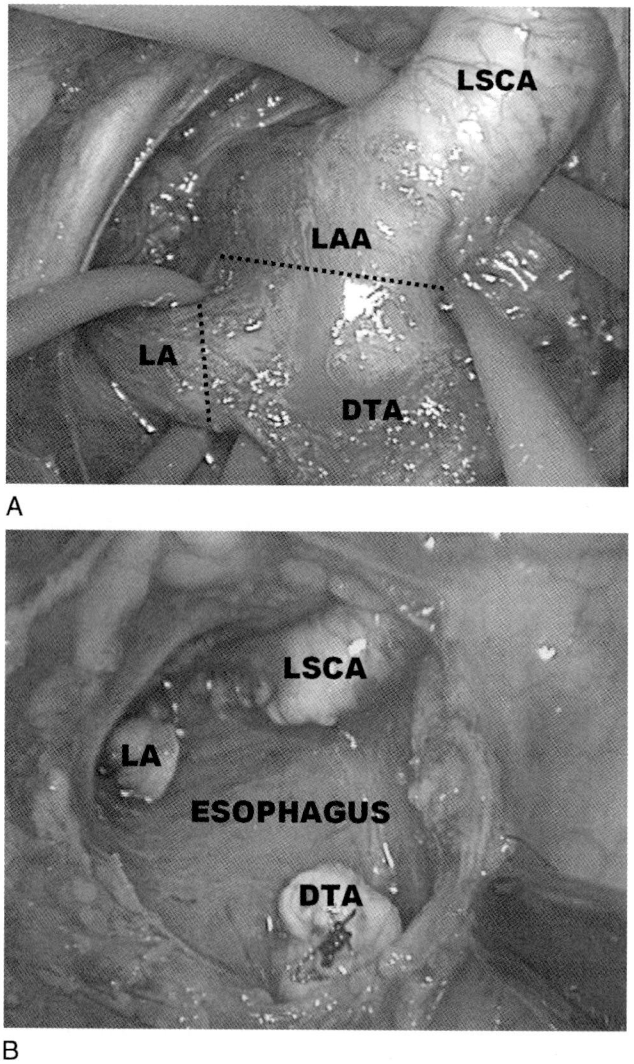

Figure 107–6 Operative image of double aortic arch and division (A and B).

Right Aortic Arch with Retroesophageal Left Ligamentum

The right aortic arch with retroesophageal left ligamentum may occur in two forms, with an aberrant left subclavian artery in 70% of patients and with mirror image branching in 30%. Rare forms of right aortic arch, right ligamentum, and absent left pulmonary artery have been described.[40] In the most frequent form of vascular ring with a right aortic arch, an aberrant origin of the left subclavian artery from a retroesophageal diverticulum (Kommerel's diverticulum) is present, which originates as the last branch of the aortic arch, distal to the right subclavian artery. The ring is completed by a left-sided ductus arteriosus, or a ligamentum arteriosum, passing from the aberrant left subclavian artery to the proximal left pulmonary artery. The retroesophageal diverticulum is distinguished from the aberrant left subclavian artery by its larger caliber. On anterior barium esophagram the arch creates an indentation on the right, with a smaller indentation from the left ligamentum, and a posterior indentation is visible on the lateral film.

A right aortic arch with mirror-image branching forms a vascular ring when the ligamentum originates from the descending aorta; however, no ring is formed when the ligamentum arises from the innominate artery. This arrangement may be seen in patients with tetralogy of Fallot and truncus arteriosus. Vascular ring with right aortic arch rarely has been associated with coarctation and has been corrected through the left side of the chest with Dacron graft interposition.[52] Other unusual forms of right aortic arch producing a vascular ring have been described.[40] With right aortic arch the course of the descending thoracic aorta varies, descending on the right, or crossing gradually to the left of the vertebral column to pass through the diaphragm in the usual location of the aortic hiatus. Symptomatic compression of the trachea seems to occur slightly later in life, with vascular rings having a right aortic arch when compared with vascular rings with double aortic arch. The pathophysiology of vascular rings with a right aortic arch does not differ among the various anatomical forms. Some patients may develop recurrent respiratory infections, and some may exhibit failure to thrive because of the combination of increased metabolic requirements from respiratory and feeding work and relatively poor oral intake. The surgical approach is through the left side of the chest, where the left-sided ligamentum is divided.

Left Aortic Arch, Right Descending Aorta, and Right Ligament

With regression of the right fourth arch, a left aortic arch with a right descending aorta and a right-sided ligamentum may create a complete ring.[13] This type of ring may be associated with other congenital heart defects. This is the rare vascular ring approached from the right side of the chest, through which the right-sided ligamentum is divided.

Partial Vascular Rings

Two forms of partial vascular ring may develop in the presence of a left aortic arch. These include a left aortic arch with an aberrant right subclavian artery and an anomalous innominate artery with anterior tracheal compression. Retroesophageal aberrant right subclavian artery may produce significant dysphagia. The barium esophagram shows a high-angled (going up from the patient's left to right), posterior impression. This arrangement may be found at the time of coarctation repair or during interrupted arch repair. In neonates this vessel is often divided without reimplantation. Surgical relief also can be achieved by relocating the subclavian artery to the carotid, innominate, or ascending aorta via median sternotomy or right thoracotomy.

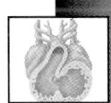

Malposition of the innominate artery, usually characterized as a "late takeof," more to the patient's left than usual, may produce anterior tracheal compression. This anomaly may be associated with chest wall deformities such as pectus excavatum. Bronchoscopy is an essential diagnostic tool. Innominate compression can be demonstrated visually at bronchoscopy and confirmed by tilting the bronchoscope anteriorly in the trachea, occluding the innominate artery, and ablating the distal radial artery pulse.

The innominate artery compression syndrome may lead to life-threatening airway occlusion. Many of these patients have apnea, severe hypoxic episodes, and seizures. Tracheal compression and resultant tracheomalacia can be effectively approached by aortopexy via left thoracotomy or a right submammary incision and suture fixation of the aorta and innominate artery to the posterior sternum (Figure 107-7).[3,57] It also is possible to detach the innominate artery from the leftward position and reimplant it on the right side of the ascending aorta.[39] Intraoperative bronchoscopy should show marked improvement in airway caliber. Forced expiratory volume may improve from 52–82% predicted, and symptomatic relief may be complete.[137]

Pulmonary Artery Sling

The embryological left pulmonary artery may migrate posteriorly around the trachea, anterior to the esophagus, and insert into the distal posterosuperior right pulmonary artery, creating a pulmonary artery sling. The right upper lobe branch may arise from the proximal left pulmonary artery. There is not a complete ring, but a "sling" forms around the right main stem bronchus and the distal trachea, appearing like a vaudevillian hook pulling the trachea offstage to the left. This lesion is frequently associated with tracheal stenosis and complete tracheal rings (33–50%), which may involve part or all of the trachea, giving rise to the term "ring–sling complex."[15] Infants display episodic stridor soon after birth and have visible suprasternal retractions. They may be misdiagnosed with asthma and suffer repeated respiratory infections. Examination findings are similar to those for other forms of vascular ring. Chest radiography may show hyperinflation of the right lung and anterior bowing of the right main bronchus, with carinal deviation to the left. Barium esophagram shows an anterior indentation in the esophageal wall just above the carina, distinct from the posterior and lateral compressions seen with vascular rings. The only other anomaly creating this anterior compression is the ductus arteriosus sling. A variety of noninvasive imaging techniques may be used to characterize the pulmonary artery sling and prepare for surgical correction.[83] Echocardiography may document the abnormal path of the left pulmonary artery, and MRI[42] provides information on the degree and extent of tracheal and pulmonary artery stenosis. Tracheal anatomy may be abnormal, including the potential for a bronchus suis, with independent takeoff of the eparterial right upper lobe bronchus.[16] Half of these patients may have associated congenital heart defects, including left superior vena cava, atrial septal defect, and tetralogy of Fallot.

Surgical approaches vary and generally include relocating the left pulmonary artery with tracheoplasty, versus resecting the tracheal stenosis and repositioning the left pulmonary artery anteriorly (Figure 107-8). Median sternotomy provides optimal exposure, enhances airway management, and enables cardiopulmonary bypass if needed.[9] In both repairs, residual stenosis of both the left pulmonary artery and the trachea is possible. The tracheal stenosis is resected when the complete rings are limited to a short segment of trachea. Anterior tracheoplasty with rib or pericardium,[64] or slide tracheoplasty, is used for patients with long-segment stenosis. Left pulmonary artery thrombosis may occur early after repair, even in patients who are symptomatically improved. Early postoperative surveillance catheterization and transcatheter intervention may be indicated to improve the long-term patency of

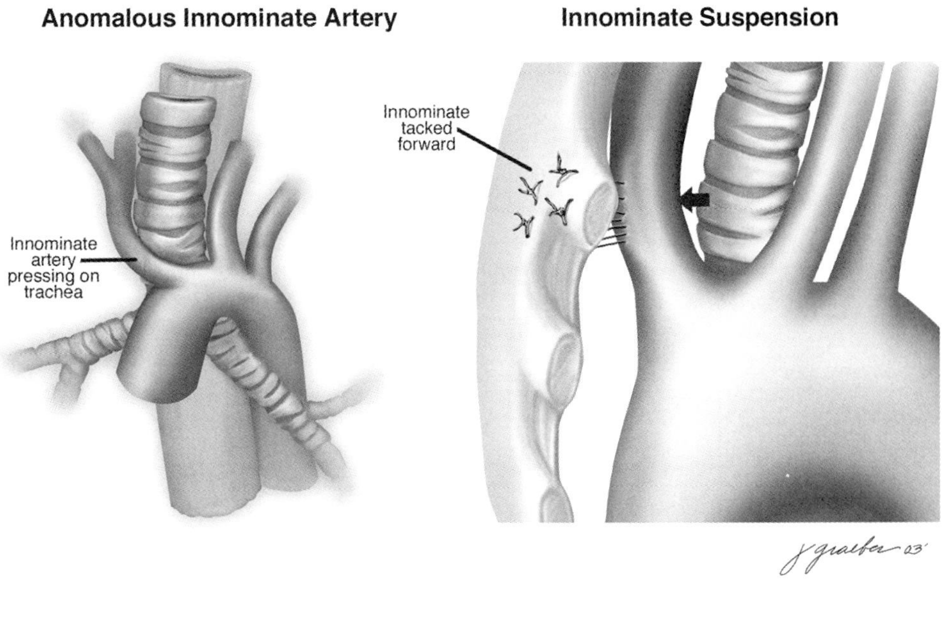

Figure 107–7 Innominate artery compression syndrome produced by late takeoff of the innominate artery.

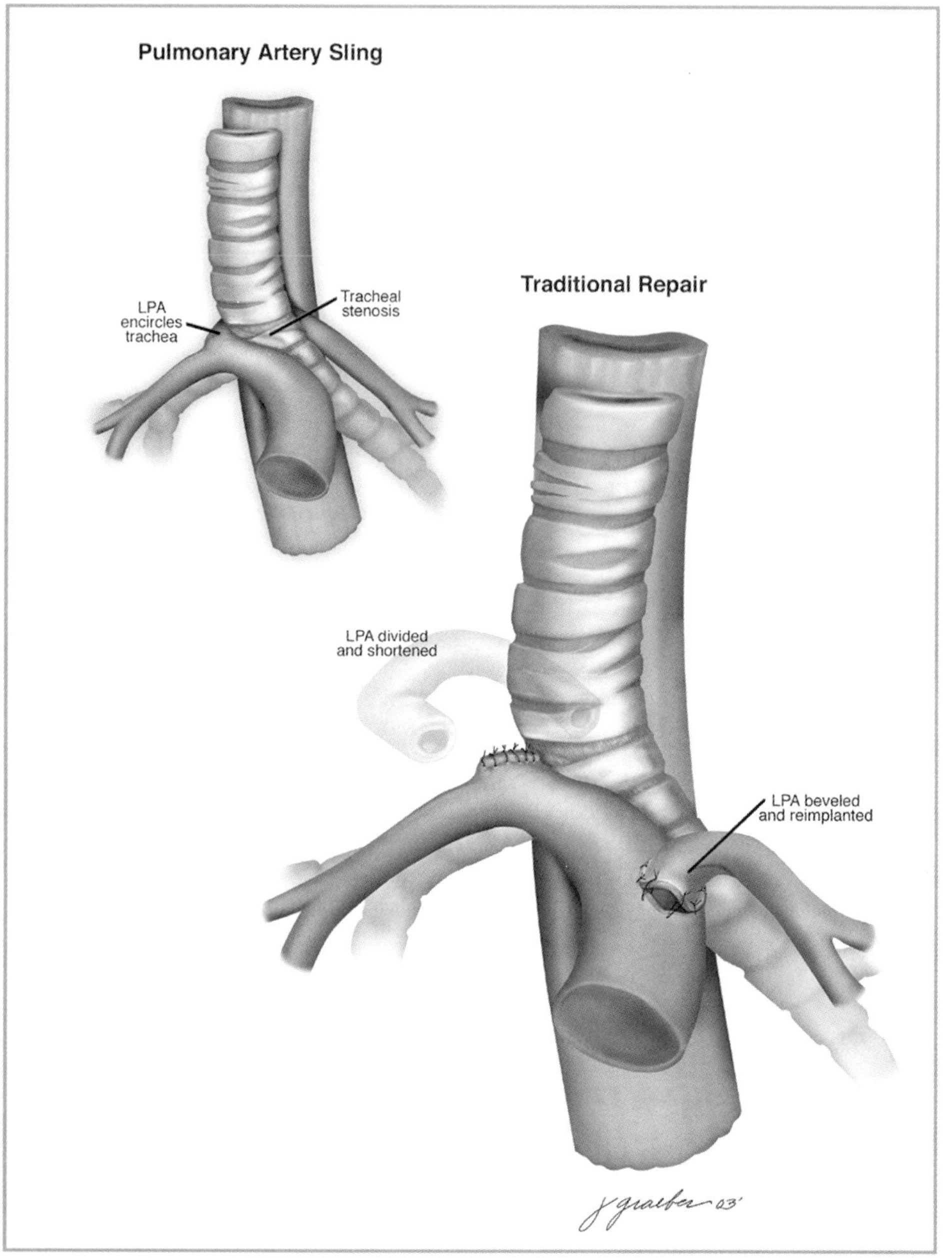

Figure 107–8 Surgical approach to pulmonary artery reimplantation for ring–sling complex.

the relocated or repositioned left pulmonary artery. Outcomes appear to depend mainly on the effectiveness of the tracheal reconstruction.[63]

Surgical Considerations

Preoperative preparation for vascular ring surgery is usually short—focused on early surgical intervention with optimal nutrition and pulmonary toilet. Parents are counseled that mild symptoms will probably persist for months after surgery while the airway and esophagus recover from prolonged compression. Patients generally are approached via lateral thoracotomy through the left fourth interspace under general anesthesia, with single or double lung ventilation. The left subclavian artery is used to orient the dissection and guide the surgeon down to the ring elements. The vagus, phrenic, and recurrent nerves are at risk during these dissections and must be protected. For double aortic arch the nondominant arch is divided through the atretic segment, or at the descending aortic insertion, taking care not to stenose the origins of adjacent vessels. The ligamentum or ductus is lower than the arch and may be embedded in the wall of the underlying esophagus. Missing the ligamentum leaves an intact vascular ring and necessitates reoperation.

For right aortic arch with aberrant left subclavian and left ligamentum, the ligament is divided. Again, the ligament may be embedded in the wall of the underlying esophagus and must be elevated off the esophagus to achieve length for division. Bands of scar tissue around the ligamentum impression on the esophageal wall should be divided. Surgeons vary in their approach to the Kommerel's diverticulum in patients with right aortic arch and aberrant left subclavian artery, with some choosing to pexy the diverticulum to the posterior chest wall, others resecting the diverticulum, and some leaving the diverticulum intact after dividing the ring. Persistent airway or esophageal obstruction after vascular ring division has been related to the diverticulum. In selected patients, reoperation with resection of the Kommerel's diverticulum and transfer of the retroesophageal left subclavian artery to the carotid artery has produced symptomatic relief.[7] Reported complications after vascular ring division include recurrent and phrenic nerve injury and chylothorax. Surgical outcomes after vascular ring division have been outstanding in institutions with large series.[8,18] Mortality should be extremely rare, and morbidity should be limited.

The thoracoscopic or VATS approach to vascular ring division evolved from a growing effort to reduce the trauma of congenital heart surgery.[22,125] VATS vascular ring division can be performed with the same instrumentation and operative techniques as PDA interruption. Patients with vascular rings composed of nonpatent vascular structures are considered ideal candidates. Vascular rings composed of large patent vascular structures are better approached by thoracotomy. Four trocars are placed as for PDA interruption, and arch elements are dissected free using the left subclavian artery as an initial landmark. The appropriate ring elements are divided between thoracoscopic sutures or vascular clips. Patients undergoing VATS and conventional thoracotomy for vascular ring division have similar outcomes.[24] Long-term airway dysfunction has been shown in patients repaired after onset of symptoms,[92] but early surgery in asymptomatic patients has not yet been shown to mitigate this chronic airway damage.

REFERENCES

1. Achiron R, Rotstein Z, Heggesh J, et al: Anomalies of the fetal aortic arch: A novel sonographic approach to in-utero diagnosis. Ultrasound Obstet Gynecol 20:553–557, 2002.
2. Adamska E: [Ibuprofen—a new application for pharmacological closure of patent ductus arteriosus in preterm infants. Preliminary report]. Med Wieku Rozwoj 4:65–71, 2000.
3. Adler SC, Isaacson G, Balsara RK: Innominate artery compression of the trachea: Diagnosis and treatment by anterior suspension. A 25-year experience. Ann Otol Rhinol Laryngol 104:924–927, 1995.
4. Angelini A, Dimoponlos K, Frescura C, et al: Fatal aortoesophageal fistula in two cases of tight vascular ring. Cardiol Young 12:172–176, 2002.
5. Arlettaz R, Archer N, Wilkinson AR: Closure of the ductus arteriosus and development of pulmonary branch stenosis in babies of less than 32 weeks gestation. Arch Dis Child Fetal Neonatal Ed 85:F197–F200, 2001.
6. Backer CL, Mavroudis C: Congenital Heart Surgery Nomenclature and Database Project: Vascular rings, tracheal stenosis, pectus excavatum. Ann Thorac Surg 69:S308–S318, 2000.
7. Backer CL, Hillman N, Mavroudis C, Holinger LD: Resection of Kommerell's diverticulum and left subclavian artery transfer for recurrent symptoms after vascular ring division. Eur J Cardiothorac Surg 22:64–69, 2002.
8. Backer CL, Ilbawi MN, Idriss FS, DeLeon SY: Vascular anomalies causing tracheoesophageal compression. Review of experience in children. J Thorac Cardiovasc Surg 97:725–731, 1989.
9. Backer CL, Mavroudis C, Dunham ME, Holinger LD: Pulmonary artery sling: Results with median sternotomy, cardiopulmonary bypass, and reimplantation. Ann Thorac Surg 67:1738–1744, 1999.
10. Balzer DT, Spray TL, McMullin D, et al: Endarteritis associated with a clinically silent patent ductus arteriosus. Am Heart J 125:1192–1193, 1993.
11. Bancalari E: Changes in the pathogenesis and prevention of chronic lung disease of prematurity. Am J Perinatol 18:1–9, 2001.
12. Bayford D: An account of a singular case of obstructed deglutition. Mem Med Soc Lond 2:275, 1794.
13. Belarbi N, Sebag G, Holvoet L, et al: [Left aortic arch with right descending aorta and right ligamentum arteriosum in an infant]. J Radiol 79:61–63, 1998.
14. Bensky AS, Raines KH, Hines MH: Late follow-up after thoracoscopic ductal ligation. Am J Cardiol 86:360–361, 2000.
15. Berdon WE, et al: Complete cartilage-ring tracheal stenosis associated with anomalous left pulmonary artery: The ring-sling complex. Radiology 152:57–64, 1984.
16. Berlin SC, Morrison SC, Myers MT, et al: Pediatric case of the day. Pulmonary sling with tracheal stenosis and bronchus suis. AJR Am J Roentgenol 169:305, 308, 1997.
17. Bertrand JM, Chartrand C, Lamarre A, Lapierre JG: Vascular ring: Clinical and physiological assessment of pulmonary function following surgical correction. Pediatr Pulmonol 2:378–383, 1986.
18. Binet JP, Langlois J, Planche C, et al: [Abnormal aortic arches in infants and children (experience with 322 cases)]. C R Acad Sci III 299:107–114, 1984.
19. Boorman CJ, Shimeld SM: The evolution of left-right asymmetry in chordates. Bioessays 24:1004–1011, 2002.
20. Borini I, Dalmonte P, Cervo G, et al: [Closure of patent ductus arteriosus in thoracoscopy: Analysis of the experience in the Gaslini Institute of Genoa]. G Ital Cardiol 27:786–789, 1997.
21. Brandt B, Marvin WJ, Ehrenhaft JL, et al: Ligation of patent ductus arteriosus in premature infants. Ann Thorac Surg 32:166–172, 1981.
22. Burke RP, Chang AC: Video-assisted thoracoscopic division of a vascular ring in an infant: a new operative technique. J Card Surg 8:537–540, 1993.
23. Burke RP, Jacobs JP, Cheng W, et al: Video-assisted thoracoscopic surgery for patent ductus arteriosus in low birth weight neonates and infants. Pediatrics 104:227–230, 1999.
24. Burke RP, Rosenfeld HM, Wernovsky G, Jonas RA: Video-assisted thoracoscopic vascular ring division in infants and children. J Am Coll Cardiol 25:943–947, 1995.
25. Burke RP, Wernovsky G, van der Velde M, et al: Video-assisted thoracoscopic surgery for congenital heart disease. J Thorac Cardiovasc Surg 109:499–507, discussion 508, 1995.
26. Campbell M: Natural history of persistent ductus arteriosus. Br Heart J 30:4–13, 1968.
27. Cherup LL, Siewers RD, Futrell JW: Breast and pectoral muscle maldevelopment after anterolateral and posterolateral thoracotomies in children. Ann Thorac Surg 41:492–497, 1986.
28. Chisholm JC, Salmon AP, Keeton BR, et al: Persistent hemolysis after transcatheter occlusion of a patent ductus arteriosus: Surgical ligation of the duct over the occlusion device. Pediatr Cardiol 16:194–196, 1995.
29. Christmann V, Liem KD, Semmekrot BA van de Bor, M: Changes in cerebral, renal and mesenteric blood flow velocity during continuous and bolus infusion of indomethacin. Acta Paediatr 91:440–446, 2002.

30. Chu JJ, Chang CH, Lin PJ, et al: Video-assisted thoracoscopic operation for interruption of patent ductus arteriosus in adults. Ann Thorac Surg 63:175–178, discussion 178–179, 1997.
31. Currarino G, Nikaidoh H: Esophageal foreign bodies in children with vascular ring or aberrant right subclavian artery: Coincidence or causation? Pediatr Radiol 21:406–408, 1991.
32. Cuzzolin L, Dal Cere M, Fanos V: NSAID-induced nephrotoxicity from the fetus to the child. Drug Saf 24:9–18, 2001.
33. Daft PA, Johnston MC, Sulik KK: Abnormal heart and great vessel development following acute ethanol exposure in mice. Teratology 33:93–104, 1986.
34. Dagar KS, Hsaia TY, Yates R, et al: Concurrent vascular ring and occult left pulmonary artery associated with ventricular septal defect: A report of an uncommon constellation. J Thorac Cardiovasc Surg 118:1127–1129, 1999.
35. Daher AH, Berkowitz FE: Infective endocarditis in neonates. Clin Pediatr (Phila) 34:198–206, 1995.
36. Dajczman E, Gordon A, Kreisman H, Wolkove N: Long-term postthoracotomy pain. Chest 99:270–274, 1991.
37. Das MB, Kapoor L, Moulick A, et al: Video-assisted thoracoscopic surgery for closure of patent ductus arteriosus in children. Indian Heart J 49:300–302, 1997.
38. DeCampli WM: Video-assisted thoracic surgical procedures in children. Semin Thorac Cardiovasc Surg Pediatr Card Surg Annu 1:61–74, 1998.
39. DeLeon SY, Quinones JA, Pifarre R: Aortoinnominopexy versus innominate artery reimplantation for displaced innominate artery. J Thorac Cardiovasc Surg 107:947–948, 1994.
40. Dodge-Khatami A, Backer CL, Dunham ME, Mavroudis C: Right aortic arch, right ligamentum, absent left pulmonary artery: A rare vascular ring. Ann Thorac Surg 67:1472–1474, 1999.
41. Edwards JE: Anomalies of the derivatives of the aortic arch system. Med Clin North Am 925, 1948.
42. Eichhorn J, Fink C, Bock M, et al: Images in cardiovascular medicine. Time-resolved three-dimensional magnetic resonance angiography for assessing a pulmonary artery sling in a pediatric patient. Circulation 106:e61–e62, 2002.
43. Ellison RC, Peckham GJ, Lang P, et al: Evaluation of the preterm infant for patent ductus arteriosus. Pediatrics 71:364–372, 1983.
44. Fan LL, Campbell DN, Clarke DR, et al: Paralyzed left vocal cord associated with ligation of patent ductus arteriosus. J Thorac Cardiovasc Surg 98:611–613, 1989.
45. Feingold B, O'Sullivan B, del Nido P, Pollack P: Situs inversus totalis and corrected transposition of the great arteries [I,D,D] in association with a previously unreported vascular ring. Pediatr Cardiol 22:338–342, 2001.
46. Fleenor JT, Weinberg PM, Kramer SS, Fogel M: Vascular rings and their effect on tracheal geometry. Pediatr Cardiol 24:430–435, 2003.
47. Friedman WF, Hirschklau MJ, Printz MP. Pharmacologic closure of patent ductus arteriosus in the premature infant. N Engl J Med 295:526–529, 2003.
48. Fujii AM, Brown E, Mirochnick M, et al: Neonatal necrotizing enterocolitis with intestinal perforation in extremely premature infants receiving early indomethacin treatment for patent ductus arteriosus. J Perinatol 22:535–540, 2002.
49. Galvin IF, Shepherd DR, Gibbons JR: Tracheal stenosis caused by congenital vascular ring anomaly misinterpreted as asthma for 45 years. Thorac Cardiovasc Surg 38:42–44, 1990.
50. Garza JJ, Shew SB, Keshen TH, et al: Energy expenditure in ill premature neonates. J Pediatr Surg 37:289–293, 2002.
51. Gentile R, Stevenson G, Dooley T: Pulsed Doppler echocardiographic determination of time of ductal closure in normal newborn infants. J Pediatr 98:443, 1981.
52. Gil-Jaurena JM, Murtra M, Goncalves A, Miro L: Aortic coarctation, vascular ring, and right aortic arch with aberrant subclavian artery. Ann Thorac Surg 73:1640–1642, 2002.
53. Glaevecke, Doehle: Ueber eine seltene angeborene Anomalie der Pulmonalarterie. Munchen Med Wochenschr 44:950, 1897.
54. Grathwohl KW, Afifi AY, Dillard TA, et al: Vascular rings of the thoracic aorta in adults. Am Surg 65:1077–1083, 1999.
55. Gross RE: Surgical relief for tracheal obstruction from a vascular ring. N Engl J Med 233:586–590, 1945.
56. Gross RE, Hubbard JP: Surgical ligation of a patent ductus arteriosus. Report of first successful case. JAMA 112:729, 1939.
57. Gross RE, Neuhauser EB: Compression of the trachea by an anomalous innominate artery. An operation for its relief. Am J Dis Child 75:570–574, 1948.
58. Haramati LB, Glickstein JS, Issenberg HJ, et al: MR imaging and CT of vascular anomalies and connections in patients with congenital heart disease: Significance in surgical planning. Radiographics 22:337–347, 2002.
59. Helund GL, Bisset GS 3rd: Esophageal duplication cyst and aberrant right subclavian artery mimicking a symptomatic vascular ring. Pediatr Radiol 19:543–544, 1989.
60. Hernandez RJ: Magnetic resonance imaging of mediastinal vessels. Magn Reson Imaging Clin N Am 10:237–251, 2002.
61. Hines MH, Bensky AS, Hammon JW, Pennington DG: Video-assisted thoracoscopic ligation of patent ductus arteriosus: Safe and outpatient. Ann Thorac Surg 66:853–858, 1998.
62. Ho SY, Anderson RH: Anatomical closure of the ductus arteriosus: A study in 35 specimens. J Anat 128:829–836, 1979.
63. Hodina M, Wicky S, Payot M, et al: Non-invasive imaging of the ring-sling complex in children. Pediatr Cardiol 22:333–337, 2001.
64. Idriss FS, DeLeon SY, Ilbawi MN, et al: Tracheoplasty with pericardial patch for extensive tracheal stenosis in infants and children. J Thorac Cardiovasc Surg 88:527–536, 1984.
65. James RC, Murty GE: Previously undiagnosed congenital vascular ring presenting as dysphagia in a six-week post-partum female. J Laryngol Otol 114:881–882, 2000.
66. Janorkar S, Goh T, Wilkinson J: Transcatheter closure of patent ductus arteriosus with the use of Rashkind occluders and/or Gianturco coils: Long-term follow-up in 123 patients and special reference to comparison, residual shunts, complications, and technique. Am Heart J 138:1176–1183, 1999.
67. Jaureguizar E, Vazquez J, Murcia J, Diez Pardo J: Morbid musculoskeletal sequelae of thoracotomy for tracheoesophageal fistula. J Pediatr Surg 20:511–514, 1985.
68. Jog SM, Patole SK: Diaphragmatic paralysis in extremely low birthweight neonates: Is waiting for spontaneous recovery justified? J Paediatr Child Health 38:101–103, 2002.
69. Julsrud PR, Ehman RL: Magnetic resonance imaging of vascular rings. Mayo Clin Proc 61:181–185, 1986.
70. Kim BY, Choi HH, Park YB, et al: Video assisted thoracoscopic ligation of patent ductus arteriosus. Technique of sliding loop ligation. J Cardiovasc Surg (Torino) 41:69–72, 2000.
71. Kinoshita Y, Udagawa H, Kajiyama Y, et al: Esophageal cancer and right aortic arch associated with a vascular ring. Dis Esophagus 12:216–218, 1999.
72. Kluckow M, Evans N: Ductal shunting, high pulmonary blood flow, and pulmonary hemorrhage. J Pediatr 137:68–72, 2000.
73. Knight DB: The treatment of patent ductus arteriosus in preterm infants. A review and overview of randomized trials. Semin Neonatol 6:63–73, 2001.
74. Koch A, Hofbeck M, Buheitel G, et al: Hypoparathyroidism in conotruncal heart defects. Eur J Pediatr 161:208–211, 2002.

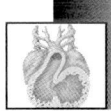

75. Kocis KC, Midgley FM, Ruckman RN: Aortic arch complex anomalies: 20-year experience with symptoms, diagnosis, associated cardiac defects, and surgical repair. Pediatr Cardiol 18:127–132, 1997.
76. Koehne PS, Bein G, Alexi-Meskhishvili V, et al: Patent ductus arteriosus in very low birthweight infants: Complications of pharmacological and surgical treatment. J Perinat Med 29:327–334, 2001.
77. Kupferschmid JP, Burns SA, Jonas RA, et al: Repair of double aortic arch associated with D-transposition of the great arteries. Ann Thorac Surg 56:570–572, 1993.
78. Laborde F, Noirhomme P, Karam J, et al: A new video-assisted thoracoscopic surgical technique for interruption of patent ductus arteriosus in infants and children. J Thorac Cardiovasc Surg 105:278–280, 1993.
79. Laborde F, Folliguet TA, Etienne PY, et al: Video-thoracoscopic surgical interruption of patent ductus arteriosus. Routine experience in 332 pediatric cases. Eur J Cardiothorac Surg 11:1052–1055, 1997.
80. Laird WP, Fixler DE: Echocardiography of premature infants with pulmonary disease: A noninvasive method for detecting large ductal left-to-right shunts. Radiology 122:455–457, 1977.
81. Lavoie J, Javorski JJ, Donahue K, et al: Detection of residual flow by transesophageal echocardiography during video-assisted thoracoscopic patent ductus arteriosus interruption. Anesth Analg 80:1071–1075, 1995.
82. Le Bret E, Papadatos S, Folliguet T, et al: Interruption of patent ductus arteriosus in children: Robotically assisted versus videothoracoscopic surgery. J Thorac Cardiovasc Surg 123:973–976, 2002.
83. Lee KH, Yoon CS, Choe KO, et al: Use of imaging for assessing anatomical relationships of tracheobronchial anomalies associated with left pulmonary artery sling. Pediatr Radiol 31:269–278, 2001.
84. Levinson MM, Dewhurst T, Han MT, et al: Cosmetic minimally invasive surgical closure of a patent foramen ovale. Report and surgical technique. Heart Surg Forum http://www.hsforum.com/HeartSurgery/Directories/Articles/L/LevinsonMM/MISASD/1996-12451.hsfhttp://www.hsforum.com/HeartSurgeery/Directories/Articles/L/LevinsonMM/MISASD/1996-12451.hsf (1996).
85. Lillehei CW, Colan S: Echocardiography in the preoperative evaluation of vascular rings. J Pediatr Surg 27:1118–1120, 1992.
86. Linna O, Hyrynkangas K, Lanning P, Nieminen P: Central airways stenosis in school-aged children: Differential diagnosis from asthma. Acta Paediatr 91:399–402, 2002.
87. Liu C, Liu W, Palie J, et al: Pitx2c patterns anterior myocardium and aortic arch vessels and is required for local cell movement into atrioventricular cushions. Development 129:5081–5091, 2002.
88. Lowe GM, Donaldson JS, Backer CL: Vascular rings: 10-year review of imaging. Radiographics 11:637–646, 1991.
89. Lund JT, Jensen MB, Hjelms E: Aneurysm of the ductus arteriosus. A review of the literature and the surgical implications. Eur J Cardiothorac Surg 5:566–570, 1991.
90. Mani A, Meraji SM, Houshyar R, et al: Finding genetic contributions to sporadic disease: A recessive locus at 12q24 commonly contributes to patent ductus arteriosus. Proc Natl Acad Sci USA 99:15054–15059, 2002.
91. Marasini M, Rimini A, Zannini L, Pongiglione G: Giant aneurysm following coil occlusion of patent ductus arteriosus. Catheter Cardiovasc Interv 50:186–189, 2000.
92. Marmon LM, Bye MR, Haas JM, Joe B: Vascular ring and slings: Long-term followup of pulmonary function. J Pediatr Surg 19:683–692, 1984.
93. McDonald-McGinn DM, Driscoll DA, Bason L, et al: Autosomal dominant "Opitz" GBBB syndrome due to a 22q11.2 deletion. Am J Med Genet 59:103–113, 1995.
94. McElhinney DB, Clark BJ 3rd, Weinberg PM, et al: Association of chromosome 22q11 deletion with isolated anomalies of aortic arch laterality and branching. J Am Coll Cardiol 37:2114–2119, 2001.
95. McElhinney DB, Jacobs I, McDonald-McGinn DM, et al: Chromosomal and cardiovascular anomalies associated with congenital laryngeal web. Int J Pediatr Otorhinolaryngol 66:23–27, 2002.
96. McElhinney DB, McDonald-McGinn D, Zackai EH, Goldmuntz E: Cardiovascular anomalies in patients diagnosed with a chromosome 22q11 deletion beyond 6 months of age. Pediatrics 108:E104, 2001.
97. McKeating J, Smith S, Kochanck P, et al: Fatal aorto-esophageal fistula due to double aortic arch: An unusual complication of prolonged nasogastric intubation. J Pediatr Surg 25:1298–1300, 1990.
98. Mizushima A, Sakai H, Hanzawa K, Horimoto Y: [Unexpected intraoperative respiratory distress; an infant who developed tracheomalacia and fatal aortoesophageal fistula due to unrecognized vascular ring]. Masui 44:1000–1004, 1995.
99. Momma K, Matsuoka R, Takao A: Aortic arch anomalies associated with chromosome 22q11 deletion (CATCH 22). Pediatr Cardiol 20:97–102, 1999.
100. Moore FD, Folkman J: Biographical Memoirs: Robert E. Gross. National Academy of Sciences, 2003.
101. Morel V, Corbineau H, Lecoz A, et al: Two cases of 'asthma' revealing a diverticulum of Kommerell. Respiration 69:456–460, 2002.
102. Nakahira M, Nakatani H, Takeda T: Left vocal cord paralysis associated with long-standing patent ductus arteriosus. AJNR Am J Neuroradiol 22:759–761, 2001.
103. Nezafati MH, Mahmoodi E, Hashemian SH, Hamedanchi A: Video-assisted thoracoscopic surgical (VATS) closure of patent ductus arteriosus: Report of three-hundred cases. Heart Surg Forum 5:57–59, 2002.
104. Niinikoski H, Alanen M, Parvinen T, et al: Surgical closure of patent ductus arteriosus in very-low-birth-weight infants. Pediatr Surg Int 17:338–341, 2001.
105. Odegard KC, Kirse DJ, del Nido PJ, et al: Intraoperative recurrent laryngeal nerve monitoring during video-assisted throracoscopic surgery for patent ductus arteriosus. J Cardiothorac Vasc Anesth 14:562–564, 2000.
106. Olley PM: Nonsurgical palliation of congenital heart malformations. N Engl J Med 292:1292, 1975.
107. Othersen HB Jr, Khalil B, Zellner J, et al: Aortoesophageal fistula and double aortic arch: Two important points in management. J Pediatr Surg 31:594–595, 1996.
108. Oto O, Hazan E, Acikel V, et al: Ligation of patent ductus arterious by the method of video-assisted thoracoscopic surgery and our other VATS experiences. J Cardiovasc Surg (Torino) 39:379–381, 1998.
109. Patel HT, Cao QL, Rhodes J, Hijazi ZM: Long-term outcome of transcatheter coil closure of small to large patent ductus arteriosus. Catheter Cardiovasc Interv 47:457–461, 1999.
110. Pontius R, Danielson G, Noonan J, Judson J: Illusions leading to surgical closure of the distal left pulmonary artery instead of the ductus arteriosus. J Thorac Cardiovasc Surg 82:107–113, 1981.
111. Porstmann W, Wierny L, Warnke H, et al: Catheter closure of patent ductus arteriosus, 62 cases treated without thoracotomy. Radiol Clin North Am 9:203–218, 1971.
112. Potts WJ, Holinger PH, Rosenblum AH: Anomalous left pulmonary artery causing obstruction to right main bronchus. Report of a case. JAMA 155:1409, 1954.
113. Pumberger W, Voitl P, Gopfrich H: Recurrent respiratory tract infections and dysphagia in a child with an aortic vascular ring. South Med J 95:265–268, 2002.

114. Reese J, Paria BC, Brown N, et al: Coordinated regulation of fetal and maternal prostaglandins directs successful birth and postnatal adaptation in the mouse. Proc Natl Acad Sci USA 97:9759–9764, 2000.
115. Rothman A, Tong AD: Percutaneous coil embolization of superfluous vascular connections in patients with congenital heart disease. Am Heart J 126:206–213, 1993.
116. Roughneen PT, Parikh P, Stark J: Bronchial obstruction secondary to aneurysm of a persistent ductus arteriosus. Eur J Cardiothorac Surg 10:146–147, 1996.
117. Schafer K, Neuhaus P, Kruse J, Braun T: The homeobox gene Lbx1 specifies a subpopulation of cardiac neural crest necessary for normal heart development. Circ Res 92:73–80, 2003.
118. Schlesinger AE, Mendeloff E, Sharkey AM, Spray TL: MR of right aortic arch with mirror-image branching and a left ligamentum arteriosum: An unusual cause of a vascular ring. Pediatr Radiol 25:455–457, 1995.
119. Sebening C, Jakob H, Tochtermann U, et al: Vascular tracheobronchial compression syndromes—experience in surgical treatment and literature review. Thorac Cardiovasc Surg 48:164–174, 2000.
120. Seghaye MC, Grabitz R, Alzen G, et al: Thoracic sequelae after surgical closure of the patent ductus arteriosus in premature infants. Acta Paediatr 86:213–216, 1997.
121. Selman E, Sosa H, Arango Casado JE, et al: [The atrioventricular canal and vascular ring. The surgical treatment of a rare anatomical association]. G Ital Cardiol 24:517–519, 1994.
122. Sielenkamper AW, Meyer J, Loick HM, Hachenberg T: Thoracoscopic interruption of patent ductus arteriosus compromises cardiopulmonary function in newborn pigs. Anesth Analg 87:1037–1040, 1998.
123. Skinner LJ, Ryan S, Russell JD: Complete vascular ring detected by barium esophagography. Ear Nose Throat J 81:554–555, 2002.
124. Sorenson K, Kristensen B, Hanson OK: Frequency of occurrence of residual ductal flow after surgical ligation by colorflow mapping. Am J Cardiol 67:653–654, 1991.
125. Stark J: Video-assisted thoracoscopic division of a vascular ring in an infant. J Card Surg 9:132–133, 1994.
126. Suetsugu F, Matsuo K, Yokayama S, et al: [Repair of D-transposition of the great arteries associated with double aortic arch]. Nippon Kyobu Geka Gakkai Zasshi 45:894–899, 1997.
127. Sugi K, Katoh T, Gohra H, et al: Progressive hyperthermia during thoracoscopic procedures in infants and children. Paediatr Anaesth 8:211–214, 1998.
128. Supapannachart S, Khowsathit P, Patchakapati B: Indomethacin prophylaxis for patent ductus arteriosus (PDA) in infants with a birth weight of less than 1250 grams. J Med Assoc Thai 82(suppl 1):S87–S92, 1999.
129. Tan TH, Wong KY, Heng JT: Echocardiographic features and management of neonatal ductal aneurysm. Ann Acad Med Singapore 29:783–788, 2000.
130. Tepper RS, Eigen H, Brown J, Hurwitz R: Use of maximal expiratory flows to evaluate central airways obstruction in infants. Pediatr Pulmonol 6:272–274, 1989.
131. Therrien J, Connelly MS, Webb GD: Patent ductus arteriosus. Curr Treat Options Cardiovasc Med 1:341–346, 1999.
132. Tsuboi H, Ikeda N, Minami Y, et al: A video-assisted thoracoscopic surgical technique for interruption of patent ductus arteriosus. Surg Today 27:439–442, 1997.
133. Virdi IS, Keeton BR, Shore DF, Monro JL: Surgical management in tetralogy of Fallot and vascular ring. Pediatr Cardiol 8:131–134, 1987.
134. Wagner HR, Ellison RC, Zierler S, et al: Surgical closure of patent ductus arteriosus in 268 preterm infants. J Thorac Cardiovasc Surg 87:870–875, 1984.
135. Watanabe M, Kawasaki S, Sato H, et al: Left aortic arch with right descending aorta and right ligamentum arteriosum associated with D-TGA and large VSD: Surgical treatment of a rare form of vascular ring. J Pediatr Surg 30:1363–1365, 1995.
136. Watterberg KL, Scott SM, Backstrom C, et al: Links between early adrenal function and respiratory outcome in preterm infants: Airway inflammation and patent ductus arteriosus. Pediatrics 105:320–324, 2000.
137. Weber TR, Keller MS, Fiore A: Aortic suspension (aortopexy) for severe tracheomalacia in infants and children. Am J Surg 184:573–577, 2002.
138. Westfelt JN, Nordwall A: Thoracotomy and scoliosis. Spine 16:1124–1125, 1991.
139. Xiao H, Zhong R, Lin J: [Video-assisted thoracoscopic surgical technique for interruption of patent ductus arteriosus]. Zhonghua Wai Ke Za Zhi 34:82–83, 1996.

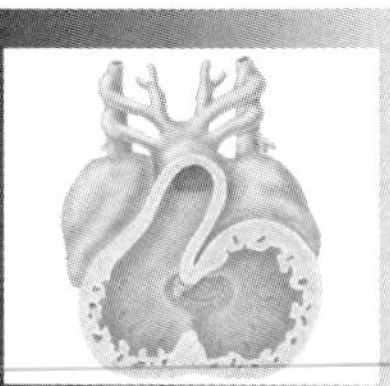

Coarctation of the Aorta, Aortopulmonary Shunts, and Aortopulmonary Collaterals

J. William Gaynor

CHAPTER 108

COARCTATION OF THE AORTA

Historical Aspects

Coarctation is derived from the Latin *coarctatio* (a drawing or pressing together). Coarctation of the aorta is defined as a narrowing that diminishes the lumen and produces an obstruction to the flow of blood. Paris first described coarctation of the aorta in 1791, although Meckel in 1750 and Morgagni in 1760 had reported finding aortic narrowing at autopsy.[73] In 1944 Crafoord performed the first surgical correction with resection of the coarctation and end-to-end anastomosis.[36] Gross independently performed a similar procedure in 1945.[60,62] Subsequently, Gross was the first to use interposition grafts (aortic homografts) to repair coarctation.[61] Repair using a prosthetic onlay graft was first performed by Vossschulte in 1957.[156] Waldhausen introduced the subclavian flap aortoplasty in 1966.[158]

Embryology and Pathological Anatomy

Coarctation may be a localized obstruction or may be associated with diffuse hypoplasia of the aortic arch. Coarctation may occur at any site within the aorta, but the most common location is at the insertion of the ductus (or ligamentum arteriosus). Externally the aorta appears to be sharply indented or constricted. Internally there is an obstructing diaphragm or shelf on the posterior wall resulting in luminal narrowing, which is usually more marked than is apparent by external appearance. The shelf consists of an infolding of the aortic media with a ridge of intimal hypoplasia and may include tissue extending from the ductus arteriosus. The aortic isthmus (the segment of aorta between the left subclavian artery and the insertion of the ductus arteriosus) is often hypoplastic. In some patients, hypoplasia of the transverse arch also is present.

The etiology of coarctation of the aorta and hypoplasia of the aortic arch remains uncertain. In the normal fetus, blood flow across the isthmus is less than flow in either the ascending or descending aorta (which receives the ductal flow), and thus the diameter of the isthmus is less than that of either the ascending or descending aorta. Adaptation of the aorta to the postnatal circulation in normal newborns is characterized by increasing diameters of the transverse arch and isthmus.[98] There are significant morphological differences between the aortas of normal patients and those with coarctation and arch hypoplasia. The hypoplastic arch is characterized by an increased number of elastin lamellae and a decrease in α-actin positive cells.[99] This decrease in α-actin positive cells may result from a decrease in smooth muscle cells or a change in phenotype, possibly resulting in decreased growth potential.

In some patients with coarctation, tissue from the ductus arteriosus (a muscular artery) extends circumferentially into the aortic wall (an elastic artery). Contraction and fibrosis of this ductal tissue at the time of ductal closure may lead to a localized narrowing. Extension of ductal tissue into the aortic wall has been shown histologically by Wielenga and Dankmeijer,[162] by Ho and Anderson,[67] and by Elzenga and Gittenberger-deGroot[47] (Figure 108-1). Russell and colleagues[131] performed pathological examination of tissue resected during coarctation repair in patients younger than 3 months of age and found a circumferential sling of ductal tissue extending from the ductus arteriosus into the aorta at the level of the coarctation shelf in 22 of 23 specimens. In 15 of the patients there were one or two tongue-like protrusions of ductal tissue that arose from the circumferential sling (opposite the ductal insertion) and extended into the descending aorta below the insertion of the ductus. Van Son[153] reported proximal extension of similar tongues of ductal tissue into the isthmus.

Other investigators have not found abnormal ductal tissue and hypothesized that coarctation results from abnormal fetal blood flow patterns.[130,143] An increased incidence of coarctation is seen with lesions that produce left ventricular outflow tract obstruction (ventricular septal defects [VSDs], aortic stenosis, mitral valve anomalies), thus diminishing antegrade aortic flow, which might lead to an abnormal narrowing of the isthmus. Coarctation is rarely associated with anomalies that decrease ductal flow and increase antegrade aortic flow (e.g., tetralogy of Fallot). Both abnormal extension of ductal tissue and hemodynamic factors likely have a role in the pathogenesis of coarctation. Increased ductal flow with decreased flow through the aortic arch may facilitate proliferation of the ductal tissue into the aorta.

There is increasing evidence that genetic factors are important in the development of coarctation and arch hypoplasia.[149] The association of coarctation with Turner's syndrome and the occurrence of familial cases provides evidence of the role of genetic factors. Coarctation may occur in 15–36% of patients with Turner's syndrome.[125] Familial inheritance is usually via autosomal dominant transmission with incomplete penetrance.[149] There is likely a significant interplay between genetic factors, abnormal blood flow patterns, and abnormal extension of ductal tissue, producing the wide spectrum of arch anatomy found in patients with coarctation.

Pseudocoarctation is a buckling or kinking of the aorta that does not produce an obstruction to flow. The chest film usually reveals an abnormal aortic contour mimicking a left superior mediastinal mass. There is no evidence of collateral circulation. Imaging studies demonstrate a tortuous kinked aorta with no measurable pressure gradient. Pseudocoarctation was thought to be a benign entity; however, aneurysmal dilatation can occur in the segment distal to the buckled area.

Incidence and Associated Anomalies

Coarctation of the aorta represents 5–10% of congenital heart disease, and the autopsy incidence is 1 in 3000–4000 autopsies. With isolated coarctation, males predominate, but there is no sex predisposition in patients with more complex lesions. Anomalies commonly found in patients with coarctation of the aorta include bicuspid aortic valve,

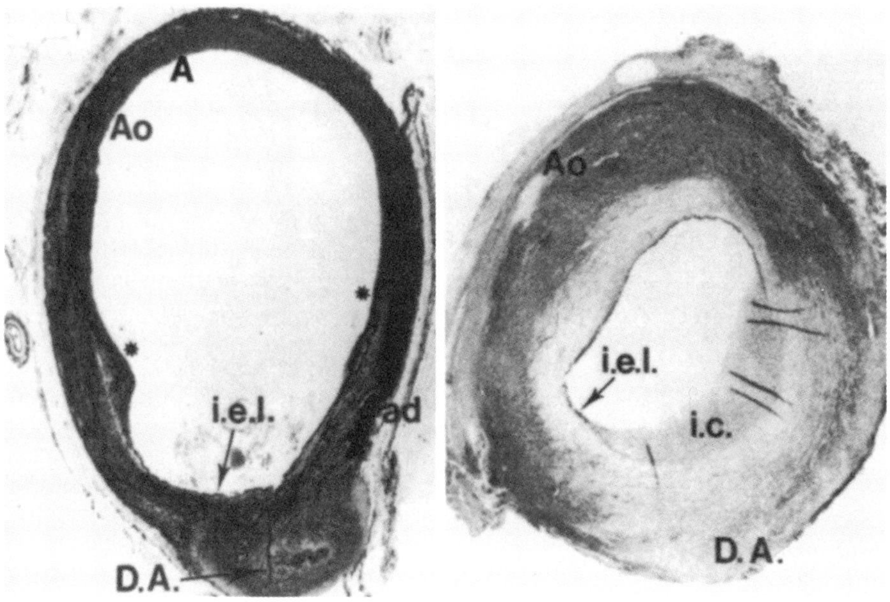

Figure 108–1 **A,** Transverse section of a normal aorta of a newborn at the level of the ductus arteriosus (DA). Ductal tissue stains lighter than aortic tissue because it is relatively poor in elastin. The inner third of the elastic lamellae of the aorta (Ao) merges onto the internal elastic lamina (iel) of the ductus, whereas the outer two thirds merges onto the adventitia (ad), resulting in a fishtail-like (*asterisk*) connection of the walls of the two vessels (more clearly visible on the right side of the figure than on the left). Ductal tissue does not extend beyond one third of the total circumference of the aorta (elastic tissue stain; original magnification × 10). **B,** Transverse section of the aorta of a young infant with preductal coarctation at the level of the ductus arteriosus. The lightly stained tissue of the ductus is clearly seen to encircle the lumen of the aorta. A small intimal cushion (ic) is present in the specimen (elastic tissue stain; original magnification × 10.).
(From Elzenga, NJ, Gittenberger-deGroot, AC: Localised coarctation of the aorta. An age dependent spectrum. Br Heart J, 49:317-323, 1983.)

VSD, patent ductus arteriosus (PDA), and various mitral valve disorders.[12] Coarctation also may occur in patients with complex forms of transposition of the great arteries and double-outlet right ventricle.[108] Patients with severe associated defects tend to have diffuse hypoplasia of the aortic arch rather than isolated coarctation. VSDs that occur with coarctation are often associated with posterior septal malalignment, compromising the left ventricular outflow tract.[107] Mitral valve anomalies with stenosis or regurgitation secondary to the abnormalities of the chordae tendineae and papillary muscles are frequently seen in patients with coarctation.[28,51,129] Shone's syndrome is a complex of parachute mitral valve, cor triatriatum, subaortic stenosis, and coarctation.[144] The left ventricle may be hypoplastic in patients with coarctation and arch hypoplasia. There is a continuous spectrum of pathological anatomy from patients with true hypoplastic left heart syndrome (HLHS) with aortic atresia and mitral atresia to those with a slightly hypoplastic but adequate left ventricle in the presence of isolated coarctation with or without arch hypoplasia. Determination of the appropriate therapeutic strategy (single ventricle versus two-ventricle reconstruction) may be difficult in patients with coarctation and a small left ventricle.

Clinical Manifestations

The age at presentation and symptoms at presentation depend on the location and severity of the coarctation, as well as the associated anomalies. Presence of a coarctation may not seriously alter the normal fetal circulation and therefore does not provide a stimulus to development of a collateral circulation in utero. Infants with severe narrowing may appear normal at birth and have palpable femoral pulses if a PDA allows blood flow past the obstructive shelf. Symptoms develop as the ductus closes, resulting in significant aortic obstruction. The infants become irritable, tachypneic, and disinterested in feeding. A systolic murmur may be present over the left precordium and posteriorly between the scapulae. Although blood pressure is difficult to record accurately in neonates, moderate upper extremity hypertension and an arm–leg systolic pressure gradient or absent femoral pulses are usually present. These findings may be absent in critically ill infants with a low cardiac output. Hypotension, oliguria, and severe metabolic acidosis are frequently present in critically ill infants, and cardiovascular collapse may occur. In some patients with severe obstruction or even complete aortic interruption, a pulmonary artery pulse may be felt in the femoral arteries when the ductus is open, obscuring the diagnosis. Differential cyanosis may be present between the upper and lower extremities. Left-to-right shunting may occur though a patent foramen ovale. Signs of a collateral circulation are not present in infants.

Older children and adults often have unexplained hypertension or complications of hypertension. Some may be asymptomatic for many years and lead an active life. Presenting complaints include headache, epistaxis, visual disturbances, and exertional dyspnea. Some patients have a cerebrovascular accident (secondary to an aneurysm of the circle of Willis), aortic rupture, dissecting aneurysm, or bacterial endocarditis.[142] Many cases are discovered during evaluation of hypertension or of a murmur heard on routine examination.

Diagnosis

Diagnosis of a coarctation of the aorta usually can be made clinically and depends on evidence of obstruction to blood flow in the thoracic aorta. The findings include hypertension, a systolic pressure gradient between the arms and legs, a systolic murmur heard over the left precordium and posteriorly between the scapulas, and diminished or absent femoral pulses with a delayed upstroke. Anomalous origin of the right subclavian artery can occur with the origin distal to the coarctation; therefore the blood pressure must be obtained in both arms as the orifice of either subclavian artery may be involved in the coarctation. Evidence of a collateral circulation may be found in older children and adults, involving branches of the subclavian arteries proximal to the obstruction (the internal mammary, vertebral, thyrocervical, and costocervical arteries) that anastomose with intercostal arteries and other arteries below the obstruction. Aneurysmal dilatation of the intercostal arteries can occur and may complicate surgical reconstruction. Poststenotic dilatation of the descending aorta is common. Rarely, an aneurysm of the ascending or descending aorta may be present.

The electrocardiogram (ECG) in infancy may show right ventricular, left ventricular, or biventricular hypertrophy. In older children and adults the ECG may be normal or show evidence of left ventricular hypertrophy, often with a strain pattern. The chest film may reveal cardiomegaly with left ventricular hypertrophy. Infants with heart failure may demonstrate extreme cardiomegaly and pulmonary congestion. Rib notching secondary to the enlarged tortuous intercostal vessels is almost pathognomonic and was first described by Meckel in 1827.[74] These are erosions that occur on the underside of the rib. The notching may be unilateral if the orifice of the left subclavian artery is narrowed by the coarctation or if there is anomalous origin of the right subclavian artery distal to the coarctation. Absence of rib notching in older patients may indicate a poor collateral circulation.

Echocardiography is the diagnostic method of choice in neonates and infants with suspected coarctation (Figure 108-2). Two-dimensional echocardiography with color-flow Doppler echocardiography is useful to show the site of the obstruction, suggest or exclude associated anomalies, and provide an estimate of the arterial pressure gradient (Figure 108-2B). In some neonates it may be difficult to confirm a diagnosis of coarctation by echocardiography with the presence of a PDA, and the ductus must be allowed to close under close evaluation to confirm the diagnosis. It is important to realize that Doppler echocardiography may not accurately estimate the magnitude of the pressure gradient either preoperatively or postoperatively. Computed tomography (CT) and magnetic resonance imaging (MRI) are useful to evaluate arch anatomy, particularly in older patients in whom echocardiographic imaging may be suboptimal. MRI provides excellent delineation of complex arch anatomy and is the imaging modality of choice in older children and adults (Figure 108-3). Cardiac catheterization is rarely used in patients with coarctation, except to evaluate associated anomalies or if transcatheter intervention is placed. Increased utilization of obstetrical ultrasound has led to an increased antenatal diagnosis of coarctation. There is

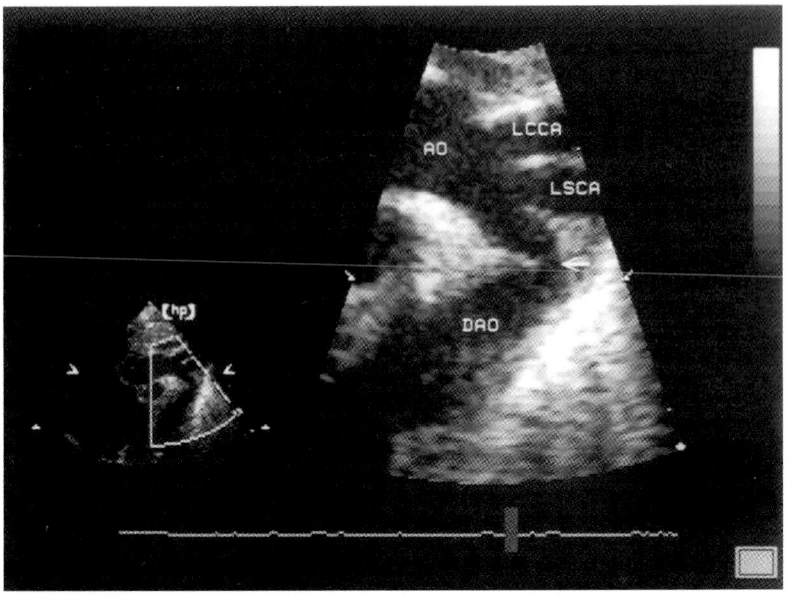

A

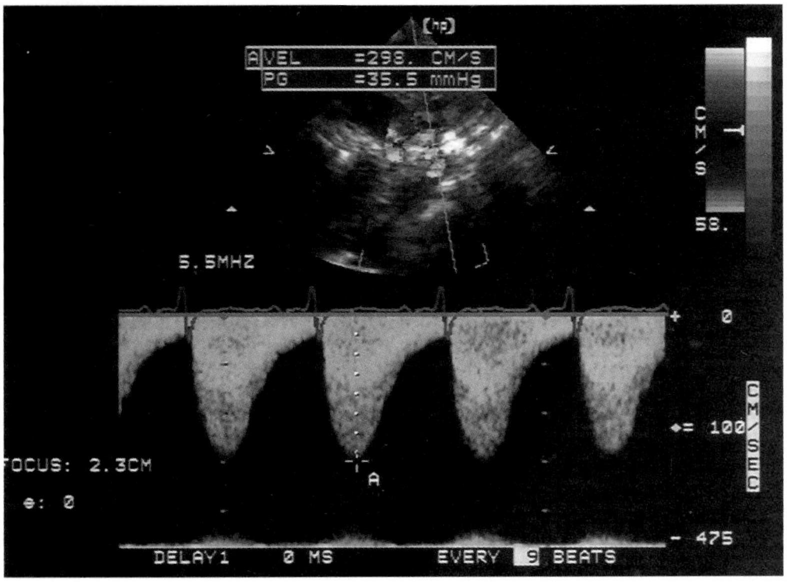

B

Figure 108–2 **A,** Two-dimensional echocardiogram demonstrating discrete juxtaductal coarctation. Arrow marks site of coarctation. Ao, Ascending aorta; LCCA, left common carotid artery; LSCA, left subclavian artery; DAO, descending aorta. **B,** Color flow Doppler echocardiogram of coarctation demonstrating turbulent flow *(upper image)* with continuous-wave Doppler demonstrating typical coarctation pattern with diastolic runoff.
(Courtesy Dr. Jack Rychik, The Children's Hospital of Philadelphia.)

evidence that antenatal diagnosis allows earlier initiation of prostaglandin therapy, resulting in a decreased risk of cardiovascular collapse secondary to ductal closure and an improved preoperative clinical condition.[23]

Natural History

The natural history of untreated coarctation of the aorta depends on the age at presentation and associated anomalies. Symptomatic infants have a high mortality, depending on the severity of the coarctation and the presence of associated defects. Patients surviving until adulthood have a greatly decreased life expectancy. In 1928, before the development of antibiotics and surgical correction of coarctation, Abbott[1] reviewed 200 cases of coarctation confirmed at autopsy in patients older than 2 years of age. Death occurred in 34% of the patients by 40 years of age, and the average age at death was 42 years. The most common causes of death were spontaneous rupture of the aorta, bacterial endocarditis, and cerebral hemorrhage. Reifenstein and colleagues[126] reported 104 cases of coarctation in 1947. The average age at death was 35 years, with 23% of the patients dying of aortic rupture, 22% of bacterial endocarditis or aortitis, 18% of congestive heart failure, and 11% of cerebrovascular accident. Rupture of the aorta or an intracranial aneurysm usually occurred in the second or third decade of life. Endocarditis was most commonly associated with a bicuspid aortic valve. Campbell[26] calculated that of patients with coarctation surviving the first 2 years of life, 25% would die by 20 years of age, 50% by 32 years of age, 75% by 46 years of age, and 90% by 58 years of age. However, the presence of a coarctation does not exclude prolonged survival because one patient is known to have lived to the age of 92. The coronary arteries in patients with untreated coarctation

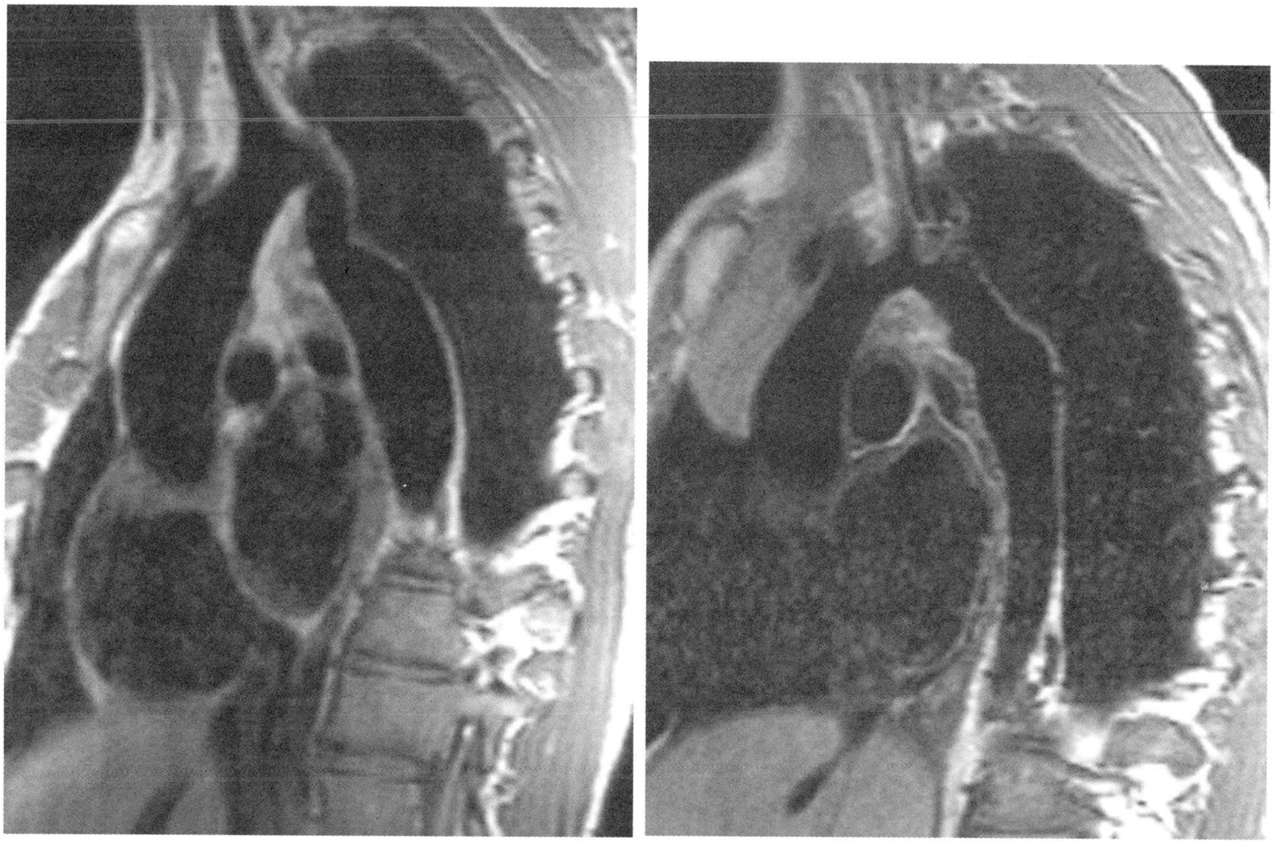

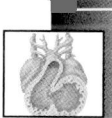

Figure 108–3 **Magnetic resonance images of coarctation. A,** Parasagittal section of native coarctation. **B,** Parasagittal section showing postoperative coarctation with arch hypoplasia and mild aneurysmal dilatation at the site of repair. *(Courtesy Dr. Mark Fogel, The Children's Hospital of Philadelphia.)*

show striking changes such as intimal degeneration, medial thickening, and an increase in mineralization. These changes can be demonstrated even in young children and may predispose patients to early atherosclerosis. The advent of surgical therapy has significantly increased the life expectancy of patients with coarctation, although they do not become fully normal.

Hypertension

The pathogenesis of hypertension in coarctation is multifactorial. The most prominent causes appear to be mechanical obstruction and renal factors, although recent investigations suggest that abnormal endothelial function in the upper body also may be important. Scott and Bahnson[139] were the first to definitively demonstrate the role of the kidneys in the pathogenesis of the hypertension of coarctation and experimental coarctation. In experimental coarctation, hypertension could be eliminated by transplanting one kidney to the neck (proximal to the obstruction) with contralateral nephrectomy. Renal blood flow is usually normal in patients with coarctation, and studies of the renin–angiotensin system have yielded conflicting results. Renin and angiotensin levels have been reported to be normal both in experimental animals and patients with coarctation. However, Bagby and co-workers,[7,8] using a canine model of coarctation, were able to show greater than expected elevation of plasma renin activity during sodium restriction. During low, normal, and high sodium intake, plasma volume, extracellular volume, and plasma renin activity were higher in animals with coarctation than in control animals. Alpert and colleagues[4] showed significant increases in plasma renin activity during volume depletion in coarctation patients compared with normal controls. These findings suggest that the hypertension of coarctation is similar to a one-kidney one-clip Goldblatt model of hypertension. Plasma renin activity is initially elevated, leading to an increase in plasma volume, which restores renal perfusion to normal levels. The stimulus for increased renin secretion is diminished, and plasma renin activity returns to normal levels, with the hypertension maintained by volume expansion.[114] Angiotensin blockade has not been consistently useful in treating the hypertension of coarctation. Ferguson and co-workers,[48] using a model of coarctation similar to Scott and Bahnson, showed that animals with coarctation developed generalized hypertension, but when a graft was used to reestablish renal blood flow, hypertension developed only proximal to the stenosis. Other investigators have shown abnormal stiffness of the prestenotic aortic wall[141] and abnormal baroreceptor function.[13] Gardiner and co-workers[53] demonstrated abnormal endothelial-mediated vasodilatation in normotensive adults after coarctation repair, suggesting that abnormal endothelial function may be a factor in the pathogenesis of hypertension. de Divitiis and colleagues recently evaluated endothelial function of conduit arteries in the upper and lower limbs of patients after successful coarctation repair.[40] Flow-mediated vasodilation and dilatation after sublingual nitroglycerin were evaluated using ultrasound of the brachial and posterior tibial arteries. In addition to endothelial function, arterial stiffness was determined by pulse wave velocity in the upper extremities (between the brachial and radial artery), as well as in the lower extremities (between the femoral and dorsalis pedis arteries). Despite successful repair of aortic coarctation, there was persistent abnormal conduit artery function with abnormal vasodilation in response to both flow and nitroglycerin in the upper body. Increased arterial stiffness also was present in the upper body (proximal to the coarctation). Endothelial function and arterial stiffness in the leg (distal to the coarctation) were preserved. Interestingly, repair at an early age (in the first 4 months of life) resulted in normal arterial stiffness in the upper extremities. However; impaired endothelial function of the brachial arteries, manifested by both reduced flow-mediated dilatation and dilatation after sublingual nitroglycerin, persisted. The authors interpreted this pattern of persistent abnormalities in the conduit arteries of the upper extremities as being consistent with the hypothesis that aortic coarctation is associated with arterial dysfunction as a result of the abnormal hemodynamics in the upper body before surgical repair.[40]

Management

Medical therapy has only a small role in patients with coarctation. Presence of coarctation generally is sufficient indication for intervention. The major questions are the timing and method of repair. Symptomatic infants usually require intervention, although a few improve with conservative medical treatment of congestive heart failure and can then undergo elective surgical correction. A major advance in the treatment of critically ill neonates with coarctation and interrupted aortic arch has been the introduction of prostaglandin-E_1 therapy.[96] Infusion of prostaglandin-E_1 can reopen and maintain patency of the ductus arteriosus in many neonates, allowing perfusion in the lower body with correction of the severe metabolic acidosis and oliguria that are often present.[66] Stabilization of these severely ill infants allows surgical correction to be accomplished in more optimal conditions with decreased mortality.

The timing of elective repair of the coarctation of the aorta is perhaps the most important determinant of long-term outcome. Repair in late childhood or adulthood, although providing relief of some symptoms, has an increased incidence of persistent hypertension, with its associated morbidity. The current trend is for elective repair at an early age, and some authors believe that repair should be undertaken at the time of diagnosis in symptomatic and asymptomatic infants to prevent the development of complications. In recent years percutaneous transluminal balloon angioplasty has been introduced as an alternative therapy for coarctation. The long-term results of balloon angioplasty for a native coarctation of the aorta in terms of recoarctation are unknown.

Surgical Correction

The classic method of repair of coarctation developed by Crafoord and by Gross is resection of the area of obstruction with a primary end-to-end anastomosis. Because of early unsatisfactory results in terms of recoarctation, particularly in infants, other techniques were developed. In 1957 Vossschulte[156] introduced the prosthetic patch onlay graft technique using a prosthetic patch to enlarge the area of constriction. Subclavian flap aortoplasty was introduced by Waldhausen and Nahrwold in 1966.[158] In this repair a flap of the left subclavian artery is turned down onto the aorta to enlarge the area of constriction.[64,158,159] More extensive forms of the classic repair have been developed in recent years. Amato and associates[5] proposed anastomosis of the distal aorta to the inferior aspect of the arch with anastomosis of the contiguous walls of the left carotid and subclavian arteries, if necessary, to alleviate the obstruction. Lansman and colleagues[91] proposed an extended resection with primary anastomosis. The coarcted segment is excised and the anastomosis enlarged by an incision proximally on the inferior aspect of the arch. A more extensive procedure has been described by Elliott[46] in which the arch is completely dissected, the descending aorta is mobilized to the diaphragm, an incision is made on the inferior aspect of the arch as proximal as possible, the descending aorta is spatulated posteriorly, and the anastomosis is completed.

Methods of Repair

Resection and End-to-End Anastomosis

After induction of anesthesia, an arterial line is inserted in the right radial artery. The patient is positioned in the right lateral decubitus position, and a left posterolateral thoracotomy is performed. The lung is retracted inferiorly and anteriorly, and the pleura overlying the descending aorta is incised. The proximal aorta and left subclavian artery, area of coarctation, and ligamentum (or ductus arteriosum) are carefully dissected, avoiding damage to the recurrent laryngeal nerve (Figure 108-4). Care is taken not to injure any enlarged intercostal arteries during the dissection. Division of these arteries occasionally may be necessary, especially if aneurysm dilatation has occurred, but it is preferable to preserve all collaterals. For an optimal result to be obtained with this technique, it is necessary to resect the entire coarct segment and construct the anastomosis without tension. The extent of the dissection necessary depends on the extent of the resection planned. If an extended resection and anastomosis to the inferior aspect of the arch are planned, it is necessary to completely dissect and mobilize the aortic arch to the innominate artery (Figure 108-5). The descending aorta must be fully mobilized in order to construct an anastomosis without tension. After the dissection is completed, heparin is administered, although in neonates, some prefer to avoid heparin. The aorta is clamped proximally and distally. If an extended resection is planned, it may be necessary to place the proximal clamp so that the left carotid is occluded and the clamp extends onto the ascending aorta and innominate artery; care must be taken to ensure adequate flow into the innominate artery and right carotid artery. The ductus is ligated and divided, and the

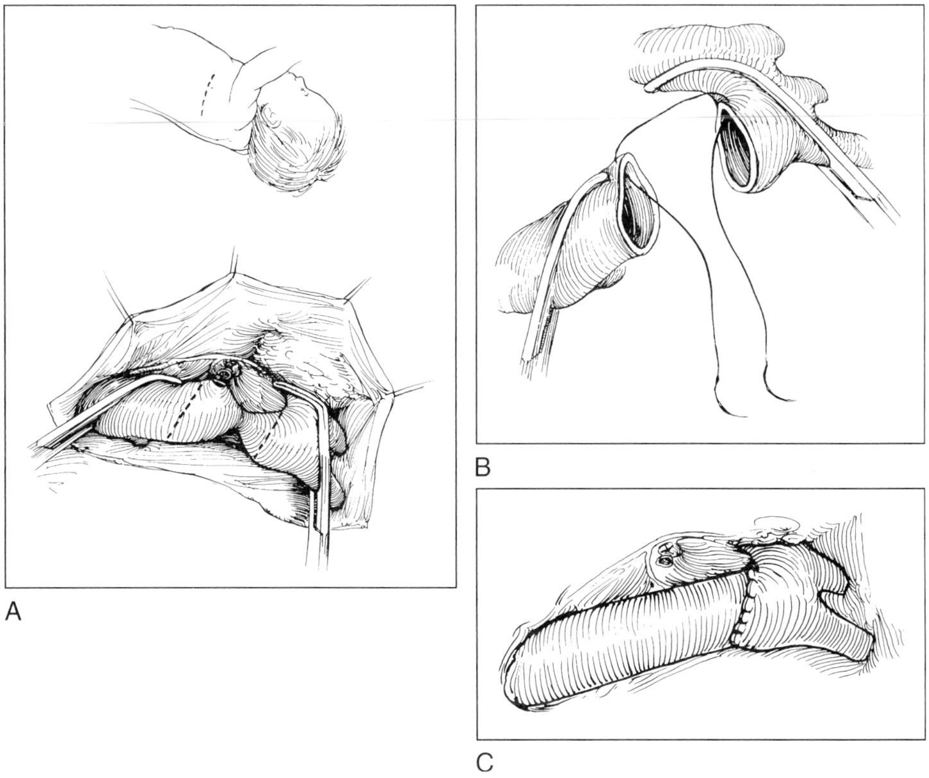

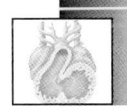

Figure 108–4 End-to-end resection and anastomosis are easily accomplished through a left thoracotomy. **A,** The proximal ductus arteriosus is securely tied. Vascular clamps control the aortic arch and the descending aorta. When present, collateral vessels can be controlled with hemoclips. The area of coarctation is excised and removed. **B,** The two ends of the aorta are then anastomosed using a continuous suture technique. **C,** This provides a normal appearance to the reconstructed aorta, and in most patients there is little difficulty in mobilizing the aorta to be reconstructed in this manner.
(From Ungerleider RM: Coarctation of the aorta. In Kaiser RL, Kron IL, Spray TL, editors: Mastery of Cardiothoracic Surgery. Philadelphia: Lippincott-Raven, 1998.)

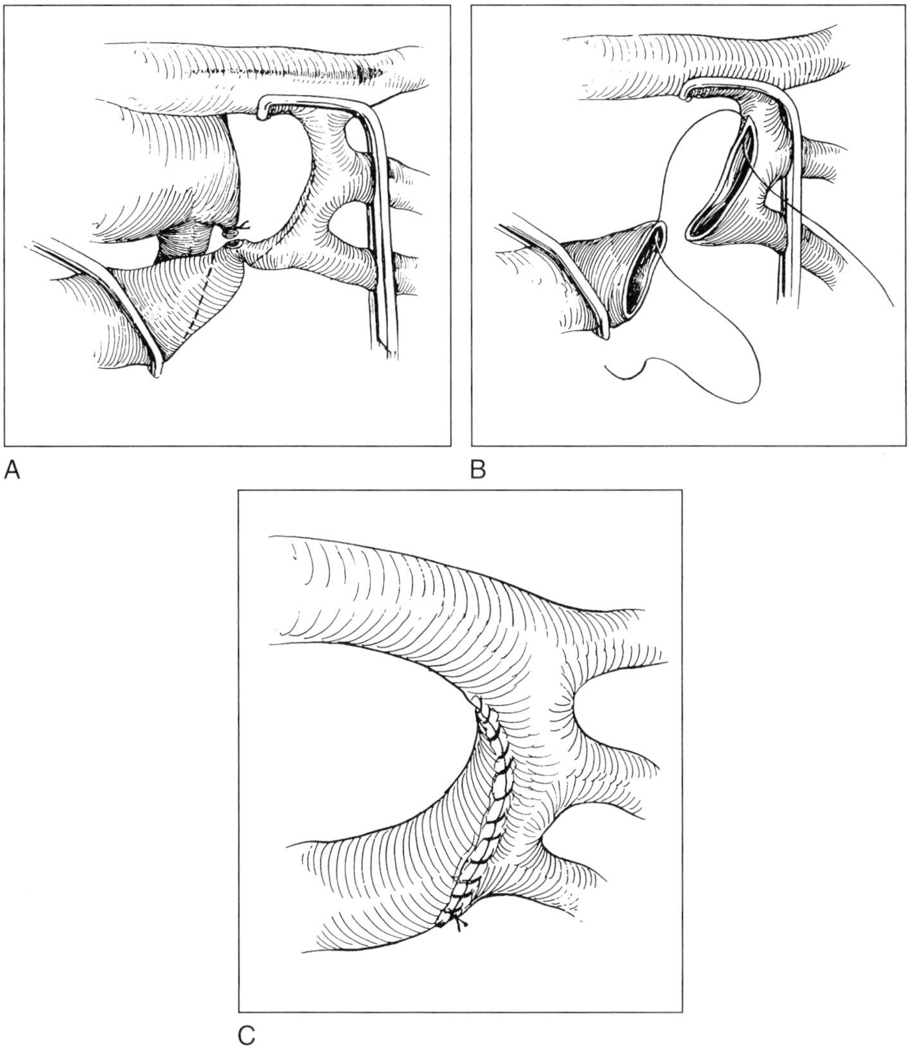

Figure 108–5 An extended end-to-end resection can also be performed through a left thoracotomy. **A,** It is necessary to place the proximal clamp across the left subclavian and left common carotid artery. The clamp should extend onto the ascending aorta and occlude part of the innominate artery so that the proximal incision on the underside of the aorta can extend proximally as far as the origin of the left common carotid (or farther, if necessary). The ductus arteriosus is ligated, and a distal clamp is placed on the descending aorta. It is important to mobilize the descending aorta as distally as possible, and hemoclips can be used to control collateral vessels. These hemoclips can be removed at the completion of the procedure. **B,** The incision on the underside of the aortic arch is carried as proximally as necessary. The incision on the descending aorta is enlarged so that it matches the size of the proximal incision. **C,** The two ends of the aorta are then anastomosed using a continuous suture, and this provides augmentation of a hypoplastic arch.
(From Ungerleider RM: Coarctation of the aorta. In Kaiser RL, Kron IL, Spray TL, editors: Mastery of Cardiothoracic Surgery. Philadelphia: Lippincott-Raven, 1998.)

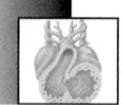

coarct segment is completely excised. Complete excision of all tissue that appears to be ductal in origin is very important. Care should be taken to preserve as much of the lateral isthmus as possible. The undersized aortic arch is incised to a point proximal to the area of hypoplasia, and the incision can be continued to the medial aspect of the ascending aorta if necessary. An incision is then made on the posterolateral aspect of the descending aorta. This incision is important because it divides any constricting ring of ductal tissue that may be present. The anastomosis is performed using a continuous polypropylene suture, and the aortic clamps are removed. After completion of the repair, the pressure should be measured in the descending aorta and compared with the right arm pressure to determine if there is any residual obstruction. Advantages of this technique of repair include complete relief of left ventricular obstruction, wide resection of ductal tissue, absence of prosthetic material, and preservation of the left subclavian artery.

Subclavian Flap Aortoplasty

Subclavian flap aortoplasty is performed through a left thoracotomy (Figure 108-6). The initial dissection and exposure is similar to that for resection and anastomosis, although less dissection is required. The left subclavian artery is fully mobilized and ligated at its first branch. The vertebral artery should be ligated to prevent a subclavian steal phenomenon. However, it is important to preserve the more distal branches to preserve an adequate collateral circulation to the left atrium. A longitudinal incision is made through the region of the coarctation and continued on to the subclavian artery, creating a flap. The posterior obstructing shelf is resected, and the flap of the subclavian artery is turned down to enlarge the area of constriction. The flap must be of sufficient length to bridge the obstruction. Advantages of this technique include avoidance of prosthetic material, decreased dissection, decreased aortic cross-clamp period, and a possible increase in anastomotic growth because there is no circumferential suture line. If the area of narrowing occurs proximal to the left subclavian artery, the flap may be directed proximally and a reversed subclavian flap aortoplasty done to enlarge the aortic arch.

Prosthetic Patch Onlay Graft

A left thoracotomy is performed. The area of constriction is incised longitudinally; however, the obstructing shelf is not excised (previous reports suggest an increased risk of aneurysm if the shelf is resected) and a prosthetic patch used to enlarge the lumen (Figure 108-7). Yee and associates[165] reported the use of Gore-Tex patches and emphasized the advantages of the technique, including decreased operative time, decreased dissection, maximal augmentation of the area of stenosis preservation of collateral vessels, and no need for sacrifice of normal vascular structures. However, there have been increasingly frequent reports of the formation of aneurysms and pseudoaneurysms[3,15,106] after prosthetic patch repairs of coarctation.

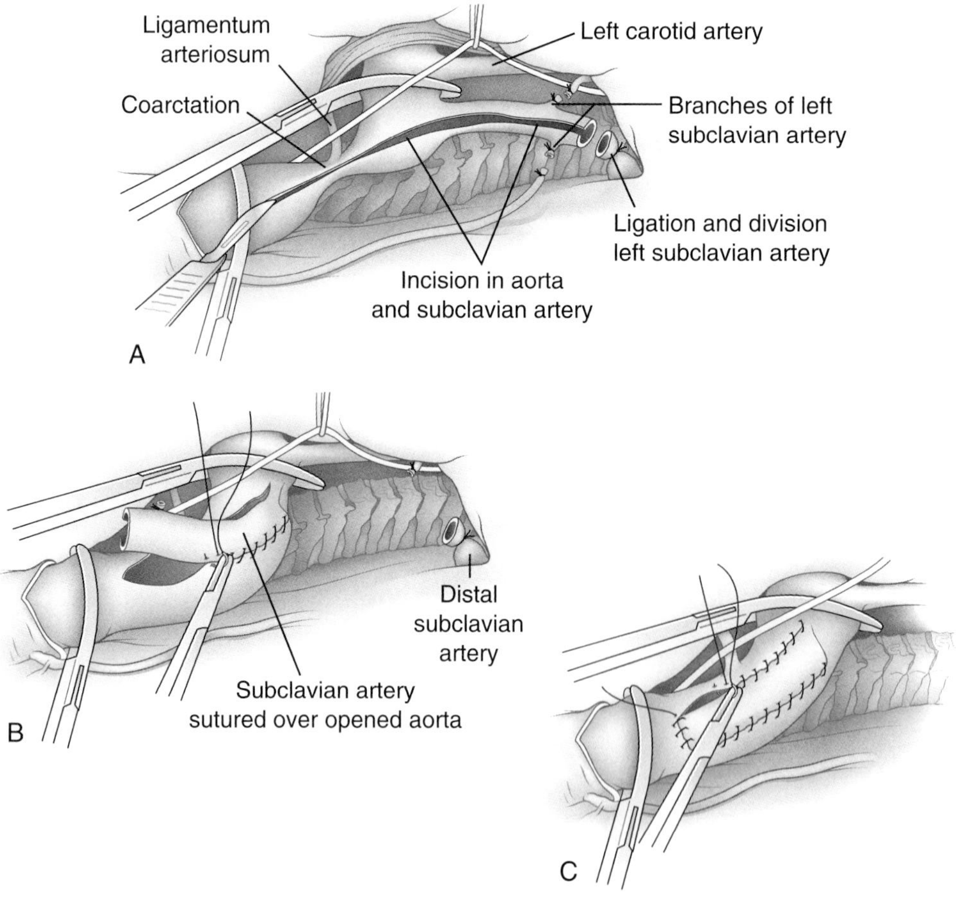

Figure 108–6 Subclavian flap aortoplasty. A, Through a left posterolateral thoracotomy, the proximal and distal aorta is mobilized and the aorta is cross-clamped between the left subclavian artery and the left carotid artery. The aorta is also clamped distally. The subclavian artery is divided, and the longitudinal incision is made through the entire length of the subclavian artery and the coarctation segment. **B,** The subclavian artery is rolled down over the coarctation to enlarge the segment. **C,** The suture line is completed. Care must be taken to ensure that the length of the subclavian artery is adequate to cover the entire coarctation segment. *(Modified from Elbert PA: Atlas of Congenital Cardiac Surgery. New York: Churchill Livingstone, 1989.)*

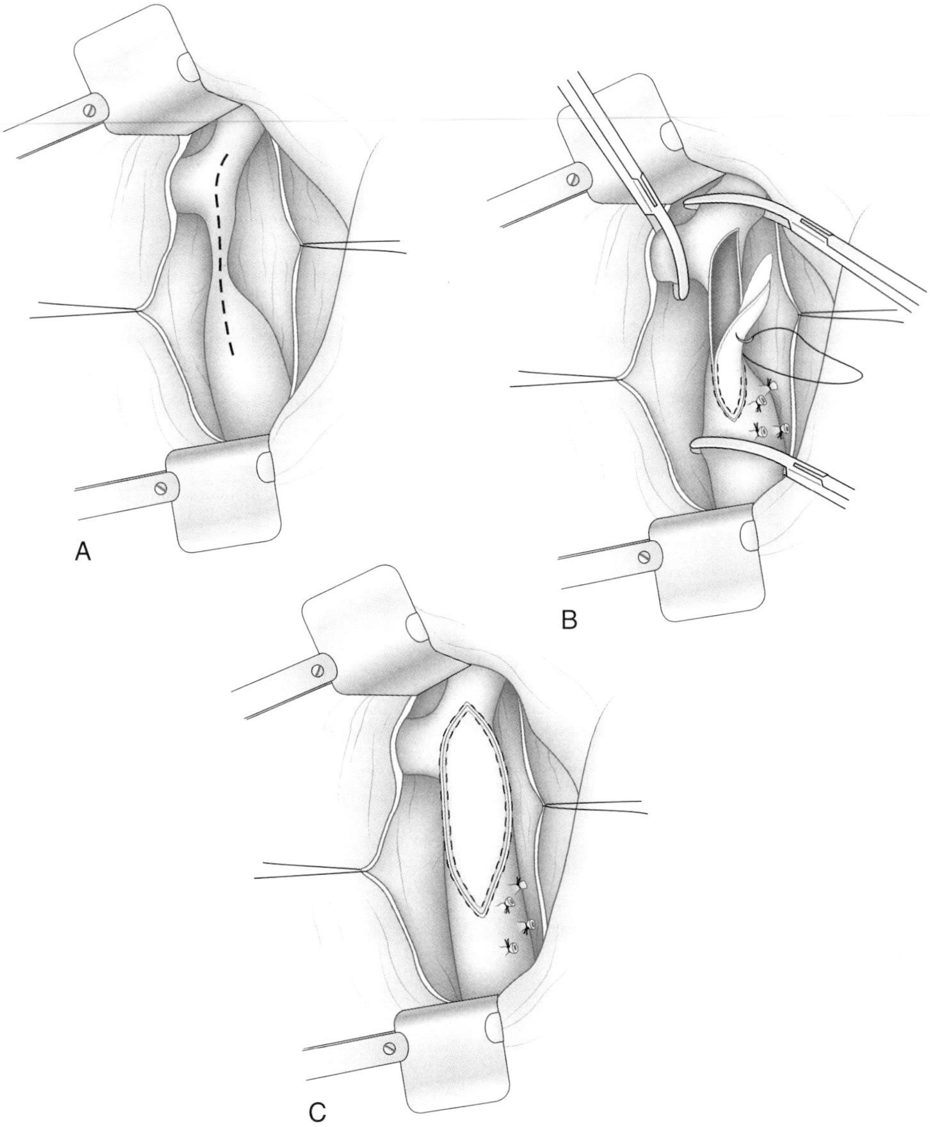

Figure 108–7 Operative technique for repair of the aorta with a synthetic patch aortoplasty. **A,** Operative view showing the line of incision across coarctation. **B,** Placement of patch to enlarge area of constriction. **C,** Completed repair. *(Modified from Vossschulte K: Surgical correction of coarctation of the aorta by an "isthmusplastic" operation. Thorax 16:338–345, 1961.)*

Interposition Grafts

In some older patients with tubular hypoplasia and inelastic aortas it may not be possible to resect the narrow segment completely and restore aortic continuity by primary anastomosis. Gross[61] pioneered the use of aortic homografts as an interposition graft in these patients and reported follow-up of 70 patients who had undergone homograft insertion.[137] No complications other than calcification of the graft (which was present in less than 50% of the patients) were reported. There were no cases of aneurysm formation. Prosthetic interposition grafts are rarely indicated, but may be useful in patients with complex coarctation, recurrent coarctation, or aneurysm formation.

Alternative Repairs

Numerous alternative procedures have been proposed for correction of coarctation. The Blalock–Park anastomosis involves division of the left subclavian artery with anastomosis to the descending aorta to bypass the obstruction.[17] Several modifications of the subclavian flap aortoplasty have been developed, including subclavian artery reimplantation, end-to-end anastomosis with use of a subclavian flap to enlarge the anastomosis, and end-to-end anastomosis with reimplantation of the subclavian artery. Ascending aorta to descending aorta bypass grafts also have been used and may be useful at the time of reoperation.

Management of Aortic Arch Hypoplasia

Hypoplasia of the aortic arch is frequently present in patients with coarctation of the aorta. This may involve only the aortic isthmus or may involve the more proximal transverse arch. Patients with proximal arch hypoplasia frequently have associated cardiac defects, including VSD. However, in some children arch hypoplasia and coarctation may occur in absence of associated intracardiac defects.

A variety of criteria have been used to define arch hypoplasia. Some authors have suggested that the ratio of transverse arch to ascending aorta diameters may be used as a measure of the severity of transverse arch hypoplasia.

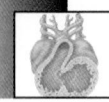

A greater than 50% reduction of the diameter of the transverse arch compared with the ascending aorta would represent significant hypoplasia. Mee and colleagues[79] suggested that the aortic arch is hypoplastic if the transverse arch diameter is less than the patient's body weight in kilograms plus 1. Other authors have used Z scores for the diameter of the transverse arch and consider the aortic arch to be hypoplastic if the Z score is −2 or less. Regardless of the exact criteria used for the definition of arch hypoplasia, infants with a hypoplastic aortic arch are often unsuitable candidates for coarctation repair alone.

A variety of techniques have been used to address arch hypoplasia in infants with coarctation. The applicability of a technique depends on the exact anatomy and the extent of the hypoplasia. In patients with distal arch hypoplasia (distal to the left common carotid artery), the repair can commonly be performed via a left thoracotomy. Some authors have suggested that arch hypoplasia can be adequately addressed using an extended resection and end-to-end anastomosis carried proximal to the left carotid artery.[152] A few authors have suggested that arch hypoplasia does not need to be addressed at the time of coarctation repair and that increased flow secondary to relief of the distal obstruction results in increased growth of a hypoplastic transverse arch.[22,72,110]

Kanter and colleagues[77] have used a repair incorporating reverse subclavian aortoplasty to enlarge the hypoplastic distal transverse arch with subsequent resection and end-to-end anastomosis repair of the coarctation. This procedure is performed through a left thoracotomy. After extensive mobilization of the arch, a clamp is placed across the arch proximal to the left carotid artery. The aortic isthmus is snared to allow perfusion of the distal body via the ductus arteriosus. The subclavian artery is ligated and divided distally. The vertebrae artery should be ligated with preservations of the distal branches. An incision is made on the medial aspect of the left subclavian artery, carried along the superior aspect of the hypoplastic distal arch, and continued onto the lateral aspect of the proximal left carotid artery. The left subclavian artery is turned down as a flap to enlarge the hypoplastic arch. After this procedure, a clamp is placed on the distal aorta and the ductus is ligated and divided. The coarct segment is excised, and an end-to-end anastomosis is performed between the enlarged distal arch and the descending aorta.

An alternative technique for management of arch hypoplasia repair through a left thoracotomy is end-to-side aortic anastomosis of the descending aorta to the proximal aortic arch.[123] In this technique the coarct segment is excised, the isthmus is ligated, and the descending aorta is anastomosed in an end-to-side fashion to the undersurface of the proximal arch. This proximal end-to-side anastomosis avoids incorporation of the distal arch in the repair, thus excluding all ductal tissue. In addition, the undersurface of the proximal arch is opened with the lengthwise incision, enlarging the anastomosis to the descending aorta. This technique can also be used in infants with coarctation without arch hypoplasia.

Arch repair in patients with extensive arch hypoplasia can be difficult via a left thoracotomy. Presence of a "bovine" aorta with common origin of the innominate and left carotid arteries may complicate proximal clamp placement, preventing adequate relief of proximal arch obstruction. Some authors have suggested that arch augmentation via a median sternotomy is a more appropriate technique. Ungerleider and Ebert[151] demonstrated the applicability of patch aortoplasty via a median sternotomy in selected infants requiring simultaneous correction of coarctation and intracardiac defects. Homograft patch enlargement and resection with end-to-end anastomosis also can be performed via a median sternotomy. Cardiopulmonary bypass with deep hypothermic circulatory arrest (DHCA) is usually used when arch augmentation is performed via a median sternotomy. Elgamal and colleagues[45] reported use of a technique similar to end-to-side anastomosis, which they termed aortic arch advancement, which they performed via a median sternotomy under DCHA. In recent years, however, there has been increasing interest in the use of regional cerebral perfusion during arch repair to avoid the need for DHCA.[117]

Management of Associated Anomalies

The optimal management of infants with associated anomalies is still controversial. A PDA is frequently present and should be divided and ligated. A bicuspid aortic valve may be present, but often requires no intervention at the time of correction of the coarctation. Occasionally coarctation occurs with complex intracardiac defects, including transposition of the great arteries with VSD and the Taussig–Bing anomaly.[107,134,154] Single-stage repair, including coarctation repair, is usually preferred for infants with complex defects.

VSD is one of the most common associated anomalies found in patients with aortic coarctation. There is considerable variation in the morphology of the aortic arch, with hypoplasia of the proximal arch often present. Additional levels of left ventricular outflow tract obstruction are often present secondary to valvar aortic stenosis or subaortic stenosis from a posterior malalignment VSD. A variety of therapeutic strategies have been used, including coarctation repair alone with later VSD closure, coarctation repair with pulmonary artery banding followed by delayed VSD closure and debanding, and single-stage repair of both defects.[54,94] Most reports have contained relatively small numbers of patients and focused on the short-term outcome of the specific strategy in terms of operative mortality and early recoarctation. Advocates of coarctation repair alone note that many VSDs close spontaneously and thus a second operation is avoided. However, many infants with moderate or large VSDs have persistent congestive heart failure after isolated coarctation repair and may remain ventilator dependent. Coarctation repair in conjunction with pulmonary artery banding provides control of pulmonary blood flow, but requires results in a second operation for removal of the pulmonary artery band, even if the VSD closes spontaneously. Advantages of single-stage repair include restoration of normal physiology and avoidance of a second operation in many children.[54,55]

A recently reported alternative approach is coarctation repair with placement of an absorbable pulmonary artery band.[19] Coarctation repair is performed via a left thoracotomy with placement of an absorbable pulmonary band. The band material is absorbed over a several-month period, thus limiting pulmonary artery blood flow during spontaneous closure of the VSD while avoiding an obligate second operation.

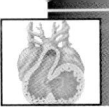

Complications of Coarctation Repair

Correction of coarctation may be complicated by hemorrhage, chylothorax, recurrent nerve paralysis, infection, and suture line thrombosis. It has been suggested that patients with Turner's syndrome may have an increased risk for hemorrhage because of friable tissues.[20,125] Several unique problems may develop in the postoperative period. Paradoxical elevation of the blood pressure to greater than preoperative levels may occur. This is a two-phase phenomenon characterized by a rise of a systolic blood pressure during the first 24–36 hours after operation and a later increase in the diastolic pressure. The first phase is characterized by activation of the sympathetic nervous system with elevation of serum catecholamines.[14] The late phase is characterized by elevation of plasma renin and angiotensin levels.[50] Postoperative elevation of blood pressure has not been described in children undergoing thoracotomy for repair of other cardiac lesions. Paradoxical hypertension may be associated with the postcoarctectomy syndrome of abdominal pain and distension first described by Sealy in 1953.[140] Up to 20% of patients undergoing repair of coarctation of the aorta experience abdominal pain and distension postoperatively. Laparotomy occasionally is indicated and may reveal evidence of mesenteric ischemia, and bowel resection may be necessary in some cases.[44] Arteriography shows changes in mesenteric vessels, and pathological examination reveals necrotizing mesenteric arteritis.[80] The syndrome is possibly related to elevated renin levels. Aggressive therapy of hypertension appears to prevent the full manifestation of the postcoarctectomy syndrome. Many drugs have been successfully used to control postoperative hypertension, and the use of vasodilators such as sodium nitroprusside with beta blockade has been useful.[163] Interestingly, a small series suggests that paradoxical hypertension may not occur after balloon angioplasty of the constructing lesion.[29] This may be related to less effective relief of the stenosis or lack of surgical manipulation of the aorta and periaortic neural fibers.

The most dreaded complication of coarctation repair is paraplegia, which occurs in 0.1–1% of patients. Poor collaterals, anomalous origin of the right subclavian artery, distal hypertension during the period of aortic cross-clamping, reoperation, or hyperthermia may predispose to paraplegia during the procedure. Brewer and colleagues[21] reviewed 66 cases of paraplegia after 12,532 procedures for repair of coarctation, an incidence of 0.41%. In this study neither sacrifice of intercostals nor duration of aortic cross-clamping could be related to the occurrence of paraplegia. Brewer emphasized the marked variation in spinal cord blood supply and suggested that measurement of distal pressure after cross-clamping of the aorta be done to assess the adequacy of the collateral circulation. A survey of surgeons in the United Kingdom and Ireland revealed that paraplegia occurred in 16 patients out of 5492 operations (an incidence of 0.3%).[81]

The exact indications for use of bypass during coarctation repair have not been defined. Hughes and Reemtsma,[68] based on results in two patients, suggested monitoring distal perfusion pressure with use of bypass if the pressure fell below 60 mm Hg. Others have recommended monitoring of the cerebrospinal fluid (CSF) pressure with the use of bypass and drainage of spinal fluid, if necessary, to maintain an adequate perfusion pressure of the spinal cord. The use of somatosensory evolved potentials (SEPs) to assess the adequacy of spinal cord perfusion has been extensively investigated.[89,92,93,119] Loss of SEP is a sensitive indicator of spinal cord ischemia. Maintenance of the distal aortic pressure above 60 mm Hg during aortic cross-clamping correlated with preservation of SEPs. Distal hypotension with the loss of SEPs for more than 30 minutes was associated with a greater than 70% incidence of paraplegia.[37] Wada and colleagues[157] evaluated 82 patients aged 17–81 years undergoing thoracic aorta surgery, including coarctation repair. They monitored SEP, distal aortic pressure, and CSF pressure. Ischemic changes of SEP occurred in 17 patients and resolved by increasing spinal cord perfusion pressure to greater than 40 mm Hg. Paraplegia developed in two patients who had complete loss of SEP.

In older children, adolescents, and adults undergoing coarctation repair, use of either left atrial to descending aorta (or femoral artery) bypass or femoral–femoral bypass with hypothermia should be considered. Use of bypass or shunts also should be considered in patients undergoing operations for recurrent coarctation.

Transcatheter Therapy

In recent years percutaneous transluminal balloon angioplasty has been introduced as an alternative therapy for coarctation. Initial results were encouraging; however, reports soon appeared of aneurysmal dilatation after balloon angioplasty of previously unoperated coarctations. Dilatation of recurrent stenosis had been more successful, and there had been fewer reports of aneurysm formation, presumably secondary to surrounding scar tissue. Morrow and co-workers[109] reported successful angioplasty in 31 of 33 patients with native coarctation. Follow-up angiography in 10 patients showed no restenosis. However, aneurysmal dilatation was present in two patients. Rao and Chopra[124] reported balloon angioplasty of native coarctation in 20 neonates and infants under the age of 1. The peak systolic gradient was reduced from 40 mm Hg to 11 mm Hg, and no patient required immediate surgical intervention. The residual gradient at a mean follow-up period of 12 months was 18 ± 15 mm Hg. No patient developed an aneurysm. Recoarctation developed in five infants and was successfully treated by surgical resection in two infants and by repeat angioplasty in three. Cystic medial necrosis has been described as a consistent histological finding in patients with coarctation, suggesting that balloon-induced tears into an abnormal media may provide the substrate for aneurysm formation.[69,97] The long-term results of balloon angioplasty for native coarctation in terms of recoarctation, and especially aneurysm formation, are unknown. Rupture of the aorta has been reported during balloon dilation of coarctation.[10] The indications for balloon angioplasty for native coarctation are uncertain, and many centers still use surgical therapy as the primary therapy. The results of angioplasty of postoperative recoarctation appear to be good, and angioplasty may be associated with less mortality and morbidity than reoperation. However, long-term follow-up is necessary.[136]

Because of concern over recoarctation after balloon dilatation, there has been increased interest in the use of endovascular shunts for both native and postoperative coarctation (Figure 108-8). Marshall and associates[102] reported early results of stent implantation in 33 children and young adults. There was an immediate decrease in the systolic pressure gradient, which persisted at short-term follow-up. Hamdan and co-workers[63] evaluated 34 patients with native and recurrent coarctation who underwent stent implantation. There was a successful outcome in 32 patients, with increase in aorta diameter and a decreased pressure gradient. Potential complications include aorta rupture, stent migration, balloon rupture, stent embolization, and vascular complications. The long-term results of endovascular stents in terms of recoarctation, relief of hypertension, and need for reintervention are not known.

Results

The results of surgical correction depend on the anatomy of the defect, including the presence or absence of hypoplasia of the aortic arch, the age at repair, the type of repair used, and the presence of associated anomalies. Operative mortality in neonates with isolated coarctation has decreased to less than 5% and is lower in older children.

Any comparison of techniques for repair of coarctation must consider the historical time frame.[64,87,167] Advances in the care of critically ill infants, including the introduction of neonatal intensive care units and the use of prostaglandin infusions, have provided dramatic improvements in the preoperative condition of the patients with coarctation, and these changes may affect mortality as much as the choice of repair. Some authors have suggested that introduction of prostaglandin therapy has altered the anatomical spectrum of coarctation in patients presenting for surgical therapy. These authors hypothesize that patients with severe arch hypoplasia who died from arch obstruction and low cardiac output before the prostaglandin era are now successfully resuscitated and undergo surgical therapy.[47] Advances in suture materials and vascular surgical technique also make it difficult to compare results from different time periods. Circumferential arterial suture lines have been effectively used in the arterial switch operation for transposition of the great vessels and other congenital cardiac anomalies and therefore should be successful in coarctation repair. Because a prospective randomized trial of the various repair techniques has not been done, long-term results with different techniques cannot be accurately compared.

Recent series of resection and primary anastomosis have shown excellent results, even in neonates. Lacour-Gayet and colleagues[90] reported results in 66 consecutive neonates treated with extended resection and anastomosis with reconstruction of the aortic arch. The overall early mortality rate was 14%, and freedom from reoperation was 89.5% at 5 years. Van Heurn and associates,[152] from the Hospital for Sick Children in London, reported 151 infants younger than the age of 3 months who underwent repair of coarctation between 1985 and 1990. More than 50% of these children had hypoplasia of a portion of the aortic arch. Subclavian flap angioplasty was used in 15 patients, resection with a traditional end-to-end anastomosis was used in 43, and an extended end-to-end anastomosis was used in 77. The actuarial freedom from recoarctation at 4 years was 57% after subclavian flap angioplasty, 83% after extended end-to-end anastomosis, and 96% after radically extended end-to-end anastomosis (proximal to the origin of the left carotid artery). These authors felt that extended end-to-end anastomosis could be successfully applied to almost all types of

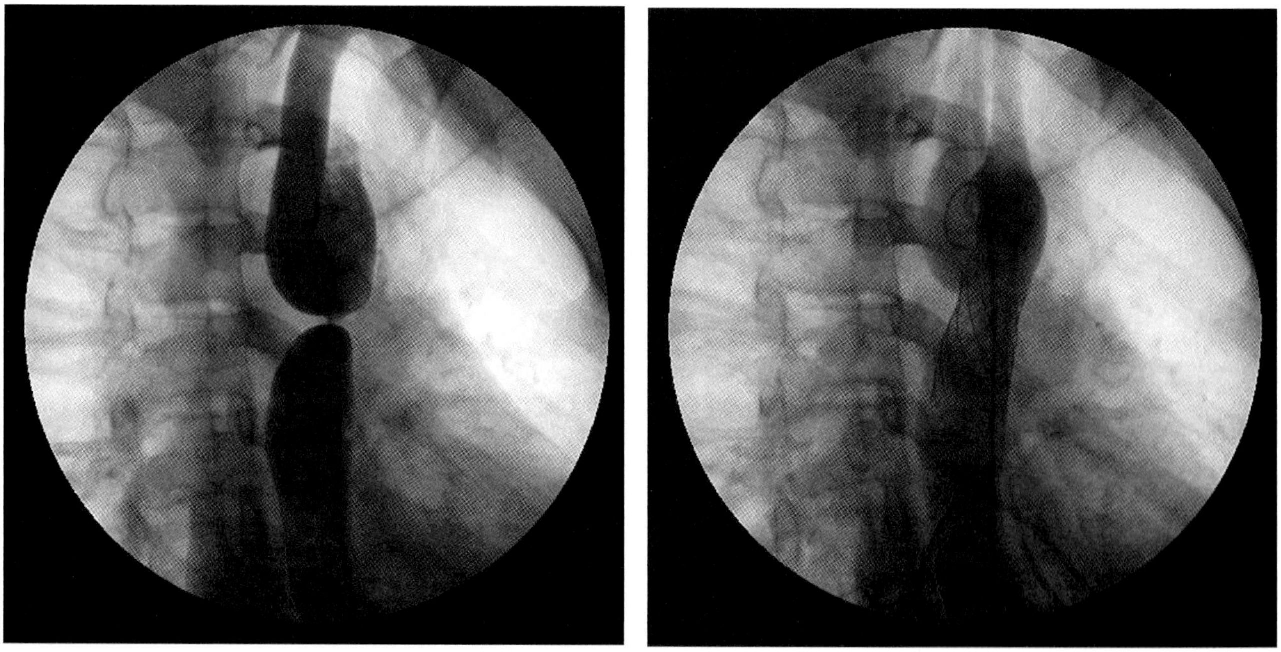

Figure 108–8 **A,** Aortogram of postoperative recurrent coarctation. **B,** Aortogram after endovascular stent placement with relief of obstruction.
(Courtesy Dr. Jonathan Rome, The Children's Hospital of Philadelphia.)

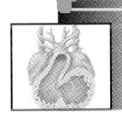

arch anomalies and produced the lowest incidence of recoarctation.

McElhinney and colleagues[104] evaluated risk factors for recurrent arch obstruction after repair of coarctation in neonates and young infants. Between 1990 and 1999, 103 patients younger than 3 months of age underwent repair of coarctation through a left thoracotomy. The median age at surgery was 18 days. Forty-five patients were younger than 2 weeks of age at the time of surgery. The median weight was 3.3 kg, and 14 patients weighed less than 2 kg. Resection with end-to-end anastomosis was used for repair of the coarctation in 64 patients, subclavian flap angioplasty was used in 34 patients, and patch augmentation of the arch was used in five patients. There was one early death and one late death, both in patients who had no evidence of recoarctation. At a median follow-up period at 24 months, reintervention for recurrent arch obstruction had been performed in 15 patients. Freedom from arch reintervention was 88 % at 1 year and 82% at 5 years. Factors associated with arch reintervention included younger age, smaller transverse arch diameter (<3.5 mm), and smaller ascending aorta. By multivariable analysis, a smaller absolute transverse arch diameter and younger age at the time of surgery were the only independent predictors of earlier need for arch reintervention. Interestingly, low weight at the time of repair, including weight less than 2 kg, and the type of repair did not correlate with the risk of recoarctation.

Bacha and associates[6] evaluated 18 consecutive neonates weighing less than 2 kg who underwent coarctation repair. All patients underwent surgery via left thoracotomy. Resection and end-to-end anastomosis were performed in 16 patients, and in two patients reverse subclavian flap augmentation of the arch and subsequent end- to end anastomosis were used. There was one early death and two late deaths. Multivariable analysis showed that associated Shone's syndrome and presence of a hypoplastic arch were associated with increased mortality. Freedom from reintervention for recurrent coarctation at 5 years was 60%.

Younoszai and colleagues[166] reported follow up of 88 patients who underwent coarctation with end-to-side anastomosis to the proximal arch. In five children the repair was performed through a median sternotomy during the repair of other defects. There were no perioperative deaths and four late deaths. No patient operated on at 1 month of age or older developed recurrent obstruction. Only three patients operated on during the neonatal period (5.5%) developed recurrent obstruction. Freedom from reintervention in the neonatal group was 95.8% at 1 and 2 years. Elgamal and colleagues[45] reported outcomes of 65 newborns who underwent repair of coarctation and arch hypoplasia using aortic arch advancement between 1995 and 2000. Isolated arch hypoplasia and coarctation was present in 13 patients, a VSD was present in 20 patients, and additional complex cardiac lesions were present in the remainder. There were three early deaths, all in patients with either VSD or complex cardiac disease, and two late deaths in patients with complex cardiac defects for an actuarial 5-year survival rate of 91%. Recurrent arch obstruction occurred in only one patient, with freedom from recurrence of 98% at 5 years. Kanter and associates[78] have reported retrospective analysis of 46 infants younger than 3 months of age undergoing coarctation repair with hypoplastic arch enlargement by reverse subclavian flap aortoplasty. At a mean follow-up period of 38 months, five patients developed recurrent aortic obstruction: three at the coarctation site and two at the site of arch augmentation.

Good results also have been reported for subclavian flap angioplasty.[24] Sciolaro and associates[138] reviewed 56 children under 4 years of age. Thirty-four had a subclavian flap angioplasty, and 22 had resection with end-to-end anastomosis. Among the 23 infants younger than 3 months of age, the 6-year actual freedom from recoarctation was 93% in the subclavian flap group compared with 53% in the end-to-end anastomosis group. These investigators recommended use of the subclavian flap angioplasty in patients younger than 3 months of age. Jahangiri and colleagues[72] retrospectively analyzed 185 consecutive patients who underwent subclavian flap angioplasty between 1974 and 1998. Aortic arch hypoplasia defined as a diameter of the distal arch of less than 50% of the ascending aorta was present in 22% of patients. Subclavian flap angioplasty was performed in all patients, with an early mortality of 3%. Recoarctation, defined as an echocardiographic gradient of 25 mm Hg or greater, occurred in 6% of the patients at a median follow-up period of 6.2 years. By multivariate analysis, the only risk factor for recoarctation was persistent arch hypoplasia after surgical repair. The authors stated that angiographic imaging of the aorta showed that the recoarctation did not occur at the site of hypoplastic transverse arch, but at the site of residual ductal tissue. Overall freedom from reoperation for recoarctation was 95% at 2 years and 92% at 5 and 15 years. These authors suggested that in the majority of patients with coarctation and distal arch hypoplasia, repair of the coarctation alone can be performed with excellent results, low mortality, and resolution of arch hypoplasia after relief of the distal obstruction.

However, there has been concern that subclavian flap aortoplasty may not be the optimum method for coarctation repaired in very young infants. Cobanoglu and colleagues[31] reported an increased incidence of early recoarctation in infants under 3 months of age after subclavian flap aortoplasty when compared with the resection of primary anastomosis. They proposed that the etiology of restenosis was inadequate resection of ductal tissue in the aortic wall with continued constriction and fibrosis. Sanchez and colleagues[135] reported a 22% incidence of early recoarctation after subclavian flap angioplasty secondary to a posterior shelf in infants younger than 3 months of age. Restenosis was strongly correlated with younger age at the time of surgical correction and was thought to be secondary to persistent ductal tissue in the aortic wall. Trinquet and associates[150] reported follow up on 178 infants undergoing coarctation repair at less than 3 months of age; 63 infants had an isolated coarctation, 47 had associated VSD, and 68 had other associated anomalies. Actuarial survival rate at 5 years was 90% for infants with isolated coarctation, 84% for those with associated VSD, and 40% for those with complex anomalies. The rate of restenosis was the same for subclavian flap angioplasty, resection with primary anastomosis, and extended resection and anastomosis. In addition, often in very young neonates, there is some concern about sacrifice of the major vascular supply to the left upper extremity. The subclavian artery is frequently divided for creation of systemic-to-pulmonary shunts, and adverse sequelae have been rare. However, there is evidence of decreased growth of the extremity, resulting in decreased length and mass, and rare reports of vascular insufficiency with gangrene of the arm,[57,105,148,161] especially if branches of the subclavian artery distal to the vertebral artery are ligated.

The prosthetic patch onlay graft technique has been used in patients of all ages for correction of coarctation of the aorta. Yee and associates[165] reported the use of Gore-Tex patches and emphasized the advantages of the technique, including decreased operative time, decreased dissection, maximal augmentation of the area of stenosis, preservation of the collateral vessels, and no need for sacrifice of normal vascular structures. A thoracotomy incision commonly has been used for synthetic patch aortoplasty. Ungerleider and Ebert[151] demonstrated the applicability of patch aortoplasty via a median sternotomy in selected infants who require simultaneous correction of coarctation of intracardiac defects. Sade and co-workers[132] documented growth of the posterior wall of the aorta after patch aortoplasty. Patch aortoplasty is highly effective in relieving the aortic obstruction[133] with a low incidence of restenosis and persistent hypertension (at rest and after exercise).[146] However, the use of prosthetic material may predispose to infection, and there are increasing frequent reports of the formation of aneurysms and pseudoaneurysms.[3,15,106] Aneurysmal dilatation of the posterior aortic wall opposite the prosthetic patch has been reported in up to 38% of patients,[30] but the true incidence is unknown. An experimental study suggested that damage to the posterior wall during excision of the obstructing shelf may predispose to aneurysm formation.[43] Microscopic examination of the aneurysm wall in patients with aneurysmal dilation after patch aortoplasty demonstrated degeneration of the media.[65] Differences in the tensile strength between the prosthetic patch and native aortic wall also may be a factor in the formation of true and false aneurysms. Aebert and associates[3] reported significant dilatation of the operative site in 35% of patients after patch graft repair for coarctation of the aorta, and reoperation was necessary in 19.5%. Mendelsohn and colleagues[106] examined the ratio of the aortic diameter at the repair site to the aortic diameter at the diaphragm in 29 patients after patch repair of coarctation of the aorta. Patients with a ratio of greater than 1.5% progressed to aneurysmal dilation within 3–5 years. All patients who have undergone synthetic patch aortoplasty must be carefully monitored to evaluate possible aneurysm formation.[42] Older age at time of coarctation repair may increase the risk of aneurysm formation.[155] Patients with bicuspid aorta valve and coarctation can develop aneurysms of the ascending aorta.[155] Aortic aneurysms also have been reported after subclavian aortoplasty and resection with end-to-end anastomosis.[16,103] Female patients who have undergone patch aortoplasty may be at increased risk for aneurysmal dilation and rupture during pregnancy.[115]

Coarctation with Ventricular Septal Defect

In 1994 the Congenital Heart Surgeons Society reported results of a multi-institutional study evaluating 326 symptomatic neonates with coarctation either with or without an associated VSD.[122] A VSD was present in 155 of these infants, and 153 underwent surgical repair. For neonates with a moderately large VSD, repair of the coarctation plus pulmonary artery banding was associated with the highest non–risk-adjusted and risk-adjusted survival. Single-stage repair of both defects was associated with the lowest non–risk-adjusted survival.

Gaynor and colleagues[55] reported outcomes of 25 infants undergoing single-stage repair of coarctation with a moderate or large VSD. Arch reconstruction was performed by means of patch aortoplasty in 21 patients, and end-to-end anastomosis was performed in four patients. There was one operative death (4%) and one late death. Freedom from reintervention for recurrent coarctation was 75% 2 years after the operation. Isomatsu and associates[70] reported short- and intermediate-term outcomes for two-stage repair of coarctation and associated ventricular septal defect in 79 patients. The initial coarctation repair was performed with subclavian flap aortoplasty, and VSD closure and removal of the pulmonary artery band was performed at a mean interval of 10 months after the initial procedure. The short- and intermediate-term outcomes were excellent, with a low operative mortality (2 of 79) and four late deaths. However, two of the late deaths occurred during the second operation for VSD closure, and the other two deaths were secondary to congestive heart failure. Freedom from recoarctation was 90% at 10 years. Ishino and colleagues reported outcomes after single-stage repair of VSD and coarctation with the use of isolated cerebral perfusion to avoid DHCA during the arch repair. They compared single-stage repair in 11 patients (5 with a hypoplastic arch) with two-stage repair and 13 patients (4 with a hypoplastic arch). There were no operative deaths and one late death in each group. They noted no neurological complications; however, formal neurodevelopmental assessments were not performed. At a mean follow-up period of 20 months for the single-stage repair, no patient had developed recurrent arch obstruction.

Bonnet and colleagues[19] have reported use of an absorbable pulmonary artery band. Eleven infants underwent coarctation repair with placement of an absorbable pulmonary artery ban. There were no hospital deaths. Absorption of the pulmonary artery band was complete after a mean follow-up period of 5.7 months in all patients. The VSD closed completely in four infants and partially in six infants in whom the pulmonary artery pressure was normal. Only one patient required surgical closure of the VSD.

Management of Recoarctation

Recoarctation usually manifests as persistent hypertension or an arm–leg pressure gradient. The arm–leg gradient should be measured in the immediate postoperative period to differentiate residual stenosis secondary to inadequate repair from true recoarctation. Causes of recoarctation include failure of growth of the anastomosis, inadequate resection of the narrowed segment, residual abnormal ductal tissue, and suture line thrombosis. Exercise testing with measurement of the arm–leg gradient can be done to evaluate postoperative repair in patients.[35] Some patients who are normotensive at rest without an arm–leg gradient develop severe hypertension with a measured gradient after exercise and may have a significant restenosis. It is important to measure the arm and leg pressure simultaneously to assess the gradient accurately, which can also be done using

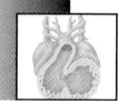

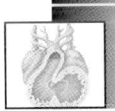

Doppler pressure measurements at rest and immediately after exercise. In infants the arm–leg gradient can be assessed before and after a noxious stimulus. The long-term consequences of exercise-induced hypertension after correction of coarctation are unknown, but this finding may adversely affect the prognosis.[52,82,95,100]

Reoperation is indicated if significant hypertension or other symptoms occur and a pressure gradient can be demonstrated.[49] Reoperation is more difficult because of scarring, and there is increased morbidity and mortality. Lack of a collateral circulation may result in the increased incidence of paraplegia. In patients who have had previous resection and end-to-end anastomosis or subclavian flap aortoplasty, a prosthetic patch onlay graft is an appropriate method repair of recoarctation.[118] Sweeney and associates[147] reported follow up of 53 patients who required reoperation. Patch aortoplasty was used in 26 patients. Bypass grafting was used in 16 patients, interposition grafts were necessary in eight patients, and three patients underwent resection with end-to-end anastomosis. Temporary shunts and bypass techniques were not used. There were no operative deaths and no neurological complications. Jacob and associates[71] reported the use of ascending aorta to descending aorta bypass in 10 patients with recoarctation without mortality or paraplegia. They used a two-incision approach via a left thoracotomy and median sternotomy without cardiopulmonary bypass. Reoperation for recurrent coarctation also may require treatment of aortic aneurysms and pseudoaneurysms. In older patients aortic valve replacement, coronary bypass surgery, mitral valve repair or replacement, and other procedures may be necessary.

In patients with complex arch obstruction, an alternative is placement of a ascending-to-descending aortic bypass graft within the pericardium. This extraanatomical bypass graft is performed through a median sternotomy using cardiopulmonary bypass. The heart is retracted cephalad, and a pericardial incision is made overlying the descending aorta. A partial occluding clamp is placed on the descending aorta, and an end-to-side anastomosis is created between a Dacron graft and the aorta. The graft is positioned along the right atrium either anterior or posterior to the inferior vena cava. An end-to-side anastomosis is performed with the ascending aorta using a partial occluding clamp. Advantages include avoidance of dissection in the region of the aortic arch and the ability to repair additional defects at the same procedure. Connolly and colleagues[34] reported 18 patients who underwent extraanatomical bypass through a median sternotomy between 1985 and 2000. All patients survived the operation and were alive with a patent graft at a mean follow-up period of 45 months. There were no graft-related complications and no cases of paraplegia. Additional procedures performed included aortic valve replacement, coronary bypass surgery, mitral valve repair and replacement, and VSD closure. If the recurrent coarctation and aneurysm involve the distal arch and proximal descending aorta, the repair may be performed through a standard posterolateral thoracotomy.[59] Some authors recommend the use of cardiopulmonary bypass with either femoral arterial and femoral venous cannulation or left-sided heart bypass with left atrial to descending aorta or femoral arterial cannulation.[62,164] Use of DHCA can facilitate the repair. Balloon angioplasty has become a frequently used technique in patients with recoarctation and may be the optimal initial therapy for recoarctation.[76]

Follow-Up after Coarctation Repair

Follow up of surgical patients indicates that they are not rendered entirely normal.[145] Some patients who have had a technically excellent repair may not have complete resolution of hypertension.[111] The etiology of persistent hypertension after repair is unclear but is related to the age at repair and the duration of preoperative hypertension. Maron and associates[101] reporting long-term follow-up of 248 patients who had correction of aortic coarctation found an increased incidence of premature death usually secondary to cardiovascular disease and related this to the duration of preoperative hypertension. There is evidence of increased coronary atherosclerosis in patients with coarctation.[33] Koller and colleagues[86] found that patients operated on between the ages of 2 and 4 years had a lower risk rate of persistent hypertension. Cohen and colleagues[32] at the Mayo Clinic reported long-term follow up on 571 patients after repair of coarctation. Age at the time of surgery was the most important predictor of survival. If the repair was performed at less than 14 years of age, survival to 20 years was 91%; however, if the repair was performed at greater than 14 years of age, 20-year survival was 79%. The best survivorship was for patients repaired before the age of 9 years. Age at the time of repair was also the most important predictor of persistent hypertension. Coronary artery disease was the most common cause of late death. Use of 24-hour ambulatory blood pressure measurements suggests that the prevalence of hypertension may be significantly greater than previously thought.[75,112] O'Sullivan and associates[112] evaluated 24-hour blood pressure measurements in 199 children who underwent coarctation repair in the first 2 years of life. Mean 24-hour systolic blood pressure was greater than the 95th percentile in 30% of the overall cohort. Importantly, mean 24-hour systolic blood pressure was elevated in 19% of patients, with no evidence of residual arch obstruction.

There is evidence of abnormal left ventricular function despite relief of the obstruction.[27] Kimball and associates[82] showed a persistent increase in ventricular contractility after successful coarctation repair possibly secondary to cardiac ultrastructural changes resulting from congenital pressure overload. They also have documented abnormal thallium scans after successful coarctation repair, suggesting persistent changes in the coronary arteries.[83] Abnormal left ventricle geometry and hypertrophy may persist even in normotensive patients after coarctation repair.[113] Pacileo and associates[113] showed that abnormal left ventricular geometry with significant hypertrophy is present in up to 40% of patients after successful coarctation repair and is associated with a hyperdynamic contractile state. Gardiner and colleagues[53] have documented abnormal endothelial response to nitroglycerin in normotensive patients after successful coarctation repair, suggesting that damage occurs early in vessels proximal to the coarctation and may persist even after successful repair in the neonatal period. The importance of abnormal endothelial function for development of persistent hypertension and coronary artery disease is unknown. Aortic stenosis and regurgitation secondary to a bicuspid aortic valve may develop and necessitate valve replacement. As has been emphasized, the long-term prognosis of many patients is determined primarily by the presence of associated anomalies.

AORTOPULMONARY SHUNTS

Historical Aspects

The first aortopulmonary shunt procedure was performed at John Hopkins University by Alfred Blalock in 1944.[18] This procedure was the first successful procedure for palliation of children with cyanotic heart disease, and success initiated a new era in the treatment of congenital heart disease. In 1946 Potts and associates[121] described creation of a descending aorta to left pulmonary artery shunt. In 1955 Davidson[38] introduced direct anastomosis of the ascending aorta to the main pulmonary artery. Waterson described creation of an ascending aorta to right pulmonary artery anastomosis.[39] Creation of a modified Blalock–Taussig shunt using an interposition graft was reported by Klinner and colleagues in 1961.[85] Gazzaniga and colleagues[56] introduced the use of the Gore-Tex interposition graft, which was subsequently popularized by de Leval and colleagues.[41]

Indications for Aortopulmonary Shunts

With the increasing use of infant and neonatal repair for complex heart defects, creation of aortopulmonary shunts as primary palliative procedures has become less common. The primary indication for creation of an aortopulmonary shunt in the current era is the presence of pulmonary atresia or severe stenosis in neonates and infants with complex defects such as single ventricle, pulmonary atresia with intact VSD and VSD with major aortopulmonary arteries (MAPCAs) undergoing staged reconstructive surgery. Shunts also are created as part of the Norwood procedure in infants with HLHS or variants. Shunts are now rarely used as palliation in infants with tetralogy of Fallot and inadequate pulmonary blood flow, and primary repair is more common even in neonates.

Blalock–Taussig Shunt

The classic Blalock–Taussig shunt is a end-to-side anastomosis of the transected subclavian artery to the pulmonary artery. A classic Blalock–Taussig shunt has the advantages of avoiding the use of prosthetic material, but it does require sacrifice of the subclavian artery. The operation is performed through a thoracotomy. The shunt is constructed on the side opposite the aortic arch so that the subclavian artery arises from the innominate artery to avoid kinking. Classic Blalock–Taussig shunts are now rarely used. The most commonly used shunt is the modified Blalock–Taussig shunt using a Gore-Tex interposition graft. This shunt can be constructed through either a lateral thoracotomy or a median sternotomy (Figure 108-9). Advantages of the median sternotomy approach include easy accessibility of the shunt for takedown and reconstruction of the right pulmonary artery, as well as the ability to use cardiopulmonary bypass if hemodynamic instability develops during the operation.

When a modified Blalock–Taussig shunt is used, shunt flow is largely regulated by the size of the subclavian or innominate artery. However, the diameter and length of the Gore-Tex graft also contributes to the resistance to pulmonary blood flow. Creation of large shunts should be avoided to prevent excessive pulmonary blood flow. In general, a 3.0-mm graft is used for neonates weighing less than 2 kg,

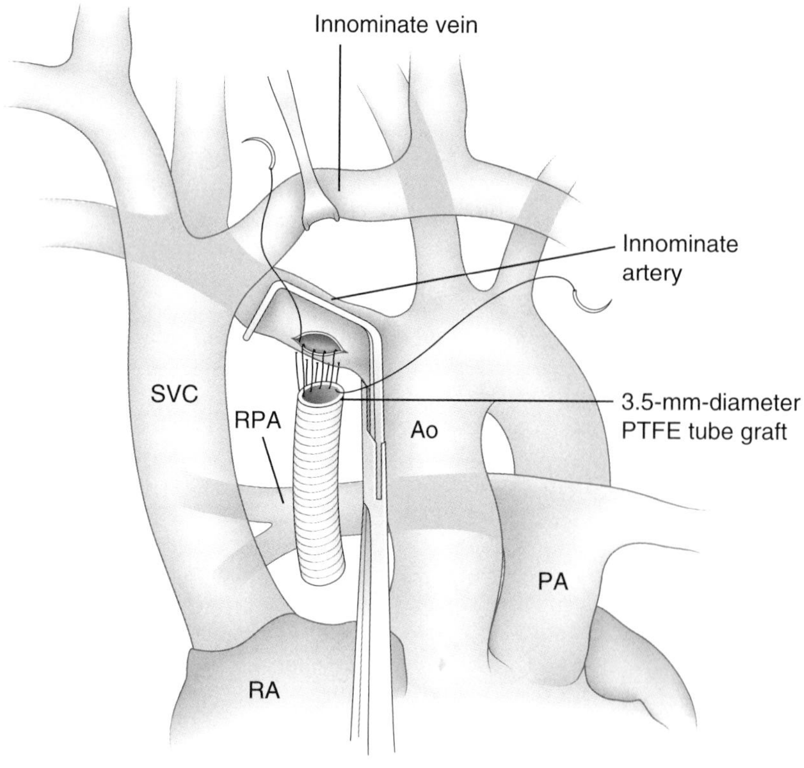

Figure 108–9 Schematic diagram of right modified Blalock–Taussig shunt (RMBTS) via sternotomy approach. SVC, superior vena cava; RPA, right pulmonary artery; RA, right atrium; PA, pulmonary artery; Ao, aorta. *(Modified from Odim J, Portzky M, Zurakowski D, et al: Sternotomy approach for a modified Blalock-Taussig shunt. Circulation 92 [suppl 9]: II-256–II-261, 1995).*

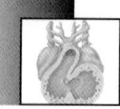

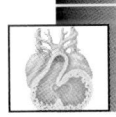

a 3.5-mm graft is used for infants weighing 2–3.5 kg, and a 4.0-mm graft is used for larger infants. A median sternotomy is performed, and the thymus is resected. The innominate artery is usually used for the proximal anastomosis; however, the graft may be placed on the subclavian artery or the ascending aorta (see Figure 108-9). If an aberrant right subclavian artery is present, the graft may be placed on the right carotid artery. The ascending aorta and proximal innominate artery are mobilized, as is the right pulmonary artery. Heparin is administered. A vascular clamp is placed on the proximal innominate artery. An arteriotomy is performed on the underside of the innominate artery. The Gore-Tex graft is beveled and the anastomosis constructed using a continuous suture of 7-0 Prolene. The clamp is removed to access inflow. The graft is then occluded with a hemoclip and cut to an appropriate length. A vascular clamp is placed on the right pulmonary artery with the artery positioned so that the arteriotomy can be performed on the superior aspect, proximal to the upper lobe branch. The patient should be observed with the pulmonary artery occluded for several minutes to ensure hemodynamic stability and adequate pulmonary blood flow. If hemodynamic instability or decreased oxygen saturation develops, the clamp can be removed and the patient cannulated for cardiopulmonary bypass. After stability is ensured, an arteriotomy is performed on the superior aspect of the right pulmonary artery and an end-to-side anastomosis is performed. The shunt is opened, and there should be an immediate fall in diastolic blood pressure with an increase in oxygen saturation. The ductus arteriosus can be snared and the patient observed to ensure adequate shunt flow. The ductus is then ligated. In some infants, particularly those with heterotaxy syndrome and single ventricle, stenosis of the pulmonary artery at the ductal insertion is common. Pulmonary arterioplasty may be necessary at the time of shunt placement to avoid the development of discontinuous pulmonary arteries.

Takedown of a modified Blalock–Taussig shunt at the time of definitive repair or subsequent palliative surgery such as a cavopulmonary connection is straightforward, particularly if the shunt was performed through a median sternotomy. The shunt is located by dissecting along the medial aspect of the superior vena cava. There is usually a thick fibrous peel around the graft. The plane between the peel and the graft is mobilized. After initiation of cardiopulmonary bypass, the graft can easily be ligated. The graft should be divided to prevent vessel distortion as the patient grows. Any stenosis of the right pulmonary artery at the shunt insertion can be repaired by removing the distal portion of the graft and performing an pulmonary arterioplasty.

Diminutive Pulmonary Arteries

Because of concern of distortion of the branch pulmonary arteries by a classic or modified Blalock–Taussig shunt, some authors have recommended central shunts with the origin of the graft on the ascending aorta and termination on the main pulmonary artery or the bifurcation. Davidson[38] initially suggested creating a direct side-to-side anastomosis, essentially creating an aortopulmonary window. Pulmonary blood flow may be difficult to regulate, and takedown can be difficult with this type of defects. Others have suggested use of an interposition graft between the ascending aorta and main pulmonary artery.[11,120] Potential advantages include avoidance of branch pulmonary artery distortion and more symmetrical distribution of pulmonary blood flow. Takedown of these shunts can be more difficult than takedown of a modified Blalock–Taussig shunt. An alternative in patients with very small pulmonary arteries is a direct central end-to-side shunt.[160] This technique has been most commonly used in patients with pulmonary atresia, VSD, MAPCAs, and small central pulmonary arteries. The procedure is performed through a median sternotomy. Cardiopulmonary bypass may not be required if there is adequate pulmonary blood flow via the MAPCAs.[160] The main and branch pulmonary arteries are mobilized. The ascending aorta is mobilized, and a partial occluding clamp is placed on the leftward aspect as far posterior as possible. A small button of aortic wall is excised. The main pulmonary artery is divided, and the incision is extended onto the right pulmonary artery. A direct anastomosis is performed between the main pulmonary artery and the posterior aorta. Preliminary results suggest that this shunt is effective in promoting growth of very small pulmonary arteries.[128,160] However, distortion of the proximal branch pulmonary arteries, particularly the right, is common. The patients must be carefully followed because excessive pulmonary blood flow may develop, resulting in congestive heart failure and early pulmonary vascular disease. Takedown can be difficult and may require transection of the ascending aorta.

Potts and Waterston Shunts

The Potts shunt is an anastomosis between the descending aorta and the left pulmonary artery. Use of the Potts shunt has been abandoned because of complications, including aneurysms of the left pulmonary artery, excessive pulmonary blood flow resulting in pulmonary vascular disease and congestive heart failure, and difficult shunt takedown at the time of definitive surgery. The Waterston shunt is an anastomosis between the ascending aorta and the right pulmonary artery. The Waterston shunt often resulted in excessive pulmonary blood flow. In addition, significant distortion and kinking of the right pulmonary artery frequently developed.

Occasionally, older patients are seen in whom a shunt of this type must be taken down at the time of corrective or further palliative surgery. Technically, takedown of a Waterston shunt is somewhat easier than a Potts anastomosis. A median sternotomy is performed. The shunt and right pulmonary artery are mobilized so that the shunt and/or pulmonary arteries can be snared or clamped before institution of cardiopulmonary bypass. The patient is cannulated, and bypass is initiated. The aorta is cross-clamped, and cardioplegia solution is administered with the shunt or pulmonary arteries occluded. Usually the anastomosis is divided and the defects in both vessels are closed either primarily or with a patch. An alternative method is closure from within the aorta if there is no pulmonary artery distortion. If visualization is poor, the ascending aorta can be divided to allow patch augmentation of the right pulmonary artery.

Takedown of a Potts shunt may be particularly difficult because of aneurysmal dilatation of the pulmonary artery and the risk of cerebral air embolism. Takedown is performed through a median sternotomy. Arterial cannulation can be performed either through the ascending aorta or the femoral artery. If possible, the pulmonary arteries are controlled with snares before the initiation of cardiopulmonary bypass; however, control of the distal left pulmonary artery may be very difficult. If necessary, the shunt is occluded with a finger during cooling. Deep hypothermic circulatory arrest is often used. After adequate cooling, the head vessels are occluded and cardioplegia solution is administered. The left pulmonary artery can safely be opened anteriorly and the shunt closed from within the pulmonary artery. All air must be evacuated from the ascending aorta before releasing the snares and reperfusing the brain.

Results and Complications

Mortality for isolated shunt placement should be low, but is dependent on the underlying defect. Mortality for infants with more complex defects is greater. Complications of shunt placement include inadequate or excessive pulmonary blood flow, pulmonary artery distortion or stenosis, shunt thrombus, damage to the recurrent laryngeal or phrenic nerves, and chylothorax. When a Gore-Tex interposition graft is used, leakage of serous fluid through the graft may result in a seroma.

AORTOPULMONARY COLLATERALS

Aortopulmonary collateral vessels are arteries arising from systemic arteries, including the aorta, which anastomose with the pulmonary circulation and drain via the pulmonary veins into the left atrium.[2,9] These vessels may be congenital and are associated with a variety of congenital heart defects, including tetralogy of Fallot and transposition of the great arteries.[58,116,128] These vessels may represent enlarged bronchial arteries or may arise from other systemic vessels. In patients with tetralogy of Fallot with pulmonary atresia, MAPCAs may provide the majority of pulmonary blood flow, particularly in children with very small true pulmonary arteries. Aortopulmonary collaterals also may be acquired, particularly in patients with chronic cyanosis. In cyanotic patients who have undergone a thoracotomy, significant collaterals may develop from the chest wall and mediastinum and connect to the pulmonary vasculature via postoperative adhesions.[88] Aortopulmonary collaterals also may develop in patients with pulmonary artery agenesis, acquired pulmonary artery stenosis, or acquired pulmonary artery occlusion.[25,127] Significant collaterals also can develop in patients with single ventricle undergoing staged reconstructive surgery and may complicate the Fontan procedure.[78] Some authors have suggested that these vessels should be embolized before the Fontan procedure. However, there is no definitive evidence that occlusion of these vessels leads to improved outcomes. During cardiac surgery, collateral flow can lead to hypotension with increased return to the left atrium and result in cardiac distention.[2] Collateral vessels may increase the risk of cerebral hypoperfusion and central nervous system injury during cardiopulmonary bypass.[84] Large collateral vessels should be controlled with snares or ligated before the institution of cardiopulmonary bypass. When significant collaterals are present, pH-stat blood gas management during cooling may improve cerebral blood flow.[84]

Enlarged bronchial arteries also may lead to severe hemoptysis, particularly in patients with unilateral pulmonary artery occlusion. Cardiac catheterization and embolization of the enlarged collaterals may be successful in controlling the hemoptysis.[25,116,127] Occasionally in some patients with recurrent severe hemoptysis, pneumonectomy may be necessary. Aortopulmonary collaterals also can complicate lung transplantation in patients with cyanotic heart disease. Pulmonary transplantation may be contraindicated in cyanotic patients who have undergone thoracotomies because of the significant risk of uncontrollable hemorrhage from the collateral vessels.[88]

REFERENCES

1. Abbott ME: Coarctation of the aorta of the adult type. Am Heart J 3:574–618, 1928.
2. Acherman RJ, Siassi B, Pratti-Madrid G, et al: Systemic to pulmonary collaterals in very low birth weight infants: Color Doppler detection of systemic to pulmonary connections during neonatal and early infancy period. Pediatrics 105:528–532, 2000.
3. Aebert H, Laas J, Bednarski P, et al: High incidence of aneurysm formation following patch plasty repair of coarctation. Eur J Cardiothorac Surg 7:200–204, 1993.
4. Alpert BS, Bain HH, Balfe JW, et al: Role of the renin-angiotensin-aldosterone system in hypertensive children with coarctation of the aorta. Am J Cardiol 43:828–834, 1979.
5. Amato JJ, Rheinlander HF, Cleveland RJ: A method of enlarging the distal transverse arch in infants with hypoplasia and coarctation of the aorta. Ann Thorac Surg 23:261–263, 1977.
6. Bacha EA, Almodovar M, Wessel DL, et al: Surgery for coarctation of the aorta in infants weighing less than 2 kg. Ann Thorac Surg 71:1260–1264, 2001.
7. Bagby SP, Mass RD: Abnormality of the renin/body-fluid-volume relationship in serially-studied inbred dogs with neonatally-induced coarctation hypertension. Hypertension 2:631–642, 1980.
8. Bagby SP, McDonald WJ, Strong DW, et al: Abnormalities of renal perfusion and the renal pressor system in dogs with chronic aortic coarctation. Circ Res 37:615–620, 1975.
9. Baile EM, Ling H, Heyworth, et al: Bronchopulmonary anastomotic and noncoronary collateral blood flow in humans during cardiopulmonary bypass. Chest 87:749–754, 1985.
10. Balaji S, Oommen R, Rees PG: Fatal aortic rupture during balloon dilatation of recoarctation. Br Heart J 65:100–101, 1991.
11. Barragry TP, Ring WS, Blatchford JW, et al: Central aorta-pulmonary artery shunts in neonates with complex cyanotic congenital heart disease. J Thorac Cardiovasc Surg 93: 767–774, 1987.
12. Becker AE, Becker MJ, Edwards JE: Anomalies associated with coarctation of aorta: Particular reference to infancy. Circulation 41:1067–1075, 1970.
13. Beekman RH, Katz BP, Moorehead-Steffens C, et al: Altered baroreceptor function in children with systolic hypertension after coarctation repair. Am J Cardiol 52:112–117, 1983.
14. Benedict CR, Phil D, Grahame-Smith DG, et al: Changes in plasma catecholamines and dopamine beta-hydroxylase after corrective surgery for coarctation of the aorta. Circulation 57:598–609, 1978.
15. Bergdahl L, Ljungqvist A: Long-term results after repair of coarctation of the aorta by patch grafting. J Thorac Cardiovasc Surg 80:177–181, 1980.

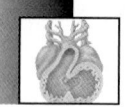

16. Berri G, Welsh P, and Capelli H: Aortic aneurysm after subclavian arterial flap angioplasty for coarctation of the aorta. J Thorac Cardiovasc Surg 1993; 105:951.
17. Blalock A, Park EA: The surgical treatment of experimental coarctation (atresia) of the aorta. Ann Surg 119:445–446, 1944.
18. Blalock A, Taussig HB: The surgical treatment of malformations of the heart. JAMA 128:189–203, 1945.
19. Bonnet D, Patkai J, Tamisier D, et al: A new strategy for the surgical treatment of aortic coarctation associated with ventricular septal defect in infants using an absorbable pulmonary artery band. J Am Coll Cardiol 34:866–870, 1999.
20. Brandt B 3rd, Heintz SE, Rose EF, et al: Repair of coarctation of the aorta in children with Turner's syndrome. Pediatr Cardiol 5:175–177, 1984.
21. Brewer LA III, Fosburg RG, Mulder GA, et al: Spinal cord complications following surgery for coarctation of the aorta: A study of 66 cases. J Thorac Cardiovasc Surg 64:368–381, 1972.
22. Brouwer MH, Cromme-Dijkhuis AH, Ebels T, et al: Growth of the hypoplastic aortic arch after simple coarctation resection and end-to-end anastomosis. J Thorac Cardiovasc Surg 104:426–433, 1992.
23. Burch FM, Manning N, Sleeman K, et al: Prenatal diagnosis of coarctation of the aorta improves survival and reduces morbidity. Heart 87:67–69, 2002.
24. Campbell DB, Waldhausen JA, Pierce WS, et al: Should elective repair of coarctation of the aorta be done in infancy? J Thorac Cardiovasc Surg 88:929–938, 1984.
25. Campbell KR, Krasuski R, Wang A: Congenital agenesis of the right pulmonary artery. Catheterization Cardiovasc Interv 51:460–463, 2000.
26. Campbell M: Natural history of coarctation of the aorta. Br Heart J 32:633–640, 1970.
27. Carpenter MA, Dammann JF, Watson DD, et al: Left ventricular hyperkinesia at rest and during exercise in normotensive patients 2 to 27 years after coarctation repair. J Am Coll Cardiol 6:879–886, 1974.
28. Celano V, Pieroni DR, Morera JA, et al: Two-dimensional echocardiographic examination of mitral valve abnormalities associated with coarctation of the aorta. Circulation 69:924–932, 1984.
29. Choy M, Rocchini AP, Beekman RH, et al: Paradoxical hypertension after repair of coarctation of the aorta in children: Balloon angioplasty versus surgical repair. Circulation 75:1186–1191, 1987.
30. Clarkson PM, Brandt PWT, Barratt-Boyes BG, et al: Prosthetic repair of coarctation of the aorta with particular reference to Dacron onlay patch grafts and late aneurysm formation. Am J Cardiol 56:342–346, 1985.
31. Cobanoglu A, Teply JF, Grunkemeier GL, et al: Coarctation of the aorta in patients younger than three months. J Thorac Cardiovasc Surg 89:128–135, 1985.
32. Cohen M, Fuster V, Steele MP, et al: Coarctation of the aorta: Long-term follow-up and prediction of outcome after surgical correction. Circulation 80:840–845, 1989.
33. Cokkinos DV, Leachman RD, Cooley DA: Increased mortality rate from coronary artery disease following operation for coarctation of the aorta at a late age. J Thorac Cardiovasc Surg 77:315–318, 1979.
34. Connolly HM, Hartzell VS, Izhar U, et al: Posterior pericardial ascending-to-descending aortic bypass. Circulation 104:I133–I137, 2001.
35. Connors TM: Evaluation of persistent coarctation of aorta after surgery with blood pressure measurement and exercise testing. Am J Cardiol 43:74–78, 1979.
36. Crafoord C, Nylin G: Congenital coarctation of the aorta and its surgical treatment. J Thorac Cardiovasc Surg 14:347–361, 1945.
37. Cunningham HN Jr, Laschinger JC, Spencer FC: Monitoring of somatosensory evoked potentials during surgical procedures on the thoracoabdominal aorta. IV: Clinical observations and results. J Thorac Cardiovasc Surg 94:275–285, 1987.
38. Davidson JS: Anastomosis between the ascending aorta and the main pulmonary artery in the tetralogy of Fallot. Thorax 10:348–350, 1955.
39. DeBoer A: Classics in thoracic surgery. The Waterson shunt: A commentary. Ann Thorac Surg 44:326–327, 1987.
40. de Divitiis M, Pilla C, Kattenhorn M, et al: Vascular dysfunction after repair of coarctation of the aorta: Impact of early surgery. Circulation 104:I165–I170, 2001.
41. de Leval MR, McKay R, Jones M, et al: Modified Blalock-Taussig shunt. Use of subclavian artery orifice as flow regulator in prosthetic systemic-pulmonary artery shunts. J Thorac Cadiovasc Surg 81:112–119, 1981.
42. del Nido PJ, Williams WG, Wilson GJ, et al: Synthetic patch angioplasty for repair of coarctation of the aorta: Experience with aneurysm formation. Circulation 74(suppl.I):32–36, 1986.
43. DeSanto A, Bills RG, King H, et al: Pathogenesis of aneurysm formation opposite prosthetic patches used for coarctation repair: An experimental study. J Thorac Cardiovasc Surg 94:720–723, 1987.
44. Downing DF, Grotzinger PJ, Weller RW: Coarctation of the aorta: The syndrome of necrotizing arteritis of the small intestine following surgical therapy. Am J Dis Child 96:711–719, 1958.
45. Elgamal MA, McKenzie ED, Fraser CD: Aortic arch advancement: The optimal one-stage approach for surgical management of neonatal coarctation with arch hypoplasia. Ann Thorac Surg 73:1267–1272, 2002.
46. Elliott MJ: Coarctation of the aorta with arch hypoplasia: Improvements on a new technique. Ann Thorac Surg 44:321–323, 1987.
47. Elzenga NJ, Gittenberger-deGroot AC: Localised coarctation of the aorta. An age dependent spectrum. Br Heart J 49:317–323, 1983.
48. Ferguson JC, Barrie WW, Schenk WG Jr: Hypertension of aortic coarctation: The role of renal and other factors. Ann Surg 185:423–428, 1977.
49. Foster ED: Reoperation for aortic coarctation. Ann Thorac Surg 38:81–89, 1984.
50. Fox S, Pierce WS, Waldausen JA: Pathogenesis of paradoxical hypertension after coarctation repair. Ann Thorac Surg 29:135–141, 1980.
51. Freed MD, Keane JF, Van Praagh R, et al: Coarctation of the aorta with congenital mitral regurgitation. Circulation 49:1175–1184, 1974.
52. Freed MD, Rocchini A, Rosenthal A, et al: Exercise-induced hypertension after surgical repair of coarctation of the aorta. Am J Cardiol 43:253–258, 1979.
53. Gardiner HM, Celermajer DS, Sorensen KE, et al: Abnormal endothelial response in the precoarctation vascular bed of young normotensive adults after successful coarctation repair. Br Heart J 69:18, 1993.
54. Gaynor JW: Management strategies for infants coarctation and an associated ventricular septal defect. J Thorac Cardiovasc Surg 122:424–426, 2001.
55. Gaynor JW, Wernovsky G, Rychik J, et al: Outcome following single-stage repair of coarctation with ventricular septal defect. Eur J Cardiothorac Surg 18:62–67, 2000.
56. Gazzaniga AB, Elliot MP, Sperling DR, et al: Microporous expanded polytetrafluoroethylene arterial prothesis for construction of aortopulmonary shunts: Experimental and clinical results. Ann Thorac Surg 21:322–327, 1976.
57. Geiss D, Williams WG, Lindsay WK, Rowe RD: Upper extremity gangrene: A complication of subclavian artery division. Ann Thorac Surg 30:487–489, 1980.
58. Golej J, Trittenwein G, Marx M, et al: Aortopulmonary collateral artery embolization during postoperative extracorporeal

membrane oxygenation after arterial switch procedure. Artif Organs 23:1938–1040, 1999.
59. Grinda JM, Mace L, Dervanian P, et al: Bypass graft for complex forms of isthmic aortic coarctation in adults. Ann Thorac Surg 60:1299–1302, 1995.
60. Gross RE: Surgical correction for coarctations of the aorta. Surgery 18:673–678, 1945.
61. Gross RE: Treatment of certain aortic coarctations by homologous grafts. Ann Surg 134:753–768, 1951.
62. Gross RE, Hufnagel CA: Coarctation of the aorta: Experimental studies regarding its surgical corrections. N Engl J Med 233:287–293, 1945.
63. Hamdan MA, Maheshwari S, Fahey JT, et al: Endovascular stents for coarctation of the aorta: Initial results and intermediate follow-up. Am J Cardiol 38:1518–1523, 2001.
64. Hamilton DI, Di Eusanio G, Sandrasagra FA, et al: Early and late results of aortoplasty with a left subclavian flap for coarctation of the aorta in infancy. J Thorac Cardiovasc Surg 75:699–704, 1978.
65. Hehrlein FW, Mulch J, Rautenburg HW, et al: Incidence and pathogenesis of late aneurysms after patch graft aortoplasty for coarctation. J Thorac Cardiovasc Surg 92:226–230, 1986.
66. Heymann MA, Berman W Jr, Rudolph AM, Whitman V: Dilatation of the ductus arteriosus by prostaglandin E_1 in aortic arch abnormalities. Circulation 59:169–173, 1979.
67. Ho SY, Anderson RH: Coarctation, tubular hypoplasia, and the ductus arteriosus: Histological study of 35 specimens. Br Heart J 41:268–274, 1979.
68. Hughes RK, Reemtsma K: Correction of coarctation of the aorta. Manometric determination of safety during test occlusion. J Thorac Cardiovasc Surg 62:31–33, 1971.
69. Isner JM, Donaldson RF, Fulton D, et al: Cystic medial necrosis in coarctation of the aorta: A potential factor contributing to adverse consequences observed after percutaneous balloon angioplasty of coarctation sites. Circulation 75:689–695, 1987.
70. Isomatsu Y, Imai Y, Shin'oka T, et al: Coarctation of the aorta and ventricular septal defect: Should we perform a single-stage repair? J Thorac Cardiovasc Surg 122:524–528, 2001.
71. Jacob T, Cobanoglu A, Starr A: Late results of ascending aorta-descending aorta bypass grafts for recurrent coarctation of the aorta. J Thorac Cardiovasc Surg 95:782–787, 1988.
72. Jahangiri M, Shinebourne EA, Zurakowski D, et al: Subclavian flap angioplasty: Does it look after itself? J Thorac Cardiocasc Surg 120:224–229, 2000.
73. Jarcho S: Coarctation of the aorta (Meckel, 1750; Paris, 1791). Am J Cardiol 7:844–852, 1961.
74. Jarcho S: Coarctation of the aorta (Albrecht Meckel, 1827). Am J Cardiol 9:307–311, 1962.
75. Johnson D, Perrault H, Vobecky SJ, et al: Influence of the postoperative period and surgical procedure on ambulatory blood pressure-determination of hypertension load after successful surgical repair of coarctation of the aorta. Eur Heart J 19:638–646, 1998.
76. Kan JS, White RI Jr, Mitchell SE, et al: Treatment of restenosis of coarctation by percutaneous transluminal angioplasty. Circulation 68:1087–1094, 1983.
77. Kanter KR, Vincent RN, Fyfe DA: Reverse subclavian flap repair of hypoplastic transverse aorta in infancy. Ann Thorac Surg 71:1530–1536, 2001.
78. Kanter KR, Vincent RN, Raviele AA, et al: Importance of acquired systemic-to-pulmonary collaterals in the Fontan operation. Ann Thorac Surg 68:969–975, 1999.
79. Karl TR, Sano S, Brawn W, Mee RBB: Repair of hypoplastic or interrupted aortic arch via sternotomy. J Thorac Cardiovasc Surg 104:688–695, 1992.
80. Kawauchi M, Tada Y, Asano K, Sudo K: Angiographic demonstration of mesenteric arterial changes in postcoarctectomy syndrome. Surgery 98:602–604, 1985.
81. Keen G: Spinal cord damage and operations for coarctation of the aorta: Aetiology, practice, and prospects. Thorax 42:11–18, 1987.
82. Kimball BP, Shurvell BL, Houle S, et al: Persistent ventricular adaptations in postoperative coarctation of the aorta. J Am Coll Cardiol 8:172–178, 1986.
83. Kimball BP, Shurvell BL, Mildenberger RR, et al: Abnormal thallium kinetics in postoperative coarctation of the aorta: Evidence for diffuse hypertension-induced vascular pathology. J Am Coll Cardiol 7:538–545, 1986.
84. Kirshbom PM, Skaryak LR, DiBernardo LR, et al: pH-stat cooling improves cerebral metabolic recovery after circulatory arrest in a piglet model of aortopulmonary collaterals. J Thorac Cardiovasc Surg 111:147–155, discussion 156–157, 1996.
85. Klinner W: Klinishe und experimentalle untersuchungen zur operativen korrektur der fallotschen tetralogie. Aus der chirirgischen Klinink der Universitat Munchen, 44:58–111, 1962.
86. Koller M, Rothlin M, Sinning A: Coarctation of the aorta: Review of 362 operated patients. Long-term follow-up and assessment of prognostic variables. Eur Heart J 8:670–679, 1987.
87. Korfer R, Meyer H, Kleikamp G, Bircks W: Early and late results after resection and end-to-end anastomosis of coarctation of the thoracic aorta in early infancy. J Thorac Cardiovasc Surg 89:616–622, 1985.
88. Koutlas TC, Bridges N, Gaynor JW, et al: Pediatric lung transplantation—Are there surgical contraindications? Transplantation 63:269–274, 1997.
89. Krieger KH, Spencer FC: Is paraplegia after repair of coarctation of the aorta due principally to distal hypotension during aortic cross-clamping? Surgery 1:2–7, 1985.
90. Lacour-Gayet F, Bruniaux J, Serraf A, et al: Hypoplastic transverse arch and coarctation in neonates. surgical reconstruction of the aortic arch: A study of sixty-six patients. J Thorac Cardiovasc Surg 100:808–816, 1990.
91. Lansman S, Shapiro AJ, Schiller MS, et al: Extended aortic arch anastomosis for repair of coarctation in infancy. Circulation 74(suppl. I):37–41, 1986.
92. Laschinger JC, Cunningham JN Jr, Baumann FG, et al: Monitoring of somatosensory evoked potentials during surgical procedures on the thoracoabdominal aorta. II. Use of somatosensory evoked potentials to assess adequacy of distal aortic bypass and perfusion after thoracic aortic cross-clamping. J Thorac Cardiovasc Surg 94:266–270, 1987.
93. Laschinger JC, Cunningham JN Jr, Baumann FG, et al: Monitoring of somatosensory evoked potentials during surgical procedures on the thoracoabdominal aorta. III. Intraoperative identification of vessels critical to spinal cord blood supply. J Thorac Cardiovasc Surg 4:271–274, 1987.
94. Leanage R, Taylor JFN, DeLeval M, et al: Surgical management of coarctation of aorta with ventricular septal defect. Br Heart J 46:269–277, 1981.
95. Leandro J, Smallhorn JF, Benson L, et al: Ambulatory blood pressure monitoring and left ventricular mass and function after successful surgical repair of coarctation of the aorta. J Am Coll Cardiol 20:197–204, 1992.
96. Leoni F, Huhta JC, Douglas J, et al: Effect of prostaglandin on early surgical mortality in obstructive lesions of the systemic circulation. Br Heart J 52:654–659, 1984.
97. Lindsay J Jr: Coarctation of the aorta, bicuspid aortic valve and abnormal ascending aortic wall. Am J Cardiol 61:182–184, 1988.
98. Machii M, Becker AE: Hypoplastic aortic arch morphology pertinent to growth after surgical correction of aortic coarctation. Ann Thorac Surg 64:516–520, 1997.
99. Machii M, Becker AE: Morphological features of the normal aortic arch in neonates, infants, and children pertinent to growth. Ann Thorac Surg 64:511–515, 1997.

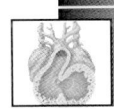

100. Markel H, Rocchini AP, Beekman RH, et al: Exercise-induced hypertension after repair of coarctation of the aorta: Arm versus leg exercise. J Am Coll Cardiol 8:165–171, 1986.
101. Maron BJ, Humphries JO, Rowe RD, et al: Prognosis of surgically corrected coarctation of the aorta: A 20-year postoperative appraisal. Circulation 47:119–126, 1973.
102. Marshall AC, Perry SB, Keane JF, et al: Early results and medium-term follow-up of stent implantation for mild residual or recurrent aortic coarctation. Am Heart J 139:9–14, 2000.
103. Martin MM, Beekman RH, Rocchini AP, et al: Aortic aneurysms after subclavian angioplasty repair of coarctation of the aorta. Am J Cardiol 61:951–953, 1988.
104. McElhinney DB, Yang SG, Hogarty AN, et al: Recurrent arch obstruction after repair of isolated coarctation of the aorta in neonates and young infants: Is low weight a risk factor? J Thorac Cardiovasc Surg 122:883–890, 2001.
105. Mellgren G, Friberg LG, Eriksson BO, et al: Neonatal surgery for coarctation of the aorta. Scand J Thorac Cardiovasc Surg 21:193–197, 1987.
106. Mendelsohn AM, Crowley DC, Lindauer A, et al: Rapid progression of aortic aneurysms after patch aortoplasty repair of coarctation of the aorta. J Am Coll Cardiol 20:381–385, 1992.
107. Moene RJ, Gittenberger-DeGroot AC, Oppenheimer-Dekker A, et al: Anatomical characteristics of ventricular septal defect associated with coarctation of the aorta. Am J Cardiol 59:952–955, 1987.
108. Moene RJ, Ottenkamp J, Oppenheimer-Dekker A, Bartelings MM: Transposition of the great arteries and narrowing of the aortic arch: Emphasis on right ventricular characteristics. Br Heart J 53:58–63, 1985.
109. Morrow WR, Vick GW, Nihill MR, et al: Balloon dilatation of unopened coarctation of the aorta: Short- and intermediate-term results. J Am Coll Cardiol 11:133–138, 1988.
110. Myers JL, McConnell BA, Waldhausen JA: Coarctation of the aorta in infants: Does the aortic arch grow after repair? Ann Thorac Surg 54:869–874, 1992.
111. Nanton MA, Olley PM: Residual hypertension after coarctectomy in children. Am J Cardiol 37:769–772, 1976.
112. O'Sullivan JJ, Derrick G, Darnell R: Prevalence of hypertension in children after early repair of coarctation of the aorta: A cohort study using casual and 24 hour blood pressure measurement. Heart 88:163–166, 2002.
113. Pacileo G, Pisacane C, Russo MG, et al: Left ventricular remodeling and mechanics after successful repair of aortic coarctation. Am J Cardiol 87:748–752, 2001.
114. Parker FB, Farrell B, Streeten DHP, et al: Hypertensive mechanisms in coarctation of the aorta: Further studies of the renin-angiotensin system. J Thorac Cardiovasc Surg 80:568–573, 1980.
115. Parks WJ, Thankg D, Plauth WH, et al: Incidence of aneurysm formation after Dacron patch aortoplasty repair coarctation of the aorta: Long-term results and assessment utilizing magnetic resonance angiography with three dimensional surface rendering. J Am Coll Cardiol 26:266–271, 1995.
116. Perry SB, Radtke W, Fellows KE, et al: Coil embolization to occlude aortopulmonary collateral vessels and shunts in patients with congenital heart disease. J Am Coll Cardiol 13:100–108, 1989.
117. Pigula FA, Gandi SK, Siewers RD, et al: Regional low-flow perfusion provides somatic circulatory support during aortic arch surgery. Ann Thorac Surg 72:401–406, discussion 406–407, 2001.
118. Pollack P, Freed MD, Castaneda AR, Norwood WI: Reoperation for isthmic coarctation of the aorta: Follow-up of 26 patients. Am J Cardiol 51:1690–1694, 1983.
119. Pollock JC, Jamieson MP, McWilliam R: Somatosensory evoked potentials in the detection of spinal cord ischemia in aortic coarctation repair. Ann Thorac Surg 41:251–254, 1986.
120. Potapov EV, Alexi-Meskishvili VV, Dahnert I, et al: Development of pulmonary arteries after central aortopulmonary shunt in newborns. Ann Thorac Surg 71:899–906, 2001.
121. Potts WJ, Smith S, Gibson S: Anastomosis of the aorta to a pulmonary artery. JAMA 132:627–631, 1946.
122. Quaegebeur JM, Jonas RA, Weinberg AD, et al: Outcomes in seriously ill neonates with coarctation of the aorta. J Thorac Cardiovasc Surg 108:841–851, discussion 852–854, 1994.
123. Rajasinghe HA, Reddy VM, van Son JA, et al: Coarctation repair using end-to-side anastomosis of descending aorta to proximal aortic arch. Ann Thorac Surg 61:840–844, 1996.
124. Rao PS, Chopra PS: Role of balloon angioplasty in the treatment of aortic coarctation. Ann Thorac Surg 52:621–631, 1991.
125. Ravelo HR, Stephenson LW, Friedman S, et al: Coarctation resection in children with Turner's syndrome: A note of caution. J Thorac Cardiovasc Surg 80:427–430, 1980.
126. Reifenstein GH, Levine SA, Gross RE: Coarctation of the aorta: A review of 104 autopsied cases of the "adult type" 2 years of age or older. Am Heart J 33:146–168, 1947.
127. Rene M, Sans J, Sancho C, et al: Unilateral pulmonary artery agenesis presenting with hemoptysis: treatment by embolization of systemic collaterals. Cardiovasc Intervent Radiol 18:251–254, 1995.
128. Rodefeld MD, Reddy VM, Thompson LD, et al: Surgical creation of aortopulmonary window in selected patients with pulmonary atresia with poorly developed aortopulmonary collaterals and hypoplastic pulmonary arteries. J Thorac Cardiovasc Surg 123:1147–1168, 2002.
129. Rosenquist GC: Congenital mitral valve disease associated with coarctation of the aorta. Circulation 49:985–993, 1974.
130. Rudolph AM, Heymann MA, Spitznas U: Hemodynamic considerations in the development of narrowing of the aorta. Am J Cardiol 30:514–525, 1972.
131. Russell GA, Berry PJ, Watterson K, et al: Patterns of ductal tissue in coarctation of the aorta in the first three months of life. J Thorac Cardiovasc Surg 102:596–601, 1991.
132. Sade RM, Crawford FA, Hohn AR, et al: Growth of the aorta after prosthetic patch aortoplasty for coarctation in infants. Ann Thorac Surg 38:21–25, 1984.
133. Sade RM, Taylor AB, Chariker EP: Aortoplasty compared with resection for coarctation of the aorta in young children. Ann Thorac Surg 28:346–353, 1979.
134. Sadow SH, Synhorst DP, Pappas G: Taussig-Bing anomaly and coarctation of the aorta in infancy. Surgical options. Pediatr Cardiol 6:83–89, 1985.
135. Sanchez GR, Balsara RK, Dunn JM, et al: Recurrent obstruction after subclavian flap repair of coarctation of the aorta in infants. J Thorac Cardiovasc Surg 91:738–746, 1986.
136. Saul JP, Keane JF, Fellows KE, et al: Balloon dilatation angioplasty of postoperative aortic obstructions. Am J Cardiol 59:943–948, 1987.
137. Schuster SR, Gross RE: Surgery for coarctation of the aorta: A review of 500 cases. J Thorac Cardiovasc Surg 43:54–70, 1962.
138. Sciolaro C, Copeland J, Cork R, et al: Long-term follow-up comparing subclavian flap angioplasty to resection with modified oblique end-to-end anastomosis. J Thorac Cardiovasc Surg 101:1–13, 1991.
139. Scott HW Jr, Bahnson HT: Evidence for a renal factor in the hypertension of experimental coarctation of the aorta. Surgery 30:206–217, 1951.
140. Sealy WC, Harris JS, Young WG Jr, et al: Paradoxical hypertension following resection of coarctation of aorta. Surgery 42:135–147, 1957.
141. Sehested J, Baandrup U, Mikkelsen E: Different reactivity and structure of the prestenotic and poststenotic aorta in human coarctation. Circulation 65:1060–1065, 1982.

142. Shearer WT, Rutman JY, Weinberg WA, et al: Coarctation of the aorta and cerebrovascular accident: A proposal for early corrective surgery. J Pediatr 77:1004–1009, 1970.
143. Shinebourne EA, Elseed AM: Relation between fetal flow patterns, coarctation of the aorta, and pulmonary blood flow. Br Heart J 36:492–498, 1974.
144. Shone JD, Sellers RD, Anderson RC, et al: The developmental complex of "parachute mitral valve" supravalvular ring of left atrium, subaortic stenosis, and coarctation of aorta. Am J Cardiol 11:714–725, 1963.
145. Simon AB, Zloto AE: Coarctation of the aorta: Longitudinal assessment of operated patients. Circulation 50: 456–464, 1974.
146. Smith RT Jr, Sade RM, Riopel DA, et al: Stress testing for comparison of synthetic patch aortoplasty with resection and end-to-end anastomosis for repair of coarctation in childhood. J Am Coll Cardiol 4:765–770, 1984.
147. Sweeney MS, Walker WE, Duncan JM, et al: Reoperation for aortic coarctation: Techniques, results, and indications for various approaches. Ann Thorac Surg 40:46–49, 1985.
148. Todd PJ, Dangerfield PH, Hamilton DI, et al: Late effects on the left upper limb of subclavian flap aortoplasty. J Thorac Cardiovasc Surg 85:678–681, 1983.
149. Towbin JA, Belmont J: Molecular determinants of left and right outflow tract obstruction. Am J Med Genet 97:297–303, 2000.
150. Trinquet F, Vouhe PR, Vernant F, et al: Coarctation of the aorta in infants: Which operation? Ann Thorac Surg 45:186–191, 1988.
151. Ungerleider RM, Ebert PE: Indications and techniques for midline approach to aortic coarctation in infants and children. Ann Thorac Surg 44:517–522, 1987.
152. Van Heurn LWE, Wong CM, Spiegelhalter DJ, et al: Surgical treatment of aortic coarctation in infants younger than three months, 1985 to 1990: Success of extended end-to-end arch aortoplasty. J Thorac Cardiovasc Surg 107:74–85, 1994.
153. Van Son JAM: Patterns of ductal tissue in coarctation of the aorta in early infancy. J Thorac Cardiovasc Surg 105:368–369, 1993.
154. Vogel M, Freedom RM, Smallhorn JF, et al: Complete transposition of the great arteries and coarctation of the aorta. Am J Cardiol 53:1627–1632, 1984.
155. von Kodolitsch YV, Muhammet AA, Aydin A, et al: Predictors of aneurysmal formation after surgical correction of aortic coarctation. J Am Coll Cardiol 39:617–624, 2003.
156. Vossschulte K: Surgical correction of coarctation of the aorta by an "isthmusplastic" operation. Thorax 16:338–345, 1961.
157. Wada T, Hideki Y, Miyamoto T, et al: Prevention and detection of spinal cord injury during thoracic and thoracoabdominal aortic repairs. Ann Thorac Surg 72:80–85, 2001.
158. Waldhausen JA, Nahrwold DL: Repair of coarctation of the aorta with a subclavian flap. J Thorac Cardiovasc Surg 51:532–533, 1966.
159. Waldhausen JA, Whitman V, Werner JC, et al: Surgical intervention in infants with coarctation of the aorta. J Thorac Cardiovasc Surg 81:323–325, 1981.
160. Watterson KG, Wilkinson JL, Karl TR, et al: Very small pulmonary arteries: Central end-to-side shunt. Ann Thorac Surg 52:1132–1137, 1991.
161. Webb WR, Burford TH: Gangrene of the arm following use of the subclavian artery in a pulmonosystemic (Blalock) anastomosis. J Thorac Surg 23:199–204, 1952.
162. Wielenga G, Dankmeijer J: Coarctation of the aorta. J Pathol Bacteriol 95:265–274, 1986.
163. Will RJ, Walker OM, Traugott RC, et al: Sodium nitroprusside and propranolol therapy for management of postcoarctectomy hypertension. J Thorac Cardiovasc Surg 75:722–724, 1978.
164. Wong CH, Watson B, Smith J, et al: The use of left heart bypass in adult and recurrent coarctation repair. Eur J Cardiovasc Surg 20:1199–1201, 2001.
165. Yee ES, Turley K, Soifer S, et al: Synthetic patch aortoplasty. Am J Surg 148:240–243, 1984.
166. Younoszai AK, Reddy VM, Hanley FL, et al: Intermediate term follow-up of the end-to-side aortic anastomosis for coarctation of the aorta. Ann Thorac Surg 74:1631–1634, 2002.
167. Ziemer G, Jonas RA, Perry SB, et al: Surgery for coarctation of the aorta in the neonate. Circulation 74(suppl. I):25–31, 1986.

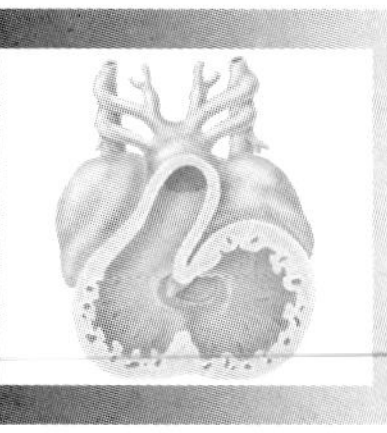

Atrial Septal Defect and Cor Triatriatum

David P. Bichell and Glenn Pelletier

CHAPTER 109

HISTORICAL CONSIDERATIONS

A variety of ingenious surgical corrections of atrial septal defect (ASD) predated the advent of cardiopulmonary bypass. Closed approaches included a blind technique in which a straight needle and suture were passed through both atria guided by palpation, and the free walls of the left and right atria were drawn together to obstruct the defect.[81] Bailey et al described the "atrio-septo-pexy" consisting of a digital invagination of the atrial appendage through the defect with external suture attachment of the atrial tissue to the perimeter of the defect.[3] Tyge Sondergaard devised a purse string external suture closure of ASDs by a near circumferential dissection around the defect in the plane of the interatrial groove and a plication of its edges.[104]

Semiopen techniques prior to cardiopulmonary bypass included notably the atrial well technique, where a right atriotomy was formed, controlled by partial atrial clamping. A 15-cm tall, open-ended rubber cone was then attached to the atriotomy to produce an open column of blood in continuity with the beating heart. Working through the "atrial well" by palpation, the defect was closed by direct suture or patch. Regional intermittent heparinization prevented blood clotting within the well.[44,58,59]

Lewis and Taufic reported the first successful open-heart ASD closure under direct visualization, employing surface cooling and circulatory arrest by inflow occlusion in 1953.[65] Further modification of this technique to include continuous coronary perfusion improved the safety of this and other early intracardiac procedures and represented a precursor to modern myocardial protection techniques.[105]

The modern era of cardiac surgery was heralded by the introduction of the pump oxygenator in 1953, and the earliest application of this technology was for ASD closure.[41] Intracardiac repairs by inflow occlusion were not uniformly replaced by extracorporeal circulation techniques until 1960.

ANATOMY/EMBRYOLOGY

Formation of the Interatrial Septum

The embryonic common atrium undergoes partitioning by the formation of two parallel, overlapping septa, starting in the fourth week of gestation. The crescentic septum primum, emerging at the superior and posterior aspect of the common atrium, begins to septate the atria as the endocardial cushion is forming below to septate the ventricles. The

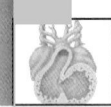

 ostium primum, a gap between the septum primum and the endocardial cushion, closes as the ostium secundum forms by a resorption of the superior aspect of the septum primum. By the end of the sixth week of gestation, the septum secundum begins to form parallel to and immediately rightward of the septum primum, obliterating the remaining ostium primum and circumscribing the fossa ovalis. In its final configuration, the atrial septum consists of the two layers, fused except for the offset openings of the fossa ovalis and the ostium secundum. The free edge of the ostium secundum forms a flap valve covering the left side of the fossa ovalis, providing free right-to-left flow through the foramen ovale until postnatal physiology favors closure of the valve (Figure 109-1). Conditions impairing the competence of the valve, or abnormalities in the formation of its components, lead to a persistent interatrial communication. Right and left omphalomesenteric and cardinal veins drain into the left and right sinus horns, which together form the sinus venosus segment of the posterior common atrium. In the fourth week of gestation, the common pulmonary vein

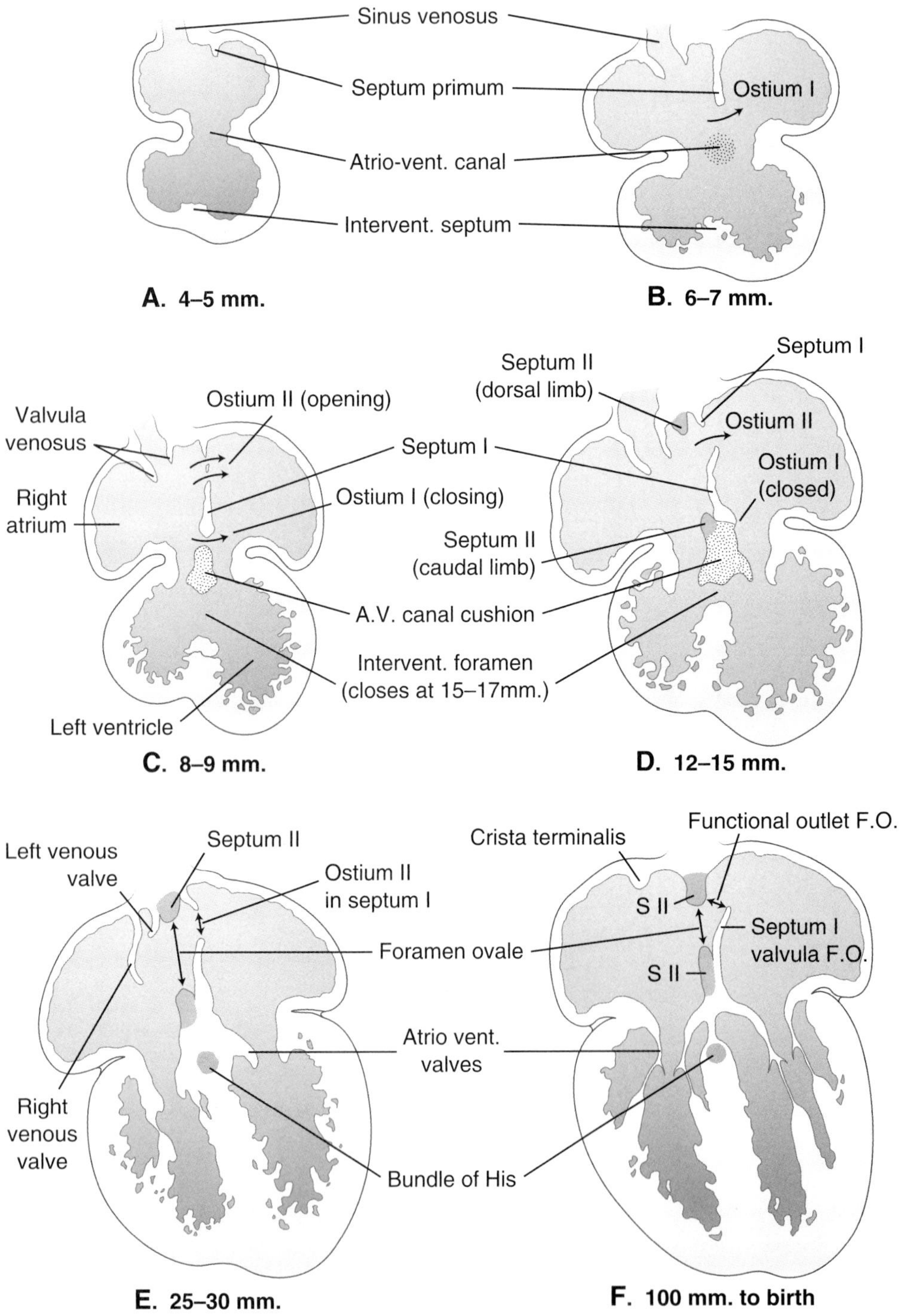

Figure 109–1 Four-chamber sectional diagrams of the fetal heart with particular attention to the morphology of the forming interatrial septum and the foramen ovale. A, The early stages in the formation of the septum primum, from the superior aspect of the common atrium. **B,** As the septum primum grows toward the endocardial cushion, the ostium primum is defined. **C,** As the ostium primum closes, the ostium secundum forms by the resorption of the cephalad portions of the septum primum. **D,** The septum secundum begins to form rightward and parallel to the septum primum, obliterating the remaining ostium primum. **E** and **F,** The septum secundum circumscribes the foramen ovale, and the septum primum creates a flap valve permitting only right-to-left flow.

(Reproduced with permission from Patten BM: Developmental defects at the foramen ovale. Am J Path 14: 135–161, 1938.)

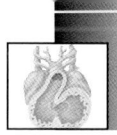

is a midline posterior invagination of the sinus venosus segment into the mesenchyme of the primitive lung buds. The formation of the septum primum directs the common pulmonary vein into the left atrium. Abnormalities in the incorporation of the common pulmonary vein into the left atrium contribute to the formation of partial anomalous pulmonary venous return (PAPVR) and cor triatriatum.

Patent Foramen Ovale

The patent foramen ovale (PFO) denotes a failure of the septum primum and septum secundum to fuse. A failure of fusion results in either a valve-competent "probe patent" PFO or valvular incompetence with or without an aneurysm of the septum primum component (Figure 109-2A). Forces producing an enlarged foramen ovale or a deficient septum primum contribute to incompetence of the valve, a physiologically significant PFO, and transseptal shunting.

Secundum Atrial Septal Defect

The secundum defect lies within the bounds of the fossa ovalis, widely ranging in morphology from the slitlike PFO at the superior aspect of the fossa, to defects involving part or all of the remainder of the fossa with a single or multiply fenestrated communication. Defects of various specific morphologies classified as secundum ASD can form as a result of underdevelopment of the septum secundum or an abnormal pattern of septum primum resorption (Figure 109-2B).[91]

Primum Atrial Septal Defect

The primum defect is a persistence of the ostium primum, and is most commonly associated with an atrioventricular septal defect (Figure 109-2C). This lesion will be discussed further with atrioventricular canal defects.

Sinus Venosus Defect

The sinus venosus interatrial defect is always associated with a partial anomalous pulmonary venous connection. The more common superior variant is an interatrial communication lying posterior and superior to the true atrial septum, and the superior vena cava (SVC) overrides the defect. The right upper pulmonary veins, usually two or more, drain to the right atrium at the superior cavoatrial junction or enter the SVC directly (Figure 109-2D). The less common inferior sinus venosus defect is a communication inferior and posterior to the fossa ovalis with the right pulmonary veins entering the right atrium near the inferior cavoatrial junction. Though the sinus venosus ASD is remote from the true inter-

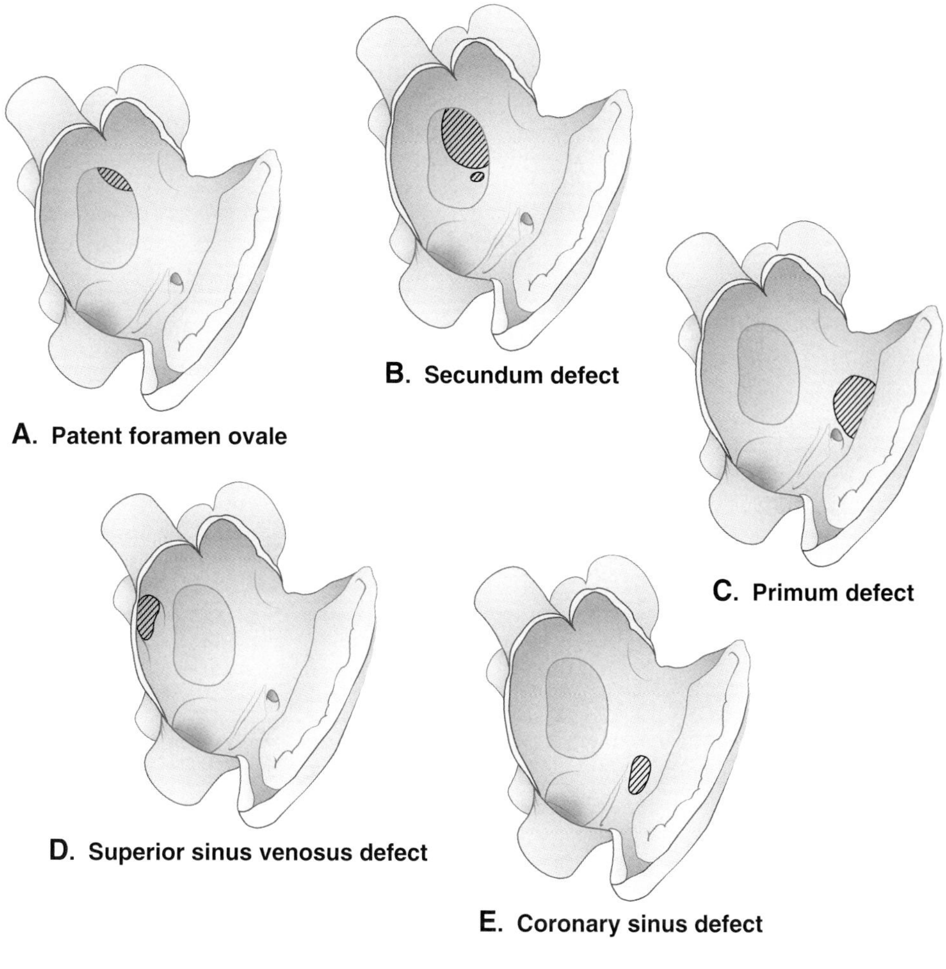

Figure 109–2 The morphological classification of atrial septal defects. A, Patent foramen ovale. **B,** Secundum atrial septal defect. **C,** Primum atrial septal defect. **D,** Superior sinus venosus defect. **E,** Coronary sinus interatrial defect.

atrial septum, a PFO or secundum ASD may additionally be present. Embryologically, the right wall of the common pulmonary vein contributes to the posterior part of the atrial septum. A deficiency in the common wall between the sinus venosus in the right atrium and the common pulmonary vein results in the development of the sinus venosus defect, associating right pulmonary veins with the right atrium.[8,113]

Atrial Septal Aneurysm

Redundant atrial septal tissue within the fossa ovalis with a respiratory excursion greater than 10 mm is termed an atrial septal aneurysm (ASA).[93] The ASA may occur with or without a PFO and has been implicated in the formation of paradoxic embolus. ASA is present in 2% to 4% of the normal population, and 70% of cases are associated with a PFO.[86]

Coronary Sinus–Type ASD

The uncommon coronary sinus–type ASD results from a complete or partial unroofing of the coronary sinus along its course through the floor of the left atrium. A communication of the coronary sinus with the left atrium results in an interatrial communication at the level of the coronary sinus ostium, the size of which is determined by the extent of unroofing and the size of the ostium (Figure 109-2, *E*).

INCIDENCE/NATURAL HISTORY

More than 60% of healthy full-term infants have a PFO.[19] With the fall in pulmonary resistance after birth, the left ventricular end diastolic pressure, and therefore the pressure in the left atrium, exceeds that in the right atrium, and the flap valve consisting of septum primum closes the foramen ovale. Fibrous adhesions form in the first year of life and seal the interatrial communication in a majority of cases. Some continued spontaneous closure of small PFOs occurs throughout life, as the incidence of PFO falls from 36% in the first decade of life to 22% in the 10th decade. The overall incidence of PFO, deduced from a study of 965 autopsy specimens, is 27.3%. A PFO is present in one third of people under 29 years of age, one fourth of those 30 to 79, and one fifth of persons older than 80.[45]

Secundum ASD occurs in 1 in 1500 live births, accounting for 10% to 15% of congenital heart defects in children and 20% to 40% of defects discovered in adults.[12] Women are affected twice as often as men. A significant number of ASDs close spontaneously within the first few years of life, but spontaneous closure after age 3 to 4 is rare.[17,39]

In contrast to children with ASDs, most patients older than 40 years of age are symptomatic and have evidence of elevated pulmonary vascular resistance. Untreated, the average life expectancy is 40–50 years. Seventy-five percent die by age 50, and 90% die by 60 years of age.[12] Even the asymptomatic adult with ASD has a measurably diminished aerobic exercise capacity, which further declines with advancing age.[34]

ASD theoretically could predispose the patient to a higher risk of subacute bacterial endocarditis, though the actual incidence of endocarditis in this setting is rare.

ASSOCIATED FEATURES

Isolated interatrial communication in infancy and childhood is seldom symptomatic even if large, and symptoms of congestive failure should prompt a careful effort to rule out additional associated abnormalities. Associated lesions found in the study of infants with ASD dying in the first year of life included left-to-right shunting lesions, such as ventricular septal defect (VSD) or patent ductus arteriosus (PDA); right-sided obstructive lesions, such as pulmonary stenosis; and left-sided obstructive lesions, such as aortic stenosis, mitral stenosis, or coarctation of the aorta. Necropsy data show that patients with VSD had an associated ASD in 18% of cases, those with left-sided obstruction had an associated ASD in 29% of cases, and those with right-sided obstructive lesions had ASD 31% of cases.[108] These associations support the hypothesis that some secundum ASDs are acquired, driven by remote lesions that favor persistent atrial level shunting and atrial dilation, in turn leading to valvar incompetence at the fossa ovalis.

Mitral valve abnormalities have long been recognized as associated with ASD, though their associated incidence is uncommon. Mitral stenosis with pulmonary artery dilation in association with ASD, known as Lutembacher's syndrome, was perhaps a more frequent association found in the era when rheumatic heart disease was more prevalent, though nonrheumatic mitral stenosis is occasionally found in association with ASD.[68,69] A cleft anterior mitral leaflet, typically associated with a primum ASD, has also been reported in uncommon association with secundum ASD.[24,42,46] Mitral regurgitation is found in 2.5% to 10% of adults with a large ASD.[53] Mitral prolapse may be present in 20% of cases, with a distribution increasing with age.[63] Mitral prolapse may be a result of septal distortion by right ventricular volume overload and a secondary effect on mitral valve geometry. As evidence in favor of this hypothesis, mitral prolapse has been shown to reverse after ASD closure.[101]

Tricuspid regurgitation in association with ASD is usually due to annular dilation from the enlarged right ventricle, and also reverses with ASD closure. In a study of 443 patients presenting with ASD or PAPVR, other associated abnormalities included left superior vena cava (5%), mild or moderate pulmonary stenosis (4%), peripheral pulmonary artery stenosis (1%), azygous extension of inferior vena cava (IVC) (1%), and VSD or PDA (<1%).[58]

HEMODYNAMICS/PATHOPHYSIOLOGY

Left-to-Right Shunt

For the newborn and infant, pulmonary resistance is high, left and right ventricular compliances are similar, and net shunting through an ASD is typically slight. As the left ventricle matures postnatally, it becomes thicker and less compliant in diastole than the right and accounts for higher left atrial pressure than right. This drives a left-to-right shunt at the atrial level in the presence of an ASD. With age, the disparity between systemic and pulmonary resistance, and in turn between left and right ventricular compliance, results in increased left-to-right shunting and advancing right ventricular volume loading. Whereas the normal

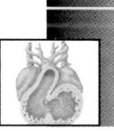

right ventricular diastolic dimension is 0.6 to 1.4 cm/m^2, a large left-to-right shunt can result in right ventricular diastolic dimensions as high as 4 cm/m^2. Over time, right ventricular volume load results in dilation and hypertrophy, eventually affecting the function of both ventricles. Atrial enlargement may contribute to the late incidence of atrial fibrillation.

Volume-induced hypertrophy of the right ventricle produces a loss of coronary reserve and eventual impairment of right ventricular systolic and diastolic function. Left ventricular functional reserve is diminished by adulthood in a majority of patients with ASD. Although left ventricular systolic function may be normal at rest, the left ventricle exhibits a subnormal diastolic dimension, and a loss of functional reserve at exercise. Mechanisms that account for left ventricular dysfunction include septal displacement secondary to right ventricular dilation and hypertrophy, and systolic anterior movement of the mitral valve. In general, the functional loss in the left and right ventricles is normalized 6 months following ASD closure in the child and young adult.[9]

Pulmonary Vascular Disease

Pulmonary hypertension associated with an isolated ASD is rare in childhood, though 35% to 50% of patients with unrepaired ASD have elevated pulmonary resistance by age 40. The development of pulmonary vascular disease is not uniformly related to age or degree of shunting across the ASD. In contrast, patients with VSD predictably develop pulmonary hypertension earlier and more severely, subjected to similar left-to-right shunting and elevated pulmonary blood flow. An explanation remains lacking for why shunts of similar volume from ASDs or VSDs, generating similar elevations in pulmonary blood flow, produce different patterns of pulmonary hypertension. In a study of 128 patients with ASD and pulmonary hypertension (all >18 years of age), one third demonstrated an elevation in PVR before 20 years of age, one third between 20 and 40, and the remainder after 40 years of age.[21]

Histopathological evidence of increased preacinar and intraacinar arterial muscularity in infants with ASD and pulmonary vascular disease suggests that the pulmonary vasculopathy is the primary disorder in the uncommon population with early pulmonary vascular disease, and the ASD may be acquired as a consequence or may be incidentally associated.[49]

Clinical Presentation

A great majority of ASDs are asymptomatic, and palpitations, atrial fibrillation, and congestive failure are late sequelae, uncommon before 40 years of age. Occasional dyspnea on extreme exertion is observed even in children. Recurrent respiratory infection in the presence of a large ASD is not uncommon. Chylothorax has been reported as a presenting manifestation of ASD, cured by ASD closure.[75]

Rarely, ASDs may be associated with cyanosis. Bidirectional shunting across the ASD without an elevation in the pulmonary resistance has been demonstrated as a source of cyanosis.[35] An alternate anatomical source for cyanosis is a streaming of desaturated IVC blood across the ASD, caused by a persistently enlarged Eustachian valve that baffles blood flow into the left atrium.[78,79] More ominously, cyanosis can develop in the setting of advanced irreversible pulmonary hypertension.

Diagnostics/Examination

Findings consistent with ASD at physical exam largely reflect the left-to-right shunting and elevated right ventricular volume and flow. A prominent right ventricle (RV) impulse is present, with a precordial RV lift, leftward displacement of the apex and possible left chest wall prominence.

Auscultatory findings include a systolic flow murmur heard over the left upper sternal border from elevated flow across the pulmonary valve, a split S2, fixed throughout the respiratory cycle, with a prominent pulmonary valve component. An apical mid-diastolic murmur, especially at inspiration, reflects increased flow across the tricuspid valve.

The chest X-ray demonstrates cardiomegaly with prominent pulmonary vascularity and a prominent pulmonary artery bulb.

The electrocardiogram in ASD shows right ventricular hypertrophy, lengthened PR interval, incomplete right bundle branch block and an RSR[81] pattern in V1. The traditional teaching is that a secundum ASD is associated with right axis deviation and incomplete right bundle branch block, whereas a primum defect exhibits left axis deviation with right bundle branch block. Though some of these electrocardiographic findings are reported as useful in children, they are not sensitive diagnostic features in adults[18,43,120] and are seldom referenced in an era when an echocardiographic diagnosis is sensitive, specific, and readily available.

Cardiac catheterization is likewise seldom employed in the diagnosis of ASD, but, when performed, an SVC to RA O_2 saturation step-up is reflective of the left-to-right shunting at the atrial level. A gradient may be detected across the pulmonary valve that is physiological, reflecting the elevated pulmonary blood flow.

SURGICAL INTERVENTION

Indications

The patients benefiting most from ASD closure are those for whom pulmonary hypertension will develop, but once pulmonary hypertension is present, surgical risk increases. This principle is the basis for the recommendation to close all significant ASDs.[40] Elective closure of ASD is generally recommended when the Qp:Qs is 1.5:1 or greater, ideally performed at age 2 to 5 years, before exercise capacity changes, while chest wall compliance is optimal, and before school age. An echo diagnosis of a significant defect with right ventricular volume overload is common and sufficient indication to close an ASD. Long-term follow-up data after surgical ASD closure show survival equal to the normal population when repair is performed early in life, with age-related diminution in survival. Twenty-seven-year survival for those operated on after 40 years of age is only 40%.[80]

Irreversible pulmonary hypertension is the only contraindication to ASD closure. It is important to consider that, in a high flow state, with a large Qp:Qs, high pulmonary artery

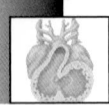

pressure may not represent fixed pulmonary hypertension. Generally, irreversible pulmonary hypertension is characterized by a pulmonary vascular resistance (PVR) 8-12 wood units/m^2, with Qp:Qs <1.2:1, despite a vasodilator challenge.

Moderate pulmonary hypertension with a reactive component is not a contraindication to ASD closure, though pulmonary hypertension may progress in these patients regardless of closure. Guidelines for inoperability are largely based on VSD data. Generally, the PVR must fall below 7 u/m2 with vasodilator therapy at cardiac catheterization for ASD closure risk to be less than prohibitive.[76,84] Vasodilators used at cardiac catheterization to determine the reversible component of pulmonary hypertension include hyperoxia, inhaled nitric oxide, and isoproterenol.[67]

Device versus Surgical Closure

A majority of ASDs today are closed by a variety of catheter-based devices, although the Amplatzer ASD occluder is the only Food and Drug Administration (FDA)-approved device at this time. The success rate and morbidity are nearly equal with the two approaches. Current published studies comparing device closure versus surgical closure with anatomically similar defects show a device success rate of 80% to 95.7%, compared with 95% to 100% success of surgical closure, though the success of device closures continues to evolve. Complications requiring treatment occur in 0% to 8% of device closures and 23% to 24% of surgical closures, and mean length of hospital stay is 1 day in the device group versus 3.4 days in the surgical group.[20,28] Continual advances in the hardware and experience with device closures are improving the success rate of these catheter-based approaches.

Conflicting cost data currently fail to definitively favor device or surgical closure as the more cost-effective approach. The major cost at present for the surgically closed ASD is intensive care unit cost, whereas the major cost of the device closure is the device itself.[4,52] Cost advantage may or may not favor device closure, particularly in light of strategies of early extubation and accelerated postoperative management protocols.

Anatomical determinants that prohibit device closure remain the major indications for surgical ASD closure in the current era. Defects unsuitable for device closure include those that have failed attempted device closure, common atria or those without sufficient septal rim to engage the device, and sinus venosus defects for which device closure would threaten obstruction of pulmonary veins, IVC, or SVC. Anterior-inferior septal deficiency can be prohibitive of device closure, as the device can interfere with the tricuspid valve, mitral valve, or coronary sinus. Individual deficient septal rims, while originally constituting contraindication to device closure, no longer are absolute contraindications but may reduce success rates.[29] The largest Amplatzer septal occlusion device presently available in the United States is 38 mm, and defects exceeding this size would require surgical closure. Multiple defects can be closed with multiple devices, though the cost of multiple device closures may exceed the cost of surgery. Determinants of the limitations to device closure are under evolution as devices and their delivery systems continue to undergo refinements.[94]

Operative Technique

Secundum ASD

The standard surgical incision for the repair of ASD is the median sternotomy. A portion of the anterior pericardium is preserved for use as a patch. Although other materials can be used, we prefer an autologous pericardial patch, treated with glutaraldehyde. Bicaval venous cannulation, mild hypothermia, and antegrade cardioplegia are employed to provide a still, blood-free field through which to expose the interatrial septum via right atriotomy made in parallel to the atrioventricular groove. A careful examination of the interatrial septum is carried out to ensure the correct identification of the margins of the defect. The SVC and IVC are identified, with special attention to any structures that might represent partial anomalous pulmonary venous return to the right atrium or vena cavae. The Eustachian valve is carefully identified to avoid the error of baffling the IVC to the left atrium. The coronary sinus is identified and protected from inclusion in the suture line, as impaired venous effluent from the coronary circulation can result in precipitous cardiac edema and heart failure after separation from cardiopulmonary bypass. A determination is made to close the defect primarily where there is sufficient septum primum tissue, or with a patch. Care is exercised to place sutures firmly into surrounding tissue but without interfering with the adjacent noncoronary sinus of the aorta superiorly, the tricuspid or mitral valves anteriorly, the coronary sinus and atrioventricular AV node inferoanteriorly, the IVC and right lower pulmonary vein orifice inferiorly and posteriorly, or the right upper pulmonary vein and SVC superoposteriorly (Figure 109-3).

Sinus Venosus ASD with PAPVR

The most common variant is superior, bringing the right upper pulmonary vein in association with the right atrium or SVC. A simple patch can be positioned to baffle the pulmonary vein through the septal defect into the left atrium in a majority of cases. When one or more pulmonary veins empty into the SVC sufficiently cephalad to prohibit such baffle without obstruction of the SVC, an adjunctive patch plasty of the lateral SVC must be carried out. Care is exercised to place the superior vena cavotomy sufficiently laterally as to avoid damage to the SA node. Anticipating such geometry, an atriotomy can be planned at the lateral base of the SVC to start with, and the septal patch and caval patch plasty can both be placed through a single atriotomy that can be extended as far as necessary onto the SVC (Figure 109-4). When the right upper pulmonary vein enters the SVC too high to baffle, a Warden procedure is performed. The Warden procedure consists of division and oversewing of the SVC cephalad to the entry of the pulmonary vein, an intraatrial patch baffling the entire SVC orifice to the left atrium, and a reimplantation of the cephalad SVC to the right atrial appendage by direct anastomosis (Figure 109-5).

Primum ASD

Characterized by the absence of any septal tissue between the AV valves, the primum defect closure requires that the

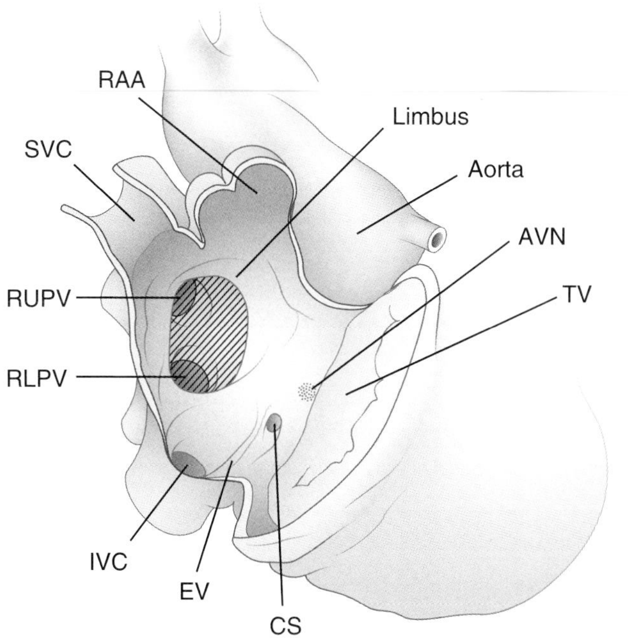

Figure 109–3 Surgical anatomy of the interatrial septum with atrial septal defect. AVN, Atrioventricular node; CS, coronary sinus; EV, eustachian valve; IVC, inferior vena cava; RAA, right atrial appendage; RLPV, right lower pulmonary vein; RUPV, right upper pulmonary vein; SVC, superior vena cava; TV, tricuspid valve.

patch be sutured directly to mitral or tricuspid tissue anteriorly, avoiding the subjacent ventricular septum and the His bundle, and sometimes leaving the coronary sinus on the left atrial side to avoid the AV node. An examination of the mitral valve and closure of the associated cleft is indicated. The primum defect will be discussed fully with AV septal defects.

Minimally Invasive Approaches

A variety of alternatives to the median sternotomy have been described for the repair of numerous cardiac defects, most notably the ASD. An inframammary incision with right anterolateral thoracotomy, bilateral anterior thoracotomy, or median sternotomy provides exposure of the right atrium with a scar that is more easily concealed than the full median sternotomy,[74] though these approaches may risk phrenic nerve palsy, lung herniation, scoliosis, and breast or chest muscle deformity.[14] The subxiphoid "ministernotomy" or partial lower sternotomy can be performed safely through incisions as small as 3.5 cm, with cannulation through the incision.[7] Smaller incisions still, without any sternotomy, have been described, with video-assistance and femoral cannulation.[5] Video-assist technology also permits ASD closure through a small right thoracotomy.[13] Though these alternative incisions may confer a cosmetic advantage over the standard midline incision and median sternotomy, it has been difficult to demonstrate objective advantages in chest wall stability, pulmonary physiology, pain, or length of hospital stay.[62] Robotic-assisted closure of ASD is not widespread, but advances in the field of robotics promise to introduce newer approaches to ASD repair as well as other cardiac procedures through diminishing invasive incisions.

Complications of Surgery

Complications following the surgical closure of ASD include early- or late-patch dehiscence, thromboembolism, and arrhythmias such as heart block, sinus node dysfunction, and atrial fibrillation or flutter. In the rare context of ASD closure with pulmonary hypertension, systemic venous hypertension, right ventricular failure, and low cardiac output can result acutely, necessitating a return to cardiopulmonary bypass to fenestrate the closure.

Though early sinus node dysfunction occurs in 9% of patients undergoing repair of superior sinus venosus defects by either Warden procedure or baffle and SVC patch, 8-year follow-up data show no persistent late sinus node dysfunction following these procedures.[115]

At examination of outcome 27 to 32 years after surgical repair of ASD, age at the time of repair is an independent risk factor for late complications, including late cardiac failure, stroke, and atrial fibrillation, all of which are more frequent when the age at repair is older than 25 years.[80] Independent risk factors for the development of atrial fibrillation with ASD, repaired or not, include age over 25 years, left atrial enlargement, and mitral or tricuspid regurgitation.[87] Thirty to forty percent of patients over 40 who exhibit atrial fibrillation after ASD repair may have an embolic event within 10 years of ASD repair, and systemic anticoagulation is recommended in this group.[48]

Catheter-Based Treatment

King and Mills reported the first catheter-delivered ASD closure in 1976, using a double umbrella device and a 23-Fr delivery catheter. The large-delivery catheter size precluded its use in children.[57] The clamshell occlusion device, reported in 1990, could be delivered through an 11-Fr sheath, bringing device closures to the pediatric population.[99] Device arm fracture resulted in its redesign, and a variety of other devices appeared and remain in use. Current devices include the CardioSEAL (Nitenol Medical, Boston, MA), the Amplatzer (AGA Medical Corp., Golden Valley, MN),[51] the Sideris buttoned occluder (Custom Medical devices, Amarillo, TX),[95] the Das Angel Wings device (Microventa Corp., White Bear Lake, MN),[23] the ASDOS device (Osypka Corp., Rheinfeldon, Germany),[103] the Helix septal occluder (W.L. Gore & associates, Inc., Flagstaff, AZ),[119] and a transcatheter polyurethane foam patch.[102]

Complications of Device Closure

The reported overall complication rate following catheter-deployed ASD closure devices is about 8%. Included among cardiac complications are device malposition or dislocation, early or late embolization, arrhythmia, pericardial effusion, left or right atrial thrombus, atrial or ventricular perforation, mitral or tricuspid regurgitation, aortoatrial fistula, eustachian valve entrapment, and sudden death. Mitral or tricuspid regurgitation can result from device entrapment within chordae, chordal rupture, or leaflet perforation by the device or the delivery system. Reported noncardiac

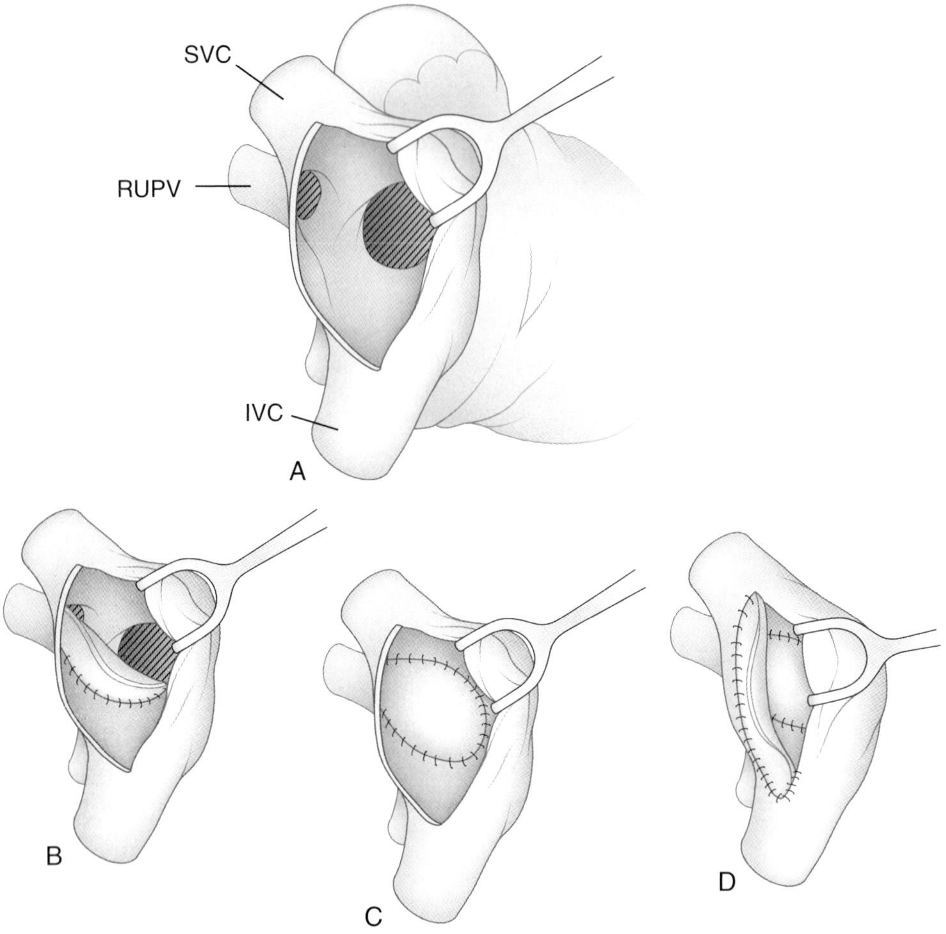

Figure 109–4 **Repair of superior sinus venosus atrial septal defect. A,** A lateral atriotomy provides exposure to the anomalous right upper pulmonary vein. **B,** A pericardial baffle is constructed to direct right upper pulmonary vein flow to the left atrium, through a created or enlarged secundum defect. **C,** Completed intraatrial baffle. **D,** A patch plasty of the atriotomy extends sufficiently cephalad on the superior vena cava to avert caval obstruction. IVC, inferior vena cava; RuPV, right upper pulmonary vein(s); SVC, superior vena cava.

complications include iliac vein dissection, retroperitoneal or groin hematoma, and leg ischemia.[6,15,88,112]

OUTCOME

Physiology of ASD Closure

Subtle changes in exercise performance in ASD patients can be measured even in childhood. An abnormal ventilatory threshold during submaximal exercise returns to normal by 6 months after repair of ASD in patients under 5 years of age, but remains subnormal for patients repaired older than 5 years.[96] Most patients older than 5 years old at the time of repair have at least some residual RV dilation and abnormal septal wall motion after ASD closure, not predicted by preoperative shunt or ASD size.[92] The clinical significance of this finding is unclear. These data may further support a strategy of ASD closure before school age.

Adult

Though the adult with ASD clearly benefits by improvement in exercise physiology and reduction of RV dilation after closure of ASD, the improvements are less pronounced with advancing age.[11,40] There is a clear survival advantage and a reduction in the incidence of cardiovascular events for ASD closure to the age of 40, compared to medical management.[60] Some controversy remains as to the best treatment strategy in the older adult population.

Regardless of the presence of symptoms, RV and RA enlargement in adults decreases after surgical or device closure of ASD, though right atrial enlargement persists proportional to the age at repair.[27,61,107] Though younger adults demonstrate an improved VO2 max within months of ASD closure, patients older than 40 years who undergo repair may take several years to show exercise improvement.[50] The incidence of atrial fibrillation is similar for the patient older than 40 years, whether surgically or medically treated. Though its onset is sooner after surgical closure of ASD, the arrhythmia has a higher relation to long-term mortality in the medically treated group.[2] The significant incidence of sustained postoperative atrial fibrillation suggests that a Maze procedure concurrent with ASD closure may be advisable for the patient older than 40.[36]

Prior to ASD closure, >60% of patients older than 40 are NYHA class III to IV, whereas after ASD closure, >80% are NYHA class I to II.[54] Patients older than 60 show functional class improvement, immediate and late reduction in pulmonary artery pressure, and improved 5- and 10-year survival after ASD closure, by comparison to medical management.[25,106] These data support a strategy of ASD closure regardless of age for the symptomatic patient, though some controversy remains over the closure of the

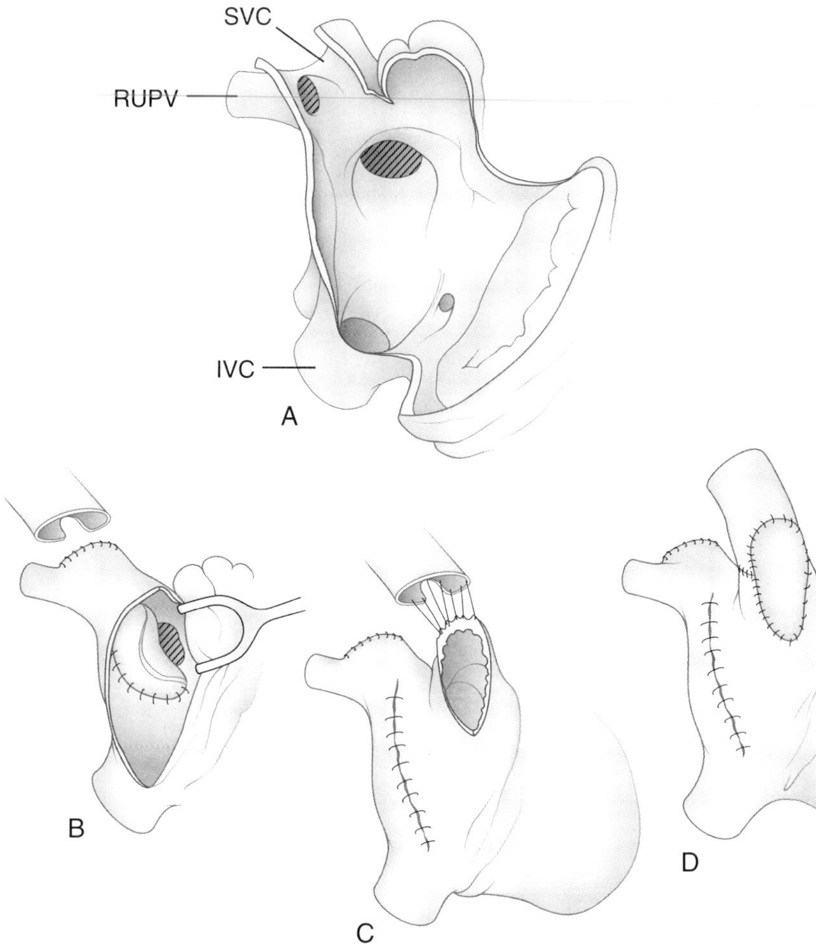

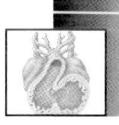

Figure 109–5 The Warden procedure. **A,** Cutaway view of the right atrium, showing the relationship of the displaced right upper pulmonary vein and its distance from the ASD and left atrium. **B,** Superior vena cava transected above the abnormal pulmonary vein. The right upper pulmonary vein with the SVC orifice is baffled to the left atrium. **C,** The transected SVC is anastomosed directly to the right atrial appendage, with **(D)** patch augmentation of the anastomosis averts cavo-atrial obstruction. IVC, inferior vena cava; RUPV, right upper pulmonary vein(s); SVC, superior vena cava.

asymptomatic ASD after age 40, as functional class deterioration and arrhythmia has been observed in this group after ASD closure.[116]

PFO MANAGEMENT

The overall risk of adverse events arising from a PFO is small, and some controversy exists surrounding the indications for intervening in the asymptomatic, incidentally diagnosed case. Adverse events attributed to the presence of a PFO or associated ASA include embolic stroke or peripheral embolus,[47] brain abscess,[26] gas embolization in diver's decompression illness,[77] platypnea-orthodeoxia syndrome,[56] and exacerbated hypoxia in settings of pulmonary embolus or elevated right heart pressures following an RV infarct. The prevention of these events has been the major rationale for interventions to close the hemodynamically insignificant PFO.[1]

Cryptogenic Stroke and PFO

The etiology of stroke in the young adult is unknown in 35% to 50% of cases.[64,117] Evidence supporting the role of PFO in cryptogenic stroke is convincing. Though PFO is thought to be present in 10% to 20% of the general population, it is present in 40% to 70% of patients suffering cryptogenic stroke. For patients under the age of 55 years, the odds ratio of ischemic stroke over controls is 3.1 in the presence of a PFO, 6.14 for ASA alone, and 16 for ASA and PFO. Causality in the over-55 group is less clear, owing likely to various other sources for ischemic stroke that occur concurrently in the older population, though odds ratios remain higher with PFO and/or ASA than without.[89] The presence of untreated PFO predicts a 2.3% risk of recurrent cerebrovascular event by 4 years following the initial event, whereas the presence of ASA and PFO predicts a 15.2% recurrence risk at 4 years.[73] These findings further indict the pocketlike septal aneurysm itself as the likely anatomical substrate for the formation of in situ thromboembolus.

Strategies for treatment of PFO after an ischemic event include PFO closure or medical management with aspirin or Coumadin. Medical management is associated with a 3.4% to 3.8% per year risk of recurrent event, and 2% to 12% risk of hemorrhagic complication.[72] Following device closure of PFO after an ischemic event, the yearly risk of recurrence is reduced to 0% to 3.4%.[10,110,118] Recurrent events following device closures were all within 10 months of device placement, suggesting that a strategy of systemic anticoagulation for 1 year following device closure is prudent.[71]

COR TRIATRIATUM

Cor triatriatum sinistrum, one of the most rare cardiac anomalies, comprises 0.1% of congenital heart defects. In the classic form, described by Church in 1868, cor triatriatum is a separation of the pulmonary veins from the left atrium by a fibromuscular membrane. The anatomical elements of the left atrium, including the atrial appendage, are all ventral to the membrane, and the communication between pulmonary veins and left atrium is restricted to an orifice in the membrane.[16] The membrane can contain single or multiple fenestrations and can also communicate with the right atrium directly, through an ASD or indirectly, through an ascending or descending vertical vein. A variety of classifications have been devised to characterize the various drainage patterns of the pulmonary venous chamber into the heart (Figure 109-6).[30,66]

A subdivided right atrium, sometimes referred to as cor triatriatum dexter, is a membranous division of the right atrium consisting of abnormally attached and persistently enlarged eustachian and thebesian valves, and is unrelated to cor triatriatum sinistrum. The subdividing right atrial membrane may take on a variety of forms, subdividing the right atrium or prolapsing through the tricuspid valve, even to the extent that right ventricular outflow is obstructed.[111]

Embryology

The cor triatriatum sinistrum membrane contains elements of the embryonic common pulmonary vein and the wall of the left atrium. Van Praagh suggests that the dorsal chamber is the embryonic common pulmonary vein, and that entrapment of the left atrial ostium of the common pulmonary vein by sinus venosus tissue results in a failure of the normal course of incorporation into the ventral left atrial chamber during the fifth embryonic week.[113] Van Praagh's explanation is the most widely accepted, though other theories postulate a malformation of the septum primum or an incomplete incorporation of the common pulmonary vein into the left atrium.[33,90]

The partially obstructed pulmonary venous chamber of cor triatriatum may have an ascending or descending vertical vein decompressing it into the systemic venous circulation at the IVC or SVC, similar to that of supracardiac or infracardiac total anomalous pulmonary venous connection.

Associated Abnormalities

Combinations of cor triatriatum and partial anomalous pulmonary venous drainage have been described, with normally draining left- or right-sided veins to the proper left atrium, and contralateral veins connecting to a dorsal venous chamber. Associated partial anomalous pulmonary venous drainage to a vertical vein or to the coronary sinus has been described.[37,97,109] Cor triatriatum has a high association with the presence of a left SVC, an association theorized to be involved in the pathogenesis of cor triatriatum.[38] Additional associations include VSD, tetralogy of Fallot, AV septal defect, and hypoplastic left heart.[70]

Clinical Presentation

The clinical presentation of cor triatriatum is usually in infancy and is manifested by symptoms and signs of pulmonary venous congestion and pulmonary hypertension. Poor growth, episodic exacerbations of pulmonary edema, and frequent pulmonary infections are common. The severity of the presentation is dependent on the degree of pulmonary venous obstruction. Those with a communication to the right atrium generally have a milder progression of symptoms, as the pulmonary venous chamber decompresses into the right atrium. Patients presenting later in life may additionally have syncope, hemoptysis, atrial fibrillation, embolic complications, and right heart failure.[82] The progression of symptoms in the adult with cor triatriatum may be owing to the development of mitral regurgitation.[32] Calcification of the membrane is found in adults and can account for a narrowing of the perforation in the membrane, with a resultant exacerbation of symptoms. In a study of 31 necropsy specimens from untreated patients prior to 1960, the mean age at death was 3.3 months if the ostial diameter was <3 mm, and 16 years for an ostial diameter >3 mm.[85] Patients presenting as adults may exhibit progressive dyspnea and palpitations as presenting symptoms.

The physical exam is remarkable for congested lungs and a prominent second pulmonary sound on auscultation. Findings in patients presenting late with longstanding pulmonary hypertension and right heart failure additionally include liver enlargement and jugular venous distension with a *v* wave. A systolic murmur at the left sternal border may be present.

The electrocardiogram demonstrates peaked p waves, suggesting right atrial enlargement. Right axis deviation and voltage is consistent with right ventricular enlargement.

The chest radiograph shows cardiomegaly consistent with right ventricular enlargement, prominent pulmonary artery and vascular markings.

The diagnosis of cor triatriatum is typically made by echocardiogram, and cardiac catheterization is seldom necessary. Findings at cardiac catheterization include a gradient from pulmonary capillary wedge pressure to left atrium, pulmonary hypertension, venous phase angiographic imaging of an upper chamber, prolonged pulmonary transit time, differential opacification of upper chamber and left atrium, and an occasional linear definition of the membrane.

Pathophysiology

In the anatomical subtype where the orifice of the membrane communicates exclusively with the left atrium, the physiology of cor triatriatum is similar to that of mitral stenosis, with pulmonary congestion and/or edema depending on the degree of restriction at the membrane. For the subtypes with communication to the right atrium, a convoluted pathway of pulmonary venous flow delivers pulmonary venous effluent to the right atrium then back to the left atrium through an interatrial communication below the membrane. Restricted filling of the left heart, low cardiac output, and pulmonary edema results, dependent on the degree of restriction along the pathway to the left atrium.

Pulmonary vein obstruction from cor triatriatum has been demonstrated to produce progressive medial thickening

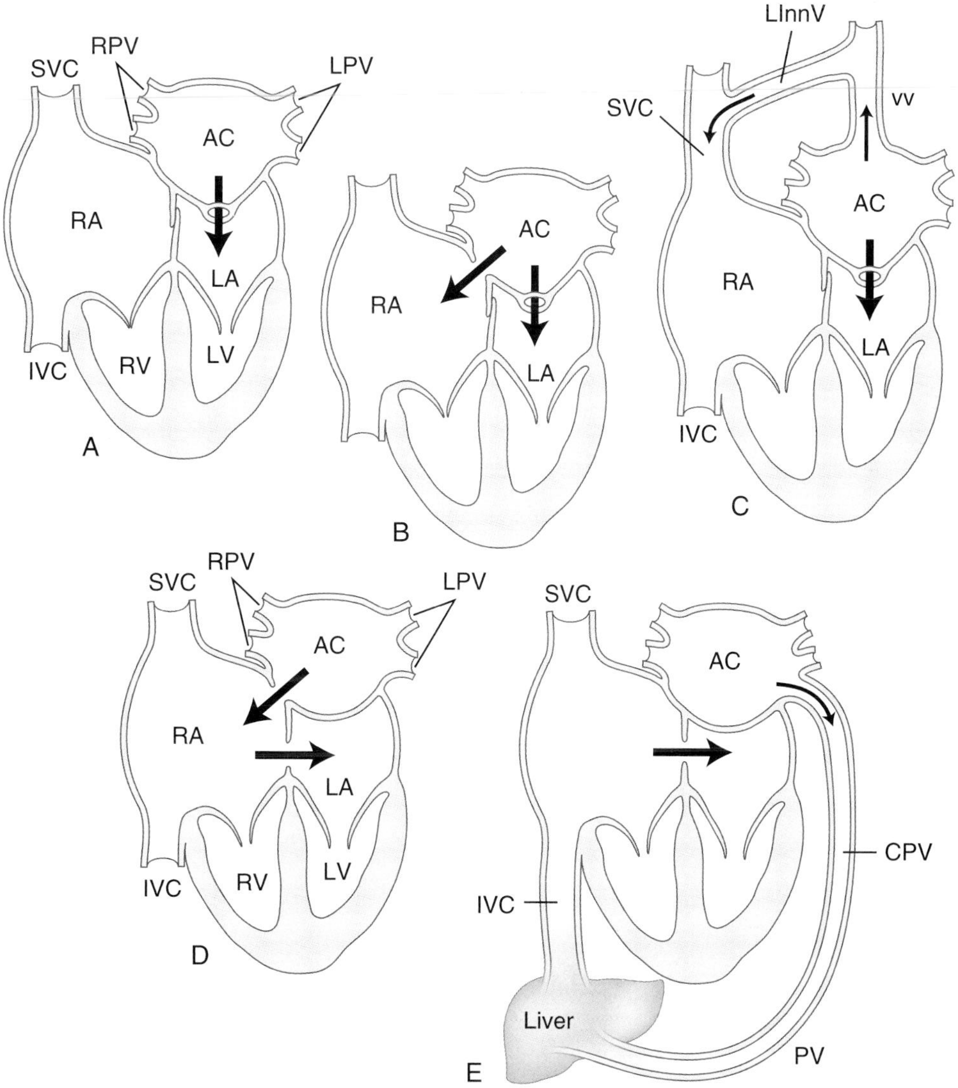

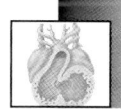

Figure 109–6 The subtypes of cor triatriatum. A, The classic cor triatriatum, with the common pulmonary chamber draining through a restrictive membrane perforation, into the true left atrium. **B,** Communications between the common pulmonary venous chamber and both right and left atria. **C,** A vertical decompressing vein from the common pulmonary venous chamber to the innominate vein. **D,** Pulmonary venous effluent entering the right atrium through a direct communication, and to the left atrium through a secundum atrial septal defect. **E,** An infracardiac vertical decompressing vein from the pulmonary venous chamber to the systemic venous system. *(Reproduced with permission from Hammon JW, Bender HW: Major anomalies of pulmonary and thoracic systemic veins. In: Sabiston DC, Spencer FC [eds]: Surgery of the Chest, 6th ed. Philadelphia: W.B. Saunders Company, 1995, p. 1422.)*

and intimal fibrosis in pulmonary veins and arteries, and lymphangiectasia, though neither as early nor as severe as is the progression of pulmonary vascular disease in VSD. The cellular intimal proliferation and advanced irreversible vascular changes characteristic of VSD or other left to right shunting lesions is not seen with pulmonary venous obstruction, and reversibility is the rule.[31]

When an interatrial communication exists between the proximal chamber and the right atrium, a left-to-right shunt exists. When a communication exists between the right atrium and the underfilled left atrial chamber, a right-to-left shunt can occur.

Treatment and Outcome

Operative Technique

The surgical repair of cor triatriatum is performed with bicaval venous cannulation, moderate hypothermia, and cardioplegic arrest. An examination of the surface anatomy of the heart often confirms the presence of a dilated pulmonary venous chamber behind the heart. The repair is typically performed through a right atriotomy and a subsequent incision into the left atrium across the interatrial septum. Caution is exercised to identify the mitral valve and protect it from injury during the resection of the membrane. Time taken to fully define the membrane prevents injury to adjacent structures, notably the mitral valve. The membrane is widely excised, so as to leave no flow gradient from the pulmonary vein orifices to the mitral inflow region of the left atrium. A careful external examination of the heart exposes any ascending or descending venous structures for ligation.

Small series of surgically treated cor triatriatum report 8% to 20% mortality, though these series are from the early 1990s, and mortality in the present era is likely lower.[99,100,114]

A concomitant Maze procedure has been described for the treatment of adults with cor triatriatum and atrial fibrillation.[83]

Though the standard of care is complete surgical resection of the obstructing membrane, a percutaneous balloon dilation of cor triatriatum membranes by a transseptal approach has been reported.[55]

REFERENCES

1. Alp N, Clarke N, Banning AP: How should patients with patent foramen ovale be managed? Heart 85:242–244, 2001.
2. Attie F, Rosas M, Granados N, et al: Surgical treatment for secundum atrial septal defects in patients >40 years old. J Am Coll Cardiol 38:2035–2042, 2001.
3. Bailey CP, Nichols HT, Bolton HE, et al: Surgical treatment of forty-six interatrial septal defects by atrio-septo-pexy. Ann Surg 140:805–820, 1954.
4. Baker SS, O'Laughlin MP, Jollis JG, et al: Cost implications of closure of atrial septal defect. Cathet Cardiovasc Intervent 55:83–87, 2002.
5. Barbero-Marcial M, Tanamati C, Jatene MB, et al: Transxiphoid approach without median sternotomy for the repair of atrial septal defects. Ann Thorac Surg 65:771–774, 1998.
6. Berdat PA, Chatterjee T, Pfammatter P, et al: Surgical management of complications after transcatheter closure of an atrial septal defect or patent foramen ovale. J Thorac Cardiovasc Surg 120:1034–1039, 2000.
7. Bichell DP, Geva T, Mayer JE, et al: Minimal access approach for the repair of atrial septal defect: the initial 135 patients. Ann Thorac Surg 70:115–118, 2000.
8. Blom NA, Gittenberger-de Groot AC, Jongeneel TH, et al: Normal development of the pulmonary veins in human embryos and formulation of a morphogenetic concept for sinus venosus defects. Am J Cardiol 87:305–309, 2001.
9. Bonow RO, Borer JS, Rosing DR, et al: Left ventricular functional reserve in adult patients with atrial septal defect: Pre- and postoperative studies. Circulation 63:1315-1322, 1981.
10. Bridges ND, Hellenbrand W, Latson L, et al: Transcatheter closure of patent foramen ovale after presumed paradoxic embolism. Circulation 86:1902–1908, 1992.
11. Brochu M-C, Baril J-F, Dore A, et al: Improvement in exercise capacity in asymptomatic and mildly symptomatic adults after atrial septal defect percutaneous closure. Circulation 106:1821–1826, 2002.
12. Campbell M: Natural history of atrial septal defect. Br Heart J 32:820–826, 1970.
13. Chang CH, Lin PJ, Chu JJ, et al: Video-assisted cardiac surgery in closure of atrial septal defects. Ann Thorac Surg 62:697–701, 1996.
14. Cherup LL, Siewers RD, Futrell JW, et al: Breast and pectoral muscle development after anterolateral and posterolateral thoracotomies in children. Ann Thorac Surg 41:492–497, 1986.
15. Chessa M, Carminati M, Butera G, et al: Early and late complications associated with transcatheter occlusion of secundum atrial, septal defect. J Am Coll Cardiol 39:1061–1065, 2002.
16. Church WS: Congenital malformations of the heart: Abnormal septum in the left auricle. Trans Pathol Soc Lond 19:188–190, 1868.
17. Cockerham JT, Martin TC, Gutierrez FR, et al: Spontaneous closure of secundum atrial septal defect in infants and young children. Am J Cardiol 52:1267–1271, 1983.
18. Cohen JS, Patton DJ, Giuffre RM: The crochetage pattern in electrocardiograms of pediatric atrial septal defect patients. Can J Cardiol 16:1241–1247, 2000.
19. Connuck D, Sun JP, Super DM, et al: Incidence of patent ductus arteriosus and patent foramen ovale in normal infants. Am J Cardiol 89:244–247, 2002.
20. Cowley CG, Lloyd TR, Bove EL, et al: Comparison of results of closure of secundum atrial septal defect by surgery versus Amplatzer septal occluder. Am J Cardiol 88:589–591, 2001.
21. Craig RJ, Selzer A: A natural history and prognosis of atrial septal defect. Circulation 37:805–815, 1968.
22. Dalen JE, Haynes FW, Dexter L: Life expectancy with atrial septal defect. Influence of complicating pulmonary vascular disease. JAMA 200:442–446, 1967.
23. Das GS, Harrison JK, O'Laughlin MP: The Angel Wings Das devices for atrial septal defect closure. Curr Interv Cardiol Rep 2:78–85, 2000.
24. Davies RS, Green DC, Brott WH. Secundum atrial septal defect and cleft mitral valve. Ann Thorac Surg 24:28–33, 1977.
25. de Lezo JS, Medina A, Romero M, et al: Effectiveness of percutaneous device occlusion for atrial septal defect in adult patients with pulmonary hypertension. Am Heart J 144: 877–880, 2002.
26. Dethy S, Manto M, Kentos A, et al: PET findings in a brain abscess associated with a silent atrial septal defect. Clin Neurol Neurosurg 97:349–353, 1995.
27. Du Z-D, Cao Q-L, Koenig P, et al: Speed of normalization of right ventricular volume overload after transcatheter closure of atrial septal defect in children and adults. Am J Cardiol 88: 1450–1453, 2001.
28. Du Z-D, Hijazi ZM, Kleinman CS, et al: Comparison between transcatheter and surgical closure of secundum atrial septal defect in children and adults. J Am Coll Cardiol 39:1836–1844, 2002.
29. Du Z-D, Koenig P, Cao Q-L, et al: Comparison of transcatheter closure of secundum atrial septal defect using the Amplatzer septal occluder associated with deficient versus sufficient rims. Am J Cardiol 90:865–869, 2002.
30. Edwards JE: Malformations of the thoracic veins. In: Gould SE (ed): Pathology of the Heart, 2nd ed. Springfield, IL: Charles C Thomas, 1960, p. 484.
31. Endo M, Yamaki S, Ohmi M, et al: Pulmonary vascular changes induced by congenital obstruction of pulmonary venous return. Ann Thorac Surg 69:193–197, 2000.
32. Feld H, Shani J, Rudansky HW, et al: Initial presentation of cor triatriatum in a 55-year old woman. Am Heart J 124: 788–791, 1992.
33. Fowler JK: Membranous band in the left auricle. Trans Pathol Soc London 33:77–94, 1881.
34. Fredriksen PM, Veldtman G, Hechter S, et al: Aerobic capacity in adults with various congenital heart diseases. Am J Cardiol 87:310–314, 2001.
35. Galve E, Angel J, Evangelista A, et al: Bidirectional shunt in uncomplicated atrial septal defect. Br Heart J 51:480–484, 1984.
36. Gatzoulis MA, Freeman MA, Siu SC, et al: Atrial arrhythmia and surgical closure of atrial septal defects in adults. N Engl J Med 340:839–846, 1999.
37. Geggel RL, Fulton DR, Chernoff HL, et al: Cor triatriatum associated with partial anomalous pulmonary venous connection to the coronary sinus: echocardiographic and angiocardiographic features. Pediatr Cardiol 8:279–283, 1987.
38. Gharagozloo F, Bulkley BH, Hutchins GM: A proposed pathogenesis of cor triatriatum: impingement of the left superior vena cava on the developing left atrium. Am Heart J 94:618–626, 1977.
39. Ghisla RP, Hannon DW, Meyer RA, et al: Spontaneous closure of isolated secundum atrial septal defects in infants: An echocardiographic study. Am Heart J 109:1327–1333, 1985.
40. Ghosh S, Chatterjee S, Black E, Firmin RK: Surgical closure of atrial septal defects in adults: Effect of age at operation and outcome. Heart 88:485–487, 2002.
41. Gibbon JH: Application of a mechanical heart and lung apparatus to cardiac surgery. Minn Med 37:171–180, 1954.
42. Goodman DJ, Hancock EW: Secundum atrial septal defect associated with a cleft mitral valve. Br Heart J 35:1315–1320, 1973.
43. Greenstein R, Naaz G, Armstrong WF: Usefulness of electrocardiographic abnormalities for the detection of atrial septal defects in adults. Am J Cardiol 88:1054–1056, 2001.

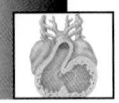

44. Gross RE, Pomeranz AA, Watkins E, et al: Surgical closure of defects of the interauricular septum by use of an atrial well. N Engl J Med 247:455–460, 1952.
45. Hagen PT, Scholz DG, Edwards WD: Incidence and size of patent foramen ovale during the first 10 decades of life: an autopsy study of 965 normal hearts. Mayo Clin Proc 59:17–20, 1984.
46. Hara M, Char F: Partial cleft of septal mitral leaflet associated with atrial septal defect of the secundum type. Am J Cardiol 17:282–285, 1966.
47. Hausmann D, Mugge A, Becht I, et al: Diagnosis of patent foramen ovale by transesophageal echocardiography and association with cerebral and peripheral embolic events. Am J Cardiol 70:668–672, 1992.
48. Hawe A, Rastelli GC, Brandenburg RO, et al: Embolic complications following repair of atrial septal defects. Circulation 39(Suppl I):I-185–191, 1969.
49. Haworth SG: Pulmonary vascular disease in secundum atrial septal defect in childhood. Am J Cardiol 51:265–272, 1983.
50. Helber U, Baumann R, Seboldt H, et al: Atrial septal defects in adults: Cardiorespiratory exercise capacity before and 4 months and 10 years after defect closure. J Am Coll Cardiol 29:1345–1350, 1997.
51. Hijazi ZM, Cao Q, Patel H, et al: Transcatheter closure of atrial communications using the Amplatzer™ septal occluder. J Intervent Cardiol 12:51–58, 1999.
52. Hughes ML, Maskell G, Goh TH, Wilkinson JL: Prospective comparison of costs and short-term health outcomes of surgical versus device closure of atrial septal defect in children. Heart 88:67–70, 2002.
53. Hynes KM, Frye RL, Brandenburg RO, et al: Atrial septal defect (secundum) associated with mitral regurgitation. Am J Cardiol 34:333–338, 1974.
54. Jemielity M, Dyszkiewicz W, Paluszkiewicz L, et al: Do patients over 40 years of age benefit from surgical closure of atrial septal defects? Heart 85:300–303, 2001.
55. Kerkar P, Vora A, Kulkarni H, et al. Percutaneous balloon dilatation of cor triatriatum sinister. Am Heart J 132:888—891, 1996.
56. Kerut EK, Norfleet WT, Plotnick GD: Patent foramen ovale: A review of associated conditions and the impact of physiological size. J Am Coll Cardiol 38:613–623, 2001.
57. King TD, Mills NL: Secundum atrial septal defects: Non-operative closure during cardiac catheterization. JAMA 235: 2506–2509, 1976.
58. Kirklin JW, Barratt-Boyes BG: Cardiac Surgery, 2nd ed. New York: Churchill-Livingstone, 1993, p. 617.
59. Kirklin JW, Ellis FH, Barratt-Boyes BG: Technique for repair of atrial septal defect using the atrial well. Surg Gynecol Obstet 103:646–649, 1956.
60. Konstantinides S, Geibel A, Olschewsky M, et al: A comparison of surgical and medical therapy for atrial septal defect in adults. N Engl J Med 333:469–473, 1995.
61. Kort HW, Balzer DT, Johnson MC: Resolution of right heart enlargement after closure of secundum atrial septal defect with transcatheter technique. J Am Coll Cardiol 38: 1528–1532, 2001.
62. Laussen PC, Bichell DP, McGowan FX, et al: Postoperative recovery in children after minimum versus full-length sternotomy. Ann Thorac Surg 69:591–596, 2000.
63. Leachman RD, Cokkinos DV, Cooley DA: Association of ostium secundum atrial septal defects with mitral valve prolapse. Am J Cardiol 38:167–169, 1976.
64. Lechat P, et al: Prevalence of patent foramen ovale in patients with stroke. N Engl J Med 318:1148–1152, 1988.
65. Lewis FJ, Taufic M: Closure of atrial septal defects with the aid of hypothermia: Experimental accomplishments and the report of the one successful case. Surgery 33:52–59, 1953.
66. Loeffler E: Unusual malformation of the left atrium: Pulmonary sinus. Arch Pathol 48:371–376, 1949.
67. Lupi-Herrera E, Sandoval J, Seoane M, et al: The role of isoproterenol in the preoperative evaluation of high-pressure high-resistance ventricular septal defect. Chest 81:42–46, 1982.
68. Lutembacher R: De la stenose mitrale avec communication interauriculaire. Arch Dis Mal Coeur 9:237–260, 1916.
69. Lutembacher R: Stenose mitral et communication interauriculaire. Arch Dis Mal Coeur 29:229–236, 1936.
70. Marin-Garcia J, Tandon R, Lucas RV Jr, et al: Cor triatriatum: study of 20 cases. Am J Cardiol 35:59–66, 1975.
71. Martin F, Sanchez PL, Doherty E, et al: Percutaneous transcatheter closure of patent foramen ovale in patients with paradoxical embolis. Circulation 106:1121–1126, 2002.
72. Mas JL, Zuber M: Recurrent cerebrovascular events in patients with patent foramen ovale, atrial septal aneurysm, or both and cryptogenic stroke or transient ischemic attack. French Study Group on Patent Foramen Ovale and Atrial Septal Aneurysm. Am Heart J 130:1083–1088, 1995.
73. Mas JL, Arquizan C, Lamy C, et al: Recurrent cerebrovascular events associated with patent foramen ovale, atrial septal aneurysm, or both. N Engl J Med 345:1740–1746, 2001.
74. Massetti M, Babatasi G, Rossi A, et al: Operation for atrial septal defect through a right anterolateral thoracotomy. Ann Thorac Surg 62:1100–1103, 1996.
75. Mignosa C, Vincenzo D, Ferlazzo G, et al: Chylothorax: An unusual manifestation of a large atrial septal defect. J Thorac Cardiovasc Surg 122:1252–1253, 2001.
76. Momma K, Takao H, Ando M, et al: Natural and postoperative history of pulmonary vascular obstruction associated with ventricular septal defect. Jpn Circ J 45:230–237, 1981.
77. Moon RE, Camporesi EM, Kisslo JA, et al: Patent foramen ovale and decompression sickness in divers. Lancet 1:513–514, 1989.
78. Morishita Y, Yamashita M, Yamada K, et al: Cyanosis in atrial septal defect due to persistent eustachian valve. Ann Thorac Surg 40:614–616, 1985.
79. Morrison JG, Merrill WH, Friesinger GC, et al: Cyanosis, interatrial communication, and normal pulmonary vascular resistance in adults. Am J Cardiol 58:1128–1129, 1986.
80. Murphy JG, Gersh BJ, McGoon MD, et al: Long-term outcome after surgical repair of isolated atrial septal defect. Follow-up at 27-32 years. N Engl J Med 323(24):1645–1650, 1990.
81. Murray G: Closure of defects in cardiac septa. Ann Surg 128:843–853, 1948.
82. Nagatsu M: Clinical classification and surgical treatment of cor triatriatum Jpn J Cardiothorac Surg 40:473–484, 1992.
83. Nakajima H, Kobayashi J, Kurita T, Kitamura S. Maze procedure and cor triatriatum repair. Ann Thorac Surg74:251–253, 2002.
84. Neutze JM, Ishikawa T, Clarkson PM, et al: Assessment and follow-up of patients with ventricular septal defect and elevated pulmonary vascular resistance. J Am Coll Cardiol 63: 327–331, 1989.
85. Niwayama G: Cor triatriatum, a review. Am Heart J 59:291–317, 1960.
86. Olivares-Reyes A, Chan S, Lazar EJ, et al: Atrial septal aneurysm: a new classification in two hundred five adults. J Am Soc Echocardiogr 10:644–656, 1997.
87. Olivier JM, Gallego P, Gonzalez A, et al: Predisposing conditions for atrial fibrillation in atrial septal defect with and without operative closure. Am J Cardiol 89:39–43, 2002.
88. Onorato E, Pera IG, Melzi G, et al: Persistent redundant Eustachian valve interfering with Amplatzer PFO occluder placement: Anatomico-clinical and technical implications. Cathet Cardiovasc Intervent 55:521–524, 2002.
89. Overell JR, Bone I, Lees KR: Interatrial septal abnormalities and stroke. A meta-analysis of case control studies. Neurology 55:1172–1179, 2000.

90. Parsons CG. Cor triatriatum: Concerning the nature of an anomalous septum in the left auricle. Br Heart J 12:327–338, 1950.
91. Patten BM: Developmental defects at the foramen ovale. Am J Path 14:135–161, 1938.
92. Pearlman AS, Borer JS, Clark CE, et al: Abnormal right ventricular size and ventricular septal motion after atrial septal defect closure. Am J Cardiol 41:295–301, 1978.
93. Pearson AC, Nagelhout D, Castello R, et al: Atrial septal aneurysm and stroke: a transesophageal echocardiographic study. J Am Coll Cardiol 18:1223–1229, 1991.
94. Podnar T, Martanovic P, Gavora P, et al: Morphological variations of secundum-type atrial septal defects: feasibility for percutaneous closure using the Amplatzer septal occluders. Cathet Cardiovasc Intervent 53:386–391, 2001.
95. Rao PS, Berger F, Rey C, et al: Results of transvenous occlusion of secundum atrial septal defects with the fourth generation buttoned device: Comparison with first, second, and third generation devices. J Am Coll Cardiol 36:583–592, 2000.
96. Reybrouck T, Bisschop A, Dumoulin M, et al: Cardiorespiratory exercise capacity after surgical closure of atrial septal defect is influenced by the age at surgery. Am Heart J 122:1073–1078, 1991.
97. Richardson JV, Doty DB, Siewers RD, et al: Cor triatriatum (subdivided left atrium). J Thorac Cardiovasc Surg 81:232, 1981.
98. Rodefeld MD, Brown JW, Heimansohn DA, et al: Cor triatriatum: Clinical presentation and surgical results in 12 patients. Ann Thorac Surg 50:562–568, 1990.
99. Rome JJ, Keane JF, Perry SB, et al: Double umbrella closure of atrial septal defects: initial clinical applications. Circulation 82:751–758, 1990.
100. Salamone G, Tiraboschi R, Bianchi T, et al: Cor triatriatum: Clinical presentation and operative results. J Thorac Cardiovasc Surg 101:1088–1092, 1991.
101. Schreiber TL, Feigenbaum H, Weyman AE: Effect of atrial septal defect repair on left ventricular geometry and degree of mitral valve prolapse. Circulation 61:888–896, 1980.
102. Sideris EB, Toumanides S, Macuil B, et al: Transcatheter patch correction of secundum atrial septal defects. Am J Cardiol 89:1082–1086, 2002.
103. Sievart H, Babic UU, Hausdorf G, et al: Transcatheter closure of atrial septal defect and patent foramen ovale with the ASDOS device (a multi-institutional European trial). Am J Cardiol 82:1405–1413, 1998.
104. Sondergaard T: Closure of atrial septal defects: Report of three cases. Acta Chir Scand 107:492–498, 1954.
105. Spencer FC, Bahnson HT: Intracardiac surgery employing hypothermia and coronary perfusion performed on 100 patients. Surgery 46:987–995, 1959.
106. St. John-Sutton MG, Tajik AJ, McGoon DC: Atrial septal defects in patients ages 60 years or older: Operative results and long-term postoperative follow-up. Circulation 64: 402–409, 1981.
107. Steele PM, Fuster V, Cohen M, et al: Isolated atrial septal defect with pulmonary vascular obstructive disease: long-term follow-up and prediction of outcome after surgical correction. Circulation 76:1037–1042, 1987.
108. Tandon R, Edwards JE: Atrial septal defect in infancy. Common association with other anomalies. Circulation 49:1005–1010, 1974.
109. Thilenius OG, Bharati S, Lev M: Subdivided left atrium: an expanded concept of cor triatriatum sinistrum. Am J Cardiol 37:743–752, 1976.
110. Tobis J: The case for closing PFOs. Cathet Cardiovasc Intervent 55:195–196, 2002.
111. Trento A, Zuberbuhler JR, Anderson RH, et al: Divided right atrium (prominence of the eustachian and thebesian valves). J Thorac Cardiovasc Surg 96:457–463, 1988.
112. Vanderheyden M, Willaert W, Claessens P, et al: Thrombosis of a patent foramen ovale closure device: Thrombolytic management. Cathet Cardiovasc Intervent 56: 522–526, 2002.
113. Van Praagh R, Corsini I: Cor Triatriatum: Pathologic anatomy and a consideration of morphogenesis based on 13 post mortem cases and a study of normal development of the pulmonary vein and atrial septum in 83 human embryos. Am Heart J 78:379–405, 1969.
114. Van Son JAM, Danielson GK, Schaff HV, et al: Cor triatriatum: Diagnosis, operative approach, and late results. Mayo Clin Proc 68:854–859, 1993.
115. Walker RE, Mayer JE, Alexander ME, et al: Paucity of sinus node dysfunction following repair of sinus venosus defects in children. Am J Cardiol 87:1223–1226, 2001.
116. Webb G: Do patients over 40 years of age benefit from closure of an atrial septal defect? Heart 85:249–250, 2001.
117. Webster MW, Chancellor AM, Smith AM, et al: Patent foramen ovale in young stroke patients. Lancet 2:11–12, 1988.
118. Windecker S, Wahl A, Chatterjee T, et al: Percutaneous closure of patent foramen ovale in patients with paradoxic embolism: Long-term risk of recurrent thromboembolic events. Circulation 101:893–898, 2000.
119. Zahn EM, Wilson N, Cutright W, et al: Development and testing of the Helix septal occluder, a new expanded polytetrafluoroethylene atrial septal defect occlusion system. Circulation 104:711–716, 2001.
120. Zufelt K, Rosenberg HC, Li MD, et al: The electrocardiogram and the secundum atrial septal defect. A reexamination in the era of echocardiography. Can J Cardiol 14:227–232, 1998.

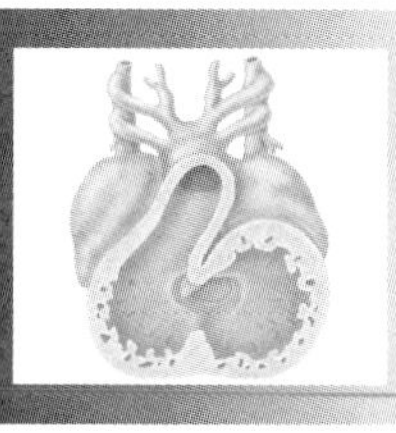

CHAPTER 110

Surgical Considerations in Pulmonary Vein Anomalies

Christopher A. Caldarone

ETIOLOGY

Normal embryological development of the pulmonary venous system involves creation of a connection between the left atrium and the pulmonary venous plexus and subsequent regression of systemic-to-pulmonary venous connections. Inappropriate connection of the pulmonary venous system to the systemic venous system is termed anomalous pulmonary venous drainage.

As part of normal embryological development, the lungs form as buds arising from the primitive foregut. During the initial stages of pulmonary development, the pulmonary venous drainage is through the cardinal and umbilical–vitelline venous systems (systemic veins). During later stages of development, an outpouching of the common atrium forms to the leftward of the developing septum primum.[31] This structure, termed the common pulmonary vein, primordial pulmonary vein, or pulmonary pit, extends and bifurcates into the pulmonary venous plexus and establishes venous draining of the developing lung buds (Figure 110-1).[30] Thereafter, the connections between the lung buds and the systemic venous system regress, leaving the developing lungs with direct drainage to the left atrium.

Anomalous pulmonary venous drainage can result from failure of fusion between the left atrial outpouching and the pulmonary venous plexus or from malposition of the relationship between the atrial outpouching and the developing atrial septum. If all of the pulmonary veins maintain an anomalous connection to a single systemic venous site, the lesion is termed total anomalous pulmonary venous drainage. In contradistinction, if all the pulmonary veins drain anomalously to multiple discrete systemic veins, the lesion is called mixed total anomalous pulmonary venous drainage. If one to three pulmonary veins drain via an anomalous pathway and at least one pulmonary vein drains to the left atrium, the lesion is termed partial anomalous pulmonary venous drainage.

PARTIAL ANOMALOUS PULMONARY VENOUS DRAINAGE

Anatomy

Partial anomalous pulmonary venous drainage is characterized by a failure of one to three of the pulmonary veins to connect with the left atrium during fetal development. Typically the pulmonary vein has an abnormal connection to the superior vena cava near the cavoatrial junction. In more than 80% of patients, the lesion is associated with another congenital heart defect, the most common of which is an atrial septal defect, although in a minority of patients, the atrial septum is intact.[15] Most commonly a combination of right-upper and middle lobe drainage occurs at once,

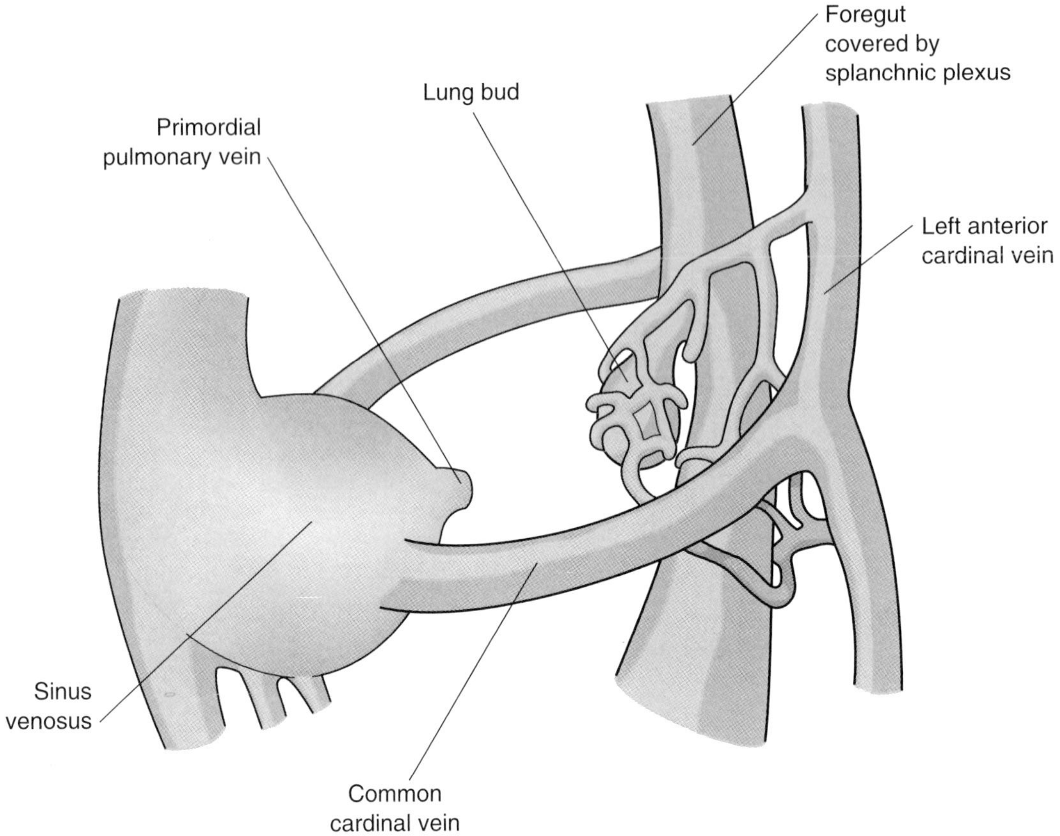

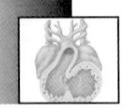

Figure 110–1 During embryological development, lung buds arise from the primitive foregut with systemic venous drainage. In later stages an outpouching from the common atrium extends and bifurcates into the pulmonary venous plexus to establish drainage to the atrium, followed by regression of the systemic venous drainage.
(Modified from Jonas RA, Smolinsky A, Mayer JE, et al: Obstructed pulmonary venous drainage with total anomalous pulmonary venous connection to the coronary sinus. Am J Cardiol 59:431–435, 1987.)

draining to the superior vena caval–right atrial junction. Less commonly, isolated anomalous right upper lobe venous drainage is present. Least commonly, the entire right lung drains via an anomalous vein.[11] Other less common sites of anomalous venous drainage include the inferior vena cava (e.g., as part of the scimitar syndrome), the left-sided superior vena cava, and the innominate vein.

Presentation

Patients often are asymptomatic and display a murmur noted on routine examination caused by increased flow across the pulmonic valve. A split and prominent second heart sound also is present. Symptomatic patients display the sequelae of a left-to-right shunt and, consequently, have symptoms including decreased exercise tolerance and poor growth. Patients are not cyanotic unless they have developed pulmonary hypertension as a late manifestation of a large left-to-right shunt. In such patients, Eisenmenger's syndrome is manifested by the reversal of the shunt (right to left) in association with an atrial septal defect.

Pathophysiology

The dominant hemodynamic abnormality is related to the left-to-right shunt imposed by pulmonary venous drainage into the right atrium. In the absence of an atrial septal defect, the left-to-right shunt is determined by the amount of flow in the anomalous pulmonary vein. An associated atrial septal defect adds potential for increased left-to-right shunting at the atrial level. Increased right-sided flow can lead to right ventricular dilation, tricuspid insufficiency, and supraventricular arrhythmias.

Surgical Repair

The goal of surgical therapy is to divert the anomalous pulmonary venous effluent to the left atrium in an unobstructed fashion. In the presence of a sinus venosus atrial septal defect and an anomalous right upper pulmonary vein, the flow is diverted with a baffle constructed along the edge of the sinus venosus atrial septal defect (see Chapter 109). In the absence of an atrial septal defect (e.g., intact atrial septum), a septal defect must be created and a similar baffle constructed to divert flow from the anomalous pulmonary vein to the newly created atrial septal defect.

Planning the Superior Vena Caval Cannulation

Careful review of anatomy with preoperative echocardiogram, computed tomography (CT) scan, or magnetic resonance imaging (MRI) is the single most important component in developing an operative plan. Definition of the pulmonary venous anatomy and associated defects allows assessment of options for cannulation techniques and surgical approaches. This point is especially pertinent in partial anomalous pulmonary venous drainage, in which the location of the anomalous pulmonary venous drainage influences the feasibility of a minimally invasive sternotomy incision and placement of venous cannulas. A common clinical scenario involves an anomalous right upper pulmonary vein inserting high into the superior vena cava at or above the level of the pulmonary artery. Options for control of the superior vena cava include a high cannulation of the superior vena cava, cannulation of the innominate vein, or percutaneous cannulation via the internal jugular vein with vacuum-assisted venous drainage. A minimally invasive approach through a lower midline partial sternal split can be difficult when a high insertion of an anomalous pulmonary vein is present. A final technique to consider is to cannulate the right atrium and direct the catheter into the superior vena cava. After snaring the cava around the cannula (above the anomalous pulmonary vein insertion), an atrial incision allows access to the origin of the anomalous pulmonary vein from within the atrium. Although this technique is easily accomplished with a minimally invasive lower midline partial sternal split, working around the cannula through the right atrial–superior vena caval junction can be challenging.

Before initiation of cardiopulmonary bypass, the location of the pulmonary veins is confirmed. Drainage to the superior vena cava requires dissection of the lateral margin of the superior vena cava to identify all pulmonary vein branches. Frequently, multiple branches drain into the vena cava through a large confluence. The source of the veins is not always clear, and the identification of any systemic veins draining into the region must be clarified. In ambiguous cases, a needle aspiration determines the oxygen saturation of the effluent and hence its origin.

After heparinization, cannulation, and initiation of normothermic cardiopulmonary bypass, the aorta is clamped and blood cardioplegic arrest is obtained. It often is helpful to place a vent into the left atrium for later deairing. A lateral right atriotomy is made and the atrium explored for identification of any additional anomalies (Figure 110-2). If the atrial septum is intact, an atrial septal defect is created by incising the region of the foramen ovale and extending the incision across the limbus in the direction of the anomalous pulmonary vein. Resection within the region of the limbus allows enlargement of the newly created atrial septal defect. Injury to the sinus node artery can occur when creating the atrial septal defect in patients whose artery courses through the superior portion of the interatrial septum. Typically a glutaraldehyde-treated pericardial patch can be used to create a baffle so that pulmonary venous blood flows beneath the baffle and through the atrial septal defect into the left atrium.

Systemic venous blood from the superior vena cava must pass over this baffle into the right atrium without obstruction. If the origin of the pulmonary vein is high in the superior vena cava, the baffle must be carefully constructed to avoid obstruction to flow on either side of the baffle. A longitudinal incision in the lateral aspect of the superior vena cava allows the baffle construction to be better visualized. Placement of the incision on the lateral aspect of the superior vena cava is important to diminish the risk of injury to the sinus node. Closure of the superior vena cava incision with a generous patch to augment its diameter allows unobstructed flow on both sides of the baffle.

Alternatively, a new anastomosis between the superior vena cava and right atrial appendage is established by dividing the superior vena cava cephalad to the anomalous pulmonary venous entry and translocating the cephalad end of the superior vena cava to the right atrial appendage. The divided cardiac end of the superior vena cava (bearing the anomalous pulmonary venous connection) is closed, and within the right atrium, a baffle is created from the orifice of the superior vena cava to the newly created atrial septal defect.[11] By creating a new superior vena caval–right atrial junction, this procedure eliminates the need to partition the superior vena cava with a baffle dividing the systemic and pulmonary venous flow paths. This approach may be particularly helpful in infants and small children with a high insertion of an anomalous pulmonary vein into the superior vena cava.

Results

Long-term prognosis for patients after repair is excellent. In children, closure of an associated atrial septal defect almost eliminates the risk of late development of atrial arrhythmias. However, in adults, closure of an atrial septal defect is associated with persistent risk of late development of atrial arrhythmias.[9] Although extrapolation of these data for atrial septal defect closure to patients with partial anomalous pulmonary venous drainage and intact atrial septum has not been specifically validated, it seems reasonable to conclude that early removal of a left-to-right shunt associated with right ventricular overload is appropriate.

Pertinent complications after repair of partial anomalous pulmonary venous drainage include stenosis of the superior vena cava or the anomalous pulmonary vein, residual atrial septal defects, and atrial arrhythmias. Failure to include all pulmonary veins in the newly constructed baffle to the left atrium can result in a residual left-to-right shunt. Conversely, incorporation of a systemic vein into the newly constructed baffle results in a residual right-to-left shunt. Finally, injury to the sinus node or sinus node artery can lead to the requirement for pacemaker insertion in patients with severe sinus node dysfunction.

SCIMITAR SYNDROME

Anatomy

Scimitar syndrome is an unusual congenital anomaly that is manifested by partial anomalous pulmonary venous drainage of the right lung to the inferior vena cava and is often associated with hypoplasia of the right lung, dextrocardia, systemic pulmonary arterial supply from the abdominal aorta to the lower lobe of the right lung, and bronchial abnormalities. Other commonly associated anomalies include atrial septal defect, aortic coarctation, and a left-sided superior vena cava.[16] The morphology of the anomalous pulmonary venous drainage to the right lower lobe creates a characteristic appearance to the right-sided heart border suggestive of a Turkish sword, hence the term “scimitar syndrome”

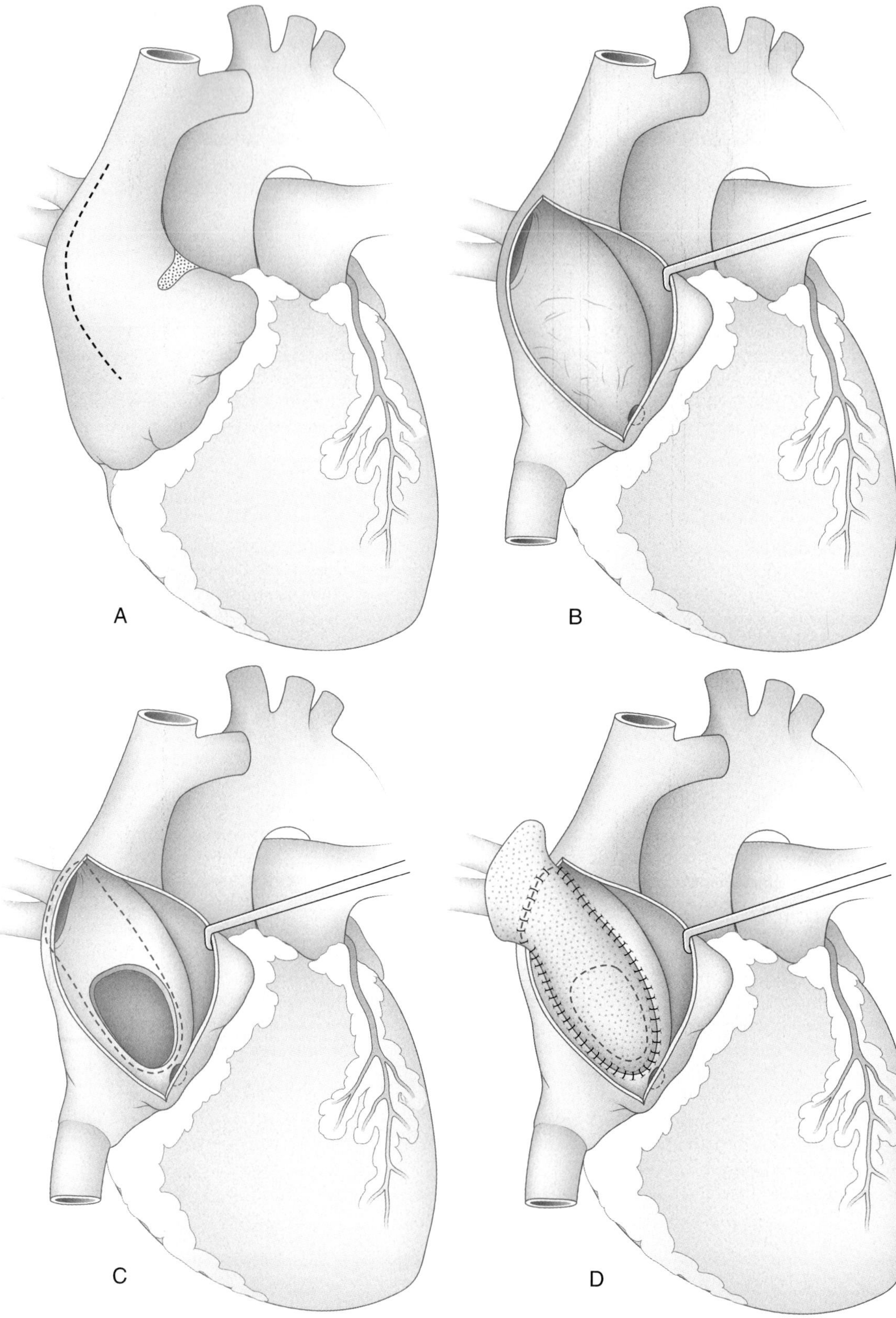

Figure 110–2 Surgical exposure for repair of partial anomalous drainage of the right upper pulmonary vein with intact atrial septum. After initiation of cardiopulmonary bypass and cardioplegic arrest, a right atrial incision is made as shown in the dashed line in **A**. The stippled area represents the approximate location of the sinoatrial node. Retraction of the atrial wall (**B**) reveals the intact atrial septum and the combined orifice of the anomalous right upper pulmonary veins. A secundum type of atrial septal defect is created by excising the septum primum in the region of the limbus, with care taken to avoid potential injury to the conduction system by keeping well clear of the triangle of Koch (**C**). The limbus can be resected cephalad to increase the diameter of the orifice. A patch of glutaraldehyde-treated pericardium is sutured in place along the rim of the newly created defect, thereby creating a tunnel from the pulmonary vein orifice to the left atrium (**D**).

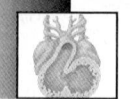

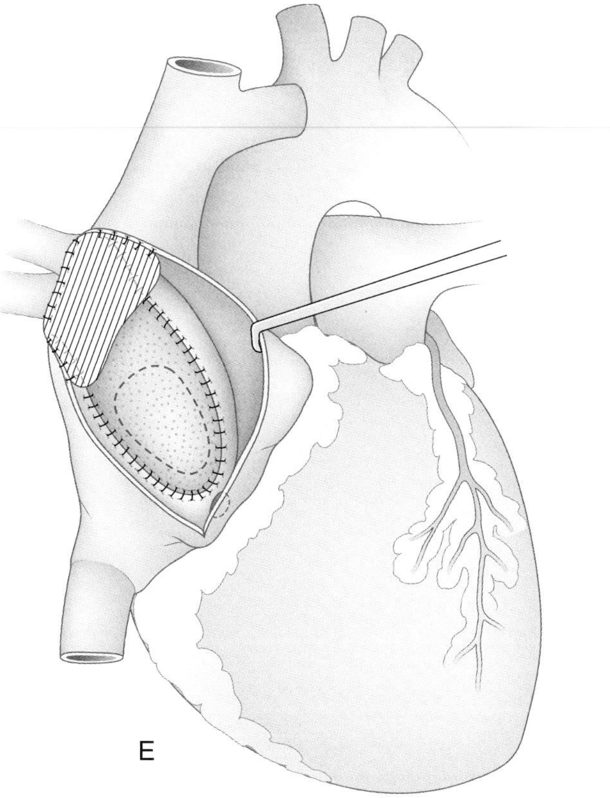

Figure 110–2 cont'd The patch is deliberately longer than necessary to reach the pulmonary vein orifice, and the redundant portion is left unattached as the suture line is extended across the edge of the divided pulmonary vein–atrial edge. The redundant portion of the patch is then folded anteriorly to augment the diameter of the superior cavoatrial junction, thereby preventing superior vena cava syndrome (**E**).

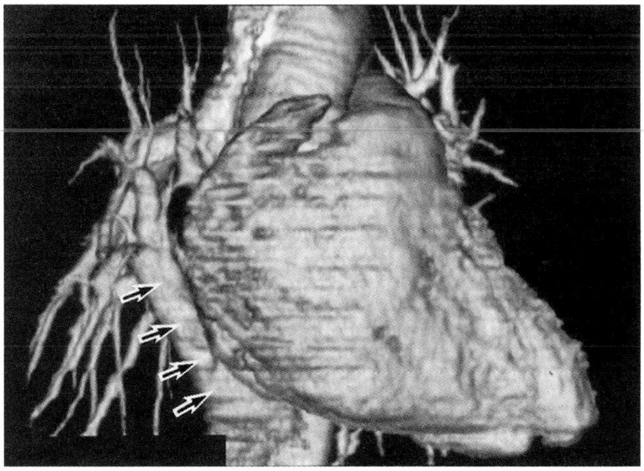

Figure 110–3 Magnetic resonance image of scimitar syndrome. The anomalous right-sided pulmonary venous drainage *(arrows)* draining to the inferior vena cava contributes to the "scimitar" shadow on routine chest X-ray.
(From Inoue T, Ichihara M, Uchida T, et al: Three-dimensional computed tomography showing partial anomalous pulmonary venous connection complicated by the scimitar syndrome. Circulation 105:663, 2002.).

(Figure 110-3). The right-sided pulmonary veins drain to the inferior portions of the right atrium, the inferior vena caval–right atrial junction, or, more commonly, the inferior vena cava below the diaphragm. There frequently is some stenosis present at the junction of the anomalous pulmonary vein and the vena cava.

The presentation of patients with scimitar syndrome can be variable and depends on the severity of the associated lesions. At the most benign end of the spectrum, patients can display an asymptomatic flow murmur on physical examination as a result of increased pulmonary flow secondary to the left-to-right shunt caused by the anomalous pulmonary venous drainage to the inferior vena cava. At the most severe end of the spectrum, infants can have presenting symptoms of severe congestive heart failure, failure to thrive, tachypnea, and occasionally cyanosis. Infantile pulmonary artery pressures are often elevated (e.g., >40% of the systemic pressure) with a Qp/Qs of ~2:1.[24]

Surgical Management

The management strategy for patients with scimitar syndrome is determined by the degree of right lung hypoplasia, the presence of aortopulmonary sources of blood flow to the right lung, and the location and pattern of the right-sided pulmonary venous drainage. The degree of right lung hypoplasia is an important determinant of the likelihood of salvaging a functional right lung, and in cases of severe hypoplasia, a right pneumonectomy has been advocated.[16] In cases with less severe hypoplasia, attention is turned to correction of the pulmonary venous drainage patterns, control of aortopulmonary sources of blood flow, and correction of associated anomalies. Control of the aortopulmonary sources of blood flow can be achieved through coil embolization in the catheterization laboratory or by ligation in the operating room.

Surgical repair of the pulmonary venous drainage is designed to create unobstructed flow from the anomalous pulmonary vein to the left atrium. For this objective to be accomplished, a direct surgical approach is to place a long baffle within the lumen of the inferior vena cava to channel the anomalous pulmonary vein effluent to the right atrium, and then through an atrial septal defect to the left atrium. It can be challenging to create an unobstructed baffle when the anomalous pulmonary venous connection is relatively caudad in the inferior vena cava. In such a case a period of circulatory arrest is necessary to segregate the pulmonary vein orifice from the hepatic veins that may be in proximity. A right atrial incision can be carried down to the level of the anomalous pulmonary vein orifice, and the orifice is augmented with a patch of autologous pericardium if it is stenotic. The baffle is then created within the lumen of the inferior vena cava, and, if necessary, the inferior vena cava diameter can be augmented with a patch to ensure that there is no residual obstruction in the vena cava or the pulmonary venous flow pathway. This technique has a relatively high incidence of late stenosis, presumably because of the length of the baffle and because the blood must pass through a near-180° turn as it travels caudally to the inferior vena cava and then cephalad up through the baffle to the atrial septal defect.[16]

A second approach is to divide the anomalous pulmonary vein and reimplant it at a convenient location in the right atrium and then create a baffle to divert flow to the left atrium through an atrial septal incision or atrial septal defect (if present). This approach has an advantage in that it provides a shorter, more direct pathway for the pulmonary venous effluent. It is difficult to use this approach, however, when the anomalous pulmonary vein courses in the posterior portion of the lung and necessitates a great deal of angulation to create an anastomosis with the atrium. In cases where the pulmonary vein passes through the posterior mediastinum, Huddleston et al[16] have recommended pneumonectomy because of the high incidence of late stenosis with reimplantation techniques. As further justification of pneumonectomy in this setting, Huddleston et al point out that the right lung is often hypoplastic and that the left lung typically has undergone some compensatory growth. Furthermore, perfusion scans typically demonstrate that only ~25% of the pulmonary blood flow perfuses the right lung in patients with scimitar syndrome.[24]

Results and Complications

Survival after complete repair (embolization or ligation of anomalous pulmonary arterial flow with correction of the anomalous pulmonary venous return) is anticipated in older children and adults. In recent series, 5-year survival rates have reached 100%, although a significant incidence of late pulmonary vein obstruction remains. In the infantile form of the lesion, hospital mortality is higher, depending on the degree of lung hypoplasia and the presence of pulmonary hypertension. Even with a technically perfect repair, blood flow to the right lung often remains diminished. The left-to-right shunt, however, is abolished. Pulmonary venous obstruction is a prevalent late finding in up to 50% of patients.[24] Pneumonectomy remains an option in patients with persistently compromised pulmonary blood flow resulting from pulmonary hypertension or pulmonary venous obstruction.[16,17]

▸ TOTAL ANOMALOUS PULMONARY VENOUS DRAINAGE

In patients with total anomalous pulmonary venous drainage, all the venous effluent from the lungs drains to the systemic venous system, creating a large left-to-right shunt. A right-to-left shunt must be present to allow blood to reach the left ventricle and contribute to systemic cardiac output. Commonly this shunt is at the atrial level as an atrial septal defect or patent foramen ovale (PFO). The shunt also may be present as a ventricular septal defect or a patent ductus arteriosus. The absence of this shunt is incompatible with survival, and the magnitude of this shunt determines the systemic cardiac output.

Anatomy

Although well palliated in utero, infants with total anomalous pulmonary venous drainage have abnormalities in the pulmonary vascular system. There is often hypertrophy of the media of the pulmonary veins and arteries, intimal fibrous thickening of the pulmonary veins, and lymphangiectasia. These findings are accentuated in patients with pulmonary hypertension and evidence of pulmonary venous obstruction.[33] The various types of total anomalous pulmonary venous drainage are classified by the site of connection to the systemic venous system.

Supracardiac

Supracardiac drainage is the most common anatomical variant, occurring in 45–55% of patients with total anomalous pulmonary venous drainage.[2,32] The venous connection is typically through a pulmonary venous confluence behind the left atrium to a connecting vein (often termed a vertical vein) to the innominate vein. Other sites of pulmonary–systemic connection can be to a left- or right-sided superior vena cava (Figures 110-4 and 110-5).

Cardiac

The pulmonary–systemic pulmonary venous connection can be present at the cardiac level in 15–20% of patients. In this setting the pulmonary veins typically drain to a pulmonary venous confluence behind the left atrium. The confluence then drains to the coronary sinus or, less commonly, to the right atrium. In some patients the right- and left-sided pulmonary veins converge into a short vertical vein before draining into the coronary sinus. This latter variant may be more susceptible to late obstruction.[20]

Infracardiac

The systemic–pulmonary venous connection is present at the infracardiac level in 15–20% of patients. In this setting the pulmonary veins drain to a confluence behind the left atrium, which drains via a descending vertical vein to the portal vein, to the ductus venosus, or directly to the inferior vena cava. This subset displays obstruction in the pulmonary venous circuit in the majority of patients (Figure 110-6).

Mixed

In the 5–10% of patients with mixed anomalous pulmonary venous drainage, the systemic–pulmonary venous connection is at multiple sites at the supracardiac, cardiac, and/or infracardiac level.

Presentation

Patients without significant pulmonary venous obstruction present in infancy or early childhood with signs and symptoms related to the presence of a large left-to-right shunt. These patients have dyspnea, poor feeding, and poor growth. They may have cyanosis on examination, but this manifestation is usually mild. Other findings include a second heart sound that is split and a systolic flow murmur caused by increased flow across the pulmonary valve.

Obstruction in the pulmonary venous pathway in patients with total anomalous pulmonary venous drainage constitutes a surgical emergency. Medical measures to stabilize and

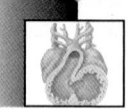

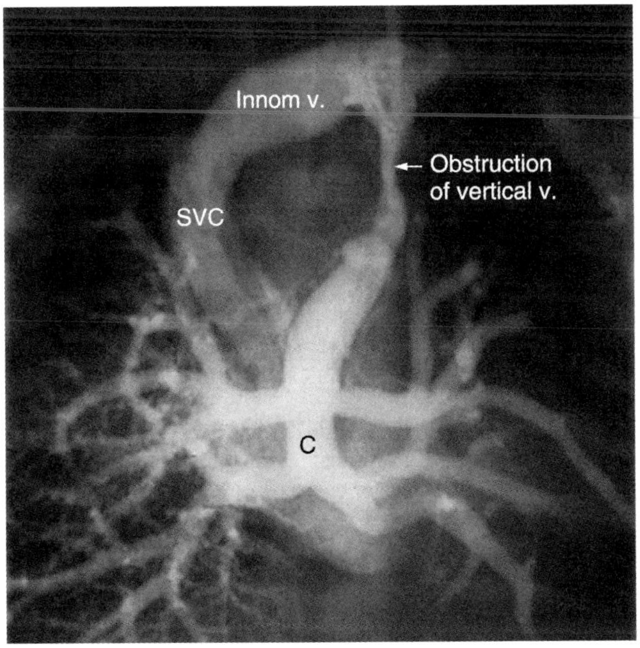

Figure 110–4 Catheterization demonstrating pulmonary venous phase of patient with total anomalous pulmonary venous drainage through a vertical vein to the innominate vein. There is some stenosis in the vertical vein in association with its passage between the left pulmonary artery and the left main stem bronchus. C, pulmonary vein confluence; Innom V, innominate vein; SVC, superior vena cava.
(Courtesy Dr. Yang Min Kim, Sejong Heart Institute, Seoul, Korea.)

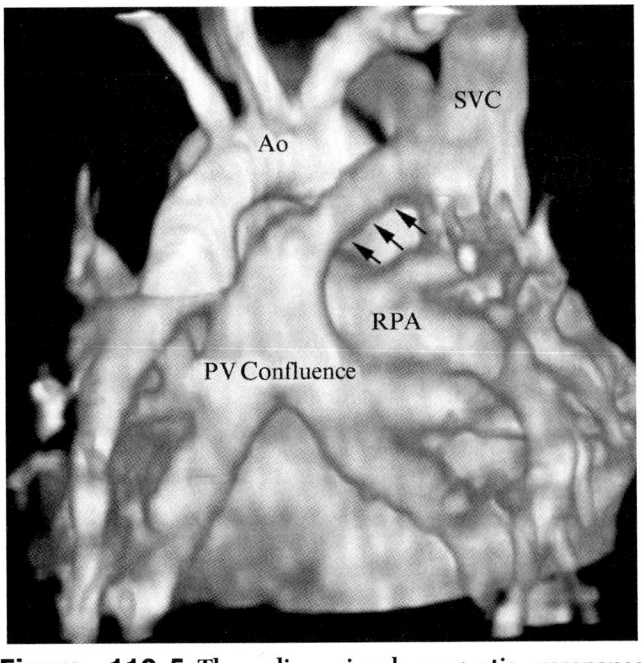

Figure 110–5 Three-dimensional magnetic resonance imaging (MRI) reconstruction of total anomalous pulmonary venous drainage with a vertical vein *(arrows)* to the innominate vein viewed from the posterior mediastinum. Ao, aorta; SVC, superior vena cava; RPA, right pulmonary artery; PV, pulmonary vein.
(Courtesy Dr. Yang Min Kim, Sejong Heart Institute, Seoul, Korea.)

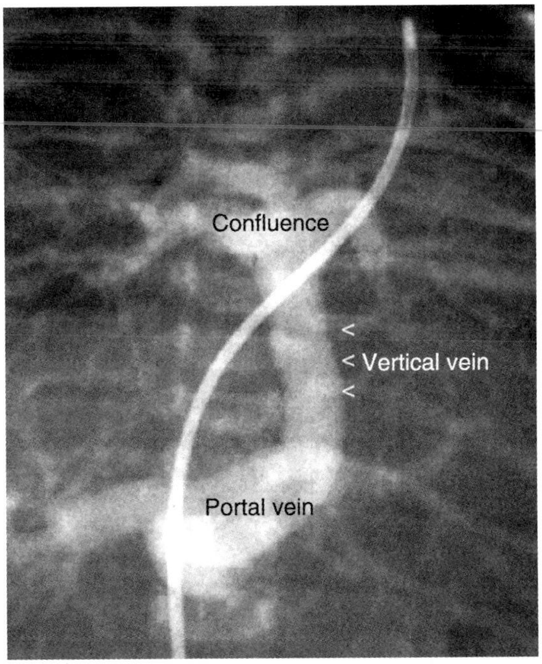

Figure 110–6 Catheterization demonstrating pulmonary venous phase of patient with total anomalous pulmonary venous drainage through a descending vertical vein to a portal vein.
(Courtesy Dr. Yang Min Kim, Sejong Heart Institute, Seoul, Korea.)

resuscitate the patient are minimally effective and include intubation, ventilation with 100% oxygen, hyperventilation, correction of pH, and inotropic support. Administration of prostaglandin E_1 has been reported to open the ductus venosus in an attempt to decompress the pulmonary veins in patients with infracardiac total anomalous pulmonary venous drainage and obstruction.[28] The common therapeutic goal of these strategies is relief of pulmonary venous obstruction, which can be accomplished only by surgical repair.

Clinical presentation is largely determined by the degree of pulmonary venous obstruction. Patients with high-grade obstruction present as in the neonatal period with cyanosis, respiratory distress, and poor growth. On examination the infant is tachypneic, is cyanotic, and has poor systemic perfusion. The second heart sound is prominent and split as a result of pulmonary arterial hypertension.

Pathophysiology

The hemodynamic abnormality in patients with total anomalous pulmonary venous drainage is related to the complete diversion of pulmonary venous blood away from the left atrium to a systemic vein. Consequently, the anatomical factors most important in determining the clinical status of the patient include the presence and location of a right-to-left shunt and the presence or absence of obstruction in the pulmonary venous circuit.

Because pulmonary venous blood is diverted from the left atrium, blood cannot reach the left ventricle in the absence of a right-to-left shunt. Therefore, to sustain life, a right-to-left shunt must be present. Most commonly a PFO or atrial septal defect is present to allow entry of blood into the left atrium and then to the left ventricle for systemic output.

The cardiac output of the patient is therefore limited by the amount of blood that can cross the atrial septum. Thus the characteristics of the obligatory right-to-left shunt determine the systemic cardiac output.

A second important anatomical factor determining the clinical status of the patient is the presence or absence of obstruction in the pulmonary venous pathway. When obstruction is present, egress of blood from the lungs is limited and results in pulmonary venous congestion and impairment of oxygenation. This can lead to life-threatening cyanosis in neonates. In addition to deficits in oxygenation and pulmonary blood flow, restriction at the level of the atrial septal defect reduces systemic cardiac output and further exacerbates the patient's precarious clinical status.

In patients with supracardiac anomalous pulmonary venous drainage, obstruction can occur in the ascending vertical vein connecting the pulmonary venous confluence to the innominate vein. In this situation the passage of the vertical vein between the pulmonary artery and the left bronchus can cause compression within the vertical vein. As the egress of blood from the lungs is restricted, the pulmonary artery pressure rises, causing further distention of the pulmonary artery and further compression of the vertical vein. This can create a repeating cycle of pulmonary artery distention and further obstruction (see Figure 110-4). Obstruction also can occur at the site of connection between the pulmonary venous confluence and the systemic vein. This is a common feature of infracardiac total anomalous pulmonary venous drainage.

Diagnostic Techniques

Arterial blood gas determinations assist in resuscitation of a neonate with obstruction and total anomalous pulmonary venous drainage. Often severe metabolic acidosis and mild hypoxemia are seen.

Chest Radiography

The appearance of the lung fields on chest radiographs is determined by the presence or absence of obstruction to pulmonary venous drainage. In patients without obstruction, pulmonary vascularity is increased as a result of the large left-to-right shunt created by drainage of pulmonary venous return into the right side of the heart. In patients with obstruction, the lung fields may be extremely congested because of obstruction of the egress of blood from the pulmonary veins and the left-to-right shunt. A prominence of the pulmonary artery shadow and the right atrium silhouette often exists. In supracardiac drainage the prominence of the upper mediastinal silhouette can create the classic "snowman" or "figure-eight" appearance.

Echocardiography

Echocardiography is the study of choice in diagnosing total anomalous pulmonary venous drainage. The pulmonary venous confluence, pulmonary veins, and connection to the systemic venous system typically can be defined, allowing an expeditious and noninvasive diagnosis in critically ill infants, as well as in asymptomatic children. Consequently, echocardiography has largely replaced angiography as the principal diagnostic study in patients with total anomalous pulmonary venous drainage. Echocardiography also can offer important prognostic data. Jenkins et al[19] correlated operative survival to the size of the pulmonary venous confluence and the sum of the pulmonary venous diameters (Figure 110-7).

Echocardiography also is helpful in monitoring the pulmonary veins for obstruction in both preoperative and long-term postoperative follow-up. The demonstration of turbulence in the pulmonary veins can be used as a sensitive marker for the presence of obstruction in the pulmonary venous circuit. Because obstruction in the pulmonary veins late after surgical repair can progress in a clinically silent fashion, the sensitivity of the echocardiogram to detect the presence of turbulence in the pulmonary veins may allow early detection and correction of pulmonary vein stenosis after repair.

Cardiac Catheterization

In the current era, cardiac catheterization infrequently is used for diagnosis in routine total anomalous pulmonary venous drainage or partial anomalous pulmonary venous drainage. Cardiac catheterization is helpful in patients in whom echocardiograph findings are ambiguous or in patients with other complex defects. A classical finding at catheterization associated with total anomalous pulmonary venous drainage is identical oxygen saturations in all chambers of the heart. This occurs as a result of upstream mixing of oxygenated pulmonary venous effluent and deoxygenated systemic venous blood and subsequent delivery of partially saturated blood to the right side of the heart, as well as to the left side of the heart through the atrial septal defect. Catheterization also is helpful in defining the anatomy of pulmonary vein stenosis, which may develop after repair of total anomalous pulmonary venous drainage.

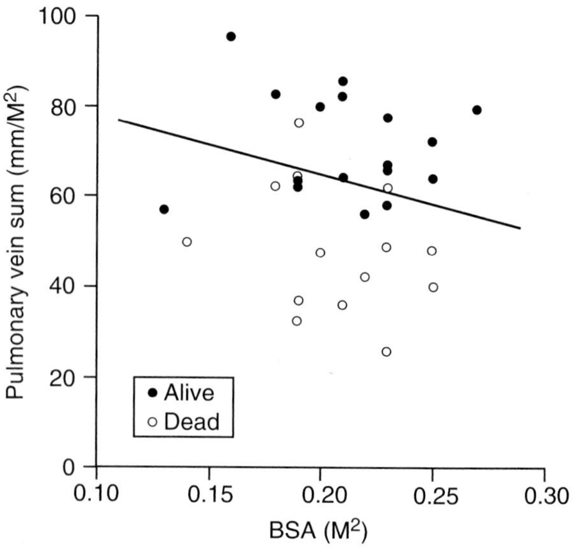

Figure 110–7 A smaller sum of pulmonary vein diameters is associated with higher surgical mortality after repair of total anomalous pulmonary venous drainage. BSA, body surface area. *(Modified from Jenkins KJ, Sanders SP, Orav EJ, et al: Individual pulmonary vein size and survival in infants with totally anomalous pulmonary venous connection. J Am Coll Cardiol 22:201–206, 1993.)*

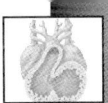

Balloon atrial septostomy may be helpful in hemodynamic stabilization before surgical repair in patients with obstruction of pulmonary venous return at the level of a restrictive atrial septal defect. In this situation the relief of obstruction at the atrial septal defect allows increased right-to-left shunting and improved systemic cardiac output.

Surgical Repair

The goal of surgical therapy is to create unobstructed egress of blood from the pulmonary veins into the left atrium. Aortal–bicaval cannulation offers flexibility to repair all forms of total anomalous pulmonary venous drainage. In some centers, deep hypothermic circulatory arrest is preferred to allow improved visualization of the pulmonary veins in a bloodless field. Continuous perfusion techniques require the use of cardiotomy suction devices in the pulmonary veins to allow proper visualization during the repair. For this reason, systemic hypothermia allows for safely decreasing perfusion flow rates during the critical portions of the anastomosis.

After initiation of cardiopulmonary bypass, ductus arteriosus ligation, and systemic cooling to 18–20° C, the aorta is cross-clamped and cold antegrade blood cardioplegia is administered. The vertical vein is ligated. The pulmonary venous confluence is seen in the posterior pericardium by retracting the heart anteriorly and to the right. Because of the lack of pulmonary vein attachments to the left atrium, the heart is unusually mobile and retraction of the heart out of the mediastinum offers excellent exposure of the pulmonary vein confluence. A longitudinal incision is created in the pulmonary venous confluence to match a corresponding incision in the posterior left atrium extended out to the left atrial appendage. With care to avoid distortion, a left-atrial-to-pulmonary confluence anastomosis is created using fine sutures. Controversy exists over the use of absorbable versus nonabsorbable sutures, as well as interrupted versus continuous techniques.[13,32] With all techniques the primary goal is a large, unobstructed anastomosis, and the superiority of any one of these techniques has not been convincingly demonstrated. A short period of low-flow cardiopulmonary bypass may be helpful for improved visualization during construction of a meticulous anastomosis.

The use of the approach described in the preceding paragraph is applicable to all types of total anomalous pulmonary venous drainage. It can be challenging, however, to orient the left atrial and pulmonary vein confluence incisions while simultaneously retracting the heart. Furthermore, the retraction required to visualize the anastomosis can place tension on the developing suture line during construction of the anastomosis. Finally, the left atrium tends to be small in patients with total anomalous pulmonary venous drainage, and, consequently, the limitation to rightward extension of the anastomosis by the atrial septum can limit the size of the anastomosis. The limitation imposed by the location of the atrial septum is a greater issue in patients in whom the pulmonary venous confluence is oriented rightward with respect to the left atrium.

An alternative approach is to create the anastomosis through a generous atriotomy extended transversely across the right atrium and then across the atrial septum (Figure 110-8). This approach allows visualization of the posterior wall of the left atrium to place the incision precisely over the pulmonary venous confluence. Furthermore, in patients with small left atria and rightward displacement of the pulmonary vein confluence, the approach allows patch augmentation of the left atrium when reconstructing the atrial septum and right atrial incision.

A third operative approach to construction of a pulmonary-vein-to-left-atrial anastomosis is between the aorta and superior vena cava. Using this technique, the aorta and superior vena cava are retracted laterally, exposing the dome of the left atrium and the pulmonary vein confluence. This approach is especially helpful in patients with supracardiac variants of total anomalous pulmonary venous drainage. Further exposure can easily be obtained by dividing the aorta.[27]

A technique limited to patients with total anomalous pulmonary venous drainage to the coronary sinus involves unroofing the coronary sinus with an incision between the coronary sinus and the foramen ovale. A glutaraldehyde-treated pericardial patch is used to reconstruct the atrial septum, leaving the pulmonary venous drainage to flow through the unroofed coronary sinus into the left atrium. Concern has been expressed that this unroofing technique may have a higher risk of late stenosis in patients who have a short segment of vein interposed between the pulmonary venous confluence and the coronary sinus.[20] In this situation, direct anastomosis of the pulmonary veins to the left atrial wall may be more appropriate at the initial repair.

In patients with infracardiac pulmonary venous connections, the pulmonary venous confluence tends to be oriented more vertically, creating a Y-shaped confluence that drains through a vertical vein to the portal system. Consequently, the incision into the left atrium is more vertical or Y-shaped to maximize the size of the newly created left atrium. Some surgeons leave the vertical vein intact to provide a pressure relief "pop-off" if left atrial pressure is high in the early postoperative period because of small left atrial size or poor ventricular compliance.[6]

Poor hemodynamics in the early postoperative period should raise concern for potential obstruction at the site of the venous anastomosis and/or pulmonary hypertensive crisis. Any suspicion of residual postoperative pulmonary venous obstruction should prompt an ECG to examine and interrogate the pulmonary venous anastomosis. In patients with preoperative pulmonary venous obstruction, chest radiograph findings of pulmonary vascular obstruction often persist for several days despite normal hemodynamics. Therefore the presence of congestion on chest X-ray cannot be used to rule out the presence of a pulmonary hypertensive crisis (which normally would be associated with relatively dark lung fields). Pulmonary hypertensive crises are a common feature in the postoperative management of infants after repair of total anomalous pulmonary venous drainage. In many centers routine postoperative pulmonary artery pressure monitoring has allowed early recognition and treatment of pulmonary hypertensive events with deep sedation, prolonged intubation, and inotropic support for right-sided heart failure. Inhaled nitric oxide also can be used for postoperative pulmonary hypertension, although caution must exercised because of the potential to create paradoxical pulmonary hypertension caused by rapidly increasing the left ventricular preload in patients with noncompliant or small left ventricles.[25]

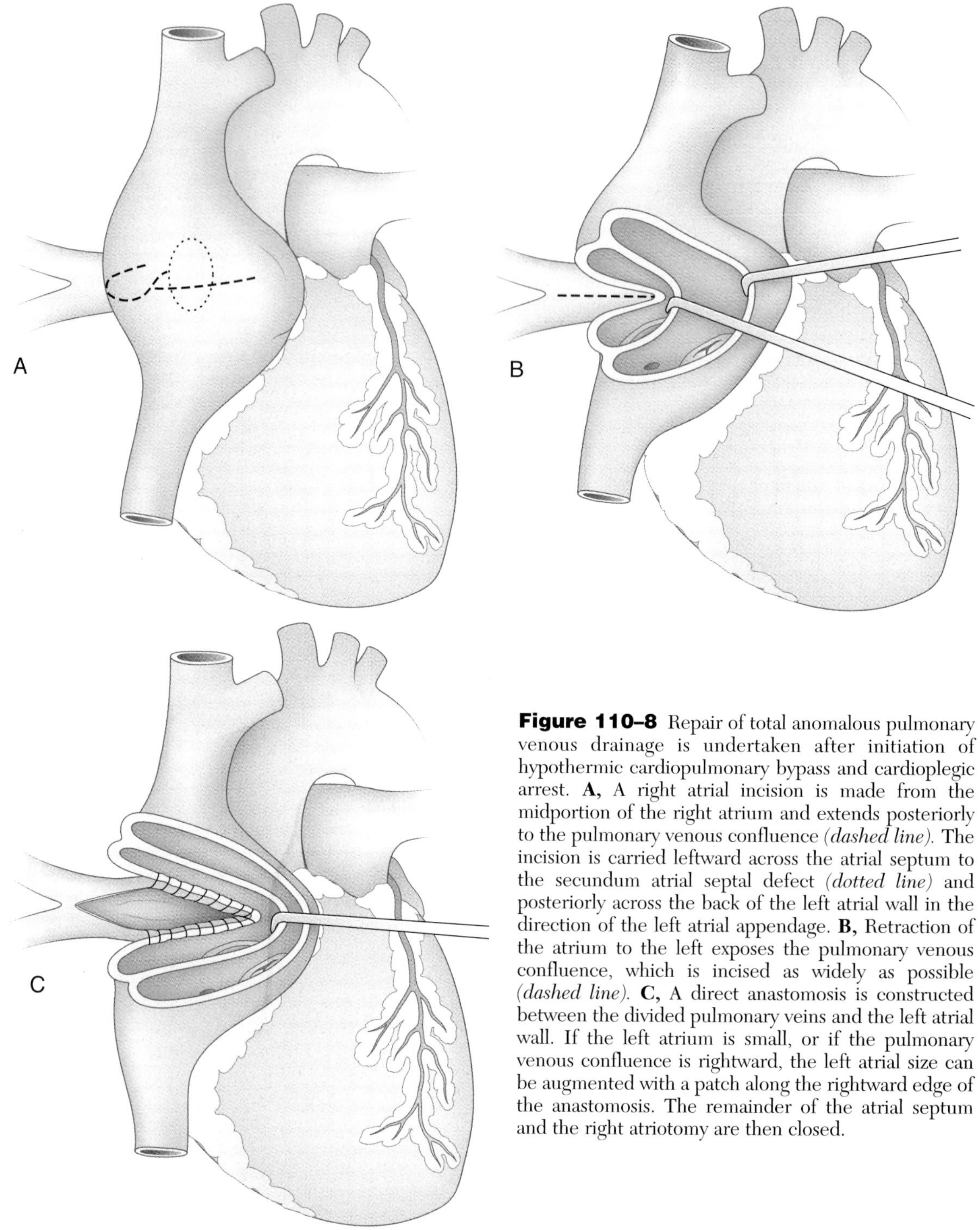

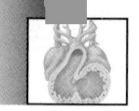

Figure 110–8 Repair of total anomalous pulmonary venous drainage is undertaken after initiation of hypothermic cardiopulmonary bypass and cardioplegic arrest. **A,** A right atrial incision is made from the midportion of the right atrium and extends posteriorly to the pulmonary venous confluence *(dashed line)*. The incision is carried leftward across the atrial septum to the secundum atrial septal defect *(dotted line)* and posteriorly across the back of the left atrial wall in the direction of the left atrial appendage. **B,** Retraction of the atrium to the left exposes the pulmonary venous confluence, which is incised as widely as possible *(dashed line)*. **C,** A direct anastomosis is constructed between the divided pulmonary veins and the left atrial wall. If the left atrium is small, or if the pulmonary venous confluence is rightward, the left atrial size can be augmented with a patch along the rightward edge of the anastomosis. The remainder of the atrial septum and the right atriotomy are then closed.

In patients with a small pulmonary venous confluence and small pulmonary veins, direct anastomosis of the divided edge of the pulmonary veins to the left atrial wall can lead to geometric distortion of the pulmonary vein anastomosis, local trauma from handling the delicate pulmonary veins, and local reaction from suture-related ischemia. For these potential problems to be avoided in patients with small pulmonary vein confluences, the preferred anastomotic technique at the Hospital for Sick Children in Toronto has evolved into a "sutureless" anastomosis. With this technique, a longitudinal incision is made in the posterior pericardium, the underlying pulmonary venous confluence, and the corresponding portion of the left atrium. In contrast to direct suture techniques, however, the left atrium is sutured to the pericardium circumferentially around the pericardial incision, avoiding direct suturing to the pulmonary veins. A "neo-atrium" is created into which the pulmonary veins bleed in a controlled fashion, and from which pulmonary venous effluent drains into the remainder of the left atrium and the left ventricle (Figure 110-9).

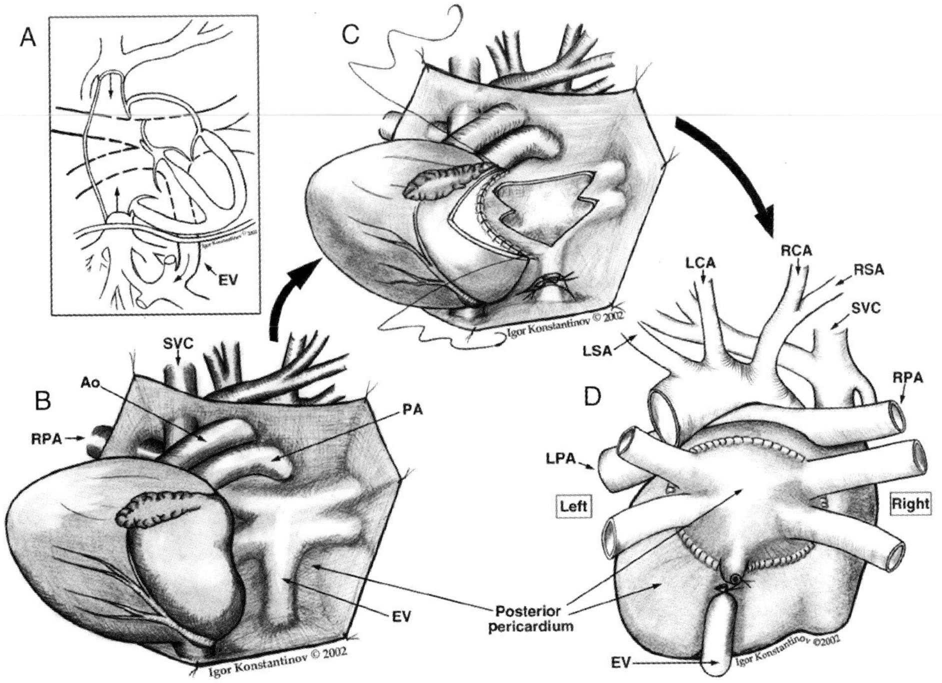

Figure 110–9 Repair of recurrent pulmonary vein stenosis after repair of total anomalous pulmonary venous drainage can be accomplished using a "sutureless" technique. A broad incision is made in the stenotic pulmonary veins, and the left atrium is sutured to the pericardium to create a "controlled bleed" into a neo-atrium. Complete avoidance of direct suturing of the pulmonary veins minimizes surgery-induced trauma to the pulmonary veins and the potential for distortion of the pulmonary veins as a result of suturing-related alterations in local geometry. **A,** Schematic demonstrates infracardiac total anomalous pulmonary renew drainage. EV, vertical vein. **B,** The heart is retracted anteriorly and rightward. Ao, aorta; SVC, superior vena cava; PA, main pulmonary artery. **C,** The vertical vein has been ligated, and the divided edges of the left atrial wall are sutured to the posterior pericardium using a suture line that is remote from the incised pulmonary venous confluence. **D,** Posterior view of completed anastomosis. RPA, right pulmonary artery; LPA, left pulmonary artery; LCA, left carotid artery; RCA, right carotid artery; RSA, right subclavian artery.
(Courtesy Dr. Igor E. Konstantinov, The Hospital for Sick Children, Toronto, Ontario, Canada.)

Results

Operative survival for patients with total anomalous pulmonary venous drainage has markedly improved in the most recent decade, with survival rates of >90% often reported.[2,4,23] Long-term prognosis for patients after repair of total anomalous pulmonary venous drainage is also favorable, with relatively few late deaths.[2,4] Approximately 10–15% of patients have some evidence of late pulmonary vein obstruction, and, for this reason, long-term surveillance is important.

Special Considerations

Mixed Type

Patients with a mixed type of total anomalous pulmonary venous drainage have pulmonary venous drainage to a combination of systemic venous, cardiac, and left atrial sites. The pulmonary venous drainage pattern tends to fall into two different patterns. In one pattern, three of the pulmonary veins drain to a horizontal confluence behind the left atrium, whereas one vein drains to another systemic site. A second pattern is results in pulmonary venous drainage to at least two separate systemic venous sites with an absence of a horizontal confluence behind the heart.[8] Repair of this lesion is accomplished using a combination of the techniques described earlier. Connection of the horizontal confluence to the left atrium is accomplished a retrocardiac, transatrial, or supracardiac approach as described earlier. In the absence of a horizontal confluence, the individual pulmonary veins are anastomosed to the left atrium for left-sided veins using the left atrial appendage. For right-sided connections, the repair is accomplished using techniques described earlier for partial anomalous pulmonary venous drainage.

Total Anomalous Pulmonary Venous Drainage in Heterotaxy

Visceral heterotaxy is manifested by abnormalities of multiple organ systems, including the lungs, liver, spleen, and systemic veins, as well as cardiac manifestations, including anomalous pulmonary venous drainage. In the subset of patients with asplenia, or right atrial isomerism, other cardiac anomalies include a common atrium, common atrioventricular valves, pulmonary outflow tract obstruction, and hypoplastic left or right ventricles resulting in functional univentricular hearts. Total anomalous pulmonary venous drainage is present in approximately 90% of patients.[12]

Patients with the common combination of total anomalous pulmonary venous drainage and functional single ventricles typically present within the first month of life for palliation.[12,14] The type of palliation required is determined by the presence of uncontrolled pulmonary blood flow (e.g., functional single ventricle with unrestrictive pulmonary valve) or restricted pulmonary blood flow (e.g., pulmonary stenosis or atresia). Superimposed on the alterations of pulmonary arterial flow is the frequent presence of pulmonary venous obstruction, which may be present in up to 30% of patients.[12] The presence of obstruction, however, may not be readily apparent until after augmentation of pulmonary blood flow (e.g., arteriopulmonary shunting) in patients initially displaying pulmonary stenosis or atresia.[4,14] The majority of these patients have "arterialization" of the pulmonary veins and increased muscularity of the pulmonary arteries.[10]

Patients who require palliation as neonates, including repair of obstructed total anomalous pulmonary drainage and control of pulmonary blood flow with either pulmonary artery banding or arteriopulmonary shunting, have an extremely poor prognosis.[4,10,12] The poor prognosis in this subset may be a reflection of the pathological changes occurring in the pulmonary vasculature and the inability of the relatively crude mechanisms used to control pulmonary blood flow (e.g., bands or shunts) to effectively provide a stable source of pulmonary blood flow in the early and late postoperative periods.[4] Consequently, cardiac transplantation has been advocated for this patient subset.[10]

Patients who do not require repair of obstructed pulmonary veins in the first month of life tend to have a better long-term prognosis.[26] Of these survivors, those with functional single ventricles eventually require palliation with the Fontan procedure. Short- and mid-term survival after the Fontan procedure in this subset is improving in the current era, with a 10–15% operative mortality and very little late mortality.[1]

Postrepair Pulmonary Vein Stenosis

Development of stenosis after repair of total anomalous pulmonary venous drainage occurs in 5–15% of patients after initial repair,[2,3,22] often within the first year after repair. The obstruction can occur in one of three general patterns. The simplest form involves a ring of inflammatory fibrosis stenosis limited to the site of the anastomotic area. The next, more complex, form involves the distal pulmonary veins in a similar localized region of intimal proliferation. The most complex of the processes involves diffuse retrograde pulmonary vein stenosis extending far into the proximal pulmonary veins. These types of obstruction can occur in a unilateral fashion, progressing to complete occlusion of the pulmonary venous drainage of the involved lung.[3] Survival is greater in patients with unilateral pulmonary vein stenosis.[3,22] Diffuse postrepair pulmonary vein stenosis is a dreaded complication of total anomalous pulmonary venous drainage and is associated with a high mortality rate.

Obstruction at the site of pulmonary venous repair is manifested by poor cardiac output and chest radiograph findings of pulmonary congestion. The principal diagnostic feature is the presence of turbulence at the pulmonary venous anastomotic site, as noted on echocardiograph images.[29] Because the stenosis often progresses in a clinically silent manner, periodic ECGs after repair of anomalous pulmonary venous return are recommended.

The presence of turbulence at the site of anastomosis has been postulated to create a cycle of local injury leading to hyperplasia and increasing turbulence, thereby perpetuating a process of diffuse pulmonary vein stenosis. Improved understanding of the vascular biology responsible for diffuse pulmonary vein stenosis in this group will lead to better therapy. At present, surgical revision of the pulmonary venous anastomosis and lung transplantation are commonly offered. Pulmonary vein stenting has been uniformly unsuccessful, although innovation in terms of newer-generation covered stents, as well as stents delivering local doses of radiation or chemotherapy, may offer benefit in the future.

Surgical revision of postrepair pulmonary vein stenosis can be accomplished by creating a "sutureless neo-atrium" as described previously (Figure 110-9). The pulmonary veins are incised longitudinally through all stenotic areas, and the incision is extended distally until nonstenotic segments of pulmonary vein are reached. This may require incision of the veins well into secondary or tertiary branches within the pulmonary hilum and parenchyma. Because of previous surgery, retrocardiac adhesions are helpful to maintain hemostasis and are left intact where possible. Long-term follow up is not yet available for the use of the sutureless neo-atrium, but short-term results have been favorable.[3,21,34]

REFERENCES

1. Azakie A, Merklinger SL, Williams WG, et al: Improving outcomes of the Fontan operation in children with atrial isomerism and heterotaxy. Ann Thorac Surg 72(5):1636–1640, 2001.
2. Bando K, Turrentine MW, Ensing GJ, et al: Surgical management of total anomalous pulmonary venous connection: Thirty-year trends. Circulation 94(suppl II):12–16, 1996.
3. Caldarone CA, Najm HK, Kadletz M, et al: Relentless pulmonary vein stenosis after repair of total anomalous pulmonary venous drainage. Ann Thorac Surg 66(5):1514–1520, 1998.
4. Caldarone CA, Najm HK, Kadletz M, et al: Surgical management of total anomalous pulmonary venous drainage: Impact of coexisting cardiac anomalies. Ann Thorac Surg 66(5):1521–1526, 1998.
5. Coles JG, Yemets I, Najm HK, et al: Experience with repair of congenital heart defects using adjunctive endovascular devices. J Thorac Cardiovasc Surg 110:1513–1520, 1995.
6. Cope JT, Banks D, McDaniel NL, et al: Is vertical vein ligation necessary in repair of total anomalous pulmonary venous connection? Ann Thorac Surg 64(1):23–28; discussion 29, 1997.
8. Delius RE, de Leval MR, Elliot MJ, et al: Mixed total anomalous pulmonary venous drainage: Still a surgical challenge. J Thorac Cardiovasc Surg 112:1581–1588, 1996.
9. Gatzoulis MA, Freeman MA, Siu SC, et al: Atrial arrhythmia after surgical closure of atrial septal defects in adults. N Engl J Med 340(11):839–846, 1999.

10. Gaynor JW, Collins MH, Rychik J, et al: Long-term outcome of infants with single ventricle and total anomalous pulmonary venous connection. J Thorac Cardiovasc Surg 117(3):506–513; discussion 513–514, 1999.
11. Gustafson RA, Warden HE, Murray GF, et al: Partial anomalous pulmonary venous connection to the right side of the heart. J Thorac Cardiovasc Surg 98:861–868, 1989.
12. Hashmi A, Abu-Sulaiman R, McCrindle BW, et al: Management and outcomes of right atrial isomerism: A 26-year experience. J Am Coll Cardiol 31(5)1120–1126, 1998.
13. Hawkins JA, Minich LL, Tani LY, et al: Absorbable polydioxanone suture and results in total anomalous pulmonary venous connection. Ann Thorac Surg 60(1):55–59, 1995.
14. Heinemann MK, Hanley FL, Van Praagh S, et al: Total anomalous pulmonary venous drainage in newborns with visceral heterotaxy. Ann Thorac Surg 57:88–91, 1994.
15. Hijii T, Fukushige J, Hara T: Diagnosis and management of partial anomalous pulmonary venous connection. Cardiology 89:148–151, 1998.
16. Huddleston CB, Exil V, Canter CE, et al: Scimitar syndrome presenting in infancy. Ann Thorac Surg 67:154–160, 1999.
17. Huddleston CB, Mendeloff EN: Scimitar syndrome. Adv Card Surg 11:161–178, 1999.
18. Inoue T, Ichihara M, Uchida T, et al: Three-dimensional computed tomography showing partial anomalous pulmonary venous connection complicated by the scimitar syndrome. Circulation 105(5):663, 2002.
19. Jenkins KJ, Sanders SP, Orav EJ, et al: Individual pulmonary vein size and survival in infants with totally anomalous pulmonary venous connection. J Am Coll Cardiol 22(1):201–206, 1993.
20. Jonas RA, Smolinsky A, Mayer JE, et al: Obstructed pulmonary venous drainage with total anomalous pulmonary venous connection to the coronary sinus. Am J Cardiol 59:431–435, 1987.
21. Lacour-Gayet F, Rey C, Planché C: Sténose des veines pulmonaires. Description d'une technique chirurgicale sans suture utilisant le péricarde in situ. Arch Mal Coeur 89(5):633–636, 1996.
22. Lacour-Gayet F, Zoghbi J, Serraf AE, et al: Surgical management of progressive pulmonary venous obstruction after repair of total anomalous pulmonary venous connection. J Thorac Cardiovasc Surg 117:679–687, 1999.
23. Lupinetti FM, Kulik TJ, Beekman RH, et al: Correction of total anomalous pulmonary venous connection in infancy. J Thorac Cardiovasc Surg 106:880–885, 1993.
24. Najm HK, Williams WG, Coles JG, et al: Scimitar syndrome: Twenty years' experience and results of repair. J Thorac Cardiovasc Surg 112:1161–1169, 1996.
25. Rosales AM, Bolivar J, Burke RP, et al: Adverse hemodynamic effects observed with inhaled nitric oxide after surgical repair of total anomalous pulmonary venous return. Pediatr Cardiol 20(3):224–226, 1999.
26. Sadiq M, Stumper O, De Giovanni JV, et al: Management and outcome of infants and children with right atrial isomerism. Heart 75:314–319, 1996.
27. Serraf A, Belli E, Roux D, et al: Modified superior approach for repair of supracardiac and mixed total anomalous pulmonary venous drainage. Ann Thorac Surg 65:1391–1393, 1998.
28. Serraf A, Bruniaux J, Lacour-Gayet F, et al: Obstructed total anomalous pulmonary venous return. J Thorac Cardiovasc Surg 101:601–606, 1991.
29. Smallhorn JF, Burrows P, Wilson G, et al: Two-dimensional and pulsed Doppler echocardiography in the postoperative evaluation of total anomalous pulmonary venous connection. Circulation 76(2):298–305, 1987.
30. Tasaka H, Krug EL, Markwald RR: Origin of the pulmonary venous orifice in the mouse and its relation to the morphogenesis of the sinus venosus, extracardiac mesenchyme (spina vestibuli), and atrium. Anat Rec 246:107–113, 1996.
31. Webb S, Brown NA, Wessels A, et al: Development of the murine pulmonary vein and its relationship to the embryonic venous sinus. Anat Rec 250:325–334, 1998.
32. Wilson WR Jr, Ilbawi MN, DeLeon SY, et al: Technical modifications for improved results in total anomalous pulmonary venous drainage. J Thorac Cardiovasc Surg 103(5):861–870; discussion 870–871, 1992.
33. Yamaki S, Tsunemoto M, Shimada M, et al: Quantitative analysis of pulmonary vascular disease in total anomalous pulmonary venous connection in sixty infants. J Thorac Cardiovasc Surg 104(3):728–735, 1992.
34. Yun TJ, Coles JG, Konstantines IE, et al: Conventional and sutureless techniques for management of the pulmonary veins: Evolution and indications from postrepair pulmonary vein stenosis to primary pulmonary vein anomalies. J Thor Cardiovasc Surg 2004 (inpress).

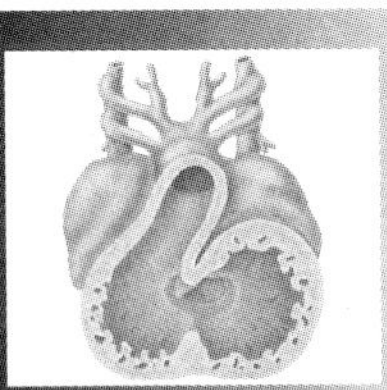

CHAPTER 111

Atrioventricular Canal Defects

Bassem N. Mora, Sabine H. Daebritz, and Pedro J. del Nido

INTRODUCTION

Atrioventricular (AV) canal defects encompass a spectrum of lesions in which the common etiology appears to be abnormal development of the endocardial cushions, resulting in a defect in the AV septum. This group of lesions forms approximately 3% of all major congenital cardiac defects, and approximately one half of the patients have Down syndrome.[29] In children with Down syndrome, AV canal defects are seen in 20–25% or a 1000-fold increased risk when compared with the incidence in the general population.[73]

Although AV canal defects constitute a continuum of related anatomical lesions, they can be arbitrarily divided into the following three main groups[37] (partial, transitional, and complete AV canal defects), based on the extent of the interventricular communication:

- *Partial AV canal defects* consist of a large ostium primum atrial septal defect (ASD) and a cleft between the left superior and inferior leaflets, without an interventricular communication. There are generally two distinct AV valve orifices, corresponding to the mitral and tricuspid valves. Leaflet tissue joins the left superior and inferior leaflets together at the crest of the interventricular septum, eliminating the interventricular communication. In general, partial AV canal defects constitute approximately 5–10% of all ASDs.
- *Transitional AV canal defects* consist of an ostium primum ASD, a left-sided cleft, and a restrictive ventricular septal defect (VSD) that is usually small, partially closed by the attachments of chordae from the superior and inferior bridging leaflets to the crest of the interventricular septum. Two AV valves are present, forming two separate orifices. At one extreme the VSD may consist of a very small communication located at the point of apposition of the left superior and inferior leaflets. In these cases the pathophysiology resembles partial AV canal defects. In other cases of transitional AV canal defect, the interventricular communication is larger, but is still restrictive to flow, with a measurable gradient by echocardiography or cardiac catheterization.
- *Complete AV canal defects* constitute the other end of the spectrum and are the most common form of AV canal defects. There is generally an ostium primum ASD and a nonrestrictive VSD in the inlet portion of the interventricular septum. One common AV valve orifice is present, with left and right components. An inlet-septal VSD alone does not fall under AV canal defects because the AV septum is intact in these malformations. On the other hand, some patients have an inlet-septal VSD and a cleft mitral valve with a restrictive or absent interatrial communication; these should be considered to be within the spectrum of AV canal defects.

In this chapter we describe the principal anatomical features relevant to the preoperative evaluation and surgical management of defects amenable to a two-ventricle repair and briefly discuss the features that may preclude such an approach. Surgical techniques with early and late results are described. Various associated cardiac lesions are discussed, in addition to the management of recurrent mitral regurgitation. We will not discuss the management of AV canal defects associated with heterotaxy syndrome because the AV canal defect is not the primary pathophysiological abnormality; these patients are generally managed along a single-ventricle pathway.

ANATOMY

The anatomical malformation that is common to all forms of AV canal defects is a deficiency in the AV septum caused by incomplete embryonic development of superior and inferior endocardial cushion tissue. The common AV canal is normally present during the early tubular stage of fetal life and constitutes the sole connection between the primitive common atrium and primitive common ventricle. After looping and septation, the AV junction expands rightward to allow direct inflow into the right ventricle. Projections of the endocardial jelly develop at the AV junction, which then differentiate into the AV valves and the AV septum (Figure 111-1). Abnormal differentiation and remodeling of the cushion mesenchyme into valvuloseptal tissue is thought to be a mechanism for the development of AV canal defects.[25] The resultant anatomical defect involves the abnormal development of AV valves and the persistence of interatrial and interventricular communications.[77]

The wide variability in the degree of development of the endocardial cushions explains the variability in size and extent of the septal defects and the degree of involvement of the AV valves. Nevertheless, several anatomical features are shared between all types of AV canal defects. These include the following:

- Shortened dimension of the inlet septum-to-ventricular apex, giving the interventricular septum a "scooped-out" appearance. This deficiency in the inlet septum is typically deeper in complete AV canal defects than in partial AV canal defects.
- Lengthened dimension of the outlet septum-to-ventricular apex, resulting in a "goose-neck" appearance and anterior displacement of the left ventricular (LV) outflow tract. Although the LV outflow tract is narrowed, true LV outflow tract obstruction (LVOTO) is rare. In the normal heart, the inlet septum-to-ventricular apex length and the outlet septum-to-ventricular apex length are equal.
- Absence of the usual wedged position of the aortic valve between the AV valves, caused by maldevelopment of the endocardial cushions. This results in elevation and anterior deviation of the aortic valve.
- Apical displacement of the attachments of the AV valves to the crest of the interventricular septum, caused by the deficiency in the inlet septum.
- Decreased contribution of the left lateral leaflet to AV valve circumference. In the normal situation the posterior mitral leaflet forms two thirds of the mitral valve circumference. In AV canal defects the left lateral leaflet, which corresponds to the posterior mitral leaflet in the normal heart, forms only one third of the circumference of the AV valve.

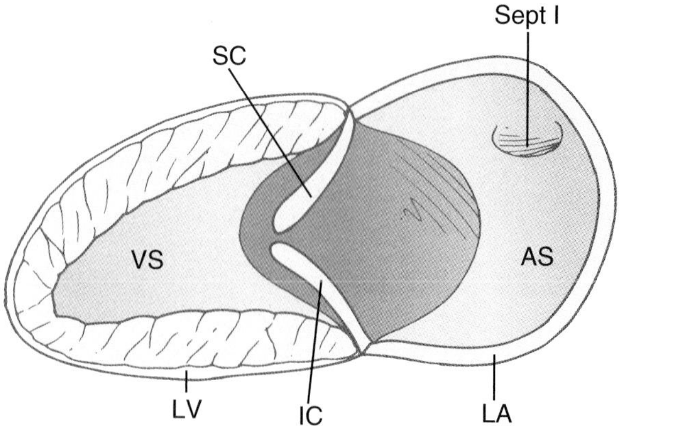

Figure 111-1 Schematic of complete atrioventricular (AV) canal defect during morphogenesis, with the AV canal region shown in dark gray. Projections from the superior and inferior endocardial cushions normally differentiate into the AV valves and AV septum. AS, Atrial septum; IC, inferior endocardial cushion; LA, left atrium; LV, left ventricle; SC, superior endocardial cushion; Sept 1, septum primum; VS, ventricular septum.
(Modified from Van Praagh R, Litovsky S: Pathology and embryology of common atrioventricular canal. Prog Pediatr Cardiol 10:115–127, 1999.)

- Inferior displacement of the AV node and coronary sinus. The bundle of His is also displaced inferiorly, coursing at the inferior rim of the scooped-out basal portion of the interventricular septum.
- Variable degree of underdevelopment of the inlet portion of the interventricular septum, resulting in absence of a VSD (partial AV canal defects), a restrictive VSD (transitional AV canal defects), or a large VSD (complete AV canal defects).

In addition to these fundamental concepts, anatomical features of significance to the surgeon include the following:

- Size and extent of the interventricular and interatrial communications.
- Valve leaflet morphology, including papillary muscle anatomy, valve regurgitation, and presence of chordal attachments to the septum.
- Relative balance of the common AV valve orifice over the two ventricles.
- Other major associated cardiac and noncardiac defects.

The left-sided AV valve has a cleft between the left superior and inferior leaflets. This cleft is not a commissure,[82] as was once thought,[4,14,75] for two reasons. First, a commissure is generally supported by chordae on either side of the defect, whereas a cleft is unsupported, with paucity of chordae at the edges. Second, the chordae that arise from the two adjacent leaflets in a commissure usually attach to a single papillary muscle, which promotes coaptation and prevents regurgitation. The chordae that arise from the left superior and inferior leaflets attach to two different papillary muscles. This increases the distracting force during ventricular systole and predisposes to regurgitation through the cleft. The extent of regurgitation is generally mild to moderate, although severe regurgitation can be present.

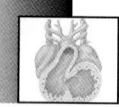

In 1966 Rastelli and Kirklin[62] described a classification of complete AV canal defect based on the extent of bridging of the left superior leaflet (LSL) across the interventricular septum (Figure 111-2). In complete AV canal defects the left inferior leaflet (LIL) is not well developed; it is usually short and immobile with rolled edges. The Rastelli classification does not take into consideration the LIL, which displays greater anatomical variation. No clear morphological relationship exists between the LSL and the LIL.

The most common Rastelli type, present in approximately 75% of patients, is the Rastelli A defect, which is also the most common form of complete AV canal in patients with Down syndrome. There is no bridging of the LSL; instead, its chordae attach to the crest of the interventricular septum. The superior bridging leaflet can be divided into left and right components over the crest of the interventricular septum. The inferior bridging leaflet is rarely divided and is often attached by short dense chordae to the crest of the interventricular septum. The size of the interventricular communication is often larger under the LSL than under the LIL.

In the rare Rastelli B defect the superior bridging leaflet is often partially divided into right and left components, with associated mild to moderate bridging of the LSL. Its chordae attach either to the right of the crest of the interventricular septum or to a prominent papillary muscle in the right ventricle (RV), depending on the extent of bridging. The moderator band is often short. The Rastelli B subtype is often associated with unbalanced AV canal defect.

In the Rastelli C defect there is extensive bridging of the LSL. Its chordae are free floating and are not attached to the underlying crest of the interventricular septum, but rather attach to the anterolateral papillary muscle of the RV. The Rastelli C type of complete AV canal defect can be seen in association with other complex heart lesions such as tetralogy of Fallot (TOF), transposition of the great arteries (TGA), and double-outlet right ventricle (DORV).

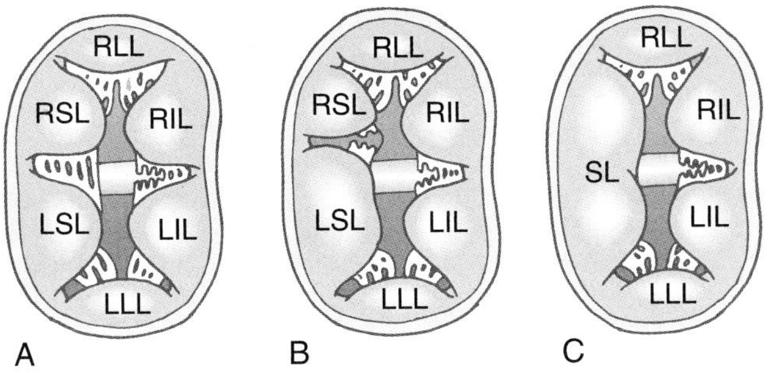

Figure 111-2 The Rastelli classification for complete atrioventricular (AV) canal defects. A, In the Rastelli type A defect the superior bridging leaflet is divided into two leaflets at the crest of the interventricular septum, corresponding to the right superior leaflet (RSL) and the left superior leaflet (LSL). **B,** In the Rastelli type B defect the LSL bridges across the septum and attaches to a papillary muscle within the right ventricle. **C,** In the Rastelli type C defect there is marked bridging of the superior bridging leaflet, making it free floating and unattached to the underlying interventricular septum. LIL, Left inferior leaflet; LLL, left lateral leaflet; LSL, left superior leaflet; RIL, right inferior leaflet; RLL, right lateral leaflet; RSL, right superior leaflet; SL, superior leaflet.

(Modified from Jacobs JP, Burke RP, Quintessenza JA, Mavroudis C: Congenital Heart Surgery Nomenclature and Database Project: Atrioventricular canal defect. Ann Thorac Surg 69:S36–S43, 2000.)

The development of the Rastelli classification facilitated the widespread application of corrective surgery for this defect. Although it is an oversimplification and represents categorization of a continuum of leaflet abnormalities, it may still have a limited role in the repair of complete AV canal defects using the classic single-patch technique. In that setting, recognition of whether the bridging leaflets are undivided over the crest of the interventricular septum is important because undivided leaflets need to be surgically incised into right and left components to allow placement of a patch to close the interventricular and interatrial communications. Even in those settings, however, the Rastelli classification may have limited applications because neither the extent nor the location of naturally occurring divisions in the bridging leaflets is taken into account. The Rastelli classification is of less importance in the double-patch or modified single-patch techniques that are described later in the chapter.

Lev's description of the location of the conduction tissue[42] was another important contribution in the field because it facilitated the development of surgical techniques that avoided injury to the His bundle and the AV node. The coronary sinus ostium and the AV node are displaced inferiorly in AV canal defects. The AV node lies at the junction of the interatrial septum and the hinge point of the AV valve. This places the AV node between the coronary sinus ostium and the crest of the interventricular septum, in the so-called nodal triangle, which is not at the tip of Koch's triangle. The nodal triangle is bound by the inferior extent of the right AV valve annulus, the coronary sinus orifice, and the inferior edge of the interatrial septum (Figure 111-3). The bundle of His then passes superiorly and anteriorly from the AV node to the crest of the interventricular septum, reaching it where the crest is fused posteriorly with the AV valve annulus. The bundle then travels along the crest of the interventricular septum, in an inferior-to-superior direction, giving rise to the left bundle branches. Before reaching the midpoint of the interventricular crest, it becomes the right bundle branch and heads toward the moderator band and the muscle of Lancisi.[28] The superior aspect of the interventricular septum is devoid of conduction fibers. In patients with complete AV canal defects and heterotaxy syndrome, two AV nodes may be found.[39]

The relationship between the common AV valve and the ventricles varies. If the AV valve is situated primarily over one ventricle, associated hypoplasia of the contralateral ventricle frequently occurs, which in extreme cases precludes a two-ventricle repair. Abnormal papillary muscle development, such as two closely spaced papillary muscles or a single papillary muscle, is seen in RV-dominant forms of complete AV canal defect. This can result in left AV valve stenosis postoperatively if the cleft is fully closed, because after cleft closure, the orifice of the left AV valve is determined by the narrow width of the left lateral leaflet.

Approximately 50–75% of patients with complete AV canal have Down syndrome, whereas Down syndrome is rare in patients with partial AV canal defects,[29] occurring in less than 10% of patients. AV canal defects form approximately 3% of all major congenital cardiac defects and are seen in approximately 25% of patients with Down syndrome. This represents a 1000-fold higher rate compared with the general population.[73] AV canal defects represent the most common congenital heart anomaly in Down syndrome. Other less frequent cardiac lesions seen in patients

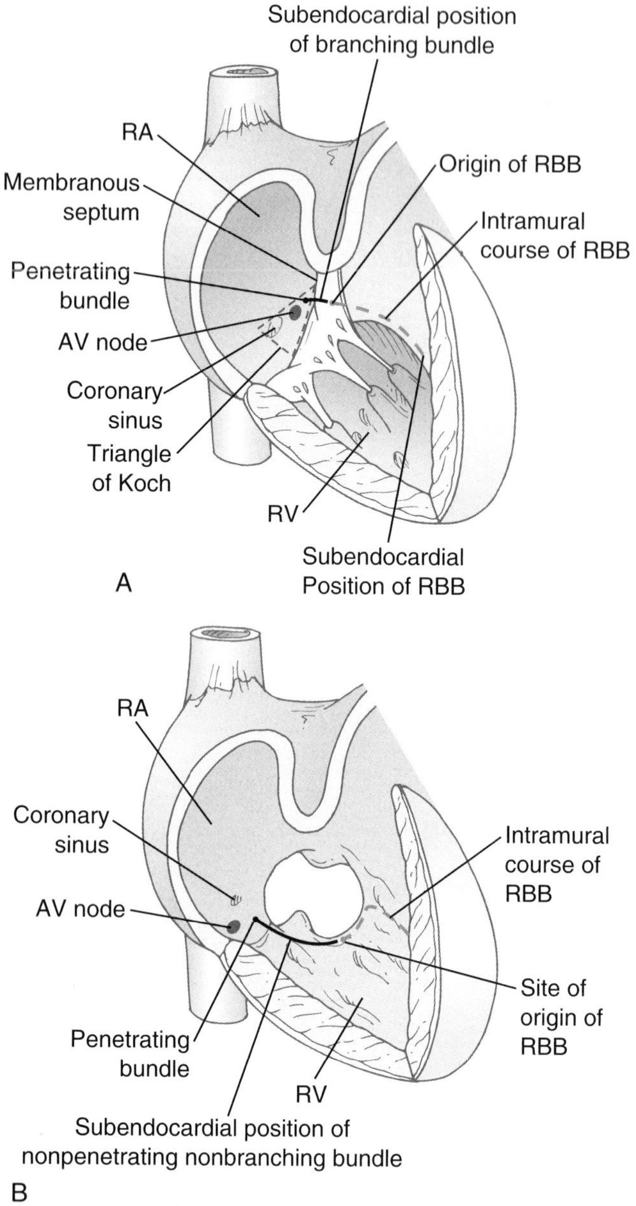

Figure 111–3 The location of the atrioventricular (AV) node and the conduction tissue. A, Normal heart. Note the location of the AV node at the tip of the triangle of Koch. **B,** AV canal heart: The AV node is now located within the nodal triangle, not at the tip of the triangle of Koch. The coronary sinus, AV node, and bundle of His are displaced inferiorly compared with the normal heart. *RA,* Right atrium; *RBB,* right bundle branch; *RV,* right ventricle.

(Modified from Kertesz NJ: The conduction system and arrhythmias in common atrioventricular canal. Prog Pediatr Cardiol 10:153–159, 1999.)

with Down syndrome include VSD, ASD, patent ductus arteriosus (PDA), and TOF.[46] Interestingly, the presence of Down syndrome seems to be protective from more complex cardiac lesions such as univentricular connections, TGA, and atrial situs abnormalities. The presence of Down syndrome is thought to accelerate the development of pulmonary vascular obstructive disease (PVOD), especially in the setting of complete AV canal and a left ventricle-to-right atrial shunt. An additional 15–20% of fetuses with AV canal syndrome have heterotaxy syndrome: AV canal defects are present in almost all patients with asplenia and a high number of patients with polysplenia.

Although an underlying genetic mechanism has not been identified, some intriguing evidence exists in that regard. First, there is a strong association between AV canal defects and Down syndrome. Second, a weaker association exists with heterotaxy syndrome. Third, familial clustering of AV canal defects has been reported.[71] Fourth, the incidence of recurrent congenital heart disease in offspring of patients with AV canal defects is approximately 10%.[12] In another study, approximately 14% of offspring of mothers with isolated AV canal defects had congenital heart disease, usually either TOF or AV canal defects.[27] This contrasts with the 2–4% probability of congenital heart disease in children of parents with other congenital cardiac lesions.

PATHOPHYSIOLOGY

A left-to-right shunt is present in patients with AV canal defects, unless PVOD or coexistent RV outflow tract obstruction is present. Patient presentation depends on the extent of left-to-right shunting, which in turn depends on the amount of pulmonary blood flow and pulmonary vascular resistance. The amount of left-to-right shunting increases in the first few weeks of life, paralleling the fall in pulmonary vascular resistance.

In partial AV canal defects, where an interventricular communication is absent, the shunt is located only at atrial level. Patients with partial AV canal defects with little or no regurgitation through the AV valves have a clinical presentation similar to secundum ASDs. The degree of shunting depends on the size of the ostium primum ASD defect and the relative diastolic compliance of the two ventricles. RV stroke volume is increased, whereas RV systolic pressure may be normal or only slightly increased. Patients may remain asymptomatic for years. An exception is the presence of significant left AV valve regurgitation in the setting of an ostium primum ASD, which is the case in 10–15% of patients. The LIL in this situation is often severely hypoplastic. The regurgitation increases left-to-right shunting considerably; a left ventricle-to-right atrium shunt may also be present. This results in increased RV and LV stroke volume, cardiomegaly, tachypnea, tachycardia, poor feeding, and failure to thrive, leading to progressive heart failure in infancy. Without treatment, patients with partial AV canal defects rarely survive beyond 40 years of age, although older patients have been reported.[36] Atrial arrhythmias are common, increase in frequency with advancing age, and are a poor prognostic sign.

Patients with complete AV canal defects exhibit left-to-right shunting because the VSD is large and nonrestrictive. The extent of the shunt at ventricular level primarily depends on pulmonary vascular resistance. The pathophysiology in complete AV canal defects is similar to a large nonrestrictive VSD with two additional features. First, an atrial level shunt is present, with the potential for a left ventricle-to-right atrium shunt and increased volume loading of the ventricle. Second, AV valve regurgitation may be present, further increasing the volume load. These factors accelerate the development of heart failure symptoms in early infancy.

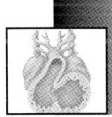

In many patients, particularly those with Down syndrome, pulmonary vascular resistance remains elevated after birth, which decreases the magnitude of left-to-right shunting. In other infants, pulmonary vascular resistance drops in the first few weeks of life, resulting in a large left-to-right shunt. This results in elevations of RV and pulmonary artery pressures to systemic levels. Patients typically display tachypnea, failure to thrive, cardiomegaly, and diminished distal perfusion in the first few months of life. If AV valve regurgitation is coexistent, the extent of left-to-right shunting is increased because of shunting at both atrial and ventricular levels, resulting in biventricular volume overload. This accelerates the development of heart failure. In one study, moderate AV valve regurgitation was present in approximately 20% of complete AV canal defects, whereas severe regurgitation was present in 15% of such lesions.[16] In our experience,[35] mild AV valve regurgitation is common, occurring in approximately 35% of patients in the first year of life, although the incidence of severe AV valve regurgitation is less frequent, occurring in approximately 4% of patients.

Irreversible changes in the pulmonary vasculature are seen as early as 6 months in unrepaired complete AV canal defects.[57] The presence of Down syndrome accelerates the development of PVOD.[17] This may be due in part to increased bronchial secretions, decreased number of distal bronchi, inherent abnormalities of the lung parenchyma, and the thick tongue that predisposes to oropharyngeal airway obstruction, hypoventilation, sleep apnea, tracheobronchomalacia, and CO_2 retention. These factors accelerate the development of respiratory infections and PVOD. Over time, PVOD leads to decreased left-to-right shunting, which prolongs life but precludes successful surgical intervention. Eventually the shunt reverses to a right-to-left shunt and the Eisenmenger complex develops, with progressive cyanosis in later stages.

Without surgery, patients with complete AV canal defects and Down syndrome had an 80% survival rate at 10 and 15 years.[11] The primary causes of death within the first several years of life are heart failure and recurrent pulmonary infections. Subsequently, PVOD becomes an increasingly prevalent cause of death. Toward the end of the second decade of life, exercise tolerance progressively decreases, leading to premature death from PVOD by the third to fourth decades of life. One of the more dramatic causes of death in patients with PVOD is massive hemoptysis, which can occur as early as the third decade of life.

TIMING OF SURGERY

The development of surgical techniques to treat AV canal defects parallels the evolution of cardiac surgery for congenital hearts defects. Initial attempts at repair were complicated by limited knowledge of the anatomical features, particularly with respect to the conduction tissue.

The first cardiac operation using a pump oxygenator was attempted by Dennis and Varco in 1952 in a patient with a preoperative diagnosis of an ASD. The patient did not survive surgery. Postmortem examination revealed a partial AV canal defect. In 1955 Lillehei et al[44] were the first to report repair of complete AV canal using cross-circulation. Successful repair of an ostium primum defect using cardiopulmonary bypass was first reported by Kirklin et al in 1955.[41]

Complete Atrioventricular Canal

Two different techniques have been proposed for repair of complete AV canal defects. A single patch covering atrial and ventricular defects with partition of the superior bridging leaflet was originally developed by Rastelli and Kirklin at the Mayo Clinic.[63] Separate atrial and ventricular patches were proposed by Trusler[51] in 1975 and advocated by others.[2,14,79] A recent modification of the single-patch technique has been introduced.[59,81]

Management of the cleft has evolved over the years. Carpentier,[14] Anderson and associates,[4] and others[75] had recommended that the cleft be viewed as a commissure. They advocated leaving the cleft open to result in a "trifoliate" left AV valve and prevent the development of stenosis. However, the left-sided cleft is not a normal commissure, as discussed earlier. Left AV valve regurgitation frequently originates at the cleft; in later stages, as the regurgitation progresses, a central regurgitant jet may also be seen. Many surgeons in the 1980s left the cleft open only to have a sizable number of patients return with significant mitral regurgitation (MR) primarily through the cleft. For this reason, most surgeons today close the cleft completely. However, the cleft should be left open or only partially closed in patients with double-orifice mitral valve or unbalanced AV canal defects, because mitral stenosis can result when complete cleft closure is undertaken in these settings.

Many surgeons during the 1970s and early 1980s advocated palliation with pulmonary artery banding to delay surgical repair beyond infancy. However, as surgical techniques improved and cardiopulmonary bypass in infants became safer and more widely applied, most centers abandoned this practice and opted for elective repair before 6–9 months of age. One exception is children with partial and transitional AV canal defects who frequently are asymptomatic; repair can generally be deferred until the first few years of life unless AV valve regurgitation is severe. Although we advocate primary repair of complete AV canal in early infancy, there may be a very limited role for the use of a palliative pulmonary artery band in patients with very complex anatomy, such as unbalanced complete AV canal defects in which single ventricle management is planned. Palliation by construction of a modified Blalock–Taussig shunt has been proposed in patients with complete AV canal defects and TOF to avoid early repair, although we do not advocate this approach, as will be discussed later.

We advocate elective repair within the first 2–4 months of age in asymptomatic infants with complete AV canal defects. Delay beyond this age is unnecessary and is potentially hazardous. Repair of AV canal defects beyond 3 months of age recently has been shown to be an incremental risk factor for death.[69] The chronic volume overload from left-to-right shunting increases common AV valve annular dilatation and results in increased left AV valve regurgitation. Freedom from reoperation for left AV valve regurgitation is higher when patients are repaired at a younger age.[69]

Another sequela of delaying surgery is the development of pulmonary hypertension with elevated pulmonary vascular resistance, predisposing to postoperative pulmonary hypertensive crises, which are serious and life-threatening postoperative complications. Although pulmonary hypertension can, in most cases, be treated with sedation, hyperventilation, and inhaled nitric oxide, prevention by timely elective repair is far safer and avoids the risk of development of irreversible PVOD, which can occur within the first year of life, especially in the presence of Down syndrome. In fact, by 1 year of age, Heath–Edwards grade III and IV pathological changes in the lung have been noted in the majority of patients with complete AV canal defects who had not undergone surgical correction.[57]

Infants with failure to thrive and symptoms of heart failure requiring multiple medications should undergo surgery as soon as possible to permit normal growth and development. This is particularly true in young infants with recurrent upper respiratory tract infections who are at higher risk for significant morbidity and mortality if a severe respiratory infection complicates unrepaired AV canal defect. Prematurity or severe AV valve regurgitation should not be contraindications for corrective surgery because the results with palliation in these groups are particularly poor.

Partial Atrioventricular Canal

Patients with partial AV canal defects should be repaired by 1–3 years of age in the majority of patients. This is similar to the recommendation for closure of isolated secundum atrial septal defects. If significant left AV valve regurgitation is present, then earlier repair is recommended.

Sommerville[67] reviewed the outcome of 122 unoperated patients with ostium primum atrial septal defects between 1958 and 1964. Increasing morbidity and mortality occurred with increasing age. The presence of significant mitral regurgitation correlated with increasing symptoms. Fourteen percent of 96 patients younger than 30 years of age either had died (n = 5) or had significant disabling symptoms (n = 8).

A subgroup of patients with partial AV canal defects display heart failure symptoms that are unresponsive to medical management in the first year of life.[45] They require early surgical correction. Frequent associated findings include the presence of several left-sided obstructive lesions such as hypoplasia of the left AV valve, LV, aortic valve, and aortic arch, in addition to aortic coarctation. Complex mitral valve anomalies also have been documented in this subset of patients.[32]

Transitional Atrioventricular Canal

Patients with transitional AV canal defects fall between partial and complete AV canal because of the restrictive nature of the VSD, which protects against the harmful sequelae of torrential pulmonary blood flow. Usually the restrictive VSD is small, which allows transitional AV canal defects to be repaired in the first 1–2 years of life. If the restrictive VSD is moderate in size, then repair should proceed earlier to prevent the complications of PVOD.

PREOPERATIVE EVALUATION

Because of the nearly continuous spectrum of lesions involving the atrial, ventricular, and valvular portions of the AV canal defects, preoperative definition of the anatomical features in each case is helpful. Information regarding the mechanism of valve regurgitation and LVOTO are especially valuable in planning operative intervention. Needless to say, intraoperative confirmation of the anatomical features is imperative to guide decisions regarding patch size, position of valve leaflets, and extent of cleft closure.

Physical examination correlates with the type of AV canal defect. In partial AV canal defects a systolic pulmonary flow murmur is heard along with fixed wide splitting of the second heart sound, as in a secundum ASD. An apical blowing systolic murmur of mitral regurgitation may be present. If a VSD is present, as in transitional or complete AV canal defects, then a holosystolic murmur is present, best heard at the left lower sternal border or the ventricular apex. A hyperactive precordium may be present. P_2 is often loud, with fixed splitting of the second heart sound. Often a mid-diastolic low-pitched rumble is present. A pulmonary flow murmur may also be present.

The electrocardiogram reveals marked RV hypertrophy and sometimes may reveal LV hypertrophy and biatrial enlargement. The PR interval is often prolonged. The vectorcardiogram reveals a counterclockwise frontal plane loop that is anterior and to the right. This results in a QRS axis that is leftward and superior, with Q waves in leads I and AVL and deep S waves in lead AVF. There is left-axis deviation, with a QRS axis between −30 and −150 degrees. This can be useful in distinguishing ostium primum ASDs from secundum ASDs, where the loop is clockwise.

The chest X-ray shows evidence of increased pulmonary blood flow, along with cardiomegaly. The presence of left AV valve regurgitation accentuates these findings; the left atrium may be severely dilated, with resultant elevation of the left main stem bronchus.

In nearly all cases the anatomical features, associated defects, and mechanism of valve dysfunction can be obtained from two-dimensional echocardiography, along with Doppler evaluation of blood flow direction and velocity.[43] The four-chamber view shows the left and right AV valves at the same horizontal level, which is in contradistinction to the normal situation where the tricuspid valve is attached to the AV septum more toward the apex of the heart than is the mitral valve. Other features on echocardiography include the elongated LV outflow tract and the unwedged aortic valve. It is important to assess the presence of chordal attachments to the LV outflow tract, because this is a substrate for the development of LVOTO. The AV valve leaflets should be examined, and the mechanism of AV valve regurgitation should be assessed carefully. The presence of a double-orifice mitral valve is not easily seen by echocardiography; it is often diagnosed by intraoperative inspection.

Cardiac catheterization and angiography rarely add information not obtained by echocardiography in the majority of patients. One notable exception is the unoperated patient older than 1 year of age in whom measurement of pulmonary vascular resistance is needed to determine operability. Another exception is the postoperative patient in whom quantification of residual postoperative lesions such as residual VSDs and LVOTO are required to assess the need for reoperation.

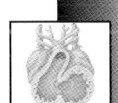

SURGICAL TECHNIQUE

Median sternotomy, either partial or complete, has been the standard technique for exposing the heart and great vessels. Some have advocated a right anterior thoracotomy for partial AV canal defects in older female children to improve cosmesis. More recently, however, techniques to minimize surgical trauma by limiting the extent of the sternotomy have been used, such as a lower ministernotomy (Figure 111-4).[58] This approach can be applied to infants and children of all ages and may be helpful in decreasing postoperative pain and development of chest wall deformities such as pectus carinatum. We are now using this ministernotomy approach for nearly all AV canal defects, except in cases where there are major associated cardiac lesions such as aortic coarctation, TOF, or TGA, where a full sternotomy is required for optimal exposure.

Cardiopulmonary bypass with moderate hypothermia and bicaval cannulation is used in nearly all cases; deep hypothermic circulatory arrest should be considered for patients weighing less than 2 kg. Bicaval cannulation is usually achieved with small-angled metal cannulas inserted directly into the venae cavae to provide adequate exposure to the right atrium. Aortic cross-clamping and cardioplegia are used in all cases to facilitate repair, particularly during the attachment of the septal patches near the AV node and coronary sinus.

In the setting of a large ostium primum ASD, both AV valves and intraventricular anatomy can be readily visualized. If a small or absent interatrial communication is present, then an incision in the septum primum provides access to the left AV valve for valve testing and cleft closure. This also aids in securing the VSD patch to the crest of the interventricular septum.

Complete Atrioventricular Canal

In complete AV canal defects there is usually a large ostium primum defect and a moderate to large nonrestrictive VSD under the superior and inferior bridging leaflets (Figure 111-5). There may be chordal attachments of either or both bridging leaflets to the crest of the septum, and these leaflets may be partitioned into right and left components or may form a single bridging leaflet over the crest of the septum. Two surgical approaches have been developed and are commonly used in this setting. A double-patch technique involves the placement of two separate patches, one to close the VSD and the other to close the ASD. In the classic single-patch technique a single autologous pericardial patch is used to close the VSD and ASD components, often with division of the superior and inferior bridging leaflets. More recently a modified single-patch technique has been introduced, where the VSD is obliterated by suturing the bridging leaflets to the crest of the interventricular septum; a single pericardial patch is then used to close the ASD. Although there are advantages and disadvantages to each technique, excellent results have been reported with all three methods.

Double-Patch Technique

In the double-patch technique, separate patches are used for closure of the ventricular and atrial septal defects. The ventricular patch is made of synthetic material such as Dacron. The atrial patch is usually autologous pericardium, either untreated or treated with glutaraldehyde. The use of a synthetic atrial patch should be avoided because hemolysis can result when a left AV valve regurgitant jet strikes the patch.

Initial inspection of the AV valve and filling of the LV with cold saline facilitates the delineation of the point of

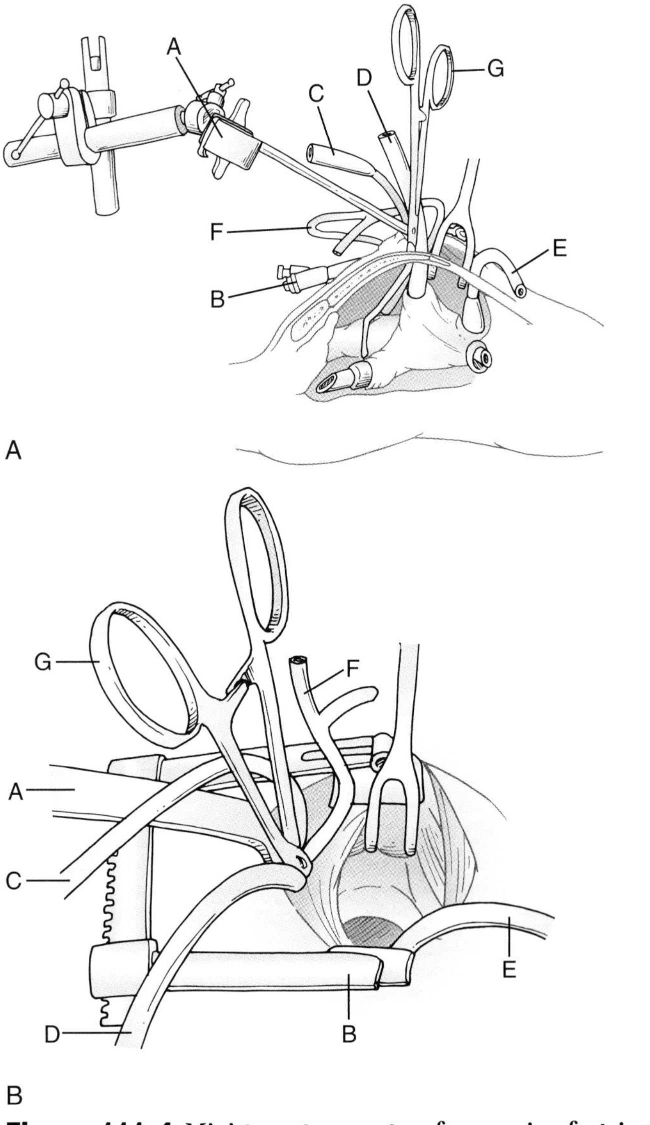

Figure 111–4 Ministernotomy setup for repair of atrioventricular (AV) canal defects. A, Representative parasagittal cross section with bicaval cannulation and aortic cross-clamping. **B,** Surgeon's view of the operative field. The inside of the atrium is well visualized for AV canal repair. A, Bookwalter retractor arm connected to an Army–Navy retractor; B, pediatric sternal retractor; C, aortic cannula; D, superior vena cava cannula via the right atrium, although direct cannulation is preferred for complete AV canal repair; E, Inferior vena cava cannula; F, cardioplegia cannula; G, aortic cross-clamp.
(Modified from del Nido PJ, Bichell DP: Minimal-access surgery for congenital heart defects. Semin Thorac Cardiovasc Surg Pediatr Card Surg Annu 1:75–80, 1998.)

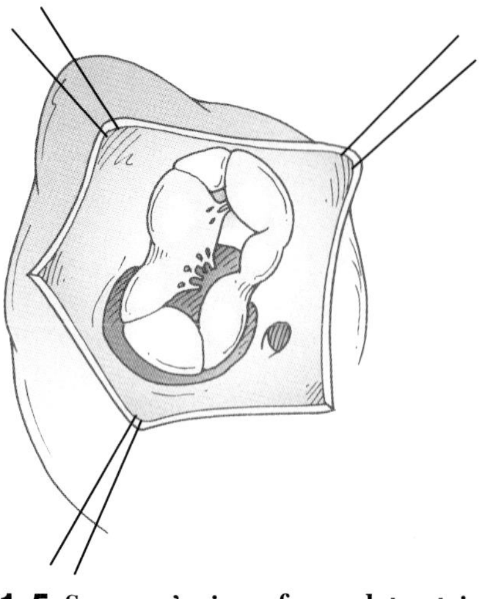

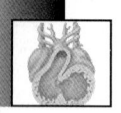

Figure 111–5 Surgeon's view of complete atrioventricular (AV) canal defect. The superior bridging leaflet (to the viewer's left) is undivided and unattached to the underlying crest of the interventricular septum, as in a Rastelli type C defect. The AV node and coronary sinus ostium are displaced inferiorly as shown. There is a cleft between the left superior and inferior leaflets. A large ostium primum defect is present, allowing good visualization into the left atrium.
(Modified from Daebritz S, del Nido PJ: Surgical management of common atrioventricular canal. Prog Pediatr Cardiol 10:161–171, 1999.)

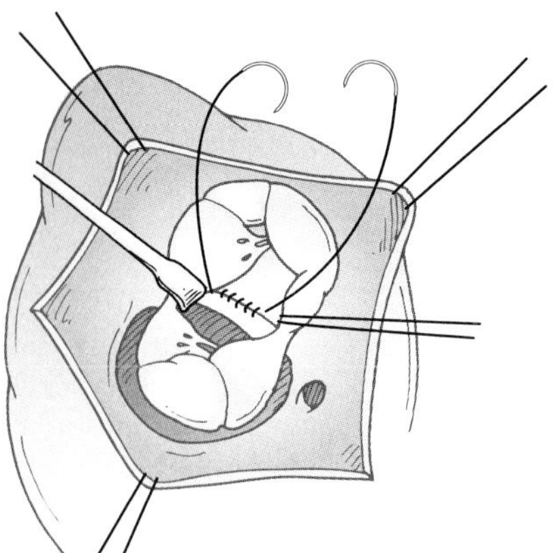

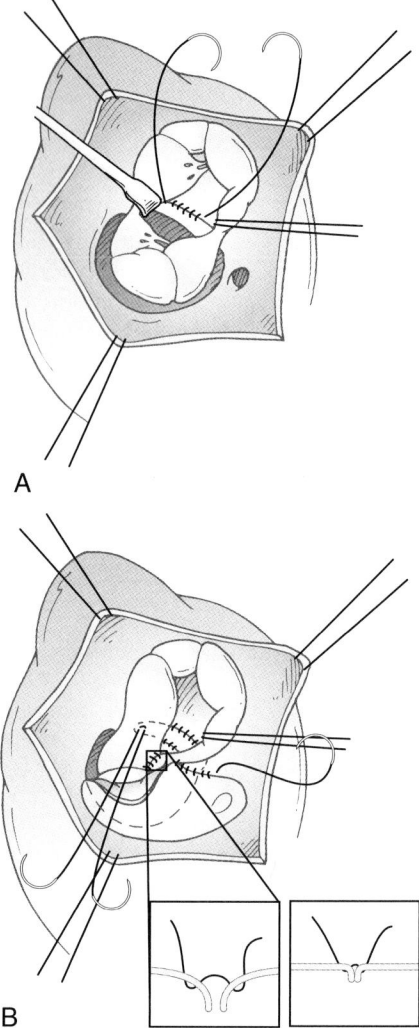

Figure 111–6 The double-patch technique for repair of complete atrioventricular (AV) canal defects. A, Placement of the crescent-shaped ventricular septal defect (VSD) patch, showing suturing to the crest of the interventricular septum. The superior leaflet is retracted cephalad to allow accurate suturing without entrapment of chordae. Similar retraction is used at the inferior leaflet, where the patch is sewn to the right of the crest of the interventricular septum to avoid iatrogenic injury to the AV node. **B,** Completion of the double-patch repair is achieved by inserting the atrial septal defect (ASD) patch. Sutures are passed through the VSD patch, valve leaflets, and ASD patch, thereby sandwiching the valve between the two patches. In this example the ASD patch is sewn to the right of the AV node and coronary sinus. If a secundum defect or patent foramen is present, the ASD patch can be extended to cover both defects. Cleft closure is usually done once the valve leaflets are attached to the ASD and VSD patches. The insert shows apposition of the cleft edges during systole.
(Modified from Daebritz S, del Nido PJ: Surgical management of common atrioventricular canal. Prog Pediatr Cardiol 10:161–171, 1999.)

coaptation of the left superior and inferior bridging leaflets. This permits measurement of the base-to-apex dimension of the VSD at the point of leaflet coaptation, corresponding to the height of the VSD patch. The distance between the two junction points of the interventricular septum and the AV valve annulus, at the aortic valve cephalad and AV node caudad, should also be determined. This is helpful in determining the width of the VSD patch.

The patch shape is that of a crescent rather than a half-circle because of the apical displacement of the point of coaptation of the superior and inferior bridging leaflets (Figure 111-6A). The VSD patch is attached to the right of the crest of the interventricular septum using running or horizontal mattress interrupted pledgeted sutures. Care should be taken to avoid distortion of valve chordae that attach to the septum. As the suture line approaches the AV node area, the patch is attached more to the right of the septum, fixed 3–4 mm away from the junction of the interventricular septum and the AV valve.

The superior and inferior leaflets are then draped over the edge of the VSD patch. The pericardial patch is cut to an appropriate width, made narrower than the true distance between the aortic valve and the AV node to perform an annuloplasty of the AV valve, thereby decreasing the incidence of MR. A running horizontal suture line is performed to sandwich the AV valve leaflets between the VSD and ASD patches. These sutures pass through the pericardial patch, the left AV valve leaflets, the VSD Dacron patch, and the right AV valve leaflets.

The mitral valve cleft, created by coaptation of the superior and inferior bridging leaflets, is then closed, using either running or interrupted horizontal mattress or simple sutures. The extent of cleft closure is determined in great part by the position of the papillary muscles and the size of the left lateral leaflet. Because closure of the cleft limits mobility of the superior and inferior leaflets, the greater the valve orifice area that is covered by these two leaflets, the greater the chance for creating valve stenosis. In cases where the papillary muscles are close together or a single

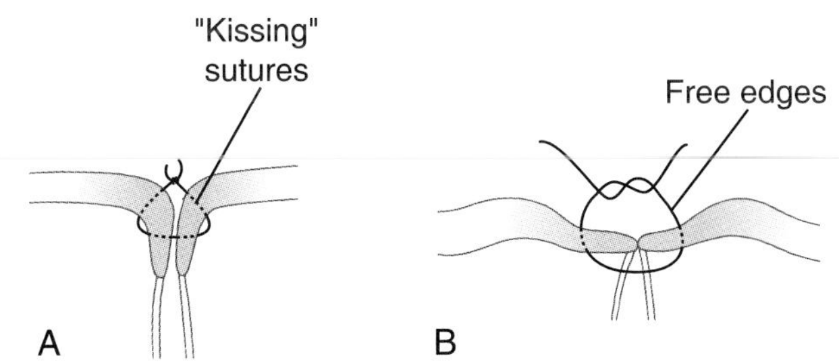

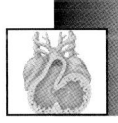

Figure 111-7 Cleft closure sutures. A, Placement of sutures at the zone of apposition of the cleft edges, so-called kissing sutures, decreases the probability of mitral regurgitation (MR). **B,** If the sutures are taken through the free edges of the valve leaflets, the leaflets have less support during ventricular systole, predisposing to MR.
(Modified from Khonsari S, Sintek CF: Atrioventricular septal defects. In Khonsari S, Sintek CF, editors: Cardiac Surgery: Safeguards and Pitfalls in Operative Technique, 3rd ed., pp. 243–251. Philadelphia: Lippincott Williams & Wilkins, 2003.)

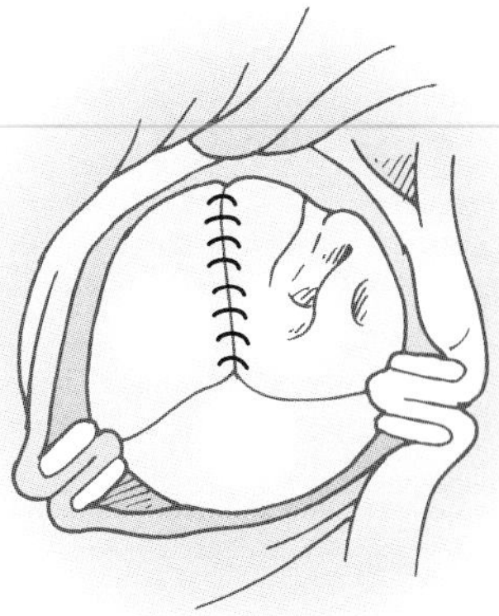

Figure 111-8 Commissuroplasty sutures at the two junctions of the left lateral leaflet with the left superior leaflet (LSL) and left inferior leaflet (LIL). These decrease the degree of residual mitral regurgitation (MR) after cleft closure. Care should be taken to avoid narrowing the mitral annulus to a sufficient extent that mitral stenosis ensues.
(Modified from Castaneda AR, Jonas RA, Meyer JE Jr, Hanley FL: Atrioventricular canal defect. In Castaneda AR, Jonas RA, Mayer JE Jr, Hanley FL, editors: Cardiac Surgery of the Neonate and Infant. Philadelphia: W B. Saunders, 1994.)

papillary muscle is present, closure of the cleft creates a slitlike orifice of the mitral valve, resulting in significant stenosis. In these cases the cleft must be left open to facilitate leaflet mobility. Frequently the edges of the leaflets creating the cleft are rolled and coapt over a small surface area. Care must be taken to preserve this degree of coaptation in closing the cleft and not to unroll the leaflet edges, because leaflet coaptation adds strength to the cleft closure, particularly during systole, thereby minimizing MR (Figure 111-7).

The degree of MR is determined by injecting cold normal saline into the LV cavity. If significant regurgitation is present after cleft closure, then central regurgitation from poor leaflet coaptation is the usual culprit. This is managed by narrowing the commissure between the LSL and the left lateral leaflet with pledgeted mattress sutures. The valve is tested again; if residual regurgitation is still present, a similar commissuroplasty suture is placed at the commissure between the LIL and the left lateral leaflet. This brings the left lateral leaflet closer to the interventricular septum and improves central leaflet coaptation. Care should be taken to avoid mitral stenosis from the placement of generous commissuroplasty sutures (Figure 111-8).

The ASD patch is then sutured to the remnants of the interatrial septum. The two surgical options available for avoiding injury to the AV node are attachment of the patch to the right or to the left of the AV node. Most surgeons attach the ASD patch to the right of the AV node. This involves suturing to the *right* inferior leaflet, where superficial bites are taken. The suturing continues to the right of the coronary sinus orifice, leaving the coronary sinus draining into the left atrium. Alternatively, the suturing can be extended to the edge of the coronary sinus orifice, leaving the orifice on the right atrial side. The advantage of placing the patch to the right of the coronary sinus ostium is that the suture line remains far from conduction tissue. The disadvantage is that the coronary sinus is left draining to the left atrium. This may cause a variable degree of obstruction to coronary sinus drainage unless the coronary sinus is surgically unroofed. The arterial saturation is typically not affected. Alternatively, the ASD patch can be attached to the *left* inferior leaflet, gradually returning to the edge of the interatrial septum, as initially advocated by McGoon and colleagues.[63] This leaves the coronary sinus draining into the right atrium. The disadvantage of this technique is that sutures must be placed through the LIL; in small infants these sutures may tear through the delicate leaflet tissue or may distort the leaflet enough to cause significant MR.

Our preference is to place the pericardial ASD patch to the right of the coronary sinus ostium while also unroofing the coronary sinus into the left atrium. In ostium primum defects in older children, we prefer to place the patch on the LIL, leaving the AV node and coronary sinus ostium on the right atrial side. In patients with complete AV canal and a left superior vena cava draining to the coronary sinus, we prefer to place the patch to the right of the AV node and suture it to the edge of the coronary sinus ostium, leaving the ostium draining into the right atrium.

Classic Single-Patch Technique

In the classic single-patch technique the same patch of autologous pericardium, usually treated with glutaraldehyde, is used to cover both the ventricular and atrial septal defects. It is critically important to determine the position of the mitral cleft and superior bridging leaflet with respect to the crest of the interventricular septum. In cases where the right and left components of the AV valve are already partitioned with chordal attachments to the crest of the septum, then only the position of the mitral valve cleft needs to be determined. Often incisions must be made in the superior and inferior bridging leaflets parallel and to the right of the interventricular septum to permit proper positioning of the single patch. The extent of leaflet division depends

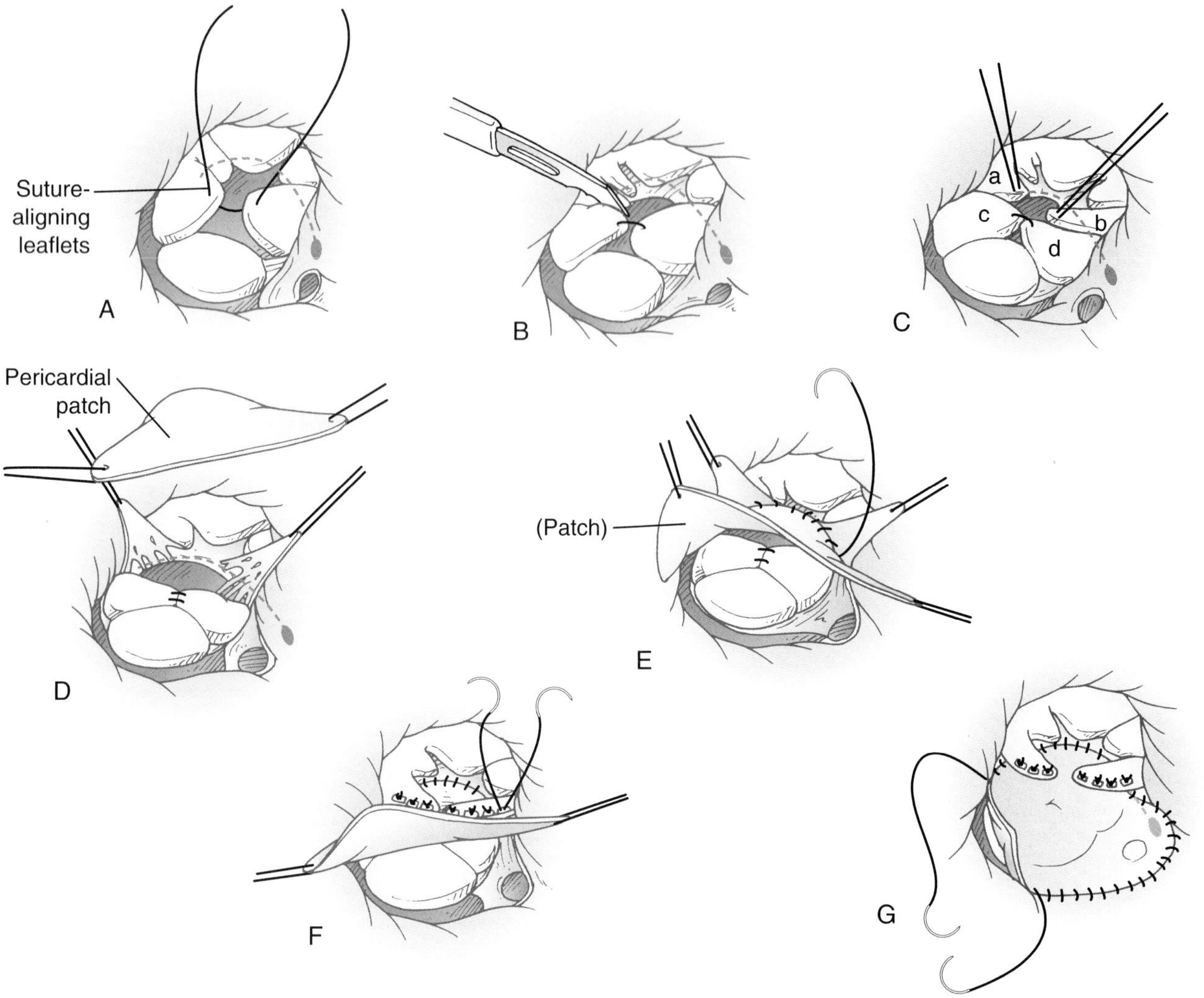

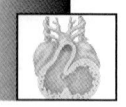

Figure 111–9 Classic single-patch technique for repair of complete atrioventricular (AV) canal defects. A, Alignment sutures placed through the left superior leaflet (LSL) and left inferior leaflet (LIL) at the crest of the interventricular septum. **B,** The superior bridging leaflet is incised. **C,** Two portions of the superior bridging leaflet (a and c) and two portions of the inferior bridging leaflet (b and d) are shown after division of the corresponding leaflets. The division of the inferior bridging leaflet need not extend beyond the underlying interventricular communication. **D,** The left-sided cleft is closed. **E,** The pericardial patch is sewn to the crest of the interventricular septum. **F,** The right and left AV valve leaflets are suspended onto the pericardial patch. **G,** Completion of the repair by closure of the atrial septal defect (ASD). The AV node and coronary sinus ostium are shown draining on the left atrial side.
(Modified from Castaneda AR, Jonas RA, Meyer JE Jr, Hanley FL: Atrioventricular canal defect. In Castaneda AR, Jonas RA, Mayer JE Jr, Hanley FL, editors: Cardiac Surgery of the Neonate and Infant. Philadelphia: W B. Saunders, 1994.)

on the extent of the underlying VSD. Because the VSD under the superior bridging leaflet often extends to the AV valve annulus, the leaflet incision has to extend to the AV annulus as well. This is often not the case for the inferior bridging leaflet, especially in the Rastelli A subtype where the underlying VSD may not extend to the AV valve annulus because of variable fibrous fusion between the LIL and the crest of the interventricular septum. The leaflet incision in that case is only partial, without extension to the AV valve annulus. This protects the conduction tissue and AV node from iatrogenic injury. In patients in whom the VSD under the inferior bridging leaflet extends to the AV valve annulus, the division of the leaflet should be to the right of the crest of the interventricular septum. This allows placement of the patch toward the right, thereby avoiding injury to the underlying conduction tissue at the crest of the interventricular septum (Figure 111-9).

As with the double-patch technique, precise measurement of the width of the patch with respect to the width of the AV canal defect is necessary to prevent MR from distortion of valve leaflets. If the patch is too wide, then the AV valve annulus size will increase, particularly over the interventricular septum; the superior and inferior bridging leaflet tissue available may not be sufficient to cover the orifice, resulting in MR.

Once the AV valve is partitioned into the right and left components, the VSD patch is attached to the right of the crest of the interventricular septum using running or interrupted pledgeted sutures. As with the double-patch technique, the suture line is placed to the right of the crest of the interventricular septum to avoid injury to the bundle of His.

Once the patch is attached to the ventricular septum, the AV valve leaflets must be reattached to the patch. This maneuver is greatly facilitated by prior placement of a suture marking the coaptation point of the LSL and LIL at the base of the cleft at the crest of the interventricular septum. The valve leaflets should not be reattached too far to the atrial side of the patch because this will tether the leaflets and limit coaptation, resulting in MR. Attachment of valve leaflets to the patch is done with pledgeted sutures because these valve leaflets are thin and friable, particularly in infants, predisposing to tearing if attached with nonpledgeted sutures.

The mitral cleft is closed next. The same considerations regarding cleft closure as described for the double-patch technique are applicable here. Similarly, individual commissuroplasty sutures can be placed for the treatment of central left AV valve regurgitation. The patch is then sutured to close the interatrial communication. As discussed earlier for double-patch repair, the coronary sinus may be left draining into the right or left atrium.

The most common causes of MR after single-patch repair of complete AV canal defects are listed as follows. These are applicable to the other two methods of repair as well.

- Partitioning the valve too far to the left of the interventricular septum, which leaves too little AV valve leaflet tissue on the mitral side, preventing leaflet apposition.
- Gathering too much leaflet tissue in the suture line while reattaching the leaflets to the single patch, which decreases the amount of leaflet tissue available.
- Positioning the reattached leaflets too far onto the atrial side. This is the reason why we advocate a crescent-shaped patch rather than a semicircle patch in the double-patch repair method.
- Making the septal patch too wide, resulting in an increased AV valve diameter and preventing good leaflet apposition.
- Unrolling the cleft edges during cleft closure so that the sutures are taken through the true leaflet edges rather than through the edges of apposition of the leaflets. This decreases the amount of leaflet tissue that is in apposition during ventricular systole.
- Closing the cleft only partially, which results in regurgitation through the remaining cleft.
- Closing the cleft too extensively, beyond the first chordal insertions, which tethers the left superior and inferior leaflets, resulting in central MR.
- Deficiency of the AV valve leaflets. This is rarely seen, particularly if no significant preoperative AV valve regurgitation was present.

Modified Single-Patch Technique

The original description of complete AV canal repair by Dr. Lillehei involved attaching the AV valve leaflets to the crest of the interventricular septum primarily, because patch material was not readily available at the time; the ASD was also closed primarily.[44] Recently Wilcox and colleagues[81] reintroduced this method of repair for patients with small VSDs. Nicholson, Nunn, and colleagues[59] have broadened the indications to those with moderate and large VSDs. Other reports have confirmed their findings.[5,52]

In this technique, several pledgeted horizontal mattress sutures are brought through the crest of the interventricular septum, the AV valve leaflets, the autologous pericardial patch, and a narrow strip of Dacron, in that order (Figure 111-10). Care should be taken to avoid damage to the bundle of His by keeping the sutures to the right of the crest of the interventricular septum, especially inferiorly. Suturing through AV valve leaflets effectively partitions the bridging superior and inferior leaflets into right and left components. The strip of Dacron acts as an annuloplasty because its superior–inferior dimension is approximately 80% of the superior–inferior dimension of the AV canal defect, thereby bringing the left-sided AV valve leaflets into closer apposition, minimizing MR. Some have advocated avoiding the use of a strip of Dacron because of concerns about the impact of fixation of the mitral annulus on its long-term growth potential. One potential disadvantage of this technique is the development of LVOTO because the interventricular communication is closed primarily, without patch material. So far, based on limited follow up, this has not been seen. The amount of MR appears similar to that seen with the classic single-patch and double-patch methods, although long-term follow up is not yet available.

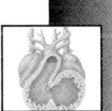

Partial Atrioventricular Canal

The surgical approach to repair ostium primum AV canal defects is similar to that for complete AV canal defects. We use a midline incision extending only into the lower one third of the sternum to provide access to the heart and great vessels. Bicaval cannulation with continuous cardiopulmonary bypass at moderate hypothermia is used, except in

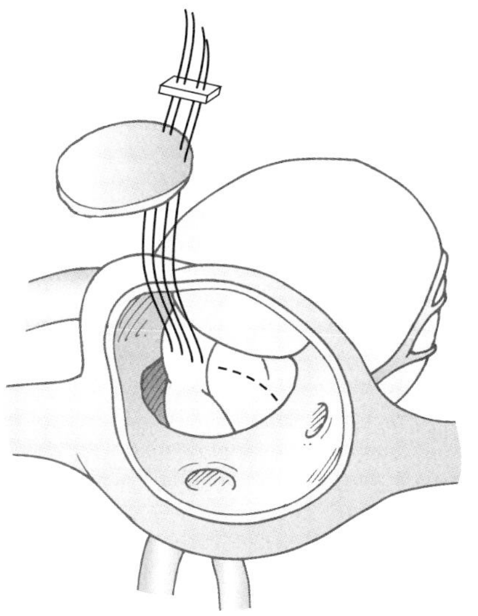

Figure 111-10 Modified single-patch technique for repair of complete atrioventricular (AV) canal defects. Horizontal mattress pledgeted sutures are passed through the crest of the interventricular septum, the AV valve leaflets, and the pericardial patch, and then through a Dacron strip annuloplasty.
(Modified from Nicholson IA, Nunn GR, Sholler GF, et al: Simplified single patch technique for the repair of atrioventricular septal defect. J Thorac Cardiovasc Surg 118:642–646, 1999.)

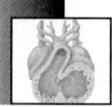

cases where extensive repair of the mitral valve is required, for which lower core temperatures are used. Right atriotomy provides access to the ASD and the mitral valve. If the ostium primum defect is small, an incision is made in the septum primum in a superior–inferior direction to provide adequate visualization of the mitral valve.

As with repair of complete AV canal, initial inspection and testing of the mitral valve is done. The presence of a partial or complete cleft is noted; in the majority of cases the cleft extends to the interventricular septum. The technique for cleft closure is similar to that described earlier, with emphasis on maintaining leaflet coaptation. The ostium primum ASD is closed using autologous pericardium because this tissue is more pliable than synthetic material and less likely to distort valve leaflets; it also results in less hemolysis from residual postoperative MR. A secundum ASD or patent foramen ovale, if present, is closed, either separately or with the same patch (Figure 111-11).

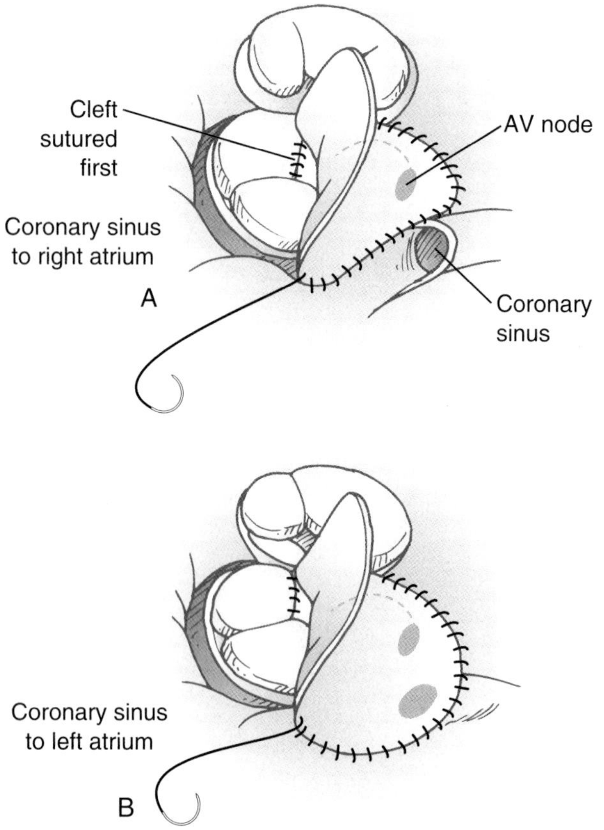

Figure 111–11 Repair of partial atrioventricular (AV) canal defect by closure of the mitral cleft, then pericardial patch closure of the ostium primum defect. A, The coronary sinus drains into the right atrium. The patch is sutured to the right inferior leaflet tissue, and then heads down toward the coronary sinus. An alternative technique (not shown) is suturing to the left inferior leaflet tissue, at the rim of the ostium primum defect. **B,** The coronary sinus drains into the left atrium. This technique decreases injury to the AV node.
(Modified from Castaneda AR, Jonas RA, Meyer JE Jr, Hanley FL: Atrioventricular canal defect. In Castaneda AR, Jonas RA, Mayer JE Jr, Hanley FL, editors: Cardiac Surgery of the Neonate and Infant. Philadelphia: W B. Saunders, 1994.)

Transitional Atrioventricular Canal

Whereas the VSD is nonrestrictive in complete AV canal defects, it is small and restrictive in transitional AV canal defects, is usually centrally located, and is caused by incomplete fusion of the point of coaptation between the LSL and LIL. There is usually a large ostium primum defect and a cleft mitral valve.

Additional small VSDs may be found under the superior or inferior leaflets in cases where the leaflets have not completely fused to the crest of the interventricular septum. In cases where the VSDs are small, they can be difficult to identify intraoperatively. Retraction of the right superior leaflet can provide adequate access to these small defects, and a small 1–2-mm probe can be used to identify residual interventricular communications.

These small VSDs can usually be closed primarily with double-pledgeted sutures. Closure of the central VSD is usually done with the same suture that is used to close the portion of the cleft at the crest of the interventricular septum. Closure of the interatrial communication is done in a manner similar to ostium primum defects (Figure 111-12). Alternatively, a modified single-patch technique could be used, whereby the AV valve leaflets are brought to the crest of the interventricular septum to obliterate the restrictive interventricular communications.

ASSOCIATED CARDIAC LESIONS

Associated cardiovascular lesions are not uncommon, particularly with complete AV canal defects. Extracardiac defects such as PDA and aortic coarctation are usually treated during the same operative procedure for repair of the AV canal defect. The surgical techniques for repair of associated defects are usually not different in the presence of an AV canal defect than when the lesions are isolated defects. Exceptions to this include the presence of secundum ASDs or additional muscular VSDs that are close to the AV canal defect; these can be repaired by extension of the septal patch to cover both lesions. Lesions that include conotruncal abnormalities such as TOF require significant modifications to the surgical approach and are discussed separately.

Patent Ductus Arteriosus

A small PDA is not an uncommon associated defect, particularly in younger infants. The overall incidence is approximately 10%. It is more often present in the setting of complete AV canal defects compared with partial AV canal defects.

Routine ligation of the ductal ligament at the time of operative repair of the canal defect is done in all infants under 3 months of age. In cases where there is a large PDA and the infant has signs of congestive heart failure, our recommendation is to repair both defects simultaneously because ductal ligation alone via left thoracotomy is unlikely to provide symptomatic relief.

Tetralogy of Fallot

TOF complicates approximately 5% of patients with complete AV canal defects. The LSL is typically free floating

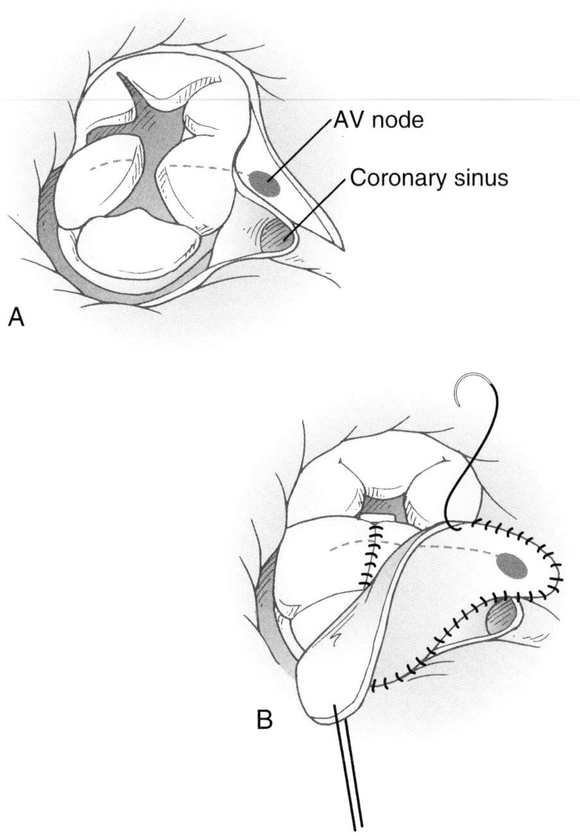

Figure 111–12 Repair of transitional atrioventricular (AV) canal defect. A, Transitional AV canal defect with a small restrictive interventricular communication at the crest of the interventricular septum, between the left superior leaflet (LSL) and the left inferior leaflet (LIL). **B,** A pledgeted suture is taken through the crest of the interventricular septum, then through the LSL and LIL, to close the ventricular septal defect (VSD). The mitral valve cleft is closed. Repair is completed by closure of the ostium primum atrial septal defect (ASD) with a pericardial patch. *(Modified from Castaneda AR, Jonas RA, Meyer JE Jr, Hanley FL: Atrioventricular canal defect. In Castaneda AR, Jonas RA, Mayer JE Jr, Hanley FL, editors: Cardiac Surgery of the Neonate and Infant. Philadelphia: W B. Saunders, 1994.)*

over the interventricular crest of the septum, as in a Rastelli type C defect, resulting in a large VSD with outlet extension. In contrast to heart failure symptoms seen in the majority of isolated complete AV canal defects, the main symptom in the combined lesion is cyanosis. This occurs because of right-to-left intracardiac shunting, which depends primarily on the degree of RV outflow tract obstruction. Cyanosis is often severe and progressive. On the extreme end of this spectrum are patients who have both cyanosis and severe AV valve regurgitation. In a minority of patients the degree of RV outflow tract obstruction is minimal; these patients display heart failure symptoms in early infancy, similar to isolated complete AV canal defects.

The operative management of complete AV canal defects associated with TOF requires modification of the VSD patch because it has to extend to cover the conoventricular anteriorly malaligned VSD. As with most forms of TOF, there is frequently infundibular obstruction, along with pulmonary valvar hypoplasia and stenosis requiring augmentation of the entire RV outflow tract. Because of the anterior position of the aortic valve annulus in this defect, visualization of the anterosuperior edge of the VSD is best accomplished through a small right infundibulotomy. As with cases of uncomplicated AV canal defects, the width of the VSD patch at the AV valve annulus level must be chosen carefully to prevent enlarging the AV valve annulus and resulting in MR.

When the single-patch technique is used to repair complete AV canal in association with TOF, an incision in the superior bridging leaflet is usually needed and is particularly critical. This incision should be further toward the right of the crest of the interventricular septum, toward the right AV valve, to accommodate the underlying anterior deviation of the conal septum. This prevents the development of subaortic obstruction and LVOTO seen when the patch is placed too far to the left of the interventricular septum. This is less of an issue with the double-patch method of repair, although correct positioning of the VSD patch under the superior leaflet is still required. The shape of the VSD patch for the combined lesion resembles a teardrop rather than the typical crescent shape in isolated complete AV canal defect. The modified single-patch technique as originally described is not applicable to canal defects with TOF because the large malalignment defect precludes direct suturing of the LSL to the crest of the interventricular septum.

Repair of the RV outflow tract obstruction is managed in a manner similar to that of isolated TOF, often with an incision in the RV outflow tract. The major difference in the combined lesion is that MR can result in left atrial hypertension with subsequent pulmonary arterial hypertension. If a transannular patch is used, the regurgitant fraction across the enlarged RV outflow tract is increased, leading to RV distention and dysfunction. The right ventriculotomy combined with division of RV muscle bundles in the outflow tract further exacerbate RV dysfunction. In such cases consideration should be given to insertion of a valved conduit such as a homograft or creation of a temporary single-leaflet valve made from autologous pericardium. Careful testing of the tricuspid valve should be undertaken to rule out the presence of significant tricuspid regurgitation. If present, this can be often repaired by closure of the cleft between the right superior and inferior leaflets while avoiding the underlying conduction tissue.

Some have advocated the placement of a systemic-to-pulmonary shunt (such as a right modified Blalock–Taussig shunt) in the neonatal period in patients with severe cyanosis, with subsequent repair at 1–3 years of age, which potentially decreases the need for a transannular patch.[38] An exception is the patient with both cyanosis and severe AV valve regurgitation. The placement of a systemic-to-pulmonary shunt results in worsening ventricular dysfunction and heart failure symptoms. Definitive repair is advocated in that setting.

With the combined lesion, we usually close the interatrial communication completely. A small patent foramen ovale in an infant with isolated TOF is very likely to close spontaneously, whereas a residual interatrial communication in a patient with AV canal defect and TOF is unlikely to close and may result in a persistent atrial-level shunt.

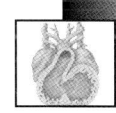

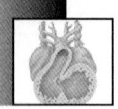

The outcomes of patients with the combined lesion appear to be inferior to those with either isolated TOF or isolated complete AV canal. This is based on a small number of patients reported in various studies. The largest study to date demonstrated no significant difference in mortality,[38] although the degree of technical complexity was increased. Residual MR appears to be the predominant reason for reoperation. Long-term studies are currently lacking because of the small number of long-term survivors with the combined lesion.

Double-Outlet Right Ventricle

An anatomical scenario that can be similar to TOF is DORV, which is differentiated from TOF by the degree of aortic override. When more than 50% of the aortic valve is located over the RV, the lesion is defined as DORV rather than TOF. DORV is present in approximately 1–2% of patients with complete AV canal defects.[70] Typically DORV in this setting is associated with heterotaxy syndrome and unbalanced AV canal defects, increasing the likelihood of univentricular palliation.

Two-ventricle repair of DORV and complete AV canal defects parallels the repair of the two separate lesions. If the VSD is in the subaortic position, the repair is similar to TOF with complete AV canal defect. The patch is more complex because the left ventricle has to be baffled through the VSD to the aortic valve.

Coarctation of the Aorta

If aortic coarctation is present, the left-sided cardiac structures need to be studied carefully to ensure that they are of adequate size and rule out unbalanced AV canal with RV dominance. Aortic coarctation has been associated with hypoplasia of left-sided structures, including left AV valve hypoplasia, single papillary muscle, subaortic stenosis, aortic valve hypoplasia, and aortic arch narrowing. In balanced AV canal defects, a sternotomy approach is used to repair the coarctation by resection and end-to-end anastomosis in conjunction with AV canal repair.

If significant MR is present after repair of complete AV canal defects, an exhaustive search should be performed to rule out the presence of residual LVOTO or aortic coarctation. If present, this increases LV afterload, which increases the distracting pressure on the thin and friable mitral leaflets and worsens the degree of MR. Repair of aortic coarctation in this setting often decreases the degree of MR.

Left Ventricular Outflow Tract Obstruction

Hemodynamically significant LVOTO is relatively rare in the setting of AV canal defects. Interestingly, LVOTO is very rare in the presence of Down syndrome.[22] It is more common in partial AV canal defects than in complete AV canal defects,[34] unless ventricular imbalance is present. This may be due to the modification of the LV outflow tract in complete AV canal repair through the insertion of a VSD patch, whereas no such patch is needed during partial AV canal repair because no VSD is present. LVOTO results in an increased left-to-right shunt with accelerated development of heart failure symptoms. LVOTO appears to be more commonly associated with the Rastelli A subtype of complete AV canal.[76] The development of LVOTO can be acquired, progressive, and recurrent.[65]

The normal LV outflow tract has an angle of almost 90° between the plane of the crest of the interventricular septum and the plane of the outlet septum. This angle is significantly decreased in AV canal defects, measuring 22° in one study.[76] In the Rastelli C subtype the angle is nearly normal after repair of complete AV canal, accounting for the decreased incidence of LVOTO in this setting.

Several anatomical substrates can result in LVOTO:

- Short thickened leaflet chordae may attach the LSL to the left-sided outlet septum, resulting in subaortic fibrous obstruction.
- The anterolateral muscle of the LV, the muscle of Moulaert, may bulge into the LV outflow tract, causing muscular subaortic obstruction.
- Discrete fibrous narrowing, as in an isolated subaortic membrane, may be present.
- Excrescences of accessory AV valve tissue may form in the LV outflow tract, causing obstruction. These may be excised without incident.
- The papillary muscles may have an abnormal position within the ventricle, predisposing to LVOTO.
- Malalignment of the aorta over the interventricular septum may occur, causing obstruction to flow.
- Asymmetrical ventricular hypertrophy also may contribute.

The mechanism and severity of LVOTO usually can be delineated by two-dimensional echocardiography. Cardiac catheterization is reserved to confirm the degree of obstruction, particularly in patients presenting late after AV canal repair.

The surgical treatment is usually determined by the mechanism of obstruction. If there is a discrete subaortic membrane, it may be resected by performing an aortotomy and working through the aortic valve; a myectomy is recommended in this setting. Obstructing primary AV valve chordal attachments can be divided off the crest of the septum, and then reattached to the VSD patch. These primary chordae originate from the free margins of the superior and inferior leaflets and attach onto papillary muscles. Division of these chordae should be done in conjunction with mitral valve repair, because chordal resection alone results in unsupported mitral valve leaflets, leading to MR.[68] Secondary AV valve chordae may be divided, if necessary. These typically originate from the undersurface of the leaflets and attach to the ventricular surface. As a result, the risk of MR after division of secondary chordae is much less than after division of primary chordae. In tunnel-like LVOTO, more extensive enlargement of the LV outflow tract is required, such as a modified Konno procedure. Unlike the more common forms of tunnel-like LVOTO, in AV canal defects the conduction tissue is farther away from the area of enlargement and therefore injury to the AV node is rare. In more extreme cases where the extent of LV outflow obstruction and aortic hypoplasia is thought to preclude a two-ventricle repair, surgical management as a single-ventricle lesion is advised, ultimately leading to a Fontan circulation.

Subaortic obstruction may be recurrent. In one study of 19 patients with subaortic stenosis associated with AV canal defects, 27 operations for LVOTO were performed.[76] The most common procedure was fibrous resection of a subaortic membrane with myectomy. Mean time to reoperation for recurrent LVOTO was 4.9 years at a median follow-up period of 5.6 years. This resulted in a 6-year actuarial freedom from reoperation of 66%. Leaflet augmentation with pericardium, and fibromyectomy, have been suggested in order to decrease the incidence of reoperation.

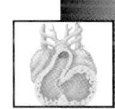

Transposition of the Great Arteries

Management of TGA associated with complete AV canal defect is similar to the surgical treatment of each isolated defect. The AV canal defect is repaired, and an arterial switch procedure is performed. The AV canal repair is more challenging because valve leaflets are very friable in the first week of life compared with the first few months of life. All heart structures are smaller as well, which increases the technical complexity of the procedure. We recommend reinforcement of all sutures through AV valve leaflets with autologous pericardial pledgets, especially those placed for cleft closure. If the superior bridging leaflet is undivided, we recommend avoiding the classic single-patch technique because leaflet division is necessary. Resuspension of the leaflets onto the single patch may gather too much precious leaflet tissue, predisposing to the development of MR.

Double-Orifice Mitral Valve

Another unusual abnormality of the left-sided AV valve is double-orifice mitral valve, present in approximately 5% of cases. A second accessory orifice is present, usually on the inferior aspect of the left lateral leaflet, which can vary substantially in size. If the second orifice is small, it may be left open without consequence.

If large, the papillary muscles need to be examined because one papillary muscle may be related to each orifice, resulting in a parachute mitral valve of the major orifice. In these situations the cleft should be closed only partially, because postoperative mitral stenosis results with complete cleft closure. Splitting the bridging leaflet tissue between the two orifices is not advised; this may result in significant MR because the leaflet tissue becomes unsupported. In some cases where regurgitation is present at the accessory orifice, addition of a triangular-shaped patch made from glutaraldehyde-treated autologous pericardium has been advocated in an attempt to extend the width of the leaflets and improve coaptation.

Parachute Mitral Valve

A single papillary muscle is present in 5% of cases of complete AV canal defect. The presence of two closely spaced papillary muscles or a single papillary muscle can result in all chordal structures attaching to a single point, referred to as parachute mitral valve. This is especially the case if the chordae are thick and the interchordal spaces are small.

The surgical management of mitral valve abnormalities in common AV canal defects remains a challenging area. Because of wide variability in leaflet and papillary muscle morphology and position, no single approach is applicable to all cases. Careful preoperative echocardiographic analysis of the number and spacing of the papillary muscles and the extent of chordal attachments is essential to successful outcomes.

Closure of the cleft between the LSL and LIL frequently results in postoperative mitral stenosis in this setting. We elect to leave the cleft either partially or fully open, depending on the degree of separation of the papillary muscles, the thickness of the chordae, and the width of the interchordal spaces. If this still results in significant regurgitation, valve replacement may be the only option. Although techniques have been described for improving leaflet mobility by separating the chordae, inflow to the ventricle is still dependent on the size of the interchordal spaces, which remains narrow when the chordae attach to a relatively narrow area within the ventricle. In cases where there are two separate but closely spaced papillary muscles, mobilizing the papillary muscles away from each other may be effective in improving the effective orifice of the mitral valve.

Unbalanced Atrioventricular Canal

Bharati, Lev, and colleagues[10] pointed out that the AV junction may be committed primarily to one ventricle in some cases of complete AV canal defects, resulting in associated hypoplasia of the contralateral ventricular cavity and outflow structures. This occurs in approximately 5–7% of patients with complete AV canal defects. In the more common RV-dominant form there is significant hypoplasia of the LV, aortic valve, ascending aorta, and aortic arch. Conversely, in the LV-dominant type, hypoplasia of the RV, pulmonary valve, and pulmonary artery is seen.

Management decisions regarding the potential use of the hypoplastic chamber as part of a two-ventricle repair should be based on objective criteria because this group of patients is at higher risk for operative mortality and morbidity in most series. Several preoperative indexes of ventricular dominance have been proposed, although most are based on a small number of patients.[19,78] Measurement of relative ventricular cavity volume to compare RV versus LV volume is frequently unreliable in the RV-dominant form because the RV is larger than the LV even in the balanced forms, as a result of RV volume overload from left-to-right shunting. Absolute LV volume calculations have been proposed as useful predictive indexes with values of 15 ml/m^2 or greater as sufficient criteria for successful two-ventricle repair. The relative size of the right versus left component of the AV junction as measured from a subcostal left anterior oblique view has also been proposed as a predictive index. This AV valve index has been shown to be superior to ratio measurements of ventricular cavity size because it is less affected by volume load differences resulting from left-to-right shunting.

There are no standardized criteria that favor one-ventricle versus two-ventricle repair in the majority of equivocal patients.[24] If the canal is only mildly unbalanced, then a two-ventricle repair can often be performed. If the canal is grossly unbalanced with severe hypoplasia of one ventricular cavity, then a single-ventricle approach should be followed. For the remainder of patients with unbalanced AV canal, we use the following criteria, in aggregate, to favor a two-ventricle repair. They involve a determination of relative ventricular size, AV valve architecture and function, outflow tract size and position, and the presence of associated cardiac lesions:

- The LV reaches the apex or near the apex.
- The calculated postoperative LV volume is 15 ml/m^2 or greater.
- The calculated postoperative mitral valve annulus Z-score is −2 or greater.
- Two papillary muscles are present, although a single papillary muscle is not an absolute contraindication for two-ventricle repair.
- AV valve chordae attaching to the conal septum, which is a substrate for LVOTO, are absent. Associated aortic coarctation is often present.
- Heterotaxy syndrome is absent, although rarely, a patient with polysplenia will have two well-balanced ventricles that are amenable to two-ventricle repair.

These criteria, however, do not take into account the growth potential that exists, particularly in very young infants. Recent reports have described growth of the LV cavity after closure of interatrial communications by forcing blood flow across the left AV valve.[30] However, because of the limited experience with this technique and the inherent errors in LV cavity calculations, confirmation of the findings of LV cavity growth is needed before wide adoption can be recommended.

Single Ventricle

In cases where more complex malformations are present, such as heterotaxy syndrome or severely unbalanced AV canal defects, consideration should be given to managing these patients along a single-ventricle pathway. In patients with complete AV canal defects and heterotaxy syndrome, associated lesions include a common atrium, cor triatriatum, interrupted inferior vena cava with hemiazygos continuation into a left superior vena cava draining into the roof of the left atrium, and a small right superior vena cava. These further increase the surgical complexity of two-ventricle repair.[60]

Similar considerations should be given to patients with DORV and complete AV canal defect with an inlet-septal VSD. In these cases the VSD is remote from the semilunar valves. Baffling the LV to the aorta, or baffling the LV to the pulmonary artery along with a concomitant arterial switch procedure, requires enlarging the VSD. Complications include baffle obstruction and complete heart block. A single-ventricle approach may be less risky in this setting.

Recurrent Mitral Regurgitation

Significant postoperative MR requiring reoperation is present in 4–15% of patients after repair of AV canal defects.[53,56] In our experience, those at highest risk had at least moderate MR early postoperatively.[35] Other factors associated with progressive late postoperative MR include parachute mitral valve,[9] double-orifice mitral valve,[35,50,55] patients without Down syndrome,[79] no closure of the cleft at primary repair,[55,79,80] and preoperative MR.[50,56] Although mild deterioration is fairly common after complete AV canal repair, serious deterioration is rare, especially after the first 30 postoperative months, as reported in one recent study of 39 patients.[66] Another recent study followed two groups of patients, one in whom the cleft was closed at the time of initial AV canal surgery, and the other in whom the cleft was deliberately left open as part of a trifoliate repair.[80] Overall survival and freedom from reoperation for MR were significantly better when the mitral valve cleft was closed at the time of initial AV canal surgery. One confounding variable was the earlier date of surgery in the group in whom the cleft was left open; improvements in myocardial preservation and postoperative care could have contributed to the improved results seen in the more recent group of patients in whom the cleft was closed.

The mechanism of late MR in the majority of cases has been regurgitation through the cleft, either because it was left open initially or because it reopened after complete or partial closure. Annular dilatation with central regurgitation is frequently an associated finding. Worsening MR leads to worsening LV volume overload, and eccentric LV hypertrophy, ultimately leading to LV dysfunction and failure.

Preoperative echocardiographic studies should delineate the mechanism of regurgitation and the location of the regurgitant jet (either centrally or through the cleft or both). A direct measurement of the diameter of the mitral annulus should be performed and compared to the expected annular diameter for the patient's age, corresponding to a Z-score of 0.

Reoperative mitral valve repair depends on the underlying anatomical abnormality. If the regurgitation is through a cleft, then closure of the cleft, along with reduction of the mitral annular diameter to an appropriate size (Z-score between −2 and +2), is often effective. More complex mechanisms such as immobile, thickened, or retracted mitral leaflets are more difficult to repair and frequently require leaflet augmentation with autologous pericardium, along with reduction of the annular diameter. Rarely regurgitation may be through a tear in the LSL or LIL. This can occur if sutures through thin and friable leaflets were not reinforced with autologous pericardial pledgets at the time of initial surgery as a neonate. The presence of MR thickens the leaflets, allowing for closure of the tear either primarily or using a small pericardial patch. In the older child a flexible annuloplasty ring should be implanted, which provides support for the repaired valve, especially during ventricular systole.

In some cases, mitral repair is not possible. Mitral valve replacement becomes necessary, typically using a mechanical prosthesis. Because the native left AV valve encroaches on the LV outflow tract, valve replacement may result in significant LVOTO. This can be avoided by first suturing a rectangular Dacron patch to the left AV valve annulus in the subaortic region. The mitral prosthesis can then be attached to the Dacron patch superiorly.[48] The conduction tissue is located at the anteroinferior aspect of the left AV valve annulus. The native AV valve leaflet tissue should be preserved in that location and not excised. Sutures can be passed through these native leaflets rather than through the mitral annulus in that location to minimize the incidence of heart block. Care should also be taken to avoid injury to the left circumflex coronary artery, which can be surprisingly close in small patients.

Outcomes after surgical management of recurrent MR are inferior to those reported after initial AV canal defects. In a study from our institution representing the largest series to date, 46 patients underwent reoperation between 1988 and 1998 for recurrent hemodynamically significant MR.[53] Survival at 10 years was 86.6%. Three of nine patients undergoing mitral valve replacement developed complete heart block. Significant improvements in clinical status were present after mitral valve surgery. Overall freedom from reoperation at 5 years was 78.5% for mitral valve repair and 85.7% for mitral valve replacement.

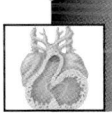

POSTOPERATIVE CARE

Postoperative management of patients after repair of complete AV canal defects is similar to the management of other patients after complex cardiac surgery. Intraoperative confirmation of complete closure of the VSD and ASD should be obtained. Our preference is to use measurements of right atrial and pulmonary artery oxygen saturations to detect residual left-to-right shunts. A step-up in oxygen saturation greater than 10 mmHg or an absolute pulmonary artery oxygen saturation greater than 80% while on 50% inspired oxygen is suspicious for the presence of a hemodynamically significant residual VSD ($\dot{Q}p:\dot{Q}s$ >1.5). This should prompt intraoperative confirmation by echocardiography before return to cardiopulmonary bypass and closure of the residual VSD.

Intraoperative transesophageal echocardiogram (TEE) is highly recommended for patients weighing more than 5 kg. TEE can be performed in patients as small as 2.5 kg, albeit with a higher risk of esophageal trauma and perforation coupled with a higher probability of left atrial compression by the posteriorly positioned TEE probe, which raises left atrial pressure. TEE is especially useful in evaluating AV valve function, particularly if significant MR is suspected. Monitoring left atrial and pulmonary artery pressure aids in the postoperative care of these patients, especially in cases where preoperative pulmonary hypertension is present.

Low cardiac output state should be judiciously managed by aggressive use of inotropic support rather than volume resuscitation because excessive volume infusion can result in ventricular distention and valvar dilation, resulting in worsening MR. The atrial filling pressures should be kept low, not significantly higher than 10 mm Hg, especially in the first 24 hours postoperatively. Use of afterload reduction, particularly with phosphodiesterase inhibitors such as milrinone, is particularly valuable in the early postoperative period. Typically the milrinone loading dose of 50 μg/kg is followed by a milrinone infusion at 0.5 μg/kg/min (range: 0.25–1.0 μg/kg/min). If significant hypotension is present, then the loading dose may be held and the drip may be decreased to 0.25 μg/kg/min. An aggressive search should be undertaken to exclude anatomical causes of low cardiac output syndrome.

The insertion of temporary atrial and ventricular pacing wires at the time of surgery is strongly recommended to allow for postoperative atrial pacing if junctional rhythm develops. Pacing, in addition to cooling and neuromuscular blockage, usually allows the resolution of junctional rhythm over several days. Because the AV node is displaced inferiorly in AV canal defects, iatrogenic injury to the conduction tissue is possible. Atrial and ventricular pacing is recommended in that setting because ventricular pacing alone can worsen left AV valve regurgitation.

Early postoperative pulmonary hypertension can be seen in patients with complete AV canal defects, and it is more prevalent with increasing age at the time of definitive repair and correlates with surgical mortality. Patients with Down syndrome usually have both increased pulmonary artery pressure and increased pulmonary vascular resistance in the perioperative period.[54] The insertion of a pulmonary artery line at the time of surgery aids in making the diagnosis. Anatomical causes that mimic pulmonary hypertension need to be excluded, such as severe MR, severe mitral stenosis, and residual VSD. Echocardiography is helpful in differentiating anatomical from nonanatomical causes of postoperative pulmonary hypertension.

Patients with complete AV canal defects, especially in association with Down syndrome, are prone to develop pulmonary hypertensive crises postoperatively because of elevated pulmonary vascular resistance. Suctioning of the endotracheal tube may trigger such crises. This is manifested by a sudden rise in pulmonary artery pressure, sometimes to suprasystemic levels, along with an elevation in RV pressure and a fall in systemic arterial blood pressure. Treatment is by hyperventilation with 100% oxygen, and judicious use of sedation, neuromuscular blockade, and inhaled nitric oxide. Although some have advocated the use of phenoxybenzamine in this setting, we have not found this to be necessary.

OUTCOMES

During the period between January 1990 and December 1998, 365 patients with various forms of AV canal defects have undergone two-ventricle repair at Children's Hospital Boston.[21] Of these, 191 had a complete AV canal defect where the VSD was deemed at least moderate in size and required patch closure. Among the 365 patients, 19 had associated TOF (5%) and 140 had either an ostium primum atrial septal defect alone or a transitional AV canal defect. Five patients had associated coarctation of the aorta, and seven had preoperative LVOTO. Trivial to mild AV valve regurgitation was present preoperatively in 159 patients (83%), and 26 (13%) had moderate to severe AV valve regurgitation. Of the patients with complete AV canal defects, 11% had at least moderate hypoplasia of one ventricle, with 4% having a dominant LV and 7% having a dominant RV.

The classic one-patch technique was used in 83% of children with complete AV canal defects; the remaining 16% were repaired using the two-patch technique, depending on surgeon preference. The median age at repair was 4.6 months, and median weight was 4.5 kg.

In the 191 patients with complete AV canal defects undergoing biventricular repair, there were three early deaths, for an operative mortality of 1.5%. Three patients had complete heart block postoperatively, which required pacemaker insertion during the initial hospitalization. Trivial to mild MR was present on postoperative echocardiographic follow up in 66% of the patients, whereas 10% had at least moderate MR at the time of discharge. There was no correlation between the presence of MR preoperatively and postoperatively.

Complete Atrioventricular Canal Defect

Several factors have contributed to decreasing mortality for repair of complete AV canal defects over the past 2 decades.

Mortality currently ranges between 2.5–13% in various recent studies.[2,49,72,74] Risk factors that affect overall survival and the need for reoperation include the following:

- *Earlier era of operation*[8,33,35,74]: This has been a consistent risk factor for both early death and late reoperation in a variety of studies. Improvements in myocardial preservation, intraoperative anesthetic management, perfusion methods, intraoperative transesophageal echocardiography, postoperative care, and better understanding of lesion anatomy, along with better surgical techniques, have contributed to decreasing mortality over time.
- *Older age at surgery:* Repair beyond age 3–4 months has been correlated with increased perioperative mortality.[50,69] This may be related to higher incidence of pulmonary hypertensive crises seen with increasing patient age at the time of definitive surgery.[7] Postoperative pulmonary hypertensive crises have been correlated with increased operative mortality and need for reoperation.[2,8] Increasing age as a risk factor for mortality has not been shown to be the case in all studies.[3,33] In fact, in one study of 274 patients, repair at less than 6 months of age was an incremental risk factor for perioperative mortality.[33]
- *Postoperative left AV valve regurgitation:* This has been identified in most series to be a key risk factor for the subsequent need for reoperation[8,13,47,55] and death.[8,35] The overall incidence of significant postoperative MR has slowly decreased over the years as surgical techniques have improved and a better understanding of the underlying anatomy has evolved. A review from our institution revealed a reoperation rate of 7% in recent years.[35] Other contemporary series have noted an incidence of 16% for at least moderate postoperative MR.[31]
- *Preoperative AV valve regurgitation:* A higher incidence of postoperative MR is seen in patients with higher degrees of preoperative AV valve regurgitation.[31] Leaflet division may exacerbate this association.[31] This has not been a consistent finding, with one recent study of 115 patients reporting that moderate to severe preoperative left AV valve regurgitation, present in 21 patients, was not a risk factor for operative mortality.[74] In the same study, moderate or severe late MR was present in 17% of patients with mild or less preoperative left AV valve regurgitation compared with 33% of patients with moderate or severe preoperative left AV valve regurgitation, although this difference was not statistically significant. An earlier study of 62 infants operated on before 1987 also failed to show the correlation between preoperative and postoperative MR.[79]
- *Double-orifice mitral valve*[*]: This adversely affects both survival and freedom from reoperation. It may be associated with unbalanced AV canal with RV dominance, a single papillary muscle, LVOTO, and aortic coarctation. If the cleft is closed completely, postoperative mitral stenosis may result. Some have recommended leaving a fenestration in the interatrial septum to allow for decompression of the left atrium as needed.[55]

Double-Patch Technique

There are more reports in the literature with the use of the double-patch technique compared with the single-patch technique for repair of complete AV canal defects. In one representative study of 203 patients[8] operated on between 1974 and 1995, operative mortality was 7.9%, which decreased to 3% after 1990. Cleft closure was performed in 93% of patients. All deaths in patients with moderate or severe postoperative MR occurred within the first year after surgery. At a median follow-up period of 4.9 years, late mitral valve function was available in 72% of patients, with trivial or mild MR present in 94% of patients. In another study of 115 patients[6] repaired between 1983 and 1994, operative mortality was 6%. At a mean follow-up period of 2.4 years, eight patients (7%) underwent reoperation for MR. Bando and colleagues[8] reviewed 203 patients treated between 1974 and 1995 using a double-patch technique without division of the leaflets. Operative mortality decreased from 19% before 1980 to 3% after 1990. Important risk factors for early mortality included postoperative severe MR, double-orifice mitral valve, and postoperative pulmonary hypertensive crises.

The use of one or two patches has been studied. In a series of 363 children with transitional and complete AV canal defects repaired between July 1982 and February 1995 in Toronto, 243 patients underwent repair with a double-patch technique and 99 underwent repair using the classic single-patch method.[55] Median age at surgery was 8.3 months. Early mortality was 10.5%, whereas 10-year survival was 83%. Freedom from reoperation for left AV valve repair was 86% at 10 years. The use of one or two patches did not affect operative mortality, a conclusion supported by others.[74] A total of 114 patients (31%) had one or both leaflets divided to place the VSD patch. In that study, leaflet division was not a risk factor for reoperation or mortality.

This conclusion has been questioned recently when a later group of 209 patients with complete and transitional AV canal defects repaired at the same institution between 1995 and 2002 were examined.[31] Median age at repair was 5 months. All patients were treated with the double-patch technique. Bridging leaflets were divided in 73% of patients to better visualize the VSD and subaortic region. Division of valve leaflets was a risk factor for the development of moderate or greater MR within the first postoperative year. This may be due to the gathering of precious leaflet tissue during resuspension of the leaflets. An alternative explanation is that leaflet division may make it easier to insert a wider-than-usual VSD patch, thereby pulling the leaflets farther apart during systole and decreasing the area of leaflet coaptation, predisposing to MR. Interestingly, the incidence of reoperation for residual VSDs (2.9%) was unchanged in this series compared with the earlier series of patients (2.5%) from the same institution.

Classic Single-Patch Technique

Similar results have been obtained with the classic single-patch technique. Overall mortality has been decreasing with time. In a study of 301 patients from our institution operated on between 1972 and 1992, 30-day operative mortality decreased from 25% before 1976 to 3% after 1987.[35] The majority of patients (97%) underwent repair using a classic single-patch technique. The incidence of reoperation for residual MR decreased over time, but remained at 7% in recent years. An earlier year of operation, double-orifice

*References 3, 8, 18, 35, 55, 70.

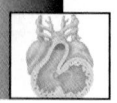

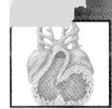

mitral valve and significant residual postoperative MR were risk factors for operative mortality. Only 61% of patients had cleft closure at the time of initial AV canal surgery.

In a follow-up study from our institution,[21] a total of 365 patients with AV canal defects were repaired between January 1990 and December 1998. Isolated complete AV canal defect was present in 191 patients, 73% of whom had a Rastelli type A defect, 5% had a Rastelli type B defect, and 22% had a Rastelli type C defect. An additional 30 patients had complete AV canal defects associated with complex congenital heart disease, including 19 patients with TOF. The remaining 140 patients had partial AV canal defects (n = 88) or transitional AV canal defects (n = 52). Down syndrome was present in 54% of the study cohort. It was most commonly associated with complete AV canal defects, present in 75% of patients. Down syndrome was present in 53% of patients with complete AV canal defects and other complex heart lesions and was present in only 30% of patients with either partial or transitional AV canal defects. Survival for patients with complete AV canal defects in association with other complex congenital heart defects was lower compared with patients with isolated complete AV canal defects: Operative survival was 89% versus 97%, 1-year survival was 77% versus 96%, and 5-year survival was 77% versus 96%, respectively. Incomplete mitral cleft closure and absence of Down syndrome were the risk factors identified by multivariate analysis for the late development of moderate or severe MR or the need for mitral valve reoperation.

Decreasing operative mortality was documented in another study of 172 consecutive patients with AV canal defects,[20] operated on with the classic single-patch technique at a mean age of 10.8 months between 1981 and 2000. Mortality decreased from 16.4% to 3% in the second decade of the study. Factors contributing to this include earlier age at repair with avoidance of initial palliative procedures, decreased incidence of postoperative low cardiac output syndrome, fewer residual defects of hemodynamic significance, and a lower incidence of complete heart block. The incidence of late reoperation for recurrent MR was 6.4%. Freedom from late reoperation for severe MR was 90% at 15 years, which did not significantly improve in the second decade of the study.

Earlier age at surgery has been advocated in an effort to decrease the incidence of late MR. Reddy and colleagues,[64] using a single-patch technique, reported excellent results using this technique in a group of 72 patients operated on at a median age of 3.9 months. Forty percent of patients underwent surgery at less than 3 months of age. Moderate MR was present in three patients at hospital discharge. At a median follow-up period of 2 years, age was not related to postoperative MR, death, or the need for reoperation. This study emphasizes the excellent outcomes possible in operating on younger patients. Delaying surgery increases the risks of heart failure, failure to thrive, PVOD, and damage to the AV valve tissues.

Modified Single-Patch Technique

In early follow-up, the results in patients treated with the modified single-patch technique mirror those with the classic single-patch and double-patch techniques. Specifically, the incidence of operative death, MR, and LVOTO appear similar.

Wilcox and colleagues[81] initially reported 21 patients with complete AV canal defect, of whom 12 had small VSD components and were repaired with the modified single-patch technique; the rest were repaired with either a classic single-patch or double-patch technique. At 34 months of follow-up, comparable results were obtained using the various techniques in this small cohort of patients.

Nicholson, Nunn, and colleagues[59] adopted this modified single-patch technique and expanded its indications to include those with moderate and large interventricular communications. They reported 47 consecutive patients operated on between 1995 and 1998, with a 4% operative mortality. No significant LVOTO was noted on intermediate-term follow up. Mild MR was present in 26% of patients, whereas moderate MR was seen in 6% of patients at a mean follow-up period of 1.9 years. The absence of LVOTO at 1-year follow-up was recently reported in another group of 15 consecutive complete AV canal patients repaired using the modified single-patch technique.[5] There was no operative mortality. One patient developed severe MR requiring mitral valve replacement.

Results from our institution with this technique[52] mirror those published elsewhere. In a series of 33 patients, most of whom had moderate or large interventricular communications repaired between 1998 and 2002, outcomes differed based on the extent of ventricular imbalance. In patients with balanced AV canal defects, no operative mortality was present. One patient required mitral valve repair at 1 year postoperatively because of cleft dehiscence. In patients with unbalanced AV canal defects who underwent biventricular repair (n = 9), two died and an additional patient required a short course of extracorporeal membrane oxygenation. Follow-up echocardiograms in 66% of patients revealed trivial to no MR in 12%, mild MR in 55%, moderate MR in 21%, and severe MR in 6%. There has been no significant LVOTO to date.

Partial Atrioventricular Canal Defect

The operative mortality for partial AV canal defects is low, less than 1–2% in most series.[49] A small subset of patients displays heart failure symptoms and several left-sided obstructive lesions within the first year of life.[45] These represent a higher-risk subgroup.

In a study of 180 patients repaired between 1982 and 1996,[56] early mortality was 1.6%. The mean age at repair was 4.6 years; repair at less than 1 year of age was a significant risk factor for mortality. With a mean follow-up period of 6 years, 10-year actuarial survival was 98%. Important long-term sequelae were the development of late MR and subaortic obstruction.

Similar findings were reported recently in the largest series to date of patients with ostium primum ASD.[26] A total of 334 patients who underwent repair over a 40-year period between 1955 and 1995 were studied, with a median follow-up period of 19 years. Thirty-day perioperative mortality was 2%, whereas 20-year and 40-year survival rates were 87% and 76%, respectively. Although this long-term survival was good, it was lower than that for the general population. Reoperation occurred in 11% of patients, most commonly for mitral stenosis or MR. LVOTO occurred in 11% of patients (n = 36), although only seven patients required reoperation. Postoperative supraventricular arrhythmias were common, especially in older patients. Although the study was descriptive, with important limitations with respect to data collection and analysis, it does provide long-term insight with respect to outcomes in these patients.

Late MR, although rare, correlates with late morbidity, similar to the situation for complete AV canal defects. In partial AV canal defects, the incidence of significant MR requiring reoperation ranges between 7–10%, depending on the study and the length of follow up.[49,61] This may be correlated with a more frequent need for valve replacement than in complete AV canal defects,[1,61] possibly related to the fixation of the superior leaflet to the crest of the interventricular septum and the association of subvalvar abnormalities.

SUMMARY

AV canal defects represent a continuum of lesions with varying degrees of AV valvar abnormalities and interatrial and interventricular communications. In complete AV canal defects, complete elective repair should be performed early in infancy, preferably between 2 and 4 months of age. Equivalent results have been obtained with the three standard techniques of repair. Surgical intervention results in low mortality and morbidity, both in the short term and the long term. In cases where congestive heart failure or moderate to severe MR is present, complete repair should be undertaken at the time of presentation, because further delay or use of palliative procedures only increases the risks of subsequent definitive surgical therapy.

Surgical management of transitional and partial AV canal defects should include elective repair in early childhood. In cases where left AV valve regurgitation is significant, repair should be undertaken earlier to prevent further deterioration of valve function and LV dilation and dysfunction.

Associated cardiac surgical lesions should be repaired at the time of complete AV canal repair. A remaining management dilemma is the patient with unbalanced AV canal defect, where surgical options include biventricular correction versus univentricular palliation.

Outcomes of patients with complete AV canal defects have improved steadily over the years. This reflects not only better intraoperative management, but also improved preoperative and postoperative care and follow up in these patients.

REFERENCES

1. Abbruzzese PA, Napoleone A, Bini RM, et al: Late left atrioventricular valve insufficiency after repair of partial atrioventricular septal defects: Anatomical and surgical determinants. Ann Thorac Surg 49:111–114, 1990.
2. Alexi-Meskishvili V, Ishino K, Dahnert I, et al: Correction of complete atrioventricular septal defects with the double-patch technique and cleft closure. Ann Thorac Surg 62:519–524, 1996.
3. Al-Hay AA, MacNeill SJ, Yacoub M, et al: Complete atrioventricular septal defect, Down syndrome, and surgical outcome: Risk factors. Ann Thorac Surg 75:412–421, 2003.
4. Anderson RH, Zuberbuhler JR, Penkoske PA, Neches WH: Of clefts, commissures, and things. J Thorac Cardiovasc Surg 90: 605–610, 1985.
5. Anil Kumar D, Suresh Kumar RN, Rao PN, et al: Complete atrioventricular septal defect repair: Simplified single patch technique. Ind J Thorac Cardiovasc Surg 19:102–107, 2003.
6. Backer CL, Mavroudis C, Alboliras ET, Zales VR: Repair of complete atrioventricular canal defects: Results with the two-patch technique. Ann Thorac Surg 60:530–537, 1995.
7. Bando K, Turrentine MW, Sharp TG, et al: Pulmonary hypertension after operations for congenital heart disease: Analysis of risk factors and management. J Thorac Cardiovasc Surg 112:1600–1607, 1996.
8. Bando K, Turrentine MW, Sun K, et al: Surgical management of complete atrioventricular septal defects. A twenty-year experience. J Thorac Cardiovasc Surg 110:1543–1554, 1995.
9. Baufreton C, Journois D, Leca F, et al: Ten-year experience with surgical treatment of partial atrioventricular septal defect: Risk factors in the early postoperative period. J Thorac Cardiovasc Surg 112:14–20, 1996.
10. Bharati S, Lev M, McAllister HA Jr, Kirklin JW: Surgical anatomy of the atrioventricular valve in the intermediate type of common atrioventricular orifice. J Thorac Cardiovasc Surg 79:884–889, 1980.
11. Bull C, Rigby ML, Shinebourne EA: Should management of complete atrioventricular canal defect be influenced by coexistent Down syndrome? Lancet 1:1147–1149, 1985.
12. Burn J, Brennan P, Little J, et al: Recurrence risks in offspring of adults with major heart defects: Results from first cohort of British collaborative study. Lancet 351:311–316, 1998.
13. Capouya ER, Laks H, Drinkwater DC Jr, et al: Management of the left atrioventricular valve in the repair of complete atrioventricular septal defects. J Thorac Cardiovasc Surg 104: 196–201, 1992.
14. Carpentier A: Surgical anatomy and management of the mitral component of the atrioventricular canal defects. In Anderson RH, Shinebourne EA, editors: Pediatric Cardiology, pp. 466–490. London: Churchill Livingstone, 1979.
15. Castaneda AR, Jonas RA, Mayer JE Jr, Hanley FL: Atrioventricular canal defect. In Castaneda AR, Jonas RA, Mayer JE Jr, Hanley FL, editors: Cardiac Surgery of the Neonate and Infant. Philadelphia: W B. Saunders, 1994.
16. Chin AJ, Keane JF, Norwood WI, Castaneda AR: Repair of complete common atrioventricular canal in infancy. J Thorac Cardiovasc Surg 84:437–445, 1982.
17. Clapp S, Perry BL, Farooki ZQ, et al: Down's syndrome, complete atrioventricular canal, and pulmonary vascular obstructive disease. J Thorac Cardiovasc Surg 100:115–121, 1990.
18. Clapp SK, Perry BL, Farooki ZQ, et al: Surgical and medical results of complete atrioventricular canal: A ten-year review. Am J Cardiol 59:454–458, 1987.
19. Cohen MS, Jacobs ML, Weinberg PM, Rychik J: Morphometric analysis of unbalanced common atrioventricular canal using two-dimensional echocardiography. J Am Coll Cardiol 28:1017–1023, 1996.
20. Crawford FA Jr, Stroud MR: Surgical repair of complete atrioventricular septal defect. Ann Thorac Surg 72:1621–1629, 2001.
21. Daebritz S, del Nido PJ: Surgical management of common atrioventricular canal. Prog Pediatr Cardiol 10:161–171, 1999.
22. De Biase L, Di Ciommo V, Ballerini L, et al: Prevalence of left-sided obstructive lesions in patients with atrioventricular canal without Down's syndrome. J Thorac Cardiovasc Surg 91: 467–469, 1986.
23. del Nido PJ, Bichell DP: Minimal-access surgery for congenital heart defects. Semin Thorac Cardiovasc Surg Pediatr Card Surg Annu 1:75–80, 1998.
24. Drinkwater DC Jr, Laks H: Unbalanced atrioventricular septal defects. Semin Thorac Cardiovasc Surg 9:21–25, 1997.

25. Eisenberg LM, Markwald RR: Molecular regulation of atrioventricular valvuloseptal morphogenesis. Circ Res 77:1–6, 1995.
26. El-Najdawi EK, Driscoll DJ, Puga FJ, et al: Operation for partial atrioventricular septal defect: A forty-year review. J Thorac Cardiovasc Surg 119:880–889, 2000.
27. Emanuel R, Somerville J, Inns A, Withers R: Evidence of congenital heart disease in the offspring of parents with atrioventricular defects. Br Heart J 49:144–147, 1983.
28. Feldt RH, DuShane JW, Titus JL: The atrioventricular conduction system in persistent common atrioventricular canal defect: Correlations with electrocardiogram. Circulation 42:437–444, 1970.
29. Flyer DC, Buckley LP, Hellenbrand WE, et al: Report of the New England Regional Infant Cardiac Program. Pediatrics 65:375–461, 1980.
30. Foker JE, Berry J, Steinberger J: Ventricular growth stimulation to achieve two-ventricle repair in unbalanced common atrioventricular canal. Prog Pediatr Cardiol 10:173–186, 1999.
31. Fortuna RS, Ashburn DA, Carias De Oliveira N, et al: Atrioventricular septal defects: Effect of bridging leaflet division on early valve function. Ann Thorac Surg 77:895–902, 2004.
32. Giamberti A, Marino B, di Carlo D, et al: Partial atrioventricular canal with congestive heart failure in the first year of life: Surgical options. Ann Thorac Surg 62:151–154, 1996.
33. Gunther T, Mazzitelli D, Haehnel CJ, et al: Long-term results after repair of complete atrioventricular septal defects: Analysis of risk factors. Ann Thorac Surg 65:754–759, 1998.
34. Gurbuz AT, Novick WM, Pierce CA, Watson DC: Left ventricular outflow tract obstruction after partial atrioventricular septal defect repair. Ann Thorac Surg 68: 1723–1726, 1999.
35. Hanley FL, Fenton KN, Jonas RA, et al: Surgical repair of complete atrioventricular canal defects in infancy. Twenty-year trends. J Thorac Cardiovasc Surg 106:387–397, 1993.
36. Hynes JK, Tajik AJ, Seward JB, et al: Partial atrioventricular canal defect in adults. Circulation 66:284–287, 1982.
37. Jacobs JP, Burke RP, Quintessenza JA, Mavroudis C: Congenital Heart Surgery Nomenclature and Database Project: Atrioventricular canal defect. Ann Thorac Surg 69: S36–S43, 2000.
38. Karl TR: Atrioventricular septal defect with tetralogy of Fallot or double-outlet right ventricle: Surgical considerations. Semin Thorac Cardiovasc Surg 9:26–34, 1997.
39. Kertesz NJ: The conduction system and arrhythmias in common atrioventricular canal. Prog Pediatr Cardiol 10: 153–159, 1999.
40. Khonsari S, Sintek CF: Atrioventricular septal defects. In Khonsari S, Sintek CF, editors: Cardiac Surgery: Safeguards and Pitfalls in Operative Technique, 3rd ed., pp. 243–251. Philadelphia: Lippincott Williams & Wilkins, 2003.
41. Kirklin JW, Daugherty GW, Burchell HB, et al: Repair of the partial form of persistent common atrioventricular canal: Ventricular communication. Ann Surg 142:858, 1955.
42. Lev M: The architecture of the conduction system in congenital heart disease. I. Common atrioventricular orifice. Arch Pathol 65:174, 1958.
43. Levine JC, Geva T: Echocardiographic assessment of common atrioventricular canal. Prog Pediatr Cardiol 10:137–151, 1999.
44. Lillehei C, Cohen M, Warden H, Varco R: The direct-vision intracardiac correction of congenital anomalies by controlled cross-circulation. Surgery 38:11–29, 1955.
45. Manning PB, Mayer JE Jr, Sanders SP, et al: Unique features and prognosis of primum ASD presenting in the first year of life. Circulation 90:II30–II35, 1994.
46. Marino B: Congenital heart disease in patients with Down's syndrome: Anatomic and genetic aspects. Biomed Pharmacother 47:197–200, 1993.
47. McGrath LB, Gonzalez-Lavin L: Actuarial survival, freedom from reoperation, and other events after repair of atrioventricular septal defects. J Thorac Cardiovasc Surg 94: 582–590, 1987.
48. McGrath LB, Kirklin JW, Soto B, Bargeron LM Jr: Secondary left atrioventricular valve replacement in atrioventricular septal (AV canal) defect: A method to avoid left ventricular outflow tract obstruction. J Thorac Cardiovasc Surg 89: 632–635, 1985.
49. Meisner H, Guenther T: Atrioventricular septal defect. Pediatr Cardiol 19:276–281, 1998.
50. Michielon G, Stellin G, Rizzoli G, Casarotto DC: Repair of complete common atrioventricular canal defects in patients younger than four months of age. Circulation 96:II316–II322, 1997.
51. Mills NL, Ochsner JL, King TD: Correction of Type C complete atrioventricular canal. Surgical considerations. J Thorac Cardiovasc Surg 71:20–28, 1976.
52. Mora BN, Marx GR, Roth SJ, et al: Modified single-patch repair of complete atrioventricular canal defect. J Thorac Cardiovasc Surg 2004 (in press).
53. Moran AM, Daebritz S, Keane JF, Mayer JE: Surgical management of mitral regurgitation after repair of endocardial cushion defects: Early and midterm results. Circulation 102:III160–III165, 2000.
54. Morris CD, Magilke D, Reller M. Down's syndrome affects results of surgical correction of complete atrioventricular canal. Pediatr Cardiol 13:80–84, 1992.
55. Najm HK, Coles JG, Endo M, et al: Complete atrioventricular septal defects: Results of repair, risk factors, and freedom from reoperation. Circulation 96(suppl II):II311–II315, 1997.
56. Najm HK, Williams WG, Chuaratanaphong S, et al: Primum atrial septal defect in children: Early results, risk factors, and freedom from reoperation. Ann Thorac Surg 66:829–835, 1998.
57. Newfeld EA, Sher M, Paul MH, Nikaidoh H: Pulmonary vascular disease in complete atrioventricular canal defect. Am J Cardiol 39:721–726, 1977.
58. Nicholson IA, Bichell DP, Bacha EA, del Nido PJ: Minimal sternotomy approach for congenital heart operations. Ann Thorac Surg 71:469–472, 2001.
59. Nicholson IA, Nunn GR, Sholler GF, et al: Simplified single patch technique for the repair of atrioventricular septal defect. J Thorac Cardiovasc Surg 118:642–646, 1999.
60. Oshima Y, Yamaguchi M, Yoshimura N, et al: Anatomically corrective repair of complete atrioventricular septal defects and major cardiac anomalies. Ann Thorac Surg 72:424–429, 2001.
61. Permut LC, Mehta V: Late results and reoperation after repair of complete and partial atrioventricular canal defect. Semin Thorac Cardiovasc Surg 9:44–54, 1997.
62. Rastelli G, Kirklin JW, Titus JL: Anatomic observations on complete form of persistent common atrioventricular canal with special reference to atrioventricular valves. Mayo Clin Proc 41:296–308, 1966.
63. Rastelli GC, Ongley PA, McGoon DC: Surgical repair of complete atrioventricular canal with anterior common leaflet undivided and unattached to ventricular septum. Mayo Clin Proc 44:335–341, 1969.
64. Reddy VM, McElhinney DB, Brook MM, et al: Atrioventricular valve function after single patch repair of complete atrioventricular septal defect in infancy: How early should repair be attempted? J Thorac Cardiovasc Surg 115:1032–1040, 1998.
65. Reeder GS, Danielson GK, Seward JB, et al: Fixed subaortic stenosis in atrioventricular canal defect: A Doppler echocardiographic study. J Am Coll Cardiol 20:386–394, 1992.

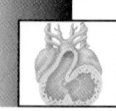

66. Rhodes J, Warner KG, Fulton DR, et al: Fate of mitral regurgitation following repair of atrioventricular septal defect. Am J Cardiol 80:1194–1197, 1997.
67. Sommerville J: Ostium primum defect: Factors causing deterioration in the natural history. Br Heart J 27:413–419, 1965.
68. Starr A, Hovaguimian H: Surgical repair of subaortic stenosis in atrioventricular canal defects. J Thorac Cardiovasc Surg 108:373–376, 1994.
69. Stellin G, Vida VL, Milanesi O, et al: Surgical treatment of complete A-V canal defects in children before 3 months of age. Eur J Cardiothorac Surg 23:187–193, 2003.
70. Studer M, Blackstone EH, Kirklin JW, et al. Determinants of early and late results of repair of atrioventricular septal (canal) defects. J Thorac Cardiovasc Surg 84:523–542, 1982.
71. Tennant SN, Hammon JW Jr, Bender HW Jr, et al: Familial clustering of atrioventricular canal defects. Am Heart J 108: 175–177, 1984.
72. Thies WR, Breymann T, Matthies W, et al: Primary repair of complete atrioventricular septal defect in infancy. Eur J Cardiothorac Surg 5:571–574, 1991.
73. Torfs CP, Christianson RE: Anomalies in Down syndrome individuals in a large population-based registry. Am J Med Genet 77:431–438, 1998.
74. Tweddell JS, Litwin SB, Berger S, et al: Twenty-year experience with repair of complete atrioventricular septal defects. Ann Thorac Surg 62:419–424, 1996.
75. Ugarte M, Enriquez de Salamanca F, Quero M: Endocardial cushion defects: An anatomical study of 54 specimens. Br Heart J 38:674–682, 1976.
76. Van Arsdell GS, Williams WG, Boutin C, et al: Subaortic stenosis in the spectrum of atrioventricular septal defects. Solutions may be complex and palliative. J Thorac Cardiovasc Surg 110:1534–1541, 1995.
77. Van Praagh R, Litovsky S: Pathology and embryology of common atrioventricular canal. Prog Pediatr Cardiol 10: 115–127, 1999.
78. van Son JA, Phoon CK, Silverman NH, Haas GS: Predicting feasibility of biventricular repair of right-dominant unbalanced atrioventricular canal. Ann Thorac Surg 63:1657–1663, 1997.
79. Weintraub RG, Brawn WJ, Venables AW, Mee RB: Two-patch repair of complete atrioventricular septal defect in the first year of life. Results and sequential assessment of atrioventricular valve function. J Thorac Cardiovasc Surg 99:320–326, 1990.
80. Wetter J, Sinzobahamvya N, Blaschczok C, et al: Closure of the zone of apposition at correction of complete atrioventricular septal defect improves outcome. Eur J Cardiothorac Surg 17: 146–153, 2000.
81. Wilcox BR, Jones DR, Frantz EG, et al: Anatomically sound, simplified approach to repair of "complete" atrioventricular septal defect. Ann Thorac Surg 64:487–494, 1997.
82. Yilmaz AT, Arslan M, Kuralay E, et al: Repair of the left AV valve in atrioventricular septal defect in adults. J Card Surg 11:363–367, 1996.

Ventricular Septal Defect and Double-Outlet Right Ventricle

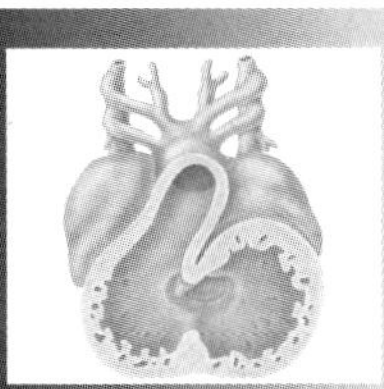

CHAPTER 112

Emile A. Bacha

VENTRICULAR SEPTAL DEFECT

Definition

A ventricular septal defect (VSD) is a hole between the left and right ventricles. A VSD may occur as an isolated anomaly or with a wide variety of intracardiac anomalies, such as tetralogy of Fallot, transposition of the great arteries, and others. This chapter deals with isolated VSD.

Historical Aspects

Banding of the pulmonary artery as a palliative maneuver was first described in 1952.[19] This decreased left-to-right shunting and as a consequence prevented the development of pulmonary vascular obstructive disease and left-sided volume overload. Until the mid-1960s when primary VSD closure became safer, pulmonary artery banding was the procedure of choice in managing VSDs. The first VSD closure was performed in 1954 by Lillehei and associates[17] at the University of Minnesota, using controlled cross-circulation between the child and parent. Nineteen of the 27 patients who underwent this procedure survived. In 1955 Kirklin and associates[13] at the Mayo Clinic closed a VSD using a heart–lung machine. In 1958 transatrial VSD closure was performed,[23] followed in 1969 by the popularization of primary repair in symptomatic infants by Barratt-Boyes and associates[5] using cardiopulmonary bypass, deep hypothermia, and circulatory arrest.

Anatomy

Anatomy of the Tricuspid Valve, Conduction System, and Right Ventricular Septum

Surgeons planning VSD surgery must have intimate knowledge of the tricuspid valve, the conduction system, and the right ventricular septal anatomy.

Tricuspid Valve

The tricuspid valve has three leaflets: anterior, septal, and posterior. The anterior leaflet is connected via the chordae tendineae cordis to the anterior papillary muscle (located on the anterior right ventricular free wall) and to the septal papillary muscle (sometimes called muscle of Lancisi). The septal papillary muscle is itself part of the septal band of the septomarginal trabecula. The posterior leaflet is attached to the anterior and posterior papillary muscles, and the septal leaflet attaches to the posterior and septal papillary muscles.

Right Ventricular Septum

The right ventricular septum has five components (Figure 112-1):

1. The membranous septum
2. The atrioventricular (AV) canal or inlet septum
3. The muscular septum (apical trabecular septum or sinus septum)
4. The trabecula septomarginalis (septal band and moderator band)
5. The conal septum (infundibular septum and parietal band)

Unlike the left ventricular septum, which is free of any papillary muscle attachment (the mitral valve can be called "septophobic," whereas the tricuspid valve can be called "septophilic"), the right ventricular septum is where the septal (sometimes called medial) papillary muscle and part of the posterior papillary muscle originate. The septal papillary muscle is a portion of the septal band, which runs along the septum (hence its name). The septal band itself is a portion of the septomarginal trabecula, which also comprises the moderator band. The moderator band itself links the septum to the anterior papillary muscle (called moderator band because it was erroneously thought to "moderate" the right ventricular free wall, that is, keep in sync with the rest of the ventricle). The membranous septum is the only fibrous component of the septum. It is wedged between the aortic valve, tricuspid valve, and mitral valve. Because the tricuspid valve is normally apically displaced vis-à-vis the mitral valve, a portion of membranous septum ends up between the right atrium and the left ventricle, called the atrioventricular part of the membranous septum. The portion of membranous septum located between both ventricles is called the interventricular part.

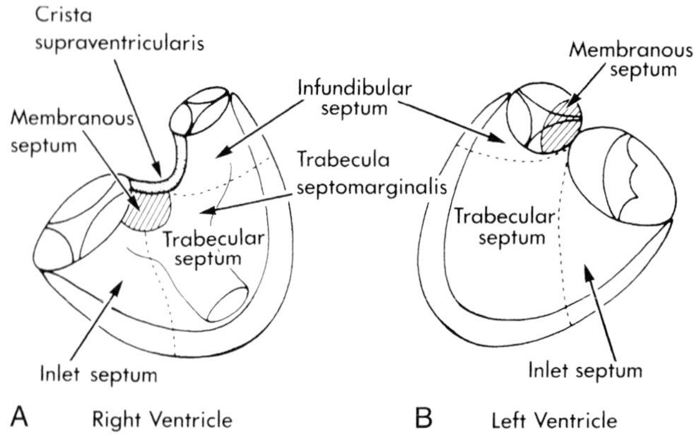

Figure 112–1 The components of the ventricular septum as seen from the right ventricle (A) and left ventricle (B). *(Modified from Soto B, Becker AE, Moulaert AJ, et al: Classification of ventricular septal defects. Br Heart J 43: 332, 1980.)*

Conduction System

Knowledge of the conduction system of the heart also is critical when approaching VSDs in order to avoid damaging it (Figure 112-2). The various atrial conduction tracts all converge toward the AV node of Aschoff–Tawara. The AV node is located in the inferior posterior portion of the membranous septum, just inferior to the anteroseptal commissure of the tricuspid valve. A different description of its location is that it occupies the apex of the triangle of Koch, which is limited by the ligament of Todaro posteriorly, the orifice of the coronary sinus inferiorly, and the tricuspid valve annulus superiorly (see Figure 112-2). From the AV node, the common AV bundle of His descends within the interventricular part of the membranous septum (in case of a membranous VSD, the posteroinferior rim of the VSD), traverses the septum, and then courses along the left ventricular aspect of the septum. It then separates into a right bundle branch, which travels back to the right ventricular surface, as well as a left bundle branch. At the anteroinferior border at the level of the muscle of Lancisi, the right bundle branch descends toward the right ventricular apex.

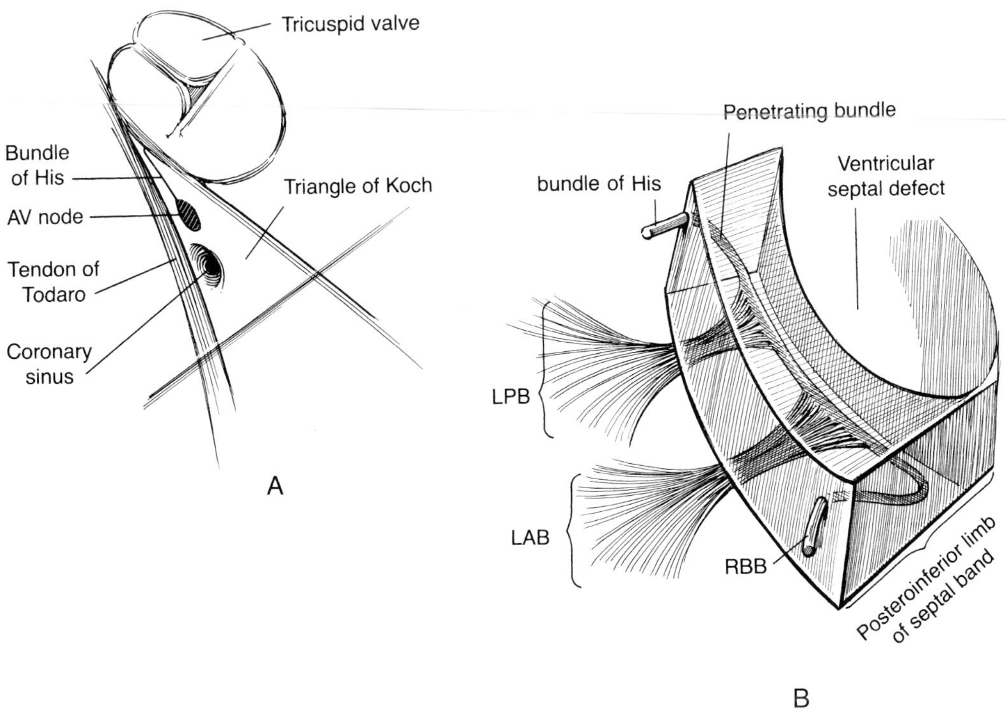

Figure 112–2 Schematic representation of the conduction system. A, The atrioventricular (AV) node lies embedded within the triangle of Koch, close to the orifice of the coronary sinus and between the annulus of the tricuspid valve and the tendon of Todaro. The bundle of His originates from the AV node, extends toward the commissure between the septal and anterior leaflets of the tricuspid valve, and penetrates along the posteroinferior margin of the membranous septum and across the muscular ventricular septum, giving rise to the left posterior branch (LPB) and left anterior branch (LAB); the right bundle branch (RBB) then travels back along the ventricular septum toward the right ventricular septal surface (**B**). At the level of the muscle of Lancisi, the right bundle branch descends toward the right ventricular apex.
(Modified from Castaneda AR, Jonas RA, Mayer JE Jr, Hanley FL: Double outlet right ventricle. In Castaneda AR, Jonas RA, Mayer JE Jr, Hanley FL, editors: Cardiac Surgery of the Neonate and Infant, pp. 445–449. Philadelphia: W.B. Saunders, 1994.)

Anatomical classification of VSDs

A useful surgical classification of VSDs was initially developed in 1980 by Soto and associates[22] (Figure 112-3) and then further modified by Van Praagh and associates[24] (Figure 112-4). Variations of this classification are used in most pediatric cardiac centers. Ventricular septal defects can be classified as:

- Conoventricular (or membranous) defects
- Conal (or outlet) VSD
- Inlet (or AV canal type) VSD
- Muscular VSD (single or multiple)

Conoventricular (or Membranous) Defects

Conoventricular defects are located between the conal septum and the ventricular septum. They are centered in or around the membranous septum and comprise 80% of all VSDs. They may be located exclusively within the membranous septum, or they also can extend beyond the boundaries of the membranous septum toward inferior, posterior, or anterior directions, and are then sometimes called "perimembranous" or "paramembranous" VSDs. The prefix "peri-," appearing in loan words from the Greek, means "surrounding" (i.e., perimeter). As such, a truly perimembranous ventricular septal defect would surround the membranous septum. In contrast, the prefix "para-," also from the Greek, means "adjacent to" or "beside" and more accurately reflects the notion of a

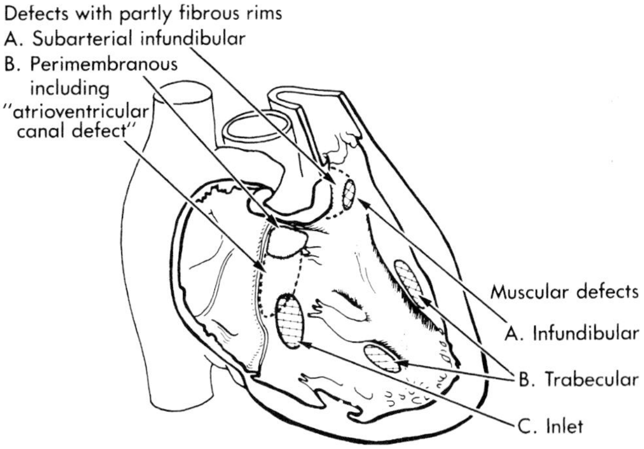

Figure 112–3 Classification of ventricular septal defects (VSDs) according to their location within the septum. *(Modified from Soto B, Becker AE, Moulaert AJ, et al: Classification of ventricular septal defects. Br Heart J 43:332, 1980.)*

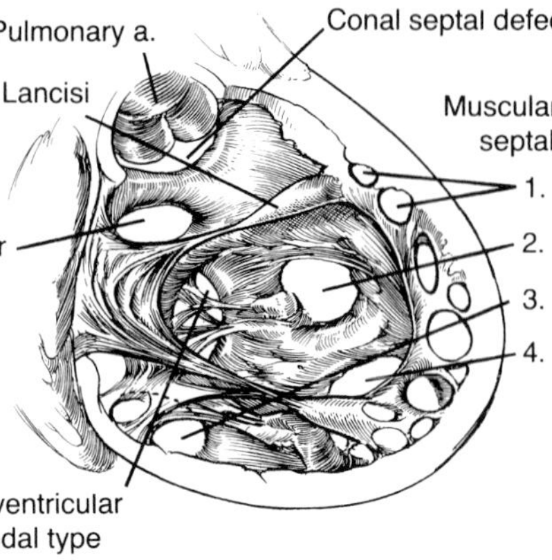

Figure 112–4 Classification of ventricular septal defects (VSDs): VSD, atrioventricular canal type; muscular VSDs: midventricular (1), apical (2), anterior (3), and posterior (4); conoventricular septal defect, which includes paramembranous and malalignment conoventricular septal defects; and conal septal defects.
(Modified from Castaneda AR, Jonas RA, Mayer JE Jr, Hanley FL: Double outlet right ventricle. In Castaneda AR, Jonas RA, Mayer JE Jr, Hanley FL, editors: Cardiac Surgery of the Neonate and Infant, pp. 445–449. Philadelphia: W.B. Saunders, 1994.)

defect adjacent to the membranous septum. Neither *perimembranous* nor *paramembranous* correctly describes the typical defect involving the membranous septum *and* extending into the adjacent septum. The current recommendation is to call these defects either membranous VSDs or conoventricular defects. Malalignment of the conal septal plane vis-à-vis the ventricular septal plane results in the typical conoventricular defect. The malalignment can be anterior, as seen in tetralogy of Fallot, for example, or posterior, as seen in interrupted aortic arch. In addition to resulting in a VSD, anterior conal septal malalignment also results in right ventricular outflow tract obstruction, whereas posterior malalignment of the conal septum results in left ventricular outflow tract obstruction. Important landmarks in conoventricular septal defects are the anteroseptal commissure of the tricuspid valve inferiorly and the noncoronary cusp of the aortic valve. When the ventricular portion of the membranous septum is entirely absent, the VSD extends to the base of the aortic valve (sometimes called "subaortic" VSD). The medial papillary muscle (muscle of Lancisi) located at the inferior–posterior border of the defect is also an important landmark. Both the septal and anterior tricuspid valve leaflets are attached to it.

Conal Septal Defects

Approximately 8% of VSDs are located in the conal (infundibulum or outlet) septum. They also are called supracristal VSDs. They are either entirely surrounded by muscle (muscular conal VSDs) or limited upstream by the aortic or pulmonary annuli (sometimes called subarterial VSDs).

Inlet (or Atrioventricular Canal Type) VSD

This defect is characterized by the absence of part or all of the AV canal (inlet) septum. The VSD is located immediately underneath the septal leaflet of the tricuspid valve with no tissue in between. Approximately 6% of all VSDs are inlet-type VSDs.

Muscular VSDs

Muscular VSDs (10% of all VSDs) are entirely surrounded by muscle. They can occur anywhere in the trabecular portion of the septum and can be isolated or multiple. They are described by their location, that is, anterior, midventricular (between the muscular septum and the septal band), posterior, or apical. When inspected through the left side of the septum, what appeared to be multiple muscular defects often converge into either a single hole or two separate holes.

Commonly Associated Defects

VSDs are an intrinsic portion of many, if not most, complex cardiac malformations. These VSDs are discussed separately with their respective entities (see other chapters). Almost one half of patients who undergo surgical treatment of "primary" VSD have an associated lesion.

Patent Ductus Arteriosus

In symptomatic neonates or infants with VSDs, a large patent ductus arteriosus (PDA) is present in about 25% of cases.[5] This is important to know because preoperative echocardiography may fail to show a PDA in the presence of a large amount of left-to-right shunting. Furthermore, intraoperative transesophageal echocardiogram (TEE) is notoriously unreliable in excluding PDAs. Therefore the possibility of a PDA should be kept in mind while approaching a VSD, and if there is any doubt, or if there is a large amount of backflow through the pulmonary arteries on cardiopulmonary bypass, the PDA should be ligated or clipped.

Aortic Coarctation

A hemodynamically significant aortic coarctation is present in approximately 10% of cases. Because of the unique pathophysiology here (more left-to-right shunting across the VSD because of increased afterload caused by the coarctation), these patients usually have presenting symptoms before 3 months of age.[10]

Left Ventricular Outflow Tract Obstruction

Congenital valvar or subvalvar aortic stenosis is seen in approximately 4% of patients requiring an operation for VSD.[15] The most common type of subaortic stenosis associated with VSDs is the discrete fibromuscular membrane of the VSD that is located inferior or upstream to it. Congenital mitral valve stenosis is rare and occurs in about 2% of patients.

Other significant anomalies include large atrial septal defects (ASDs), right ventricular outflow tract obstruction, vascular ring, or persistent left superior vena cava.

Pathophysiology

Shunt Direction and Magnitude

The magnitude and direction of the shunt across a VSD depend on the size of the defect and the pressure gradient across it during the various phases of the cardiac cycle. Large VSDs offer little or no resistance to blood flow and are therefore called "nonrestrictive." The right ventricular pressure equals the left ventricular pressure, and the pulmonary/systemic flow ratio ("shunt") (Qp/Qs) is dependent on the ratio of pulmonary vascular resistance (PVR) to systemic vascular resistance (SVR). On the other hand, small VSDs offer resistance to flow across the defect and are therefore termed "restrictive" VSDs. The Qp/Qs rarely exceeds 1.5. Moderate-sized VSDs fall between these two categories, and the Qp/Qs usually ranges between 2.5 and 3. To a lesser degree, further determinants of shunt magnitude also include the relative compliance of both ventricles and the pressure relations during the various phases of the cardiac cycle. The size of the VSD, in particular muscular VSDs, also may vary during various phases of the cardiac cycle. Because the PVR is elevated during the first few weeks of life, it is unusual to have to close an isolated VSD. As the PVR falls with increasing age, left-to-right shunting increases, necessitating treatment.

Sequelae of Left-to-Right Shunting

Left-to-right shunting at the ventricular level implies increased pulmonary blood flow. Thus left ventricular preload is similarly increased, resulting in increased workload for both the left and right ventricles. The left atrium is enlarged, and the left atrial pressure is elevated. The left ventricle dilates. The raised left atrial pressure causes many infants with VSD to have an increased accumulation of interstitial fluid in the lungs, resulting sometimes in repeated pulmonary infections. The work of breathing is increased as the lung compliance is decreased. This increases energy expenditure, which, along with the relatively low systemic blood flow, causes these infants to have striking failure to thrive. When pulmonary resistance rises as a result of the development of pulmonary vascular disease, pulmonary blood flow is reduced and the child appears to improve. Unfortunately, further increases in PVR occur, and the classic Eisenmenger complex results. These patients are characterized by fixed pulmonary hypertension, bidirectional shunting, right ventricular hypertrophy, and a normal-sized left ventricle. They are often inoperable and require heart–lung transplantation for further survival.

Pulmonary Vascular Disease

The classic description of the pathology of hypertensive pulmonary vascular disease is that of Heath and Edwards.[11] They correlated the PVR of patients with large VSDs with the histological severity of pulmonary vascular changes. Grade 1 changes were defined as medial hypertrophy without intimal proliferation; grade 2 as medial hypertrophy with cellular intimal reaction; grade 3 as intimal fibrosis and medial hypertrophy; grade 4 as generalized vascular dilation, an area of vascular occlusion by intimal fibrosis and plexiform lesions; grade 5 as other "dilatation lesions" such as cavernous and angiomatoid lesions; and grade 6 as necrotizing arteritis. It is assumed that Heath–Edwards grade 3 or greater is not reversible.

Natural History and Indications for Surgery

Symptoms

Approximately 30% of infants with severe symptoms such as intractable congestive heart failure or failure to thrive require surgery within the first year of life.[9] The remainder usually can be managed medically because the natural history of VSDs is well known.[12] Aggressive medical management is indicated because a majority of membranous and muscular VSDs tend to close spontaneously.[12] Malalignment of conoventricular VSDs or inlet-type VSDs are unlikely to close spontaneously, and therefore closure at the time of diagnosis is recommended, regardless of age or weight. Asymptomatic children with isolated small restrictive VSDs can be followed safely by serial echocardiograms.

Pulmonary Vascular Disease

It is important to remember that the development of pulmonary vascular disease is a tragedy that can be prevented with virtually no mortality by VSD closure. If in doubt, cardiac catheterization and measurement of PVR-to-SVR ratio should help with decision making. In addition, pulmonary artery (PA) pressures greater than one half systemic in a child older than 1 year indicate the need for surgery. If PA pressures are greater than one half systemic, the response of the pulmonary vasculature to inhaled nitric oxide and 100% inspired oxygen should be studied during catheterization. Children who even have significant pulmonary hypertension with a reversible component to it can become operative candidates.

Development of Aortic Regurgitation

During the first decade of life, a small proportion (5%) of patients with membranous or outlet VSDs develop prolapse of an aortic cusp into the VSD. This usually results in gradual decrease of the effective orifice and shunt flow, but also in increasing aortic regurgitation. Increasing aortic cusp prolapse and regurgitation is an indication to operate.

Diagnosis and Workup

Physical examination, chest X-ray, and electrocardiogram (ECG) depend on the underlying pathophysiology. Patients with large VSDs and increased pulmonary blood flow usually have presenting symptoms such as tachypnea, growth failure, profuse sweating during feeding, a bulging precordium, a pansystolic murmur, an enlarged liver, and thready pulses. Chest X-ray shows large central and peripheral PAs and an enlarged left atrium and ventricles (Figure 112-5). ECG shows signs of biventricular enlargement. In contrast, patients with small VSDs and small left-to-right shunts have only a systolic murmur. Chest X-ray and ECG may be entirely normal (Figure 112-6). Two-dimensional (2D) echocardiography and color Doppler flow studies have

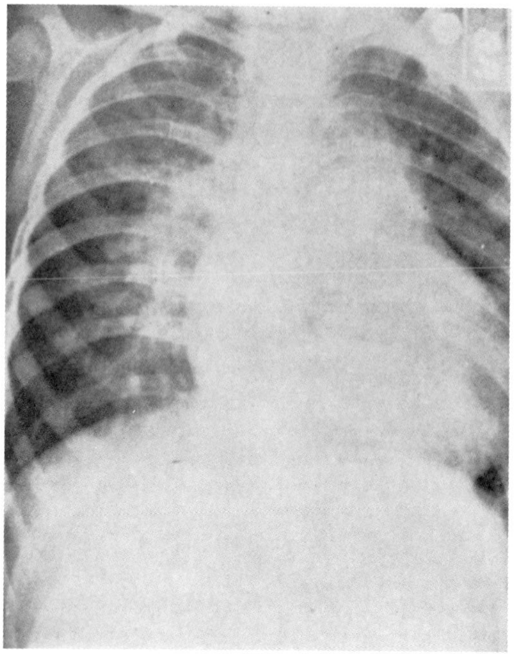

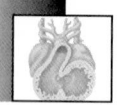

Figure 112–5 Chest film of a child with a large ventricular septal defect (VSD), large pulmonary blood flow, and pulmonary hypertension, but only mildly elevated pulmonary vascular resistance. This is reflected in the evidence of left and right ventricular enlargement, enlargement of the main pulmonary artery, and a sharp increase in pulmonary vascular pattern.

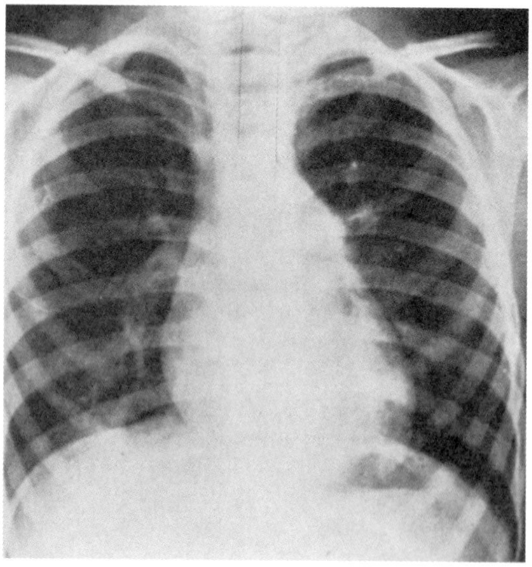

Figure 112–6 This chest film is in contrast to that shown in Figure 112–5. The heart is not enlarged overall. The main pulmonary artery is enlarged; there is no evidence of increased pulmonary blood flow. This patient has a large ventricular septal defect (VSD), pulmonary hypertension, severe elevation of pulmonary vascular resistance, and pulmonary blood flow that is less than systemic blood flow. The condition is inoperable and usually requires a heart–lung transplant.
(Modified from Dushane JW, Kirklin JW: Selection for surgery of patients with ventricular septal defects and pulmonary hypertension. Circulation 21:13, 1960. By permission of the American Heart Association, Inc.)

essentially replaced cardiac catheterization in most patients with isolated VSDs. Cardiac catheterization is needed only when PVR and PA pressure need to be measured.

Surgical Technique

Closure of Conoventricular Septal Defects

The PDA is routinely dissected and ligated as soon as cardiopulmonary bypass is instituted. The left branch PA and distal aortic arch should be positively identified before ligation. Moderate hypothermia (rectal temperature 28–32° C) is usually sufficient. Small infants weighing less than 2.5 kg may require lower temperatures (18–25° C) in order to safely institute low-flow bypass. Deep hypothermic circulatory arrest is very rarely used for closure of VSDs. After cross-clamping the aorta and delivering the cardioplegia solution, the caval tapes are tightened. A right atriotomy approach is preferred for the vast majority of VSDs. The atrium is opened obliquely (Figure 112-7) to avoid the area of the sinus node. The atrial septum is inspected first, and if a patent foramen ovale (PFO) is present, a left atrial vent sucker can be placed. Retraction of the septal and anterior leaflets of the tricuspid valve usually provides adequate exposure. Commonly the area located behind the anteroseptal commissure of the tricuspid valve is the most difficult to expose. If the tricuspid valve attachments are in the way, the surgeon may detach the septal or anterior leaflet by making an incision that parallels the tricuspid annulus (see Figure 112-7). Some surgeons perform this maneuver routinely. If VSD exposure remains poor despite rearranging the field, an infundibular incision is the usual fallback option for exposure. Interrupted mattressed or running nonabsorbable sutures are used. Teflon pledgets are very useful in neonates and infants, in whom the myocardium is very friable. The first suture is usually placed into the midportion of the defect, approximately 3 mm from the rim of the defect. When the inferior margin is reached (about the level of the muscle of Lancisi), sutures should be placed further away from the edge and become more superficial. At the tricuspid annulus, sutures are passed through its fibrous tissue. Because conduction tissue is composed of specialized muscle cells, fibrous tissue offers a safe area to place sutures. There is usually very little tissue separating the aortic valve from the posterosuperior margin of the defect. Therefore several sutures are usually placed from the right atrial side through the tricuspid valve annulus to avoid damage to the aortic valve cusp. Infusion of cardioplegic solution fills the aortic root and allows accurate delineation of the insertion of the aortic valve cusps. All sutures are then passed through an appropriately tailored patch (Dacron, Gore-Tex, or pericardium) and tied in place. The tricuspid valve should be routinely inspected and passively inflated with saline to ensure that no significant tricuspid valve regurgitation has been inadvertently created.

Closure of Atrioventricular Canal Type of VSD (Figure 112-8)

Exposure is usually straightforward. A continuous suture technique is often preferred, because it allows for weaving in and out between the various chordae and papillary mus-

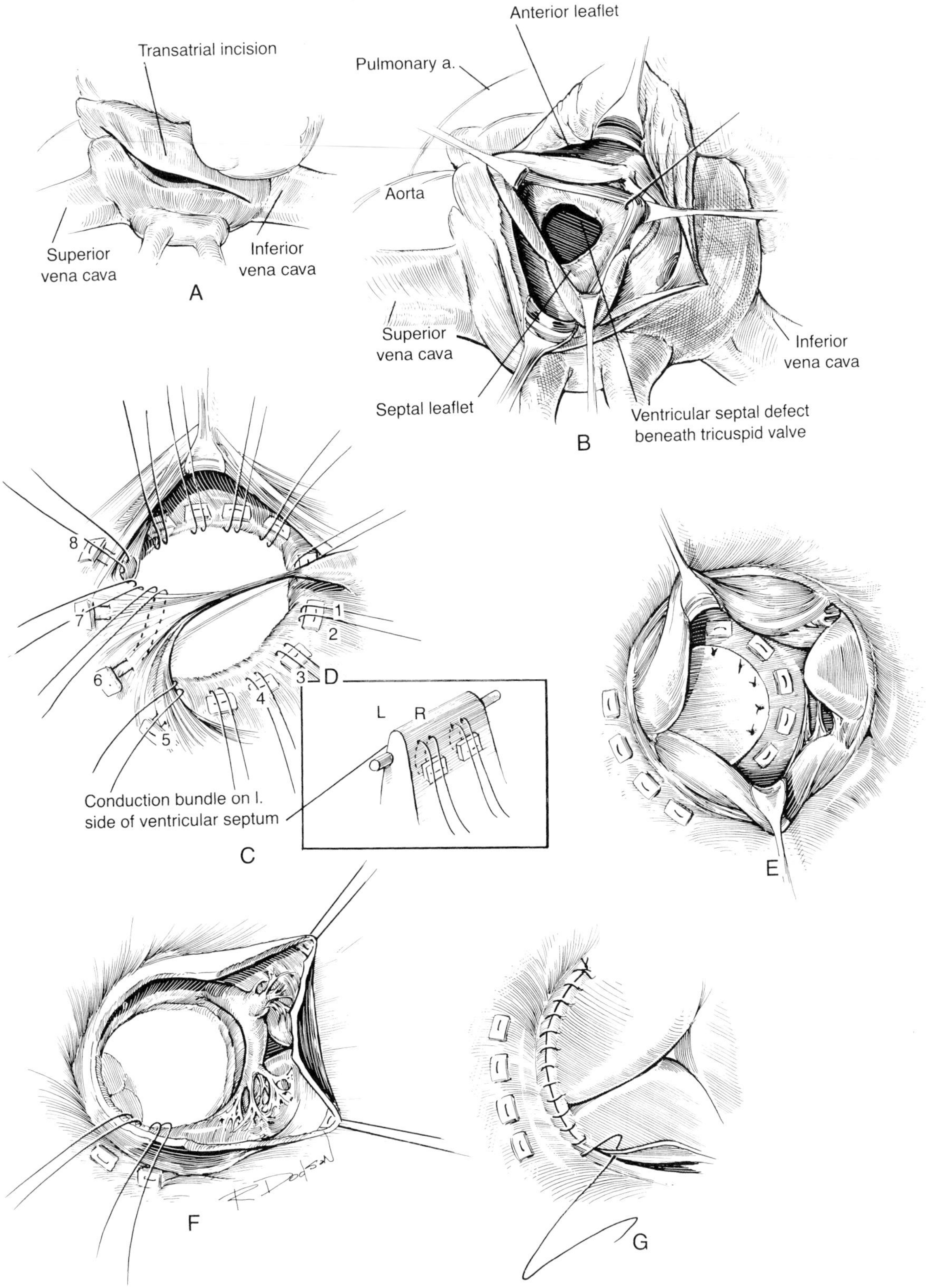

Figure 112–7 Trans–right atrial exposure of conoventricular ventricular septal defect (VSD). A, Incision in the right atrium. **B,** Exposure of conoventricular VSD with retraction of the anterior and septal leaflets of the tricuspid valve. **C,** Sutures 1, 2, 3, and 4 are placed within the ventricular septal wall, approximately 3 mm from the rim of the defect. **D,** Suture 5 is placed where the leaflet fuses with the crest of the VSD, and sutures 6, 7, and 8 are passed from the right atrial side through the tricuspid annulus; the rest of the sutures are placed within the anterosuperior rim of the VSD. **E,** Completed closure of the VSD with a Dacron patch and pledgeted sutures. **F,** If chordae and papillary muscles obliterate the view of the VSD, the septal and anterior leaflets of the tricuspid valve are incised along the base, permitting complete exposure of the VSD. **G,** Septal and anterior leaflets of the tricuspid valve resutured after closure of the VSD with a patch.
(Modified from Castaneda AR, Jonas RA, Mayer JE Jr, Hanley FL: Double outlet right ventricle. In Castaneda AR, Jonas RA, Mayer JE Jr, Hanley FL, editors: Cardiac Surgery of the Neonate and Infant, pp. 445–449. Philadelphia: W.B. Saunders, 1994.)

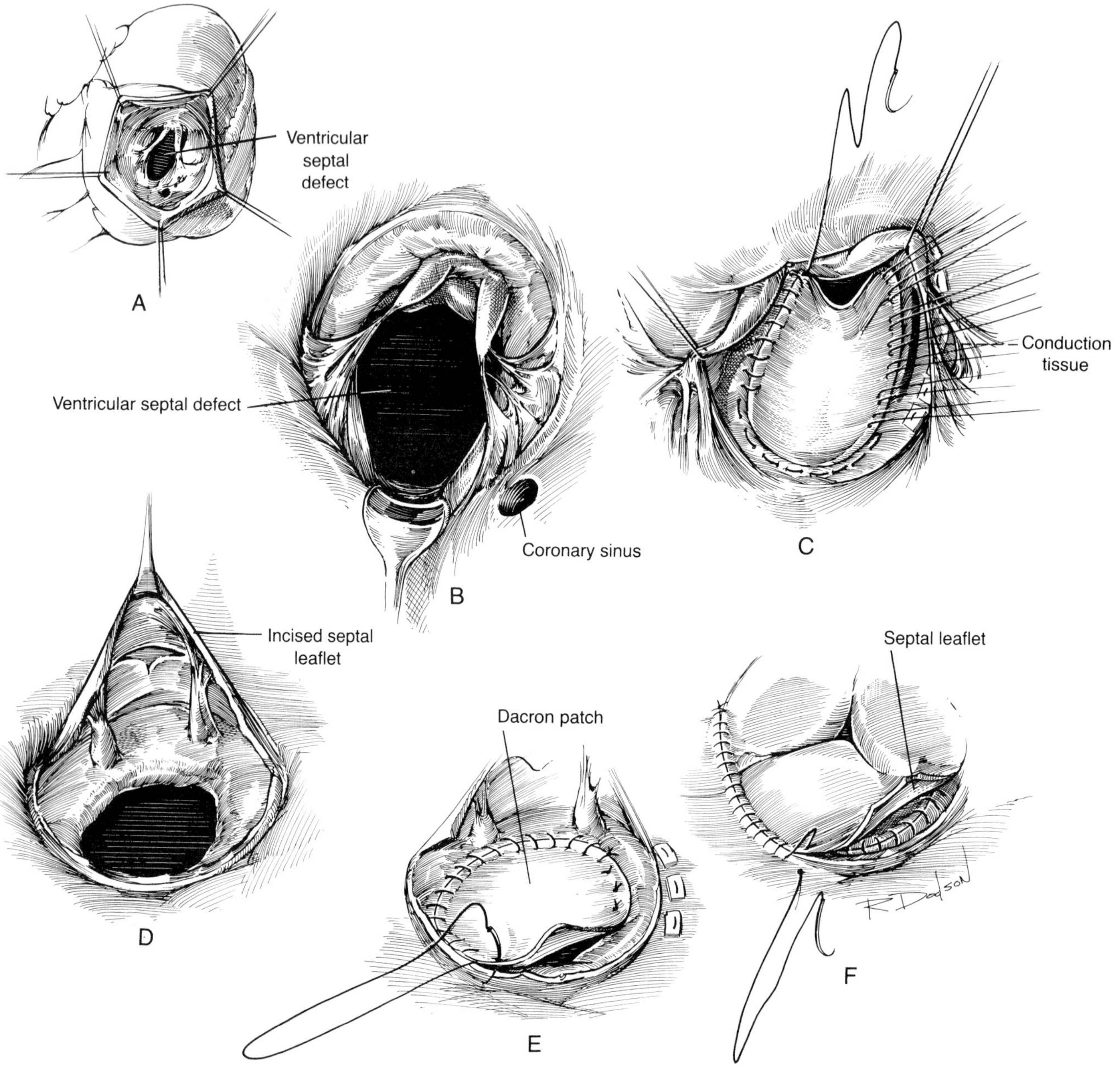

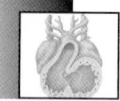

Figure 112–8 **Closure of atrioventricular (AV) canal type of ventricular septal defect (VSD). A,** Transatrial view of AV canal type of VSD. **B,** Retraction of the septal leaflet of the tricuspid valve exposes the defect to the tricuspid valve annulus. **C,** Closure of AV canal defect with the continuous suture technique. (Note the continuous horizontal mattress suture with the septal leaflet tissue and also the interrupted horizontal mattress sutures along the posteroinferior portion of the VSD, placed approximately 4 mm from the VSD to avoid damage of the conduction bundle.) **D,** If dense chordae obstruct the view of the defect, the septal leaflet of the tricuspid valve is incised along its base, providing exposure of the entire circumference of the AV canal type of VSD. **E,** Patch closure of the AV canal type of VSD. **(F)** The incised leaflet is reattached with continuous suture.
(Modified from Castaneda AR, Jonas RA, Mayer JE Jr, Hanley FL: Double outlet right ventricle. In Castaneda AR, Jonas RA, Mayer JE Jr, Hanley FL, editors: Cardiac Surgery of the Neonate and Infant, pp. 445–449. Philadelphia: W.B. Saunders, 1994.)

cles that usually crowd the edge of these defects. To avoid damage to the bundle of His and the right bundle branch that course along the posteroinferior edge, stitches in that area are placed farther away from the edge of the VSD.

Closure of Conal VSD (Figure 112-9)

Exposure is obtained through the infundibulum, the pulmonary artery, or the aorta. There is often no muscle between the superior edge of the defect and the pulmonary valve. Again, it can be useful to fill the aortic root with cardioplegic solution to determine the exact position of the cusps. The initial sutures are placed either within the fibrous rim separating the two semilunar valves or within the left and right pulmonary sinuses of Valsalva. The remaining sutures can be placed with no fear of injury to the conduction tissue as it travels farther caudally between the infundibular and trabecular ventricular septum.

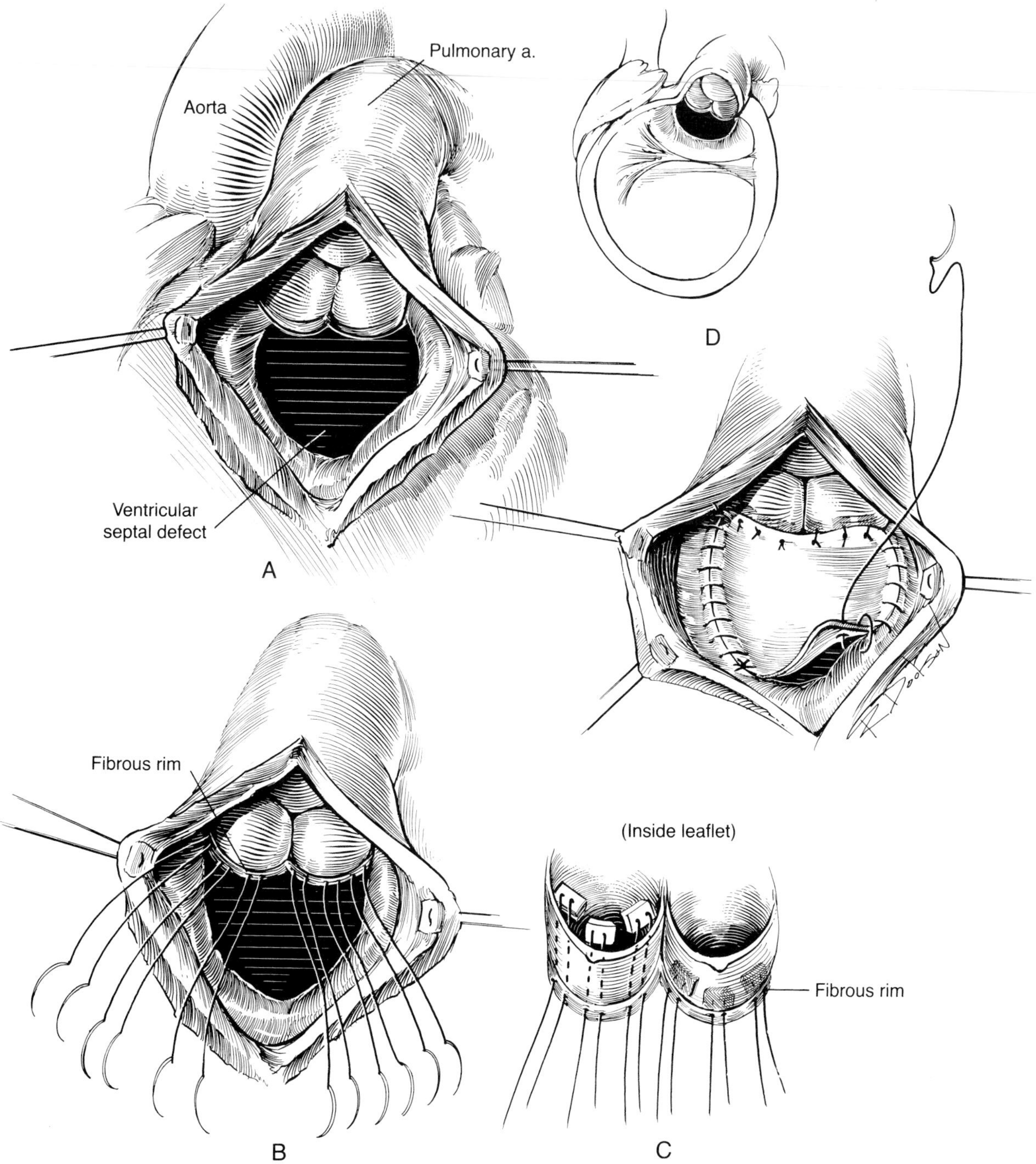

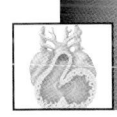

Figure 112–9 Transventricular approach for closure of conal septal defect. A, Commonly there is no intervening muscle between the superior edge of the defect and the pulmonary valve. **B,** Initial sutures placed within the fibrous rim separating the two semilunar valves. **C,** If the area between the aorta and the pulmonary cusps is tenuous, interrupted pledgeted mattress sutures are passed within the right and left pulmonary sinuses. **D,** The Dacron patch is anchored to the remainder of the ventricular septal defect with a continuous suture.
(Modified from Castaneda AR, Jonas RA, Mayer JE Jr, Hanley FL: Double outlet right ventricle. In Castaneda AR, Jonas RA, Mayer JE Jr, Hanley FL, editors: Cardiac Surgery of the Neonate and Infant, pp. 445–449. Philadelphia: W.B. Saunders, 1994.)

Closure of Muscular VSDs

Midmuscular defects are preferably closed through a right atriotomy. A single patch can cover several separate defects. Posterior muscular defects are hidden behind the posterior leaflet of the tricuspid valve. Anterior muscular defects are often difficult to find, because they are hidden behind the septal band and hypertrophied trabeculae of the right ventricular free wall. It is important to divide the muscle bundles binding the septal band to the septum to adequately expose the true margins of the VSD. A patch is used, with

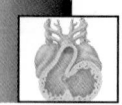

the surgeon paying close attention to avoid distortion of the left anterior descending coronary artery. Apical defects are among the most difficult defects to expose. The coarse trabeculations located in the right ventricular apex make the exact determination of the true margins difficult. An apical right ventriculotomy is helpful. Left ventricular apical incisions are essentially obsolete because of the high prevalence of left ventricular dyskinesia and apical aneurysms after this incision. Percutaneous transcatheter closure of muscular VSDs with occluding devices is rapidly becoming the preferred approach in patients with apical VSDs or multiple muscular VSDs. In patients for whom the percutaneous approach is not possible, intraoperative deployment of the devices on the beating heart via a right ventricular puncture has been employed successfully.[3]

Surgical Management of Ventricular Septal Defect with Associated Anomalies

VSD with Coarctation of the Aorta

The vast majority of these patients are young infants. The traditional approach has been to simultaneously repair the coarctation and band the pulmonary artery. This evolved into aortic coarctation repair followed by VSD repair during the same hospitalization, if symptoms of heart failure persisted, in the form of failure to extubate, for example. As techniques for complex neonatal repairs matured and results improved, many centers today favor a single-stage method of simultaneously repairing the coarctation and the VSD via a midline approach.[10] Of course, this is done only if the VSD is judged to be not likely to close spontaneously, whether by size or location.

VSD with Aortic Insufficiency

These patients usually are older children. The right or noncoronary cusp is prolapsing into the VSD secondary to the Bernoulli effect. In case of mild to mild-moderate aortic regurgitation with little scarring or fibrosis of the cusps, VSD closure alone is required. Patients with more than moderate aortic incompetence (AI) and cusp retraction usually require commissural resuspension of the affected cusp via an aortotomy (see chapter on aortic valve surgery).

VSD with Prior Banding

These are most often patients with multiple muscular VSDs (so-called Swiss-cheese septum). The resulting right ventricular hypertrophy makes the intraoperative identification of these VSDs even more difficult. Intraoperative device closure via right ventricular puncture has been employed successfully, along with removal of the PA band and PA plasty in one setting.[3]

Postoperative Care

Most infants convalesce normally after VSD repair, and special treatment usually is not required. Patients are generally extubated within 24 hours of operation and recover rapidly. In the unusual case of low cardiac output after operation, in addition to the usual supportive treatment, it should be stressed that it is the surgeon's responsibility to prove that there are no technical issues causing the unusual postoperative course. This can range from a large residual VSD to injury to the aortic cusp during suture placement or tricuspid regurgitation. Bedside echocardiography usually quickly diagnoses these problems. If complete AV dissociation occurs after cardiopulmonary bypass, temporary pacing wires are used until sinus rhythm reappears. AV block can last up to 10–14 days, beyond which it is usually permanent and a permanent pacemaker should be placed. Pulmonary hypertensive crisis is a severe postoperative complication that can occur in older patients with a reactive pulmonary vasculature. If the patient is at risk, then a pulmonary arterial line should be placed in the operating room, introduced via an infundibular puncture. A pulmonary hypertensive crisis can occur without a precipitating factor; however, tracheal suctioning, respiratory or metabolic acidosis, hypoxemia, and high-dose inotropes can be precipitating factors. Patients benefit from increased sedation, muscular paralysis, and hyperventilation with high inspired oxygen. Inhaled nitric oxide, at doses ranging from 5–40 ppm, is the preferred agent in managing pulmonary hypertension. Ideally it is started prophylactically in the operating room as soon as ventilation resumes while still on cardiopulmonary bypass.[6]

Results of Surgical Treatment

Early Results

Because of improvements in intraoperative and postoperative management and minimization of human error, the hospital mortality rate for repair of isolated VSD now approaches 0% in most pediatric cardiac centers. Since the late 1980s, along with marked improvement in survival after complex neonatal cardiac surgery, very small-weight or very young babies with isolated VSDs also have a mortality rate below 5%.[27] Prematurity, significant preexisting respiratory problems such as bronchopulmonary dysplasia, or unrecognized respiratory syncytial virus infection does increase morbidity and mortality slightly, but not significantly so. In an operable patient, elevated pulmonary vascular resistance is a risk factor for complications or prolonged hospital stay, but is not a determinant of hospital mortality. Unrecognized additional cardiac lesions can lead to significant problems if reoperation is required. Although complete AV dissociation is uncommon after isolated VSD repair, it remains a complication that occurs in 0.5–3% of patients after VSD closure. Right bundle branch block occurs in a majority of patients after VSD closure and is usually very well tolerated. Its implications in the long term are unclear. Significant residual postoperative left-to-right shunting is uncommon when proper techniques are used. Most often it results from suture dehiscence, seen most often in small babies with friable myocardium. When it is hemodynamically significant, reoperation should be performed expeditiously. When the patient is asymptomatic and progressing well during his or her postoperative course, the leak is usually smaller and the surgeon may elect to observe the patient with serial echocardiograms for a period of several weeks. Most small residual VSDs (<3 mm) close spontaneously over a period of months because of scar formation at the edge of the patch.

Late Results

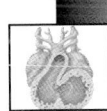

Repair of VSD in the first year or two of life cures most patients and results in full functional activity and normal or almost normal life expectancy. Normal or near-normal long-term growth and cardiac function is expected in most patients.[26] Late deaths virtually never occur in patients with normal or near-normal PVR. Detailed studies of PA pressure and PVR were performed in infants undergoing VSD closure at the Boston Children's Hospital. Ninety-six percent of infants had a mean PA pressure of greater than 40 mm Hg. Fifty-one percent continued to have elevated PA pressures at 24 hours postoperatively. Postoperative catheterization studies taken 1 year later showed that mean PA pressure in this group had decreased to a mean of 14 mm Hg.[8,20] Severe pulmonary hypertension postoperatively can increase with time and cause premature death, usually within 3–10 years of operation. Other patients with pulmonary hypertension have a stabilization of their pulmonary vascular process with neither increase nor decrease of the PVR. They usually have limitations in their exercise tolerance. In a study of 296 surviving patients after VSD closure followed for 30–35 years postoperatively, higher mortality was observed in those undergoing surgery after the age of 5 years, those with PVR greater than 7 U/m^2, and those with transient or permanent complete heart block.[18]

DOUBLE-OUTLET RIGHT VENTRICLE WITH NORMALLY RELATED GREAT ARTERIES

Definition

Simply defined, double-outlet right ventricle (DORV) refers to a heterogeneous group of cardiac malformations in which both great arteries arise from the right ventricle.[23,24] Although the term DORV can be correctly applied to single-ventricle hearts or hearts with AV discordance (e.g., congenitally corrected transposition of the great arteries), for simplicity of discussion, only hearts with AV concordance and two adequate ventricles are discussed in this chapter. Furthermore, the management of DORV with transposition for the great arteries is discussed in greater detail in Chapter 23. Two definitions, not mutually exclusive and best employed concurrently, are usually used[8,16]: The "50%-rule" states that a heart is termed DORV if, in addition to the PA, >50% of the aorta (or the PA in DORV with transposition) arises from the right ventricle. The other definition is that a "double conus" (subaortic and subpulmonary conal tube, also called infundibulum) is present. This means that there should be no aortic-to-mitral continuity.

Classification of DORV by VSD Location and Other Anatomical Determinants of Physiology

DORV is virtually always associated with a VSD. The physiology of DORV encompasses a spectrum that extends from a tetralogy type of DORV to a transposition type of DORV (Figure 112-10). The classic pathological classification of DORV centers on the location of the VSD[16] (Figure 112-11) and differentiates between subaortic, subpulmonic, doubly committed, and noncommitted types of VSD. VSD location alone, although important, does not define the physiology nor is enough to select the optimal method of repair. The presence or absence of right ventricular outflow tract obstruction is critical to the physiology and clinical presentation (Table 112–1). Furthermore, the great artery relationship, the distance between the pulmonary and tricuspid valves, the prominence of the conal septum, and the coronary artery anatomy are all important factors that also determine what type of repair should be performed.[25]

Subaortic VSD (see Figure 112-11)

DORV with subaortic VSD is the most common type of DORV, comprising approximately 50% of all patients.[25] With right ventricular outflow tract obstruction, the presentation is similar to tetralogy of Fallot, where a subaortic anterior malalignment VSD is also present. However, tetralogy of Fallot patients will not have a subaortic conus. The presentation and physiology without pulmonary stenosis is similar to that of a child with a large VSD.

Subpulmonic VSD (see Figure 112-11)

DORV with subpulmonary VSD is the second most common type of DORV, occurring in 30% of patients.[25] Because of the location of the VSD, oxygenated left ventricular blood preferentially streams through the VSD into the pulmonary artery while desaturated right ventricular blood streams into the aorta, thereby resulting in a transposition type of physiology. Association with subaortic stenosis, aortic coarctation, or interrupted aortic arch is common. The term *Taussig–Bing heart* is usually applied for hearts presenting subaortic and subpulmonary coni, side-by-side great arteries, and a subpulmonary VSD (Taussig–Bing).[25]

Doubly Committed VSD

The VSD is immediately beneath both the PA and the aorta. The conal septum is absent or hypoplastic. Clinical presentation is usually similar to that of a subaortic VSD with or without pulmonary stenosis.

Noncommitted VSD Type

Any VSD that is located below the conal septum (subpulmonary VSD) or the junction of conal and muscular interventricular septa (conoventricular or subaortic VSD) is likely to be so remote from the semilunar valves that it is very difficult to create a baffle that directs left ventricular blood flow into the aortic valve. These VSDs are frequently located in the inlet septum (AV canal type), or they can be midmuscular or apical VSDs. Clinical presentation is similar to DORV with subaortic VSD and depends on the presence or absence of pulmonary stenosis.[7]

Other Important Anatomical Features and Impact on the Type of Repair

Distance Between Tricuspid and Pulmonary Valve

The judgment as to which type of repair is best in a specific anatomical situation constitutes the fundamental complexity

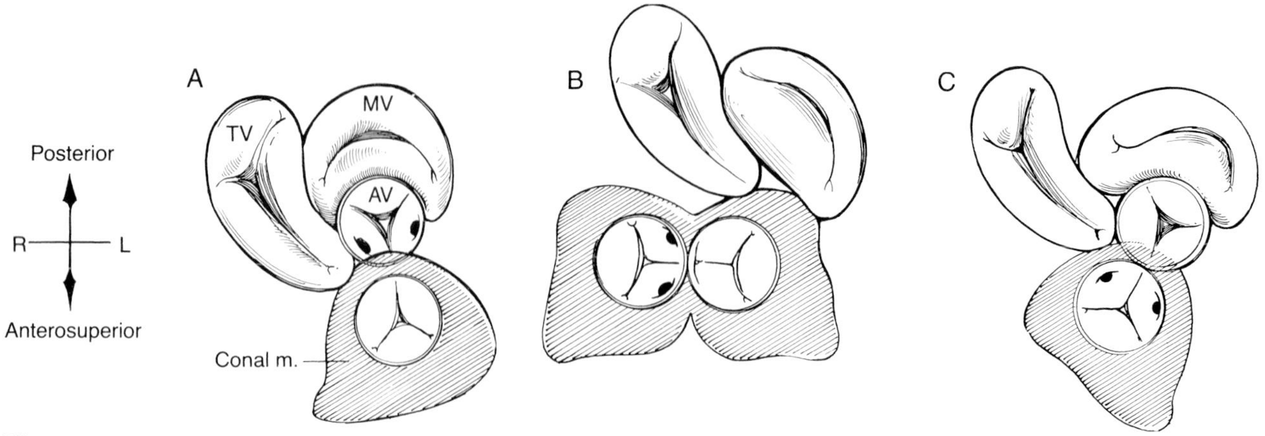

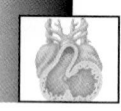

Figure 112–10 The spectrum of conus development between the tetralogy and transposition ends of the double-outlet right ventricle (DORV) spectrum. A, Tetralogy of Fallot: There is a subpulmonary conus with fibrous continuity between the aortic and mitral valve. **B,** The middle of the DORV spectrum: There are both subpulmonary and subaortic coni. **C,** Transposition of the great arteries: There is a subaortic conus with fibrous continuity between the pulmonary and mitral valves. In all diaphragms, the aortic valve is indicated by the coronary ostia, the tricuspid valve by three leaflets, and the mitral valve by two leaflets; hatching indicates conal myocardium. AV, aortic valve; MV, mitral valve; TV, tricuspid valve.
(Modified from Castaneda AR, Jonas RA, Mayer JE Jr, Hanley FL: Double outlet right ventricle. In Castaneda AR, Jonas RA, Mayer JE Jr, Hanley FL, editors: Cardiac Surgery of the Neonate and Infant, Philadelphia: W.B. Saunders, 1994, pp. 445–449.)

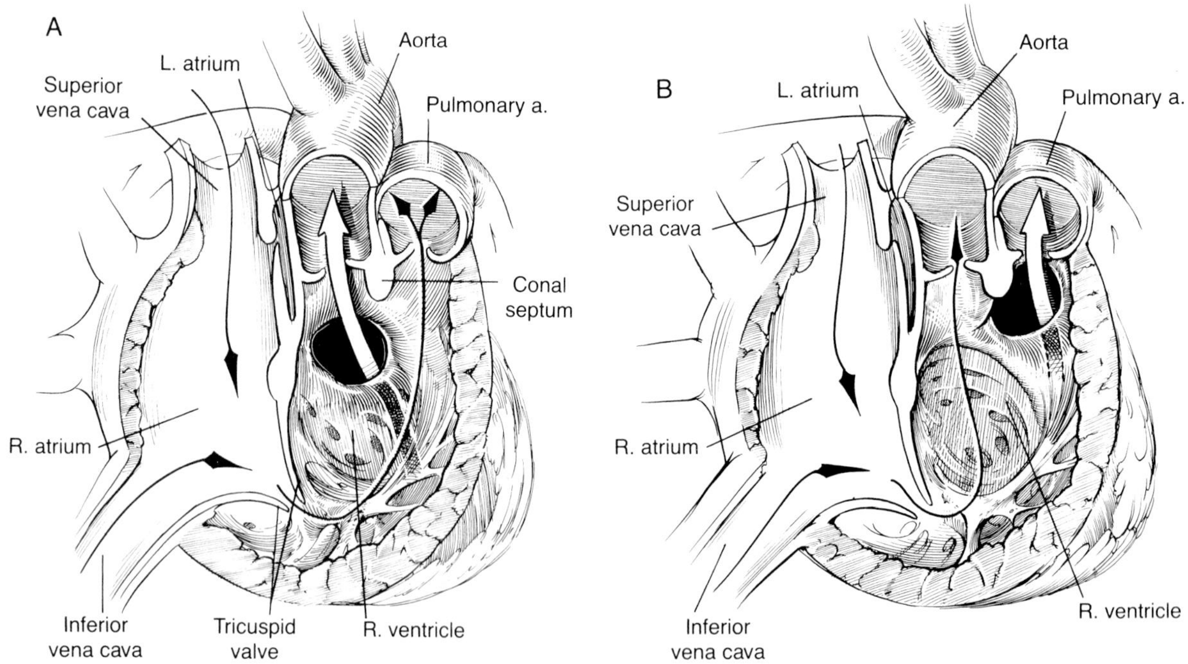

Figure 112–11 A, Double-outlet right ventricle (DORV) with a subaortic ventricular septal defect (VSD). Flow from the left ventricle preferentially enters the aorta. This is similar to what occurs in tetralogy of Fallot. **B,** DORV with a subpulmonary VSD. Left ventricular blood preferentially enters the pulmonary artery, resulting in physiology similar to that seen in transposition of the great arteries.
(Modified from Castaneda AR, Jonas RA, Mayer JE Jr, Hanley FL: Double outlet right ventricle. In Castaneda AR, Jonas RA, Mayer JE Jr, Hanley FL, editors: Cardiac Surgery of the Neonate and Infant, Philadelphia: W.B. Saunders, 1994, pp. 445–449.)

of the surgical management of DORV. An *intraventricular repair* denotes a baffle that is entirely within the right ventricle. The baffle is constructed around the VSD and creates a pathway from the left ventricle to the aorta. The right ventricular outflow thus curves around the left ventricular baffle. When the aorta is pushed away from the left ventricle by a very prominent subaortic conus or if the VSD is remote, a longer tunnel must be created. This often results in D-malposition of the aorta, where the aortic valve moves superior and anterior to the tricuspid valve, allowing the pulmonary valve to move closer to the tricuspid valve. Because the baffle must pass between the tricuspid and

Table 112–1

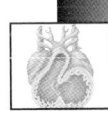

Pathophysiology of Double-Outlet Right Ventricle

VSD location	*RVOTO*	*Clinical presentation*
Subaortic	Absent	VSD
Subaortic	Present	TOF
Subpulmonary	Absent	TGA/VSD
Subpulmonary/ TGA	Present (subaortic stenosis)	Ductal-dependent lesion
Doubly or noncommitted	Absent	VSD
Doubly or noncommitted	Present	TOF

RVOTO, Right ventricular outflow tract obstruction; TOF, tetralogy of Fallot; TGA, transposition of the great arteries.

pulmonary valves, there is a point when this is no longer possible without either creating baffle obstruction (subaortic stenosis) or occluding the pulmonary valve, thus creating the need for a right ventricle–to–PA conduit. Thus the distance between the tricuspid valve and pulmonary valve must be carefully studied on multiple views by echocardiography and angiography (ventriculogram) when planning an intraventricular repair.

Conal Septum

A prominent conal septum also may be in the way of a successful intraventricular baffle. The length of the conal septum is determined by the development of the subaortic and subpulmonary coni. The conal septum may be resected if there are no important atrioventricular valve chordae attached to it (Figure 112-12). A long conal septum may be associated with a closer proximity between the tricuspid valve and the pulmonary valve. It also may be a substrate for the development of future subaortic stenosis, which in turn can be associated with aortic arch hypoplasia.[21]

Pulmonary Outflow Tract Obstruction

The presence of pulmonary outflow tract obstruction also needs to be carefully dealt with during surgery. Intraventricular repair must include relief of any subpulmonary stenosis, usually by means of division of hypertrophied muscle bands and placement of an infundibular outflow patch. Even in mild forms of subpulmonary stenosis, an infundibular patch may be needed because by definition an intraventricular baffle protrudes to some extent into the right ventricular outflow tract, thus crowding the right ventricular outflow. An infundibular patch thus prevents the creation of iatrogenic subpulmonary stenosis. Pulmonary stenosis is dealt with as during tetralogy surgery, by transannular patch, or by valvuloplasty. A Rastelli type of repair is sometimes required when the space between the tricuspid valve and pulmonary annulus is not sufficient and there is significant pulmonary annular hypoplasia. It is best to then incorporate the entire pulmonary annulus into the baffle, thus creating a generous subaortic passage; divide the main PA; and place a conduit (usually a homograft) between the right ventricle and distal main PA. If the pulmonary annulus is of normal size but an intraventricular baffle is not possible for the reasons cited previously, an arterial switch operation with baffling of the VSD to the pulmonary valve should be performed.[14]

Coronary Artery Anatomy

Knowledge of the coronary artery anatomy is also critical to successful management of DORV, because a left anterior descending coronary artery passing anterior to the right ventricular outflow in the tetralogy end of the spectrum excludes an intraventricular repair and requires a conduit. Complex coronary artery anatomy, frequently seen in Taussig–Bing hearts, renders an arterial switch operation more challenging.

Great Artery Relationship

Most hearts with DORV have normally related great arteries spiraling around each other, with the aorta posterior and to the right of the pulmonary artery. The VSD is usually subaortic. When the great arteries are parallel to each other without a spiral, the aorta can be found side-by-side rightward of the pulmonary artery (D-malposition), anterior to the PA, or side-by-side leftward (L-malposition). The VSD is usually subpulmonary, but can also be noncommitted. Great artery relationship gives an indication of VSD location, but both can also be independent of each other.[25]

Preoperative Evaluation

The presenting age and symptoms are mostly determined by the degree of pulmonary stenosis. Most cases are diagnosed during the neonatal period. Echocardiography is the test of choice in the neonate and young infant and is usually sufficient. At the transposition end of the spectrum, a balloon atrial septostomy may be needed to improve mixing. Catheterization also may be necessary in the older child to exclude pulmonary vascular disease. A left ventricular injection is helpful to follow the dye as it is ejected by the left ventricle (preferentially into the aorta or pulmonary artery) to plan (or exclude) a potential intraventricular baffle. Important echocardiographic details include the annular sizes of all valves; the size of the left and right ventricles; the relative position of both great arteries to each other; the degree of development of the conal septum; the chordal attachment to the conal septum; the level and degree of subpulmonary or pulmonary stenosis; the position of the VSD; and the status of the remainder of the septum, the coronary artery anatomy, and the aortic arch anatomy.

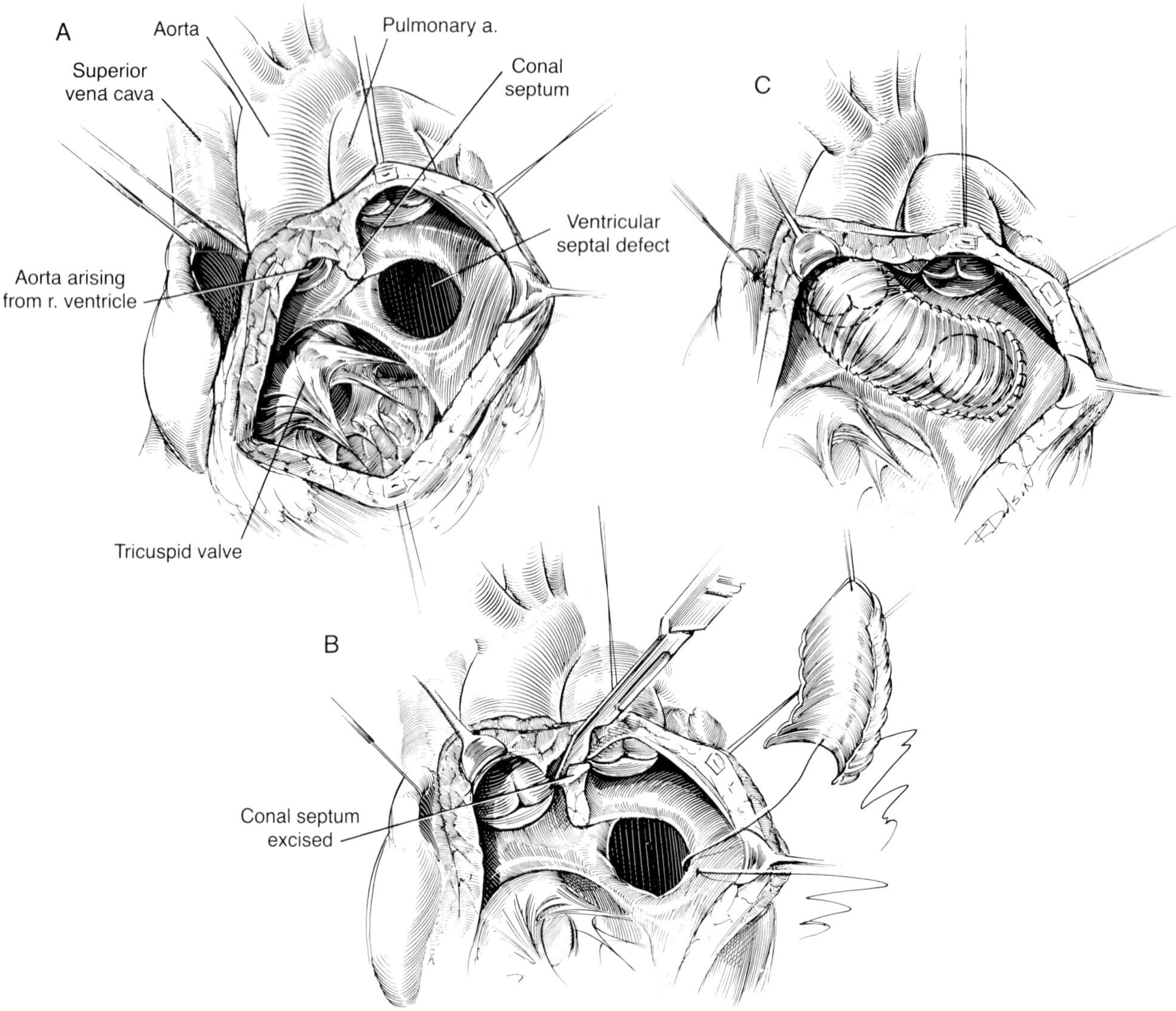

Figure 112–12 **A,** Prominent conal septum may project into the intraventricular baffle pathway. **B,** Resection of the conal septum may be necessary to prevent subaortic stenosis. **C,** Completion of intraventricular repair with a baffle.
(Modified from Castaneda AR, Jonas RA, Mayer JE Jr, Hanley FL: Double outlet right ventricle. In Castaneda AR, Jonas RA, Mayer JE Jr, Hanley FL, editors: Cardiac Surgery of the Neonate and Infant, pp. 445–449. Philadelphia: W.B. Saunders, 1994.)

Surgical Management

Management of DORV is always surgical. Medical management may be indicated in relatively asymptomatic neonates with tetralogy-type physiology until they are a few months old. Because of markedly improved results with neonatal repairs, surgical palliation in the form of pulmonary artery banding in VSD-type physiology or aortopulmonary shunting in tetralogy-type physiology is rarely performed. Routine cardiopulmonary bypass with bicaval cannulation is usually used.

Intraventricular Repair of DORV with Subaortic VSD or Doubly Committed VSD without Pulmonary Stenosis

Patients without pulmonary stenosis generally can be managed by placement of a patch baffle around the VSD, thus connecting the left ventricle to the aorta. The relationship of the aortic valve annulus to the VSD rims and to the conal septum has to be carefully studied. If there appears to be a need for a larger subaortic circumference, a portion of a synthetic tube graft rather than a flat patch can be used, thus giving the baffle more of a tunnel appearance (Figure 112-13).[8] If the VSD appears restrictive, it should be enlarged by making an incision anterosuperiorly and/or by resecting a wedge of the conal septum.

Intraventricular Repair of DORV with Subaortic VSD or Doubly Committed VSD with Pulmonary Stenosis

Techniques of repair are generally similar to those described for repair of tetralogy of Fallot. However, the VSD is closed by creation of a tunnel rather than a straight patch. It is generally recommended to perform an infundibulotomy because subpulmonary stenosis is almost always present. The site of the infundibulotomy has to be carefully planned,

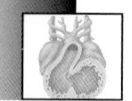

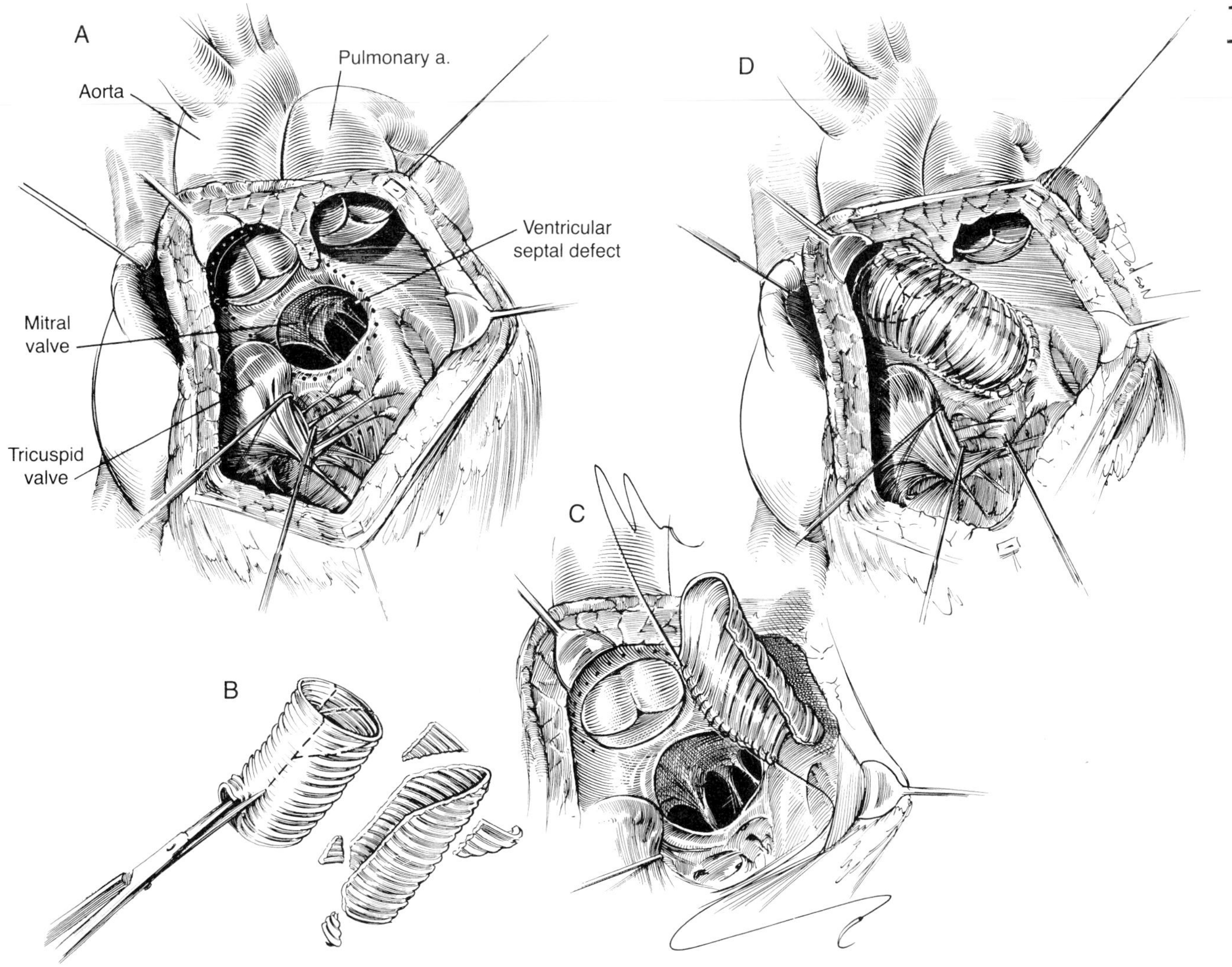

Figure 112–13 The long synthetic baffle used to direct left ventricular blood to the aorta is best constructed from a partial tube graft. A, The suture line is indicated by a *dotted line*. **B,** Tailoring of the baffle from a tube graft. **C,** A continuous suture technique may be necessary for a very long baffle. **D,** Completion of intraventricular baffle repair of tetralogy of Fallot type of DORV. *(Modified from Castaneda AR, Jonas RA, Mayer JE Jr, Hanley FL: Double outlet right ventricle. In Castaneda AR, Jonas RA, Mayer JE Jr, Hanley FL, editors: Cardiac Surgery of the Neonate and Infant, pp. 445–449. Philadelphia: W.B. Saunders, 1994.)*

staying away from any major coronary arteries. In case of an anomalous coronary artery crossing the right ventricular outflow tract, a conduit may sometimes be necessary. Division of parietal and septal bands is always performed, along with placement of an infundibular outflow patch. Stenoses at the level of the pulmonary annulus, pulmonary valve, or branch pulmonary arteries can be handled as in tetralogy of Fallot (see Chapter 114).

Repair of DORV with Noncommitted VSD

The VSD is generally of the inlet type. Intraventricular (and thus biventricular) repair is difficult, but can sometimes be accomplished by creation of a tunnel from the left ventricle to the aorta. Anatomical variations generally considered to contraindicate a biventricular repair are multiple muscular VSDs, straddling AV valve tissue, or an inability to reliably channel the remote VSD to the aorta. If it is easier to baffle left ventricular blood to the pulmonary valve, or if the pulmonary valve is in the pathway of the baffle, and there is no pulmonary stenosis, consideration should be given to performing an arterial switch procedure along with the intraventricular repair.[14] It is always necessary to enlarge the VSD superoanteriorly. If the tunnel obstructs the right ventricular outflow tract, an infundibular patch or transannular patch should be placed. If there are significant tricuspid valve attachments to the anterior and superior edge of the VSD, or if a straddling tricuspid or mitral valve is present, it is generally contraindicated to attempt intraventricular repair. However, there have been reports of successful division and reimplantation of the tricuspid chordae on the patch. In the long term the problem of subaortic stenosis with these complex baffles is real. A double-patch technique has been described that may mitigate this problem.[4]

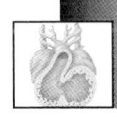

A noncommitted muscular trabecular defect also can sometimes be enlarged anteriorly and inferiorly, because the conduction system courses on the superior–posterior aspect of the defect. However, these baffles are often very bulky, do not grow with the child, and are generally not very satisfactory. With the improving medium-term outcome for the single ventricle approach in recent years, it is generally preferable to perform a straightforward single ventricle repair with preservation of excellent ventricular function rather than a less-than-satisfactory higher-risk biventricular repair in which multiple and usually complex reoperations will be necessary.[25] This approach might also be extended to patients who are at increased operative risk with a conventional biventricular repair.

Repair of DORV with Subpulmonary VSD

At the transposition end of the DORV spectrum, an arterial switch operation is usually preferred. A Taussig–Bing type of DORV can be repaired by an arterial switch operation (the most commonly employed repair), a Rastelli procedure with Damus–Kaye–Stansel anastomosis, a Nikaidoh procedure, or a REV (reparation à l'etage ventriculaire) procedure. Surgical management of DORV-transposition of the great arteries (TGA) is discussed in Chapter 121.

Results of Surgical Treatment

The early mortality is low among patients with noncomplex forms of DORV, but is higher in patients with complicating anatomical features.[2] Most complications are mechanical in nature and should be routinely sought out by TEE before the patient leaves the operating room. As with VSD surgery, complete heart block and residual VSDs can occur. Inadequate enlargement of VSD or poor baffle configuration can result in subaortic obstruction. Direct measurements in the operating room can help elucidate cases in which TEE is not definitive. Residual muscular obstruction often can be resected through the aortic valve, and an aortotomy is generally a good first approach when approaching this problem. A separate patch also can be placed inside the original patch if it is too narrowing or if there is a waist created by a tortuous course. In cases of DORV with noncommitted VSD, it sometimes may be necessary to convert an acutely failed biventricular repair to a single ventricle strategy. Significant right ventricular outflow tract obstruction can occur and should be managed as for tetralogy of Fallot. Patients with preoperative pulmonary hypertension are usually better served with implantation of a pulmonary valve. Because of prolonged myocardial ischemic times needed for these complex repairs, myocardial protection should be carefully attended to and myocardial dysfunction can be a significant problem. Delayed sternal closure and mechanical assistance are important fallback measures that can be lifesaving.

REFERENCES

1. Anderson RH, Pickering D, Brown T: Double outlet right ventricle with L-malposition and noncommitted ventricular septal defect. Eur J Cardiol 32:133–138, 1975.
2. Aoki M, Forbess JM, Jonas RA, et al: Results of biventricular repair for double-outlet right ventricle. J Thorac Cardiovasc Surg 107:338–350, 1994.
3. Bacha EA, Cao QL, Starr J, et al: Periventricular closure of muscular ventricular septal defects on the beating heart: Technique and results. J Thorac Cardiovasc Surg 126: 1718–1723, 2003.
4. Barbero-Marcial M, Tanamati C, Atik E, et al: Intraventricular repair of double-outlet right ventricle with non-committed ventricular septal defect: Advantages of multiple patches. J Thorac Cardiovasc Surg 118:1056–1067, 1999.
5. Barratt-Boyes BG, Simpson M, Neutze JM: Intracardiac surgery in neonates and infants using deep hypothermia with surface cooling and limited cardiopulmonary bypass. Circulation 43(suppl I):25–31, 1971.
6. Berner M, Behetti M, Ricou B, et al: Relief of severe pulmonary hypertension after closure of a large ventricular septal defect using low dose inhaled nitric oxide. Intensive Care Med 19:75-79, 1993.
7. Brown JW, Ruzmetov M, Okada Y, et al: Surgical results in patients with double outlet right ventricle: A 20-year experience. Ann Thorac Surg 72:1630–1635, 2001.
8. Castaneda AR, Jonas RA, Mayer JE Jr, Hanley FL: Double outlet right ventricle. In Castaneda AR, Jonas RA, Mayer JE Jr, Hanley FL, editors: Cardiac Surgery of the Neonate and Infant, pp. 445–449. Philadelphia: W.B. Saunders, 1994.
9. Collins G, Calder L, Rose V, et al: Ventricular septal defect: clinical and hemodynamic changes in the first five years of life. Am Heart J 84:695–701, 1972.
10. Gaynor JW: Management strategies for infants with coarctation and an associated ventricular septal defect. J Thorac Cardiovasc Surg 122:424–426, 2001.
11. Heath D, Edwards JE: The pathology of hypertensive pulmonary vascular disease: A description of 6 grades of structural changes in the pulmonary arteries with special reference to congenital cardiac septal defects. Circulation 18:533–543, 1958.
12. Hoffman JIE, Rudolph AM: The natural history of ventricular septal defects in infancy. Am J Cardiol 16:634–638, 1965.
13. Kirklin JW, Harshbarger HG, Donald DE, et al: Surgical correction of ventricular septal defect: Anatomic and technical considerations. J Thorac Surg 33:45–53, 1957.
14. Lacour-Gayet F, Haun C, Ntalakoura K, et al: Biventricular repair of double-outlet-right ventricle with non committed ventricular septal defect by VSD rerouting to the pulmonary artery and arterial switch. Eur J Cardiothorac Surg 21:1042–1048, 2002.
15. Lauer RM, Dushane JW, Edwards JE: Obstruction of the left ventricular outlet in association with ventricular septal defect. Circulation 22:110–117, 1960.
16. Lev M, Bharati S, Meng CCL, et al: A concept of double outlet right ventricle. J Thorac Cardiovasc Surg 64:271–279, 1972.
17. Lillehei CW, Corden M, Warden HE, et al: The results of direct vision closure of ventricular septal defects in eight patients by means of controlled cross circulation. Surg Gynecol Obstet 101:446–450, 1955.
18. Moller JH, Patton C, Varco RL, et al: Late results (30 to 35 years) after operative closure of isolated ventricular septal defect from 1954 to 1960. Am J Cardiol 68:1491–1496, 1991.
19. Muller WH Jr, Damman JF Jr: The treatment of certain congenital malformations of the heart by the creation of pulmonary stenosis to reduce pulmonary hypertension and excessive pulmonary blood flow: A preliminary report. Surg Gynecol Obstet 95:213–216, 1952.
20. Rein JG, Freed MD, Norwood WI, et al: Early and late results of closure of ventricular septal defect in infancy. Ann Thorac Surg 24:19–26, 1977.

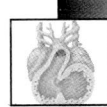

21. Sondheimer HM, Freedom RM, Olley PM: Double outlet right ventricle: Clinical spectrum and prognosis. Am J Cardiol 709:39–45, 1977.
22. Soto B, Becker AE, Moulaert AJ, et al: Classification of ventricular septal defects. Br Heart J 43:332–337, 1980.
23. Stirling GR, Stanley PH, Lilehei CW: The effects of cardiac bypass and ventriculotomy upon right ventricular function with report of successful closure of ventricular septal defect by use of atriotomy. Surg Forum 8:433–437, 1958.
24. Van Praagh R, Geva T, Kreutzer J: Ventricular septal defects: How shall we describe, name and classify them? J Am Coll Cardiol 14:1298–1303, 1989.
25. Walters HL, Mavroudis C, Tchervenkov CI, et al: Congenital heart surgery nomenclature and database project: Double outlet right ventricle. Ann Thorac Surg 69:249–263, 2000.
26. Weintraub RG, Menahem S: Early surgical closure of a large ventricular septal defect: Influence on long-term growth. J Am Coll Cardiol 18:552–557, 1991.
27. Yeager SB, Freed MD, Keane JF, et al: Primary surgical closure of ventricular septal defect in the first year of life: Results in 128 infants. J Am Coll Cardiol 3:1269–1273, 1984.

Pulmonary Atresia with Intact Ventricular Septum

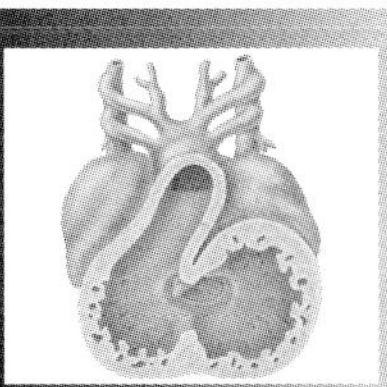

CHAPTER 113

Erle H. Austin, III

INTRODUCTION

Pulmonary atresia with intact ventricular septum (PA/IVS) is a rare congenital heart defect occurring at a rate of 4–10 per 100,000 live births.[10,11] This malformation is characterized by a variably sized right ventricle that has no exit, failing to provide pulmonary blood flow and unable to decompress itself through the interventricular septum. Blood flow through the ductus arteriosus permits survival at birth, but within hours, hypoxemia progresses to death as the ductus closes. Thus without early diagnosis and treatment, PA/IVS is uniformly fatal. Before 1970, reported survival to 3 years of age was less than 3%.[14] By the early 1990s, improvements in diagnosis and management resulted in a 3-year survival rate greater than 60%.[18] More recent reports indicate that careful initial evaluation and selective management of these patients can achieve survival rates in excess of 90%.[20]

Because this anomaly is rare and its morphology is heterogeneous, the majority of reports and recommendations have been derived from small series with variable morphological compositions. Although a great deal has been learned from the experiences of individual centers,[8,27,33,39] much more has been learned from a prospective multi-institutional study initiated by the Congenital Heart Surgeons Society in 1987[18] and from more recent population-based studies from the United Kingdom and Ireland[9,10] and from Sweden.[11] Data acquired from these studies have provided important new insights into the spectrum of morphology, as well as the outcome of surgical treatment of this malformation.

ANATOMY

Characteristically, PA/IVS occurs in hearts with situs solitus and atrioventricular and ventriculoarterial concordance. The essential feature of this lesion is an absent communication between the right ventricle and the pulmonary trunk (Figure 113-1). The character of the atretic segment ranges from a thin imperforate membrane to a long section of infundibular muscle without a definable lumen. In contrast to pulmonary atresia with ventricular septal defect, the pulmonary trunk and branch pulmonary arteries are usually near-normal in size and configuration. The size and morphology of the right ventricle varies significantly in this condition, and in most patients, the right ventricular cavity is reduced in size. There is a continuum from tiny "unipartite" chambers that have only an inlet component to larger-than-normal "tripartite" ventricles that have well-defined inlet, trabecular, and infundibular portions. The rare patients with enlarged right ventricular cavities also may have Ebstein's anomaly with severe tricuspid regurgitation. More typically the cavity is small and marked hypertrophy of the right ventricular wall is present, often contributing to obliteration of the outflow (infundibular) portion of the cavity. The tricuspid valve is usually small with thickened leaflets and abnormal chordae. The diameter of the tricuspid valve correlates with the size of the right ventricular cavity and provides a useful index of right ventricular size. The right atrium is enlarged, and an interatrial communication, usually a patent foramen ovale, is present. At birth the ductus arteriosus is patent, providing the only blood flow to the lungs. Significant aortopulmonary collateral arteries are uncommon.

An important anatomical feature of PA/IVS is the presence in some patients of connections between the right ventricle and the coronary circulation (Figures 113-2 and 113-3). Sinusoids or "intermuscular spaces" in the right ventricular myocardium occur in about 50% of patients.[18] In 90% of these patients, the sinusoids communicate with the coronary arteries. The smaller the tricuspid valve (and thus the right ventricular cavity), the more likely it is that right ventricle–coronary arterial fistulas are present. In 20% of patients with these fistulas, significant proximal coronary

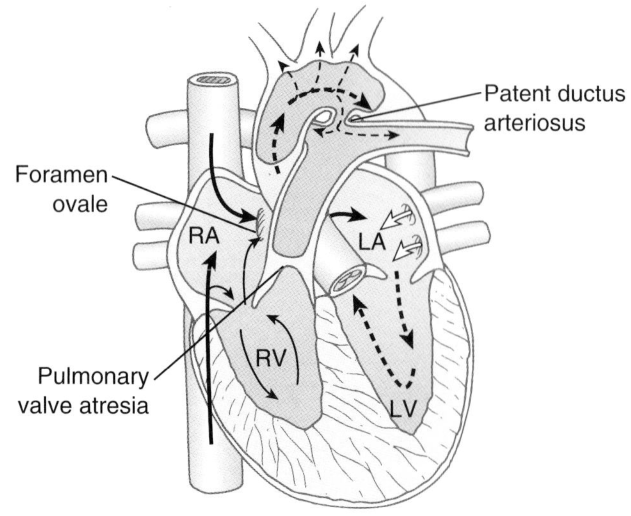

Figure 113–1 Schematic representation of blood flow in pulmonary atresia with intact ventricular septum (PA/IVS). An obligatory right-to-left shunt occurs at the atrial level. Peripheral oxygenation is dependent on flow through the ductus arteriosus. RA, right atrium; RV, right ventricle; LA, left atrium; LV, left ventricle.

artery stenoses exist, making myocardial blood flow dependent on blood from the right ventricle.[18] Knowledge of the presence of a right ventricle–dependent coronary circulation is important in deciding on surgical therapy, because in these cases decompression of the right ventricle may cause myocardial ischemia or infarction.[16]

PATHOPHYSIOLOGY

In PA/IVS, desaturated systemic venous blood is obliged to cross the interatrial septum to mix with saturated pulmonary venous blood in the left atrium (see Figure 113-1). The resultant admixture is ejected into the systemic arterial circulation, and the systemic arterial saturation is dependent on adequate pulmonary blood flow. Closure of the ductus arteriosus soon after birth markedly reduces pulmonary blood flow, and progressive hypoxemia and tissue acidosis leads to death. Expeditious administration of prostaglandin E_1 can temporarily reverse ductal closure until a surgical procedure to increase pulmonary blood flow can be performed.

INITIAL CLINICAL PRESENTATION AND MANAGEMENT

Infants with PA/IVS are typically full-term, well-developed babies without other anomalies. Delivery is usually uncomplicated, but cyanosis develops on the first day of life and rapidly progresses to respiratory distress and metabolic acidosis. A murmur is unusual unless significant tricuspid regurgitation exists. There is no splitting of the second heart sound. Chest radiography demonstrates clear lung fields with decreased vascular markings. The electrocardiogram (ECG) is often normal, although the typical neonatal pattern of right ventricular hypertrophy may be absent. Definitive diagnosis is made using two-dimensional (2D) echocardiography, which reveals the right ventricular outflow obstruction and the size of the right ventricle and tricuspid valve and, combined with color-flow Doppler techniques, can identify right ventricle–coronary artery fistulas.[26,38]

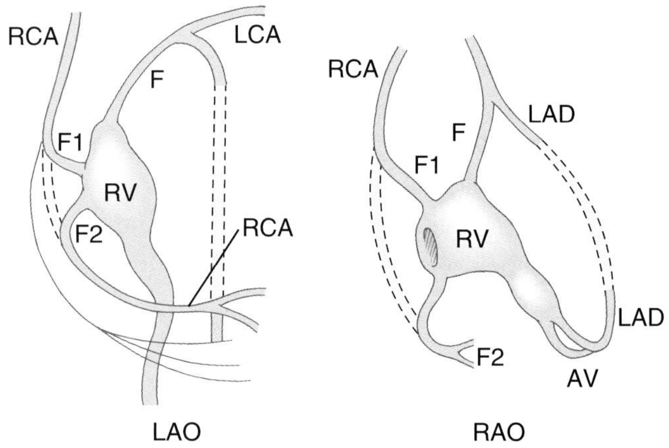

Figure 113–3 Outlines of right ventricular cineangiograms in a patient with right ventricle–dependent coronary circulation. RCA, right coronary artery; LCA left coronary artery; RAO, right anterior oblique; LAO, left anterior oblique; AV, apical vessels; F, fistula locations. The *dashed lines* indicate coronary occlusion.
(Modified from Giglia TM, Mandell S, Connor AR, et al: Diagnosis and management of right ventricle-dependent coronary circulation in pulmonary atresia with intact ventricular septum. Circulation 86:1516–1528, 1992.)

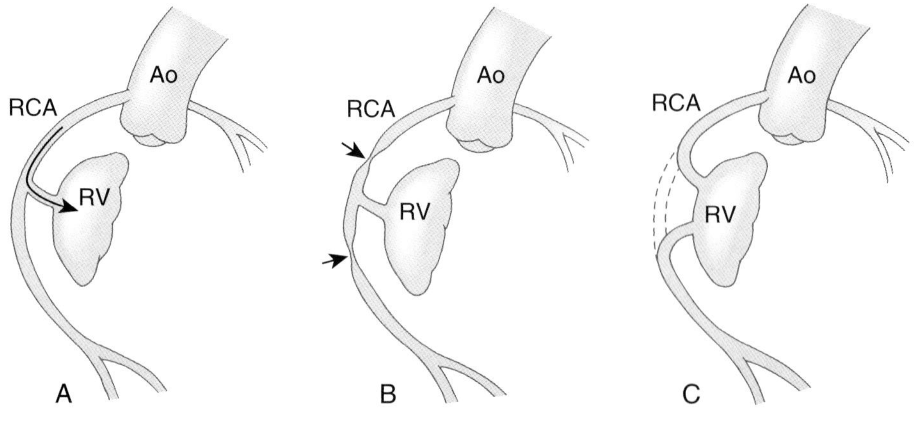

Figure 113–2 Right ventricle–coronary artery fistulas in pulmonary atresia with intact ventricular septum. **A,** Without coronary stenosis: potential right ventricular "steal" phenomenon. **B,** With proximal and/or distal coronary stenosis: potential "steal" and/or ischemia. **C,** With coronary occlusion/atresia: potential isolation and myocardial infarction. Ao, aorta; RCA, right coronary artery; RV, right ventricle.
(Modified from Giglia TM, Mandell S, Connor AR, et al: Diagnosis and management of right ventricle-dependent coronary circulation in pulmonary atresia with intact ventricular septum. Circulation 86:1516–1528, 1992.)

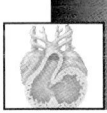

As soon as the diagnosis of PA/IVS is suspected, an infusion of prostaglandin E_1 is begun. Elective intubation and controlled ventilation may be advisable, especially if the infant is to be transported to a tertiary treatment center, because apnea is a common complication of prostaglandin E_1 infusion.

Cardiac catheterization and cineangiography are recommended for the majority of these patients, especially in those with moderate or severe right ventricular hypoplasia. Right ventriculography, aortography, and when indicated, selective coronary angiography are performed to determine the presence and extent of right ventricle–to–coronary artery fistulas and the presence of coronary artery obstructions[7,16] (see Figures 113-2 and 113-3). At catheterization an adequate atrial communication must be ensured. If echocardiography and catheterization indicate that right ventricle to pulmonary artery decompression cannot be performed and a flow gradient exists between the right and left atrium, a balloon atrial septostomy is performed at this catheterization.

SURGICAL MANAGEMENT

The ideal long-term outcome for all infants with PA/IVS would be to achieve a two-ventricle circulation with the right ventricle providing all blood flow to the lungs at a low filling pressure without residual right-to-left shunt. The anatomical heterogeneity of this group of patients, however, prevents the achievement of this goal in all patients. In fact, this ideal is achieved in only one third of patients surviving infancy.[18] A more realistic outcome for the remaining patients is the elimination of cyanosis by separating the systemic and pulmonary circulations without limiting cardiac output or inducing excessively elevated systemic venous pressures. Such an outcome can be achieved with a one-ventricle repair (the Fontan operation) for hearts whose right ventricle cannot contribute to pulmonary blood flow or with a one and one-half–ventricle repair for hearts whose right ventricle can provide a portion of pulmonary blood flow. Careful assessment of right ventricular size and coronary artery anatomy are crucial to selecting the appropriate strategy for each patient.

In the neonate it is useful to classify right ventricular hypoplasia into mild, moderate, and severe degrees (Table 113-1). Echocardiographic measurement of the diameter of the tricuspid valve with conversion to a Z-value provides a quantitative measurement to facilitate classification[24] (Figure 113-4). Patients with mild right ventricular hypoplasia have tricuspid valve Z-values of −2 or greater. Tricuspid Z-values between −4 and −2 indicate moderate right ventricular hypoplasia, and Z-values of −4 or less are seen in patients with severe right ventricular hypoplasia. Tripartite right ventricles with a well-developed right ventricular outflow tract fall into the mild group, whereas unipartite right ventricles without a definable infundibular or trabecular portion are classified as severe.[5] Patients with mild right ventricular hypoplasia have definite potential for

Table 113–1

Effect of Degree of Right Ventricular Hypoplasia on Surgical Management of Pulmonary Atresia with Intact Ventricular Septum

	Degree of right ventricular hypoplasia		
Parameter/surgical management	***Mild***	***Moderate***	***Severe***
Tricuspid Z-value	>-2	-2 to -4	<-4
Right ventricular morphology	Tripartite	Bipartite	Unipartite
Infundibular cavity	Present	Intermediate	Absent
Right ventricle–dependent coronary circulation	Rare	Possible	Common
Surgical palliation	Transannular patch ± shunt	Transannular patch + shunt (no right ventricular decompression if right ventricle–dependent coronary circulation)	Shunt only
Definitive operation	Two-ventricle repair	Two-ventricle repair; one and one-half–ventricle repair; Fontan if right ventricle–dependent coronary circulation	Fontan

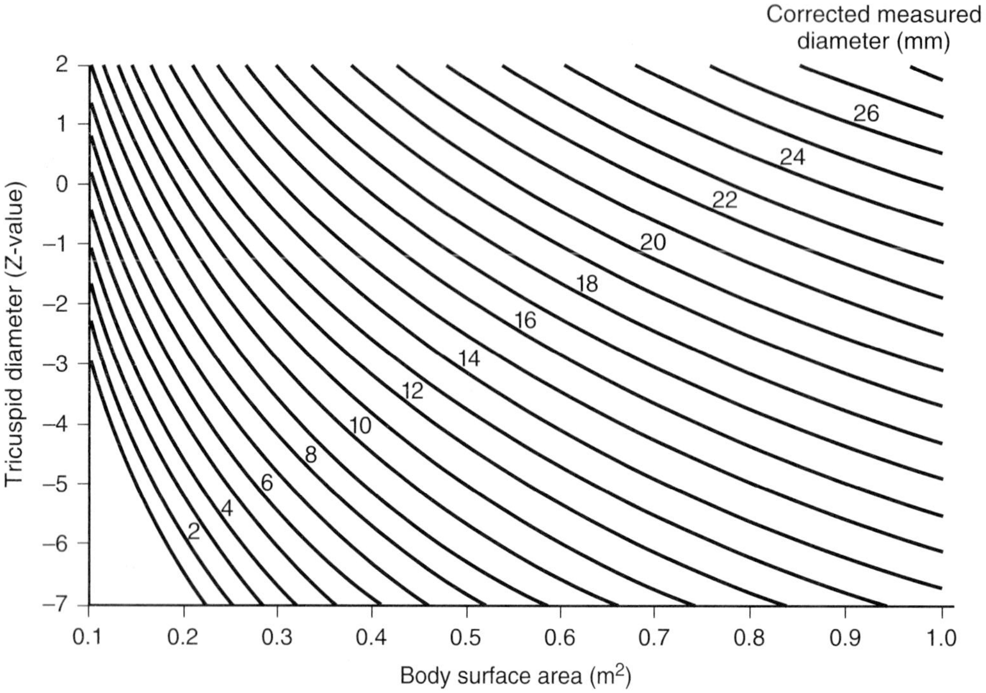

Figure 113-4 Nomogram for converting echocardiographically measured tricuspid valve diameters to the Z-value. Knowledge of the tricuspid Z-value may help select initial surgical management and predict long-term outcome.
(Modified from Hanley FL, Sade RM, Blackstone EH, et al: Outcomes in neonatal pulmonary atresia with intact ventricular septum. J Thorac Cardiovasc Surg 105:406–427, 1993.)

conversion to a two-ventricle system at the time of definitive repair, whereas those with severe right ventricular hypoplasia can achieve only separation of systemic and pulmonary circulations with a one-ventricle repair (a Fontan operation). Patients with moderate right ventricular hypoplasia are also potential candidates for two-ventricle or one and one-half–ventricle repair, provided they do not have a right ventricle–dependent coronary circulation.

Initial Palliation

The surgical management of PA/IVS is typically undertaken in two stages, the first for palliation and the second for definitive repair. To ensure early survival, pulmonary blood flow must be maintained after ductal closure. Although the creation of a systemic-to-pulmonary shunt can ensure continued pulmonary blood flow, the right ventricle must be assessed for its potential recruitment into the circulation. When possible, decompressing the right ventricle into the pulmonary artery permits right ventricular growth such that a two-ventricle repair may become feasible. Failure to decompress the right ventricle at initial palliation essentially eliminates the possibility of ever achieving a definitive two-ventricle repair.[6]

Thus neonates with mild to moderate right ventricular hypoplasia are best served by relieving the right ventricle–to–pulmonary artery obstruction and creating a systemic-to-pulmonary shunt. This may be accomplished with or without cardiopulmonary bypass. Without bypass, a pulmonary valvotomy can be performed blindly with a transventricular dilator[19] or under direct vision through the main pulmonary artery[22] (Figure 113-5). The use of cardiopulmonary bypass allows more controlled access into the right ventricular outflow tract so that obstructing infundibular muscle can be excised under direct vision and a transannular outflow patch can be placed (Figure 113-6). By maximizing unobstructed forward flow, transannular patching provides the greatest possibility for right ventricular growth.[13,18] Because early postoperative right ventricular failure may cause increased right-to-left shunting across the patent foramen ovale and antegrade flow from the right ventricle may be limited, a systemic–to–pulmonary artery shunt (a 3.5- or 4-mm polytetrafluoroethylene [PTFE] tube graft) also should be placed to prevent life-threatening hypoxia. Initial results from the Congenital Heart Surgeons Society's study

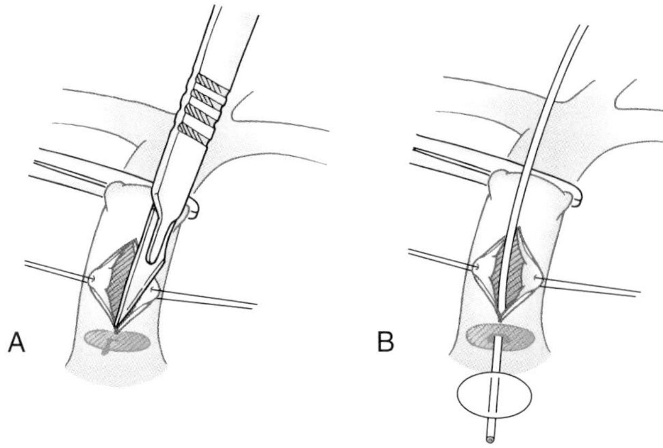

Figure 113-5 Open pulmonary valvotomy without cardiopulmonary bypass can be performed via median sternotomy or left thoracotomy. A, After clamping the pulmonary trunk just proximal to the bifurcation, the pulmonary artery is opened and the atretic pulmonary valve is opened sharply. **B,** A Fogarty catheter positioned in the infundibulum provides hemostasis as the atretic valve is excised.
(Modified from Kanter KR, Pennington DG, Nouri S, et al: Concomitant valvotomy and subclavian–main pulmonary artery shunt in neonates with pulmonary atresia and intact ventricular septum. Ann Thorac Surg 43:490–494, 1987.)

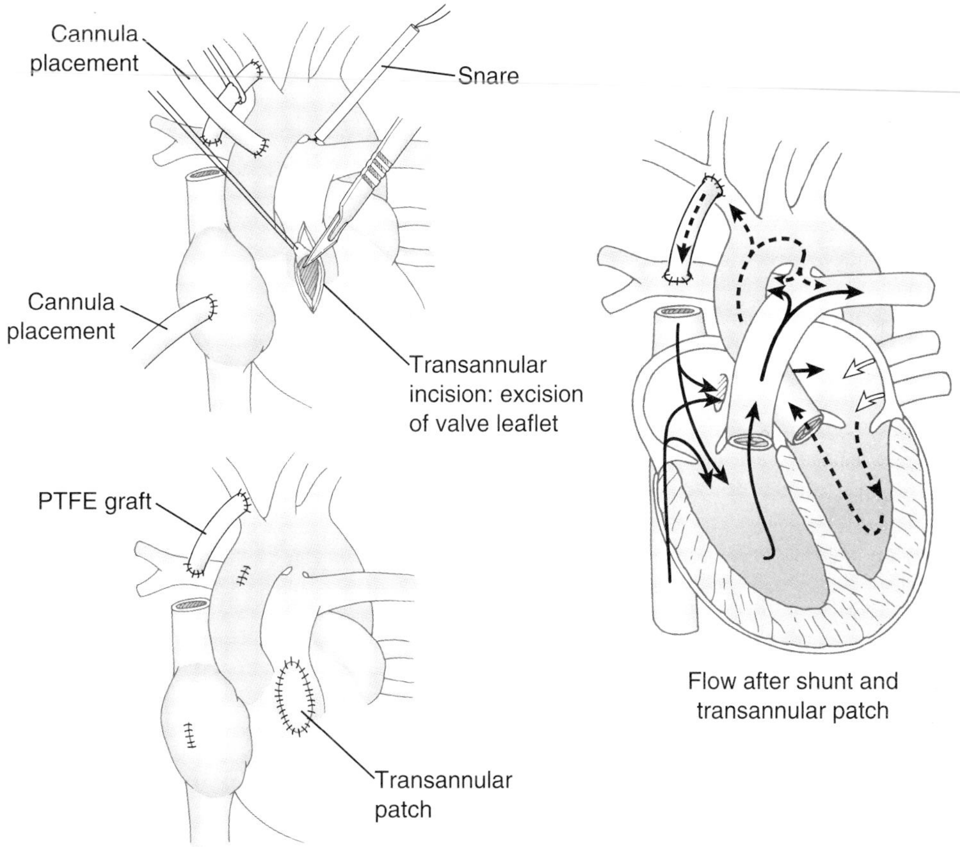

Figure 113–6 Placement of a transannular patch and a systemic–to–pulmonary artery shunt. A 3.5-mm polytetrafluoroethylene (PTFE) tube graft is placed from the innominate artery to right pulmonary artery. Cardiopulmonary bypass is established and the shunt and ductus are temporarily occluded. A pulmonary artery incision is extended into the right ventricular outflow tract. Obstructing tissue is excised, and a pericardial patch is sewn in place. Separation from bypass is done with the shunt open and the ductus occluded. If peripheral oxygen saturations exceed 80%, the ductus is ligated. If peripheral oxygen saturations are less than 80%, the ductus is unsnared as demonstrated at right.

suggest that concomitant insertion of a transannular patch and placement of a systemic–to–pulmonary artery shunt is the optimal initial treatment for neonates with tricuspid valve Z-values between −1.5 and −4[18] (Figure 113-7). On the other hand, any form of right ventricular decompression is contraindicated if a right ventricle–dependent coronary circulation exists.

Neonates with severe right ventricular hypoplasia and/or a right ventricle–dependent coronary circulation are best placed on a definitive one-ventricle (Fontan) tract. As such, initial surgical therapy should be limited to a systemic–to–pulmonary artery shunt[18] (see Figure 113-7). A 3.5- or 4-mm PTFE tube graft placed via a median sternotomy or a right thoracotomy from the innominate or right subclavian artery to the right pulmonary artery provides adequate pulmonary blood flow and facilitates shunt access at the time of definitive one-ventricle repair. Shunts greater than 4 mm should be avoided because they may result in excessive pulmonary blood flow and low diastolic arterial blood pressure, causing life-threatening myocardial ischemia.

Definitive Procedures

Two-Ventricle Repair

Patients selected at initial palliation for a two-ventricle strategy should have echocardiographic evidence of satisfactory right ventricular decompression with estimated right ventricular pressure less than or equal to one half of systemic arterial pressure. Those infants treated originally with valvotomy rather than transannular patching are especially vulnerable to residual or recurrent right ventricular outflow tract obstruction,[6,18] which should be relieved by a second right ventricular outflow tract procedure (a transannular patch) before considering conversion to a two-ventricle circulation. Follow-up cardiac catheterization should be performed between 6–12 months of age. At catheterization the systemic–to–pulmonary artery shunt is temporarily occluded. If arterial saturations remain high, the atrial septal defect (patent foramen ovale) is occluded as well. If right atrial pressure remains below 15 mm Hg and cardiac output is adequate, the shunt and atrial communication can be closed permanently and a two-ventricle circulation achieved. At some centers, the shunt and atrial defect can be closed during the catheterization using percutaneous techniques.[29,36]

One and One-Half Ventricle Repair

Patients studied at 6–12 months who do not tolerate temporary occlusion of the systemic–to–pulmonary artery shunt are receiving too little pulmonary blood flow from the right ventricle to achieve a two-ventricle repair. Assuming there is no significant residual right ventricular outflow obstruction, these patients should be considered candidates for a one and one-half–ventricle repair. This repair involves takedown of the arterial systemic-to-pulmonary shunt and the creation of a bidirectional superior cavopulmonary anastomosis (a bidirectional Glenn procedure), which relieves the

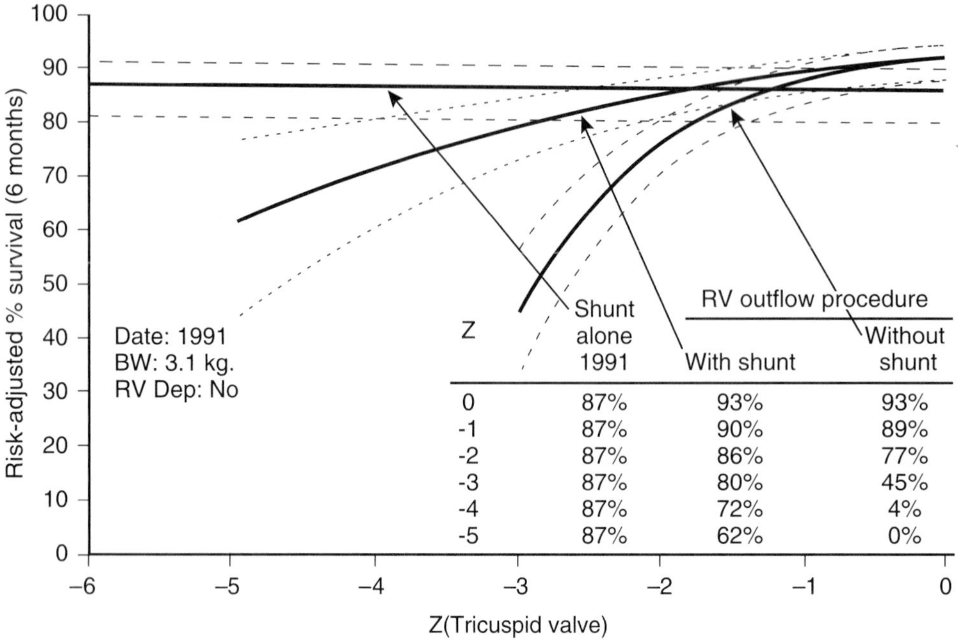

Figure 113-7 The effect of tricuspid valve diameter (Z-value) and type of initial procedure on 6-month survival in neonates with pulmonary atresia and intact septum. This nomogram was derived after analyzing 171 neonates and solving a multivariable equation setting birthweight at "3.1 kg," right ventricle–dependent circulation at "no," and date of shunt operation at "1991." Right ventricular outflow procedure includes valvotomy and transannular patch.
(Modified from Hanley FL, Sade RM, Blackstone EH, et al: Outcomes in neonatal atresia with intact ventricular septum. J Thorac Cardiovasc Surg 105:406–427, 1993.)

right ventricle of the superior vena caval blood flow. Ideally the atrial septal communication is closed at the same operation. However, if the right atrial pressure exceeds 15 mm Hg, a small (4-mm) fenestration can be left. Catheter closure of the fenestration can usually be performed within months of the surgical procedure.[36] Alternatively, a pursestring suture and an adjustable snare can permit incremental closure of the atrial septal defect in the postoperative period[2] (Figure 113-8). Patients with tricuspid Z-values as small as −6 may be definitively managed with the one and one-half–ventricle strategy.[41]

One-Ventricle Repair

Infants with severe right ventricular hypoplasia and/or right ventricle–dependent coronary circulation are typically designated for a one-ventricle strategy at initial palliation. At 4–6 months of age these patients undergo takedown of the systemic-to-pulmonary shunt and the creation of a bidirectional cavopulmonary anastomosis. At 2–4 years of age they are considered candidates for the Fontan operation. Before the Fontan operation, cardiac catheterization is essential to ensure adequate left ventricular function and low pulmonary vascular resistance. Poor left ventricular function would leave cardiac transplantation as the only alternative therapy. Heart–lung transplantation is the only alternative if pulmonary vascular resistance is elevated. Fortunately, the early creation of a bidirectional cavopulmonary anastomosis appears to help preserve ventricular function and prevent the development of pulmonary vascular disease so that those drastic measures are rarely necessary.

When the Fontan procedure is performed, inferior vena caval blood flow is directed to the pulmonary arteries. This may be performed with a lateral atrial tunnel technique wherein a baffle of PTFE is placed inside the right atrium[34] (Figure 113-9), or with an extracardiac conduit.[28] Many surgeons prefer to place a small fenestration in the baffle to permit some right-to-left shunting to maintain cardiac output in the perioperative period when pulmonary vascular resistance may be elevated.[4] Routine fenestration, however, may not be necessary when an extracardiac conduit is used.[40]

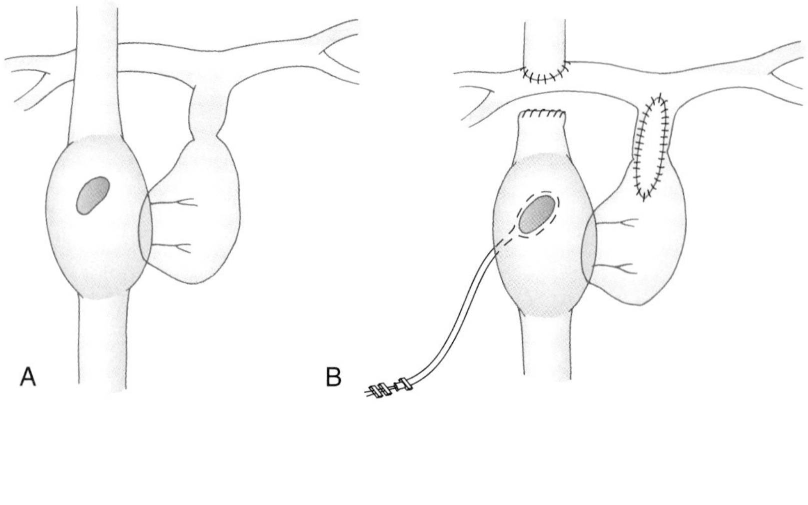

Figure 113-8 Creation of a one and one-half–ventricle circulation. Superior vena caval flow is directed to the right pulmonary artery with a bidirectional cavopulmonary anastomosis. Residual right ventricular outflow tract stenosis is relieved with a transannular patch. Placement of an adjustable snare around the atrial septal defect permits incremental closure in the postoperative period.
(Modified from Billingsley AM, Laks H, Boyce SW, et al: Definitive repair in patients with pulmonary atresia and intact ventricular septum. J Thorac Cardiovasc Surg 97:746–754, 1989.)

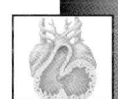

It also may be preferable to avoid fenestration when a right ventricle–dependent coronary circulation is present. Enlarging the atrial septal defect and unroofing the coronary sinus to ensure that the blood entering the right ventricle is well oxygenated also has been recommended for right ventricle–dependent coronary circulations (see Figure 113-9).

RESULTS

The report from the Congenital Heart Surgeons Society (CHSS) in 1993[18] continues to provide the best overall perspective of outcomes in neonates with PA/IVS. This prospective multi-institutional study involved 31 centers and enrolled 171 unselected neonates with this diagnosis within a 4-year period (1987–1991). The initial right ventricular morphology and tricuspid valve size (Z-value) were known for all patients, and follow-up through 1991 was complete. Techniques for surgical management were not randomized, but left to the discretion of each institution.

In this unselected group, 54% of patients were found to have severe right ventricular hypoplasia and 29% had moderate right ventricular hypoplasia. Survival at 1 month after the first intervention was 81%, with survival at 1 year of 69% and at 4 years of 64% (Figure 113-10). A more recently reported population-based study from the United Kingdom and Ireland demonstrated very similar findings, with a 1-year survival of 71% and a 3-year survival of 66%.[10] Multivariable analysis in the CHSS study indicated that small size (Z-value) of the tricuspid valve, right ventricle–dependent coronary circulation, and low birth weight were the strongest risk factors for death. Patients who initially underwent transannular patching with a systemic–to–pulmonary artery shunt were less likely to require an interim procedure before definitive correction. When a valvotomy or transannular patch was performed without a concomitant systemic–to–pulmonary artery shunt, approximately 50% of the patients required shunt placement within the first 4 weeks after the initial procedure. In addition, approximately 40% of patients treated initially with pulmonary valvotomy required a transannular patch at a subsequent operation.[18] Of patients alive 24 months after entry, 24% had received a complete two-ventricle repair with an operative mortality of 5% (1 out of 21). Eleven percent had undergone a definitive one-ventricle repair (the Fontan operation) with an operative mortality of 12.5% (1 out of 8).[18]

A recent report from one of the CHSS member institutions indicates that more favorable results are now being realized. Using information derived from the CHSS study, Boston Children's Hospital applied a policy of routine coronary angiography, right ventricular decompression with transannular patching for patients without right ventricle–dependent coronary circulations, and a systemic-to-pulmonary shunt in virtually all patients. In a consecutive group of 47 patients from 1991–1998, this institution was able to achieve an actuarial survival of 98% at 1 year, 5 years, and 7.5 years.[20] To achieve this excellent survival, a one-ventricle or a one and one-half–ventricle repair was required in the majority of patients.

CONTROVERSIAL ISSUES

Decompression of the Right Ventricle

Antegrade right ventricular decompression is required to recruit the right ventricle for an ultimate two-ventricle or one and one-half–ventricle circulation. When significant communications (fistulas) between the right ventricle and the coronary circulation are present, controversy exists regarding the advisability and technique of right ventricular decompression. Virtually all authors agree that when proximal coronary obstructions are also present that make the coronary circulation dependent on the right ventricle, decompression of the right ventricle is contraindicated. Consensus is not uniform, however, when significant right ventricle–to–coronary connections are present without proximal coronary artery obstructions. Some authors advise

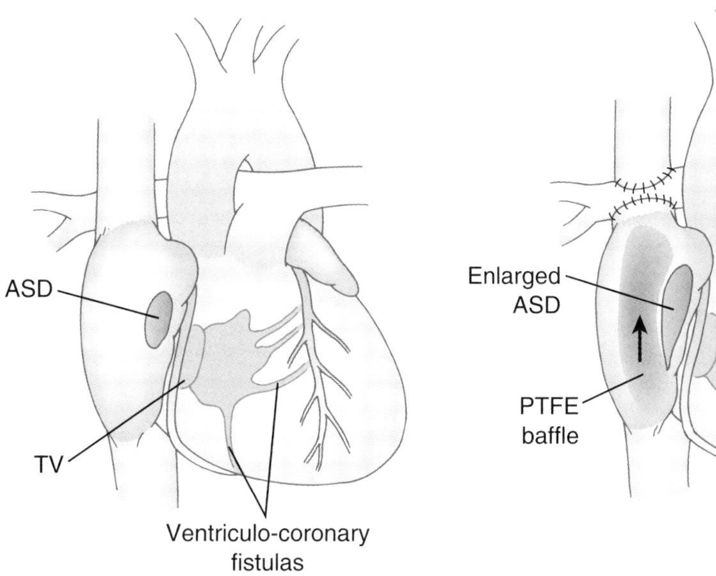

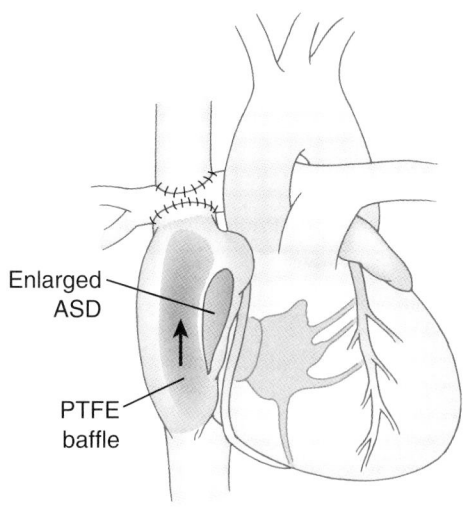

Figure 113–9 Lateral tunnel Fontan procedure in a patient with right ventricle–dependent coronary circulation. Inferior vena caval flow is directed to superior vena cava by polytetrafluoroethylene (PTFE) baffle. Atrial septal defect (ASD) is enlarged, allowing fully saturated pulmonary venous blood to enter the right ventricle (RV). TV, tricuspid valve. *(Modified from Pearl JM, Laks H, Stein DG, et al: Total cavopulmonary anastomosis versus conventional modified Fontan procedure. Ann Thorac Surg 52:189–195, 1991.)*

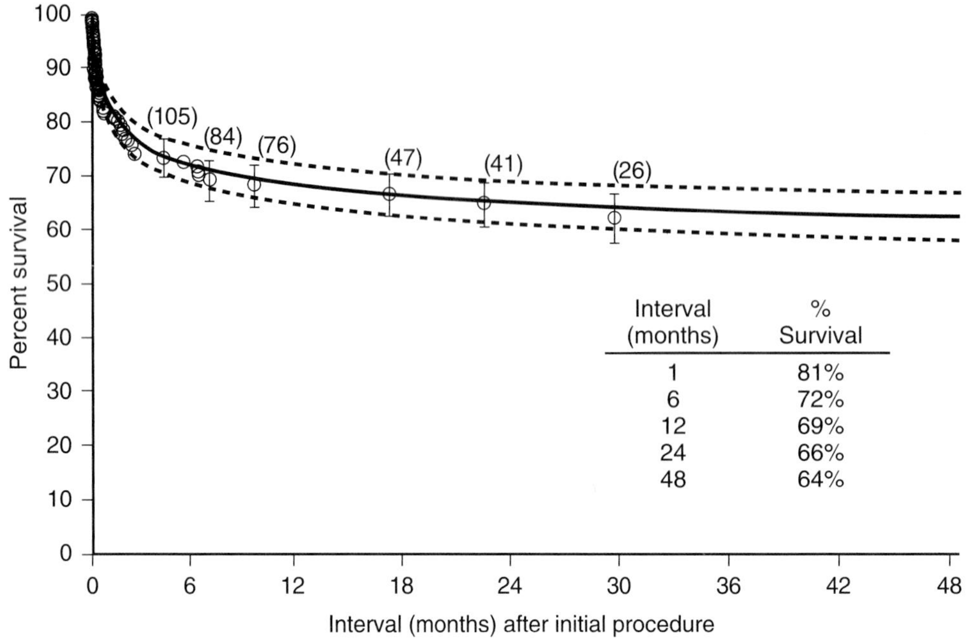

Figure 113–10 **Survival (derived from life-table and parametric methods) after the initial procedure of neonates with pulmonary atresia and intact ventricular septum.** *Circles* represent individual deaths. *Vertical bars* and *dotted lines* represent 70% confidence intervals. (*Modified from Hanley FL, Sade RM, Blackstone EH, et al: Outcomes in neonatal pulmonary atresia with intact ventricular septum. J Thorac Cardiovasc Surg 105:406–427, 1993.*)

against decompression in these cases for fear that decreasing right ventricular pressure will result in a "steal" phenomenon with compromised blood flow to portions of myocardium[1,17,31] (see Figure 113-2, *A*). Other authors express concern that failure to decompress the right ventricle will allow these fistulas to persist, resulting in ischemia and progressive myocardial fibrosis.[19,30] To encourage regression of these connections, these authors recommend antegrade decompression if an infundibular cavity is present, or retrograde decompression by tricuspid valve excision if there is no infundibulum.[19] Other authors recommend tricuspid valve closure[42] or right ventricular thromboexclusion[30] to prevent deoxygenated blood from entering the coronary circulation.

In a study of PA/IVS patients with right ventricle–to–coronary artery connections and a spectrum of coronary artery abnormalities, Giglia and associates[16] found that antegrade right ventricular decompression could be performed without jeopardizing left ventricular function when coronary stenoses were absent or involved only a single coronary artery. At present, therefore, most centers attempt right ventricular decompression in the presence of right ventricle–coronary artery connections when a right ventricle–dependent coronary circulation has been ruled out and antegrade decompression is possible.[20] When antegrade decompression is not possible, the approach to right ventricular decompression remains controversial and continues to be institution specific.[19,20,30,37,42]

Transcatheter Pulmonary Valvotomy

Advances in interventional catheter techniques now make it possible for some infants with PA/IVS to undergo antegrade decompression of the right ventricle while still in the catheterization laboratory without surgery. Using mechanical, laser, or radiofrequency energy at the tip of a catheter, the membranous atresia can be perforated and the resulting communication dilated with percutaneous balloon techniques.[12,21,32] As experience with this procedure increases, it is being considered as first-line treatment in place of surgical intervention at some centers.[15] Right ventricular growth and a definitive two-ventricle circulation have been achieved with this technique in some patients.[32,43] Use of this approach, however, does require careful selection of patients and is essentially limited to infants with a patent infundibulum and a right ventricle large enough to support the pulmonary circulation without a systemic-to-pulmonary shunt. Accordingly, after catheter valvotomy some patients have required prolonged hospitalization for continued administration of prostaglandin E_1 and/or surgery to place a systemic-to-pulmonary shunt.[21] Thus, although this technique may become appropriate therapy for a subset of PA/IVS patients, surgery is required for the greater proportion with less favorable anatomy who require a systemic-to-pulmonary shunt with or without a transannular patch.

Indications for Transplantation

Because early mortality continues to occur despite appropriate surgical management,[10,11] cardiac transplantation has been considered a suitable therapy for a small segment of patients with PA/IVS.[37] Infants with moderate or severe right ventricular hypoplasia who also demonstrate significant diminution of left ventricular function should be considered for cardiac transplantation. Infants with right ventricle–dependent coronary circulations but satisfactory left ventricular function also may be appropriate candidates because of the high early mortality in this group, even when right ventricular decompression is avoided.[1,25] Such a policy remains controversial, however, because some centers have had satisfactory results using a single-ventricle approach with these patients.[20,30] Powell and associates[35] recently reported a 5-year survival of 83% in these patients. Such survival exceeds the 65–75% that is currently being achieved for infant heart transplantation.[3,23] Nevertheless, for a specific infant with signs of ischemia and/or left ventricular dysfunction, transplantation may be the best strategy.

REFERENCES

1. Akagi T, Benson LN, Williams WG, et al: Ventriculo-coronary arterial connections in pulmonary atresia with intact ventricular septum, and their influences on ventricular performance and clinical course. Am J Cardiol 72:586–590, 1993.
2. Billingsley AM, Laks H, Boyce SW, et al: Definitive repair in patients with pulmonary atresia and intact ventricular septum. J Thorac Cardiovasc Surg 97:746–754, 1989.
3. Boucek MM, Edwards LB, Keck BM, et al: The Registry of the International Society for Heart and Lung Transplantation: Fifth Official Pediatric Report—2001 to 2002. J Heart Lung Transplant 21:827–840, 2002.
4. Bridges ND, Mayer JE, Lock JE, et al: Effect of baffle fenestration on outcome of the modified Fontan operation. Circulation 86:1762–1769, 1992.
5. Bull C, de Leval MR, Mercanti C, et al: Pulmonary atresia and intact ventricular septum: A revised classification. Circulation 66:266–272, 1982.
6. Bull C, Kostelka M, Sorensen K, et al: Outcome measures for the neonatal management of pulmonary atresia with intact ventricular septum. J Thorac Cardiovasc Surg 107:359–366, 1994.
7. Burrows PE, Freedom RM, Benson LN, et al: Coronary angiographic abnormalities in infants and children with pulmonary atresia, hypoplastic right ventricle, and ventriculo-coronary communications. Am J Radiol 154:789–795, 1990.
8. Coles JG, Freedom RM, Lightfoot NE, et al: Long-term results in neonates with pulmonary atresia and intact ventricular septum. Ann Thorac Surg 47:213–217, 1989.
9. Daubeney PE, Delany DJ, Anderson RH, et al: Pulmonary atresia with intact ventricular septum: Range of morphology in a population-based study. J Am Coll Cardiol 39:1670–1679, 2002.
10. Daubeney PE, Webber SA: The UK and Eire collaborative study of pulmonary atresia with intact ventricular septum. In Redington AN, Brawn WJ, Deanfield JE, Anderson RH, editors: The Right Heart in Congenital Heart Disease, pp. 35–40. London: Greenwich Medical Media Ltd, 1998.
11. Ekman Joelsson BM, Sunnegardh J, Hanseus K, et al: The outcome of children born with pulmonary atresia and intact ventricular septum in Sweden from 1980 to 1999. Scand Cardiovasc J 35:192–198, 2001.
12. Fedderly RT, Lloyd TR, Mendelsohn AM, et al: Determinants of successful balloon valvotomy in infants with critical pulmonary stenosis or membranous pulmonary atresia with intact ventricular septum. J Am Coll Cardiol 25:460–465, 1995.
13. Foker JE, Braunlin EA, St Cyr JA, et al: Management of pulmonary atresia with intact ventricular septum. J Thorac Cardiovasc Surg 92:706–715, 1986.
14. Gersony WM, Bernhard WF, Nadas AS, et al: Diagnosis and surgical treatment of infants with critical pulmonary outflow obstruction: Study of 34 infants with pulmonary stenosis or atresia, and intact ventricular septum. Circulation 35:765, 1967.
15. Gibbs JL, Blackburn ME, Uzun O, et al: Laser valvotomy with balloon valvoplasty for pulmonary atresia with intact ventricular septum: Five years' experience. Heart 77:225–228, 1997.
16. Giglia TM, Mandell VS, Connor AR, et al: Diagnosis and management of right ventricle-dependent coronary circulation in pulmonary atresia with intact ventricular septum. Circulation 86:1516–1528, 1992.
17. Gittenberger-de Groot AC, Sauer U, Bindl L, et al: Competition of coronary arteries and ventriculo-coronary arterial communications in pulmonary atresia with intact ventricular septum. Int J Cardiol 18:243–258, 1988.
18. Hanley FL, Sade RM, Blackstone EH, et al: Outcomes in neonatal pulmonary atresia with intact ventricular septum. A multiinstitutional study. J Thorac Cardiovasc Surg 105: 406–407, 1993.
19. Hawkins JA, Thorne JK, Boucek MM, et al: Early and late results in pulmonary atresia and intact ventricular septum. J Thorac Cardiovasc Surg 100:492–497, 1990.
20. Jahangiri M, Zurakowski D, Bichell D, et al: Improved results with selective management in pulmonary atresia with intact ventricular septum. J Thorac Cardiovasc Surg 118:1046–1055, 1999.
21. Justo RN, Nykanen DG, Williams WG, et al: Transcatheter perforation of the right ventricular outflow tract as initial therapy for pulmonary valve atresia and intact ventricular septum in the newborn. Cathet Cardiovasc Diagn 40:408–413, 1997.
22. Kanter KR, Pennington DG, Nouri S, et al: Concomitant valvotomy and subclavian-main pulmonary artery shunt in neonates with pulmonary atresia and intact ventricular septum. Ann Thorac Surg 43:490, 1987.
23. Kanter KR, Tam VK, Vincent RN, et al: Current results with pediatric heart transplantation. Ann Thorac Surg 68:527–530, 1999.
24. Kirklin JW, Barratt-Boyes BG: Anatomy, dimensions, and terminology. In Kirklin JW, Barratt-Boyes BG, editors: Cardiac Surgery, pp. 3–60. New York: Churchill Livingstone, 1993.
25. L'Ecuyer TJ, Poulik JM, Vincent JA: Myocardial infarction due to coronary abnormalities in pulmonary atresia with intact ventricular septum. Pediatr Cardiol 22:68–70, 2001.
26. Leung MP, Mok C, Hue P: Echocardiographic assessment of neonates with pulmonary atresia and intact ventricular septum. J Am Coll Cardiol 12:719, 1988.
27. Mainwaring RD, Lamberti JJ: Pulmonary atresia with intact ventricular septum. Surgical approach based on ventricular size and coronary anatomy. J Thorac Cardiovasc Surg 106: 733–738, 1993.
28. Marcelletti CF, Iorio FS, Abella RF: Late results of extracardiac Fontan repair. Semin Thorac Cardiovasc Surg Pediatr Card Surg 2:131–142, 1999.
29. Moore JM, Ing FF, Drummond D, et al: Transcatheter closure of surgical shunts in patients with congenital heart disease. Am J Cardiol 85:636–640, 2000.
30. Najm HK, Williams WG, Coles JG, et al: Pulmonary atresia with intact ventricular septum: Results of the Fontan procedure. Ann Thorac Surg 63:669–675, 1997.
31. O'Connor WN, Cottrill CM, Johnson GL, et al: Pulmonary atresia with intact ventricular septum and ventriculocoronary communications: Surgical significance. Circulation 65: 805–809, 1982.
32. Ovaert C, Qureshi SA, Rosenthal E, et al: Growth of the right ventricle after successful transcatheter pulmonary valvotomy in neonates and infants with pulmonary atresia and intact ventricular septum. J Thorac Cardiovasc Surg 115:1055–1062, 1998.
33. Pawade A, Capuani A, Penny DJ, et al: Pulmonary atresia with intact ventricular septum: Surgical management based on right ventricular infundibulum. J Card Surg 8:371–383, 1993.
34. Pearl JM, Laks H, Stein DG, et al: Total cavopulmonary anastomosis versus conventional modified Fontan procedure. Ann Thorac Surg 52:189–195, 1991.
35. Powell AJ, Mayer JE, Lang P, et al: Outcome in infants with pulmonary atresia, intact ventricular septum, and right ventricle-dependent coronary circulation. Am J Cardiol 86: 1272–1274, 2000.
36. Rao PS: Summary and comparison of atrial septal defect closure devices. Curr Intervent Cardiol Rep 2:367–376, 2000.
37. Rychik J, Levy H, Gaynor JW, et al: Outcome after operations for pulmonary atresia with intact ventricular septum. J Thorac Cardiovasc Surg 116:924–931, 1998.

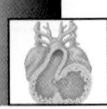

38. Sanders SP, Parness IA, Colan SD: Recognition of abnormal connections of coronary arteries with the use of Doppler color-flow mapping. J Am Coll Cardiol 13:922, 1989.
39. Steinberger J, Berry JM, Bass JL, et al: Results of a right ventricular outflow patch for pulmonary atresia with intact ventricular septum. Circulation 86:II167–II175, 1992.
40. Thompson LD, Petrossian E, McElhinney DB, et al: Is it necessary to routinely fenestrate an extracardiac Fontan? J Am Coll Cardiol 34:539–544, 1999.
41. VanArsdell GS: One and one half ventricle repairs. Pediatr Card Surg Ann Semin Thorac Cardiovasc Surg 3:173–178, 2000.
42. Waldman JD, Karp RB, Lamberti JJ, et al: Tricuspid valve closure in pulmonary atresia and important RV-to-coronary artery connections. Ann Thorac Surg 59:933–940, 1995.
43. Wang JK, Wu MH, Chang CI, et al: Outcomes of transcatheter valvotomy in patients with pulmonary atresia and intact ventricular septum. Am J Cardiol 84:1055–1060, 1999.

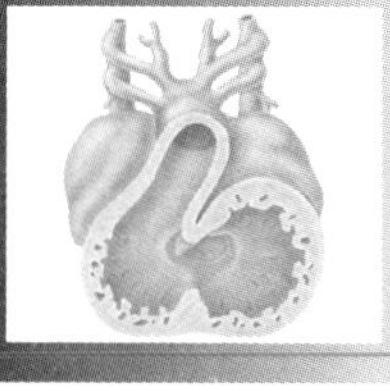

CHAPTER 114

Tetralogy of Fallot with Pulmonary Stenosis

Brian W. Duncan and Roger B. B. Mee

HISTORY

In 1888, Etienne-Louis Arthur Fallot described the four features of the congenital cardiac anomaly that bears his name: (1) ventricular septal defect (VSD), (2) infundibular pulmonic stenosis, (3) right ventricular hypertrophy, and (4) dextroposition of the aorta.[32] More than 50 years later, the first successful surgical therapy for tetralogy of Fallot (TOF) was reported by Blalock and Taussig in 1945 when they performed a palliative subclavian-to-pulmonary artery shunt.[7] Potts and Waterston also devised systemic-to-pulmonary arterial shunts with anastomoses between the descending aorta and left pulmonary artery or between the ascending aorta and right pulmonary artery, respectively.[104,134] The first successful repair of this condition was performed by Lillehei and Varco at the University of Minnesota in 1954 using "controlled cross circulation," with another patient serving as the oxygenator and blood reservoir.[84,85] Kirklin reported the first repair of TOF using a pump oxygenator at the Mayo Clinic in 1955.[72] Kirklin, Warden, Ross, Barrett-Boyes, Castaneda, and others[5,11,73,109,133] made important contributions to the surgical management of TOF, including timing of operative repair, indications for the use of a transannular patch to relieve right ventricular outflow tract obstruction, and the use of grafts to reconstruct the right ventricular outflow tract.

ANATOMY AND PHYSIOLOGY

Infundibular Septum

The four anatomical components originally described for TOF can actually be direct consequences of a single anatomical abnormality: anterior and leftward displacement of the infundibulum or infundibular septum.[128] This anomaly of the infundibular septum variably narrows the right ventricular outflow tract, leading to subpulmonic obstruction, which may be complete (atresia). Displacement of the infundibular septum away from the anterior and posterior limbs of the trabecula septomarginalis results in typical "anterior malalignment" VSD (see subsequent discussion). Because of the location of the aortic valve directly behind the infundibular septum, with anterior displacement of the infundibular septum, the aortic valve overrides the interventricular septum and attains some degree of association with the right ventricular cavity (Figures 114-1 and 114-2). Right ventricular hypertrophy is a consequence of equalization of pressures in the right and left ventricles by virtue of an unrestrictive VSD.

Muscular extensions from the free wall of the right ventricle (parietal bands) or the interventricular septum (septal bands) contribute to obstruction of right ventricular outflow and must be divided at the time of repair. In some cases, the infundibular septum is significantly hypoplastic or even completely absent. In these cases, right ventricular outflow tract obstruction is caused by the small size of the pulmonic valve annulus. The VSD extends to a subpulmonary location in these patients, with the superior-most margin of the defect being composed of the confluence of the fibrous portions of the aortic and pulmonary valve annuli.

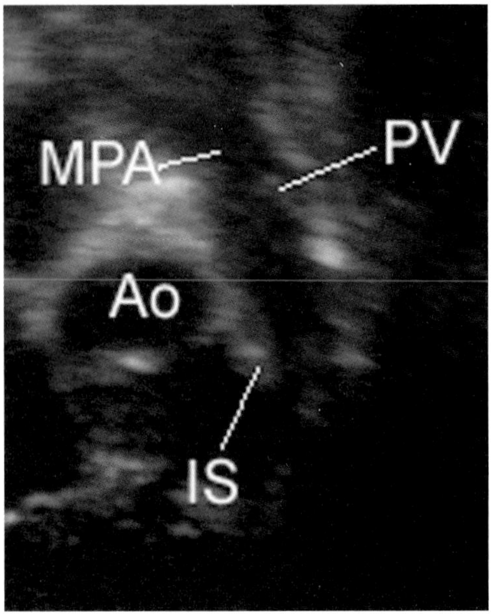

Figure 114–2 Long-axis echocardiographic view of the right ventricular outflow tract in similar orientation as Figure 114-1. MPA, main pulmonary artery; PV, pulmonary valve; Ao, aorta; IS, infundibular septum.

Pulmonary Valve and Pulmonary Valve Annulus

The pulmonary valve is stenotic in 75% of cases; in one half to two thirds of cases, the valve is bicuspid.[3,55,76] Valve stenosis usually results from hypoplasia and fusion of bicuspid leaflets, supravalvar tethering, or a combination of these factors. Tethering of the leaflets often distorts the main pulmonary artery at the sinotubular junction, forming a ridge that may be obstructive, producing supravalvar stenosis. The leaflets themselves are often thickened with myxomatous excrescences, and when most severely affected, the leaflets may have a rigid, cartilaginous appearance (Figure 114-3). The pulmonary valve annulus is invariably smaller than the aorta (the opposite of normal); however, it is not necessarily significantly obstructive. In symptomatic infants, the pulmonary valve annulus usually contributes to multilevel right ventricular outflow tract obstruction.

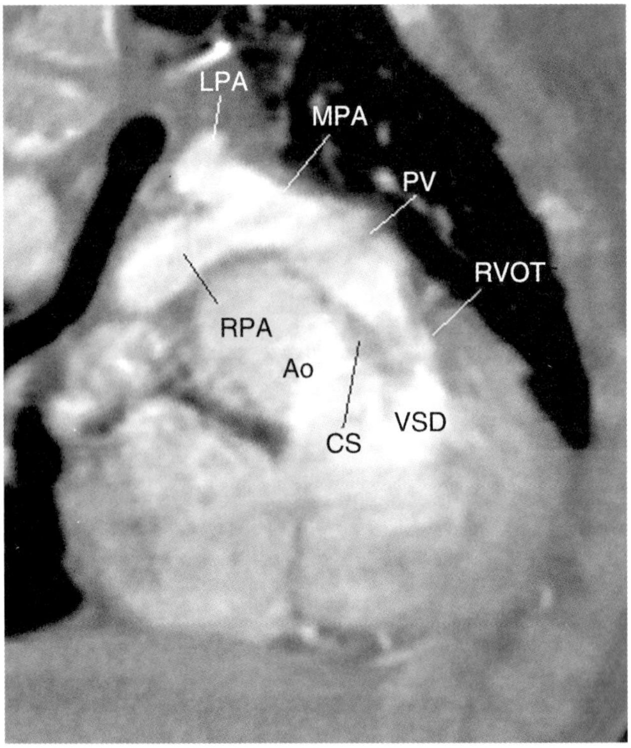

Figure 114–1 Computed tomography reconstruction demonstrating right ventricular outflow tract in tetralogy of Fallot. Subvalvar narrowing is evident in the right ventricular outflow tract (RVOT). Note the relationship between the ventricular septal defect (VSD) and the overriding aorta (Ao). Anterior deviation of the conal septum (CS) into the RVOT is also shown. LPA, left pulmonary artery; RPA, right pulmonary artery; MPA, main pulmonary artery; PV, pulmonary valve.

Main Pulmonary Artery and Branch Pulmonary Arteries

The main pulmonary artery is usually somewhat diffusely small and is often short with a posterior angulation above the valve. The narrowest portion of the main pulmonary artery is often at the sinotubular junction because of the previously mentioned valvar narrowing at that level (Figures 114-4 and 114-5).

The left pulmonary artery usually appears as a direct continuation of the main pulmonary artery, with the right pulmonary artery branching at nearly a right angle; however, important stenoses of the branch pulmonary arteries occur relatively infrequently. Analysis performed at the Green Lane Hospital demonstrated that branch pulmonary artery abnormalities occurred in only 10% of cases.[76] Bilateral branch pulmonary artery stenosis made up approximately half of these cases, with juxtaductal stenosis of the left pulmonary artery occurring next most frequently. The branch pulmonary arteries themselves beyond their origins are not abnormally small on average; however, within the pulmonary parenchyma, the sizes of the intraacinar arteries, alveolar size and number, and lung volumes are reduced.[53,62]

Ventricular Septal Defect

As noted previously, the classical description of the VSD typically seen in TOF is an anterior malalignment VSD aris-

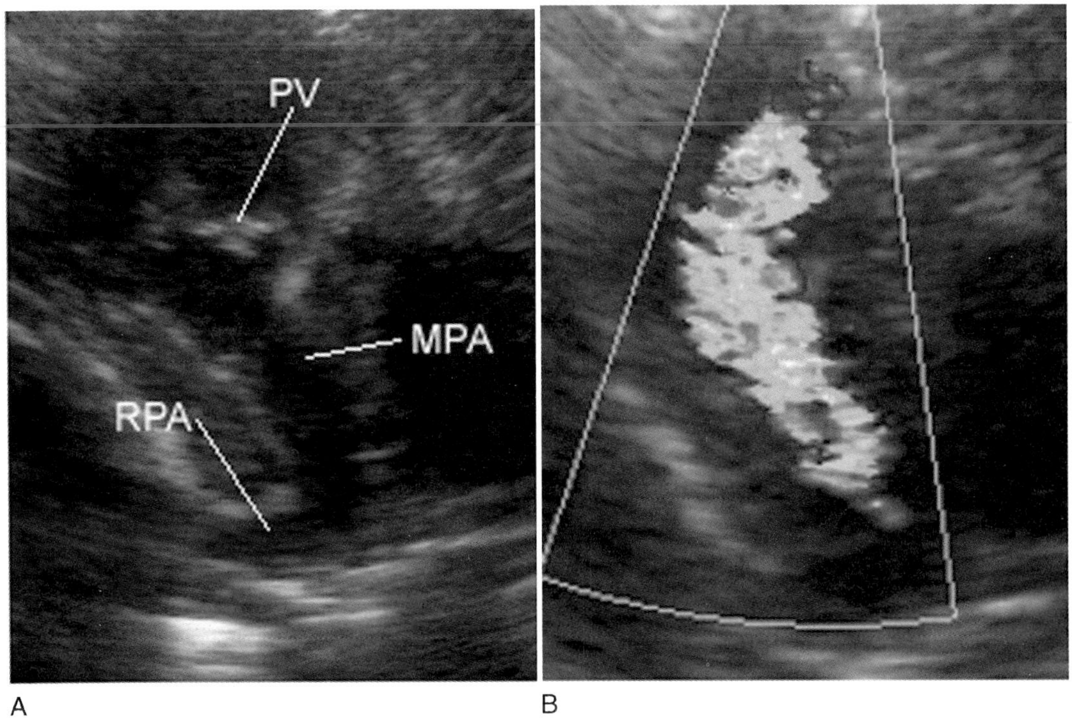

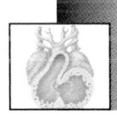

Figure 114–3 **A,** Echocardiographic view of the main pulmonary artery (MPA), right pulmonary artery (RPA), and pulmonary valve (PV). PV is echodense, suggesting the presence of a thickened, dysplastic valve. **B,** Doppler flow study demonstrating turbulence and flow acceleration across PV.

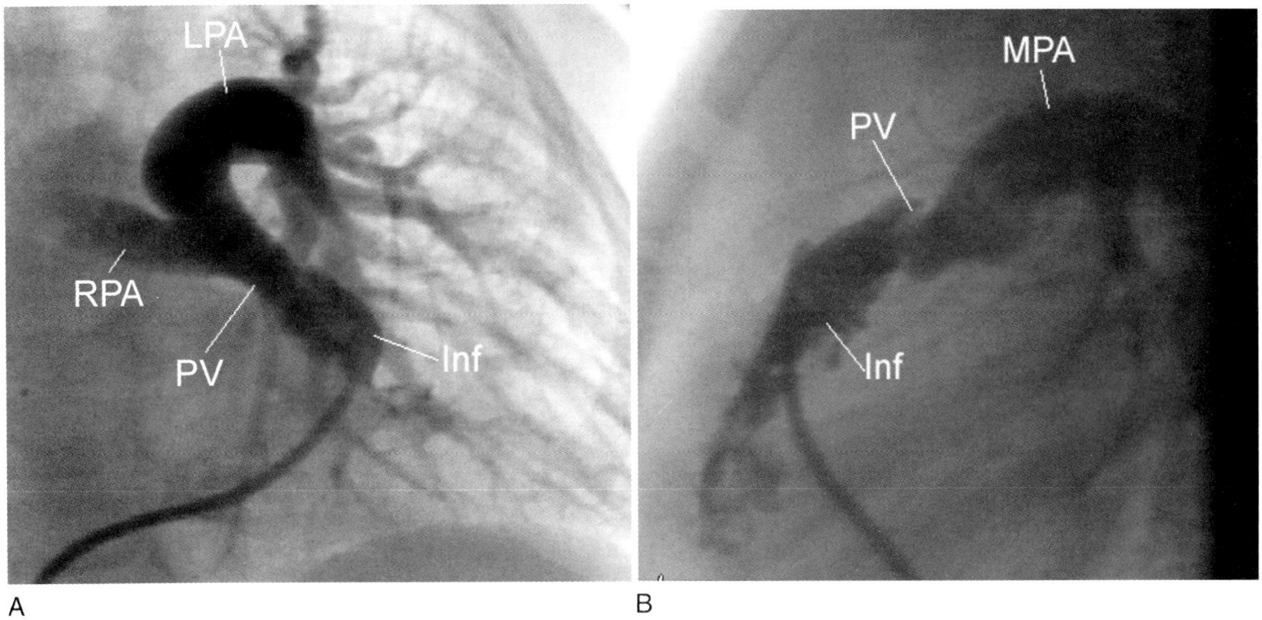

Figure 114–4 **A,** Right anterior oblique projection of angiogram made by injection in right ventricular infundibulum (Inf) demonstrating subvalvar stenosis. Pulmonary valve (PV) is also small. LPA, left pulmonary artery; RPA, right pulmonary artery. **B,** Lateral projection. MPA, main pulmonary artery.

ing because of anterior displacement of the infundibular septum away from the trabecula septomarginalis. Because of its close association with the posterior infundibular septum, the aortic valve overrides the interventricular septum associating with the anterior and superior extent of the defect. The membranous septum is usually absent or attenuated, with the defect usually extending under the septal leaflet of the tricuspid valve and at times into the inlet portion of the interventricular septum. The superior margin of the VSD usually consists of fibrous tissue composed of the anteroseptal commissure of the tricuspid valve and the right fibrous trigone at the nadir of the right coronary cusp of the

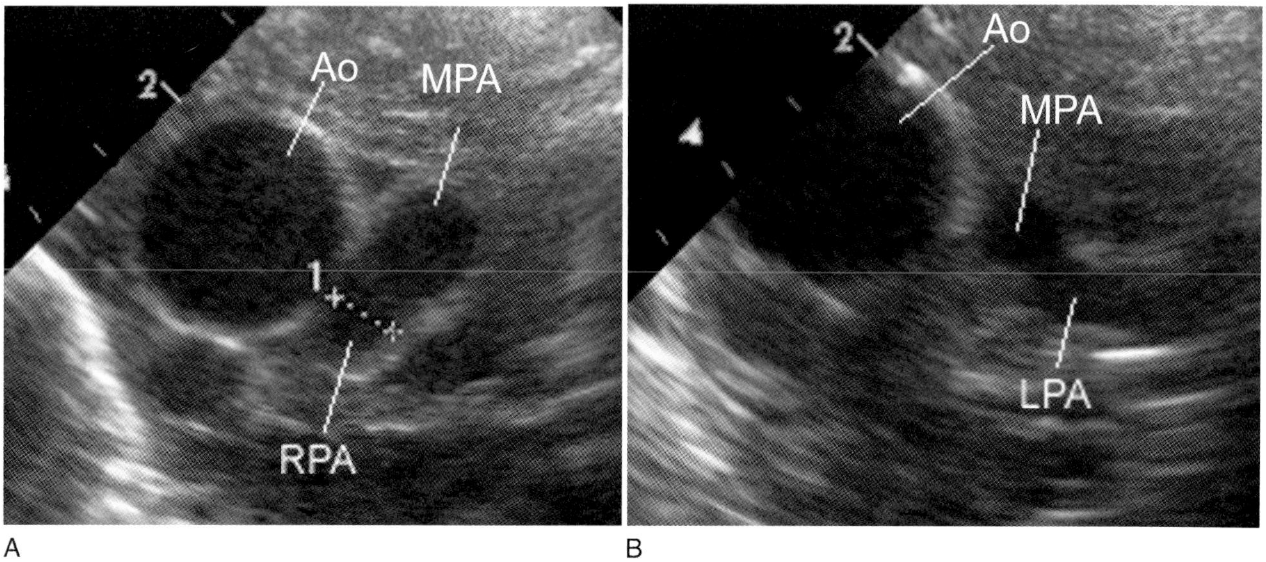

Figure 114–5 **A,** Short-axis echocardiographic view of small main pulmonary artery (MPA) with adequate-sized right pulmonary artery (RPA). Ao, aorta. **B,** Same view demonstrating relationship of slightly small left pulmonary artery (LPA) to MPA.

aortic valve. The posterior limb of the trabecula septomarginalis forms the posteroinferior border of the VSD, which buries the conducting bundle under a muscular rim and gives rise to the papillary muscle of the conus, which provides a marker for the course of the right bundle branch of the conducting bundle. In approximately 25% of cases, the ventriculo-infundibular fold extends inferiorly, separating the VSD from the tricuspid annulus, and with the posterior limb of the trabecula septomarginalis forms an additional muscle layer over the conducting bundle.[3,81] Anteriorly, the muscular margin of the VSD is composed of the anterior limb of the trabecula septomarginalis.

The VSD is usually large and unrestrictive with a diameter equal to or greater than that of the aortic annulus; therefore the direction of shunting at the level of the defect depends on the degree of right ventricular outflow tract obstruction (Figures 114-6 to 114-8). Typically, shunting is bidirectional but with a significant right-to-left component throughout much of the cardiac cycle. Systemic arterial desaturation occurs because of the limitation of blood flow into the pulmonary arteries and because of intracardiac right-to-left shunting with the extent of clinically evident cyanosis being inversely proportional to the amount of pulmonary blood flow. Patients with a good-sized pulmonary valve annulus and relatively mild infundibular stenosis may have systemic arterial saturations that approach normal or may even present with congestive heart failure. Conversely, children with severe obstruction to pulmonary blood flow may be severely cyanotic in the neonatal period. Anatomically, these children typically have multilevel right ventricular outflow tract

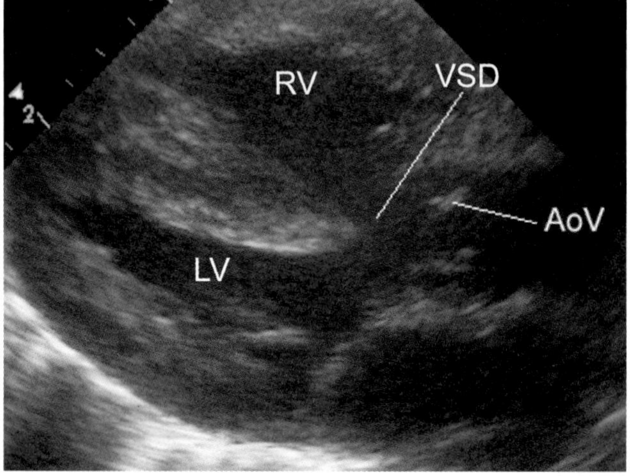

Figure 114–6 **Long-axis echocardiographic view demonstrating the aorta (Ao) overriding ventricular septal defect (VSD).** RV, right ventricle; LV, left ventricle.

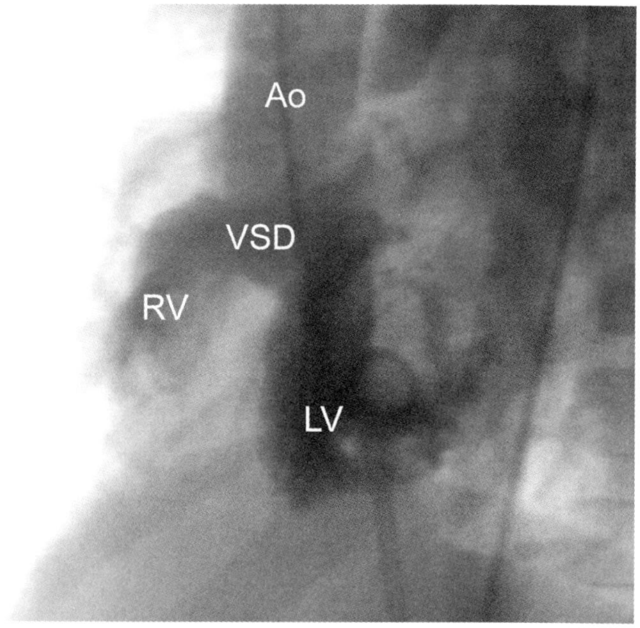

Figure 114–7 **Lateral left ventriculogram demonstrating relationship of aorta (Ao) and ventricular septal defect (VSD).** RV, right ventricle; LV, left ventricle.

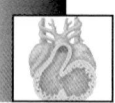

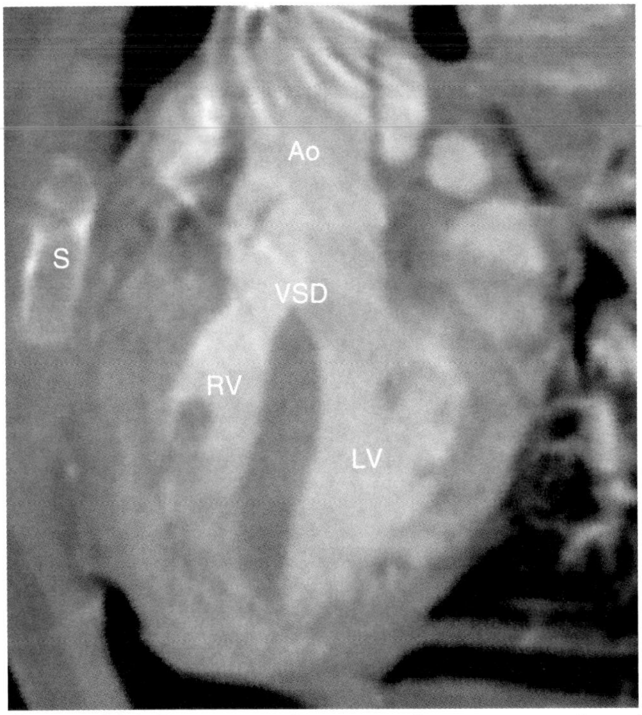

Figure 114–8 Computed tomography reconstruction of patient with TOF demonstrating relationship of aorta (Ao) and ventricular septal defect (VSD). RV, right ventricle; LV, left ventricle; S, sternum.

obstruction with narrowing of the infundibulum, hypoplasia of the pulmonary valve annulus, a small main pulmonary artery, and possibly, small branch pulmonary arteries.

Up to 15% of cases have additional VSDs, which are usually single and muscular, residing in the anterior portion of the septum.[33,76] In some cases, an additional VSD exists in the inlet portion of the septum; multiple VSDs are occasionally seen and may be located anywhere in the interventricular septum.

Conduction System

The positions of the sinus and atrioventricular (AV) nodes are normal in TOF, whereas the bundle of His follows the same general course as seen in isolated perimembranous VSDs.[3] The bundle of His passes close to the crest of the interventricular septum or slightly to the left of the inferior margin of the VSD. The proximity of the bundle to the crest of the inferior VSD margin is determined by the degree of additional layering in the presence of an extended ventriculo-infundibular fold. When well developed, the ventriculo-infundibular fold and the posterior limb of the trabecula septomarginalis form a continuous muscle border separating the tricuspid annulus from the VSD covering the membranous septum. In these cases, the bundle lies deeply imbedded in muscle away from the crest of the inferior margin of the VSD, and sutures may be safely placed within this muscle to anchor the patch. When the posterior limb is hypoplastic, the bundle of His comes very close to the crest of the septum, and in these cases, the placement of sutures should be determined by the presence or absence of residual membranous septum. In cases in which a generous portion of fibrous membranous septal tissue is present, a so-called membranous flap suture may be safely placed through this fibrous tissue.[81,118] In cases in which there is a true perimembranous VSD without a membranous flap, sutures must be placed further down onto the right ventricular aspect of the interventricular septum to avoid the bundle of His. Suture placement in this area contributes to the presence of a right bundle branch block pattern on the postoperative electrocardiogram (ECG), because the bundle of His divides at this point with the right bundle branch continuing on the rightward aspect of the interventricular septum.[48]

Coronary Arteries

Significant anomalies of the coronary arteries occur in approximately 5% of patients with TOF.[44,76,93,98] Single coronary arteries arising from the right or left coronary sinuses occur rarely. A single left coronary artery may give rise to the right coronary artery, which may cross the distal right ventricular outflow tract (Figure 114-9). The most clinically important coronary anomalies occur when large branches from the right coronary artery cross the right ventricular outflow tract. Usually, these are moderate-sized conal branches of the right coronary artery; however, when these reach the anterior interventricular groove, they may contribute to the coronary arterial supply of the interventricular septum and left ventricle. In rare instances the anterior descending coronary artery is derived in its entirety from the right coronary artery crossing the right ventricular outflow tract (Figure 114-10). Rarely, significant anterior descending coronary branches from the right coronary artery cross the right ventricular outflow tract in the infundibular muscle and are not visible on the epicardial surface, making injury to these vessels at the time of TOF repair particularly likely. These anomalies of the coronary

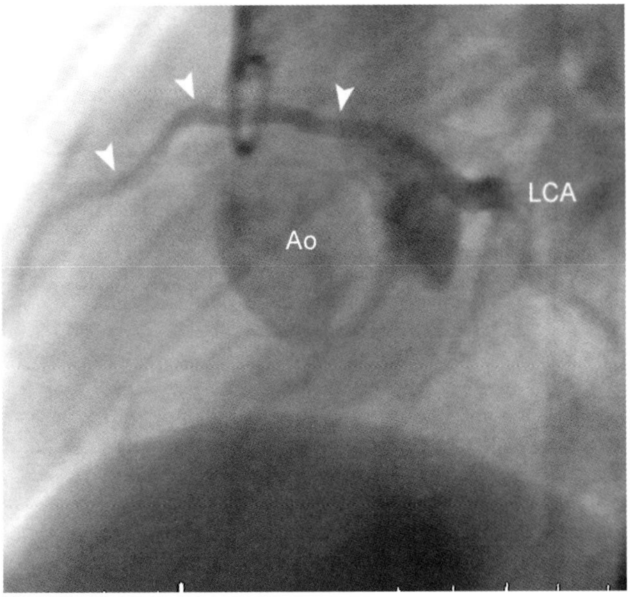

A

Figure 114–9 A, Aortogram demonstrating single left coronary artery (LCA) giving rise to right coronary artery *(arrowheads)*. Ao, aorta.

(Continued)

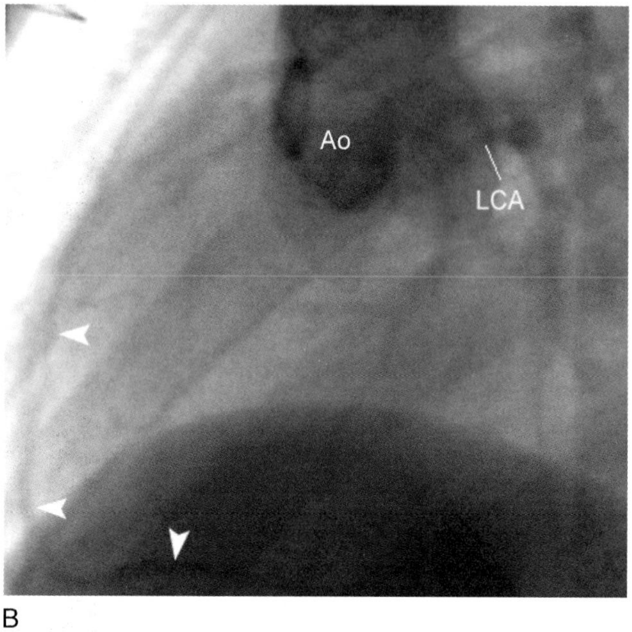

Figure 114–9 cont'd B, Later after aortic injection demonstrating course of right coronary artery *(arrowheads)*.

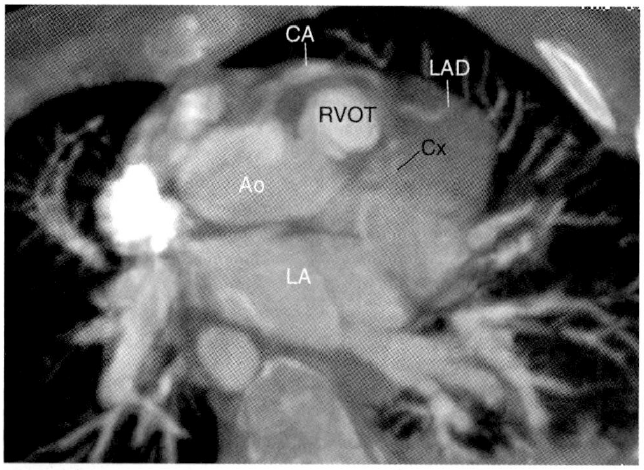

Figure 114–10 Computed tomography demonstrating single right coronary artery giving rise to left coronary artery with branching into left anterior descending (LAD) and circumflex coronary arteries (Cx). Notice course of coronary artery (CA) anterior to right ventricular outflow tract (RVOT). Ao, aorta; LA, left atrium.

arteries have been reported to be more likely in cases in which there is anterior and lateral rotation of the aorta in relation to the pulmonary artery.[13] Significant crossing vessels usually can be detected preoperatively by echocardiography, and surgical management can be modified during TOF repair to avoid injury to vessels supplying significant amounts of myocardium.[98]

Other Anatomical Features

There is a right aortic arch in approximately 25% of cases.[76] A patent foramen ovale is commonly seen, whereas a true atrial septal defect (ASD) is probably present only 10% of the time. Major associated lesions are relatively uncommon; multiple VSDs, patent ductus arteriosus, and complete AV septal defects are among the most common.[76]

CLINICAL FEATURES AND DIAGNOSIS

Presentation

Most children with TOF have some degree of cyanosis. The severity of obstruction of the right ventricular outflow tract determines the degree of right-to-left shunting, which usually determines the degree of cyanosis and the age of presentation. Patients with significant cyanosis early in infancy usually have severe and multilevel obstruction of the right ventricular outflow tract. At the other end of the clinical spectrum, patients with mild right-sided obstruction may have normal room air saturations and congestive heart failure resulting from predominant left-to-right shunting through the unrestrictive VSD—so-called acyanotic or pink tetralogy. If patients with severe right-sided obstruction fail to demonstrate a proportionately severe degree of cyanosis, additional sources of pulmonary blood flow, such as a patent ductus arteriosus or aortopulmonary collateral arteries, should be suspected and their presence ruled out.

Previously, patients often presented because of complications of long-standing cyanosis. At present, with the widespread use of pulse oximetry in nurseries and careful clinical evaluation, most affected children are detected in the newborn period or in infancy. For this reason, late presentation because of complications arising from chronic cyanosis, such as polycythemia leading to cerebrovascular thrombosis, should rarely occur. In addition, other presentations resulting from advanced untreated cyanotic congenital heart disease, such as hemoptysis secondary to enlarged bronchial arteries, paradoxical embolism, or brain abscess, are currently uncommon. Squatting, a classical behavioral adaptation of older children with TOF whereby systemic vascular resistance is increased, producing more pulmonary blood flow, is also rarely seen because of early diagnosis and treatment.

Hypercyanotic episodes ("tet spells") remain a serious clinical occurrence during the workup and treatment of patients with TOF. These episodes are characterized by intense cyanosis that may last minutes to hours, during which time oxygen delivery may be so compromised as to cause loss of consciousness or impairment of myocardial function. A reduction of cardiac afterload or preload and tachycardia (reduced diastolic filling and right ventricular ejection) are the mechanisms of spell initiation. Dehydration, viral respiratory infection, and the injudicious administration of medications that lead to peripheral vasodilation all may cause a hypercyanotic episode in a patient who has been previously stable. Medical management of hypercyanosis is discussed subsequently; however, the occurrence of these episodes should prompt consideration for urgent operation to avoid end-organ damage resulting from repeated episodes of profound hypoxemia.

Physical Examination

In addition to cyanosis of variable degree, the physical examination typically reveals a moderate-intensity, midsystolic ejection murmur heard loudest in the second and third left intercostal spaces that may radiate into the axilla. The intensity of the murmur may actually decrease with increasing obstruction and may be absent during hypercyanotic episodes. The second heart sound may be single when cyanosis is severe because of advanced disease of the pulmonary valve, whereas it may be split if cyanosis is not severe, especially in the presence of branch pulmonary artery stenoses and a relatively normal pulmonary valve. Other stigmata of chronic cyanosis observed on physical examination (e.g., digital clubbing) are seen only in advanced cases, and it is hoped that they are now rare. Pink tetralogy patients may have findings more typical of pulmonary overcirculation and congestive heart failure.

Chest X-Ray and Electrocardiogram

The classical appearance of the cardiomediastinal silhouette is that of a boot-shaped heart *(coeur en sabot)*. This typical, but not universal, radiographic appearance is due to right ventricular hypertrophy and tends to become more exaggerated with time as hypertrophy progresses. In addition, the lung fields usually appear to be oligemic in proportion to the degree of cyanosis. Normal pulmonary vascular markings in the presence of severe obstruction of the right ventricular outflow tract suggest that other sources of pulmonary blood flow, such as aortopulmonary collateral arteries, are present. A right aortic arch occurs in approximately 25% of cases. The ECG demonstrates right ventricular hypertrophy, which may be difficult to differentiate from normal in newborns.

Laboratory Studies

Polycythemia is present in most children with chronic cyanosis, and when it is absent, the presence of iron-deficiency anemia should be suspected. Blood sampling to determine the presence of a deletion on the long arm of chromosome 22 (22qll.2) has become routine during the workup of patients with conotruncal abnormalities. In current practice, this relatively large deletion is detected by fluorescent *in situ* hybridization; however, a single gene in the ubiquitin-proteasome pathway involved in apoptosis during embryogenesis may be responsible for the multisystem involvement often observed in these patients.[86] Perhaps 10% of patients with TOF and pulmonic stenosis have such a chromosomal deletion, making this the most common syndromic cause of TOF.[21,86] There is an even higher incidence of this deletion in patients with TOF and pulmonary atresia, especially in the presence of a right aortic arch and anomalous origin of the left subclavian artery. The chief importance of demonstrating this deletion in a given patient is to provide the opportunity for genetic counseling for future pregnancies and to identify the need for workup of other organ systems that are commonly involved, which are summarized by the acronym CATCH-22 (*c*ardiac disease, *a*bnormal faces, *t*hymic hypoplasia, *c*left palate, and *h*ypocalcemia associated with a deletion in chromosome 22). Variants of this syndrome have been referred to by several names, including velocardiofacial syndrome, conotruncal anomaly face syndrome, and others; however, the term used to describe its most severe form, *DiGeorge syndrome*, is usually reserved for patients with absent thymus, accompanying T-lymphocyte dysfunction, hypocalcemia, and developmental delay.

Echocardiography

As in most congenital cardiac diagnoses, echocardiography has become the most common and usually the definitive diagnostic modality for TOF with pulmonic stenosis. Detailed elucidation of the important anatomical features, including the number and location of VSDs, the nature of the right ventricular outflow tract obstruction, the anatomy of the proximal branch pulmonary arteries, and the coronary artery pattern, can be accomplished with a high degree of accuracy.[63,98,111,125] The ability to acquire definitive anatomical images noninvasively without having to transport the patient is especially important in critically ill neonates, such as those suffering hypercyanotic episodes.

An increasing number of patients are identified *in utero* with fetal echocardiography[71,83,122,136] (Figure 114-11). Prenatal echocardiography can accurately diagnose conotruncal defects such as TOF by the late or, at the earliest, middle second trimester.[122] Still, most cases remain undetected until after birth, which reflects the fact that many pregnancies are not evaluated by prenatal ultrasound and those that are may miss the diagnosis with a simple screening scan. The ultimate impact of the prenatal diagnosis of TOF on survival has not been clearly established; however, identification of these infants prenatally allows delivery to be performed with the appropriate medical and surgical support. Perhaps most importantly, prenatal diagnosis of a serious cardiac condition allows the presence of associated conditions such as chromosomal anomalies to be identified, which may have a significant impact on an affected child's prognosis.

Cardiac Catheterization

Angiography remains a highly accurate diagnostic modality that can identify all of the important anatomical features of TOF. The anatomy of the branch pulmonary arteries and

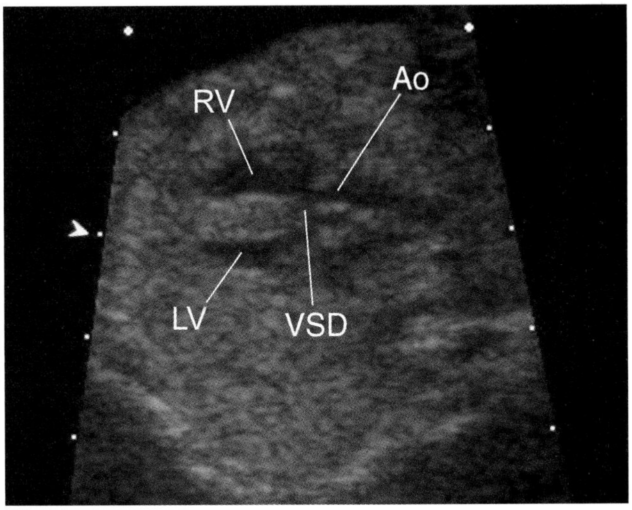

Figure 114-11 Fetal echocardiogram (22 weeks of gestation) of TOF demonstrating ventricular septal defect (VSD) with aortic (Ao) override. RV, right ventricle; LV, left ventricle.

the coronary arteries is particularly well demonstrated angiographically. However, in current practice, angiography is rarely indicated, having been replaced by echocardiography in most cases of TOF. Angiography is invasive and usually requires transport of patients who may be critically ill; however, angiography remains the diagnostic modality of choice if there is any suggestion that multiple sources of pulmonary blood supply exist. The presence of aortopulmonary collateral arteries arising from the ascending aorta, descending aorta, transverse arch, or brachiocephalic vessels should be determined angiographically in these cases. Cardiac catheterization may also be performed if an attempt at balloon pulmonary valvuloplasty is to be performed (see *Balloon Pulmonary Valvuloplasty* later).

MEDICAL MANAGEMENT

Outpatient Management

TOF is a disease remedied only by surgical intervention with medical management designed to optimize a patient's surgical candidacy. The goals of medical management are to allow growth and development of the child until surgical repair is undertaken while hypercyanotic episodes or complications arising from the condition are prevented. Children who maintain systemic arterial saturations with normal growth and development can safely await elective surgical repair. If this status cannot be maintained, a more urgent surgical plan should be undertaken.

A cornerstone of preoperative management is maintaining these infants in a well-hydrated state. Ensuring that these children are on an adequate feeding regimen is extremely important, and prolonged periods without adequate oral intake should be avoided. Every effort should be made to protect affected infants from contacts who have known viral infections. Respiratory viruses such as respiratory syncytial virus can trigger unrelenting hypercyanotic episodes that necessitate emergency surgery. Similarly, dehydration accompanying diarrheal illnesses caused by enteroviruses can also trigger hypercyanotic episodes. Emergency surgery in the face of an ongoing viral process considerably increases the morbidity and mortality rates of the procedure. In the absence of underlying pulmonary disease, prolonged oxygen therapy usually is not necessary, and, in fact, a new oxygen requirement in a child with previously stable oxygen saturations should suggest that the need for surgery is imminent. β-Blockers such as propranolol (Inderal) have been used in the outpatient management of children with TOF. The salutary effects of β-blockers can be attributed to their negative chronotropic effects with increased ventricular filling at slower heart rates. In general, β-blockers probably provide little additional margin of safety in the outpatient management of these children, and their perceived need should suggest a more urgent approach to surgery. Diuretics are contraindicated in cyanotic tetralogy, although "pink tets" with relatively unrestricted pulmonary blood flow may require diuretics to treat congestive heart failure.

Management of Hypercyanotic Episodes

Hypercyanotic episodes are true clinical emergencies in which end-organ, particularly cerebral, oxygenation is critically low. Basic treatment principles include administration of intravenous fluids, morphine or other intravenous sedatives, and oxygen. Placing the infant in a knee-chest position can elevate systemic vascular resistance with a resultant increase in pulmonary blood flow. Intravenous β-blockers such as esmolol and α-agonists such as phenylephrine may also be used to temporize; however, the need for such agents suggests that urgent surgery is needed. Intubation and positive pressure ventilation may also be used to attempt to increase oxygenation, but the requirement for intubation further underscores the need for prompt surgical repair unless there is a known significant intercurrent illness that may need treatment first.

Balloon Pulmonary Valvuloplasty

Several groups have demonstrated that balloon pulmonary valvuloplasty can be safely performed to palliate infants and children with TOF and pulmonary stenosis.[8,106,115] Most cases in these reports had improvement in oxygen saturation, and a delay in surgical intervention was often possible for months after the procedure. Although balloon pulmonary valvuloplasty provides reasonable palliation in select cases, its role in TOF remains limited. Balloon pulmonary valvuloplasty may not relieve the multiple levels of obstruction to pulmonary blood flow that are commonly seen in tetralogy patients, especially in those who are most symptomatic in infancy. In addition, postprocedural pulmonic insufficiency and catheter-related complications may be significant in these patients. Most infants and children with TOF and severe cyanosis should undergo surgical intervention as described in the next section; however, balloon pulmonary valvuloplasty may occupy a palliative role when immediate surgery is best deferred, such as in those patients with concomitant viral respiratory infection.

SURGICAL MANAGEMENT

The goals of surgical therapy are to (1) close intracardiac shunts, (2) provide relatively unobstructed pulmonary blood flow, (3) maintain normal function of the right ventricle, (4) maintain normal function of the pulmonary and tricuspid valves, and (5) maintain normal sinus rhythm with minimal cumulative morbidity or mortality. Differences in philosophy exist between centers regarding specific details of surgery, such as the anatomical approach (transventricular or transatrial/transpulmonary) or the need for selective interval systemic-to-pulmonary arterial shunting. These areas of controversy are discussed in the next section.

Cardiopulmonary Bypass

The complete repair can usually be performed with bicaval cannulation and continuous cardiopulmonary bypass. A median sternotomy is performed, and the pericardium is opened to the left of the midline and remains unharvested. The aorta is separated from the main and right pulmonary artery, and existing shunts are dissected out with electrocautery. The aorta is cannulated high with a soft, flexible cannula, whereas both cavae are cannulated directly with right-angled metal-tipped cannulas; cardiopulmonary bypass is commenced and systemic cooling to moderate levels of hypothermia is performed. During cooling, caval snares are passed, systemic-to-pulmonary arterial shunts are divided, and a patent ductus arteriosus is ligated. During cooling, the aorta is cross-clamped, and blood-containing or crystalloid cardioplegia is administered into the aortic root. The left side of the heart is vented either by direct cannulation of the left atrium or with a sucker placed through the foramen ovale.

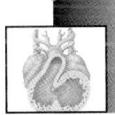

Intracardiac Portion of the Repair

Access to the VSD and obstructing muscle bundles in the right ventricular outflow tract is easily achieved by an incision either in the right atrium or in the right ventricular infundibulum.[76] Viewed through a right atrial incision, the VSD is directly under the septal leaflet of the tricuspid valve with a view underneath the parietal muscle bundles and infundibular septum (Figure 114-12). Through a right ventricular incision, the infundibular septum is visualized with the VSD deep to the inferior tip of the infundibular septum and the aortic valve on its posterior surface. When approached through a ventriculotomy, the parietal and septal muscle bundles reside in the lateral recesses above the infundibular septum to the patient's right and left, respectively. Obstructing parietal muscle bundles are dissected off the ventricular infundibular fold and transected 4 to 5 mm away from the VSD and aortic annulus (toward the right ventricular free wall). A wedge of muscle is removed from this location, particularly in older patients who may possess a large amount of hypertrophy of these obstructing muscle bands; simple incision of this area may suffice in infants. Obstructing muscle bundle extensions from the infundibular septum along the septal (patient's left) aspect of the right ventricular outflow tract may also be incised or resected as needed.

The VSD may then be closed with patch material of either polytetrafluoroethylene (PTFE or Teflon) or stretch-knitted polyethylene terephthalate (Dacron) after trimming to the appropriate shape. Interrupted pledgetted polypropylene (Figure 114-12B) or braided nonabsorbable sutures or a running polypropylene suture may be used to sew in the patch. Several critical points of anatomy must be appreciated to ensure complete VSD closure and to minimize the chances for complications. Anteriorly and superiorly, stitches are placed in the fibrous tissue of the aortic annulus to avoid a residual VSD in this region. Inferiorly, if there is a fibrous membranous flap or a prominent muscle bundle from the posterior limb of the trabecula septomarginalis, sutures may be safely placed in these structures. In the absence of these structures, sutures must be placed onto the right ventricular aspect of the interventricular septum to avoid the bundle of His. In the absence of a well-developed posterior limb of the trabecula septomarginalis, sutures must be placed in the septal leaflet of the tricuspid valve. If

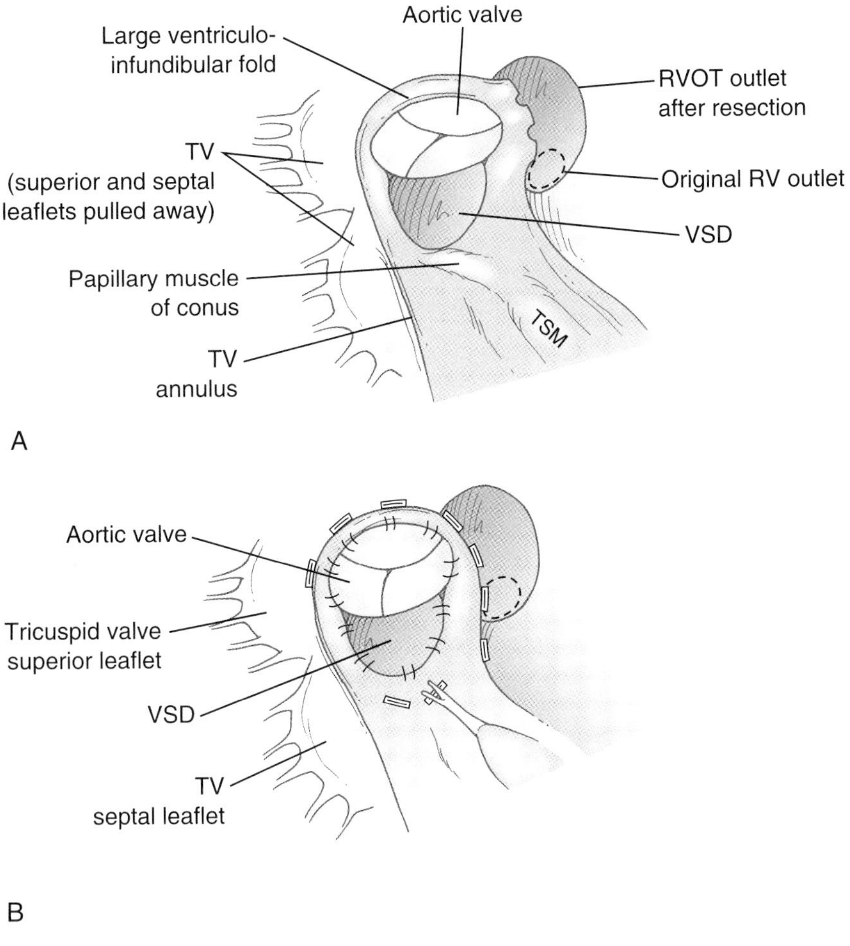

Figure 114–12 **A,** The appearance of the ventricular septal defect (VSD), aortic valve (AV), and right ventricular outflow tract (RVOT) as seen from below through the right atrium with the right ventricle cut away. (Note: In this view, the anterior and septal leaflets of the tricuspid valve [TV] have been detached and flapped to the right.) TSM, trabecula septomarginalis. **B,** Appearance after placement of interrupted, pledgetted sutures for VSD closure.
(From Mee RBB: Transatrial transpulmonary repair of tetralogy of Fallot. In Yacoub, M, ed.: Annual of Cardiac Surgery, ed 8. Philadelphia: Lippincott Williams & Wilkins, 1995, pp. 141–147.)

interrupted sutures are used, the sutures should be placed through the tricuspid annulus except in the region of the conducting bundle. This suture is placed a few millimeters from the annulus to avoid impingement on the AV node by the pledgets. If a continuous suture is used for VSD closure, this portion of the suture line should be performed as a mattress suture to ensure complete closure in this region.

Pulmonary Artery Portion of the Repair

After resection of obstructing muscle bundles in the right ventricular outflow tract, the pulmonary valve is probed using graded dilators. Probing of the pulmonary valve is easily accomplished through either a transatrial approach or a right ventriculotomy. If the pulmonary valve is too small, a longitudinal incision is made in the main pulmonary artery between fine-stay sutures (Figure 114-13). The valve is inspected, full commissurotomies are performed, and the pulmonary valve is probed again, and if it is still inadequate (see following discussion), a transannular patch will be required and the valve annulus is incised through the most anterior commissure. If the VSD has been closed through a ventriculotomy, the incision in the pulmonary artery and the incision in the infundibulum are joined through the anterior commissure. If a transatrial approach to the VSD has been used, the incision through the pulmonary valve annulus can often be limited to 2–8 mm below the annulus, and further resection of muscle from the right ventricular outflow tract can be performed through the pulmonary artery at that point.

The decision to perform transannular patching of the right ventricular outflow tract is based on a determination of the Z-value, obtained by transforming the pulmonary annulus in millimeters to the number of standard deviations from the mean normal value of the pulmonary valve annulus for the body surface area of the patient. Historically, a pulmonary annulus Z-value of –3 or less obtained angiographically was statistically associated with an unacceptably high right ventricle/left ventricle pressure ratio without transannular patching.[74–76] In the relaxed heart after cardioplegia, the ability to pass a dilator through the right ventricular outflow tract 1–2 mm larger than the predicted Z-value of zero for that patient usually ensures that no significant fixed anatomical obstruction exists in the outflow tract.[91] If the pulmonary valve annulus is less than 1–2 mm greater than the predicted Z-value of zero, a minimal transannular patch should be considered.

It should be noted that much of the reconstruction of the pulmonary artery and right ventricular outflow tract may be performed after removal of the aortic cross clamp using cardiotomy suction in the distal pulmonary artery and in the right ventricular outflow tract. The incision in the pulmonary artery and any transannular extension is closed with a patch of fresh autologous pericardium. Branch pulmonary artery stenoses are also dealt with at this time, as depicted in Figure 114-14. The general surgical approach is to straighten the line from the apex of the incision through the branch pulmonary artery stenoses to the pulmonary valve to avoid placing pericardial patches with sharp angulations.[91] Otherwise, these areas of angulation often become the site of patch kinking and stenoses. Straightening of these suture lines can be accomplished by suturing adjacent edges of pulmonary artery wall together, which effectively extends the width of

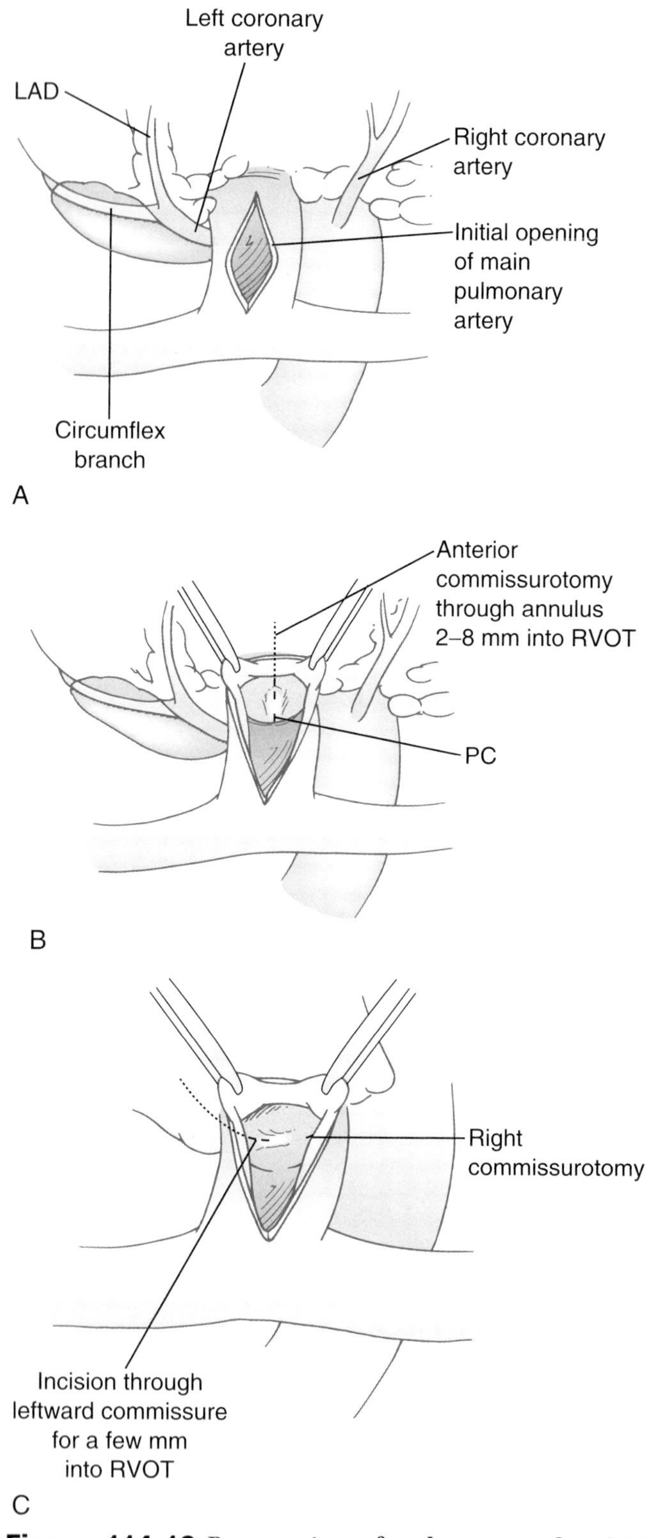

Figure 114–13 Preservation of pulmonary valve (PV) cusps in small PV. A, Initial pulmonary arteriotomy. LAD, left anterior descending coronary artery. **B,** Placement of anterior and posterior commissurotomies (PC). RVOT, right ventricular outflow tract. **C,** Left and right commissurotomies are performed if necessary.

(From Mee RBB: Transatrial transpulmonary repair of tetralogy of Fallot. In Yacoub, M, ed.: Annual of Cardiac Surgery, ed 8. Philadelphia: Lippincott Williams & Wilkins, 1995, pp. 141–147.)

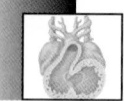

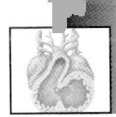

the back wall. For example, stenosis of the left pulmonary artery origin can be dealt with by suturing the adjacent inferior walls of the main pulmonary artery and the left pulmonary artery, which creates a nearly straight line from the apex of the incision in the left pulmonary artery and the apex of the incision in the right ventricular outflow tract (Figure 114-14B and C). In this case, the pericardial patch used for reconstruction forms a gentle D-shape without a sharp angulation. Other pulmonary artery reconstructions may also be required for bifurcation stenosis (Figures 114-15 and 114-16) or if there is right ventricular outflow tract obstruction caused by a small main pulmonary artery directly above the valve (Figure 114-17). Fine polypropylene suture (7-0) is used for all distal branch pulmonary artery reconstructions.

With the approach described, revision of the reconstruction of the right ventricular outflow tract or branch pulmonary arteries should be unusual. Transesophageal echocardiography and direct measurements of the ratio between the right and left ventricular pressure may be helpful to rule out significant residual obstruction of the right ventricular outflow tract. However, if the right atrial pressure is low, the right ventricle appears to be vigorous, and the appropriate-size dilator has been passed in the relaxed heart, residual obstruction is probably dynamic and can be predicted to decrease with time.

SPECIAL TOPICS IN SURGICAL MANAGEMENT

Use of a Monocusp Valve in Reconstruction of the Right Ventricular Outflow Tract

Monocusp reconstruction of the right ventricular outflow tract may be easily accomplished with autologous pericardium. Bovine pericardium may also be used if native pericardium is insufficient. PTFE is yet another material that can be used to provide a more durable monocusp valve. Reports vary regarding the usefulness of monocusp valve reconstruction of the right ventricular outflow tract.[6,42,110,124] If extensive reconstruction of the branch pulmonary arteries is required or if there is distal disease of the pulmonary vasculature, inclusion of a monocusp in the repair may improve hemodynamics in the immediate postoperative state. When pericardium is used to create a monocusp, the valve function is probably limited to the first weeks to months after repair, but the mode of valve failure (adherence of the monocusp to the right ventricular outflow tract patch) is nonobstructive.[6,42]

Anomalous Coronary Patterns

Conventional repair is complicated by the occurrence of the left anterior descending coronary artery originating totally or

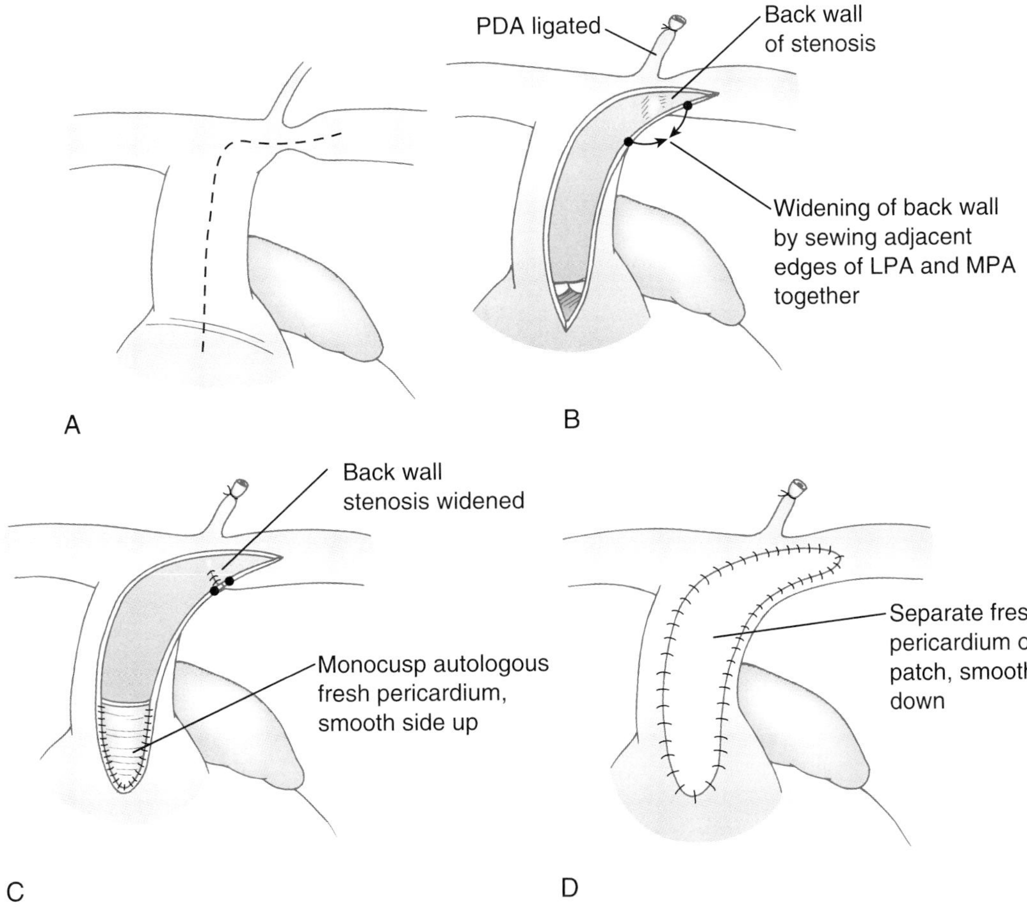

Figure 114–14 A–D, Reconstruction of proximal left pulmonary artery (LPA) stenosis resulting from ductal involution with accompanying small pulmonary valve. Notice insertion of monocusp valve constructed from fresh autologous pericardium (**C**). MPA, main pulmonary artery; PDA, patent ductus arteriosus.
(From Mee RBB: Transatrial transpulmonary repair of tetralogy of Fallot. In Yacoub, M, ed.: Annual of Cardiac Surgery, ed 8. Philadelphia: Lippincott Williams & Wilkins, 1995, pp. 141–147.)

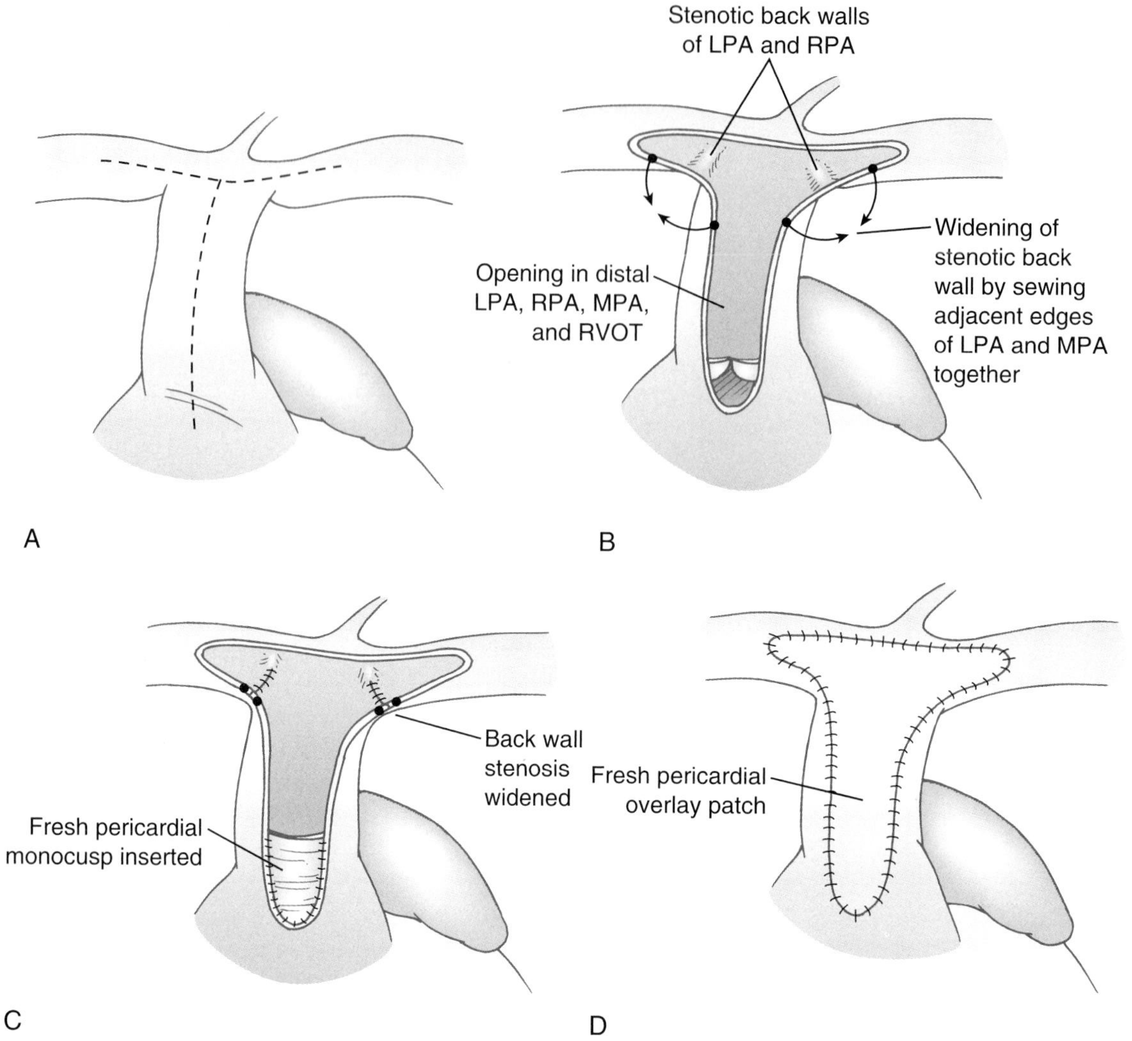

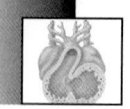

Figure 114-15 **A–D,** Reconstruction of pulmonary artery bifurcation stenosis with small main pulmonary artery (MPA) and pulmonic valve (PV). RPA, right pulmonary artery; LPA, left pulmonary artery; RVOT, right ventricular outflow tract. *(From Mee RBB: Transatrial transpulmonary repair of tetralogy of Fallot. In Yacoub, M, ed.: Annual of Cardiac Surgery, ed 8. Philadelphia: Lippincott Williams & Wilkins, 1995, pp. 141–147.)*

in part (dual left anterior descending coronary pattern) from the right coronary artery with the arterial supply from the right coronary artery crossing the right ventricular outflow tract.* Achieving adequate relief of the right ventricular outflow tract obstruction while maintaining the integrity of the coronary supply requires an understanding of different surgical options and flexibility in their application. Conduit reconstruction of the right ventricular outflow tract with origin from a ventriculotomy placed below the anomalous coronary has given reliable results but ultimately necessitates reoperation for conduit replacement. Translocation of the pulmonary artery to a distal ventriculotomy and use of the native pulmonary artery as a composite conduit to create a double outflow from the right ventricle have also been successfully completed[19,119] The transatrial/transpulmonary approach has been especially successful in dealing with this difficult anatomy.[9,64] Brizard[9] reported on Duncan's approach in 36 patients, which allowed a conduit to be avoided in all but two cases (Figure 114-18). Twenty-five patients required a limited transannular patch that was slightly deviated when necessary to avoid injuring the anomalous coronary artery. There were no perioperative or long-term deaths, and postoperative right ventricular pressures were low and equivalent to those obtained in contemporaneous patients undergoing TOF repair without coronary anomalies. There was also no difference in reoperation rates for patients with or without anomalous coronaries.[9]

*References 9, 19, 57, 58, 64, 119.

CONTROVERSIES IN SURGICAL MANAGEMENT

Ventriculotomy Versus Transatrial/Transpulmonary Approach

Excellent exposure of the VSD and obstructive muscle bundles in the right ventricular outflow tract can be achieved through either a right ventriculotomy or an incision in the right atrium.[76] Approach through a right ventriculotomy has been advocated in cases in which placement of a transannular patch is likely. In addition,

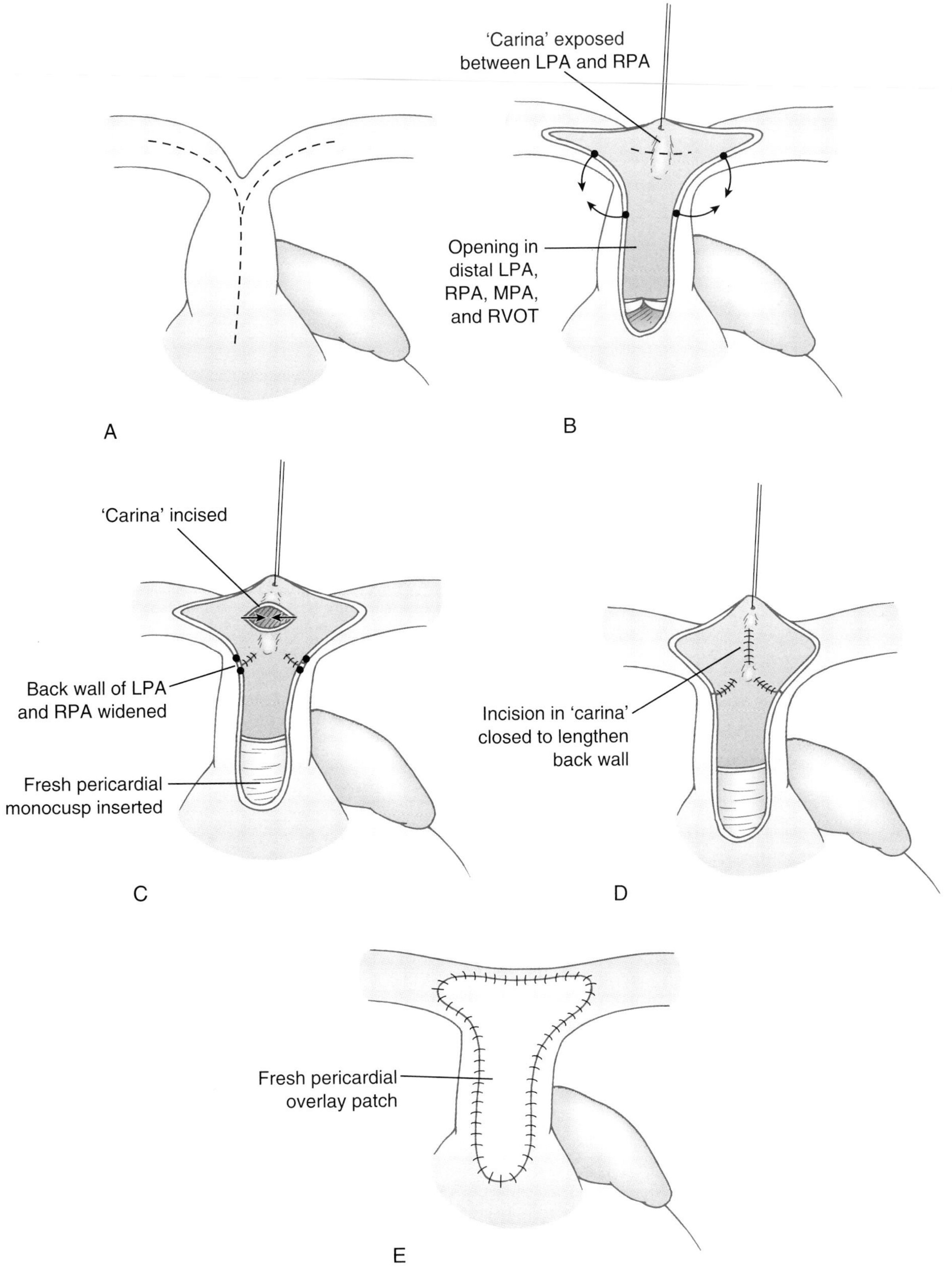

Figure 114–16 **A–E,** Reconstruction of early bifurcation stenosis with small pulmonary valve. MPA, main pulmonary artery; LPA, left pulmonary artery; RPA, right pulmonary artery; RVOT, right ventricular outflow tract.
(From Mee RBB: Transatrial transpulmonary repair of tetralogy of Fallot. In Yacoub, M, ed.: Annual of Cardiac Surgery, ed 8. Philadelphia: Lippincott Williams & Wilkins, 1995, pp. 141–147.)

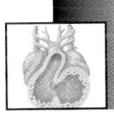

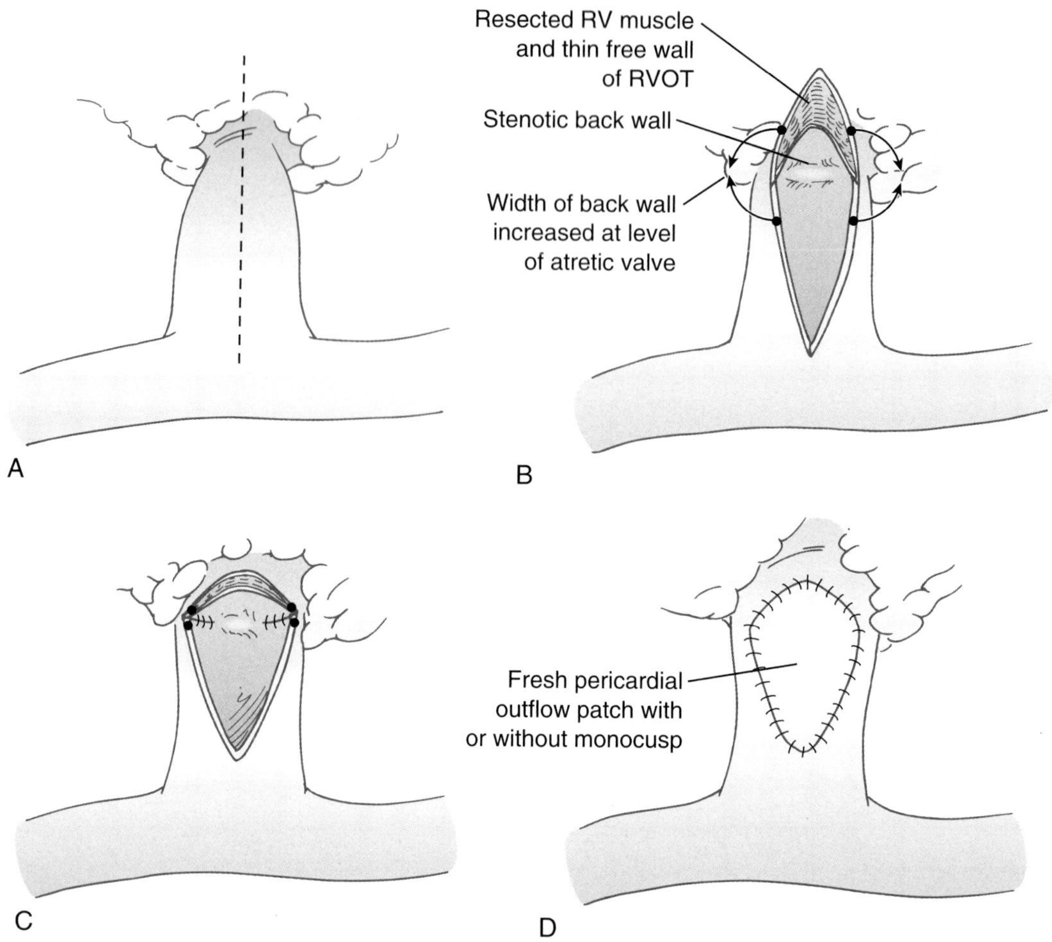

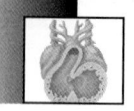

Figure 114–17 **A–D,** Surgical approach for managing small main pulmonary artery with significant obstruction directly above the valve. RVOT, right ventricular outflow tract; RV, right ventricle.
(From Mee RBB: Transatrial transpulmonary repair of tetralogy of Fallot. In Yacoub, M, ed.: Annual of Cardiac Surgery, ed 8. Philadelphia: Lippincott Williams & Wilkins, 1995, pp. 141–147.)

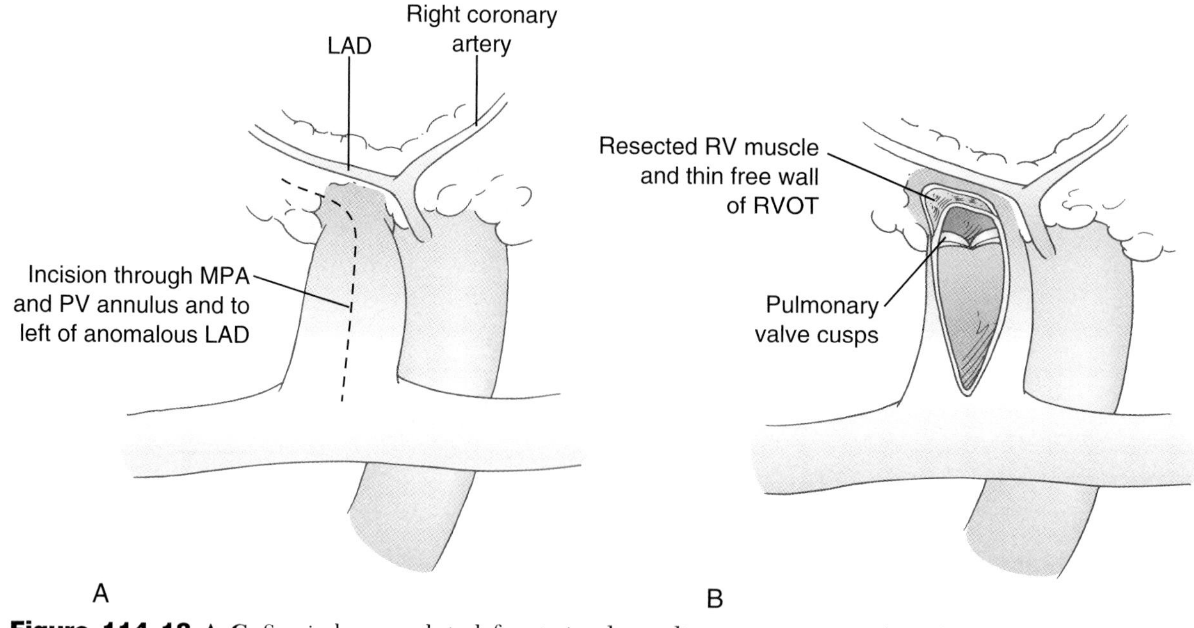

Figure 114–18 **A–C,** Surgical approach to left anterior descending coronary artery (LAD) arising from the right coronary artery and passing anterior to the right ventricular outflow tract (RVOT). MPA, main pulmonary artery; PV, pulmonary valve; RV, right ventricle.

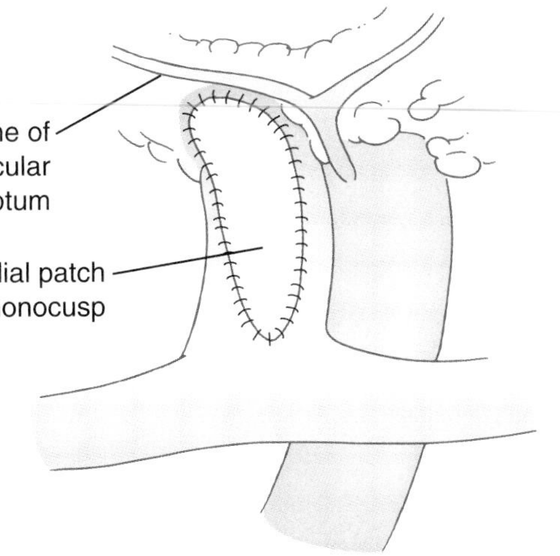

Figure 114–18 cont'd

some groups have reported a lower incidence of recurrent right ventricular outflow tract obstruction in patients corrected with ventriculotomy.[2]

Approach through a combined right atrial incision, and when necessary an incision in the pulmonary artery, avoids a ventriculotomy and may help avoid right ventricular dysfunction after repair, especially in the immediate postoperative period and in the very young heart.* Miura and others[94] demonstrated better preservation of right ventricular function at baseline and in response to catecholamine infusion in patients who had undergone a transatrial/transpulmonary approach compared with those with a right ventriculotomy. If a transannular patch is required, a limited right ventriculotomy extending only a few millimeters below the pulmonary annulus is possible. Minimizing or eliminating a right ventriculotomy altogether by using a transatrial/transpulmonary approach may also reduce the substrate for ventricular arrhythmias arising from incisions in the right ventricle.[67]

Timing of Operation

The predominant trend in the timing of surgical intervention has been toward earlier intervention with elective repair within the first 4–6 months of life.† There is less consensus regarding how best to treat patients who become symptomatic in early infancy or as neonates. Some advocate primary repair of symptomatic infants regardless of age, whereas some centers have adopted a policy of elective repair of all infants at the time of presentation, even in neonates.[101,107] Advocates of early primary repair note that this approach limits the duration of exposure of these children to cyanosis and its attendant cumulative complications. In addition, initial complete repair avoids attrition that may occur during the period between initial placement of a systemic-to-pulmonary arterial shunt and full repair in patients who undergo a staged approach. Furthermore, it has been postulated that ongoing pressure loading of the right ventricle in combination with chronic hypoxia creates a substrate in the right ventricular myocardium that predisposes to arrhythmia and diastolic dysfunction in patients who undergo later complete repair.[95] Two recent reports using primary repair of TOF in early infancy, such as those by Parry and Pigula, reported mortality rates of 0% (90% C.I. 0–6%) and 3% (90% C.I. 0–7%), respectively, with low rates of reoperation.[101,103] Kirklin and coauthors[75] compared results between two institutions: one institution that performed primary repair in all cases, even in neonates, if they became symptomatic, and one institution that performed initial systemic-to-pulmonary arterial shunting in the youngest patients. This study found no clear survival advantage in children who had undergone an initial shunt procedure; however, mortality was highest in the youngest patients (<3 months of age) who underwent primary repair.

Excellent results have also been reported with approaches that selectively use systemic-to-pulmonary arterial shunting as initial palliation for symptomatic neonates and young infants, and this remains the authors' strong preference.[35,67] Proponents of this approach cite the fact that mortality and morbidity are relatively higher in the youngest infants in many series that report success with early primary repair. The neonatal myocardium may be less capable of handling the right ventricular volume load that follows VSD closure in a cyanotic patient exacerbated by the additional volume loading from pulmonary incompetence and possible tricuspid valve incompetence in a heart that has undergone an ischemic period required for surgical repair. Deferring complete repair until after the neonatal period may in fact result in a reduced need for transannular patching. In addition, well-executed shunting for TOF in early infancy carries a very low risk of pulmonary artery distortion or early or interval mortality.[35,60,67] Fraser[35] recently reported an experience with selective application of primary repair to patients larger than 4 kg with initial shunting of smaller patients who required earlier attention because of symptoms or anatomy. Although most patients had TOF with pulmonic stenosis, this series also included patients with TOF and pulmonary atresia and patients with TOF and an AV septal defect. One shunted patient with TOF and a complete AV septal defect died in the interval before primary repair, but there were no perioperative deaths at the time of complete repair. Karl[67] reported an 11-year experience, which was overseen by this chapter's senior author, using initial palliation in neonates and young infants followed by complete repair at 10–15 months of age. With this approach in more than 360 patients, there was a requirement for shunting in 10–15% of patients with negligible interval mortality after shunting and 0.5% perioperative mortality at the time of complete repair.

POSTOPERATIVE MANAGEMENT

Most patients have relatively uncomplicated postoperative courses. Inotropic support is usually provided with low doses of dopamine, and extubation is usually possible in the first 12–48 h after surgery. Right ventricular dysfunction as a cause of low cardiac output in the immediate postoperative period is occasionally seen.[114] Significant diastolic dysfunction of the right ventricle after TOF repair may produce a

*References 25, 35, 39, 67, 69, 70, 91, 94, 100.
†References 1, 11, 14, 24, 29, 41, 45, 52, 95, 101, 103, 105, 107, 113, 116, 123, 127.

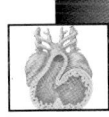

"restrictive physiology" in which the stiff right ventricle demonstrates little true filling and may behave as an almost passive conduit for pulmonary blood flow.[12,18] The causes of right ventricular dysfunction include pulmonic regurgitation, the presence of a right ventriculotomy, and residual lesions such as a hemodynamically significant VSD or right ventricular outflow tract obstruction. Right ventricular dysfunction is apparent as an elevation in the right atrial pressure along with the accompanying clinical manifestations of liver enlargement, edema, and effusions in a patient with evidence of low cardiac output (decreased cutaneous temperature, elevated lactate, decreased urine output). Right ventricular dysfunction after TOF repair is usually transient and responds to increased inotropic support and diuretics. In addition, a strategy of ventilatory support that produces mild respiratory alkalosis and low ventilatory pressures can be used to decrease pulmonary vascular resistance and right ventricular afterload.[114] Right-sided heart failure is more common after early primary repair but may be offset by the routine creation of a small interatrial communication.

Junctional ectopic tachycardia (JET) is not uncommon after TOF repair, especially in the first several hours after surgery.[28,102,114] When it does occur, postoperative JET is characterized by AV dissociation with rapid junctional rates of up to 230 bpm. A recent report found that JET occurred in 22% of patients who had undergone TOF repair.[28] In this report, resection rather than simple transection of muscle bundles in the right ventricular outflow tract, higher bypass temperatures, and a transatrial approach to VSD closure were all associated with a higher incidence of postoperative JET. The authors concluded that avoidance of excessive muscle resection in the right ventricular outflow tract and minimizing traction during VSD exposure should be attempted to reduce the incidence of postoperative JET. Treatment of JET includes core cooling (34–35° C), reduction in inotrope dosages, atrial pacing above the junctional rate, and the administration of antiarrhythmics.[114] Loading with amiodarone over 2–4 h followed by continuous infusion is a useful pharmacological approach to JET after TOF repair.

Residual lesions after TOF repair include residual VSDs and significant right ventricular outflow tract obstruction. Even small residual VSDs (3–4 mm) that would be well tolerated in patients with repaired large left-to-right shunts (VSD, truncus arteriosus) may be poorly tolerated after TOF repair. Poor tolerance of residual left-to-right shunts after TOF repair may result from a combination of factors including coexisting pulmonic regurgitation, noncompliant ventricles, and sudden volume loading of the left ventricle, particularly in neonates and young infants.[114] The presence of a residual VSD should be ruled out using intraoperative transesophageal echocardiography. Patients with significant VSDs demonstrate a higher-than-expected left atrial pressure. If a pulmonary artery catheter is in place, an oxygen saturation of greater than 80% in pulmonary arterial blood is predictive of a hemodynamically significant residual VSD.[82] Significant residual right ventricular outflow tract obstruction is usually tolerated in the immediate postoperative period; however, late problems including ventricular tachyarrhythmias and the need for late reoperation occur more commonly.[114] Hemodynamic instability arising from residual VSDs or right ventricular outflow tract obstruction may be attributed to postoperative right ventricular dysfunction alone; therefore, these residual lesions should be aggressively ruled out in patients with poor postoperative hemodynamics.

LONG-TERM FOLLOW-UP

Right Ventricular Performance and Functional Status

Decisions made at the time of surgery have a definite impact on the performance of TOF repair over the subsequent 20–30 years and beyond. Several reports now exist that detail the outcomes of patients who have undergone TOF repair, with follow-up into the third and fourth decades in some cases.* Despite institutional differences in surgical approach, timing of surgery, and many other aspects of management, long-term outcomes in survivors of TOF repair are uniformly favorable. Alexiou[1] reported a 20-year survival of 98% after TOF repair, with 99% of survivors in New York Heart Association (NYHA) functional class I. Knott-Craig[77] reported a 20-year survival of 98% with freedom from reintervention on the right ventricular outflow tract of 86% after 20 years of follow-up. Katz and coauthors[68] demonstrated an 8-year actuarial survival of 96% after TOF repair with 98% freedom from reoperation. In this study, older age at surgery, an increased right ventricular/left ventricular pressure ratio, and the use of a preceding Potts shunt were all risk factors for late events. The use of a transannular patch during repair or a Blalock-Taussig shunt before repair was not associated with adverse late events. Murphy[96] found a 32-year actuarial survival of 86%, which was less than the expected rate of 96% in age-matched controls. This report also found age at operation beyond 12 years and an elevated right ventricular/left ventricular pressure ratio to be associated with late mortality, whereas the presence of a transannular patch or a Blalock-Taussig shunt was not associated with late mortality. Kobayashi[78] reported that 85% of patients had no more than mild tricuspid regurgitation during a mean follow-up of 7 years after repair and that the development of moderate to severe tricuspid regurgitation was independent of the operative approach used (transatrial versus transventricular) but was associated with significant pulmonic regurgitation and elevated right ventricular pressure.

The performance of patients who have undergone TOF repair during exercise testing is also well maintained in most reports.[54,79,87,92,131] Mahle[87] reported that the mean maximal $\dot{V}O_2$ of patients after TOF repair was 95% of the predicted mean value for a control population, whereas the mean maximal work rate was 98% of what was predicted. In this study, the age of repair (<1 year of age versus >1 year of age) had no impact on exercise performance, which is an important finding for decisions regarding timing of repair. Kondo et al[79] found that cardiac output was normal at rest and during exercise in patients after repair; however, the incremental increase in left ventricular ejection fraction during exercise was reduced. The authors hypothesized that right ventricular enlargement with pathological changes in the septum

*References 1, 4, 15, 31, 36, 51, 54, 68, 77–79, 87, 92, 96, 131.

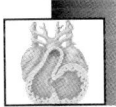

such as fibrosis causes latent left ventricular dysfunction during exercise in these patients.

Late Pulmonary Valve Replacement

Pulmonary valve replacement for pulmonic insufficiency after TOF repair has been reported to be necessary in approximately 2% of patients at 10-year follow-up and increases to 12% after 20 years.[76] Rates of replacement will undoubtedly increase as patients are followed for even longer periods after repair. Pulmonary valve replacement secondary to pulmonic insufficiency is rarely necessary in the absence of a transannular patch; often some obstruction at the level of the pulmonary artery or its branches is present as well in cases in which pulmonary valve replacement is necessary. Indications for pulmonary valve replacement for pulmonic insufficiency after TOF repair are not well established, but the procedure should be considered when there is documentation of progressive right ventricular enlargement and right ventricular dysfunction, especially with progressive tricuspid regurgitation or decreased exercise tolerance. Ventricular or supraventricular arrhythmias in the presence of enlargement of the corresponding cardiac chamber (right ventricle or right atrium, respectively) should also be considered as indications for pulmonary valve replacement to treat significant postrepair pulmonic insufficiency.

Several reports have detailed various clinical aspects of pulmonary valve replacement in patients after TOF repair.* Discigil and coauthors[27] reported 42 patients who underwent pulmonary valve replacement an average of 11 years after TOF repair. Decreased exercise tolerance (58%), right-sided heart failure (21%), arrhythmias (14%), syncope (10%), and right ventricular dilation (7%) were all indications for replacement. Ninety-eight percent of patients were hospital survivors with 5- and 10-year survival of 95% and 76%, respectively. Before surgery, 27% of patients were in NYHA class I or II, whereas after pulmonary valve replacement, 97% were in NYHA class I or II. Significant atrial arrhythmias were present in 14% preoperatively and 2% postoperatively. Freedom from repeat valve replacement was 93% at 5 years and 70% at 10 years. Vliegen and coworkers[130] used magnetic resonance imaging to evaluate patients before and after pulmonary valve replacement and found that right ventricular end-diastolic volume and right ventricular end-systolic volume decreased, whereas right ventricular ejection fraction increased after valve replacement. As a functional correlate, NYHA class was also found to improve substantially after pulmonary valve replacement. Despite demonstrating improvement in right ventricular volumes and functional status after pulmonary valve replacement, several studies demonstrate improvement only if valve replacement is performed appropriately early.[22,59,120] De Ruijter[22] reported an incidence of severe pulmonary insufficiency of 31% at an average of nearly 10 years after TOF repair, with significant right ventricular dilation in 38%. Of patients treated with pulmonary valve replacement, only 44% had normalization of right ventricular size and symptomatic relief. Therrien[120] reported no improvement in right ventricular volumes after pulmonary valve replacement. In addition, right ventricular ejection fraction remained depressed (<0.4) in 87% of patients in whom prereplacement right ventricular ejection was less than 0.4, whereas 50% of patients with prereplacement right ventricular ejection fraction of greater than 0.4 maintained postreplacement right ventricular ejection fractions greater than 0.4. These authors concluded that late pulmonary valve replacement failed to normalize right ventricular volumes and that the best chance of maintaining right ventricular function was to perform valve replacement before significant right ventricular dysfunction had occurred.

*References 22, 27, 30, 34, 49, 59, 65, 120, 130.

Arrhythmias

Supraventricular and ventricular arrhythmias are a relatively uncommon occurrence late after TOF repair, but they occur with increasing frequency as the duration of follow-up increases.* Studies have reported the incidence of arrhythmias requiring treatment in patients followed for more than 20 years after TOF repair to be 2% to 4% for atrial fibrillation/flutter, 3% to 4% for sustained ventricular tachycardia, and 2% to 4% for sudden cardiac death.[38,46] Holter monitoring detects a higher percentage of arrhythmias, with one recent report demonstrating that 19% of patients had sustained ventricular tachycardia, whereas 23% of patients had atrial fibrillation/flutter on 24-hour Holter monitoring.[108] Following TOF repair, the occurrence of arrhythmias is associated with elevated right ventricular volumes and pressure, decreased right and left ventricular ejection fractions, pulmonic regurgitation, and other disease of the right ventricular outflow tract such as aneurysm or significant stenosis.[20,38,47,88,137] Gatzoulis[38] found that pulmonic regurgitation was associated with ventricular tachycardia and sudden death, whereas tricuspid regurgitation was associated with atrial fibrillation/flutter. These same workers demonstrated that a substantially widened QRS complex on ECG is a prognostic marker of ventricular tachycardia and sudden cardiac death, with a QRS duration greater than 180 msec sensitively predicting the occurrence of life-threatening ventricular ectopy.[37,38] Dietl and coauthors[26] found that the original operative approach was associated with significant ventricular ectopy after repair. These workers found that 39% of patients had significant ventricular ectopy after a ventricular approach to TOF repair, whereas only 2.8% had significant ventricular ectopy after a transatrial approach. In this report, the incidence of moderate to severe pulmonic regurgitation was nearly twice as high in the ventricular repair group (25.9%) versus the transatrial repair group (12.5%). Therrien et al[121] found that pulmonary valve replacement, when performed in the presence of substantial pulmonic regurgitation and right ventricular enlargement, was associated with a substantial decrease in arrhythmias and stabilization of the QRS duration. These authors used intraoperative electrophysiological mapping and cryoablation in addition to pulmonary valve replacement in selected cases. In this series, atrial arrhythmias decreased from 17% to 12% postoperatively, whereas ventricular tachyarrhythmias decreased from 22% to 9%. In the 15 patients who underwent intraoperative cryoablation, there were no postoperative recurrences of significant arrhythmia. All of these studies underline that residual hemodynamic abnormalities

*References 17, 20, 26, 37, 38, 46, 47, 61, 88, 108, 121, 126, 132, 137, 138.

drive postoperative arrhythmias after TOF repair and that all efforts should be made at the time of repair to provide the anatomical substrate to minimize long-term hemodynamic problems. Volume and pressure loading of the right ventricle caused by residual abnormalities of the right ventricular outflow tract, such as pulmonic insufficiency, should be treated with replacement of the pulmonary valve to minimize the development of potentially lethal arrhythmias.

ATRIOVENTRICULAR CANAL AND TETRALOGY OF FALLOT

The presence of a common AV valve, ostium primum atrial septal defect, and nonrestrictive inlet ventricular septal defect occurs in combination with an anterior malalignment VSD and right ventricular outflow tract obstruction typical of TOF in perhaps 2% of all cases of TOF.[76,97] Repair may be accomplished by a single- or two-patch technique; in addition, transventricular or transatrial/transpulmonary approaches may be used successfully.* In general, most or all of the VSD can be closed through the right atrium, as is standard for repair of an AV septal defect; however, the patch must be elongated and wide enough anteriorly to close the anterior extension of the VSD without causing subaortic obstruction. Closure of the cleft in the left-sided AV valve and closure of the ostium primum ASD are performed in a standard fashion, and relief of the right ventricular outflow tract obstruction is performed as would normally be done for TOF. Some controversy exists regarding the timing of repair for combined AV septal defect and TOF, similar to timing issues in the management of simple TOF. There is consensus that children older than 6 months of age can safely undergo primary repair; however, the management of symptomatic neonates and younger infants remains in some dispute. Fifteen years ago repair of this condition carried a high risk. Currently, programs have reported success either with primary repair in children regardless of age or with selective management using initial shunting in the youngest patients with little or no increased risk over repair of simple TOF.[23,90,97,99] The authors' preference is to repair while the heart is volume loaded, either early in the presence of inadequate right ventricular outflow tract obstruction or later after interval systemic-to-pulmonary arterial shunt in patients who have significant cyanosis.

TETRALOGY OF FALLOT WITH ABSENT PULMONARY VALVE

The anatomical features of TOF with absent pulmonary valve include massively enlarged pulmonary arteries, anterior malalignment VSD, aplasia or rudimentary development of the pulmonary valve, a relatively small pulmonary valve ring, and absence of the ductus arteriosus. The cause of the aneurysmal enlargement of the pulmonary arteries may result from the effects of pulmonic insufficiency throughout fetal development or abnormalities within the vessel wall. Alternatively, the destroyed pulmonic valve and dilated pulmonary arteries may arise secondary to severe pulmonary hypertension in the absence of a decompressing patent ductus arteriosus. Massive enlargement of the pulmonary arteries often causes obstruction of the central bronchi, and the degree of airway obstruction dictates the clinical course observed in affected patients. Presentation varies from asymptomatic patients without clinically significant airway obstruction to severe bronchial obstruction requiring mechanical ventilation and operative correction in the newborn period.

Operative repair requires intracardiac correction typical of simple TOF with some type of surgical reduction in the size of the dilated main and branch pulmonary arteries.* In most cases, both the main and the branch pulmonary artery are massively enlarged and must be surgically reduced. The main pulmonary artery may be plicated or transected with a portion excised posteriorly, which effectively pulls the pulmonary arteries anteriorly away from the tracheobronchial tree. The branch pulmonary arteries are reduced in diameter by removing portions of the anterior wall, often with plication of the posterior wall.[40,89,112,135] In most cases, a transannular incision is necessary; reconstruction of the right ventricular outflow tract may then be performed with a homograft valve insertion[80,112]; however, right ventricular outflow tract reconstruction may also be performed with a monocusp or, often, without any valve implantation.[16,40,89,135] McDonnell[89] recently reported an experience with surgical management for 28 patients with TOF and absent pulmonary valve. Thirteen patients (46%) required preoperative intubation and mechanical ventilation. There was a 21% in-hospital mortality, whereas freedom from death or reintervention at 1 and 10 years was 68% and 52%, respectively. The requirement for preoperative mechanical ventilation was the only risk factor for mortality in this series. Hraska[56] reported a novel approach to this problem that includes transection and removal of a wedge-shaped portion of the ascending aorta to bring the aorta caudally and to the left. A LeCompte maneuver bringing the pulmonary arteries anterior to the aorta is then performed with or without concomitant plication of the branch pulmonary arteries. This approach pulls the pulmonary arteries off the tracheobronchial tree without requiring extensive suture lines, whereas the method of resection of the aorta creates a space for the new location of the pulmonary arteries while minimizing the risk of compression of the right coronary artery. Although experience with this technique is limited, it has provided good intermediate-term results in a small number of patients.

*References 23, 43, 90, 97, 99, 129.

*References 10, 16, 40, 50, 56, 66, 80, 89, 112, 117, 135.

REFERENCES

1. Alexiou C, Mahmoud H, Al-Khaddour A, et al: Outcome after repair of tetralogy of Fallot in the first year of life, *Ann Thorac Surg* 71:494–500, 2001.
2. Alexiou C, Chen Q, Galogavrou M, et al: Repair of tetralogy of Fallot in infancy with a transventricular or a transatrial approach, *Eur J Cardiothorac Surg* 22:174–183, 2002.
3. Anderson RH, Allwork SP, Ho SY, et al: Surgical anatomy of tetralogy of Fallot, *J Thorac Cardiovasc Surg* 81:887–896, 1981.

4. Bacha EA, Scheule AM, Zurakowski D, et al: Long-term results after early primary repair of tetralogy of Fallot, *J Thorac Cardiovasc Surg* 122:154–161, 2001.
5. Barrett-Boyes BG, Neutze JM: Primary repair of tetralogy of Fallot in infancy using profound hypothermia with circulatory arrest and limited cardiopulmonary bypass: a comparison with conventional two-stage management, *Ann Surg* 178:406, 1973.
6. Bigras JL, Boutin C, McCrindle BW, et al: Short-term effect of monocuspid valves on pulmonary insufficiency and clinical outcome after surgical repair of tetralogy of Fallot (comment), *J Thorac Cardiovasc Surg* 112:33–37, 1996.
7. Blalock A, Taussig HB: The surgical treatment of malformations of the heart in which there is pulmonary stenosis or pulmonary atresia, *JAMA* 128:189, 1945.
8. Boucek MM, Webster HE, Orsmond GS, et al: Balloon pulmonary valvotomy: palliation for cyanotic heart disease, *Am Heart J* 115:318–322, 1988.
9. Brizard CP, Mas C, Sohn YS, et al: Transatrial-transpulmonary tetralogy of Fallot repair is effective in the presence of anomalous coronary arteries, *J Thorac Cardiovasc Surg* 116:770–779, 1998.
10. Byrne JP, Hawkins JA, Battiste CE, et al: Palliative procedures in tetralogy of Fallot with absent pulmonary valve: a new approach, *Ann Thorac Surg* 33:499–502, 1982.
11. Castaneda AR: Classical repair of tetralogy of Fallot: timing, technique, and results, *Semin Thorac Cardiovasc Surg* 2:70–75, 1990.
12. Chaturvedi RR, Shore DF, Lincoln C, et al: Acute right ventricular restrictive physiology after repair of tetralogy of Fallot: association with myocardial injury and oxidative stress, *Circulation* 100:1540–1547, 1999.
13. Chiu IS, Wu CS, Wang JK, et al: Influence of aortopulmonary rotation on the anomalous coronary artery pattern in tetralogy of Fallot, *Am J Cardiol* 85:780–784, 2000.
14. Cobanoglu A, Schultz JM: Total correction of tetralogy of Fallot in the first year of life: late results, *Ann Thorac Surg* 74:133–138, 2002.
15. Cobanoglu A, Schultz JM: Total correction of tetralogy of Fallot in the first year of life: late results, *Ann Thorac Surg* 74:133–138, 2002.
16. Conte S, Serraf A, Godart F, et al: Technique to repair tetralogy of Fallot with absent pulmonary valve, *Ann Thorac Surg* 63:1489–1491, 1997.
17. Cullen S, Celermajer DS, Franklin RC, et al: Prognostic significance of ventricular arrhythmia after repair of tetralogy of Fallot: a 12-year prospective study, *J Am Coll Cardiol* 23:1151–1155, 1994.
18. Cullen S, Shore D, Redington A: Characterization of right ventricular diastolic performance after complete repair of tetralogy of Fallot. Restrictive physiology predicts slow postoperative recovery, *Circulation* 91:1782–1789, 1995.
19. Dandolu BR, Baldwin HS, Norwood WI, Jr, et al: Tetralogy of Fallot with anomalous coronary artery: double outflow technique, *Ann Thorac Surg* 67:1178–1180, 1999.
20. Davos CH, Davlouros PA, Wensel R, et al: Global impairment of cardiac autonomic nervous activity late after repair of tetralogy of Fallot, *Circulation* 106(Suppl I):I69–I75, 2002.
21. De Decker HP, Lawrenson JB: The 22q11.2 deletion: from diversity to a single gene theory, *Genet Med* 3:2–5, 2001.
22. de Ruijter FT, Weenink I, Hitchcock FJ, et al: Right ventricular dysfunction and pulmonary valve replacement after correction of tetralogy of Fallot, *Ann Thorac Surg* 73:1794–1800, 2002.
23. Delius RE, Kumar RV, Elliott MJ, et al: Atrioventricular septal defect and tetralogy of Fallot: a 15-year experience (comment), *Eur J Cardiothorac Surg* 12:171–176, 1997.
24. Di Donato RM, Jonas RA, Lang P, et al: Neonatal repair of tetralogy of Fallot with and without pulmonary atresia, *J Thorac Cardiovasc Surg* 101:126–137, 1991.
25. Dietl CA, Torres AR, Cazzaniga ME, et al: Right atrial approach for surgical correction of tetralogy of Fallot, *Ann Thorac Surg* 47:546–551, 1989.
26. Dietl CA, Cazzaniga ME, Dubner SJ, et al: Life-threatening arrhythmias and RV dysfunction after surgical repair of tetralogy of Fallot. Comparison between transventricular and transatrial approaches, *Circulation* 90(Suppl II):II7–II12, 1994.
27. Discigil B, Dearani JA, Puga FJ, et al: Late pulmonary valve replacement after repair of tetralogy of Fallot, *J Thorac Cardiovasc Surg* 121:344–351, 2001.
28. Dodge-Khatami A, Miller OI, Anderson RH, et al: Surgical substrates of postoperative junctional ectopic tachycardia in congenital heart defects, *J Thorac Cardiovasc Surg* 123:624–630, 2002.
29. Dyamenahalli U, McCrindle BW, Barker GA, et al: Influence of perioperative factors on outcomes in children younger than 18 months after repair of tetralogy of Fallot, *Ann Thorac Surg* 69:1236–1242, 2000.
30. Eyskens B, Reybrouck T, Bogaert J, et al: Homograft insertion for pulmonary regurgitation after repair of tetralogy of Fallot improves cardiorespiratory exercise performance, *Am J Cardiol* 85:221–225, 2000.
31. Faidutti B, Christenson JT, Beghetti M, et al: How to diminish reoperation rates after initial repair of tetralogy of Fallot? *Ann Thorac Surg* 73:96–101, 2002.
32. Fallot ELA: Contribution a l'anatomie pathologique de la maladie bleue (cyanose cardiaque), *Marseilles Med* 25:77, 138, 207, 270, 341, 403, 1888.
33. Fellowes KE, Freed MK, Keane JR: Preoperative angiocardiography in infants with tetrad of Fallot: review of 36 cases, *Am J Cardiol* 47:1279, 1981.
34. Finck SJ, Puga FJ, Danielson GK: Pulmonary valve insertion during reoperation for tetralogy of Fallot, *Ann Thorac Surg* 45:610–613, 1988.
35. Fraser CD, Jr, McKenzie ED, Cooley DA: Tetralogy of Fallot: surgical management individualized to the patient, *Ann Thorac Surg* 71:1556–1561, 2001.
36. Gatzoulis MA, Clark AL, Cullen S, et al: Right ventricular diastolic function 15 to 35 years after repair of tetralogy of Fallot. Restrictive physiology predicts superior exercise performance, *Circulation* 91:1775–1781, 1995.
37. Gatzoulis MA, Till JA, Somerville J, et al: Mechanoelectrical interaction in tetralogy of Fallot. QRS prolongation relates to right ventricular size and predicts malignant ventricular arrhythmias and sudden death (comment), *Circulation* 92:231–237, 1995.
38. Gatzoulis MA, Balaji S, Webber SA, et al: Risk factors for arrhythmia and sudden cardiac death late after repair of tetralogy of Fallot: a multicentre study, *Lancet* 356:975–981, 2000.
39. Giannopoulos NM, Chatzis AK, Karros P, et al: Early results after transatrial/transpulmonary repair of tetralogy of Fallot, *Eur J Cardiothorac Surg* 22:582–586, 2002.
40. Godart F, Houyel L, Lacour-Guyette F, et al: Absent pulmonary valve syndrome: surgical treatment and considerations, *Ann Thorac Surg* 62:136–142, 1996.
41. Groh MA, Meliones JN, Bove EL, et al: Repair of tetralogy of Fallot in infancy. Effect of pulmonary artery size on outcome, *Circulation* 84(Suppl III):III206–III212, 1991.
42. Gundry SR, Razzouk AJ, Boskind JF, et al: Fate of the pericardial monocusp pulmonary valve for right ventricular outflow tract reconstruction. Early function, late failure without obstruction, *J Thorac Cardiovasc Surg* 107:908–912, 1994.
43. Guo-wei H, Mee RBB: Complete atrioventricular canal associated with tetralogy of Fallot or double-outlet right ventricle and right ventricular outflow tract obstruction: a report of successful surgical treatment, *Ann Thorac Surg* 41:612–615, 1986.

44. Gupta D, Saxena A, Kothari SS, et al: Detection of coronary artery anomalies in tetralogy of Fallot using a specific angiographic protocol, *Am J Cardiol* 87:241–244, 2001.
45. Gustafson RA, Murray GF, Warden HE, et al: Early primary repair of tetralogy of Fallot, *Ann Thorac Surg* 45:235–241, 1988.
46. Hamada H, Terai M, Jibiki T, et al: Influence of early repair of tetralogy of Fallot without an outflow patch on late arrhythmias and sudden death: a 27-year follow-up study following a uniform surgical approach, *Cardiol Young* 12:345–351, 2002.
47. Harrison DA, Harris L, Siu SC, et al: Sustained ventricular tachycardia in adult patients late after tetralogy of Fallot repair, *J Am Coll Cardiol* 30:1368–1373, 1997.
48. Hazan E, Bical O, Bex JP, et al: Is right bundle branch block avoidable in surgical correction of tetralogy of Fallot? *Circulation* 62:852–854, 1980.
49. Hazekamp MG, Kurvers MM, Schoof PH, et al: Pulmonary valve insertion late after repair of Fallot's tetralogy, *Eur J Cardiothorac Surg* 19:667–670, 2001.
50. Heinemann MK, Hanley FL: Preoperative management of neonatal tetralogy of Fallot with absent pulmonary valve syndrome, *Ann Thorac Surg* 55:172–174, 1993.
51. Hennein HA, Mosca RS, Urcelay G, et al: Intermediate results after complete repair of tetralogy of Fallot in neonates, *J Thorac Cardiovasc Surg* 109:332–342, 1995.
52. Hirsch JC, Mosca RS: Complete repair of tetralogy of Fallot in the neonate, *Ann Surg* 232:508–514, 2000.
53. Hislop A, Reid L: Structural changes in the pulmonary arteries and veins in tetralogy of Fallot, *Br Heart J* 35:1178, 1973.
54. Horneffer PJ, Zahka KG, Rowe SA, et al: Long-term results of total repair of tetralogy of Fallot in childhood, *Ann Thorac Surg* 50:179–83, 1990.
55. Howell CE, Ho SY, Anderson RH, et al: Variations within the fibrous skeleton and ventricular outflow tracts in tetralogy of Fallot, *Ann Thorac Surg* 50:450–457, 1990.
56. Hraska V, Kantorova A, Kunovsky P, et al: Intermediate results with correction of tetralogy of Fallot with absent pulmonary valve using a new approach, *Eur J Cardiothorac Surg* 21:711–714, 2002.
57. Humes RA, Driscoll DJ, Danielson GK, et al: Tetralogy of Fallot with anomalous origin of left anterior descending coronary artery, *J Thorac Cardiovasc Surg* 94:784–787, 1987.
58. Hurwitz RA, Smith W, King H, et al: Tetralogy of Fallot with abnormal coronary artery: 1967–1977, *J Thorac Cardiovasc Surg* 80:129–134, 1980.
59. Ilbawi MN, Idriss FS, DeLeon SY, et al: Factors that exaggerate the deleterious effects of pulmonary insufficiency on the right ventricle after tetralogy repair. Surgical implications, *J Thorac Cardiovasc Surg* 93:36–44, 1987.
60. Jahangiri M, Lincoln C, Shinebourne EA: Does the modified Blalock-Taussig shunt cause growth of the contralateral pulmonary artery? *Ann Thorac Surg* 67:1397–1399, 1999.
61. Joffe H, Georgakopoulos D, Celermajer DS, et al: Late ventricular arrhythmia is rare after early repair of tetralogy of Fallot (comment), *J Am Coll Cardiol* 23:1146–1150, 1994.
62. Johnson RJ, Haworth SG: Pulmonary vascular and alveolar development in tetralogy of Fallot: a recommendation for early correction, *Thorax* 37:893, 1982.
63. Jureidini SB, Appleton RS, Nouri S: Detection of coronary artery abnormalities in tetralogy of Fallot by two-dimensional echocardiography, *J Am Coll Cardiol* 14:960–967, 1989.
64. Kalra S, Sharma R, Choudhary SK, et al: Right ventricular outflow tract after non-conduit repair of tetralogy of Fallot with coronary anomaly, *Ann Thorac Surg* 70:723–726, 2000.
65. Kanter KR, Budde JM, Parks WJ, et al: One hundred pulmonary valve replacements in children after relief of right ventricular outflow tract obstruction, *Ann Thorac Surg* 73:1801–1806, 2002.
66. Karl TR, de Leval M, Pincott JR, et al: Surgical treatment of absent pulmonary valve syndrome, *J Thorac Cardiovasc Surg* 91:590–597, 1986.
67. Karl TR, Sano S, Pornviliwan S, et al: Tetralogy of Fallot: favorable outcome of nonneonatal transatrial, transpulmonary repair, *Ann Thorac Surg* 54:903–907, 1992.
68. Katz NM, Blackstone EH, Kirklin JW, et al: Late survival and symptoms after repair of tetralogy of Fallot, *Circulation* 65:403–410, 1982.
69. Kawashima Y, Kitamura S, Nakano S, et al: Corrective surgery for tetralogy of Fallot without or with minimal right ventriculotomy and with repair of the pulmonary valve, *Circulation* 64(Suppl II):II147–II153, 1981.
70. Kawashima Y, Matsuda H, Hirose H, et al: Ninety consecutive corrective operations for tetralogy of Fallot with or without minimal right ventriculotomy, *J Thorac Cardiovasc Surg* 90:856–863, 1985.
71. Kirk JS, Comstock CH, Lee W, et al: Sonographic screening to detect fetal cardiac anomalies: a 5-year experience with 111 abnormal cases, *Obstet Gynecol* 89:227–232, 1997.
72. Kirklin JW, Dushane JW, Patrick RT, et al: Intracardiac surgery with the aid of a mechanical pump-oxygenator (Gibbon type): report of eight cases, *Mayo Clin Proc* 30:201, 1955.
73. Kirklin JW, Ellis FH, McGoon DC, et al: Surgical treatment for the treatment of tetralogy of Fallot by open intracardiac repair, *J Thorac Surg* 37:22, 1959.
74. Kirklin JW, Blackstone EH, Kirklin JK, et al: Surgical results and protocols in the spectrum of tetralogy of Fallot, *Ann Surg* 198:251–265, 1983.
75. Kirklin JW, Blackstone EH, Jonas RA, et al: Morphologic and surgical determinants of outcome events after repair of tetralogy of Fallot and pulmonary stenosis, *J Thorac Cardiovasc Surg* 103:706–723, 1992.
76. Kirklin JW, Barratt-Boyes BG: Ventricular septal defect and pulmonary stenosis or atresia. In Kirklin JW, Barratt-Boyes BG, (eds): *Cardiac surgery*, ed 2, New York, 1993, Churchill Livingstone, p 861.
77. Knott-Craig CJ, Elkins RC, Lane MM, et al: A 26-year experience with surgical management of tetralogy of Fallot: risk analysis for mortality or late reintervention, *Ann Thorac Surg* 66:506–511, 1998.
78. Kobayashi J, Kawashima Y, Matsuda H, et al: Prevalence and risk factors of tricuspid regurgitation after correction of tetralogy of Fallot, *J Thorac Cardiovasc Surg* 102:611–616, 1991.
79. Kondo C, Nakazawa M, Kusakabe K, et al: Left ventricular dysfunction on exercise long-term after total repair of tetralogy of Fallot, *Circulation* 92(Suppl II):II250–II255, 1995.
80. Kron IL, Johnson AM, Carpenter MA, et al: Treatment of absent pulmonary valve syndrome with homograft, *Ann Thorac Surg* 46:579–581, 1988.
81. Kurosawa H, Imai Y, Becker AE: Surgical anatomy of the atrioventricular conduction bundle in tetralogy of Fallot, *J Thorac Cardiovasc Surg* 95:586–591, 1988.
82. Lang P, Chipman CW, Siden H, et al: Early assessment of hemodynamic status after repair of tetralogy of Fallot: a comparison of 24 hour (intensive care unit) and 1 year postoperative data in 98 patients, *Am J Cardiol* 50:795–799, 1982.
83. Lee W, Smith RS, Comstock CH, et al: Tetralogy of Fallot: prenatal diagnosis and postnatal survival, *Obstet Gynecol* 86:583–588, 1995.
84. Lillehei CW, Cohen M, Warden HE, et al: The direct-vision intracardiac correction of congenital anomalies by controlled cross-circulation: results in 32 patients with ventricular septal defects, tetralogy of Fallot, and atrioventricular communis defects, *Surgery* 38:11, 1955.
85. Lillehei CW, Varco RL, Cohen M: The first open-heart repairs of ventricular septal defect, atrioventricular commu-

nis, and tetralogy of Fallot using extracorporeal circulation by cross-circulation: a thirty-year follow-up, *Ann Thorac Surg* 41:4, 1986.

86. Maeda J, Yamagishi H, Matsuoka R, et al: Frequent association of 22q11.2 deletion with tetralogy of Fallot, *Am J Med Genet* 92:269–272, 2000.
87. Mahle WT, McBride MG, Paridon SM: Exercise performance in tetralogy of Fallot: the impact of primary complete repair in infancy, *Pediatr Cardiol* 23:224–229, 2002.
88. Marie PY, Marcon F, Brunotte F, et al: Right ventricular overload and induced sustained ventricular tachycardia in operatively "repaired" tetralogy of Fallot, *Am J Cardiol* 69: 785–789, 1992.
89. McDonnell BE, Raff GW, Gaynor JW, et al: Outcome after repair of tetralogy of Fallot with absent pulmonary valve, *Ann Thorac Surg* 67:1391–1395, 1999.
90. McElhinney DB, Reddy VM, Silverman NH, et al: Atrioventricular septal defect with common valvar orifice and tetralogy of Fallot revisited: making a case for primary repair in infancy, *Cardiol Young* 8:455–461, 1998.
91. Mee RBB: Transatrial transpulmonary repair of tetralogy of Fallot. In Yacoub M, ed.: *Annual of cardiac surgery*, ed 8, Philadelphia, 1995, Lippincott Williams & Wilkins, pp. 141–147.
92. Meijboom F, Szatmari A, Deckers JW, et al: Cardiac status and health-related quality of life in the long term after surgical repair of tetralogy of Fallot in infancy and childhood, *J Thorac Cardiovasc Surg* 110:883–891, 1995.
93. Meng CCL, Eckner FA, Lev M: Coronary artery distribution in tetralogy of Fallot, *Arch Surg* 90:363–366, 1965.
94. Miura T, Nakano S, Shimazaki Y, et al: Evaluation of right ventricular function by regional wall motion analysis in patients after correction of tetralogy of Fallot, *J Thorac Cardiovasc Surg* 104:917–923, 1992.
95. Munkhammar P, Cullen S, Jogi P, et al: Early age at repair prevents restrictive right ventricular physiology after surgery for tetralogy of Fallot, *J Am Coll Cardiol* 32:1083–1087, 1998.
96. Murphy JG, Gersh BJ, Mair DD, et al: Long-term outcome in patients undergoing surgical repair of tetralogy of Fallot (comment), *N Engl J Med* 329:593–599, 1993.
97. Najm HK, Van Arsdell GS, Watzka S, et al: Primary repair is superior to initial palliation in children with atrioventricular septal defect and tetralogy of Fallot, *J Thorac Cardiovasc Surg* 116:905–913, 1998.
98. Need LR, Powell AJ, del Nido P, et al: Coronary echocardiography in tetralogy of Fallot: diagnostic accuracy, resource utilization and surgical implications over 13 years, *J Am Coll Cardiol* 36:1371–1377, 2000.
99. O'Blenes SB, Ross DB, Nanton MA, et al: Atrioventricular septal defect with tetralogy of Fallot: results of surgical correction, *Ann Thorac Surg* 66:2078–2082, 1998.
100. Pacifico AD, Sand ME, Bargeron LM Jr, Colvin EC: Transatrial-transpulmonary repair of tetralogy of Fallot, *J Thorac Cardiovasc Surg* 93:919–924, 1987.
101. Parry AJ, McElhinney DB, Kung GC, et al: Elective primary repair of acyanotic tetralogy of Fallot in early infancy: overall outcome and impact on the pulmonary valve, *J Am Coll Cardiol* 36:2279–2283, 2000.
102. Pfammatter J, Wagner B, Berdat P, et al: Procedural factors associated with early postoperative arrhythmias after repair of congenital heart defects, *J Thorac Cardiovasc Surg* 123:258–262, 2002.
103. Pigula FA, Khalil PN, Mayer JE, et al: Repair of tetralogy of Fallot in neonates and young infants, *Circulation* 100(Suppl II):II157–II161, 1999.
104. Potts WJ, Smith S, Gibson S: Anastomosis of the aorta to a pulmonary artery, *JAMA* 132:627, 1946.
105. Pozzi M, Trivedi DB, Kitchiner D, et al: Tetralogy of Fallot: what operation, at which age, *Eur J Cardiothorac Surg* 17:631–636, 2000.
106. Rao PS, Brais M: Balloon pulmonary valvuloplasty for congenital cyanotic heart defects, *Am Heart J* 115:1105–1110, 1988.
107. Reddy VM, Liddicoat JR, McElhinney DB, et al: Routine primary repair of tetralogy of Fallot in neonates and infants less than three months of age, *Ann Thorac Surg* 60:S592–S596, 1995.
108. Roos-Hesselink J, Perlroth MG, McGhie J, et al: Atrial arrhythmias in adults after repair of tetralogy of Fallot. Correlations with clinical, exercise, and echocardiographic findings (comment), *Circulation* 91:2214–2219, 1995.
109. Ross DN, Somerville J: Correction of pulmonary atresia with a homograft aortic valve, *Lancet* 2:1446, 1966.
110. Roughneen PT, DeLeon SY, Parvathaneni S, et al: The pericardial membrane pulmonary monocusp: surgical technique and early results. *J Card Surg* 14:370–374, 1999.
111. Santoro G, Marino B, DiCarlo D, et al: Echocardiographically guided repair of tetralogy of Fallot, *Am J Cardiol* 73:808–811, 1994.
112. Snir E, de Leval MR, Elliott MJ, et al: Current surgical technique to repair Fallot's tetralogy with absent pulmonary valve syndrome (comment), *Ann Thorac Surg* 51:979–982, 1991.
113. Sousa Uva M, Lacour-Gayet F, Komiya T, et al: Surgery for tetralogy of Fallot at less than six months of age, *J Thorac Cardiovasc Surg* 107:1291–1300, 1994.
114. Spray TL, Wernovsky G: Right ventricular outflow tract obstruction. In Chang AC, Hanley FL, Wernovsky G, Wessel DL, (eds): Pediatric cardiac intensive care, Baltimore, 1998, Williams & Wilkins, pp 257–264.
115. Sreeram N, Saleem M, Jackson M, et al: Results of balloon pulmonary valvuloplasty as a palliative procedure in tetralogy of Fallot (comment), *J Am Coll Cardiol* 18:159–165, 1991.
116. Starnes VA, Luciani GB, Latter DA, Griffin ML: Current surgical management of tetralogy of Fallot, *Ann Thorac Surg* 58:211–215, 1994.
117. Stellin G, Jonas RA, Goh TH, et al: Surgical treatment of absent pulmonary valve syndrome in infants: relief of bronchial obstruction, *Ann Thorac Surg* 36:468–475, 1983.
118. Suzuki A, Ho SY, Anderson RH, et al: Further morphologic studies on tetralogy of Fallot, with particular emphasis on the prevalence and structure of the membranous flap, *J Thorac Cardiovasc Surg* 99:528–535, 1990.
119. Tchervenkov CI, Pelletier MP, Shum-Tim D, et al: Primary repair minimizing the use of conduits in neonates and infants with tetralogy or double-outlet right ventricle and anomalous coronary arteries, *J Thorac Cardiovasc Surg* 119:314–323, 2000.
120. Therrien J, Siu SC, McLaughlin PR, et al: Pulmonary valve replacement in adults late after repair of tetralogy of Fallot: are we operating too late? (comment), *J Am Coll Cardiol* 36:1670–1675, 2000.
121. Therrien J, Siu SC, Harris L, et al: Impact of pulmonary valve replacement on arrhythmia propensity late after repair of tetralogy of Fallot, *Circulation* 103:2489–2494, 2001.
122. Tometzki AJ, Suda K, Kohl T, et al: Accuracy of prenatal echocardiographic diagnosis and prognosis of fetuses with conotruncal anomalies, *J Am Coll Cardiol* 33:1696–1701, 1999.
123. Touati GD, Vouhe PR, Amodeo A, et al: Primary repair of tetralogy of Fallot in infancy, *J Thorac Cardiovasc Surg* 99:396–403, 1990.
124. Turrentine MW, McCarthy RP, Vijay P, et al: PTFE monocusp valve reconstruction of the right ventricular outflow tract, *Ann Thorac Surg* 73:871–879, 2002.
125. Tworetzky W, McElhinney DB, Brook MM, et al: Echocardiographic diagnosis alone for the complete repair of

major congenital heart defects, *J Am Coll Cardiol* 33:228–233, 1999.

126. Vaksmann G, Fournier A, Davignon A, et al: Frequency and prognosis of arrhythmias after operative "correction" of tetralogy of Fallot, *Am J Cardiol* 66:346–349, 1990.
127. Van Arsdell GS, Maharaj GS, Tom J, et al: What is the optimal age for repair of tetralogy of Fallot? *Circulation* 102(Suppl III):III123–III129, 2000.
128. Van Praagh R, Van Praagh S, Nebesar RA, et al: Tetralogy of Fallot: underdevelopment of the pulmonary infundibulum and its sequelae, *Am J Cardiol* 26:25–33, 1970.
129. Vargas FJ, Coto EO, Mayer JE Jr, et al: Complete atrioventricular canal and tetralogy of Fallot: surgical considerations, *Ann Thorac Surg* 42:258–263, 1986.
130. Vliegen HW, van Straten A, de Roos A, et al: Magnetic resonance imaging to assess the hemodynamic effects of pulmonary valve replacement in adults late after repair of tetralogy of Fallot, *Circulation* 106:1703–1707, 2002.
131. Waien SA, Liu PP, Ross BL, et al: Serial follow-up of adults with repaired tetralogy of Fallot, *J Am Coll Cardiol* 20:295–300, 1992.
132. Walsh EP, Rockenmacher S, Keane JF, et al: Late results in patients with tetralogy of Fallot repaired during infancy, *Circulation* 77:1062–1067, 1988.
133. Warden HE, DeWall RA, Choen M, et al: A surgical-pathologic classification for isolated ventricular septal defects and for those in Fallot's tetralogy based on observations made on 120 patients during repair under direct vision, *J Thorac Surg* 33:21, 1957.
134. Waterston DJ: Treatment of Fallot's tetralogy in children under one year of age, *Rozhl Chir* 41:181, 1962.
135. Watterson KG, Malm TK, Karl TR, et al: Absent pulmonary valve syndrome: operation in infants with airway obstruction, *Ann Thorac Surg* 54:1116–1119, 1992.
136. Yoo SJ, Lee YH, Kim ES, et al: Tetralogy of Fallot in the fetus: findings at targeted sonography, *Ultrasound Obstet Gynecol* 14:29–37, 1999.
137. Zahka KG, Horneffer PJ, Rowe SA, et al: Long-term valvular function after total repair of tetralogy of Fallot. Relation to ventricular arrhythmias, *Circulation* 78(Suppl III):III14–III19, 1988.
138. Zimmermann M, Friedli B, Adamec R, et al: Ventricular late potentials and induced ventricular arrhythmias after surgical repair of tetralogy of Fallot, *Am J Cardiol* 67:873–878, 1991.

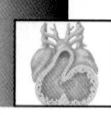

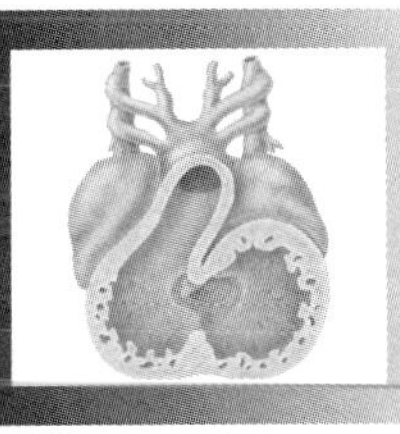

Pulmonary Atresia and Ventricular Septal Defect

CHAPTER 115

Glen S. Van Arsdell

INTRODUCTION

Pulmonary atresia occurs in association with a wide variety of lesions involving one or more segments of the heart. It may occur in hearts that will ultimately carry either a single or biventricular configuration. It may occur with or without the presence of genetic syndromes. Pulmonary atresia, in the context of this chapter, focuses on those hearts that have normal venous connections, atrioventricular and ventricular arterial concordance, and normal-sized ventricles. There is an associated ventricular septal defect and a varying degree of infundibular septal and trabecular septal malalignment. Some would refer to this anatomy as tetralogy of Fallot with pulmonary atresia. The nomenclature chosen for this chapter is pulmonary atresia with a ventricular septal defect (PA/ VSD).

PA/ VSD is frequently associated with abnormalities of the peripheral pulmonary vascular bed. In the discussion and management of PA/ VSD, with normal-sized ventricles, there are a number of important questions. Are there central pulmonary arteries? Are they of normal size? Are the central pulmonary arteries confluent? Are there major collaterals arising from the systemic vasculature? How many segments of lung are attached to the central pulmonary arteries? How many segments of lung are attached to the major systemic collateral arteries? Is there segmental or global pulmonary hypertension? Treatment strategies are devised around the answers to these questions. Irrespective of the anatomy at birth, the final goal is to close the ventricular septal defect and create a right ventricle to pulmonary artery connection. If the branch pulmonary vasculature is abnormal it is "normalized" through an operation or series of operations so that all segments of the lung blood supply arise from confluent central pulmonary arteries. Such procedures are known as unifocalization procedures.

As is the case with many congenital heart lesions, the treatment of PA/VSD is in recent evolution. Because the solutions for this congenital malformation are not ideal, the philosophy and application of repair techniques are subject to revision. Substantial controversy exists. The broad concepts for repair and varying strategies will be discussed. Results are continuously changing and must therefore be evaluated with the perspective of technique and era. Many complex congenital lesions can be repaired with mortality of 1% to 2% or less. Progress in PA/VSD is substantial but outcomes for severe cases of PA/VSD with major aortopulmonary collateral arteries continue to be a challenge.

ANATOMY AND EMBRYOLOGY

PA/VSD, as discussed in this chapter, presents with normal systemic and pulmonary venous connections and atrioventricular and ventriculoarterial concordance. There is a large perimembranous VSD with outlet extension. The VSD sits between the limbs of the trabeculae septomarginalis. The infundibular septum is anteriorly deviated. A varying degree of aortic override onto the right ventricle is present. There may occasionally be multiple VSDs. Figure 115-1 demonstrates normal-sized ventricles, a large VSD, pulmonary atresia, and mild aortic override of the VSD. Aortopulmonary collaterals can be seen coming off the descending aorta.

Conduction pathways are similar to those in perimembranous VSDs. The bundle of His penetrates from atrium to ventricle along the left side of the ventricular septum adjacent to the rightward margin of the VSD where the muscle and tricuspid annulus meet.

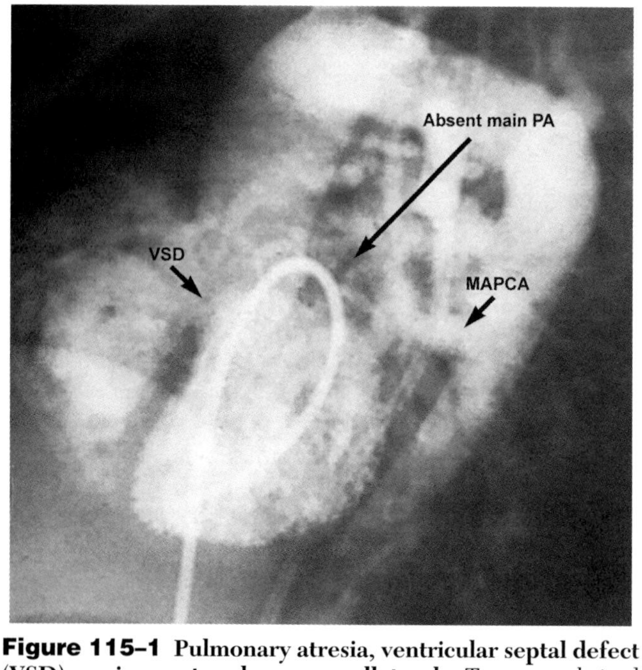

Figure 115–1 Pulmonary atresia, ventricular septal defect (VSD), major aortopulmonary collaterals. Two normal-sized ventricles connected by a large VSD. There is no main pulmonary artery (PA). Aortopulmonary collaterals can be seen coming off the descending aorta. MAPCA, Major aortopulmonary collateral.

Pulmonary Atresia

Atresia of the pulmonary outlet can occur at the level of the infundibulum (conus) or as a plate atresia of the pulmonary valve in the presence of an infundibular outlet. There is no forward flow of blood from the right ventricle to the pulmonary arteries. Plate-type atresia is commonly associated with a well-developed main pulmonary artery.

Pulmonary Arteries and Aortopulmonary Collaterals

Development of the pulmonary vasculature occurs both in the lung and from the heart.[7,10] Initially, the lung buds of the foregut receive blood via arteries originating from the dorsal aorta. The main pulmonary artery originates from septation of the truncus arteriosus. A dual supply then develops between the central pulmonary arteries derived from the sixth arch and the systemic arteries. Involution of the systemic arteries occurs by the eighth week of gestation. Failure to coalesce and/or failure to involute can lead to a wide range of anatomical sources of blood supply to the pulmonary bed. The supply to any given segment may be solely derived from systemic arteries, the central pulmonary arteries, or a combination of both. The findings of abnormal pulmonary blood supply and branching are termed abnormalities of arborization.

Central Pulmonary Arteries

The central pulmonary arteries may be confluent (Figure 115-2), nonconfluent, or absent (Figure 115-3). If present, the size of the central pulmonary arteries can vary from just over a millimeter (Figure 115-4) to normal size. Small confluent pulmonary arteries have a characteristic appearance of a "gull wing" as shown in Figures 115-2 and 115-4. Nonconfluent central pulmonary arteries receive blood supply from an ipsilateral ductus arteriosus or intraparenchymal connections from an aortopulmonary collateral. Bilateral patent ducti with supply to the ipsilateral central PA may also occur. Nonconfluence may be acquired from ductal insertion site stenosis or from surgical complications.

Aortopulmonary Artery Collaterals

The systemic to pulmonary collaterals are known by the acronym of MAPCAs (major or multiple aortopulmonary collateral artery or arteries).

Rabinovitch and colleagues[16] reported three different types of collaterals: (1) primitive intersegmental arteries that have not involuted. They usually number from two to six and are what most surgeons would think of as a MAPCA (see Figure 115-3); (2) indirect arteries from arch vessels, usually the subclavian artery (Figure 115-5); (3) bronchial arteries which preexist, follow the major bronchi, and subsequently develop intraparenchymal connections to the pulmonary artery. Bronchial arteries are small and not utilized in unifocalization procedures.

MAPCAs are systemic arteries that have a muscular media. Within the lung parenchyma they become typical

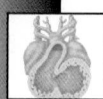

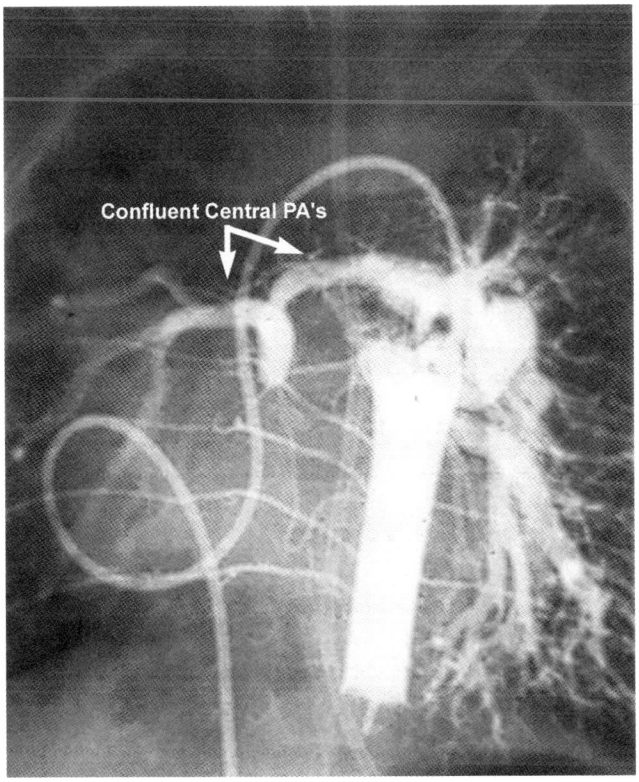

Figure 115–2 Small confluent central pulmonary arteries. Characteristic "gull wing" appearance fed by collateral connections in the left lung parenchyma.

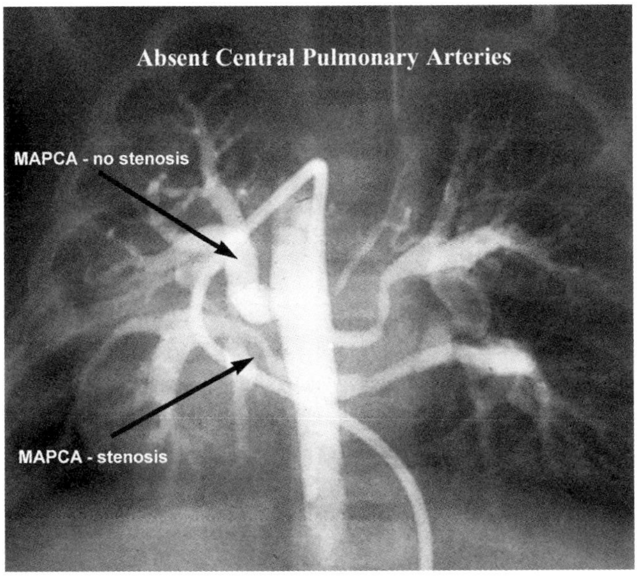

Figure 115–3 Five aortopulmonary collaterals supplying the lung parenchyma. No central pulmonary arteries (gull wing) are seen. The right upper collateral shows no stenosis, that portion of lung is at risk for pulmonary vascular occlusive disease. The right lower collateral and others show proximal stenosis. Individual collateral hemodynamic measurements would be needed for a child presenting at greater than 6 months of age.

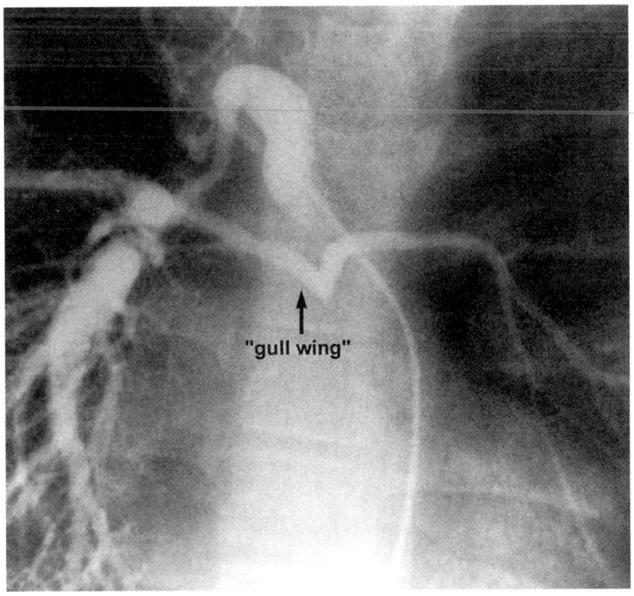

Figure 115–4 Very small central pulmonary arteries seen as a "gull wing."

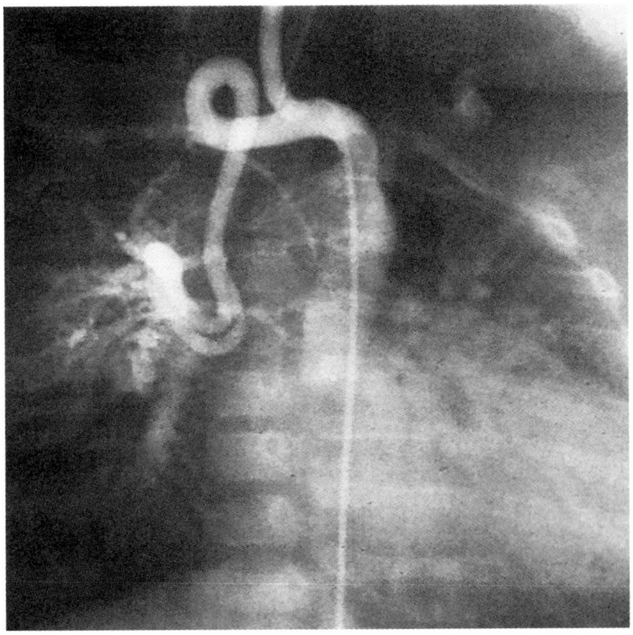

Figure 115–5 A collateral arising from the right subclavian artery.

pulmonary arteries without muscularization. MAPCAs may cause local pulmonary vascular changes. That is, the lung segments supplied by an MAPCA may see systemic pressure and thereby develop medial hypertrophy or even luminal obliteration. Paradoxically, many MAPCAs develop significant proximal stenosis over time thereby preventing the development of pulmonary vascular hypertensive changes.

Other collaterals to the pulmonary vasculature may arise directly from the chest wall as small collaterals related to cyanosis or even from coronary arteries and other places. Some have described an unusual situation in which the collateral arises as a persistence of the fifth vascular arch.[27]

NATURAL HISTORY

Unrepaired PA/VSD has a variable history dependent on the anatomy of the pulmonary arteries. Neonates with ductus arteriosus–dependent circulation and confluent pulmonary arteries without MAPCAs suffer an early hypoxic death as a result of ductus arteriosus closure. Children with MAPCAs that communicate with a central pulmonary artery may have adequate pulmonary blood flow, despite ductal closure, and be only mildly cyanotic into their second decade of life. In contrast, infants without restriction to MAPCA-derived pulmonary blood flow may have excessive pulmonary circulation and present with heart failure in early infancy. With a fortuitously well-balanced pulmonary blood flow, survival without treatment may extend into their third and fourth decades of life. Rarely would individuals survive into their fifth decade of life.[15]

Pulmonary hypertension may develop in segments of lung which have unobstructed flow from an MAPCA. There are also patients who lose "normal" antegrade flow to some segments of lung because of acquired occlusion or stenosis in an MAPCA thereby worsening cyanosis.

In a study published in 1995 on PA/VSD/MAPCAs, Bull and colleagues[3] reviewed 218 patients presenting at two institutions over the course of 26 years. Including those receiving intervention and those not receiving intervention, the survival at 1 year was 60%. Of those alive at 1 year, 65% survived to their 10th birthday. From age 10 to 35 only 16% survived.

Sixty-five percent of children presented in infancy with 50% being cyanotic, 25% having heart failure, and 25% having "well-balanced" circulation. Subsequent death was most commonly associated with a cardiac operation although cyanosis and heart failure were also causes of death. Sudden unexpected death occurred in a rare older patient. Estimated overall survival at 1 year, 10 years, 20 years, and 30 years was 60%, 40%, 25%, and 20%, respectively. Although the preceding data do not fully reflect current strategies and outcomes, it illustrates how morbid the treatment of PA/VSD/MAPCAs may be.

HISTORY OF REPAIR

PA/VSD was first repaired by Lillehei and reported in his series of controlled cross circulation in 1955.[14] Problems of repairing PA/VSD with small pulmonary arteries and abnormal pulmonary vasculature arborization were apparent in the 1960s and 1970s. Reports of RV to PA conduits or central shunts to establish antegrade flow to the pulmonary arteries in order to achieve growth of the central PAs were encouraging.[8,13] Details of MAPCAs and their characteristics became increasingly clear in the 1970s. Haworth and Macartney[9] reported the concept of connecting MAPCAs together (unifocalization) as a preliminary step to achieving complete repair. Sequential unifocalization of each lungs MAPCAs followed by central connection and complete repair was the treatment modality of the 1980s and early 1990s. In some institutions staged unifocalization continues to be the treatment of choice.

In 1995 Reddy et al[17] reported single-stage bilateral unifocalization and complete repair in infants and children as a standard course of treatment. This was an extension of the concept of primary single-stage repair to patients with increasingly complex lesions.

ASSOCIATED ABNORMALITIES

Other biventricular lesions that may be present with PA/VSD are congenitally corrected transposition, double outlet right ventricle, d-transposition of the great vessels, and complete atrioventricular septal defect. Specifics of these associated lesions are discussed in their respective chapters.

Velo-cardio-facial syndrome characterized by developmental delay, typical facial and ear anomalies, nasal speech, and palate anomalies occurs in about 10% of PA/VSD.[12] There is a predilection for a right aortic arch and aberrant subclavian arteries in the subset with velo-cardio-facial syndrome. As a group a right aortic arch occurs in 20% of those having PA/VSD.

DiGeorge syndrome may also be associated with PA/VSD. The majority of those having Di George syndrome and some of those with velo-cardio-facial syndrome have associated microdeletion of chromosome 22q11. The acronym for this complex is CATCH 22—*c*ardiac defects, *a*bnormal facies, *t*hymic hypoplasia, *c*left palate and *h*ypocalcemia along with microdeletion of chromosome 22 q11. Deletion of chromosome 22 q11 is present in 30% of patients with PA/VSD and has a slightly higher prevalence in those having MAPCAs.[1]

PULMONARY ARTERY CLASSIFICATION

No single classification system has been identified although a useful one is illustrated in Figure 115-6 and has been adopted by the Congenital Heart Surgery Nomenclature and Database Project.[25]

CLINICAL PRESENTATION

Increasingly diagnosis of PA/VSD is being made in utero allowing for elective postnatal workup and development of a treatment plan. Presentation by natural history may be with cyanosis, heart failure, or a balanced circulation as described in the natural history section.

Ductus Arteriosus Dependent Circulation

Those children with ductal dependent pulmonary circulation present within the first few hours to weeks of life with profound cyanosis that correlates to ductal closure. Treatment with prostaglandin E1 usually reopens the duct and allows for an elective workup and planning for an operation.

Physical examination reveals mildly increased precordial activity. There is no split in the second heart sound. A continuous ductal murmur may be present. For very cyanotic infants only a soft early systolic murmur may be heard at the left sternal border. There may be a systolic ejection click at the apex related to a dilated ascending aorta. Pulses are full.

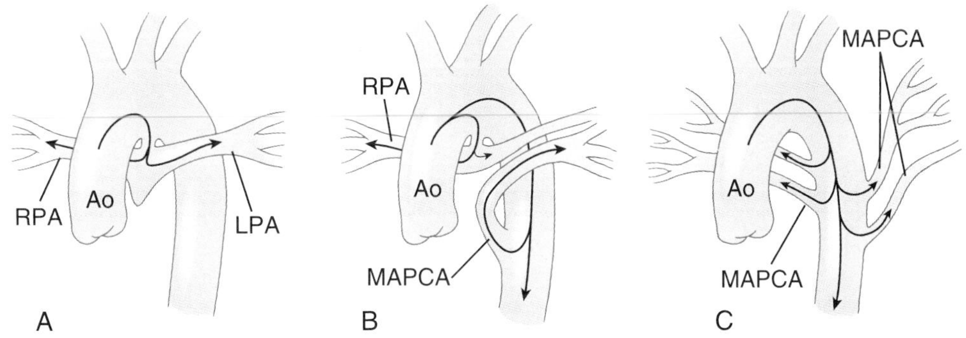

Figure 115–6 A useful pulmonary artery classification for PA/VSD. A, Presence of central pulmonary arteries without MAPCAs. **B,** Presence of central pulmonary arteries and MAPCAs. **C,** Absent central pulmonary arteries, lung blood supply primarily from MAPCAs. Within the first two categories are the potential for spectrum of size of the pulmonary arteries and confluence of the pulmonary arteries. The number of and size of MAPCAs usually varies from two to six.

Chest Radiography

There is an absent main pulmonary artery manifested as an exaggerated notch between the aorta and left heart border (Figure 115-7). The arch may be right sided. The lung fields are oligemic.

Electrocardiography

Assuming situs solitus and levocardia, the QRS axis is deviated rightward and can be as much as +180 degrees. Right ventricular hypertrophy is present. Peaked p waves associate with right atrial enlargement may be present.

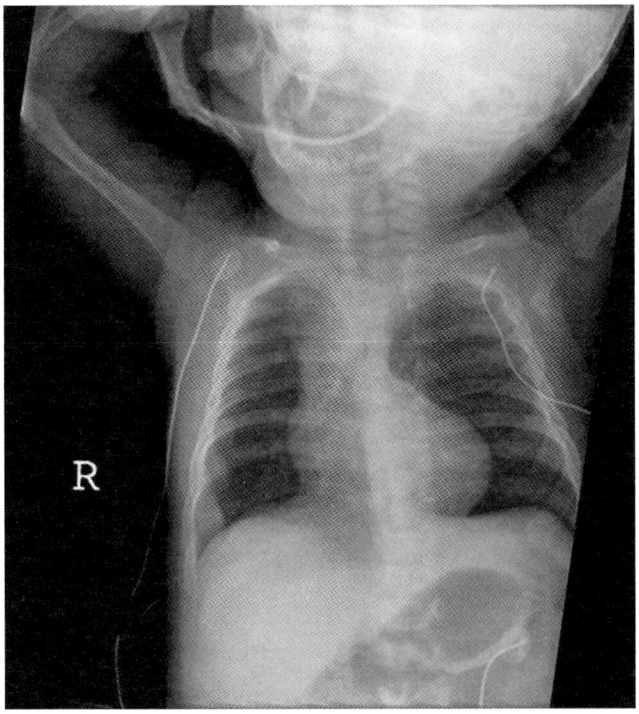

Figure 115–7 PA/VSD chest roentgenography. An exaggerated notch between the aorta and left heart is seen and is indicative of pulmonary atresia.

PA/VSD/MAPCAs

Children with MAPCAs may be "asymptomatic" for several years, if the pulmonary blood flow is appropriate, and present with only a mild degree of cyanosis or heart failure. Depending on the amount of pulmonary blood flow they may present with cyanosis, or tachypnea, dyspnea and an engorged liver. Those children in heart failure have a hyperdynamic precordium which may protrude because of an enlarged heart.

Cardiac sounds are that of a single second heart sound. There may be a continuous murmur in multiple locations related to the multiple positions of the MAPCAs. A diastolic flow murmur may be heard at the apex if the left-to-right shunt is substantial. An apical ejection click related to the large ascending aorta is common. Peripheral pulses may be strong just as one sees in aortic insufficiency.

Chest Radiography

Pulmonary vascular markings may be increased. The main pulmonary artery segment may be absent or small. The heart is generous in size.

Electrocardiography

Findings are similar to the ductal dependent child. There may be biventricular hypertrophy.

DIAGNOSTIC TECHNIQUES

Echocardiography

An experienced echocardiographer can reliably delineate intracardiac anatomy in a newborn. The finding of PA/VSD then leads to the question of the source of pulmonary blood flow and the status of the pulmonary arteries. In the majority of cases echocardiography is able to delineate the presence or absence of central pulmonary arteries and whether the pulmonary arteries are confluent. Central pulmonary size is also measured. Multiple sources of pulmonary blood flow can be identified although details of the multiple sources may not be well defined.

If confluent pulmonary arteries are present and there are no MAPCAs, no further diagnostic tests are needed. For the child who initially presents at age 2–3 months or older there are usually MAPCAs, and therefore further diagnostic workup is necessary.

Cardiac Catheterization

Cardiac catheterization continues to be the central diagnostic tool in the treatment of PA/VSD/MAPCAs. Multiplane cineangiography of balloon occlusion and retrograde injection of the aorta provides detailed views of the MAPCAs. Data elicited are number of collaterals, size of collaterals, stenosis in the collaterals, connections of collaterals to normal intraparenchymal pulmonary arteries, size of the central pulmonary arteries if present, and which lung segments are supplied by what origin of pulmonary blood flow.

Direct individual collateral injections may be necessary. In older children direct hemodynamic measurements of individual collaterals beyond stenosis can help to determine whether the supplied segments have been protected from the risk of pulmonary vascular hypertensive changes.

Catheterization with interventional occlusion of collaterals that are redundant in their supply of blood to various lung segments has been shown to be a useful tool to simplify later operations. Occlusion preoperatively should only be performed if the blood supply is clearly redundant and only if profound cyanosis will not occur. Test balloon occlusion assists in the decision making.

Magnetic Resonance Imaging

Magnetic resonance imaging (MRI) has emerged as a useful additive diagnostic measure. It is excellent for defining the number, location, and course of MAPCAs (Figure 115-8). Three-dimensional reconstructions can be achieved. Details of individual MAPCAs that are sometimes not clear on angiography, such as whether there is a single orifice at the level of the aorta, can sometimes be delineated with the additive findings in the MRI. Functional studies such as percentage of flow to a given lung or percentage of regurgitation in pulmonary insufficiency are emerging as useful evaluative tools.

Lung Perfusion Scan

Following unifocalization and repair, it is not unusual to have problems with stenosis of various arterial segments. Lung perfusion scans are useful to determine the functional extent of major branch pulmonary artery stenosis and to guide the timing and need for intervention. Both before and after surgery flow to areas of each lung can be delineated. Lung areas supplied by large nonstenotic collaterals that demonstrate paradoxically poor perfusion can be assumed to have localized pulmonary hypertension.

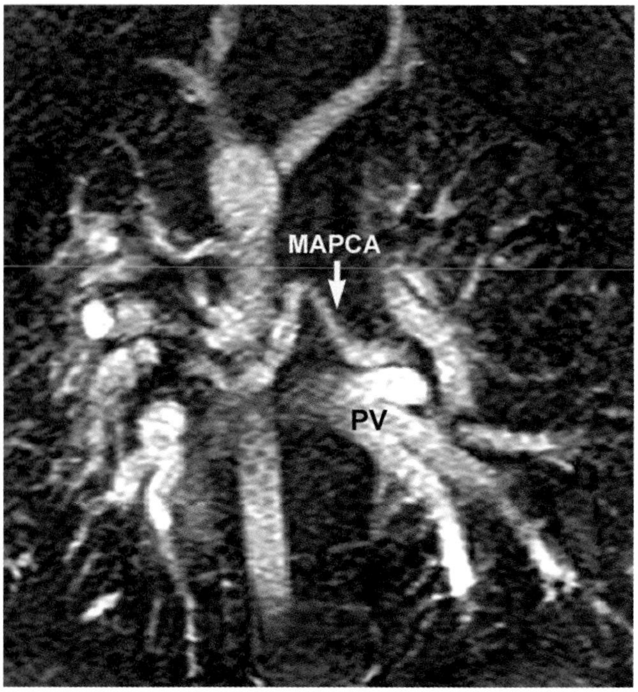

Figure 115-8 A magnetic resonance image (MRI) of PA/VSD provides additional information beyond catheterization. It is also a good for follow up as a noninvasive screen tool for development of stenosis and to characterize percentages of flow to each lung.

REPAIR STRATEGIES

Current repair strategies at our institution follow a decision-making algorithm as outlined in Figure 115-9. Most, but not all children, diagnosed today will be diagnosed either in utero or soon after birth. The first questions we seek to answer would be: What is the source of pulmonary blood flow, and is it reliable? Subsequently details of the pulmonary vasculature can be outlined using the previously described modalities.

Pulmonary Atresia/VSD/Absent MAPCAs/ Present Ductus Arteriosus

If a child has normal central pulmonary arteries that are supplied by a ductus arteriosus (see Figure 115-6) (referred to as "simple" PA/VSD), we would perform a primary repair within the first 2 weeks of life. Repair consists of ductal closure, closure of the VSD via a right ventriculotomy, and creation of a right ventricle to pulmonary artery (RV to PA) connection (Figure 115-10). Pulmonary valvar atresia associated with a main pulmonary artery is repaired with a transannular patch. Neonates with conal atresia are repaired with a RV to PA conduit of either homograft or bovine jugular vein material. The patent foramen ovale is narrowed to 3–4 mm. Conduit size is chosen by availability but we prefer a size that is a few millimeters larger than normal for that heart.

Repair is achieved with bicaval venous cannulation thereby obviating the need for circulatory arrest. In the neonate the sternum is frequently left open for a few days until myocardial and peripheral swelling subside. In some,

DECISION ALGORITHM

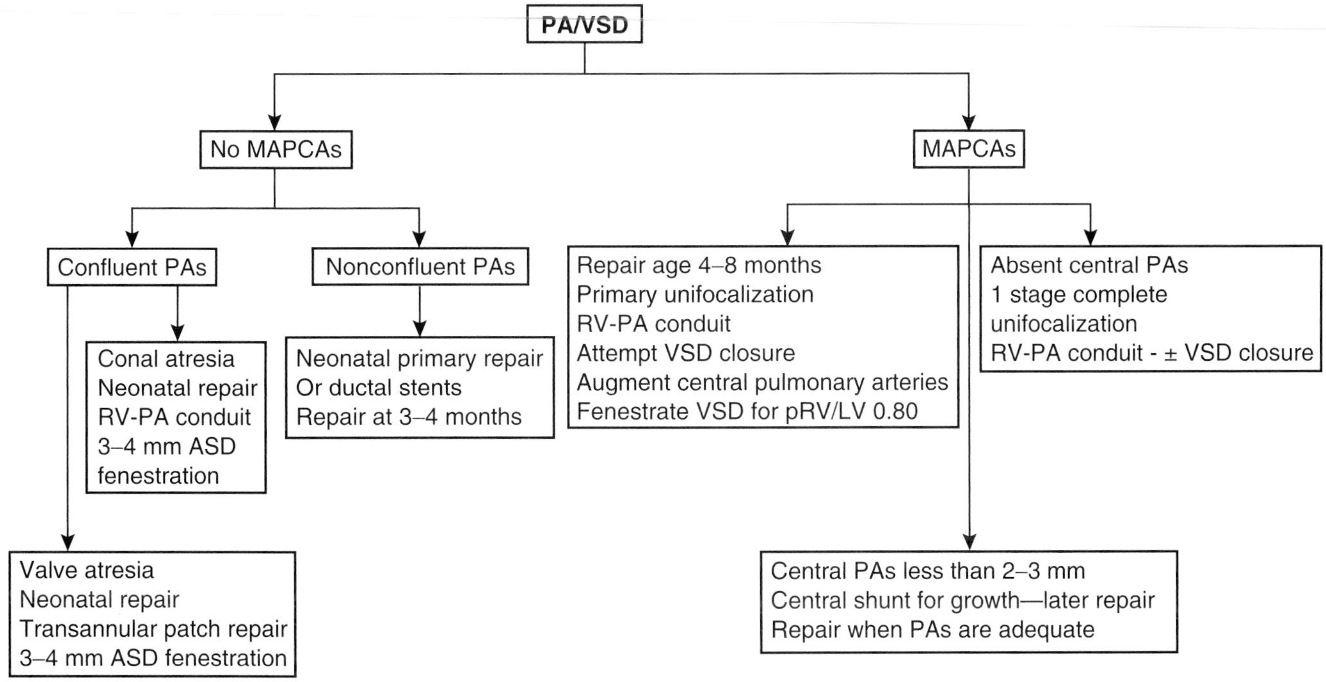

Figure 115–9 Decision algorithm for PA/VSD.

the position of the RV to PA conduit may be anterior and bulky making early sternal closure cause compression of the conduit. Myocardial swelling may make sternal closure cause a tissue-related tamponade effect. Both of these causes for delayed sternal closure resolve with decreased myocardial swelling over the course of a few days.

A peritoneal drain is left in place as a means of preventing abdominal compartment syndrome. The need for dialysis has been rare.

A second alternative for repair of "simple" PA/VSD is to perform a neonatal modified Blalock-Taussig shunt shortly after birth. The patent ductus is allowed to close or it is ligated. Full repair with VSD closure, a RV to PA conduit, and takedown of the BT shunts is then performed around 6–10 months of age. While there has been a broad trend toward primary repair, a number of programs continue the two-step approach with good outcomes.

Rationale for Single Stage or Two-Stage Repair in "Simple" PA/VSD

The rationale supporting a strategy of a systemic to pulmonary artery shunt followed by repair for simple PA/VSD is that neonatal right heart repair is associated with prolonged need for intensive care. Such morbidity may be associated with increased mortality. A Blalock-Taussig shunt for a neonate with a biventricular heart should be associated with little morbidity or mortality. If the pulmonary arteries are small they will grow because of increased pulmonary artery flow from the shunt.

The rationale for a single stage approach is that there is some mortality associated with neonatal shunts and there is risk of shunt thrombosis causing interval death. Shunts are also associated with pulmonary artery stenosis that may require augmentation. In an era of excellent arterial switch outcomes and markedly improved neonatal palliative outcomes for hypoplastic left heart surgery, enough has been learned about neonatal management to preclude significant mortality with primary repair of "simple" PA/VSD.

While era outcomes are clearly different, in recent years in our institution, outcomes for "simple" PA/VSD are markedly better with primary repair.

It is unusual but conceivable that the native pulmonary arteries in "simple" PA/VSD may be only 2–3 mm in size for a normal-weight term baby. In such instances complete repair may not be possible. Growth of the pulmonary arteries can be achieved by an attempt at primary repair with subsequent VSD fenestration if needed or alternatively by a Blalock-Taussig shunt. We have not found small pulmonary arteries in "simple" PA/VSD that preclude complete primary repair.

Pulmonary Atresia/VSD/MAPCAs

Surgical therapy for repair of infants with MAPCAs associated with PA/VSD is much more complex. The long-term goal of therapy is to achieve blood supply to all segments of lung, from central branch pulmonary arteries. The process is known as unifocalization (see Figure 115-10A)—a descriptive term of anastomosing MAPCAs to a confluence with a single source of blood supply. Unifocalization and complete repair may be achieved in one operation or may occur in multiple stages using a variety of techniques.

Our practice has evolved to performing single stage unifocalization of all pulmonary artery segments even if there is redundant supply. An RV to PA conduit is placed at the same

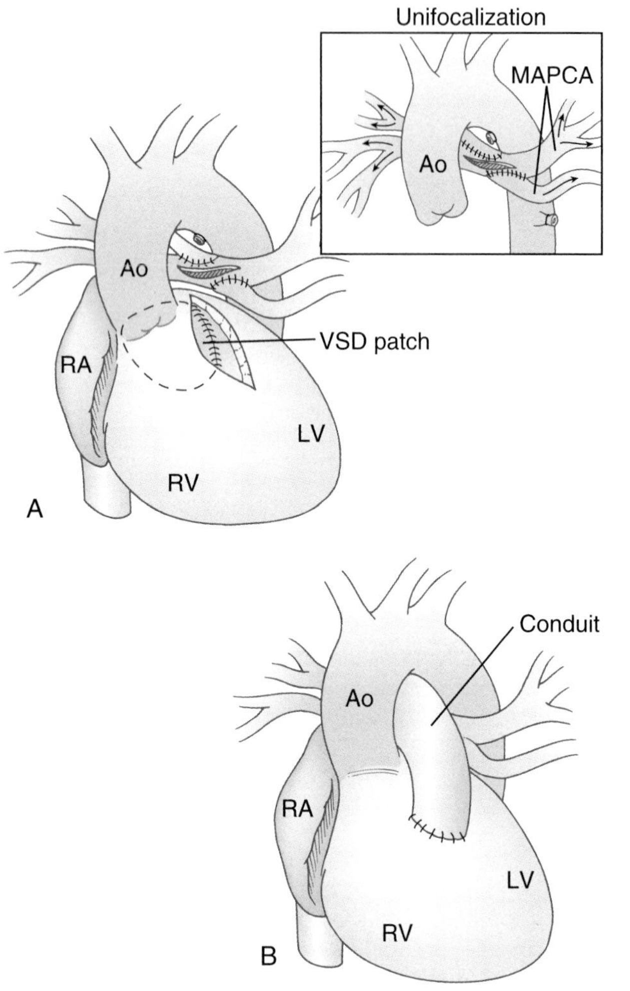

Figure 115–10 **A,** Ventriculotomy and patch closure of the VSD. **B,** RV-PA conduit. **Inset:** Unifocalization of two MAPCAs (no need for "simple" PA/VSD).

setting and the VSD is closed. Right ventricular pressures as high as 70% to 80% of systemic pressures are accepted following repair. For higher pressures, with or without hemodynamic instability, the VSD patch is fenestrated. Fenestrating the VSD allows for good systemic cardiac output. Without fenestration for systemic or suprasystemic RV pressures, the risk of death increases, causes of death are RV failure and/or inadequate systemic cardiac output because of poor LV preload volume. The VSD is fenestrated by cutting out the central portion of the patch and leaving a rim of patch material so that there is potential for future interventional catheterization closure of the created defect.

Rationale for Early Single Stage Unifocalization for PA/VSD/MAPCAs

The rationale for single stage early unifocalization and repair is that one can incorporate all segments of blood supply to the lung before stenosis develop in the MAPCAs and before potential changes of pulmonary hypertension occur. Our preferred age for single staged repairs would be in the range of 4 to 8 months of age. Reasons for repair at that age are an improved tolerance of long operations as compared to younger infancy, and it is typically prior to the development of risks of pulmonary hypertensive vascular changes or the development of MAPCA stenosis. Earlier repair would be indicated for saturations percentages below 70 or if there is an unreliable source of pulmonary blood flow.

Technique for Single Stage Complete Unifocalization

The approach for single stage unifocalization and complete repair is by a sternotomy or clamshell anterior bilateral thoracotomy. Our choice has been a sternotomy. Mobilization of the central pulmonary arteries is achieved. The MAPCAs are isolated by dissection of the posterior mediastinum through "windows" cephalad and caudad to both the left and right bronchus. Retraction of the aorta leftward allows for dissection of the posterior mediastinum. Detailed knowledge of the MAPCAs is required to ensure that control of each is obtained prior to initiating cardiopulmonary bypass. Without vascular control of the MAPCAs, blood flow to the lungs may "steal" cerebral and systemic flow and also prevent adequate perfusion pressure—a potentially morbid or lethal problem. Figure 115-11 shows a "map" that we take to the operating room to guide dissection.

Following dissection of all MAPCAs, cardiopulmonary bypass is instituted and the proximal portion of each MAPCA is snared. If the central pulmonary arteries are small they are opened from hilum to hilum. Each MAPCA is divided adjacent to the aorta, shortened to the appropriate length and sometimes rerouted under a bronchus or the esophagus so that there is minimal distance to the lung from the anastomotic site. The MAPCA is spatulated open. A back or side wall anastomosis to the nearest portion of the central pulmonary arteries is achieved with fine monofilament suture (see Figure 115-10). Shortening of the MAPCAs allows exclusion of some areas of narrowing. Occasionally stenosis in the MAPCAs requires placement of a stent or patch angioplasty. Following unifocalization the

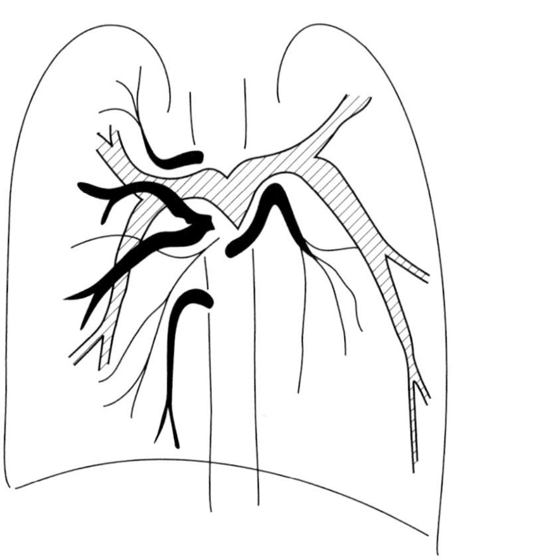

Figure 115–11 **Synthesized drawing of angiographic and MRI data for a patient with PA/VSD/MAPCAs.** Nonshaded arteries are the pulmonary arteries. Shaded arteries are MAPCAs. This drawing is posted in the operating room for the surgeon to use as a map.

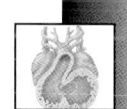

anterior aspect of the central pulmonary arteries is augmented with autologous pericardium if needed.

Single stage unifocalization and repair require long bypass times. Reddy and colleagues[17] reported a median cardiopulmonary bypass time of 265 minutes and median cross clamp time of 58 minutes.

Rationale for Staged Unifocalization

The rationale for staged unifocalization centers around the fact that central pulmonary arteries in PA/VSD/MAPCAs are frequently small and need to be "rehabilitated" to normal size by augmenting central pulmonary artery flow with an aortopulmonary artery shunt or a RV to PA conduit. MAPCAs that have peripheral stenosis need to be addressed at the time of unifocalization. To gain exposure to the distal MAPCA, hilar and intraparenchymal dissection is facilitated through unilateral or staged bilateral thoracotomies. Identification and mobilization of MAPCAs is much easier through a posterolateral thoracotomy than a sternotomy approach. Single stage unifocalization is a long and tedious procedure that can be very physiologically stressful to a child. Staged unifocalization simplifies each individual case and breaks it up into more physiologically tolerated segments.

Staged Unifocalization

More than one approach is advocated for staged unifocalization.* Staged repairs are broadly based on two strategies: (1) central pulmonary artery-based repairs achieved by first inducing growth of the central PAs with a central shunt or with an RV to PA conduit (Figure 115-12). Staged unifocalization and VSD closure is subsequently performed. (2) Staged thoracotomy-based unifocalization of MAPCAs with insertion of a systemic to pulmonary artery shunt to the created ipsilateral pulmonary arterial confluence (Figure 115-13). The final procedure of the latter approach entails creating central pulmonary arteries, if needed, to connect the blood supply to each hilum, a RV to PA conduit, and VSD closure.

*References 5, 6, 11, 15, 21, 22.

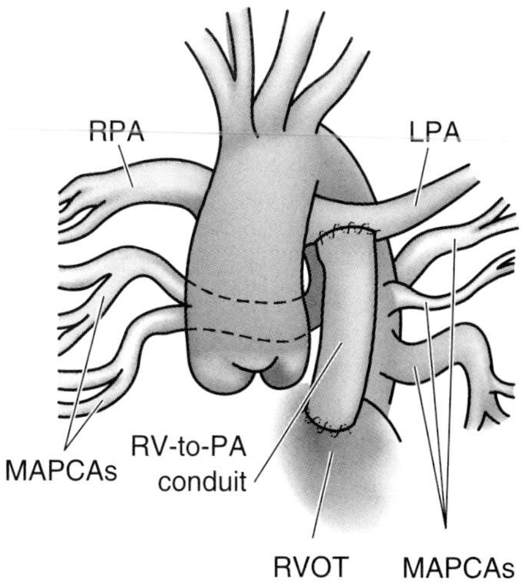

Figure 115-12 Right ventricle to pulmonary artery conduit inserted to achieve central pulmonary artery growth. The RV to PA connection allows access for balloon angioplasty of more peripheral pulmonary arteries. Following adequate pulmonary artery growth, staged unifocalization is achieved along with VSD closure and replacement of the RV-PA connection. Subsequent completion of the repair can be performed as one or two procedures.

Those who perform central pulmonary artery-based repairs for PA/VSD/MAPCAs perform some single stage complete repairs in highly selected cases.[6,15] However, they argue that near normal-sized central branch pulmonary arteries are needed and the unifocalization should be simple. Small central pulmonary arteries are seen as unfavorable and need to be "rehabilitated." Central shunts and RV to PA conduits have both been shown to effectively increase central pulmonary artery size. Catheter-based interventions are subsequently used to rehabilitate local areas of stenosis with either balloon dilation or stent insertion.

Following growth of the central pulmonary arteries, redundant MAPCAs are coiled or surgically ligated at the time of staged unifocalization. Staged sequential thoracotomies (or sometimes through a sternotomy or both) are

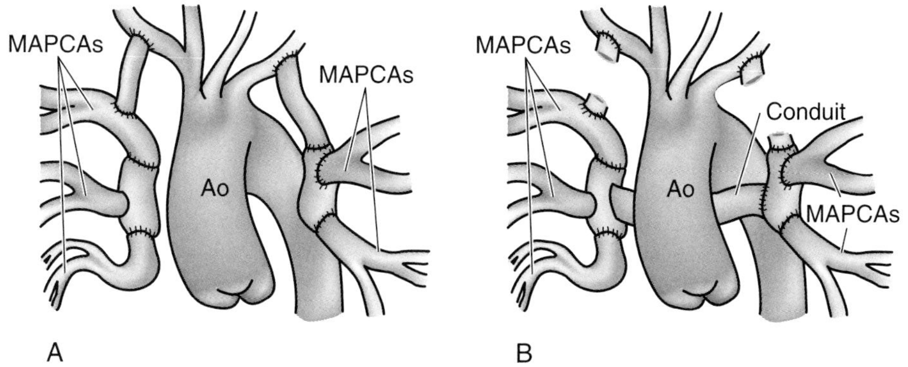

Figure 115-13 A, Sequential thoracotomies are used to unifocalize all pulmonary arterial supply. If the central branch pulmonary arterial branch is too small for unifocalization anastomosis, a pericardial tube may be created. A central or Blalock-Taussig shunt is placed as the source of ipsilateral pulmonary blood flow. **B,** Creation of central pulmonary arteries with a homograft or polytetrafluoroethylene tube is done as a third procedure. The shunts are taken down and VSD closure is performed along with insertion of an RV-PA conduit.

performed to unifocalize each lung's nonredundant MAPCAs to the corresponding pulmonary artery. Subsequent VSD closure with establishment of an appropriate RV to PA connection is done as a separate operation. Decisions in staged unifocalization are individualized for each case making combining one stage with another possible, for example, unifocalizing one lung's MAPCAs may be combined with VSD closure and an RV to PA conduit.

Sequential unifocalization based on the MAPCAs approach is performed through sequential thoracotomies.[5] All the blood supply to all the segments of lung on that side are anastomosed to a common vascular confluence that might be the ipsilateral native pulmonary artery (if it is of suitable size for use) or a created pericardial channel. A systemic to pulmonary artery shunt is placed to augment the blood supply to the ipsilateral lung. In a second operation unifocalization is performed for the other lung. If the native central pulmonary arteries are an inadequate connection between the unifocalized vasculature of the right and left lung, this is achieved with an interpulmonary conduit (essentially new central pulmonary arteries) at the time of the RV-PA conduit insertion and VSD closure.

Irrespective of the strategy for repair, proponents of a given strategy have demonstrated a crossover to another strategy if it appeared to be in the patient's best interest.[6,21]

Anatomical Predictors of Successful VSD Closure

Independent of how many stages it takes to achieve final unifocalization and an appropriate RV to PA connection, the ability of the pulmonary vascular bed to accept a full cardiac output at an RV pressure of 60% to 70% of systemic determines whether one can successfully close the VSD. Most surgeons suggest that a minimum of 12 to 14 lung segments are required.

Absolute size of the arteries is also important. Two methods of quantifying size of the pulmonary arteries are used. One is to calculate the pulmonary artery area index for all MAPCAs and central pulmonary arteries, a useful technique for the MAPCA based unifocalization procedures. If the index is greater that 150 mm2/m2 then successful closure is likely.[5]

Another technique of determining whether the central pulmonary arteries are large enough for complete repairs is to use the Birmingham formula that predicts a postoperative RV to LV pressure ratio.[2,11]

$$pRV/LV = 0.484[\text{dia. RPA/dia. Ao} + \text{dia. LPA/dia. A Ao}] + 0.2007$$

where p = pressure, dia. = diameter, Ao = aorta, RPA = right pulmonary artery, and LPA = left pulmonary artery. Measurements of the pulmonary arteries are at the hilum.

Successful repair is thought to be achievable for predicted pressure ratios of less than 70%.[11]

However, success of VSD closure may not be predictable. There is a component of anatomical analysis that is based on assumptions of normal flow, normal pulmonary intraparenchymal architecture, and perfect anatomical repair. Assumptions may be wrong and in the end, successful closure of the VSD is dependent on the physiological findings of systolic RV pressure less than 80% of systolic systemic pressure (preferably less than two-thirds of systemic) along with good systemic hemodynamics. Near systemic, suprasystemic RV pressures, or systemic pressure instability attributable to left ventricular filling, require creating an ample fenestration in the VSD to prevent acute right ventricular failure or later sudden death.

Functional Predictors of Successful VSD Closure

Evidence of a net left-to-right shunt across the VSD, following unifocalization in children who failed one stage primary repair or who have undergone intentional multistage repairs, is a good indicator that the pulmonary vascular bed is receptive to high pulmonary flow with low right ventricular pressures. Saturation percentages are typically in the high 80s or low 90s. There may be evidence of fluid retention and congestive heart failure on chest roentgenography.

Reddy and Hanley[18] have described an intraoperative functional technique for prediction of successful closure of a VSD. Following unifocalization and while still on cardiopulmonary bypass, flow is introduced to the pulmonary vasculature at a cardiac index of 2.5 liters/min. A pressure, for that flow rate, of less the 30 mm Hg was predictive of successful closure of the VSD.

SPECIAL SITUATIONS

Extremely Small Central Pulmonary Arteries

Those who advocate single-stage unifocalization and repair recognize that the approach requires a minimum pulmonary artery size. The central pulmonary arteries may be confluent but only about 2 mm in size. Single stage unifocalization is unlikely to be successful. A direct aorta to pulmonary artery connection can facilitate growth of the central pulmonary arteries and allow for later repair.[11,21] The likelihood of undergoing subsequent complete repair has been reported to be as high as 61%.[21]

Alternatively, an RV to PA rigid nonvalved conduit (such as Gore-Tex or Dacron) has been shown to also increase central pulmonary artery size.[11,22]

Nonconfluent Central Pulmonary Arteries

Nonconfluent central pulmonary arteries by necessity have differing sources of blood flow. Usually the left pulmonary artery arises from a patent ductus arteriosus. The right pulmonary artery may be supplied by a second ductus arteriosus or an aortopulmonary collateral. Nonconfluent pulmonary arteries are at risk of becoming atretic and thereby not being present for use in unifocalization. Early establishment of confluence with a reliable source of central pulmonary blood flow is mandatory.[23,24] Occasionally, stents in the ductus may allow for reliable flow to the associated pulmonary artery preserving it for unifocalization at an appropriate elective date.

Age at Repair for PA/VSD/MAPCAs

When the diagnosis is known at birth, we currently attempt single stage repair at 4–8 months of age. Repair at an earlier age is possible but only necessary for profound cyanosis. Timing of repair may be dependent on age of referral—some children are not recognized to have the disease until an older age. Our choice of age for repair is intended to achieve unifocalization prior to the development of any pulmonary vascular hypertensive changes and on achieving unifocalization prior to loosing segments of lung to stenosis or atresia of MAPCAs or central pulmonary arteries.

HSC Experience

At the Hospital for Sick Children in Toronto between July 1982 and March 2003, 251 infants and children under the age of 18 years were operated for PA/VSD. Of those, 182 (72.5%) had "simple" PA/VSD and 69 (27.5%) had PA/VSD/MAPCAs. Actuarial survival for the entire operated cohort is seen in Figure 115-14.

"Simple" PA/VSD

Operative survival for the entire cohort of "simple PA/VSD" was 86.1%. Ninety children (49.4%) had multiple stage complete repair. Forty-seven (26%) had a single stage complete repair. Of those without complete repair (45 children, 24.7%) 20 patients died prior to complete repair, 15 were lost to follow-up in their country of origin, 4 are awaiting complete repair, and 6 have other reasons for lack of follow-up or incomplete repair. Survival for primary repair versus staged repair for "simple" PA/VSD is shown in Figure 115-15. The difference in survival is not statistically significant but the curves do not reflect data relating to era. Operative survival for single stage repair in the past 7 years has been 100% (n = 33).

PA/VSD/MAPCAs

Of the 69 children with PA/VSD/MAPCAs, 57 (82.6%) have undergone attempts at complete repair with either multiple-stage unifocalization and VSD closure or single-stage unifocalization and VSD closure. Multiple-stage attempted

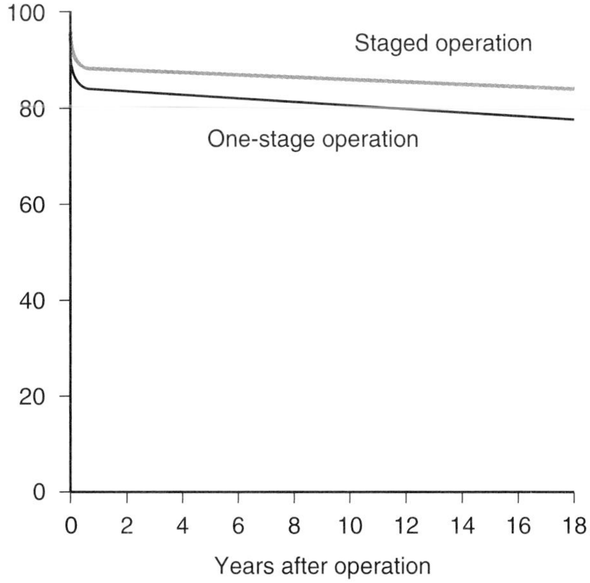

Figure 115–15 Actuarial survival of single stage repair and multi-stage repair for "simple" PA/VSD. There is no difference between the groups. The curves do not reflect era. Survival for single stage repair in the past 7 years is 100% (n = 33).

complete repair was performed in 25 children (36%) of whom 2 (8%) had a hemodynamic need for a residual VSD. Operative mortality was 12% (n = 3). Attempted single stage complete repair was performed in 32 children of whom 12 had a hemodynamic need for a residual VSD (37.5%). Operative mortality was 21.8%. Twelve children were not considered candidates for complete repair and received palliation only. Survival curves for single- versus multiple-stage attempts at repair of PA/VSD/MAPCAs are shown in Figure 115-16. Operative mortality for attempted single-stage repair

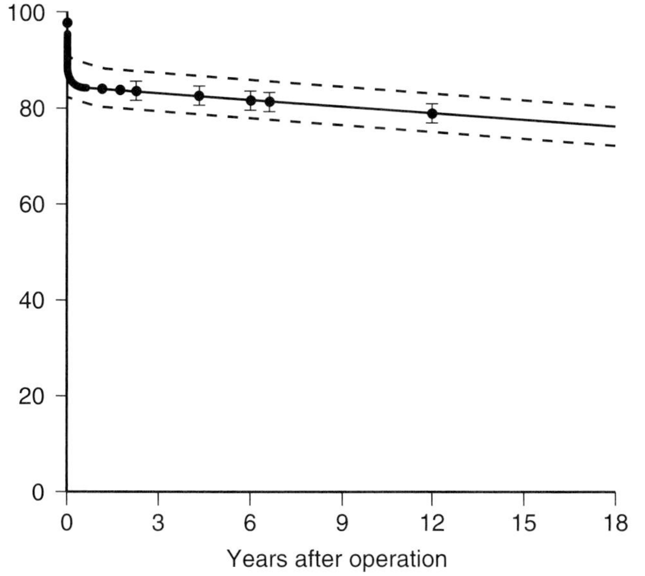

Figure 115–14 Actuarial survival curve for "simple" PA/VSD and PA/VSD/MAPCAs combined. Ninety-five percent confidence intervals are shown.
(Data from the Hospital for Sick Children, Toronto, July 1982 to March 2003.)

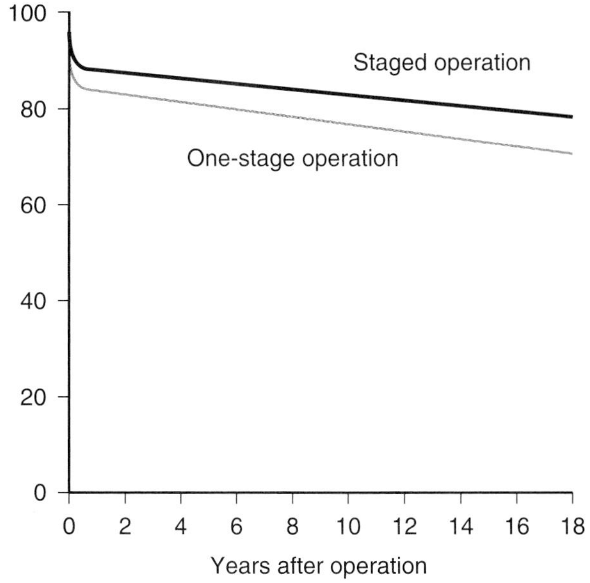

Figure 115–16 Actuarial survival curve for single- versus multiple-stage repair of PA/VSD/MAPCAs. There was no difference between groups.

in the past 7 years was 14% (4 of 28 children). One third (32%) of those children required a residual VSD.

COMPLICATIONS

Early

Operative mortality in the current era for primary repair "simple" PA/VSD is 0% to 3%. Operative mortality for primary unifocalization and repair for PA/VSD/MAPCAs is 10% to 20%.[19] Despite complete unifocalization of all available segments, some children having PA/VSD/MAPCAs will never have an appropriate pulmonary vascular bed to allow closure of the VSD. Reasons for an inability to tolerate VSD closure would be irreversible pulmonary hypertensive changes, inadequate growth of the unifocalized pulmonary arteries, or diffuse pulmonary arterial stenosis not amenable to surgical or catheter-based therapy.

Some children having unifocalization without VSD closure may suffer from profound cyanosis. Increasing intraventricular pressure by elevating systemic vascular resistance may improve pulmonary blood flow.

On the other end of the spectrum are children who have a nearly adequate pulmonary vasculature but not quite sufficient to avoid a fenestrated VSD. These children may have saturations that increase over 90% in the first few weeks following repair and require early closure of the VSD by reoperation or catheter-based device closure.

Complete repair of simple or complex PA/VSD may be associated with impaired right ventricular diastolic function. Restrictive right ventricular physiology is characterized by antegrade flow in the pulmonary artery during diastole as a result of atrial contraction (i.e., the right ventricle is stiff and lacks compliance for diastolic filling). Consequently the atrium assists in pulmonary blood flow. Maintenance of sinus rhythm is important in the presence of restrictive physiology. A patent foramen ovale allows for right-to-left shunting at the atrial level. We routinely leave a patent foramen for neonatal repairs. Despite poor RV compliance a good systemic cardiac output can be maintained. This intracardiac shunt may cause desaturation to percentages as low as the middle 70s. Although desaturation is not ideal, it is well tolerated in patients with satisfactory systemic cardiac output. In contrast, avoidance of cyanosis by eliminating a potential right-to-left shunt, may occur at the expense of inadequate systemic cardiac output that may be lethal. Full saturation returns when RV compliance improves.

Heart block can occur related to the VSD closure in about 1%. Phrenic nerve palsy related to extensive mediastinal dissection occasionally complicates recovery. Ipsilateral diaphragm plication is performed if respiratory mechanics are significantly impaired. Chylothorax caused by the extensive mediastinal dissection may occur. Expectant management with a median chain triglyceride diet or with parenteral nutrition is usually all that is required. Occasionally thoracic duct ligation through a right thoracotomy may be beneficial. Recalcitrant chylothorax can sometimes successfully be treated with a somatostatin analog. Pleurodesis should be avoided particularly if future thoracotomy might be needed.

Systemic pressure or near-systemic pressure in the reconstructed right ventricular outflow may lead to the development of a pseudoaneurysm in the right ventricular outflow tract. We perform echocardiographic screening for pseudoaneurysms in all children with high RV pressures prior to discharge and at a postoperative visit. Rupture of a pseudoaneurysm may be catastrophic.

Late

Later complications include failure to achieve, at anytime, an adequate pulmonary vascular bed for VSD closure. Children with persistent right-to-left shunts through a VSD or increasing RV pressures following closure need cardiac catheterization to determine whether portions of the vascular tree may be rehabilitated using interventional techniques. Figure 115-17 shows a unifocalized portion of the right pulmonary vasculature before and after balloon rehabilitation techniques. Placement of pulmonary artery stents may also be useful.[26]

Planned postoperative surveillance with echocardiographic estimates of right ventricular pressure can help to determine when cardiac catheterization investigation is needed.

Nearly all children undergoing implantation of an RV to PA conduit will need conduit replacement. Most homografts develop stenosis overtime. Stenosis is related to conduit shrinkage/fibrosis and/or calcification. Longevity of the con-

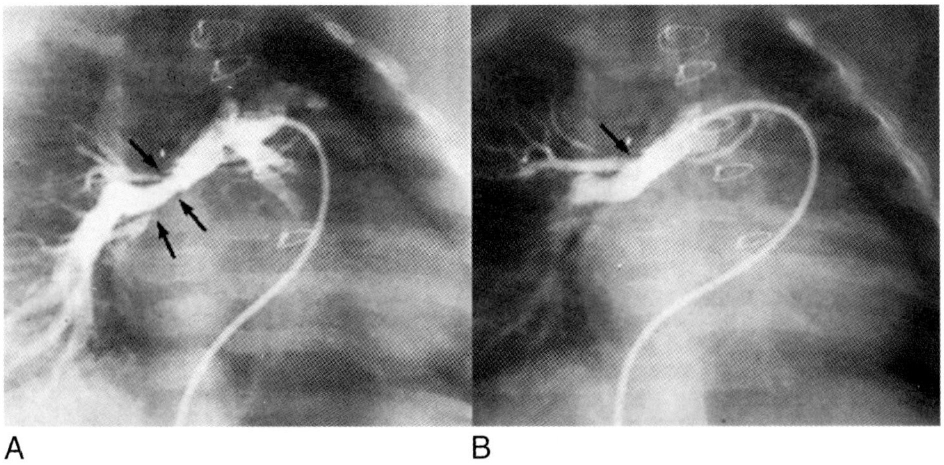

Figure 115–17 **A,** Stenosed unifocalized segments to the right pulmonary artery. **B,** Improved right pulmonary artery and segmental branches following balloon angioplasty. The lower branches are not well seen but also improved with balloon angioplasty.

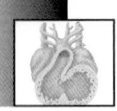

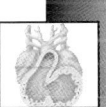

duit may be improved by a few years with stent implantation within the conduit. Nevertheless, the most important predictor for need of conduit replacement is younger age of insertion.[4] Cho and colleagues[6] reported the need for reoperation of 55% at 10 years for those having a complete repair of PA/VSD.

One to two percent of patients will develop late aortic insufficiency and in some cases aortic root dilation requiring valve and root replacement.[6]

Our experience suggests the potential impact of segmental or regional stenosis can be delineated with lung perfusion scans and/or a MRI. For example, a stenosis identified by MRI to be present in a major segment feeding the left lung can have its functional impact evaluated with MRI-based flow studies and/or a perfusion scan. Findings of a flow ratio to the left lung of 15% would indicate that elevated right ventricular pressures might improve dramatically with successful treatment of stenosis. On the other hand, a flow ratio to the left lung of 35% would indicate that the stenosis is a less important cause of elevated right ventricular pressure.

OTHER SELECTED INSTITUTIONAL OUTCOMES

In a series of 495 patients with PA/VSD with or without MAPCAs operated over a 22-year period, the Mayo Clinic reported complete repair in 63% of patients.[6] An additional 9% had the possibility of complete repair. Complete repair was performed as a one-stage procedure in 29%, the remaining complete repair patients had a mean of 1.5 surgical procedures prior to the complete repair. Average RV/LV pressure ratio at the completion of repair was 0.66. Surgical mortality for those having complete repair was 4.5 %. Of those who survived complete repair, actuarial survival was 83% at 15 years. Risks for operative mortality were need for reopening the VSD, an RV/LV pressure ratio of greater that 0.7, male sex, and need for a pulmonary artery confluence graft. Late follow-up causes of death were primarily cardiac failure, arrhythmia, bronchospasm-respiratory failure, and conduit change.

In the same Mayo Clinic series, the most recent era mortality for palliated patients was 7.6%. Those who survived palliation had an actuarial survival of 61% at 15 years.

Reddy and Hanley[19] reported intermediate term outcomes with early primary repair of PA/VSD/MAPCAs in 85 patients with a median age of 7 months. One-stage unifocalization was performed in 90% of children. Complete one-stage repair (with VSD closure) was performed in 66%. Operative mortality was 10%. Actuarial survival was 80% at 3 years for the entire group. For those children who underwent complete repair, actuarial survival was 88% at 2 years. Nearly 30% required reintervention on the newly reconstructed pulmonary arteries.

Heart–Lung Transplantation

Heart–lung transplantation is theoretically an attractive solution for unsuccessfully palliated cases of PA/VSD/MAPCAs. While case reports or small series of successful transplants have been published,[20] there are no successful large series of heart/lung transplantation in PA/VSD/MAPCAs.

SUMMARY

These two large series and the experience in Toronto illustrate that ideal solutions for PA/VSD remain to be found. Operative mortality for "simple" PA/VSD is low but the RV to PA conduit requires replacement. Unifocalization of PA/VSD/MAPCAs in one or more stages improves the chances for complete repair; however, one-third or more of these children are unable to undergo complete repair. Operative mortality for the complex cases still ranges from 5% to 20%.

REFERENCES

1. Anaclerio S, Marino B, Carotti A, et al: Pulmonary atresia with ventricular septal defect: prevalence of deletion 22q11 in the different anatomic patterns. Ital Heart J 2:384–387, 2001.
2. Blackstone EH, Kirklin JW, Bertranou EG, et al: Preoperative prediction from cineangiograms of post repair right ventricular pressure in tetralogy of Fallot. J Thorac Cardiovasc Surg 78:542–552, 1979.
3. Bull K, Somerville J, Ty E, Spiegelhalter D: Presentation and attrition in complex pulmonary atresia. J Am Coll Cardiol 25:491–499, 1995.
4. Caldarone CA, McCrindle BW, Van Arsdell GS, et al: Independent factors associated with longevity of prosthetic valves and valved conduits. J Thorac Cardiovasc Surg 120:1022–1030, 2000.
5. Carotti A, Di Donato RM, Squiteri C, et al: Total repair of pulmonary atresia with ventricular septal defect and major aortopulmonary collaterals: an integrated approach. J Thorac Cardiovasc Surg 116:914–923, 1998.
6. Cho JM, Puga FJ, Danielson GK, et al: Early and long-term results of the surgical treatment of tetralogy of Fallot with pulmonary atresia, with or without major aortopulmonary collateral arteries. J Thorac Cardiovasc Surg 124:70–81, 2002.
7. DeRiuiter MC, Gittenberger-deGroot A, Poelmann RE, et al: Development of the pharyngeal arch system related to the pulmonary and bronchial vessels in the avian embryo. Circulation 87:1306–1319, 1993.
8. Gill CC, Moodie DS, McGoon DC: Stage surgical management of pulmonary atresia with diminutive pulmonary arteries. J Thorac Cardiovasc Surg 73:436, 1977.
9. Haworth SG, Macartney FJ: Growth and development of pulmonary circulation in pulmonary atresia with ventricular septal defect and major aortopulmonary collateral arteries. Br Heart J 44:14, 1980.
10. Haworth SG: Pulmonary vascular development. In: Long WA (ed): Fetal and Neonatal Cardiology. Philadelphia: WB Saunders, 1990, pp. 51–63.
11. Iyer KS, Mee RBB: Staged repair of pulmonary atresia with ventricular septal defect and major systemic to pulmonary artery collaterals. Ann Thorac Surg 51:65–72, 1991.
12. Jedele KB, Michels VV, Puga FJ, Feldt RH: Velo-cardio-facial syndrome associated with ventricular septal defect, pulmonary atresia, and hypoplastic pulmonary arteries. Pediatrics 89:915–919, 1992.
13. Kirklin JW, Bargeron LM Jr, Pacifico AD: The enlargement of small pulmonary arteries by preliminary palliative operations. Circulation 56:612, 1977.
14. Lillehei CW, Cohen M, Warden HE, et al: Direct vision intracardiac surgical correction of the tetralogy of Fallot, pentalogy of Fallot, and pulmonary atresia defects: report of first 10 cases. Ann Surg 142:418, 1955.

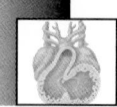

15. Marelli AJ, Perloff JK, Child JS, Laks H: Pulmonary atresia with ventricular septal defects in adults. Circulation 89:243–251, 1994.
16. Rabinovitch M, Herrera-DeLeon V, Castaneda AR, Reid L: Growth and development of the pulmonary vascular bed in patients with tetralogy of Fallot with or without pulmonary atresia. Circulation 64:1234–1249, 1981.
17. Reddy VM, Liddicoat JR, Hanley FL: Midline one-stage complete unifocalization and repair of pulmonary atresia with ventricular septal defect and major aortopulmonary collaterals. J Thorac Cardiovasc Surg 109:832–845, 1995.
18. Reddy VM, Petrossian E, McElhinney DB, et al: One-stage complete unifocalization in infants: when should the ventricular septal defect be closed? J Thorac Cardiovasc Surg 113:858–868, 1997.
19. Reddy MV, McElhinney DB, Amin Z, et al: Early and intermediate outcomes after repair of pulmonary atresia with ventricular septal defect and major aortopulmonary collateral arteries. Circ 101:1826–1832, 2000.
20. Reichart B, Gulbins H, Meiser BM, et al: Improved results after heart-lung transplantation: a 17 year experience. Transplantation 75:127–132, 2003.
21. Rodefeld MD, Reddy VM, Thompson LD, et al: Surgical creation of aortopulmonary window in selected patients with pulmonary atresia with poorly developed aortopulmonary collaterals and hypoplastic pulmonary arteries. J Thorac Cardiovasc Surg 123:1147–1154, 2002.
22. Rome JJ, Mayer JE, Castaneda AR, Lock JE: Tetralogy of Fallot with pulmonary atresia. Circulation 88:1691–1698, 1993.
23. Shanley CJ, Lupinetti FM, Shah NL, et al: Primary unifocalization for the absence of intrapericardial pulmonary arteries in the neonate. J Thorac Cardiovasc Surg 106:237–247, 1993.
24. Stamm C, Friehs I, Zurakowski D, et al: Outcome after reconstruction of discontinuous pulmonary arteries. J Thorac Cardiovasc Surg 123:246–257, 2002.
25. Tchervenkov CI, Roy N: Congenital heart surgery nomenclature and database project: pulmonary atresia - ventricular septal defect. Ann Thorac Surg 69:S97–105, 2000.
26. Vranicar M, Teitel DF, Moore P: Use of small stents for rehabilitation of hypoplastic pulmonary arteries in pulmonary atresia with ventricular septal defect. Cath Cardiovasc Intervent 55:78–82, 2002.
27. Yoo SJ, Moes CA, Burrows PE, et al: Pulmonary blood supply by a branch from the distal ascending aorta in pulmonary atresia with ventricular septal defect. Pediatr Cardiol 14:230–233, 1993.

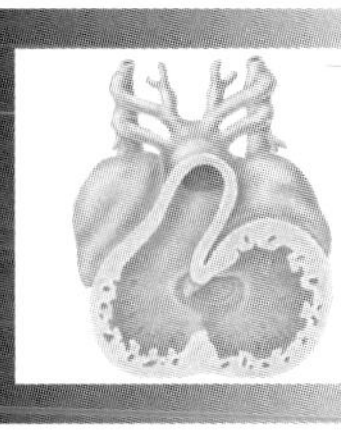

Right Ventricle-to-Pulmonary Artery Conduits

Jess M. Schultz, Irving Shen, and Ross M. Ungerleider

CHAPTER 116

INTRODUCTION

Extracardiac conduits between the right ventricle (RV) and pulmonary artery (PA) allow reconstruction of several congenital heart malformations, as well as replacement of the pulmonary explant during the Ross procedure (Box 116-1). Historically, a variety of conduits have been used as RV-to-PA conduits (Box 116-2). Rastelli et al reported the use of a nonvalved, Teflon RV-to-PA conduit in the treatment of truncus arteriosus in 1965.[83] The same year, Klinner and Zenker described implantation of a nonvalved conduit to reconstruct the right ventricular outflow tract (RVOT) for tetralogy of Fallot.[59] Ross and Summerville documented the first use of an aortic allograft to correct pulmonary atresia in 1966; and McGoon et al described the use of an aortic allograft as an RV-PA conduit in the treatment of truncus arteriosus in 1968.[72,86] The 1973 report by Bowman et al demonstrated that a Dacron conduit with a porcine valve could be used to repair a variety of congenital heart defects.[19]

Advancements in perioperative care and surgical technique have been accompanied by the increased use of RV-to-PA conduits in neonates. The use of RV-to-PA conduits in these young patients allows an early biventricular repair, which ensures normal pulmonary blood flow and pressure, and minimizes volume and pressure loading on the developing RV.[18,44,70,80] An earlier age of repair may be associated with improved long-term survival[36] (Figure 116-1). Additionally, the early use of RV-to-PA conduits can eliminate the risks of palliation, which include PA distortion, the morbidity and mortality of the palliative procedure, and finally the attrition rate prior to definitive surgery.

In the 1970s, aortic and pulmonary allografts were sterilized by irradiation, which resulted in early calcification and valvular degeneration.* These results led to the abandonment of irradiated allograft in favor of porcine-valved Dacron conduits. However, cryopreserved allografts did appear to possess adequate long-term function in the RV-to-PA position.[7] These findings led to the refinement of cryopreservation techniques and the emergence of cryopreserved allografts as the most common conduit used to restore RV-to-PA continuity.[42,55] In the current era, xenograft conduits from a variety of sources have also been used as an alternative for reconstruction of the RVOT.

The variety of materials available indicate the lack of one superior conduit for reconstruction of the RVOT. An ideal RV-to-PA conduit would be durable, with long-term patency and growth potential, and would provide an adequate supply of blood to the pulmonary circulation during all phases of the patient's growth.[24,30,32,45,56] This conduit would also have excellent handling characteristics to facilitate implantation, and be available in ample numbers and sizes to allow flexibility during surgery. Valve function would ideally be maintained without the need for anticoagulants and without degeneration resulting in valvular insufficiency or stenosis. Unfortunately, no ideal vascular replacement for the pulmonary outflow tract has been developed. Synthetic conduits are plagued with neointimal growth and thrombus formation. Allografts continue to suffer from limited lifespans resulting from valve degeneration and conduit stenosis. All conduits currently available are incapable of growing with the patient.[56,60]

SYNTHETIC CONDUITS

Synthetic Conduits with Valves

In the early 1970s, a woven Dacron conduit with low porosity became available for cardiac surgery.[19] These Dacron conduits can be combined with either mechanical or biologic valves for extracardiac reconstructions. These synthetic-valved conduits are available in numerous sizes and have an indefinite shelf life. Porcine-valved synthetic conduits, such as the Hancock conduit and the Carpentier–Edwards conduit, are popular options in the treatment of congenital heart defects. These conduits combine a glutaraldehyde-treated porcine valve with a Dacron tube graft and do not require anticoagulation of the patient.[26,85] Dacron conduits with pericardial valves are also available, but these have not been found to offer any

*References 18, 20, 24, 35, 44, 71.

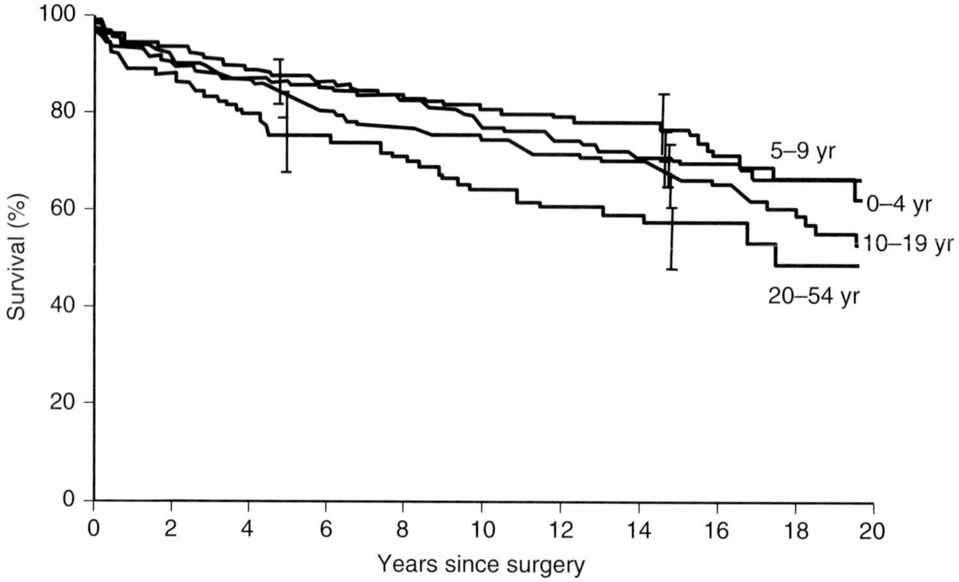

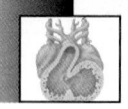

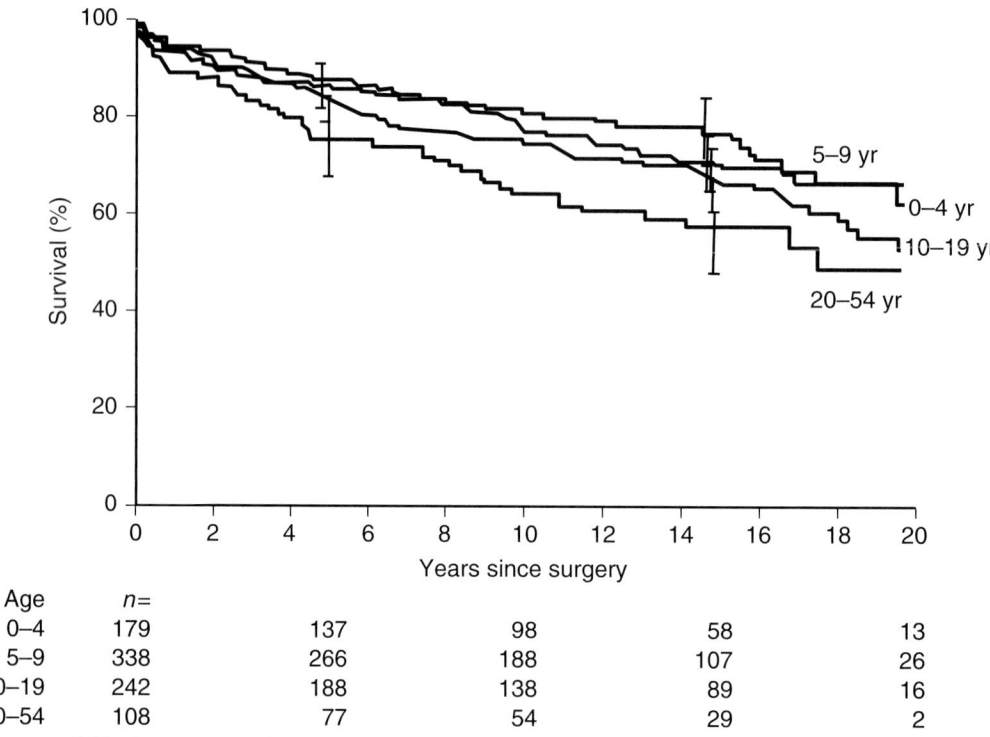

Age	*n*=				
0–4	179	137	98	58	13
5–9	338	266	188	107	26
10–19	242	188	138	89	16
20–54	108	77	54	29	2

Figure 116–1 **Survival of patients after placement of a right ventricle-to-pulmonary artery stratified according to age (excludes early deaths).**
(Modified with permission from Dearani JA, Danielson GK, Puga FJ, et al: Late follow-up of 1095 patients undergoing operation for complex congenital heart disease utilizing pulmonary ventricle to pulmonary artery conduits. Ann Thorac Surg 75:406, 2003).

long-term advantage compared to the Hancock conduits.[36] Unfortunately, synthetic-valved conduits appear to be associated with an increased risk of postoperative hemorrhage.[5,36,43,88,95] In general, the synthetic-valved conduits have poor handling characteristics that make implantation in infants and neonates technically challenging.[42,85] However, a 12-mm

Box 116–1. Congenital Heart Diseases That May Require a Right Ventricle-to-Pulmonary Artery Conduit During Surgical Reconstruction.

- Tetralogy of Fallot
- Pulmonary Atresia
  - with Ventricular Septal Defect
  - with Intact Ventricular Septum
- D-Transposition of the Great Arteries
  - with Pulmonary Stenosis and Ventricular Septal Defect
  - with Chronic LV Outflow Obstruction After Atrial Switch (LV-PA Conduit)
- Corrected Transposition (L-TGA)
  - with Ventricular Septal Defect and Pulmonary Stenosis
  - with Chronic Pulmonary Stenosis (LV-to-PA Conduit)
- Double-Outlet Right Ventricle
- Truncus Arteriosus
- LV Outflow Obstruction Requiring Ross Procedure
- Interrupted Aortic Arch with VSD and Severe Subaortic Outflow Obstruction

Box 116–2. Materials Used as Right Ventricle-to-Pulmonary Artery Conduits.

- Nonvalved Conduits
  - Synthetic
    - Dacron
    - Gore-Tex
    - Tascon Conduit (nonvalved)
  - Autologous
    - Vein Graft
    - Pericardial
    - Atrial
- Valved Conduits
  - Porcine-valved Dacron Conduit
    - Hancock Conduit
    - Ionescu–Shiley Conduit
    - Carpentier–Edwards Conduit
    - Tascon Conduit (valved)
  - Allografts (Cryopreserved or Irradiated)
    - Aortic Homograft
    - Pulmonary Homograft
  - Xenografts
    - Contegra
    - Equine Pericardium
    - Bovine Pericardium
    - Porcine Aortic Root
    - Ovine Aortic Root

porcine valve conduit is available, and it remains an option in small patients with complex congenital heart diseases.[20,85]

In selected patients with pulmonary insufficiency, pulmonary valve replacement with a heterograft valve alone, without the need for a conduit, can produce very satisfying results. It should be recognized that a pulmonary valve is a conduit, albeit a very short one, and thus its use is considered in this chapter. Heterograft pulmonary valves can have excellent intermediate-term function with a more likely failure mode that results in gradual stenosis (from valve calcification or degeneration) rather than insufficiency, and this makes them particularly attractive for implantation in patients whose primary problems relate to long-standing pulmonary insufficiency, such as patients with tetralogy of Fallot when the primary operation included a transannular RV outflow patch.

Conduit Longevity

Synthetic conduits with valves are reported to possess a longer life span, and a prolonged freedom from reoperation, when compared to allograft conduits.[36,71,84,88] Razzouk et al compared 126 patients who received porcine-valved Dacron RV-to-PA conduits against 130 patients who received cryopreserved aortic or pulmonary allografts prior to 1991.[84] Patients with porcine-valved Dacron conduits had a freedom from conduit replacement of 89% at 5 years, compared to those patients with allografts, who had a 46% freedom from conduit replacement over the same interval.[84] However, a systematic evaluation of conduit function or patient cardiovascular status was not reported within this study. Dearani, et al corroborated these findings, and reported a freedom from reoperation after placement of the Hancock conduit in the RV-to-PA position to be 60.7 % at 10 years, and 45.1 % at 15 years.[36] This recent series reported that the Hancock conduit had a greater freedom from reoperation than either irradiated or cryopreserved allografts[36] (Figure 116-2).

Several reports have documented the development of significant transvalvular gradients in synthetic-valved conduits.[52,73] The indication for conduit replacement is usually either conduit stenosis or obstruction.[10,36,52,60] One major source of stenosis or occlusion is the formation of thick pseudointimal fibrous peels within the Dacron graft. These peels can dissect free from the tightly woven conduit fibers, and result in occlusion.[1,2,15,40] The clinicopathologic study presented by Agarwal, et al reported that the level of obstruction in synthetic conduits occurs within the tube graft in one-third of patients, the valve in one-third of the patients, and with a combination of tube graft and the valve obstruction in the remaining one-third of the patients.[1] Additionally, early calcification of the porcine valve can result in valvular dysfunction and occlusion.[60,73,87] Endovascular stent implantation has

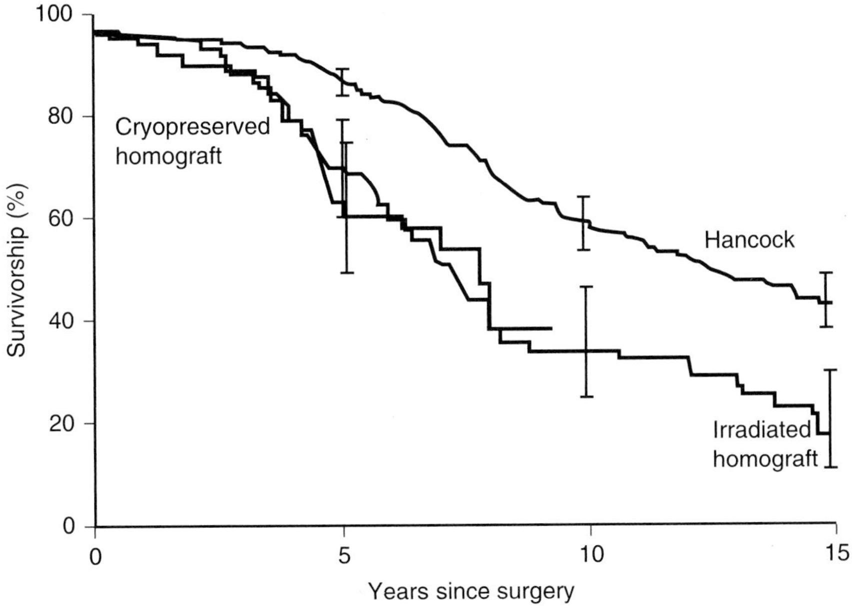

	$n =$			
Irradiated homograft	90	54	23	9
Cryopreserved homograft	90	9	0	0
Hancock	444	332	198	101

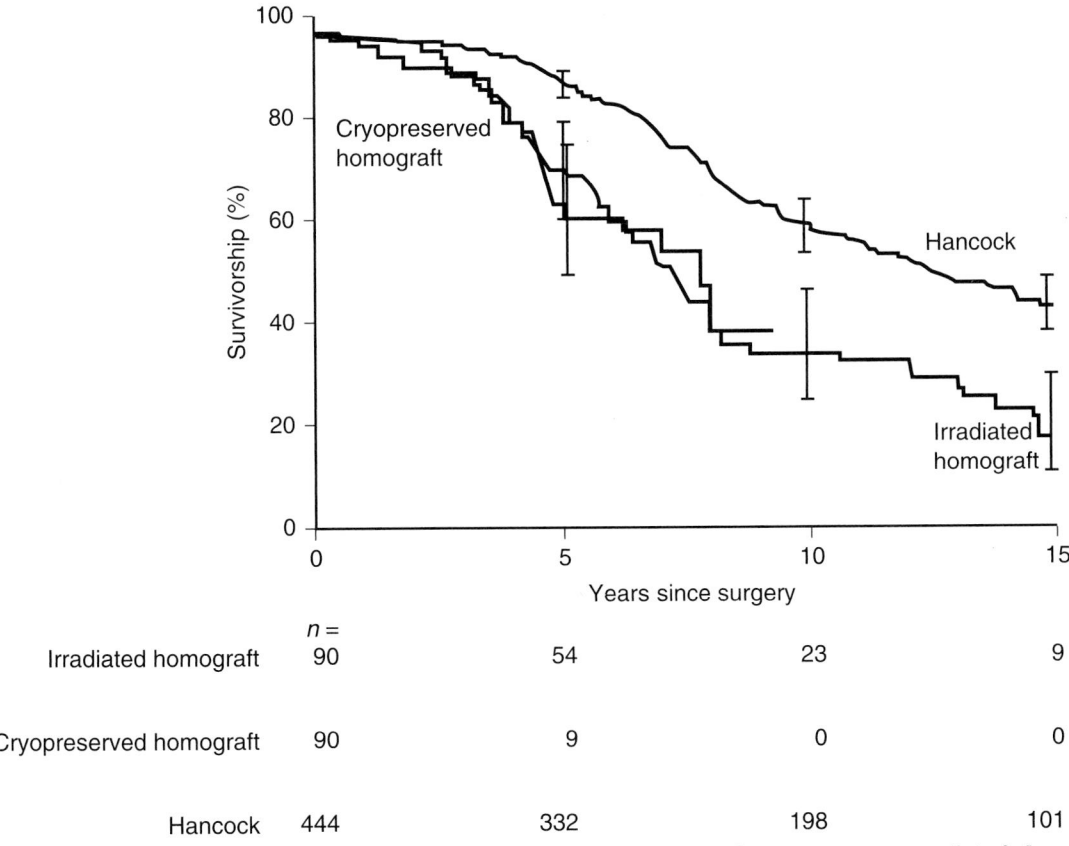

Figure 116–2 Freedom from reoperation for right ventricle-to-pulmonary artery conduit failure, stratified according to conduit type.
(Modified with permission from Dearani JA, Danielson GK, Puga FJ, et al: Late follow-up of 1095 patients undergoing operation for complex congenital heart disease utilizing pulmonary ventricle to pulmonary artery conduits. Ann Thorac Surg 75:408, 2003.)

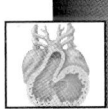

been successfully used to manage stenosis and obstruction of both the valve and tube graft components of synthetic-valved RV-to-PA conduits.[78,81] Endovascular stent placement can prolong the interval to reoperation at all three of these levels of obstruction.[78] Unfortunately, placement of a stent in a conduit will result in complete loss of valve function, which may have undesirable consequences in certain patients.

Synthetic Conduits Without Valves

Synthetic tube grafts without valves, constructed of either Dacron or expanded polytetrafluoroethylene, have also been used as RV-to-PA conduits.[35,36,38,52] Contraindications to the use of a nonvalved conduit include elevated pulmonary vascular resistance, PA hypoplasia, advanced pulmonary-ventricular failure, or unrepaired tricuspid valve regurgitation.[36,38] Downing described the use of nonvalved Dacron conduits to replace obstructed valved RV-to-PA conduits in 15 patients. At 19.6 months, no deaths had occurred and NYHA functional class was good to excellent. The authors concluded that selective use of nonvalved conduits in children may reduce the incidence of reoperation for conduit obstruction, which appeared to have occurred with greater frequency in valved conduits as compared to nonvalved conduits.[38] However, the recent series reported by Dearani et al did not detect a difference in the rate of reoperation for conduit failure between valved and nonvalved conduits.[36] Currently, most centers will use a valved RV-to-PA conduit, which should reduce injury to the pulmonary ventricle caused by long-term exposure to pulmonary regurgitation.[16,56] However, the nonvalved synthetic conduit remains an important option for certain congenital heart defects.[36]

BIOLOGIC CONDUITS

Allografts

The advantages of cryopreserved allografts include availability in a wide number of sizes, handling characteristics that conform well to native tissue and encourage hemostasis, and excellent short- and mid-term performance as RV-to-PA conduits.* Additionally, some reports have demonstrated that the long-term function of allografts in the pulmonary position may match synthetic conduits with valves.[49,63,85,92] The primary disadvantages of this material are a potential limitation of the supply, (particularly in pediatric sizes); and higher cost. The limited supply of smaller allografts is compounded by their limited shelf life. Liquid nitrogen–cryopreserved allografts have a safe storage time of up to 2 years; however, allografts stored in an antibiotic solution have an effective shelf life of only 4 weeks.[55] Size reduction of a larger allograft, by incising the conduit and excising one leaflet of the allograft valve, is one method that could increase the number of allografts available in smaller sizes.[58,93] The function of these "bicuspid" allograft conduits has been reported to be equivalent to standard tricuspid allografts.[61]

Both aortic and pulmonary allografts can be obtained during autopsy or multiple organ retrieval.[23] Controversy exists whether the pulmonary or aortic cryopreserved allograft is better suited as an RV-PA conduit.† Many series conclude that no difference in allograft longevity exists between aortic and pulmonary allografts.‡ Other series have demonstrated that pulmonary allografts have a superior freedom from reopera-

*References 5, 42, 45, 57, 67, 85.
†References 12, 42, 45, 25, 47.
‡References 32, 45, 63, 64, 94, 97.

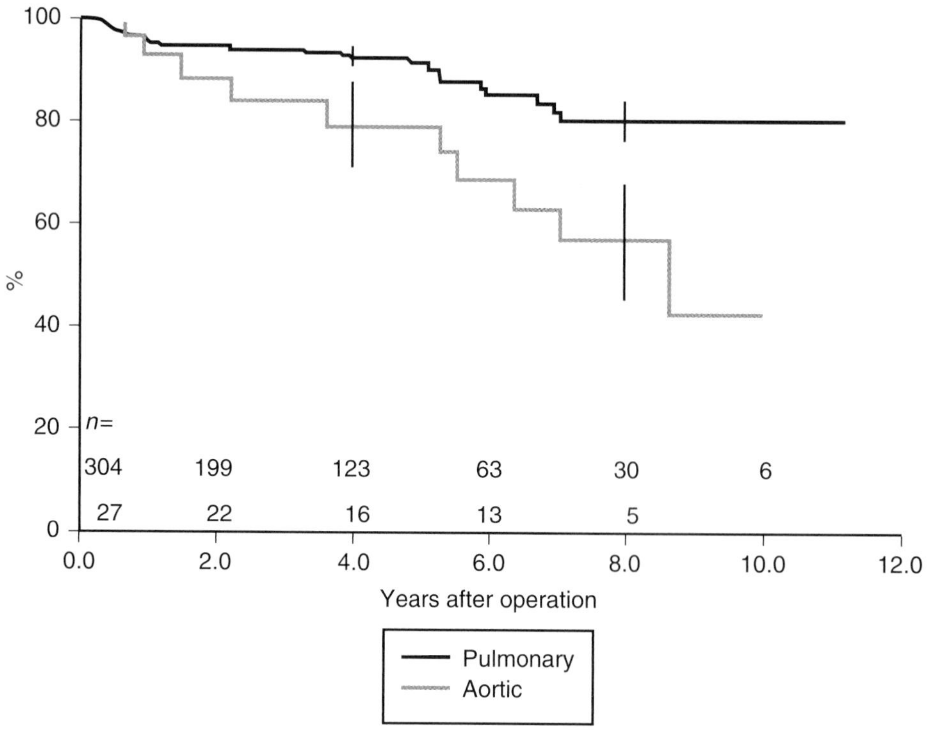

Figure 116–3 **Freedom from reoperation for right ventricle-to-pulmonary artery conduit failure stratified according to allograft source.**
(Modified from Niwaya K, Knott-Craig CJ, Lane MM, et al: Cryopreserved homograft valves in the pulmonary position: risk analysis for intermediate-term failure. J Thorac Cardiovasc Surg 117:145, 1999.)

tion compared to aortic allografts, when implanted into the RV-to-PA position* (Figure 116-3). The cause of this disparity is unknown. Aortic allografts may be prone to calcification, which results in a relatively high rate of conduit failure, compared to pulmonary allografts.[12,75,91] However, the longevity of pulmonary allografts can be reduced in an environment of elevated PA pressure or an elevated PA to right ventricular pressure gradient.[37,47,54,74] A more recent series described by Danielson, et al challenged this conclusion, and documented that isolated elevated pulmonary vascular resistance does not result in a higher failure rate for pulmonary allografts.[35] Regardless, under exposure to high pressures, both aortic and pulmonary allografts are at higher risk of aneurysm formation.[54,67] The formation of pseudoaneurysms in either the allograft, or at the RV to allograft anastomosis have also been reported to occur with elevated and normal PA pressures.[67]

Patient anatomy could influence the choice to use either an aortic or pulmonary allograft. Aortic allografts are longer, which may reduce the need for synthetic extensions to more distal anastomoses. Pulmonary allografts may also be preferable in those patients who require distal anastomoses to branch pulmonary arteries, as the tissue match is similar between pulmonary allografts and native pulmonary arteries. In small patients, the wall thickness of the pulmonary allograft is also a better match to the native pulmonary arteries.[23] The pulmonary allograft bifurcation can also be used to enlarge stenotic branch pulmonary arteries.[23,45] Additionally, more pulmonary allografts are available for older patients, because the larger sizes of aortic allografts are often used in the reconstruction of left ventricular outflow tracts.[66]

*References 5, 12, 31, 34, 36, 47, 68.

Allograft Longevity

Cryopreserved allografts appear to possess better short- and mid-term function and a greater freedom from reoperation at early follow-up than synthetic valved conduits.[63,66,85] Series that describe the results for patients receiving cryopreserved allografts as RV-to-PA conduits are increasing in enrollment numbers as well as length of follow-up. In 1987, Kirklin, et al reported a freedom from reoperation after implantation of an aortic allograft was 94% for 147 patients at a mean follow-up of 3.5 years.[57] A recent series of 290 patients, which included the use of both aortic and pulmonary conduits demonstrated 5- and 10-year freedom from conduit replacement at 85% and 69% respectively, was described by Weipert et al.[97] Primary reasons for cryopreserved allograft failure include stenosis, valvular calcification or degeneration, patient somatic growth.[35,36,43,47] Endovascular stents have been used to prolong the interval to reoperation for RV-to-PA conduit failure for both allograft stenosis and conduit–patient size mismatch.[42,78,81]

The type of congenital heart defect influences the rate of allograft failure. The longevity of RV-to-PA allografts is decreased in the congenital heart diseases that have higher incidence of pulmonary arterial stenosis or distortion, leading to increased resistance distal to the conduit.[37,42] In support of this conclusion, excellent allograft longevity

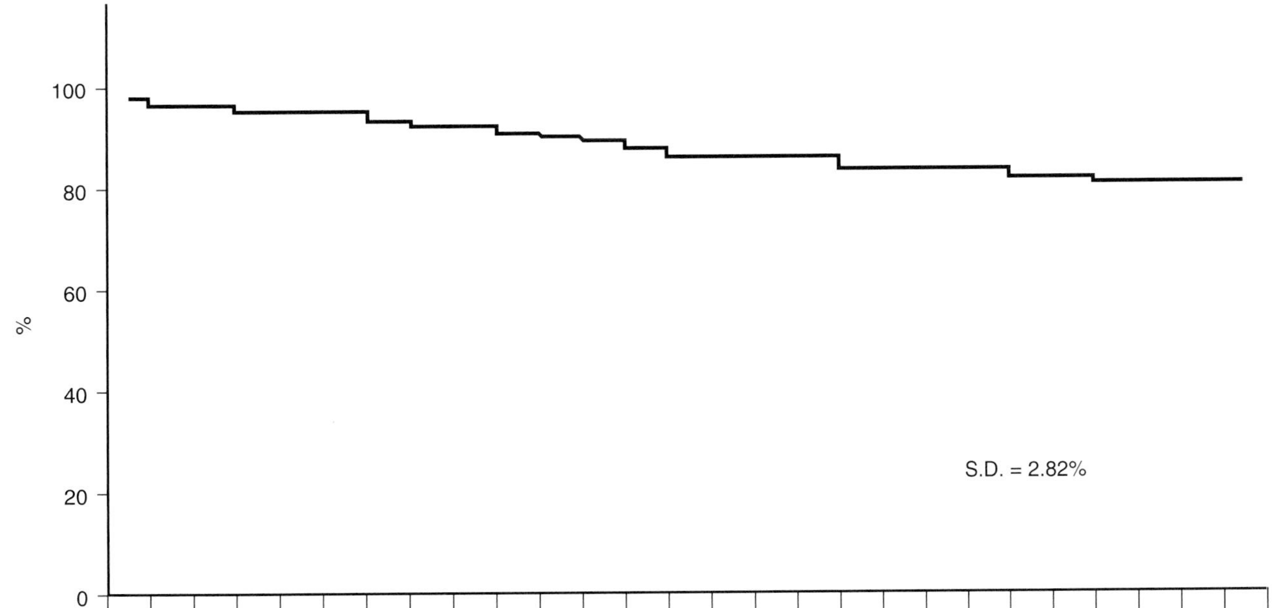

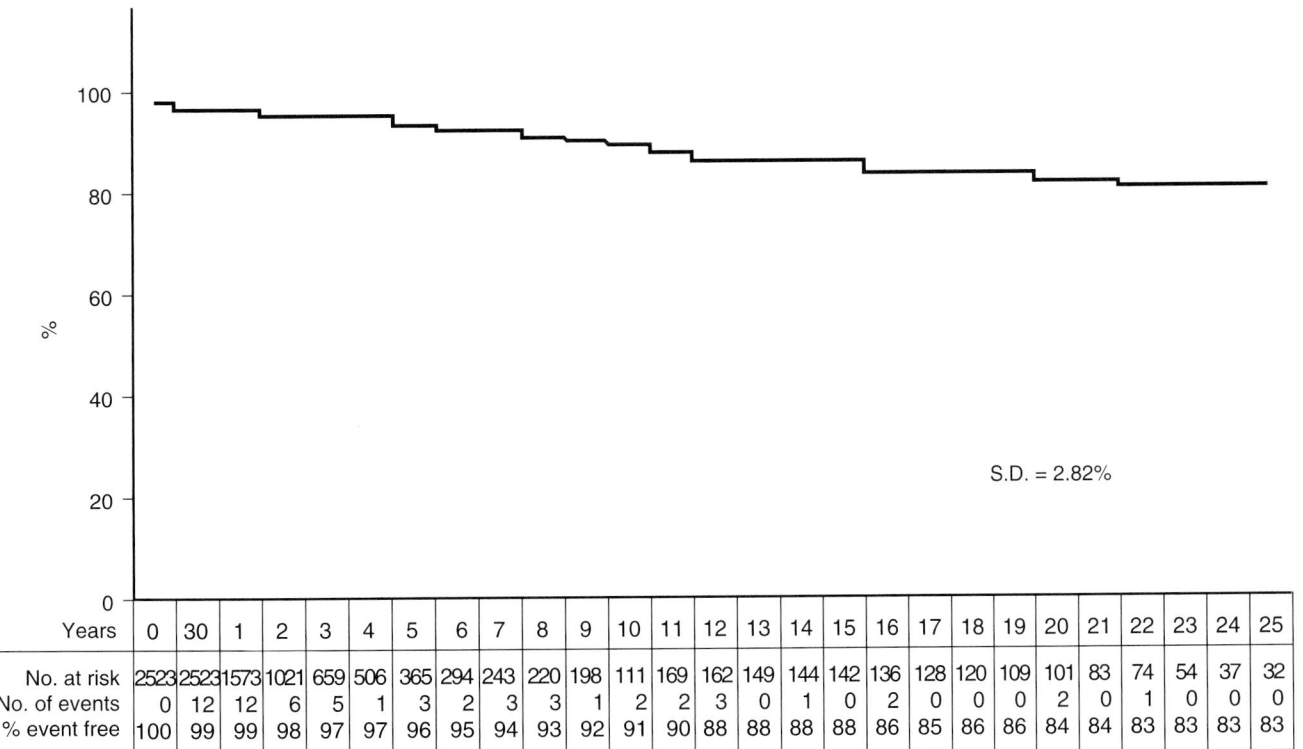

Years	0	30	1	2	3	4	5	6	7	8	9	10	11	12	13	14	15	16	17	18	19	20	21	22	23	24	25
No. at risk	2523	2523	1573	1021	659	506	365	294	243	220	198	111	169	162	149	144	142	136	128	120	109	101	83	74	54	37	32
No. of events	0	12	12	6	5	1	3	2	3	3	1	2	2	3	0	1	0	2	0	0	0	2	0	1	0	0	0
% event free	100	99	99	98	97	97	96	95	94	93	92	91	90	88	88	88	88	86	85	86	86	84	84	83	83	83	83

Time (years)

Figure 116–4 **Freedom from right ventricular outflow tract revision or repair, after Ross Procedure, life table analysis (*n* = 2523).**
(Modified with permission from Oury JH, Hiro SP, Maxwell JM, et al: The Ross Procedure: current registry results. Ann Thorac Surg 66:S164, 1998.)

has been found in patients with normal PA anatomy and pulmonary vascular resistance.[39,42,75,77]

An important use of allograft pulmonary valves is in RV-PA reconstruction during the Ross Procedure (pulmonary autograft) to replace the aortic valve. Interestingly, if a perfect experiment were designed to test the durability of a pulmonary allograft in the pulmonary position, the design would be to remove the pulmonary valve from a patient with a normal pulmonary valve and pulmonary arterial tree and to replace that valve with an allograft valve. Ironically, this is precisely what is done in the Ross Procedure, where the normal pulmonary valve is harvested to replace a diseased aortic valve and an allograft pulmonary valve is placed in the pulmonary position. The outcome for pulmonary allografts placed in such patients is excellent, with allograft survival of greater than 80% at 25 years[77] (Figure 116-4). These results are so vastly superior to the results of allograft survival in all other patients that it is reasonable to speculate that factors leading to allograft failure are related to the recipient and the underlying disease, not to the allograft itself. These factors may be anatomic (the anterior position of an allograft in many patients when it is used to create an extraanatomic connection between the RV and the PA, or distal PA stenosis, as is seen in some patients with tetralogy of Fallot) or physiologic (abnormally high pulmonary resistance seen in some patients with long standing congenital heart disease). Regardless, the outcome for pulmonary allografts in the RV-to-PA position following a Ross Procedure seem to be distinctly and uniquely better than a pulmonary allografts for all other indications of RV-to-PA reconstruction.[42,76]

Several sources have also indicated that small or young patients, or the use of small diameter allografts, are risk factors associated with reduced freedom from reoperation for RV-to-PA conduit failure[42,45,64,75,80] (Figure 116-5). These findings are likely the result of allograft implantation into neonates or infants, followed by patient growth and the need for increased pulmonary flow.[42] This phenomenon was highlighted by Perron et al, who found that freedom from reoperation for neonates receiving RV-to-PA allografts was 22% at 5 years.[8] Implanting oversized allografts into neonates and infants has been done to reduce the rate of reoperation. However, care should be taken at oversizing the conduit, because either kinking of the conduit or compression of the conduit or valve against the sternum can occur.[9,10]

Allograft longevity may also be affected by immune responses against the transplanted allograft initiated by the patient.[14,82] Early reports indicated that ABO incompatibility between the allograft and the recipient could result in reduced allograft longevity.[48,98] An antibody response to both Heart and Lung Association (HLA) class I and II antigens of cryopreserved allografts has also been demonstrated *in vivo*.[46] Cellular viability of the allograft endothelium is affected by both the method of preservation, as well as the antibiotic media used for sterilization prior to cryopreservation.[3,4,53] It is possible that antigen expression by the allograft endothelium, or any adherent cardiac tissue, initiates a recipient immune

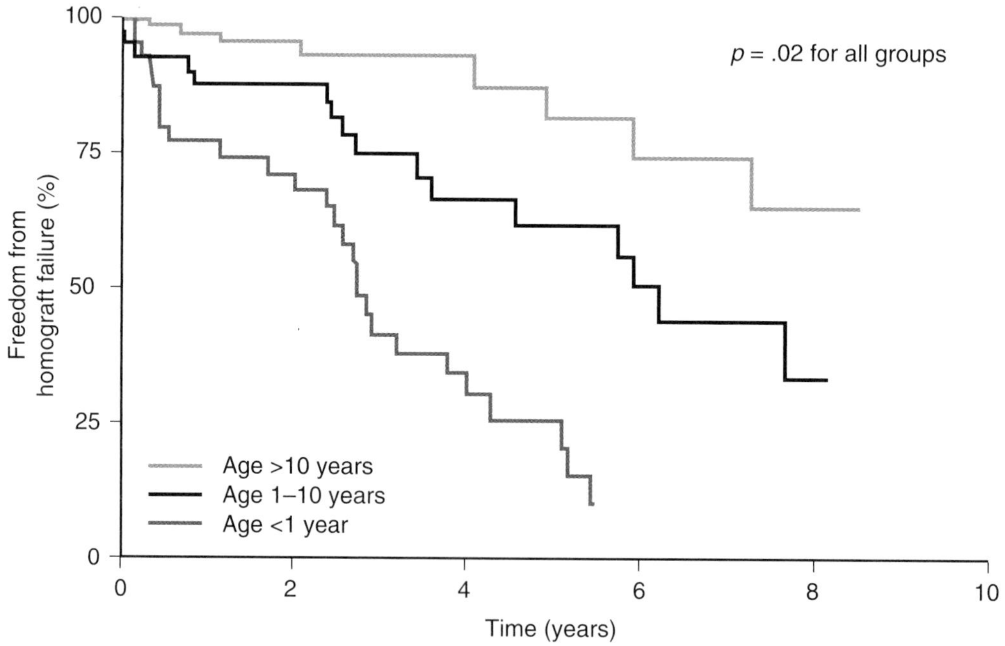

Number at risk

<1yr	53	28	12	1	0
1–10 yrs	46	29	20	10	4
>10 yrs	85	49	18	10	7

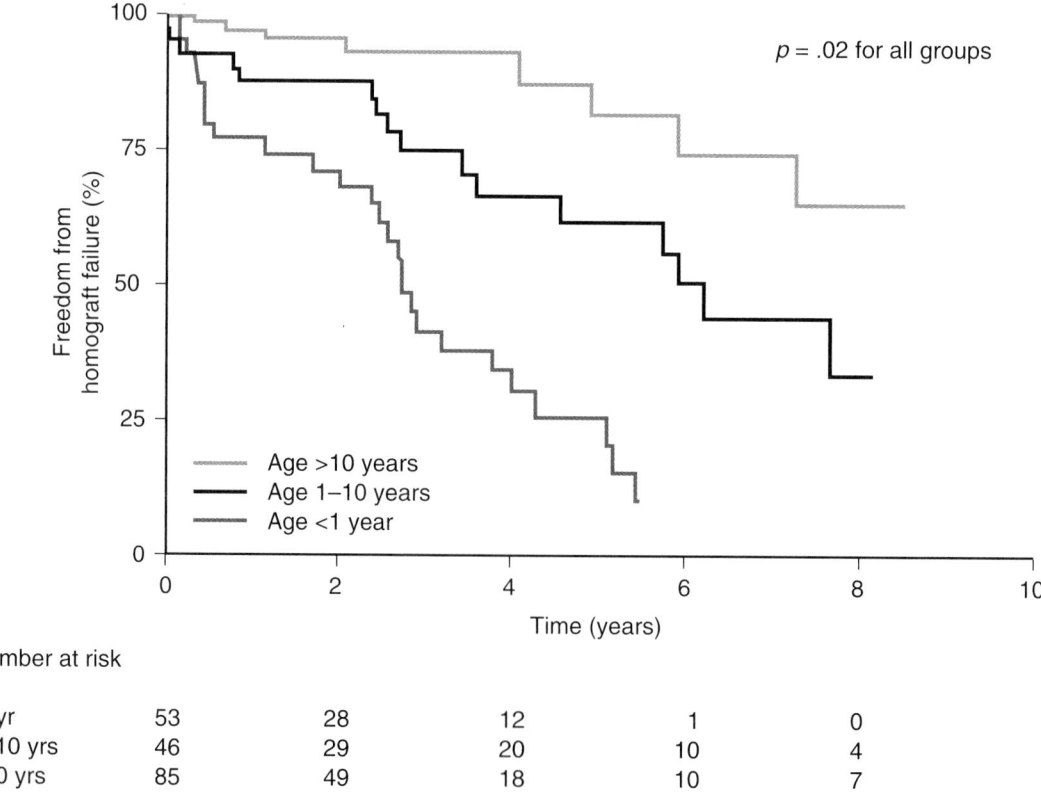

Figure 116–5 Freedom from reoperation for right ventricle to pulmonary artery conduit failure stratified according age at first operation.
(Modified with permission from Forbess JM, Shah AS, St. Louis JD, et al: Cryopreserved homografts in the pulmonary position: determinants of durability. Ann Thorac Surg 71:56, 2001.)

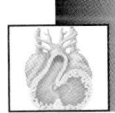

response resulting in early conduit calcification and valve degeneration. However, Cleveland et al compared four different cryopreservation techniques and found no difference in late outcomes of conduit function.[32] Additionally, several series have demonstrated that ABO incompatibility between the allograft and the recipient has no effect on the longevity of the allograft.[11,41,53,63] Despite these findings, some centers are exploring the use of immunosuppressants as a therapy to reduce the rate of allograft failure.[65,89,90]

Autogenous Tissue

Autogenous tissue can be used to create both valved and nonvalved RV-to-PA conduits.[6,28,51,89] Schlicter et al reported the results of a valved conduit manufactured from the patient's pericardium immediately prior to conduit implantation. The mean time to construct the conduit was 35 minutes, and conduit diameters varied from 12–20 mm. In this series of 55 patients, the freedom from reoperation for conduit failure was 90% at 5 years. Interestingly, at the most recent follow-up, the conduit diameter had increased by 1–7 mm in 27 of the patients.

Autologous pericardium has been repeatedly used as a nonvalved conduit during replacement of obstructed RV-to-PA conduits.[28,35] Other sources of autogenous tissue used in the reconstruction of the RVOT include jugular vein, homograft dura mater, and atrial tissue.[28,35]

Xenograft Conduits

Xenograft RV-to-PA conduits have been procured from porcine, bovine, ovine, and equine sources.[8,13,21,50,96] Xenograft conduits, like allografts, have handling characteristics that match native tissues, and they may be available in small sizes when allograft availability is limited.* Unfortunately, the durability of many xenograft conduits may be less than the allograft conduits (Table 116-1). However, this disadvantage may be irrelevant if the expected conduit replacement interval is short, for example in infants and neonates.[97]

The most popular xenograft conduits for children include the Contegra bovine jugular vein and the Shelhigh porcine PA. The Contegra conduit, a xenograft obtained from bovine jugular vein with a naturally integrated trileaflet venous valve, has been used for the reconstruction of the RVOT.[17,22,27,33] The Contegra conduit is available in diameters from 12–22 mm and possesses tissue characteristics that are comparable to allograft tissue.[22,27] It should be noted that in small patients, the length of the venous valve within the conduit may necessitate implantation of the entire length of the Contegra conduit, but this does not seem to create technical difficulties during surgery.[27] At short- and mid-term follow-up, the Contegra conduit in the RV-to-PA position appears to match or surpass the freedom from reintervention seen with allografts[17,22,33] (Figure 116-6). The slow rate of valve degeneration, as well as the potential for unlimited supply, could make the Contegra conduit an excellent alternative to allografts for the reconstruction of the RVOT.[22]

The Shelhigh PA may be an excellent choice for infants and children, particularly if there are multiple distal stenoses in the branch pulmonary arteries, because this option combines the advantages of a heterograft pulmonary valve with the features of a tissue-type conduit.[69] The valve may hold up better against the distal pressures, and the conduit material, while not as easy to handle as homograft tissue, is superior in handling to Dacron or Gore-Tex. Initial reports of marked foreign body reactions causing early stenosis and failure in infants[79] have resulted in improvements in processing of these valves with more encouraging results in recent, unreported experiences.

OPERATIVE TECHNIQUES

Insertion of RV-to-PA conduits requires the use of cardiopulmonary bypass. In many cases of primary conduit insertion, there is no continuity between the RV and the PA,

*References 8, 13, 21, 49, 66, 92.

Table 116–1

Xenografts Used as Right Ventricle-to-Pulmonary Artery Conduits[8,13,21,50,96]

Series	*Source of conduit*	*n*	*Conduit diameter*	*Freedom from reintervention for conduit failure*
Vrandecic et al	Porcine valve, bovine pericardial conduit	33	11–23 mm	82 (± 19)% at 5 years
Aupecle et al	Porcine valve bovine pericardial conduit	55	11–17 mm	64 (± 18)% at 5 years
Barbero-Marciel et al	Bovine pericardial	29	12–20 mm	100% at 21 months
Brawn	Ovine	4	12–13 mm	0% at 5 years
Imai et al	Equine pericardial	143	12–35 mm	97% at 5 years

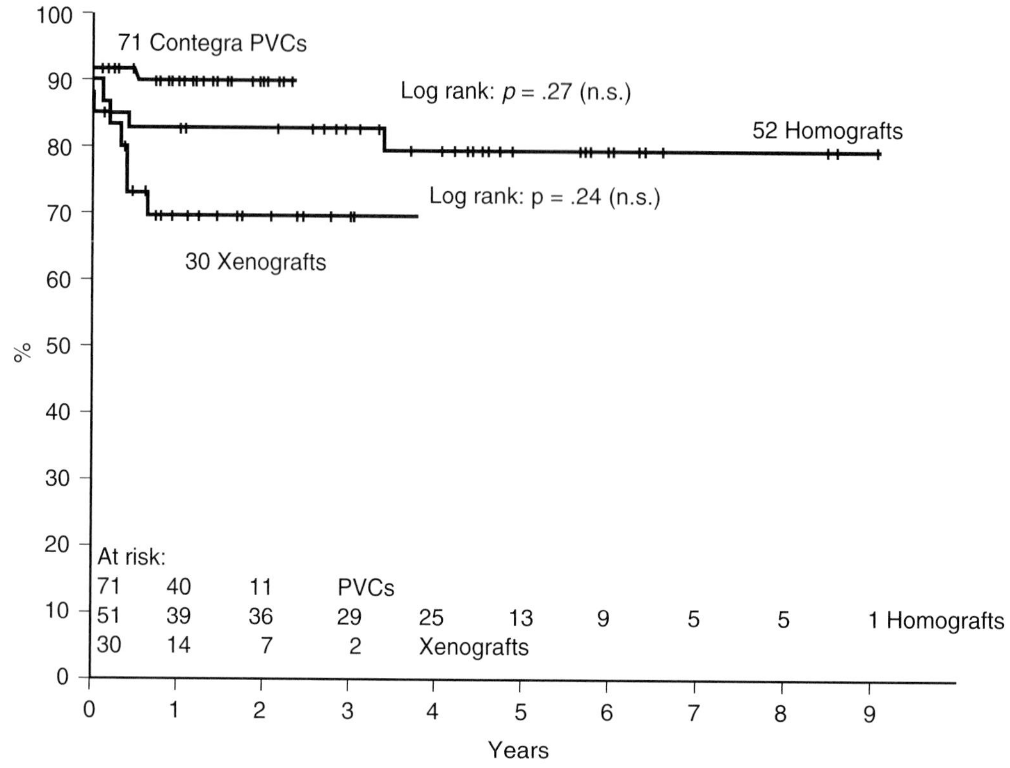

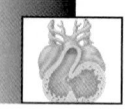

Figure 116–6 Freedom from explantation of right ventricle-to-pulmonary artery conduit for conduit failure comparison among the Contegra conduit, allograft conduit, and porcine-valved Dacron conduit.
(Modified with permission from Breymann T, Thies WR, Boethig D, et al: Bovine valved venous xenografts for RVOT reconstruction: results after 71 implantations. Eur J Cardio-Thorac Surg 21:708, 2001.)

and a ventricular septal defect (VSD) is often present. In these circumstances, the VSD is closed through a right ventriculotomy and this ventriculotomy then provides the outflow from the RV and the site of proximal conduit anastomosis (Figure 116-7). The distal PAs are prepared in a variety of ways for conduit anastomosis. If the PAs are not contiguous, they are "unifocalized" to create a central PA whenever possible. Confluent PAs, which are more common, are opened at the bifurcation between the right and left PA, and this opening is enlarged to provide ample inflow from the RV conduit. Once both the RV outflow and PA inflow sites are prepared, the conduit can be cut to appropriate size and anastomosis is usually performed first to the PA, which can usually be accomplished with a continuous suture of monofilament and then completed (Figure 116-8). The insertion of the RV-to-PA conduit next requires anastomosing the proximal conduit to the RV (Figure 116-9). The proximal anastomosis may require a "hood" of pericardium or prosthetic material (often Gore-Tex) to provide adequate RV outflow with limited valve distortion (Figure 116-10).

A pulmonary valve can be inserted into a previously placed RV-to-PA conduit. The outflow tract is opened distally onto the left PA (Figure 116-11). The posterior portion of the valve-sewing ring can be anastomosed to the back wall of the RV-to-PA conduit using continuous sutures (Figure 116-12). The valve is seated within the conduits in Figure 116-13. A hood of Gore-Tex is used as a patch over the incised RV-to-PA conduit and the valve is secured to this hood (Figure 116-14). This technique allows for the implantation of "oversized" valves because the anterior hood can accommodate valves that are larger than what would normally fit in the outflow tract.

Conduit placement can be performed with the heart cardioplegically arrested or fibrillating. In conduit replacement operations, when intracardiac defects have been previously repaired, and especially in circumstances in which it is difficult to get control of the aorta and there is significant aortic insufficiency, it can be desirable and practical to perform conduit replacement on a beating heart. Regardless of the technique, it is important to try to select a site for the conduit that prevents it from lying directly behind the sternum. When a conduit is directly beneath the sternum, it is more likely to be compressed by the sternum and result in early, if not immediate, conduit dysfunction. Furthermore, a location directly behind the sternum increases the risk of inadvertent conduit reentry during repeat sternotomy. It may be advantageous to cover the conduit with a pericardial membrane to protect it from injury on a repeat sternotomy. Whenever it is necessary to place the conduit in an unusual position, the surgeon should indicate the conduit course in the operative report so that the future surgeon can be prepared to deal with unexpected circumstances.

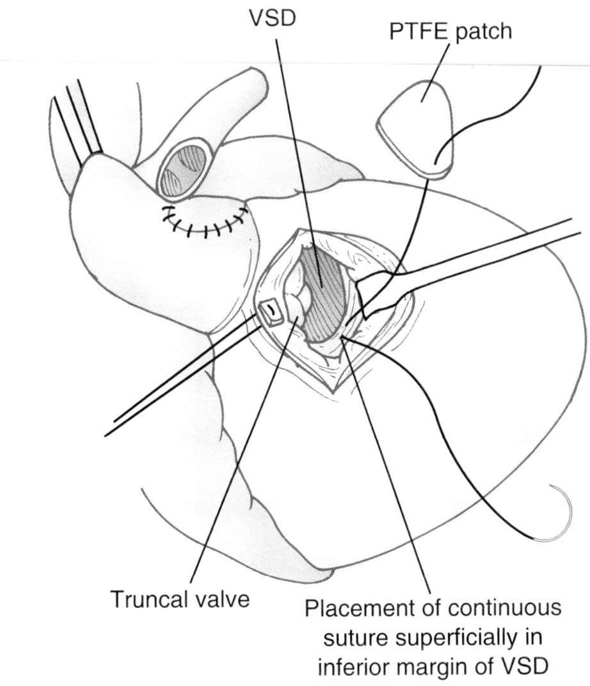

Figure 116–7 The ventricular septal defect (VSD) is closed through a right ventriculotomy, and this ventriculotomy, then provides the outflow from the RV and the site of proximal conduit anastomosis.
(Modified from Ungerleider RM: Truncus arteriosus. In Sabiston DC, editor: Atlas of Cardiothoracic Surgery, 1st ed. Philadelphia: WB Saunders,1995, p. 321.)

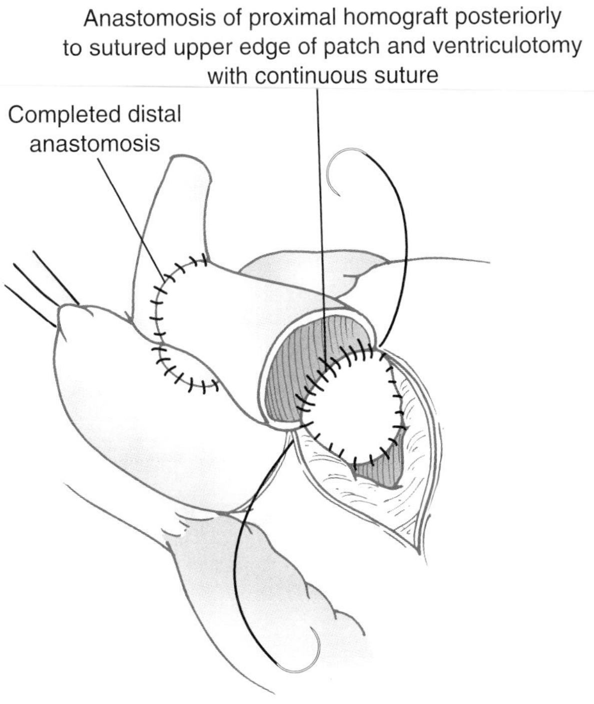

Figure 116–9 The insertion of the RV-to-PA conduit next requires an anastomosis between the proximal conduit and the right ventricle.
(Modified with permission from Ungerleider RM: Truncus arteriosus. In Sabiston DC, editor: Atlas of Cardiothoracic Surgery, 1st ed. Philadelphia: WB Saunders, 1995, p. 323.)

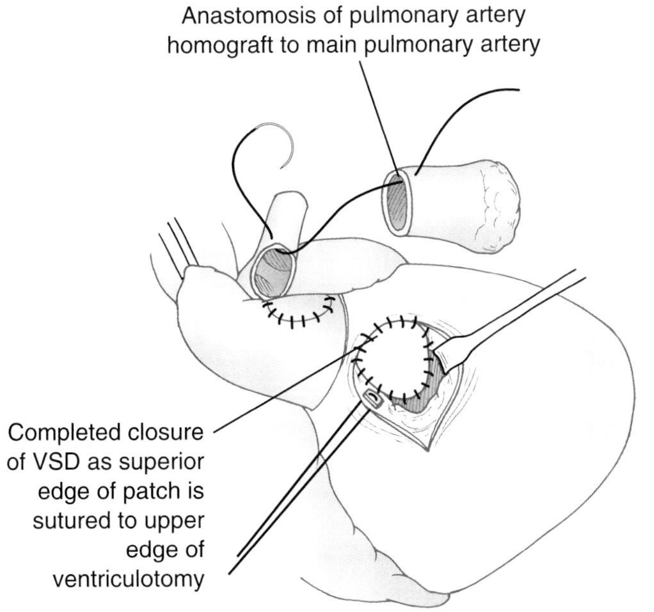

Figure 116–8 The conduit can be cut to appropriate size, and anastomosis is usually performed first between the conduit and the pulmonary artery. VSD, ventricular septal defect.
(Modified from Ungerleider RM: Truncus arteriosus. In Sabiston DC, editor: Atlas of Cardiothoracic Surgery, 1st ed. Philadelphia: WB Saunders, 1995, p. 322.)

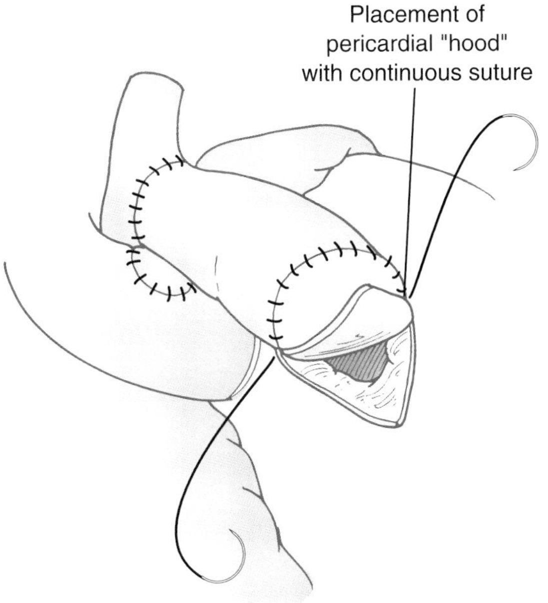

Figure 116–10 The proximal anastomosis may require a "hood" to provide adequate RV outflow with limited valve distortion.
(Modified from Ungerleider RM: Truncus arteriosus. In Sabiston DC, editor: Atlas of Cardiothoracic Surgery, 1st ed. Philadelphia: WB Saunders , 1995, p. 323).

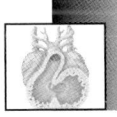

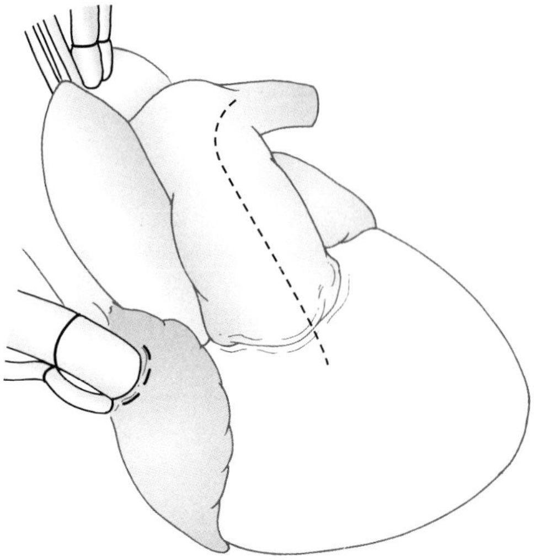

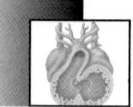

Figure 116–11 The RV-to-PA conduit is opened onto the left pulmonary artery.

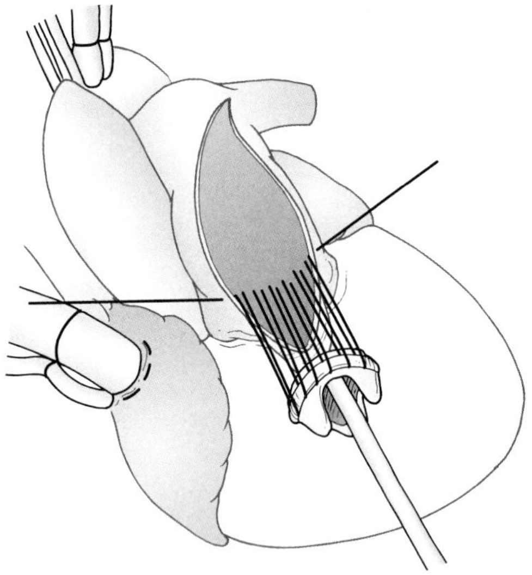

Figure 116–12 The posterior portion of the valve sewing ring is anastomosed to the back wall of the RV-to-PA conduit with a continuous suture.

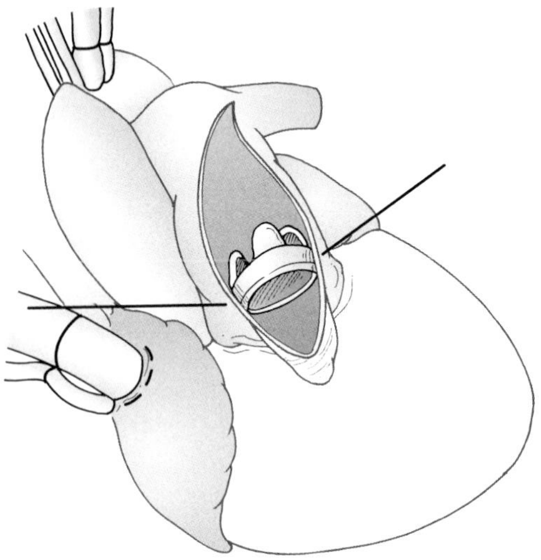

Figure 116–13 The valve is seated within the RV-to-PA conduit.

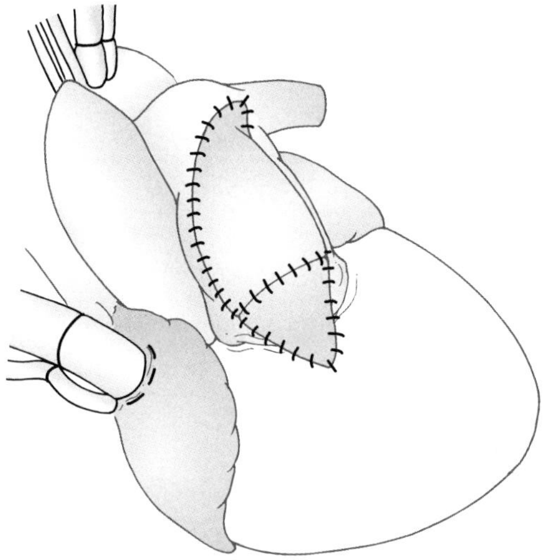

Figure 116–14 A hood of Gore-Tex is used as a patch over the incised RV-to-PA conduit and the valve is secured to this hood.

PATIENT MORTALITY

Operative Mortality

The operative mortality following placement of an RV-to-PA conduit is highly dependent on the severity of the underlying congenital heart defect. The greatest early mortality rates have been reported for patients with truncus arteriosus, transposition of the great arteries, and univentricular hearts, when compared to those patients with tetralogy of Fallot or pulmonary atresia.* A steady decrease in the early or operative mortality rate has occurred over time.[29,36,50] Series from the 1970s and early 1980s commonly described operative mortality rates between 20% and 50%.[24,52,55] These earlier series were largely comprised of patients greater than 1 year of age who possessed some form of palliation before receiving an RV-to-PA conduit. Later series demonstrated a significant improvement in operative mortality in patients over a wide distribution of ages.[47,64,95] However, survival continued to be disappointing in those patients operated on at less than 1 year of age, with 5-year mortality rates reported to be as high as 25%.[45] Series from the current era have demonstrated that the operative mortality in infants and neonates can be low. For example,

*References 24, 29, 36, 52, 63, 84, 97.

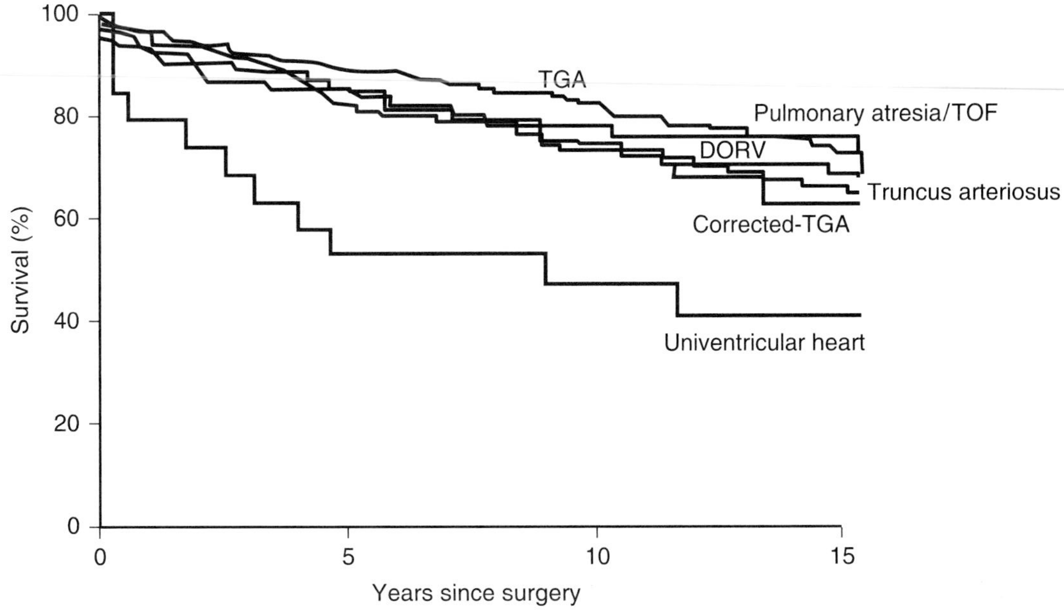

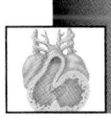

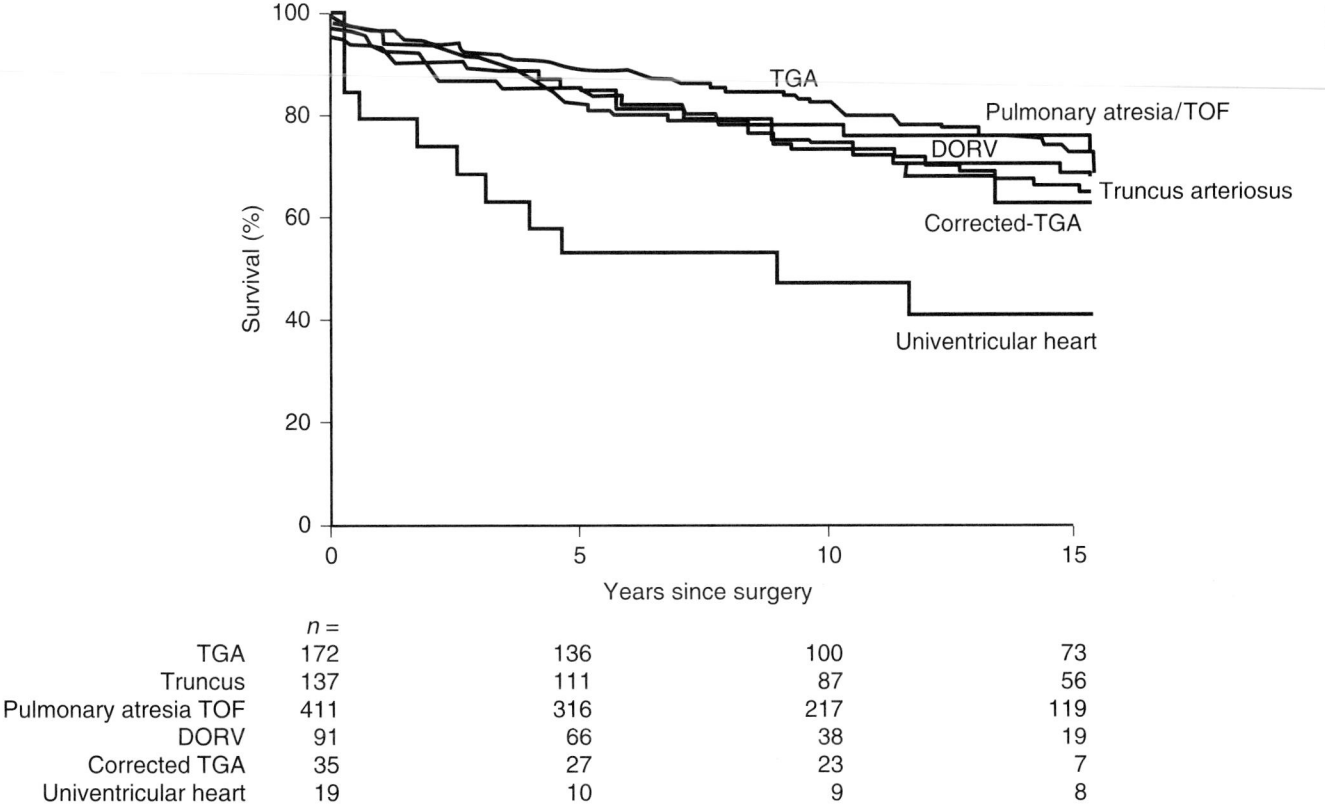

	n =			
TGA	172	136	100	73
Truncus	137	111	87	56
Pulmonary atresia TOF	411	316	217	119
DORV	91	66	38	19
Corrected TGA	35	27	23	7
Univentricular heart	19	10	9	8

Figure 116–15 Survival of patients after placement of a right ventricle to pulmonary artery stratified according to initial diagnosis (excludes early deaths).
(Modified from Dearani JA, Danielson GK, Puga FJ, et al: Late follow-up of 1095 patients undergoing operation for complex congenital heart disease utilizing pulmonary ventricle to pulmonary artery conduits. Ann Thorac Surg 75:406, 2003).

Dearani, et al reported an early mortality rate of 3.7% for those patients operated on after 1993.[36]

Long-term Survival

Long-term survival after implantation of RV-PA conduits is also related to the severity of the underlying congenital heart defect.[24,29,36,84] The extended series from the Mayo clinic, which includes porcine-valved Dacron conduits, nonvalved conduits, and allografts, has reported the 10-year survival to be 77% and 20-year survival to exceed 59% for all diagnoses.[36] It is unclear whether the type of conduit plays a role in long-term survival, because most large series combine several types of conduits within their survival data.[36,52] However, some reports detailing survival with specific conduit types are available.[29,42,52,55,97] Those series that provide comparisons in survival between the different types of conduits generally find no large differences in long-term survival (Figure 116-15).*

SUMMARY

The need for an improved RV-to-PA conduit exists. The number of neonates receiving RV-to-PA conduits will likely continue to increase, resulting in more children and adults requiring conduit replacement for patient-conduit size mismatch. Furthermore, as patient mortality continues to decline, the number of reinterventions each patient receives for conduit failure will increase. Methods to improve the longevity of RV-to-PA conduits will focus on the production of materials that provide an optimal tissue match between the conduit and patient, which should facilitate conduit implantation, provide flow characteristics to minimize valve stress, and reduce the risk of immune response to foreign antigens present within the conduit. Future research may provide a conduit with these characteristics, which most importantly will be capable of growing with the patient.

*References 5, 24, 35, 36, 50, 62, 63, 66, 84, 85.

REFERENCES

1. Agarwal KC, Edwards WD, Feldt RH, et al: Clinicopathological correlates of obstructed right-sided porcine-valved extracardiac conduits. J Thorac Cardiovasc Surg 81:591–601,1981.
2. Agarwal KC, Edwards WD, Feldt RH, et al: Pathogenesis of nonobstructive fibrous peels in right-sided porcine-valved extracardiac conduits. J Thorac Cardiovasc Surg. 83:584–589, 1982.
3. Armiger LC, Gavin JB, Barratt-Boyes BG: Histological assessment of orthotopic aortic valve leaflet allografts: its role in selecting graft pre-treatment. Pathology 15:67–73, 1983.

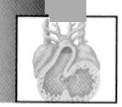

4. Armiger LC, Thomson RW, Strickett MG, Barratt-Boyes BG: Morphology of heart valves preserved by liquid nitrogen freezing. Thorax 40:778–786, 1985.
5. Albert JD, Bishop DA, Fullerton DA, et al: Conduit reconstruction of the right ventricular outflow tract. Lessons learned in a twelve-year experience. J Thorac Cardiovasc Surg 106:228–235,1993; discussion 235–236.
6. Ando M, Imai Y, Takanashi Y, et al: Fate of trileaflet equine pericardial extracardiac conduit used for the correction of anomalies having pulmonic ventricle–pulmonary arterial discontinuity. Ann Thorac Surg 64:154–158, 1997.
7. Angell JD, Christopher BS, Hawtrey O, Angell WM: A fresh, viable human heart valve bank: sterilization, sterility testing, and cryogenic preservation. Transplant Proc 82:139–147, 1976.
8. Aupecle B, Serraf A, Belli E, et al:Intermediate follow-up of a composite stentless porcine valved conduit of bovine pericardium in the pulmonary circulation. AnnThorac Surg 74:127–132, 2002.
9. Bailey WW: Cryopreserved pulmonary homograft valved external conduits: early results. J Cardiac Surg 2:199–204, 1987.
10. Bailey WW, Kirklin JW, Bargeron LM Jr., et al: Late results with synthetic valved external conduits from venous ventricle to pulmonary arteries. Circulation 56:1173–1179, 1977.
11. Balch CM, Karp RB: Blood group compatibility and aortic valve allotransplantation in man. J Thorac Cardiovasc Surg 70:256–259, 1975.
12. Bando K, Danielson GK, Schaff HV, et al: Outcome of pulmonary and aortic homografts for right ventricular outflow tract reconstruction. J Thorac Cardiovasc Surg 109:509–517, 1995; discussion 517–518.
13. Barbero-Marcial M, Baucia JA, Jatene A: Valved conduits of bovine pericardium for right ventricle to pulmonary artery connections. Semin Thorac Cardiovasc Surg 7:148–153, 1995.
14. Baskett RJ, Nanton MA, Warren AE, Ross DB: Human leukocyte antigen-DR and ABO mismatch are associated with accelerated homograft valve failure in children: implications for therapeutic interventions. J Thorac Cardiovasc Surg 126:232–239, 2003.
15. Ben-Shachar G, Nicoloff DM, Edwards JE: Separation of neointima from Dacron graft causing obstruction. Case following Fontan procedure for tricuspid atresia. J Thorac Cardiovasc Surg 82:268–271, 1981.
16. Bove EL, Byrum CJ, Thomas FD, et al: The influence of pulmonary insufficiency on ventricular function following repair of tetralogy of Fallot. Evaluation using radionuclide ventriculography. J Thorac Cardiovasc Surg 85:691–696, 1983.
17. Bove T, Demanet H, Wauthy P, et al: Early results of valved bovine jugular vein conduit versus bicuspid homograft for right ventricular outflow tract reconstruction. Ann Thorac Surg 74:536–541, 2002; discussion 541.
18. Bove EL, Lupinetti FM, Pridjian AK, et al: Results of a policy of primary repair of truncus arteriosus in the neonate. J ThoracCardiovasc Surg 105:1057–1065, 1993; discussion 1065–1066.
19. Bowman FO Jr., Hancock WD, Malm JR: A valve-containing Dacron prosthesis. Its use in restoring pulmonary artery-right ventricular continuity. Arch Surg 107:724–728, 1973.
20. Boyce SW, Turley K, Yee ES, et al: The fate of the 12 mm porcine valved conduit from the right ventricle to the pulmonary artery. A ten-year experience. J Thorac Cardiovasc Surg 95:201–207, 1988.
21. Brawn WJ: The use of a glutaraldehyde-preserved ovine pulmonary valve as a pulmonary valve substitute in infants. Semin Thorac Cardiovasc Surg 7:154–156, 1995.
22. Breymann T, Thies WR, Boethig D, et al: Bovine valved venous xenografts for RVOT reconstruction: results after 71 implantations. Eur J Cardio-Thorac Surg 21:703–710, 2002; discussion 710.
23. Brown JW, Aufiero TX, Sun K: Conduits in the pulmonary circulation. Adv Cardiac Surg 8:109–129, 1996.
24. Bull C, Macartney FJ, Horvath P, et al: Evaluation of long-term results of homograft and heterograft valves in extracardiac conduits. J Thorac Cardiovasc Surg 94:12–19, 1987.
25. Campbell DN Clark DR: Use of the allograft aortic valved conduit. Ann Thorac Surg 50:320–322, 1990.
26. Carpentier A, Lemaigre G, Robert L, et al: Biological factors affecting long-term results of valvular heterografts. J Thorac Cardiovasc Surg 58:467–483, 1969.
27. Carrel T, Berdat P, Pavlovic M, Pfammatter JP: The bovine jugular vein: a totally integrated valved conduit to repair the right ventricular outflow. J Heart Valve Dis 11:552–556, 2002.
28. Cerfolio RJ, Danielson GK, Warnes CA, et al: Results of an autologous tissue reconstruction for replacement of obstructed extracardiac conduits. J Thorac Cardiovasc Surg 110:1359–1366, 1995; discussion 1366–1368.
29. Champsaur G, Robin J, Curtil A, et al: Long-term clinical and hemodynamic evaluation of porcine valved conduits implanted from the right ventricle to the pulmonary artery. J Thorac Cardiovasc Surg 116:793–804, 1998.
30. Chan KC, Fyfe DA, McKay CA, et al: Right ventricular outflow reconstruction with cryopreserved homografts in pediatric patients: intermediate-term follow-up with serial echocardiographic assessment. J Am Coll Cardiol 24:483–489, 1994.
31. Clarke DR, Campbell DN, Pappas G: Pulmonary allograft conduit repair of tetralogy of Fallot. An alternative to transannular patch repair. J Thorac Cardiovasc Surg 98:730–736, 1989; discussion 736–737.
32. Cleveland DC, Williams WG, Razzouk AJ, et al:, Failure of cryopreserved homograft valved conduits in the pulmonary circulation. Circulation 86:11150–11153, 1992.
33. Corno AF, Hurni M, Griffin H, et al: Bovine jugular vein as right ventricle-to-pulmonary artery valved conduit. J Heart Valve Dis 11:242–247, 2002; discussion 248.
34. Daenen W, Narine K, Goffin Y, Gewillig M: Right ventricular outflow reconstruction with homografts. Eur J Cardio-Thorac Surg 9:448–451, 1995; discussion 451–452.
35. Danielson GK, Anderson BJ, Schleck CD, Ilstrup DM: Late results of pulmonary ventricle to pulmonary artery conduits. Semin Thorac Cardiovasc Surg 7:162–167, 1995.
36. Dearani JA, Danielson GK, Puga FJ, et al: Late follow-up of 1095 patients undergoing operation for complex congenital heart disease utilizing pulmonary ventricle to pulmonary artery conduits. Ann Thorac Surg 75:399–410, 2003; discussion 410–411.
37. DeLeon SY, Tuchek JM, Bell TJ, et al: Early pulmonary homograft failure from dilatation due to distal pulmonary artery stenosis. Ann Thorac Surg 61:234–236, 1996; discussion 236–237.
38. Downing TP, Danielson GK, Schaff HV, et al: Replacement of obstructed right ventricular-pulmonary arterial valved conduits with nonvalved conduits in children. Circulation 72:1184–1187, 1985.
39. Elkins RC, Lane MM, McCue C, Ward KE: Pulmonary autograft root replacement: mid-term results. J Heart Valve Dis 8:499–503, 1999; discussion 503–506.
40. Fiore AC, Peigh PS, Robison RJ, et al: Valved and nonvalved right ventricular–pulmonary arterial extracardiac conduits. An experimental comparison. J Thorac Cardiovasc Surg 86:490–497, 1983.
41. Fischlein T, Schutz A, Haushofer M, et al:, Immunologic reaction and viability of cryopreserved homografts. Ann Thorac Surg 60:S122–S125, 1995; discussion S125–126.

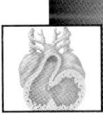

42. Forbess JM, Shah AS, St. Louis JD, et al: Cryopreserved homografts in the pulmonary position: determinants of durability. Ann Thorac Surg 71:54–59, 2001; discussion 59–60.
43. Hanley FL: Clinical experience with the autologous pulmonary valve in the systemic circulation. Semin Thorac Cardiovasc Surg 6:41–47, 1994.
44. Hanley FL, Heinemann MK, Jonas RA, et al: Repair of truncus arteriosus in the neonate. J Thorac Cardiovasc Surg 105:1047–1056, 1993.
45. Hawkins JA, Bailey WW, Dillon T, Schwartz DC: Midterm results with cryopreserved allograft valved conduits from the right ventricle to the pulmonary arteries. J Thorac Cardiovasc Surg 104:910–916, 1992.
46. Hawkins JA, Breinholt JP, Lambert LM, et al: Class I and class II anti-HLA antibodies after implantation of cryopreserved allograft material in pediatric patients. J Thorac Cardiovasc Surg 119:324–330, 2000.
47. Heinemann MK, Hanley FL, Fenton KN, et al: Fate of small homograft conduits after early repair of truncus arteriosus. Ann Thorac Surg 55:1409–1411, 1993; discussion 1411–1412.
48. Heslop BF, Wilson SE, Hardy BE: Antigenicity of aortic valve allografts. Ann Surg 177:301–306, 1973.
49. Homann M, Haehnel JC, Mendler N, et al: Reconstruction of the RVOT with valved biological conduits: 25 years experience with allografts and xenografts. Eur J Cardio-Thorac Surg 17:624–630, 2000.
50. Imai Y, Takanashi Y, Hoshino S, Nakata S: The equine pericardial valved conduit and current strategies for pulmonary reconstruction. Semin Thorac Cardiovasc Surg 7:157–161, 1995.
51. Iyer KS, Sharma R: The right ventricle to pulmonary artery connection: when homografts are not always available. Semin Thorac Cardiovasc Surg 7:145–147, 1995.
52. Jonas RA, Freed MD, Mayer JE Jr., Castaneda AR: Long-term follow-up of patients with synthetic right heart conduits. Circulation 72:1177–1183, 1985.
53. Kadner A, Chen RH, Mitchell RN, Adams DH: Hemograft crossmatching is unnecessary due to the absence of blood group antigens. Ann Thorac Surg 71:S349–S352, 2001.
54. Kadoba K, Armiger LC, Sawatari K, Jonas RA: Mechanical durability of pulmonary allograft conduits at systemic pressure. Angiographic and histologic study in lambs. J Thorac Cardiovasc Surg 105:132–141, 1993.
55. Kay PH, Ross DN: Fifteen years' experience with the aortic homograft: the conduit of choice for right ventricular outflow tract reconstruction. Ann ThoracSurg 40:360–364, 1985.
56. Kirklin JW: Ventricular to pulmonary artery connections: generalizations. Semin Thorac Cardiovasc Surg 7:168–171, 1995.
57. Kirklin JW, Blackstone EH, Maehara T, et al: Intermediate-term fate of cryopreserved allograft and xenograft valved conduits. Ann Thorac Surg 44:598–606, 1987.
58. Kitamura S, Kawachi K, Niwaya K, et al: Size-reduced cryopreserved pulmonary valve allograft for an RV-PA conduit: technical modification and functional evaluation. J Cardiac Surg 10:14–20, 1995.
59. Klinner W: Experience with correction of Fallot's tetralogy in 178 cases. Surgery 57:353–357, 1965.
60. Klovekorn WP, Meisner H, Paek SU, Sebening F: Long-term results after right ventricular outflow tract reconstruction with porcine and allograft conduits. Thorac Cardiovasc Surg 39:225–227, 1991.
61. Koirala B, Merklinger SL, Van A, et al: Extending the usable size range of homografts in the pulmonary circulation: outcome of bicuspid homografts. Ann Thorac Surg 73:866–869, 2002; discussion 869–870.
62. Lacour-Gayet F, Serraf A, Komiya T, et al: Truncus arteriosus repair: influence of techniques of right ventricular outflow tract reconstruction. J Thorac Cardiovasc Surg 111:849–856, 1996.
63. Lange R, Weipert J, Homann M, et al: Performance of allografts and xenografts for right ventricular outflow tract reconstruction. Ann Thorac Surg 71:S365S367, 2001.
64. LeBlanc JG, Russell JL, Sett SS, Potts JE: Intermediate follow-up of right ventricular outflow tract reconstruction with allograft conduits. Ann Thorac Surg 66:S174–S148, 1998.
65. Legare JF, Ross DB, Issekutz TB, et al: Prevention of allograft heart valve failure in a rat model. J Thorac Cardiovasc Surg 122:310–317, 2001.
66. Levine AJ, Miller PA, Stumper OS, et al: Early results of right ventricular-pulmonary artery conduits in patients under 1 year of age. Eur J Cardio-Thorac Surg 19:122–126, 2001.
67. Levine JC, Mayer JE Jr., Keane JF, et al: Anastomotic pseudoaneurysm of the ventricle after homograft placement in children. Ann Thorac Surg 59:60–66, 1995.
68. Livi U, Abdulla AK, Parker R, et al: Viability and morphology of aortic and pulmonary homografts. A comparative study. J Thorac Cardiovasc Surg 93:755–760, 1987.
69. Marianeschi SM, Iacona GM, Seddio F, et al: Shelhigh No-React porcine pulmonic valve conduit: a new alternative to the homograft. Ann Thorac Surg 71:619–623, 2001.
70. Mayer JE Jr: Uses of homograft conduits for right ventricle to pulmonary artery connections in the neonatal period. Semin Thorac Cardiovasc Surg 7:130–132, 1995.
71. McGoon DC, Danielson GK, Puga FJ, et al: Late results after extracardiac conduit repair for congenital cardiac defects. Am J Cardiol 49:1741–1749, 1982.
72. McGoon DC, Rastelli GC, Ongley PA: An operation for the correction of truncus arteriosus. JAMA 205:69–73, 1968.
73. Miller DC, Stinson EB, Oyer PE, et al: The durability of porcine xenograft valves and conduits in children. Circulation 66:1172–1185, 1982.
74. Molina JE, Edwards J, Bianco R, et al: Growth of fresh-frozen pulmonary allograft conduit in growing lambs. Circulation 80:1183–1190, 1989.
75. Niwaya K, Knott-Craig CJ, Lane MM, et al: Cryopreserved homograft valves in the pulmonary position: risk analysis for intermediate-term failure. J Thorac Cardiovasc Surg 117:141–146, 1999; discussion 46–47.
76. Oury JH, Doty DB, Oswalt JD, et al: Cardiopulmonary response to maximal exercise in young athletes following the Ross procedure. Ann Thorac Surg 66:S153–S154, 1998.
77. Oury JH, Hiro SP, Maxwell JM, et al: The Ross Procedure: current registry results. Ann Thorac Surg. 66:S162–S165, 1998.
78. Ovaert C, Caldarone CA, McCrindle BW, et al: Endovascular stent implantation for the management of postoperative right ventricular outflow tract obstruction: clinical efficacy. J Thorac Cardiovasc Surg 118:886–893, 1999.
79. Pearl JM, Manning PB: The use of the Shelhigh porcine valve conduit in infants. Ann Thorac Surg 73:697–698, 2002.
80. Perron J, Moran AM, Gauvreau K, et al: Valved homograft conduit repair of the right heart in early infancy. Ann Thorac Surg 68:542–548, 1999.
81. Powell AJ, Lock JE, Keane JF, Perry SB: Prolongation of RV-PA conduit life span by percutaneous stent implantation. Intermediate-term results. Circulation 92:3282–3288, 1995.
82. Rajani B, Mee RB, Ratliff NB: Evidence for rejection of homograft cardiac valves in infants.[comment]. J Thorac Cardiovasc Surg 115: 111–117, 1998.
83. Rasteli GC, Davis GD: Surgical repair for pulmonary valve atresia with coronary-pulmonary artery fistula: Report of case. Mayo Clin Proc 40:521–527, 1965.
84. Razzouk AJ, Williams WG, Cleveland DC, et al: Surgical connections from ventricle to pulmonary artery. Comparison

of four types of valved implants. Circulation 86:11154–11158, 1992.
85. Reddy VM, Rajasinghe HA, McElhinney DB, Hanley FL: Performance of right ventricle to pulmonary artery conduits after repair of truncus arteriosus: a comparison of Dacron-housed porcine valves and cryopreserved allografts. Semin Thorac Cardiovasc Surg 7:133–138, 1995.
86. Ross DN, Somerville J: Correction of pulmonary atresia with a homograft aortic valve. Lancet 2:1446–1447, 1966.
87. Sanders SP, Levy RJ, Freed MD, et al: Use of Hancock porcine xenografts in children and adolescents. Am J Cardiol 46:429–438, 1980.
88. Sano S, Karl TR, Mee RB: Extracardiac valved conduits in the pulmonary circuit. Ann Thorac Surg 52:285–290, 1991.
89. Schlichter AJ, Kreutzer C, Mayorquim RC, et al: Long-term follow-up of autologous pericardial valved conduits. Ann Thorac Surg 62:155–160, 1996.
90. Shaddy RE, Lambert LM, Fuller TC, et al: Prospective randomized trial of azathioprine in cryopreserved valved allografts in children. Ann Thorac Surg 71:43–47, 2001; discussion 47–48.
91. Shaddy RE, Tani LY, Sturtevant JE, et al: Effects of homograft blood type and anatomic type on stenosis, regurgitation and calcium in homografts in the pulmonary position. Am J Cardiol 70:392–393, 1992.
92. Stark J: The use of valved conduits in pediatric cardiac surgery. Pediatr Cardiol 19:282–288, 1998.
93. Santini F, Mazzucco A: Bicuspid homograft reconstruction of the right ventricular outflow tract in infants. Ann Thorac Surg 60:S624–S625, 1995.
94. Sung HW, Witzel TH, Hata C, et al: Development and evaluation of a pliable biological valved conduit. Part II: Functional and hemodynamic evaluation. Intl J Artif Organs 16:199–204, 1993.
95. Turley K, Ebert PA: Aortic allografts: reconstruction of right ventricle-pulmonary artery continuity. Ann Thorac Surg 47:278–281, 1989.
96. Vrandecic MO, Fantini FA, Gontijo BF, et al: Porcine stentless valve/bovine pericardial conduit for right ventricle to pulmonary artery. Ann Thorac Surg 66:S179–S182, 1998.
97. Weipert J, Meisner H, Mendler N, et al: Allograft implantation in pediatric cardiac surgery: surgical experience from 1982 to 1994. Ann Thorac Surg 60:S101–S104, 1995.
98. Yankah AC, Alexi-Meskhishvili V, Weng Y, et al: Accelerated degeneration of allografts in the first two years of life. Ann ThoracSurg 60:S71–S76, 1995; discussion 576–577.
99. Yankah AC, Wottge HU, Muller-Ruchholtz W: Short-course cyclosporin A therapy for definite allograft valve survival immunosuppression in allograft valve operations. Ann Thorac Surg 60:S146–S150, 1995.

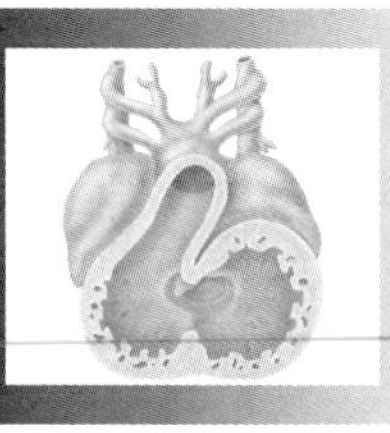

CHAPTER 117

Truncus Arteriosus and Aortopulmonary Window

Richard G. Ohye, Eric J. Devaney, and Edward L. Bove

TRUNCUS ARTERIOSUS

Truncus arteriosus is a relatively rare congenital heart defect in which there is a single vascular trunk arising from the heart, giving origin to the true pulmonary arteries, aorta, coronary arteries, and brachiocephalic vessels. The lesion accounts for approximately 0.4–4.0% of all congenital heart lesions.[14,64,71] Truncus arteriosus was first described by Wilson[81] in 1798. Subsequently, in 1942, Lev and Saphir[46] defined the anatomy currently associated with truncus arteriosus.

Embryology

During the fifth week of gestation, paired lateral ridges appear in the cephalic portion of the truncus. These truncal swellings will ultimately form the aorticopulmonary septum. The right superior truncus swelling, located on the right superior wall of the truncus, grows distally and leftward, while the left inferior truncus swelling, located on the left inferior wall, moves distally and rightward. The opposing movement of the swellings as they grow toward the aortic sac results in the spiraling of the aorticopulmonary septum. The most proximal portions of the swellings form parts of the infundibular or conal septum. Hence, variable deficiency of these truncal swellings results in the various forms of truncus arteriosus and the commonly present ventricular septal defect (VSD).

Pluripotent neural crest cells play an important role in the development of the conotruncus and aortic arch. Selective ablation of neural crest cells in chick embryos before migration results in a number of congenital heart defects.[39] These anomalies include truncus arteriosus and interrupted aortic arch, explaining their coexistence in approximately 10–20% of patients with truncus arteriosus.[13,54]

Animal models provide further insight into the genetic basis for truncus arteriosus. The mouse mutant, *Splotch*, which has a mutation in the homeobox gene *Pax3*, has a phenotype with truncus arteriosus and aortic arch abnormalities.[25] In human beings, monoallelic microdeletion of chromosome *22qll* is associated with multiple defects of neural crest origin, including typical facies, cleft palate, thyroid and parathyroid gland aplasia, and conotruncal and aortic arch abnormalities. The resulting phenotypical syndromes include DiGeorge, velocardiofacial, and Shprintzen syndromes, which are associated with truncus arteriosus. One candidate gene identified within the area of the microdeletion is *HIRA*. *HIRA* interacts with *Pax3* and thus may be integral to *Pax3* regulation of neural crest cells.[26] Environmental risk factors for the development of truncus arteriosus include maternal diabetes and exposure to retinoic acid.

Anatomy

In truncus arteriosus, there is generally *situs solitus* and d-looping of the ventricles. A single great vessel arises from the base of the heart, giving origin to the pulmonary, systemic, and coronary arteries. Classifications of truncus arteriosus were proposed by Collett and Edwards[16] in 1949 and by Van Praagh and Van Praagh[77] in 1965 (Figure 117-1). The system described by Collett and Edwards (Table 117-1) is based upon the site of origin of the pulmonary arteries, while the Van Praagh classification (Table 117-2) is based upon the degree of separation of the trunk and the presence or absence of a VSD. The Van Praagh scheme also requires that at least one of the pulmonary arteries arise from the common trunk. This stipulation appropriately relegates Collett and Edwards type IV, or *pseudotruncus,* to the spectrum of pulmonary atresia with aortopulmonary collaterals. The Van Praagh classification also provides for the inclusion of the relatively common association of hypoplastic or interrupted aortic arch. The term *hernitruncus* is frequently encountered in the literature to describe the anomalous origin of the right pulmonary artery from the ascending aorta with a normal origin of the left pulmonary artery from the main pulmonary artery, usually in the absence of a VSD. This lesion is distinct from Van Praagh type B3 and should not be considered a form of truncus arteriosus.

A VSD is nearly always present. It results from the deficiency of the infundibular septum and is generally nonrestrictive. The VSD is cradled by the two limbs of the septal band and bounded superiorly by the truncal valve (Figure 117-2). The posterior (inferior) limb of the septal band usually inserts into the parietal band, resulting in discontinuity of the tricuspid and truncal valves, maintaining a muscular rim between the conduction system and the VSD. When there is failure of insertion, the VSD extends into the membranous septum, with the conduction system running along the posterior–inferior rim of the defect.

The truncal valve may be tricuspid (69%), quadricuspid (22%), bicuspid (9%), or rarely unicuspid or pentacuspid.[28] The valve is usually in continuity with the mitral valve but infrequently with the tricuspid valve. The truncus equally overrides both ventricles in 68–83% of cases, is deviated over the right ventricle in 11–29%, and is deviated to the left in 4–6%.[8,39] The valve may be stenotic or regurgitant, which can complicate management of the patient with truncus arteriosus. A moderate or greater degree of truncal insufficiency is present in 20–26% of patients.[45,75] Mild stenosis is generally detected on preoperative evaluation because of increased flow across the truncal valve. Significant stenosis is present in only 4–7%.[45,75] Gradients of greater than 30 mm Hg are concerning for residual stenosis after complete repair.[10]

The branch pulmonary arteries generally originate from the left posterolateral aspect of the truncus, just distal to the truncal valve. They are usually of good size without ostial or branch stenosis. Collett and Edwards type I is most frequently encountered, occurring in 48–68% of cases, followed by type II (29–48%) and type III (6–10%).[8,39] In practice, most cases seem to fall into a category of "type 1½," with the branch pulmonary arteries arising not from a main pulmonary artery, but in proximity from the posterior aspect of the truncus. Origin of one pulmonary artery from a systemic artery other than the truncus (Van Praagh type A3/B3) is relatively rare, with an incidence of 2–5%.[45,72]

Associated Anomalies

An interrupted aortic arch, most commonly type B, is present in association with truncus arteriosus (Van Praagh type A4/B4) in approximately 10–20% of patients[13,54] The arch is

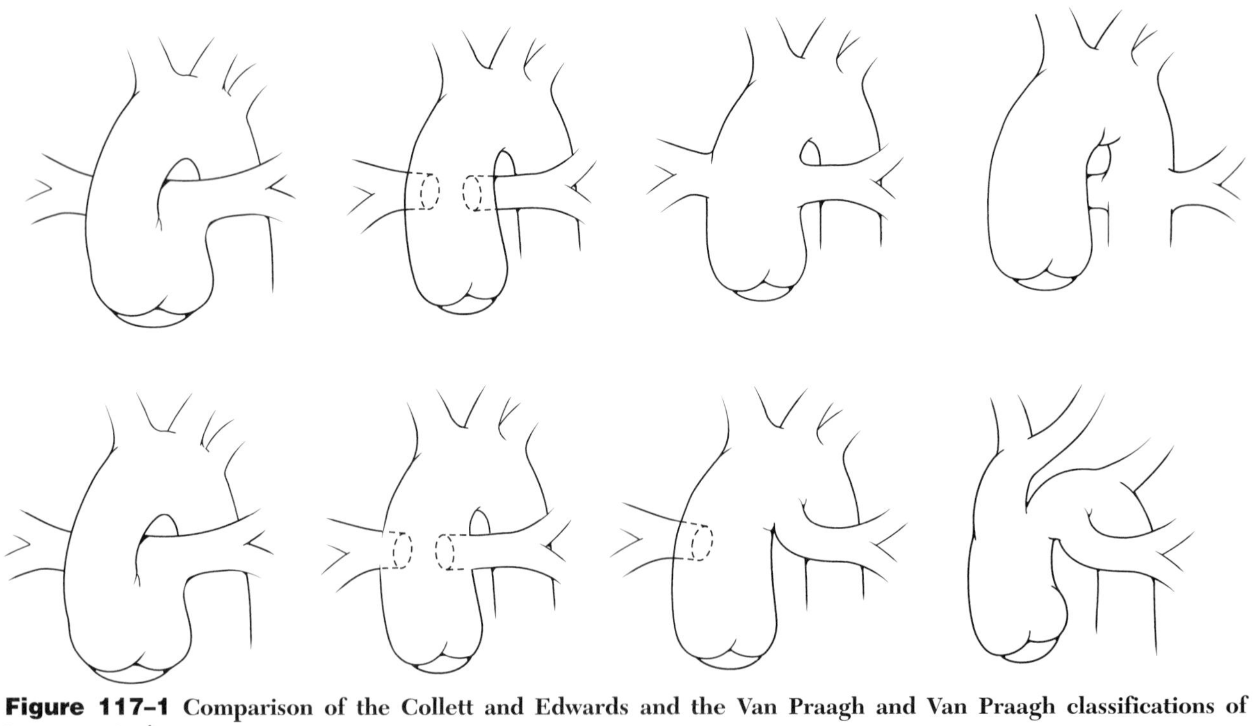

Figure 117–1 Comparison of the Collett and Edwards and the Van Praagh and Van Praagh classifications of truncus arteriosus.

Table 117–1

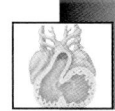

Collett and Edwards classification

Type I	Branch pulmonary arteries arise from a segment of main pulmonary artery off of the common trunk.
Type II	Branch pulmonary arteries arise in close proximity from the posterior aspect of the common trunk.
Type III	Branch pulmonary arteries arise from separate widely spaced origins.
Type IV	Absent "true" branch pulmonary arteries with aortopulmonary collaterals.

Table 117–2

Van Praagh and Van Praagh Classifications

Type A	Ventricular septal defect present
Type B	Ventricular septal defect absent
1	Partial development of the aorticopulmonary septum
2	Absence of the aorticopulmonary septum
3	Absence of one of the branch pulmonary arteries
4	Coarctation, hypoplasia, or interruption of the aortic arch with a patent ductus arteriosus

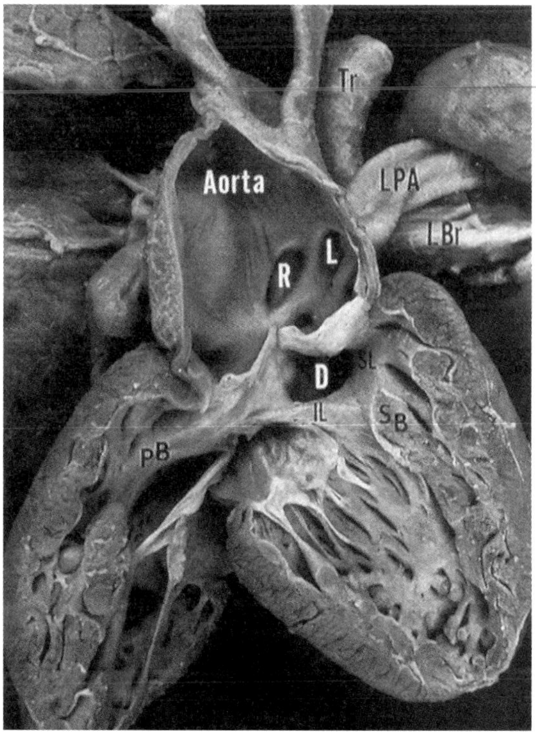

Figure 117–2 Right ventricular view of the pathological anatomy of truncus arteriosus. The truncal origins of the aorta and left (L) and right (R) pulmonary arteries are apparent. The ventricular septal defect (D) is cradled between the inferior (IL) and superior (SL) limbs of the septal band (SB). Insertion of the inferior limb (IL) into the parietal band (PB) provides muscular discontinuity between the tricuspid and truncal valves. Tr, trachea; LPA, left pulmonary artery; LBr, left bronchus.
(Reprinted with permission from Mair DD, Edwards WD, Julsrud PR, et al: Truncus arteriosus. In Allen HD, Gutgesell HP, Clark EB, Driscoll DJ, editors: Moss and Adams' Heart Disease in Infants, Children, and Adolescents. Philadelphia: Lippincott, Williams & Wilkins, 2001.)

rightward, generally with mirror image branching, in 21–36%.[13,47] Aberrant origins of the brachiocephalic vessels are reported, most commonly an aberrant right subclavian artery in 4–10%.[8,47]

Coronary variations are common in truncus arteriosus and are of potential importance in surgical repair of the lesion. The left anterior descending artery is often small, with prominent conal branches from the right coronary artery supplying the right ventricular infundibulum.[20] Origin of the left anterior descending from the right coronary can occur with the obvious surgical ramifications for the right ventricular infundibulotomy. There is left coronary dominance in 27%, which is approximately three times the incidence found in the general population.[67] Coronary ostial abnormalities are of particular surgical significance and occur in 37–49% of cases.[67] The usual arrangement, regardless of the number of cusps, is for the left coronary artery to arise from the left posterolateral cusp and the right to originate from the right anterolateral cusp. Coronaries may arise from a single orifice or from two ostia in a single cusp.[13] There may be ostial stenosis, often described as a slit-like orifice, or obstruction from abnormal valve tissue. The left coronary artery is frequently noted to have a high origin, not uncommonly near the takeoff of the pulmonary arteries. Rarely, the left coronary can originate from the main pulmonary trunk or a branch pulmonary artery.[8]

Other cardiac anomalies are common, with a patent foramen ovale (PFO) usually present. A true atrial septal defect is found in 9–20%, a persistent left superior vena cava in 4–9%, and mild tricuspid valve stenosis in 6%.[8,47] Mitral valve abnormalities are reported in 5–10% of patients. Tricuspid atresia, complete atrioventricular septal defect, anomalies of pulmonary venous return, mitral atresia, ventricular inversion, and heterotaxy syndrome have all been reported in association with truncus arteriosus.

Extracardiac anomalies are reported in approximately 28% of patients with truncus arteriosus.[75] Described abnormalities include skeletal, genitourinary, and gastrointestinal deformities. As mentioned earlier, monoallelic microdeletion of chromosome *22qll* is common, with DiGeorge syndrome diagnosed in at least 11%.[75]

Pathophysiology

The pathophysiology of truncus arteriosus is one of a total admixture lesion, with mixing occurring at the level of the VSD and proximal truncus. While there is cyanosis, systemic oxygen saturations are frequently 85–90% in the newborn period because of elevated pulmonary blood flow. In the absence of pulmonary artery stenosis or systemic outflow obstruction, the amount of pulmonary blood flow is mainly affected by the pulmonary vascular resistance (PVR). In the first few days of life, PVR remains relatively high, limiting pulmonary blood flow. As PVR decreases, the amount of pulmonary blood flow increases, leading to pulmonary overcirculation and signs and symptoms of congestive heart failure. The unrestricted left-to-right shunt results in both pressure and volume overload to the pulmonary circuit. In addition, truncus arteriosus is distinguished from other left-to-right shunt lesions by both systolic and diastolic shunting. These factors lead to the early development of irreversible pulmonary vascular occlusive disease in truncus arteriosus.

Truncal valve regurgitation and, less frequently, stenosis can exacerbate the hemodynamic stresses placed upon the heart in truncus arteriosus. Regurgitation adds an additional volume overload to the ventricles, worsening the signs and symptoms of congestive heart failure. The diastolic run-off, which occurs not only because of the insufficient valve but also as a result of the low-resistance pulmonary vascular bed, can lead to poor systemic perfusion, most notably to the coronary arteries. Stenosis increases the afterload on the ventricles and thereby increases myocardial oxygen demand. Significant stenosis can limit systemic perfusion, again compounded by the run-off into the pulmonary circuit.

Diagnosis

Clinical Features

The diagnosis of truncus arteriosus is generally made in early infancy, often during the neonatal period. The lesion may also be recognized antenatally on fetal echocardiography. The degree of cyanosis or congestive heart failure is dependent on the pulmonary vascular resistance and the resultant volume of pulmonary blood flow. The clinical manifestations may be exacerbated by associated lesions, such as truncal valve insufficiency or interrupted aortic arch, or may be ameliorated by pulmonary artery stenosis.

Physical findings are dependent upon the amount of pulmonary blood flow and the degree of truncal valve insufficiency. In general, the neonate with truncus arteriosus may show only mild cyanosis at the time of birth. As the pulmonary vascular resistance falls and pulmonary blood flow increases, signs of congestive heart failure become manifest and cyanosis decreases. Truncal regurgitation will accelerate the onset and increase the severity of congestive failure. The infant will show the typical findings of tachypnea, tachycardia, diaphoresis, and poor feeding. The precordium is hyperactive and a thrill may be palpable over the left sternal border.

There is a normal S1 and a single loud S2, which may be associated with an opening click. An S3 is not uncommon as the degree of failure progresses. A pansystolic murmur is common at the left sternal border. A low-pitch diastolic murmur at the apex, representing increased flow across the mitral valve, may be present. A high-pitched diastolic murmur along the left sternal border is indicative of truncal valve regurgitation. In the absence of the rarely encountered pulmonary artery stenosis, a continuous murmur is distinctly uncommon. The detection of a continuous murmur is consistent with other diagnoses, notably pulmonary atresia with a patent ductus or aortopulmonary collaterals. The peripheral pulse pressure is increased because of the diastolic run-off into the pulmonary bed and is further widened by truncal insufficiency.

Diagnostic Studies

The chest radiograph generally shows moderate cardiomegaly with increased pulmonary vascular markings. The arch is rightward in approximately one third of patients, and the thymus gland may be absent in those with *22qll* microdeletion. The combination of a right arch and increased pulmonary vascular markings is strongly suggestive of truncus arteriosus. The two-dimensional and Doppler echocardiography examinations are the diagnostic modalities of choice. The echocardiogram can define the anatomy of truncus arteriosus at birth or *in utero*. A parasternal long-axis view will demonstrate the large truncal valve overriding the VSD (Figure 117-3A). The addition of Doppler interrogation will reveal truncal valve stenosis or regurgitation (Figure 117-3B). Suprasternal notch views can further define the anatomy of the pulmonary arteries and aortic arch (Figure 117-4). Cardiac catheterization is generally reserved for the delineation of the anatomy in complex forms of truncus arteriosus, such as truncus arteriosus with a single pulmonary artery (Van Praagh type A3/B3). Cardiac catheterization is also indicated to assess PVR in the patient presenting late with truncus arteriosus. Magnetic resonance imaging (MRI) is a useful alternative or adjunct to cardiac catheterization for defining the anatomy of complex truncus arteriosus.

Natural History

The typical natural history of truncus arteriosus is characterized by early demise because of congestive heart failure. Approximately 40% of infants are dead within one month, 70% by three months, and 90% by one year.[40] Those patients who survive infancy generally succumb by childhood or early adolescence because of congestive heart failure or, more commonly, pulmonary vascular obstructive disease. Rarely, patients may survive infancy without the development of pulmonary vascular obstructive disease, although those who do are estimated to be less than 5% of all patients.[40]

Treatment

Because of the inherent high early mortality, truncus arteriosus warrants early intervention. Initially, the surgical treatment of truncus arteriosus was limited to the banding

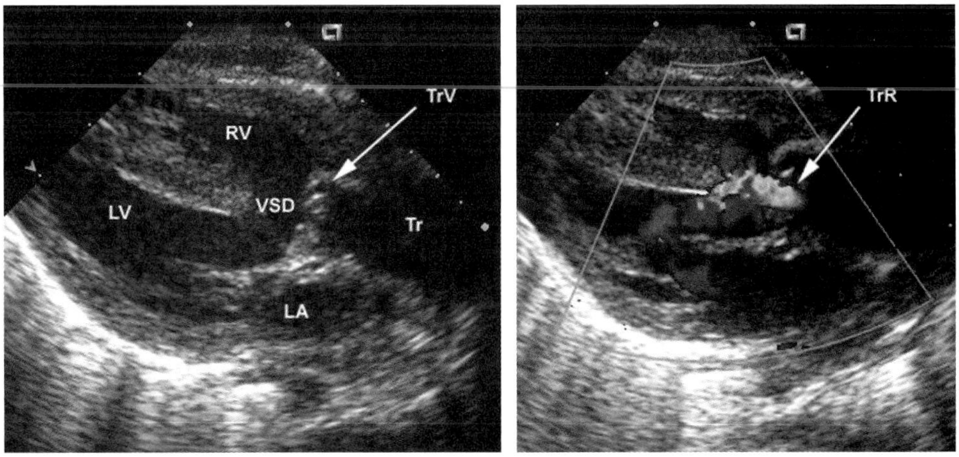

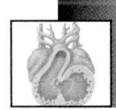

Figure 117-3 **Parasternal long-axis view of a patient with truncus arteriosus.** **A,** The large truncus (Tr) overriding the ventricular septal defect (VSD) is demonstrated. **B,** The addition of Doppler reveals a jet of truncal regurgitation (TrR). LA, left atrium; LV, left ventricle; RV, right ventricle; TrV, truncal valve. (See color plate.)

of one or both of the branch pulmonary arteries. The first successful intracardiac repair was accomplished by Sloan at the University of Michigan in 1962 using an unvalved polytetrafluoroethylene (PTFE) conduit for the pulmonary reconstruction.[6] In 1967, McGoon[51] performed the first valved conduit repair, using an aortic allograft. During this period, complete repair was often undertaken as a staged procedure following initial pulmonary artery banding. However, complications of pulmonary artery banding, including pulmonary artery distortion, band migration, and failure to prevent the development of pulmonary vascular obstructive disease, resulted in a continued high mortality with this strategy. Ebert[22] published the first series of patients undergoing repair of truncus arteriosus in infancy in 1984. With continued improvements in neonatal operative techniques, as well as in perioperative care, management has evolved to earlier complete repair. Following the early reports of neonatal repair from the University of Michigan[10] and the Children's Hospital of Boston,[31] neonatal repair has become the treatment of choice for truncus arteriosus.

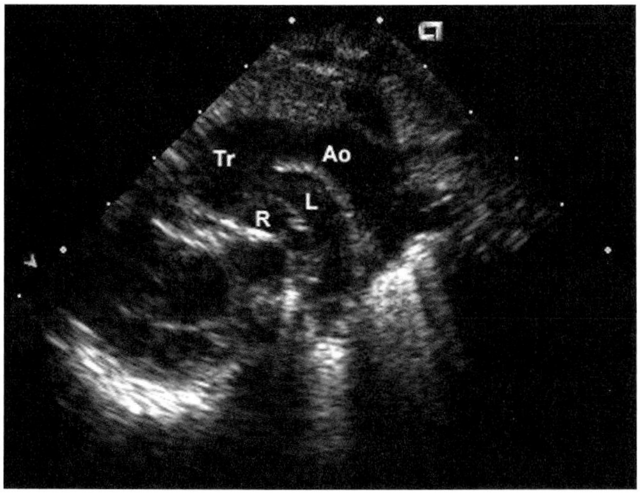

Figure 117-4 **Suprasternal notch view demonstrating close but separate origins of the right (R) and left (L) pulmonary arteries from the truncus (Tr) with continuation at the aorta (Ao).**

Surgical Technique

The repair is performed via a standard median sternotomy. While deep hypothermia with circulatory arrest or low-flow bypass has been advocated by some authors, the repair of simple forms of truncus arteriosus can easily be done on full flow with moderate hypothermia. More complex forms, such as Van Praagh type A3/B3 (one pulmonary artery absent) or A4/B4 (with interrupted aortic arch), may require periods of deep hypothermic circulatory arrest. The arterial cannula is placed distally in the ascending aorta at the base of the innominate artery. Bicaval cannulation is utilized for venous return, with an additional left ventricular vent placed through the right upper pulmonary vein. The pulmonary arteries are mobilized and snared to direct cardiopulmonary bypass flow to the systemic circulation.

The heart is arrested with antegrade cardioplegia, with the aortic cross clamp placed as distally as possible. Significant truncal valve regurgitation may necessitate the use of retrograde cardioplegia. Once the cardioplegia is delivered, the pulmonary arteries are removed. If the coronary arteries can be positively identified and the exposure is adequate, the pulmonary arteries can be directly removed from the posterior aspect of the truncus, particularly for Collett and Edwards type I truncus arteriosus. Often, it is helpful to open the aorta anteriorly to aid in the removal of the pulmonary arteries and to identify the origins of the coronary arteries (Figure 117-5A). Transection of the aorta, just distal to the origins of the branch pulmonary arteries, is another useful technique to facilitate pulmonary artery and coronary exposure (Figure 117-5B). The pulmonary arteries are removed together with a small rim of adjacent truncal wall. Care is taken to avoid injuring the left coronary artery and truncal valve, which are often in close proximity to the pulmonary arteries. The defect is then repaired directly or with a patch of PTFE. At this point, additional doses of cardioplegia can be given at intervals, depending on the surgeon's preference.

An inspection of the heart for the presence of any large conal branches, location of the left anterior descending artery, and possibility of aberrant coronary arteries is performed. A right infundibulotomy is then made in an avascular area of the right ventricular outflow tract. The infundibulotomy is

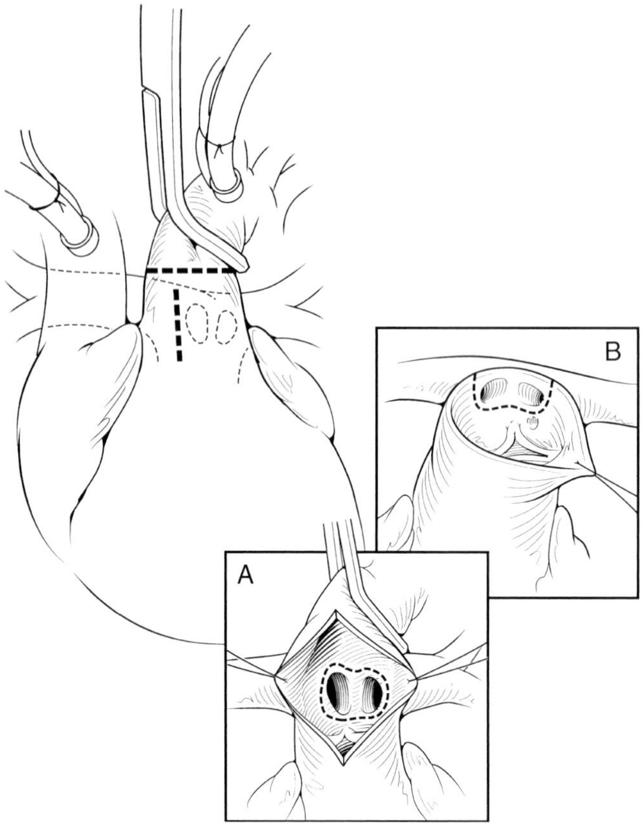

Figure 117–5 Repair of truncus arteriosus. Removal of the pulmonary arteries from the truncus is facilitated by an anterior longitudinal aortotomy **(A)** or by transection of the aorta **(B)**.

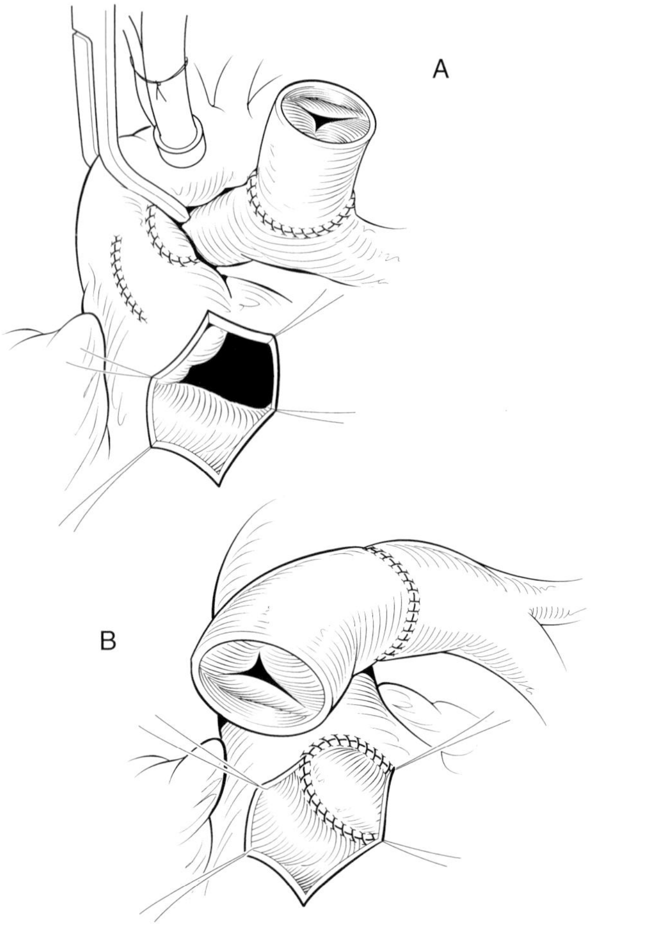

Figure 117–6 Repair of truncus arteriosus. The ventricular septal defect (VSD) is exposed through a right infundibulotomy **(A)**. The VSD patch is transitioned to the epicardium at the superiormost portion of the infundibulotomy. The posterior aspect of the pulmonary allograft is sewn directly to the superior portion of the infundibulotomy **(B)**.

carried cranially toward the truncal valve and is limited to the size necessary to allow unobstructed output from the right ventricle through the anticipated conduit (Figure 117-6A). Through the infundibulotomy, the VSD is closed with a patch of PTFE. We employ a running suture technique, although an interrupted technique may be used as well. When there is membranous or inlet extension of the VSD, care is taken not to injure the conduction tissue in the posteroinferior aspect of the VSD. It is helpful to transition from the endocardium of the right ventricular outflow tract to the epicardium in the anterosuperiormost portion of the infundibulotomy to avoid injuring the truncal valve and to ensure a widely patent left ventricular outflow tract (Figure 117-6B). If present, the atrial septal defect is then closed. A small patent foramen ovale may be left as a "pop-off valve" to aid in the postoperative management.

Once the VSD is closed, the remainder of the procedure may be performed with the cross clamp off and the heart beating. We prefer to use cryopreserved pulmonary allograft for reconstruction of the pulmonary outflow tract, although heterograft-valved conduit and cryopreserved aortic allograft are viable alternatives. The distal anastomosis of the allograft is performed to the confluence of the native branch pulmonary arteries. The posterior aspect of the allograft is then approximated to the superior portion of the right infundibulotomy. Anteriorly, the conduit is augmented with a patch of PTFE or additional allograft material (Figure 117-7).

Other Surgical Considerations

Interrupted Aortic Arch

The surgical repair of truncus arteriosus with interrupted aortic arch (Figure 117-8) requires several modifications to the basic operative procedure. The aortic cannulation is performed proximally in the truncus to perfuse all of the brachiocephalic vessels and the distal aorta. Bicaval cannulation is utilized for venous return, with a left ventricular vent placed through the right upper pulmonary vein. The patient is placed on cardiopulmonary bypass and cooled to 18° C over a minimum of 20 min. The pulmonary arteries are snared to prevent pulmonary overcirculation. During cooling, the ascending aorta, arch, proximal descending aorta, brachiocephalic vessels, and pulmonary arteries are mobilized. The arch repair can be performed under deep hypothermic circulatory arrest. Alternatively, regional cerebral perfusion, as described by Pigula[57] and others, can be delivered by anastomosing a PTFE tube graft to the innominate artery or by directly cannulating the aorta at the base of the innominate artery and advancing the cannula into the innominate. After adequate cooling, the head vessels are

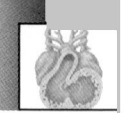

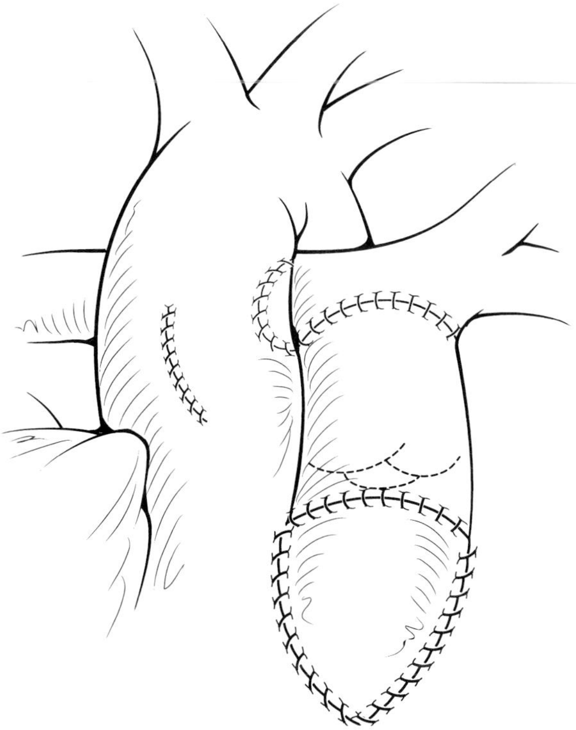

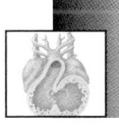

Figure 117–7 Repair of the truncus arteriosus. Right ventricle-to-pulmonary artery continuity is then completed with a hood of polytetrafluoroethylene.

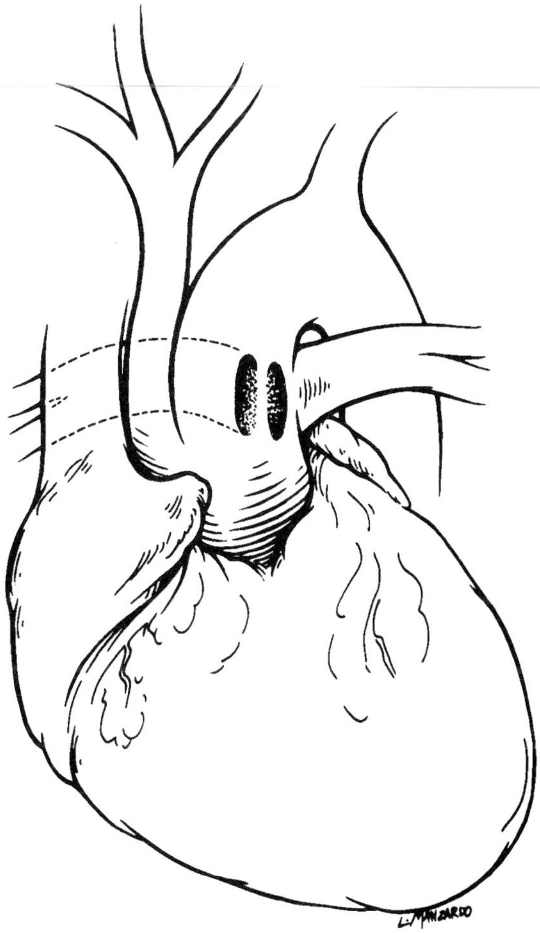

Figure 117–8 Truncus arteriosus (Collett and Edwards type II) with a type B interrupted aortic arch.
(Reprinted from Mosca RS, Bove EL: Truncus arteriosus. In Baue AE, Geha AS, Hammond GL, et al, editors: Glenn's Thoracic and Cardiovascular Surgery. Stamford: Connecticut: Appleton and Lange, 1996.)

snared, bypass is stopped, and regional cerebral perfusion is initiated, if desired. The ductus arteriosus is ligated just distal to the origin of the pulmonary arteries and divided. All residual ductal tissue is resected from the proximal descending aorta. The ascending aorta and proximal descending aorta are spatulated (Figure 117-9). The back walls of the distal ascending aorta and proximal descending aorta are approximated, and the repair is augmented with a patch of cryopreserved pulmonary allograft (Figure 117-10). Once the arch reconstruction is completed, the aorta may be recannulated and de-aired, an aortic cross clamp placed, and cardiopulmonary bypass resumed. Then, additional doses of cardioplegia may be administered and rewarming begun. The remainder of the repair, including VSD closure and pulmonary outflow tract reconstruction, is similar to simple truncus arteriosus surgical procedure.

Truncal Valve Regurgitation or Stenosis

Significant truncal valve regurgitation, or less frequently stenosis, can complicate the operative management of truncus arteriosus in approximately one quarter of cases. A conservative approach is warranted, as frequently both regurgitation and stenosis improve after corrective surgery and relief of the volume overload. Gradients of less than 30 mm Hg generally do not require intervention.[10] In addition, even moderate degrees of truncal regurgitation are well tolerated, and delay of valve repair or replacement can often be accomplished. In the face of severe truncal regurgitation, many patients may not survive to operation. For those patients who do survive, options include root replacement with cryopreserved aortic allograft, mechanical valve replacement, or truncal valve repair. Truncal valve replacement may be facilitated by enlargement of the valve annulus by the VSD patch. For truncal valve repair, several techniques have been described in small series of patients with reasonable survivals. These techniques include annuloplasty, resection of cusps, closure of commissures, resuspension of cusps, and cusp repair.[9,23] Older children and adults have a greater number of options for valve replacement, including aortic allograft, stented or stentless tissue valves, and mechanical valves, or they may undergo repair.

Pulmonary Outflow Tract Reconstruction

While the majority of surgeons utilize valved heterograft or allograft conduits, several other techniques have been described. These other techniques include the use of unvalved conduits, fresh autologous pericardial valved conduits, monocusps, and various methods for achieving native tissue apposition between the right ventricle and pulmonary artery.

Unvalved tube grafts have been used in the past with good results but have been largely abandoned with the

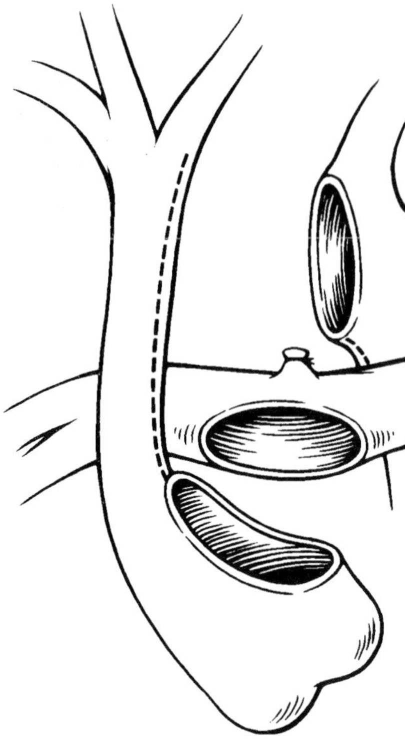

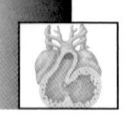

Figure 117–9 Repair of truncus arteriosus with interrupted aortic arch. The ductus arteriosus has been ligated and divided and the pulmonary arteries removed from the truncus. The areas for spatulation on the ascending aorta and proximal descending aorta are indicated (*dashed lines*).
(Reprinted from Mosca RS, Bove EL: Truncus arteriosus. In Baue AE, Geha AS, Hammond GL, et al, editors: Glenn's thoracic and cardiovascular surgery. Stamford, Connecticut: Appleton and Lange, 1996.)

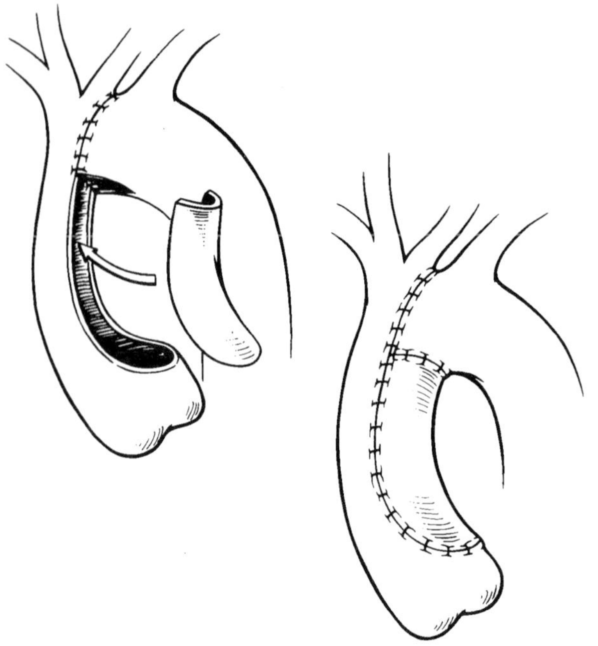

Figure 117–10 Repair of truncus arteriosus with interrupted aortic arch. The distal ascending and proximal descending aorta are reapproximated and augmented with cryopreserved pulmonary allograft.
(Reprinted from Mosca RS, Bove EL: Truncus arteriosus. In Baue AE, Geha AS, Hammond GL, et al, editors: Glenn's thoracic and cardiovascular surgery. Stamford, Connecticut: Appleton and Lange, 1996.)

development of appropriately sized valved conduits.[69] Advantages include availability and lower risk of stenosis related to valve dysfunction or calcification. The obvious disadvantage is the lack of a valve in the immediate postoperative period, with free regurgitation into a right ventricle compromised by a ventriculotomy and periods of ischemia and cardiopulmonary bypass. In addition, a valve may be advantageous in the neonate with labile pulmonary vascular resistance or the older patient with pulmonary vascular obstructive disease.

Options for valved conduits include heterografts and allografts. Porcine heterografts within Dacron tube grafts are available in sizes as small as 12 mm. Advantages include their ready availability. Disadvantages are primarily related to the stiff Dacron tube graft, which is less hemostatic and less forgiving, with a greater risk of distortion of the branch pulmonary arteries. Dacron also tends to form a neointimal peel, potentially leading to stenosis. In addition, the rigid metal ring of the heterograft valve can be compressed beneath the sternum, obstructing the left anterior descending artery. Recently, valved bovine jugular vein grafts have been introduced in sizes down to 12 mm. Bovine jugular vein grafts handle well because they are hemostatic and forgiving; however, long-term data on conduit performance are pending. Cryopreserved pulmonary allografts have the advantages of excellent tissue handling characteristics and ease of implantation. Aortic allografts can also be used, although they appear to be less durable than their pulmonary counterparts.[33,75] The disadvantage of these conduits is primarily related to their limited availability in the very small sizes, although allografts in the range of 12–16 mm can generally be placed in neonates without difficulty. A larger pulmonary allograft can be downsized by removal of one of the cusps, creating a bicuspid valve. The authors' group and others[42] have successfully used this technique when appropriately sized allografts are unavailable.

Whether heterografts or allografts have superior longevity remains controversial. Several published studies, including the authors' own experience, have shown that pulmonary allografts are the optimal conduit in neonates and infants.[33,60,75] The authors' results for the placement of a right ventricle-to-pulmonary artery conduit in a series of 155 infants demonstrated a significantly greater 5-year freedom from reoperation for cryopreserved pulmonary allograft (50%) compared to aortic allograft (24%, $p = .02$) and heterograft (26%, $p = .05$). Others have found no significant difference in longevity between heterografts and allografts for the repair of truncus arteriosus.[59]

In an effort to decrease the need for reoperation, several groups have suggested methods of achieving native tissue apposition in the right ventricular outflow tract to allow for growth. In 1990, Barbero-Marcial and associates[4] introduced a technique for anastomosing the pulmonary bifurcation directly to the superior margin of the infundibulotomy. The anterior aspect of the anastomosis is then augmented

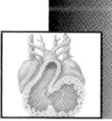

with a patch, which includes a monocusp. One patient in the series had the interposition of a flap of left atrium between the right ventricle and pulmonary artery, a technique that has since been more widely applied by others. Late follow-up of 45 patients by Barbero-Marcial and Tanamati[5] demonstrated that this technique resulted in a reintervention rate of 12% over a mean follow-up of 47 months, with an 11.4-year actuarial survival rate of 67.5%. In addition, 44.4% had moderate to severe pulmonary regurgitation, and 23.3% had pulmonary stenosis. Lacour-Gayet and colleagues[45] reported their experience with 56 consecutive patients undergoing repair for truncus arteriosus using a number of different techniques for pulmonary outflow tract reconstruction. They found an equivalent rate of reintervention for heterograft and direct anastomosis of approximately 80%. Danton and associates[19] published a series of 61 patients with truncus arteriosus, 38 repaired with a conduit and 23 with direct anastomosis. While mortality was not influenced (conduit group 8%, direct anastomosis 22%; $p = .23$), 10-year actuarial freedom from reoperation was 89% in the direct anastomosis group, compared to 56% in the conduit group ($p = .023$).

Right ventricular outflow tract reconstruction utilizing fresh autologous pericardial valved conduits has been described by Kreutzer and associates.[43] Their series of 86 patients undergoing this technique included 23 cases of truncus arteriosus. Operative mortality for the patients with truncus arteriosus was 26%. Among the entire group, moderate to severe conduit regurgitation was present immediately after surgery in 12.7%. By 6 months following surgery, no valve tissue could be identified in any patient either by echocardiography or by visual inspection in those patients requiring reoperation. For the entire cohort, the need for conduit-related reintervention was 83% at 5 years and 60% at 10 years for conduits less than 16 mm at the time of implantation. These findings did not vary by diagnostic group. By contrast, in the report by Lacour-Gayet et al,[45] freedom from reoperation or angioplasty at 7 years was 100% for patients receiving a pericardial conduit in the repair of truncus arteriosus. However, the authors also found the use of direct anastomosis or pericardial conduit to be a significant risk factor for operative mortality (43%), when compared to heterograft or allograft (7.1%, $p = .015$).

Postoperative Management

Most patients will require low doses of inotropic support with standard postoperative care techniques. The placement of a left atrial transthoracic monitoring line is helpful, as the central venous pressure may not accurately reflect left-sided filling pressures because of right ventricular dysfunction. Early operation has virtually eliminated the postoperative pulmonary hypertensive crisis seen in earlier studies. For older patients in whom pulmonary vascular hypertensive crisis or pulmonary vascular obstructive disease can be anticipated, the placement of a transthoracic pulmonary artery line can aid in postoperative management. Avoiding acidosis, hypercarbia, and hypoxia can minimize pulmonary vascular resistance. Sedation and paralysis are also utilized to minimize fluctuations in pulmonary vascular resistance. The use of nitric oxide, and more recently sildenafil, can induce pulmonary vascular smooth muscle relaxation and may be particularly useful in the older patient with reversible pulmonary vascular obstructive disease.

Results

Because the first large series of truncus arteriosus repair in infants by Ebert[22] in 1984, the management has evolved to earlier neonatal repair with a continual improvement in survival. Current hospital mortality for the neonatal repair of truncus arteriosus ranges between 4.3 and 17%, with the majority of deaths occurring in complex truncus arteriosus or in truncus arteriosus with associated severe truncal valve regurgitation.[10,12,45,72,75] Risk factors for poor outcome identified in various studies include significant truncal regurgitation, need for truncal valve replacement, birth weight less than 2.5 kg, presence of interrupted aortic arch or coronary artery anomalies, pulmonary reconstruction with a technique other than valved heterograft or allograft, and age greater than 100 days.* Other recent studies have demonstrated that interrupted aortic arch has been neutralized as a risk factor.[10,72]

Long-term survivals for patients with truncus arteriosus are also encouraging. Reddy[60] and Danton[19] both reported 2-year actuarial survivals of 73%, while Lacour-Gayet[45] achieved an 80% actuarial survival at 7 years. Examination of the Kaplan–Meier survival curves reveals that the majority of mortality is associated with the operative repair. Thus, the outlook is good for those survivors of the initial operation, with actuarial survivals of 90% at 5 years, 85% at 10 years, and 83% at 15 years; the majority of survivors (97%) in New York Heart Association Class 1-11.[47,59]

AORTOPULMONARY WINDOW

Aortopulmonary window is an uncommon malformation which is characterized by an anomalous communication between the adjacent portions of the ascending aorta and main pulmonary artery. Distinctively, the aortic and pulmonary semilunar valves are both present, and the ventricular septum is typically intact. This lesion represents between 0.2 and 0.3% of all congenital heart lesions.[1,44] Aortopulmonary window was first described by Eliotson in a clinicopathological discussion given at St. Thomas' Hospital in London in 1830.[24]

Embryology

Descriptions of cardiac embryology can be confusing because of varying terminology used by different authors. For the purpose of this discussion, the embryonic cardiac outflow tract may be considered as that portion of the primitive heart tube, which connects the ventricles with the aortic arch arteries. This outflow tract comprises the conus, the truncus, and the aortic sac. Histologically, the conotruncus has an external muscle layer and internal cardiac jelly (which is cellular), while the aortic sac has a wall consisting of endothelium surrounded by loose mesenchyme. Septation of the outflow tract seems to occur in a craniocaudal direction by two mechanisms.[80] Initial septation occurs by an ingrowth of mesenchyme (principally neural crest tissue), which separates the aortic sac into the definitive aorta and

*References 10, 12, 31, 45, 59, 72, 75.

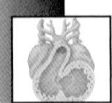

pulmonary artery. This aorticopulmonary septum then extends caudally to divide the distal truncus. Meanwhile, within the proximal conotruncus, paired ridges (consisting of both neural crest and non-neural crest tissue) bulge into the lumen and meet. The caudal portion of the aorticopulmonary septum ultimately fuses with the cranial extent of the conotruncal ridges to complete septation. This entire process occurs in human embryos beginning at 6-mm crown–rump length and is completed by the 9-mm stage over a period of about 5 days.[56]

The embryological defect in aortopulmonary window is presumed to be related to nonfusion of the aorticopulmonary septum with the conotruncal septum, malalignment of the two septa, or complete absence of the aorticopulmonary septum.[44] The defects leading to truncus arteriosus and aortopulmonary window are thought to be distinct. While a number of gene mutations that lead to a phenotype of truncus arteriosus have been identified, none of these has resulted in isolated aortopulmonary window. Additionally, isolated aortopulmonary window is generally not seen within the constellation of conotruncal abnormalities that occur in conjunction with DiGeorge syndrome.

Anatomy

The defect in aortopulmonary window is usually oval-shaped and solitary, although its precise location may vary. Many classification schemes have been proposed to describe the variation in morphology of this anomaly. One widely utilized classification was proposed by Richardson et al and describes three variants.[62] Type I defects represent the classic proximal window involving the posteromedial wall of the ascending aorta just above the left sinus of Valsalva and the adjacent wall of the main pulmonary artery. The inferior extent of the proximal defect may be close to the origin of the left coronary artery. Type II defects are more distal communications occurring near the origin of the right pulmonary artery. Distal windows may be associated with a variable degree of "unroofing" of the right pulmonary artery that may lead to the apparent origin of this vessel from the posterolateral aspect of the ascending aorta. Finally, type III defects describe anomalous origin of the right pulmonary artery from the posterolateral wall of the ascending aorta (without an associated window). The type III defect has also been called "hemitruncus," although the use of this term has been discouraged in favor of the more descriptive appellation "anomalous origin of the right pulmonary artery from the aorta."

A more useful scheme was advanced by Mori and associates.[53] In the Mori classification, type I and II defects are analogous to their counterparts in the Richardson classification, with type I (proximal) defects occurring between the adjacent portions of the proximal ascending aorta and main pulmonary artery, and type II (distal) defects located more distally near the origin of the right pulmonary artery. Mori type III (total) defects are large defects representing a combination of types I and II.

Recently, Jacobs and members of the Congenital Heart Surgery Nomenclature and Database Project proposed general use of the Mori classification (proximal, distal, and total) with the addition of a fourth type termed "intermediate" and representing a window similar to the total defect but slightly smaller, with well-defined superior and inferior rims.[35] The remainder of this chapter will adhere to this terminology. Figure 117-11 illustrates the anatomical subtypes of aortopulmonary window.

Associated Anomalies

Associated anomalies may occur in 25–65% of cases of aortopulmonary window.[2,27,32,44,55] These associated defects may be considered minor or major.[50] Common minor defects include right aortic arch, patent ductus arteriosus, atrial septal defect, and patent foramen ovale. Major defects commonly seen with aortopulmonary window include interrupted aortic arch (usually type A), tetralogy of Fallot, ventricular septal defect, anomalous coronary artery, coarctation of the aorta, and univentricular heart lesions. Berry and colleagues described a syndrome characterized by a distal aortopulmonary window, aortic origin of the right pulmonary artery, intact ventricular septum, patent ductus arteriosus, and interruption or coarctation of the aortic isthmus.[7] Braunlin et al emphasized the frequency of arch

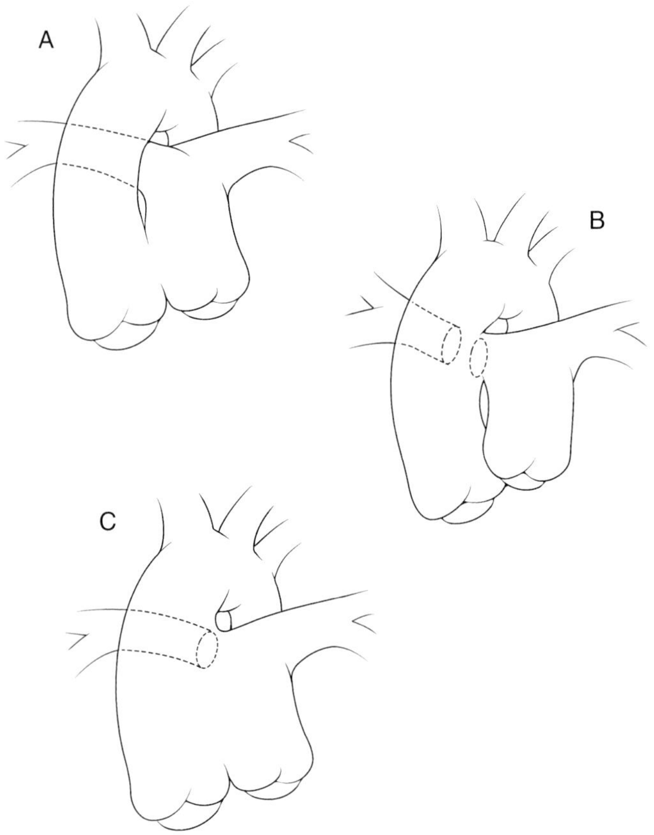

Figure 117-11 Anatomy and classification of aortopulmonary window as recommended by the Congenital Heart Surgery Nomenclature and Database Project. A, Type I (proximal) defects occur between the adjacent portions of the proximal ascending aorta and main pulmonary artery. **B,** Type II (distal) defects are located more distally near the origin of the right pulmonary artery. **C,** Type III (total) defects are large defects with poorly defined margins representing a combination of types I and II. Intermediate defects (not illustrated) are similar to total defects but are slightly smaller with well-defined superior and inferior rims.

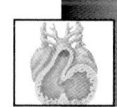

obstruction in patients with an aortopulmonary window, reporting interrupted aortic arch in 43% and coarctation in 14%.[11] The presence of an aortopulmonary window must always be excluded in infants with an interrupted aortic arch and intact ventricular septum.

Pathophysiology

An aortopulmonary window invariably leads to excessive pulmonary blood flow secondary to a large-volume left-to-right shunt that occurs during both systole and diastole. The degree of shunting is, of course, determined by the size of the window and the ratio of systemic to pulmonary vascular resistance. The window is usually nonrestrictive in nature, thereby leading to equalization of pressures within the aorta and pulmonary arteries. As pulmonary vascular resistance decreases following birth, shunt volume increases. The end result is left ventricular volume overload, as well as a pressure load on the right ventricle. Excessive pulmonary blood flow may acutely lead to the development of interstitial pulmonary edema. Over time, pulmonary overcirculation may lead to the development of pulmonary vascular obstructive disease.

The presence of associated defects may, of course, affect the physiology of this condition. Most importantly, the presence of aortic arch obstruction will exacerbate left-to-right shunting across the aortopulmonary window. In cases of severe coarctation or arch interruption, in which systemic perfusion is ductal-dependent, closure of the ductus will precipitate severe systemic malperfusion and divert even more blood flow to the lungs.

Diagnosis

Clinical Features

As with truncus arteriosus, the diagnosis of aortopulmonary window is generally made during infancy. A loud continuous murmur with systolic accentuation is heard best at the left upper sternal border and may be confused with the murmur associated with a patent ductus arteriosus. The second heart sound may be accentuated and narrowly split. The diastolic blood pressure is usually reduced with a concomitant widened pulse pressure and, on occasion, a water-hammer pulse. Patients typically present with symptoms of congestive heart failure (viz., tachypnea, diaphoresis, failure to thrive, or recurrent respiratory infections).

The differential diagnosis of aortopulmonary window includes patent ductus arteriosus, truncus arteriosus, ventricular septal defect with aortic insufficiency, and ruptured sinus of Valsalva's aneurysm.

Diagnostic Studies

A chest radiograph demonstrates moderate cardiomegaly and increased pulmonary vascular markings. A right aortic arch may be present.

Echocardiography is generally diagnostic and has replaced angiography as the gold standard.[3,38,61,65,68] The margins of the window can be imaged by two-dimensional echo, and Doppler color-flow mapping can confirm flow across the communication. The most useful echocardiographic views to delineate the margins of the window include the suprasternal long axis, the subcostal coronal plane through the pulmonary trunk, and the high parasternal short plane cephalad to the aortic valve (see Figure 117-12). Additional echocardiographic findings include left atrial and left ventricular enlargement, which are usually in proportion to the degree of volume overload. Continuous forward flow in the distal main or branch pulmonary arteries is evident. When a jet of tricuspid or pulmonary insufficiency is present, pulmonary hypertension can be confirmed. The diagnosis of aortopulmonary window can also be made during fetal echocardiography.[76]

MRI is an emerging technique that is capable of clarifying anatomy with great detail.[29,34]

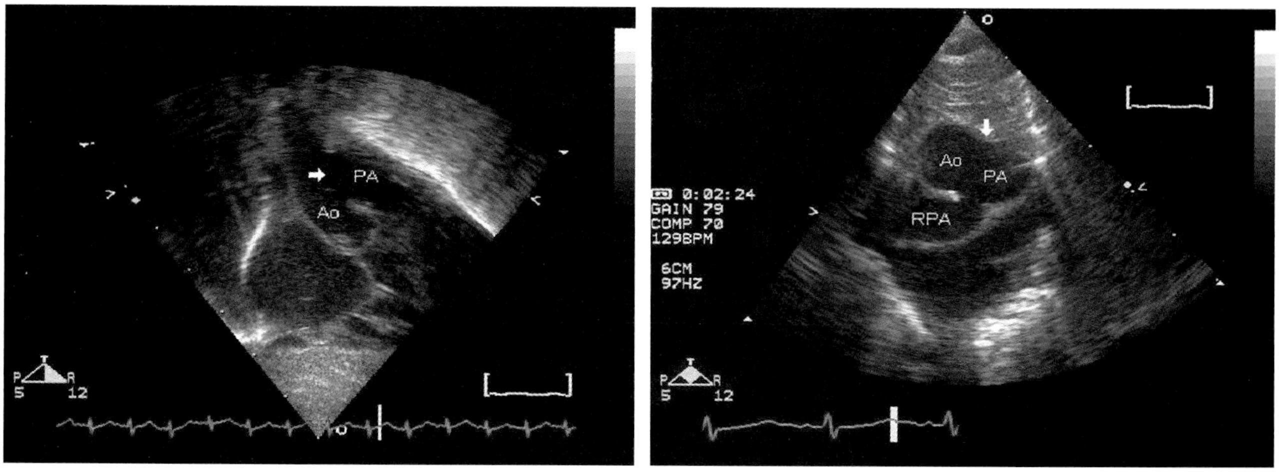

A B

Figure 117–12 Echocardiographic views in a patient with a large (total type) aortopulmonary window (as well as a type A interrupted aortic arch). A, Subcostal coronal view illustrates the large communication (*arrow*) between the ascending aorta (Ao) and main pulmonary artery (PA). **B,** Parasternal short axis view demonstrates that the distal extent of the aortopulmonary window involves the origin of the right pulmonary artery (RPA). The anterior border of the window is identified by the arrow.

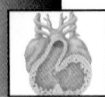

Cardiac catheterization is currently reserved for the clarification of the anatomy of the window or associated defects, including the origins of the coronary arteries. In patients who present beyond infancy, catheterization allows for the calculation of pulmonary vascular resistance.

Natural History

Patients with large aortopulmonary windows generally do not survive beyond childhood. Forty percent of untreated patients will die within the first year of life.[73] Untreated patients generally develop pulmonary vascular obstructive disease. Because of the poor prognosis associated with this condition, it is recommended that all patients with aortopulmonary window undergo repair.

Treatment

Robert Gross performed the first surgical closure of an aortopulmonary window in 1948.[30] The patient was a 4-year-old girl who was explored via a left thoracotomy for a presumptive patent ductus arteriosus. The correct diagnosis was made at operation. Gross successfully ligated the window but acknowledged the potential risks and limitations of this technique. Scott and Sabiston developed an animal model for aortopulmonary window and then devised techniques for closed division and suture closure using partial occluding clamps; they subsequently successfully applied these techniques clinically in 1951.[66] Cooley et al were the first to employ cardiopulmonary bypass to facilitate division and oversewing of an aortopulmonary window in 1956.[17] Since this time, most published reports have emphasized the adjunctive use of cardiopulmonary bypass. In 1966, Putnam and Gross suggested a transpulmonary approach to repair, whereby the defect could be sutured closed from within the lumen of the main pulmonary artery via a longitudinal arteriotomy.[58] Whereas most early repairs were performed in older children, Cordell et al reported the first closure of an aortopulmonary window in an infant (6 months of age) in 1967.[18] Wright et al described suture closure of the defect via a transaortic approach.[82] This approach provided excellent exposure of the margins of the defect as well as the origins of the left coronary artery and right pulmonary artery. In 1969, Deverall and colleagues reported their experience using a transaortic approach with closure of the defect using a Dacron patch.[21] The advantages of patching the defect via a transaortic approach were emphasized in a report from Clarke and Richardson.[15] This became the early standard approach for most cases of aortopulmonary window.

The initial approach to the repair of aortopulmonary window, by necessity, utilized closed techniques. This was associated with several major limitations. First, dissection of the window was fairly risky because of potential bleeding complications. Second, division and primary closure of the window could lead to significant narrowing of both the aorta and the pulmonary artery and potential distortion of the semilunar valves. Third, the closed approach did not allow for visualization of the coronary ostia, and therefore, coronary perfusion might be compromised following repair. The introduction of cardiopulmonary bypass brought a greater margin of safety to the closed approach, but more importantly, cardiopulmonary bypass permitted the development of open techniques which could be applied to the repair of all types of aortopulmonary window defects as well as their associated defects.

The preoperative care of patients with aortopulmonary window primarily involves management of associated congestive heart failure using standard techniques. Patients with significant aortic arch obstruction will require infusion of PGE1.

All symptomatic patients should undergo prompt repair, once the diagnosis is confirmed. Asymptomatic patients should undergo repair by 3–4 months of age in order to avert the development of pulmonary vascular obstructive disease, which may occur in some patients as early as 6 months of age. Older patients should undergo preoperative catheterization to assess pulmonary vascular resistance and its response to oxygen and nitric oxide. An R_p/R_s of greater than 0.4 has been shown to be a risk factor for perioperative death.[79] A PVR greater than 8–10 and an R_p/R_s greater than 0.7 probably represent absolute contraindications for repair.

Surgical Technique

The repair is performed via standard median sternotomy. Bicaval venous and distal aortic cannulation is recommended. Snares are placed around both branch pulmonary arteries. Cardiopulmonary bypass with moderate hypothermia is initiated and pulmonary arterial snares are tightened. Following aortic cross clamping, standard cardioplegia is delivered via the aortic root. Subsequent doses of cardioplegia (if necessary) are readily given by retrograde or direct antegrade approach.

Many centers continue to utilize the transaortic approach for the repair of aortopulmonary window. A longitudinal aortotomy is made in the ascending aorta. For simple proximal (type I) defects, closure is readily accomplished using a polytetrafluoroethylene patch (Figure 117-13). Care must be taken to identify the left coronary orifice. For distal (type II) defects, a more extensive patch must be fashioned (Figure 117-14). When there is considerable unroofing of the right pulmonary artery, the creation of an intraaortic baffle may result in aortic obstruction; this may be alleviated by simply closing the aortotomy with an elliptical patch (Figure 117-15). Total (type III) and intermediate type defects are repaired using analogous techniques (Figure 117-16).

Johansson and colleagues described a transwindow approach (also called a sandwich-type repair), which has gained wide acceptance as the optimal approach for the repair of aortopulmonary window.[36] In this technique (see Figure 117-17), an incision is made in the anterior wall of the communication between the aorta and pulmonary trunk. A patch is then sutured to the posterior wall of the defect. The suture line is subsequently carried anteriorly to incorporate the patch in the closure of the arteriotomy. This approach has the advantage of being slightly quicker to perform, as there is no need to close a separate aortotomy.

Several authors have utilized a pulmonary flap technique in order to avoid the use of prosthetic patch material to reconstruct the ascending aorta.[48,49,52,78] In this approach, an anterior flap of pulmonary artery is incised in continuity with the aorta along the anterior border of the window. The

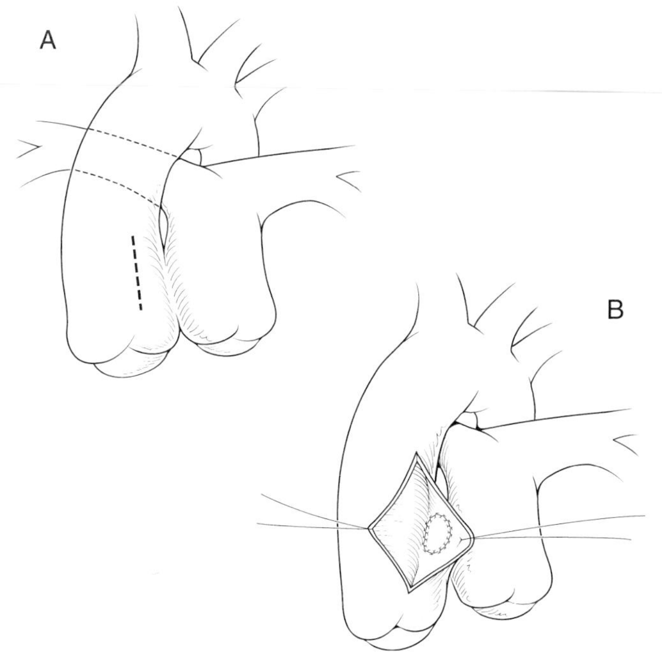

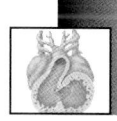

Figure 117–13 **Transaortic patch repair of a proximal aortopulmonary window. A,** A vertical aortotomy in the proximal ascending aorta provides excellent exposure. **B,** Patch closure of the defect is illustrated. Care must be taken to identify and protect the origin of the left coronary artery.

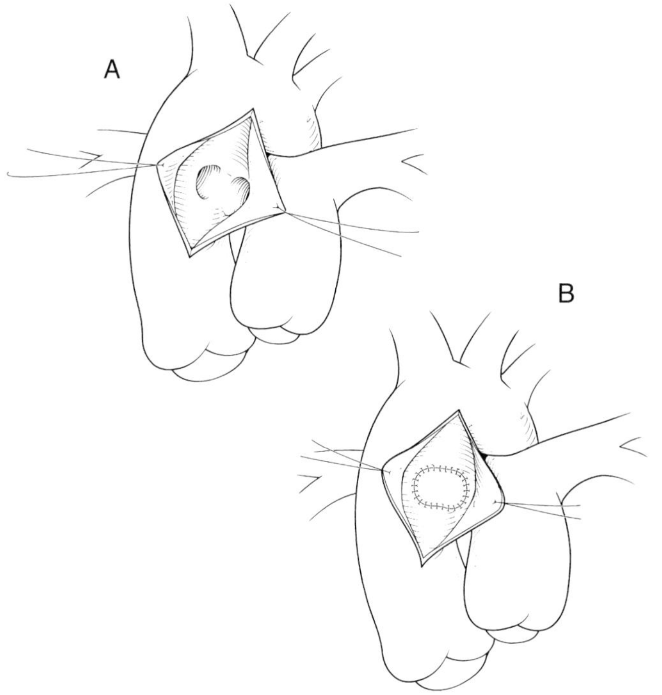

Figure 117–14 **Repair of a distal aortopulmonary window. A,** A more distal aortotomy exposes the defect that is related to the origin of the right pulmonary artery. **B,** Use of a generous patch avoids stenosis of the origin of the right pulmonary artery.

anterior flap is then sewn to the posterior margin of the aortopulmonary window, thereby closing the defect in the aorta. The resultant defect in the pulmonary artery is then closed with a patch (autologous or heterologous).

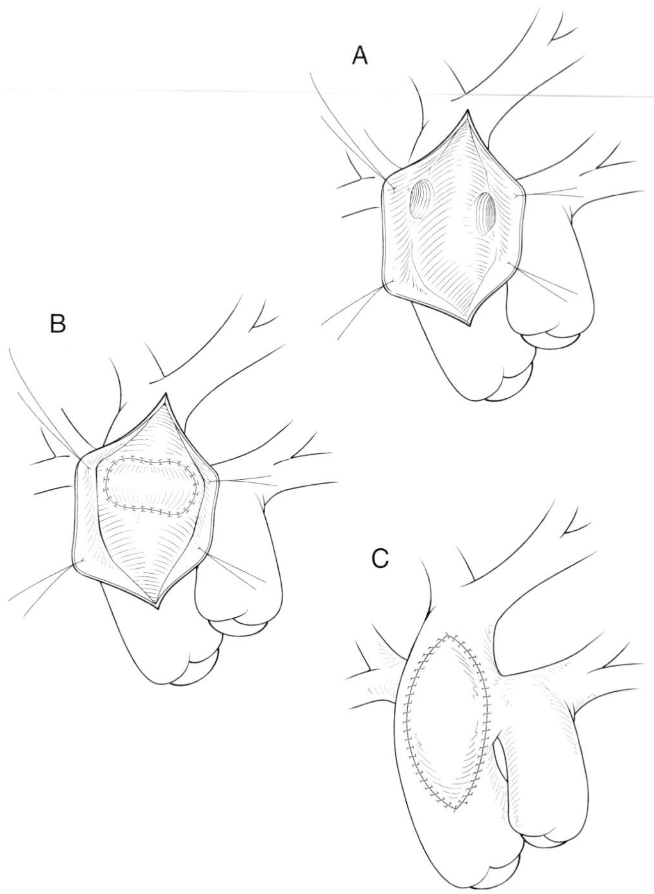

Figure 117–15 **Repair of a distal aortopulmonary window with extensive unroofing of the right pulmonary artery. A,** Extensive unroofing leads to the appearance of anomalous origin of the right pulmonary artery from the ascending aorta. **B,** An extensive intra-aortic baffle is created to join the window to the origin of the right pulmonary artery. **C,** Obstruction of the lumen of the ascending aorta can be obviated by closing the aortotomy with an elliptical patch.

Kitagawa has reported an alternative technique to repair a distal aortopulmonary window with extensive unroofing of the right pulmonary artery.[41] In this approach, the ascending aorta is transected at the distal extent of the window, and the right pulmonary artery is excised along with a strip of posterior aorta in continuity with the window and pulmonary trunk. The defect in the pulmonary artery is then repaired either primarily or using a patch, while the aorta is reconnected primarily. This technique has the advantage of avoiding any potential problems resulting from an intraaortic baffle.

Other Surgical Considerations

Associated defects are generally repaired concurrently. Special consideration should be given to repair of defects associated with arch interruption. Because of the presence of the window, single arterial cannulation of the ascending aorta is sufficient. Cardiopulmonary bypass with deep hypothermia is utilized (with occlusion of the branch pulmonary arteries). The repair is typically performed under

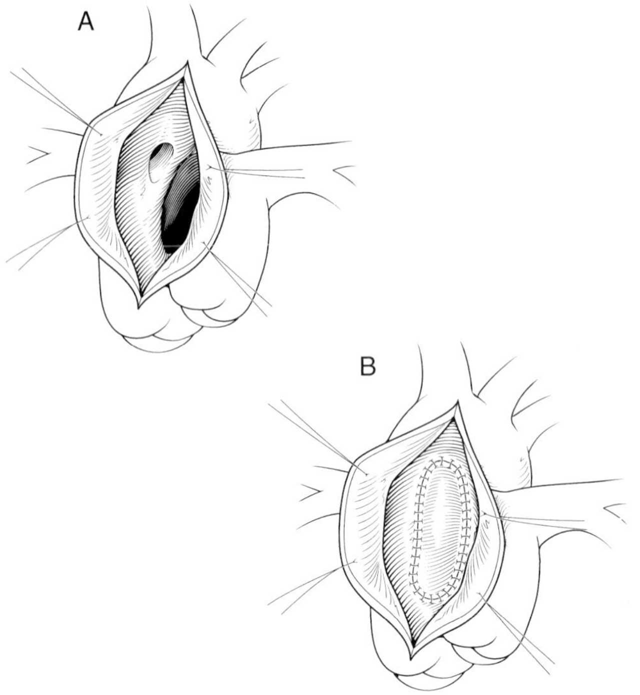

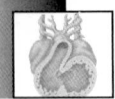

Figure 117–16 **Repair of a total- (or immediate-) type aortopulmonary window. A,** Exposure is achieved with an extensive aortotomy. **B,** A large patch is used to close the defect.

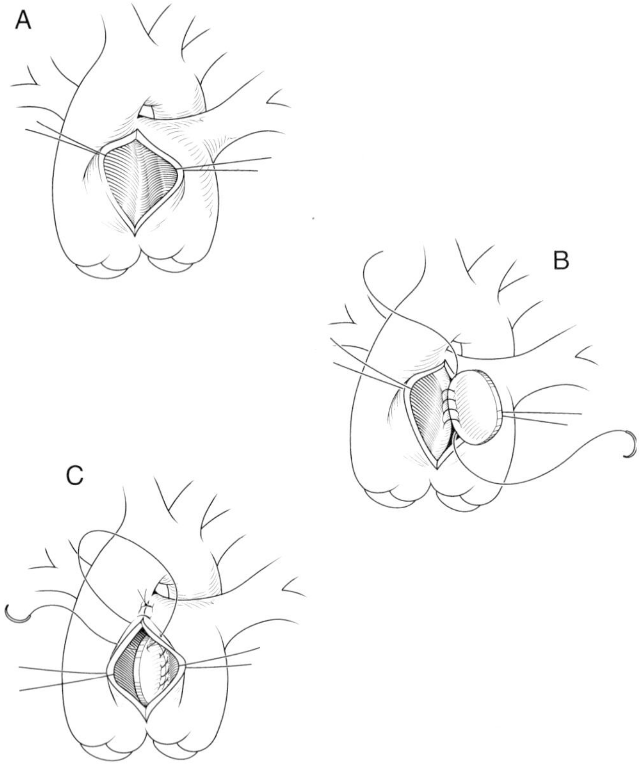

Figure 117–17 **Transwindow (sandwich) repair of aortopulmonary window. A,** An incision is made in the anterior wall of the window. **B,** A patch is then sewn to the posterior border of the defect. **C,** Finally, the anterior portion of the defect is closed by incorporating the patch in the closure of the arteriotomy.

circulatory arrest or with adjunctive regional cerebral perfusion. The ductus is ligated proximally and ductal tissue is resected distally. Two operative strategies may then be considered. Using a conventional approach, the arch interruption may be repaired first (using standard techniques), followed by repair of the window (transaortic patch or sandwich type repair). Alternatively, the ascending aorta may be separated from the pulmonary artery at the level of the window, leaving defects in both vessels. The aortic arch is then reconstructed with patching of the defect in the ascending aorta, if necessary. Finally, the defect in the pulmonary artery is repaired with a patch.

Interventional Techniques

On rare occasions, a native aortopulmonary window or residual aortopulmonary defect following surgical closure may be small enough in size to allow an interventional approach. Several groups have reported success using percutaneously placed devices to close such defects.[37,63,70,74]

Postoperative Management

Currently, as the diagnosis and treatment of aortopulmonary window are accomplished in early infancy, pulmonary hypertensive crises are rare. However, in patients presenting later in life, management of pulmonary hypertension is the most critical aspect of postoperative care of patients undergoing repair of aortopulmonary window. A pulmonary arterial catheter may be placed via a purse string in the right ventricular infundibulum in selected patients. Conventional methods for the control and prevention of pulmonary hypertension include the use of inhaled nitric oxide, administration of other pulmonary vasodilators, liberal use of fentanyl and muscle relaxants, and mild hyperventilation.

Results

Modern results associated with the closure of isolated aortopulmonary window have been good. Tkebuchova and colleagues reported a 92% operative survival and actuarial survival of 90% at 10 years' follow-up.[73] In one of the largest series, Hew et al observed an early survival of 92% and an actuarial survival of 88% at 10 years.[32] Reviewing a series of nineteen patients repaired from 1953 to 1990, van Son et al reported an overall early mortality of 21%.[79] The authors noted that all deaths occurred in patients repaired before 1962. The authors additionally observed that the long-term outcome following repair was dependent upon the pulmonary vascular resistance at the time of closure of the defect. Backer et al reported a similar improvement in results.[2] The authors reported an operative mortality of 33% when the repair was performed using the technique of closed division of the window. Since changing the operative technique to the transaortic approach, they have seen no mortality. McElhinney and colleagues emphasized the significant effect of complex associated defects on survival in their series of infants undergoing repair of aortopulmonary window under the age of 6 months.[50] Their data (excluding patients with Richardson type III defects) suggest a mortality of 36% for patients with complex associated defects.

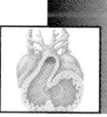

Selected Bibliography

Hew CC, Bacha EA, Zurakowski D, et al: Optimal surgical approach for repair of aortopulmonary window. Cardiol Young 11: 385–390, 2001.

This report describes the largest single-institution experience with surgical repair of aortopulmonary window in 38 patients treated over a period from 1973 to 1999. Associated lesions were present in 65% of patients, making this a high risk group of patients. Operative survival was 92%, and actuarial survival was 88% at 10 years' follow-up.

Kutsche LM, and Van Mierop LH: Anatomy and pathogenesis of aorticopulmonary septal defect. Am J Cardiol 59:443–447, 1987.

This paper provides a thorough review of the anatomy, embryology, and incidence of aortopulmonary window in a large hospital population.

Rajasinghe HA, McElhinney DB, et al: Long-term follow-up of truncus arteriosus repaired in infancy: A twenty-year experience. J Thorac Cardiovasc Surg 113:869–879, 1997.

This report is a retrospective review assessing the long-term outcomes of patients surviving a repair of truncus arteriosus at a single institution. There were 165 survivors followed up for a median of 10.5 years (range, 0.1–20.4 years). Median age at operation was 3.5 months (range, 2 days–36 years). Actuarial survival among all of the hospital survivors was 90% at 5 years, 85% at 10 years, and 83% at 15 years. All survivors, except 3 patients, were in New York Heart Association class I. An independent risk factor for death was moderate to severe truncal regurgitation at initial operation. Median time to conduit replacement was 5.5 years.

Thompson L, McElhinney DB, et al: Neonatal repair of truncus arteriosus: Continuing improvement in outcomes. Ann Thorac Surg 72:391–395, 2001.

This manuscript reviews one institution's results with the neonatal repair of truncus arteriosus over a 6.5-year period. Sixty-five patients underwent repair at a median age of 10 days (range, 2–30 days) and a median weight of 3.2 kg (range, 2.1–4.3 kg). Hospital mortality was 5%, with an additional two deaths during a median follow-up of 32 months (range, 6–92 months). Factors associated with poor survival were weight <2.4 kg at the time of operation (p = .01) and truncal valve replacement (p = .009). Actuarial freedom from reoperation for the conduit was 57% at 3 years.

Urban AE, Sinzobahamvya N, et al: Truncus arteriosus: Ten-year experience with homograft repair in neonates and infants. Ann Thorac Surg 66:5183–5188,1998.

This retrospective study reviews 46 consecutive patients undergoing repair of truncus arteriosus over a 10-year period. The median age was 62 days (range, 21 days–7.2 years) and median weight was 3.4 kg (range, 1.8–21.5 kg). There were 2 hospital deaths (4.3%) and 1 late death, for an actuarial survival at 4 months and beyond of 93%. Actuarial freedom from conduit reintervention was 43% at 75 months for aortic homograft and 73% at 62 months for pulmonary homograft.

Waldo K, Miyagawa-Tomita S, Kumiski D, et al: Cardiac neural crest cells provide new insight into septation of the cardiac outflow tract: Aortic sac to ventricular septal closure. Dev Biol l96:129–144, 1998.

This is an important paper that provides experimental evidence demonstrating the role of cardiac neural crest in the septation of the cardiac outflow tract.

REFERENCES

1. Report of the New England Regional Infant Cardiac Program. Pediatrics 65:375–461, 1980.
2. Backer CL, Mavroudis C: Surgical management of aortopulmonary window: a 40-year experience. Eur J Cardiothorac Surg 21:773–779, 2002.
3. Balaji S, Burch M, Sullivan ID: Accuracy of cross-sectional echocardiography in diagnosis of aortopulmonary window. Am J Cardiol 67:650–653, 1991.
4. Barbero-Marcial M, Riso A, et al: A technique for correction of truncus arteriosus types I and II without extracardiac conduits. J Thorac Cardiovasc Surg 99:364–369, 1990.
5. Barbero-Marcial M, Tanamati C: Alternative nonvalved techniques for repair of truncus arteriosus: Long-term results. Semin Thorac Cardiovasc Surg Pediatr Card Surg Annual 2:121–130, 1999.
6. Bedhrendt DM, Kirsh MM, et al: The surgical therapy for pulmonary artery–right ventricular discontinuity. Ann Thorac Surg 18:122–137, 1974.
7. Berry TE, Bharati S, Muster AJ, et al.: Distal aortopulmonary septal defect, aortic origin of the right pulmonary artery, intact ventricular septum, patent ductus arteriosus, and hypoplasia of the aortic isthmus: a newly recognized syndrome. Am J Cardiol 49:108–116, 1982.
8. Bharati S, McAllister HA, et al: The surgical anatomy of truncus arteriosus communis. J Thorac Cardiovasc Surg 67:501–510, 1974.
9. Black MD, Adatia I, Freedom RM: Truncal valve repair: Initial experience in neonates. Ann Thorac Surg 67:299–300, 1999.
10. Bove EL, Lupinetti FM, et al: Results of a policy of primary repair of truncus arteriosus in the neonate. J Thorac Cardiovasc Surg 105:1057–1065, 1993.
11. Braunlin E, Peoples WM, Freedom RM, et al: Interruption of the aortic arch with aorticopulmonary septal defect. An anatomic review. Pediatr Cardiol 3:329–335, 1982.
12. Brown JW, Ruzmetov M, et al: Truncus arteriosus repair; outcomes, risk factors, reoperation, and management. Eur J Cardio-Thorac Surg 20:221–227, 2001.
13. Butto F, Lucas RV, Edwards JE: Persistent truncus arteriosus: Pathologic anatomy in 54 cases. Pediatr Cardiol 7:95–101, 1986.
14. Calder L, Van Praagh R, Van Praagh S, et al: Truncus arteriosus communis: Clinical angiocardiographic and pathologic findings in 100 patients. Ann Heart J 92:23, 1976.
15. Clarke CP, Richardson JP: The management of aortopulmonary window: advantages of transaortic closure with a Dacron patch. J Thorac Cardiovasc Surg 72:48–51, 1976.
16. Collett RW, Edwards JE: Persistent truncus arteriosus: A classification according to anatomic types. Surg Clin North Am 29:1245, 1949.
17. Cooley DA, McNamara DG, Latson JR: Aorticopulmonary septal defect: diagnosis and surgical treatment. Surgery 42:101–120, 1957.
18. Cordell AR, McKone RC, Wilson HV: Management of aorticopulmonary septal defect in early infancy. Am Surg 33:962–964, 1967.
19. Danton MHD, Barron DJ, et al: Repair of truncus arteriosus: a considered approach to right ventricular outflow tract reconstruction. Eur J Cardio-Thorac Surg 20:95–104, 2001.
20. de la Cruz MV, Cayre R, et al: Coronary arteries in truncus arteriosus. Am J Cardiol 66:1482–1486, 1990.
21. Deverall PB, Lincoln JC, Aberdeen E, et al: Aortopulmonary window. J Thorac Cardiovasc Surg 57:479–486,1969.

22. Ebert PA, Turley K, et al: Surgical treatment of truncus arteriosus in the first 6 months of life. Ann Surg 200:451–456, 1984.
23. Elami A, Laks H, Pearl JM: Truncal valve repair: initial experience with infants and children. Ann Thorac Surg 57:397–401, 1994.
24. Elliotson J: Case of malformation of the pulmonary artery and aorta. Lancet 1:247–248, 1830.
25. Epstein DJ, Vogan KJ, Trasler DG, Gros P: A mutation within intron 3 of the Pax-3 gene produces aberrantly spliced mRNA transcripts in the splotch (SP) mouse mutant. Proc Nat Acad Sci 90:532–536, 1993.
26. Farrell MJ, Stadt H, Wallis KT, et al: HIRA, a DiGeorge syndrome candidate gene is required for cardiac outflow tract septation. Circ Res 84:127–135, 1999.
27. Faulkner SL, Oldham RR, Atwood GF, et al: Aortopulmonary window, ventricular septal defect, and membranous pulmonary atresia with a diagnosis of truncus arteriosus. Chest 65:351–353, 1974.
28. Fuglestad SJ, Puga FJ, et al: Surgical pathology of the truncal valve: a study of 12 cases. Am J Cardiovasc Pathol 2:39–47, 1988.
29. Garver KA, Hernandez RJ, Vermilion RP, et al: Images in cardiovascular medicine. Correlative imaging of aortopulmonary window: demonstration with echocardiography, angiography, and MRI. Circulation 96:1036–1037, 1997.
30. Gross RE: Surgical closure of an aortic septal defect. Circulation 5:858–863, 1952.
31. Hanley FLY, Heinemann MK, et al: Repair of truncus arteriosus in the neonate. J Thorac Cardiovasc Surg 1047-1056, 1993.
32. Hew CC, Bacha EA, Zurakowski D, et al: Optimal surgical approach for repair of aortopulmonary window. Cardiol Young 11:385–390, 2001.
33. Hirsch JC, Sasson L, et al: Long-term outcome of right ventricle to pulmonary artery conduits for the repair of congenital heart defects in infants. Midwest Pediatric Cardiology Society 25th Annual Meeting, Omaha, September 13, 2001.
34. Incesu L, Baysal K, Kalayci AG, et al: Magnetic resonance imaging of proximal aortopulmonary window. Clin Imaging 22:23–25, 1998
35. Jacobs JP, Quintessenza JAY, Gaynor JW, et al: Congenital Heart Surgery Nomenclature and Database Project: Aortopulmonary window. Ann Thorac Surg 69:S44–49, 2000.
36. Johansson L, Michaelsson MY, Westerholm CJ, et al: Aortopulmonary window: a new operative approach. Ann Thorac Surg 25:564–567, 1978.
37. Jureidini SB, Spadaro JJ, and Rao PS: Successful transcatheter closure with the buttoned device of aortopulmonary window in an adult. Am J Cardiol 81:371–372, 1998.
38. King DH, Huhta JC, Gutgesell HP, et al: Two-dimensional echocardiographic diagnosis of anomalous origin of the right pulmonary artery from the aorta: Differentiation from aortopulmonary window. J Am Coll Cardiol 4:351–355, 1984.
39. Kirby ML, Waldo KL: Role of neural crest in congenital heart disease. Circulation 82:332–340, 1990.
40. Kirklin JW, Barrat-Boyes BG (Eds): Truncus arteriosus. In Cardiac Surgery. New York: Churchill Livingstone, 1993.
41. Kitagawa T, Katoh I, Taki H, et al: New operative method for distal aortopulmonary septal defect. Ann Thorac Surg 51:680–682, 1991.
42. Koirala B, Merklinger SL, et al: Extending the useable size range of homografts in the pulmonary circulation: outcome of bicuspid homografts. Ann Thorac Surg 73:866–869, 2002.
43. Kreutzer C, Kreutzer GO, et al: Early and late results of fresh autologous pericardial valved conduits. Ped Card Surg 2:65–75, 1999.
44. Kutsche LM, Van Mierop LH: Anatomy and pathogenesis of aorticopulmonary septal defect. Am J Cardiol 59:443–447, 1987.
45. Lacour-Gayet F, Serraf A, et al: Truncus arteriosus repair: influence of techniques of right ventricular outflow tract reconstruction. J Thorac Cardiovasc Surg 111:849–856, 1996.
46. Lev M, Saphir O: Truncus arteriosus communis persistens. J Pediatr 20:74, 1943.
47. Marcelletti C, McGoon DC, et al: Early and late results of surgical repair of truncus arteriosus. Circulation 55:636-41, 1977.
48. Matsuki O, Yagihara T, Yamamoto F, et al: New surgical technique for total-defect aortopulmonary window. Ann Thorac Surg 54:991–992, 1992
49. Matsuki O, Yagihara T, Yamamoto F, et al: As originally published in 1992: New surgical technique for total-defect aortopulmonary window. Updated in 1999. Ann Thorac Surg 67:891, 1999.
50. McElhinney DB, Reddy VM, Tworetzky W, et al: Early and late results after repair of aortopulmonary septal defect and associated anomalies in infants 6 months of age. Am J Cardiol 81:195–201, 1998.
51. McGoon DC, Rastelli GC, Ongley PA: An operation for correction of truncus arteriosus. JAMA 205:69–73, 1968.
52. Messmer BJ: Pulmonary artery flap for closure of aortopulmonary window. Ann Thorac Surg 57:498–501, 1994.
53. Mori K, Ando M, Takao A, et al: Distal type of aortopulmonary window. Report of 4 cases. Br Heart J 40:681–689, 1978.
54. Nath PH, Zollikofer C, Castaneda-Zuniga, et al: Persistent truncus arteriosis associated with interruption of the aortic arch. Br J Radiol 53:853–859, 1980.
55. Neufeld HN, Lester RG, Adams P, Jr, et al: Aorticopulmonary septal defect. Am J Cardiol 9:12–25, 1962.
56. Orts-Llorca F, Puerta Fonolla J, Sobrado J: The formation, septation, and fate of the truncus arteriosus in man. J Anat 134:41–56, 1982.
57. Pigula FA, Namoton EM, et al: Regional low-flow perfusion provides cerebral circulatory support during neonatal aortic arch reconstruction. J Thorac Cardiovasc Surg 119:33 1–9, 2000.
58. Putnam TC, Gross RE: Surgical management of aortopulmonary fenestration. Surgery 59:727–735, 1966.
59. Rajasinghe HA, McElhinney DB, et al: Long-term follow-up of truncus arteriosus repaired in infancy: A twenty year experience. J Thorac Cardiovasc Surg 113:869–879, 1997.
60. Reddy VM, Rajasinghe HA, et al: Performance of right ventricle to pulmonary artery conduits after repair of truncus arteriosus: a comparison of Dacron-housed porcine valves and cryopreserved allografts. Seminars in Thorac and Cardiovasc Surg 7:133–138, 1995.
61. Rice MJ, Seward JB, Hagler DJ, et al: Visualization of aortopulmonary window by two-dimensional echocardiography. Mayo Clin Proc 57:482–487, 1982.
62. Richardson JV, Doty DB, Rossi NP, et al: The spectrum of anomalies of aortopulmonary septation. J Thorac Cardiovasc Surg 78:21–27, 1979.
63. Richens T, Wilson N: Amplatzer device closure of a residual aortopulmonary window. Catheter Cardiovasc Interv 50:431–433, 2000.
64. Rowe RD, Freedom RM, Mehrizi A, et al: The neonate with congenital heart disease. Philadelphia: WB Saunders, 1981.
65. Satomi G, Nakamura K, Imai Y, et al: Two-dimensional echocardiographic diagnosis of aorticopulmonary window. Br Heart J 43: 351-356, 1980.
66. Scott HW Jr, and Sabiston DC Jr: Surgical treatment for congenital aorticopulmonary fistula. J Thorac Surg 25:26–39, 1953.

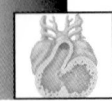

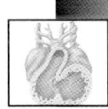

67. Shrivastava S, Edwards JE: Coronary arterial origin in persistent truncus arteriosus. Circulation 55:551–554, 1977.
68. Smallhorn JF, Anderson RH, Macartney FJ: Two-dimensional echocardiographic assessment of communications between ascending aorta and pulmonary trunk or individual pulmonary arteries. Br Heart J 47:563–572, 1982.
69. Spicer RL, Brendt D, Crowley DC, et al: Repair of truncus arteriosus in neonates with the use of a valveless conduit. Circulation 70(3pt2):126–129, 1984.
70. Stamato T, Benson LN, Smallhorn JF, et al: Transcatheter closure of an aortopulmonary window with a modified double umbrella occluder system. Cathet Cardiovasc Diagn 35:165–167, 1995.
71. Tandon R, Hanck AJ, Nadas AS: Persistent truncus arteriosus: A clinical hemodynamic and autopsy study of 19 cases. Circulation 28:1050, 1963.
72. Thompson L, McElhinney DB, et al: Neonatal repair of truncus arteriosus: Continuing improvement in outcomes. Ann Thorac Surg 72:391–395, 2001.
73. Tkebuchava T, von Segesser LK, Vogt PR, et al: Congenital aortopulmonary window: Diagnosis, surgical technique, and long-term results. Eur J Curdiothoruc Surg 11: 293–297, 1997.
74. Tulloh RM, Rigby ML: Transcatheter umbrella closure of aortopulmonary window. Heart 77:479–480, 1997.
75. Urban AE, Sinzobahamvya N, et al: Truncus arteriosus: Ten-year experience with homograft repair in neonates and infants. Ann Thorac Surg 66:5183–5188, 1998.
76. Valsangiacomo ER, Smallhorn JF: Images in cardiovascular medicine. Prenatal diagnosis of aortopulmonary window by fetal echocardiography. Circulation 105:El92, 2002.
77. Van Praagh R, Van Praagh S: The anatomy of common aorticopulmonary trunk (truncus arteriosus communis) and its embryologic implications: A study of 57 necropsy cases. Am J Cardiol 16:406, 1965.
78. van Son JA, Hambsch J, Mohr FW: Anatomical reconstruction of aorta and pulmonary trunk in patients with an aortopulmonary window. Ann Thoruc Surg 70:674–675, discussion 676, 2000.
79. van Son JA, Puga FJ, Danielson GK, et al: Aortopulmonary window: Factors associated with early and late success after surgical treatment. Mayo Clin Proc 68:128–133, 1993.
80. Waldo K, Miyagawa-Tomita S, Kumiski D, et al: Cardiac neural crest cells provide new insight into septation of the cardiac outflow tract: Aortic sac to ventricular septal closure. Dev Biol 196:129–144, 1998.
81. Wilson J: A description of a very unusual malformation of the human heart. Phil Trans R Soc London (Biol) 18:346, 1798.
82. Wright JS, Freeman R, Johnston JB: Aortopulmonary fenestration. A technique of surgical management. J Thorac Cardiovasc Surg 55:280–283, 1968.

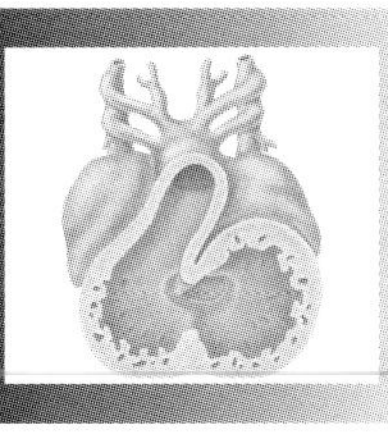

Interrupted Aortic Arch

Gary K. Lofland and James E. O'Brien, Jr.

CHAPTER 118

INTRODUCTION

Interrupted aortic arch is a rare but serious disorder that continues to provide therapeutic challenges. Indeed, our understanding of effective management of this condition is less than two decades old. Prior to the advent of prostaglandin E1 (PGE_1) in 1975 by Elliott et al,[8] interrupted aortic arch was associated with an extremely high mortality in the neonatal period. Further advances throughout the 1980s in our understanding of neonatal cardiopulmonary physiology enabled caregivers to optimize post-diagnostic and preoperative resuscitation in these patients. Ventilatory and other parameters could be manipulated to optimize systemic blood flow. Advances in echocardiography and two dimensional color Doppler enabled noninvasive diagnosis, largely supplanting cardiac catheterization as a diagnostic necessity. Instead of taking an infant in extremis to the operating room emergently following a stressful cardiac catheterization, an infant could be resuscitated and stabilized, and all organ systems normalized. These measures and this improved understanding, translated into better clinical outcomes.

HISTORICAL NOTES

The first description of interrupted aortic arch was by Steidele in 1778.[40] In this reported case, the aortic isthmus was absent. Interruption between the left common carotid and left subclavian arteries was described by Seidel in 1818.[37] Interruption between the innominate artery and left common carotid artery was described by Weisman and Kesten in 1948.[47] In 1959 Celoria and Patten had collected 28 cases which were classified according to the site of obstruction into types A, B, and C,[4] establishing a classification system that has persisted.

The first reported correction of interrupted aortic arch was by Samson in 1955.[28] The patient was a 3 year-old child with a Type A interruption and a widely patent ductus arteriosus adjacent to the left subclavian artery. The child had two ventricular septal defects (VSDs). A primary anastomosis was possible leaving the VSDs open, which were then closed 4 years later. For the next two decades, sporadic case reports of successful outcomes were reported.

One stage repair using a Dacron graft to bridge the interruption was reported by Barrett-Boyes and associates in 1970.[2] Single stage repair utilizing direct anastomosis was reported by Trusler and Izakawa in 1975.[42]

ANATOMY AND ANATOMICAL PATHOLOGY

The aortic arch is divided taxonomically into three different segments (Figure 118-1). The proximal segment extends from the medial origin of the innominate artery to the left common carotid artery. The distal segment extends from the left common carotid artery to the left subclavian artery. The segment of the aortic arch distal to the left subclavian artery that connects the distal aortic arch to the juxtaductal region of the proximal descending thoracic aorta is called the aortic isthmus. It is this isthmal segment that is absent in Type A interruption and is usually significantly hypoplastic in neonatal coarctation. Indeed in neonatal coarctation, the isthmus may be a fibrous cord without luminal continuity, and is not uncommon in our series of patients. This is sometimes called aortic arch atresia.

About 40% of aortic arch interruptions are Type A.[11,44] Type B interruption occurs between the left common carotid artery and the left subclavian artery. It is the most common type, occurring between 55% and 70% of the time in most series.[11,44] Type C interruption occurs between the innominate artery and the left common carotid artery. It is extremely rare, occurring in less that 4% of cases. It was reported in only one of 53 cases in the Baltimore Washington Infant Study.[10,11,25]

Each of the arch segments has a different embryological origin. The proximal arch is derived from the aortic sac, the distal arch from the fourth embryonic arch, and the isthmus from the junction of the sixth embryonic arch (ductus) with the left dorsal aorta and the fourth embryonic arch. This diversity in the origins of the arch segments is felt to contribute to the anatomical variation one encounters in interrupted aortic arch anatomy. Anomalies of the origins of the brachiocephalic vessels are frequent in association with interrupted arch.[33] Thus an aberrant right subclavian artery originating as a branch from the upper descending thoracic aorta is not uncommon in type B but can also occur in Type A.[1] The right subclavian artery may arise in the neck from the right common carotid artery.[24] A right-sided ductus may also persist from the right pulmonary artery and give rise to the right subclavian artery. The pulmonary arteries may be discontinuous, with the right pulmonary artery arising from the ascending aorta. Interrupted arch may occur with a right aortic arch, with both left and right ducti remaining patent and giving origin to the subclavian arteries.[33]

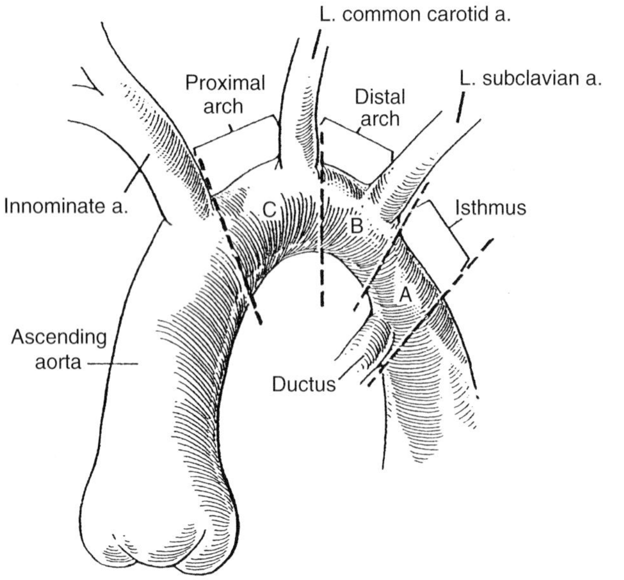

Figure 118–1 The aortic arch described in three segments. The proximal arch beginning at the innominate artery and extending to the left common carotid artery, the distal arch beginning at the left common carotid artery and extending to the left subclavian artery, and the aortic isthmus connecting the distal aortic arch to the proximal descending thoracic aorta. The classification by Celoria and Patton into interrupted arch types A, B, and C is indicated. *(From Castaneda, Jones, Mayer, et al. Cardiac surgery of the neonate and infant, Philadephia: W.B. Saunders, 1994, p. 353.)*

Typically, the ascending aorta is approximately half its normal diameter and is straight, dividing into two branches of approximately equal size. The main pulmonary artery is extremely large. The ductus is likewise large in the neonate, and the descending thoracic aorta exists as a direct continuation of the ductus arteriosus.

VENTRICULAR SEPTAL DEFECT

A large ventricular septal defect (VSD) is almost always present, and frequently the outlet or conal septum is malaligned and displaced posteriorly and leftward.

Most of the VSDs are conotruncal in type, although all types may occur. Some of the conotruncal defects have perimembranous extension.

CONAL SEPTUM

Frequently there is posterior malalignment of the conal septum relative to the ventricular septum that contributes to obstruction of the left ventricular outflow tract. The malaligned and displaced outlet septum usually produces subaortic obstruction of variable severity.[13,15,17,38] There are other constituents that can potentially contribute to obstruction of the left ventricular outflow tract.[20] Figure 118-2 illustrates some of these components. The aortic annulus itself may be hypoplastic. Frequently the aortic valve is bicuspid, with associated commissural fusion. Opposite the septum, there may be a prominent bundle of muscle that extends from the anterolateral papillary muscle into the outflow tract (muscle of Moulaert). Some authors have suggested that aortic valve diameter is the most important predictor of left ventricular outflow tract obstruction.[35] Other authors feel that potential obstruction may exist at multiple levels.

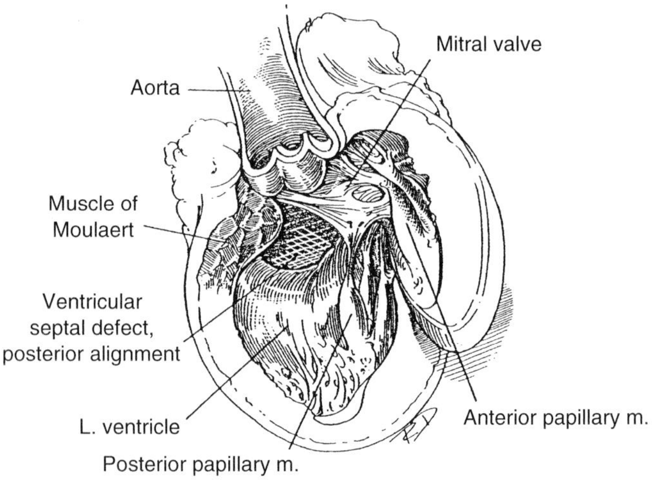

Figure 118–2 Morphological factors contributing to obstruction of the left ventricular outflow tract with an interrupted arch include posterior malalignment of the conal septum relative to the ventricular septum, a prominent muscle of Moulaert, hypoplasia of the aortic annulus, and a bicuspid aortic valve. *(From Castaneda AR, Jones RA, Mayer JE, et al. Cardiac surgery of the neonate and infant, Philadephia: W.B. Saunders, 1994, p. 355.)*

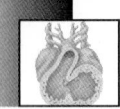

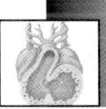

In a recent study, Kreutzer and Van Praagh[23] examined 60 postmortem cases of interrupted aortic arch with ventricular septal defect and coarctation of the aorta with ventricular septal defect with 30 cases in each diagnostic group. A morphometric comparison of the anatomical causes of left ventricular outflow tract obstruction was undertaken. This study revealed that posterior malalignment of the conal septum with a conoventricular VSD was significantly more prevalent with interruption (93%) than with coarctation (47%) ($p < .001$). In addition, the ratio of the aortic valve diameter to the pulmonary valve diameter, which provided a quantitative index of the degree of posterior conal septal malalignment and of the consequent LV outflow tract obstruction at and immediately below the level of the aortic valve, was significantly smaller with interruption (</=0.50 in 67%) than with coarctation (</=0.50 in 17%) ($p < .001$). A bicuspid or unicuspid aortic valve, both with interruption and with coarctation, was more prevalent with posterior conal septal malalignment than with normal conal septal alignment. Posterior conal septal malalignment was associated with LV outflow tract obstruction at three different sites: subvalvar, annular, and leaflet. These anatomical findings may help explain the incidence of postoperative LV outflow tract obstruction in patients with interrupted aortic arch after simple VSD closure.

Table 118–1

Coexisting Cardiac Anomalies in Patients with Interrupted Aortic Arch[a]

Morphology of Patient	*n*	*% of 97*
Ventricular septal defect	70	72%
Truncus arteriosus	9	9%
Transposition of the great arteries	4	4%
Double outlet right ventricle	4	4%
Double outlet right ventricle with common AV valve	1	1%
Double inlet left ventricle	2	2%
Mitral atresia	1	1%
Tricuspid atresia	1	1%
Without other major cardiac anomaly		
Aortopulmonary window	3	3%
Mildly stenotic mitral valve	1	1%
Moderately hypoplastic LV	1	1%
Subtotal	97	
Unknown	2	
Total	99	

[a]The data are from the multi-institutional study of the Congenital Heart Surgeons Society, 1987 – January 1990.
Adapted from Kirklin JW, Barratt-Boyes BG: Cardiac Surgery, 2nd ed. New York: Churchill Livingstone, 1993, p. 1305.

CO-EXISTING CARDIAC ANOMALIES

Other cardiac lesions may coexist with interrupted aortic arch. These are shown in Table 118-1. There is quite frequently an associated atrial septal defect, although this is usually merely a stretched patent foramen ovale. Of note, however, is that truncus arteriosus may coexist in approximately 9-10% of patients.

ASSOCIATED SYNDROMES

Absence of thymic tissue (DiGeorge Syndrome) is frequently associated[5,14,44] and should be looked for routinely. Van Microp and Kutsche found this association only in type B interrupted arch.[43] In the Baltimore Washington Infant Study, however, DiGeorge Syndrome was found in all three types of interrupted aortic arch, although much more frequently in type B.[25]

A more recent association has been a recognition of abnormalities involving chromosome 22q11.[*] These abnormalities may take the form of microdeletions of the twenty-second chromosome, and should prove to be an exciting new venue for research.

When DiGeorge syndrome is indeed present, calcium metabolism and hypocalcemia will need to be addressed in the newborn, and possible immunological problems will need to be addressed throughout the patient's life.

PATHOPHYSIOLOGY AND CLINICAL PRESENTATION

The pathophysiology and clinical presentation of a patient with interrupted aortic arch, especially those with the most common form of interrupted aortic arch (associated PDA and conoventricular VSD) are similar to those of any patient with a left-sided atretic lesion and ductal dependent systemic circulation. In the typical neonate with the a conoventricular septal defect and a large ductus arteriosus associated with interrupted aortic arch, there may be no indication of any pathology early in the neonatal period, as long as the ductus remains open. It is only upon closure of the ductus arteriosus that symptoms and problems arise. Perfusion of the lower two thirds of the body is dependent upon ductal patency. With ductal closure, perfusion is dependent upon collateral circulation. With abrupt ductal closure, there is virtually no chance for the development of collateralization. This will result in profound acidosis, anuria, hepatic failure and poor perfusion of the gut. The level of interruption of the arch will be reflected in physical findings in the upper extremities. For instance in a patient with a type A interruption, ductal closure will result in physical findings identical to that of a neonate with coarctation of the aorta (i.e., palpable pulses in both upper extremities, with non palpable pulses in the lower extremities). Interruption of the arch proximal to the left subclavian artery will result in no pulses in the left arm and lower extremities upon closure of the ductus arteriosus. Hepatic injury is reflected in marked elevation of hepatic enzymes. Renal injury is reflected by the levels of BUN and creatinine. Injury to the gut is followed by evidence of necrotizing enterocolitis (abdominal distention, bloody stools).

[*]References 7, 12, 18, 27, 30, 32, 34, 41, 46.

Although a neonate may tolerate short periods of acidosis much better than a more mature patient, a severe degree of systemic acidosis will ultimately result in injury to all bodily tissues, including the central nervous system and the myocardium. Injury to these organs may be manifested by seizures and poor myocardial contractility. Pulmonary blood flow is preserved, however, and the neonate may hyperventilate as a compensatory mechanism for the profound metabolic acidosis.

If a ductus closes more slowly, the child will manifest signs of increasing congestive heart failure over the ensuing weeks, as neonatal pulmonary vascular resistance begins to fall.

EARLY PREOPERATIVE MANAGEMENT

Early preoperative medical management of these patients is predicated upon timelines and accuracy of diagnosis. In patients diagnosed prior to ductal closure, maintenance of ductal patency is of paramount importance. If the ductus is closed, reestablishment of ductal patency and reversal of multiorgan system dysfunction are necessities. Even if a ductus closes abruptly, the ductus in a neonate can virtually always be reopened with appropriate pharmacological management. There should never be an excuse for an emergency operation for interrupted aortic arch.

The mainstay of medical management is prostaglandin (PGE_1). PGE_1 must be infused through a secure intravenous line. If ductal patency does not become apparent in any neonate within 1 hour after administration of PGE_1, a therapeutic error has occurred. This may be either a dosage error or a technical problem with medication delivery into the central bloodstream. Establishing ductal patency through the use of PGE_1 is the all important first step in medically resuscitating these neonates.

Because the lower two thirds of the body is dependent upon perfusion through the ductus, pulmonary vascular resistance can be manipulated in order to optimize systemic perfusion. High levels of inspired oxygen and respiratory alkalosis through hyperventilation should be avoided. Indeed, endotracheal intubation and mechanical ventilation should be an important next step in these patients. Depending upon levels of infusion, prostaglandin can be a respiratory depressant. Endotracheal intubation and mechanical ventilation eliminates this as a concern. Endotracheal intubation and mechanical ventilation can decrease cardiac workload by eliminating the work of respiration thereby improving cardiac performance. Mechanical ventilation also enables manipulation of ventilatory parameters to achieve a PCO_2 level of 40-50 mm Hg, thereby decreasing pulmonary blood flow while improving systemic blood flow.

Metabolic acidosis should be aggressively treated with appropriate doses of sodium bicarbonate. Inotropic support may be necessary. Dopamine may be routinely employed but high doses should be avoided. Dopamine at approximately 3 µg/kg/min has the added advantage of maximizing renal perfusion within the context of an ischemic renal insult.

Medical management may need to persist for 2 to 3 days or even longer before surgery is undertaken. It should not be necessary for a neonate to be taken for corrective surgery with any acid base, renal, or hepatic abnormalities. During the medical management phase, a head ultrasound should be obtained as a baseline study. Blood for appropriate chromosomal studies should also be obtained during this period.

DIAGNOSTIC TECHNIQUES

Echocardiography

Accurate diagnosis is essential prior to operative intervention. Echocardiography has emerged as the diagnostic modality of choice in interrupted aortic arch. The use of echocardiography alone is especially advantageous in the critically ill neonate, because the additional risks associated with cardiac catheterization can be avoided. Echocardiography must be able to achieve several objectives, however. In addition to defining the site of interruption, echocardiography should measure the distance between the discontinuous aortic segments. The left ventricular outflow tract must be precisely described, including accurate definition of posterior displacement of the conal septum. The diameter of the aortic annulus, the diameter of the ascending aorta at the sino-tubular junction, and the diameter of the ascending aorta should be measured. Accurate definition of the conal septum must be achieved. The conal septum is often severely hypoplastic, making approach to the superior margin of the defect working through the tricuspid valve quite difficult. The types of quantitative echocardiographic measurements that must be obtained are outlined in detail in a paper from the Congenital Heart Surgeons' Society utilizing echocardiographic assessment of the left ventricular outflow tract in neonates with critical aortic stenosis.[26] Hemodynamic assessment using echocardiography can sometimes be difficult, because the VSD is almost always nonrestrictive. This makes attempts to quantitate the degree of obstruction of the left ventricular outflow tract by measuring a pressure gradient extremely difficult because of a lack of information regarding the amount of flow passing through the left ventricular outflow tract. Therefore, morphology and dimensions of the left ventricular outflow tract obtained by echocardiography are even more essential. In a study by Kaulitz and associates,[21] preoperative echocardiography was found to offer accurate and complete diagnosis in the critically ill neonate in all but 2 of 45 patients.

CARDIAC CATHETERIZATION

In spite of some statements to the contrary, cardiac catheterization remains an important adjunct if anatomical definition is incomplete or uncertain using echocardiography alone. This is usually due to additional cardiac or extra cardiac anomalies unassociated with the arch interruption. For instance, discontinuous pulmonary arteries can be very difficult to assess echocardiographically. Likewise, anomalous pulmonary venous connections can be suggested but incompletely defined. Finally, in the patient with interrupted arch and transposition of the great arteries, cardiac catheterization can provide the opportunity to perform a balloon atrial septostomy, thereby allowing better mixing at the level of the atrial septum while surgical intervention is being planned.

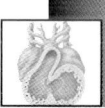

Cardiac catheterization may be utilized in the postoperative period if the child's clinical performance suggests hemodynamic compromise or persistent left ventricular outflow tract obstruction. While echocardiography may suggest persistence left ventricular outflow tract obstruction, this can be confirmed or excluded through cardiac catheterization. Finally, cardiac catheterization is frequently useful in the later postoperative period if a residual or recurrent pressure gradient across the aortic arch is identified. Balloon dilation of stenoses can be accomplished at the time of cardiac catheterization.

MAGNETIC RESONANCE IMAGING AND COMPUTED TOMOGRAPHY

Conventional magnetic resonance imaging (MRI) and computed tomography (CT) have never achieved prominence in the diagnosis or management of the neonate with interrupted aortic arch, primarily because of the cumbersome logistical problems inherent in their use. While echocardiography can be performed at the bedside, both MRI and CT require transport of a neonate to the imaging suite. During imaging, the neonate would need to be anesthetized because of the length of time associated with obtaining the images. During the past several years, however, three-dimensional (3D) imaging technology, including MRI,[6,45] helical computed tomography,[16,22] and electron beam CT,[48] has markedly progressed and allows 3D visualization of congenital heart anomalies from any angle of view and perspective. Even with these modalities it is sometimes difficult to define accurately the morphology of these conditions because the anomalous components are generally intricate and tortuous. Shiraishi and associates[39] have utilized a differential color imaging technique of helical CT angiography. The subsequent 3D reconstruction can be modified to allow for appropriate coloring of the vascular structures. More importantly, the helical CT examinations can be accomplished in approximately 15 seconds in a neonate. Such technology will undoubtedly assume a more prominent role in the diagnosis of these neonates in the future.

SURGICAL MANAGEMENT

Indication for Surgery

Interrupted aortic arch is incompatible with life without patency of the ductus arteriosus. Consequently, surgical intervention should be undertaken as soon as resuscitation measures are deemed complete and all organ systems have returned to normal function.

ONE-STAGE REPAIR

One-stage repair has emerged as the surgical method of choice in many institutions, including our own. No matter if one-chooses a one stage repair or a two-stage repair, however, all of the principles and techniques employed in the resuscitation and preoperative medical management of the patient should be continued during transport to the operating room and throughout anesthesia induction. Specifically, hyperventilation and high oxygen saturations indicating pulmonary overperfusion should be avoided.

Most of the neonates will arrive in the operating room with umbilical arterial catheters, umbilical venous catheters, or both already in place. These should be maintained, as the umbilical arterial catheter will allow for direct measurements of arterial pressure below the level of the arch anastomosis. During anesthesia induction, we insert percutaneous double lumen internal jugular or subclavian lines, plus a right radial arterial catheter. Single-stage repair has been nicely described by Casteneda and associates[3] and is illustrated in Figure 118-3. Their technique is described.

Approach is via a median sternotomy alone. If a thymus is present, it is largely excised. Pericardium is not usually harvested, as there is no need to utilize this in any portion of the reconstruction. Accurate arterial cannulation is an essential key to the success of the procedure. Although a single arterial cannula will ultimately achieve complete cooling, cannulation of both the ascending aorta and the pulmonary artery optimizes tissue perfusion, particularly of the brain and heart, in the critical early phase of cooling when all organs are still warm. Generally, a number eight French arterial cannula is used for the ascending aorta. As indicated by Figure 118-3, this cannula should be inserted in the right lateral aspect of the ascending aorta, opposite the anticipated location of the anastomosis. This decreases the chance that either retrograde flow to the coronary arteries or antegrade flow to the brain will be compromised. The second arterial cannula is connected to the arterial tubing by a Y connector and inserted into the anterior surface of the main pulmonary artery. Immediately after the start of bypass, tourniquets are tightened around the right and left pulmonary arteries so that flow will be entirely directed through the ductus arteriosus to the descending aorta. (PGE infusion must be continued during the cooling phase of cardiopulmonary bypass.) Venous cannulation is routine with a single straight cannula in the right atrium. During cooling, the ascending aorta and its branches are thoroughly mobilized. The ductus and descending aorta are also mobilized to minimize tension on the anastomosis. If an aberrant right subclavian artery is present, it should be ligated and divided at its origin from the descending aorta to improve mobility of the distal aortic segment. Also, in a Type B interruption, it is often useful to divide the left subclavian artery to further minimize anastomotic tension as well as to simplify the anastomosis, thereby decreasing the risk of bleeding and stenosis. When both rectal and tympanic temperatures are less than 18°C, bypass is ceased. Tourniquets are tightened around the innominate and left common carotid arteries, and pulmonary artery tourniquets are removed. Cardioplegic solution is infused through a side arm on the ascending arterial cannula connector. This same side arm can be used to monitor ascending aortic pressure during the early post bypass phase. Both arterial cannula are then removed along with the venous cannula.

The ductus is ligated and divided at its junction with the descending aorta. Any residual ductal tissue is excised from the descending aorta. A c-clamp applied across the descend-

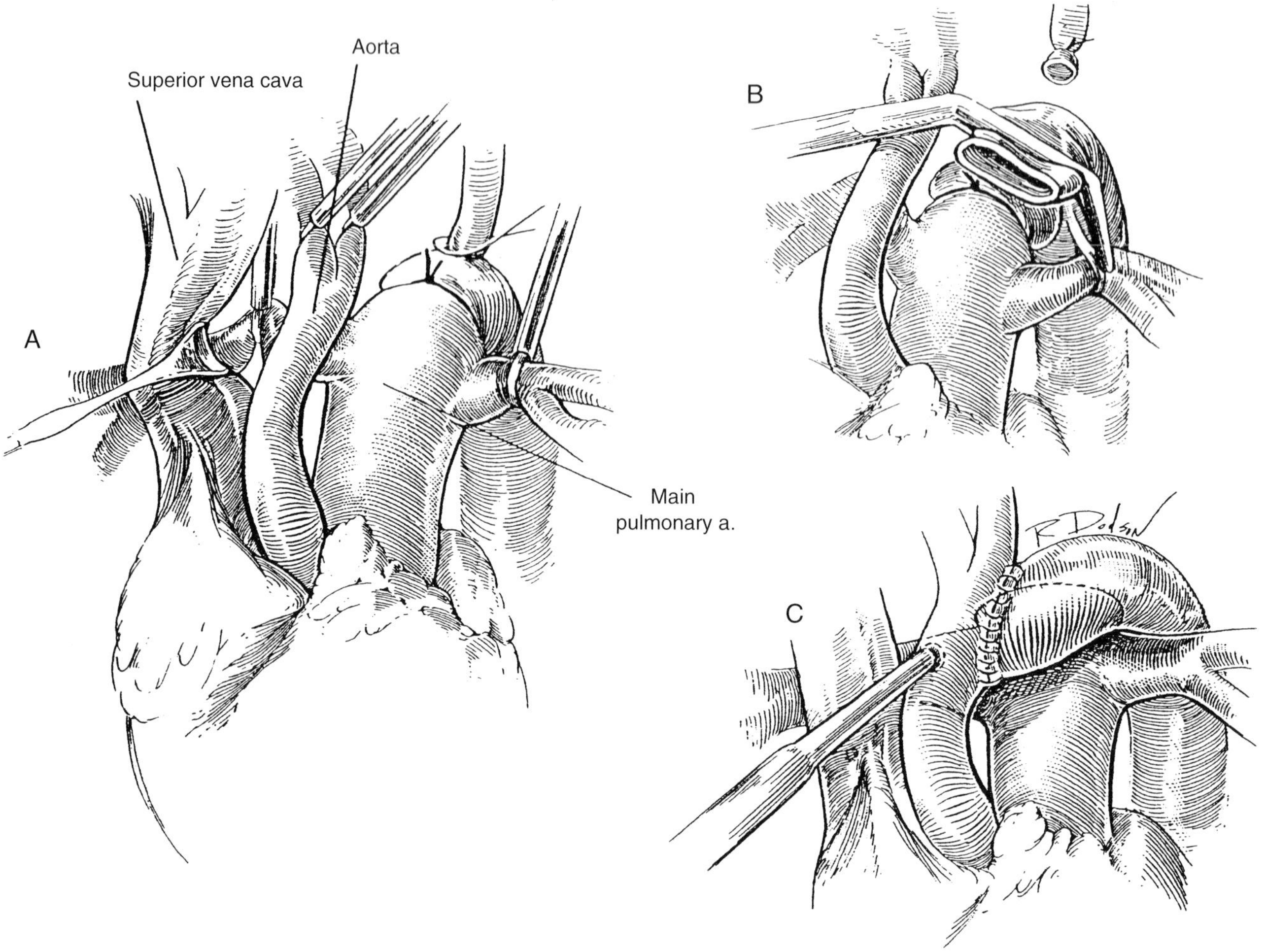

Figure 118–3 Schematic representation of the technique for repair by direct anastomosis of interrupted arch type B. **A,** Tourniquets control the branch pulmonary arteries during core cooling. During circulatory arrest, tourniquets control the carotid arteries to prevent cerebral air embolism. **B,** Following wide mobilization of the ascending and descending aorta, including division of the left subclavian artery, if necessary, in addition to the ductus arteriosus, the descending aorta is approximated to the ascending aorta with a C-clamp. **C,** The completed arch anastomosis. Note that in this technique the anastomosis does not extend up the left common carotid artery. Note also, the precise placement of the aortic perfusion cannula opposite the midpoint of the anastomosis.
(From Castaneda AR, Jones RA, Mayer JE, et al. Cardiac surgery of the neonate and infant, Philadephia: W.B. Saunders, 1994, p. 357.)

ing aorta helps to draw it to the level of the anastomosis, which can then be performed with the opposing tissues under no tension. The anastomosis should be situated on the ascending aorta, where tension will be minimized. Although many surgeons believe that this requires the site of the anastomosis to be partially on the left common carotid artery, we generally prefer it to be completely on the ascending aorta. The anastomosis will be exactly opposite the site of the ascending aortic cannulation. Absorbable polydioxanone 6-0 continuous suture may be used, although there is no evidence that the use of this suture results in a lower incidence of anastomotic stenosis. Many surgeons continue to prefer polypropylene suture. Its lesser tissue drag distributes tension more evenly through the suture line, which appears to enhance hemostasis.

The approach to the VSD will depend on the preoperative echocardiographic assessment. When there is extreme hypoplasia of the conal septum, the best approach is via a transverse incision in the proximal main pulmonary artery, immediately distal to the pulmonary valve. At the superior margin, sutures are passed through the pulmonary annulus with the pledgets lying above the pulmonary valve leaflets in the sinus of Valsalva. If the conal septum is well developed, the VSD is approached through the right atrium.

A decision should be made preoperatively regarding the need to close an atrial septal defect. If there is any doubt, the atrial septum should be examined through a short right atrial incision. Because of the poor left-sided compliance that often persists for some time postoperatively, even a small atrial septal defect can result in a large left to right shunt.

One arterial cannula is carefully reinserted (in the ascending aorta only) for rewarming after filling the heart with saline to exclude air. Routine monitoring lines (i.e., a left atrial, pulmonary artery, and right atrial line) are placed during rewarming.

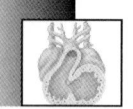

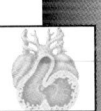

ALTERNATIVE TECHNIQUE

While respecting and utilizing many of the principles outlined by Casteneda and associates in the preceding description, we employ in our institution a modified version of this technique to obtain the same objective. We also employ a median sternotomy with a subthymectomy or near total thymectomy and creation of a pericardial cradle without harvesting of any pericardium. As much dissection as possible of the arch segments is accomplished prior to initiating cardiopulmonary bypass. Dual arterial cannulation is employed, with accurate placement of the ascending aortic cannula of vital importance. We, however, employ dual caval cannulation and vacuum assisted bypass, instead of a single atrial cannula. Once bypass is established, cooling to 18° C is accomplished. We do not employ snares around the pulmonary arteries but simply collapse the lungs, and allow them to remain in continuity to achieve cooling of the pulmonary parenchyma. After cooling is complete, flow is reduced to approximately one third, the pulmonary artery cannula is removed, and the ductus is ligated at its junction with the pulmonary arterial confluence. The aorta is then cross clamped proximal to the single remaining aortic cannula, and cardioplegic solution is infused into the aortic root via a small cardioplegic cannula. The right atrium is then opened, and the ventricular septal defect closed while working through the tricuspid valve. A continuous suture technique using 5-0 polypropylene suture and a very small fully curved needle are usually utilized for this, with pericardial pledgets used on the tricuspid annular portion of the closure to further bolster the security of the closure. During this time, a vent is placed across the patent foramen to decompress the left ventricle. An additional dose of cardioplegic solution is then administered following completion of the VSD closure. A c-clamp is then placed across the proximal descending thoracic aorta, extending up the left subclavian artery. Flow continues through the ascending aortic cannula at approximately one third of calculated full flow. All ductal tissue is then excised from its junction with the descending thoracic aorta, and the aortotomy extended several millimeters down the descending thoracic aorta. The aortotomy is likewise extended for approximately 5 mm up the left subclavian artery. A short segment of cryopreserved aortic allograft is then anastomosed end to side to these arteriotomies. A continuous 6-0 polypropylene suture technique is utilized. The proximal end of the aortic allograft is then brought up to the ascending aortic segment, in order to determine how much of the graft should be excised, to allow both anastomoses to be under no tension. Allograft sizes vary from 10–14 mm, depending upon the size of the patient. Excision of the proximal portion of the allograft usually results in a trapezoidally shaped segment of the aortic allograft, which functions as the reconstructed arch. Circulatory arrest is then utilized to create the aortotomy on the ascending aorta. This usually extends several millimeters up the left common carotid. The proximal anastomosis is then accomplished with a continuous 6-0 polypropylene suture technique. During the period of circulatory arrest, the head and neck vessels are ensnared with Silastic vessel loops placed as Potts ties. The period of circulatory arrest becomes only that necessary to accomplish the proximal anastomosis, no more than 6-8 minutes. The graft is then back-bled by the removal of the c-clamp to allow for evacuation of all air, flow is resumed through the ascending aortic cannula, the aortic cross clamp is released, and the vessel loops are removed.

The ASD is then reduced in size to approximately 2 to 3 mm leaving the LV vent in place. The atriotomy is then closed with 6-0 polypropylene suture. As a precaution against air, the patient is placed in the Trendelenburg position following removal of the aortic cross clamp. At 18° C, however, there is no cardiac ejection, and once the atriotomy is closed, the combination of the vent, plus vacuum-assisted bypass, succeeds in removing all residual air. Flow is then restored to normal and the patient is rewarmed. During rewarming and once ventricular contractility has resumed, the vent is then removed and the atriotomy closure completed. Prior to removal from cardiopulmonary bypass, transesophageal echocardiography is utilized to assess the integrity of the intracardiac repair, the probe having been placed during anesthesia induction. We do not routinely place intracardiac lines, but rely on the lines placed percutaneously during anesthesia induction.

While this technique does interpose a short segment (1–2 cm) of cryopreserved allograft, it offers the advantages of not sacrificing any arch vessels (subclavian arteries) and of minimizing the period of circulatory arrest.

Postoperative management should be routine and identical to that of any neonate undergoing a biventricular repair. We prefer to keep the patient heavily sedated and mechanically ventilated for the first 24–48 h postoperatively as prophylaxis against pulmonary hypertensive crises. Otherwise, failure to adequately progress after 3–4 days should prompt a search for an underlying cause: residual VSD, left ventricular outflow tract obstruction, or problems with the arch reconstruction. Echocardiography and, if need be, cardiac catheterization can be utilized for assessment and diagnosis.

TWO-STAGE APPROACH

A two-stage approach involves establishment of arch continuity with an interposition graft, usually a synthetic conduit, with placement of a pulmonary artery band if the VSD is deemed nonrestrictive. The VSD is then closed at a later date.[31] The arch reconstruction is accomplished through a left thoracotomy, although some surgeons utilize a combination of left thoracotomy and median sternotomy, the latter incision used for the proximal anastomosis. This approach is still used in many centers worldwide and is felt by many surgeons to be an especially attractive option for a Type A interruption.

IAA WITH LEFT VENTRICULAR OUTFLOW TRACT OBSTRUCTION

The presence of significant left ventricular outflow tract obstruction may necessitate consideration of more radical, and somewhat creative, alternative approaches. If the ventricular septal defect is large and nonrestrictive, a biventricular repair can be achieved using an operative technique described by Yasui and associates.[49] With this technique, a Damus-Kaye-Stansel/Norwood reconstruction of the aortic arch and ascending aorta is accomplished using the proximal main pulmonary artery. Through a right ventriculotomy, an intracardiac baffle is then created to direct left ventricular outflow into the main pulmonary artery. Finally, an extracardiac right ventricular to pulmonary arterial conduit is placed (Rastelli type repair). This approach will obviously necessitate periodic conduit changes throughout the life of the patient.

If there are questions about the adequacy of the VSD in association with the left ventricular outflow tract obstruction, a DKS/Norwood type palliative approach can be utilized in the neonatal period. This approach does not preclude the possibility of a subsequent biventricular repair. Erez and associates have recently reported using the approach in 13 neonates, with 6 ultimately achieving biventricular repair.[9]

RESULTS: MORTALITY AND COMPLICATIONS

The results of surgery improved steadily over the past 2 decades. The reasons for this are multifactorial, and some reasons have been alluded to earlier in the chapter. The availability of prostaglandin enabled better resuscitation correction of acidosis and normalization of all organ system function. The advent of echocardiography and two dimensional color Doppler enabled noninvasive diagnosis to be accomplished. There was steady improvement in image quality with improved technology over this time period. Improved knowledge of neonatal physiology enabled caregivers to manipulate cardiopulmonary physiology to achieve better systemic perfusion. Technical improvements in ventilators enabled caregivers to provide a far more refined approach to ventilatory management. Improvement in surgical and cardiopulmonary bypass techniques enabled a much safer journey through the surgical period, and much better technical results. The experience of Children's Hospital Boston throughout the decade of the 1980s in nicely summarized in Figure 118-4 and is outlined in publication.[38]

The largest and most comprehensive analysis of surgical outcomes is the result of a multiinstitutional study conducted by the Congenital Heart Surgeons Society.[19] This study examined 250 neonates with interrupted aortic arch, 183 of whom had coexisting VSD. Nine of these infants died before repair was accomplished. Survival at 1 month was 73%, indicating an early mortality of approximately 27%. Survival at 1, 3, and 4 years after repair did not change appreciably. Risk factors for death in this study were low birth weight, younger age at repair, interrupted arch Type B, outlet and trabecular ventricular septal defects, smaller size of the ventricular septal defect, and subaortic narrowing.

A more recent summary of a single institution's experience was published by Schrieber and associates.[36] Between 1975 and 1999, these authors treated 94 patients with interrupted arch. In this series, early mortality for patients undergoing a two-stage procedure was 37% and late mortality was 26%. Early mortality for patients undergoing a single-stage procedure was 12%, with a late mortality of 20%.

All of these series indicate that interrupted aortic arch continues to be a challenge and that a late risk factor appears to be persistent or acquired obstruction of the left ventricular outflow tract.

EARLY COMPLICATIONS

Persistent obstruction of the left ventricular outflow tract has been mentioned earlier in the chapter. An additional early complication, seen at the time of surgery or in the immediate postoperative period, is persistent bleeding. When it is seen, bleeding invariably occurs somewhere along the arch anastomosis and is usually associated with the friability of arch tissue. No matter which technique one uses for reconstructing the arch, it is vitally important to excise all ductal tissue. Ductal tissue consists mostly of intima and adventitia, with very little in the way of media. It does not hold sutures well. In addition, it is vasoactive tissue, and left behind, will contribute to recurrent stenosis as the tissue shrinks and scars. Friability of the aortic tissue can be seen after extreme preoperative acidosis or after prolonged administration of prostaglandins. It is certainly a phenome-

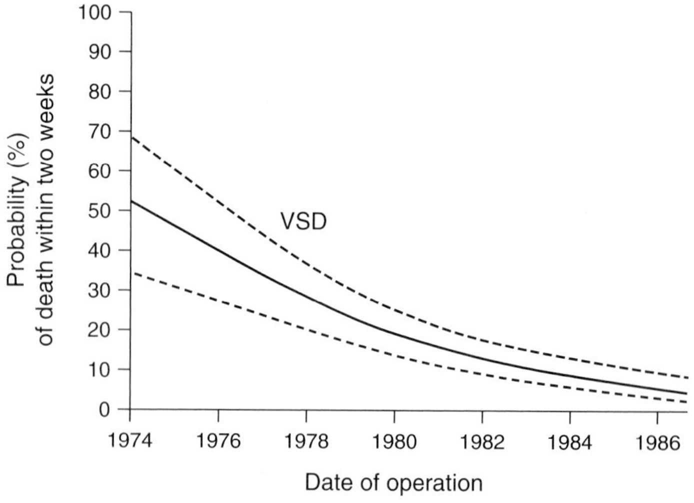

Figure 118–4 Probability of death within 2 weeks of repair of an interrupted aortic arch with a ventricular septal defect (VSD) as the only associated anomaly, according to year of operation at Children's Hospital, Boston, from 1974-1987. Note the progressive increase in anticipated survival.
(From Castaneda AR, Jones RA, Mayer JE, et al. Cardiac surgery of the neonate and infant, Philadelphia: W.B. Saunders, 1994, p. 359.)

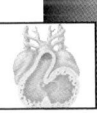

non that every surgeon correcting interrupted aortic arch has encountered.

Injury to the recurrent laryngeal nerve and phrenic nerves can be seen after correction of interrupted aortic arch. These are usually stretch injuries, and the nerves will eventually recover, as regeneration proceeds at 1–3 mm per day from the point of injury. Injury to the recurrent laryngeal nerve is usually of little consequence, as having one vocal cord injured will result merely in a change in the baby's cry.

Injury to the phrenic nerve is more problematic, as it will either interfere with a baby's ability to be weaned from the ventilator or prevent the baby from remaining off the ventilator once extubated. If phrenic nerve injury and diaphragmatic paralysis is suspected, fluoroscopic examination of the baby's diaphragms while the baby is breathing spontaneously should be undertaken. If paradoxical movement is seen, the patient should undergo plication of the left hemidiaphragm. This is a very straightforward procedure and usually results in the child being weaned from the ventilator within 1 day.

LATE COMPLICATIONS

Late complications following correction of interrupted aortic arch and closure of ventricular septal defect may include recurrent stenosis of the arch reconstruction, obstruction of the left ventricular outflow tract, left bronchial obstruction, and long-term sequelae of DiGeorge syndrome.

RECURRENT OBSTRUCTION OF THE AORTIC ARCH

Recurrent obstruction of the aortic arch can occur as early as several months following arch reconstruction. Usually this takes the form of stenosis at a suture line. All patients, however, who have had their arch reconstructed with a tube graft will eventually develop a pressure gradient across the aortic arch as the synthetic tube graft does not allow for growth of arch structures.

Patients who have had a direct reconstruction of the aortic arch using as much autologous tissue as possible can usually have the gradient relieved by interventional cardiac catheterization with balloon dilation of the area of obstruction. This has proven to be ever more useful as technology has advanced. Patients who have had the arch reconstruction with interposition of a synthetic tube graft will need replacement of the graft, bypass of the graft, or enlargement of the existing graft.

LEFT VENTRICULAR OUTFLOW TRACT OBSTRUCTION

Although obstruction of the left ventricular outflow tract is something that is monitored early after initial repair, it usually does not require intervention early in the patient's life. It does become more problematic after the patient grows out of infancy. Because of the variability in the morphology of the left ventricular outflow tract in these patients, obstruction can occur at several levels.

If the obstruction is in the subvalvar region at the level of the conal septum or exists as a fibromuscular ridge contiguous with the VSD closure, this can sometimes be resected by working down through the aortic valve. One must be prepared to close an additional ventricular septal defect if one is created in order to achieve an adequate resection. If the aortic valve is dysplastic or the annulus small, an aortic valve or root replacement with an annular enlargement procedure may be necessary to correct this. This may also be the case if the obstruction is a tunnel type subaortic stenosis extending up to the level of the annulus. The annulus can be enlarged posteriorly by extending an incision onto the anterior leaflet of the mitral valve when the stenosis is not severe, or it may be enlarged through a Konno-type procedure with an extended aortic root replacement, extending the ventriculotomy through the conal septum in order to enlarge the entire left ventricular outflow tract. Depending upon what the morphology of the conal septum was and how close the upper rim of the ventricular septal defect was to the pulmonary valve annulus, utilization of a pulmonary autograft may be impossible. There may have been very little separation between aortic and pulmonic valve annuli. In these cases, either an allograft or a mechanical prosthesis may need to be used. Alternative techniques that have been used historically when the degree of left ventricular outflow tract obstruction is especially severe include the use of a conduit from the left ventricular apex to the descending aorta. This should rarely be necessary with the availability of allografts.

OBSTRUCTION OF THE LEFT MAIN STEM BRONCHUS

The left main stem bronchus passes beneath the arch of the aorta. An interposition graft may impinge upon the left main stem bronchus. Likewise, a direct anastomosis performed without mobilization may result in a bowstring effect over the left main stem bronchus. Symptoms may include wheezing or recurrent respiratory infections. Radiographic findings may include air trapping in the left lung with a degree of hyperexpansion. The diagnosis can be confirmed by bronchoscopy and airways imaging using CT or MRI. Management may necessitate dividing the arch and placement of a ascending to descending aortic conduit. Mitchell and associates[29] reported a successful correction of bronchial compression and severe bronchomalacia using transverse aortic arch extension with a pulmonary artery autograft and left bronchial sleeve resection. With adequate mobilization of the ascending and descending aorta, however, these sorts of radical approaches to late complications should not be necessary.

DIGEORGE SYNDROME

While DiGeorge syndrome may present problems with calcium metabolism early in the neonatal period, management after this period usually just includes vitamin D and calcium supplementation. Long term immunological sequelae associated with DiGeorge syndrome have not yet emerged as major problems. The immunological consequences of DiGeorge syndrome will certainly need to be monitored as these patients grow into adulthood.

REFERENCES

1. Bailey LL, Jacobson JG, Vyhmeister E, et al. Interrupted aortic arch complex. Successful total correction in the neonate. Ann Thorac Surg 25:66, 1978.
2. Barratt-Boyes BG, Nicholls TT, Brandt PWT, Neutze JM: Aortic arch interruption associated with patent ductus arteriosus, ventricular septal defect, and total anomalous pulmonary venous connection. J Thorac Cardiovasc Surg 63:367, 1972.
3. Castaneda AR, Jones RA, Mayer JE, et al. Cardiac Surgery of the Neonate and infant, Philadelphia: W.B. Saunders, 1994, p. 357.
4. Celoria GC, Patton RB: Congenital absence of the aortic arch. Am Heart J 58:407, 1959.
5. Collins-Nakai RL, Dick M, Parisi-Buckley L, et al. Interrupted aortic arch in infancy. J. Pediatr 88:959, 1976.
6. Didier D, Ratib O, Beghetti M, et al. Morphologic and functional evaluation of congenital heart disease by magnetic resonance imaging. J Magn Reson Imaging. 10:639–655, 1999.
7. Driscoll DA, Budarf ML, Emanuel BS. 1992. A genetic etiology for DiGeorge syndrome: Consistent deletions and micro deletion of 22q11. Am J Hum Genet 50:924–933.
8. Elliott RB, Starling MB, Neutze JM. Medical management of the ductus. Lancet 1:140, 1975.
9. Erez E, Tam VK, Kanter KR, et al. Successful biventricular repair alter initial Norwood operation for interrupted aortic arch with severe left ventricular outflow tract obstruction. Ann Thorac Surg 2001 Jun 71(6):1974–7.
10. Ferencz C, Loffredo CA, Correa-Villasenor A, et al. Genetic and Environmental Risk Factors of Major Cardiovascular Malformations: The Baltimore-Washington Infant Study 1981-1989. Armonk, NY: Futura, 1997.
11. Ferencz C, Rubin JD, Loffredo C, Magee C: Epidemiology of Congenital Heart Disease: The Baltimore-Washington Infant Study, 1981–1989. Mt. Kisco, NY: Futura, 1993.
12. Fibison WJ, Budarf M, McDermid H, et al: Molecular studies of DiGeorge syndrome. Am J Hum Genet 46:888–895, 1990.
13. Fleming WH, Sarafian LB, Clarke ED, et al. Critical aortic coarctation: Patch aortoplasty in infants less than age 3 months. Am J Cardiol 44:687, 1979.
14. Freedom RM, Rosen FS, Nadas AS: Congenital cardiovascular disease and anomalies of the third and fourth pharyngeal pouch. Circulatio 46:165, 1972.
15. Freedom RM, Bain HH, Esplugas E, et al. Ventricular septal defect in interruption of aortic arch. Am J Cardiol 39:572, 1977.
16. Hamaoka K, Ozawa S, Sutou F, et al. Spiral CR angiography for assessing systemic-to-pulmonary shunt in children. Lancet 348:341, 1996.
17. Ho Sy, Wilcox BR, Anderson RH, et al. Interrupted aortic arch–Anatomical features of surgical significance. Thorac Cardiovasc Surg 31:199, 1983.
18. Ito T, Okubo T, Sato H: Familial 22q11.2 deletion: an infant with interrupted aortic arch and DiGeorge syndrome delivered from by a mother with tetralogy of Fallot. Eur J Cardiothorac Surg 13(3):310–312, 1998.
19. Jonas RA, Quaegebeur JM, Kirklin JW, et al. Outcomes in patients with interrupted aortic arch and ventricular septal defect. J Thorac Cardiovasc Surg 107:1099–1113, 1994.
20. Jonas RA, Sell JE, Van Praagh R, et al. Left ventricular outflow obstruction associated with interrupted aortic arch and ventricular septal defect. In Crupi G, Parenzan L, Anderson RH (eds). Perspectives in Pediatric Cardiology. New York, Futura, 1989, pp. 61–65.
21. Kaulitz R, Jonas RA, van der Velde ME: Echocardiographic assessment of interrupted aortic arch. Cardiol Young. 9:562–571, 1999.
22. Kawano T, Ishii M, Takagi J, et al. Three-dimensional helical computed tomographic angiography in neonates and infants with complex congenital heart disease. Am Heart J 139:654–660, 2000.
23. Kreutzer J, Van Praagh R: Comparison of left ventricular outflow tract obstruction in interruption of the aortic arch and in coarctation of the aorta, with diagnostic, developmental, and surgical implications. Am J Cardiol 86:856–862, 2000.
24. Kutsche LM, Van Mierop LHS: Cervical origin of the right subclavian artery in aortic arch interruption: Pathogenesis and significance. Am J Cardiol 53:892, 1984.
25. Loffredo CA, Ferencz C, Wilson PD, et al. Interrupted aortic arch: an epidemiologic study, Teratology 61:368–375, 2000.
26. Lofland GK, McCrindle BW, Williams WG, et al. Critical aortic stenosis in the neonate: a multi-institutional study of management, outcomes, and risk factors. J Thorac Cardiovasc Surg; 121:10–27, 2001.
27. Marino B, Digilio MC, Persiani M, et al. Deletion 22q11 in patients with interrupted aortic arch. Am J Cardiol. 84:360–1, A9, 1999.
28. Merrill DL, Webster CA, Samson PC: Congenital absence of the aortic isthmus. J Thorac Surg 33:311, 1957.
29. Mitchell MB, Campbell DN, Toews WH, et al. Autograft aortic arch extension and sleeve resection for bronchial compression after interrupted aortic arch repair. Ann Thorac Surg 73:1969–1971, 2002.
30. Momma K, Ando M, Matsuoka R, et al. Interruption of the aortic arch associated with deletion of chromosome 22q11 is associated with a subarterial and doubly committed ventricular septal defect in Japanese patients. Cardiol Young. 9:463–467, 1999.
31. Norwood WI, Lang P, Castaneda AR, et al. Reparative operations for interrupted aortic arch with ventricular septal defect. J Thorac Cardiovasc Surg 86:837, 1983.
32. Rauch A, Hofbeck M, Leipold G: Incidence and significance of 22q11.2 hemizygosity in patients with interrupted aortic arch. Am J Med Genet. 78:322–331, 1998.
33. Roberts WC, Morrow AG, Braunwald E: Complete interruption of the aortic arch. Circulation 26:39, 1962.
34. Ryan AK, Goodship JA, Wilson DI, et al. Spectrum of clinical features associated with interstitial chromosome 22q11 deletions: a European collaborative study. J Med Genet 34:798–804, 1997.
35. Salem MM, Starnes VA, Wells WJ, et al. Predictors of left ventricular outflow obstruction following single stage repair of interrupted aortic arch and ventricular septal defect. Am J Cardiol. 86:1044–1047, A11, 2000.
36. Schreiber C, Eicken A, Vogt M, et al. Repair of interrupted aortic arch: results after more than 20 years. Ann Thorac Surg 70:1896–1899; discussion 1899–1900, 2000.
37. Seidel JF: Index Musei Anatomici Kiliensis. Kiel: CF Mohr, 1818, p. 61.
38. Sell JE, Jonas RA, Mayer JE, et al. The results of a surgical program for interrupted aortic arch. J Thorac Cardiovasc Surg 96:864, 1988.
39. Shiraishi I, Yamamoto Y, Ozawa S, et al. Application of helical computed tomographic angiography with differential color imaging three-dimensional reconstruction in the diagnosis of complicated congenital heart diseases. J Thorac Cardiovasc Surg 125:36–39, 2003.
40. Steidele RJ: Samml Chir Med Beob. Vienna: 1778. Vol.2, p. 114.
41. Takahashi K, Kuwahara T, Nagatsu M: Interruption of the aortic arch at the isthmus with DiGeorge syndrome and 22q11.2 deletion. Cardiol Young. 9:516–518, 1999.
42. Trusler GA, Izakawa T. Interrupted aortic arch and ventricular septal defect. Direct repair through a median sternotomy

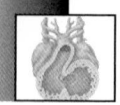

incision in a 13-day-old infant. J Thorac Cardiovasc Surg 69:126, 1975.

43. Van Mierop LHS, Kutsche LM: Interruption of the aortic arch and coarctation of the aorta: Pathogenetic relations. Am J Cardiol 54:829, 1984.

44. Van Praagh R, Bernhard WF, Rosenthal A, Parisi LF, Fyler DC: Interrupted aortic arch: Surgical treatment. Am J Cardiol 27:200, 1971.

45. Vick GW III. Three-and four-dimensional visualization of magnetic resonance imaging data sets in pediatric cardiology. Pediatr Cardiol. 21:27–36, 2000.

46. Volpe P, Gentile M, Marasini M: Interrupted aortic arch type A with 22q11 deletion: prenatal detection of an unusual association. Prenat Diagn 22:371–374, 2002.

47. Weisman D, Kesten HD: Absence of transverse aortic arch with defects of cardiac septums. Report of a case simulating acute abdominal disease in a newborn infant. Am J DisChild 76:326, 1948.

48. Westra SJ, Hurteau J, Galindo A, et al. Cardiac electron-beam CT in children undergoing surgical repair for pulmonary atresia. Radiology 213:502–512, 1999.

49. Yasui H, Kado H, Nakano E, et al. Primary repair of interrupted aortic arch with severe aortic stenosis in neonates. J Thorac Cardiovasc Surg 93:539, 1987.

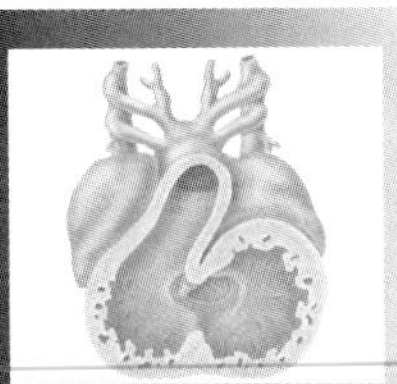

Surgery for Congenital Anomalies of the Aortic Valve and Root

CHAPTER 119

Frank A. Pigula

INTRODUCTION

Congenital aortic valve disease is one of the more commonly encountered congenital cardiac defects, occurring in about 3–6% of children born with congenital heart disease. Manifesting primarily as aortic stenosis, congenital aortic valve disease tends to be a progressive disease, with morbidity and mortality resulting from the hemodynamic burden imposed on the left ventricle. Although the same pathological mechanisms are operational in both congenital and acquired aortic valve disease, the context differs dramatically. Congenital aortic valve pathology often presents alongside multiple associated cardiovascular lesions, and multiple levels of the left ventricular outflow tract may be involved. Competing treatment paradigms (e.g., interventional and surgical, single ventricle versus biventricular repair) may require consideration. Growth, behavior, and anticoagulation may present special concerns. Thus, the evaluation and treatment of congenital aortic valve disease may present unique anatomical and physiological considerations. This chapter will address these considerations and the related challenges encountered during the surgical treatment of congenital heart disease.

SURGICAL ANATOMY OF THE AORTIC VALVE AND ROOT

The aortic valve and root span the transition from the left ventricular chamber to the systemic circulation, including the subaortic left ventricular outflow tract, the aortic valve, and the aortic wall up to the level of the sinotubular junction. Congenital heart disease can involve one or more levels of the atrioventricular complex. A thorough understanding and appreciation of these inconspicuous anatomical relationships form the basis of successful surgical treatment of congenital aortic valve disease, and these relationships will be referred to throughout this chapter.

The normal aortic valve sits wedged into the left ventricular outflow tract. In addition to supporting the coronary circulation, this central location places the aortic valve at the nexus of several critical intracardiac structures. Among these are the anterior leaflet of the mitral valve, the membranous interventricular septum, and the conduction apparatus. Because multiple levels of the atrioventricular complex may be involved in congenital heart disease, it is helpful to consider the normal anatomy with regard to its subvalvular, valvular, and supravalvular components.

The subvalvular anatomy is dominated by the anatomical relationships between the aortic valve, the interventricular septum, the membranous septum, the mitral valve, and the conduction apparatus (Figure 119-1). Parts of the aortic leaflets are in fibrous continuity with the anterior leaflet of the mitral valve and also with the tricuspid valve (via the membranous septum). These structures contribute to the central supporting structure of the heart, known as the fibrous skeleton. In addition to providing points of fixation for the atrioventricular valves, the fibrous skeleton also provides electrical insulation between the atria and the ventricles, thereby restricting impulse conduction to the bundle of His. After arising from the atrioventricular node, the bundle of His penetrates the membranous septum, emerging on the surface of the left ventricular septum immediately below the aortic annulus. Looking through the aortic valve, the bundle will lie beneath the annulus, just below the commissure between the noncoronary and the right coronary leaflet. From the surgeon's perspective, important radiations of the bundle reach to the nadir of the right coronary leaflet as they fall away toward the apex of the heart.

Valvular anatomy is dominated by the semilunar leaflets, commissures, and the sinuses of Valsalva. The leaflets and their sinuses are identified by the associated coronary artery. The right coronary artery ostium is found in the right coronary sinus, which is almost directly anterior when viewed by the surgeon. The left coronary artery emerges posteriorly from the left coronary sinus. The leaflets themselves are made up of a fibrous core lined with endothelium.

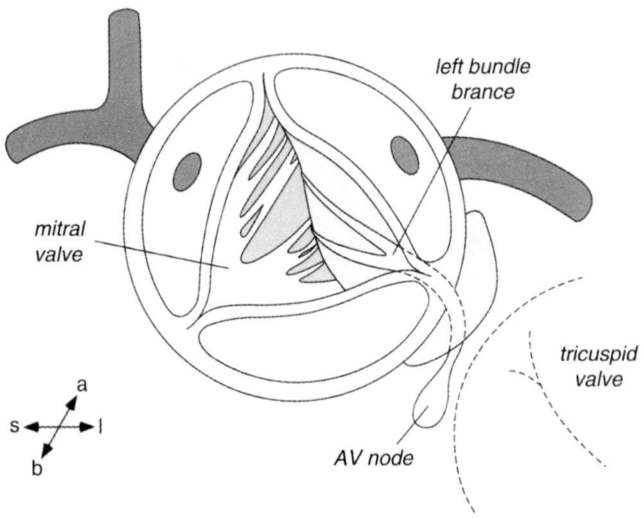

Figure 119–1 Anatomical relationships within the aortic valve.

The commissures, along with the free-edge coaptation provided by the leaflets themselves, provide the strength necessary to ensure a competent valve.

The aortic sinuses are dilatations of the aortic wall above distal to the insertion of the semilunar leaflets, and they are well suited to support the coronary ostia. Although the leaflets retract during systole, eddy currents developing within the sinuses prevent occlusion of the coronary ostia by the retracted aortic leaflets. Their presence is probably important to the long-term function of the aortic valve leaflets.[56,75]

Finally, the supravalvular area denotes the transition from the left ventricle–aorta complex to the aorta proper. For practical purposes, this area includes the sinotubular junction, which is the area just distal to the tips of the commissural posts and the dilatations of the aortic sinuses.

Abnormalities at any level may be expected in congenital heart disease, and a discussion of the various forms of congenital aortic valve pathology will be categorized by level: subvalvular, valvular, or supravalvular.

AORTIC STENOSIS

Prevalence

Congenital aortic stenosis has been reported to be present in between 3% and 6% of children with congenital heart disease.[70] Males are affected more commonly than females, with an incidence ratio of 3:1.[52] Although aortic insufficiency may afflict congenitally abnormal valves later in life, it is a decidedly uncommon lesion during infancy and early childhood. When present in these age groups, it is usually an iatrogenic consequence of a procedure designed to relieve congenital aortic stenosis.

Clinical Characteristics

The clinical presentation varies with the severity of the lesion and the age at presentation. In the neonate, critical aortic stenosis may present rapidly and dramatically, with abrupt hemodynamic deterioration, cardiovascular collapse, and shock. The cardiogram may reveal left ventricular hypertrophy with S-T and T wave abnormalities. The chest X-ray may demonstrate cardiomegaly and pulmonary edema. Transthoracic echocardiogram will rapidly establish the diagnosis, and it is useful for determining the presence of associated abnormalities of the left ventricle, the mitral valve, or the aortic arch. Aggressive resuscitation with inotropes and prostaglandin is required to support the circulation.

Older children may be asymptomatic, and aortic stenosis may be suspected as a result of physical examination. Chest pain and exercise intolerance are possible but uncommon. As is the case for the neonate, the diagnosis may be confirmed by echocardiography.

Diagnosis

Physical examination may be very suggestive of the diagnosis of congenital aortic valve disease. There may be a harsh crescendo-decrescendo murmur heard best at the right second interspace, with transmission into the neck. A thrill will be present in the suprasternal notch and over the right second intercostal spaces in severe aortic stenosis. Because ventricular systole is prolonged in the setting of aortic stenosis, the second heart sound may be prolonged, thus resulting in a narrowly split second heart sound. An associated diastolic murmur would suggest an element of aortic insufficiency.

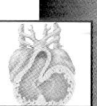

Electrocardiographic changes are consistent with ventricular hypertrophy as evidenced by increased left-sided R wave voltage. Changes in S-T segment and T wave in the left precordial leads may denote left ventricle strain. Except in the situation of obvious congestive heart failure, the chest X-ray is usually unremarkable.

Echocardiography

Echocardiography is the mainstay for contemporary diagnosis of congenital aortic valve disease. This noninvasive test provides important anatomical and physiological information, such as the number and anatomy of the aortic leaflets, the size of the aortic annulus and ascending aorta, the location of the coronary arteries, the adequacy of the subaortic left ventricular outflow tract, and the site of the hemodynamic stenosis. The peak instantaneous gradient may be estimated by measuring the velocity of blood flow across the stenosis and by employing a modification of the Bernoulli equation (velocity $[m/s]^2 \times 4$).[110]

Stress Testing

Stress testing may be helpful in the older patient with mild/moderate aortic stenosis in whom symptoms may be vague or suspicious and not clearly related to the aortic valve disease. Stress-related changes in the S-T segment or T wave morphology would suggest important stenosis, with myocardium in jeopardy. In these instances, relief of the stenosis should be seriously considered, despite mild/moderate resting peak gradients.

Cardiac Catheterization

At the present time, the major role of catheterization is to provide access for catheter-based interventions that are designed to relieve stenosis (e.g., balloon valvotomy). In selected cases, catheterization may also be helpful to assess left ventricular diastolic function and pulmonary artery pressure, to identify associated vascular lesions, and to evaluate patients with multiple levels of left ventricular outflow tract obstruction.

Natural History

Neonates with critical aortic stenosis make up a unique group that may suffer from immediate life-threatening left ventricular outflow tract obstruction. Without prompt treatment, these infants may succumb to cardiovascular collapse.

By contrast, older children with aortic stenosis are often asymptomatic. Given the important considerations pertaining to pediatric aortic valve replacement, the timing of the operation becomes an important consideration. Understanding the natural history and progression of asymptomatic children is useful.

Aortic valve disease in children tends to be a progressive disease, with stenosis increasing over time; the condition can be classified as mild, moderate, or severe. As categorized by Hossack and colleagues,[65] patients with mild stenosis are those with normal pulse volumes and with a resting peak systolic gradient (measured at catheterization) between the left ventricle–aorta of less than 40 mm Hg.[65] Patients are considered to suffer from moderate aortic stenosis when they present with diminished pulse volumes by palpation and resting peak systolic gradients of 40–75 mm Hg at rest. Severe stenosis is demonstrated when the patients present with abnormal pulse volumes and a resting peak systolic pressure gradient in excess of 75 mm Hg.

It should be noted that these gradient criteria were obtained by direct pullback measurements obtained at catheterization. Currently gradients across the left ventricular outflow tract are most often obtained by echocardiography. In most cases, the Doppler-derived peak instantaneous gradient correlates well with catheter-derived data; however, at lower gradients, Doppler may result in an overestimation.[5,120]

Because aortic valve disease in children is progressive, the natural history of this progression is of some interest. Among children presenting with nonobstructive aortic lesions, Mills and others[93] reported that 7% progressed to mild obstruction after 7–15 years.

When mild stenosis was present on the initial evaluation, progression was more rapid. Twenty percent of patients developed moderate or severe stenosis within 10 years, with 45% progressing within 20 years. Finally, about 60% of patients presenting with moderate stenosis will progress to severe stenosis within 10 years.[65]

TREATMENT

Critical Aortic Stenosis in the Neonate

Aortic stenosis presenting during the neonatal period may be a very severe hemodynamic lesion that is life-threatening (Figure 119-2). These children often present in shock as a consequence of ductal closure in the setting of left heart structures that are inadequate to support the systemic circulation; their systemic circulation is "ductal dependent." These children require urgent medical stabilization, including assisted ventilation and inotropic support. Prostaglandin E_1 is administered to reopen the duct and to maintain ductal patency. After the patient is stabilized, a thorough echocardiographic examination of the left-sided structures is required to determine their suitability to support the systemic circulation.

When approaching critical aortic stenosis in the neonate, the single most important decision involved in treatment is deciding which patients will benefit from biventricular repair and which are better suited to a single-ventricle approach. The importance of proper treatment selection is reflected by the high mortality in older, unstratified series of neonates undergoing valvotomy for critical aortic stenosis.[54] An accurate determination of which patients will benefit from a single-ventricle treatment pathway (Norwood operation) is critical and has been the impetus for the Congenital Heart Surgeons Society (CHSS)-sponsored study designed to accomplish this.[76] An estimate of survival benefit for

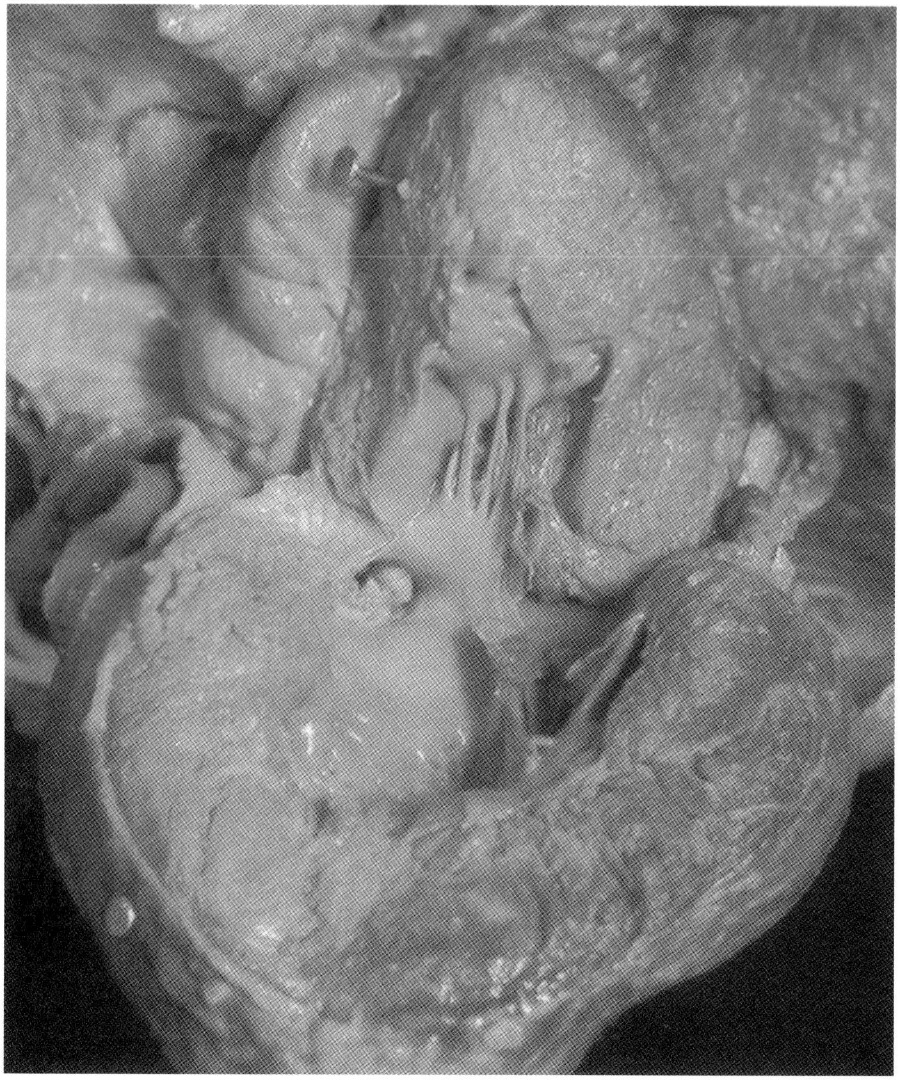

Figure 119–2 Pathological specimen showing aortic stenosis in the neonatal heart.

specific left heart morphology can be obtained at the CHSS Web site (www.chssdc.org). The management of these patients has been detailed in Chapter 125. This discussion will focus on patients with aortic stenosis as the dominant lesion in the setting of two adequate ventricles.

For patients with anatomy deemed suitable to support a two-ventricle circulation, aortic valvotomy provides very effective relief of aortic stenosis. Two techniques of aortic valvotomy have been developed: (1) balloon dilatation of the stenotic valve and (2) surgical valvotomy (open and closed). Although balloon valvotomy is the favored technique at many institutions, surgical valvotomy remains preferred by some. Proponents of balloon valvotomy cite avoidance of potential surgical morbidity, whereas advocates of surgical valvotomy maintain that a more accurate valvotomy is possible under direct vision.

Although there are no prospective randomized studies that directly compare these two techniques, some data are available. McCrindle and colleagues[89] described a CHSS-sponsored multiinstitutional review of 110 neonates undergoing either surgical (28) or balloon (82) valvotomy for critical aortic valve stenosis during the neonatal period.[89] Survival was similar between the 2 procedures (82% at 1 month, 72% at 5 years). Although balloon valvotomy was more effective for relieving stenosis (mean residual gradient, 20 versus 36 mm Hg), it was accomplished at the expense of a higher incidence of important aortic insufficiency (18% after balloon valvotomy versus 3% after surgical valvotomy). Despite these differences, the outcome data between the two techniques are quite comparable. Overall freedom from reintervention was similar for both groups (91% at 1 month, 48% at 5 years). The need for subsequent procedures—regardless of technique—emphasizes the palliative nature of valvotomy for critical aortic stenosis.

Although balloon valvotomy has assumed a prominent role in the treatment of congenital aortic stenosis in many institutions, its role vis-à-vis surgical valvotomy remains controversial. Hawkins and colleagues[59] have estimated the incidence of aortic valve operation after balloon valvotomy to be 5–7% per year; others have reported the risk of surgery to be lower, but the incidence of reintervention, including subsequent balloon dilatation, remains high (60% at

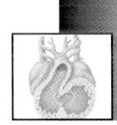

8 years).[95] It may be, however, that specific aortic valvular substrates may lend themselves to one treatment or the other. For a group of 54 infants (57% neonates) undergoing surgical aortic valvotomy, Bhabra and others[8] reported significant differences in the long-term outcomes based on leaflet morphology. When valvotomy resulted in a trileaflet structure, patients did significantly better than when only a bileaflet valve was achieved. At 10 years, the actuarial freedom from reintervention was 92% among trileaflet valves but only 33% among bileaflet valves ($P = .01$). Similar differences were reported for freedom from aortic valve reoperation ($P = .04$). Freedom from aortic valve replacement was 100% in trileaflet valves and 57% in bileaflet valves. However, by echocardiogram, the authors were only able to retrospectively identify 14 out of 28 bileaflet valves, whereas 7 out of 8 valves with trileaflet potential could be identified (sensitivity, 88%; specificity, 50%). These results have yet to be confirmed, but closer examination of the anatomical subtypes of aortic valve stenosis may be justified before selecting the appropriate technique. At the present time, there appears to be little if any role for surgical transventricular (closed) aortic valvotomy.

Catheter Versus Surgical Relief in Infancy

A few studies have compared balloon aortic valvotomy to surgical valvotomy in older children. McCrindle and colleagues[88] reported their analysis of 630 balloon valvotomies on 606 patients from 23 institutions. They reported a median age of 6.8 years, with a range of 1 day to 18 years. Because of technical issues, the procedure was abandoned 4.1% of the time, and procedural mortality was 1.9%. A suboptimal result (failure to complete procedure, residual gradient >60 mm Hg, left ventricle:aortic pressure = 1.6, or major morbidity or mortality) was reported in 17% of patients. Independent risk factors for poor outcomes were age of less than 3 months, earlier procedure date, higher preoperative gradient, unrepaired aortic coarctation, and the use of undersized balloons.

Other groups have reported similar results with balloon valvotomy in non-neonates. Moore and others[95] reported successful dilatation in 87% of patients (129 out of 148), with a very low procedural mortality (0.7%) and good long-term survival (95% at 8 years). Freedom from reintervention at 8 years was 50%, a figure that is consistent with other studies.[37]

In these patients, the risk of repeat intervention was related to the degree of regurgitation and to residual gradients following initial balloon valvotomy. Similar to the report by Bhabra and colleagues,[8] the authors reported differential results based on the angiographic morphology of the stenotic aortic valve.

However, as is the case in non-neonates, it is difficult to clearly demonstrate the superiority of balloon or surgical aortic valvotomy. Chartrand and colleagues[20] reported their experience with 67 children (age, >6 months) undergoing surgical valvotomy between 1960 and 1992. There was no operative mortality, and the 20-year freedom from death, reoperation, and aortic valve replacement was 94%, 63%, and 73%, respectively. The authors concluded that surgical valvuloplasty is a safe and effective procedure with durable results. In summary, as is seen in neonates, aortic valve morphology appears to influence the response to intervention, and further characterization may be justified. At the present time there appear to be institutional preferences for balloon or surgical valvotomy that can be defended on the basis of experience.

Aortic Stenosis in the Older Child

In contrast with the clinical presentation of the neonate with critical aortic stenosis, older children are commonly asymptomatic. For them, durable preservation of left ventricular function becomes the primary goal of treatment. The etiology of aortic stenosis in the older child (>1 year of age) is most commonly to the result of valvular aortic stenosis (79%), with subvalvular aortic stenosis 7%, and supravalvular stenosis 6% being much less common.[52] When present, aortic regurgitation is often associated with congenital aortic stenosis, and it may be the consequence of previous interventions for the relief of stenosis.

Most older children with aortic stenosis enjoy normal growth and development. When present, symptoms such as chest pain, exercise intolerance, or syncope constitute clear surgical indications. For asymptomatic patients, the indications for intervention are more subtle. For patients with severe stenosis (left ventricle-aortic gradient, >75 mm Hg), operation is recommended. For children thought to have moderate stenosis (left ventricle-aortic gradient, 40–75 mm Hg), more information may be needed before a recommendation can be made. In this setting, electro-cardiographic changes (e.g., ST-T wave changes consistent with left ventricle strain, left ventricle hypertrophy) or a positive stress test would be indications for operation. For these asymptomatic patients, somatic growth, surgical options, and timing of intervention become important concerns.

Because of the progressive nature of the disease, older children thought to have mild aortic stenosis (left ventricle-aortic gradient, <40 mm Hg) should be followed with periodic examinations and echocardiograms. It should be remembered that the gradient is dependent on the cardiac output, and, in a severely dysfunctional left ventricle, the gradient may be unimpressive.

The management options for older children depend on the context of their disease. Older children who are newly diagnosed with important aortic stenosis with minimal insufficiency may be well served by balloon valvotomy. The more common scenario, however, is several years of excellent palliation after an initial valvotomy, during which time the child grows and develops normally. However, with time and/or repeated interventions, many patients will develop important aortic insufficiency. Any residual valvular stenosis is magnified by the resulting volume load, and the combinations of these lesions conspire to threaten left ventricle function. However, by virtue of their older age and larger size, these children are better candidates for durable surgical palliation, usually including valve replacement.

SUBVALVULAR AORTIC STENOSIS

Fixed subaortic stenosis is a heterogeneous lesion that can take the form of a discrete membrane, tunnel-like stenosis, or muscular obstruction (Figure 119-3). A variety of surgical approaches have been designed to address each of these variants.

Subaortic Membrane

This lesion is found in association with other congenital lesions in 60–70% of cases, with ventricular septal defect (VSD) being the most common (35%).[100] Membranous subaortic stenosis results from the proliferation of fibrous tissue just beneath the leaflets of the aortic valve. This tissue may be very thin and tough, and it is often circumferential, involving the underside of the anterior leaflet of the mitral valve. In fact, careful examination of the echocardiogram may suggest a hinge point that represents tethering on the leaflet by the membrane.[22,103] Although the etiology of this form of aortic pathology is not known, studies have implicated that shear stress, precipitated by abnormal angles between the ventricular septum and the aortic barrel, may play an important role. The addition of a VSD adds to the generation of shear stress in this setting.[17]

The surgical approach to this lesion requires cardiopulmonary bypass. A single right atrial venous cannula is usually adequate. The aortic valve is exposed through a transverse aortotomy, which may be carried down into the noncoronary sinus, if needed. Careful retraction of the aortic leaflets will reveal the subaortic membrane. The distance between the aortic valve and the membrane may vary slightly, but it can usually be well visualized. The membrane is incised in the safe zone of the ventricular septum, just left of the nadir of the right coronary sinus. In many instances, the membrane can be peeled or endarterectomized from the endocardium anteriorly and to the right and from the anterior leaflet of the mitral valve posteriorly. In severe cases, this membrane may encroach on and even involve the belly of the aortic valve leaflets. When this happens, the leaflets require careful débridement of the tenacious fibrous tissue.

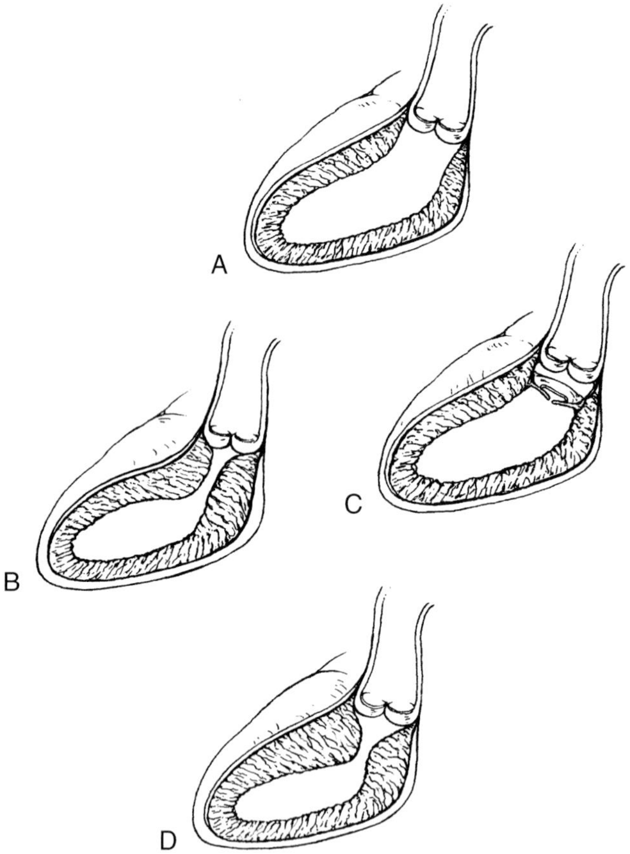

Figure 119–3 **Examples of forms of fixed aortic stenosis (A); discrete membrane (B), tunnel-like stenosis (C), muscular obstruction (D).**

Surgical Indications

In general, the surgical indications for membranous subaortic stenosis adhere to the general recommendations for aortic stenosis. However, citing a lower incidence of recurrence, some centers advocate earlier surgical resection for subaortic stenosis. Brauner and others[11] reported that the recurrence rate of subaortic stenosis (predominately composed of membranous stenosis but with a few instances of tunnel-like stenosis) was related to a preoperative gradient of at least 40 mm Hg, and they argued that surgical resection at lower gradients was justified. Some groups have advocated repair at the time of diagnosis, irrespective of the gradient.[111,125] However, the advantages of early intervention have not been confirmed; other investigators have reported no benefit of early surgery on recurrence.[32]

Because the timing of surgery remains controversial, it is helpful to examine the natural history of membranous subaortic stenosis. There are data that suggest that some children with mild subaortic stenosis (peak systolic gradient, <40 mm Hg) may not require surgery for at least several years. A large representative study of the rate of progression of subvalvular aortic stenosis was reported by Rohlicek and others,[112] who studied children from several centers in eastern Canada. To document the natural history and surgical outcomes, they followed 92 children from the time of diagnosis. There was a slight male preponderance (1.6:1), and the mean age at diagnosis was 5.3 years. Thirteen patients had bicuspid aortic valves; 42 of these children ultimately came to surgery an average of 2.2 ± 0.4 years after diagnosis, and 44 were followed medically and never came to operation (mean follow-up, 4 years). Children ultimately requiring surgery presented with higher initial gradients (40 ± 5 mm Hg versus 21 ± 2 mm Hg), and they were more likely to present with AI at diagnosis (35% versus 13%). Analysis showed the echo gradient at diagnosis to be predictive of subsequent gradient progression and of the appearance of aortic insufficiency. Eight children undergoing surgery required reoperation for recurrent subaortic stenosis an average of 4.9 ± 0.9 years after initial resection. These patients initially presented with significantly higher gradients (66 ± 10 mm Hg).

In contrast with a more aggressive approach of aggressive surgical resection of membranous subaortic stenosis at the time of diagnosis, these data suggest that a significant proportion of these patients will have stable or at least slowly progressive gradients. Although the management approach to patients remains variable, it seems reasonable to pursue surgical resection for peak systolic gradients of 40 mm Hg or greater (obtained by echocardiography). The new onset of aortic insufficiency should probably be considered an important indication for surgery, regardless of the gradient. Although these authors did not discern any improvement in aortic insufficiency after operation, it has been the experi-

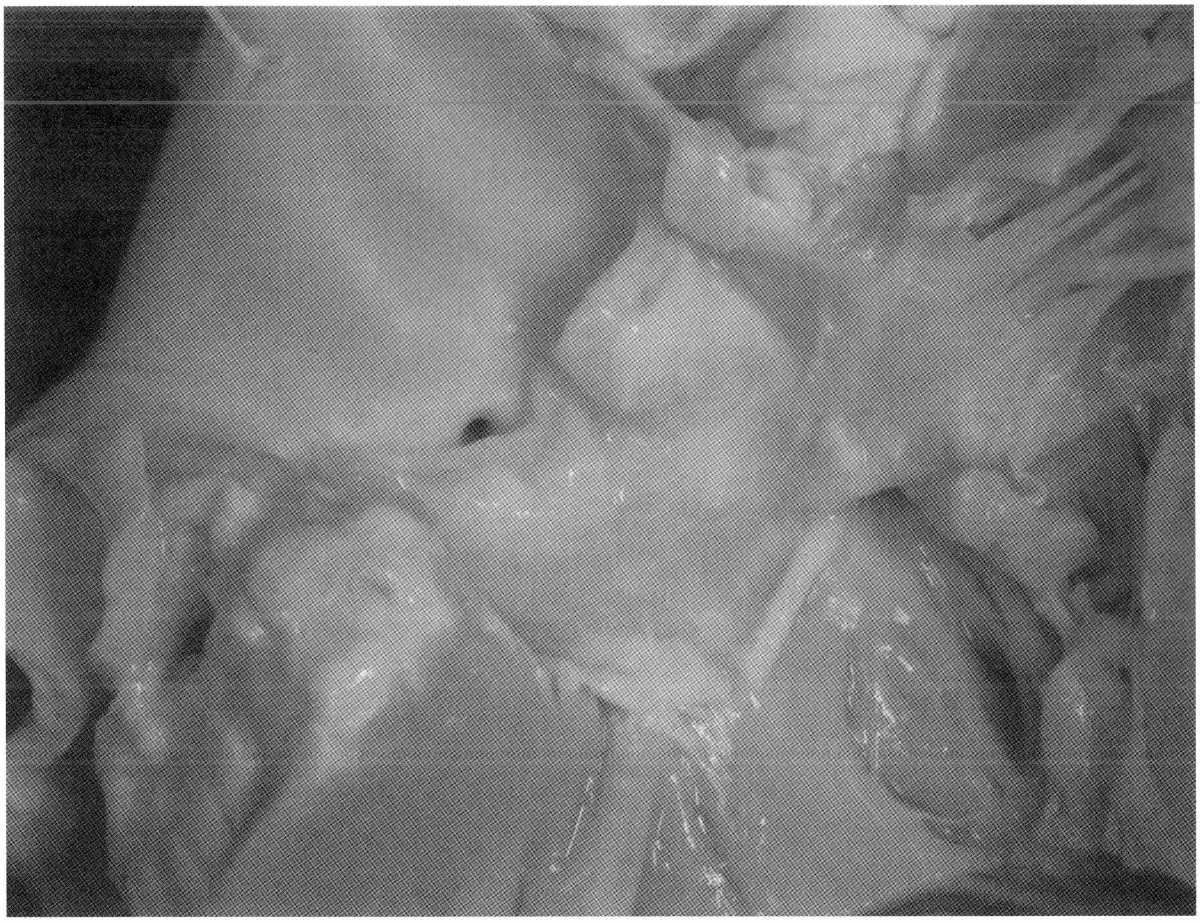

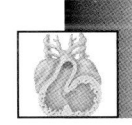

Figure 119–4 **Pathological specimen showing fibrous tissue in growth at the insertion of the anterior leaflet of the mitral valve into the left ventricle.**

ence of others that careful débridement of fibrous tissue encroaching on the aortic leaflets often results in significant improvement in aortic insufficiency.[104]

Results of Membranous Subaortic Stenosis

Membranous subaortic stenosis has been the subject of intense scrutiny, because of both its incidence and its propensity for recurrence after seemingly completely adequate surgical resection.

The reported recurrence rate for membranous subaortic stenosis has been reported to be between 0 and 55%, with most reports documenting a recurrence rate of 15–21%.* Septal myotomy, in addition to membrane resection, has been reported to reduce the incidence of recurrence. Lupinetti and others[79] reported a recurrence rate of 4% when a septal myomectomy was performed in addition to membrane resection; however, this finding has not been confirmed by other studies.[11,27]

Other surgeons advocate an even more aggressive approach. Yacoub and colleagues[135] have suggested that an important pathological feature of membranous subaortic stenosis is fibrous tissue in growth at the point of insertion of the anterior leaflet of the mitral valve into the left ventricular myocardium (Figure 119-4). This ingrowth interferes with the dynamic widening of the outflow tract (including posterior displacement of the mitral apparatus) during systole.

Adding resection of the fibrous tissue from the mitral valve trigones to membrane resection and septal myomectomy, the authors reported excellent relief of left ventricular outflow tract (LVOT) gradient (mean, 8 mm Hg) in 57 patients.[135] Over an average follow-up of 15 years, 7 patients had mild to moderate aortic regurgitation. Most notable was that no patient has required reoperation for recurrent stenosis.

Although periodic attempts at balloon dilatation have been performed, the resulting gradients are generally high (approximately 30 mm Hg), and subsequent surgery is required in the majority of patients. Among 13 patients undergoing dilatation, Moskowitz and colleagues[98] reported that 9 required subsequent surgery. Suarez de Lezo and colleagues[117,118] reported a 50% recurrence rate within 3 years. At this time, balloon dilatation should not be considered as a primary treatment of discrete subaortic stenosis.

Tunnel-like Stenosis

Long-segment or tunnel-like stenosis has been defined as a muscular or fibromuscular subaortic stenosis, the length of which is more than a third of the aortic diameter.[49] Although

*References 13, 32, 50, 60, 68, 135.

tunnel-like stenosis may be associated with other lesions (e.g., interrupted aortic arch, atrioventricular septal defect), this discussion will confine itself to long-segment stenosis in the setting of concordant atrioventricular and ventriculoarterial connections with an intact ventricular septum.

Surgical Indications

The indications for operation for subaortic tunnel are similar to those described for membranous subaortic obstruction.

Treatment

Modified Konno Operation

The degree of hypoplasia encountered in tunnel-like subaortic stenosis does not lend itself to transaortic resection, which might be performed for membranous subaortic stenosis; the surgical treatment of tunnel-like stenosis requires a more extensive procedure. In the presence of a suitable aortic valve, the modified Konno operation has become a favored technique for approaching tunnel-like subaortic stenosis; it has the great appeal of enlarging the left ventricular outflow tract while preserving the native aortic valve. Excellent technical reviews of this technique are available.[16,67]

Briefly, under moderate hypothermia with bicaval cannulation, an aortotomy is performed, and the aortic valve and subaortic area are examined. Only if the aortic valve is satisfactory should the valve-sparing modified Konno operation be performed. If the valve is inadequate, a more extensive procedure designed to enlarge the LVOT and to replace the aortic valve will be necessary, such as the Konno-Rastan or the Ross-Konno operation.

After inspection of the aortic valve, the infundibulum of the right ventricle is incised in a transverse fashion. Visualization of the ventricular septum from these two perspectives (i.e., through the aortic valve and through the infundibulum) allows an accurate incision through the ventricular septum (Figure 119-5). Indentation of the safe area of the ventricular septum (left of the nadir of the right coronary leaflet) with a right-angled clamp placed through the aortic valve allows for an accurate incision through the septum via the infundibulotomy. It is important that the trajectory of this incision be directed toward the apex of the left ventricle (which, from the surgeon's perspective, is almost directly to the left) and carried as distally as necessary to relieve the obstruction. Proximally, the incision may be carried up to—and, if necessary, into—the commissure between the right and left aortic leaflets. Septal tissue may be débrided from the left ventricular side of the septum, but this should be on the left portion of the incision to spare the left-sided conduction apparatus as it courses down the ventricular septum. The resulting VSD is then closed with a generous Gore-Tex patch, which augments the LVOT. The aortic valve is carefully débrided of any fibrous tissue, and the incisions are closed.

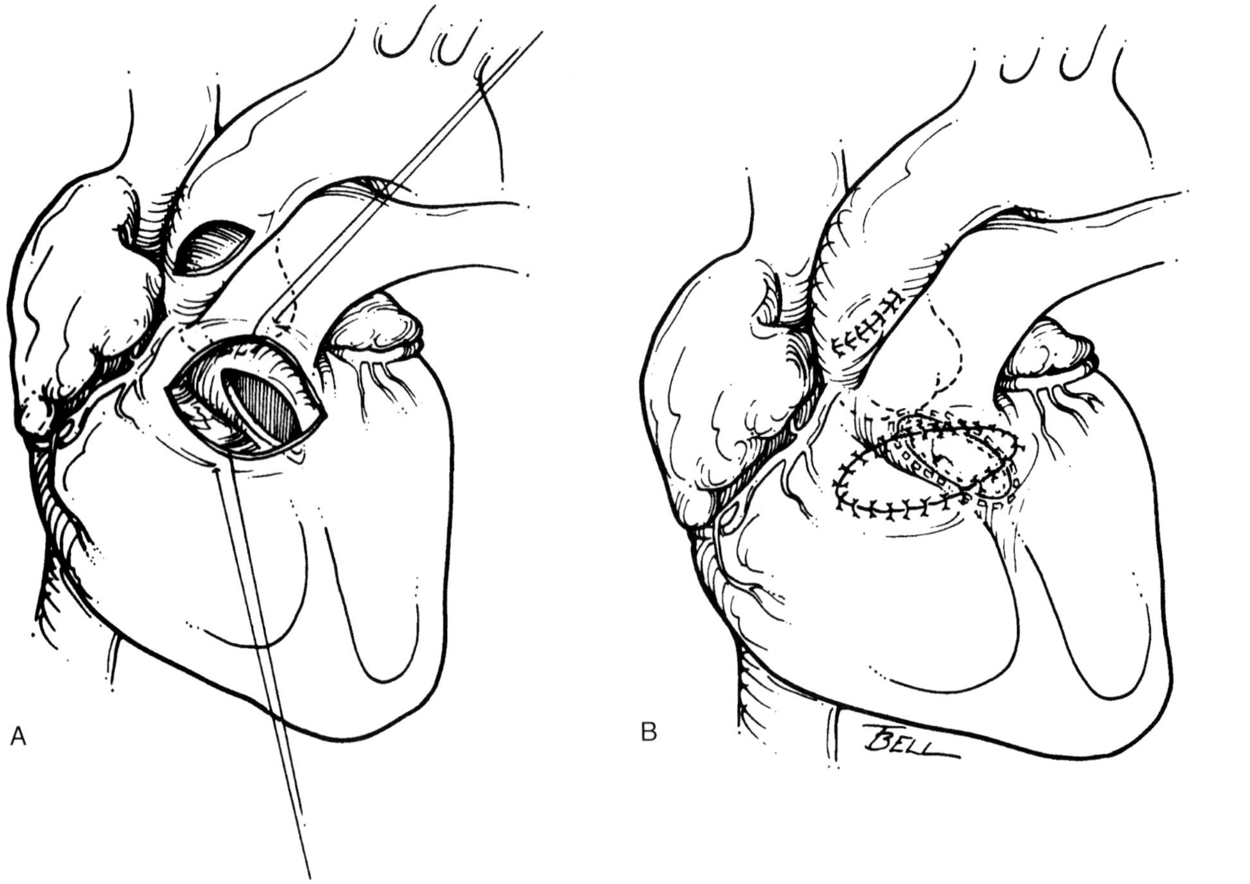

Figure 119-5 Modified Konno operation. Transverse incision of the infundibulum showing the perspective of the ventricle septum through the aortic valve and the infundibulum.

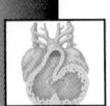

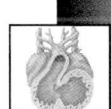

Indications for and Results of the Modified Konno Operation

The indications for the modified Konno operation for the relief of subaortic obstruction are evolving. Roughneen and others[116] described their experience with the operation in 15 children. Indications for the operation were recurrent subaortic stenosis (3), hypertrophic subaortic stenosis (3), tunnel stenosis of the LVOT (2), and subaortic stenosis after atrioventricular septal defect (AVSD) (2) or ventricular septal defect (VSD) (5). The modified Konno operation was very effective for reducing the LVOT gradient (mean, 50 mm Hg to 3 mm Hg). Caldarone and colleagues[15] reported similar results among 18 patients. Although the technique is very effective for relieving subaortic stenosis that results from a variety of lesions, complications can occur. In general, operative mortality among published reports has been negligible. However, right bundle branch block has been commonly noted after the modified Konno operation; this is significant in the setting of preexisting left bundle branch blocks, such as those that may exist after the transaortic resection of subaortic stenosis, and complete heart block has been noted in up to 12.5% of cases. Although the aortic valve is at risk and residual VSDs may occur, with careful technique, these complications are uncommon.

Given these results, some surgeons have advocated this operation for recurrent membranous subaortic stenosis. Although the modified Konno operation certainly alters the geometry of the LVOT (which is thought to contribute to the genesis of membrane), its impact on additional recurrences is unknown.

Konno-Rastan Aortoventriculoplasty

The Konno-Rastan operation, which was described independently by both Konno and Rastan in 1975 and 1976,[71,109] is required when tunnel-like subaortic stenosis coexists with significant aortic valve pathology. Incision of the ventricular septum as performed in the modified Konno operation, which involves going through the aortic annulus and the ascending aorta, provides effective relief of all levels of obstruction. This operation requires bicaval cannulation. A vertical aortotomy to the left of the right coronary artery is made. At this point, an incision in the infundibulum of the right ventricle is helpful for guiding the septal incision. The annulus of the aortic valve is incised to the left of the nadir of the right coronary leaflet, and it is extended into the interventricular septum, thus relieving the subaortic stenosis. The aortic annulus is débrided, and an appropriate-sized mechanical prosthesis is inserted and fixed into the posterior annulus. A patch (Dacron or polytetrafluoroethylene [PTFE]) is fashioned such that it enlarges the LVOT, and it is sutured into place up to the aortic annulus, thus enlarging the subaortic dimensions. Sutures are then passed through the valve sewing ring and through the patch, thereby reestablishing annular continuity. The patch is then carried distally, enlarging and closing the ascending aorta (Figure 119-6). The right

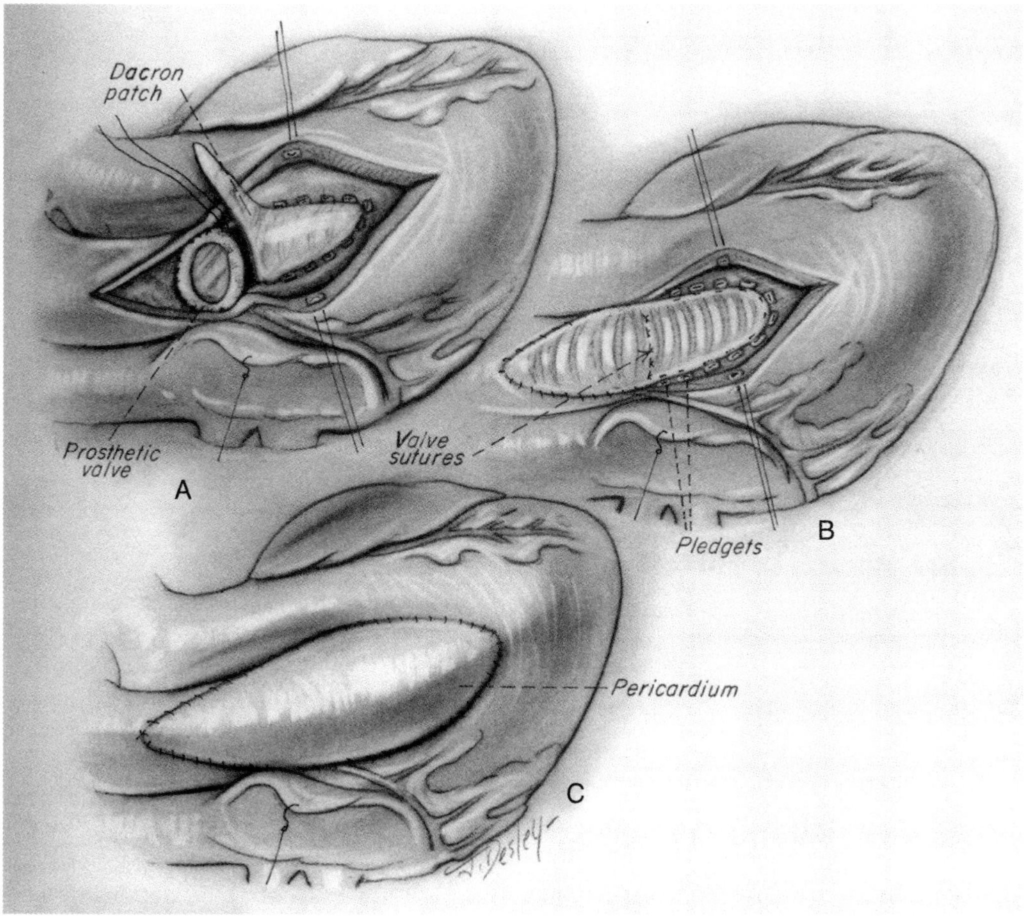

Figure 119–6 Konno-Rastan aortoventriculoplasty.

ventricular outflow tract is repaired, which allows for adequate clearance for the underlying augmented left ventricular outflow tract. Fixed bovine pericardium works well for this application.

Results

The results of the Konno operation have improved since its introduction in 1975. Erez and others[44] reported their experience with the Konno operation in 60 pediatric patients between 1982 and 2000. Forty-two mechanical valves, 9 homografts, 6 xenografts, and 15 autografts were placed. Operative mortality declined from 25% early in the experience to about 10%, which was comparable with other contemporary pediatric series.[26,51,114] Although mortality has declined, complications remain common, with 16% of prosthetic-valve Konno patients requiring surgical exploration for bleeding and 1 out of 15 (6.8%) patients undergoing the Ross-Konno procedure requiring reoperation for bleeding. Heart block occurred in 8.8% of prosthetic-valve Konno operations and in 6.7% of Ross-Konno operations. Long-term survival for the Konno operation has been related to the underlying pathology and to recurrent or residual LVOT obstruction that may require complex reoperation. The experience with homografts or xenografts in conjunction with the Konno operation has not been satisfactory. Among patients receiving biological valves, freedom from reoperation at 10 years was 0% (Figure 119-7). Repeat Konno operation was required for valve failure. Among the patients with mechanical valves who required reoperation, valve outgrowth (6) and endocarditis (3) were the indications.

Among the 15 patients undergoing the Ross-Konno operation between 1997 and 2000, 1 operative death occurred (6.7%), and there were 2 late deaths in syndromic children. Although the authors concluded that the Ross-Konno operation was less morbid than mechanical valve, the durability of the autograft in the aortic position remains a concern, especially in the very young. Reporting their neonatal/infant experience with the Ross-Konno operation, Ohye and others[102] reported no operative mortality among 10 patients. With a median follow-up of 48 months, the authors reported no reoperations on the autograft, although 2 patients had developed significant autograft insufficiency. Despite concerns about the durability of the autograft, the Ross-Konno operation probably presents the best available option for relief of complex LVOT obstruction in the very small child (Figure 119-8).

HYPERTROPHIC OBSTRUCTIVE CARDIOMYOPATHY

Hypertrophic obstructive cardiomyopathy is a dynamic form of subaortic LVOT obstruction that results from myocardial hypertrophy prominently affecting the interventricular septum. A variety of treatments, including calcium-channel blockers, beta blockers, and dual-chamber pacing, have met with mixed success.[83,113,121,126]

Surgical relief can be accomplished by transaortic septal myotomy designed to relieve the subaortic septal muscular

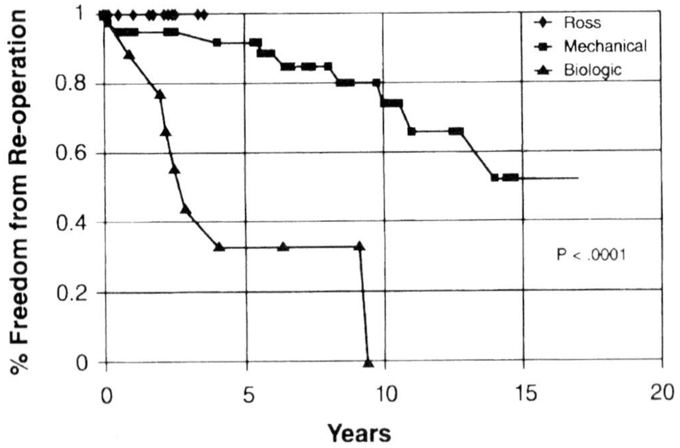

Figure 119–7 Comparison of failure rate percentage of Ross, mechanical, and biological procedures and time to reoperation.

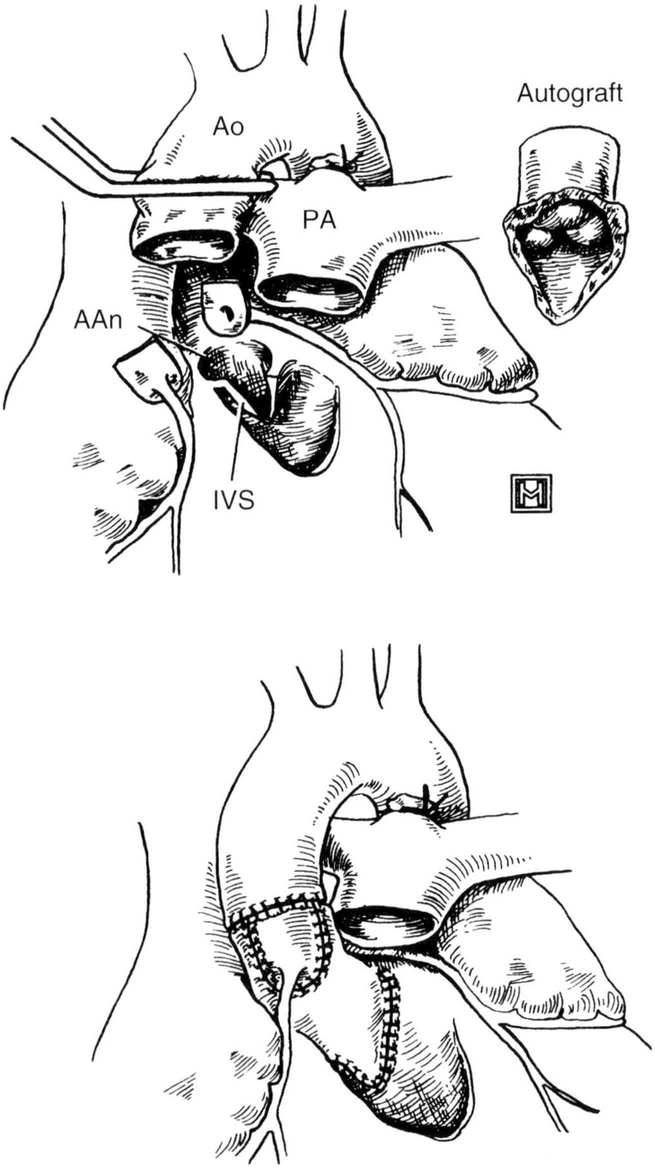

Figure 119–8 Ross-Konno operation for complex left ventricular outflow tract (LVOT) obstruction in a small child.

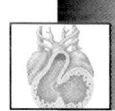

obstruction. Originally described by Morrow and colleagues,[96] septal myotomy provides effective hemodynamic relief of the obstruction, and it can be expected to provide both symptomatic relief and improvement in New York Heart Association (NYHA) class. Improvement in survival, however, has been more difficult to document. Despite an operative mortality of 1–2%, the subsequent annual mortality rate approaches 2%, which is comparable with that reported in patients who are treated nonsurgically.[91] Recently, the modified Konno operation has also been successfully applied to hypertrophic obstructive cardiomyopathy.

Surgical Indications

Surgical indications for this condition remain controversial. In general, operation has been advocated for symptomatic patients (NYHA III and IV) with peak instantaneous gradients exceeding 50 mm Hg or asymptomatic patients with gradients exceeding 100 mm HG, despite medical management.[94,97]

More recently, attenuation of the interventricular septum has been induced by the injection of absolute ethanol into the proximal septal coronary artery.[72] Although this technique has been successful for lowering the outflow tract gradient by 60–80%, 11–29% of these patients develop complete heart block.[23,48] Although alcohol ablation holds promise, it represents a selective alternative to surgical therapy, and it currently has no place in the treatment of young children. At the present time, septal myomectomy remains the gold standard for medically refractory symptomatic patients with high-grade LVOT obstruction.[84]

Aortoapical Conduit

The aortoapical conduit (ACC) is largely of historical interest. Brown and colleagues[13] reported their experience with the ACC conduit in 22 children with tunnel-like stenosis between 1978 and 1992. They reported 1 early death and 6 late deaths, for an overall mortality of 32%. The ACC was also associated with a high rate of reoperation. This technique has largely been abandoned in favor of surgical alternatives, such as the modified Konno and the Konno-Rastan procedures.

SUPRAVALVULAR STENOSIS

Supravalvular aortic stenosis is the least common form of aortic stenosis, accounting for 6–7% aortic outflow abnormalities. First described by Mencarelli in 1930,[92] supravalvular aortic stenosis is the result of narrowing of the aorta beginning just above the aortic valve, usually at the level of the sinotubular junction. The gender incidence is more equitable than most forms of aortic stenosis, with about a 1:1 male-to-female ratio. In 1961, Williams and others[134] described the common association of several other features, including characteristic facial features (e.g., elfin facies), mental retardation, and, infrequently, hypercalcemia. Soon afterwards, an association with Williams' syndrome and peripheral pulmonary stenosis was identified.[7,10]

In addition to its association with Williams' syndrome, supravalvular aortic stenosis occurs in a familial form that is transmitted by autosomal dominant inheritance and also in a sporadic form. Microdeletion of chromosome 7q11.23 has been identified in patients suffering from all three forms of supravalvular stenosis.[29,47,49] Affected individuals express only about 50% of the normal amount of tropoelastin, which results in reduced elastin deposition and fiber disorganization within the arterial wall.

Clinical Presentation

Williams' syndrome may be suspected on the basis of characteristic facies, and all suspected Williams' patients should be evaluated for supravalvular aortic stenosis. Any asymptomatic patient with a familial history should be evaluated and, in the presence of a cardiac murmur of thrill, should undergo echocardiography.

Other, nonaortic vascular lesions are commonly present and should be sought. These lesions include pulmonary arterial stenosis (30%), renal artery stenosis (5%), and coarctation of the aorta (15%).[53] The degree of involvement in the aorta may vary from localized disease at the sinotubular junction to diffuse involvement of the aortic arch and the brachiocephalic vessels. Thus, patients diagnosed with supravalvular aortic stenosis should undergo catheterization to fully delineate the extent of vascular involvement (Figure 119-9).

Surgical Indications

As is the case with other forms of aortic obstruction, supravalvular aortic stenosis tends to be a progressive lesion. Indications for operation are generally consistent with those that are advocated for other forms of aortic stenosis (symptoms; gradient of >40–50 mm Hg). Syncope or chest pain may represent cusp adherence to the sinotubular junction and episodic coronary ischemia; it is a clear indication for surgery.[127]

Significant pulmonary artery stenosis is often present in patients who require the relief of supravalvular aortic stenosis. Surgery should not be delayed in these patients, because the natural history of associated pulmonary stenosis is generally indolent, with regression of these lesions over time. However, a few patients will present with severe central pulmonary artery stenosis, and, in the presence of markedly elevated right ventricular pressures, relief of the pulmonary stenosis should also be performed if the lesions are surgically accessible.

Surgical Treatment

The surgical treatment of supravalvular aortic stenosis is determined by the extent of the stenosis. A variety of techniques have been used to relieve this condition when it is localized. A single-patch technique, which involves the placement of a teardrop- or diamond-shaped patch across the sinotubular junction and extending between the base of the noncoronary sinus and into the ascending aorta, was initially described by McGoon and colleagues[90] at the Mayo Clinic in 1961. Doty and others[35] extended the aortoplasty by fashioning a bifurcated, pantaloon-shaped patch that straddled the commissure between the right-noncoronary leaflet, thus enlarging both the noncoronary and the right coronary sinuses (Figure 119-10). Concern about an untreated left

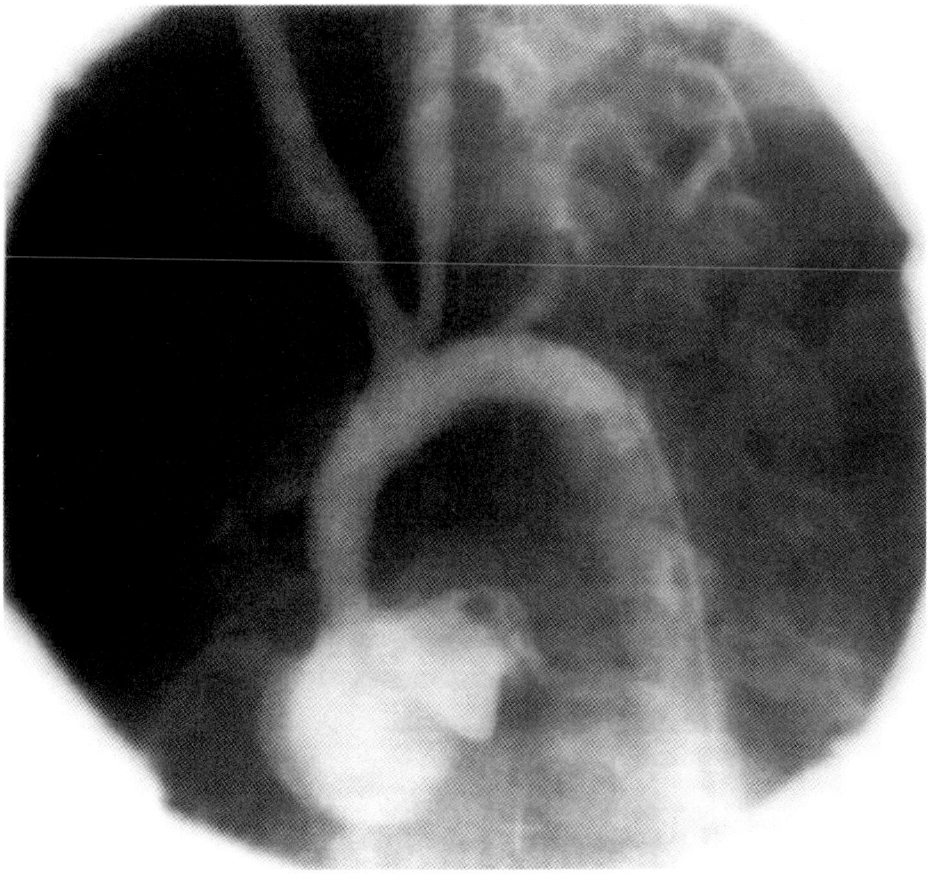

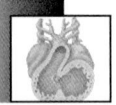

Figure 119-9 Extent of supravalvular aortic stenosis determined by catheterization.

coronary sinus as well as the functional effect of an asymmetrical augmentation on the aortic valve led Brom[12] to propose a three-sinus repair. A modification of this technique proposed by Myers and colleagues[99] accomplishes a three-sinus augmentation by placing counterincisions into the ascending aorta, thereby enlarging the sinuses without prosthetic tissue.

About 30% of patients will present with diffuse stenosis involving the ascending aorta, sometimes with extension into the arch.[133] The diffuse form of supravalvular aortic stenosis has been shown to be an independent risk factor for death and reoperation.[124] In cases in which the lesion is limited to the ascending aorta, patch enlargement is usually possible using cardiopulmonary bypass. When the stenosis involves the arch, deep hypothermic circulatory arrest is used to patch across the entire area. Patients presenting with lesions in the origins of the brachiocephalic vessels may require patch augmentation of these vessels as well.[106,131]

Supravalvular aortic stenosis may also involve the coronary ostia. This may take the form of restricted coronary inflow as a result of leaflet fusion along the narrowed and exaggerated sinotubular ridge or, less commonly, as a result of encroachment on the ostial lumen by the disease. Although relief of the supravalvular stenosis treats the former, true ostial involvement may require specific attention. Modest encroachment on the coronary ostium by sinus tissue may be amenable to simple débridement, whereas severe cases may require patching of the ostium or bypass grafting.[85,86,122]

Results

There has been a gradual evolution from the single-patch repair to the double-patch repair and, ultimately, to the three-sinus repair for the relief of discrete supravalvular aortic stenosis.

In a review of 75 patients with supravalvular aortic stenosis, Stamm and colleagues[124] reviewed the impact of surgical technique on long-term outcomes. A comparison of single-versus multiple-sinus augmentations (inverted bifurcated aortoplasty, 35; three-sinus technique, 6) showed that patients undergoing single-sinus augmentation had significantly higher gradients (mean, 20 mm Hg versus 10 mm Hg; $p = .008$) at long-term follow-up (mean, 12.8 years). Similar results have been reported by others.[13] Analysis showed single-sinus augmentation to be an independent risk factor for both death and reoperation; these findings were independent of the year of operation (Figure 119-11A and B).

The authors concluded that multiple-sinus augmentation was superior to single-sinus augmentation. Although not proven, it seems reasonable to expect that augmentation of all three sinuses using techniques developed by Brom,[12] Myers,[99] and others may provide further long-term advantages by allowing for a more complete restoration of aortic root geometry.

The prognosis of diffuse supravalvular aortic stenosis appears to be worse than that of the discreet variant, and it has been identified as an independent risk factor for reoperation as well as death (Figure 119-12A and B).

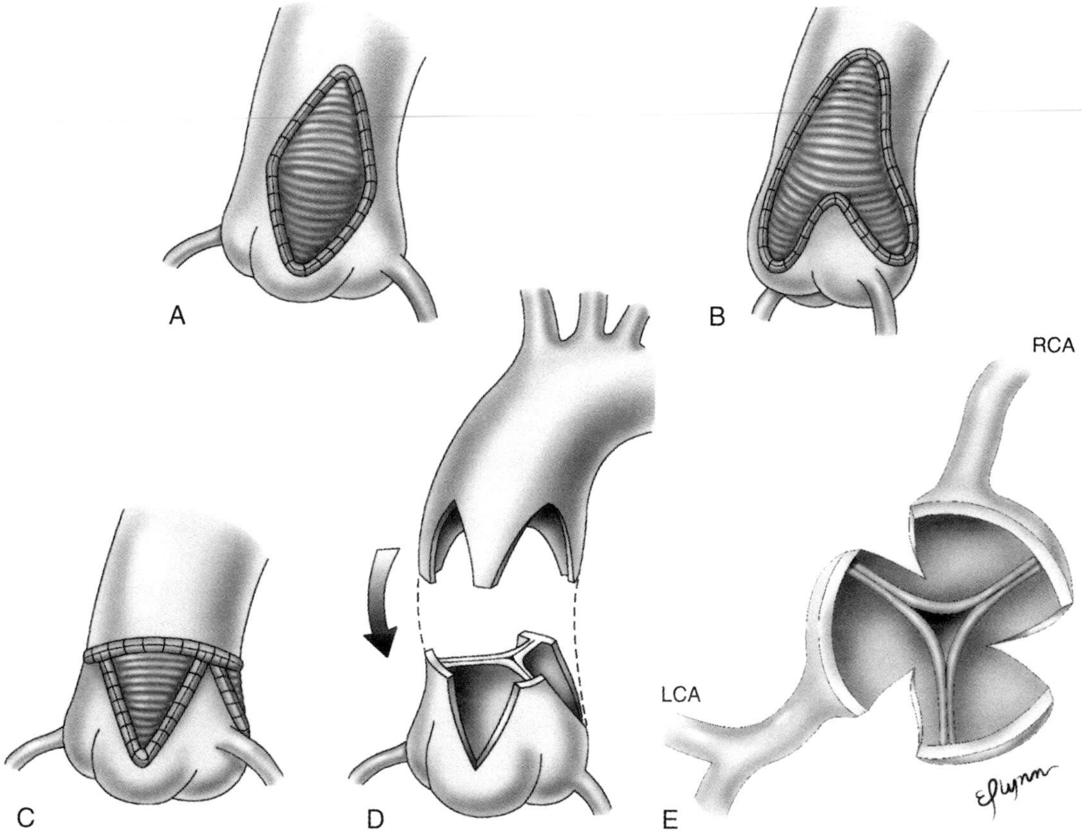

Figure 119–10 Surgical treatment of supravalvular aortic stenosis.

AORTIC INSUFFICIENCY

Although it is a recognized lesion, isolated congenital aortic insufficiency is very rare, and it is usually the consequence of efforts designed to relieve aortic stenosis.[33] It is commonly seen clinically that efforts to relieve aortic stenosis early in life come at the expense of introducing aortic insufficiency. Patients with these conditions may present years later with ventricular dysfunction in the setting of mixed aortic valve pathology. Determining the appropriate timing for operation in these asymptomatic patients can be difficult. Accepted guidelines for aortic valve replacement in the adolescent and young adult include the appearance of symptoms, asymptomatic left ventricular systolic dysfunction, or asymptomatic progressive left ventricular enlargement with a Z score of 4.[9]

The timing of operation for aortic insufficiency in children has been addressed by Cheung and colleagues.[21] The authors studied a group of 21 asymptomatic young patients (median age, 13 years) with aortic insufficiency undergoing the Ross operation. Eighteen of these patients had previously undergone aortic valvotomy (surgical or balloon) for aortic stenosis. In this particular experience, the Z score of the preoperative left ventricular end-diastolic dimension was the most sensitive predictor of postoperative left ventricular performance. This type of performance was significantly impaired in patients with a preoperative Z score of 4, and the authors recommended aortic valve replacement in asymptomatic patients when the left ventricular end-diastolic Z scores exceeded 3.

MARFAN'S SYNDROME

Marfan's syndrome is a systemic collagen vascular disorder that may affect the aortic valve early in life. van Karnebeck and colleagues[130] reported the natural history of Marfan's syndrome in 52 pediatric patients. There were 25 male and 27 females, with a mean age at presentation of 7.9 years (range, 1–16 years); follow-up was 7.7 years (range, 2–15 years). Sixty-three percent of patients represented familial cases, and 33% were sporadic. Aortic dilatation was present in 80% of patients, and aortic regurgitation developed in 13 (25%); 10 out of 13 (77%) patients required aortic operation. The authors concluded that childhood and adolescence are crucial periods in the development of the cardiovascular manifestations associated with Marfan's syndrome. When the condition is diagnosed during the newborn period, mortality from cardiac causes is high (33% 1-year mortality) and is reported to result from multivalve disease.[1,128]

With the potential for aortic dissection in older Marfan's patients, attempts have been made to identify patients that would benefit from preemptive surgery. Legget and others[74] reported that patients with an aortic ratio (normalized for age and body surface area) of at least 1.3 or a rate of progression exceeding 5% per year were at increased risk for aortic root complications. In cases of aortic valve disease presenting with a dilated ascending aorta, Elkins[39] has suggested that replacement of the aorta exceeding 3.5 cm in small patients and 4.5 cm in older patients is reasonable. No published guidelines are available for children,

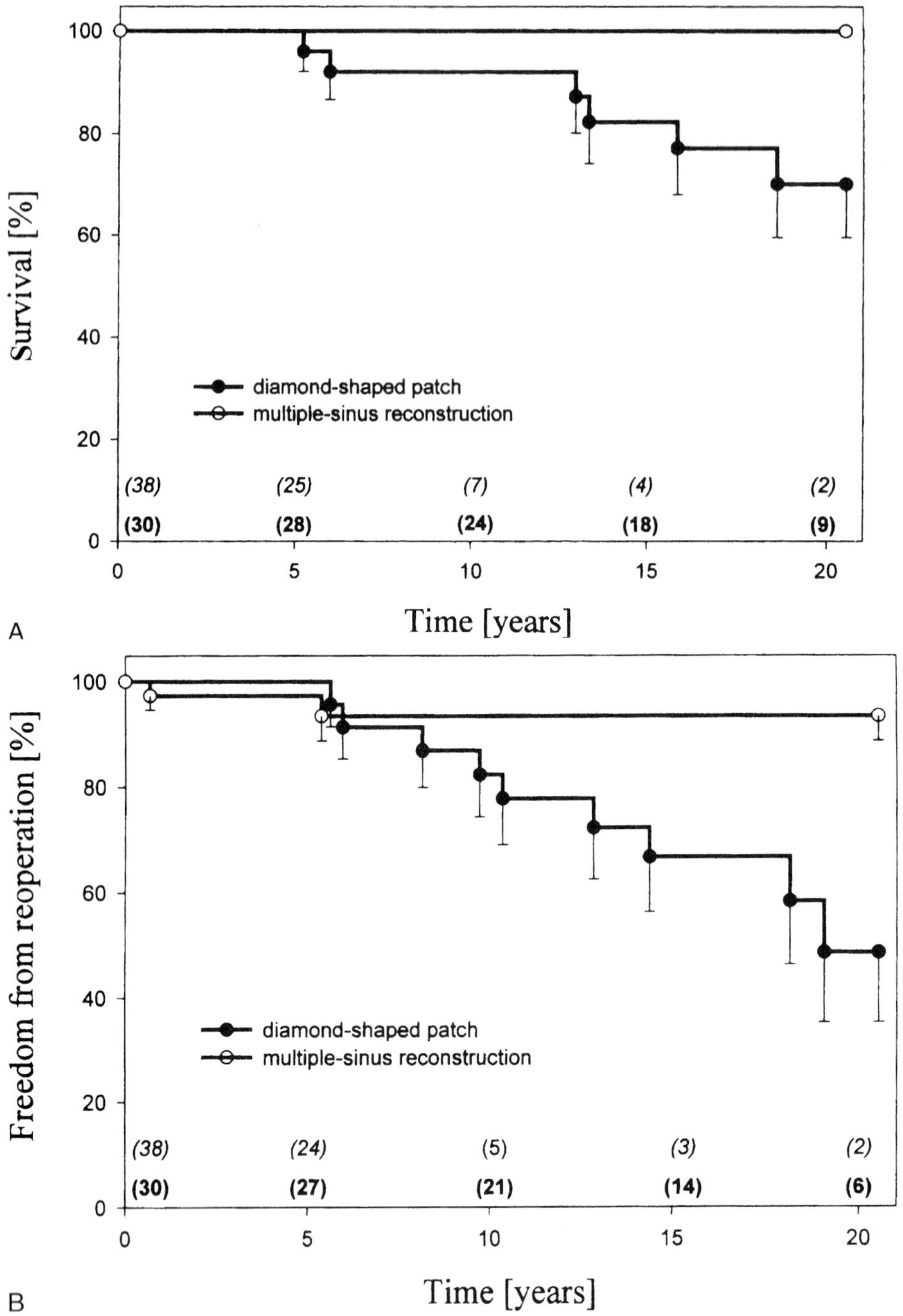

Figure 119–11 **A,** Comparison of long term survival in patients with single or multiple reconstructions. **B,** Free from reoperation percentage by type of operation and length of time to first reoperation.

but when aortic root Z scores exceed 8–10, operation is probably justified.

AORTIC VALVE RECONSTRUCTIVE TECHNIQUES

The effectiveness of reconstructive techniques for aortic insufficiency has been variable, and it is related to the etiology of the underlying aortic valve disease. In some specific instances (e.g., in association with a VSD), repair can be successful and durable.

In the setting of a perimembranous or subarterial VSD, associated aortic valve prolapse is an indication for surgery. Eroglu and colleauges[45] reported that 38% of these patients with prolapse will develop aortic insufficiency within 1 year. Once present, the progression of aortic insufficiency was relatively rapid, with 31% of patients progressing from mild to moderate insufficiency within 1.1 years. VSD closure in the setting of severe aortic insufficiency is less successful than when the insufficiency is judged to be mild or moderate (freedom from reoperation, 64% versus 77% at 10 years, respectively; $p < .05$).[63] Thus, repair of perimembranous or subarterial VSDs presenting with aortic valve prolapse is justified, even in the setting of hemodynamically small defects.

As noted, simple VSD closure in the face of severe prolapse and aortic insufficiency may be inadequate. In these

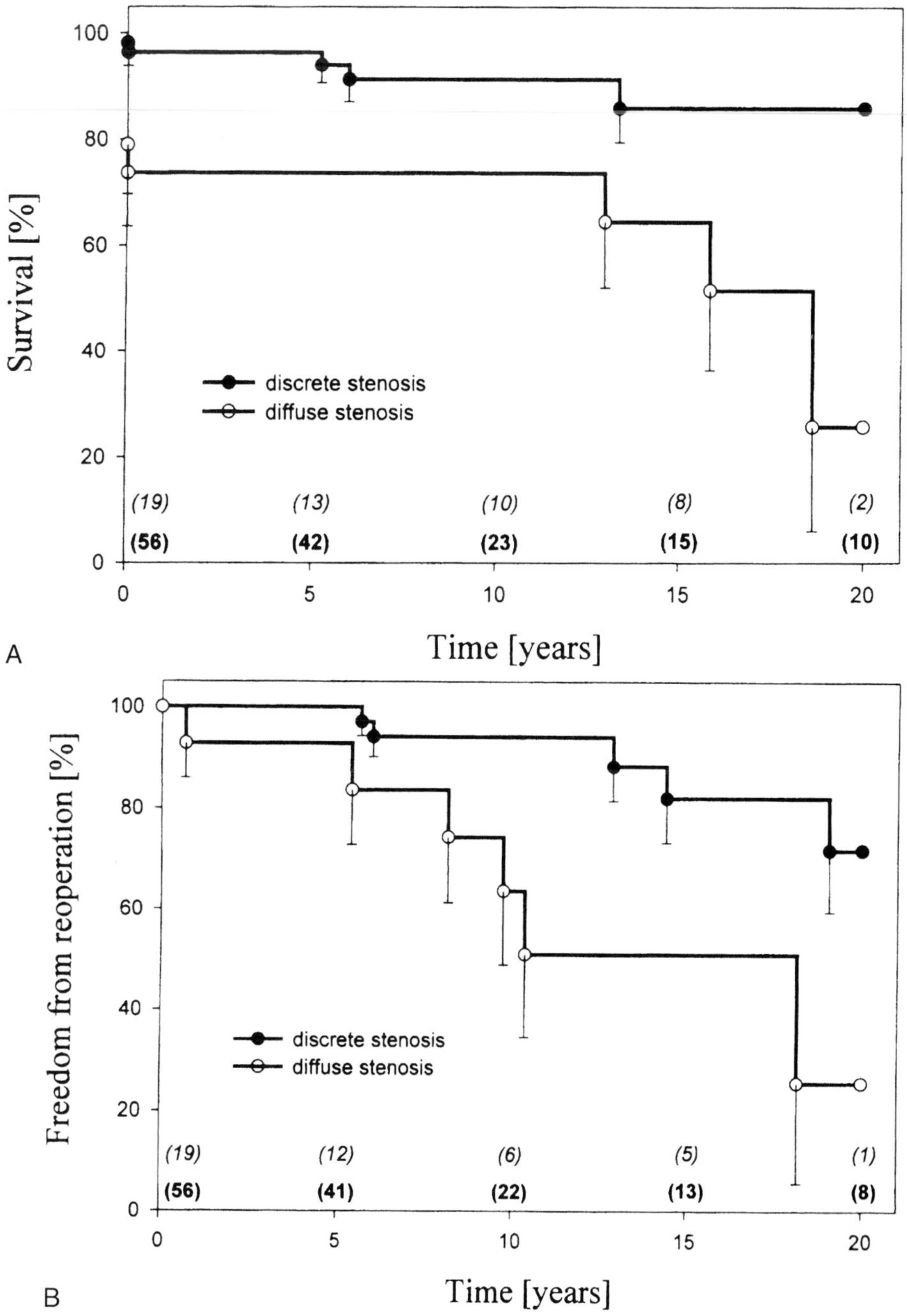

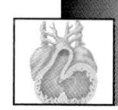

Figure 119–12 **A,** Survival rate comparison of discrete and diffuse stenosis, in years. **B,** Freedom from reoperation of discrete and diffuse stenosis, in years.

instances, repair of the aortic valve, including plication of the aortic sinus, may be effective (Figure 119-13). Yacoub and others[136] reported their results in 46 such patients, with an average follow-up of 8.4 years. Under these circumstances, VSD closure with aortic sinus plication has proven to be effective and durable.

When aortic insufficiency results from a lack of central leaflet coaptation, reparative techniques usually employ some variant of leaflet extension. Fixed pericardium—either bovine or autologous—has been used to extend the diseased leaflets, thereby increasing the area of coaptation. Duran and colleagues[36] have reported their experience with leaflet extension in 72 patients, many of which suffered from a rheumatic etiology. Over a limited follow-up (5 years), there were 2 late deaths (2.8%) and 4 (5.5%) reoperations between 4 and 38 months postoperatively. Similar results have been reported by Grinda and colleagues.[57] Among 89 patients (mean age, 16 years) undergoing leaflet extension, the 5-year survival and freedom from reoperation rates were 96% and 92%, respectively. Although reparative techniques may be effective for short term, the durability of the repair remains a concern. The role of these techniques may be best appreciated in young rheumatics in whom the results of the Ross operation have been suboptimal and in whom other valve substitutes are not practical.

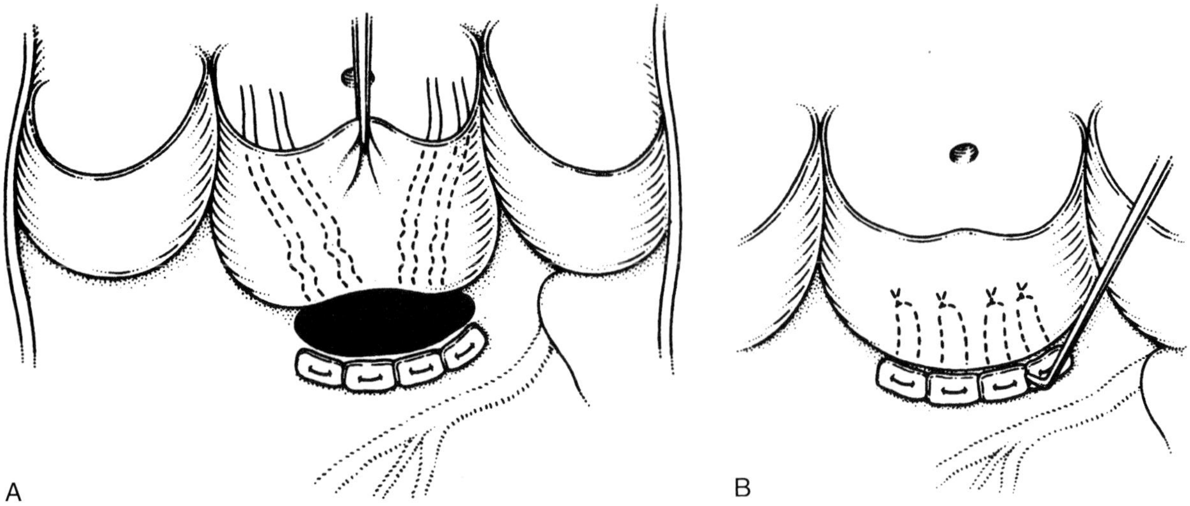

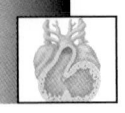

Figure 119–13 Repair of the aortic valve including placation of the aortic sinus.

VALVE REPLACEMENT

Available aortic valve substitutes include mechanical and biological valves. Among the available options for biological valve replacement are xenografts, homografts, and autografts. The choice of valve substitute in the pediatric population must balance several competing factors: durability, size, growth potential, and the need for anticoagulation.

Mechanical versus Tissue Valves

The surgeon is faced with several options for aortic valve replacement in the pediatric patient. Each option presents a unique profile of advantages, disadvantages, and performance characteristics, which will be reviewed later.

A major decision point when it comes to valve selection for pediatric aortic valve replacement is whether to choose a mechanical or a biological (xenograft, homograft, or autograft) graft. The early mortality of mechanical aortic valve replacements has been placed between 0% and 13%, and the late mortality is between 0% and 11%. The incidence of reoperation on these valves is between 6% and 16%.[19,80,87] Patients receiving xenografts appear to have a lower mortality (early and late mortality, 0%) but a higher risk of reoperation; about 50% of these grafts will require replacement within 6 years. In general, homografts and autografts have superior resistance to postoperative endocarditis as compared with mechanical valves. Mechanical valves demonstrate a higher risk of prosthesis endocarditis during the early postoperative period, but this declines within a year and then approximates the low-level hazard of biological valves.[69] The risks of endocarditis with autografts and homografts appear to be comparable, and these are preferred over other prostheses in the setting of active endocarditis.

Because of their tendency to degenerate, xenograft valves have generally been avoided among pediatric patients. Turrentine and colleagues[129] compared the results of mechanical versus biological valves in the aortic position. They reported a lower incidence of valve-related complications in the autograft group as compared with all other valve options. The homograft and xenograft performed particularly poorly in terms of freedom from reoperation, with 70% (7 out of 10) of xenografts and 50% (1 out of 2) of homografts requiring replacement for deterioration within 9 years (Figure 119-14A and B). Although efforts to develop xenografts suitable for the pediatric population continue, the follow-up is short.[6] Thus, in the absence of compelling indications for their use, homografts and xenografts in the aortic position in children should probably be avoided.

Comparisons between the autograft (Ross operation) and mechanical aortic valve replacement AVR have also been reported. Elkins[39] has reported an 89% freedom from reoperation or death at 6 years when using the Ross operation as compared with only 49% among children receiving a mechanical AVR. However, these populations were from different time periods, with the mechanical AVR operations being performed before 1986. A more contemporary study reported by Alexiou and colleagues[3] reported results from mechanical AVR that were more consistent with those obtained with the Ross operation. These authors performed mechanical AVR on 56 children between 1972 and 1999. Freedom from late events, including thrombosis, hemorrhage, and reoperation, was about 90% at 6 years (Figure 119-15). Although this group presented excellent results with pediatric AVR, it should be noted that the majority of these patients were more than 10 years old, and 50% underwent aortic root enlargement at the time of valve insertion. There were 2 major (valve thrombosis, stroke) and 4 minor (nosebleeds) complications related to anticoagulation.

The indications for valve replacement may also have an impact on outcomes. Lubiszewska and others[77] found mechanical valves in the aortic position to be satisfactory substitutes, especially for aortic insufficiency. Children with these valves often present with a normal-sized or enlarged aortic annulus, and adult-sized valves are readily accepted.

In a review of 50 patients undergoing aortic valve replacement (25 mechanical, 19 autografts, 6 homografts), Lupinetti and colleagues[81] reported a significantly higher incidence of late complications in those who received

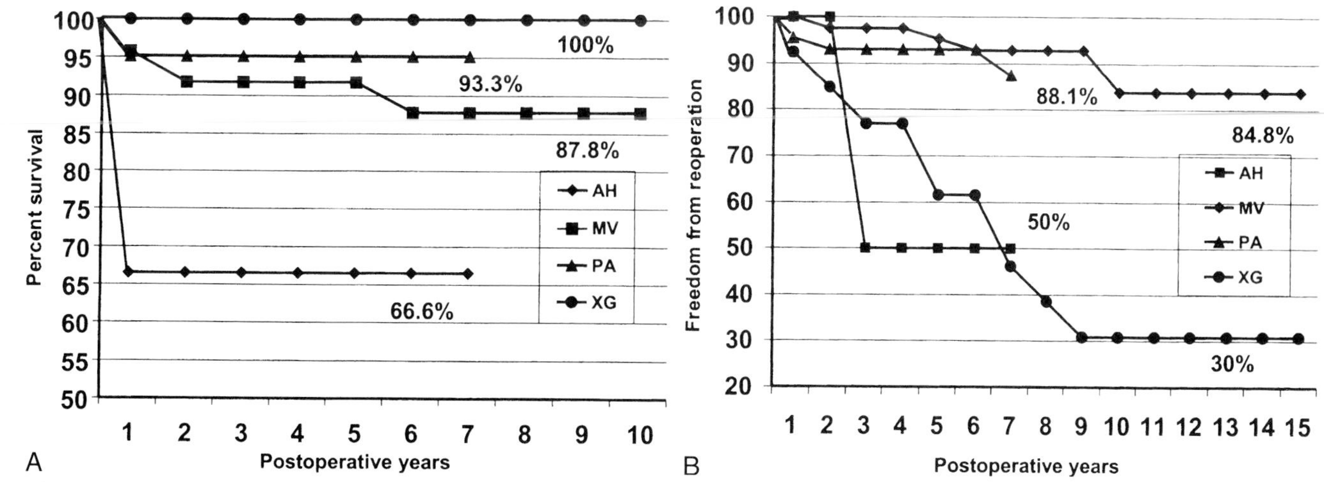

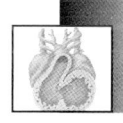

Figure 119–14 Survival (A) and freedom from reoperation (B) rates comparing mechanical and biological valve replacements in postoperative years.

mechanical valves. The most common long-term complication reported in this group was the development of subaortic stenosis due to pannus ingrowth. Although these authors reported no serious complications related to anticoagulation, others have. Cabalka and others[14] reported 6 serious complications among 36 patients undergoing isolated aortic valve replacements between 1982 and 1994; all occurred in the setting of supratherapeutic prothrombin times. Freedom from anticoagulation-related bleeding for isolated AVR was about 80% at 4 years.

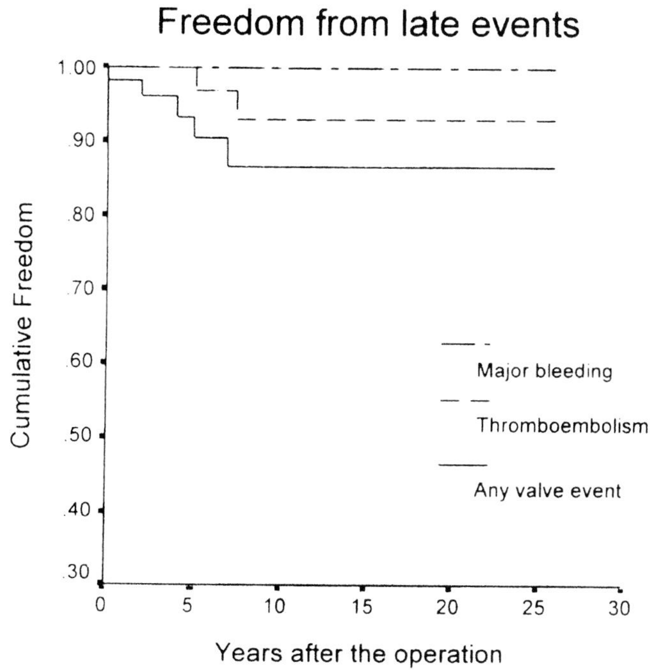

Figure 119–15 Freedom from late events in mechanical aortic valve replacements.

Autograft versus Homograft

Although homografts share some of the advantages that are provided by autografts, they also present serious disadvantages. Besides a lack of growth potential, early degeneration requiring replacement has been documented, especially among young patients, and some authors have reported inferior hemodynamics as compared with autograft.[25,101] This has led some investigators to compare the outcomes of the Ross procedure with those of its most comparable alternative: the homograft.

In the earliest and largest series comparing the autograft with the homograft in young patients, Gerosa and others[55] compared the results of 103 young patients receiving homografts in the aortic position with 43 receiving autografts. The 15-year freedom from reoperation was 54% ± 8% versus 68% ± 11%; freedom from endocarditis was 97% ± 2% versus 75% ±10%; and freedom from any complication was 41% ± 7% versus 50% ± 10%. Primary tissue failure was identified in 19 homografts but in none of the autografts.

Aklog and colleagues[2] have examined the performance of these two options in a prospective randomized trial. A total of 182 patients with a mean age of 37 years (range, 2–64 years) were randomized. Ninety-seven patients received a pulmonary autograft, and 85 received a homograft. Thirty-day mortality was 1% for autografts and 4% for homografts, and actuarial survival was 97.8% and 95.3% at 48 months, respectively. There were no autograft-related reoperations. Freedom from reoperation was slightly higher in the autograft group (94.2% versus 87.7%; P = not significant). With respect to the pediatric age group, the authors reported that 2 out of 6 (33%) children required reoperation on the homograft as compared with none of the 10 children in the autograft group. Furthermore, there was echocardiographic evidence of progressive, subclinical deterioration in the homograft group that was absent in the autograft group. The authors concluded that the autograft appeared to be superior to the homograft in the pediatric population, and they suggested that longer follow-up will reveal a durability advantage in the autograft's favor. The long-term follow-up of these patients may be instructive.

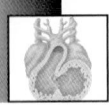

Lupinetti and colleagues[82] examined the comparative effects of these autografts and those of the homograft on left ventricular remodeling in the pediatric population. Although the authors reported that initial left ventricular outflow tract gradients and left ventricular wall thickness (surrogates for hemodynamic efficiency) were comparable among 78 children undergoing the Ross operation (25 of whom were receiving homografts), a divergence was noted over time. Whereas peak left ventricular outflow tract velocities decreased over time after the Ross operation, they increased significantly over a similar time period in the homograft group. The decrease in left ventricular wall thickness seen in those undergoing the Ross operation was absent in the homograft group. This effect may be most operative in young patients in whom significant somatic growth may be expected.

Thus, although the homograft may provide excellent palliation among older patients, its lack of durability appears to be a serious disadvantage, especially among younger children. Under these circumstances, its use should probably be relegated to an option for children who are deemed unsuitable for an autograft or for a mechanical valve.

THE ROSS OPERATION (PULMONARY AUTOGRAFT)

The transplantation of the pulmonary valve to the aortic position, which was introduced by Donald Ross in 1967,[115] has several potential advantages over other valve-replacement options. Most notably, among children, the growth potential of the autograft is a unique feature, especially in the infant population, in which small-caliber homografts are the only alternative. In addition, superior hemodynamics are obtainable without the need for systemic anticoagulation.

The autograft may be inserted into the aortic position using a variety of techniques, including the subcoronary technique, the root-inclusion technique, and the root-replacement technique. Excellent reviews of each technique are available.[43,124] The most commonly performed and reproducible technique is that of root replacement (Figure 119-16). The autograft root replacement is usually performed with bicaval cannulation. The aortic valve is inspected and, if it is deemed irreparable, the pulmonary artery is opened at the bifurcation. The pulmonary valve is inspected, valves with important anatomical abnormalities (e.g., bicuspid valve, significant leaflet fenestrations) are not suitable for use in the aortic position, and an alternative valve replacement is chosen. Small leaflet fenestrations, particularly near the valve commissures, are probably acceptable.

The autograft is excised with a rim of infundibular muscle. Posteriorly care must be taken to avoid the first septal perforated, because significant ventricular dysfunction may accompany its injury. After débridement of the aortic annulus, the autograft is oriented anatomically and sutured into the aortic position. The coronary arteries are inserted into the appropriate sinus, and the distal anastomosis between the autograft and the ascending aorta is performed. The right ventricular outflow tract is reconstructed with the aid of a cryopreserved homograft. Although some groups have advocated the direct approximation of the pulmonary arteries to the right ventricle (similar to the REV technique),[28] oversized homografts provide excellent durability and are probably a superior option.

Disadvantages of the Ross operation include increased technical complexity, homograft reconstruction of the right ventricular outflow tract (RVOT), and potential autograft failure.

To date, the Ross operation has been performed in at least 1749 patients younger than the age of 20 and in 5578 patients total. These figures, which were obtained from the International Registry for the Ross Procedure (www.RossRegistry.com), surely represent an underestimation, because not all centers submit data to this registry. However, the Registry represents the largest compilation of Ross outcomes available at the present time. With a median follow-up of 7261 days, there is a 3.6% incidence of autograft explant (Figure 119-17) and a 2.2% incidence of autograft repair. Reoperation on the right ventricle to pulmonary artery (RV-PA) homograft has been required in 2.8% of patients (Figure 119-18). It should be noted, however, that these undistilled data include all age groups; small-caliber homografts in children will almost certainly require earlier reoperation.

For the pediatric age group specifically, Elkins and others[41] reported midterm and late results with the Ross operation between 1986 and 2001. Operative mortality was 4.5%, with a 12-year actuarial survival of 92 ± 3%. Actuarial freedom from autograft replacement and from RV homograft replacement was 93 ± 3% and 90 ± 4% at 12 years, respectively. Most contemporary series place the operative mortality between 0% and 4%.[64,105,108]

In a recent large series reported by Pessotto and colleagues,[105] 67 children underwent the Ross operation. Two (3%) neonates undergoing the Ross-Konno procedure after failed attempt at balloon dilatation for critical aortic stenosis died of multisystem organ failure. Two others (3%) have required reoperation for progressive autograft insufficiency; in one of these patients, annular reduction successfully salvaged the autograft.

The question of durability is a concern that continues to be examined. The longest follow-up to date has been reported by Chambers and colleagues,[18] who have described the experience of the 131 hospital survivors who underwent the Ross operation between 1967 and 1984. Of the survivors, the reported freedom from autograft replacement was 88% and 75% at 10 and 20 years, respectively. Interestingly, this was quite similar to the freedom from reoperation rate found for the RVOT (89% and 80%). Of the 30 autografts explanted, only 3 showed histological signs of focal degenerative changes; all others showed evidence of transmural cellular viability.

Contraindications to the Ross Operation

The Ross operation requires careful patient selection. Systemic collagen vascular disorders constitute a clear contraindication to the Ross operation, as do anatomical abnormalities of the pulmonary valve.

In addition, the Ross operation should also be avoided in the setting of systemic inflammatory conditions such as rheumatoid arthritis, lupus, and rheumatic heart disease.[31,132] Autograft involvement and deterioration have been noted under these circumstances.[107]

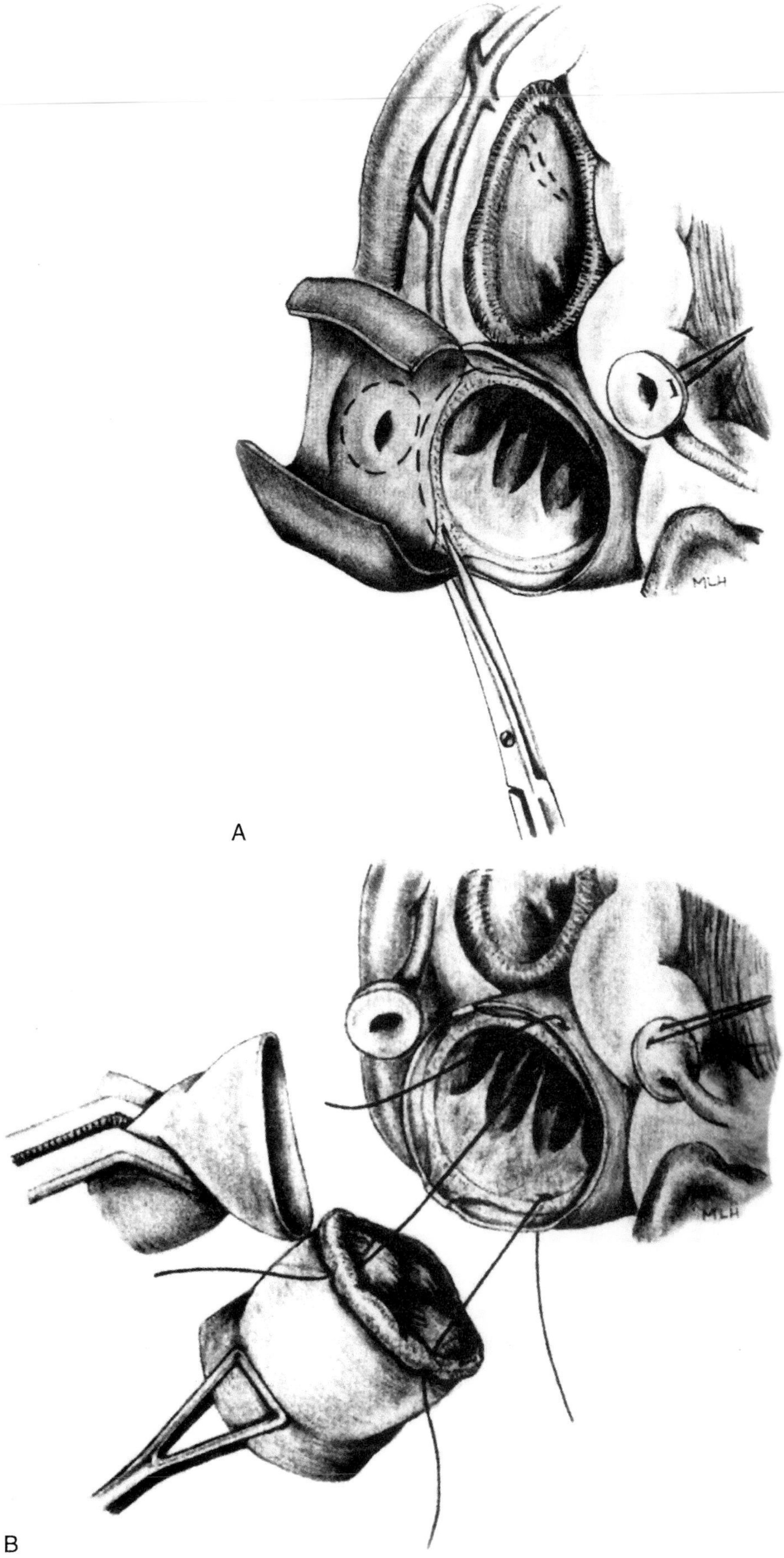

Figure 119–16 Autograft root replacement.

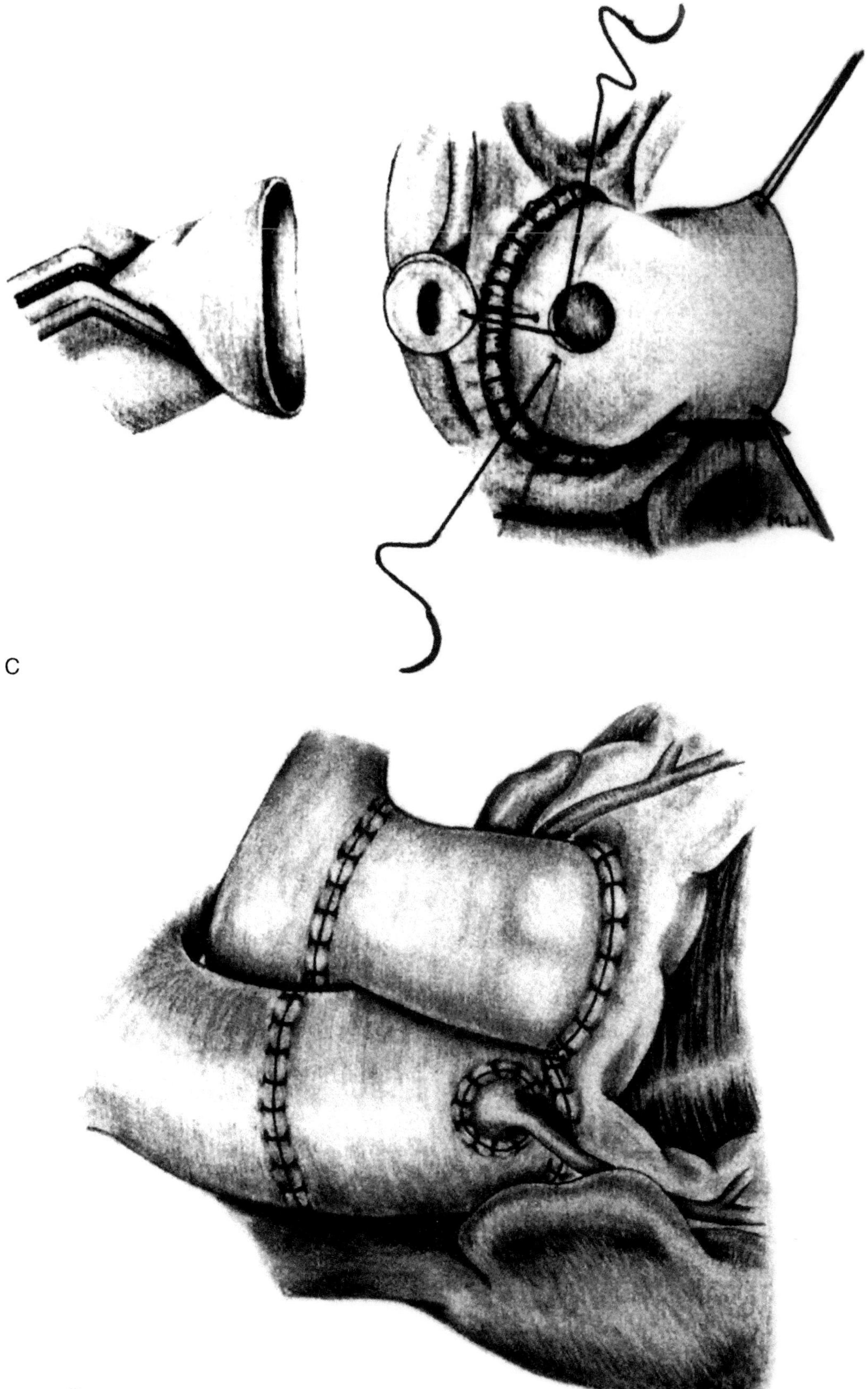

Figure 119–16 cont'd

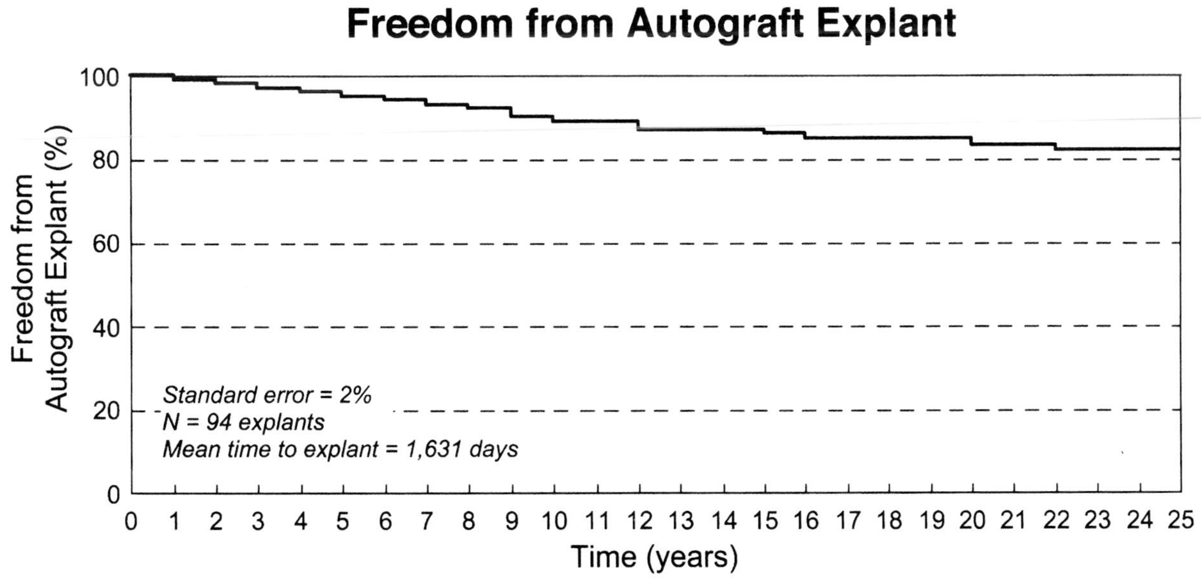

Years	0	1	2	3	4	5	6	7	8	9	10	11	12	13	14	15	16	17	18	19	20	21	22	23	24	25
# at Risk	2758	2758	1815	1242	936	671	484	376	305	250	219	195	178	154	144	142	136	128	120	109	101	83	74	54	38	33
# of Events	0	29	12	12	4	7	6	4	4	3	2	2	3	0	1	0	2	0	0	0	2	0	1	0	0	0
% Event Free	100	99	98	97	96	95	94	93	92	90	89	89	87	87	87	86	85	85	85	85	83	83	82	82	82	82

Figure 119–17 Figures from the International Registry for the Ross Procedure showing time of freedom from autograft explant.

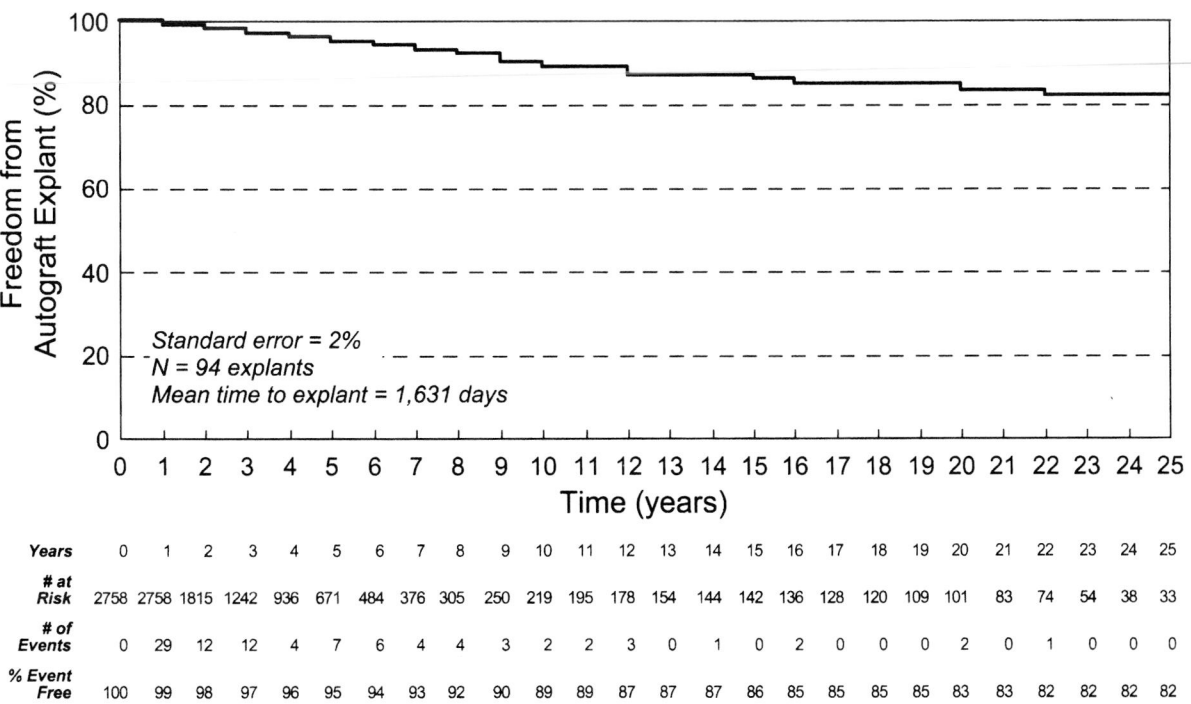

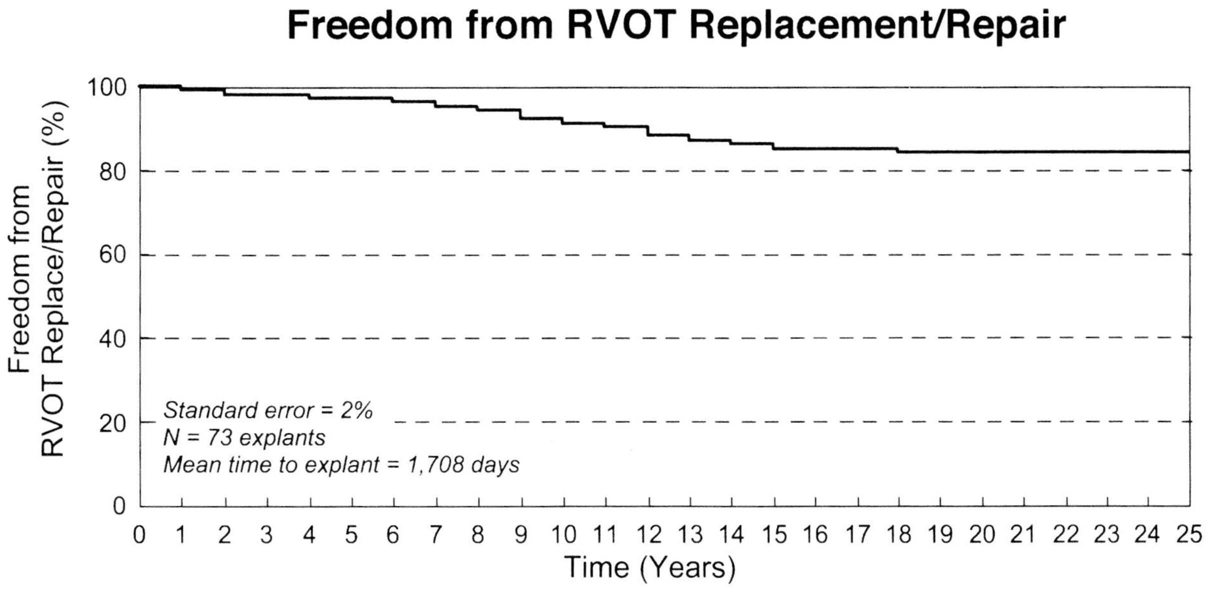

Years	0	1	2	3	4	5	6	7	8	9	10	11	12	13	14	15	16	17	18	19	20	21	22	23	24	25
# at Risk	2758	2758	1815	1237	935	669	482	372	300	247	214	191	178	154	142	139	132	125	116	106	99	85	75	56	36	32
# of Events	0	20	11	7	3	2	6	3	4	3	3	2	4	1	2	1	0	1	0	0	0	0	0	0	0	0
% Event Free	100	99	98	98	97	97	96	95	94	92	91	90	88	87	86	85	85	84	84	84	84	84	84	84	84	84

Figure 119–18 Figures from the International Registry for the Ross Procedure showing time of freedom from right ventricular outflow tract (RVOT) replacement or repair.

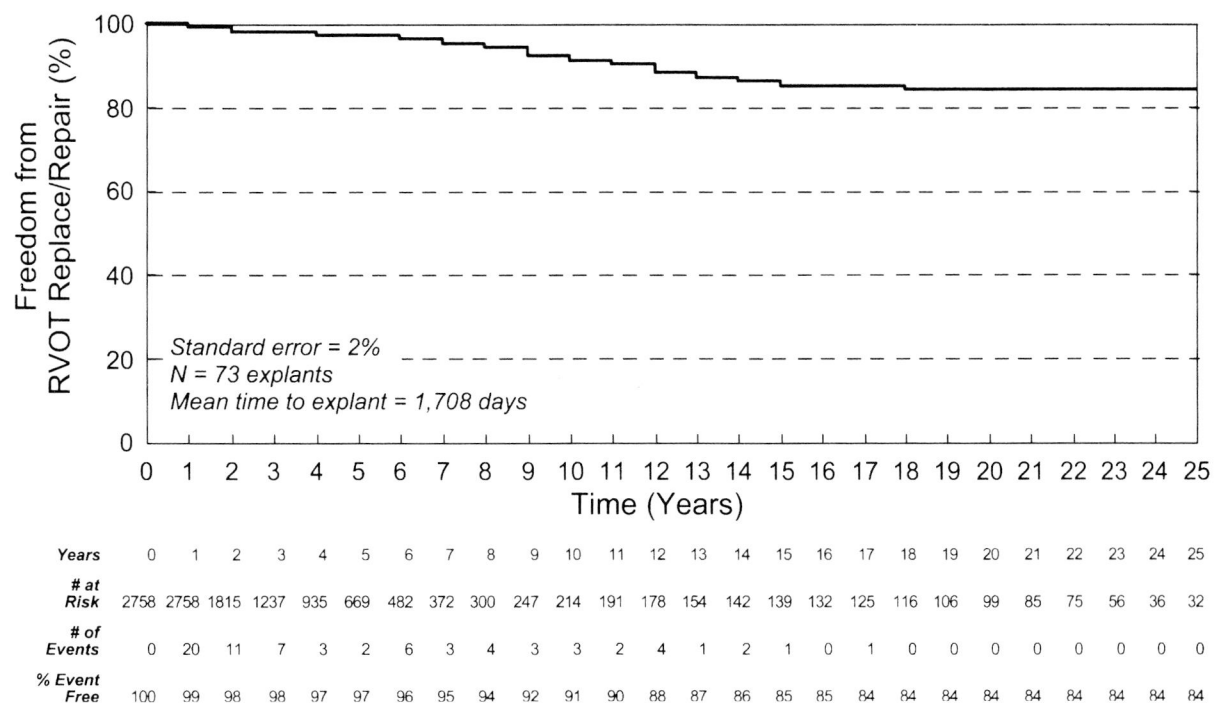

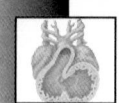

Al-Halees and colleagues[4] reviewed their results with 78 patients undergoing the Ross operation in the Middle East. Eighty percent of these patients suffered from rheumatic disease of the aortic valve, and 28% presented with significant mitral regurgitation. Five (8%) of these patients have required reoperation between 20 and 26 months postoperatively: 4 for autograft failure and 1 for recurrent mitral regurgitation. One autograft demonstrated histological evidence of valvulitis that was consistent with rheumatic disease. Choudhary and colleagues[24] performed the Ross operation in 75 patients suffering from rheumatic aortic valve disease. Two patients required reoperation for autograft failure, and 13 showed evidence of moderate or severe autograft insufficiency with leaflet thickening, generally between 12 and 24 months after the operation. Autograft function was significantly inferior in rheumatic patients.

Bicuspid aortic valve disease is considered by some to be a contraindication for the Ross procedure; however, the data supporting this remain controversial. Examining the pulmonary trunk in patients with bicuspid aortic valve disease, de Sa and others[30] reported histological evidence of cystic medial necrosis, elastic fragmentation, and smooth muscle cell abnormalities. They suggested that these findings manifest themselves as subsequent autograft dilatation.

However, conflicting results have also been reported.[42,78] Luciani and colleagues[78] have reported no histopathology of the pulmonary trunk in the setting of bicuspid aortic valve disease, and they noted no greater tendency for autografts in this setting to dilate. Likewise, in a large pediatric experience, Elkins and others[42] reported that preoperative aortic regurgitation—but not valve morphology—was associated with autograft degeneration.

PROSTHETIC VALVES, ANTICOAGULATION, AND PREGNANCY

Prosthetic valves, systemic anticoagulation, and pregnancy are important issues for young women with aortic valve disease. Edmunds[38] reported that women with mechanical valves were at risk for thrombotic complications if anticoagulation was interrupted. However, it has been suggested that as many as 30% of fetuses exposed to warfarin between the sixth and ninth week of gestation will develop warfarin embryopathy (nasal hypoplasia, stippled epiphyses).[66] Warfarin exposure during the second trimester has been implicated in central nervous system abnormalities in about 3% of fetuses.[58] In 1994, major European centers were asked about their clinical approaches to anticoagulation, prosthetic valves, and pregnancy.[119] There were 214 pregnancies in 182 women; 151 were in 133 women with mechanical valves, and 63 were in 45 women with bioprosthetic valves. Including abortions (spontaneous and therapeutic), 83% of pregnancies among women with bioprosthetic valves and 73% among women with mechanical prostheses resulted in healthy children; this is consistent with other reports.[73]

Anticoagulation medication was administered in 150 of the 151 pregnancies among 133 women with mechanical valves. Thirty-four received subcutaneous heparin throughout the pregnancy, 50 received warfarin for the duration of gestation, and 66 received subcutaneous heparin for the first trimester and Warfarin thereafter. Warfarin was discontinued and subcutaneous heparin was restarted 2–4 weeks before the estimated date of confinement. No cases of warfarin embryopathies were reported. There were 13 mechanical valve thromboses; 12 occurred when the patient was in the mitral position, and 10 of these women were taking heparin ($p < .05$). The single woman who suffered aortic valve thrombosis refused all anticoagulation efforts and died from valve thrombosis. Of the 7 major bleeding complications, 5 occurred in women taking heparin, and 2 occurred in women taking Warfarin ($p < .05$) The incidence of spontaneous abortions did not differ between the two groups (10% and 12%). Among the 45 women with bioprosthetic valves, pregnancy tended to accelerate deterioration of these valves. Thirty-one percent of these women required valve replacement during pregnancy or shortly thereafter.

In conclusion, these authors suggested that mechanical valves were preferable in women with childbearing potential and that oral Warfarin therapy for the duration of gestation (except during the last 2 weeks) was most appropriate.

Potential discrepancies between these bodies of data may be related to techniques used for monitoring Coumadin anticoagulation. During the early 1990s, the United States adopted the International Normalized Ratio (INR), which stands for the patient's prothrombin time divided by the control time using the thromboplastin standard of the World Health Organization. Before the adoption of the INR, the use of thromboplastins of low responsiveness may have contributed to over-anticoagulation, which was equivalent to an INR of up to nine in some preparations.[61,62] Warfarin embryopathy is thought to be a dose-related phenomenon, and it may have been exacerbated by these discrepancies.

Finally, the Ross operation has been proposed as an excellent option for young women who are anticipating future motherhood. In a retrospective review of pregnancy in 8 women after they had undergone the Ross operation, there were 14 uncomplicated pregnancies, and no deterioration in autograft function occurred during or after pregnancy.[34]

SUMMARY

Congenital aortic valve disease is a progressive, lifelong condition that can be palliated but not cured. The surgical management of congenital disease of the aortic valve and root remains challenging. In general, there has been a movement away from indirect surgical therapies (e.g., apical-aortic conduits) and toward more direct surgical procedures that are designed to address the pathology directly (e.g., Konno-Rastan, modified Konno, Ross). Despite the development of techniques designed to relieve stenosis at all levels, the ultimate success of palliation will often depend on the suitability of associated left heart structures.

Areas such as patient selection (particularly in the neonatal population) and the long-term results of procedures such as the Ross operation remain subjects for investigation. The development of catheter-based interventions that are designed to treat specific forms of aortic root and valve pathology will continue. Lifelong surveillance is mandatory to provide long-lasting preservation of left ventricular function.

REFERENCES

1. Abdel-Massih T, Goldenberg A, Vouhe P, et al: Marfan syndrome in the newborn and infants less than 4 months: a series on 9 patients. Arch Mal Coeur Vaiss 95:469–472, 2002.
2. Aklog L, Carr-White GS, Birks EJ, Yacoub MH: Pulmonary autograft versus aortic homograft for aortic valve replacement: interim results from a prospective randomized trial. J Heart Valve Dis 9:176–189, 2000.
3. Alexiou C, McDonald A, Langley SM, et al: Aortic valve replacement in children: are mechanical prosthesis a good option? Eur J Cardiothorac Surg 17:125–133, 2000.
4. Al-Halees Z, Kumar N, Gallo R, et al: Pulmonary autograft for aortic valve replacement in rheumatic disease: a caveat. Ann Thorac Surg 60:S172–S176, 1995.
5. Barker PC, Ensing G, Ludomirsky A, et al: Comparison of simultaneous invasive and noninvasive measurements of pressure gradients in congenital aortic stenosis. J Am Soc Echocardiogr 15:1496–1502, 2002.
6. Berrebi AC, Carpentier SM, Phan P, et al: Results of up to 9 years of high-temperature-fixed valvular bioprosthesis in a young population. Ann Thorac Surg 71:S353–S355, 2001.
7. Beuren AJ, Schulze C, Eberle P, et al: The syndrome of supravalvular aortic stenosis, peripheral pulmonary stenosis, mental retardation and facial appearance. Am J Cardiol 13:471–483, 1964.
8. Bhabra MS, Dhillon R, Bhudia S, et al: Surgical aortic valvotomy in infancy: impact of leaflet morphology on long-term outcomes. Ann Thorac Surg 76:1412–1416, 2003.
9. Bonow RO, Carabello B, de Leon AC Jr, et al: Guidelines for the management of patients with valvular heart disease: executive summary. A report of the American College of Cardiology/American Heart Association Task Force on Practice Guidelines (Committee on Management of Patients with Valvular Heart Disease). Circulation 98:1949–1984, 1998.
10. Bourassa MG, Campeau L: Combined supravalvular aortic and pulmonic stenosis. Circulation 28:572–581, 1963.
11. Brauner R, Laks H, Drinkwater DC, et al: Benefits of early surgical repair in fixed subaortic stenosis. J Am Coll Cardiol 30:1835–1842, 1997.
12. Brom AG: In Khonsari S (editor): Cardiac Surgery: Safeguards and Pitfalls in Operative Technique. Rockville, MD: Aspen, 1988, pp. 276–280.
13. Brown JW, Ruzmetov M, Palaniswamy V, et al: Surgery for aortic stenosis in children: a 40 year experience. Ann Thorac Surg 76:1398–1411, 2003.
14. Cabalka AK, Emery RW, Petersen RJ, et al: Long-term follow-up of the St. Jude medical prosthesis in pediatric patients. Ann Thorac Surg 60:S618–S623, 1995.
15. Caldarone CA, Van Natta TL, Frazer JR, et al: The modified Konno procedure for complex left ventricular outflow tract obstruction. Ann Thorac Surg 75:147–151, 2003.
16. Caldarone CA: Left ventricular outflow tract obstruction: the role of the modified Konno procedure. Semin Thorac Cardiovasc Surg Pediatr Card Surg Annu 6:98–107, 2003.
17. Cape EG, Vanauker MD, Sigfusson G, et al: Potential role of shear stress in the etiology of pediatric heart disease: septal shear stress in subaortic stenosis. J Am Coll Cardiol 30:247–254, 1997.
18. Chambers JC, Somerville J, Stone S, Ross DN: Pulmonary autograft procedure for aortic valve disease: long-term results of the pioneer series. Circulation 96:2206–2214, 1997.
19. Champsaur G, Robin J, Tronc F, et al: Mechanical valve in aortic position is a valid option in children and adolescents. Eur J Cardiothorac Surg 11:117–122, 1997.
20. Chartrand CC, Saro-Servando E, Vobecky JS: Long-term results of surgical valvuloplasty for congenital valvar aortic stenosis in children. Ann Thorac Surg 68:1356–1359, 1999.
21. Cheung MMH, Sullivan ID, de Leval MR, et al: Optimal timing of the Ross procedure in the management of chronic aortic incompetence in the young. Cardiol Young 13:253–257, 2003.
22. Choi JY, Sullivan ID: Fixed subaortic stenosis; anatomical spectrum and nature of progression. Br Heart J 65:280–286, 1991.
23. Chojnowska L, Ruzyllo W, Witkowski A, et al: Early and long-term results of non-surgical septal reduction in patients with hypertrophic cardiomyopathy. Kardiol Pol 59:269–282, 2003.
24. Choudary SK, Mathur A, Sharma R, et al: Pulmonary autograft: should it be used in young patients with rheumatic disease? J Thorac Cardiovasc Surg 118:483–490, 1999.
25. Clarke DR, Campbell DN, Hayward AR, Bishop DA: Degeneration of aortic valve allografts in young recipients. J Thorac Cardiovasc Surg 103:934–941, 1993.
26. Cobanoglu A, Thyagarajan GK, Dobbs J: Konno-aortoventriculoplasty with a mechanical prosthesis in dealing with small aortic root: a good surgical option. Eur J Cardiothorac Surg 12:766–770, 1997.
27. Coleman DM, Smallhorn JF, McCrindle BW, et al: Postoperative follow-up of fibromuscular subaortic stenosis. J Am Coll Cardiol 24:1558–1564, 1994.
28. Couetil JP, Berrebi A, Ferdinand FD, et al: New approach for reconstruction of the pulmonary outflow tract during the Ross procedure. Circulation 98(19 Suppl):II368–II371, 1998.
29. Curran ME, Atkinson DL, Ewart AK, et al: The elastin gene is disrupted by a translocation associated with supravalvular aortic stenosis. Cell 73:159–168, 1993.
30. de Sa M, Moshkovitz Y, Butany J, David TE: Histologic abnormalities of the ascending aorta and pulmonary trunk in patients with bicuspid aortic valve disease: clinical relevance to the Ross procedure. J Thorac Cardiovasc Surg 118:588–594, 1999.
31. de Vries H, Bogers AJ, Schoof PH, et al: Pulmonary autograft failure caused by a relapse of rheumatic fever. Ann Thorac Surg 57:750–751, 1994.
32. DeVries AG, Hess J, Witsengurg M, et al: Management of fixed subaortic stenosis: a retrospective study of 57 cases. J Am Coll Cardiol 19:1013–1017, 1992.
33. Donofrio MT, Engle MA, O'Loughlin JE, et al: Congenital aortic regurgitation: natural history and management. J Am Coll Cardiol 20:366–372, 1992.
34. Dore A, Somerville J: Pregnancy in patients with pulmonary autograft valve replacement. Eur Heart J 18:1659–1661, 1997.
35. Doty DB, Polansky DB, Jenson CB. Supravalvular aortic stenosis. Repair by extended aortoplasty. J Thorac Cardiovasc Surg 74:362–371, 1977.
36. Duran CMG, Gometza B: Aortic valve reconstruction in the young. J Card Surg 9(Suppl):204–208, 1994.
37. Echigo S: Balloon valvuloplasty for congenital heart disease: immediate and long-term results of multi-institutional study. Pediatr Int 43:542–547, 2001.
38. Edmunds LH Jr: Thrombotic and bleeding complications of prosthetic heart valves. Ann Thorac Surg 44:430–445, 1987.
39. Elkins RC: Congenital aortic valve disease: evolving management. Ann Thorac Surg 59:269–274, 1995.
40. Elkins RC, Lane MM, McCue C: Ross procedure for ascending aortic replacement. Ann Thorac Surg 67:1843–1845; discussion 1853–1856, 1999.
41. Elkins RC, Lane MM, McCue C: Ross operation in children: late results. J Heart Valve Dis 10:736–741, 2001.
42. Elkins RC, Lane MM, McCue C, et al: Ross operation and aneurysm or dilatation of the ascending aorta. Semin Thoracic Cardiovasc Surg 11(Suppl I):50–54, 1999.
43. Elkins RC: The Ross operation: applications to children. Semin Thorac Cardiovasc Surg 8:345–349, 1996.

44. Erez E, Kanter KR, Tam VK, et al: Konno aortoventriculoplasty in children and adolescents: from prosthetic valves to the Ross operation. Ann Thorac Surg 74:122–126, 2002.
45. Eroglu AG, Oztunc F, Saltik L, et al: Aortic valve prolapse and aortic regurgitation in patients with ventricular septal defect. Pediatr Cardiol 24:36–39, 2003.
46. Ewart AK, Morris CA, Atkinson D, et al: Hemizygosity at the elastin locus in a developmental disorder, Williams Syndrome. Nat Genet 5:11–16, 1993.
47. Ewart AK, Morris CA, Ensing CA, et al: A human vascular disorder, supravalvular aortic stenosis, maps to chromosome 7. Proc Natl Acad Sci U S A 90:3226–3230, 1993.
48. Faber L, Seggewiss H, Gleichman U: Percutaneous transluminal septal myocardial ablation in hypertrophic obstructive cardiomyopathy: results with respect to intraprocedural myocardial contrast echocardiography. Circulation 98:2415–2421, 1998.
49. Feigl A, Feigl D, Lucas RV Jr, et al: Involvement of the aortic valve cusps in discrete subaortic stenosis. Pediatr Cardiol 5:185–190, 1984.
50. Frommelt MA, Snider R, Bove EL, et al: Echocardiographic assessment of subvalvular aortic stenosis before and after operation. J Am Coll Cardiol 19:1018–1023, 1992.
51. Frommelt PC, Lupinetti FM, Bove EL: Aortoventriculoplasty in infants and children. Circulation 86(Suppl II):176–180, 1992.
52. Fyler DC (editor): Nadas' Pediatric Cardiology. Philadelphia: Hanley & Belfus, Inc, 1992, pp. 494–495.
53. Fyler DC (editor): Nadas' Pediatric Cardiology. Philadelphia: Hanley & Belfus, Inc, 1992, pp. 506.
54. Gaynor JW, Bull C, Sullivan UID, et al: Late outcome of survivors of intervention for neonatal aortic valve stenosis. Ann Thorac Surg 60:122–125, 1995.
55. Gerosa G, McKay R, Davies J, Ross DN: Comparison of the aortic homograft and the pulmonary autograft for aortic valve or root replacement in children. J Thorac Cardiovasc Surg 102:51–61, 1991.
56. Grande-Allen KJ, Cochran RP, Reinhall PG, et al: Re-creation of sinuses is important for sparing the aortic valve: a finite element study. J Thorac Cardiovasc Surg 119:753–763, 2000.
57. Grinda JM, Latremouille C, Berrebi AJ, et al: Aortic cusp extension for rheumatic aortic valve disease: midterm results. Ann Thorac Surg 74:438–443, 2002.
58. Hall JG, Pauli RM, Wilson KM: Maternal and fetal sequelae of anticoagulation during pregnancy. Am J Med 68:122–140, 1980.
59. Hawkins JA, Minich LL, Shaddy RE, et al: Aortic valve repair and replacement after balloon aortic valvuloplasty in children. Ann Thorac Surg 61:1355–1358, 1996.
60. Hazekamp MG, Frank M, Hardjowijono FM, et al: Surgery for membranous subaortic stenosis. Long-term follow-up. Eur J Cardiothorac Surg 7:356–359, 1993.
61. Hirsh J, Deykin D, Poller L: "Therapeutic range" for oral anticoagulant therapy. Chest 89(2 Suppl):11S-15S, 1986.
62. Hirsh J: Is the dose of warfarin prescribed by American physicians unnecessarily high? Arch Intern Med 147:769–771, 1987.
63. Hisatomi K, Isomura T, Sato T, et al: Long-term results after conservative aortic valve repair for aortic regurgitation with ventricular septal defect. J Cardiovasc Surg 36:541–544, 1995.
64. Hokken RB, Cromme-Dijkhuis AH, Bogers AJ, et al: Clinical outcome and left ventricular function after pulmonary autograft implantation in children. Ann Thorac Surg 63:1713–1717, 1997.
65. Hossack KF, Neutze JM, Lowe JB, Barrat-Boyes BG: Congenital aortic valvar stenosis. Natural history and assessment for operation. Br Heart J 43:561–573, 1980.
66. Iturbe-Alessio I, Fonseca M, Mutchinik O, et al: Risks of anticoagulant therapy in pregnant women with artificial heart valves. N Engl J Med 315:1390–1393, 1986.
67. Jahangiri M, Nicholson IA, del Nido PJ, et al: Surgical management of complex and tunnel-like subaortic stenosis. Eur J Cardiothorac Surg 17:637–642, 2000.
68. Jaumin P, Rubay J, Lintermans J, et al: Surgical treatment of subvalvular aortic stenosis: long-term results. J Cardiovasc Surg (Torino) 31:31–35, 1990.
69. Kirklin JW, Barratt-Boyes BG (editors): Cardiac Surgery, ed 2, vol 1. New York: Churchill Livingstone, 1993, pp. 546.
70. Kitchiner DJ, Jackson M, Walsh K, et al: Incidence and prognosis of congenital aortic valve stenosis in Liverpool (1960-1990). Br Heart J 69:71–79, 1993.
71. Konno S, Imai Y, Iida Y, et al: A new method for prosthetic valve replacement in congenital aortic stenosis associated with hypoplasia of the aortic valve ring. J Thorac Cardiovasc Surg 70:909–917, 1975.
72. Kuhn H, Gietzen F, Leuner C, et al: Induction of subaortic septal ischemia to reduce obstruction in hypertrophic obstructive cardiomyopathy. Studies to develop a new catheter-based concept of treatment. Eur Heart J 18: 846–851, 1997.
73. Larrea JL, Nunez L, Reque JA, et al: Pregnancy and mechanical valve prosthesis: a high-risk situation for the mother and the fetus. Ann Thorac Surg 36:459–463, 1983.
74. Legget ME, Unger TA, O'Sullivan CK, et al: Aortic root complications in Marfan's syndrome: identification of a lower risk group. Heart 75:389–395, 1996.
75. Leyh RG, Schmidtke C, Sievers HH, et al: Opening and closing characteristics of the aortic valve after different types of valve-preserving surgery. Circulation 100:2153–2160, 1999.
76. Lofland GK, McCrindle BW, Williams WG, et al: Critical aortic stenosis in the neonate: a multi-institutional study of management, outcomes and risk factors. J Thorac Cardiovasc Surg 121:10–27, 2001.
77. Lubiszewska B, Rozanski J, Szufladowicz M, et al: Mechanical valve replacement in congenital heart disease in children. J Heart Valve Dis 8:74–79, 1999.
78. Luciani GB, Barozzi L, Tomezzoli A, et al: Bicuspid aortic valve disease and pulmonary autograft root dilatation after the Ross procedure: a clinicopathologic study. J Thorac Cardiovasc Surg 122:74–79, 2001.
79. Lupinetti FM, Duncan BW, Lewin M, et al: Comparison of autograft and allograft aortic valve replacement in children. J Thorac Cardiovasc Surg 126:240–246, 2003.
80. Lupinetti FM, Marner J, Jones TK, Herndon SP: Comparison of human and mechanical prostheses for aortic valve replacement in children. Circulation 96:321–325, 1997.
81. Lupinetti FM, Pridjian AK, Callow MB, et al: Optimum treatment of discrete subaortic stenosis. Ann Thorac Surg 54:467–471, 1992.
82. Lupinetti FM, Warner J, Jones TK, et al: Comparison of human tissues and mechanical prostheses for aortic valve replacement in children. Circulation 96:321–325, 1997.
83. Maron BJ, McKenna WJ, Danielson GK, et al: American College of Cardiology/European Society of Cardiology clinical expert consensus document on hypertrophic cardiomyopathy. A report of the American College of Cardiology Foundation Task Force on Clinical Expert Consensus Documents and the European Society of Cardiology Committee for Practice Guidelines. J Am Coll Cardiol 42:1687–1713, 2003.
84. Maron BJ, Nishimura RA, McKenna WJ, et al: Assessment of permanent dual-chamber pacing as a treatment for drug-refractory symptomatic patients with obstructive hypertrophic cardiomyopathy. A randomized, double blind, crossover study (M-PATHY). Circulation 99:2927–2933, 1999.

85. Martin MM, Lemmer JH, Shaffer E, et al: Obstruction to the left coronary artery blood flow secondary to obliteration of the coronary ostium in supravalvular aortic stenosis. Ann Thorac Surg 45:16–20, 1988.
86. Matsuda H, Miyamoto Y, Takahashi T, et al: Extended aortic and left main coronary angioplasty with a single pericardial patch in a patient with Williams syndrome. Ann Thorac Surg 52:1331–1333, 1991.
87. Mazzitelli DF, Guenther T, Schreiber C, et al: Aortic valve replacement in children: are we on the right track? Eur J Cardiothorac Surg 13:565–571, 1998.
88. McCrindle BW: Independent predictors of immediate results of percutaneous balloon aortic valvotomy in children. Valvuloplasty and Angiopalsty on Congenital Anomalies (VACA) Registry Investigators. Am J Cardiol 77:286–293, 1996.
89. McCrindle BW, Blackstone EH, Williams WG, et al: Are outcomes of surgical versus transcatheter balloon valvotomy equivalent in neonatal critical aortic stenosis? Circulation 2001;104:I-152–I-158.
90. McGoon DC, Mankin HT, Vlad P, Kirklin JW: The surgical treatment of supravalvular aortic stenosis. J Thorac Cardiovasc Surg 41:125–133, 1961.
91. McKenna W, Deabfield J, Faruqui A, et al: Prognosis in hypertrophic cardiomyopathy: role of age and clinical, echocardiographic and hemodynamic features. Am J Cardiol 47:532–538, 1981.
92. Mencarelli L. Stenosis sopravalvolare aortica ad ancello. Arch Ital Anat Patol 1:829, 1930.
93. Mills P, Leech G, Davies M, Leatham A: The natural history of a non-stenotic bicuspid aortic valve. Br Heart J 40:951–957, 1978.
94. Mohr R, Schaff HV, Danielson GK, et al: The outcome of surgical treatment of hypertrophic obstructive cardiomyopathy. Experience over 15 years. J Thorac Cardiovasc Surg 97:666–674, 1989.
95. Moore P, Egito E, Mowrey H, et al: Midterm results of balloon dilatation of congenital aortic stenosis: predictors of success. J Am Coll Cardiol 27:1257–1263, 1996.
96. Morrow AG, Koch JP, Maron BJ, et al: Left ventricular myotomy and myomectomy in patients with obstructive hypertrophic cardiomyopathy and previous cardiac arrest. Am J Cardiol 46:313–316, 1980.
97. Morrow AG, Reitz BA, Epstein SE, et al: Operative treatment in hypertrophic subaortic stenosis. Techniques and the results of pre and postoperative assessments in 83 patients. Circulation 52:88–102, 1975.
98. Moskowitz WB, Schieken RM: Balloon dilatation of discrete subaortic stenosis associated with other cardiac defects in children. J Invasive Cardiol 11:116–120, 1999.
99. Myers JL, Waldhausen JA, Cyran SE, et al: Results of surgical repair of congenital supravalvular aortic stenosis. J Thorac Cardiovasc Surg 105:281–288, 1993.
100. Newfield EA, Muster AJ, Paul MH, et al: Discrete subvalvar aortic stenosis in childhood. Am J Cardiol 38:53–61, 1976.
101. Ng SK, O'Brien MF, Harrocks S, et al: Influence of patient age and implantation technique on the probability of re-replacement of the homograft aortic valve. J Heart Valve Dis 11:217–223, 2002.
102. Ohye RG, Gomez CA, Ohye BJ, et al: The Ross/Konno procedure in neonates and infants: intermediate-term survival and autograft function. Ann Thorac Surg 72:823–830, 2001.
103. Orie JD, Beerman LB, Ettedgui JA, et al: Discrete subaortic stenosis in children: natural and unnatural history [abstract]. J Am Coll Cardiol 23:119A, 1994.
104. Parry AJ, Kovalchin JP, Suda K, et al: Resection of subaortic stenosis; can a more aggressive approach be justified? Eur J Cardiothorac Surg 15:631–638, 1999.
105. Pessotto R, Wells WJ, Baker CJ, et al: Midterm results of the Ross procedure. Ann Thorac Surg 71:S336–S339, 2001.
106. Petre R, Arbenz U, Vogt PR, Turina MI: Application of successive principles to correct supravalvular aortic stenosis. Ann Thorac Surg 67:1167–1169, 1999.
107. Pieters F, Al-Halees Z, Zwann F, et al: Autograft failure after the Ross operation in a rheumatic population: pre and postoperative echocardiographic observation. J Heart Valve Dis 5:404–409, 1996.
108. Pigula FA, Paolillo J, McGrath M, et al: Aortopulmonary size discrepancy is not a contraindication to the pediatric Ross operation. Ann Thorac Surg 72:1610–1614, 2001.
109. Rastan H, Koncz J: Aortoventriculoplasty: a new technique for the treatment of left ventricular outflow tract obstruction. J Thorac Cardiovasc Surg 71:920–927, 1976.
110. Requarth JA, Goldberg SJ, Vasko SD, et al: In vitro verification of Doppler prediction of transvalve pressure gradient and orifice area in stenosis. Am J Cardiol 53:1369–1373, 1984.
111. Rizzoli G, Tiso E, Mazzucco A, et al: Discrete subaortic stenosis. Operative age and gradient as predictors of late aortic valve incompetence. J Thorac Cardiovasc Surg 106:95–104, 1993.
112. Rohlicek CV, Font del Pino S, Hosking M, et al: Natural history and surgical outcomes for isolated discrete subaortic stenosis in children. Heart 82:708–713, 1999.
113. Rosing DR, Kent KN, Borer JS, et al: Verapamil therapy: a new approach to the pharmacologic treatment of hypertrophic cardiomyopathy. I. Hemodynamic effects. Circulation 60:1201–1207, 1979.
114. Ross DB, Trusler GA, Coles JG, et al: Small aortic root in childhood: surgical options. Ann Thorac Surg 58:1617–1624, 1994.
115. Ross DN: Replacement of the aortic and mitral valves with a pulmonary autograft. Lancet 11:956–958, 1967.
116. Roughneen PT, DeLeon SY, Cetta F, et al: Modified Konno-Rastan procedure for subaortic stenosis: indications, operative techniques, and results. Ann Thorac Surg 65:1368–1375, 1998.
117. Saurez de Lezo J, Pan M, Medina A, et al: Immediate and follow-up results of transluminal balloon dilatation for discrete subaortic stenosis. J Am Coll Cardiol 18:1309–1315, 1991.
118. Saurez de Lezo J, Pan M, Sancho M, et al: Percutaneous transluminal balloon dilatation. For discrete subaortic stenosis. Am J Cardiol 58:619–621, 1986.
119. Sbarouni E, Oakley CM: Outcomes of pregnancy in women with valve prostheses. Br Heart J 71:196–201, 1994.
120. Scholler GF, Colan SD, Sanders SP, et al: Noninvasive estimation of the left ventricular pressure waveform throughout ejection in young patients with aortic stenosis. J Am Coll Cardiol 12:492–497, 1988.
121. Sherrid M, Delia E, Dwyer E: Oral disopyramide therapy for obstructive hypertrophic cardiomyopathy. Am J Cardiol 62:1085–1088, 1988.
122. Shin H, Katogi T, Yozu R, et al: Surgical angioplasty of left main coronary stenosis complicating supravalvular aortic stenosis. Ann Thorac Surg 67:1147–1148, 1999.
123. Spray TL: Technique of pulmonary autograft aortic valve replacement in children (the Ross procedure). Semin Thorac Cardiovasc Surg Pediatr Card Surg Annu 1:165–178, 1998.
124. Stamm C, Kreutzer C, Zurakowski D, et al: Forty-one years of surgical experience with congenital supravalvular aortic stenosis. J Thorac Cardiovasc Surg 118:874–885, 1999.
125. Stellin G, Mazzucco A, Bartolotti U, et al: Late results after resection of discrete and tunnel subaortic stenosis. Eur J Cardiothorac Surg 3:325–340, 1989.
126. Stenson RE, Flamm MD Jr, Harrison DC, et al: Hypertrophic subaortic stenosis. Clinical and hemodynamic

effects of long-term propranolol therapy. Am J Cardiol 31:763–773, 1973.
127. Sun CC, Jacot J, Brenner JI: Sudden death in supravalvular aortic stenosis: fusion of coronary leaflet to the sinus ridge, dysplasia and stenosis of aortic and pulmonary leaflets. Pediatr Pathol 12:751–759, 1992.
128. Tsang VT, Pawade A, Karl TR, Mee RB: Surgical management of Marfan syndrome in children. J Card Surg 9:50–54, 1994.
129. Turrentine MW, Ruzmetov M, Vijay P, et al: Biological versus mechanical aortic valve replacement in children. Ann Thorac Surg 71:S356–S360, 2001.
130. van Karnebeck CDM, Naeff MSJ, Mulder BJM, et al: Natural history of cardiovascular manifestations in Marfan syndrome. Arch Dis Child 84:129–137, 2001.
131. van Son JAM, Danielson GK, Puga FJ, et al: Supravalvular aortic stenosis. Long-term results of surgical treatment. J Cardiovasc Thorac Surg 107:103–115, 1994.
132. van Suylen RJ, Schoof PH, Bos E, et al: Pulmonary autograft failure after aortic root replacement in a patient with juvenile rheumatoid arthritis. Eur J Cardiothorac Surg 6:571–572, 1992.
133. Wessel A, Pankau R, Kececioglu D, et al: Three decades of follow-up of aortic and pulmonary vascular lesions in the Williams-Beuren Syndrome. Am J Med Genet 52:297–301, 1994.
134. Williams JCP, Barrat-Boyes BG, Lowe JB: Supravalvular aortic stenosis. Circulation 24:1311–1318, 1961.
135. Yacoub M, Onuzo O, Riedel B, Radley-Smith R: Mobilization of the left and right fibrous trigones for relief of severe left ventricular outflow obstruction. J Thorac Cardiovasc Surg 117:126–133, 1999.
136. Yacoub MH, Khan H, Stavri G, et al: Anatomic correction of the sinus of prolapsing right coronary aortic cusp, dilatation of the sinus of Valsalva, and ventricular septal defect. J Thorac Cardiovasc Surg 113:253–261, 1997.

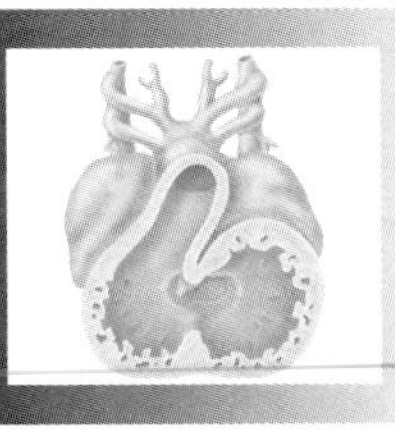

CHAPTER 120

Surgery for Congenital Anomalies of the Coronary Arteries

Andrew D. Cochrane

INTRODUCTION

Congenital coronary artery abnormalities fall into two groups. Firstly, there are variations in coronary origin from the aorta, in their course and their distribution, which are relatively common, being present in almost 1% of the population,[38] and the majority of which are benign. Secondly, there are major defects that are rare but potentially fatal either in infancy or by leading to premature death in adult life.

These abnormalities of congenital origin can be anatomically classified into four groups: anomalous left coronary artery (LCA) from the pulmonary artery (PA) and its variants, coronary–cameral fistulas, abnormalities of aortic origin of the coronary arteries in structurally normal hearts, and abnormalities of aortic origin in association with structural defects such as transposition of the great arteries and tetralogy of Fallot. The first two anatomical defects are discussed in detail in this chapter.

An important acquired coronary defect, but commonly manifest in the pediatric age group, is arterial disease due to Kawasaki disease,[37] first described in 1967. This will not be discussed here, but is well reviewed by others.[40,41]

ANOMALOUS ORIGIN OF THE LEFT CORONARY ARTERY FROM THE PULMONARY ARTERY

Origin of a major coronary artery from the PA is an uncommon congenital defect that is often lethal if not diagnosed and treated. The main LCA is the vessel most commonly involved, but it can involve the left anterior descending artery (LAD) alone, the circumflex artery alone, the right coronary artery (RCA), or very rarely may affect the origin of both coronary arteries. Anomalous origin of the RCA from the main pulmonary artery may cause sudden death.[13] Origin of both coronary arteries from the pulmonary artery usually results in death in the newborn period.[28]

Anomalous origin of the left coronary artery from the pulmonary artery (ALCAPA) is the most common variant, with a reported incidence between 1 in 30,000 and 1 in 300,000 infants.[82] It is reported to account for 0.25–0.5% of all congenital cardiac defects. It is the most common cause of myocardial infarction in the pediatric age group.[82]

Surgical Anatomy

The anomalous LCA arises either from the main PA (MPA) or less commonly from the right pulmonary artery (RPA). In the case of origin from the main PA, the abnormal ostium is most commonly found arising from the left posterior sinus, and then following the course and distribution of the normal LCA; less commonly it may arise from the right posterior sinus or from the posterior wall of the main PA.[75]

Associated anomalies with ALCAPA are uncommon, but they are well described and occur in approximately 15% of cases. The associated defect may be important in reducing the degree of myocardial ischemia if they lead to an elevated PA pressure. It has been described together with ventricular septal defect (VSD),[20] patent ductus arteriosus (PDA),[62,76] Fallot's tetralogy, pulmonary valvar stenosis,[50] and together with coarctation. A single case has been described in association with hypoplastic left heart syndrome, the coronary artery arising from the RPA, and presenting at 9 months of age with a patent ductus maintaining systemic perfusion.[72]

Origin from the RPA is rare, but in this subgroup 70% of patients have other defects. The combination of coarctation in association with anomalous LCA from the RPA has been described in several cases.[24,52] Origin from the RPA is also associated with an intramural course through the aortic wall.[3,83]

The largest series of patients described in the literature came from Toronto, with 67 children over a 48-year period; 64 had anomalous origin of the whole LCA, two had anomalous circumflex coronary, and one had anomalous RCA from the PA.[7] Another large series was described from the Texas Heart Institute, and among 60 cases of coronary anomaly there were 56 patients in whom the LCA arose from the main PA, two patients with RCA from the main PA, and two patients with a branch of the LCA arising from the MPA.[26]

In a series of 26 cases seen at Royal Children's Hospital (RCH Melbourne) over 23 years, there were 25 patients with origin of the whole LCA from the PA (21 from the MPA and 4 cases from the RPA) and one patient with origin of the left circumflex alone from the MPA.[26]

Pathophysiology

The effect of ALCAPA depends upon the pressure difference between the systemic and pulmonary circulations and on the adequacy of the collateral vessels between the right and left coronary systems, as proposed by Edwards.[25] During fetal life, the pulmonary vascular resistance is elevated, the pulmonary artery pressure is systemic, and the LCA perfusion pressure is adequate although the blood is desaturated. This explains why the lesion is rarely if ever symptomatic in the newborn period.

When the pulmonary vascular resistance and the pulmonary arterial pressure fall in the first few weeks of life, the antegrade LCA flow declines, and the perfusion of the LCA increasingly depends upon collateral circulation from the RCA. If the collaterals are adequate, then the (left ventricle) LV myocardium remains viable and there will be significant retrograde flow into the main PA. If the collateral flow is inadequate, then there is resultant myocardial ischemia and infarction of the anterior and lateral walls of the LV, and the degree of retrograde flow into the PA is minimal. The infarction commences at the subendocardium, and is often patchy in distribution, because of the gradual onset and chronic nature of the ischemia, but in the most severe cases becomes transmural and confluent (Figure 120-1). If the PA pressure is maintained at an elevated level and at a higher oxygen saturation by the presence of a VSD or PDA, then the coronary defect is masked and may not become clinically evident until after closure of the left-to-right shunt, with potentially fatal outcome.

Histologically, there is usually evidence of ischemia of the LV myocardium, both acute and chronic, with necrosis and fibrosis. The continuing development of collaterals may limit these changes to the subendocardium and stabilize cardiac function, but result inevitably in a left-to-right shunt or coronary "steal" with retrograde flow into the main PA. There is commonly mitral regurgitation, due to papillary muscle and subendocardial infarction. If the collateral development is inadequate, then transmural infarction develops, resulting in marked LV dilation, severely impaired function, and rarely in LV free wall rupture.[17]

Clinical Presentation

Clinical signs and symptoms usually begin from 4–6 weeks of age, when the pulmonary vascular resistance has fallen, but it may be another few weeks before the infant is recognized to be unwell and the diagnosis is made. The typical features are tachypnea, sweating, poor feeding, poor weight gain, and pallor. The infant is often diagnosed as having heart failure due to a cardiomyopathy, but the presence of this diagnosis in a young infant should always arouse suspicion of a coronary artery anomaly. A syndrome of "anginal equivalent" has been described, which includes severe pallor, sweating, and irritability following a feeding; this can be misdiagnosed as infantile colic.[48] Older infants may present with a heart murmur and findings of mitral valve regurgitation (MR). A small number of patients do not have symptoms recognized until teenage or early adult life, presenting with angina pectoris, dyspnea, and fatigue from impaired LV function, or with arrhythmia or sudden death. There are very rare reports of adults who remain asymptomatic.[32]

Examination of the infant with ALCAPA may reveal evidence of heart failure with tachypnea, tachycardia, hepatomegaly, cardiomegaly, a murmur of mitral regurgitation, and a gallop rhythm. Chest radiography in most infants demonstrates marked cardiomegaly and pulmonary congestion, but may appear normal in older children or adults with less marked symptoms.

The electrocardiogram (ECG) is a very important clue to the diagnosis in the sick infant. It classically shows lateral wall or anterolateral infarction, with Q waves and ST elevation (Figure 120-2). Older children and adults may have less prominent Q waves because of less severe ischemic injury or because of compensatory hypertrophy of the posterobasal LV wall.[82]

Diagnostic Techniques

Echocardiography usually shows a dilated and poorly contracting LV, mitral regurgitation due to reduced movement of the posterior leaflet of the mitral valve, enlargement of the RCA, and sometimes the anomalous origin of the artery can be seen with retrograde flow into the PA. The enlargement of the RCA is a very important clue to the diagnosis. However, there may still be uncertainty in the diagnosis, particularly early in the evolution of the pathological

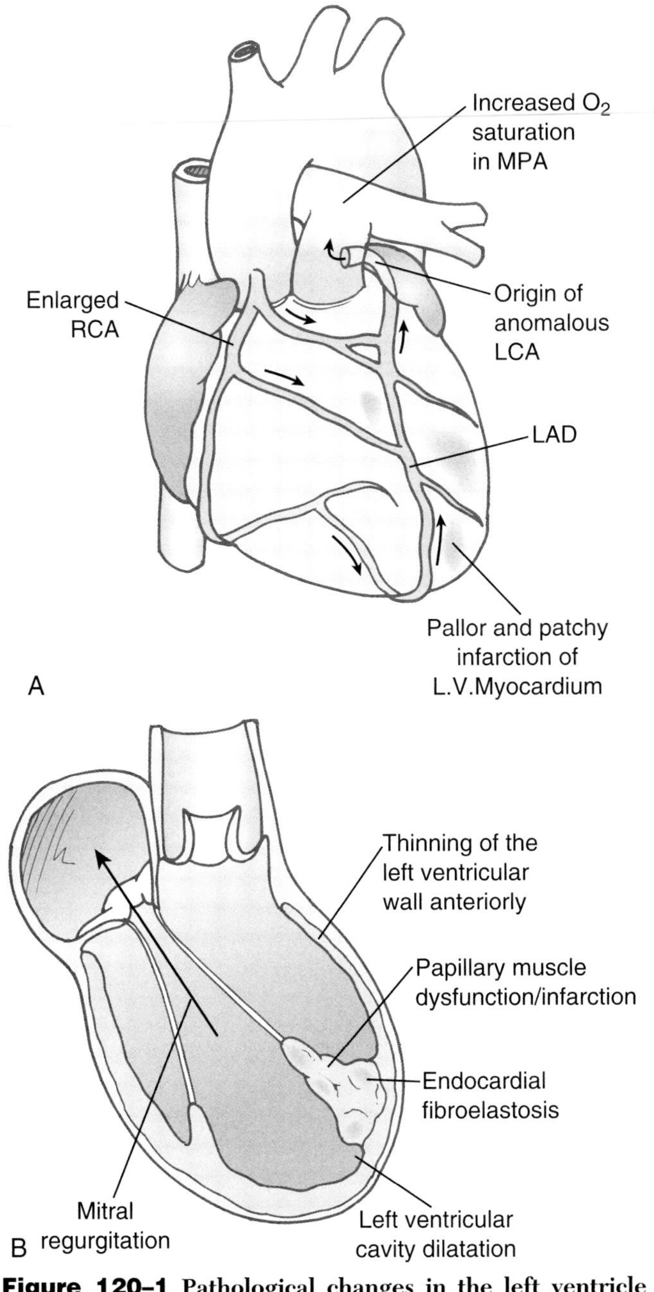

Figure 120–1 Pathological changes in the left ventricle from ALCAPA. A, The common coronary anatomy with blood draining into the pulmonary artery. **B,** Pathological changes in the LV myocardium.
(Modified from Karl TR, Cochrane AD: Anomalous origin of the left coronary artery from the pulmonary artery. In: Buxton B, Frazier OH, Westaby S [eds]: Ischemic Heart Disease: Surgical Management, St Louis: Mosby, 1999, p. 273).

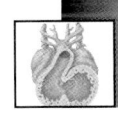

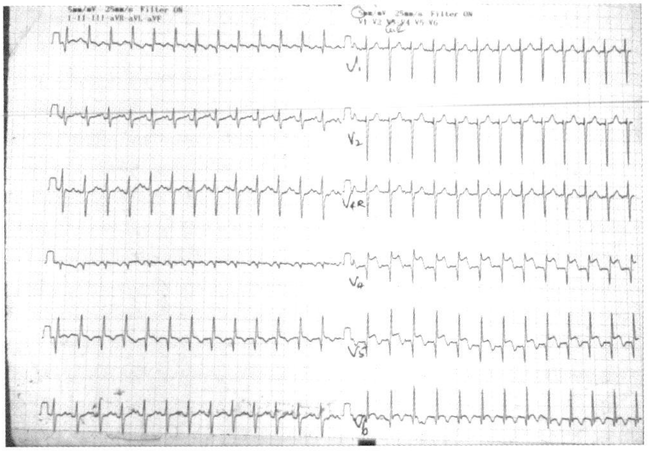

Figure 120–2 The ECG of an infant with an anomalous left coronary artery, demonstrating anterolateral infarction.

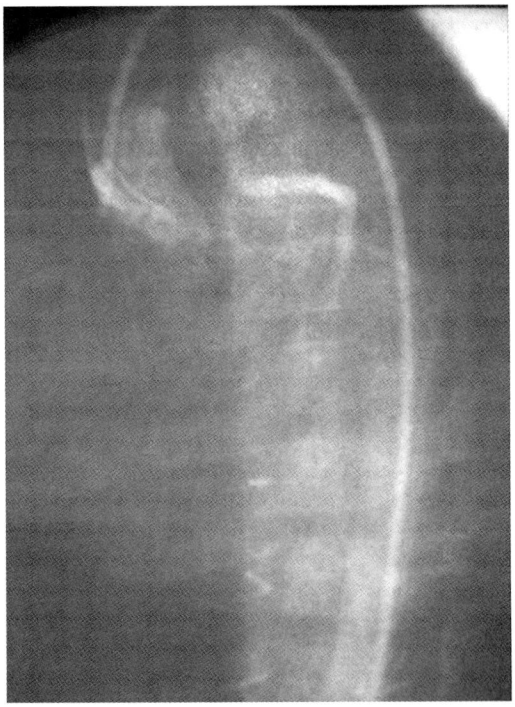

Figure 120–3 Angiogram, demonstrating anomalous origin of the left coronary artery.

changes, or at a later age in a child with minimal symptoms, reasonably preserved LV function and mitral regurgitation as the dominant defect.

Cardiac catheterization demonstrates elevated LV end-diastolic, left atrial, and PA pressures. An aortogram shows only the single, dilated RCA arising from the aorta and may show numerous collaterals providing late and retrograde filling of the LCA, with a blush of contrast in the main PA (Figure 120-3). If there is a large run-off, a step-up in oxygen saturation may be detected in the PA. If doubt remains about the diagnosis or about the position of the ostium of the LCA, pulmonary angiography can be performed in the main PA; to aid the delineation of the anomalous LCA, distal balloon occlusion may be advantageous.[66]

MRI is increasingly reported to be useful in the diagnosis of individual cases,[22,56] but no major series with this defect have been studied. Taylor et al[81] studied 25 patients with congenital cardiac defects often associated with coronary anomalies, and respiratory gated magnetic resonance angiography (MRA) was compared with conventional angiography. Coronary MRA had a sensitivity of 92% and a specificity of 100% in this situation. Coronary MRA was particularly useful for defining the proximal course of the vessels, confirming the findings of other groups.[67]

Differential Diagnosis

Misdiagnosis of ALCAPA may occur because of its rarity, and because the secondary effects may dominate the diagnostic options considered by the cardiologist. In early infancy the diagnosis of myocarditis or cardiomyopathy is the most common error; in some cases echocardiography has mistakenly demonstrated the LCA to be arising normally from the aorta. At a later stage it may be misdiagnosed as primary or congenital mitral valve disease. At RCH Melbourne, we have seen examples of both errors resulting in delayed diagnosis. In infants with a severe, dilated cardiomyopathy there is a strong argument for routine aortography to exclude origin of the whole LCA or the origin of an isolated LAD or circumflex artery from the aorta.

Surgical Management

Indications for Surgery

Surgery is indicated in all cases of ALCAPA—in infants it requires intervention within days of diagnosis, since the symptomatic infant is at risk of death from continuing myocardial ischemia, while in adults the surgery can generally be done electively. Nearly 90% of untreated infants will die in the first year of life.[88,90] Medical treatment alone, while awaiting delayed surgery is associated with high mortality[31]; surgery was delayed in this series until after 12 months of age, and five of the 12 infants died while waiting. Even in adults, if any symptoms are present, it has been shown that sudden death is a common outcome, often after physical exertion.[27,60,90] George[27] reviewed 14 adult cases reported in the literature, of whom 10 died suddenly, the majority in young adult life. Wesselhoeft[90] reported a cohort of 11 adults with only minimal symptoms; sudden death occurred in nine of the patients during long-term follow-up, five of these in relation to exertion. The establishment of the diagnosis is therefore a strong indication for surgery.

In the sick infant with myocardial ischemia and infarction, severe heart failure and very poor LV function, preoperative stabilization for 24 hours with mechanical ventilation, inotropes, and vasodilators may be beneficial.

Although a small number of infants with ALCAPA and severely impaired LV function have been treated primarily with cardiac transplantation, reconstruction of a two-coronary circulation is the preferred option, and even patients with severe global LV dysfunction have been shown to have the potential for excellent recovery. This coronary defect provides an excellent example of "hibernating myocardium," with areas of viable but nonfunctioning myocardium that can rapidly recover function with restoration of adequate blood supply.[12] The one caveat to this recommendation is that a number of infants with severely impaired LV function will require LVAD support for a few days after surgery, and this support facility should be available before embarking on reconstruction; in its absence, the infant should be referred to a pediatric center with the ability to provide mechanical support.

Anesthesia and Cardiopulmonary Bypass

Because ALCAPA is a rare disease and the affected infant is often severely ill with low cardiac output and minimal cardiac reserve, the involvement of an experienced pediatric cardiac anesthetist is important. The main aims are to maintain adequate systemic blood pressure and as a result ensure adequate collateral coronary perfusion, and to avoid major decreases in pulmonary vascular resistance, which could acutely increase the coronary "steal." Therefore normocapnia is ensured to maintain the pulmonary resistance, and high inflation pressures are avoided to minimize any reduction in cardiac output. The selection of anesthetic drugs is important to minimize myocardial depression. Inotropic support and careful volume infusion are important adjuncts. The surgeon needs to be expeditious in achieving cardiopulmonary bypass (CPB), and minimizing delay.

Techniques of CPB vary, and the surgeon will generally follow that established in the treating center. The entire operation can be performed on full flow bypass (150 ml/kg/min) with moderate hypothermia (26° to 30° C). Circulatory arrest or marked reduction in flow is unnecessary, even in small infants. Once bypass is established, the pulmonary arteries should be mobilized and snared to improve diastolic perfusion of the myocardium, because the emptying of the pulmonary circulation once on bypass may increase the coronary "steal," and also to aid delivery of cardioplegia to the coronary arteries. During bypass, the mean perfusion pressure is usually maintained at 35 to 50 mm Hg. Vasodilators are often used, in particular, phentolamine or phenoxybenzamine, isoflurane or nitroprusside.

Optimal myocardial protection is important, in order to protect the remaining functioning myocardium which will support the infant through the early postoperative period until recovery of the ischemic areas can occur. In addition to antegrade aortic cardioplegia, the additional techniques to achieve optimum delivery to the LCA include a second cardioplegic cannula placed in the MPA, immediate opening of the MPA and administration into the ostium of the LCA, or retrograde infusion via the coronary sinus.

Techniques of Repair

ALCAPA: History of Various Techniques

The two main procedures in current use are coronary transfer or translocation to the aorta and the intrapulmonary baffle (Takeuchi operation).[79] However, numerous procedures have been described in the past.

Early operations were designed to increase the PA pressure and LCA perfusion either by banding the PA or creating an aortopulmonary window.[4] Ligation of the LCA at its origin to abolish the coronary "steal" into the MPA was widely used, but there was a significant early mortality and reviews of the late results of ligation alone suggest that the LV remains dilated with only partial recovery of function, suggesting continued ischemia.[14]

The first successful revascularization appears to have been performed by Denton Cooley, describing two children who underwent a bypass graft from the aorta to the left coronary artery, after mobilization of the ostium from the MPA, one with a Dacron graft and the other with saphenous vein.[19] Other early methods of revascularization in infants that were used effectively in the past but are used rarely now included subclavian to LCA bypass[55] and aortocoronary

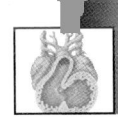

bypass with saphenous vein, together with ligation of the proximal LCA. Arciniegas and colleagues[1] described an intrapulmonary graft to the anomalous ostium, which was refined as an intrapulmonary baffle by Takeuchi.[79]

The first report of direct aortic implantation or transfer was from Neches and colleagues[59] in 1974; however, this procedure can be technically challenging and did not become popular until pediatric surgeons were regularly performing the arterial switch and other forms of major aortic root surgery, and became comfortable with the surgical technique.

Coronary Transfer to the Aorta

This is technically possible in most patients, sometimes in conjunction with a technique to lengthen the LCA and achieve an anastomosis free of tension. The principles of the procedure are similar to those of the arterial switch (Figure 120-4).

Through a median sternotomy, cardiopulmonary bypass is achieved with arterial cannulation of the aorta and bicaval venous cannulation. A single venous cannula in the right atrium is an alternative technique, but is less favored by the author because of the annoying development of "airlock" in the venous line, and because the atrial cannula lying adjacent to the aorta in a small infant can clutter the operative field. The PA branches are mobilized and snared. The main PA and aorta are separated. Two cardioplegic cannulae can be placed, in the aorta and main PA. The aorta is clamped and cardioplegia is administered into both great arteries, leaving the PA branches occluded. (An alternative is to place a single cardioplegic cannula in the aorta, and to open the MPA rapidly after the heart arrests, in order to administer cardioplegia into the coronary ostium. However, if the ostium is in an unexpected position, such as the proximal RPA, this technique may become very difficult). The right atrium is opened, and the left atrium vented via the foramen ovale (in older patients a vent catheter can be placed in the left atrium).

The main PA is opened transversely at its midpoint. The ostium of the anomalous LCA is identified and can then be excised with a generous cuff of sinus wall. If the ostium is very close to the commissure of the pulmonary valve, the commissure can be detached from the PA wall, as described for the arterial switch operation.[6]

The exact site and method of implantation on the aorta depends on the length of the coronary pedicle, the pulmonary

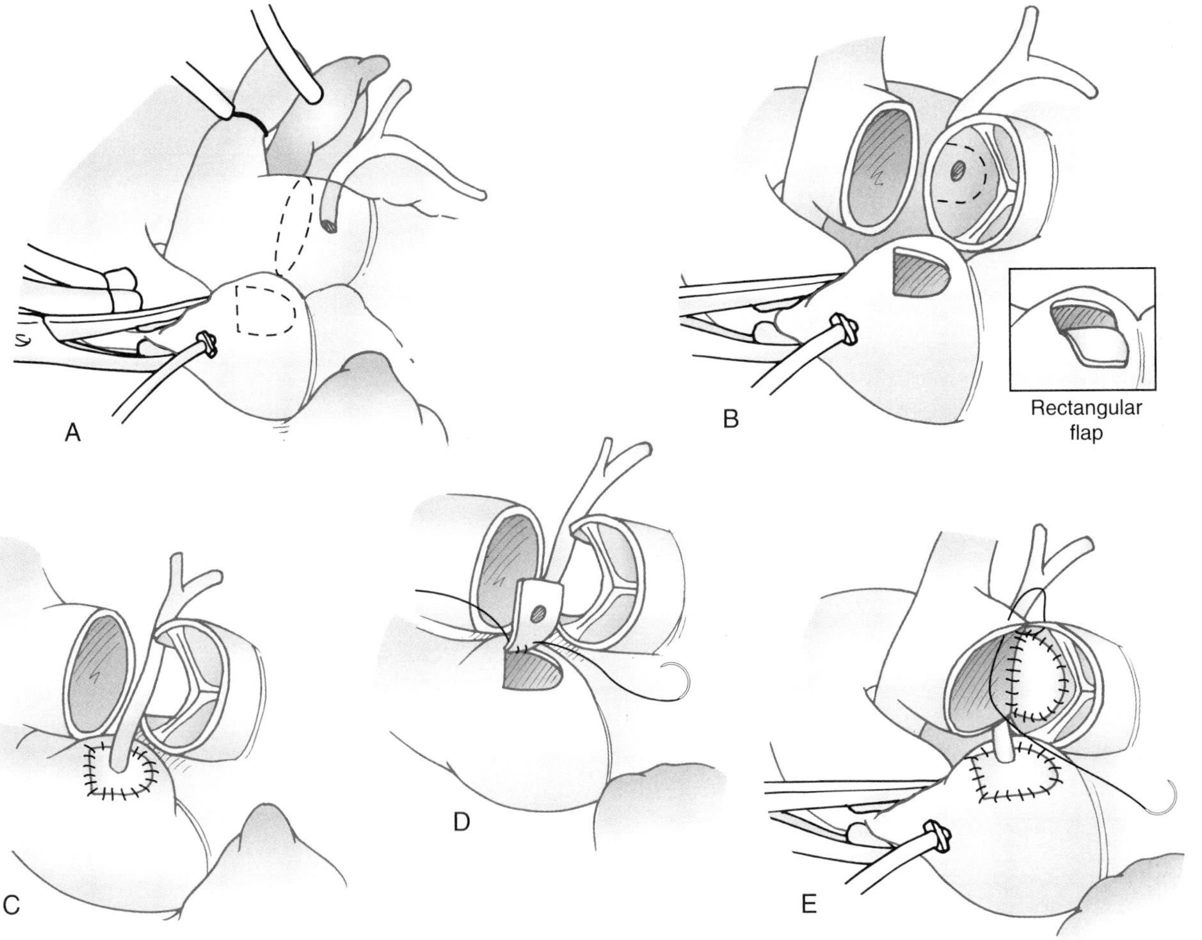

Figure 120–4 Reimplantation of the anomalous left coronary artery.
(Modified from Karl TR, Cochrane AD: Anomalous origin of the left coronary artery from the pulmonary artery. In: Buxton B, Frazier OH, Westaby S [eds]: Ischemic Heart Disease: Surgical Management, St Louis: Mosby, 1999, p. 277.)

sinus of origin, and the experience and preference of the surgeon. A window can be created on the left posterolateral aspect of the aorta; alternatively, an anteriorly based rectangular flap of aortic wall can be used, which decreases the arc of rotation of the coronary button and reduces the tension on the anastomosis (see Figure 120-4). In some cases, the coronary anastomosis is made easier by division of the ascending aorta above the sino-tubular junction. The coronary button is reimplanted with continuous 7/0 Prolene in the infant, or 6/0 Prolene in older children and adults.

The defect in the PA sinus is then repaired using a generous patch of autologous pericardium, and the main PA segments are then anastomosed. These steps, or part of them, can be performed once the heart is beating again, to minimize the cross-clamp time, after closure of the atrial septum and evacuation of air from the left heart chambers.

After completion of the repair, left heart venting is sometimes required for a period to prevent LV distention. The vent can then be removed, pressure lines placed and pacing wires attached. Weaning from bypass is usually slow and graduated, carefully assessing the LV function, the degree of LV distention, and adjusting inotrope administration.

A good hemoglobin level is essential (>100 gm/L) to wean these impaired hearts, and subsequent modified ultrafiltration may be beneficial.

Potential surgical complications include ischemia (excessive tension on the coronary pedicle or torsion of the pedicle), valve damage, and in particular bleeding from the suture lines that may be inaccessible on the posterior aspect of the aorta.

Coronary Lengthening Procedures

If the distance for transfer of the ostium to the aorta appears excessive, then a number of techniques have been described to lengthen the coronary artery in a tubular fashion (Figure 120-5). The ostium can be mobilized with transverse flaps of the MPA wall, and the flaps can be sutured to lengthen the coronary artery.

Sese and Imoto[74] described the combination of a cuff of PA wall anteriorly and a door-shaped flap of aortic wall posteriorly to create a prolongation of the LCA. Tashiro et al[80] described the excision of a circumferential cuff of MPA wall with the ostium, the upper and lower edges of which were closed to create a tunnel. A variety of techniques were described by Turley.[83] The combination of aortic and pulmonary flaps has also been described by others.[2,36,58]

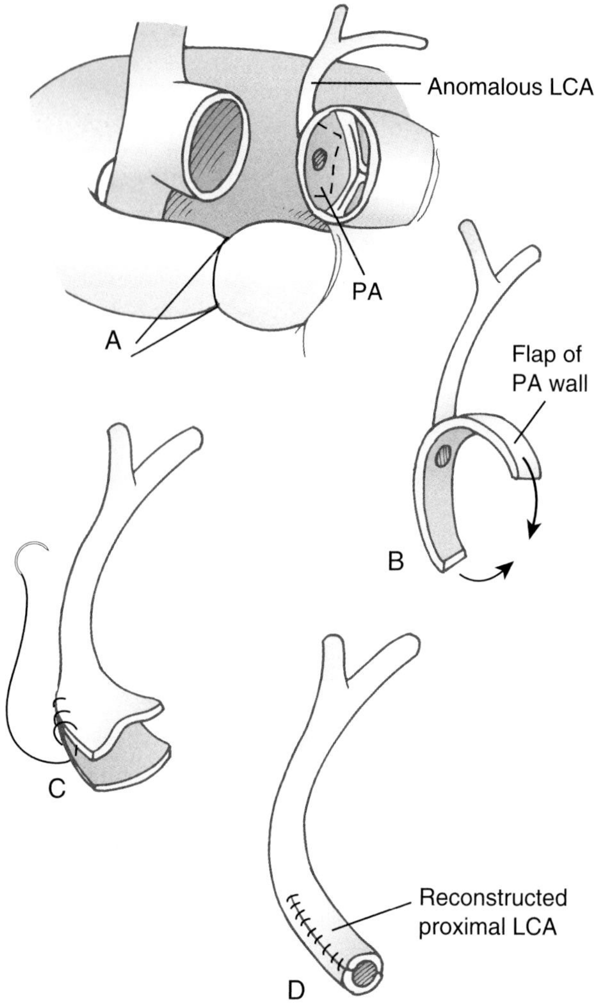

Figure 120-5 Lengthening of the left coronary pedicle using a flap of pulmonary wall. A, Transection of the pulmonary artery (PA). **B,** Mobilization of the anomalous coronary artery with flaps of pulmonary artery wall. **C,** The flaps of PA wall are sutured together to lengthen the vessel. **D,** The elongated left coronary artery is ready for anastomosis to the aorta.
(Modified from Karl TR, Cochrane AD: Anomalous origin of the left coronary artery from the pulmonary artery. In: Buxton B, Frazier OH, Westaby S [eds]: Ischemic Heart Disease: Surgical Management, St Louis: Mosby, 1999, p. 278.)

Takeuchi Operation

This technique preceded the common application of direct transfer, being first described in 1979 (Takeuchi[79]). Its advantage is that no coronary mobilization and transfer is required, and the procedure can generally be completed with a shorter aortic cross-clamp time, but it has the disadvantages of potential supravalvar pulmonary stenosis and for a residual coronary artery–pulmonary artery fistula to occur. It may be preferred if the surgeon has limited experience with the arterial switch operation and coronary transfer, or if the anomalous coronary arises from the leftward extent of the nonfacing pulmonary sinus and there is likely to be excessive tension without a coronary lengthening procedure (Figure 120-6).

After application of the aortic cross-clamp and administration of cardioplegia, a transverse incision is made on the MPA, the site of the coronary ostium identified, and the incision is extended close to the ostium (assuming that it lies in the usual position). The incision is then extended to create a medially based flap, sufficiently wide to provide an adequate tunnel. An aortopulmonary "window" is created at the base of the tunnel, using a 5-mm punch on both the aorta and the MPA and performing a direct anastomosis with continuous Prolene. The flap of anterior PA wall is then sutured along the posterior PA wall and around the coronary ostium, to create the tunnel connecting the aorta with the anomalous coronary artery. Warming of the patient can be commenced,

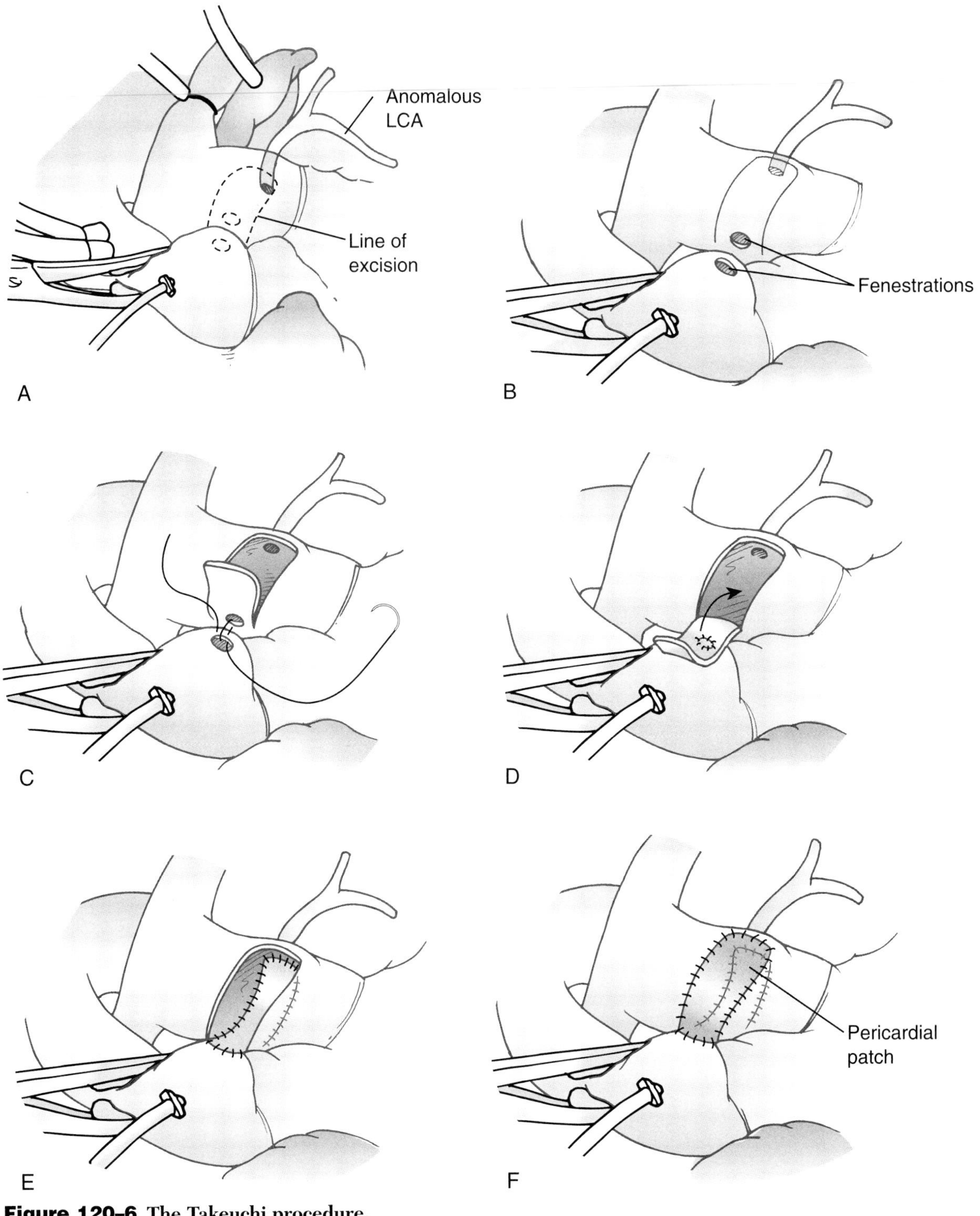

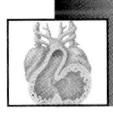

Figure 120–6 The Takeuchi procedure.
(Modified from Karl TR, Cochrane AD: Anomalous origin of the left coronary artery from the pulmonary artery. In: Buxton B, Frazier OH, Westaby S [eds]: Ischemic Heart Disease: Surgical Management, St Louis: Mosby, 1999, p. 279).

the heart can be de-aired, and the cross-clamp removed. The anterior defect in the MPA is then repaired with an autologous pericardial patch; this patch should be generous in size to prevent late supravalvar pulmonary stenosis. The operation is then completed as described for coronary transfer.

Potential surgical complications include making the PA wall flap for the tunnel too narrow, damage to the pulmonary valve, making the pericardial patch to the MPA too small, and leaving a residual coronary–pulmonary artery fistula. Bleeding is not a common problem, because the suture lines are either internal or readily accessible. Schwartz and colleagues from Boston[73] described moderate or severe supravalvar pulmonary stenosis (>26 mm Hg gradient) in 8 of 21 patients, of whom two required reoperation. At RCH

Melbourne, reoperation was necessary for one patient (8% incidence) over a follow-up period of 13 to 23 years.

Postoperative Management

Low cardiac output and hypotension related to the preoperative myocardial injury is by far the most common complication, irrespective of the method of repair. Weaning from bypass can be difficult and slow, requiring patience and attention to detail. It is very important to optimize the hemoglobin, electrolytes, acid-base status, cardiac filling, and the combination of inotropes and vasodilators.

The choice of inotropic agents is guided more by the preference and experience of the particular unit and the clinicians, and their personal beliefs, than by any scientific basis. Our preference in the first instance is a combination of dopamine with a vasodilator such as glyceryl trinitrate (GTN), or dobutamine alone. If further vasodilation appears appropriate, a phentolamine infusion or phenoxybenzamine (given very slowly over 1 to 2 hours, each 8 to 12 hours) may be added. If the infant appears excessively vasodilated as a result of the inflammatory response to CPB and the use of intraoperative vasodilators, then a low dose of noradrenaline may sometimes be necessary. The use of mechanical support may be necessary, as discussed later.

Bleeding is the second most common complication, particularly in small infants, aggravated by prolonged bypass and particularly if left ventricular assist devices (LVAD) or extracorporeal membrane oxygenation (ECMO) support is required. Administration of aprotinin may be effective in reducing the time to achieve hemostasis intraoperatively and the amount of continued bleeding, and it can be continued as an infusion postoperatively for 6 to 12 hours at 10,000 to 20,000 U/kg/hr if there is ongoing excessive loss. Aggressive replacement with platelets and FFP is often required.

In infants with either or both of these problems it is often necessary to delay sternal closure for 48–72 hours, using a Gore-Tex or Silastic membrane to close the wound. Temporary deterioration in renal function can be managed with a frusemide infusion or peritoneal dialysis. Once the inotropic dose is weaning, the urine output is established and the infant's edema is resolving, the sternum can usually be safely closed.

Indications for Mechanical Support

Some patients, despite a well-performed operation and good myocardial protection, cannot be weaned from CPB, the left ventricle quickly failing, with falling blood pressure, rising atrial pressures, and progressive cardiac distention and bradycardia. Others can be weaned, but only with high doses of inotropes and vasoconstrictors, creating the potential for multi-organ failure, acidosis, poor cerebral perfusion, and a high risk of cardiac arrest in the ICU. For patients in these two groups, the use of mechanical support for 48–96 hours is preferable, ensuring adequate organ perfusion and minimizing the chance of cardiac arrest and adverse cerebral outcomes.

At RCH Melbourne our preference is LVAD with a centrifugal pump, using cannulation of the left atrium and aorta, usually with the same cannulae that have been used for CPB.[34,35] Initially, while still on bypass, one of the two venous cannulae is transferred to the left atrium, usually behind the interatrial groove, and then the remaining right-sided venous cannula progressively clamped, while ventilating the lungs fully. This allows a gradual conversion from CPB to LVAD, and allows assessment of the adequacy of lung function and right ventricular function without any irreversible maneuvers. If the heart remains stable on LVAD circulation for 10–15 minutes, then the bypass circuit is rapidly cut out and changed to the centrifugal pump circuit. The inotropic support can then be reduced, sufficient to support the RV function adequately, as judged by central venous pressure, the visual appearance of the RV, and the adequacy of flow reaching the left atrium and the centrifugal pump.

Other cardiac units have reported good success with ECMO support in this situation. However, we believe that the advantages of LVAD are the simplicity of the circuit, and the lower anticoagulation requirement without an oxygenator.

Early Results: Mortality and Complications

Table 120-1 has a summary of early results. Historically, the early results of surgery were disappointing, not unexpected in view of the severe LV impairment often seen.[23,39] In 1980, Arciniegas and colleagues[1] reported no deaths from 15 revascularization operations. In 1987 the Boston Children's Hospital[14] reported their experience with 24 cases; in 12 patients undergoing ligation there were four early deaths, while in a later group of 12 infants undergoing revascularization there were no deaths (0%). In 1992, Backer and colleagues[8] from Chicago reported on 20 infants undergoing surgery over a 20-year period; in 9 patients a coronary ligation was performed with three early deaths and one late death, while in the later period 10 patients underwent revascularization using a variety of procedures with no early or late deaths. One patient in their series underwent primary cardiac transplantation, an approach also described by Starnes.[77]

Vouhe and others[88] from Paris reported on 31 patients undergoing direct reimplantation between 1983 and 1991, with three hospital deaths (10%) and two deaths early after discharge. The Texas Heart Institute[26] reported 60 patients, the major technique being direct reimplantation. There were four early deaths with no late deaths.

Toronto reported a series of 47 patients undergoing aortic implantation, with early survival of 92%.[7] Five infants required postoperative ECMO for a median of 4 days, but had normal ejection fraction and LV dimensions at follow-up.

At RCH Melbourne, 26 patients have undergone revascularization between 1980 and 2003. There have been no early deaths and no late deaths. Other recent but smaller series have also reported no mortality.[3,10]

Late Results

In general the late results have remained very satisfactory for both of the commonly used methods of revascularization. Our late results at RCH Melbourne suggest no difference between aortic transfer and the intrapulmonary baffle.[18]

Recovery of LV Function

The late follow-up from many centers demonstrates that there is excellent recovery of LV function and exercise

Table 120–1

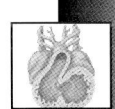

Early (Operative) Mortality Results from Major Series Reported in the Literature

Author	*Year of report*	*Surgical procedure*	*Number of patients*	*Mortality %*	*95% CI range*
Askenazi & Nadas, Boston	1975	Ligation	9	33% plus 2 late deaths	7%–70%
Arciniegas et al, Chicago	1980	Ligation Revascularization	4 15	50% 0%	7%–93% 0%–22%
Laborde et al, Paris	1981	Revascularization: variety of types	20	30%	12%–54%
Bunton et al, Boston	1987	Ligation Revascularization	12 12	33% 0%	10%–65% 0%–26%
Backer et al, Chicago	1992	Ligation Revascularization	9 10	33% 0%	7-70 % 0-31 %
Vouhe et al, Paris	1992	Reimplantation	31	10%	2-26%
Fernandes et al, Houston	1992	Revascularization: variety of types	60	7%	2%–16%
Schwartz et al, Boston	1997	Revascularization – variety of types	42	14%	5%–29%
Huddleston et al, St.Louis	2001	Reimplantation	17	6%	0%–30%
Azakie et al, Toronto	2003	Reimplantation	47	8%	2%–20%
RCH, Melbourne	2003	Takeuchi and reimplantation	26	0%	0%–13%

capacity, despite severe impairment at presentation.[7,18,69,73] The recovery begins in the first few days after surgery, demonstrated by the good results in infants requiring mechanical support, and is usually complete by one year after surgery.[7,18]

In studies from RCH Melbourne[18] the LV size rapidly diminishes within a week of surgery, with the left ventricular end-diagnostic dimension (LVEDD) falling from 48 mm (SD 5.8 mm) before surgery to 37 mm (SD 6.2 mm) at one week after surgery ($p < .001$). The LV fractional shortening initially remained unchanged, but then returned to normal over 6 to 12 months (Figures 120-7 and 120-8).

Azakie et al[7] from Toronto have reported 47 patients who underwent aortic reimplantation. There were no late deaths, with a maximum follow-up of 15 years, and actuarial survival of 91% at 5 and 10 years. On ECG, there was excellent and sustained improvement in mean ejection fraction (64% vs 33% preoperatively) and significant reduction in mitral regurgitation. The LVEDD returned to normal.

Special Considerations

Mitral Regurgitation with ALCAPA

The management of MR at the time of presentation and primary surgery is a controversial topic, with advocates for both conservative and aggressive surgical approaches. There is no doubt that MR is a prominent feature at presentation, often at least moderate in degree, due to a combination of papillary muscle ischemia or permanent fibrosis, LV free

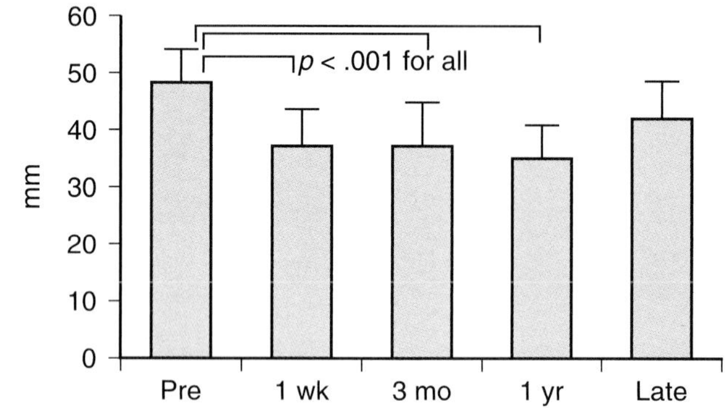

Figure 120-7 Time-related changes in LVEDD, before surgery, and at 1 week, 1 to 6 months, 1 year, and beyond 2 years from surgery. * $p < .05$, ** $p < .01$, *** $p < .001$.

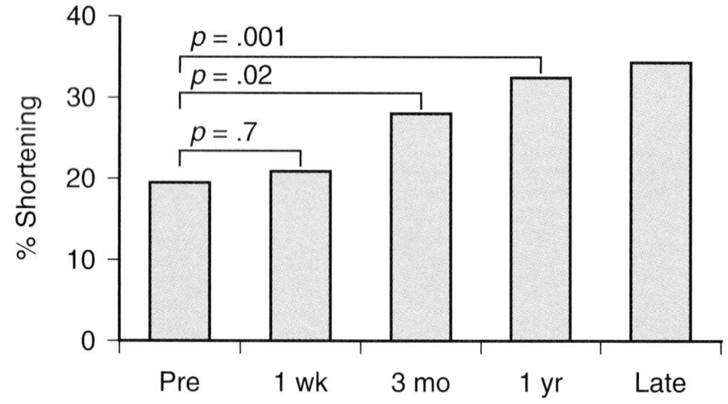

Figure 120-8 Time-related changes in LV fractional shortening percentage, before surgery, and then at 1 week, 1 to 6 months, 1 year, and beyond 2 years after surgery. * $p < .05$, ** $p < .01$, *** $p < .001$.

wall dyskinesis due to ischemia and LV chamber dilation. In general, we have observed that the degree of MR becomes significantly less in two thirds of patients, without any attempt to repair the valve, probably because of resolution of the LV free wall dyskinesis and reduction of LV diameter.[18] We do not repair the valve because this would be likely to increase the cardiac cross-clamp time in a damaged heart, it can be technically difficult in an infant's heart, and in view of the documented resolution of MR with time it would be unnecessary in many patients. However, significant MR may persist in one third of patients, despite good recovery of LV function, probably reflecting the permanent papillary muscle damage and scarring.

Other groups share this approach.[59,88] Among 47 patients in the Toronto series, only one underwent concomitant mitral valve repair, and at late follow-up only 9% had important MR.[7] Huddleston[30] reported the late valve status in 17 infants undergoing aortic transfer without mitral repair—moderate or severe MR was present in only two patients postoperatively, both of whom had developed LCA obstruction, and required a second revascularization procedure and mitral repair.

Other groups adopt a different approach. Imai from Japan performs a routine Kay annuloplasty in all cases at the time of revascularization. Similarly, Alexi-Meskishvili reports concomitant mitral repair in all cases, with no need for late mitral valve surgery.[18] Clearly there are different philosophies and methods, and no one correct method of management.

In summary, we believe that early repair of the mitral valve is not required in the majority of cases. Late valve repair in a small number of patients is more likely to be technically feasible and more successful, and can be done completely electively with low risk. The persistence of severe MR should prompt full re-investigation because it may be a marker of persisting coronary stenosis and residual ischemia,[18,30] and coronary angiography should be performed before performing mitral valve surgery. However, if an older child presents with ALCAPA and significant MR as the dominant feature, concomitant valve repair is warranted.

Late Presentation of ALCAPA in the Adult

Recognition of this cardiac defect in adult life appears to be increasing, or certainly reported more often.* As discussed previously, surgery is indicated in adults with any symptoms or with objective evidence of ischemia, in view of the relatively high incidence of sudden death with exercise.

In these cases, coronary bypass grafting with the left internal thoracic artery (LITA) and ligation of the left coronary origin would appear to be the simplest and safest option, which all adult cardiac surgeons would be able to perform with low mortality.[16] The excellent long-term patency of the LITA graft suggests that this is a reasonable option, despite the expectation that patency would be required for almost 50 years in a young adult. It is arguable whether a second graft to the circumflex system is necessary, using a right internal thoracic artery (RITA) graft, radial artery, or saphenous vein graft.

CORONARY—CAMERAL FISTULA

A coronary artery fistula is an abnormal connection between a coronary artery and any of the four chambers of the heart or any of the great vessels (superior vena cava, pulmonary artery, pulmonary veins, or coronary sinus). Coronary fistulas make up 0.2–0.4% of congenital cardiac defects, and comprise up to one half of congenital coro-nary anomalies.[26,53]

Usually the fistula is congenital in origin, found either in isolation or in association with structural heart disease. Fistulas may also be acquired, as a result of cardiac surgery, coronary angioplasty, and other transcatheter procedures,[33] endomyocardial biopsy, penetrating trauma, and as a complication of Kawasaki disease.[42]

Many fistulas are small, present as incidental findings on angiography, and do not require attention; coronary fistulas have been reported in 0.1–0.26% of patients undergoing coronary angiography.[64] Therefore, the findings of angiographic series are often different from surgical series (Figure 120-9).

Surgical Anatomy

The RCA or its branches are the site of origin in 55% of surgical cases, the LCA in 40%, and both arteries are involved

*References 22, 32, 54, 63, 70, 78.

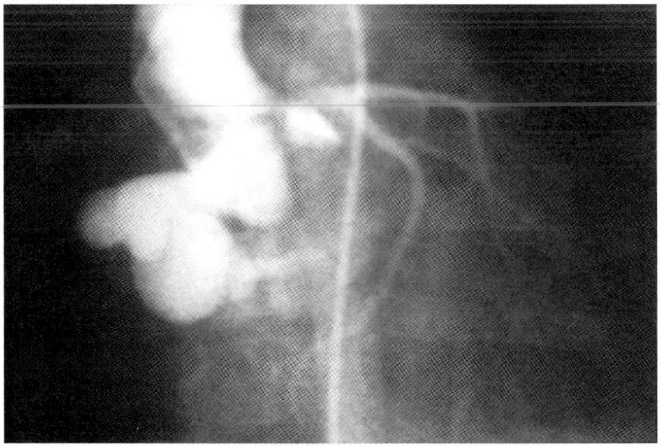

A

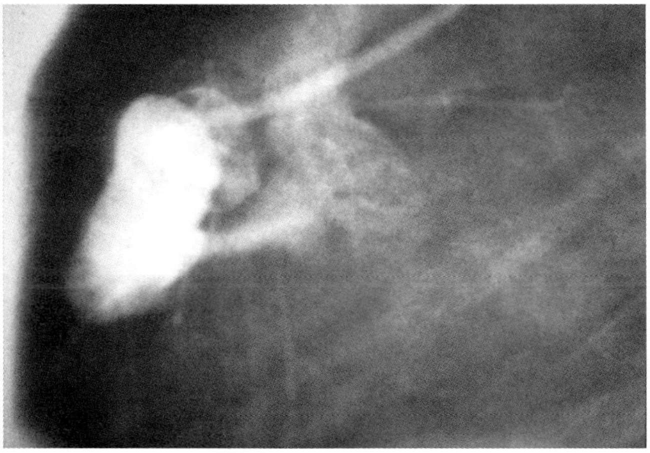

B

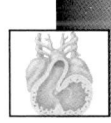

Figure 120–9 **A** and **B,** Coronary artery fistula from the midright coronary artery (RCA) to the right ventricle (RV) in oblique and lateral projections.

in 5% of patients.[46] The fistula originates either from the side of the vessel of origin or at the termination of the vessel. The affected artery is dilated and elongated proximal to the fistula, roughly proportional in diameter to the size of the shunt across the fistula. Where the artery continues beyond the fistula, it usually abruptly returns to a small diameter. The proximal dilation is usually uniform, but aneurysmal change may occur.

The distal connection of the fistula more commonly involves the right-sided heart structures than the left-sided heart.[47] In surgical series, 40% drain to the RV, 25% to the RA, 20% to the PA, 7% to the coronary sinus, and 1% to the SVC. However, in angiographic series, fistulas to the MPA and to the left side of the heart are more common.[9]

Pathophysiology

The pathophysiological effects are related to the volume of blood flowing through the fistula, the chamber into which the fistula drains, and the presence of myocardial ischemia that may result from a coronary steal.

Coronary fistulas to the right side of the circulation result in a left-to-right shunt. This is commonly modest in size, rarely greater than 1.8 to 1. When the fistula enters a left-sided chamber it produces run-off from the aorta mimicking aortic valve regurgitation.

Clinical Presentation

The majority of infants and children with coronary fistulas are asymptomatic, and symptoms tend to occur in adult life. In the Green Lane series, 15 of 27 patients presented in adult life.[9] In another surgical series, 80% of patients under 20 years of age were asymptomatic compared with only 40% older than 20 years of age.[46] Spontaneous closure is rare, occurring in only 1–2% of fistulas.[64]

The most common symptoms are exertional dyspnea and fatigue. Congestive heart failure is much more common in patients with a fistula to the coronary sinus[61] and in older patients. The onset of atrial fibrillation in older patients as a result of right atrial dilation from a fistula to the right atrium may also precipitate symptoms.

Examination usually reveals a continuous murmur. There may be evidence of cardiomegaly and ventricular hypertrophy. Large fistulas to the left-sided heart chambers may be associated with a collapsing pulse.

Complications of Fistulas

A variety of complications may occur before the onset of heart failure. *Bacterial endocarditis* at the fistula is reported in 5–10% of cases, presumably related to the turbulent flow.[21] This figure is derived from surgical series in an earlier era and may significantly overstate the current risk, particularly for a small fistula. *Rupture of a fistula* may occur, but is a rare complication, usually the result of aneurysmal dilation of the arterial wall weakened by atherosclerosis or a congenital defect.[5,11,29] *Myocardial infarction*, *aneurysm formation*, and *congestive heart failure* may occur.

Diagnostic Techniques

The *ECG* is normal in about 50% of the surgical patients described in the literature. In the remainder, it may show right or left ventricular hypertrophy from volume overload. Atrial fibrillation may be present in older patients with fistulas to the right atrium. An ischemic pattern is more likely if the coronary steal involves a major branch of the LCA.

The *chest radiograph* may show cardiomegaly and pulmonary plethora.

2-D ECG may establish the diagnosis, demonstrating the origin and drainage site, or provide clues such as coronary dilation or chamber enlargement.

MRI is increasingly utilized to achieve noninvasive diagnosis, but most reports so far are case reports or small series.[85,89] However, with increasingly detailed scans, it will probably reduce the need for cardiac catheterization.

Role of Cardiac Catheter

Catheterization and coronary angiography are still usually required for definitive diagnosis and planning management, and increasingly the interventional cardiologist is able to occlude fistulas at the time of catheter study.

Surgical Management

The conduct of the operation has changed little over time. The approach is generally through a median sternotomy, with the bypass circuit available if needed. About 50% of fistulas can be exposed and either ligated or divided epicardially in the beating heart. Intraoperative transesophageal echocardiography (TOE) can be used to assess the resolution of the fistula and to detect any regional wall motion abnormalities related to induced ischemia.

There are three main surgical techniques utilized, or a combination of these methods. The first and most common one is epicardial identification and mobilization of the fistula, with ligation or division of the fistula. Secondly, an arteriotomy can be performed in the dilated proximal coronary artery, close to the fistula site, to oversew the fistula from within the lumen. Last, the fistulous connection(s) can be exposed from within the cardiac chambers and closed by direct suture.

Indications for CPB include the following:

1. Fistulas that are inaccessible, such as in the left atrioventricular groove or on the posterior surface of the heart
2. Aneurysms of the coronary artery requiring excision
3. For treatment of coexisting cardiac lesions that require repair

When necessary, CPB is performed with aortic and bicaval cannulation, because access to the right heart chambers is usually necessary. The fistula may be approached while the heart is beating, which allows better confirmation of complete closure at the time of ablation. If cardioplegic arrest is instituted, the fistula should be temporarily occluded to minimize run-off through the fistula, thereby ensuring delivery to the myocardium. The fistula may then be exposed by opening the dilated coronary artery on the epicardial surface, in order to oversew the fistula from within the artery, or the fistula can be exposed from within the heart and the opening closed off.

Transcatheter Occlusion

Fistulas have been closed by a number of techniques—coils,[65,68] detachable balloons,[43] and umbrella devices.[65] However, many fistulas cannot be closed by this approach, and there is an important incidence of device embolization. The requirements for safe and satisfactory closure include the ability to cannulate the coronary artery supplying the fistula, absence of large branches that might be inadvertently embolized, and a single, narrow fistula site.

The major contraindications to catheter occlusion include very young age, a large and wide fistula, a fistula with multiple communications, a distal fistula, an adjacent vessel at risk, and the need for other concomitant surgical repair.[51]

Results of Surgery

Mortality in current series is very low. Recent studies[9,47,51] all report no mortality and a very low rate of recurrence.

Complications of surgery are uncommon, but can include myocardial ischemia, either temporary or rarely progressing to infarction, arrhythmias, and fistula recurrence in 4% of cases.

REFERENCES

1. Arciniegas E, Farooki ZQ, Hakimi M, Green E: Management of anomalous left coronary artery from the pulmonary artery. Circulation 62(Suppl I):180–189, 1980.
2. Amanullah MM, Hamilton JR, Hasan A: Anomalous left coronary artery from the pulmonary artery: creating an autogenous arterial conduit for aortic implantation. Eur J Cardiothor Surg 20:853–855, 2001.
3. Ando M, Mee RBB, Duncan BW, et al: Creation of a dual-coronary system for anomalous origin of the left coronary artery from the pulmonary artery utilizing the trapdoor flap method. Eur J Cardiothor Surg 22:576–581, 2002.
4. Apley J, Horton RE, Wilson MG: The possible role of surgery in the treatment of anomalous left coronary artery. Thorax 12: 28–33, 1957.
5. Arraya I, Oda Y, Yamamoto K, et al: Surgical experience with congenital coronary AV fistula. Jpn J Thorac Surg 19:281–284, 1966.
6. Asou T, Karl TR, Pawade A, Mee RB: Arterial switch: translocation of intramural coronary arteries. Ann Thorac Surg 57:461–465, 1993.
7. Azakie A, Russell JL, McCrindle BW, et al: Anatomic repair of anomalous left coronary artery from the pulmonary artery by aortic reimplantation: early survival, patterns of ventricular recovery and late outcome. Ann Thor Surg 75:1535–1541, 2003.
8. Backer CL, Stout MJ, Zales VR, et al: Anomalous origin of the left coronary artery. A twenty year review of surgical management. J Thorac Cardiovasc Surg 103:1049–1058, 1992.
9. Barrett-Boyes BG, Kirklin JW: Congenital anomalies of the coronary arteries. In: Kirklin JW, Barratt-Boyes BG, eds. Cardiac Surgery, 2nd ed. New York: Churchill Livingstone, 1993, pp. 1167–1177.
10. Barth MJ, Allen BS, Gulecyuz M, et al: Experience with an alternative technique for the management of anomalous left coronary artery from the pulmonary artery. Ann Thor Surg 761429–1434, 2003.
11. Bauer HH, Allmendinger PD, Flaherty J, et al: Congenital coronary arteriovenous fistula: spontaneous rupture and cardiac tamponade. Ann Thor Surg 62:1521–1523, 1996.
12. Braunwald E, Rutherford JD: Reversible ischemic left ventricular dysfunction: evidence for the "hibernating myocardium." J Am Coll Cardiol 8:1467–1470, 1986.
13. Bregman D, Brennan FJ, Singer A, et al: Anomalous origin of the right coronary artery from the pulmonary artery. J Thorac Cardiovasc Surg72:626–630, 1976.
14. Bunton R, Jonas RA, Lang P, et al: Anomalous origin of left coronary artery from pulmonary artery. Ligation versus establishment of a two coronary system. J Thorac Cardiovasc Surg 93:103–108, 1987.
15. Chaitman BR, Bourassa MG, Lesperance J, Grondin P: Anomalous left coronary artery from pulmonary artery: an eight year angiographic follow-up after saphenous vein bypass graft. Circulation 51:552–555, 1975.
16. Chan RK, Hare DL, Buxton BF: Anomalous left main coronary artery arising from the pulmonary artery in an adult: treatment by internal mammary artery grafting. J Thorac Cardiovasc Surg 109:393–394, 1995.
17. Cochrane AD, Austin C, Goh TH, Karl TR: Incipient left ventricular rupture complicating anomalous left coronary artery. Ann Thorac Surg 67:254–256, 1999.
18. Cochrane AD, Coleman DM, Davis AM, et al: Excellent long-term functional outcome after an operation for anomalous left coronary artery from the pulmonary artery. J Thorac Cardiovasc Surg 117:332–342, 1999.
19. Cooley DA, Hallman GL, Bloodwell RD: Definitive surgical treatment of anomalous origin of left coronary artery from pulmonary artery: indications and results. J Thorac Cardiovasc Surg 52:798–808, 1966.
20. Cottrill CM, Davis D, McMillen M, et al: Anomalous left coronary artery from the pulmonary artery: significance of associated intracardiac defects. J Am Coll Cardiol 6:237–242, 1985.

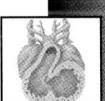

21. Daniel TM, Graham TP, Sabiston DC. Coronary artery- right ventricular fistula with congestive heart failure: surgical correction in the neonatal period. Surgery 67:985–994, 1970.
22. Douard H, Barat JL, Laurent F, et al: Magnetic resonance imaging of an anomalous origin of the left coronary artery from the pulmonary artery. Eur Heart J 9:1356–1360, 1988.
23. Driscoll DJ, Nihill MR, Mullins CE, et al: Management of symptomatic infants with anomalous origin of the left coronary artery from the pulmonary artery. Am J Cardiol 47:642–648, 1981.
24. Driscoll DJ, Garson A Jr, McNamara DG: Anomalous origin of the left coronary artery from the right pulmonary artery in association with complex congenital heart disease. Cathet Cardiovasc Diagn 1:55–61, 1982.
25. Edwards JE: The direction of blood flow in coronary arteries arising from the pulmonary trunk. Circulation 29:163–166, 1964.
26. Fernandes ED, Kadivar H, Hallman GL, et al: Congenital malformations of the coronary arteries: the Texas Heart Institute experience. Ann Thorac Surg 54:732–740, 1992.
27. George JM, Knowlan DM: Anomalous origin of the left coronary artery from the pulmonary artery in an adult. N Engl J Med 261:993–998, 1959.
28. Goldblatt E, Adams AP, Ross IK, et al: Single-trunk anomalous origin of both coronary arteries from the pulmonary artery. J Thorac Cardiovasc Surg 87:59–65, 1984.
29. Habermann JH, Howard ML, Johnson ES: Rupture of the coronary sinus with hemopericardium. A rare complication of coronary arteriovenous fistula. Circulation 28:1143–1144, 1963.
30. Huddleston CB, Balzer DT, Mendeloff EN: Repair of anomalous left main coronary artery arising from the pulmonary artery in infants: long-term impact on the mitral valve. Ann Thor Surg 71:1985–1989, 2001.
31. Kakou Guikahue M, Sidi D, Kachaner J, et al: Anomalous left coronary artery arising from the pulmonary artery in infancy: is early operation better? Brit Heart J60:522–526, 1988.
32. Kandzari DE, Harrison JK, Behar VS: An anomalous left coronary artery originating from the pulmonary artery in a 72-year old woman: diagnosis by colour flow myocardial blush and coronary arteriography. J Invasive Cardiol 14:96–99, 2002.
33. Karim MA: Coronary artery aneurysmal fistula: a late complication of stent deployment. Int J Cardiol 57:207–209, 1996.
34. Karl TR: Extracorporeal circulatory support in infants and children. Semin Thorac Cardiovasc Surg 6:154–160, 1994.
35. Karl TR, Cochrane AD: Anomalous origin of the left coronary artery from the pulmonary artery. In: Buxton B, Frazier OH, Westaby S, (eds): Ischemic Heart Disease: Surgical Management, St Louis: Mosby, 1999.
36. Katsumata T, Westaby S: Anomalous left coronary artery from the pulmonary artery: a simple method for aortic implantation with autogenous arterial tissue. Ann Thor Surg 68:1090–1091, 1999.
37. Kawasaki T: Acute febrile mucocutaneous syndrome with lymphoid involvement with specific desquamation of the fingers and toes in children. Jpn J Allergy 16: 178-222, 1967.
38. Kimbiris D, Iskandrian AS, Segal BL, Bemis CE. Anomalous origin of coronary arteries. Circulation 58:606–615, 1978.
39. Kirklin JW, Barratt-Boyes BG (eds): Cardiac Surgery, 2nd ed. New York: Churchill Livingstone, 1993, pp. 1167–1193.
40. Kitamura S: Kawasaki disease. In: Buxton B, Frazier OH, Westaby S (eds): Ischemic Heart Disease: Surgical Management, St Louis: Mosby, 1999, pp. 267–270.
41. Kitamura S, Kameda Y, Seki T, et al: Long-term outcome of myocardial revascularization in patients with Kawasaki coronary artery disease: A multi-centre cooperative study. J Thorac Cardiovasc Surg 107:663–674, 1994.
42. Koenig PR, Kimball TR, Schwartz DC: Coronary artery fistula complicating the evaluation of Kawasaki disease. Pediatr Cardiol 14:179–180, 1993.
43. Krabill KA, Hunter DW: Transcatheter closure of congenital coronary arterial fistula with a detachable balloon. Pediatr Cardiol 14:176–178, 1993.
44. Levin SE, Dansky R, Kinsley RH: Origin of left coronary artery from right pulmonary artery co-existing with coarctation of the aorta. Int J Cardiol 27:31–36, 1990.
45. Levin DC, Fellows KE, Abrams HL: Hemodynamically significant primary anomalies of the coronary arteries. Circulation 58:25–34, 1978.
46. Liberthson RR, Sagar K, Berkoben JP, et al: Congenital coronary arteriovenous fistula. Report of 13 patients, review of the literature and delineation of management. Circulation 59:849–854, 1979.
47. Lowe JE, Oldham HN Jr, Sabiston DC Jr. Surgical management of congenital coronary artery fistulas. Ann Surg 194:373–380, 1981.
48. Mahle WT: A dangerous case of colic: anomalous left coronary artery presenting with paroxysms of irritability. Pediatr Emerg Care 14:24–27, 1998.
49. Makoto A, Mee RBB, Duncan BW, et al: Creation of a dual-coronary system for anomalous origin of the left coronary artery from the pulmonary artery utilizing the trapdoor flap method. Eur J Cardiothor Surg 22:576–581, 2002.
50. Masel, LF: Tetralogy of Fallot with origin of the left coronary from the right pulmonary artery. Med J Aust 1:213–217, 1960.
51. Mavroudis C, Backer CL, Rocchini AP, et al: Coronary artery fistulas in infants and children : a surgical review and discussion of coil embolization. Ann Thorac Surg 63:1235–1242, 1997.
52. McMahon CJ, Di Bardino DJ, Undar A, Fraser CD Jr: Anomalous origin of the left coronary artery from the right pulmonary artery in association with type three aortopulmonary window and interrupted aortic arch. Ann Thor Surg 74:919–921, 2002.
53. McNamara JJ, Gross RE: Congenital coronary artery fistula. Surgery 65:59–69, 1969.
54. Mesurolle B, Qanadli SD, Merad M, et al: Anomalous origin of the left coronary artery arising from the pulmonary trunk: report of an adult case with long-term follow-up after surgery. Eur Radiol 9:1570–1573, 1999.
55. Meyer BW, Stefanik G, Stiles QR, et al: A method of definitive surgical treatment of anomalous origin of left coronary artery. J Thorac Cardiovasc Surg 56:104–107, 1968.
56. Molinari G, Balbi M, Bertero G, et al: Magnetic resonance imaging in Bland-White-Garland syndrome. Am Heart J 129:1040–1042, 1995.
57. Montigny M, Stanley P, Chartrand C, et al: Postoperative evaluation after end-to-end subclavian-left coronary artery anastomosis in anomalous left coronary artery. J Thorac Cardiovasc Surg 100:270–273, 1990.
58. Murthy KS, Krishnanaik S, Mohanty SR, et al: A new repair for anomalous left coronary artery. Ann Thorac Surg 71:1384–1386, 2001.
59. Neches WH, Mathews RA, Park SC, et al: Anomalous origin of the left coronary artery from the pulmonary artery. Circulation 50:582–587, 1974.
60. Nielsen HB, Perko M, Aldershvile J, Saunamaki K: Cardiac arrest during exercise: anomalous left coronary artery from the pulmonary trunk. Scand Cardiovasc J 33:369–371, 1999.
61. Ogden JA, Stansel HC: Coronary artery fistulas terminating in the coronary venous system. J Thorac Cardiovasc Surg 63: 172–182, 1972.
62. Ortiz E, de Leval M, Somerville J: Ductus arteriosus associated with an anomalous left coronary artery arising from the pulmonary artery: catastrophe after duct ligation. Br Heart J55:415–417, 1986.

63. Ortiz de Salazar A, Gonzalez JA, Zuazo J, et al: Anomalous left coronary artery originating from the pulmonary artery in an adult. Texas Heart Inst J 23:296–297, 1996.
64. Perloff JK: Congenital coronary arterial fistula. In: Clinical Recognition of Congenital Heart Disease. Philadelphia: WB Saunders, 2003, pp.443–456.
65. Perry SB, Rome J, Keane JF, et al: Transcatheter closure of coronary artery fistulas. J Am Coll Cardiol 20:205–209, 1992.
66. Piechaud JF, Shalaby L, Kachaner J, et al: Pulmonary artery "stop-flow" angiography to visualize the anomalous origin of the left coronary artery from the pulmonary artery in infants. Pediatr Cardiol 8:11–15, 1987.
67. Post JC, vanRossum AC, Bronzwaer JGF, et al: Magnetic resonance angiography of anomalous coronary arteries. A new gold standard for delineating the proximal course? Circulation 92:3163–3171, 1995.
68. Reidy JF, Anjos RT, Qureshi SA, et al: Transcatheter embolization in the treatment of coronary artery fistulas. J Am Coll Cardiol 18:187–192, 1991.
69. Rein AJJT, Colan SD, Parness IA, et al: Regional and global left ventricular function in infants with anomalous origin of the left coronary artery from the pulmonary trunk: preoperative and postoperative assessment. Circulation 75:115–123, 1987.
70. Saito T, Fuse K, Kato M, et al: Anomalous left main coronary artery arising from the pulmonary artery in an adult: treatment by direct reimplantation. Surgery Today 26:453–456, 1996.
71. Santoro G, di Carlo D, Carotti A, et al: Origin of both coronary arteries from the right pulmonary artery and coarctation. Ann Thor Surg 60:706–708, 1995.
72. Sarris GE, Drummond-Webb JJ, Ebeid MR, et al: Anomalous origin of left coronary from right pulmonary artery in hypoplastic left heart syndrome. Ann Thor Surg 64:836–838, 1997.
73. Schwartz ML, Jonas RA, Colan SD: Anomalous origin of left coronary artery from pulmonary artery: recovery of left ventricular function after dual coronary repair. J Am Coll Cardiol 30:547–553, 1997.
74. Sese A, Imoto Y: New technique in the transfer of an anomalously originated left coronary artery to the aorta. Ann Thorac Surg 53:527–529, 1992.
75. Smith A, Arnold R, Anderson RH, et al: Anomalous origin of the left coronary artery from the pulmonary trunk. Anatomic findings in relation to pathophysiology and surgical repair. J Thorac Cardiovasc Surg 98:16–24, 1989.
76. Sreeram N, Hunter S, Wren C: Acute myocardial infarction in infancy: unmasking of anomalous origin of the left coronary artery from the pulmonary artery by ligation of an arterial duct. Br Heart J 61:307–308, 1989.
77. Starnes VA, Bernstein D, Oyer PE, et al: Heart transplantation in children. J Heart Transplant 8:20–26, 1989.
78. Takenaga M, Matsuda J, Miyamoto N, et al: Magnetic resonance imaging of Bland-White-Garland syndrome: a case of anomalous origin of the left coronary artery from the pulmonary trunk in a 22-year old woman. Jpn Circ J62:219–221, 1998.
79. Takeuchi S, Imamura H, Katsumoto K, et al: New surgical method for repair of anomalous left coronary artery from pulmonary artery. J Thorac Cardiovasc Surg 78:7, 1979.
80. Tashiro T, Todo K, Haruta Y, et al: Anomalous origin of the left coronary artery from the pulmonary artery: New operative technique. J Thorac Cardiovasc Surg 106:718–722, 1993.
81. Taylor AM, Thorne SA, Rubens P, et al: Coronary artery imaging in grown up congenital heart disease: Complementary role of magnetic resonance and X-ray coronary angiography. Circulation 101:1670, 2000.
82. Towbin JA: Myocardial infarction in childhood. In: Garson A, Bricker JT, McNamara DG (eds.): The science and practice of pediatric cardiology. Philadelphia: Lea & Febiger, 1990, p. 1684.
83. Turley K, Szarnicki RJ, Flachbart KD, et al: Aortic implantation is possible in all cases of anomalous origin of the left coronary artery from the pulmonary artery. Ann Thorac Surg 60:84–89, 1995.
84. Tyrrell MJ, Duncan WJ, Hayton RC, Bharadwaj BB: Anomalous left coronary artery from the pulmonary artery: effect of coronary anatomy on clinical course. Angiology 38: 833–840, 1987.
85. Vandenbossche JL, Felice H, Grivegnee A, et al: Noninvasive imaging of left coronary arteriovenous fistula. Chest 93: 885–887, 1988.
86. Vigneswaran WT, Campbell DN, Pappas G, et al: Evolution of the management of anomalous left coronary artery: a new surgical approach. Ann Thorac Surg 48:560–564, 1989.
87. Vouhe PR, Bailloot-Vernant F, Trinquet F, et al: Anomalous left coronary artery from the pulmonary artery in infants. Which operation? When? J Thorac Cardiovasc Surg 94: 192–199, 1987.
88. Vouhe PR, Tamisier D, Sidi D, et al: Anomalous left coronary artery from the pulmonary artery: results of isolated aortic reimplantation. Ann Thorac Surg 54:621–626, 1992.
89. Wertheimer JH, Toto A, Goldman A, et al: Magnetic resonance imaging and two-dimensional and Doppler echocardiography in the diagnosis of coronary cameral fistula. Am Heart J 114(I Pt 1):159–162, 1987.
90. Wesselhoeft H, Fawcett JS, Johnson AL: Anomalous origin of the left coronary artery from the pulmonary trunk. Its clinical spectrum, pathology, and pathophysiology, based on a review of 140 cases with seven further cases. Circulation 38:403–425, 1968.

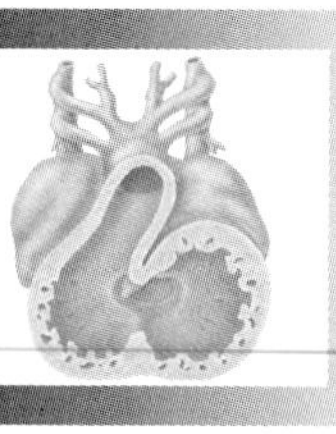

CHAPTER 121

Transposition of the Great Arteries

Andrew J. Lodge and Thomas L. Spray

HISTORY

Transposition of the great arteries (TGA) was first recognized and described over two centuries ago. Although reference was made to malposition of the aorta and pulmonary artery (PA) by Steno in 1672 and Morgagni in 1761, the anatomical description of TGA is credited to Baillie in 1797.[4] It was Farre in 1814 who introduced the term transposition of aorta and PA, meaning that the aorta and PA are displaced across the ventricular septum.[23] An attempt to classify the various types of transposition was reported by Von Rokitansky,[77] and the first clinical recognition of TGA in life was noted by Fanconi in 1932.[22] In 1938, Taussig described the pathological anatomy and hemodynamic and clinical characteristics of the cardiac defect.[72]

With the development of cardiac surgery in the 1950s, effective therapy for this disease has only become available relatively recently. Initial treatments were palliative and included atrial septectomy, first described by Blalock and Hanlon.[6] The first successful attempts to re-route the circulations were at the atrial level. These were followed later by successful arterial level repair and correction of TGA and ventricular septal defect (VSD). These developments are further described in the following section.

EPIDEMIOLOGY

Today TGA is known to be relatively common, accounting for 9.9% of infants with congenital heart disease, or 0.206 per 1000 live births, in one New England study.[27] There is a 2:1 male-to-female ratio that increases to 3.3:1 when the ventricular septum is intact.[44] In complex forms of transposition, gender predominance has not been noted. If TGA is not treated, 90% of children with D-TGA and intact septum will die by 1 year of age.

CLASSIFICATION AND EMBRYOLOGY

TGA is generally classified as a type of conotruncal abnormality, a group of abnormalities that has a common theme of deranged development of the cardiac outflow tract. In this disease there is ventriculoarterial (VA) discordance—the aorta arises from the right ventricle and the PA from the left ventricle. The more common form of the disease is associated with otherwise normal cardiac structural relationships, including normal ventricular (D) looping. There is atrioventricular (AV) concordance but VA discordance {S,D,D}. This set of relationships is commonly referred to as D-transposition (D-TGA). In this form of TGA the aorta is, by definition, anterior and to the right of the PA. This pattern results in the systemic and pulmonary circulations occurring in parallel rather than in series. As a consequence, deoxygenated blood is continuously pumped to the body and never passes through the lungs, and oxygenated blood is recirculated through the lungs and does not supply the rest of the body. For the patient to survive there is an obligatory shunt elsewhere, usually at the level of the atrial septum that allows mixing of oxygenated and deoxygenated blood.

Although some have used the term transposition to describe a discordant VA connection, other authors have used transposition to describe any heart in which the aorta is anterior to the PA. Use of the term TGA is confused by the use of this definition in some patients with double inlet ventricle or absent AV connection and in patients with nonlateralized atrial arrangements (some heterotaxy syndromes). D-TGA has also been used to describe a concordant AV and discordant VA arrangement, but this nomenclature does not adequately describe patients in whom the aorta is anterior and to the left of the PA. Thus, in this section complete TGA is defined as normal atrial situs, AV concordance, and VA discordance.

Several theories have been advanced regarding the morphogenesis of the abnormal relationship between the great arteries and the ventricles in TGA. It has been suggested that the subaortic conus persists and develops during normal looping of the ventricles while the subpulmonary conus undergoes absorption and thus establishes eventual fibrous continuity between the mitral and pulmonary valves, the reverse of the normal situation.[75] In the normal heart the subaortic conus does not grow, and dominant growth of the pulmonary conus forces the pulmonary valve anterior, superior, and to the left. In transposition, differential growth of the subaortic conus pushes the aorta anteriorly and disrupts aortic to mitral valve continuity. If the subpulmonary conus fails to develop, the PA will maintain a posterior location and pulmonary to mitral valve continuity will occur. As a consequence of this relationship, the aortic valve becomes anterior to the pulmonary valve, permitting both semilunar valves to connect with the distal great vessels without the rotation that is hypothesized to occur in normal cardiac development. Because conal development determines rotation of the truncus arteriosus, the great arteries are similar in relationship at the semilunar valves as they are at the arch, resulting in no twist in the great arteries.

Some debate also exists about the relationship between the various conotruncal abnormalities, which also include tetralogy of Fallot and double outlet right ventricle. Recent evidence suggests that TGA may be unique in that it is not seen in the spectrum of conotruncal abnormalities generated from the most common experimental model of these disorders.[41] A new animal model, which is the most reliable to date for producing isolated D-TGA, suggests that TGA may be due to abnormal migration of neural crest cells during a critical phase of outflow tract development.[13]

ANATOMY

Anatomical variations in TGA are often encountered. Normal atrial situs occurs in 95% of patients, while left-to-right juxtaposition of the atrial appendages signals the presence of other intracardiac anomalies. Although a true ostium secundum atrial septal defect (ASD) is present in 10% to 20% of cases, the majority of atrial communications are through a patent foramen ovale. Right aortic arch is present in 4% of patients with intact ventricular septum and up to 16% of those with VSD.[50] Up to 50% of patients with TGA have an associated VSD, many of which spontaneously close.[52] The VSDs are commonly perimembranous, although they may be found anywhere in the ventricular septum. Pulmonary stenosis (PS) or atresia, overriding or straddling AV valves, coarctation of the aorta, and interruption of the aortic arch have all been noted in association with transposition and VSD.

The spatial relationship of the great vessels is quite variable; however, the aorta is most frequently to the right and anterior to the PA. In almost all cases, the sinuses of Valsalva and the coronary artery ostia face the corresponding pulmonary arterial sinuses. This situation is favorable for transfer of the coronary arteries with the arterial switch operation (ASO), although the origin of a coronary artery from a nonfacing sinus poses a problem for arterial switch in only a small number of patients. Many classification systems have been used to describe the coronary anatomy in TGA. The most widely accepted scheme within the surgical community is the Leiden classification system, which is depicted with the other common systems of classification in Figure 121-1. The most common coronary pattern in D-TGA (68%) consists of the left main coronary arising from the leftward coronary sinus, giving rise to the left anterior descending and circumflex coronary arteries.[30] The right coronary arises as a separate ostium from the rightward posterior-facing sinus. Occasionally, there is no true circumflex coronary artery but separate branches arise from the left coronary to supply the corresponding portion of the left ventricle. In up to 20% of cases, the circumflex coronary arises from the right coronary artery off the rightward posterior-facing sinus and passes behind the PA. The left anterior descending artery then arises from a separate coronary ostium off the left coronary sinus. More rare coronary patterns involve a single right coronary artery from the rightward posterior sinus (4.5%) or a single left coronary artery from the leftward coronary sinus (1.5%).[18] Intramural coronary arteries that proceed in the aortic wall for a distance before exiting to the epicardial surface have been described and commonly occur at the commissural attachment of the semilunar valve.[42] Single coronary ostium or separate ostia close together arising from a single sinus have also been described. Abnormal coronary anatomy is more commonly seen in transposition with VSD than in the intact septum variety. Abnormal coronary patterns have also been found to be more common when the relationship of the great arterial trunks is not usual (aorta anterior and to the right).[48]

Important left ventricular outflow tract obstruction is unusual in association with TGA but has significant implications for the management of these neonates. The most common type of left ventricular outflow tract obstruction is dynamic, developing in patients with TGA and an intact ventricular septum as a result of leftward displacement of the muscular ventricular septum secondary to the development of higher systemic right ventricular pressures. The septum may then narrow the outflow tract, resulting in abnormal systolic anterior mitral leaflet motion and a situation similar to that noted in hypertrophic obstructive cardiomyopathy. Occasionally, a subvalvular fibrous ridge may produce subvalvular obstruction. Posterior malalignment of the ventricular septum may produce a more tunnel-type obstruction. In addition, fibrous tags arising from the mitral apparatus or membranous septum may result in significant subvalvular obstruction, more commonly when a VSD is present. Valvular stenosis is uncommon, although a bicuspid pulmonary valve has frequently been noted. In rare cases,

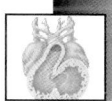

		G.*	Q.	Y.
Usual coronary anatomy in TGA 68%	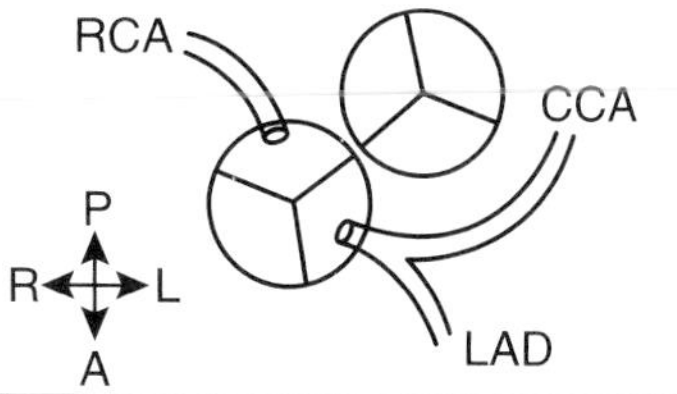	A I	1LCx–2R	A
Circumflex coronary from the right coronary artery 14%	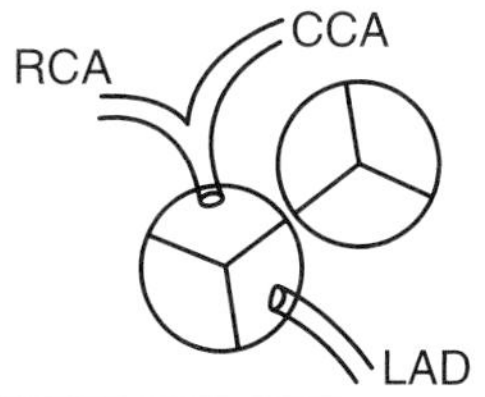	AB I	1L–2CxR	D
Single right coronary artery 4.5%	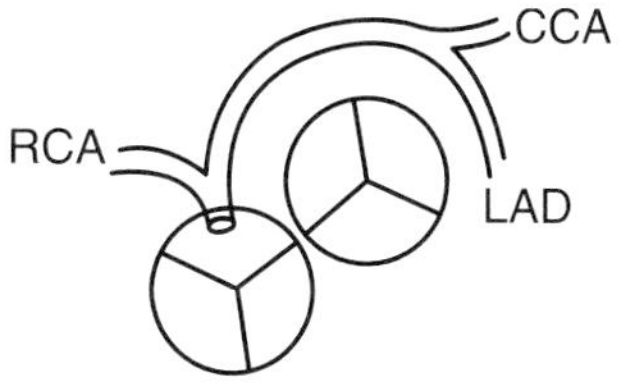	B I	2LCxR	—
Single left coronary artery 1.5%	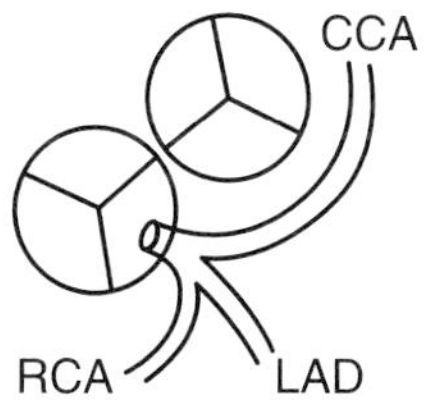	A II	1RLCx	—
Inverted origin of the coronary arteries 3%	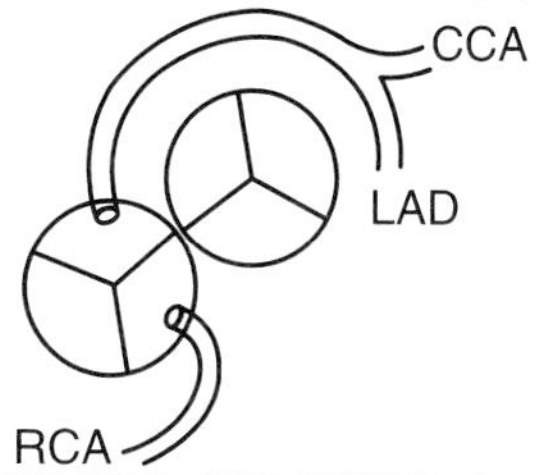	B II	1R–2LCx	—
Inverted origin of the circumflex and right coronary artery 7%	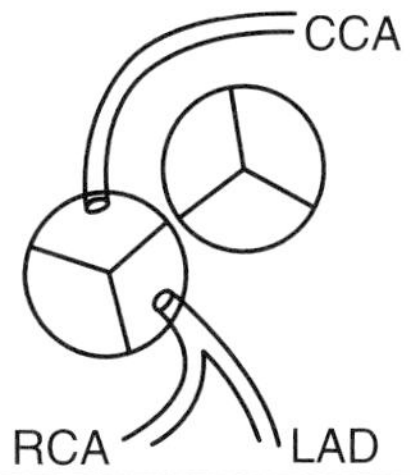	AB II	1RL–2Cx	E

* G., Gittenberger-de-Groot; Q., Quaegebeur; Y., Yacoub

Figure 121–1 The six most common types of coronary artery anatomy in TGA. Descriptive classification is on the left, and three simplified classification codes are described on the right. *(From DiDonato RM, Castañeda AR: Anatomic correction of transposition of the great arteries at the arterial level. In: Sabiston DC Jr., Spencer FC [eds.]: Surgery of the Chest, 5th ed. Philadelphia: WB Saunders, 1990, pp. 1435–1451.)*

aortic arch obstruction with coarctation or true interruption of the aortic arch has been observed in patients with TGA, left ventricular outflow tract obstruction, and VSD.[11]

CLINICAL FEATURES

In complete TGA the pulmonary and systemic circulations exist in parallel instead of in series. This results in nonoxygenated venous blood passing through the right ventricle to the aorta while the oxygenated pulmonary venous blood passes through the left ventricle back to the pulmonary arterial circulation. Mixing between the pulmonary and systemic circulations through a patent foramen ovale or ASD, a VSD, or a patent ductus arteriosus (PDA) is mandatory for survival. Patients with TGA and an intact ventricular septum survive initially because of aortopulmonary flow through a PDA. After birth, both ventricles are relatively noncompliant, and infants with TGA often have an increased pulmonary blood flow, which causes enlargement of the left atrium and functional incompetence of the foramen ovale, resulting in atrial-level mixing of oxygenated and nonoxygenated blood. Inadequacy of this mixing, however, may result in only marginal tissue oxygenation, which does not improve with oxygen administration.

Patients with TGA and significant VSD often have higher oxygen saturations by virtue of greater pulmonary blood flow and greater mixing at both atrial and ventricular levels. In children with high pulmonary blood flow, pulmonary resistance may progressively increase throughout infancy. Ferenz has observed significant histological changes in children older than 2 years of age with TGA, and children as young as 1 month of age have had intimal fibrosis noted in the PAs.[24] This early development of severe pulmonary vascular disease in children with TGA is exacerbated in patients with associated VSD, but early important pulmonary vascular disease can occur in patients with TGA regardless of the presence of a VSD as demonstrated by Ferguson in 1960[25] and Ferenz in 1966.[24] The rapidity of development of pulmonary obstructive disease may be related to hypoxemia associated with increased sympathetic activity and in association with excessive pulmonary blood flow.[21]

Although neonatal pulmonary vascular resistance is normal in infants with TGA, the resistance falls progressively during the neonatal period with associated changes in the pulmonary and systemic ventricular compliance. Shortly after birth in the normal infant there is an increase in the left ventricular volume load and pressure load and a decrease in right ventricular volume and pressure load. These physiologic changes result in a rapid increase in the left ventricular myocardial mass.[5] This normal development of the left ventricle is lost in infants with D-TGA where the left ventricle ejects to the lower resistance pulmonary vascular bed (Figure 121-2). Thus, the left ventricle does not increase muscle mass relative to the right ventricle and within a few weeks it loses the ability to maintain adequate cardiac output against significant afterload. This change occurs despite the fact that the left ventricle still maintains a volume load in patients with transposition and intact ventricular septum. When, however, a VSD or large PDA is present, both volume and pressure overload of the left ventricle is maintained, and in D-TGA with left ventricular outflow tract obstruction without a VSD a ventricular pressure load is imposed without a significant volume load. These physiological changes in the neonatal heart are important for the consideration of surgical approaches because after a few weeks to months of postuterine life, the left ventricle in D-TGA with intact ventricular septum takes on the characteristics and wall thickness of a pulmonary ventricle and may not be adequate to support the systemic circulation.

The most common clinical finding in the infant with TGA is cyanosis (arterial PO_2 of 25–40 mm Hg), which will vary in degree depending on associated anomalies. Typically, the cyanosis is more pronounced when the ventricular septum is intact and is often present at birth. The development of cyanosis later in infancy is usually associated with the presence of a significant VSD. Congestive heart failure may be the predominant clinical finding in patients with large VSD or PDA, and the combination of cyanosis and increased pulmonary blood flow is almost pathognomonic of TGA in the infant. Symptoms of cardiac failure rarely present in the first week of life, but commonly appear by 1 month of age as pulmonary vascular resistance decreases and pulmonary blood flow becomes excessive, even in the patient with an intact ventricular septum.

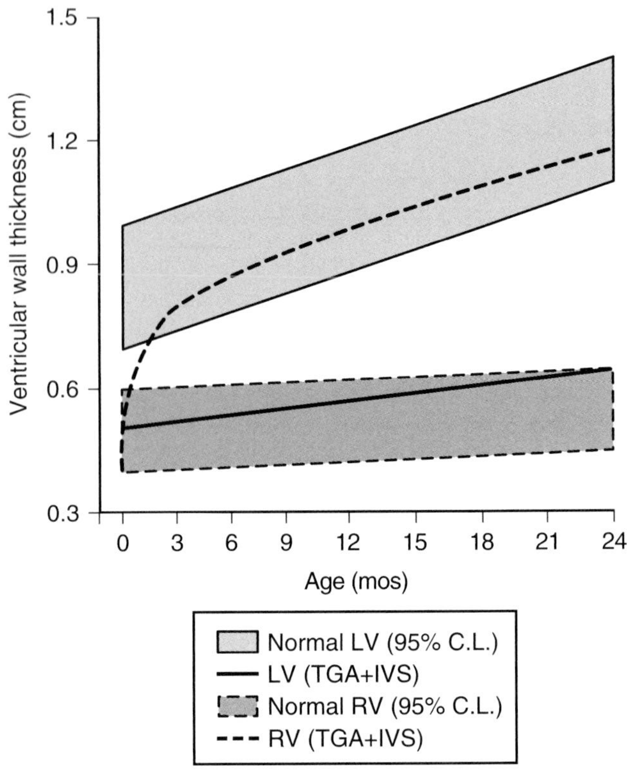

Figure 121–2 The normal left ventricular wall thickness in TGA at birth. The solid line shows the decreased development of left ventricular muscle mass in TGA that results from a rapid decrease in pulmonary vascular resistance and drop in left ventricular pressure. The upper bar shows increase in left ventricular thickness with normally related great arteries. The dashed line shows the similar increase in right ventricular muscle mass over time in TGA.
(From Castañeda AR, Jonas RA, Mayer JE Jr., Hanley FL.: D-transposition of the great arteries. In: Cardiac Surgery of the Neonate and Infant. Philadelphia: WB Saunders, 1994, pp. 409–438.)

DIAGNOSIS

Physical Examination

Cardiac examination typically reveals a mildly overactive precordium, and 75% of patients with TGA and intact ventricular septum have a soft systolic murmur. The second heart sound is typically single and loud because of the proximity of the aorta to the anterior chest wall, which may make assessment of pulmonary vascular resistance difficult.[21] End-diastolic gallop rhythms are often noted in patients with associated VSD. In the presence of a large PDA, the femoral pulses are often bounding. The liver may be enlarged in patients with a large systemic-to-pulmonary shunt and may be associated with tachypnea, intercostal retractions, and inability to successfully nurse. Children with significant valvular or subvalvular PS often have a crescendo/decrescendo cardiac murmur along the left sternal border transmitted to the right clavicular area.

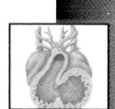

Diagnostic Studies

The electrocardiogram may be normal at birth but over time shows signs of increasing right ventricular or biventricular hypertrophy. Electrocardiographic findings vary depending on age, the presence or absence of a VSD, and the development of pulmonary vascular resistance. The axis may be normal in patients with a VSD, but typically right-axis deviation is noted in children with an intact ventricular septum. Chest X-ray findings in D-TGA include an egg-shaped cardiac configuration, narrow superior mediastinum, and increased pulmonary markings with cardiomegaly. Asymmetry of pulmonary blood flow due to preferential right pulmonary arterial flow may result in right-sided congestive changes. The chest roentgenogram may be normal at birth, although progressive development of prominent pulmonary markings usually occurs along with progressive cardiomegaly.

The widespread use of fetal ultrasound techniques has resulted in the common antenatal diagnosis of TGA. This fact and the fact that the majority of children with TGA are cyanotic in the first week of life have led to the initiation of treatment at a very early age. While in the past cardiac catheterization was generally necessary to confirm the diagnosis of TGA and to demonstrate the position of the cardiac chambers and the associated lesions, echocardiography is now usually all that is necessary in the majority of patients. Echocardiographic views confirming a posterior great vessel that divides into right and left PAs and arises from the left ventricle in association with an anterior aorta arising from a right ventricle confirms the diagnosis of TGA (Figure 121-3). The intracavitary shunts can be determined by Doppler echocardiography techniques, and several echo views can determine the size and location of VSDs with reference to the infundibular septum, the nature and size of atrial communications, the anatomy of the AV valves, and the presence and location of significant degrees of subpulmonary stenosis. In addition, in the majority of cases the origins and anatomical distributions of the coronary arteries can be adequately visualized by echocardiography (Figure 121-4). Because the majority of coronary arterial variations can be successfully addressed at operation, identification of the origins of the coronary arteries is usually sufficient by echocardiography to preclude angiography. Cardiac catheterization is now indicated only in infants in whom inadequate shunting is noted or infants with associated intracardiac or extracardiac abnormalities that require clarification. It is usually reserved for the purpose of enlarging the interatrial septal communication in those patients with significant clinical instability characterized by acidemia or severe hypoxemia (see following).

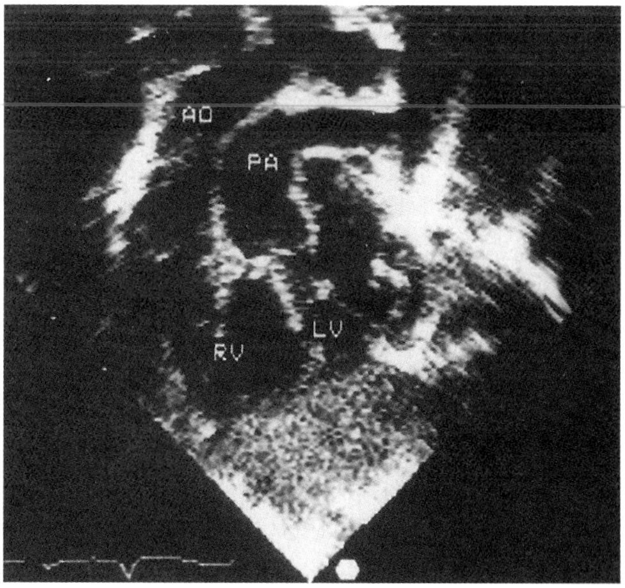

Figure 121–3 Subcostal sagittal view of the heart in D-TGA and intact ventricular septum. The anterior great vessel (AO) is the aorta, and the posterior great vessel that bifurcates is the pulmonary artery (PA). LV, left ventricle; RV, right ventricle. *(From Mavroudis C, Backer CL: D-transposition of the great arteries. In: Mavroudis C, Backer CL [eds.]: Pediatric Cardiac Surgery, 2nd ed. St. Louis: Mosby, 1994, pp. 339–366.)*

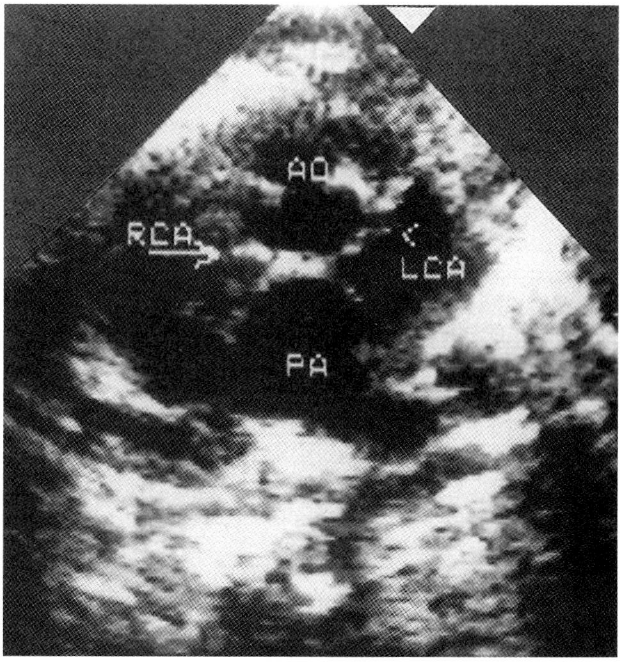

Figure 121–4 Parasternal short-axis view of the heart in D-TGA and intact ventricular septum with usual coronary anatomy. Coronary arteries are noted to arise from the left and right coronary cusps, and the pulmonary artery is posterior. AO, aorta; LCA, left coronary artery; PA, pulmonary artery; RCA, right coronary artery. *(From Mavroudis C, Backer CL: D-transposition of the great arteries. In: Mavroudis C, Backer CL [eds.]: Pediatric Cardiac Surgery, 2nd ed. St. Louis: Mosby, 1994, pp. 339–366.)*

PREOPERATIVE MEDICAL MANAGEMENT

Patients who are good anatomical candidates for an arterial switch procedure and have acceptable arterial oxygen saturation are generally referred for early operation if the clinical condition permits. Prostaglandin E1 is usually administered to maintain ductal patency, increase pulmonary blood flow, and improve stabilization of patients before early operative repair. Because relative dehydration may decrease the degree of interatrial shunting, volume infusions may improve hemodynamics in infants presenting with TGA and intact septum early in life. A major development in the treatment of TGA occurred in 1966 when Rashkind and Miller reported the use of a balloon catheter technique to enlarge the ASD in patients with TGA, causing improved early physiological stability.[63] If there is significant instability as evidenced by persistent acidemia or hypoxemia despite conservative measures, the mainstay of management has become a Rashkind balloon atrial septostomy.

In the neonate with TGA, left atrial pressure is usually greater than the right atrial pressure. The pressure in the pulmonary (left) ventricle is dependent on the presence or absence of a VSD, valvar or subvalvar stenosis, the age of the patient, and the magnitude of elevation of pulmonary vascular resistance. If inadequate interatrial shunting is noted, a Rashkind atrial septostomy is performed.[63] A balloon-tipped catheter is passed through the systemic veins, through the right atrium and foramen ovale, and into the left atrium; the balloon is inflated and pulled vigorously across the atrial septum to tear the foramen ovale, improving admixture of pulmonary and systemic venous blood and an improving tissue oxygen delivery. Although this procedure is usually performed at cardiac catheterization, it may be performed in the intensive care unit with echocardiographic guidance in children who are very unstable. Performance of a Rashkind atrial septostomy results in decompression of the left ventricle and therefore may result in poor left ventricular performance if a subsequent arterial switch procedure is delayed.

SURGICAL MANAGEMENT

Surgical Correction

Satisfactory correction of TGA results in rerouting of systemic venous blood to the pulmonary circulation and the pulmonary venous blood into the systemic arterial circulation. This may be accomplished at the atrial, the ventricular, or the great arterial level. The earliest repairs of TGA involve rerouting of the systemic and pulmonary venous returns at the atrial level, resulting in an adequate physiological repair but not an anatomical repair because the morphological right ventricle continues to be the systemic ventricle. Both ventricular (Rastelli) and great arterial (arterial switch) repairs are more anatomical corrections, resulting in a morphological left ventricle as the systemic ventricle.

Palliative Operations

Initial surgical therapy for TGA involved creation of an ASD using a closed technique to increase the mixing between systemic venous and pulmonary venous circulations by Blalock and Hanlon in 1950.[6] Although the early mortality was high with this operative approach, successful creation of an ASD resulted in significant palliation in many of these children. The introduction of the balloon atrial septostomy has essentially eliminated the need for operative atrial septectomy. Infants with associated cardiac abnormalities and a thick atrial septum who are considered for later atrial baffle repair may benefit from the Blalock-Hanlon technique, although the safety of cardiopulmonary bypass (CPB) has resulted in the common use of open atrial septectomy in these patients.

Pulmonary arterial banding has been used for palliation in patients with TGA and VSD in young infants who have intractable congestive heart failure until operative repair at 3 to 6 months of age. As the results with arterial switch procedure and VSD closure in infancy have improved, banding in most instances is unnecessary because complete repair can be accomplished in infancy. Therefore, banding of the PA has now been limited to very small neonates who might benefit from delay in corrective operation, those patients with TGA and intact ventricular septum who present late for arterial switch repair and require preparation of the left ventricle to become the systemic ventricle, and in patients who develop right ventricular dysfunction and failure after atrial baffle operations as a component of staged conversion to an arterial switch repair (see below). Pulmonary arterial banding in TGA is a delicate procedure, because limitation of pulmonary blood flow results in significant hypoxia and metabolic acidosis, and loose banding results in inadequate protection of the pulmonary vascular bed and poor development of the left (pulmonary) ventricle. Thus, in many situations where preparation of the left ventricle is undertaken for conversion to an arterial switch procedure, banding must be associated with creation of an aortopulmonary shunt to maintain adequate pulmonary blood flow and prevent hypoxemia and ventricular dysfunction.

Atrial Repairs

Initial attempts to reverse the transposed vessels in patients with TGA by both Mustard and Bailey and their colleagues were frustrated by their inability to maintain coronary perfusion and by poor function of the anatomic left ventricle.[3,54] Thus, initial surgical therapy was directed toward atrial transposition of pulmonary and systemic venous returns. In 1952, Lillehei and Varco transferred the right-sided pulmonary veins to the right atrium and connected the inferior vena cava to the left atrium.[45] A successful modification of this technique using an allograft to connect the inferior vena cava to the left atrium was described by Baffes in 1956.[2] In 1954 Albert suggested the concept of switching the atrial septum so that caval return was directed to the left ventricle and pulmonary venous return to the right ventricle at the atrial level.[1] This atrial switch concept was first successfully accomplished by Senning in 1959, using an ingenious technique for relocating the walls of the right atrium and the atrial septum.[68] In this operation, pulmonary and systemic venous return was rerouted by incising and realigning the atrial septum over the pulmonary veins and using the free right atrial wall to create a pulmonary venous baffle (Figure 121-5). The Senning operation was not associated with high survival at first because of its complexity and by the fact that the operation was performed in children between 1 and 2 years of age or with a VSD, and significant pulmonary vascular obstructive disease had already developed in many of these children.

In 1964, Mustard described an alternate procedure for intraatrial repair excising the atrial septum and creating a large interatrial baffle of pericardium to redirect pulmonary

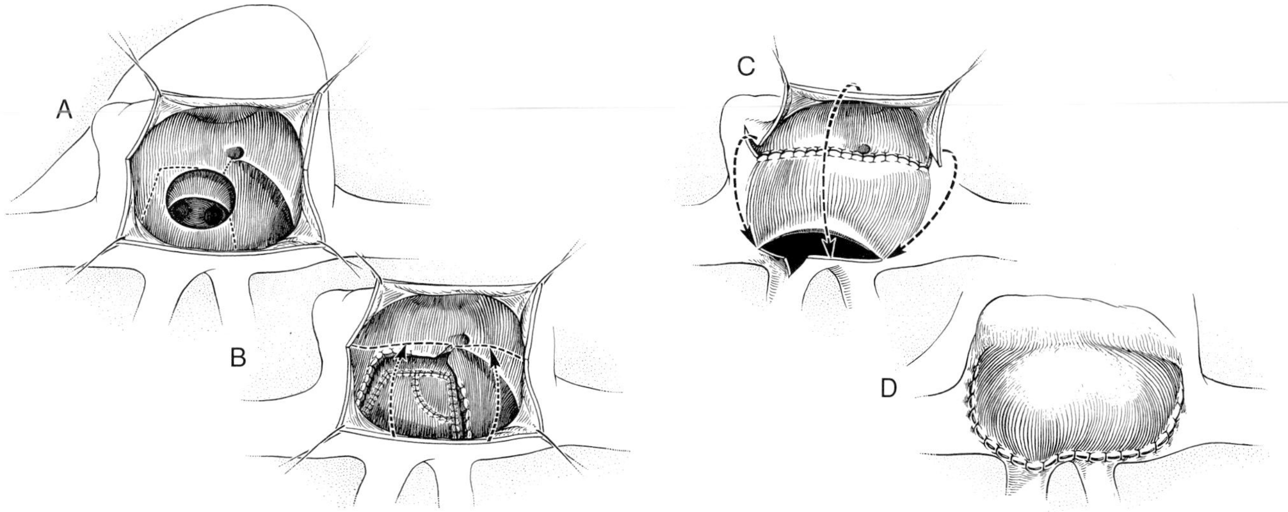

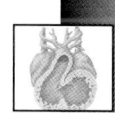

Figure 121–5 The Senning operation. A, View from the right atrium showing incision lines *(dashed lines)* to create a flap of the posterior atrial septum and an incision into the base of the coronary sinus. **B,** The posterior flap of atrial septum is augmented with a piece of pericardium and sutured inferiorly over the origins of the pulmonary veins in the left atrium. The posterior wall of the right atrium is then sutured to the anterior portion of the atrial septum, baffling the vena caval return across the septum to the mitral valve. **C,** After completion of the venous baffle, the anterior wall of the right atrium is sutured to an opening made in the left atrium posterior to the interatrial septum at the entrance point of the right pulmonary veins, baffling the pulmonary venous blood over the systemic venous pathway into the right ventricle. **D,** Completed suture line showing repair with autologous tissue.
(From Mavroudis C, Backer CL: D-transposition of the great arteries. In: Mavroudis C, Backer CL [eds.]: Pediatric Cardiac Surgery, 2nd ed. St. Louis: Mosby, 1994, pp. 339–366.)

and systemic venous blood (Figure 121-6).[53] This repair resulted in a larger atrial size than the Senning operation. In the Mustard operation, creation of a virtual common atrium is necessary with resection of the atrial septum and the ridge of tissue between the superior vena caval entrance and the superior aspect of the atrial septum. Inadequate resection of the atrial septum has resulted in the occurrence of baffle obstruction of the systemic venous return to the heart. Early results with the Mustard operation were markedly improved over the previously reported Senning repairs and reflected the significant number of patients in Toronto who had had successful Blalock-Hanlon atrial septectomies early in life. Because of its technical simplicity, the Mustard operation became the most commonly performed procedure for transposition over the decade of the 1960s, and it became clear that repair in the first few months of life could be accomplished with a low operative mortality and improved results compared with repair at a later age. In 1970, the Senning procedure reemerged as the persistent problems of baffle obstruction and arrhythmias following the Mustard operation became well defined, and the ability to use autologous tissue for the atrial reconstruction became a preferred approach. Performing the Senning operation in infancy after successful balloon atrial septostomy became the preferred technique in many centers.

Outcome After Senning and Mustard Operations

The Senning and Mustard operations share the feature of placing the right ventricle and the tricuspid valve in the systemic circulation. These children who undergo the operations are physiologically, but not anatomically, repaired. Both of these operations theoretically create the substrate for late complications. As the first atrial switch type operation was described in the 1950s, ample time has passed to observe and evaluate the results.

Overall outcomes of these two operations have been good. As techniques improved the use of either Senning- or Mustard-type repairs in infancy was noted to be associated with a lower incidence of cerebral thrombosis and hypoxic injury due to cyanosis and peripheral emboli from right-to-left shunting. A standard approach developed using balloon atrial septostomy in infancy followed by the elective repair in infants between the ages of 3 and 8 months. Operative mortality in many larger series ranged between 2 and 10% even for patients in early infancy.[10,56,74] Long-term actuarial survival for all patients with TGA undergoing atrial switch procedures is reported to be 88% at 10 years, 76–82% at 20 years and 74–77% at 25 years.[55] Results are slightly better in isolated TGA compared to TGA associated with VSD or other complicating conditions.

Late systemic (right) ventricular dysfunction occurs in between 5 and 25% of patients. It is the most common cause of late mortality, being the cause of death in approximately 6% of patients in one large series.[10] Several challenges exist in following these patients. The reported incidence of late RV dysfunction is variable. This reflects the difficulty in quantitating RV function. One of the problems is that ejection fraction, which is widely used to estimate left ventricular function, is more difficult to measure in the right ventricle, and does not always correlate with other measures of RV function. However, if RV function is evaluated objectively the systemic right ventricle virtually always functions abnormally compared to controls. One of the more recent studies using echocardiographic analysis of RV longitudinal shortening showed that RV function could be judged abnormal in

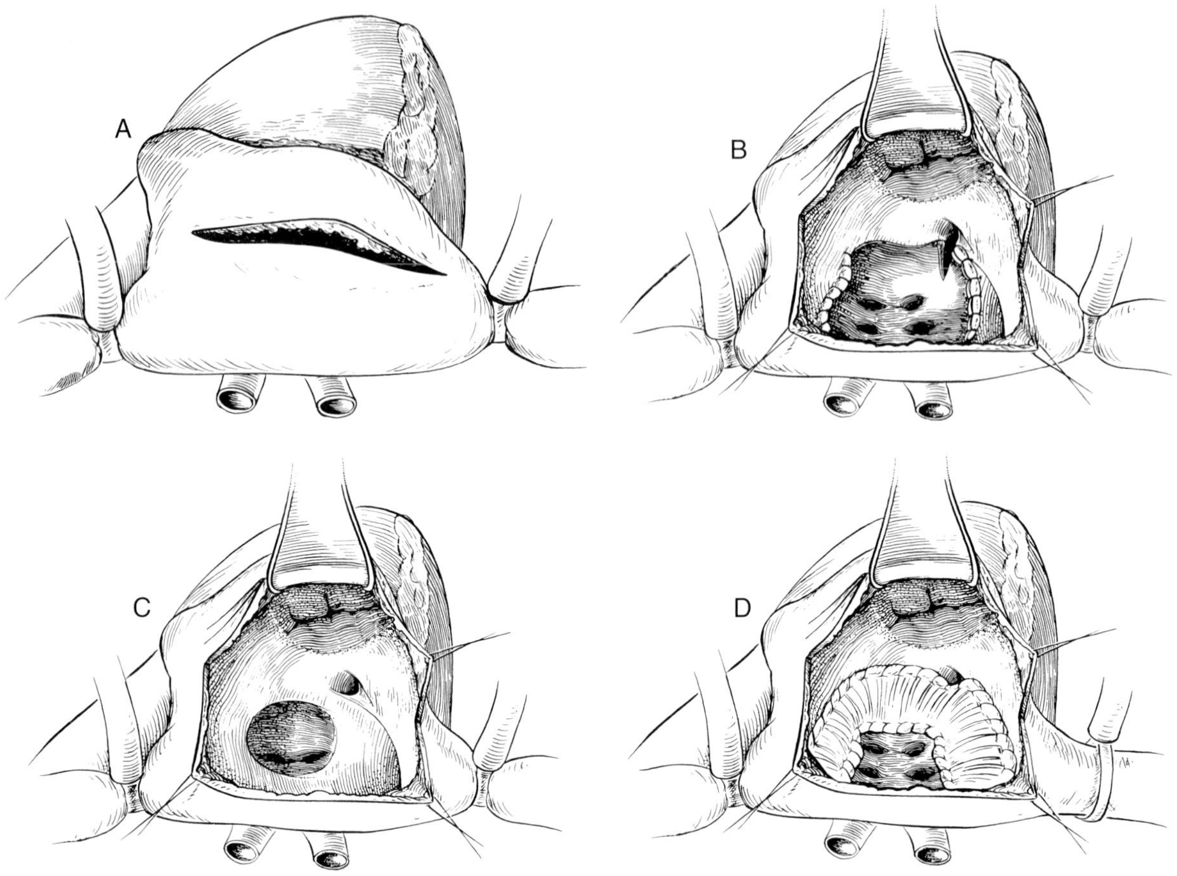

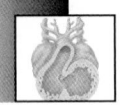

Figure 121–6 The Mustard operation. A, A longitudinal incision is made in the right atrium away from the sinus node. **B,** The posterior aspect of the atrial septum is excised, creating a wide opening for baffling the venous blood into the left atrium *(dotted lines).* **C,** The coronary sinus is cut back into the left atrium to avoid suturing near the AV node. Raw margins of atrial septum may be oversewn. The suture line for the placement of the baffle around the pulmonary veins is noted with the dotted line. **D,** A baffle of Dacron or pericardium is used to baffle the vena caval blood flow to the left atrium across the mitral valve. Completion of this baffle allows venous blood to enter the right atrium and cross the tricuspid valve to the aorta.
(From Trusler GA, Freedom RM: Transposition of the great arteries: The Mustard procedure. In: Sabiston DC Jr., Spencer FC [eds.]: Gibbons Surgery of the Chest. Philadelphia: WB Saunders, 1983, p. 1138.)

all 20 patients depending on the parameter evaluated.[16] There has also been some difficulty in predicting those patients with measurable RV dysfunction that will progress and require further intervention. It has been suggested that late RV dysfunction may be at least partially due to perfusion defects, which are common in these patients, although the etiology is unclear.[51] Another group suggests that marked increase of the RV muscle mass (hypertrophy) in response to systemic afterload may be a contributor.[32]

Late functional outcome has been reported to be good. One series with good long-term follow-up reported 66% of patients in New York Heart Association (NYHA) class I and 29% in class II.[55] It should be noted that even in the asymptomatic patients, a significant percentage had suboptimal maximal oxygen uptake (MVO_2) when tested. A similar finding was noted by Ebenroth who looked at patients an average of 14 years after surgery and found that 75% had normal RV ejection fractions and 84% perceived themselves to be in good health, but only 51% had normal exercise tolerance.[20] Varied results from exercise testing in these patients have been reported. One study showed a decrease in the normal cardiovascular response to exercise over time.[69] Another showed no decrease in MVO_2 with aging, but maximal oxygen consumption in these patients was significantly less than that of individuals without congenital heart disease.[26] This finding was corroborated by a study using magnetic resonance imaging in a group of adult patients after atrial level repair.[65] Abnormal cardiac recovery after exercise was found despite the patients being in NYHA class I and on no medications. An echocardiographic study suggested that abnormalities in function during exercise might be due to impaired AV transport leading to reduced stroke volumes with stress.[17]

Late arrhythmias are common after the atrial switch procedures. At a median follow up of 23 years only two thirds of patients are in sinus rhythm, and two thirds have experienced supraventricular (SVT) arrhythmias.[55] Risk factors for SVT include pulmonary hypertension and a history of junctional rhythm. A separate study found arrhythmias in 22% of patients an average of 23 years after the Mustard procedure and found that ventricular function was compromised in these patients compared to Mustard patients without

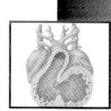

arrhythmias suggesting that late arrhythmias are a marker for systemic ventricular dysfunction.[29] By 14 years after surgery, pacemakers were required in 22% of patients for either sick sinus syndrome or bradycardia because of heart block.[20]

Treatment for right ventricular dysfunction in these patients is evolving. Because of the hypertrophy of the RV, some have suggested angiotensin converting enzyme (ACE) inhibition, which has been shown to be beneficial in LV remodeling. Although there is some encouraging data for this patient population, results have not been consistent.[31] There are several surgical options to deal with late right ventricular failure after atrial switch: tricuspid valve repair or replacement if the ventricular dysfunction is associated with severe tricuspid regurgitation, conversion to an arterial switch, or heart transplantation. As severe RV dysfunction is frequently, if not always, associated with severe TR in these patients, the first option seems an attractive one. The results however have been disappointing, with no significant improvement in function after surgery.[10] Discussion of conversion to an arterial switch follows.

In summary overall functional results after atrial switch procedures have been good after mid- and long-term follow up. However, assessment of the systemic RV reveals that its function is not normal in the systemic circulation. There are significant risks for progressive late RV dysfunction and late arrhythmias, and for heart failure. As patients age they must be followed closely for these complications and means of treatment must be refined.

Arterial Repairs

In spite of the excellent results with the Mustard and Senning procedures, both operations are associated with physiological and not anatomical correction. The morphological RV remains the systemic ventricle in these patients, and although most patients have had many years of successful function of the RV as the systemic ventricle, there remain concerns about its long-term function. The RV is typically thin walled and heavily trabeculated, and the geometric configuration of the ventricle is different from a morphological left ventricle. The tricuspid AV valve also is not anatomically designed to maintain competency at systemic pressure like the mitral valve. Although it may not be inevitable that systemic morphological RVs will fail with time, a considerable number of patients have now returned after an atrial baffle operation with complications of intractable atrial arrhythmias and right ventricular failure. Thus there has been increasing interest in the more anatomical correction by the ASO in hopes of preventing late ventricular dysfunction and arrhythmias.

The success with the atrial switch operations for TGA with intact septum did not translate to repair of transposition with large VSD. Disappointing results with VSD closure and atrial repair in this group of patients continued to be a stimulus for development of an arterial switch procedure that was first successfully performed by Jatene and colleagues in 1975,[40] and subsequently reported by Yacoub.[79] The success of the arterial switch procedure with reimplantation of the coronary arteries in some patients with TGA and VSD led to reintroduction of this technique for patients with intact ventricular septum. Yacoub's initial attempts in patients with TGA and an intact ventricular septum were unsuccessful in 1972; however, additional reports by 1976 suggested that such repair was possible in infancy.[79] Early mortality with the arterial switch in infancy was related to the development of pulmonary vascular obstructive disease and the complexity of the operation, and to the fact that the left (pulmonary) ventricle was not prepared to sustain systemic pressure. Therefore initial approaches included pulmonary arterial banding as a first stage, followed by arterial switch at a later time.[80] However, improvements in the techniques of coronary transfer, myocardial protection, and neonatal vessel reconstruction have resulted in improved survival statistics in the arterial switch. Brawn, Castañeda, Quaegebeur, Yacoub, and their associates subsequently demonstrated the feasibility of repair of simple transposition in the first few days of life by ASO while the pulmonary ventricle has a relatively high pressure producing results that rival or exceed those of atrial baffle operations.[8,12,62,79]

Technique

The principles of successful anatomical correction include dividing the aorta and PA, excising the origins of the coronary arteries with a button of aortic wall, repositioning the coronary arteries to the posterior great vessel (pulmonary artery), and reconstructing each ventricular outflow to the appropriate distal vessel (Figure 121-7). The details of the operative techniques, however, vary from one institution to another. The procedures are performed with a median sternotomy incision and the use of CPB and hypothermia, although hypothermic circulatory arrest is used for the procedure in varying degrees in many institutions. After the median sternotomy is made, a portion of the anterior pericardium is excised for autologous patch reconstruction of the defects in the anterior great vessel. The pericardium may be used fresh or fixed in glutaraldehyde to make it easier to manipulate during the operation. The ligamentum arteriosum or ductus arteriosus is dissected and the PAs are mobilized to the bifurcation of the vessels in the hilum of the lung bilaterally. It is important to mobilize the PAs freely to permit anterior relocation of the pulmonary bifurcation without distortion of the pulmonary artery or aorta. The aorta is typically cannulated for bypass distally to allow room for manipulation of the proximal aorta during the reconstruction. After bypass is established, the ductus arteriosus is ligated and divided and the aortic end and pulmonary arterial end oversewn as necessary. The aorta is then clamped close to the aortic cannula and cardioplegia administered into the aortic root.

If a VSD is present, it is approached either through the right atrium across the tricuspid valve or occasionally through the anterior great vessel. The aorta is then transected above the level of the coronary ostia and the PA is transected just below the bifurcation, with care not to carry the incision into the left PA. The PA bifurcation is brought anterior to the aorta (the Lecompte maneuver). The coronary ostia are examined and excised from the anterior great vessel with a button of aortic wall extending down into the base of the sinuses of Valsalva. The epicardial course of the coronaries is then mobilized adequately to allow turning the coronary ostia to the posterior great vessel without kinking of the epicardial course. On occasion, the small conal branches of the

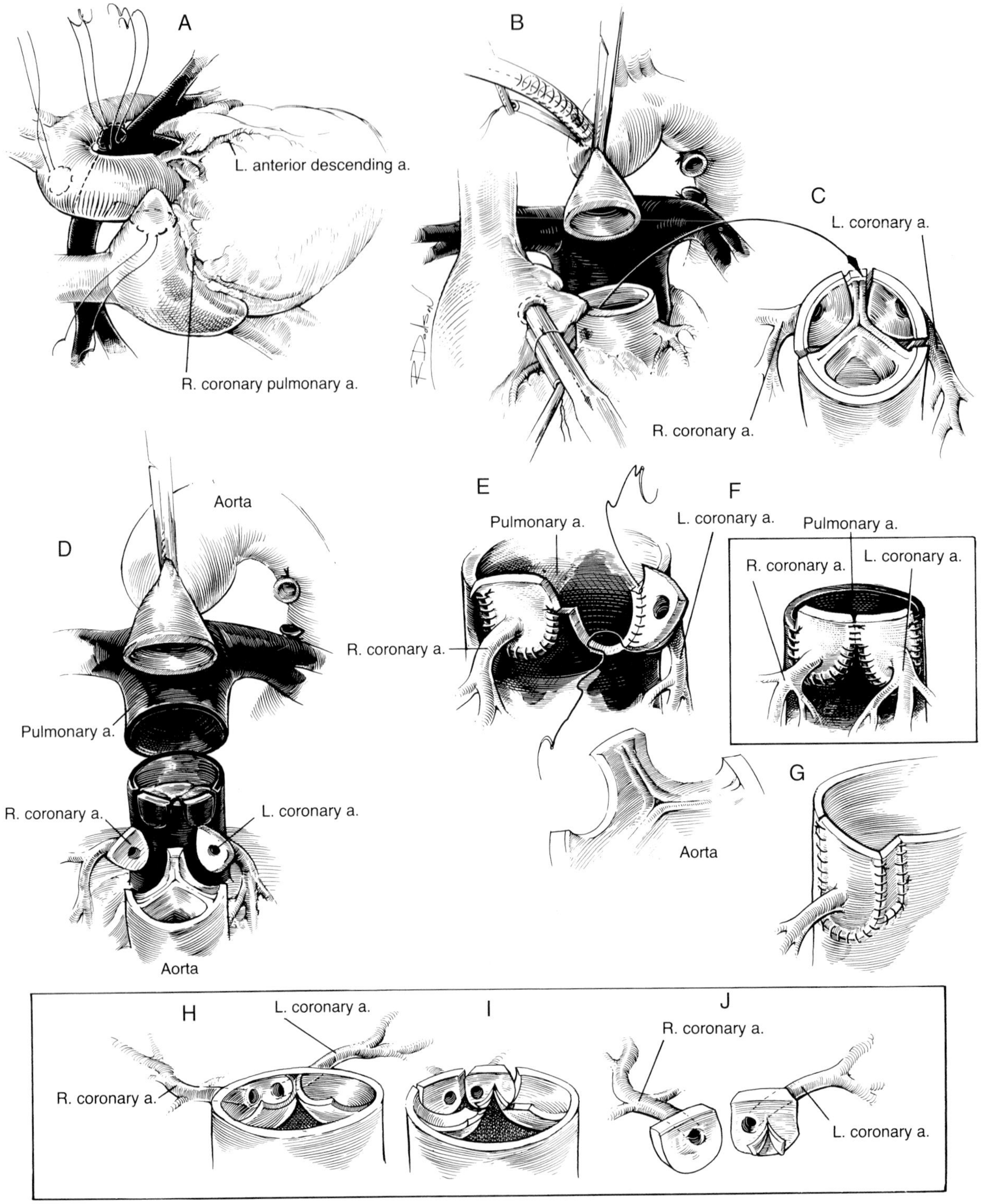

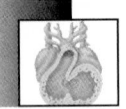

Figure 121–7 **A,** Cannulation sites for cardiopulmonary bypass in the arterial switch operation. Single atrial or bicaval venous cannulation can be utilized. The ductus arteriosus is ligated and divided between sutures. **B,** Division of the ductus arteriosus and ascending aorta after initiation of cardioplegic arrest. **C,** Excision of the left and right coronary ostia with a button of aortic wall. **D,** Excision of corresponding segments of the posterior great vessel wall to which the coronary arteries will be re-implanted. Alternatively, medially based flap incisions can be used. **E,** Suturing of the coronary ostial buttons to the posterior great vessel. **F,** Completed anastomoses of the reimplanted coronary arteries. In some cases, the coronary buttons can be approximated together in the midline. **G,** Augmentation of the medial aspect of the anastomosis to prevent kinking is occasionally necessary, although less common if medially based flap incisions are used for coronary reimplantation. **H,** If juxtacommissural origins of either or both coronary arteries from the facing sinuses are present, excision of a portion of the native aortic valve may be necessary to allow mobilization. **I** and **J,** Separation of the coronary arteries is done, if possible, to prevent distortion and provide easier implantation.

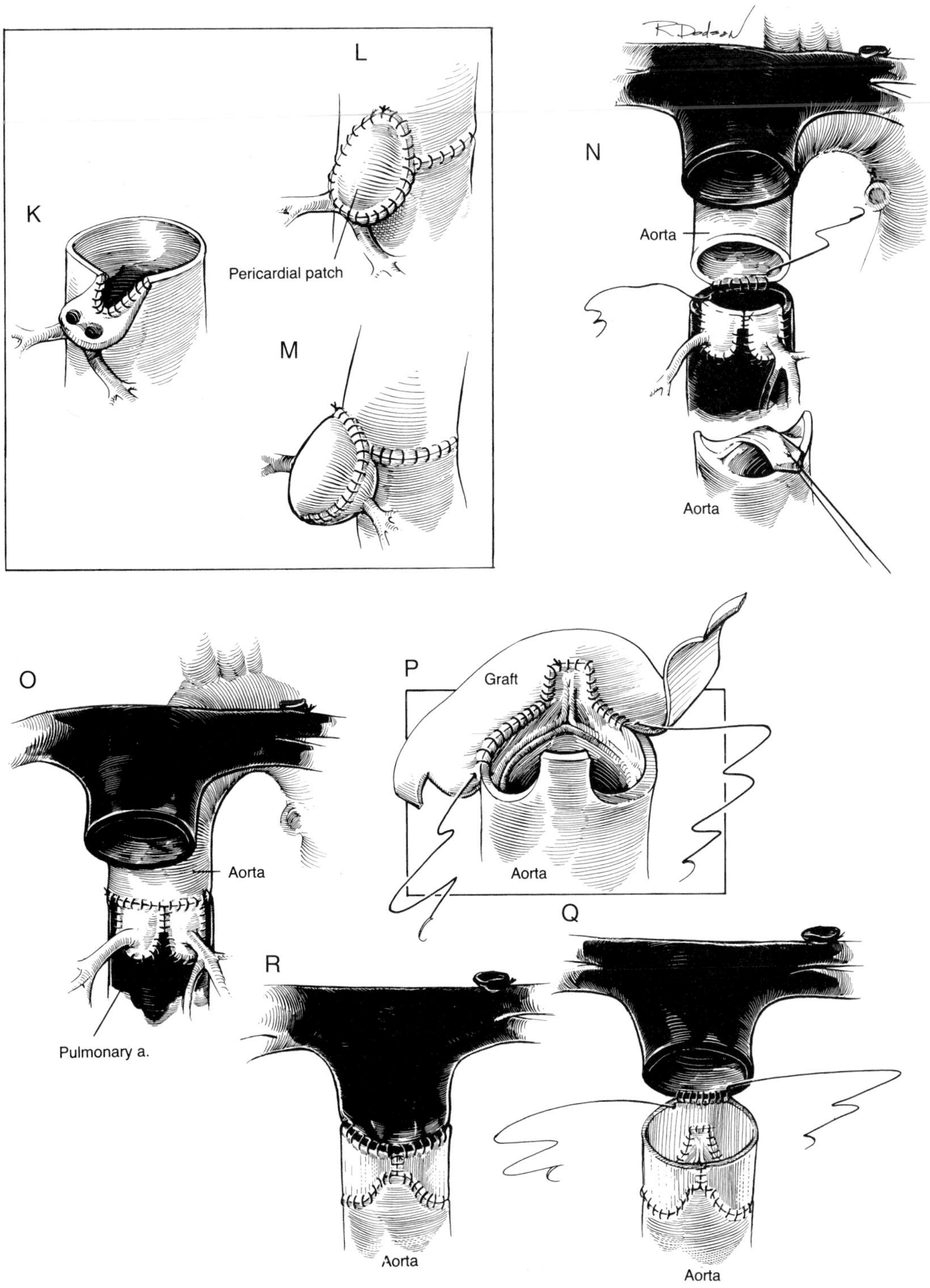

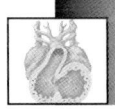

Figure 121–7 cont'd **K,** If right and left intramural coronary arteries are present, the aortic coronary flap is left in place and sutured along the cephalic border to an incision in the anterior neoaorta. **L** and **M,** A pericardial patch is then used to provide unrestricted entrance of blood into the coronary ostia. **N,** After completion of the coronary transfer, the distal aorta is anastomosed to the neoaorta. **O,** The pulmonary bifurcation is brought anterior to the aorta in the Lecompte maneuver. **P,** The defects in the aorta from which the coronary arteries have been excised is augmented with a pantaloon-shaped patch of pericardium. **Q,** The pulmonary bifurcation is then anastomosed to the augmented aorta. In most cases pericardium is not sutured completely around the aorta to create a complete pericardial tube. **R,** Completed anastomosis of the pulmonary artery anterior to the new aorta.
(From Castañeda AR, Jonas RA, Mayer JE Jr., Hanley FL: D-transposition of the great arteries. In: Cardiac Surgery of the Neonate and Infant. Philadelphia: WB Saunders, 1994, pp. 409–438.)

coronaries may need to be sacrificed to permit adequate mobilization. An incision is then made in the posterior great vessel at the site for reattachment of the coronary ostia, and a medially based flap incision is created to allow takeoff of the coronary ostia without tension or kinking. The coronary ostia are then sewn to the incisions in the posterior great vessel using an absorbable suture to allow for maximum growth.

Although transfer of the coronary arteries is one of the most technically challenging and important parts of the arterial switch procedure, experience and refinements in technique have made it possible to deal with most variations in coronary anatomy. When both coronaries come off a single sinus with the left coronary orifice near the commissural attachment of the aortic valve, it is possible to mobilize the commissure and excise the coronary arteries in the usual fashion. Alternatively, if the coronary ostia are close together or if there is a single coronary artery, a single button containing the adjacent ostia or common orifice can be excised and transferred to the posterior great vessel. This is done in a side-to-side fashion and the distal aorta is fashioned to create an anterior flap that is sewn over the button to complete the anastomosis (see Figure 121-7K–M). Another concept that is helpful in dealing with single coronary arteries is to translocate the button higher onto the posterior great vessel to alleviate any kinking that may occur with rotation of the flap.

After completion of the coronary anastomoses the distal aorta is anastomosed to the posterior great vessel to which the coronary arteries have been transferred. Additional cardioplegia may be administered at this time to check for hemostasis of the suture lines and to confirm good myocardial perfusion without kinking of the coronary anastomoses. The defects in the anterior great vessels from which the coronary arteries have been excised are then repaired with a generous portion of pericardium. The anterior great vessel is sutured to the PA bifurcation, with care being taken to avoid tension on the PAs that may interfere with symmetrical pulmonary blood flow. Finally, the ASD is closed either primarily or with a small patch of pericardium, and the atrium is closed. In the situation in which the great vessels are side to side rather than anteroposterior, it may be advisable to leave the pulmonary confluence posterior to the aorta and open the right PA, closing the pulmonary bifurcation to transpose the opening in the PA more to the right than usual. This may facilitate reconstruction to the RV.

After completion of the repair, left atrial and right atrial lines are placed for postoperative monitoring and temporary pacemaker wires applied. The infant is weaned from bypass, maintaining a systemic pressure of approximately 60 mm Hg to prevent distention of the newly systemic LV.

Postoperative Management

Continuous sedation with mechanical ventilation and moderate inotropic support are usually used in the first 12–18 hours postrepair, as in other infants undergoing complex congenital heart repair. Neuromuscular blockade may be administered continuously during this period, or in patients who are anticipated to have a more stable course and may be candidates for earlier extubation it may be used intermittently on an as needed basis. If stable after the initial postoperative period, sedation is reduced and the patient is weaned from the ventilator over the next 24–48 hours. After extubation, inotropic support is discontinued, umbilical lines are removed if they are present, and enteral feeding is commenced. Once enteral intake is satisfactory the rest of the support equipment can be removed in preparation for discharge. The current usual hospital stay for correction of TGA is 10–12 days.[39,67,78]

Outcome After Arterial Switch Operation

Initial results of the ASO would be considered poor by today's standards. Jatene's original series included a mortality of approximately 60%. This high early mortality was duplicated in other series, yet surgeons pressed on with this operation with the belief that it was physiologically superior to atrial level switch procedures.

More long-term follow-up data are now available on children undergoing neonatal arterial switch. Prifti et al reported the results of a large series of patients with a mean follow up of 3.5 years. Early mortality was 12.7%, but significantly lower (5.7%) for those children with isolated TGA. Actuarial survival was 98%, 93%, and 91.5% at 1, 3, and 5 years, respectively, after surgery. Freedom from reoperation was 95%, 90.5%, and 83% at the same time points. The presence of a VSD adversely affected survival. Predictors of reintervention included VSD, coronary anomalies, aortic coarctation, and left ventricular outflow tract obstruction or moderate PS.[61] Another series of 181 patients with a mean follow-up of 5.8 years revealed a 5.5% early mortality and 92% survival at 5 and 10 years. VSD was a risk factor for early and late death.[76] The largest series in the literature with long-term follow-up was reported in 2001 and included data on 1095 patients from a single institution. Mean follow-up was approximately 5 years. Early mortality was 8.6%. Survival was 89% at 1 year and 88% at 10 and 15 years (including those patients who died early) (Figure 121-8). Simple TGA was found to be associated with improved survival (92% versus 80% for complex TGA). Freedom from reintervention was 90%, 83%, and 82% at 5, 10, and 15 years, respectively, of follow-up (Figure 121-9).[46]

Although early mortality seems high in some of the larger series that include earlier results, current operative mortality is approximately 2% to 3%.[14,37,59] Analysis of large series found complex anatomy (large VSD, multiple VSDs, Taussig-Bing anomaly but not aortic coarctation), coronary anomalies, previous operation, and prolonged bypass time to be risk factors for early death.[14] Another study also identified female gender and preoperative instability as risk factors for operative mortality, and suggested that in the current era abnormal coronary patterns were less of a factor.[9] Although this seems to be true, a single coronary ostium and intramural coronary course are still risk factors for mortality.[57] Coronary artery-related problems are the most common cause of early death, followed by right ventricular failure and pulmonary hypertension.[59] It has been suggested that risk factors for late death include an unusual relationship of the great vessels, single coronary ostium, prolonged bypass time, and coarctation of the aorta, although none of these proved to be significant in multivariate analysis.[14]

Cardiac rhythm abnormalities are unusual after ASO with over 90% of patients in normal sinus rhythm. Left ventricular function is generally normal. The vast majority of

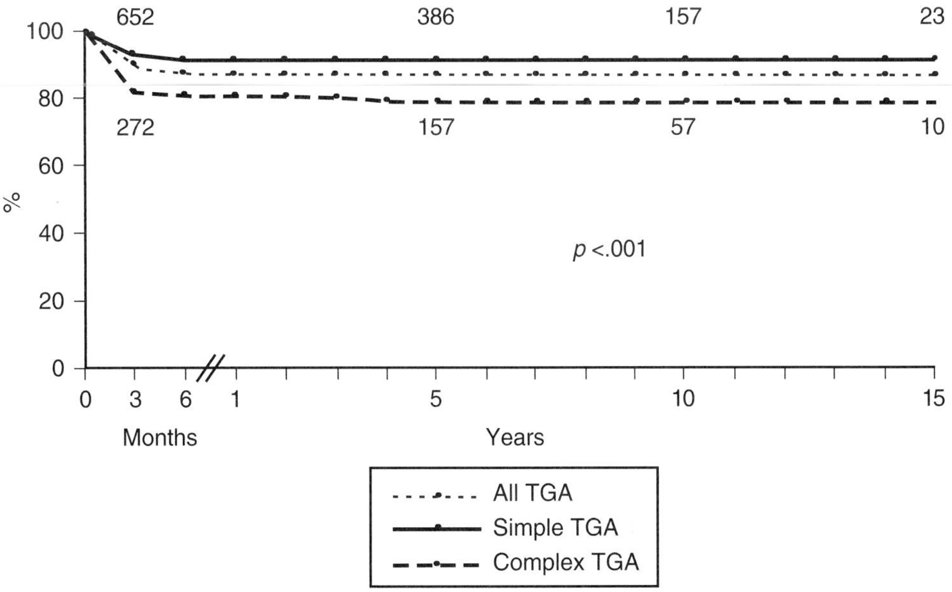

Figure 121–8 Actuarial survival for 1200 patients who underwent ASO. Curves for the total group *(dotted line)*, and curves for simple *(solid line)*, and complex TGA *(dashed line)* are shown. Numbers shown indicate number of patients observed at beginning of interval. *(From Losay J, Touchot A, Serraf A et al: Late outcome after arterial switch operation for transposition of the great arteries. Circulation 104[suppl I]:I-121–I-126, 2001.)*

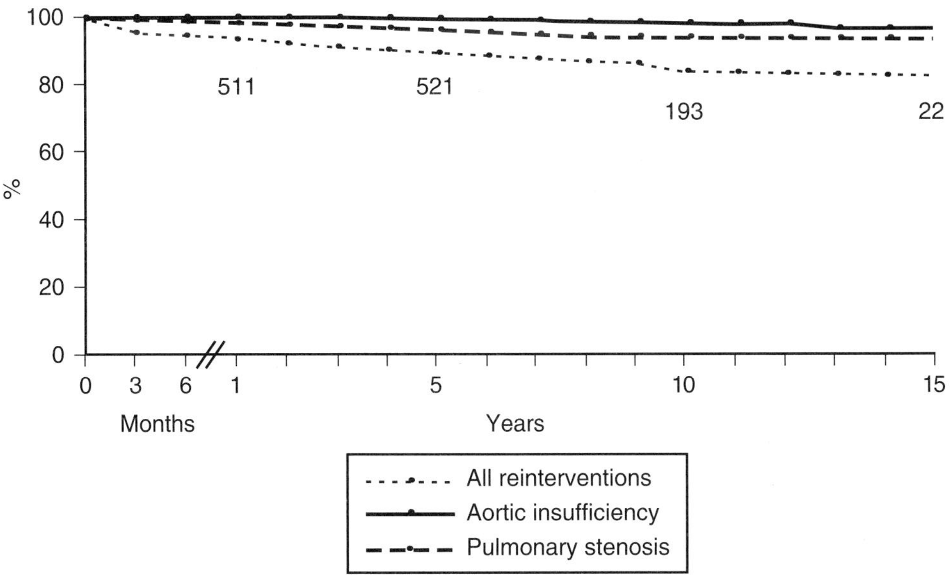

Figure 121–9 Graph showing actuarial freedom from reoperation in 1095 survivors of the ASO. Curves are shown for all reoperations *(dotted line)*, and reoperations for aortic insufficiency *(solid line)* and pulmonary stenosis *(dashed line)*. Numbers shown indicate number of patients observed at beginning of interval. *(From Losay J, Touchot A, Serraf A, et al: Late outcome after arterial switch operation for transposition of the great arteries. Circulation 104[suppl I]:I-121–I-126, 2001.)*

patients (>95%) are in NYHA functional class I at long-term follow-up.[37] Aortic stenosis is very rare, and mild aortic insufficiency is seen approximately 10%. Although there was initial concern that the neoaortic root dilated disproportionately, raising the concern of progressive aortic insufficiency, longitudinal analysis has shown that the neoaorta undergoes dilation during the first year of life, but then tends toward the normal size as further growth occurs.[38] PS is seen slightly more frequently.[76] Very few patients are taking cardiac medications at midterm follow-up.[34,59] Late coronary artery problems are rare.

Several studies have also documented late functional outcome. Somatic growth after operation has been found to be normal.[19] Head circumference has been noted to be slightly less than normal up to 2 years postoperatively, but the significance of this is unclear.[66] At the age of 8 years, average general health as assessed by standardized testing was found to be similar to that of the general population, although in the same study parents reported more problems with attention, learning, and speech than those of the general population.[19] Although exercise capacity has been found to be compromised in children having undergone an atrial switch operation, exercise testing of patients at a mean of 11 years after ASO showed a normal exercise capacity.[47] This finding is corroborated by another study that showed 96% of children to be without limitation of their physical activity.[34]

Late neurological outcome has also been investigated. Some evidence of neurological impairment, but not reduced development, has been found 3–4 years after ASO.[36] Another study reported the neurologic outcomes of a cohort of 60 patients who underwent arterial switch as neonates for TGA. The operative technique included a combination of circulatory arrest and low flow CPB. Follow-up data 8–14 years after operation indicated some impairment in school performance and more behavioral problems in children operated on for TGA compared to normal children, but the results were not well quantitated[33]. Neurological status and cognitive and motor development have been found to be normal in 74% of children having undergone ASO. Some concern is raised by a follow-up study of the same cohort of children at a mean of 10 years after ASO that suggests further neurological impairment at this stage with only 45% having no measurable neurological dysfunction. Risk factors for poor neurological outcome include severe preoperative acidosis or hypoxia. Although these studies have demonstrated some differences in testing between children after ASO compared to normal children, the magnitude and significance of these differences is not clear.

In summary, outcomes after arterial switch are generally very good. Follow-up to date suggests that, as expected, the results are superior to atrial switches in terms of late ventricular function, freedom from arrhythmias, and functional status. Further follow-up will be necessary to confirm these observations over the long term. The rapidly decreasing mortality for ASOs has resulted in this surgical approach becoming the standard corrective surgical procedure at the present time and results in both an anatomical and physiological reconstruction of this cardiac defect.

POSTOPERATIVE COMPLICATIONS

One of the most common complications after the arterial switch is supravalvar PS, and it is the most common reason for reoperation.[46] In one series 23% of patients required reintervention at some point after the arterial switch, the majority of which were for PS.[28] In this series about half of the patients were managed operatively, with the other half being managed by percutaneous dilation. Age at operation was found to be a significant risk factor for the development of postoperative PS with younger children having higher gradients.[61] The use of a pantaloon patch was found to be advantageous, with patients having had this method of PA reconstruction having lower gradients than others.[61] Other reasons for late reintervention include residual VSD, residual ASD, aortic arch obstruction, aortic stenosis, and coronary artery stenosis but each of these is rare.[28] Evidence of previously unsuspected coronary artery abnormalities in asymptomatic patients were found in only 3% of patients studied.[71] These abnormalities were not associated with evidence of ventricular dysfunction and their long-term significance is unclear. In rare cases in which there is evidence of postoperative coronary ischemia, revascularization can be successfully accomplished either by bypass grafting with the internal mammary artery or by surgical angioplasty.[60]

SPECIAL SITUATIONS

TGA with LV Outflow Tract Obstruction

Infants with significant left ventricular outflow tract obstruction represent a small proportion of children presenting with TGA. Because left ventricular outflow tract obstruction is often dynamic, the relative contributions of the dynamic components of obstruction and the more fixed components such as subvalvular fibrous rings and mitral valve leaflet tags are often difficult to ascertain. Although it may be possible to resect fixed forms of left ventricular outflow tract obstruction with exposure across the pulmonary valve at the time of ASO, complete relief of obstruction is not often possible. However, mild to moderate residual left ventricular outflow tract obstruction can usually be tolerated after the arterial switch procedure because the pulmonary ventricle has been preconditioned to elevated intracavitary pressure.

In the rare forms of severe left ventricular outflow tract obstruction presenting in infancy, creation of an interatrial communication and a systemic-to-pulmonary arterial shunt may be the best early approach, followed by later repair, although in some centers early complete repair is preferred. Repair is by the Rastelli operation, first described in 1969, which involves the combination of an intraventricular tunnel repair, closing the VSD and baffling the pulmonary venous blood from the LV to the aorta, closing the PA exit from the LV and creating an extracardiac conduit from the anatomical RV to the pulmonary bifurcation (Figure 121-10). This results in an anatomical repair for TGA/VSD and left ventricular outflow tract obstruction.[64]

In patients with an intact ventricular septum and significant left ventricular outflow tract obstruction, atrial baffle repair and creation of a conduit from the left ventricular cavity to the pulmonary bifurcation may also be considered. Obstruction of the reconstructed left ventricular outflow tract remains a common complication of the Rastelli-type repair. This has led to the development of a variation of the intraventricular repair by Lecompte's réparation à l'etage ventriculaire (REV) procedure.[64] This procedure results in a more anatomical repair by transposing the aorta to a more normal location over the left ventricular outflow tract, in some cases precluding the need for a valved conduit from the RV to the pulmonary bifurcation and the subsequent necessity for replacement of this nonviable conduit (Figure 121-11).

Taussig-Bing Anomaly

The Taussig-Bing anomaly is a form of double outlet RV with dextroposition of the aorta and a subpulmonary VSD. Because of the position of the VSD, flow from the LV is preferentially directed to the PA making the physiology of this lesion similar to that of TGA with VSD. Anatomical repair of this lesion, as with TGA, is now favored early in life. This may be accomplished either by intraventricular means with a Rastelli-like procedure or by arterial switch with VSD closure. The intraventricular method involves baffling the left ventricular outflow through the VSD to the aorta. This technique is limited by the propensity for late outflow tract obstruction, so only patients with the most favorable anatomy are considered candidates.[49] The arterial switch procedure is more widely applicable. This involves closure of the VSD with a prosthetic patch through a right atriotomy with rearrangement of the great arteries and standard coronary artery transfer. This procedure can be performed with an operative mortality of approximately 7%.[7] The presence of side-by-side great vessels, which is associated with abnormal coronary patterns, is a risk factor for repair.[70] Some patients with associated abnormalities

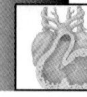

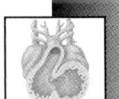

such as hypoplastic or straddling AV valves may not be candidates for biventricular repair and are best served by staging to a Fontan procedure.

TGA with Aortic Arch Obstruction

Hypoplasia of the aortic arch, interrupted aortic arch, or aortic coarctation is associated with TGA in up to 12% of patients.[7] These conditions occur more frequently with the Taussig-Bing anomaly. Previously, the presence of aortic arch obstruction has been noted to be an independent risk factor for mortality in TGA.[78] Repair of this combination of defects was first approached using a two-staged strategy. The first stage consisted of repair of the arch anomaly or coarctation with a PA band through a thoracotomy. The second stage consisted of removal of the band and intracardiac repair. This method was associated with a relatively high mortality prompting interest in repair of both defects during a single operation. Single-stage repair with arterial switch and repair of the aortic arch has now become the preferred approach, and can be accomplished with a low mortality.[73]

Arterial Switch After LV Retraining

There are two situations when LV "retraining" might be necessary prior to ASO: in patients with TGA and intact ventricular septum who present late and in patients that present with RV dysfunction after atrial switch that is refractory to medical management. Surgical options to address the latter issue include tricuspid valve repair or replacement if there is significant TR, which has not had encouraging results, and heart transplantation, which is limited by donor availability and long-term complications. Perhaps the best option for these patients is conversion to an arterial switch. In both of these sets of patients the LV must be retrained to handle the systemic afterload in order for arterial switch to be successful. This is accomplished with the application of a PA band. Banding is performed via sternotomy without the use of CPB. One to three bandings are typically required to adequately prepare the LV. The status of the LV during banding must be closely assessed. Monitoring of the LV is done with echocardiography, magnetic resonance imaging, and cardiac catheterization, and various criteria have been developed to assess for adequate preparation of the ventricle. These

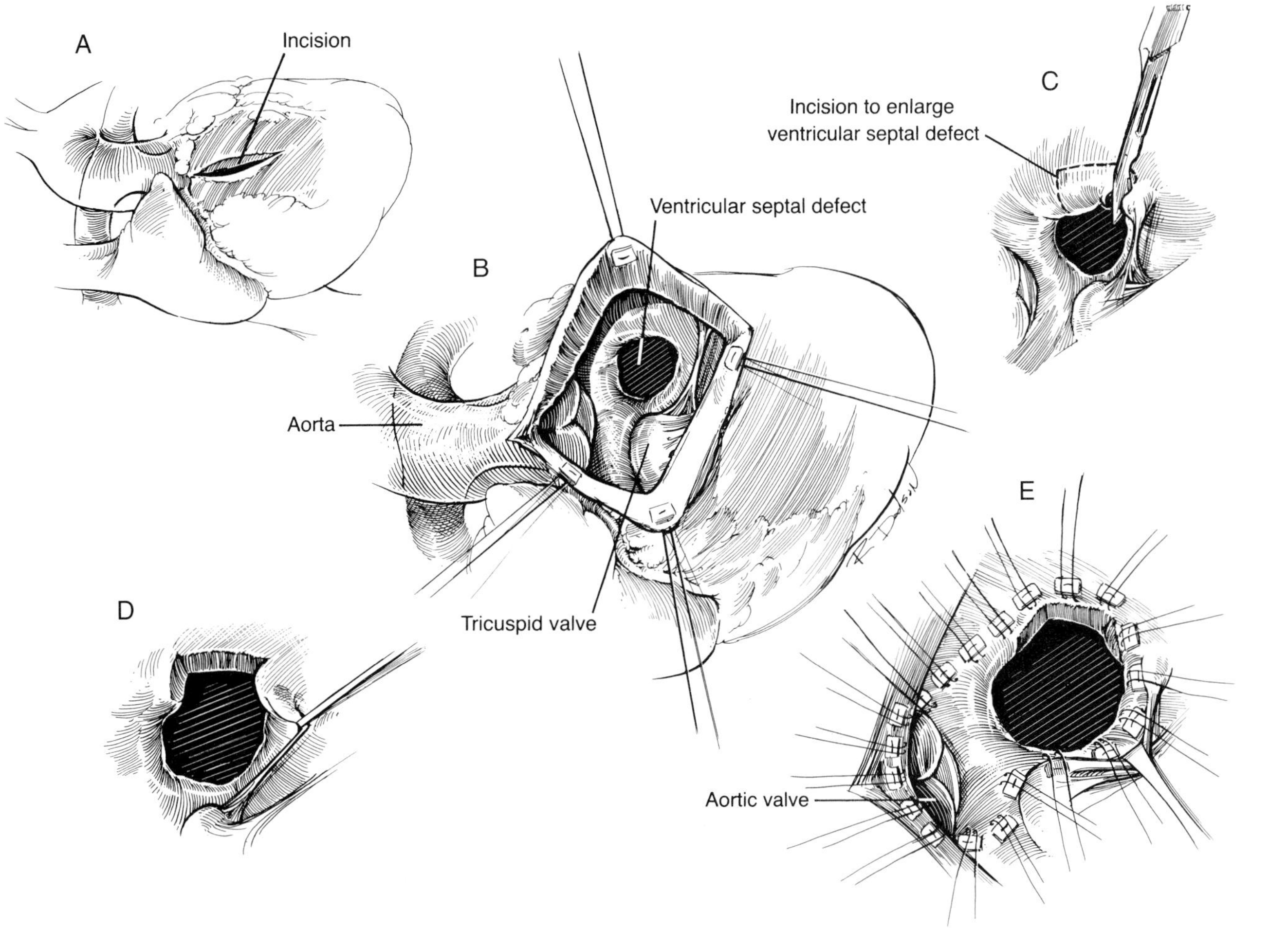

Figure 121–10 The Rastelli operation for TGA with VSD and left ventricular outflow tract obstruction. A, An incision is made in the right ventricular muscle, avoiding major coronary branches. **B,** The VSD is exposed through the right ventricle. **C** and **D,** Excision of the anterior-superior limb of the septal band enlarges the VSD to provide unobstructed flow from the left ventricle to the aorta. **E,** Mattress sutures are used to place the VSD patch that will direct blood across the defect to the anteriorly located aorta.

(Continued)

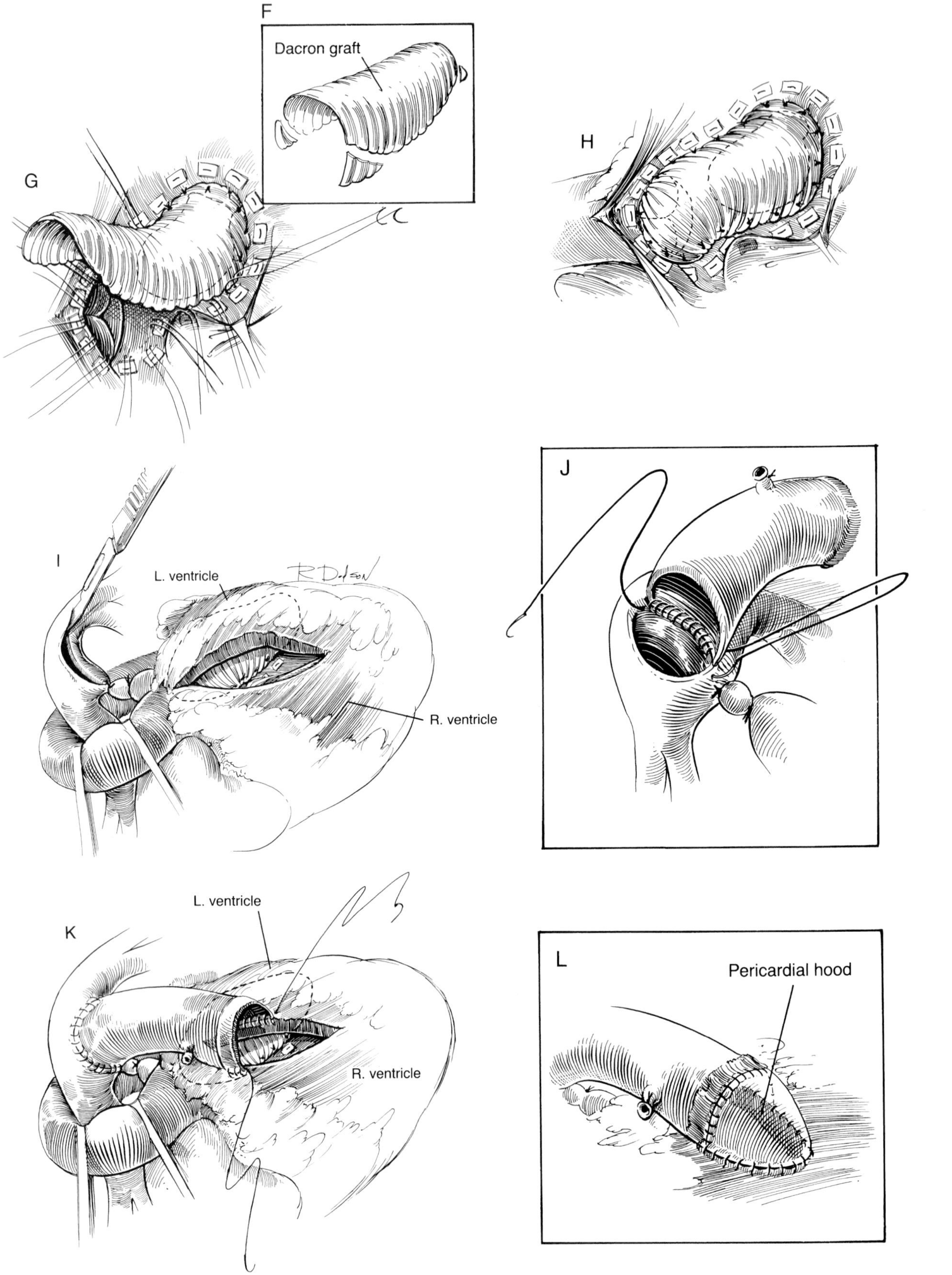

Figure 121–10 cont'd F, A baffle is created from a Dacron graft to prevent compression against the conal muscle and obstruction of the outflow tract and secured in place with the previously placed sutures **(G)**. **H,** Completed VSD closure with the Dacron baffle. **I** and **J,** Ligation of the main pulmonary artery proximal to the bifurcation and suturing of a homograft conduit to the pulmonary artery bifurcation. **K,** Proximal anastomosis of the valved homograft conduit to the incision in the right ventricle. **L,** Augmentation of the takeoff of the pulmonary homograft with a pericardial hood to prevent compression and obstruction.
(From Castañeda AR, Jonas RA, Mayer JE Jr., Hanley FL: D-transposition of the great arteries. In: Cardiac Surgery of the Neonate and Infant. Philadelphia: WB Saunders, 1994, pp. 409–438.)

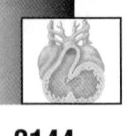

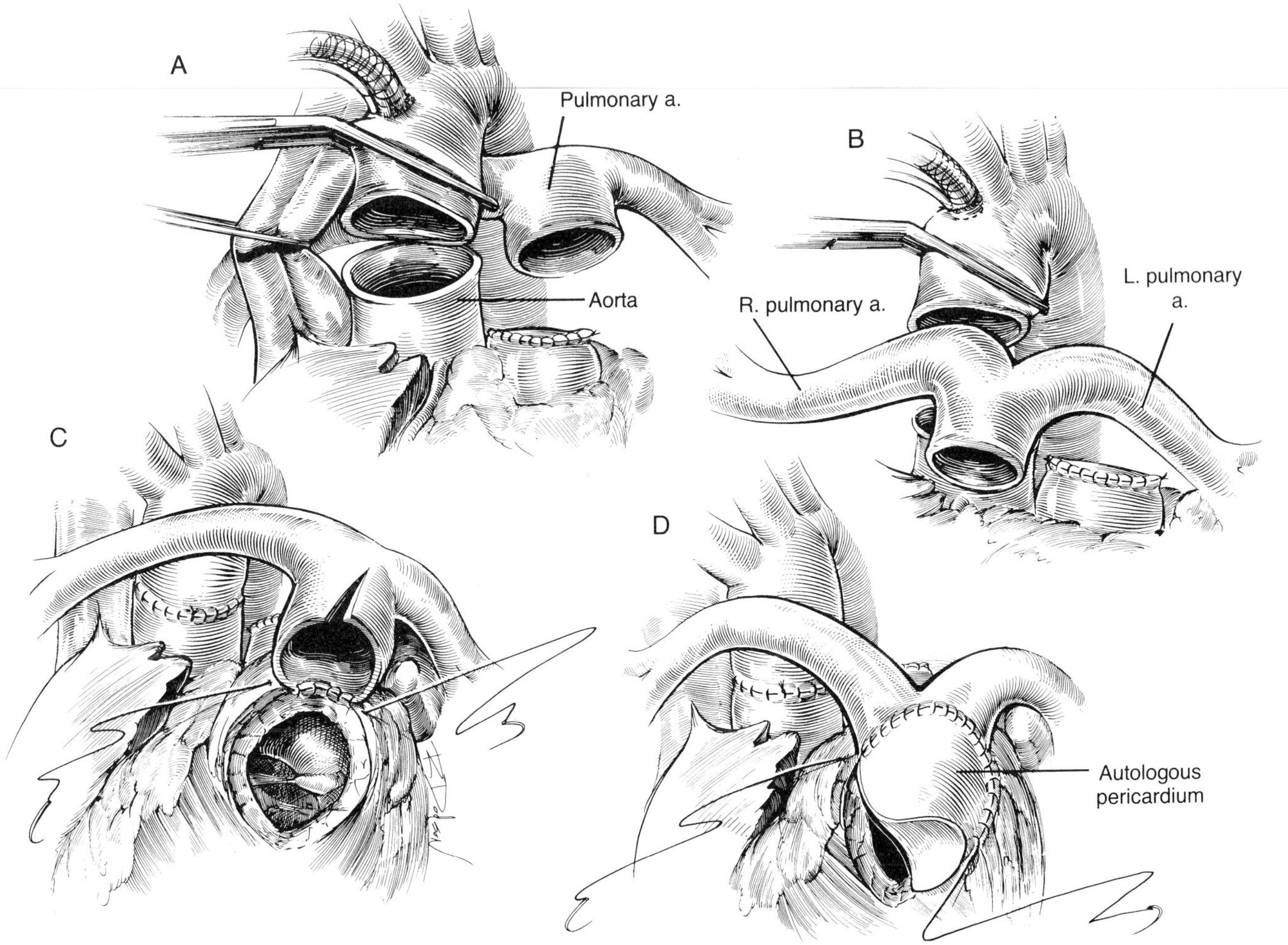

Figure 121–11 Lecompte's REV procedure (réparation à l'etage ventriculaire). A, Division of ascending aorta and pulmonary artery. The pulmonary artery is oversewn, eliminating the egress of blood from the left ventricle. The VSD is closed as in a Rastelli operation, baffling blood to the aorta. **B,** The Lecompte maneuver is performed, bringing the pulmonary artery bifurcation anterior to the great vessels. **C,** The aorta is reconstructed after anterior translocation of the pulmonary bifurcation, and the pulmonary bifurcation is sewn to an incision in the right ventricular infundibulum. **D,** Completion of the repair with augmentation of the outflow tract with autologous pericardium prevents outflow tract with autologous pericardium prevents outflow tract obstruction.
(From Castañeda AR, Jonas RA, Mayer JE Jr., Hanley FL: Double outlet right ventricle. In: Cardiac Surgery of the Neonate and Infant. Philadelphia: WB Saunders, 1994, pp. 445–459.)

include LV mass index and LV/RV pressure ratio. In unoperated infants who present after the early neonatal period, this retraining can usually be accomplished more rapidly, that is, after a single PA band and an average of 10 days,[43] and PA banding is usually accompanied by a systemic-pulmonary shunt. In patients being converted from an atrial switch, preparation typically occurs over a longer period of time, that is, after an average of 19 months.[15] These procedures are significant undertakings, with substantial intensive care unit and hospital stays, but when accomplished successfully can offer good long term outcomes. Poirer and Mee reported a series of 84 patients who underwent arterial switch conversion with an 85% overall survival. Normal late LV and RV function were seen in approximately 90% of these patients. The best results were obtained in patients undergoing conversion prior to adolescence, with less predictable results and higher mortality rates observed in adult patients.[58]

SUMMARY

The treatment of TGA has evolved rapidly. Current results with the ASO are excellent and make this procedure the standard of care for neonates with this diagnosis. Experience is being gained with complicating anatomical variations, allowing safe anatomical repair for these patients as well. Continued surveillance of patients following repair is necessary to detect and deal with complications of the various surgical procedures.

REFERENCES

1. Albert HM: Surgical correction of transposition of the great arteries. Surg Forum 5:74, 1954.
2. Baffes TG: A new method for surgical correction of transposition of the aorta and pulmonary artery. Surg Gynecol Obstet 102:227, 1956.

3. Bailey CP, Cookson BA, Downing DF, et al: Cardiac surgery under hypothermia. J Thorac Cardiovasc Surg 27:73, 1954.
4. Baillie M: The Morbid Anatomy of Some of the More Important Parts of the Human Body London: Johnson & Nichol, 1797, p. 38.
5. Bano-Rodrigo A, Quero-Jiminez M, Moreno-Granado F: Wall thickness of ventricular chambers in transposition of the great arteries: surgical implications. J Thorac Cardiovasc Surg 79:592, 1980.
6. Blalock A, Hanlon CR: The surgical treatment of complete transposition of the aorta and pulmonary artery. Surg Gynecol Obstet 90:1, 1950.
7. Blume ED, Altmann K, Mayer J, et al: Evolution of risk factors influencing early mortality of the arterial switch operation. J Am Coll Cardiol 33:1702–1709, 1999.
8. Brawn WJ, Mee RBB: Early results for anatomic correction of transposition of the great arteries and for double-outlet right ventricle with subpulmonary ventricular septal defect. J Thorac Cardiovasc Surg 95:230, 1988.
9. Brown JW, Park HJ, Turrentine MW: Arterial switch operation: factors impacting survival in the current era. Ann Thorac Surg 71:1978–1984, 2001.
10. Carrel T, Pfammatter JP. Complete transposition of the great arteries: surgical concepts for patients with systemic right ventricular failure following intraatrial repair. Thorac Cardiov Surg 48:224–227, 2000.
11. Castañeda AR, Jonas RA, Mayer JE, Jr, et al: D-transposition of the great arteries. In: Cardiac Surgery of the Neonate and Infant,. Philadelphia: WB Saunders, 1994, pp. 409–438.
12. Castañeda AR, Trusler GA, Paul MH, et al: Congenital Heart Surgeons Society: The early results of treatment of simple transposition in the current era. J Thorac Cardiovasc Surg 95:14, 1988.
13. Costell M, Carmona R, Gustafsson E, et al: Hyperplastic conotruncal endocardial cushions and transposition of great arteries in perlecan-null mice. Circ Res 91:158–164, 2002.
14. Daebritz SH, Nollert G, Sachweh JS, et al: Anatomical risk factors for mortality and cardiac morbidity after arterial switch operation. Ann Thorac Surg 69:1880–1886, 2000.
15. Daebritz SH, Tiete AR, Sachweh JS, et al: Systemic right ventricular failure after atrial switch operation: midterm results of conversion to an arterial switch. Ann Thorac Surg 71:1255–1259, 2001.
16. Derrick GP, Josen M, Vogel M, et al: Abnormalities of right ventricular long axis function after atrial repair of transposition of the great arteries. Heart 86(2):203–206, 2001.
17. Derrick GP, Narang I, White PA, et al: Failure of stroke volume augmentation during exercise and dobutamine stress is unrelated to load-independent indexes of right ventricular performance after the Mustard operation. Circ 102[suppl III]:III-154–III-159, 2000.
18. DiDonato RM, Castañeda AR: Anatomic correction of transposition of the great arteries at the arterial level. In: Sabiston DC, Jr., Spencer FC (eds): Surgery of the Chest, 5th ed. Philadelphia: WB Saunders, 1990, pp. 1435–1451.
19. Dunbar-Masterson C, Wypij D, Bellinger D. et al: General health status of children with D-transposition of the great arteries after the arterial switch operation. Circ 104[suppl I]: I-138–I-142, 2001.
20. Ebenroth ES, Hurwitz RA: Functional outcome of patients operated for d-transposition of the great arteries with the Mustard procedure. Am J Cardiol 89:353–356, 2002.
21. Ebert PA: Transposition of the great arteries. In: Sabiston DC Jr., (ed): Textbook of Surgery, 14th ed. Philadelphia: WB Saunders, 1986, pp. 2249–2259.
22. Fanconi G: Die Transposition der grossen Gefuse (das Charakteristische Rontgenbild). Arch. Kinderheilkd 95:202, 1932.
23. Farre JR: Pathological Researches. Essay 1: On Malformations of the Human Heart,. London: Longman, Hurst, Rees, Orme, Brown, 1814, p. 28.
24. Ferencz C: Transposition of the great vessels: Pathophysiologic considerations based upon a study of the lungs. Circ 33:232, 1966.
25. Ferguson DJ, Adams P, Watson D: Pulmonary arteriosclerosis in transposition of the great vessels. Am J Dis Child 99:653, 1960.
26. Fredriksen PM, Veldtman G, Hechter S, et al: Aerobic capacity in adults with various congenital heart diseases. Am J Cardiol 87:310–314, 2001.
27. Fyler DC: Report of the New England Regional Infant Cardiac Program, Pediatrics 65:375, 1980.
28. Gandhi SK, Pigula FA, Siewers RD: Successful late reintervention after the arterial switch procedure. Ann Thorac Surg 73:88–95, 2002.
29. Gatzoulis MA, Walters J, McLaughlin PR, et al. Late arrhythmia in adults with the Mustard procedure for transposition of the great arteries: a surrogate marker for right ventricular dysfunction? Heart 84(4):409–415, 2000.
30. Gittenberger-de Groot AC, Sauer U, Oppenheimer-Dekker A, et al: Coronary arterial anatomy in transposition of the great arteries: A morphologic study. Pediatr Cardiol (Suppl)4:15, 1983.
31. Hechter SJ, Fredriksen PM, Liu P, et al: Angiotensin-converting enzyme inhibitors in adults after the Mustard procedure. Am J Cardiol 87:660–663, 2001.
32. Hornung TS, Kilner PJ, Davlouros PA, et al: Excessive right ventricular hypertrophic response in adults with the Mustard procedure for transposition of the great arteries. Am J Cardiol 90:800–803, 2002.
33. Hovels-Gurich HH, Konrad K, Wiesner M, et al: Long term behavioral outcome after neonatal arterial switch operation for transposition of the great arteries. Arch Dis Child 87:506–510, 2002.
34. Hovels-Gurich HH, Seghaye MC, Dabritz S, et al: Cardiological and general health status in preschool and school-age children after neonatal arterial switch operation. Eur J Cardiothorac Surg 12:593–601, 1997.
35. Hovels-Gurich HH, Seghaye MC, Dabritz S, et al: Cognitive and motor development in preschool and school-age children after neonatal arterial switch operation. J Thorac Cardiovasc Surg 114:578–585, 1997.
36. Hovels-Gurich HH, Seghaye M-C, Sigler M, et al: Neurodevelopmental outcome related to cerebral risk factors in children after neonatal arterial switch operation. Ann Thorac Surg 71:881–888, 2001.
37. Hutter PA, Kreb DL, Mantel SF, et al. Twenty-five years' experience with the arterial switch operation. J Thorac Cardiovasc Surg 124:790–797, 2002.
38. Hutter PA, Thomeer BJM, Jansen P, et al: Fate of the aortic root after arterial switch operation. Eur J Cardiothor Surg 20:82–88, 2001.
39. Imura H, Modi P, Pawade A, et al: Cardiac Troponin I in neonates undergoing the arterial switch operation. Ann Thorac Surg 74:1998–2002, 2002.
40. Jatene A, Fontes VF, Paulista PP, et al: Anatomic correction of transposition of the great vessels. J Thorac Cardiovasc Surg 72:364, 1976.
41. Kirby M. Embryogenesis of transposition of the great arteries: A lesson from the heart. Circ Res 91:87-89, 2002.
42. Kurasawa H., Imai Y, Kawada M: Coronary arterial anatomy in regard to the arterial switch procedure. Cardiol Young 1:54, 1991.
43. Lacour-Gayet F, Piot D, Zoghbi J, et al: Surgical management and indication of left ventricular retraining in arterial switch for transposition of the great arteries with intact ventricular septum. Eur J Cardiothor Surg 20:824–829, 2001.

44. Liebman J, Cullum L, Belloc NB: Natural history of transposition of the great arteries: Anatomy and birth and death characteristics. Circ 40:237, 1969.
45. Lillehei CW, Varco RL: Certain physiologic, pathologic and surgical features of complete transposition of the great vessels. Surgery 34:376, 1953.
46. Losay J, Touchot A, Serraf A, et al: Late outcome after arterial switch operation for transposition of the great arteries. Circ 104[suppl I]:I-121–I-126, 2001.
47. Mahle WT, McBride MG, Paridon SM: Exercise performance after the arterial switch operation for D-transposition of the great arteries. Am J Cardiol 87:753–758, 2001.
48. Massoudy P, Baltalarli A, de Leval MR, et al: Anatomic variability in coronary arterial distribution with regard to the arterial switch procedure. Circ 106:1980–1984, 2002.
49. Masuda M, Kado H, Shiokawa Y, et al: Clinical results of arterial switch operation for double-outlet right ventricle with subpulmonary VSD. Eur J Cardiothorac Surg 15:283–288, 1999.
50. Mathew R, Rosenthal A, Fellows KE: The significance of right aortic arch in d-transposition of the great arteries. Am Heart J 87:314, 1974.
51. Millane T, Bernard EJ, Jaeggi E, et al: Role of ischemia and infarction in late right ventricular dysfunction after atrial repair of transposition of the great arteries. J Am Coll Cardiol 35:1661–1668, 2000.
52. Moene RJ, Oppenheimer-Dekker A, Wenink ACG, et al: Morphology of ventricular septal defect in complete transposition of the great arteries. Am J Cardiol 55:1566, 1985.
53. Mustard WT: Successful two-stage correction of transposition of the great vessels. Surgery 55:469, 1964.
54. Mustard WT, Chute AL, Keith JD, et al: A surgical approach to transposition of the great vessels with extracorporeal circuit. Surgery 36:39, 1954.
55. Oechslin E, Jenni R: 40 years after the first atrial switch procedure in patients with transposition of the great arteries: long term results in Toronto and Zurich. Thorac Cardiov Surg 48:233–237, 2000.
56. Pacifico AD: Concordant transposition: Senning operation. In: Stark J, DeLeval M (eds.): Surgery for Congenital Heart Defects. New York: Grune & Stratton, 1983, pp. 345–361.
57. Pasquali SK, Hasselblad V, Li JS, et al: Coronary artery pattern and outcome of arterial switch operation for transposition of the great arteries: a meta-analysis. Circ 106:2575–2580, 2002.
58. Poirier NC, Mee RB: Left ventricular reconditioning and anatomical correction for systemic right ventricular dysfunction. Semin Thorac Cardiovasc Surg Pediatr Card Surg Annu 3:198–215, 2000.
59. Pretre R, Tamisier D, Bonhoeffer P, et al: Results of the arterial switch operation in neonates with transposed great arteries. Lancet 357:1826–1830, 2001.
60. Prifti E, Bonacchi, Luisi SV, et al: Coronary revascularization after arterial switch operation. Eur J Cardiothorac Surg 21:111–113, 2002.
61. Prifti E, Crucean A, Bonacchi M, et al: Early and long term outcome of the arterial switch operation for transposition of the great arteries: predictors and functional evaluation. Eur J Cardiothor Surg 22:864–873, 2002.
62. Quaegebeur JM, Rohmer J, Ottenkamp J, et al: The arterial switch operation. J Thorac Cardiovasc Surg 92:361, 1986.
63. Rashkind WJ, Miller WW: Creation of an atrial septal defect without thoracotomy: A palliative approach to complete transposition of the great arteries. JAMA 96:991, 1966.
64. Rastelli GC, Wallace RB, Ongley PA: Complete repair of transposition of the great arteries with pulmonary stenosis: A review and report of a case corrected by using a new surgical technique. Circ 39:83, 1969.
65. Roest AAW, Kunz P, Helbing WA, et al: Prolonged cardiac recovery from exercise in asymptomatic adults late after atrial correction of transposition of the great arteries: evaluation with magnetic resonance flow mapping. Am J Cardiol 88:1011–1017, 2001.
66. Rosti L, Frigiola A, Bini RM, et al: Growth after neonatal arterial switch operation for D-transposition of the great arteries. Pediatr Cardiol 23:32–35, 2002.
67. Scott WA, Fixler DE: Effect of center volume on outcome of ventricular septal defect closure and arterial switch operation. Am J Cardiol 88:1259–1263, 2001.
68. Senning A. Surgical correction of transposition of the great vessels. Surgery 45:966, 1959.
69. Singh TP, Wolfe RR, Sullivan NM, et al: Assessment of progressive changes in exercise performance in patients with a systemic right ventricle following the atrial switch repair. Pediatr Cardiol 22:210–214, 2001.
70. Takeuchi K, McGowan FX, Moran AM, et al: Surgical outcome of double-outlet right ventricle with subpulmonary VSD. Ann Thorac Surg 71:49–53, 2001.
71. Tanel RE, Wernovsky G, Landzberg MJ, et al: Coronary artery abnormalities detected at cardiac catheterization following the arterial switch operation for transposition of the great arteries. Am J Cardiol 76:153–157, 1995.
72. Taussig HB: Complete transposition of the great vessels. Am Heart J 16:728, 1938.
73. Tchervenkov CI, Tahta SA, Cecere R, et al: Single-stage arterial switch with aortic arch enlargement for transposition complexes with aortic arch obstruction. Ann Thorac Surg 64:1776–1781, 1997.
74. Trusler GA, Williams WG, Duncan KF, et al: Results with the Mustard operation in simple transposition of the great arteries. Ann Surg 206:251, 1987.
75. Van Praagh R, Van Praagh S: Isolated ventricular inversion: A consideration of the morphogenesis, definition and diagnosis of nontransposed and transposed great arteries. Am J Cardiol 17:395, 1966.
76. Von Bernuth G. 25 years after the first arterial switch procedure: mid-term results. Thorac Cardiov Surg 48:228–232, 2000.
77. Von Rokitansky C: Die Defekte der Scheidewande der Herzens. Vienna: Braumuller, 1875.
78. Wernovsky G, Mayer JE, Jonas RA, et al: Factors influencing early and late outcome of the arterial switch operation for transposition of the great arteries. J Thorac Cardiovasc Surg 109:289–302, 1995.
79. Yacoub MH, Radley-Smith R, Hilton CJ: Anatomical correction of complete transposition of the great arteries and ventricular septal defect in infancy. Br Med J 1:1112, 1976.
80. Yacoub MH, Radley-Smith R, MacLaurin R: Two-stage operation for anatomical correction of transposition of the great arteries with intact interventricular septum. Lancet 1:1275, 1977.

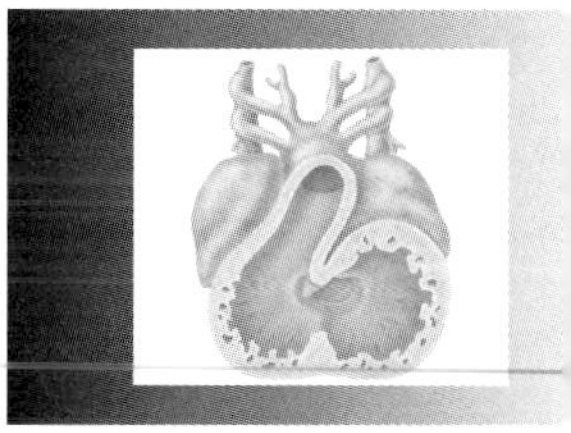

Transposition of the Great Arteries (Complex Forms)

CHAPTER 122

Pedro J. del Nido

INTRODUCTION

Transposition of the great arteries can exist in association with a number of intracardiac defects resulting in complex anatomy that provides a significant challenge to the cardiologist defining the anatomy and the surgeon who has to achieve a hemodynamically satisfactory repair. In particular, associated conotruncal anomalies have important consequences for the development of downstream structures such as semilunar valves and great vessels, which impact the surgical correction and even the timing of surgical intervention. In this chapter, the diagnosis and surgical management of some of these complex forms of transposition will be discussed. The management of "simple" transposition of the great arteries with or without a ventricular septal defect is covered in the previous chapter (see Chapter 121). Also, I will not cover complex forms that are associated with hypoplasia of one of the ventricles or where atrioventricular (AV) valve morphology, such as straddling or atresia, precludes an anatomical two-ventricle repair.

ANATOMICAL VARIANTS OF TRANSPOSITION OF THE GREAT ARTERIES

Discordant connections between the ventricles and the great vessels are the hallmark of transposition and the physiological consequence is the creation of two parallel circulations, the pulmonary circuit (left ventricle [LV]→pulmonary artery→left atrium→LV) and the systemic circuit (right ventricle [RV]→aorta→right atrium→RV), resulting in profound cyanosis if there is no mixing of blood between these two circuits. Although this discordant relationship between the ventricles and great vessels is an integral component of transposition with associated conotruncal anomalies, often the associated defects dominate the clinical presentation and management of these infants (Figure 122-1). For the purposes of this chapter we shall use the term "complex" transposition to refer to those defects in which there are additional conotruncal anomalies besides transposition of the great arteries. The associated conotruncal defects include malalignment or deviation of the conal septum either into the left ventricular or right ventricular outflow tract or persistence of a conus over the LV separating the mitral valve from the semilunar valve, also called the Taussig-Bing anomaly. Together these complex forms account for 10% to 15% of all transposition cases.[3]

Conal Septum

The conal septum separates the two semilunar valves and forms part of the septation of the common arterial trunk, present early in fetal cardiac development, into aorta and pulmonary trunk. Although abnormal development of the conus with regression of the subpulmonary component rather than the subaortic component has been proposed as the etiology of transposition, the position, orientation, and

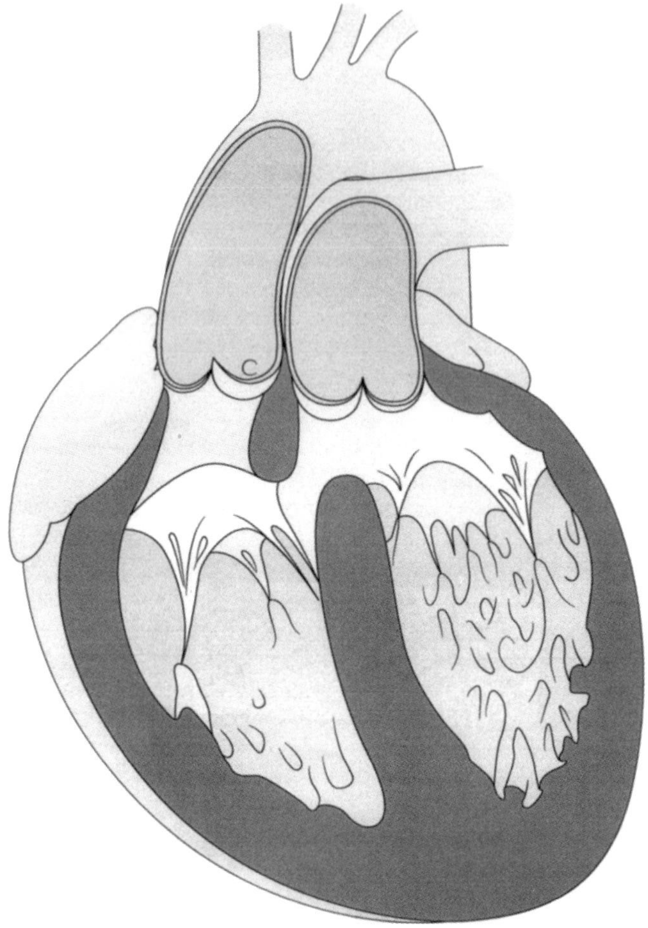

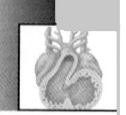

Figure 122–1 Transposition with double outlet right ventricle. The conal septum is positioned over the right ventricle. In cases in which there is deviation of the conal septum from this neutral position, the outflow semilunar valve and great artery often are hypoplastic.

size of the conal septum may vary independent of ventriculoarterial connection.[13] Thus a prominent conal septum that deviates posteriorly can cause LV outflow obstruction; similarly, anterior deviation of the conal septum can result in RV outflow obstruction. In hearts with normally related great arteries, when the conal deviation is associated with a conoventricular septal defect, the downstream consequences of the ventricular outflow obstruction are hypoplasia or atresia of the affected great artery as seen in interrupted aortic arch (LV outflow obstruction) and tetralogy of Fallot (RV outflow obstruction). In transposition, however, the affected downstream circulation is the inverse with LV outflow obstruction resulting in decreased pulmonary trunk blood flow and RV outflow obstruction resulting in aortic arch hypoplasia and/or interruption.[12,21]

Transposition and Left Ventricular Outflow Tract Obstruction

Left ventricular outflow tract obstruction (LVOTO) in an infant with transposition of the great arteries can occur in the presence or absence of a ventricular septal defect. In intact ventricular septum, most often the pressure gradient measured across the outflow tract is a result of dynamic displacement of the interventricular septum posteriorly due to the pressure difference between the right (systemic) and left (pulmonary) ventricles, with the latter functioning at lower pressures. Once the LV assumes the systemic circulation following an arterial switch, the septum usually bows toward the RV and the pressure gradient disappears. A fixed obstruction from a prominent conal septum deviated posteriorly or a fibrous ridge or muscle bundle is uncommon in the absence of a conoventricular septal defect and in most cases, can be resected and does not preclude an arterial switch operation (see Chapter 121 Simple TGA).

LVOTO in the presence of a conoventricular septal defect most often results from posterior deviation of the conal septum. In long-standing obstruction, a fibrous ridge or even fibromuscular tunnel can develop, further increasing the degree of obstruction. The obstruction is usually subvalvar but can be associated with pulmonary valve hypoplasia or dysplasia (bicuspid valve and/or thickened leaflets) precluding the use of this valve for an arterial switch procedure. The degree of obstruction in LVOTO with a VSD is often more severe than in TGA with intact septum and the obstruction often progresses early in infancy during the first few months of life requiring surgical intervention because of progressive cyanosis.

Transposition and Right Ventricular Outflow Tract Obstruction

Similar to LVOTO, deviation of the conal septum, in this case anteriorly into the RV outflow tract, is the most common cause of obstruction to flow into the systemic circulation. In transposition, RVOTO is almost always associated with a malalignment-type conoventricular septal defect and is also frequently associated with double outlet RV, also called Taussig-Bing anomaly. In this latter defect, there is persistence of a conus or infundibulum under the pulmonary trunk, resulting in muscular separation between the mitral and pulmonary valve annulus. This complex lesion accounts for 5% to 7% of transposition cases based on autopsy series.[14] There are a number of associated defects including downstream hypoplasia of the aortic valve and aortic arch with coarctation. In some infants, the degree of aortic valve and arch hypoplasia is severe, requiring maintenance of a patent arterial duct to achieve adequate systemic perfusion. Hypoplasia of the RV and tricuspid valve has also been described in this complex to a degree that a two-ventricle repair was not possible.[22] Often enlargement of the RV outflow tract is necessary in conjunction with an arterial switch operation to prevent the development of subpulmonary obstruction. Hypoplasia of the aortic valve annulus can vary in degree and in severe forms requires a transannular patch to relieve RV outflow obstruction.

In most cases of RVOTO and transposition, there is a significant mismatch in diameter between the pulmonary trunk and the ascending aorta. This fact complicates the arterial switch procedure because enlargement of the ascending aorta and, if aortic arch hypoplasia is present, enlargement of the entire transverse arch and isthmus is required to achieve a hemodynamically satisfactory result.

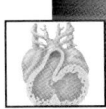

Double Outlet Right Ventricle with Transposition

Double outlet right ventricle (DORV) with transposition of the great arteries is often termed "DORV with subpulmonary VSD" to describe the great vessel relationship to the RV and to the VSD. Unlike DORV with normally related great arteries, the vessel closest to the VSD in this case is the pulmonary trunk and determines the method of anatomical repair required for correction. Subpulmonary or subaortic obstruction can be associated with transposition and DORV, usually resulting in hypoplasia of the downstream semilunar valve and great vessel. The great vessel relationship to each other often is that of a side-by-side arrangement with the aorta most commonly to the right of the pulmonary valve.

The VSD is described as malalignment type because the conal septum does not meet the septomarginal trabecula, similar to double outlet RV with normally related great vessels. The VSD can extend to the annulus of the tricuspid valve and in these cases, the conduction tissue runs on the edge of the VSD in the posterocaudal margin of the defect starting at the junction with the tricuspid valve annulus.[6] In some cases the VSD can extend to the inlet septum complicating the repair because the defect is partially covered by the septal leaflet of the tricuspid valve. In such cases, chordae from the tricuspid valve can attach to the crest of the septum and even straddle into the LV. In most cases however, the degree of straddling is limited and does not preclude a two-ventricle repair. Rarely, additional septal defects are present in the muscular septum or apical trabecular area and these can be difficult to identify and close, particularly in the apical posterior septum.

Coronary Artery Anatomy

Coronary artery anatomy can also be variable with complex forms of transposition. Transposition and DORV in particular is associated with unusual patterns of coronary artery anatomy including a relatively high incidence of single coronary giving rise to branches to both ventricles. The high association between side-by-side great vessels and unusual coronary artery pattern has been emphasized previously. In a detailed pathological study, Uemura and associates,[20] found that a single coronary artery was present in 27% of hearts with a side-by-side great artery relationship. Gordillo and colleagues have also described a higher incidence of unusual coronary artery pattern in DORV with a subpulmonary VSD.[5] Coronary anatomy continues to be an important factor in anatomical repair of transposition, however, only when an arterial switch is contemplated as part of the repair. Although in most larger centers, coronary artery pattern is no longer a significant risk factor for death, it can complicate the surgical procedure and may result in a higher rate of complications.

Aortic Arch Anatomy

Aortic arch anomalies occur in 7% to 10% of infants with transposition and VSD. This association is more common when the pulmonary valve overrides the ventricular septum particularly in DORV and transposition. A wide spectrum of arch obstruction exists from discrete coarctation at the level of the ductus to hypoplasia of the distal arch, and even aortic arch interruption. The degree of severity of arch hypoplasia is thought to be associated with the degree of subaortic obstruction, usually from deviation of the outlet or conal septum into the RV outflow. Additionally, there can be relative hypoplasia of the tricuspid valve in comparison to the mitral valve and in extreme cases, the degree of hypoplasia of the tricuspid valve can preclude a two-ventricle repair. It is important to recognize this association and preoperative measurements of the AV valves normalized to body surface area can be most helpful in deciding surgical management.

DIAGNOSIS AND PREOPERATIVE MANAGEMENT

The clinical presentation of infants with complex transposition can vary widely depending primarily on the severity of associated defects such as pulmonary obstruction or aortic arch hypoplasia and coarctation. Because an unrestrictive VSD is present in nearly all of these infants, there is the potential for adequate mixing of blood from the pulmonary and systemic circuits, thus cyanosis from lack of mixing of the two circulations is uncommon. If cyanosis is the most prominent symptom at presentation, then inadequate pulmonary blood flow from subvalvar or valvar pulmonary stenosis is the most common cause in conjunction with closure of the arterial duct after birth. In infants with subaortic obstruction and aortic arch hypoplasia, the initial presentation is similar to that of infants with isolated coarctation of the aorta, with decreased systemic perfusion, metabolic acidosis, and if unrecognized and untreated, severe shock with end organ injury. In both clinical presentations, initiation of prostaglandins can rapidly reverse the signs of severe cyanosis or inadequate systemic perfusion, by opening the arterial duct and augmenting pulmonary blood flow in infants with pulmonary obstruction, or systemic blood flow in infants with aortic arch obstruction.

Echocardiography is usually the initial diagnostic study performed when complex congenital heart defects are detected because it provides not only anatomical detail required to plan surgical repair but also physiological information on valve function, presence, location, and severity of obstructions to flow particularly in the outflow tracts of the ventricles as well as the pulmonary arteries and arch vessels. As with all echocardiographic studies, a systematic evaluation of chambers, connections, inflow and outflow valves, and ventricular size and function is imperative, particularly with difficult defects such as complex transposition. In addition, specific anatomical details such as relationship of the pulmonary root to the VSD, conal septal position, coronary artery pattern, and chordal attachments of the AV valves with respect to the septum are important to define to develop a plan for surgical correction.

Cardiac catheterization is not required in most cases of complex transposition because echocardiography is usually sufficient to detail the anatomy and important physiological features. Cardiac catheterization and angiography are therefore utilized to resolve any unanswered anatomical questions the echocardiography has not resolved and in specific circumstances in which accurate pressure measurements are required, such as pulmonary artery pressures for calculation of pulmonary vascular resistance, to measure the pressure gradient across a potentially restrictive VSD. Also, in cases in which a palliative procedure has been performed, catheterization and angiography is needed to identify potential anatomical distortion from the previous surgical interventions such as systemic-to-pulmonary shunts. Rarely is interventional catheterization required in infants unless there is a restrictive interatrial communication and inadequate mixing of blood from the pulmonary and systemic circuits, a situation more common in transposition with intact septum.

SURGICAL MANAGEMENT

TGA with LVOTO

Palliative Procedures

The pathophysiology of transposition results in cyanosis that often is unresponsive to oxygen therapy. When transposition is complicated by obstruction to the LV outflow tract, cyanosis can be more severe, frequently worsening in the first few months of life. In the extreme, when there is atresia of the LV outflow tract, pulmonary blood flow is entirely dependent on a patent arterial duct and/or systemic-to-pulmonary collaterals. In these cases, repair of this defect can be delayed by placing a systemic-to-pulmonary shunt and ligating collaterals or the arterial duct. The corrective procedure can then be deferred several months. In cases in which cyanosis is not severe, a systemic-to-pulmonary shunt is not indicated and if delayed repair is contemplated, this can usually be deferred several weeks or months. The most common reason for delaying the corrective procedure is when resection of the LV outflow is not feasible and a conduit will be required to establish RV to pulmonary artery continuity (see Rastelli repair). The institutional philosophy at Children's Hospital of Boston, however, is to achieve anatomical and physiological correction of the cardiac defect as early in life as possible.

Surgical Technique

The preferred shunt procedure for TGA with LVOTO is a modified Blalock shunt with an expanded PTFE tube graft. In infants with a left aortic arch, the origin of the shunt is the base of the right subclavian artery and the distal end connects to the right pulmonary artery. In transposition, the pulmonary trunk is often short with the ductus arising centrally as a direct extension of the main pulmonary artery. Insertion of the distal end of the shunt into the pulmonary trunk is often difficult because of its short length and proximity to the ductus. The surgical approach for a shunt is usually through a median sternotomy that provides access to the arch vessels and branch pulmonary arteries. The thymus gland is mobilized and innominate vein freed from attachments to the pericardium and aorta. Because the course of the shunt will be parallel to the superior vena cava, tissue between the ascending aorta and superior cava must be cleared. Once the innominate artery and right subclavian origin are dissected, the right pulmonary artery is mobilized from its origin to the bifurcation of the upper lobe. Heparin (50 u/kg) is administered to prevent thrombus formation in the vessels or the graft during insertion. The caudal side of the innominate-subclavian artery junction is identified for the anastomosis and a curved vascular clamp used for occlusion. The anastomosis is done with fine monofilament sutures (7-0 polypropylene), and care is taken not to damage the fragile intima of the innominate artery. The distal end is sewn to the cephalad side of the pulmonary artery, also with fine monofilament sutures. Deairing of the graft is performed and brisk flow through the graft should be confirmed prior to completing the distal anastomosis. The graft is usually 3.5 mm in diameter for neonates and young infants and provides adequate pulmonary blood flow for several months until corrective surgery is performed. In some centers, a larger shunt (4.0 mm) is chosen in an effort to gain more time with palliation. This approach, although effective, runs the risk of producing pulmonary overcirculation in the early period after shunt insertion with complications such as inadequate renal perfusion and renal insufficiency or necrotizing enterocolitis. If a larger shunt is used, great care must be taken in the early postoperative period to maintain adequate systemic perfusion to avoid these complications.

Once the shunt is unclamped, the oxygen saturations should rise within seconds confirming adequate shunt flow. An additional indicator is a modest fall in diastolic pressure. If the diastolic pressure is low (usually below 25 mm Hg), consideration should be given to ligation of the arterial duct to prevent complications of pulmonary overcirculation. Once stable, a single chest drain is left in the pericardial space and the sternum is closed. Low-dose heparin (10–15 u/kg/hr) can be continued in the postoperative period once mediastinal bleeding has subsided.

Corrective Procedures

Management of the LVOTO in transposition depends on the severity and location of the obstruction. In cases in which the obstruction appears dynamic from leftward deviation of the interventricular septum because of systemic pressure in the RV, then an arterial switch procedure with closure of a ventricular septal defect, when present, is the preferred method of correction (see Chapter 121, Transposition of the Great Arteries). In these cases, the pulmonary valve annulus is within the normal range for the child's size, and instantaneous gradient across the LV outflow, as estimated by echodoppler, is less than 35–40 mm Hg in the presence of a small or closed arterial duct.

TGA with Posterior Deviation of Conal Septum

In cases in which the conal septum is the major source of LV outflow obstruction and the pulmonary valve is adequate (Z-score of –2 or better) then resection of the conal septum with closure of the VSD (when present) and an arterial switch procedure is the best option in most cases. This approach establishes anatomical repair and avoids the use of conduits, although there is a small but present risk of developing more severe LVOTO late. Resection of the subpulmonary obstruction is most often possible through the pulmonary trunk, by retracting the pulmonary valve leaflets. This approach also ensures adequate visualization of the hinge points of the leaflets as these can attach to the conal septum directly. The LV outflow can also be seen through the mitral valve although this approach is rarely better than through the pulmonary artery.

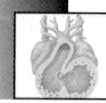

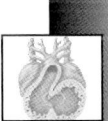

coarctation involves only the isthmus and junction with the arterial duct, then a simple resection with end-to-end anastomosis is sufficient. Frequently in infants with DORV, the transverse arch is hypoplastic to varying degrees and requires patch augmentation. Furthermore, there is almost always a significant size discrepancy between the ascending aorta and pulmonary trunk, with the latter being substantially larger (Figure 122-6). In these cases, patch augmentation of the entire ascending aorta and arch, similar to the augmentation done for hypoplastic left heart syndrome, facilitates the arterial switch by eliminating the size discrepancy with the neoaorta (Figures 122-7 and 122-8).

Arterial cannulation through the ascending aorta is usually sufficient to perfuse the lower half of the body. Rarely is a second arterial cannula via the arterial duct required for adequate perfusion. Deep hypothermia to 18° C is used although in cases with simple coarctation, circulatory arrest is not required and coarctectomy with end-to-end repair can be done with moderate hypothermia, decreased flow (~50–75 ml/kg/min) and proximal and distal clamps. If arch augmentation is required, then a period of circulatory arrest is usually necessary. For short-segment augmentation, a glutaraldehyde-treated autologous pericardial patch can be used for arch augmentation. For extensive patches, a segment of pulmonary artery homograft works well and is less likely to calcify late. The rest of the arterial switch procedure is similar to that for simple transposition. The VSD is best closed through a ventriculotomy in most cases similar to the approach for DORV, and this approach permits patch enlargement of the RV outflow if obstruction is suspected.

In cases in which the RV is hypoplastic, then careful evaluation of tricuspid valve annulus size and RV volume should be done prior to surgery. In cases where the tricuspid valve Z score is less than –2.5 or the RV volume is less than 15 ml/m^2, then single ventricle management is probably the better option rather than attempted two-ventricle repair. If the RV is borderline in size or there is concern that the combination of a mildly hypoplastic and/or the infundibular incision will result in diminished RV diastolic compliance, then leaving a small (~3–4 mm) interatrial communication will permit right-to-left shunting, preserving systemic flow at the expense of mild cyanosis similar to repair of tetralogy of Fallot in infants.

Results

TGA with LVOTO

Surgical repair of complex forms of transposition carries a significantly higher risk for morbidity and mortality than repair of simpler forms. Nevertheless, improvement in results with complex forms parallels those of simple transposition over the last two decades. In a review of the 25-year

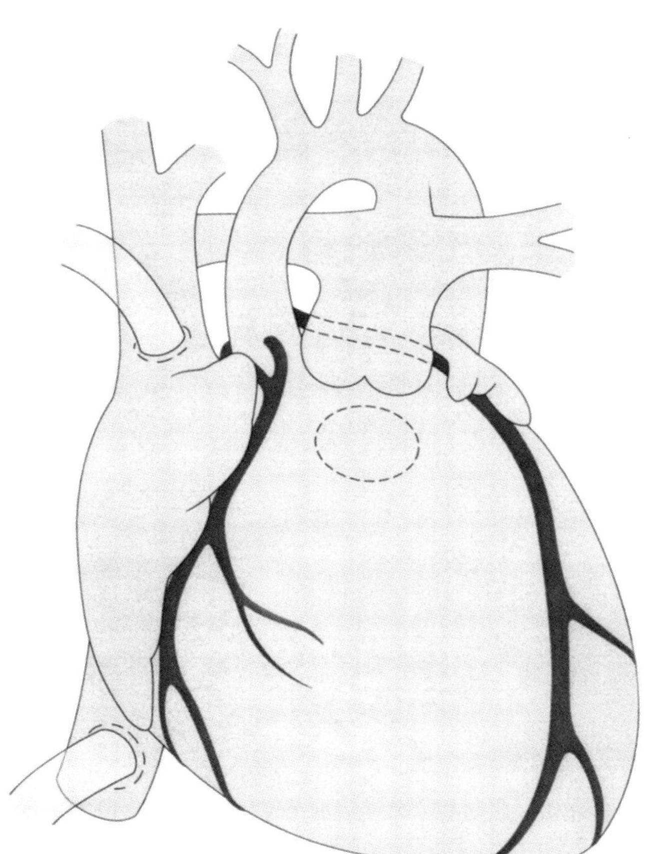

Figure 122-6 Transposition of the great arteries with aortic arch hypoplasia. There is usually a significant size discrepancy between the two semilunar valves and trunks, with the pulmonary being much larger than the aorta.

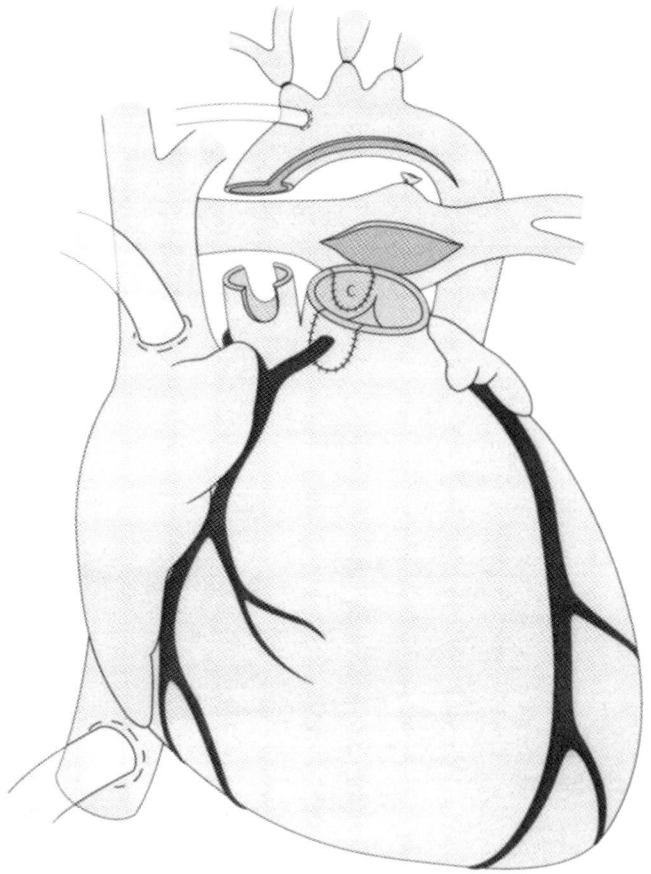

Figure 122-7 Transposition with aortic arch hypoplasia. Aortic arch augmentation is extended to the ascending aorta to account for the size discrepancy between the pulmonary artery and aorta.

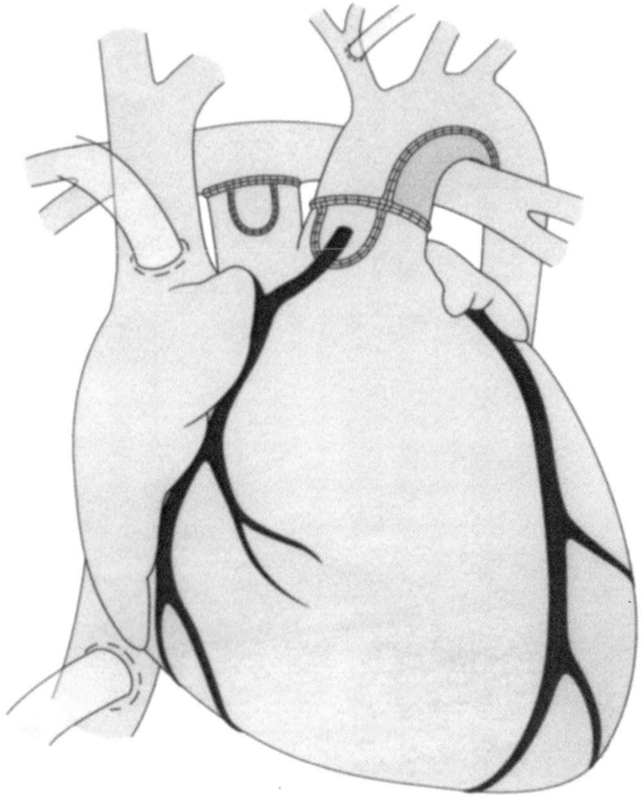

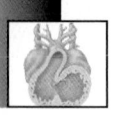

Figure 122–8 **Transposition with aortic arch hypoplasia.** Completion of the arterial switch procedure. In side-by-side configuration, the pulmonary arteries are usually mobilized to the right side without repositioning anterior to the aorta.

experience with the Rastelli operation at Children's Hospital of Boston, Kreutzer, et al reported an overall mortality of 7% for the entire review period and no deaths in the most recent 7-year period.[8] Risk factors for early death were straddling tricuspid valve and longer cross-clamp time. On late follow-up, freedom from death or transplantation was 82%, 80%, 68%, and 52% at 5, 10, 15, and 20 years, respectively. Arrhythmias and sudden death accounted for nearly one third of the late deaths and LV dysfunction accounted for another third. Freedom from death or reintervention was 53%, 24%, and 21% at 5, 10, and 15 years of follow-up, respectively. The most common indication for reintervention was conduit obstruction, but LV outflow tract obstruction was also prevalent throughout the follow-up period .

Results with Lecompte's procedure for TGA and LVOTO are similar to the Rastelli procedure with respect to early mortality with 3 of 42 patients dying early.[15] On late follow-up, however, there were no late deaths with a median follow-up of 5.4 years. Freedom from reoperation was 86 ± 8% and 51 ± 22% at 5 and 10 years, respectively, with the indication for reintervention being RV outflow obstruction in all patients.

TGA with DORV

Transposition with double outlet RV or the Taussig-Bing anomaly still represents a significant surgical challenge with respect to early morbidity and mortality. In a recent review, Takeuchi et al reported a 20% early mortality with side-by-side great vessel relationship and associated single coronary as a significant risk factor for death.[17] In the same report, infants that were managed as single ventricle with initial Glenn connection followed by Fontan had no operative deaths and no late deaths. Of the children undergoing an arterial switch, three required reoperation late, two for subaortic stenosis and one for supravalvar pulmonary stenosis. There were no late deaths in either group at an average of 24-months' follow-up. Mavroudis et al reported a series of 20 infants with Taussig-Bing anomaly comparing the arterial switch procedure with intracardiac tunneling technique described by Kawashima.[10] The operative mortality was 6% for the arterial switch group, and in the four children undergoing intracardiac baffle there were no deaths. Of importance however, was the fact that the average age at operation in these patients was 1.4 years with most requiring at least one palliative procedure prior to repair. There was a high incidence of reoperation in the arterial switch group with aortic valve regurgitation a frequent complication late, likely reflecting the effects of pulmonary artery banding as a preswitch palliation resulting in distortion of the neoaortic root.

TGA with Aortic Arch Obstruction

In recent reports, aortic arch hypoplasia or discrete coarctation have not been associated with increased mortality when the arterial switch and arch repair are undertaken together. Blume et al reported a significant increase in overall mortality in children who had arch repair prior to arterial switch although the reasons for this were unclear.[2] Tchervenkov, et al have reported no operative deaths in 12 patients undergoing arterial switch procedure for TGA with aortic arch obstruction and no late deaths after a mean follow-up time of 42 months.[19] Other centers have reported a small but present incidence of aortic arch obstruction requiring reintervention with balloon dilation late.[4]

SUMMARY

Complex transposition includes a number of associated intracardiac and great vessel anomalies, which significantly impact the symptoms at presentation, operative, and postoperative risks as compared to simple transposition with or without a VSD. Accurate diagnostic evaluation and increased experience with early single-stage repair have reduced overall mortality and morbidity in this patient group. New procedures to avoid late complications continue to be developed and continued follow up is mandatory in patients with complex repairs. Requirement for late reintervention is common with conduit obstruction remaining the most common indication for reoperation.

REFERENCES

1. Barbero-Marcial M, Tamanati C, Jatene MB, et al: Double-outlet right ventricle with nonrelated ventricular septal defect: surgical results using the multiple patches technique. Heart Surg Forum 1:125–129, 1998.
2. Blume ED, Altmann K, Mayer JE, et al: Evolution of risk factors influencing early mortality of the arterial switch operation. J Am Coll Cardiol 33:1702–1709, 1999.

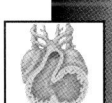

3. Fyler DC: Report of the New England regional infant cardiac program. Pediatrics 65:375, 1980.
4. Gandhi SK, Pigula FA, Siewers RD: Successful late reintervention after the arterial switch procedure. Ann Thorac Surg 73:88–93, 2002.
5. Gordillo L, Faye-Petersen O, de la Cruz MV, Soto B: Coronary arterial patterns in double-outlet right ventricle. Am J Cardiol 71:1108–1110 1993.
6. Hoyer MH, Zuberbuhler JR, Anderson RH, del Nido P: Morphology of ventricular septal defects in complete transposition. Surgical implications. J Thorac Cardiovasc Surg 104:1203–1211, 1992.
7. Konno S, Imai Y, Iida Y, et al: A new method for prosthetic valve replacement in congenital aortic stenosis associated with hypoplasia of the aortic valve ring. J. Thorac Cardiovasc Surg 70:909–917, 1975.
8. Kreutzer C, De Vive J, Oppido G, et al: Twenty-five-year experience with Rastelli repair for transposition of the great arteries. J Thorac Cardiovasc Surg 120:211–223, 2000.
9. Lecompte Y, Neveux JY, Leca F, et al: Reconstruction of the pulmonary outflow tract without a prosthetic conduit. J Thorac Cardiovasc Surg 84:727–733, 1982.
10. Mavroudis C, Backer CL, Muster AJ, et al: Taussig-Bing anomaly: arterial switch versus Kawashima intraventricular repair. Ann Thorac Surg 61:1330–1338, 1996.
11. McGoon DC: Intraventricular repair of transposition of the great arteries. J Thorac Cardiovasc Surg 64:430–434, 1972.
12. Milanesi O, Ho SY, Thiene G, et al: The ventricular septal defect in complete transposition of the great arteries: pathologic anatomy in 57 cases with emphasis on subaortic, subpulmonary, and aortic arch obstruction. Hum Pathol 18:392–396, 1987.
13. Pasquini L, Sanders SP, Parness IA, et al: Conal anatomy in 119 patients with d-loop transposition of the great arteries and ventricular septal defect: an echocardiographic and pathologic study. J Am Coll Cardiol 21:1712–1721, 1993.
14. Pigott JD, Chin AJ, Weinberg PM, et al: Transposition of the great arteries with aortic arch obstruction. Anatomical review and report of surgical management. J Thorac Cardiovasc Surg 94:82–86, 1987
15. Petre R, Gendron G, Tamisier D, et al: Results of the Lecompte procedure in malposition of the great arteries and pulmonary obstruction. Eur J Cardiothorac Surg 19:283–289, 2001.
16. Rastelli GC, MaGoon DC, Wallace RB: Anatomic correction of transposition of the great arteries with ventricular septal defect and subpulmonary stenosis. J Thorac Cardiovasc Surg 58:545–552, 1969.
17. Takeuchi K, McGowan FX Jr, Moran AM, et al: Surgical outcome of double-outlet right ventricle with subpulmonary VSD. Ann Thorac Surg 71:49–52, 2001.
18. Tchervenkov CI, Korkola SJ: Transposition complexes with systemic obstruction. Semin Thorac Cardiovasc Surg Pediatr Card Surg Annu 4:71–82, 2001.
19. Tchervenkov CI, Tahta SA, Cecere R, Beland MJ: Single-stage arterial switch with aortic arch enlargement for transposition complexes with aortic arch obstruction. Ann Thorac Surg 64:1776–1781,1997.
20. Uemura H, Yagihara T, Kawashima Y, et al: Coronary arterial anatomy in double-outlet right ventricle with subpulmonary VSD. Ann Thorac Surg 59:591–597, 1995.
21. Van Praagh R, Jung WK The arterial switch operation in transposition of the great arteries: anatomic indications and contraindications. Thorac Cardiovasc Surg Dec;39 Suppl 2:138–150, 1991.
22. Vogel M, Freedom RM, Smallhorn JF, et al: Complete transposition of the great arteries and coarctation of the aorta Am J Cardiol 53:1627–1632, Jun 1, 1984.
23. Vouhé PR, Tamisier D, Leca F, et al: Transposition of the great arteries, ventricular septal defect, and pulmonary outflow tract obstruction: Rastelli or Lecompte procedure? J Thorac Cardiovasc Surg 103:428–436, 1992.

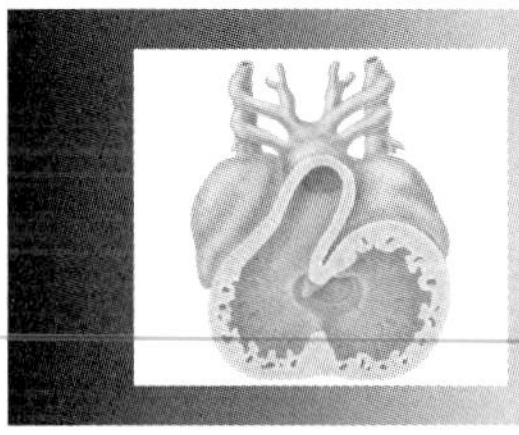

CHAPTER 123

Surgery for Congenitally Corrected Transposition of the Great Arteries

William J. Brawn and David J. Barron

INTRODUCTION

Congenitally corrected transposition of the great arteries is a rare defect (approximately 0.5% of patients with congenital heart defects),[15,17] comprising discordance of the atrioventricular (AV) connections and discordance of the ventricular arterial connections that is double discordance. The morphology of the heart is distinctly abnormal but the circulatory system is physiologically normal. Commonly congenitally corrected transposition is associated with ventricular septal defects (VSDs), pulmonary stenosis, dysplasia of the tricuspid valve, and conduction abnormalities, usually the development of heart block.[5,26,39] Whilst this condition can be compatible with a normal life span,[4,32] the majority of patients require surgery to repair the associated cardiac anomalies, and many develop heart failure due to systemic morphological right ventricular (RV) dysfunction usually with tricuspid valve regurgitation.[10,34,38,43] Historically, surgery has been directed to managing the associated cardiac anomalies, closure of the VSD, relief of pulmonary stenosis, repair or replacement of the tricuspid valve, and placement of pacemakers to manage the conduction abnormalities. This so-called classical or conventional (physiological) repair maintains the morphological right ventricle as the systemic ventricle. More recently the morphological left ventricle has been restored to the systemic circulation by an atrial switch (Senning or Mustard procedure) and an arterial switch or Rastelli procedure to connect the aorta to the morphologic left ventricle.[13,19,37,42]

GENERAL DESCRIPTION AND MORPHOLOGY

In the usual situs solitus arrangement with normal systemic and pulmonary venous drainage the ventricular apex of the heart usually points to the left side of the patient but mesocardia and dextrocardia are common, occurring in up to 20% of cases.[9,26] Malposition of the ventricular mass so it comes to lie in front of the atria and venous drainage to the heart can make surgical access to these structures difficult. In situs inversus, which can occur in about 5% of cases, mesocardia and levocardia can occur. It seems that extreme malposition of the ventricular mass is commonly associated with severe pulmonary stenosis or pulmonary atresia in association with a large VSD.[9] Characteristically the aorta is anterior and to the left side of the more deeply placed pulmonary artery hence the older term for this condition, L transposition. However, the aorta can be more anterior to the pulmonary artery and even right-sided. Likewise the morphological left ventricle is usually to the right and slightly inferior to the morphological right ventricle; however, the position of the ventricles relative to each other can show great variability.[5] The ascending aorta is often quite short and well over to the left side of the mediastinum in situs solitus, again making surgical access difficult. In the rarer form of situs inversus the aorta lies anterior and to the right of the posterior pulmonary artery and is usually more accessible.

In congenitally corrected transposition of the great arteries without associated cardiac anomalies, the circulation is physiologically normal with systemic venous return passing through the right atrium, mitral valve, and then into the morphological left ventricle. Here the morphological left ventricle pumps blood through the pulmonary arteries into the lungs where it returns to the pulmonary veins and to the left atrium. The blood flow continues through the tricuspid valve and into the morphologic right ventricle where it is pumped around the systemic circulation via the aorta (Figure 123-1). Without other cardiac anomalies patients with congenitally corrected transposition can survive well into adult life without symptoms. It is the associated anomalies of VSD, pulmonary stenosis, abnormalities of the tricuspid valve, and development of arrhythmias or complete heart block, which seem to predispose the patient to the development of cardiac failure early in life.

Ventricular Septal Defect

VSD can occur in about 70% of cases.[26] It is usually isolated and in the perimembranous region. Isolated VSDs can also occur in the infundibular region and they may be multiple. When associated with severe pulmonary stenosis or pulmonary atresia the VSD is usually subaortic and large extending from the perimembranous region to beneath the aortic valve. This is important in that it allows the VSD to be tunneled to the aorta when the morphological left ventricle is committed to the aorta as a systemic ventricle.

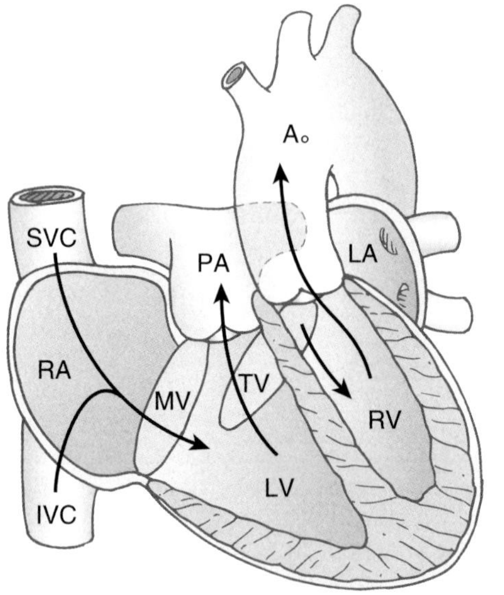

Figure 123–1 Diagram of congenitally corrected transposition. Ao, Aorta; IVC, inferior vena cava; LA, left atrium; LV, left ventricle; MV, mitral valve; PA, pulmonary artery; RA, right atrium; RV, right ventricle; SVC, superior vena cava; TV, tricuspid valve.

Pulmonary Outflow Tract Obstruction (Morphological Left Ventricular Outflow Tract Obstruction)

Obstruction to the pulmonary artery from the left ventricle is common in congenitally corrected transposition in probably up to 50% of cases.[16,26] In part this is due to the position of the pulmonary artery, it being placed between the mitral and tricuspid valves deep in toward the crux of the heart. A potential exists for hypoplasia of the subpulmonary outflow tract. When associated with a VSD there may be accessory tissue around the VSD, which can balloon into the pulmonary valve. Accessory tissue tags can prolapse into the outflow tract from either the mitral or tricuspid valve and over time fibrous tissue can be deposited in the subpulmonary area of the morphological left ventricular (LV) outflow tract. Accessory attachments of the mitral or tricuspid mitral valve through the VSD can cause obstruction beneath the pulmonary valve. The pulmonary valve itself may be stenotic.

The Mitral and Tricuspid Valves

The mitral valve is usually normal in congenitally corrected transposition. There are usually two well-formed papillary muscles on the lateral wall of the left ventricle. Occasionally we have noted a cleft in the septal component of the mitral valve.[25]

The tricuspid valve, however, is a markedly different proposition. The valve itself may be intrinsically normal but through dilation of the ventricle and the tricuspid valve annulus become progressively regurgitant over time. However, more commonly the valve is dysplastic and this predisposes to valvular regurgitation. There is a marked association with dysplasia and displacement of the septal components of the tricuspid valve well down into the body of the right ventricle, sometimes for several centimeters, and this in the setting of systemic pressures in the right ventricle can create severe tricuspid valve regurgitation. We have noted double orifices in the tricuspid valve, abnormal septal clefts as well as marked annular dilation. Because of difficult access and the great variability in the pathology in this valve, repair can be very difficult.[1,2,25]

The Ebsteinoid-like displacement of the tricuspid valve into the body of the morphological right ventricle is not associated with any atrialization of the RV free wall. Hence it is not strictly equivalent to an Ebstein tricuspid valve in a normal heart. In addition when functioning at lower pulmonary pressures after a Double Switch the regurgitation markedly reduces; that is, it is not a low-pressure regurgitant valve it tends to be a high-pressure regurgitant valve.

Rarely both straddling and override of the AV valves can occur usually in association with a degree of hypoplasia of the left or right ventricle.[6,14,30]

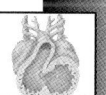

Other Associated Cardiac Anomalies

Abnormalities of the aortic arch including interruption of the aorta and coarctation can occur.

Coronary Arteries

Usually the anterior sinus of the aortic valve gives rise to what would normally be the right coronary artery (Figure 123-2). This divides to pass down the line of the interventricular septum as the anterior descending coronary artery. The other circumflex branch passes in the AV groove between the right atrium and left ventricle. The posterior sinus of the aortic valve gives rise to the morphologically right coronary artery passing in the AV groove between the left atrium and right ventricle. Almost universally the coronary artery ostia face the equivalent sinuses of the pulmonary valve. This is an important consideration in the arterial switch procedure.

The Conduction System

The abnormalities of the conduction system in congenitally corrected transposition have been well described.[3,11,24,41] Because of malalignment of the AV septum there is an anterior and superior AV node in the atrial septum adjacent to the mitral and pulmonary valve. This gives rise to a penetrating bundle that passes around the free wall of the left ventricle in a subendocardial position anterior to the pulmonary valve. The bundle then sweeps down onto the ventricular septum in the morphological left ventricle supplying a left bundle branch over the septal surface of the left ventricle and a penetrating right branch into the morphological right ventricle. The sinus node is in a normal position adjacent to the entrance of the superior vena cava into the right atrium (Figure 123-3).

In the rarer form of situs inversus the normally positioned atrioventricular node that is in the triangle of Koch superior to the coronary sinus persists and gives a penetrating branch to the ventricular septum but inferior and posterior to the pulmonary valve. These pathways are important because in situs solitus when there is a VSD in the perimembranous region, the bundle passes superior to the VSD around the pulmonary outflow tract and then down on the leftward or anterior margin of the VSD. In the rarer forms of situs inversus the bundle passes on the inferior margin of the VSD on the morphologic LV surface. Occasionally both posterior and anterior AV node exist and a loop of conduction tissue can encircle the VSD when it is present. Sutures to close the VSD are ideally placed from the morphological RV surface of the VSD to avoid damaging the conduction system.[12] The longer course of the conduction system to the ventricles associated with the malalignment of the atrioventricular septum has been given as a reason for the development of complete heart block.

CLINICAL PRESENTATION OF CONGENITALLY CORRECTED TRANSPOSITION OF THE GREAT ARTERIES

The clinical presentation of each patient is dependent on the presence or absence of associated cardiac anomalies. Without such anomalies patients may be entirely symptom-free well into late adult life. However, this is an unusual, if not rare, situation. More commonly even in the absence of associated malformations, a degree of congestive cardiac

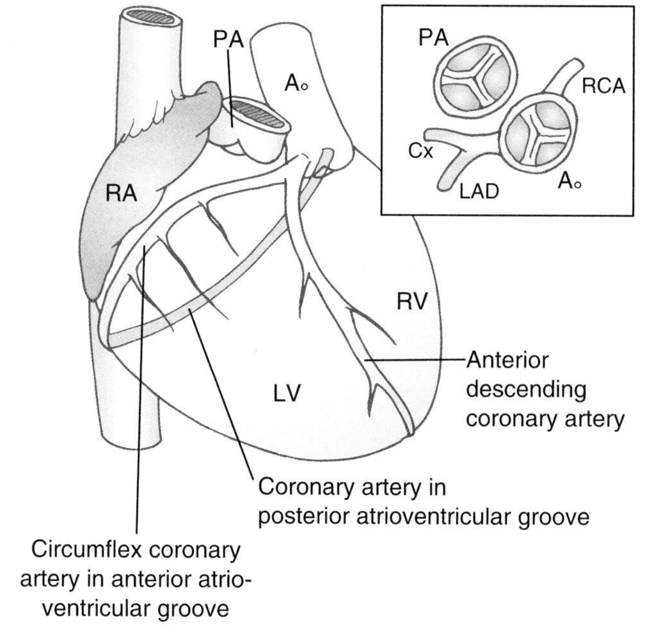

Figure 123–2 **Disposition of coronary arteries in CCTGA.** Ao, Aorta; CX, circumflex coronary artery; LAD, left anterior descending coronary artery; LV, left ventricle; PA, pulmonary artery; RA, right atrium; RV, right ventricle.

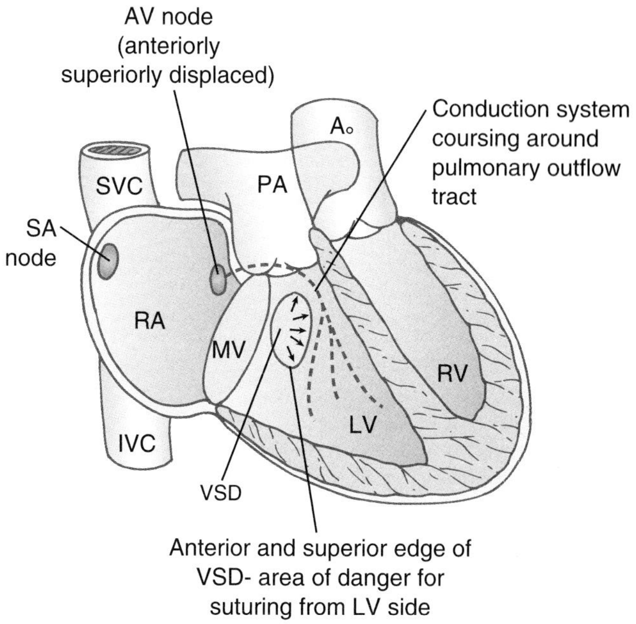

Figure 123–3 **Disposition of conduction system in CCTGA.** Relationship to VSD. AV node, Atrioventricular node; SA node, sinus atrial node.

failure develops over the lifetime of the patient usually aggravated by the development of progressive tricuspid regurgitation.[32]

When associated with a VSD, presentation in early infancy is usually with congestive cardiac failure due to pulmonary overflow from the left-to-right shunt. In view of heart failure and risk of pulmonary hypertension and progression to pulmonary vascular disease, medical management with diuretics and ACE inhibitors is usually supplemented with pulmonary artery banding. VSD in this condition usually occurs with a degree of congenital pulmonary stenosis and can produce a nicely balanced circulation without heart failure or marked cyanosis. The patient may be very well and stable for many years without the need for medical or surgical intervention. When the pulmonary stenosis progresses or is initially severe, cyanosis may be the cause of clinical presentation and early systemic-to-pulmonary shunting may be required. Pulmonary atresia with a large perimembranous VSD extending to the subaortic region is a well-recognized combination of associated cardiac anomalies, and in this situation presentation is usually with severe cyanosis as a neonate requiring an early systemic shunt.

A small percentage of patients present in early infancy with severe congestive cardiac failure sometimes associated with pulmonary hypertension. This is usually associated with marked tricuspid regurgitation secondary to dysplasia of the tricuspid valve and often associated with a VSD that may aggravate the heart failure. Early surgical management is mandatory in these critically ill infants.[25]

Thus there is whole range of possible presentations dependent on the intracardiac anatomy, ranging from the asymptomatic adults to infants in severe congestive cardiac failure. Other patients, depending on the degree of pulmonary stenosis or atresia, may vary from quite well-balanced circulation with mild cyanosis to severe cyanosis requiring systemic shunts in the neonatal period.

Throughout the patient's life, the clinical course may be complicated by the development of complete heart block and other cardiac arrhythmias.

THE PROBLEM OF THE TRICUSPID VALVE AND THE MORPHOLOGICAL RIGHT VENTRICLE IN THE SYSTEMIC CIRCULATION

The main concern highlighted in many papers* has been the unpredictable way the morphological right ventricle in association with tricuspid valve regurgitation can fail when it remains as the systemic ventricle. The development of RV failure can occur primarily without previous surgical intervention and is usually associated with dysplasia of the tricuspid valve causing tricuspid regurgitation. RV failure may also occur secondarily after conventional repair of associated cardiac defects such as VSD closure or the relief of pulmonary stenosis or atresia when the right ventricle remains in the systemic circulation.

The deterioration in the RV function associated with tricuspid regurgitation may also develop insidiously over many years without associated cardiac anomalies. There is then gradual deterioration of RV function with worsening of tricuspid regurgitation in association with the volume loading of the right ventricle. These changes may commence in childhood or even infancy and may progress at a variable rate.[1,18] When associated with dysplasia or Ebsteinoid displacement of the tricuspid valve, deterioration may be rapid. Secondary deterioration of ventricular function and development of tricuspid regurgitation are recognized to occur in an unpredictable way following conventional repair of associated cardiac anomalies. Thus VSD closure with pulmonary artery debanding may be successful with the right ventricle in the systemic circulation, although over time RV failure with tricuspid regurgitation can follow such a repair. In the situation of pulmonary atresia with VSD, closure of the VSD and placement of a valved conduit from the morphological left ventricle to the pulmonary arteries may be later associated with the development of tricuspid regurgitation and RV failure.

It therefore seems that either primarily or secondarily following conventional repair the right ventricle in the systemic circulation is prone to the development of failure and severe tricuspid regurgitation. Once the tricuspid regurgitation has developed the volume loading of the right ventricle accentuated by any systemic shunts or VSD can cause further dilation of the tricuspid valve and its annulus creating more regurgitation and so a vicious circle of heart failure with increasing tricuspid regurgitation follows. The problem is to try and recognize which patients are likely to develop these complications following a conventional repair and for those patients, what is the best surgical procedure to repair the heart.

The development of morphological RV systemic failure without previous surgical intervention is almost always associated with dysplasia of the tricuspid valve. The suggested mechanism is that dilation of the right ventricle in association with its volume loading resulting from tricuspid regurgitation displaces the ventricular septum into the morphological left ventricle. The displacement of the septal components of the tricuspid valve prevents coaptation of leaflet tissue, thus accentuating the regurgitation. This vicious circle of tricuspid valve dilation and ventricular volume overload with increasing regurgitation continues.[1] In secondary morphological RV failure following conventional closure of VSD or relief of pulmonary valve stenosis, the fall in the morphological LV pressure and realignment of ventricular septum to the pulmonary ventricle again can have the same affect by creating tricuspid regurgitation. That can then be aggravated by volume overloading of the morphological right ventricle. This is thought to be the mechanism of the development of tricuspid regurgitation and RV failure. This is supported by the observation that in placing the pulmonary artery band to train the morphological LV the tricuspid regurgitation can be acutely reduced by realignment of the ventricular septum.[1,25]

If this is the mechanism of morphological RV failure, in many cases of conventional repair of congenitally corrected transpositions, and associated cardiac anomalies, tricuspid regurgitation and RV failure can be expected to occur.

It had been suggested that the morphological left ventricle could be restored to the systemic circulation by redirecting the systemic and pulmonary venous returns, a Senning or Mustard procedure and then performing an arterial switch if the pulmonary valve and LV outflow tract were unobstructed, or a Rastelli-type procedure with rerouting of the VSD to the

*References 1, 10, 18, 27, 34, 38, 40, 43.

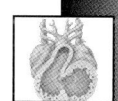

aorta when the VSD was suitably placed beneath the aortic valve.[12] Several groups reported successful double switch and Rastelli atrial switch procedures showing that the morphological left ventricle could be restored to the systemic circulation.[13,19,20,37,42] The underlying theme in these reports was that the morphological left ventricle restored to the systemic circulation could be a better long-term systemic ventricle and would have the added benefit of preventing the development of RV failure. In the double switch procedure besides restoring the morphological ventricle and mitral valve to the systemic circulation, the morphological right ventricle becomes the pulmonary ventricle, works at lower pressures and is decompressed. The amount of tricuspid regurgitation can be immediately reduced because of the lower working pressures of the right ventricle with minimal need for any repair or replacement of the tricuspid valve. Maintenance of the alignment of the ventricular septum or its displacement into the RV cavity would aid in maintaining competency of the tricuspid valve by preventing displacement of the septal leaflet of the tricuspid valve. In essence the morphological right ventricle is now working as a pulmonary ventricle at low pulmonary artery pressures and can function satisfactorily in that setting.

For two reasons double switch–type operations have become popular over the last several years. Firstly at intermediate follow-up it seems that restoration of the morphological left ventricle to the systemic circulation with the right morphological right ventricle working under lower pulmonary pressures prevents the development of RV failure and significant tricuspid regurgitation. The morphological left ventricle seems to be holding up well as the systemic ventricle. In the second situation in which RV dysfunction with associated tricuspid regurgitation exists, the recruitment of the morphological left ventricle to the systemic circulation and the delegation of the morphological right ventricle to the pulmonary circulation is appealing in that it reduces the work that the right ventricle has to do and the literature supports markedly diminished tricuspid valve regurgitation.[25] A double switch operation is possible where the morphological LV pressures had been maintained at systemic levels (e.g., in a VSD PA banded situation or when there is pulmonary atresia and VSD). However, when the morphological left ventricle has been working as a pulmonary ventricle at low pulmonary artery pressures, it is not possible to perform a primary double switch procedure expecting that the left ventricle will support the systemic circulation. The left ventricle needs some preparation to cope with the systemic work load. To create a ventricle strong enough to support the systemic circulation, many centers have first placed a pulmonary artery band to retrain the left ventricle and then later performed an arterial switch. This circumstance arises with patients who have congenitally corrected transposition without associated anomalies in whom over the first few years of life tricuspid regurgitation and a degree of RV failure has occurred in the setting of low pulmonary artery pressures. Then it is possible to retrain the left ventricle and perform a double switch once the ventricle has been retrained. It can take 6 months to 1 year or longer to accomplish this.

Training of the Left Ventricle

Training of the left ventricle has become an important aspect in congenital heart management since Mee's group[29] and others showed that it was possible to retrain the left ventricle in infants with dextrotransposition following a failing atrial repair to restore the left ventricle to the systemic circulation. This concept has been applied to the congenitally corrected transposition group of patients. Methodology of training is similar in the two groups. A pulmonary artery band is placed around the main pulmonary artery acutely to raise the morphological LV pressure to approximately 75% to 80% of the systemic pressure. Inotrope support may be necessary and band adjustment to loosen or tighten the band may be needed over the first few days or weeks after the initial procedure. It may take 6–18 months for morphological left ventricle to be adequately trained so that systolic pressures are at systemic levels and ventricular function is good with adequate thickness of the LV free wall. There is general agreement that training of the morphological left ventricle is more successful in younger patients. At the moment the probable upper age limit in which one can expect success is 15 or 16 years of age.[31]

INVESTIGATIONS AND EVALUATION

Echocardiography both transthoracic and transesophageal allows a diagnosis of congenitally corrected transposition to be made and can show the important intracardiac morphology. It can be repeated on many occasions with minimal upset to the patient to finely tune the diagnosis. Cardiac catheterization is usually performed in these patients prior to surgical intervention and is useful in confirming the morphology of the ventricular septum where there may be multiple VSDs and in clearly showing the pulmonary artery tree when previous surgery has been performed to place a pulmonary artery band or to create systemic-to-pulmonary artery shunt. It is useful to show clearly the coronary artery anatomy if an anatomical repair is to be considered. Where retraining of a morphological left ventricle with a pulmonary artery band has been performed, it is necessary to measure ventricular pressures. In patients in whom concern about pulmonary hypertension exists, cardiac catheterization with manipulation of pulmonary vascular resistance in the catheter laboratory is mandatory.

As with other forms of congenital heart disease, computerized axial tomography and magnetic resonance imaging has been increasingly used to delineate the anatomy. This, together with three-dimensional echocardiography, will undoubtedly become more widely used as it becomes more available.

SURGICAL OPTIONS

Historically the decision to surgically correct was fairly straightforward in that the associated cardiac anomalies would be repaired, the VSD could be closed, the pulmonary stenosis relieved, and the tricuspid valve repaired or replaced with or without placement of a pacemaker system. However, since the inception of the double switch procedures it is necessary to decide whether to allow the morphological right ventricle to remain in the systemic circulation or restore by the double switch the morphological left ventricle to the systemic circulation. This decision is made knowing that historically the right ventricle in the systemic circulation is known to unpredictably deteriorate even though long-term follow-up results of the double switch procedure aren't available. The algorithm in Figure 123-4 illustrates the possible surgical management for patients with congenitally corrected transposition and their associated cardiac abnormalities. Over time, with longer term results than these, indications may well change.

THE PHYSIOLOGICAL REPAIR (CONVENTIONAL OR CLASSIC)

In this operation the associated cardiac defects are repaired so that the morphological right ventricle remains as the systemic ventricle. The VSD is closed with a patch, pulmonary outflow tract obstruction is relieved directly by resection of obstructing tissues, and when this cannot be performed adequately a morphological left ventricle to pulmonary artery valve conduit is placed to relieve the obstruction (Figure 123-5). If associated with tricuspid valve regurgitation the tricuspid valve can be repaired, this can be difficult, however, because of the difficult dysplastic abnormalities associated with this valve. Clefts may be closed and annuloplasty may be performed.

CONDUCT OF CARDIOPULMONARY BYPASS IN PHYSIOLOGICAL REPAIR

Normal cardiopulmonary bypass with ascending aortic and bicaval cannulation is instituted. Core cooling is taken to 28° C or 25° C nasopharyngeal depending on the surgical complexity. Initial dissection of the heart may only be limited to the cannulation sites if this is a reoperation with further pericardial adhesions taken down on bypass. Having mobilized the heart fully, and this can be difficult because of the position of the ventricles, the aorta is cross-clamped and the heart cardiopleged with St Thomas's crystalloid cardioplegia. This is normally repeated every 30 minutes. The heart is usually irrigated with iced slush solution. Having snugged down the superior and inferior vena cava, the right atrium is opened and the left atrium drained via the intraatrial septum. The operative repair is performed, bypass rewarming

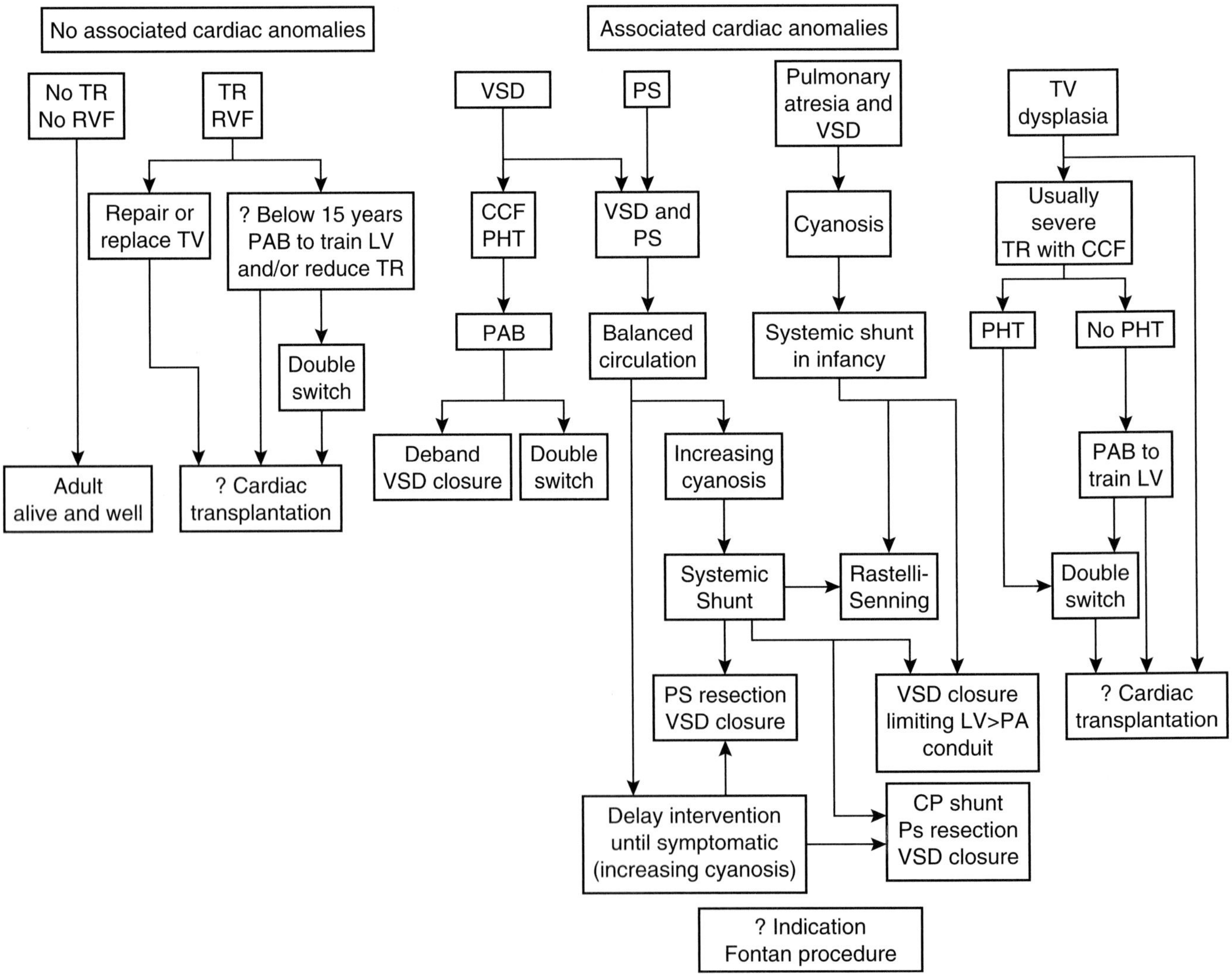

Figure 123–4 Algorithm for management of congenitally corrected transposition. TV, Tricuspid valve; TR, tricuspid regurgitation; RVF, right ventricular failure; PAB, pulmonary artery band; LV, left ventricle; CCF, congestive cardiac failure; PHT, pulmonary hypertension; VSD, ventricular septal defect; PS, pulmonary stenosis; CP shunt, cavopulmonary shunt.

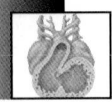

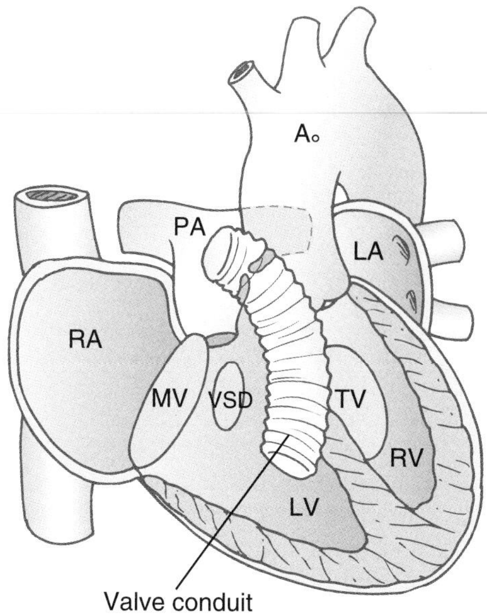

Figure 123–5 Physiological repair of congenitally corrected transposition with pulmonary stenosis and ventricular septal defects. VSD closure and placement of left ventricle to pulmonary artery valved conduit. Ao, Aorta; LA, left atrium; MV, mitral valve; PA, pulmonary artery; RA, right atrium; TV, tricuspid valve; VSD, ventricular septal defect.

commenced, and bypass discontinued having fully rewarmed in a routine way. Other techniques of cardiopulmonary bypass and cardioplegia may be equally applicable.

Closure of the Ventricular Septal Defect

In congenitally transposition the VSD is commonly perimembranous in position. In this situation the conduction system passes superiorly around the pulmonary outflow tract. Accordingly to avoid damaging the conduction system, continuous or interrupted sutures are placed through the RV margin of the VSD.[12] Access to the VSD is usually via the mitral valve or pulmonary artery. If a ventriculotomy has to be performed then access to the VSD can be gained via the ventriculotomy.

Placement of the Valved Conduit

The left ventricular to pulmonary artery valved conduit (Hancock, Medtronic Inc., Minneapolis, MN) usually passes to the right side of the aorta and is behind the sternum. Sometimes the course of the conduit can be curved away from the sternal incision, but having placed the conduit it is wise to either close the pericardium or place a protective membrane behind the sternum to allow for future reentry when the valve conduit needs replacing. Left ventriculotomy should be placed more toward the apex of the ventricle taking care to avoid the papillary muscles of the mitral valve on the inner aspect of the ventricle and superiorly the conduction system as it passes around the LV outflow tract.

Tricuspid Valve Repair or Replacement

Our own experience with repair or replacement of the tricuspid valve in congenitally corrected transposition is limited, because we would electively try to perform a double switch procedure in circumstances in which there was tricuspid valve regurgitation. Access to the tricuspid valve can be difficult if deeply seated within the right ventricle. Reparative procedures are limited unless one finds a cleft in the valve that can be directly sutured or a secondary orifice that can be closed. Various annuloplasties and reinforcing surgical rings can be placed to try and gain competence in these difficult valves. In general, however, we do not feel this is advisable and would prefer to replace the valve if a secure repair cannot be made. In general we would replace the valve with a bileaflet mechanical valve sutures with reinforced inverting mattress sutures. As much valve apparatus is preserved in suturing in the new valve to try and preserve ventricular function.

Palliative Surgical Procedures

Various palliative surgical procedures may be applicable to patients with congenitally corrected transposition. If there is cyanosis then a systemic-to-pulmonary artery shunt, usually a modified Blalock Taussig shunt is our preferred choice. When there is pulmonary overflow due to a large VSD in infancy, a pulmonary artery band is placed usually through a midline sternotomy. It may be necessary to place either temporary or permanent pacemaker systems at the time of this palliative surgery in an epicardial position.

CONDUCT OF CARDIOPULMONARY BYPASS AND GENERAL CONSIDERATIONS FOR THE ANATOMICAL REPAIR

Routine cardiopulmonary bypass techniques are used with cold crystalloid cardioplegia and topical irrigation of the heart with iced slush solution. The heart is completely mobilized by dividing all the previous adhesions. Cardiopulmonary bypass is commenced routinely cooling to 22° C nasopharyngeal or 18° C nasopharyngeal if circulatory arrest is anticipated. Often there is a considerable amount of open-heart return and short periods of low flow or even circulatory arrest are necessary to provide a clear field for the reconstructive surgery, particularly for the Senning procedure. Certain aspects of the bypass and cannulation however are particular for the anatomical repair. The superior vena cava is cannulated high underneath the innominate vein to allow room at the superior vena caval right atrial junction for placement of the superior pulmonary venous Senning suture line. The inferior vena cava is cannulated low to place the cannula below the site of the Eustachian valve. The Eustachian valve can then be incorporated into the suture line of the systemic venous pathway. Having cross-clamped the aorta and arrested the heart with St Thomas's cardioplegia, the atrium is opened.

Our practice is to use aprotinin infusion during the operation and tissue fibrin glue to help with hemostasis. Because these are long operations, we invariably do not close the sternum at the end of the operation. In addition when a valved conduit passes directly behind the sternum in front of the heart, we delay sternal closure until myocardial function has recovered, so that the heart is not compressed by the valved conduit.

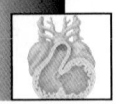

Anatomical Correction of Congenitally Corrected Transposition of the Great Arteries

As opposed to the conventional repair when the morphological right ventricle remains as the systemic ventricle, in anatomical repair the morphological left ventricle is restored to the systemic circulation. This is done by recruiting the systemic veins to the right ventricle and the pulmonary veins to the left ventricle by the Senning or Mustard procedure. Our own experience is with the Senning operation, but the Mustard procedure can also be used. An arterial switch is then performed when the pulmonary outflow tract is unobstructed, and the pulmonary valve can become the new aortic valve. If there is pulmonary stenosis and atresia with a suitable large subaortic VSD, the left ventricle can be rerouted to the aorta by baffling the VSD to the aortic valve. A valved conduit then connects the morphological right ventricle to the pulmonary artery.

The Atrial-Arterial Switch ("Double Switch")

Having commenced cardiopulmonary bypass, the interatrial groove is developed, the aorta cross-clamped and the heart cardiopleged. Cardioplegia is repeated every 30–40 minutes, either via the aortic root or directly into the coronary ostia. The Senning baffles are formed.[22,35] The right atrium is opened just anterior to the crista terminalis; this incision is extended inferiorly anterior and parallel to the crista to reach the Eustachian valve. The interatrial septum is opened adjacent to the mitral valve annulus, extending the incision superiorly and inferiorly. The superior incision is then extended deeply into the limbus back to the root of the superior vena cava and usually exits through the previously delineated interatrial groove. The atrial septum is then separated from the right pulmonary veins hinging on the wall of the right atrium to create the posterior wall of the systemic venous chamber. The interatrial septum is checked for perforations, which might need additional sutures. When there is a VSD, this is closed through the mitral valve passing sutures from the rightward side of the ventricular as in the conventional repair. However, there can be a lot of traction on the crux of the heart particularly with mesocardia or dextrocardia, and this may well create temporary or permanent heart block even if the sutures are placed carefully on the rightward side of the ventricular septum. We usually utilize a bovine pericardial patch or Gore-Tex patch held in position with multiple interrupted Teflon plegeted or native pericardial plegeted mattress sutures. The smooth patch is utilized so that if there is a neoaortic valve regurgitation the chance of hemolysis is reduced. We then turn our attention to the arterial switch. The aorta is transacted about 1–1.5 cm above the entrance of the coronary arteries. If these are not clearly visible because of adhesions, the anterior wall of the aorta is opened carefully for about one third of its circumference and the coronary arteries are visualized before aortic transection is completed. Following pulmonary banding there may be marked fibrosis between the aorta and pulmonary artery.

Careful dissection continues incising the pulmonary artery at the site of the band. Then dissection proceeds backwards and forwards between the aorta and the pulmonary artery to mobilize these vessels. The coronary arteries are then cut out with large cuffs of the aortic wall to provide good buttons of tissue around the coronary ostia. It may be necessary to release some of the commissures of the aortic valve to provide plenty of room around the ostia. The ostia must be protected by a large amount of aortic wall around them. The coronary arteries are then mobilized carefully to avoid damaging the coronary arteries. In particular, the left anterior descending coronary artery may pass quite close anteriorly to the aortic wall. Having dissected out the coronary arteries and mobilized the pulmonary arteries, the ductus ligament is ligated and divided. The pulmonary artery is transacted and completely mobilized. Then incisions are made into the sinuses facing the coronary aortic sinuses so that medially hinged flaps are created.[8]

The coronary arteries are then swung back into the facing sinuses of the pulmonary artery, and anastomosed with 6-0 or 5-0 Prolene. If the pulmonary artery is enlarged, particularly in the situation where there has been a band placed distally, it may be necessary to reduce its size by resecting tissue from the noncoronary sinus. Recently we have placed a subcommissural circumferential suture with 4-0 PDS to tailor in the new aortic root to try to prevent neoaortic valve dilation and regurgitation in this group of patients. A patch of pulmonary homograft or bovine pericardium is then sutured into the aortic defects. When the great vessels are side by side the pulmonary arteries are generally left behind the aorta. When more or less in an anterior-posterior position, the pulmonary arteries are moved anterior to the aorta. The aorta is then reconstructed with a 5-0 or 4-0 Prolene suture. At this point the heart is then recardiopleged, and we turn our attention back to the Senning procedure.

The posterior wall of the systemic venous chamber is reconstructed with continuous 5-0 Prolene starting at the posterior lip of the left atrial appendage passing superiorly leaving plenty of space superiorly between the posterior margin of the superior vena cava and the suture line. The posterior suture line is then continued inferiorly in a direct line back to the inferior vena cava. Where there is dilation of the left atrium it is important to gather quite aggressively tissue from the left atrial wall onto the posterior edge of the systemic venous baffle. The anterior wall of the systemic venous chamber is then reconstructed starting inferiorly suturing at the Eustachian valve. If that is not present then the suitable position on the internal aspect of the inferior vena cava is used extending onto the cut edge of the atrial septum. The coronary sinus drains into the systemic venous atrium. The suture line is then continued superiorly on the cut edge of the intraatrial septum between the mitral and tricuspid valves onto the extension of the crista terminalis around the atrial appendage and back so that the systemic venous chamber is completed. On occasion we have found it helpful to supplement the upper third of the systemic venous reconstruction with a small patch of bovine pericardium or native pericardium to enlarge the superior vena cava opening. It is noticeable that the tricuspid valve is set more deeply in the congenitally correct transposition and the angulation of the superior vena cava back into the tricuspid valve opening is more acute in this group of patients. When the atrial septum is intact and no dilation of the atrial chambers exists, the venous pathway may be small. Supplementation with the patch helps to open out the superior vena cava pathway. The pulmonary venous pathways are then reconstructed usually with a direct anastomosis of the free edge of the right atrium to the cut edge of the right pulmonary veins. At this point bypass rewarming is commenced and the heart deaired and with aortic root suction applied and the aortic cross-clamp removed. If heart block is a problem, temporary pacing wires are placed. The pulmonary arteries are then reconstructed anastomosing the pulmonary artery to the distal left and right pulmonary arteries. Having rewarmed, cardiac bypass is discontinued in a routine manner. Temporary pacing wires are placed, if there was heart block preoperatively permanent epicardial pacemaker wires may be placed. A left atrial line is routinely placed through the old right atrial appendage. The chest may or may not be closed postoperatively immediately. If in doubt, it is not closed (Figure 123-6).

The Rastelli-Senning Procedure

The Senning procedure is performed similarly to the double switch procedure. Having created the atrial incisions, an incision is made in the morphological right ventricle between coronary arteries and well away from the aorta. Through the ventriculotomy the VSD is visualized and baffled over to the aorta with a Dacron or Gore-Tex patch sutured with interrupted mattress, Teflon plegeted sutures. Sometimes a continuous suture is used superiorly around the infundibulum and aorta. Depending upon surgical access the valved conduit (usually a Hancock, Medtronic Inc., Minneapolis, MN) is sutured directly to the pulmonary arteries and proximally to the ventriculotomy, or the Senning procedure is completed and then the conduit placed. The ventriculotomy suture line is reinforced with Teflon plegeted mattress sutures, inside out in the heel of the graft and outside in the toe. Usually the graft is placed to the left side of the aorta, but either route allows the graft to be away from the sternum is chosen (Figure 123-7). Usually at least part of the graft is behind the sternum, and a Gore-Tex membrane is placed between the pericardial edges to allow for safer sternal opening at conduit change.[7]

Senning or Mustard Procedure (Special Note)

Our own unit utilizes the Senning procedure; however, the Mustard procedure can be used with equal validity. Sometimes because of the position of the heart in our Senning procedure, the pulmonary venous chamber is enlarged with a patch of bovine pericardium, or the Shumacker modification, utilizing in situ native pericardium.[36]

Postoperative Management

A degree of low cardiac output is not unusual after operations with these long and complex procedures. The median times for cardiac bypass were 149 minutes, aortic cross-clamp 131 minutes, and circulatory arrest 43 minutes in our own service.[25] Inotrope and ventilatory support is maintained until the cardiac output improves, and ventricular function is monitored by sequential echo evaluation. At the end of the operations, cardiac function and the pathways into and out of the heart are checked by epicardial or transesophageal echo.

After chest closure the patient is gradually weaned from all support in the intensive care unit. Recently, one patient who survived required postoperative extra corporeal membrane oxygenation (ECMO) support for 4 days at our institution.

Alternative Procedures

Alternatives to conventional and double switch repair include a one and a half operation with limited relief of LV outflow tract obstruction and a bidirectional Glen procedure.[28] This is done so that RV pressures and morphological LV pressures are maintained at a higher level, approximately 50% systemic so as to maintain alignment of the ventricular septum and hopefully prevent development of the tricuspid valve regurgitation

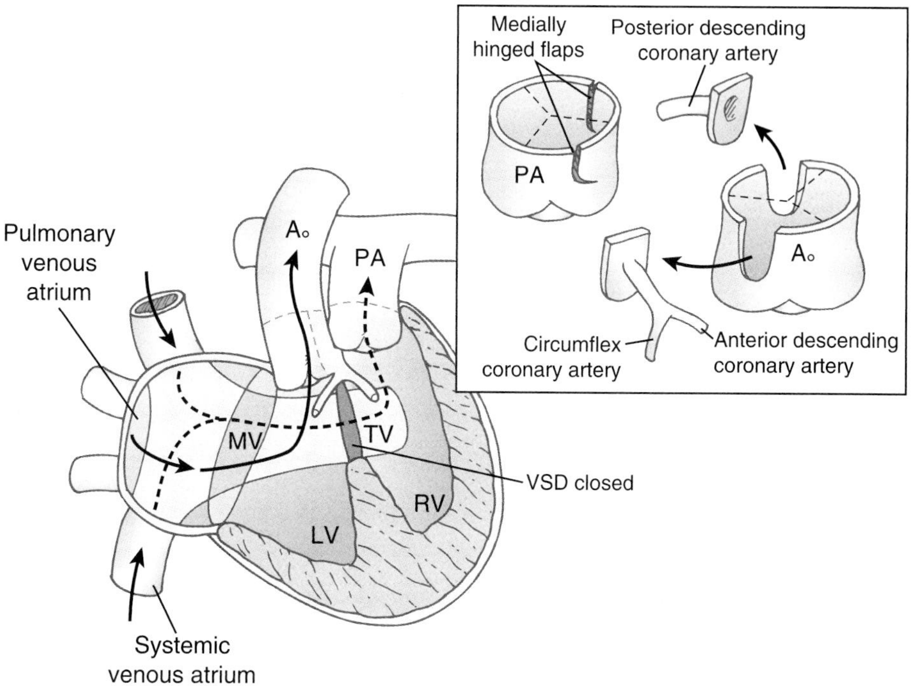

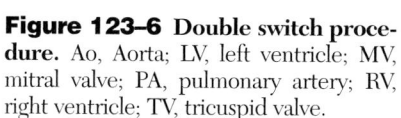

Figure 123–6 Double switch procedure. Ao, Aorta; LV, left ventricle; MV, mitral valve; PA, pulmonary artery; RV, right ventricle; TV, tricuspid valve.

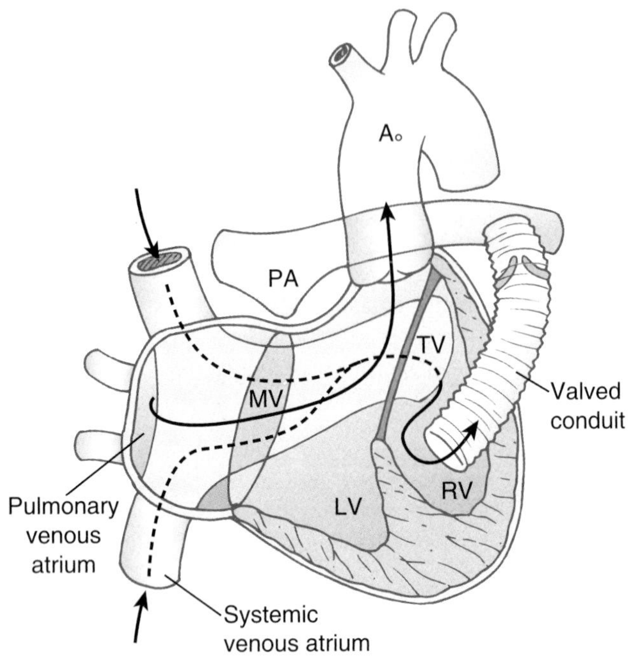

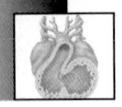

Figure 123–7 **Rastelli-Senning procedure for congenitally corrected transposition with pulmonary atresia and VSD.** Ao, Aorta; LV, left ventricle; MV, mitral valve; PA, pulmonary artery; RV, right ventricle; TV, tricuspid valve.

and systemic RV dysfunction in the longer term. This may be particularly applicable to situations in which a Rastelli Senning repair is not possible because of the position of the VSD. Finally a Fontan-type procedure may have to be considered if it is not possible by virtue of position of the heart, location of the VSD, and hypoplasia of a ventricle to perform a septation; however, this is uncommon.

RESULTS

Physiological Repair

Results from many centers throughout the world are now available.* While the early mortality is low, on the order of 5%, all groups have highlighted the long-term failure of the morphological right ventricle associated with tricuspid regurgitation. The Toronto group,[43] in particular, highlighted this long-term problem, and the Mavroudis group,[27] in their article comparing physiological as opposed to anatomical repair stated the problem clearly. Thus survival in these patients is 75% at 10 years and 50% at 20 years. In addition 56% require reoperation in the 20 years of follow-up.

Anatomical Repair

Anatomical repair has grown in popularity because of the poor long-term outcome with physiological repair. However only relatively early results for anatomical repair are available from centers in North America, Japan, and Europe.†

In our own series of 54 patients[25] the early mortality was 5.6%, with 2 of the 3 patients who died being in cardiac failure preoperatively. Seven of 54 developed new complete heart block and two were late deaths. The survival in the Birmingham UK series was 94% at 1 year, 90% at 4–9 years. Freedom from reoperation for all patients was 94% at 1 year, 85% at 5 years, and 76% at 9 years. There were no reoperations for tricuspid valve regurgitation; in fact, preoperative tricuspid regurgitation was universally improved. The reoperations as expected were for conduit change in the Rastelli group, and this will be a continuing necessity.

Disturbingly, six patients had new signs of LV dysfunction of which two had new aortic valve regurgitation in the double switch group. Others have reported this problem, though not to this degree.[21,42] Aortic regurgitation is specific to the double switch group where the old pulmonary valve becomes the new aortic valve. All of our patients had some mild degree of aortic valve insufficiency. In four patients it was moderately severe requiring aortic valve replacement in two patients. Similarly this has been reported in other series.[20,23]

Thus, with new operations, new problems and only longer-term follow-up will show whether the good early results are maintained.

Summary and Recommendations

The Algorithm (see Figure 123-4) summarizes our current management for these patients. We feel that the left ventricle in the systemic circulation will be of benefit for the majority of patients with this condition, and hence the preferred management pathways are highlighted with red arrows. Time will show whether the problems of new aortic regurgitation, LV dysfunction and the need for conduit change will increase over time. The problem of RV dysfunction and tricuspid regurgitation has been solved however. The majority of patients should be suitable for an anatomical repair. Development of heart failure in the older patient may still require tricuspid valve surgery or cardiac transplantation. At this time it is not possible to retrain the left ventricle in the older patient.[31] Debanding and closure of the VSD is not our preferred option,

When only physiological repair is possible because of the position of the VSD or in an older patient, we would agree with Mavroudis, et al[27] that the morphological left ventricle pressure should be maintained at 50% or so of systemic pressures to maintain ventricular septal alignment. This will hopefully prevent development of tricuspid regurgitation and deterioration of RV function. In the situation of hypoplasia for one of the ventricles, complex AV valve morphology with straddling, the only option may be to go down the Fontan palliative pathway. However, this is a minority of patients.

*References 1, 18, 34, 38, 40, 43.
†References 13, 19–21, 23, 25, 42.

REFERENCES

1. Acar P, Sidi D, Bonnet D, et al: Maintaining tricuspid valve competence in double discordance: A challenge for the paediatric cardiologist. Heart 80:479–483,1998.
2. Anderson KR, Danielson GK, McGoon DW, Lie JT: Ebstein's anomaly of the left-sided tricuspid valve. Pathological anatomy of the valvular malformation. Circulation 58:87–91, 1978.
3. Anderson RH, Becker AE, Arnold R, Wilkinson JL: The conducting tissues in congenitally corrected transposition. Circulation 50:911–924, Nov 1974.

4. Beauchesne LM, Warnes CA, Connolly HM, et al: Outcome of the unoperated adult who presents with congenitally corrected transposition of the great arteries. J Am Coll Cardiol 40:285–290, Jul 17, 2002.
5. Becker AE, Anderson RH: Atrioventricular Discordance in Pathology of Congenital Heart Disease. pp. 225–240. Butterworth Postgraduate Series.
6. Becker AE, Ho SY, Caruso G, et al: Straddling right atrioventricular valves in atrioventricular discordance. Circulation 61:1133, 1980.
7. Brawn WJ, Barron DJ: Technical aspects of the Rastelli and atrial switch procedure for congenitally corrected transposition of the great arteries with ventricular septal defect and pulmonary stenosis or atresia: results of therapy. Semin Thorac Cadiovasc Surg Pediatr Card Surg Ann 6:4–8 Review, 2003.
8. Brawn WJ, Mee RBB: Early results for anatomic correction of transposition of the great arteries and double outlet right ventricle (50 cases). J Thorac Cardiovasc 95:230–238, 1988.
9. Carey LS, Ruttenberg HD: Roentgenographic features of congenitally corrected transposition of the great vessels. Ann J Roentgenol 92:623, 1964.
10. Connelly M, Liu PP, Williams WG, et al: Congenitally corrected transposition of the great arteries in the adult: Functional status and complications. JACC 27:1238–1243, 1996.
11. Daliento L, Corrado D, Buja G, et al: Rhythm and conduction disturbances in isolated, congenitally corrected transposition of the great arteries. Am J Cardiol :58:314–318, 1986.
12. De Leval MR, Basto P, Stark J, et al: Surgical technique to reduce the risks of heart block following closure of ventricular septal defect in atrioventricular discordance. J Thorac Cardiovasc 78: 515–526, 1979.
13. Di Donato RM, Troconis CJ, Marino B, et al: Combined Mustard and Rastelli operations. An alternative approach for repair of associated anomalies in congenitally corrected transposition in situs inversus (IDD). J Thorac Cus 104:1246–1248, 1992.
14. Erath HG, Graham PT, Hammon JW, Smith CW: Hypoplasia of the systemic ventricle in congenitally corrected transposition of the great arteries. J Thorac Cardiovasc 79:770–775, 1980.
15. Ferencz C, Rubin JD, McCarter RJ, et al: Congenital heart disease: Prevalence at live birth. The Baltimore—Washington Infant Study. Ann J Epidemiol 121:31–36,1985.
16. Freedom RM, Benson LN, Smallhorn JF: Congenitally transposition of the great arteries. In: Moller JH, Neal WA, (eds): Fetal, Neonatal and Infant Cardiac Disease. Norwalk, CT: Appleton and Lange, 1989, pp. 555–570.
17. Fyler DC: Report of the New England Regional Infant cardiac programme. Pediatr 65(Suppl):376–461, 1980.
18. Graham TP Jr, Bernard YD, Mellen BG, et al: Long term outcome in congenitally corrected transposition of the great arteries. A multi-institutioned study. J Am Coll Cardiol 36:255–261, 2000.
19. Ilbawi MN, Deleon SY. Backer CL, et al: An alternative approach to the surgical management of physiologically corrected transposition with ventricular septal defect and pulmonary stenosis or atresia. J Thorac Cardiovasc Surg 100:410–415,1990.
20. Imai Y: The Double Switch operation for congenitally corrected transposition. Adv Cardiac Surg 9:65–86,1997.
21. Imamura M, Drummond-Webb JJ, Murphy DJ Jr, et al: Results of the Double Switch operations in the current era. Ann Thor Surg 70:100–105, Jul 2000.
22. Jonas RA, Mee RB, Sutherland HD: Reintroduction of the Senning operation for transposition of the great arteries. Med J Aust 2:260–262, 1980.
23. Karl TR, Weintraub RG, Brizard CP, et al: Senning plus arterial switch operation for discordant (congenitally corrected) transposition. Ann Thorac Surg 64:495–502, 1997.
24. Kurosawa H, Becker AE: Atrioventricular conduction in congenital heart disease. London: Springer-Verlag, 1987, pp. 225–252.
25. Langley SM, Winlaw DS, Stumper O. et al: Midterm results after restoration of the morphologically left ventricle to the systemic circulation in patients with congenitally corrected transposition of the great arteries. J Thorac Cardovasc Surg 125:1229–1241, Jun 2003.
26. Losekoot TG, Becker AE: Discordant atrioventricular connexion and congenitally corrected transposition. In: Anderson RH, MacCartney FJ, Shinebourne EA, Tynan A (eds): Paediatric Cardiology. Edinburgh: Churchill Livingstone, 1987, pp. 867–888.
27. Mavroudis C, Backer CL: Physiologic versus anatomic repair of congenitally corrected transposition of the great arteries. Pediatr Cardiac Surge Ann Semin Thorac Cardiovasc. 6:16–26, 2003.
28. Mavroudis C, Backer CL, Kohr LM, et al: Bidirectional Glenn shunt in association with congenital heart repairs: The 1½ ventricular repair. Ann Thorac Surg 68:976–981, 1999.
29. Mee RBB: Severe right ventricular failure after Mustard or Senning operation two stage repair: pulmonary artery banding and switch. J Thorac Cardiovasc 92:385–390, 1986.
30. Milo S, Ho SY, Macartney FJ, et al: Straddling and overriding atrioventricular valves. Morphology and classification. Ann J Cardiol 44:1122–1134.
31. Poirier NC, Mee RBB: Left ventricular reconditioning and anatomical correction for systemic right ventricular dysfunction. Semin Thorac Cardiovasc Pediatr Cardiac Surg Ann 3:198–215, 2000.
32. Presbitero P, Somerville J, Rabajoli F, et al: Corrected transposition of the great arteries without associated defects in adult patients: clinical profile and follow up. Br Hrt J 74:57–59, Jul 1995.
33. Reddy VM, McElhinney DB, Silverman NH, Hanley FL: The double switch procedure for anatomoical repair of congenitally corrected transposition of the great arteries in infants and children. Eur Hrt J18:1470–1477, 1997.
34. Sano T, Riesenfeld T, Karl TR, Wilkinson JL: Intermediate-Term Outcome after Intracardiac Repair of Associated Cardiac Defects in Patients with Atrioventricular and Ventriculararterial Discordance. Circulation 92:II-272–II-278, 1995.
35. Senning A: Surgical correction of transposition of the great vessels. Surgery 45:966–980, 1959.
36. Shumaker HBI: A new operation for transposition of the great vessels. Surgery 50:773–777, 1961.
37. Stumper O, Wright JG, DeGiovanni JV, et al: Combined atrial and arterial switch procedure for congenitally corrected transposition with ventricular septal defect. Br Hrt J 73:479–482, 1995.
38. Termignon JL, Leca F, Vouhé PR, et al: 'Classic' repair of congenitally corrected transposition and ventricular septal defect. Ann Thorac Surg 62:199–206, 1996.
39. Van Praagh R: What is congenitally corrected transposition (editorial) N Engl J Med 282:1097–1098,1970.
40. Van Son JA, Danielson GK, Huhta JC, et al: Late results of systemic atrioventricular valve replacement in corrected transposition. J Thorac Cardiovasc Surg 109:642–653,1995.
41. Wilkinson JL, Smith A, Linclon C, Anderson RH: Conducting tissues in congenitally corrected transposition with situs inversus. Br Hrt J. 40:41–48, 1978.
42. Yagihara T, Kishimoto H, Isobe F, et al: Double Switch operation in cardiac anomalies with atrioventricular and ventriculoarterial discordance. J Thorac Cardiovasc 107:351–358,1994.
43. Yeh TJ, Connelly MS, Coles JG, et al: Atrioventricular discordance: Results of repair in 127 patients. J Thorac Cardiovasc Surg 117:1190–1203, 1999.

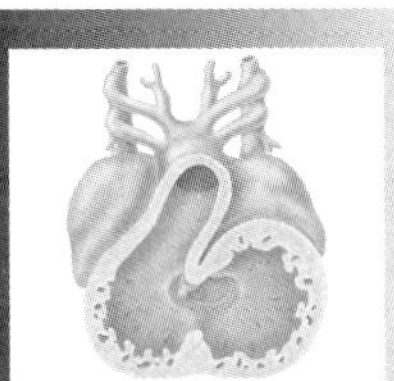

CHAPTER 124

Congenital Anomalies of the Mitral Valve

Christian P. Brizard

INTRODUCTION

This chapter will only treat the congenital anomalies of the mitral valve to the exclusion of the mitral valve in atrioventricular discordance, the mitral valve in univentricular hearts, and the mitral valve of the hypoplastic left heart syndrome. It will also exclude all acquired mitral valve disease, including the mitral valve insufficiency secondary to myocardial infarction or stunning as seen in anomalous origin of the left coronary artery from the pulmonary artery (ALCAPA). Because it is often found in congenital mitral valve materials, we have included repair of secondary or recurrent left atrioventricular (AV) valve regurgitation. Although classical and seemingly practical, we shall try to avoid the division between congenital valve stenosis and congenital mitral valve insufficiency. In effect, if they do generate different pathophysiology and mechanism of adaptation from the cardiovascular system, they have similar pathology and associated lesions, are often combined, and require similar surgical techniques for the treatment. We have also included the mitral valve anomalies associated with congenital connective tissue disorders, in which the embryology of the mitral valve itself is normal.

EMBRYOLOGY OF THE MITRAL VALVE

The embryology of the mitral valve is complex. The understanding of the formation of the leaflets and suspension apparatus has evolved,[30] and the current approach is based on immunohistochemistry, in vivo labeling of cushion tissue, and scanning electron micrograph of human and chick embryos.[46] In humans, the mitral valve develops between the fifth and the fifteenth week of embryonic life. It is established that the leaflet and chordal tissue derive from the endocardial cushion tissue laying on the inner surface of the AV junction. The separation between atrial and ventricular myocardium is dependent on the sulcus tissue located on the epicardial side of the junction. As the cushion tissue elongates and grows toward the ventricular cavity, it gets progressively delaminated from the underlying myocardium and the leaflet shapes progressively as a funnel-like structure totally attached to the myocardium. Then perforations appear into the valve leaflet. The perforations grow and form the cordae tendineae. The atrial aspect of the cushion will generate the spongy atrial layer, and the ventricular layer will generate the fibrous part of the mitral valve and the chordae. The development of the papillary muscle takes place at the same time and is originated from the myocardium. A horseshoe-shaped ridge lies within the left ventricle. Progressively the anterior and posterior parts of the ridge lose contact with the ventricular wall. They will form the papillary muscles and progressively increase their size while keeping contact with the cushion tissue at the tip of the papillary muscle. The midportion of the muscular ridge will get incorporated into the apical trabeculations of the left ventricle.[31]

Several AV cushions participate to form the final mitral valve. The most important are the superior and inferior cushion. However, there is no symmetry in the role of theses two cushion. The superior cushion tissue will give most of the anterior leaflet of the mitral valve, whereas the inferior cushion will generate most of the septal leaflet of the *tricuspid* valve. Smaller cushions are involved in the formation of the mural leaflet of the mitral valve. The wedging of the aortic root into the superior bridging leaflet mostly originated from the superior cushion will separate the forming mitral valve from its septal attachments.

PATHOLOGICAL FEATURES

Supravalvar Mitral Ring

Often considered a congenital anomaly of the mitral valve, the supravalvar mitral ring is a fibrous construction attached to the posterior annulus of the mitral valve and running from both commissures to the mid-height of the anterior leaflet. The lesion is stenotic and often more than what the extension of the ring would suggest. This is mostly due to the limitation of the opening of the anterior leaflet rather than the actual diaphragm effect of the ring (Figure 124-1). Strictly attached to the mitral valve annulus, it is to be differentiated from the cor triatriatum. Like the subaortic membrane in the left ventricular outflow tract, the supravalvular mitral ring is an acquired lesion secondary to turbulent flow through the mitral orifice. The primary lesion of the mitral valve responsible for the turbulent flow can be obvious, stenotic, regurgitant, or very discrete and difficult to identify. It can be related to a prominent coronary sinus as found in left superior vena cava draining into the coronary sinus.[2,10,18] For these reason probably, the supravalvar mitral ring is prone to reoccur after surgical resection, unless the underlying anatomical anomaly has been identified and corrected.

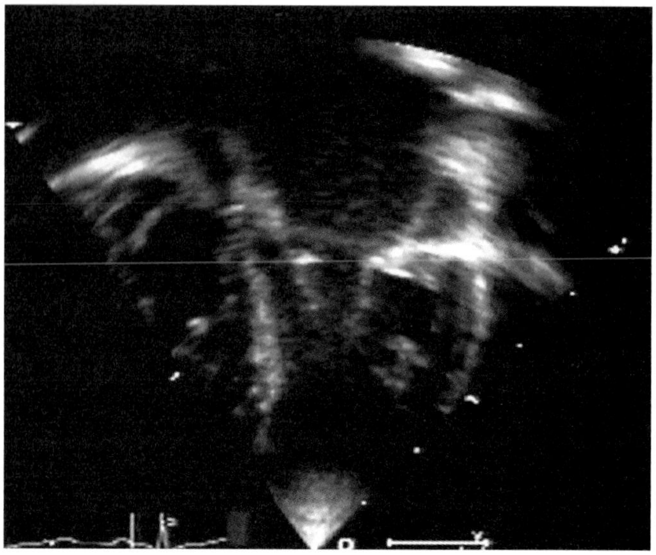

Figure 124–1 Supravalvular mitral ring. Apical view of 2D echocardiograph. Characteristic picture of the membrane attached at mid-height of the anterior leaflet whereas the posterior part of the membrane is only suggested by the hyperechogenicity of the posterior annulus.

Cleft Mitral Valve

Very often isolated, the cleft mitral valve can be easily differentiated from a left AV valve in a partial AV septal defect.[20,42] It is an actual cleft with no suspension apparatus on the edges of the defect.[7] The cleft is centered on the aortic commissure between non- and left coronary cusps.[20] Each half of the anterior leaflet at midportion bears the attachment of the strut cordae. Rarely the cleft mitral valve is associated with a leaflet tissue defect, which is an acquired defect secondary to the regurgitation through the cleft. The defect is never stenotic and may generate only little regurgitation for a long time.

Lesions Associated with Lack of Valvular Tissue

Three major anatomical types can be recognized and are worth individualizing. They are almost always associated with lack of valvar tissue of various degrees. The functional lesion can be either predominantly regurgitant or predominantly stenotic, it can be both stenotic and regurgitant. Rarely, the valve can have a normal function.

Parachute Mitral Valve

The parachute mitral valve can be found in isolation. It is, however, often integrated in a Shone syndrome.[3,39] The gross pathology is of a predominant single papillary muscle with the orifice of the mitral valve overriding the tip of the papillary muscle. There is a spectrum of lesions for the suspension apparatus starting from complete fusion of the tip of the papillary muscle to the free edge of the valve.[31] On the other end of the spectrum we can find relatively normal-looking cordae with good mobility of the leaflet (Figure 124-2). The accessory papillary muscle is usually very small and devoted to a short segment of the free edge, or even to the undersurface of the leaflet tissue, as would be a greater than normal secondary cordae. The leaflet tissue can be intact or perforated.

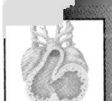

The functional anatomy depends on the interaction between the amount of tissue and mobility of the leaflet; presence and size of the fenestrations; and presence, length, and quality of the cordae.[6] The parachute mitral valve almost always has a stenotic component.

Double orifice mitral valve is a variation of the parachute mitral valve where the lesser papillary muscle is supporting a complete orifice. It is exceedingly rare. It should be differentiated from the left AV valve where an accessory orifice is often found in the instance of diminutive or absent left lateral leaflet (mural leaflet).

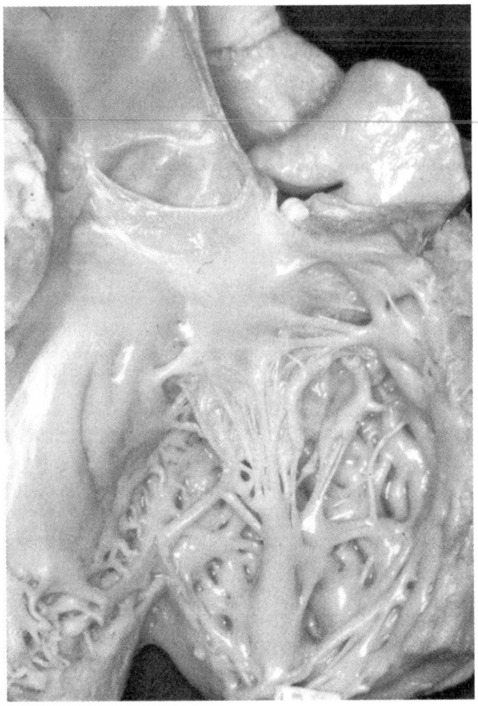

Figure 124–2 Parachute mitral valve. Macroscopic view of a parachute mitral valve. A large predominant papillary muscle distributes anomalous cordae to both commissures. A small diminutive papillary muscle can be seen to the right of the valve.

Papillary Muscle to Commissure Fusion[7]

Papillary muscle to commissure fusion is also called short chordae syndrome and is defined by the presence of very short cordae and the papillary muscle tip attached or fused to the commissural area of the free edge (Figure 124-3). In the most extreme form, the cordae are totally absent. The papillary muscles can be of normal size and volume. The valve is then generally more regurgitant than restrictive, and this is due to the lack of valvular tissue and the restriction of the leaflet motion. When the papillary muscles are hypertrophied, the bulk of their mass is generally responsible for a valve predominantly restrictive.

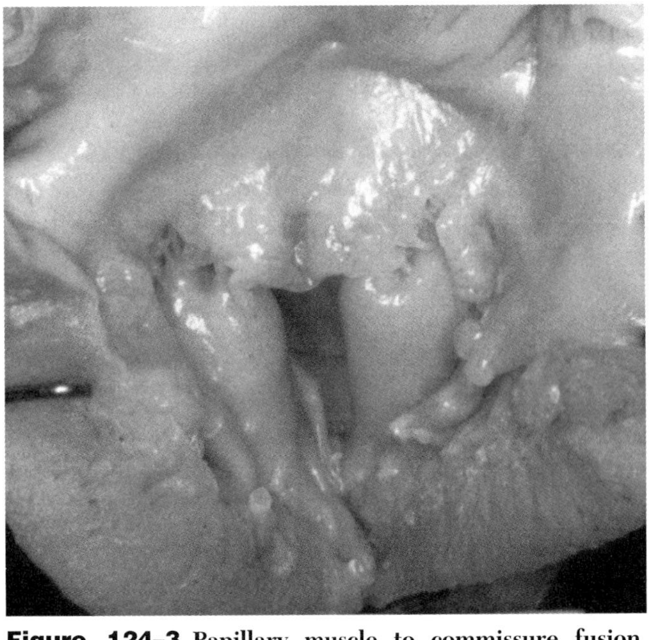

Figure 124–3 Papillary muscle to commissure fusion. Macroscopic view of a papillary muscle to commissure fusion mitral valve. Extremely short cordae are distributed to the anterior commissure *(left of the picture)*. The posterior papillary muscle is almost fused to the posterior commissure *(right of the picture)*.

Hammock Valve or Arcade Valve

In this configuration, the suspension apparatus may have lost all resemblance to the normal anatomy. There is no papillary muscle identifiable or there are multiple very small ones behind the posterior leaflet. The leaflets are suspended directly by a network of cordae directly attached to the posterior wall of the ventricle. This attachment is generally displaced toward the base of the heart with excess tension on the anterior leaflet and extreme limitation of posterior leaflet motion. The valve is most often predominantly regurgitant.

Isolated Mitral Leaflet Hypoplasia

This very rare condition is almost restricted to the middle scallop of the posterior leaflet.[6]

Isolated Dilation of the Mitral Valve Annulus and Isolated Elongation of the Cordae and/or Papillary Muscle

It is difficult to ascertain the congenital origin of these lesions when the anatomy of the mitral valve is otherwise normal. Most publications on congenital anomalies of the mitral valve include them.[6,8] However, there is no evidence of their congenital origin. They are not found at birth unlike the previously described anomalies. They are usually associated with significant volume loading of the left ventricle (e.g., large ventricular septal defect or large patent ductus arteriosus). The pathophysiology is of initial dilation of the posterior annulus under the effect of the volume loading. Secondarily the marginal cordae elongate and create the prolapse of the free edge of the anterior leaflet. Sometimes minor anomalies of the valvular tissue or the papillary muscles can give an indication toward a true congenital origin; in reality this is rare. For patients over the age of 4 with an isolated mitral regurgitation that combines anterior leaflet prolapse and various degrees of posterior leaflet retraction, especially if the latter is thickened, a rheumatic origin has to be ruled out. These lesions are not rare; they account for 15% to 40% of the patients in publications of congenital mitral valve regurgitation.[6,8,11,43,47] These mitral insufficiencies have been included in this chapter because they are often included in congenital series, and also because they are always associated with other cardiac congenital defects. On the other hand, functional mitral regurgitations secondary to cardiomyopathies are not included in this chapter.

Accessory Mitral Valve Tissue, Valvular Tags

The interchordal spaces are filled with a dense network of valve tissue. When there is continuity between the anterior and the posterior leaflet, the accessory valvular tissue may be generating a gradient directly related to the size of the perforations in the accessory tissue (Figure 124-4). When the accessory valve tissue is entrapped in the left ventricular outflow tract, the mitral valve may become regurgitant because of the traction exerted by the accessory valvular tissue on the anterior leaflet, opening the valve at mid systole[36]; however, in that case, the left ventricular outflow tract obstruction is the predominant hemodynamic lesion and is the most frequent mode of diagnosis.[37] Often,[32] the accessory mitral valve tissue does not generate significant gradient or insufficiency.

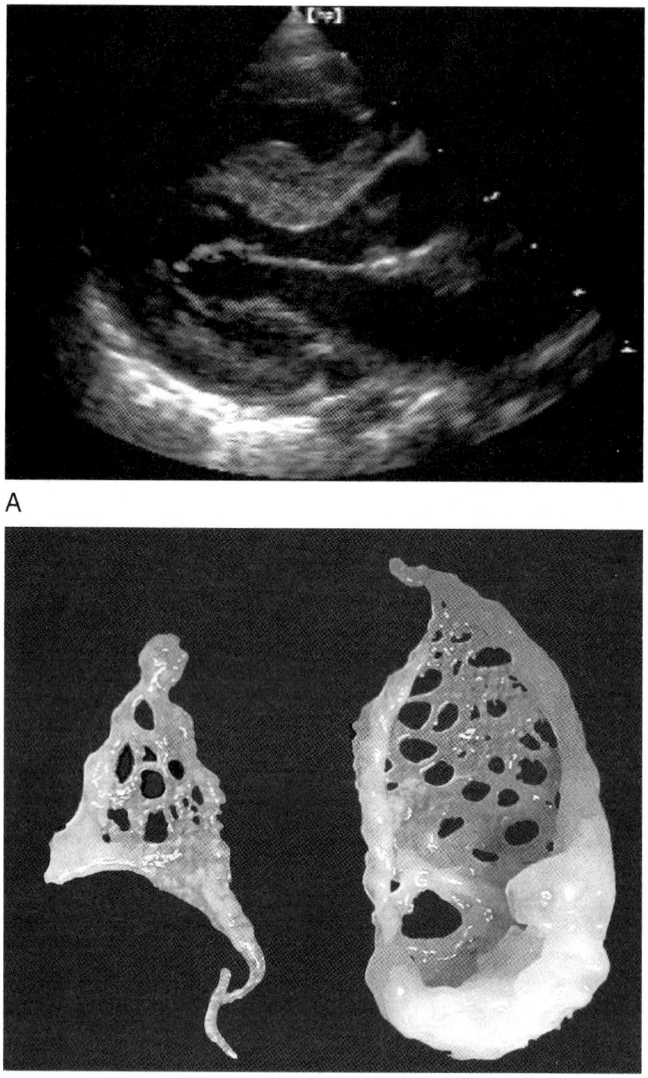

A

B

Figure 124–4 **Accessory mitral valve tissue. A,** Long axis view. The accessory mitral valve tissue is attached to the anterior and posterior leaflets of the mitral valve. The accessory mitral valve tissue is blown like a windsock. **B,** Macroscopic view of the same tissue after surgical resection. The aspect is characteristics of accessory mitral valve tissue attached to the suspension apparatus.

Mitral Valve Disease with Excess of Leaflet Tissue

Mitral Valve Prolapse and Connective Tissue Disorder

Whether to include the *mitral valve prolapse syndrome*, in its most common form, limited to the middle scallop of the posterior defect in the congenital group, is debatable. Using strict criteria, the incidence of mild bulging of the anterior leaflet was negligible, and no prolapses were detected in a large population of neonates.[27] This tends to prove that mitral valve prolapse is an acquired disease. In this form, it is exceptionally encountered in neonates and infants. In adults, the histological anomalies are limited to the middle scallop of the posterior leaflet with predominant elastic fiber alteration and myxomatous tissue proliferation.[14] In the more extensive form of mitral valve prolapse, with excess of tissue distributed to both the anterior and posterior leaflets, the histology demonstrates extensive infiltration of the spongiosa with myxomatous tissue. On the other hand, this extensive form can be seen in neonates and infants. The histological anomalies are identical to those found in *Marfan syndrome*[15,45] and *Elher-Danlos syndrome*. Marfan syndrome is autosomal dominant with varying penetrance. The mutation is found on the fibrillin gene. Ehlers-Danlos syndrome is now represented by a constellation of mutations linked to different subtypes.[35] The extensive form of the mitral valve prolapse syndrome is encountered in sporadic cases or in familial forms. No mutation has been found yet for the familial form.

Recurrent Left Atrioventricular Valve Regurgitation after Repair of Complete or Partial AVSD

In valves with normally developed left lateral leaflet, two mechanisms of the regurgitation can be found. The cleft may be open because the cleft closure performed at the time of the initial surgery has ruptured or has never been done. In that case, the regurgitation occurs through the cleft directly. Alternately, the cleft was completely closed and has remained so. The predominant mechanism for the regurgitation is then the absence of coaptation surface in front of the tip of the left lateral leaflet.

In the unrepaired atrioventricular septal defect (AVSD), the very small surface of the zone of apposition is an inherent feature of these areas of the superior and inferior bridging leaflets. For this reason, at the Royal Children's Hospital in Melbourne, we believe that the latter mechanism is always found even when the cleft closure has ruptured. The closure of the cleft does not restore a coaptation surface; in fact, the little coaptation surface that exists can be reduced and distorted by the cleft closure.

If the regurgitation has been longstanding, the secondary lesion or dysplastic lesions on the edges of the cleft are severe with thickening, sometimes calcification and severe retraction of the leaflet tissue. On the other hand, the left lateral leaflet is usually thin and pliable with no secondary or dysplastic lesion. There is no restriction of the left lateral leaflet motion and no prolapse.

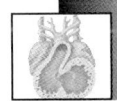

In the presence of a hypoplastic or absent left lateral leaflet, the cleft cannot be closed at the time of the primary repair without generating inflow restriction. The residual or recurrent regurgitation occurs through the cleft. The anatomy is suspected on echocardiographic study when a strong asymmetry of the papillary muscles can be seen on the short axis view of the left ventricle. The predominant papillary muscle, usually the anterior one, is connected to both superior and inferior bridging leaflets. The presence of a double orifice is also a very strong indicator. It is usually directly suspended to the posterior papillary muscle and in the body of the inferior bridging leaflet.

FUNCTIONAL CLASSIFICATION

The Carpentier's functional classification describes the leaflet motion, irrespective of the anatomy and the etiology.[5] It is an essential tool for mitral valve repair and is best studied with echocardiography. It can also give significant clues toward the lesions that will be eventually found during the surgery.

Type I. Normal leaflet motion. It can be either a perforation or a defect of one or two leaflets, or an annular dilation. Annular dilation associated with a type II of the anterior leaflet are most likely functional.

Type II. Enhanced leaflet motion. Most pediatric mitral valve regurgitations with a predominant type II started as functional and progressively elongated the suspension apparatus of the anterior leaflet.

Type III. Restricted leaflet motion. The valve can be stenotic, regurgitant, or both. Most of the patients with congenital anomalies of the mitral valve belong to this type.

Table 124-1 shows the association found between functional classification and the morphological findings adapted from Carpentier [6] and Chauvaud.[8]

Diagnosis

The diagnosis of congenital mitral valve anomaly relies on the clinical findings, the chest X-ray, the electrocardiogram (ECG), and most importantly the echocardiographic study. The positive diagnosis can often be made before the echocardiography examination in the presence of isolated mitral valve anomaly. In the presence of associated cardiac anomalies, the clinical investigation may only raise the index of suspicion or miss completely the mitral valve disease. The echocardiography is part of the initial evaluation of all pediatric patients with cardiac signs. In the presence of associated lesions, only the echocardiography will be able to ascertain the diagnosis of

Table 124–1

Most Probable Anatomical Findings According to Functional Classification and Corresponding Surgical Techniques

Functional head	*Anatomy*	*Surgical technique*
Type I	▪ Posterior leaflet defect ▪ Cleft mitral valve ▪ Annular dilation	▪ Posterior annulus plication ▪ Direct suture Patch enlargement ▪ Adult size annulus: Remodeling annuloplasty with or without leaflet enlargement ▪ Less than adult size annulus Posterior annulus annuloplasty, interrupted or continuous, leaflet enlargement
Type II	▪ Elongated cordae ▪ Absent chordae ▪ Elongated papillary muscle ▪ Excess tissue	▪ Cordal shortening, chordal transfer Wedge resection, sliding plasty ▪ Chordal transfer PTFE chordae ▪ Sliding plasty Papillary muscle shortening ▪ Chordal shortening Quadrangular resection (techniques vary with the age)
Type III	▪ Lack of valvar tissue ▪ Papillary muscle to commissure fusion ▪ Parachute mitral valve ▪ Hammock mitral valve	▪ Posterior leaflet detachment and enlargement Anterior leaflet enlargement ▪ Fenestration of papillary muscle Commissurotomy ▪ Fenestration of papillary muscle Splitting of papillary muscle; commissurotomy ▪ Posterior leaflet detachment and enlargement ▪ Mobilization of suspension apparatus, separation from posterior wall ▪ Anterior leaflet enlargement

PTFE, polytetrafluoroethylene.

the congenital mitral valve. In most patients, the echocardiography shows the congenital nature of the anomaly by demonstrating the variance with the normal anatomy. The functional evaluation of the mitral valve and the impact of the lesion on the cardiovascular system are best made by echocardiographic study. The catheter study and the ventriculogram have now no indication in the diagnosis or the preoperative assessment of a mitral valve disease. The indications for catheter study and angiography are only derived from associated lesions, mainly complex ventricular septal defects and some arch anomalies. On the other hand, the growing wealth of information both functional and morphological generated by the magnetic resonance imaging (MRI) will justify a preoperative MRI study when available.[13,23]

Clinical Examination

Mitral Stenosis

Patients rarely present during the neonatal period and in this situation the associated lesion can be predominant. Beyond the neonatal period, symptoms may include failure to thrive, dyspnea on exertion, pallor, hypotrophy, and a history of repeated chest infections. Signs of low cardiac output can be found with pallor and cold extremities, tachycardia, and dyspnea. Signs of pulmonary hypertension are present with exacerbated second heart sound and palpation of the right ventricular impulse. Diminished first sound suggests thick leaflets of limited excursion, low intensity mid-diastolic murmur is the only direct auscultation sign and can be absent low output situation.

Mitral Regurgitation

Presentation during the neonatal period is rare. At all ages patient present with various degrees of failure to thrive, dyspnea with feeding, or on exertion. Enlarged left ventricular impulse, with high-frequency, high-intensity holosystolic murmur is heard at the apex extending into the axillae.

Electrocardiogram

There are left atrial enlargement and left ventricular enlargement in mitral regurgitation; right atrial and right ventricular enlargements are seen when pulmonary hypertension is present. In the pediatric population the rhythm is almost always sinus.

Chest X-Ray

Chest X-ray demonstrates double density of the left atrial enlargement and various degree of pulmonary plethora with enlarged main pulmonary artery. Left ventricular enlargement in the presence of mitral valve regurgitation is evident.

Echocardiography

The echocardiographic study is indispensable. Systematically conducted, it provides all information necessary for the diagnosis of the mitral anomaly, its severity, and the impact on the physiology.[1] The anatomical lesion can usually be strongly suspected. It is an essential tool for surgical indication as well as assistance to the surgeon for the repair.[8]

The four-chamber view obtained with the transthoracic echocardiographic study is best to provide an accurate transvalvular gradient and define the precise amplitude of any prolapse or restriction. The short axis view of the mitral valve (en face view) gives a direct vision of the area of the mitral orifice and good location of the origin of the regurgitant jet. It allows a precise analysis of the papillary muscles (presence, size, location, and symmetry). The transesophageal echo is superior for anatomical details of the suspension apparatus and the evaluation of the functional classification. By moving the probe up and down in the esophagus, it provides a precise localization of the area of prolapse along the free edge of the anterior leaflet, using the anterior commissure (probe up) and the posterior commissure (probe down) as benchmarks.

For mitral stenoses, the peak instantaneous and mean gradients across the valve have to be interpreted according to the quality of the diastolic function of the heart and the associated lesions. The overall impact of the gradient on the surgical indication has to be weighted with the pulmonary artery pressure but mostly clinical tolerance.

TREATMENT

Medical therapy has to be vigorous when the annulus is too small to receive a mechanical prosthesis in the anatomical position. In the setting of predominant mitral regurgitation, the treatment should include an angiotensin conversion enzyme (ACE) inhibitor, diuretics and, if necessary, red cell transfusion.[24,28] In mitral stenosis, any vasodilator or afterload reduction is contraindicated.

Surgical Treatment

Indications

The indication for surgical intervention differs from the adult age. The cut-off point is more related to the size of the mitral valve annulus than to the age of the patient. When the annulus is close to an adult size, the timing of the surgical intervention is directly related to the probability of successful repair of the valve. Valves with great probability of repair should be operated as soon as the regurgitation is severe, irrespective of the severity of symptoms. This is especially valid for valves that usually do not need annular stabilization. The timing is then directly related to the experience of the surgical team.

In neonates (<28 days) and infants (>28 days and less than 1 year), repair is technically challenging, the replacement is often possible only with the use of surgical artifacts associated with significant mortality[16,19]; therefore the surgical indication should be deferred as long as the patient can be managed medically. In pediatric patients, long-term ventricular function returns to normal in severely symptomatic patients when the operation is successful.[22,26] This is in opposition with the adult population.[25,41] Two small retrospective series of mechanical valve replacements at more than 24 months of age demonstrate less than 14% hospital mortality and low late mortality.[12,29] These patients belong to the recent era with appropriate anticoagulation therapy. One important multi-institutional retrospective study[4] has demonstrated very strong risk association when there is a mismatch between the prosthetic size and the diameter of the recipient annulus.

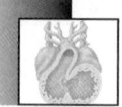

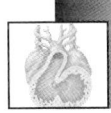

In patients older than 1 year of age, using a wide range of mitral valve repair techniques, repair of virtually all valves is an accessible goal.[8]

In small mitral annuli, the repair is difficult but replacement generates high mortality.[16,34,40] The surgery should be delayed whenever possible, but it should be conducted without hesitation when it cannot be delayed,[38] together with treatment of associated cardiac lesions. In large mitral annuli, repair is possible most of the time. If necessary, mitral valve replacements can now be done with very good long-term outcome. This is in opposition with results of earlier series.[16,44]

Mitral Valve Replacement

Mitral valve replacement in supraannular position in infants should be avoided at all cost. This type of implantation is responsible for the majority or the totality of perioperative and long-term deaths in units with experience of these patients. Mitral valve repair is often a palliation or a short-term palliation but allows for annular growth and eventually replacement in satisfactory technical condition.

Mitral valve replacement in larger anuli is possible now with excellent long-term results. Only mechanical valves should be implanted. The apparition of low profile aortic valve has proven to be very useful in the management of pediatric mitral valve replacement. Obviously the valve has to be removed from the valve holder and implanted with the opening toward the ventricular cavity. The bioprostheses have been associated with early degeneration and need for reoperation. Even if their implantation is considered a short-term palliation, they do not provide the potential benefit of repairs (growth, ease of reoperation); therefore, they should not be used in the pediatric age group.

The replacement of mechanical prosthesis is not uncommon in pediatric units. The indication is usually for apparition of a gradient with pulmonary hypertension, at rest (on Doppler study or catheter study) or on exertion (on Doppler study). A larger size can usually be implanted, but *exceptionally* more than two sizes greater than the prosthesis previously implanted.[47] This has direct implication on the indication of the initial replacement. A mitral prosthesis size 17, implanted in infancy, will generate two further valve replacements until a size 25 is implanted. On the other hand, a palliative repair should then allow for a large-size prothesis at the time of the first implantation. Technically, the replacement of a pediatric mechanical prosthesis does differ significantly from the adult size. Great care must be taken to the removal of all cuff tissue and pledgets. Everting mattress suture, especially with pledgets should be avoided as they reduce the size of the annulus. Preference should be given to simple interrupted sutures.

Mitral Valve Repair

The techniques for mitral valve repair are those described by Carpentier and others[5,7] for adult surgery with modification for the pediatric patient and small congenital mitral valves.[6,8] Cardiopulmonary bypass in Melbourne is conducted with moderate hypothermia 32° C, hemoglobin of 8 to 10 g/dcl. Pump flow of 150–200 ml/min/kg or 1 l/min/m^2. Myocardial protection with cold blood cardioplegia, administered every 20–30 min. Venous cannulation should allow as much room into the atrioventricular groove. Cannulation of the superior vena cava directly and at a distance from the cavoatrial junction and of the inferior vena cava immediately at the origin. Limited dissection of the groove is performed. After cross-clamp, the left atrium is entered into the AV groove. The exposure is enhanced with mattress sutures inserted into the posterior annulus pulling the valve upward and toward the operator. The snugger on the inferior vena cava is pulling upward and to the left. A self-retaining retractor for mitral surgery adapted to the size of the patient has to be used in all cases. We find alternatives approaches less satisfactory. If it is through the interatrial septum it then provides a lesser edge for the retractor blades to anchor and exposes the conduction tissue to more pressure. If it is through the roof of the left atrium it does not expose as well the posterior commissure and posterior papillary muscle. The preparation for bypass is used for the mandatory preoperative transesophageal echocardiographic study. Once satisfactory exposure of the mitral valve is gained, the valve is systematically analyzed integrating preoperative information. The functional classification is confirmed but the extension of mitral valve prolapse or restriction is based on echocardiographic studies. Then the morphological and anatomical examination takes place:

A supravalvular ring is confirmed or eliminated.
Diameter of the annulus.
Texture, aspect, and size of the mitral valve leaflets.
Number, aspect, and distribution of the cordae.
Presence of commissural tissue and dedicated suspension apparatus.
Presence, size, location, and morphology of the papillary muscles.

The examination finishes with a careful check for accessory mitral valve tissue in the interchordal spaces. The diameter of the anulus and of the opening of the mitral valve is compared to the reference one for the patient's body surface area. In Melbourne, we use a modification of the sizes provided by Kirklin.[21]

The treatment is adapted to the predominant functional class. Schematic correlation between functional class, pathological subgroups, and treatment is described in Table 124-1. All the techniques included in the table are identical to those of used in adult mitral valve repair surgery.[46] Few modification are dictated by the size of the pediatric patients.

Correction of Type I: Remodeling Annuloplasty

The remodeling annuloplasty is mandatory in all mitral valve insufficiency with the exception of some isolated type I without annular dilation, mostly the cleft mitral valve. Attempts to perform mitral valve repair without annuloplasty have resulted in recurrence.[3] To accommodate an adult-size device or a larger size annulus than what would be indicated from the area of the anterior leaflet, leaflet enlargement with glutaraldehyde-treated pericardium of the posterior leaflet, the anterior leaflet, or both is used.[9,17] In type III patients, the detachment of the posterior leaflet to gain access to the suspension apparatus is used for the leaflet enlargement.[46] When no device is available for the size of the patient or when the device is thought to be too small, then an annuloplasty limited to the posterior annulus is indicated. The annuloplasty has to incorporate both trigones and can be divided in the middle to allow for further growth. Several materials can be used for that purpose, for example, Dacron or PTFE. We like to use expended PTFE sheet folded three times to provide three layers and sufficient rigidity to avoid corrugating effect. Mattress sutures should not be tied too tightly (Figure 124-5).

Correction of Type II

Correction of type II is rarely necessary in congenital mitral regurgitation. Type II is mostly a secondary lesion in congenital mitral anomalies or is seen with associated lesions (mostly large volume loading of the left ventricle). Multiples techniques are available to correct the enhanced leaflet motion.[3,46] Whether techniques should be used in isolation or in combination depends on the extension in width of the prolapsus (i.e., localized or extended to the whole width of the free edge). It is the height of the prolapsus (based on the echocardiographic study) that will dictate the choice of the technique.

All techniques are extremely efficient and reliable providing that the correction is adequate (restores a large surface of apposition between anterior and posterior leaflet). An overcorrection will generate stress directly on the repaired area and void the valve of the relief of stress provided by the surface of apposition. All overcorrections eventually fail, most often very rapidly.

The chordal shortening requires thin and flexible cordae. The correction generates significant shortening of the cordae and is only adapted when significant shortening is necessary. It is time-consuming and this should be considered if multiple cordae are to be shortened.

Chordal transfer between secondary cordae and the free edge, more than cordal transfer from posterior leaflet to anterior leaflet, allows for correction of localized prolapse. The cordae should be detached from the body of the anterior leaflet with minimal amount of valvular tissue. It is then attached to the free edge directly at the required length with a small running suture.

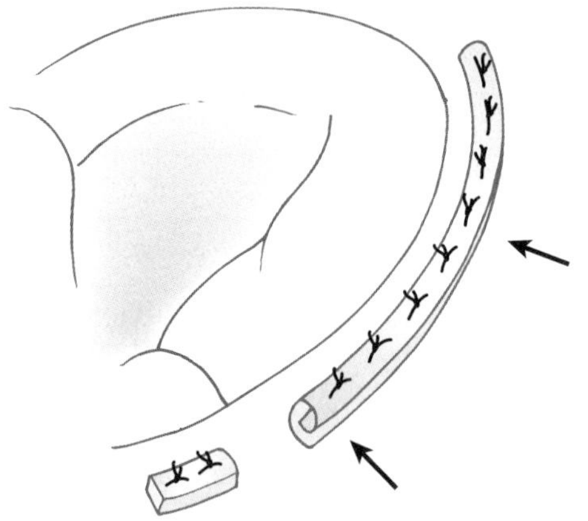

Figure 124–5 Posterior annuloplasty. Using either short strips of ePTFE or three layers of ePTFE sheet. The annuloplasty should be split once or twice *(arrows)* to allow for growth.

Wedge resection and sliding plasty generate different degree of correction of prolapsus to multiple cordae. They are very well adapted to prolapsus extended to a large segment of the anterior leaflet.

Artificial Cordae

The use of artificial cordae should be restricted to the absence of available cordae of appropriate strength and quality in the area of prolapse. The insertion requires a rigorous technique to avoid overcorrection and large knots at the free edge.

Correction of Type III

Successful correction of restricted leaflet motion and insufficient leaflet tissue is the essence of congenital mitral anomalies, especially in the first year of life.

Posterior Leaflet Mobilization and Enlargement Associated with Mobilization of the Papillary Muscles

Access to the suspension apparatus is the key to adequate mobilization of the latter. It can be done through the mitral valve orifice when it is sufficient. Most often, the mitral orifice is very small and does not allow for sufficient access to the suspension apparatus. In these situations, the detachment of the posterior leaflet generates large access to the papillary muscles. Adequate thinning, mobilization from the posterior wall, splitting and fenestration of the papillary muscles can then be performed safely with good exposure. The posterior leaflet is afterwards reconstructed with enlargement of the valvar tissue[8,9] (Figure 124-6).

Enlargement of Valvular Tissue Using Autologous Pericardium Treated with Glutaraldehyde

Augmentation of the valvular leaflet tissue is the only way to treat a lack of valvular tissue.[8,17] It can be limited to the anterior leaflet, the posterior leaflet, or used in both. The extension of the posterior leaflet should be limited to less than a half of the height of the leaflet. It can be limited to the area of the middle scallop; Alternately, when the detachment is extended from one commissure to another, the extension should reproduce a shape with three scallops and two commissures to allow for a large opening in diastole. The extension of the anterior leaflet should be done in the body of the leaflet, leaving a strip of valvar tissue close to the hinge point to avoid mechanical stress at this level. The height of the extension should not be greater than two fifth of the height of the leaflet, leaving the area close to the free edge intact to allow for supple and efficient surface of coaptation. If possible, it should be symmetrical from trigone to trigone.

Resection of Supravalvular Rings and Accessory Mitral Valve Tissue

Resection of supravalvar tissue requires an excellent exposure of the leaflet tissue. The supravalvar tissue can sometimes be peeled off the valvular tissue. More often, there will be the need for a careful cleavage with blunt dissection. Perforation to the anterior leaflet may occur and should be closed with simple figure eight suture.

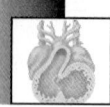

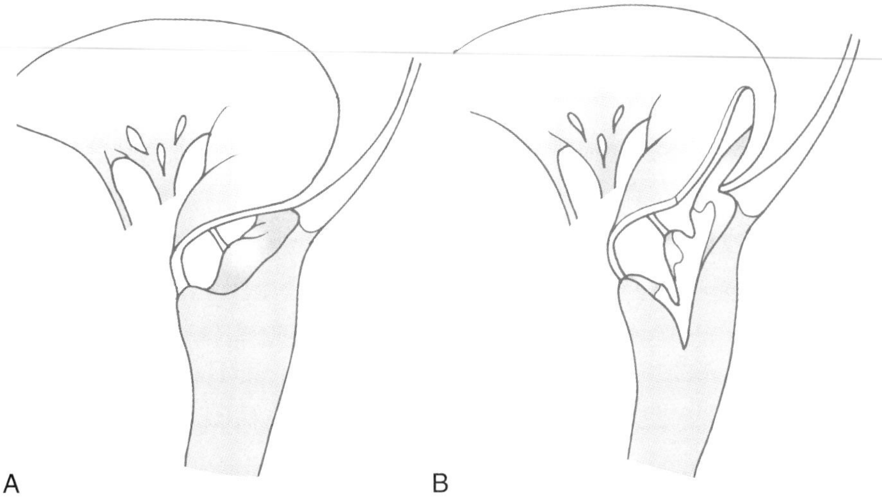

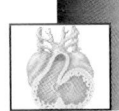

Figure 124–6 Detachment of the posterior leaflet. A, Schematic representation of a hammock/papillary commissure fusion. Access to the suspension apparatus is limited through the natural mitral orifice. **B,** After detachment of the posterior leaflet, mobilization and splitting of the suspension apparatus can easily be performed even in smallest valves.

Resection of accessory mitral valve tissue requires similarly rigorous surgical technique. A very good exposure of the subvalvar apparatus is needed to delineate perfectly the mitral valve cordae from what can be resected without compromising the integrity of the suspension apparatus. Various approaches to the suspension apparatus may have to be combined: through the mitral valve orifice and the aortic valve or detachment of the posterior leaflet.

Repair of Recurrent Left Atrioventricular Valve Regurgitation

In some cases, the valve can be repaired by resuture of the cleft. When the cleft has not ruptured, the valve should be repaired with adjunction of valvular tissue. Autologous pericardium treated with glutaraldehyde is used. The area of the combined superior and inferior bridging leaflet can be augmented.[33] At the Children's Hospital in Melbourne, we prefer to create a coaptation surface in front of the left lateral leaflet.

The area of the cleft closure is débrided of all secondary lesions around the regurgitation zone. Sufficient resection is performed to reach pliable leaflet tissue. The area of the cleft is then closed with a long and narrow patch. The patch extends into the ventricular cavity as to create a coaptation surface to face the tip of the left lateral leaflet (Figure 124-7).

In the case of hypoplastic left lateral leaflet, the cleft is reopened where it had been partially closed, and a surface of coaptation is constructed on both edges of the cleft. In this anatomy, at the Royal Children's Hospital, three different techniques are used, according to the difficulty and the anatomy; autologous pericardium treated with glutaraldehyde with ePTFE cordae on the edge of the cleft. The mid-term results have been disappointing. Alternately, we have used a partial mitral valve homograft (PMVH) of adapted size to reproduce the zone of apposition. This technique has demonstrated very good immediate and intermediate results in our experience and should allow sufficient palliation time to wait for adult-size prosthesis. Last, in relatively simple cases, the edges of the cleft can be directly suspended using ePTFE cordae.

The double orifice should not be closed, as it is never regurgitant and can produce valuable area of valve opening.

RESULTS

Mitral Valve Stenosis and Predominant Stenotic Valves

Between 1996 and 2003, ten patients were operated on for congenital mitral stenosis. The median age was 1.3 years (range 3 weeks to 13 years). The mean preoperative gradient was 13±5 mm Hg. The anatomy was papillary muscle to commissure fusion (n = 5), parachute mitral valve (n = 2), supravalvular ring (n = 3), and excess tissue (n = 1). Three patients had Shone syndrome. In these three patients, the aortic valve was treated with aortic valvotomy in two, and one had a Ross procedure. There was no early or late death. There were four reoperations in two patients with three in the same patient, leading ultimately to valve replacement with a mechanical valve diameter 23.

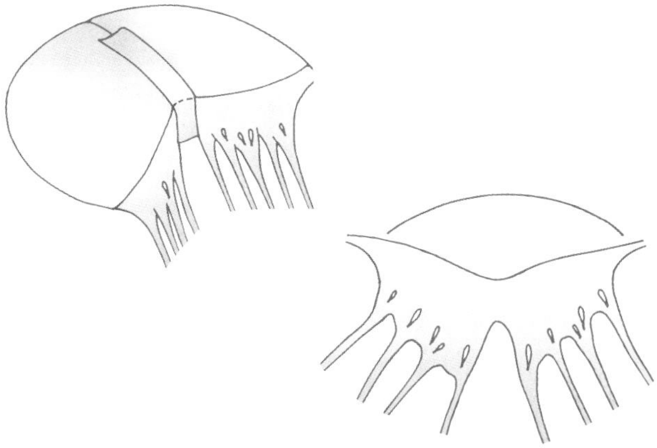

Figure 124–7 Construction of a coaptation surface at the junction between superior and inferior bridging leaflets facing the left lateral leaflet *(in caption)*.

Mitral Valve Insufficiency and Predominant Regurgitant Valves

During the same interval, 41 patients were operated on for predominant congenital mitral regurgitation. There were 15 mitral cleft and 26 complex valves. In the latter group, the median age was 4.8 years (2 weeks to 20 years). The etiology was connective tissue disorder (n = 6), anterior leaflet prolapse secondary to volume loading of the heart (n = 7), lack of valvular tissue (n = 9), and others (n = 3). At the time of initial operation, 25 repairs were done, using annuloplasty adapted to the size of the patient in 23. One valve was replaced. There were three early deaths, including one patient with mechanical valve replacement; all were infants. There was one late death. There were three late reoperations with two repairs and one mechanical replacement. At a median follow-up of 5.2 years, there were two survivors with mitral regurgitation greater than mild.

All patients with cleft mitral valve but one with moderate mitral regurgitation had a good result.

Recurrent Left Atrioventricular Valve Regurgitation

Since 1978, more than 600 patients were operated on at the Royal Children's Hospital in Melbourne for complete or partial AVSD. From 1996 to 2003, 20 patients have been reoperated on for recurrent severe mitral regurgitation with the technique described in this chapter. Before that, 41 reoperations had been performed on the same patients for the same indication with a median of two per patient. Six patients had a diminutive or absent left lateral leaflet, and 14 had a normally developed left lateral leaflet. Four patients with diminutive left lateral leaflet have received a partial mitral valve homograft. At a median follow-up of 17 months, three patients in the diminutive left lateral leaflet group had a mild regurgitation, one had a stable moderate regurgitation, and two have had mechanical valve replacement. In the normal left lateral leaflet group there was one early death. One patient, whose good postoperative result were not stable, required reoperation at 20 months. The same technique was used. Twelve patients had a stable good result.

REFERENCES

1. Barnerjee A, Kohl T, Silverman N: Echocardiographic evaluation of congenital mitral valve anomalies in children. Am J Cardiol 76:1284–1291, 1995.
2. Binet JP, Piot C, Losay J, et al: A new anatomo-clinical entity? The left superior vena cava obstructing the interior of the left atrium in association with a left-right shunt. Arch Mal Coeur Vaiss 71:104–111, 1978.
3. Braumer RA, Laks H, Drinkwater DC, et al: Multiple left heart obstructions (Shone's Anomaly) with mitral valve involvement: long-term surgical outcome. Ann Thorac Surg 64:721–729, 1997.
4. Caldarone CA, Raghuveer G, Hills CB, et al: Long term survival after mitral valve replacement in children aged less than five years: a multi-institutional study. Circulation 104(suppl I):I143—I147, 2001.
5. Carpentier A: Cardiac valve surgery—the "French correction." J Thorac Cardiovasc Surg 86:323–337, 1983.
6. Carpentier A: Congenital malformations of the mitral valve. In: Stark J, de Leval M (eds): Surgery for congenital heart defects. London: Grune & Stratton, 1983, pp. 467–482.
7. Carpentier A, Branchini B, Cour JC, et al: Congenital malformations of the mitral valve in children. J Thorac Cardiovasc Surg 72:854–866, 1976.
8. Chauvaud S, Fuzellier JF, Houel R, et al: Reconstructive surgery in congenital mitral valve insufficiency (Carpentier's techniques): Long term results. J Thorac Cardiovasc Surg 102:171–178, 1991.
9. Chauvaud S, Jebara V, Chachques JC, et al: Valve extension with glutaraldehyde-preserved autologous pericardium. J Thorac Cardiovasc Surg 102:171–178, 1991.
10. Cochrane AD, Marath A, Mee RB: Can a dilated coronary sinus produce left ventricular inflow obstruction? An unrecognized entity. Ann Thorac Surg. 58:1114–1116, 1994.
11. Coles JG, Williams WG, Watanabe T, et al: Surgical experience with reparative techniques in patients with congenital mitral valvular anomalies: Circulation 76(suppl III):III117–122, 1987.
12. Daou L, Sidi D, Mauriat P, et al: Mitral valve replacement with mechanical valves in children under two years of age. J Thorac Cardiovasc Surg 121:5, 2001.
13. Didier D, Ratib O, Lerch R, Friedli B: Detection and quantification of valvular heart disease with dynamic cardiac MR imaging. RadioGraphics 20:1279–1299, 2000.
14. Fornes P, Heudes D, Fuzellier JF, et al: Correlation between clinical and histologic patterns of degenerative mitral valve insufficiency: a histomorphometric study of 130 excised segments. Cardiovasc Pathol 8:81–92, 1999.
15. Fuzellier JF, Chauvaud SM, Fornes P, et al: Surgical management of mitral regurgitation associated with Marfan's Syndrome. Ann Thorac Surg 66:68–72, 1998.
16. Günther T, Mazzitelli D, Schreiber C, et al: Mitral-valve replacement in children under six years of age. Eur J Cardiothorac Surg 17:426–430, 2000.
17. Hisatomi K, Isomura T, Hirano A, et al: Long-term follow-up results after reconstruction of the mitral valve by leaflet advancement. Ann Thorac Surg 54:271–274, 1999.
18. Kadletz M, Black MD, Smallhorn J, et al: Total anomalous systemic venous drainage to the coronary sinus in association with hypoplastic left heart disease: More than a mere coincidence. J Thorac Cardiovasc Surg 114:282–284, 1996.
19. Kadoba K, Jonas RA, Mayer JE, Castaneda AR: Mitral valve replacement in the first year of life. J Thorac Cardiovasc Surg 100:762–768, 1990.
20. Kohl T, Silverman NH: Comparison of cleft and papillary muscle position in cleft mitral valve and atrioventricular septal defect. Am J Cardiol 77:164–169, 1996.
21. Kirklin JW, Barrat-Boyes BG: Anatomy, dimension and terminology. In: Kirklin JW Barrat-Boyes BG (eds): Cardiac Surgery, 2nd ed. Churchill Livingstone, 1993, pp. 3—60.
22. Krishnan US, Gersony WM, Berman-Rosenzweig E, Apfel HD: Late left ventricular function after surgery for children with chronic symptomatic mitral regurgitation. Circulation 96:4280–4285, 1997.
23. Kroft LJ, de Roos A: Biventricular diastolic cardiac function assessed by MR flow imaging using a single angulation. Acta Radiologica 40:563–568, 1999.
24. Lister G, Hellebrand WE, Kleinman CS, Talner NS: Physiologic effects of increasing hemoglobin concentration in left to right shunting in infants with ventricular septal defects. N Engl J Med 306:502–506, 1982.
25. Moore P, Adatia I, Spevak PJ, et al: Severe congenital mitral stenosis in infants. Circulation 89:2099–2106, 1994.
26. Murakami T, Nakazawa M, Nakanishi T, Momma K: Prediction of postoperative left ventricular pump function in congenital mitral regurgitation. Pediatr Cardiol 6:418–421, 1999.

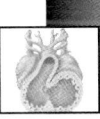

27. Nascimento R, Freitas A, Teixeira F, et al: Is mitral valve prolapse a congenital or acquired disease? Am J Cardiol 79:226–227, 1997.
28. Nihill MR, McNamara DG, Vick RL: The effect of increased blood viscosity on pulmonary vascular resistance. Am Heart J 92:65–72, 1976.
29. Ninet J, Sassolas F, Robin J, et al: Le remplacement valvulaire mitral chez le nourrisson avec la prothese mécanique Saint-Jude Medical. Arch Mal Coeur Vais 86:643–647, 1994.
30. Oosthoek PW, Wenink AC, Vrolijk BC, et al: Development of the atrioventricular valve apparatus in the human heart. Anat Embryol 198:317–329, 1998.
31. Oosthoek PW, Wenink AC, Wisse LJ, et al: Development of the papillary muscle of the mitral valve: Morphometric background of parachute like asymmetric mitral valves and other mitral valves anomalies. J Thorac Cardiovasc Surg 116:36–46, 1998.
32. Pettelot G, Gibelin P, Baudouy M, Morand P: Accessory mitral tissue in a young girl. Circulation 96:3240, 1997.
33. Poirier NC, Williams WG, Van Arsdell GS, et al: A novel repair for patients with atrioventricular septal defect requiring reoperation for left atrioventricular valve regurgitation. Eur J Cardio-thor Surg 18:54–61, 2000.
34. Pollock JC, Shawkat S, Houston A: Mitral valve replacement in the first three months of life. Br Heart J 42:549–551, 1984.
35. Pope FM, Burrows NP: Ehlers-Danlos syndrome has varied molecular mechanisms. J Med Genet 34:400–410, 1997.
36. Prifti E, Frati G, Bonacchi M, et al: Accessory mitral valve tissue causing left ventricular outflow tract obstruction: case reports and literature review. J Hrt Valve Dis 10:774–778, 2001.
37. Schmid AC, Zund G, Vogt P, Turina M: Congenital subaortic stenosis by accessory mitral valve tissue, recognition and management. Eur J Cardio Thorac Surg 15:542–544, 1999.
38. Serraf A, Zoghbi J, Belli E, et al: Congenital mitral stenosis with or without associated defects. An evolving surgical strategy. Circulation 102(suppl III):III166–171, 2000.
39. Shone JD, Sellers RD, Anderson RC, et al: The developmental complex of "parachute mitral valve" supravalvular ring of left atrium, subaortic stenosis, and coarctation of aorta. Am J Cardiol 11:714, 1963.
40. Spevak PJ, Freed M, Castaneda AR, et al: Valve replacement in children less than five years of age. JACC 8:901–908, 1986.
41. Starling MR, Kirsh MM, Montgomery DG, Gross MD: Impaired left ventricular contractile function in patients with long-term mitral regurgitation and normal ejection fraction. JACC 22:1239–1250, 1993.
42. Tamura M, Menahem S, Brizard C: Clinical features and management of isolated cleft mitral valve in childhood. JACC 35:588–594, 2000.
43. Uva MS, Galletti L, Gayet FL, et al: Surgery for congenital mitral valve disease in the first year of life. J Thorac Cardiovasc Surg 109:165–175, 1995.
44. Van Dorn K, Yates R, Tsang V, et al: Mitral valve replacement in children: mortality, morbidity, and hemodynamic status up to medium term follow up. Heart 84:636–642, 2000.
45. Van Karnebeek CD, Naeff MS, Mulder BM, et al: Natural history of cardiovascular manifestations in Marfan syndrome. Arch Dis Child 84:129–137, 2001.
46. Wessels A, Markman MWM, Vermeulen JLM, et al: The development of the atrioventricular junction in the human heart: Circulation Res 78:110–117, 1996.
47. Yoshimura N, Yamaguchi M, Oshima Y, et al: Surgery for mitral valve disease in the pediatric age group. J Thorac Cardiovasc Surg 118:99–106, 1999.

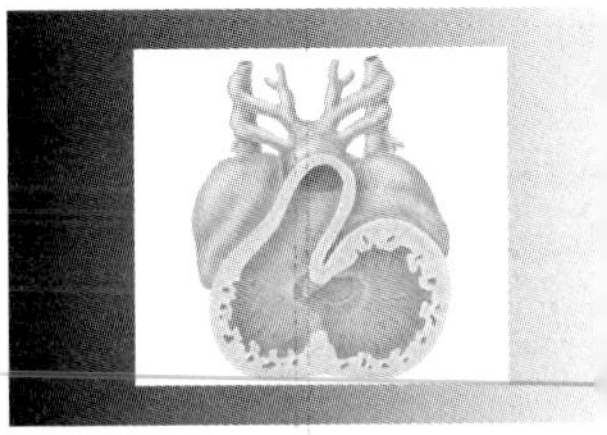

Hypoplastic Left Heart Syndrome

Frank A. Pigula

CHAPTER 125

INTRODUCTION

Hypoplastic left heart syndrome (HLHS) is characterized by a generalized underdevelopment of the left ventricle and its dependent structures; the mitral valve, the aortic valve, and the preductal/ductal aorta. Because the anatomic severity of HLHS constitutes a spectrum of disease, the value of a consistent, defined nomenclature has been recognized. Such a nomenclature has been proposed by the Congenital Heart Surgery Nomenclature and Database Project.[104] The Project has proposed an operative definition for Hypoplastic Left Heart Syndrome (HLHS) as "a spectrum of cardiac malformations, characterized by a severe underdevelopment of the left heart-aorta complex, consisting of aortic and/or mitral atresia, stenosis, or hypoplasia with marked hypoplasia or absence of the LV, and hypoplasia of the ascending aorta and the aortic arch."

The treatment of HLHS has dramatically changed over the last 2 decades. With little to offer prior to Norwood's introduction of Stage I palliation in 1983, treatment has developed into a three-stage progression to the Fontan operation. Although 1-month mortality for untreated patients is 95%, current 1-month survival among specialized centers approaches 80% to 90%.

This chapter will discuss the anatomic and physiologic challenges posed by these patients, as well as the management schemes devised to meet them.

DEMOGRAPHICS/INCIDENCE

Two large epidemiologic reports have estimated the prevalence of HLHS to be .16–.18 per 1000 live births.[29,79] Males account for 57% to 67 % of new cases, and the risk of sibling recurrence has been reported to be 0.5%.[13,75] No environmental risk factors associated with the diagnosis of HLHS have been identified.[105]

CLINICAL PRESENTATION

On physical examination these children may appear entirely normal at birth. Within hours to days however tachypnea and pallor may become apparent with nonspecific CXR and EKG findings.[93,100] Depending on the adequacy of the ductal and atrial communications, there may be rapid progress to acidosis, cyanosis, and cardiopulmonary collapse. An exception to this usual sequence occurs in neonates presenting with a restrictive atrial septum; these children will present immediately after birth in severe respiratory distress, respiratory acidosis, and cyanosis that is unresponsive to medical management.

Other congenital lesions should be sought. Natowicz, et al have reported that 28% of patients with HLHS suffered from a genetic disorder and/or major noncardiac abnormality.[74] Looking specifically at the central nervous system among infants with HLHS, Glauser and colleagues have documented anomalies in 29% and microcephaly in 27%.[34] Thus the preoperative evaluation of these neonates should also include a genetic and neurologic evaluation.

Diagnosis

Echocardiography has become the diagnostic procedure of choice in HLHS. Details such as aortic valve size and status (atretic vs. patent), aortic dimensions, origin of the coronary arteries, brachiocephalic branching, status of the atrial septum, function of the tricuspid and pulmonary valves, and presence of systemic or pulmonary venous anomalies should be sought. Coronary anomalies, while rare, are more likely encountered in the setting of mitral stenosis and aortic atresia, and may take the form of coronary-ventricular fistulas, hypoplasia, tortuosity, or single coronary arteries, anomalous left coronary from the pulmonary artery (PA).[5,21,44,67,76,96]

Cardiac Catheterization

Cardiac catheterization in HLHS should be reserved for those with equivocal anatomy who may be candidates for biventricular repair, when coronary anomalies are suspected, or to delineate abnormal pulmonary venous return.

Fetal Diagnosis

Improvements in fetal echocardiography have led to an increasing frequency of antenatal diagnoses of HLHS. Tworetzky, et al has reported that prenatal diagnosis was associated with improved preoperative clinical condition as well as improved survival after the Norwood operation.[110] Unfortunately, improved survival following Norwood palliation in children with a prenatal diagnosis has not been consistently demonstrated.[57] Mahle, et al have reported that although antenatal diagnosis improves their preoperative clinical condition, and may reduce the incidence of neurologic injury, surgical survival has not been impacted.[63]

PATHOPHYSIOLOGY

In HLHS the right ventricle must support both the systemic and pulmonary circulation. Pulmonary venous return must have access to the right atrium, either via an atrial septal defect (ASD), patent foramen ovale (PFO), or rarely via anomalous pulmonary venous connections to the systemic veins. Systemic output, delivered via the ductus arteriosus, is entirely dependent upon ductal patency (Figure 125-1). Ductal involution may be a rapid process, restricting right ventricle (RV)-dependent systemic blood flow and leading to progressive metabolic acidosis, tachypnea, and irritability prior to cardiopulmonary collapse.

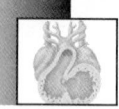

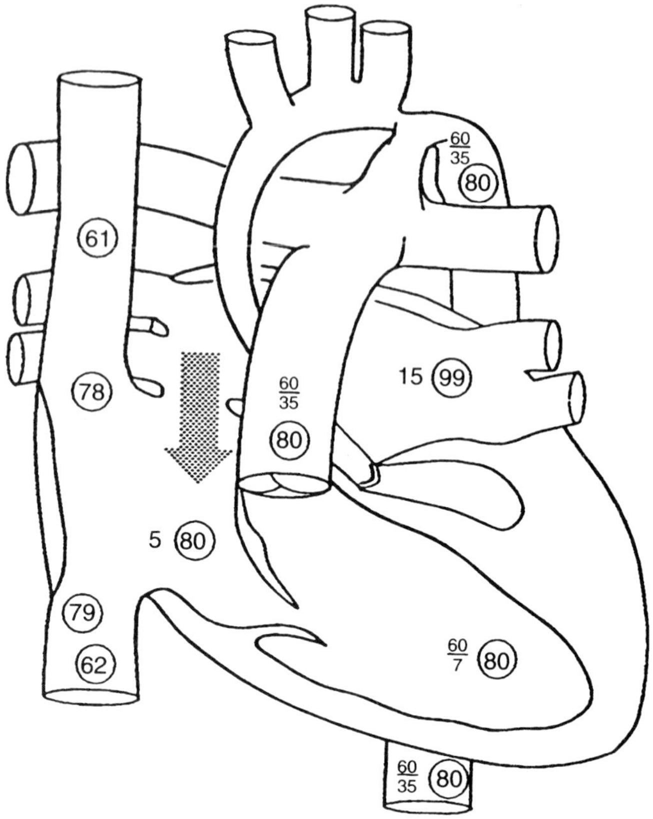

Figure 125–1 Hemodynamics and oxygen saturations *(enclosed circles)* of hypoplastic left heart syndrome in the unoperated state. Pulmonary venous return must cross the atrial septum *(shaded arrow)*, where there is mixing with systemic venous return in the right atrium. Systemic cardiac output is dependent upon a patent ductus arteriosus.
(Reprinted with permission from Jacobs ML: Hypoplastic Left Heart Syndrome, pg 859. In: Kaiser LR, Kron IL, Spray TL, (eds): Mastery of Cardiothoracic Surgery. Philadelphia: Lippincott-Raven, 1998.)

The functional size of the interatrial communication is an important physiologic determinant in these patients. In the presence of an unrestrictive atrial communication pulmonary blood flow quickly becomes excessive and the signs and symptoms of congestive heart failure predominate.

There is a subset of neonates born with a mildly restrictive interatrial septum (gradient of 2–5 mm/Hg), such that pulmonary resistance is modestly elevated. This often serves to balance systemic and pulmonary blood flow, and these children may be physiologically stable, requiring little intervention prior to surgery.

Finally, a few children will present with severe restriction of the atrial communication. These neonates suffer from a prompt and profound hypoxemia at birth, leading rapidly to a metabolic acidosis. This variant, the functional equivalent of obstructed TAPVR, represents a true hemodynamic emergency requiring immediate relief. Like obstructed TAPVR, medical management of these patients is uniformly unsuccessful. Interventions designed to enlarge and maintain the atrial communication have been successfully applied, such as balloon atrial septostomy and stenting.[2]

ETIOLOGY

HLHS can be experimentally created in the chick embryo by left atrial ligation.[98] These experimental findings were anticipated clinically by Lev and colleagues, who suggested that abnormal development of the atrial septum, including underdevelopment of the Eustachian valve and limbus, reduced right-to-left shunting at the atrial level, resulting in hypoplasia of the left heart structures.[90] Premature closure of the foramen ovale has likewise been implicated, as has primary abnormalities of the aortic valve.[59,97,99]

While identifiable genetic sequences have been reported to be associated with HLHS, their relevance remains uncertain.[80] An understanding of the developmental factors that leading to HLHS assume new relevance as intervention during the process of cardiac morphogenesis itself, that is, fetal surgery, is pursued.

SURGICAL TRIAGE

Patients satisfying all facets of the definition of HLHS are clearly destined for the Norwood operation and single ventricle palliation. However, there are patients for whom the decision between the pursuit of single ventricle palliation and biventricular repair is not so clear. Once pursued, the ability to cross over to the competing treatment is difficult, and efforts to stratify patients with equivocal anatomy have been made. Rhodes, et al combined four factors (body surface area, indexed aortic root dimension, LV length, and indexed mitral valve area) to predict death after biventricular repair for critical aortic stenosis in the neonate.[91] However application of these criteria to hypoplastic, but nonstenotic left heart structures using Rhode's criteria have proven unsatisfying, as these criteria appear to be too stringent in this setting.[103] Recognizing this, The Congenital Heart Surgeons Society sponsored a multiinstitutional study to delineate the outcomes and risk factors of critical aortic stenosis in the neonate.[60]

Presented by Lofland and colleagues, this study identified multiple morphologic and functional factors that can be used to predict which surgical approach, single ventricle palliation or biventricular repair, is more likely to result in the survival of any particular patient. This study determined that solution of a multivariable equation using these factors can predict a patient's survival. This equation:

Intercept + (age at entry) + (z-score of aortic valve at the sinuses) + (grade of EFE) + (ascending aortic diameter) + (presence of moderate or severe tricuspid regurgitation) + (z-score of the left ventricular length) = Survival benefit

can be found on the CHSS Web site at www.chssdc.org.

MANAGEMENT

The natural history of HLHS is dismal, as 95% of untreated patients die within 1 month.[30] Medically treatment modifies the natural history primarily by delaying the demise.[41]

The surgical management of HLHS represents the paradigm from which a generalized approach to the shunted single ventricle has evolved. Simply stated, the cardiovascular system in HLHS consists of a single pumping chamber supporting two parallel circulations. These parallel circulations can be considered to be in competition with each other for blood flow. For any given cardiac output, the flow apportioned to each circulation is inversely proportional to the resistance of that circulation (i.e., high pulmonary vascular resistance (PVR), low pulmonary blood flow). Thus efforts to control the circulation have focused on controlling the competing vascular resistances. These efforts have generally involved manipulation of the PVR using inspired gasses (O_2, CO_2, NO), and pressures.[53,62,70,92]

More recently, an alternative approach, one that targets manipulation of the systemic vascular resistance to maintain the balance between the pulmonary and systemic circulations, has been shown to be effective.

Manipulation of the Pulmonary Vascular Resistance

CO_2. Inspired CO_2 has been suggested to improve the hemodynamic status after the Norwood operation.[53] Clinically, Tabbutt, et al compared the use of hypoxia (17% FiO_2) to CO_2 in 10 neonates with HLHS prior to the Norwood operation under the conditions of fixed minute ventilation, anesthesia, and paralysis.[102] While both strategies reduced the Qp:Qs, Co_2 increased both superior vena cava (SVC) cooximetry and cerebral oximetry, while hypoxia reduced these indices of oxygen delivery. Bradley reported similar results among postoperative patients.[12] It is important to note however, that these benefits were only realized when the *minute ventilation* remained constant.

While thought to reflect a direct effect by some, there is evidence showing that the increase in PVR is reversed by alkalinization, suggesting that the effect is mediated by [H]+ and pH.[15]

O_2. Because the neonatal pulmonary vasculature is also sensitive to the concentration of inspired O_2, hypoxic mixtures incorporating nitrogen have also been used to control the circulation in patients with HLHS. Animal models have shown that nitrogen-induced hypoxic mixtures increase the PVR and increase systemic blood flow. However, the prolonged use of hypoxic mixtures has been shown to quickly induce anatomic changes in the pulmonary vasculature. In animals, changes in arterial wall thickness and muscularity can be seen within 24 hours, and fewer intraacinar arteries are recruited into the circulation.[38,39,69]

Clinically, Day et al have reported their experience using hypoxia to manipulate the PVR in 20 neonates with single ventricle, duct-dependent circulation awaiting heart transplant.[19] Eight patients survived; of the ten patients who underwent lung biopsy or autopsy, 9 showed medial hypertrophy in distal arterioles, and 7 (7/9) of these patients died. While the outcome cannot be completely ascribed to hypoxic management, this strategy does suggest that prolonged supportive care of the neonatal single ventricle may expose these patients to significant risks.

Systemic Vascular Resistance

Manipulation of the systemic vascular resistance is a demonstrated means of controlling the shunted circulation. In fact, our ability to pharmacologically control the systemic vascular resistance probably exceeds our current ability to selectively manage the PVR. Clinically, this approach usually employs an irreversible alpha-adrenergic antagonist, phenoxybenzamine, to achieve systemic vasodilatation. The desired systemic vascular resistance, defined at that which optimizes the QP/QS and systemic oxygen delivery, is then obtained by titrating an alpha-adrenergic agonist, usually norepinephrine. Specifics of this approach have been reported in the literature.[40,106,107]

A recent review of this strategy identified the use of phenoxybenzamine, continuous SVO2 monitoring, and the reduction of DHCA time as factors favoring survival to the Bidirectional Glenn operation.[108] To date, no studies directly comparing outcomes for these two fundamentally different management schemes has been performed.

OPERATIVE PROCEDURE STAGE I

The anatomic goals of the Stage I or Norwood operation for HLHS is threefold; 1) provide unobstructed blood flow from the systemic right ventricle to the systemic circulation; 2) assurance of an unobstructed connection between the pulmonary venous return to the systemic right ventricle; and 3) establishment of a reliable source of pulmonary blood flow. While these goals are unchanged from those originally articulated by Norwood, et al in 1980, the procedure continues to evolve.

Standard Norwood Operation

The "standard" Norwood operation is performed through a median sternotomy. The branch pulmonary arteries are dissected and controlled. We routinely anastomosis a 3.5-mm stretch Gore-Tex graft to the underside of the innominate artery. This graft, later to serve as the right modified Blalock-Taussig shunt, is left long because it is used as the primary arterial cannulation site. Venous cannulation is through the right atrial appendage, through a purse string large enough to allow subsequent atrial septectomy. Cooling to 18°C on bypass, the ductus is divided, and the brachiocephalic vessels are mobilized and loosely snared. The main PA is divided and the branch bifurcation is closed, primarily or with a patch. After at least 20 minutes of cooling and at a rectal temperature of 18°C, the brachiocephalic vessels are snared and the descending aorta clamped. For truly diminutive aortas (<2 mm), cardioplegia is administered via a side arm into the arterial cannula, while direct needle insufflation is used in the larger aorta. We perform the Norwood operation during continuous regional low flow perfusion, as previously described.[82–84]

The atrial septectomy is performed through the right atrial purse string during a period of low flow sucker bypass. The ductal remnant is amputated from the aorta, and the aorta is fillet open distally beyond the site of coarctation, and proximally to a point adjacent to the lip of the transected pulmonary valve. Proximally, a side-to-side anastomosis between the aorta and pulmonary valve is performed, while the arch is augmented using a piece of pulmonary homograft (hemi pulmonary artery) cut to the appropriate size and shape (Figure 125-2). Central bypass is resumed after cannulation of the reconstructed aorta, and the pulmonary anastomosis of the shunt is completed.

SURGICAL RESULTS

Results of Norwood Operation for HLHS

With experience, and with advances in surgical, anesthetic, and critical care management , current survival of the Norwood operation exceeds 70% at specialized centers.[10,18,108] In one of the largest single center series ever reported, Mahle et al reported their 15 year, 840 patient experience with the Norwood operation for HLHS between 1984-1999.[66] Sixty five percent were male and 35% female, a gender ratio similar to that reported elsewhere. The 1-, 2-, 5-, 10-, and 15-year survival for the group was 51%, 43%, 40%, 39%, and 39%. Risk factors identified for death were earlier era of operation, age >14 days, and weight <2.5 kg. Neither anatomic subtype, nor heterotaxy were associated with mortality.

Other investigators have cited the presence of noncardiac anomalies, longer total extracorporeal support in the operating room, and postoperative mechanical circulatory support to be predictive of death.[47,66] The incidence of subtypes has been reasonably consistent among reports, and cited as AA/MA 38%, AA/MS 24%, AS/MS 20%, and variants 18%.[26,66] While some groups have previously had better survival among patients with AS/MS, more recent reports suggest that there is no difference in outcome among the anatomic subtypes of HLHS.[18,26,66]

Low birth weight (<2.5 kg), consistently identified as a risk factor, was the subject of a subanalysis performed by Weinstein, et al.[112] They reported a 47% survival among 67 patients weighing <2.5 kg undergoing the Norwood operation between 1990–1997. While lower than the institutions overall survival of 74%, these results are very similar to that reported by Bove, Forbess, and others.[11,26,94] While they were higher risk, the authors pointed out there was no appreciable weight gain in neonates awaiting surgery, and concluded that delaying surgery in the hope of somatic growth is unwarranted.

While some reports have demonstrated poorer survival when Norwood palliation is performed beyond 2–4 weeks of life, recent reports suggest otherwise. Duncan and colleagues reported 100% survival among 9 patients, aged 36–108 days, undergoing palliation for single ventricle variants.[22] Reviewing their experience with the Norwood operation for HLHS, Rossi et al reported 90% survival among patients more than 2 weeks of age; 100% (4/4) of those over 4 weeks of age survived.[95]

Because of the continuing evolution occurring among surgical and medical management techniques applied to HLHS, contemporary experiences are important. Tweddell, et al recently reported their experience with 115 consecutive patients with HLHS undergoing the Norwood operation between 1992–2001.[108] They reported that, with the introduction of new management techniques in 1996, they were able to obtain 93% hospital survival for neonates undergoing the Norwood operation for HLHS. These strategies included the use of phenoxybenzamine, continuous SvO2 monitoring, aprotinin, modified ultrafiltration, and most recently continuous cerebral perfusion.

This report is also of interest because it attempts to quantify the influence of anatomic and operative variables on survival to Stage II palliation, rather than operative survival.

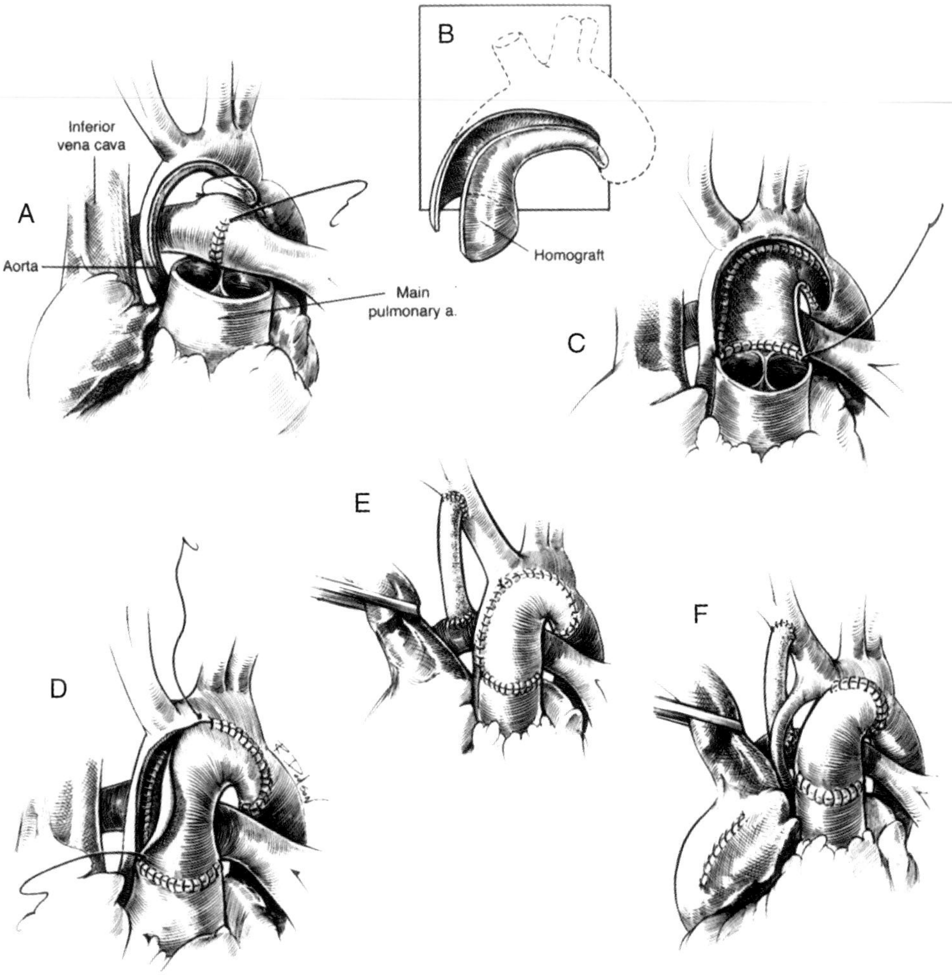

Figure 125–2 Technique of Norwood operation. A, The pulmonary artery is transected and the bifurcation closed. The hypoplastic aorta is incised and ductal tissue excised. **B** and **C,** Graft material, usually pulmonary homograft, is cut to the appropriate size and shape for arch reconstruction. **D,** Inclusion of the pulmonary valve into the systemic circulation, with completion of the arch augmentation. **E,** Pulmonary blood flow is provided by right modified Blalock-Taussig shunt. **F,** Anastomosis of the pulmonary to the arch, bypassing the diminutive ascending aorta is not recommended. Proximity of the very small ascending aorta to the shunt allows for potential coronary steal and myocardial ischemia. In these cases arch reconstruction should proceed as illustrated in **A,** or alternatively implanted into the side of the neoaorta.
(Reprinted with permission from Hypoplastic left heart syndrome,. In: Castaneda AR, Jonas RA, Mayer JE, Hanley FL (eds): Cardiac Surgery of the Neonate and Infant. Philadelphia: WB Saunders, 1994, p. 371.)

Only duration of DHCA was associated with survival to Stage II palliation; no other anatomic or physiologic variable, including weight, was predictive.

Norwood Operation for HLHS Variants

While the Norwood operation was devised specifically to treat HLHS, it has been widely applied to a variety of forms of CHD that present with systemic outflow tract obstruction and a ductal dependent systemic circulation. Because of the impact of great vessel relationships on arch reconstruction, it is useful to define these variants as those that present with normal versus abnormal relationships between the great arteries (i.e., transposition complexes; Box 125-1).

Surgical Results for HLHS Variants

While some groups have identified the presence of a well-developed morphologic left ventricle as being protective, others have not.[18,48] A recent comparison of the Norwood operation performed for HLHS (102 patients, 70 with aortic atresia) and other diagnosis (56) between 1998 and 2001

Box 125–1. Great Vessel Relationships and the Norwood Operation Anatomic Variants.

Normally related great arteries:
- Mitral atresia with VSD
- Mitral/aortic stenosis with VSD and small LV
- Interrupted aortic arch with severe subaortic obstruction
- Unbalanced AVSD

Abnormally related great arteries:
- DILV with d transposition of the great arteries
- Tricuspid atresia, VSD, transposition
- Complex DORV with arch hypoplasia

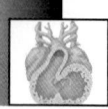

by Gaynor, et al identified no difference in survival between Norwood operation for HLHS versus other anatomic diagnosis (78% vs. 75%).[31]

Although the presence of abnormally related great arteries specifically has not been identified as a risk factor for mortality, abnormally they may render the constructed neoaorta susceptible to twists or kinks, and modifications may be required (Figures 125-3, *A* and *B*, and 125-4).[71]

EXTRACORPOREAL MEMBRANE OXYGENATION (ECMO) FOR HLHS

Once thought to be futile, perioperative support with ECMO may salvage a significant proportion of infants with postcardiotomy failure following the Norwood operation. Pizarro, et al reported that 50% (6/12) requiring ECMO support following Norwood operation were discharged home in good condition.[85] Prematurity, renal dysfunction, and the initiation of ECMO outside of the operating room were risk factors for death. In the setting of a shunt-dependent circulation, Ungerleider, et al have reported improved survival when the shunt is left open during ECMO support.[49]

MODIFICATIONS

The gradual improvement in survival for the Norwood operation is the result of continuous reappraisal of our surgical and management techniques. Bartram and colleagues have performed a systematic review of the causes of surgical mortality of 122 patients undergoing the Norwood operation between 1980 and 1995.[7] While this review is historical in nature it does bear attention, as it serves to identify the weaknesses of this operation.

They reported that inappropriate pulmonary blood flow (too much or too little) was responsible for 36% of the deaths. Second most common was impaired coronary perfusion, occurring in 27% of patients, followed by neoaortic obstruction (14%), right ventricular failure (13%), and bleeding (7%). Recently, other groups have identified an association between the duration of DHCA to both short and intermediate survival.[108] Modifications have been introduced into the procedure that attempt to nullify these weaknesses.

Control of Pulmonary Blood Flow

Control of pulmonary blood flow by pharmacologic titration of the systemic vascular resistance represents a fundamental shift in the management of palliated single ventricles. This

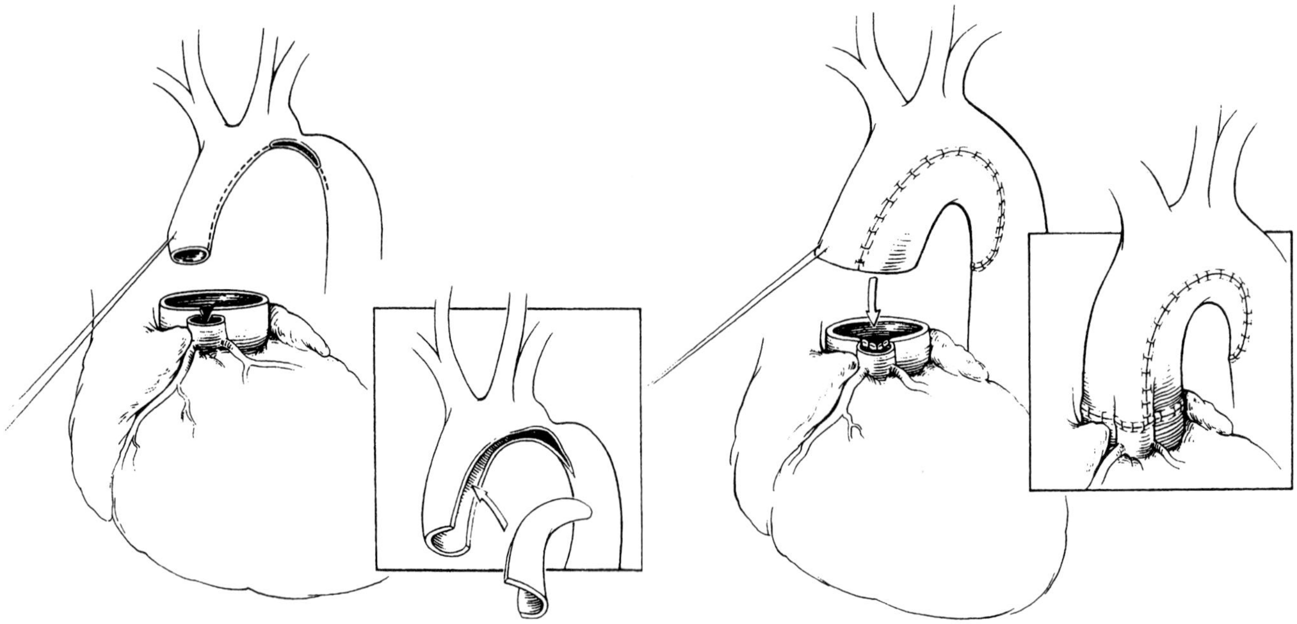

Figure 125–3 **A, Single left ventricle with ventriculoarterial discordance and a rightward and anterior aorta.** The atrial septum is excised, and both great vessels are transected just above the sinotubular junction. Augmentation of the arch is accomplished with pulmonary homograft. **B,** A side-to-side anastomosis between the aorta and pulmonary artery is fashioned. The reconstructed aorta is then anastomosed to both great vessels in an end-to-end fashion.
(Reprinted with permission from Mosca RS, Hennein HA, Kulik TJ, et al: Modified Norwood operation for single left ventricle and ventriculoarterial discordance: An improved surgical technique. Ann Thorac Surg 64:1126–1132, 1997.)

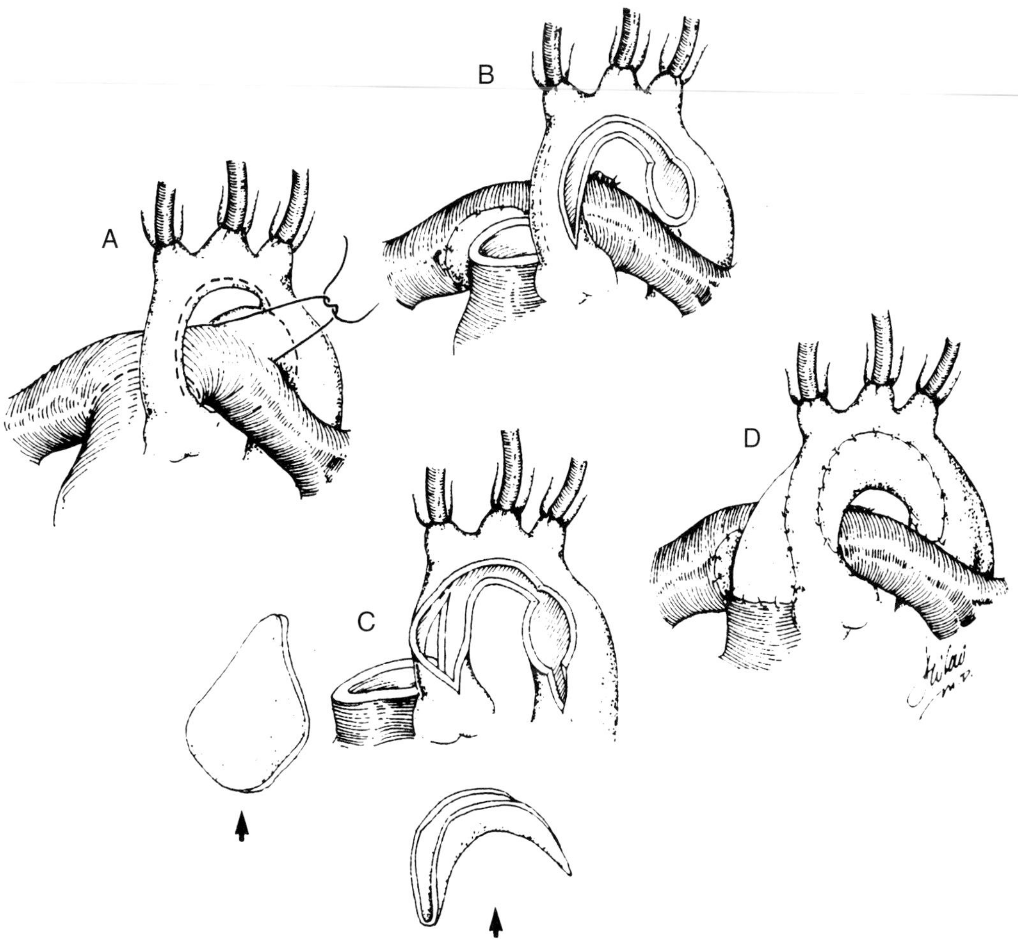

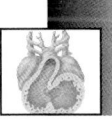

Figure 125–4 Operative technique for abnormally related great arteries as might be seen with single left ventricle and transposed great arteries, with the aorta anterior and leftward. **A,** Ligation of ductus and lines of incision. **B,** Closure of the pulmonary artery bifurcation. **C,** Overlapping incisions in ascending aorta and the arch. Augmentation is accomplished with separate patches. **D,** Completed reconstruction.
(Reprinted with permission from Jacobs ML, Rychik J, Murphy JD, et al: Results of Norwood's operation for lesions other than hypoplastic left heart syndrome. J Thorac Cardiovasc Surg 110:1555–1562, 1995.)

approach has been reported to assist in balancing the pulmonary and systemic circulations, and improving systemic oxygen delivery.[40,108] This approach appears to contribute to improved survival of neonates undergoing the Norwood operation for HLHS.

Coronary Circulation

Because of systemic runoff into the pulmonary circulation via the arteriopulmonary shunt, the myocardium is vulnerable to coronary steal and ischemia after the Norwood operation.[23] A recent technical modification of the Norwood operation designed to reduce the vulnerability of the myocardium to ischemia has been proposed by Imoto and colleagues.[42] They reasoned that with placement of shunt inflow proximal to the semilunar (pulmonary) valve, the coronary circulation would be protected from the low diastolic blood pressures that accompany continuous diastolic runoff.

In general, this technique employs a 5-mm Gore-Tex conduit anastomosed to the infundibulum of the right ventricle, coursing leftward of the pulmonary valve. The conduit is then inserted into the patch (Gore-Tex or pericardium) used to repair the pulmonary bifurcation. Technical points to be stressed using this technique include excision of RV muscle at the site of insertion, as muscular in growth with the anticipated RV hypertrophy may obstruct the conduit. Variations of this technique, interposing a valved segment of human saphenous vein between the RV and PA have also been reported.[73]

Early clinical results have been encouraging. Januszewska, et al has documented higher mean diastolic blood pressures in patients receiving the RV-PA conduit.[50] While preliminary, data based on hemodynamic data obtained prior to Stage II suggests that these patients will be excellent candidates for subsequent surgical staging, the long-term sequelae of a ventriculotomy in this setting remains unknown.[86]

Arch Modifications

Neoaortic obstruction is an important complication of the Norwood operation, occurring in about 20% of patients.[27,109] While Azaki, et al have related this complication to the size of the ascending aorta (<3 mm), Machii and Becker have suggested that longitudinal and circumferential extension of ductal tissue into the aorta also contribute.[4,61]

Despite the high incidence of recurrent coarctation, the diagnosis may remain elusive. The reliability of neonatal echocardiography is degraded as a result of thymic resection, as well as the variable position of the reconstructed aorta. Given the morbidity and mortality associated with postoperative arch obstruction, inconclusive or suggestive echocardiographic and clinical examinations are an indication for cardiac catheterization.

Both surgical and interventional techniques designed to reduce neoaortic arch obstruction have been introduced. Fraser and Mee reported their technique employing a direct anastomosis of the PA to the aortic arch (Figure 125-5).[28] They reported an operative survival of 83% among 59 patients with a median follow up of 37 months; the incidence of neoaortic arch obstruction was only 5%.[87] These and others have suggested that patients presenting with very small ascending aorta (≤ 2.5 mm) were at a higher risk using this technique, and suggested several modifications to nullify the risk in these patients.[43,87]

Recoarctation: Catheter Intervention

Soongswang and colleagues have reported a multiinstitutional experience with transcatheter balloon dilation of the neoaorta following the Norwood operation in 58 patients.[101] Although successful in 89% of patients, there were 3 early and 10 late deaths. Nine patients required reintervention for arch obstruction (6 catheter, 3 surgical), and freedom from reintervention was 78% at 1 year.

Perfusion Management

Studying 350 neonates between 1992–1997, Clancy reported that the duration of DHCA was an independent risk factor for death.[16] Among patients undergoing the Norwood operation, recent data reported by Tweddell suggests that DHCA exposure was associated with interstage mortality.[108] Once considered unavoidable for neonatal aortic arch reconstruction, newer techniques have allowed a dramatic reduction, even elimination of the need for DHCA (Figure 125-6).[82–84] The effects of limiting DHCA remain an active area of investigation.

INTERSTAGE MORTALITY

While the efforts described above have translated into improved survival following the Norwood operation, the palliated state renders these patients physiologically fragile. This vulnerability is thought to be responsible for an interstage mortality ranging between 4% and 15%.[4,65,108]

To date the only operative variable associated with interstage mortality is longer duration of DHCA.[108] Recent initiatives, such the development of home monitoring programs and/or anticoagulation protocols may also be helpful.

While earlier progression to Stage II will reduce the period of vulnerability, this approach is limited by the rate of decline in PVR. Reporting their experience with early Glenn operations, Reddy et al reported a reoperation rate of 17%, and it was more likely among patients less than 2 months of age.[89]

STAGE II

Originally, survivors of the Norwood operation were staged directly to the Fontan operation within the first year of life.

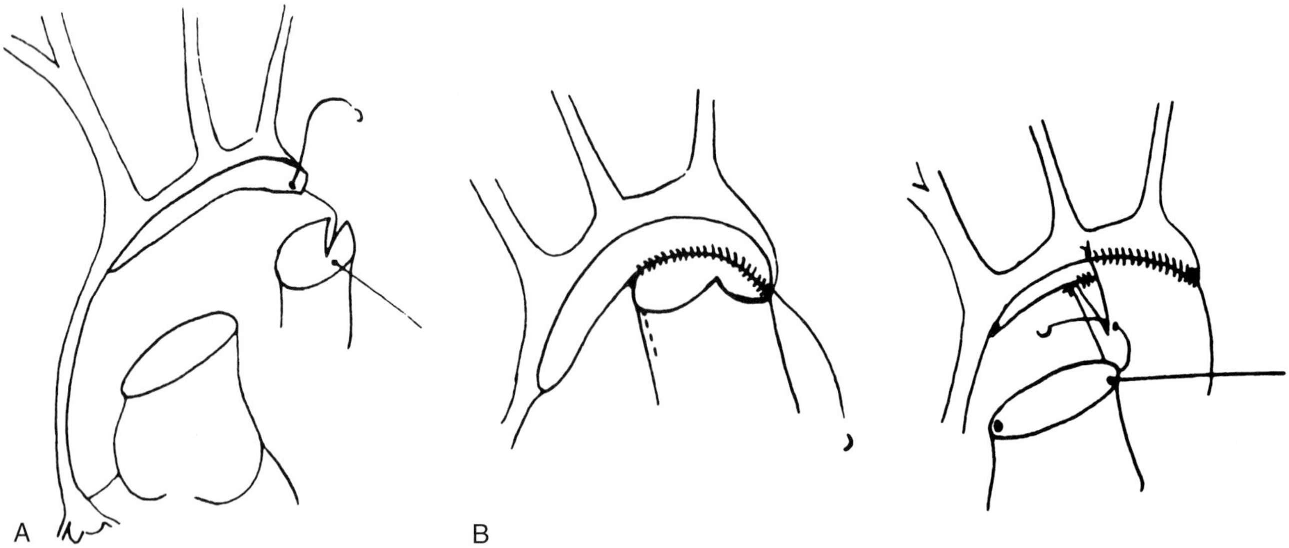

Figure 125–5 Modifications to the Norwood procedure have resulted in a reduced incidence of arch obstruction. This technique is probably unsuitable for very small ascending aorta (<2.5 mm).
(Reprinted with permission from Poirer NC, Drummond-Webb JJ, Hisamochi K, et al: Modified Norwood procedure with a high-flow cardiopulmonary strategy results in low mortality without late arch obstruction. J Thorac Cardiovasc Surg 120:875–884, 2000.)

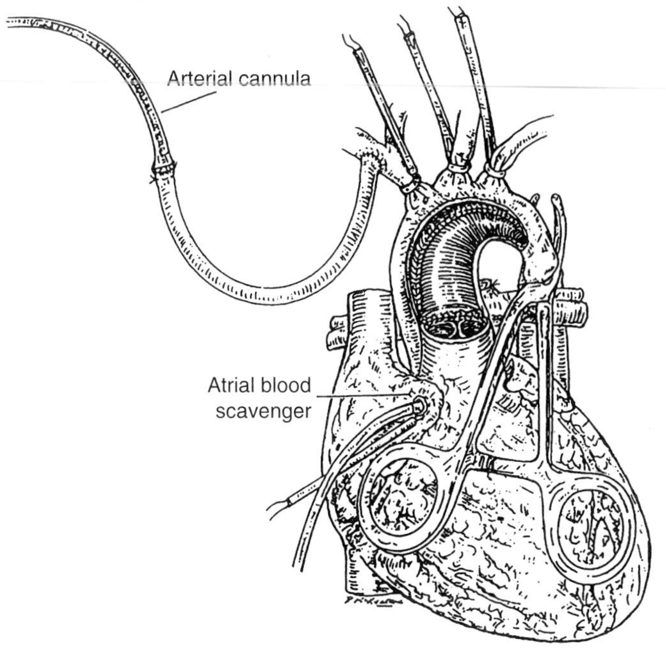

Figure 125–6 Operative field during aortic arch reconstruction during regional low flow perfusion. Arterial inflow is through the cannulated shunt after the anastomosis to the innominate artery is performed. Exposure is maintained by the brachiocephalic snares, a clamp on the descending aorta, and a right atrial scavenger. When using this technique for arch reconstruction in the setting of a two-ventricle repair, or when incorporating the right ventricle to pulmonary artery conduit into the Norwood operation, the shunt is oversewn upon completion of the procedure.
(Reprinted with permission from; Pigula FA, Nemoto EM, Griffith BP, Siewers RD: Regional low flow perfusion provides cerebral circulatory support during neonatal aortic arch reconstruction. J Thorac Cardiovasc Surg 119:331–339, 2000.)

It was soon recognized however, that this approach met with significant morbidity and mortality.[25] Consequently, the insertion of a intermediate stage, the superior bidirectional cavopulmonary anastomosis (bidirectional Glenn or Hemi-Fontan) was introduced by Norwood and Jacobs with improved survival.[46]

Currently, stage I survivors are generally evaluated at 4–6 months for progression to stage II. Anatomically, the adequacy of the arch reconstruction, the branch pulmonary arteries, and intraatrial communication should be assessed. Physiologically, catheterization is helpful to assess ventricular function and PVR.

Operative Technique: Bidirectional Glenn

The neck and the chest are prepared and draped. In the event of cavitary entry, the right neck provides ready access for peripheral cannulation. Following cannulation of the ascending aorta and with a venous cannulae in the high SVC, and right atrial appendage, the patient is cooled to 30° to 32°C. We prefer to perform a bidirectional Glenn operation with the heart beating. After division of the azygous vein the SVC is clamped at its insertion into the right atrium just above the SA node, transected, and the atrial orifice oversewn. The pulmonary remnant of the BT shunt is excised, and the pulmonary arteriotomy is enlarged to accommodate the SVC. The anastomosis is performed with a 7-0 PDS suture taking care not to purse string the anastomosis. The patient is rewarmed, ventilated, and weaned from cardiopulmonary bypass. Saturations in the 70% to 85% with SVC pressure of 10–12 mmHg, with an atrial pressure of 5–6 mmHg are expected. SVC pressure exceeding 16 or a transpulmonary gradient exceeding 8–10 mmHg should prompt critical appraisal of the anastomosis.

Hemi Fontan

Introduced by Norwood and Jacobs in 1989, the hemi Fontan operation is the preferred form of superior cavopulmonary anastomosis for some groups.[46] Briefly, the central pulmonary arteries are opened anteriorly, and anastomosed to a counter incision along the base of the right atrial appendage. Separate patches are then used to augment the central pulmonary arteries, as well as to exclude the SVC-PA anastomosis from the heart. While some surgeons have reported improved survival of the Fontan procedure following the hemi-Fontan as compared to the bidirectional Glenn, this is not uniform.[9,74]

This modification differs from the bidirectional Glenn in several important ways. Because an intraatrial patch is required to exclude the superior cavopulmonary anastomosis from the heart, cross-clamping of the aorta is required, with some authors employing a period of deep hypothermia and circulatory arrest (Figure 125-7 and 125-8).[45] Furthermore, intraatrial suture lines, implicated in the genesis of atrial arrhythmias, are required.[14]

RESULTS OF STAGE II

Regardless of which technique is preferred, the results of the stage II procedure have been reproducibly excellent, exceeding 95% in large series.[11,17] Assessments of longer term complications (i.e., sinus node dysfunction and arrhythmias) are more difficult. While Cohen and colleagues reported a higher incidence of sinus node dysfunction on postoperative day 1 in patients undergoing hemi-Fontan as compared to bidirectional Glenn, there was no difference by the time of hospital discharge. Furthermore, at the time of subsequent Fontan, the authors reported no difference in early sinus node dysfunction.[17]

FONTAN

The Fontan operation is destination therapy for HLHS. By diverting all systemic venous return to the pulmonary circuit, physiologic septation of the circulation is accomplished.[24] While HLHS has been cited as a risk factor for early Fontan failure, more recent reports have placed early survival of Fontan for HLHS as high as 98%.[32,72] Exercise performance among HLHS patients undergoing Fontan appears to be comparable to other single ventricle variants.[54]

Since its introduction in 1971, the Fontan operation has undergone a steady evolution. Progressive atrial dilation and

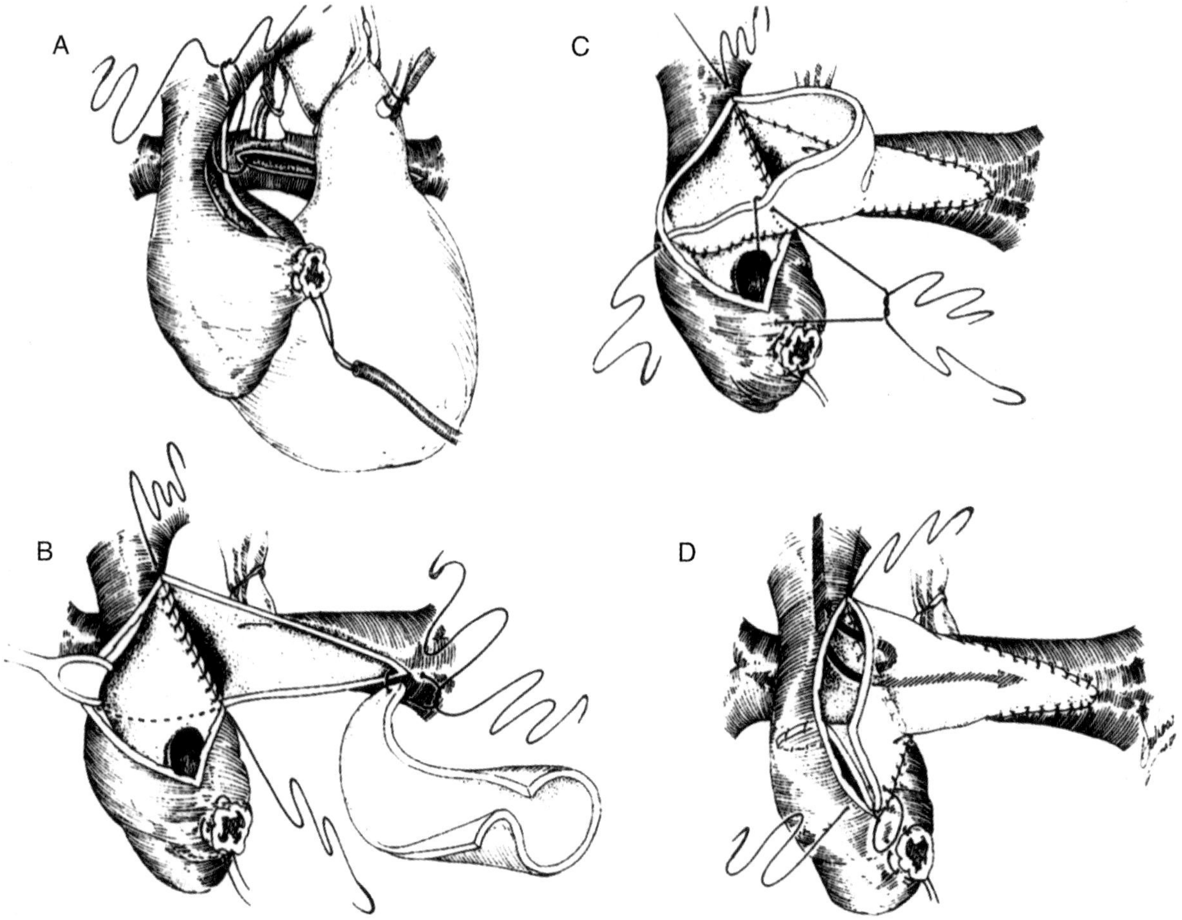

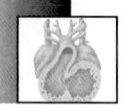

Figure 125–7 Stage II ; hemi-Fontan operation. **A,** The pulmonary arteries are opened anteriorly. **B,** The superior vena cava and the right pulmonary artery are anastomosed side to side. **C,** Pulmonary artery homograft is used to augment the confluence and to separate the anastomosis from the right atrium. **D,** Flow from the superior vena cava is into the pulmonary arteries, as indicated by the arrows.

atrial arrhythmias have led to modifications of the original operation, first to the lateral tunnel technique, and more recently to the extracardiac conduit. Experimental data suggests that the extracardiac conduit is superior to the lateral tunnel with respect to energy efficiency. Comparing to the intraatrial lateral tunnel, the extraatrial lateral tunnel, and the extracardiac conduit, Lardo, et al found the extracardiac conduit to be most hydrodynamically efficient.[58]

Short-term clinical advantages, including postoperative arrhythmias, shorter intensive care unit (ICU) stays, and earlier extubations have also been reported.[3] While little long-term data is available, there appears to be an important reduction in atrial arrhythmias over the intermediate term.[3,77] Also, the extracardiac Fontan may provide important versatility when addressing certain anatomic subsets, notably the heterotaxy variants presenting with systemic venous abnormalities. In these circumstances, unifocalization of the inferior systemic venous return to an extracardiac conduit may greatly simplify the completion Fontan. Potential disadvantages of the extracardiac conduit Fontan, including thrombogenicity and lack of growth potential, remain to be assessed over the long term.

TRANSPLANTATION

While most centers have devoted their efforts to surgical palliation using the Norwood operation, a few groups have concentrated on neonatal transplantation as the primary treatment. The technical details of heart transplantation for HLHS have been well described.[81,111]

Loma Linda has reported their experience with heart transplantation as the primary treatment for HLHS.[88] Between 1985–1995, they listed 190 infants with HLHS for heart transplant. While they reported actuarial survival at 1, 5, and 7 years to be 84%, 76%, and 70% respectively, 14 patients were delisted, and 34 of the remaining 176 (19%) patients died while awaiting transplant. Inclusion of these 34 patients listed with the intent to transplant lowers the survival of transplantation was 74% (129/176). Of note, year of transplantation was not a risk factor for death. Outcomes for transplant versus Norwood operation, on an intent-to-treat basis has been reported by Jenkins, et al.[51] Examining 231 patients born between 1989–1994, they reported that transplantation resulted in greater survival through 7 years of follow up. Multivariate analysis identified birth weight

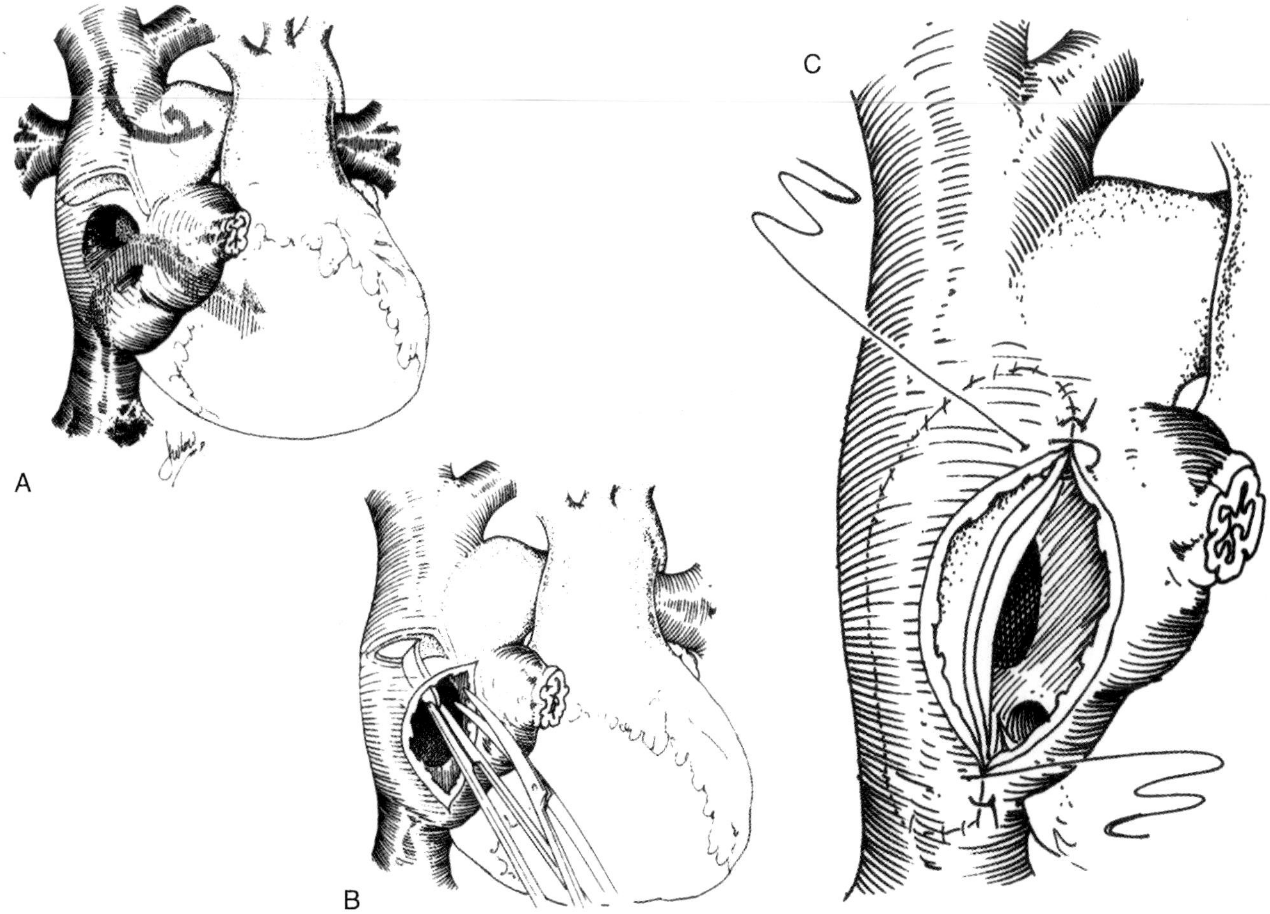

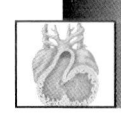

Figure 125–8 Stage III; completion Fontan. **A,** The Hemi Fontan. **B,** The previously placed homograft separating the right atrium from the superior vena cava is excised. **C,** Total cavopulmonary connection is accomplished using the lateral tunnel technique.
(Reprinted with permission from Jacobs ML: Hypoplastic left heart syndrome. In: Kaiser LR, Kron IL, Spray TL, (eds): Mastery of Cardiothoracic Surgery. Philadelphia: Lippincott-Raven, 1998, pp. 863–864.)

<3 kg, creatinine ≥2 mg/dl, and atrial septostomy were significant risk factors for death in both groups.

A decision analysis was performed on the same patients found that regional and local factors, such as organ availability and institutional dedication to a particular treatment, imparted a powerful influence on outcome.[52] Also, it is difficult to assess the rate at which improvement can be expected among the competing strategies. For instance, Jenkins, et al reported 1-year survival of the Norwood operation to be only 42% between 1989–1994, significantly lower than more contemporary results (66%, 1996–2001).[108] In contrast Razzouk, et al did not correlate improved operative survival among patients transplanted between 1985–1995.[88]

Finally, competing long-term complications of each strategy remains to be considered. For instance, it does not appear that children are particularly privileged with respect to transplant complications, as up to 35% of pediatric transplant recipients will develop diffuse graft arteriosclerosis, for which retransplantation may be required.[6,20,78]

Due in part to the special needs of a neonatal heart transplant program, the ongoing risk of transplant-related complications, as well as continued improvements in staged outcomes, staged surgery for HLHS has become the primary treatment offered at most institutions. However, transplantation for specific indications, such as coronary abnormalities and valvular disease, remains an important treatment option.

NEURODEVELOPMENTAL OUTCOMES

With improving survival after the surgical treatment for HLHS, a broader, long-term assessment of neurologic outcomes has assumed a new prominence. While studies are impaired by methodologic difficulties, most indicate that DHCA is detrimental to ultimate neurodevelopmental outcome.[8] Kern reported a negative correlation between stage I circulatory arrest time and full scale IQ an average of 4.4 years after the Norwood operation.[55]

These deficits appear to persist. Mahle, et al assessed the neurodevelopmental outcome of 115 survivors of the Norwood operation at an average age of 9 years.[64] They reported a mean IQ of 86 (range 50–118) with 18% meeting criteria for mental retardation (IQ <70). Only 3 of 23 (13%) were thought to be completely normal.

When compared to children undergoing Fontan operation for other indications, patients with HLHS demonstrated significantly lower intelligence scores than did their counterparts; the use of circulatory arrest was identified as a predictor.[35] The impact of perfusion techniques that reduce the need for DHCA during Stage I palliation remain to be studied.

FUTURE DIRECTIONS

Catheter Interventions

Catheter-based interventions designed to achieve stage I palliation without open neonatal surgery are being been pursued. One approach incorporates arch reconstruction into the stage II superior cavopulmonary connection.[1,33] Akinteurk, et al reported a series of 11 patients with HLHS treated with ductal stenting, bilateral PA banding, and balloon atrial septostomy. Two patients underwent transplantation at 66 and 331 days, and eight underwent the Norwood operation between 107 and 195 days. There were two deaths; one patient awaiting transplant, and one after Norwood operation. These represent very preliminary results, and further efforts are required to fully define the utility of this approach.

FETAL SURGERY

Even more radical departures from standard surgical approach to HLHS may be found in the pursuit of fetal intervention. This approach carries with it an important potential advantage; relief of critical hemodynamic lesions during fetal life may allow a more orderly progression of cardiac morphogenesis. For example, relief of critical aortic stenosis may allow a more normal development of dependent structures such as the left ventricle and aorta. There is some experimental support for this concept, though clinical experience remains very limited.[36,37,56,68]

While this approach may offer an exciting opportunity to understand and influence the natural history of congenital heart disease, the clinical and ethical issues of fetal intervention require careful consideration.

REFERENCES

1. Akintuerk H, Michel-Behnke I, Valeske K, et al: Stenting of the arterial duct and banding of the pulmonary arteries: Basis for combined Norwood Stage I and II repair in hypoplastic left heart. Circulation 105:1099–1103, 2002.
2. Atz AM, Feinstein JA, Jonas RA, et al: Preoperative management of pulmonary venous hypertension in hypoplastic left heart syndrome with restrictive atrial septum. Am J Cardiol 83(8):1224–1228,1999.
3. Azaki A, McCrindle BW, Van Arsdell G, et al: Extracardiac conduit versus lateral tunnel cavopulmonary connections at a single institution: Impact on outcomes. J Thorac Cardiovasc Surg 122:1219–1228, 2001.
4. Azakie A, Merklinger SL, McCrindle BW, et al: Evolving strategies and improving outcomes of the modified Norwood procedure: A 10-year single institution experience. Ann Thorac Surg 72:1349–1353, 2001.
5. Baffa JM, Chen SL, Guttenberg ME, et al: Coronary artery abnormalities and right ventricular histology in hypoplastic left heart syndrome. J Am Coll Cardiol 20:350–358, 1992.
6. Bailey LL, Zuppan CW, Chinnock RE, et al: Graft vasculopathy among recipients of heart transplantation during the first twelve years of life. Transplant Proc 27:1921–1925, 1995.
7. Bartram U, Grunenfelder J, Van Praagh R: Causes of death after the modified Norwood procedure: A study of 122 postmortem cases. Ann Thorac Surg 64:1795–1802, 1997.
8. Bellinger DC, Jonas RA, Rappaport LA, et al: Developmental and neurologic status of children after heart surgery with hypothermic circulatory arrest of low flow cardiopulmonary bypass. N Engl J Med 332:549–555, 1995.
9. Bove EL: Current status of staged reconstruction for hypoplastic left heart syndrome. Pediatr Cardiol 19:308–315, 1998.
10. Bove EL: Surgical treatment for hypoplastic left heart syndrome. Jpn J Thorac Cardiovasc Surg 47:47–56, 1999.
11. Bove EL, Lloyd TR: Staged reconstruction for hypoplastic left heart syndrome. Ann Surg 224:387–395, 1996.
12. Bradley SM, Simsic JM, Atz AM: Hemodynamic effects of inspired carbon dioxide after the Norwood procedure. Ann Thorac Surg 72:2088–2094, 2001.
13. Bridges ND, Mayer JE Jr, Lock JE, et al: Effect of baffle fenestration on outcome of the modified Fontan operation. Circulation 86:1762, 1992.
14. Bromberg BI, Schuessler RB, Gandhi SK, et al: A canine model of atrial flutter following the intra-atrial lateral tunnel Fontan operation. J Electrocardiol 30:Suppl:85–93, 1998.
15. Chang AC, Zucker HA, Hickey PR, Wessel DL: Pulmonary vascular resistance in infants after cardiac surgery: Role of carbon dioxide and hydrogen ion. Crit Care Med 23(3): 568–574,1995.
16. Clancy RR, McGaurn SA, Wernovsky G, et al: Preoperative risk-of death prediction model in heart surgery with deep hypothermic circulatory arrest in the neonate. J Thorac Cardiovasc Surg 119:347–357, 2000.
17. Cohen MI, Bridges ND, Gaynor JW, et al: Modifications to the cavopulmonary anastomosis do not eliminate early sinus node dysfunction. J Thorac Cardiovasc Surg 120:891–901, 2000.
18. Daebritz SH, Nolert GD, Zurakowski D, et al: Results of Norwood stage I operation: comparison of hypoplastic left heart syndrome with other malformations. J Thorac Cardiovasc Surg 119:358–367, 2000.
19. Day RW, Barton AJ, Pysher TJ, Shaddy RE: Pulmonary vascular resistance of children treated with nitrogen during early infancy. Ann Thorac Surg 65:1400–1404, 1998.
20. Dearani JA, Razzouk AJ, Gundry SR, et al: Pediatric cardiac retransplantation: Intermediate-term results. Ann Thorac Surg 71:66–70, 2001.
21. DeRose JJ, Corda R, Dische R, et al: Isolated left ventricular ischemia after Norwood procedure. Ann Thorac Surg 73:657–659, 2002.
22. Duncan BW, Rosenthal GL, Jones TK, et al: First-stage palliation of complex univentricular anomalies in older infants. Ann Thor Surg 72:2077–2080, 2001.
23. Fogel MA, RychkJK, VetterJ, et al: Effect of volume unloading surgery on coronary flow dynamics in patients with aortic atresia. J Thorac Cardiovasc Surg 113:1795–1802, 1997.

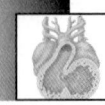

24. Fontan F, Baudet E: Surgical repair of tricuspid atresia. Thotax 26:240–248, 1971.
25. Forbess JM, Cook N, Serraf A, et al: An institutional experience with second- and third-stage palliative procedures for hypoplastic left heart syndrome: The impact of the bidirectional cavopulmonary shunt. J Am Coll Cardiol 29:665–670, 1997.
26. Forbess JM, Cook N, Roth SJ, et al: Ten-year institutional experience with palliative surgery for hypoplastic left heart syndrome; Risk factors related to stage I mortality. Circulation 92[suppl II]:II-262–II-266, 1995.
27. Fraisse A, Colan SD, Jonas RA, et al: Accuracy of echocardiography for detection of aortic arch obstruction after stage I Norwood procedure. Am Heart J 135:230–236, 1998.
28. Fraser CD, Mee RBB: Modified Norwood procedure for hypoplastic left heart syndrome. Ann Thorac Surg 60:S546–S549, 1995.
29. Fyler DC, Buckley LP, Hellenbrand WE, et al: Report of the new England regional infant cardiac program.
30. Fyler Dc, Rothman KJ, Buckley LP, et al: The determinants of 5 year survival of infants with critical congenital heart disease. In Engle MA (ed): Pediatric Cardiovascular Disease (Cardiovascular Clinics). Philadelphia:FA Davis, 1981, pp. 393–405.
31. Gaynor JW, Mahle WT, Cohen MI, et al: Risk factors for mortality after the Norwood procedure. Eur J Cardiothorac Surg 22(1):82–89, 2002.
32. Gentles TL, Mayer JE, Gauvreau K, et al: Fontan operation in five hundred consecutive patients: factors influencing early and late outcome. J Thorac Cardiovasc Surg 114:376–379, 1997.
33. Gibbs, Wren C, Watterson KG, et al: Stenting of the arterial duct combined with banding of the pulmonary arteries and atrial septostomy: a new approach to palliation for hypoplastic left heart syndrome. Br Heart J 69(6):551–555, 1993.
34. Glauser TA, Rorke LB, Weinberg PM, Clancy RR: Congenital brain abnormalities associated with the hypoplastic left heart syndrome. Pediatrics 1990.
35. Goldberg CS, Schwartz EM, Brunberg JA, et al. Neurodevelopmental outcome of patients after the Fontan operation: A comparison between children with hypoplastic left heart syndrome and other functional single ventricle lesions. J Pediatr 137:646–652,2000.
36. Hanley FL. Fetal Cardiac Surgery. Advances in Cardiac Surgery, vol 5. St. Louis: Mosby 1994, pp. 47–74.
37. Harrison MR: Surgically correctable fetal disease. Am J Surg 180(5):335–342, 2000.
38. Haworth SG, Hislop A: Effect of hypoxia on adaptation on the pulmonary circulation in the pig. Cardiovasc Research 16:293–303, 1982.
39. Hislop A, Reid L: New findings in pulmonary arteries of rat with hypoxia induced pulmonary hypertension. Br J Exp Path 57:542–554, 1976.
40. Hoffman GM, GhanayemNS, Kampine JM, et al: Venous saturation and the anaerobic threshold in neonates after the Norwood procedure for hypoplastic left heart syndrome. Ann Thorac Surg 70:1515–1521, 2000.
41. Hoshino K, Ogawa K, Hishitani T, et al: Hypoplastic left heart syndrome: Duration of survival without surgical intervention. Am Heart J 137:535–542, 1999.
42. Imoto Y, Kado H, Shiokawa Y, et al: Experience with the Norwood procedure without circulatory arrest. J Thorac Cardiovasc Surg 122:879–882, 2001.
43. Ishino K, Stumper O, De Giovanni JJV, et al: The modified Norwood procedure for hypoplastic left heart syndrome: Early to intermediate results of 120 patients with particular reference to aortic arch repair. J Thorac Cardiovasc Surg 117:920–930, 1999.
44. Ito T, Nuno M, Isiukawa J, et al: Hypoplastic left heart syndrome with a single coronary artery originating from the pulmonary artery. Acta Pediatr Jpn 37:60–63, 1995.
45. Jacobs ML: Hypoplastic left heart syndrome. In: Kaiser LR, Kron IL, Spray TL (eds): Mastery of Cardiothoracic Surgery. Philadelphia: Lippencott-Raven), 1998, pp. 862–863.
46. Jacobs ML, Norwood WI. Hypoplastic left heart syndrome. In: Jacobs M, Norwood WI (eds): Pediatric Cardiac Surgery: Current Issues. Stoneham: Butterworth, 1992, p. 182.
47. Jacobs ML, Blackstone EH, Bailey LL: Intermediate survival in neonates with aortic atresia: A multiinstitutional study. Mosby periodicals online 116(3), Sept 1998 *www.chssdc.org*.
48. Jacobs ML, Rychik J, Murphy JD, et al: Results of Norwood's operation for lesions other than hypoplastic left heart syndrome. J Thorac Cardiovasc Surg 110:15555–15562, 1995.
49. Jaggers JJ, Forbess JM, Shah AS, et al: Extracorporeal membrane oxygenation for infant postcardiotomy support: significance of shunt management. Ann Thor Surg 69(5):1476–1483, 2000.
50. Januszewska K, Malec E, Kolcz J, Mroczek T: Right ventricle to pulmonary artery shunt (RV-PA) versus modified Blalock Taussig shunt (BTS) in the Norwood procedure for hypoplastic left heart syndrome-Influence on early and late hemodynamic status. European Monte Carlo: ACTS, 2002.
51. Jenkins PC, Flanagan MF, Jenkins KJ, et al: Survival analysis and risk factors for mortality in transplantation and staged surgery for hypoplastic left heart syndrome. J Am Coll Cardiol 36:1178–1185, 2000.
52. Jenkins PC, Flanagan MF, Sargent JD, et al: A comparison of treatment strategies for hypoplastic left heart syndrome using decision analysis. J Am Coll Cardiol 38:1181–1187, 2001.
53. Jobes DR, Nicholson SC, Stevens JM, et al: Carbon dioxide prevents pulmonary overcirculation in hypoplastic left heart syndrome. Ann Thorac Surg 54:150–151, 1992.
54. Joshi VM, Carey A, Simpson P, Paridon SM: Exercise performance following repair of hypoplastic left heart syndrome: A comparison with other types of Fontan patients. Pediatr Cardiol 18:357–360, 1997.
55. Kern JH, Hinton VJ, Nereo NE, et al: Early developmental outcome after the Norwood procedure for hypoplastic left heart syndrome. Pediatrics 102:1148–1152, 1998.
56. Kohl T, Szabo Z, Suda K, et al: Fetoscopic and open transumbilical fetal cardiac catheterization in sheep: Potential approaches for human fetal cardiac intervention. Circulation 95(4):1048-53, 197.
57. Kumar RK, Newburger JW, Gauvreau K, et al: Comparison of outcome when hypoplastic left heart syndrome and transposition of the great arteries are diagnosed prenatally versus when diagnosis of these two conditions is made only postnatally. Am J Cardiopl 83:1649–1653, 1999.
58. Lardo AC, Webber SA, Friehs I, et al: Fluid dynamic comparison of intra-atrial and extracardiac total cavopulmonary connections. J Thorac Cardiovasc Surg 697–704, 1999.
59. Lev M, Arcilla R, Rimoldi HJ, et al: Premature narrowing or closure of the foramen ovale. 65:638–647, 1963.
60. Lofland GK, McCrindle BW, Williams WG, et al: Critical aortic stenosis in the neonate; A multi-institutional study of management, outcomes, and risk factors. J Thorac Cardiovasc Surg 121:10–27, 2001.
61. Machii M, Becker AE: Nature of coarctation in hypoplastic left heart syndrome. Ann Thorac Surg 59:1491–1494, 1995.
62. Maegawa Y, Mizobe T, Yamagishi M, et al: The use of nitrogen and nitric oxide to control pulmonary blood flow in the Norwood operation. J Cardiothorac Vasc Anesthes 16(2):264–266, 2002.
63. Mahle WT, Clancy RR, McGaurn SP, Goin JE, Clark BJ: Impact of prenatal diagnosis on survival and early neurologic morbidity in neonates with hypoplastic left heart syndrome. Pediatrics 107:1277–1282, 2001.

64. Mahle WT, Clancy RR, Moss EM, et al: Neurodevelopmental outcome and lifestyle assessment in school-aged and adolescent children with hypoplastic left heart syndrome. Pediatrics105:1082–1089, 2000.
65. Mahle WT, Spray TL, Gaynor JW, et al: Unexpected death after reconstructive surgery for hypoplastic left heart syndrome. Ann Thorac Surg 71:61–65, 2001.
66. Mahle WT, Spray TL, Wernovsky G, et al: Survival after reconstructive surgery for hypoplastic left heart syndrome; A fifteen-year experience from a single institution. Circulation 102[suppl III]: III-136–III-141, 2000.
67. Malec E, Mroczek T, Pajak, et al: Hypoplastic left heart syndrome with an anomalous origin of the left coronary artery. Ann Thorac Surg 72:2129–2130, 2001.
68. Maxwell D, Allen L, Tynan MJ: Balloon dilatation of the aortic valve in the fetus: a report of two cases. Br Heart J 65:256–258, 1991.
69. Meyrick B, Reid L: The effect of continued hypoxia on rat pulmonary arterial circulation. Lab Invest 38:188–200, 1978.
70. Mora GA, Pizzaro C, Jacobs ML, et al: Experimental model of single ventricle: Influence of carbon dioxide on pulmonary vascular dynamics. Circulation 90[part 2]:II-43–II-46, 1994.
71. Mosca RS, Hennien HA, Kulik TJ, et al: Modified Norwood operation for single left ventricle and ventriculoarterial discordance: An improved surgical technique. Ann Thorac Surg 64:1126–1132, 1997.
72. Mosca RS, Kulik TJ, Goldberg CS, et al: Early Results of the Fontan procedure in one hundred consecutive patients with hypoplastic left heart syndrome. J Thorac Cardiovasc Surg 119:1110–1118, 2000.
73. Murakami A, Takamoto S, Takaoka T, et al: Saphenous vein homograft containing a valve as a right ventricle-pulmonary artery conduit in the modified Norwood operation. J Thorac Cardiovasc Surg; 124:110410–110412, 2002.
74. Natowicz M, Chatten J, Clancy RR, et al: Genetic disorders and major extracardiac anomalies associated with hypoplastic left heart syndrome. Pediatrics 82:698, 1988.
75. Nora JJ, Nora AH: Genetics and counseling in cardiovascular diseases. Springfield, IL, Charles C Thomas, 1978, p. 181.)
76. O'Connor WN, Ash JB, Cottrill CM, et al: Ventriculo-coronary connections in hypoplastic left hearts: An autopsy microscopic study. Circulation 66:1078–1086, 1982.
77. Ovroutski S, Dahnert I, Alexi-meskishvili V, et al: Preliminary analysis of arrhythmias after the Fontan operation with extracardiac conduit compared with intraatrial lateral tunnel. Thorac Cardiovasc Surg 49:334–337, 2001.
78. Pahl E, Zales VR, Fricker FJ, et al: Posttransplant coronary artery disease in children: a multicenter national survey. Circulation90[part 2]:II56–II40, 1994.
79. Pediatrics 65(suppl)376–460, 1980. Laursen HB: Some epidemiologic aspects of congenital heart disease in Denmark. Acta Paediatr Scand 69:619–624, 1980.
80. Phillips HM, Renforth GL, Spalluto C, et al: Narrowing of the critical region within 11q24-qter for hypoplastic left heart and identification of a candidate gene, JAM3, expressed during cardiogenesis. Genomics 79(4):475–478, 2002.
81. Pigula FA: Heart transplantation: Surgical technique. In: Tejani AH, Harmon WE, Fine RN, (eds): Pediatric Solid Organ Transplantation, 1st ed. Copenhagen: Munksgaard, , 2000, pp. 359–370.
82. Pigula FA, Siewers RD, Nemoto EM: Regional perfusion of the brain during neonatal aortic arch reconstruction. J Thorac Cardiovasc Surg117:1023–1024, 1999.
83. Pigula FA, Gandhi SK, Siewers RD, et al: Regional low-flow perfusion provides systemic circulatory support during neonatal aortic arch surgery. Ann Thorac Surg72:401–407, 2001.
84. Pigula FA, Nomoto EM, Griffith BP, Siewers RD: Regional low-flow perfusion provides cerebral circulatory support during neonatal aortic arch reconstruction. J Thorac Cardiovasc Surg 119:331–339, 2000.
85. Pizaro C, Davis DA, Healy RM, et al: Is there a role for extracorporeal life support after stage I Norwood. Eur J Cardiothor Surg 19:294–301, 2001.
86. Pizzarro C, Maher KO, Norwood NI: Right ventricle to pulmonary artery shunt has a favorable impact on postoperative physiology after stage I Norwood for hypoplastic left heart syndrome. Presented at the EACTS, Monte Carlo, 2002.
87. Poirer NC, Drummon F, Webb JJ, et al: Modified Norwood procedure with a high-flow cardiopulmonary bypass strategy results in low mortality without late arch obstruction. J Thorac Cardiovasc Surg 120:875–884, 2000.
88. Razzouk AJ, Chinnock RE, Gundry SR, et al: Transplantation as a primary treatment for hypoplastic left heart syndrome: Intermediate term results. Ann Thorac Surg62:1–8, 1996.
89. Reddy VM, McElhinney DB, Moore P, et al: Outcomes after bidirectional cavopulmonary shunt in infants less than 6 months old. J Am Coll Cardiol 29(6):1365–1370, 1997.
90. Remmell-Dow DR, Bharati S, Davis JT, et al: Hypoplasia of the eustachian valve and abnormal orientation of the limbus of the foramen ovale in hypoplastic left heart syndrome. Am Heart J 130(1);148–152, 195.
91. Rhodes LA, Colan DS, Perry S, et al: Predictors of survival in neonates with critical aortic stenosis. Circulation 84:2325–2335, 1991.
92. Riordan CJ, Randsbaek F, Storey JH, et al: Effect of oxygen, positive end-expiratory pressure, and carbon dioxide on oxygen delivery in an animal model of the univentricular heart. J Thorac Cardiovasc Surg 112:644–654, 1996.
93. Roberts WC, Perry LW, Chandra RS, et al: Aortic valve atresia: A new classification system based on necropsy study of 73 cases. Am J Cardiol 37:753, 1976.
94. Rossi AF, Seiden HS, Sadeghi AM, et al: The outcome of cardiac operations in infants weighing two kilograms or less. J Thorac Cardiovasc Surg 116:28–35, 1998.
95. Rossi AF, Sommer RJ, Steinberg LG, et al: Effect of older age on outcome for stage one palliation of hypoplastic left heart syndrome. Am J Cardiol 77:319–321, 1996.
96. Sarris GE, Drummond-Webb JJ, Ebeid MR, et al: Anomalous origin of left coronary artery from right pulmonary artery in hypoplastic left heart syndrome. Ann Thorac Surg 64:836–838, 1997.
97. Schall SA, Dalldorf FG: Premature closure of the foramen ovale and hypoplasia of the left heart. Int J Cardiol 5(1):103–107, 1984.
98. Sedmera D, Hu N, Weiss KM, et al: Cellular changes in experimental left heart hypoplasia Anat Rec 267(2):137–456, 2002.
99. Sharland GK, Chita SK, Fagg NL, et al: Left ventricular dysfunction in the future relation to aortic valve anomalies and endocardial fibroelastosis. Br Heart J 66(6):419–424, 1991.
100. Sinha SN, Rusnak SL, Sommers HM, et al: Hypoplastic left ventricle syndrome. Analysis of thirty autopsy cases in infants with surgical consideration. Am J Cardiol 21:166, 1968.
101. Soongsswang J, McCrindle BW, Jones TK, et al: Outcomes of transcatheter balloon angioplasty of obstruction in the neoaortic arch after Norwood operation. Cardiol Young 11:54–61, 2001.
102. Tabbutt , Ramamoorthy C, Montenegro LM, et al: Impact of inspired gas mixtures on preoperative infants with hypoplastic left heart syndrome (HLHS) during controlled ventilation. Circulation 102(Suppl 2)469, 2000.
103. Tani LY, Minnich LL, Pagotto LT, et al: Left heart hypoplasia and neonatal aortic arch obstruction: Is the Rhodes left ventricular adequacy score applicable? J Thorac Cardiovasc Surg 118:81–86, 1999.
104. Tchervenkov CI, Jacobs ML, Tahta SA: Ann Thorac Surg 69:s170–179, 2000.

105. Tikkanen J, Heinonen OP: Risk factors for hypoplastic left heart syndrome. Teratology 50(2);112–117, 1994.
106. Tweddell JS, Hoffman GM, Federly RT, et al: Phenoxybenzamine improves systemic oxygen delivery after the Norwood procedure. Ann Thorac Surg 67:161–168, 1999.
107. Tweddell JS, Hoffman GM, Fedderly ,et al: Patients at risk for low systemic oxygen delivery after the Norwood procedure. Ann Thorac Surg 69:1893-99, 2000.
108. Tweddell JS, Hoffman GM, Mussatto KA, et al: Improved survival of patients undergoing palliation of hypoplastic left heart syndrome: Lessons learned from 115 consecutive patients. Circulation. 106[suppl I]:I-82–I-89, 2002.
109. Tworetzky W, Mcelhinney DB, Burch GH, et al: Balloon arterioplasty of recurrent coarctation after the modified Norwood procedure in infants. Cathet Cardiovasc Intervent 50:54–58, 2000.
110. Tworetzky W, McElhinney DB, Reddy VM, et al: Improved surgical outcome after fetal diagnosis for hypoplastic left heart syndrome. Circulation. 103:1269–1273, 2001.
111. Vricella LA, Razzouk AJ, del Rio M, et al: Heart transplantation for hypoplastic left heart syndrome: Modified technique for reducing circulatory arrest time. J Heart Lung Transplant 17:1167–1171, 1998.
112. Weinstein S, Gaynor JW, Bridges ND, et al: Early survival of infants weighing 2.5 kilograms or less undergoing first-stage reconstruction for hypoplastic left heart syndrome. Circulation 100[suppl II]:II-167–II-170, 1999.

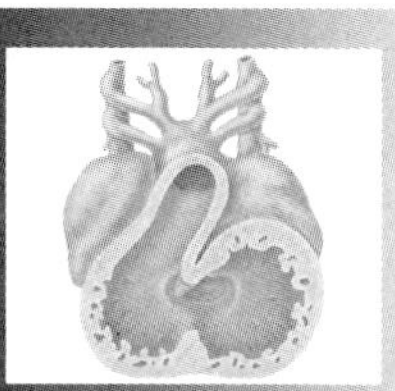

CHAPTER 126

Management of Single Ventricle and Cavopulmonary Connections

Carin van Doorn and Marc R. de Leval

INTRODUCTION

There is a wide range of structural cardiac abnormalities that effectively result in a single ventricle circulation. It is widely accepted that the definitive surgical palliation for these hearts is the Fontan circulation, whereby the pulmonary and systemic blood flow are in series with the single ventricle connected to the systemic circulation. To achieve the Fontan state, many patients will need adjustment of the pulmonary or systemic circulations. Because of the changing physiology in the early years of life, a series of operations is often necessary.

TERMINOLOGY AND ANATOMY

In this chapter we shall use the term *single ventricle* for congenital cardiac malformations that lack two completely well-developed ventricles and in which functionally there is only a single ventricular chamber that supports both the pulmonary and systemic circulations.

A truly morphological univentricular heart is rare; more often there is an additional rudimentary chamber. Over the years there have been a number of classifications and terminologies for these hearts. In the recent Congenital Heart Surgery Nomenclature and Database Project[51] the following entities were recognized: hearts with common inlet atrioventricular connection (double inlet right ventricle and double inlet left ventricle), hearts with absence of one atrioventricular connection (tricuspid atresia and mitral atresia), hearts with common atrioventricular valve and only one well-developed ventricle (unbalanced common atrioventricular canal defect), hearts with only one fully developed ventricle and heterotaxia syndrome (single ventricle heterotaxia syndrome), and finally other rare forms of univentricular hearts that do not fit in one of the above categories. Tricuspid atresia is the most common type of single ventricle with an incidence of 1–3% of all congenital heart lesions.

In addition there are some cardiac abnormalities in which in the presence of two well-developed ventricles the anatomy precludes biventricular repair. Examples include hearts with major straddling of the atrioventricular valve and double outlet right ventricle with remote ventricular septal defect. Treatment strategies for these nonseptatable hearts are the same as those applied to univentricular hearts.

In this chapter we shall not discuss the management of hypoplastic left heart syndrome, a common form of univentricular heart with a dominant right ventricle and rudimentary left ventricle. Chapter 125 is dedicated to this topic.

NATURAL HISTORY

The natural history of single ventricle circulations is greatly influenced by the degree of pulmonary blood flow and any associated lesions. Many hearts have complex anatomy, such as abnormal pulmonary and systemic venous drainage commonly seen in isomeric hearts. In addition there may be noncardiac abnormalities.

Severe obstruction to pulmonary blood flow at birth is an important determinant for early death. In pulmonary atresia with decreased pulmonary blood flow there are virtually no survivors beyond the first year of life. Patients with unobstructed pulmonary flow often die in infancy from congestive heart failure or later from pulmonary vascular disease. The clinical course may be worsened by the presence of left-sided obstructive lesions, such as coarctation of the aorta. In a small subset of patients the pulmonary and systemic circulations are well-balanced because of unrestrictive systemic blood flow and sufficient pulmonary obstruction to control pulmonary blood flow. These patients have a more favorable life expectancy.

In 101 patients with tricuspid atresia approximately 50% survived to 15 years.[25] At our institution, Franklin[36] reviewed the outcome without definitive repair of patients presenting with double-inlet ventricle in the first year of life. Actuarial survival was 57% at 1 year, 43% at 5 years, and 42% at 10 years. In a series from the Mayo Clinic, patients diagnosed between the ages of 4 and 10 years with a systemic left ventricle and rudimentary right chamber survived for a mean of 14 years after presentation.[71] The aim of surgical intervention is to improve the natural history by balancing blood flow between the pulmonary and systemic circulations and ultimately separating these circulations. In addition other significant hemodynamic abnormalities are corrected.

CLINICAL PRESENTATION AND PREOPERATIVE EVALUATION

Clinical presentation is determined by the amount of pulmonary blood flow and the associated cardiac lesions. Patients with restricted pulmonary blood flow will exhibit cyanosis. Some may have a duct-dependent pulmonary circulation and will become rapidly cyanosed as the ductus arteriosus closes after birth. In the case of a large left-to-right shunt the patient will present with congestive heart failure. Symptoms will deteriorate with falling pulmonary resistance in the first weeks after birth. Although in most single ventricles there is mixing of circulations, streaming may occur, particularly in complex hearts, resulting in differential saturations in the great arteries.

A precise anatomical diagnosis is essential to allow proper planning of the surgical procedures. In particular information on the size and course of the pulmonary arteries, degree of pulmonary blood flow, and presence of accessory lesions are required, as well as the assessment of cardiac function. History, clinical presentation, chest X-ray, and electrocardiogram all offer important, but nonspecific, information. Echocardiography provides detailed information on both the structure and function of the heart and has the advantage that it is a noninvasive investigation that can be carried out at the bedside. In particular in infants, who have excellent echo windows, enough information can often be gathered to proceed to surgery. The recent development of 3-dimensional echocardiography and tissue Doppler imaging, allows the acquisition of even more detailed structural and functional information. Angiography remains important for delineation of the great vessels and coronary arteries, and the ability to obtain direct pressure measurements. In addition interventional procedures can be carried out to supplement, or sometimes replace, surgical treatment. Magnetic resonance imaging is rapidly becoming a first-line investigation for congenital heart disease allowing 3-dimensional reconstruction of the cardiovascular system and noninvasive assessment of hemodynamic function.

SELECTION CRITERIA FOR THE FONTAN PROCEDURE

The principle of the Fontan operation as a right heart bypass procedure is based on the concept that the right atrium could replace the right ventricle as the driving force for the pulmonary circulation. In addition, placing the systemic and pulmonary circulations in series improves systemic arterial saturation and reduces the volume load on the single ventricle.

The initial selection criteria for the procedure, described by Fontan and colleagues for patients with tricuspid atresia, were stringent and known as the "ten commandments" (Box 126-1).[17] With increasing experience the criteria have been relaxed; however, because of the unique physiology that accompanies the Fontan circulation, proper patient selection remains crucial.

The age of patients undergoing the Fontan operation has been progressively lowered because of fear of deteriorating ventricular function due to long-standing cyanosis and volume overload. The optimal and minimal age for the Fontan operation remains controversial, but the best early outcome will be achieved at a time when both hemodynamics and anatomy are ideal for the Fontan state. Pulmonary vascular development carries on well into the first months of life,[49] but successful Fontan operations have been performed in patients from age 7 months onwards who presented with increasing cyanosis and suitable hemodynamics.[73] Because it is thought that muscular contraction is beneficial for venous return, the operation should perhaps not be performed before the child is at least crawling. It remains to be seen if a very early Fontan procedure has a better long-term outcome than one performed at a later age, in particular in patients with well-balanced circulations. Preoperative sinus

Box 126–1. The "Ten Commandments" for Selection of Patients with Tricuspid Atresia for the Fontan Procedure.

1. Minimum age 4 years
2. Sinus rhythm
3. Normal caval drainage
4. Right atrium of normal volume
5. Mean pulmonary artery pressure $\leq$15 mm Hg
6. Pulmonary arterial resistance <4 U/m^2
7. Pulmonary-artery-to-aorta-diameter ratio $\geq$0.75
8. Normal ventricular functions (ejection fraction >0.6)
9. Competent left atrioventricular valve
10. No impairing effects of previous shunts

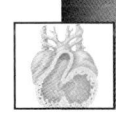

rhythm is not an absolute requirement,[3] nor is a normal volume right atrium or normal caval drainage. On the other hand, unobstructed pulmonary venous drainage is an absolute necessity.

The pulmonary vasculature and ventricular function remains the most important selection criteria for successful outcome after the Fontan operation. Pulmonary arteriolar resistance (<4 units/m^2)[60] and mean pulmonary artery pressure should be low (<15 mm Hg). Assessment of the pulmonary vascular bed can be very difficult, in particular in the presence of accessory sources of pulmonary blood flow such as aortopulmonary collateral vessels or surgical shunts.

The size of the pulmonary arteries is also a predictor of outcome after the Fontan procedure. There have been various attempts to standardize these measurements. The McGoon ratio, originally used in patients with pulmonary atresia and ventricular septal defect,[76] is obtained from the sum of the diameters of the immediately prebranching portion of the left and right pulmonary artery divided by the diameter of the descending aorta just above the diaphragm. In a retrospective study Fontan and colleagues[33] found that the risk of early death or Fontan take down rose sharply when the McGoon ratio was less than 1.8. The Nakata index[72] is derived from the sum of the diameter of the left and right pulmonary artery (measured just before the origin of the upper lobe branches) divided by the body surface area. Patients with unfavorable outcome after a modified Fontan for tricuspid atresia were shown to have a lower pulmonary artery index then those with good results (185+/−47 versus 276+/−83 mm^2/m^2),[54] but this was not confirmed by others.[79] The usefulness of these indices has been questioned because they do not take into account the compliance and maturity of the pulmonary vascular system, the peripheral and intraparenchymal pulmonary arteries, or any distortion of the central pulmonary arteries that may have occurred because of previous shunts.

Adequate ventricular function is a prime determinant for a successful Fontan circulation. Ventricular impairment, however, is not always a contraindication, in particular as it can be related to volume overload in the presence of an aortopulmonary shunt. Some of these patients may still become candidates by staging the Fontan procedure with an initial bidirectional cavopulmonary shunt (for which the indications are less critical)[38] and take down of the aortopulmonary shunt. This offloads the circulation, and if ventricular function recovers, completion of the Fontan procedure can be carried out in due course. The same applies to mild or moderate atrioventricular valve regurgitation in a volume-loaded heart. Ventricular hypertrophy has been recognized as an important risk factor for Fontan failure.[53,82] The exact mechanism for this is unknown, but it is thought that increased myocardial mass alters ventricular filling and reduces compliance while systolic ventricular function is preserved.[39] Subaortic stenosis is an important trigger for acquired ventricular hypertrophy and in particular can be found in patients who have tricuspid atresia, double inlet left ventricle, transposition of the great arteries, and ventricular septal defect and in those who have undergone pulmonary artery banding. The effects of myocardial hypertrophy are exacerbated by acute volume offloading at the time of the Fontan operation, which further increases ventricular wall thickness and diastolic dysfunction.[75]

In the absence of uniform selection criteria, most centers will use a combination of the preceding criteria and grade patients as low/medium/high risk for the Fontan procedure.

SURGICAL PREPARATION FOR THE FONTAN CIRCULATION

There is a wide variation in the distribution of pulmonary and systemic blood flow in patients with a single ventricle circulation. In the majority of patients pulmonary blood flow is restricted, some have unrestricted pulmonary flow, and very few have a naturally balanced circulation. The majority of patients, therefore, will require palliative procedures leading up to the Fontan circulation, either to restrict or to augment pulmonary flow. The choice of procedure is guided by the underlying anatomy and pulmonary vascular resistance, both of which are subject to change over time. It should always be borne in mind that improper palliative procedures can result in the loss of Fontan candidacy.

The aims of surgical procedures leading up to the Fontan circulation are (1) improve clinical symptoms, (2) provide optimal pulmonary vasculature and ventricular function, and (3) provide anatomical setup for definitive Fontan repair.

Systemic-to-Pulmonary Artery Shunt

If augmentation of pulmonary blood flow is required in the neonatal and early infantile period, when pulmonary vascular resistance is still high, a systemic-to-pulmonary artery shunt is performed. In the past direct connections between aorta and pulmonary artery were used (Potts shunt[77]: descending aorta to left pulmonary artery; Waterston shunt[98]: ascending aorta to right pulmonary artery), but these were abandoned because of unpredictability of shunt flow and high incidence of pulmonary artery distortion. The effect of a right subclavian to pulmonary artery shunt[11] was more predictable. Currently, prosthetic interposition shunts are performed that are usually placed between the subclavian artery or innominate artery and the pulmonary artery (modified Blalock-Taussig shunt).[68]

Cavopulmonary Shunt

The advantages of a venous over an arterial shunt are twofold. First, the venous blood that enters the pulmonary artery is much more desaturated, and therefore a higher take-up of oxygen per milliliter of blood is possible. Second, systemic venous return is diverted to the lungs, thus reducing the volume load on the single ventricle.

The original cavopulmonary shunt was an end-to-end anastomosis between the superior vena cava (or azygos vein) and the divided right pulmonary artery.[44] The procedure is associated with the development of pulmonary arteriovenous fistulae in the ipsilateral lung to the shunt.[67] The classical Glenn shunt was largely abandoned with the introduction of the Fontan operation in the mid-1970s.

In a bidirectional Glenn shunt the superior vena cava is connected to the (undivided) right pulmonary artery thus shunting venous blood to both lungs. This is commonly an end-to-side anastomosis of the transected superior vena cava to the right pulmonary artery (Figure 126-1).[7] The

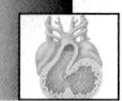

hemi-Fontan modification of the cavopulmonary shunt involves patch augmentation of the central pulmonary arteries and a connection between the right atrial-superior vena cava junction and pulmonary arteries. The hemi-Fontan operation has particularly gained popularity in patients with hypoplastic left heart syndrome where following the first stage of the Norwood operation pulmonary distortion and hypoplasia are common.[28]

Criteria for suitability for a cavopulmonary shunt are not uniformly agreed upon, but it is generally accepted that these are less strict than those for the Fontan operation. If preoperative evaluation reveals any adverse anatomical features for the Fontan circulation, such as subaortic obstruction, then this should also be addressed at the time of the cavopulmonary shunt or earlier if necessary. Whether an additional source of pulmonary blood flow (such as a patent ductus arteriosus, patent right ventricular outflow tract, or systemic-to-pulmonary artery shunt) should be taken down at the time of the cavopulmonary artery shunt remains open to discussion. A recent retrospective study from Paris reported that operative mortality at the time of the bidirectional shunt was similar for those with and without accessory pulmonary flow. There was also no difference in postoperative survival or development of pulmonary hypertension.[96]

There are a number of long-term problems associated with the bidirectional cavopulmonary shunt. As for the classic Glenn shunt, preferential perfusion of the lower parts of the lung and pulmonary arteriovenous fistulae has been documented.[18] In addition communications between superior vena cava territory and lower body veins, left atrium, and pulmonary veins may be present, promoting right-to-left shunting and increasing cyanosis.[58] Aortopulmonary collateral vessels may place an increased volume load on the heart.[93] Finally, with growth of the child the contribution of superior vena caval blood flow to total venous return decreases, the child becomes more cyanosed, and an additional source of blood flow is needed. If the patient is a Fontan candidate, completion of the cavopulmonary connection should now follow. If the patient is not suitable, another option may be to add a small arterial shunt.

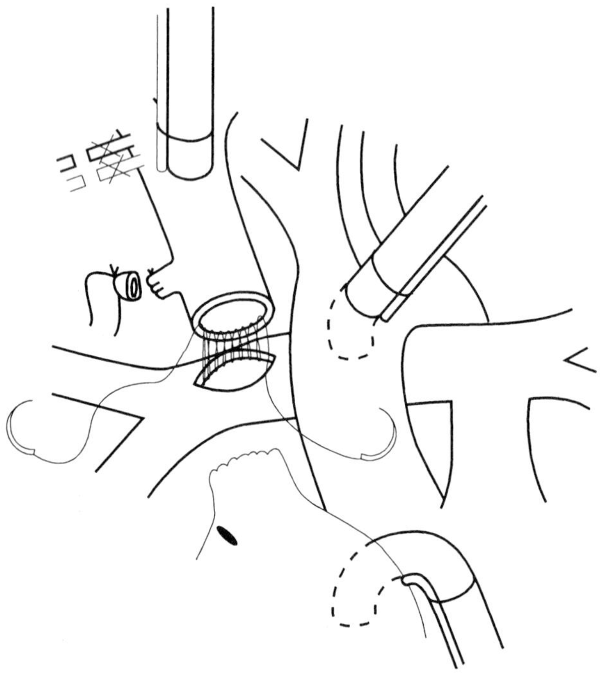

Figure 126–1 Bidirectional cavopulmonary shunt. The superior vena cava is fully mobilized, including the junction with the innominate vein. The azygos vein and small venous branches near the innominate vein junction are ligated to prevent run-off into the inferior vena cava territory. The main and right pulmonary arteries and a right systemic-to-pulmonary artery shunt, if present, are mobilized. Cardiopulmonary bypass is instituted with venous drainage from a cannula in the right atrial appendage and a further cannula in superior vena cava near the innominate junction with return via the ascending aorta. The operation is performed on a beating heart with moderate hypothermia (28° C to 32° C), but a period of aortic cross-clamping may be required for correction of other cardiac anomalies. Any right-sided systemic aortopulmonary shunt is occluded and subsequently taken down. The right and main pulmonary artery are mobilized. The superior vena cava is snugged down. A vascular clamp is applied just above the cavoatrial junction, taking care not to damage the sinus node. The superior vena cava is divided immediately above the clamp, the cardiac end is oversewn and the clamp released. The upper margin of the right pulmonary artery is incised. The superior vena cava is anastomosed end-to-side with the upper margin of the right pulmonary artery. The suture is interrupted in several places to help avoid a purse-string effect and narrowing of the anastomosis. Additional sources of pulmonary blood supply, such as forward flow over a stenosed pulmonary outflow tract or left-sided arterial pulmonary shunt, are usually left in place.

Pulmonary Artery Banding

In the case of pulmonary overflow, banding the pulmonary artery will limit the pulmonary blood flow and protect the patient from developing pulmonary vascular disease and ventricular dysfunction. Adequate tightness of the band can be difficult to achieve, and a band that is too loose initially may result in unprotected pulmonary arteries until the child grows into the band. The resultant pulmonary vascular disease may not be recognized until much later when the child is assessed for the Fontan procedure. Another complication that may result in lost Fontan candidacy is the development of subaortic stenosis,[37,90] which is thought to occur as the combined effect of myocardial hypertrophy and a reduction in volume load of the systemic ventricle. Patients at risk are those in whom the aorta arises above a small outlet chamber, such as in tricuspid atresia with double inlet left ventricle, rudimentary right ventricle, and transposition of the great arteries, particularly if the ventricular septic defect (VSD) is small or if there is coexisting aortic arch obstruction. When preexistent subaortic stenosis is present or when its development is highly likely, pulmonary artery banding is contraindicated and instead the Lamberti modification of the Damus-Kaye-Stansel procedure should be performed to establish unobstructed systemic arterial outflow. This involves transsection of both great arteries, anastomosis of the facing aortic and pulmonary walls, and connection of the distal aorta to the perimeter of the reconstructed proximal great artery. Depending on the pulmonary vascular status, blood flow to the central pulmonary arteries can be reestablished via a systemic or venous shunt or the Fontan operation.[97] Alternatively, a Norwood strategy can be followed in these patients (see Chapter 125).

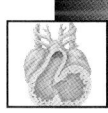

Other complications of pulmonary artery banding include distortion of the pulmonary arteries, especially if the band migrates, and erosion of the band. Over time pulmonary blood flow will become inadequate because of the fixed diameter pulmonary band and the patient needs to be evaluated for suitability for a Fontan circulation.

SURGICAL EVOLUTION OF THE FONTAN PROCEDURE

The Fontan procedure was first applied in 1968 for tricuspid atresia and was based on the principle that the right atrium could be used as a pumping chamber for the pulmonary circulation.[32] The original description of the atriopulmonary connection included the insertion of an aortic or pulmonary homograft valve, both at the inflow and the outflow of the right atrium. Kreutzer[56] described the use of the patient's native pulmonary valve between the right atrium and pulmonary artery. Because of concern of failure of the right atrium as the pulmonary pump, Gago[42] introduced an atrioventricular connection consisting of patch augmentation of the hypoplastic right ventricle and insertion of a porcine aortic valve conduit between the right atrium and right ventricle. Bjork[10] was worried about the long-term durability of conduits and valve prostheses and devised a valveless atrioventricular anastomosis whereby the right atrial appendix is anastomosed to the right ventricle with the aid of an autologous pericardial patch. He subsequently observed that in one patient the small right ventricle increased in size after the operation and now contributed to forward flow. It has since been shown, though, that incorporation of too small a right ventricle may be a hindrance rather then a help because the benefit of a forward kick in systole may be more than offset by restriction to pulmonary inflow in diastole and no net step up in mean pulmonary arterial pressure is gained.[16] For patients with subaortic obstruction undergoing the Fontan operation, Waldman[97] described the concurrent use of a modified Damus-Kaye-Stansel procedure to achieve unobstructed systemic arterial blood flow.

The efficiency of the atrium as a blood pump in the Fontan circulation has been questioned. Not only is the atrium likely to perform on the downward limb of its function curve because of elevated systemic venous pressures,[30] but more importantly, in a valveless cavo-atrio-pulmonary connection there may be little net forward flow because of backflow in the low-compliance venous system during atrial contraction.[23] In addition, studies in hydrodynamic models by de Leval and colleagues[22] revealed that the atriopulmonary connection performed poorly in terms of flow energetics because of turbulence that was further exaggerated by pulsation. In contrast a cavopulmonary connection had mainly laminar flow patterns. In this design, the superior vena cava blood drains directly into the pulmonary artery and inferior vena cava blood is baffled through a straight intraatrial conduit to the pulmonary artery (Figure 126-2). Additional theoretical advantages are a reduced risk of thrombosis because of less blood stasis (but this may be offset by the use of artificial material to construct the conduit) and exposure of only a limited portion of the right atrium to high venous pressures thus reducing the risk of arrhythmias. Also, because the coronary sinus remains in the low pressure atrium, there is unobstructed myocardial venous drainage.

Maneuvers to reduce the risk in unfavorable Fontan candidates were introduced by Bridges and colleagues. Staging the Fontan initially with a bidirectional cavopulmonary shunt and pulmonary artery reconstruction when indicated provided adequate relief of cyanosis and relieved the single ventricle from volume overload.[13] Patients may subsequently become Fontan candidates because of improved ventricular performance and pulmonary artery anatomy. Another modification was the creation of a fenestration in the Fontan baffle. The resultant right-to-left shunting will maintain systemic ventricular filling and thus cardiac output in patients with impaired pulmonary blood flow but at the costs of some cyanosis.[14] They also reported that the fenestration can be closed at a later date by a transcatheter approach (Figure 126-3). The most recent change in the design of the Fontan pathway involves the use of an extracardiac interposition graft between the transected inferior vena cava and pulmonary artery (Figure 126-4).[61] The extracardiac conduit was initially designed to avoid pulmonary and systemic venous obstruction in patients with a small atrium, and its use has the additional advantage that it avoids extensive atrial suture lines that are potentially arrhythmogenic. This procedure can be performed without cross-clamping the aorta and in some patients also without the use of cardiopulmonary bypass.[99] Thrombogenicity and lack of growth of the prosthetic conduit remain potential late problems.

Improved understanding of the Fontan physiology and evolution of surgical techniques have extended the original indication of the Fontan operation from tricuspid atresia to many single ventricle malformations.

OUTCOME AFTER THE FONTAN PROCEDURE

Early Mortality and Morbidity

More than 30 years after the introduction of the Fontan operation,[32] the operative mortality has steadily come down to around 5%.[46,95,99] This is in spite of liberating the original patient selection criteria and extending the procedure to many forms of complex univentricular hearts. These results are encouraging but merely indicate that those who underwent the Fontan procedure were suitable candidates. No current information is available on how many patients in an entire cohort either die or do not proceed to surgery because of unfavorable anatomy or physiology. In the late 1980s, this was over 40% in some cohorts,[37,90] but with modern surgical strategies it is to be expected that many more patients are now Fontan candidates. Early morbidity associated with the Fontan operation include pleural and pericardial effusions, low output state (sometimes necessitating Fontan take down), sinus node injury, and pulmonary venous and systemic venous obstruction.

Factors that have contributed to improved outcome are the more energy-efficient circulation with the use of a lateral tunnel[22] or extracardiac conduit[61] and the reduction in aortic cross-clamp and cardiopulmonary bypass time, both of which can sometimes be avoided in the extracardiac Fontan.[66,99] Other factors that have been identified by some, but disputed by others, are the use of an atrial fenestration, staging

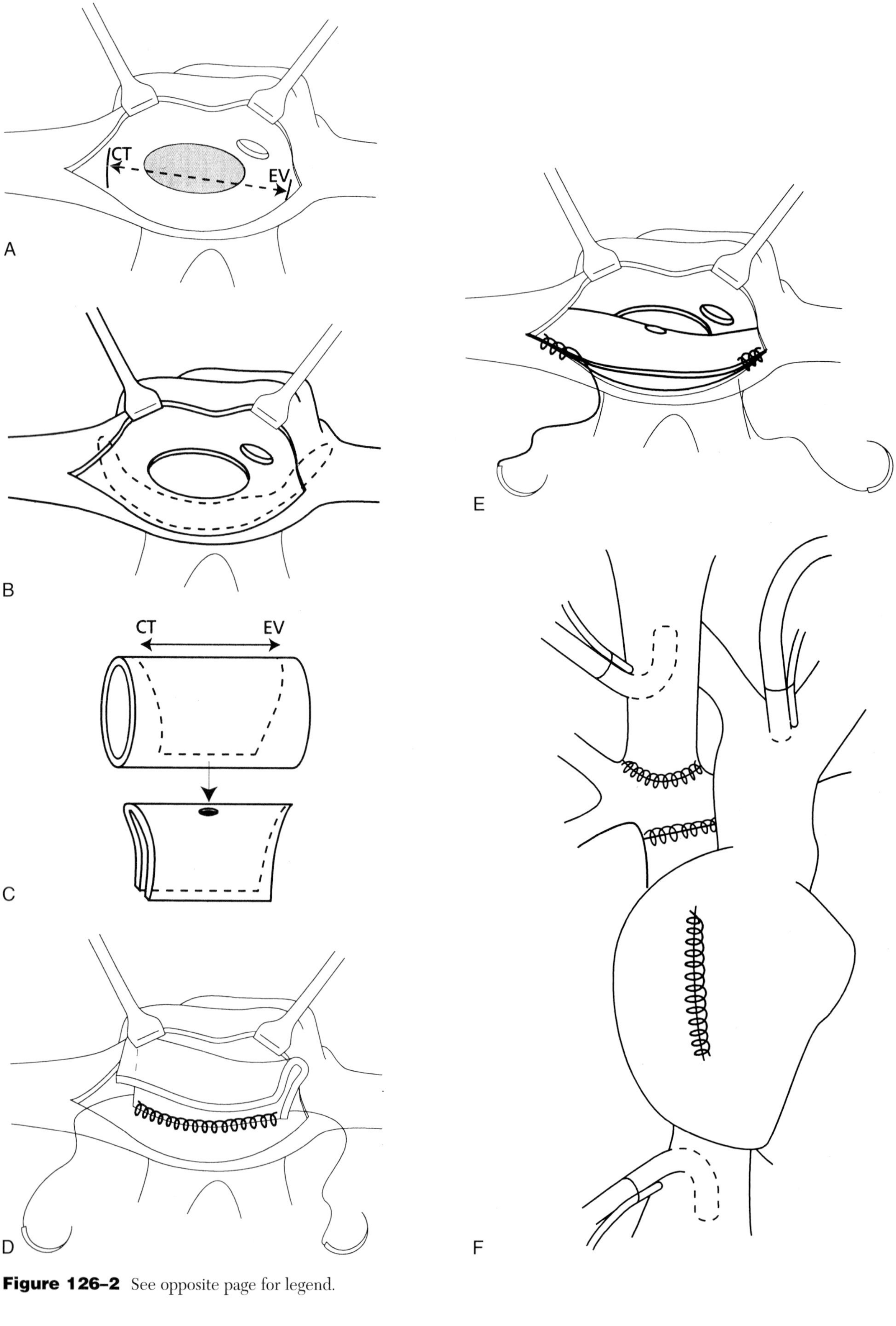

Figure 126–2 See opposite page for legend.

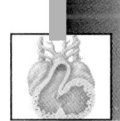

Figure 126–2 Lateral tunnel Fontan. The beginning of the operation may involve performing a bidirectional cavopulmonary anastomosis (see Figure 126-1), or this may already be in place. For cardiopulmonary bypass a venous cannula is placed low down on the inferior vena cava and a further cannula high up in the superior vena cava near the junction with the innominate vein. The ascending aorta is cannulated. The operation is performed using moderate hypothermia. Any existing systemic-to-pulmonary artery shunts are taken down. The aorta is cross-clamped and cold blood cardioplegia infused. A needle vent is placed in the ascending aorta. The main pulmonary artery is transected. To prevent bleeding or aneurysm formation after closure of the proximal pulmonary artery stump, the suture line is reinforced with two small Teflon felt strips and the pulmonary valve leaflets are included in the suture line. The distal main pulmonary artery is closed, taking care not to distort or narrow the branch pulmonary arteries. **A,** The right atrium is opened along the crest of the septum. The atrial septal defect is enlarged if necessary and the size of the intraatrial baffle measured between the Eustachian valve (EV) and crista terminalis (CT). **B,** Future site of baffle between the superior vena cava and inferior vena cava. **C,** A Gore-Tex tube of at least 16-mm diameter is cut to size and opened longitudinally, and if required, a 4–5 mm fenestration is cut. **D** and **E,** The prosthetic baffle is sewn halfway around the junction of the inferior vena cava with the right atrium, along the posterior wall of the atrial septum, crista terminalis, and halfway around the junction with the superior vena cava. Care is taken to avoid injury to the sinus node. **F,** The cardiac end of the transected superior vena cava is anastomosed end to side with the undersurface of the right pulmonary artery.

the Fontan procedure with a bidirectional cavopulmonary shunt, and preoperative occlusion of aortopulmonary collaterals.* Patients with a single ventricle and heterotaxy syndrome have always been a particularly high-risk population for the Fontan procedure because of their multiple associated cardiovascular abnormalities including variable anatomy of the sinus node and conduction system, potential for pulmonary venous obstruction, atrioventricular valve regurgitation, and recurrent or persistent cyanosis in the presence of arteriovenous shunting. In a recent paper from Toronto, surgical mortality in this difficult group had fallen to 13%, and

*References 12, 15, 47, 50, 52, 57, 95.

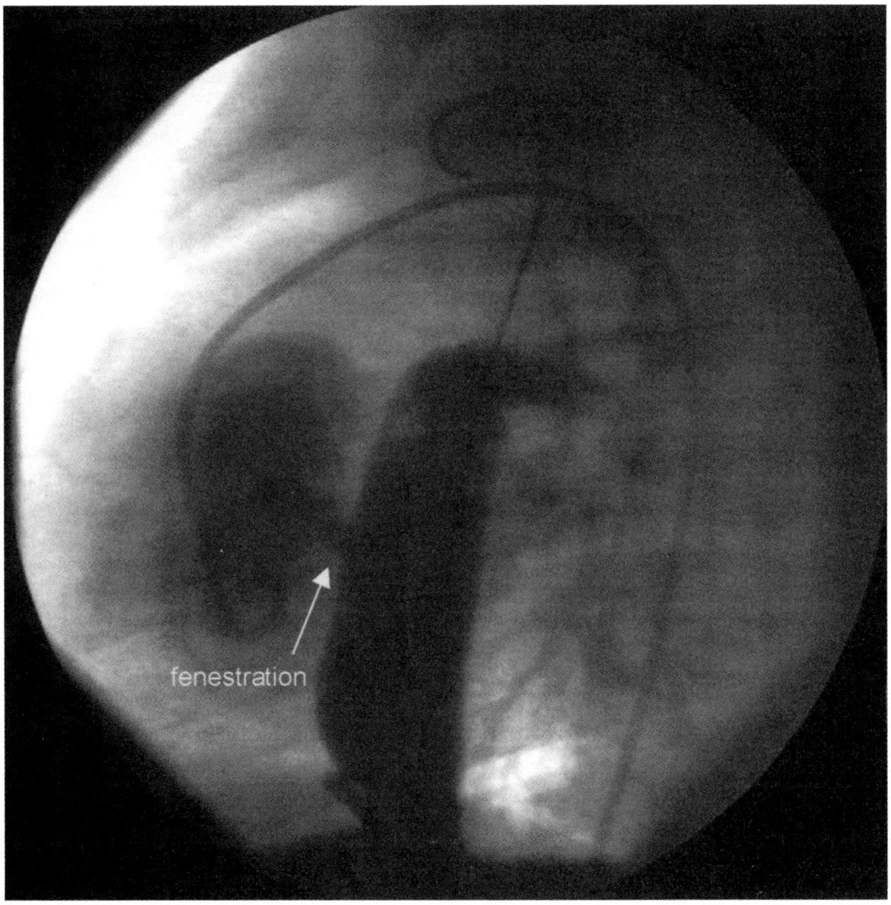

A

Figure 126–3 Fenestration in Fontan circuit closed by device. A, Injection of contrast in the extracardiac conduit of the Fontan pathway shows a communication between the pathway and the pulmonary venous atrium.

(Continued)

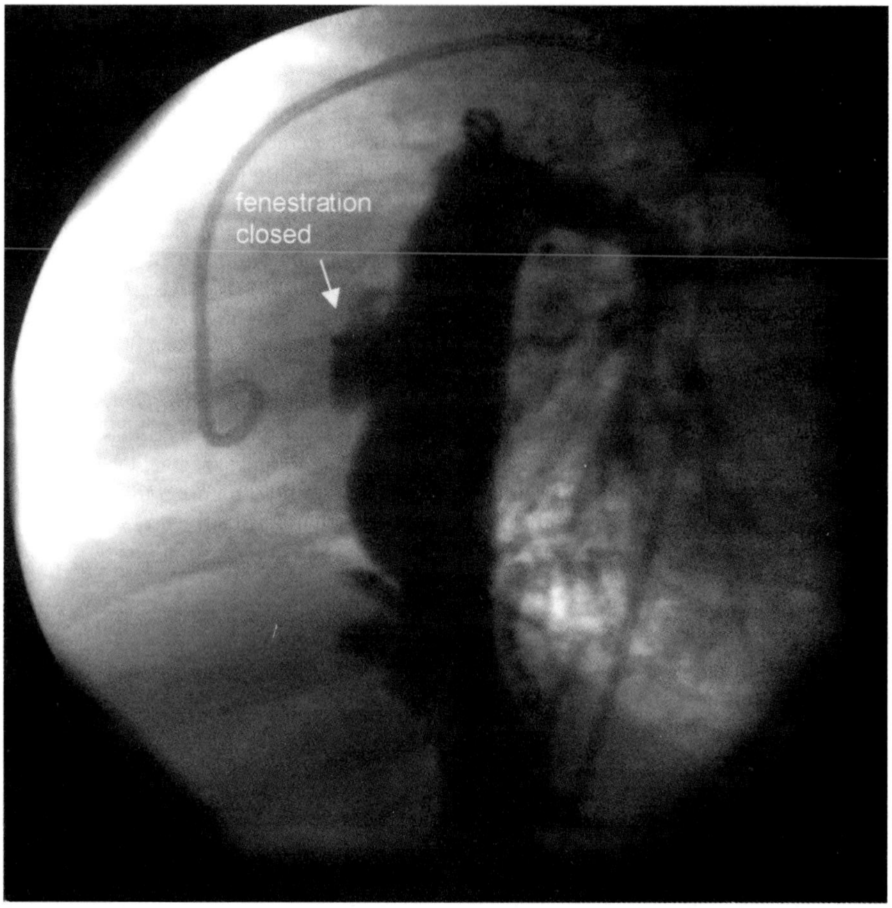

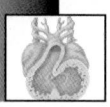

Figure 126–3 cont'd B, The fenestration has been occluded by a device. (During the same procedure a coil was also placed to occlude an aortopulmonary collateral vessel.)

the authors felt results could improve further with early detection and repair of obstructed pulmonary venous flow and correction of atriovalvular regurgitation.[6]

Late Attrition of the Fontan Circulation

With improving operative survival, late outcome after the Fontan operation is becoming increasingly important. In 1990, two decades after the introduction of the procedure, Fontan reported that the "Fontan state" was associated with a premature decline in functional status and survival.[34] Even when atriopulmonary and atrioventricular Fontan procedures were performed under perfect conditions, there was a gradual attrition with a predicted survival of 86%, 81%, and 73% at 5, 10, and 15 years, respectively, after the operation. A recent series from the Children's Hospital in Boston on the long-term results of the lateral tunnel Fontan shows 93% and 91% survival at 5 and 10 years, respectively.[88] The exact reasons for the late attrition after the Fontan operation are not known but no doubt are complex and multifactorial. Chronic elevation of systemic venous pressures is likely to play an important role and is reflected in some of the long-term complications such as right atrial distension, dilation of the coronary sinus, hepatic dysfunction, and elevated splanchnic venous pressures.

Atrial Arrhythmias

The distended atrium is prone to arrhythmias, especially in the presence of extensive suture lines. Atrial fibrillation and supraventricular reentry tachycardia may be difficult to control medically and lead to ventricular failure. Arrhythmia surgery and conversion of the Fontan circulation to a cavopulmonary connection relieves atrial arrhythmias in selected patients. Because of the high incidence of atrial arrhythmias it has been suggested that arrhythmia surgery should be incorporated in any planned Fontan conversion operation, even if sinus node function is still preserved.[20] With the introduction of lateral tunnel and extracardiac Fontan procedures, often with fenestration, the incidence of atrial arrhythmias is expected to come down. Indeed, in the recent lateral tunnel series from Boston, freedom of supraventricular tachyarrhythmias was 96% at 5 years and 91% at 10 years.[88] Risk factors for supraventricular arrhythmia were related to underlying cardiac morphology such as heterotaxy syndrome and atrioventricular valve abnormalities. Freedom of new bradyarrhythmias was 88% and 79% at 5 years and 10 years, respectively. Bradyarrhythmia, in particular slow junctional rhythm, has been noted in patients after the extracardiac Fontan operation.[85] Prophylactic treatment for atrial tachycardia has been proposed by placing lines of block across the most common

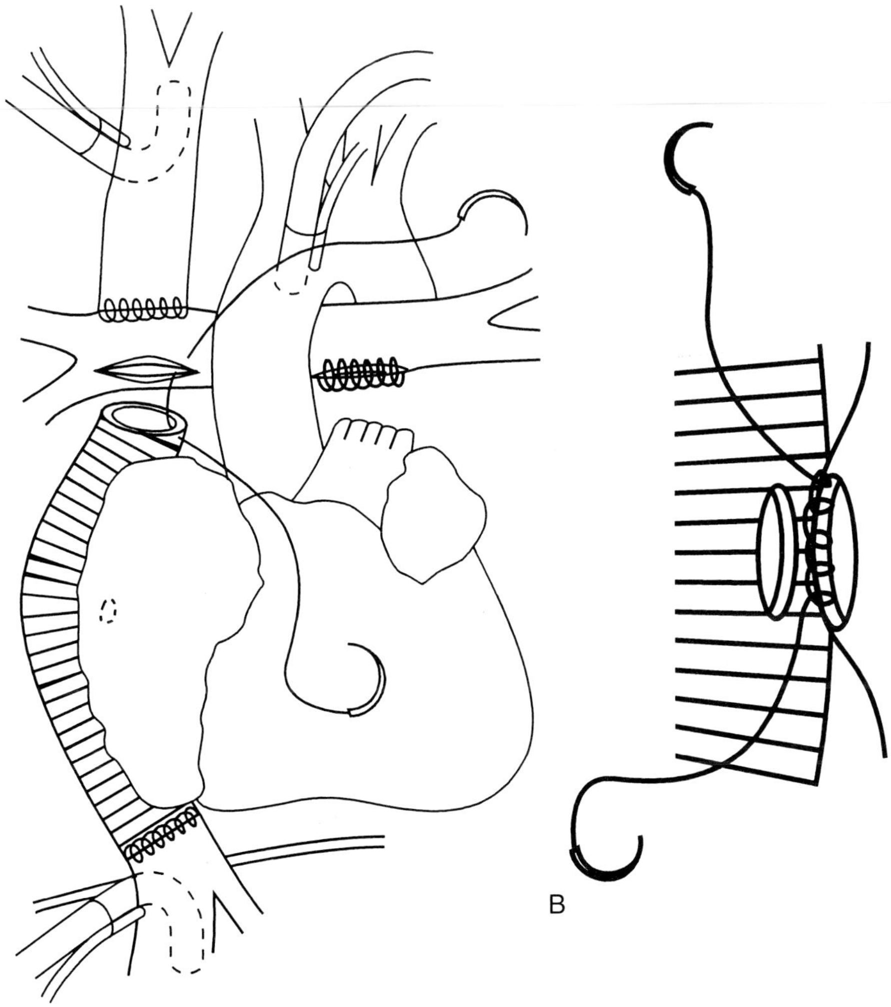

Figure 126–4 Construction of extracardiac Fontan on cardiopulmonary bypass. Cannulation for cardiopulmonary bypass is as described for the lateral tunnel Fontan operation (see Figure 126-2). It is particularly important that the inferior vena cava is cannulated low down. Any systemic-to-pulmonary artery shunts are taken down. Transection and closure of the main pulmonary artery can be facilitated by a short period of cardioplegic arrest. A needle vent is placed in the ascending aorta. The space between the right lower pulmonary vein and the inferior vena cava is dissected. The cannula in the inferior vena cava is snared and a clamp placed across the cavo-atrial junction taking care to avoid occluding the coronary sinus. **A,** The cavopulmonary junction is transected on the clamp and the cardiac end oversewn. A Gore-Tex tube of at least 16-mm diameter (22-mm diameter in adults) is anastomosed end-to-end to the transected inferior vena cava. The conduit is gently curved around the atrium toward the right pulmonary artery. The cavopulmonary shunt is temporarily occluded and the inferior surface of the right pulmonary artery incised. The top end of the prosthesis is anastomosed end-to-side to the pulmonary artery. If a fenestration is required, a side-biting clamp is placed on the free wall of the right atrium and a further clamp opposite on the prosthesis. A ~5-mm fenestration is cut in the prosthesis, and a slightly larger hole in the opposite right atrial wall. **B,** To avoid obstruction of the fenestration by atrial tissue the anastomotic suture line is placed a few millimeters away from the hole in the prosthesis.

sites of atrial reentrant circuits at the time of the initial lateral tunnel repair.[20] Another suggestion has been atrial pacing to avoid even mild degrees of atrial bradycardia to prevent prolongation of atrial refractoriness that may contribute to the development of atrial tachycardia.[86]

Collateral Circulation

Systemic venous collateral channels have been reported to occur in up to one third of patients following a cavopulmonary shunt[58,65] with communications between the higher pressure superior caval venous territory and lower pressure inferior caval veins, left atrium, or pulmonary veins. Collaterals can develop rapidly, within hours of a bidirectional cavopulmonary shunt, suggesting that they are formed by dilation of preexisting channels rather than angiogenesis.[58] Peculiar venous communications have been described in patients with isomerism of the atrial appendages after both the bilateral Glenn shunt and Fontan procedure, involving many organ systems such as liver, kidney, heart, and lungs (for review see Freedom[40]). Pulmonary atriovenous fistulae were first reported after the classic Glenn anastomosis,[67] but also occur following the bilateral cavopulmonary anastomosis and Fontan operations. Their etiology remains unclear, but exclusion of hepatic venous effluent from the pulmonary circuit may be a factor,[89] and clinically resolution of the malformations has been observed after incorporation of liver venous return in the Fontan circulation.[84] All of the above collateral channels can promote significant right-to-left shunting with resultant hypoxemia and cyanosis. Systemic-to-pulmonary collateral arteries pass from the aorta or its branches to the pulmonary vascular bed and either can be enlarged preexisting vessels or have formed de novo. These collateral vessels are common in cyanotic heart disease, and although they help increase pulmonary blood flow, significant aortopulmonary collaterals are deleterious because they act as left-to-right shunts imposing a volume load on the systemic ventricle and raising atrial pressure. This in turn increases the transpulmonary gradient and pulmonary artery pressure.

In patients with progressive cyanosis or heart failure, an aggressive search for collateral vessels should be made using cardiac catheterization and angiography followed by interruption of significant collateral channels.

Thromboembolism

Thromboembolic complications occur both early and late after the Fontan procedure. Pathway thrombosis, pulmonary artery thrombosis, and cerebral emboli or stroke may all present with clinical symptoms, but many events probably go unrecognized. The true incidence of thromboembolism is not known, but cross-sectional studies using transesophageal echocardiography have reported that 20% to 33% of patients are affected.[8,41] The etiology is multiple, including suboptimal flow patterns, arrhythmias, cyanosis, presence of foreign material in the circulation, preexistent coagulopathies, and liver dysfunction. Prophylactic long-term anticoagulation remains a contentious issue and is discussed in more detail in the following section.

Protein-Losing Enteropathy

Protein-losing enteropathy is a relatively rare but debilitating complication with a reported incidence of up to 15%. The condition involves the loss of protein within the gastrointestinal tract and can occur from weeks to years after the Fontan operation with 50% mortality at 5 years following diagnosis.[31,69] The precise reasons for its occurrence are not known, but it has been suggested that inferior vena cava hypertension causes engorgement of the liver sinusoids, thus impairing portal venous return with elevation of splanchnic venous pressure.[24] Clinical manifestations are related to the degree of hypoproteinemia and the nonselective loss of proteins may result in peripheral edema, ascites and effusions, immunodeficiency and coagulopathy. An elevated fecal alpha 1-antitrypsin level confirms enteric protein loss.[48] A detailed investigation of the cardiovascular system should take place and hemodynamics optimized if possible. This may include the creation of a fenestration, pacing, or transplantation. Symptomatic treatment is with diuretics and diet supplements. High-dose corticosteroids (1–2 mg/kg/day for a minimum of 2–3 weeks)[81] and high molecular weight heparin (5000 U/m^2/day for several weeks)[27] have been shown empirically to reduce protein loss in some patients and are thought to act through stabilizing the intestinal mucosal membrane, thus reducing the protein leak. None of the preceding treatments has been universally successful in halting protein-losing enteropathy, including—perhaps surprisingly—cardiac transplantation.[69]

Plastic Bronchitis

Plastic bronchitis is another ill-understood complication with an estimated incidence of 1% to 2%.[19] Non-inflammatory mucin-containing casts are formed in the trachea and bronchus. Symptomatic treatment is by bronchoscopic clearance. Alteration in Fontan hemodynamics may not resolve the problem. Resolution following cardiac transplantation has been reported.[40]

Pathway Problems

Complications related to the Fontan pathway are common and increase with time. In his long-term follow-up study of patients with atriopulmonary and atrioventricular connections, Fontan estimated that the freedom from reintervention for pathway problems in patients was 96%, 86%, and 59% at 5, 10, and 15 years, respectively.[34] In particular patients with a conduit placed between right atrium and right ventricle were at risk of reoperation for pathway obstruction. The recent Fontan modification involving the use of an extracardiac conduit is potentially a problem in small children because the diameter of the prosthesis may become too small with somatic growth with resultant systemic venous pathway obstruction. So far this has not been confirmed in the literature. In contrast, oversizing of the conduit has been complicated by poor hemodynamics and conduit thrombosis.[4] Baffle leaks and localized stenoses in the Fontan pathway can increasingly be managed by catheter intervention, thus avoiding reoperation in these complex cardiac patients.

Ventricular Failure

Adequate cardiac performance is a prerequisite for satisfactory function of the Fontan circulation, in particular because there is only one ventricle. There are many reasons why cardiac performance can be impaired in hearts working in a Fontan circulation. First, in some congenital abnormalities, the myocardium may be intrinsically abnormal, as has been shown for the left ventricle of hearts with pulmonary atresia and intact ventricular septum.[2] Second, the anatomical and structural characteristics of the ventricle may be inadequate for the working conditions as is suggested by the premature failure of the morphological right ventricle in the systemic

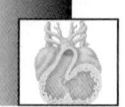

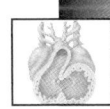

circulation following the atrial switch operation. As discussed previously, impaired ventricular function may also be related to adverse working conditions prior to the Fontan procedure such as chronic cyanosis, volume overload, subaortic stenosis, or atrioventricular valve regurgitation. Acute volume offloading at the time of the Fontan operation gives rise to a picture resembling that of hypertrophic cardiomyopathy with abnormal diastolic filling and ventricular wall motion abnormalities.[74,75] Paradoxically, at the same time the unloaded ventricle has to cope with an increased afterload because the systemic and pulmonary circulations are now in series. In a recent clinical study comparing patients with single ventricle and lateral tunnel Fontan pathway, single ventricle and Blalock-Taussig shunt, and normal two-ventricle circulation, Senzaki and colleagues[83] showed that pulsatile as well as nonpulsatile afterload was significantly higher in Fontan patients, and this was associated with decreased cardiac output. Single ventricle circulations were less energy efficient than biventricular circulations in that higher systemic ventricular power expenditure was required per unit cardiac output, and they also had less ventricular reserve capacity because of limited preload.

Preservation of ventricular function is of paramount importance for successful long-term outcome in patients with univentricular hearts. Measures to achieve this include early correction of structural abnormalities such as ventricular outflow obstruction and valvar regurgitation. The use of angiotensin-converting enzyme inhibitors has been investigated because of their beneficial effect of improving exercise capacity in adults with congestive heart failure by decreasing systemic vascular resistance and ventricular diastolic dysfunction, conditions also present in the Fontan circulation. However, a placebo-controlled, double-blind study using enalapril failed to alter elevated systemic vascular resistance, resting cardiac index, diastolic function, or exercise capacity in well-compensated patients after the Fontan procedure.[55]

MANAGEMENT OF THE FAILING FONTAN

Hemodynamic dysfunction of the Fontan circulation may be related to atrial arrhythmias, ventricular failure, structural problems, and collateral circulation, alone or in combination. Currently, most of these problems have been found in the earlier generation of Fontan patients with atriopulmonary connections that have inferior flow characteristics compared to the more recently constructed total cavopulmonary connections.

Conversion of the failing atriopulmonary Fontan to a total cavopulmonary connection with concomitant arrhythmia surgery and correction of hemodynamically significant lesions was recently introduced by Mavroudis and colleagues.[63] The group has now reported on 41 patients who underwent conversion at an average of about 11 years after their original Fontan operation.[64] There were no operative deaths, but 3 patients required transplantation at 8 days, 9 months, and 33 months. One patient died 2 years postoperatively from acute myocardial infarction. The majority of patients improved from New York Heart Association Class III to IV preoperatively to class I or II after surgery. Arrhythmia recurred in five patients, and four were on chronic antiarrhythmic treatment. The authors commented that the surgical techniques are still evolving and that the specific indications and optimal timing for the intervention were not yet known.

Significant collateral vessels can increasingly be identified in the catheter laboratory and controlled using catheter interventions (Figure 126-5). Localized stenoses in the Fontan pathway or the pulmonary arteries can be dilated and stented (Figure 126-6). Close collaboration between interventionists and surgeons is required to find the best treatment for these sick patients. If heart failure is the predominant factor in the failing Fontan, then cardiac transplantation offers the only solution. This treatment is not always successful in halting protein-losing enteropathy.[69] It is not uncommon for patients to die on the transplant waiting list.

CONTROVERSIES IN THE MANAGEMENT OF SINGLE VENTRICLE CIRCULATION

Strategies for 1-Pump, 1½-Pump, and 2-Pump Repair

For most congenitally abnormal hearts it is relatively straightforward to assess suitability for a biventricular repair. In some hearts, however, with a smaller-than-normal pulmonary ventricle, it may not be clear whether following septation the right ventricle can handle the full cardiac output. The limiting criteria for the right ventricle to successfully function as an independent pumping chamber are not strictly defined but depend on size, structure, function, and pulmonary vascular resistance. It has been suggested that in patients with pulmonary atresia and intact ventricular septum biventricular repair was likely to fail if the diameter of the tricuspid valve was below the third standard deviation of normal (z value of −3).[21] In principle, however, one would like to use the right ventricle if it still can add forward flow to the pulmonary circulation. Billingsley and colleagues[9] were the first to successfully septate these hearts and incorporate the smaller tripartite right ventricle into the circulation by adding a cavopulmonary anastomosis at the time of the repair. The principle of 1½ ventricle repair has since been extended to other abnormalities such as unbalanced atrioventricular septal defects where successful repair has been reported with right atrioventricular valve z-values as small as −10,[5] and as an adjunct to the repair of Ebstein's anomaly. D-transposition of the great arteries with VSD and small right ventricle has been repaired by arterial switch procedure and bidirectional Glenn shunt.[94] A further application has been in patients with biventricular hearts and impaired right ventricular function in which conversion to a 1½ ventricle repair was used to successfully off-load the failing right ventricle.[94]

Definitive Palliation with Fontan Versus Bidirectional Glenn Shunt with Forward Flow

Some have questioned the wisdom of a total cavopulmonary connection—especially in high-risk cases—and instead propose a bidirectional Glenn shunt with an additional source of pulmonary blood flow as definitive palliation. A recent paper from the adult congenital heart unit in Toronto reviewed the

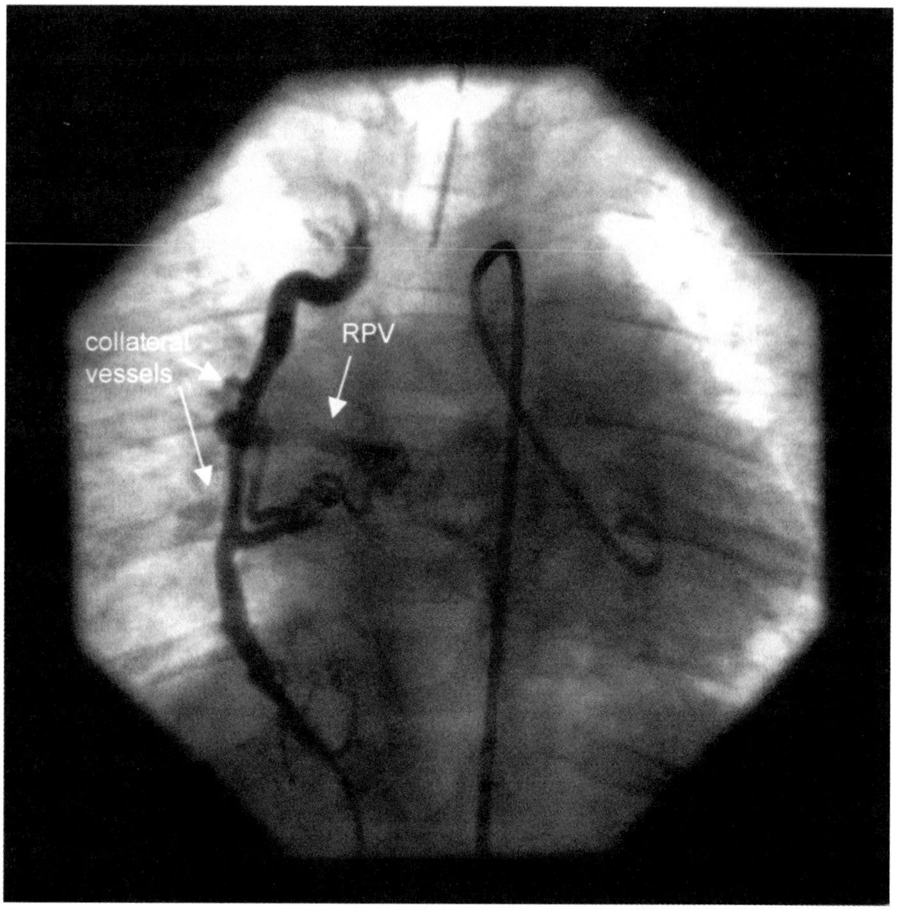

A

Figure 126–5 Occlusion of systemic to pulmonary venous collateral vessels in a patient with an extracardiac Fontan. A, Selective injection into systemic to pulmonary venous collateral vessels arising from the superior and inferior vena cava territory with contrast filling the right pulmonary vein (RPV).

outcome of 50 patients who at the time of referral had a cavopulmonary shunt, one or more aortopulmonary shunts, or both and who since had not undergone a Fontan procedure.[43] Over half of the patients had additional antegrade flow through a nondisconnected pulmonary artery trunk. Survival was 89.4% at 10 years and 51.9% at 20 years after the first clinical presentation. These results compare favorably with published Fontan series, and it was concluded that this strategy provided sustained palliation for selected patients with a single ventricle circulation. Obviously this paper reflects a different era of surgery and also is not a direct comparison with patients who underwent a Fontan strategy, but it may indicate that the Fontan route is not necessarily the universal palliation for all single ventricle circulations.

Timing and Staging of the Fontan

The ideal age for the Fontan procedure and the indications for staging the operation with a bidirectional Glenn shunt remain poorly defined. The bidirectional Glenn shunt procedure, often combined with additional reconstructive procedures, has provided excellent palliation in high-risk Fontan patients and has been useful in ameliorating risk factors for subsequent Fontan completion.[13,78] However, the routine use of staging procedures in good Fontan candidates remains open to discussion.

Increased pressure and volume load of the single ventricle, such as occurs after systemic-to-pulmonary artery shunts, is a risk factor for subsequent failure of the Fontan operation and therefore early ventricular unloading with a bidirectional Glenn shunt or Fontan procedure has been advocated. In short-term studies, regression of ventricular mass was observed in children who underwent a bidirectional Glenn shunt aged less than 3 years, but not when the procedure was performed if the child was 10 years or older.[35] Younger age at the time of bidirectional Glenn shunt or Fontan surgery was also associated with superior exercise performance compared to those in whom surgery was delayed until a later age.[59] However, the long-term outcome following establishment of an early Fontan state is not known. The unfavorable ventricular working conditions associated with the Fontan circulation and the effects of chronically elevated systemic venous pressures on the right atrium and intraabdominal organs are a case for concern.

Lateral Tunnel Versus Extracardiac Conduit

The hemodynamic superiority of cavopulmonary connections with total right heart bypass over atriopulmonary connections[24] is generally accepted, and most surgeons will now create some form of cavopulmonary connection with complete exclusion of the right heart. The lateral tunnel Fontan opti-

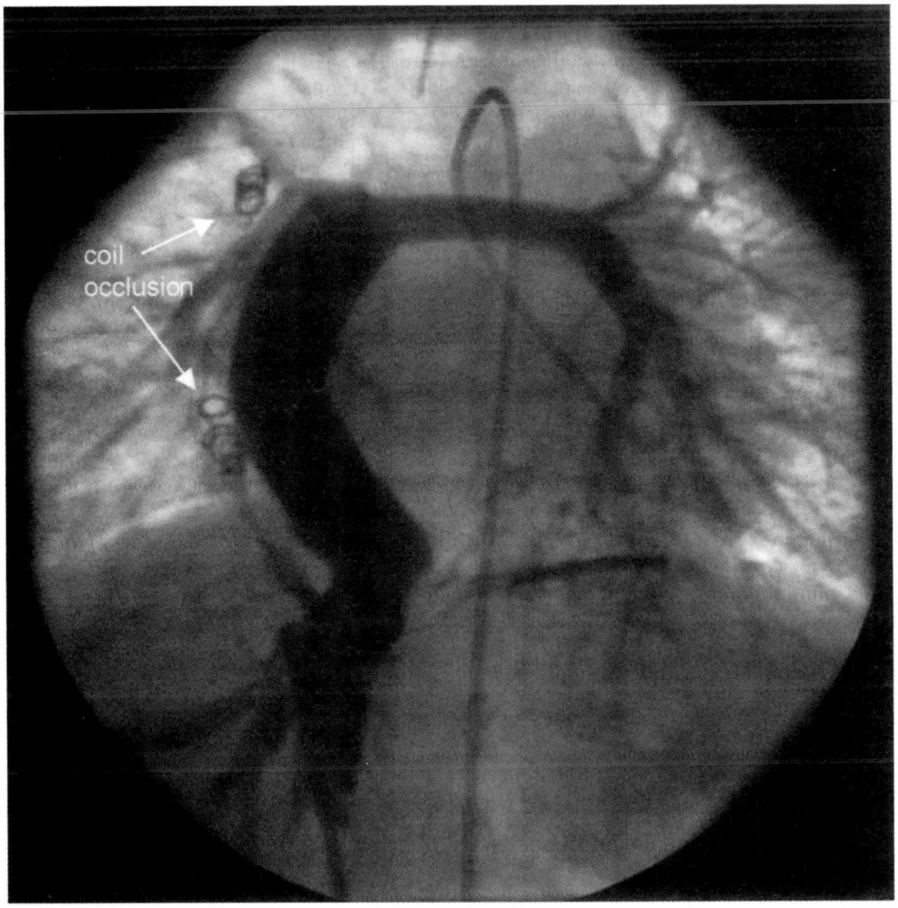

B

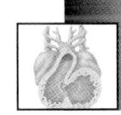

Figure 126–5 cont'd **B,** Coils have been placed in the collaterals and the pulmonary venous system no longer fills.

mizes flow dynamics in the pulmonary artery, leaves the coronary sinus in the low pressure atrium, and has a low risk of damage to the atrioventricular node. The same advantages can be attributed to the extracardiac Fontan procedure, which was originally designed to avoid pulmonary venous obstruction in patients with a small right atrium.[61] The latter procedure has the additional advantage that no intraatrial access is required and thus can be done without aortic cross-clamping and in suitable cases also without the use of cardiopulmonary bypass. In a retrospective study on 32 consecutive patients Tam and colleagues[91] reported that patients who did not go onto cardiopulmonary bypass had improved immediate postoperative hemodynamics, less use of blood products, and shorter hospital stay compared to those who underwent cardiopulmonary bypass. However, the patient groups were not comparable with regard to cardiac diagnosis and half of the patients in the cardiopulmonary bypass group underwent pulmonary artery reconstruction at the time of the Fontan operation. Another advantage of the extracardiac Fontan operation is thought to be the absence of arrhythmogenic suture lines, but bradyarrhythmias have been observed.[85] Drawbacks of the extracardiac Fontan operation include the thrombogenicity of the prosthetic conduit and lack of conduit growth, in particular with the current tendency for surgery in small children. At the age of 2–4 years and body weight of 12–15 kg, the inferior vena cava diameter and inferior vena cava-to-pulmonary artery distance are approximately 60% to 80% of adult values. Oversizing the conduit may be tempting, but has been shown to result in unfavorable Fontan hemodynamics and conduit thrombosis.[4]

Fenestrating the Fontan

The creation of a fenestration in the baffle of the Fontan circuit allows systemic venous blood to shunt to the left atrium achieving better preload for the systemic ventricle. This allows that cardiac output is maintained and limits right atrial pressure, in particular when conditions that restrict pulmonary blood flow are present. A disadvantage is the lower systemic oxygen saturation. The theoretic risk of paradoxic thromboembolism has not been confirmed.[29,57] Fenestration was first described in 1990 by Bridges et al for the high-risk Fontan patient,[14] and in a subsequent retrospective study the authors showed a significant decrease in pleural effusions and hospital stay compared to nonfenestrated patients.[15] Consequently, the fenestrated Fontan circuit has become the procedure of choice for the high-risk population. However, baffle fenestration remains controversial in standard-risk patients with a number of retrospective studies showing no benefit from fenestration,[50,92] but a decreased rate of Fontan failure and significant pleural effusions by others.[1] To help solve the issue, Lemler et al[57] carried out a prospective randomized trial and showed improved clinical outcome with less pleural drainage,

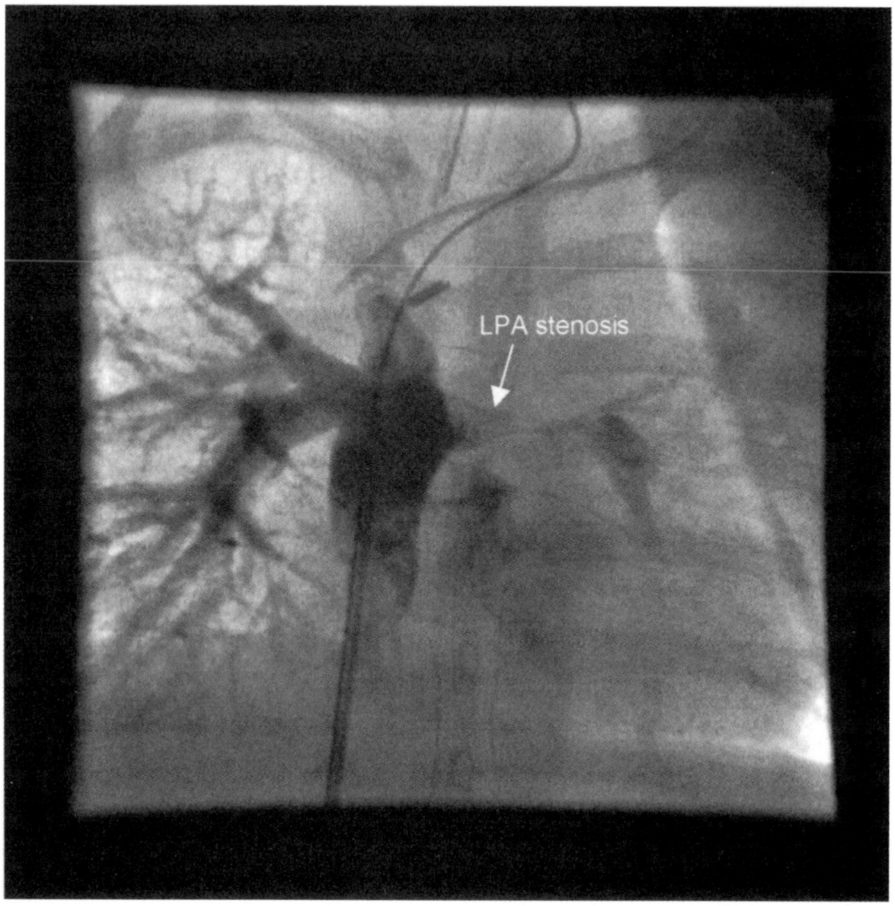

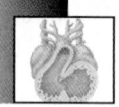

Figure 126–6 **Stenting of the left pulmonary artery in a patient with extracardiac Fontan. A,** Long-segment stenosis of the left pulmonary artery (LPA).

shorter hospital stay, and less need for additional postoperative procedures. They also reported that late fenestration in patients with persistent pleural effusions resulted in a marked clinical improvement. Interestingly, the authors commented that preoperative hemodynamic parameters were not predictive for the occurrence of postoperative effusions.

Apart from those patients in whom low saturations are a clinical indication for closure of the fenestration, it is not known whether fenestrations should be closed and if so, when. Around a third of fenestrations will close spontaneously[87] and the remainder can be relatively easily occluded by catheter intervention (see Figure 126-3). A recent follow-up of patients with a mean of 3.4 years following device closure showed improved oxygen saturation with an average increase of 9.4%, reduced need for anticongestive treatment, and improved somatic growth. Twelve percent of patients, however, had developed new arrhythmias.[45]

Prophylactic Anticoagulation

Central venous and intracardiac thrombosis, and arterial embolization to the central nervous system are an important cause of morbidity and mortality after the Fontan operation. The reported clinical incidence varies greatly, depending on outcome measure and investigations used, but has been reported up to 3% and 16% for venous thrombosis[26,80] and 3% to 19% for stroke.[29,62] The pick-up rate for thrombosis increased to 33% in cross-sectional surveys using transesophageal echocardiography.[8] The occurrence of thromboembolism was both early and late after operation at an estimated rate of 3.9 per 100 patient-years in patients not receiving anticoagulation.[80] Information on the management and outcome in the case of thromboembolism is scarce. A recent review of the literature suggests that resolution of thrombus is achieved in only 48% of cases and death occurs in 25%.[70] There is currently no agreement whether specific demographic, surgical, or hemodynamic factors predispose to thromboembolism.

The effect of prophylactic anticoagulation on the incidence of thromboembolism has not been assessed in a systematic way. The use of aspirin, warfarin, and heparin has been reported, with various dosage regimens. Thromboembolic events, however, still occurred.[70] It also has to be appreciated that anticoagulant therapy itself is not without risk. Anticoagulant-related bleeding is a cause for concern in particular in the active child and in the presence of cyanosis or heart failure when anticoagulation control may be difficult.

FUTURE DIRECTIONS

The Fontan operation has greatly improved the outcome for patients with single ventricle circulations. In the last decade important progress has been made in refining patient

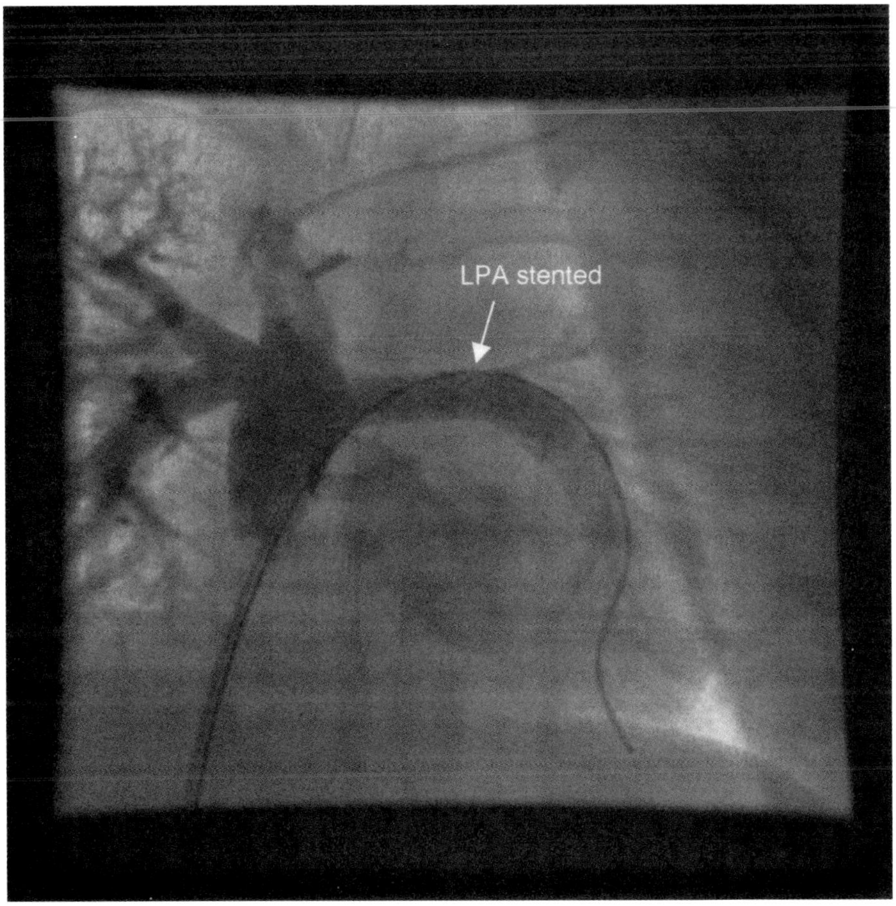

B

Figure 126–6 cont'd B, A vascular stent has been placed and the left pulmonary artery is now widely patent.

selection criteria, surgical techniques, and design of the Fontan circuit. In spite of this, our understanding of the Fontan circulation and its consequences remains limited and the late attrition of the Fontan state unexplained.

We are only just beginning to gain insight into the unique physiology associated with the Fontan state that has a decreased preload and increased afterload compared to a biventricular circulation.[83] It may be that these working conditions are ultimately detrimental to the myocardium and that entering the Fontan state starts the clock ticking toward premature cardiac failure. Conversely, it could be argued that introduction to the Fontan state at an early age may give more scope to develop adaptation mechanisms to deal with these hemodynamic challenges. To answer these questions cardiovascular interactions in the Fontan circulation need to be studied in detail, including their effects on other organ systems. This includes the state of the pulmonary vascular bed, which, although it is recognized as an important selection criterion for Fontan suitability, has not been considered in detail as a potential course for late Fontan failure. In particular the effects of long-term absence of pulsatile blood flow on the pulmonary vasculature are unknown. Finally, we have to ask ourselves whether the Fontan circulation is the universal treatment for all univentricular hearts or if some are better served by a different cardiovascular arrangement.

REFERENCES

1. Airan B, Sharma R, Choudhary SK, et al: Univentricular repair: is routine fenestration justified? Ann Thorac Surg 69:1900–1906, 2000.
2. Akiba T and Becker AE: Disease of the left ventricle in pulmonary atresia with intact ventricular septum. The limiting factor for long-lasting successful surgical intervention? J Thorac Cardiovasc Surg 108:1–8, 1994.
3. Alboliras ET, Porter CB, Danielson GK, et al: Results of the modified Fontan operation for congenital heart lesions in patients without preoperative sinus rhythm. J Am Coll Cardiol 6:228–233, 1985.
4. Alexi-Meskishvili V, Ovroutski S, Ewert P, et al: Optimal conduit size for extracardiac Fontan operation. Eur J Cardiothorac Surg 18:690–695, 2000.
5. Alvarado O, Sreeram N, McKay R, Boyd IM. Cavopulmonary connection in repair of atrioventricular septal defect with small right ventricle. Ann Thorac Surg 55:729–736, 1993.
6. Azakie A, Merklinger SL, Williams WG, et al: Improving outcomes of the Fontan operation in children with atrial isomerism and heterotaxy syndromes. Ann Thorac Surg 72:1636–1640, 2001.
7. Azzolina G, Eufrate S, Pensa P: Tricuspid atresia: experience in surgical management with a modified cavopulmonary anastomosis. Thorax 27:111–115, 1972.
8. Balling G, Vogt M, Kaemmerer H, et al: Intracardiac thrombus formation after the Fontan operation. J Thorac Cardiovasc Surg 119:745–752, 2000.

9. Billingsley AM, Laks H, Boyce SW, et al: Definitive repair in patients with pulmonary atresia and intact ventricular septum. J Thorac Cardiovasc Surg 97:746–754, 1989.
10. Bjork VO, Olin CL, Bjarke NN, Thoren CA: Right atrial-right ventricular anastomosis for correction of tricuspid atresia. J Thorac Cardiovasc Surg 77:452–458, 1979.
11. Blalock A, Taussig H: The surgical treatment of malformations of the heart in which there is pulmonary atresia. JAMA 128:189–202, 1945.
12. Bradley SM, McCall MM, Sistino JJ, Radtke WAK: Aortopulmonary collateral flow in the Fontan patient: does it matter. Ann Thorac Surg 72:408–415, 2001.
13. Bridges ND, Jonas RA, Mayer JE, et al: Bidirectional cavopulmonary anastomosis as interim palliation for high risk Fontan candidates. Early results Circulation 82(Suppl): IV170–176, 1990.
14. Bridges ND, Lock JE, Castaneda AR: Baffle fenestration with subsequent transcatheter closure: modification of the Fontan operation for patients at increased risk. Circulation 82:1681–1689, 1990.
15. Bridges ND, Mayer JE Jr., Lock JE, et al: Effect of baffle fenestration on outcome of the modified Fontan operation. Circulation 86:1762–1769, 1992.
16. Bull C, de Leval MR, Stark J, et al: Use of a subpulmonary ventricular chamber in the Fontan circulation. J Thorac Cardiovasc Surg 85:21–31, 1983.
17. Choussat A, Fontan F, Besse P, et al: Selection criteria for Fontan's procedure. In: Anderson RH, Shinebourne EA (eds): Paediatric Cardiology. Edinburgh: Churchill Livingstone, 1978, pp. 559–566.
18. Cloutier A, Ash JM, Smallhorn JF, et al: Abnormal distribution of pulmonary blood flow after the Glenn shunt or Fontan procedure: risk of development of arteriovenous fistulae. Circulation 72:471–479, 1985.
19. Colloridi V, Roggini M, Formigari R, et al: Plastic bronchitis as a rare complication of Fontan's operation. Pediatr Cardiol 11:228, 1990.
20. Deal BJ, Mavroudis C, Backer CL, et al: Comparison of anatomic isthmus block with the modified right atrial Maze procedure for late atrial tachycardia in Fontan patients. Circulation 106:575–579, 2002.
21. de Leval M, Bull C, Hopkins R, et al: Decision making in the definitive repair of the heart with a small right ventricle. Circulation 72(Suppl):II52–II60, 1985.
22. de Leval MR, Kilner P, Gewillig M, Bull C: Total cavopulmonary connection: a logical alternative to atriopulmonary connection for complex Fontan operations. J Thorac Cardiovasc Surg 96:682–695, 1988.
23. de Leval M: Right heart bypass operations. In: Stark J, de Leval M (eds): Surgery for Congenital Heart Defects, 2nd ed. Philadelphia: WB Saunders, 1994, pp. 568–569.
24. de Leval MR: The Fontan circulation: What have we learned? What to expect? Pediatr Cardiol 19:316–320, 1998.
25. Dick M, Fyler DC, Nadas AS: Tricuspid atresia: clinical course in 101 patients. Am J Cardiol 36:327–337, 1975.
26. Dobell ARC, Trusler GA, Smallhorn JF, Williams WG: Atrial thrombi after the Fontan operation. Ann Thorac Surg 42:664–667, 1986.
27. Donnelly JP, Rosenthal A, Castle VP, Holmes RD: Reversal of protein-losing enteropathy with heparin therapy in three patients with univentricular hearts and Fontan palliation. J Pediatr 130:474–478, 1997.
28. Douglas WI, Goldberg CS, Mosca RS, et al: Hemi-Fontan procedure for hypoplastic left heart syndrome: outcome and suitability for Fontan. Ann Thorac Surg 68:1361–1368, 1999.
29. du Plessis AJ, Chang AC, Wessel DL, et al: Cerebrovascular accidents following the Fontan operation. Pediatr Neurol 12:230–236, 1995.
30. Eliahou HE, Clarke SD, Bull GD: Atrial pulsation during acute distension and its possible significance in the regulation of blood volume. Clin Sci 19:377–390, 1960.
31. Feldt RH, Driscoll DJ, Offord KP, et al: Protein-losing enteropathy after Fontan operation. J Thorac Cardiovasc Surg 112:672–680, 1996.
32. Fontan F, Baudet E: Surgical repair of tricuspid atresia. Thorax 26:240–248, 1971.
33. Fontan F, Fernandez G, Costa F, et al: The size of the pulmonary arteries and the results of the Fontan operation. J Thorac Cardiovasc Surg 98:711–719, 1989.
34. Fontan F, Kirklin JW, Fernandez G, et al: Outcome after a "perfect" Fontan operation. Circulation 81:1520–1536, 1990.
35. Forbes TJ, Gajarski R, Johnson GL, et al: Influence of age on the effect of bidirectional cavopulmonary anastomosis on left ventricular volume, mass and ejection fraction. J Am Coll Cardiol 28:1301–1307, 1996.
36. Franklin RCG, Spieglhalter DJ, Anderson RH, et al: Double-inlet ventricle presenting in infancy. I. Survival without definitive repair. J Thoracic Cardiovasc Surg 101:767–776, 1991.
37. Franklin RCG, Spiegelhalter DJ, Sullivan ID, et al: Tricuspid atresia presenting in infancy: survival and suitability for the Fontan operation. Circulation 87:427–439, 1993.
38. Freedom RM: Subaortic obstruction and the Fontan operation. Ann Thorac Surg 66:649–652, 1998.
39. Freedom RM, Nykanen D, Benson LN: The physiology of the bidirectional cavopulmonary connection. Ann Thorac Surg 66:664–667, 1998.
40. Freedom RM, Hamilton R, Yoo S-J, et al: The Fontan procedure: analysis of cohorts and late complications. Cardiol Young 10:307–331, 2000.
41. Fyfe DA, Kline CH, Sade RM, Gillette PC: Transesophageal echocardiography detects thrombus formation not identified by transthoracic echocardiography after the Fontan operation. J Am Coll Cardiol 18:1733–1737, 1991.
42. Gago O, Salles CA, Stern AM, et al: A different approach for the total correction of tricuspid atresia. J Thorac Cardiovasc Surg 72:209–214, 1976.
43. Gatzoulis MA, Munk MD, Williams WG, Webb GD: Definitive palliation with cavopulmonary or aortopulmonary shunts for adults with single ventricle physiology. Heart 83:51–57, 2000.
44. Glenn WW, Patino JF: Circulatory bypass of the right heart. Preliminary observations on the direct delivery of vena caval blood into the pulmonary arterial circulation: azygos vein pulmonary artery shunt. Yale J Biol Med 24:147, 1954.
45. Goff DA, Blume ED, Gauvreau K, et al: Clinical outcome of fenestrated Fontan patients after closure. The first 10 years. Circulation 102:2094–2099, 2000.
46. Haas GS, Hess H, Black M, et al: Extracardiac conduit Fontan procedure: early and intermediate results. Eur J Cardiothorac Surg 17:648–654, 2000.
47. Harake B, Kuhn MA, Jarmakani JM, et al: Acute hemodynamic effects of adjustable atrial septal defect closure in the lateral tunnel Fontan procedure. J Am Coll Cardiol 23:1671–1676, 1994.
48. Hill RE, Hercz A, Corey ML, et al: Fecal clearance of alpha 1-antitrypsin: A reliable measure of enteric protein loss in children. J Pediatr 99:416–418, 1981.
49. Hislop A, Reid L: Development of the acinus in the human lung. Thorax 29:90–94, 1974.
50. Hsu DT, Quaegebeur JM, Ing FF, et al: Outcome after the single-stage, nonfenestrated Fontan. Circulation 96(Suppl):II335–340, 1997.
51. Jacobs ML, Mayer JE Jr: Congenital Heart Surgery Nomenclature and Database Project: Single Ventricle. Ann Thorac Surg 69(Suppl):S197–204, 2000.

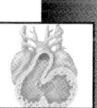

52. Kanter KR, Vincent RN, Raviele AA. Importance of acquired systemic-to-pulmonary artery collaterals in the Fontan operation. Ann Thorac Surg 68:969–974, 1999.
53. Kirklin JK, Blackstone EH, Kirklin JW, et al: The Fontan operation. Ventricular hypertrophy, age, and date of operation as risk factors. J Thorac Cardiovasc Surg 92:1049–1064, 1986.
54. Knott-Craig CJ, Julsrud PR, Schaff HV, et al: Pulmonary artery size and clinical outcome after the modified Fontan operation. Ann Thorac Surg 55:646–651, 1993.
55. Kouatli AA, Garcia JA, Zellers TM, et al: Enalapril does not enhance exercise capacity in patients after Fontan procedure. Circulation 96:1507–1512, 1997.
56. Kreutzer G, Galindez E, Bono H, et al: An operation for the correction of tricuspid atresia. J Thorac Cardiovasc Surg 66:613–621, 1973.
57. Lemler MS, Scott WA, Leonard SR, et al: Fenestration improves clinical outcome of the Fontan procedure: a prospective, randomized study. Circulation 105:207–212, 2002.
58. Magee AG, McCrindle BW, Benson LN, et al: Systemic venous collaterals after the bidirectional cavopulmonary anastomosis. Prevalence and predictors. J Am Coll Cardiol 32:502–508, 1998.
59. Mahle WT, Wernovsky G, Bridges N, et al: Impact of early ventricular unloading on exercise performance in preadolescents with single ventricle Fontan physiology. J Am Coll Cardiol 34:1637–1643, 1999.
60. Mair DD, Hagler DJ, Julsrud PR, et al: Early and late results of the modified Fontan procedure for double-inlet left ventricle: the Mayo Clinic experience. J Am Coll Cardiol 18:1727–1732, 1991.
61. Marcelletti C, Corno A, Giannico S, Marino B: Inferior vena cavopulmonary artery extracardiac conduit: a new form of right heart bypass. J Thoracic Cardiovasc Surg 100:228–232, 1990.
62. Mathews K, Bale J, Clark E, et al: Cerebral infarction complicating Fontan surgery for cyanotic congenital heart disease. Pediatr Cardiol 7:161–166, 1986.
63. Mavroudis C, Backer SL, Deal BJ, Johnsrude CL: Fontan conversion to cavopulmonary connection and arrhythmia circuit cryoablation. J Thorac Cardiovasc Surg 115:547–556, 1998.
64. Mavroudis C, Deal BJ, Backer CL: The beneficial effects of total cavopulmonary conversion and arrhythmia surgery for the failed Fontan. Semin Thorac Cardiovasc Surg Pediatr Card Surg Annu 5:12–24, 2002.
65. McElhinney DB, Reddy VM, Hanley FL, Moore P: Systemic venous collateral channels causing desaturation after bidirectional cavopulmonary anastomosis: evaluation and management. J Am Coll Cardiol 30:817–824, 1997.
66. McElhinney DB, Petrossian E, Reddy VM, Hanley FL. Extracardiac conduit Fontan procedure without cardiopulmonary bypass. Ann Thorac Surg 66:1826–1828, 1998.
67. McFaul RC, Tajik AJ, Mair DD, et al: Development of pulmonary arteriovenous shunt after superior vena cava-right pulmonary artery (Glenn) anastomosis. Report of four cases. Circulation 55:212–216, 1977.
68. McKay R, de Leval MR, Rees P, et al: Postoperative angiographic assessment of modified Blalock-Taussig shunts using expanded polytetrafluoroethylene (Gore-Tex). Ann Thorac Surg 30:137–145, 1980.
69. Mertens L, Hagler DJ, Sauer U, et al: Protein-losing enteropathy after the Fontan operation: An international multicenter study. PLE Study Group. J Thorac Cardiovasc Surg 115:1063–1073, 1998.
70. Monagle P, Cochrane A, McCrindle B, et al: Thromboembolic complications after Fontan procedures—The role of prophylactic anticoagulation (editorial). J Thorac Cardiovasc Surg 115:493–498, 1998.
71. Moodie DS, Ritter DG, Tajik AJ, et al: Long-term follow-up in the unoperated univentricular heart. Am J Cardiol 53:1124–1128, 1984.
72. Nakata S, Imai Y, Takanashi Y, et al: A new method for the quantitative standardization of cross-sectional areas of the pulmonary arteries in congenital heart diseases with decreased pulmonary blood flow. J Thorac Cardiovasc Surg 88:610–619, 1984.
73. Pearl JM, Laks H, Drinkwater DC, et al: Modified Fontan procedure in patients less than 4 years of age. Circulation 86(Suppl):II100–105, 1992.
74. Penny DJ, Rigby ML, Redington AN: Abnormal patterns of intraventricular flow and diastolic filling after the Fontan operation: evidence for incoordinate ventricular wall motion. Br Heart J 66:375–378, 1991.
75. Penny DJ, Lincoln C, Shore DF, et al: The early response of the systemic ventricle during transition to the Fontan circulation—an acute hypertrophic cardiomyopathy? Cardiol Young 2:78–84, 1992.
76. Piehler JM, Danielson GK, McGoon DC, et al: Management of pulmonary atresia with ventricular septal defect and hypoplastic pulmonary arteries by right ventricular outflow construction. J Thorac Cardiovasc Surg 80:552–567, 1980.
77. Potts W, Smith S, Gobson S: Anastomosis of aorta to pulmonary artery. Certain types in congenital heart disease. JAMA 132:627–631, 1946.
78. Pridjian AK, Mendelsohn AM, Lupinetti FM, et al: Usefulness of the bidirectional Glenn procedure as staged reconstruction for the functional single ventricle. Am J Cardiol 71:959–962, 1993.
79. Reddy VM, McElhinney DB, Moore P, et al: Pulmonary artery growth after bidirectional cavopulmonary shunt: is there a cause for concern? J Thorac Cardiovasc Surg 112:1180–1192, 1996.
80. Rosenthal D, Friedman AH, Kleinman S, et al: Thromboembolic complications after Fontan operation. Circulation 92(Suppl):II287–293, 1995.
81. Rychik J, Piccoli DA, Barber G: Usefulness of corticosteroid therapy for protein-losing enteropathy after the Fontan surgery. Am J Cardiol 68:819–821, 1991.
82. Seliem M, Muster AJ, Paul MH, Benson DW Jr.: Relation between preoperative left ventricular muscle mass and outcome of the Fontan procedure in patients with tricuspid atresia. J Am Coll Cardiol 14:750–755, 1989.
83. Senzaki H, Masutani S, Kobayashi J, et al: Ventricular afterload and ventricular work in Fontan circulation: Comparison with normal two-ventricle circulation and single-ventricle circulation with Blalock-Taussig shunts. Circulation 105:2885–2892, 2002.
84. Shah MJ, Rychik J, Fogel MA, et al: Pulmonary AV malformations after superior cavopulmonary connection: resolution after inclusion of hepatic veins in the pulmonary circulation [comment]. Ann Thorac Surg 63:960–963, 1997.
85. Shirai LK, Rosenthal DN, Reitz BA, et al: Arrhythmias and thromboembolic complications after the extracardiac Fontan operation. J Thorac Cardiovasc Surg 115:499–505, 1998.
86. Silka MJ, Manwill JR, Kron J, McAnulty JH: Bradycardia-mediated tachyarrhythmias in congenital heart disease and responses to chronic pacing at physiologic rates. Am J Cardiol 65:488–493, 1990.
87. Sommer RJ, Recto M, Golinko RJ, Griepp RB: Transcatheter coil occlusion of surgical fenestration after Fontan operation. Circulation 94:249–252, 1996.
88. Stamm C, Friehs I, Mayer JE, et al: Long-term results of the lateral tunnel Fontan operation. J Thorac Cardiovasc Surg 121:28–41, 2001.
89. Srivastava D, Preminger TJ, Lock JE, et al: Hepatic venous blood and the development of pulmonary arteriovenous

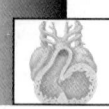

malformations in congenital heart disease. Circulation 92:1217–1222, 1995.

90. Tam CKH, Lightfoot NE, Finlay CD, et al: Course of tricuspid atresia in the Fontan era. Am J Cardiol 63:589–593, 1989.
91. Tam VKH, Miller BE, Murphy K: Modified Fontan without use of cardiopulmonary bypass. Ann Thorac Surg 68:1698–1703, 1999.
92. Thompson LD, Petrossian E, McElhinney DB, et al: Is it necessary to routinely fenestrate an extracardiac Fontan? J Am Coll Cardiol 34:539–544, 1999.
93. Triedman JK, Bridges ND, Mayer JE Jr, Lock JE: Prevalence and risk factors for aortopulmonary collateral vessels after Fontan and bidirectional Glenn procedures. J Am Coll Cardiol 22:207–215, 1993.
94. Van Arsdell GS, Williams WG, Maser CM, et al: Superior vena cava to pulmonary artery anastomosis: an adjunct to biventricular repair. J Thorac Cardiovasc Surg 112:1143–1149, 1996.
95. Van Arsdell GS, McCrindle BW, Einarson KD, et al: Interventions associated with minimal Fontan mortality. Ann Thorac Surg 70:568–574, 2000.
96. van de Wal HJCM, Oukine R, Tamisier D, et al: Bi-directional cavopulmonary shunt: is accessory pulsatile blood flow good or bad? Eur J Cardiothorac Surg 16:104–110, 1999.
97. Waldman JD, Lamberti JJ, George L, et al: Experience with Damus procedure. Circulation 78(suppl):III32–39, 1988.
98. Waterston DJ: Treatment of Fallot's tetralogy in children under 1 year of age. Rozhl Chir 41:181, 1962.
99. Yetman AT, Drummond-Webb J, Fiser WP, et al: The extracardiac Fontan procedure without cardiopulmonary bypass: technique and intermediate-term results. Ann Thorac Surg 74(Suppl):S1416–1421, 2002.

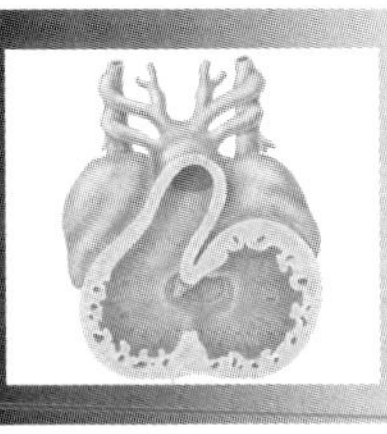

CHAPTER 127

Ebstein's Anomaly

Joseph A. Dearani and Gordon K. Danielson

Historical Aspects
Embryology and Pathological Anatomy
Pathological Physiology
Clinical Features
Diagnosis
- Electrocardiography
- Roentgenography
- Echocardiography
- Cardiac Catheterization
- Angiography

Electrophysiological Evaluation
Treatment
Indications for Operation
Operative Management
Clinical Data
Results

HISTORICAL ASPECTS

In 1866, a young physician in Breslau, Poland, Dr. Wilhelm Ebstein, described the unusual cardiac findings of a 19-year-old laborer who had died of cyanotic heart disease.[13] The anterior leaflet of the tricuspid valve was enlarged and fenestrated. There was a downward displacement of the posterior and septal leaflets in a spiral fashion below the true annulus; the leaflets were hypoplastic, thickened, and adherent to the wall of the right ventricle. The atrialized portion of the ventricle was thinned and dilated, the right atrium was enlarged, and an open foramen ovale was present.[28,35]

In addition to describing the characteristic anatomical findings in this anomaly, Dr. Ebstein accurately described the hemodynamic abnormalities and correlated them with the patient's cardiomegaly, pulsating jugular veins, and cardiac murmurs. His comprehensive report included two excellent full-size illustrations. During his lifetime, Dr. Ebstein was praised for other contributions he made to pathology and medicine, but his students and colleagues overlooked his classic description of the congenital cardiac anomaly with which his name is identified today.[28]

EMBRYOLOGY AND PATHOLOGICAL ANATOMY

The exact embryology of Ebstein's anomaly is unknown. The leaflets and the tensor apparatus of the tricuspid valve are thought to be formed at a relatively late stage in cardiac development by a process of delamination of the inner layers of the inlet zone of the right ventricle.[25,29] In Ebstein's anomaly, the insertions of the septal and posterior leaflets (and occasionally the right lateral aspect of the anterior leaflet) are displaced to the junction of the inlet and trabecular components of the ventricle, suggesting failure of delamination of these leaflets.[3] In some hearts, the endocardium is thickened and white, suggesting formation of the valve leaflets had begun but then ceased before full leaflet development and delamination had occurred. The broad spectrum of pathological changes seen in Ebstein's anomaly suggests that the mechanisms responsible for leaflet formation and right ventricular development are complex and probably related, in part, to hemodynamic forces.[3]

Ebstein's anomaly is a malformation of the tricuspid valve and right ventricle that is characterized by a spectrum of several features that include (1) adherence of the tricuspid leaflets to the underlying myocardium (failure of delamination); (2) downward (apical) displacement of the functional annulus (septal > posterior > anterior); (3) dilation of the "atrialized" portion of the right ventricle with variable degrees of hypertrophy and thinning of the wall; (4) redundancy, fenestrations, and tethering of the anterior leaflet; and (5) dilation of the right atrioventricular junction (true tricuspid annulus) (Figure 127-1).

With increasing degrees of anatomical severity of malformation, the fibrous transformation of leaflets from their muscular precursors remains incomplete, with the septal leaflet being the most severely involved and the anterior leaflet being the least severely involved. This results in a downward displacement of the hinge point of the posterior and septal leaflets in a spiral fashion below the true annulus. The tricuspid leaflets are usually bizarre and dysplastic, and are tethered by short chordae and papillary muscles or attached to the underlying myocardium directly by muscular bands. Chordae may be few to absent and leaflet fenestrations are common. The spectrum of severity is variable and no two hearts with the malformation are exactly alike. In the most severe cases, the septal leaflet is only a ridge of fibrous tissue that originates below the membranous septum and is directed toward the apex. There are varying degrees of delamination of all three leaflets. Although the anterior leaflet is the most likely to have some degree of delamination, it may also be severely deformed so that the only mobile leaflet tissue is displaced into the right ventricular outflow tract.

The malformed tricuspid valve is usually incompetent, but it may occasionally be stenotic or, rarely, imperforate.

In less severe cases, the anterior leaflet may form a large sail-like intracavitary curtain; this structure forms the basis

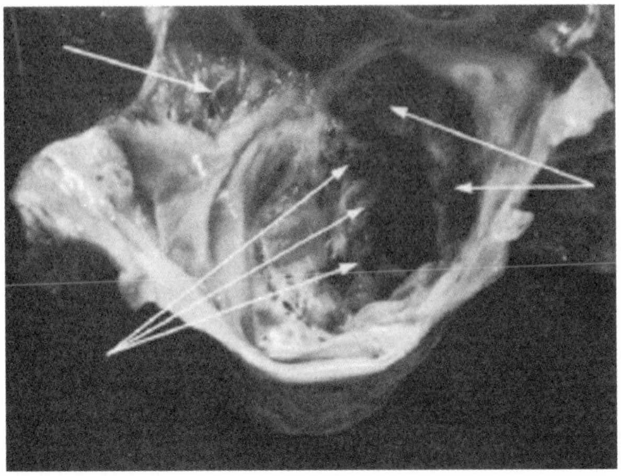

Figure 127–1 Ebstein's anomaly in a 9-day-old infant. View from the right atrium. The pathology is very similar to the original heart described by Ebstein. The single arrow indicates a patent foramen ovale. The anterior leaflet is enlarged and hooded *(double arrow)*. The posterior and septal leaflets are dysplastic and displaced in a spiral fashion toward the apex of the right ventricle *(triple arrow)*.
(Courtesy of William D. Edwards, M.D.)

of tricuspid valve repairs. A little-mentioned characteristic of the anterior leaflet that is critical to most tricuspid valve repairs is the presence of a free leading edge. The leading edge of the anterior leaflet can be free and mobile (no attachments to underlying endocardium), have hyphenated attachments (focal, segmental direct attachments to the underlying endocardium), or linear direct attachment (entire leading edge is attached to the endocardium).[26] In each case, there can be partial or complete delamination of the remaining portion of the leaflet. In the absence of a free leading edge, suboptimal repairs have been achieved.

The atrialized ventricle is characteristically thinned and dilated, but careful observation shows that the entire wall of the right ventricle, both proximal and distal to the abnormal insertion of the tricuspid leaflets, including the infundibulum, is also dilated. Dilation of the right ventricular wall is associated not only with thinning of the wall, but also with an absolute decrease in the number of myocardial fibers.[1] The atrioventricular node is located at the apex of the triangle of Koch, and the conduction system is in its normal position. Atrial septal defect and other associated anomalies are common.

In those congenital cardiac anomalies in which there is situs solitus and atrioventricular discordance with ventriculoarterial discordance (corrected transposition), Ebstein's anomaly of the left-sided (systemic, morphologically tricuspid) atrioventricular valve is a common finding. The nature of the displacement of the septal and posterior leaflets in left-sided Ebstein's anomaly is similar to that in the right-sided form, but the anterior leaflet is smaller and anatomically different.[2] Other differences relate to the functional portion of the morphologically right ventricle, which is rarely dilated in young patients, and the atrialized portion of the ventricle, which has less thinning of the wall. The atrioventricular conduction tissue in corrected transposition is right-sided and anterior, at a distance from the left-sided tricuspid valve.[4]

PATHOLOGICAL PHYSIOLOGY

The functional impairment of the right ventricle and the incompetence of the deformed tricuspid valve retard forward flow of blood through the right side of the heart. Moreover, during contraction of the atrium, the atrialized portion of the right ventricle is in diastole and balloons out (if very thin) or acts as a passive reservoir, decreasing the volume to be ejected; during ventricular systole it contracts, creating a pressure wave that impedes venous filling of the right atrium, which is in the diastolic phase. In most cases, there is a communication between the left and right atria, either due to patency of the foramen ovale caused by stretching of the atrial septum or because a distinct secundum atrial septal defect is present. The shunt of blood through the septal opening is generally from right to left but may be from left to right in some patients. The overall effect of these structural abnormalities on the right atrium is to produce gross dilation, which may reach enormous proportions, even in infancy. This dilation leads to further incompetence of the tricuspid valve and further widening of the interatrial communication. In older children and adults, significant hypertrophy of the right atrial wall is also usually present.

As a consequence of atrial dilation, atrial tachyarrhythmias are common, especially in older patients. Additionally, approximately 15% of patients will have one or more accessory conduction pathways associated with Wolff-Parkinson-White syndrome, and 1% to 2% of patients will have atrioventricular nodal reentrant tachycardia (AVNRT).[18] In end-stage heart failure, ventricular arrhythmias are common.

CLINICAL FEATURES

Ebstein's anomaly is a rare cardiac anomaly that accounts for less than 1% of all congenital heart disease. It involves both sexes nearly equally. Although a few patients reach advanced age, life expectancy for most is limited. The most common causes of death are congestive heart failure, hypoxia, and cardiac arrhythmias. When the diagnosis of Ebstein's anomaly is made in infancy, the prognosis is less favorable; one third to one half of the patients will die before 2 years of age.[16,24] When Ebstein's anomaly is diagnosed in utero by fetal echocardiography, the prognosis is even worse.[7]

Because a broad spectrum of pathological changes occurs in Ebstein's anomaly, the hemodynamic alterations vary. Symptoms are related to the severity of tricuspid regurgitation, the presence or absence of an associated atrial septal defect, the impairment of right ventricular function, and the presence of associated cardiac anomalies.

In the early neonatal period, any tricuspid regurgitation is accentuated by the normally occurring elevated pulmonary arteriolar resistance, and infants with Ebstein's anomaly may develop severe heart failure. Because the foramen ovale is patent in early infancy, severe tricuspid regurgitation, with its resultant elevation of right atrial pressure, will produce a right-to-left atrial–level shunt, and afflicted infants may be deeply cyanotic. If the infant survives this critical period, the degree of cyanosis and the symptoms often diminish as the fetal pulmonary hypertension regresses.

In older patients, the predominant symptoms are fatigability, dyspnea on exertion, and cyanosis. Palpitations in the form of paroxysmal atrial arrhythmias and premature ventricular beats are common. Less frequently, ascites and peripheral edema are present.

In an experience with 67 patients with Ebstein's anomaly and no surgical treatment who had a mean follow-up of 12 years, Giuliani and associates[16] found that 39% remained in New York Heart Association (NYHA) functional Class I or II and 61% progressed at some time into Class III or IV. Death occurred in 21% of the patients, who were characterized by one or more of the following features: (1) they were in functional Class III or IV; (2) the cardiothoracic ratio was greater than 0.65; (3) they had cyanosis or an arterial oxygen saturation of less than 90%; or (4) they were infants when the diagnosis was made.

The physical signs vary. Heart sounds are usually soft, and a multiplicity of sounds and murmurs are often heard, all originating from the right side of the heart. A systolic murmur of tricuspid regurgitation may be heard along the left sternal border. Low-intensity diastolic and presystolic murmurs, which result from anatomical or functional tricuspid stenosis, may be present; they characteristically become louder with inspiration. There is wide splitting of both the first and second heart sounds. Atrial and ventricular filling sounds are relatively common and contribute to the cadence quality that is so often found in patients with Ebstein's anomaly. Summation of these gallop sounds may result from prolongation of atrioventricular conduction.

The arterial and jugular venous pulse forms are usually normal. A large V wave can sometimes be seen in the jugular venous pulse, but this is not usual. The liver may be palpably enlarged, but it is almost never pulsatile.

DIAGNOSIS

Electrocardiography

The electrocardiogram is usually abnormal, but it is not diagnostic. Complete or incomplete right bundle branch block and right-axis deviation are typically present. The P waves are large, and the R waves in leads V1 to V2 are small. The PR interval is often prolonged, and the QRS complex is slurred. Arrhythmias are common. Ventricular preexcitation (Wolff-Parkinson-White [WPW] syndrome) is encountered in approximately 15% of patients and is almost always of the right ventricular free wall or posterior septal type; a broad band or multiple pathways may be identified at intraoperative electrophysiological mapping.[40] In addition, AVNRT is found in 1% to 2% of patients.[18]

Roentgenography

The cardiac silhouette may vary from almost normal to the typical configuration, which consists of a globular-shaped heart with a narrow waist similar to that seen with pericardial effusion. This appearance is produced by enlargement of the right atrium and displacement of the right ventricular outflow tract outward and upward. Vascularity of the pulmonary fields is either normal or decreased.

Echocardiography

Two-dimensional echocardiography has revolutionized the diagnosis of Ebstein's anomaly. Enough anatomical and hemodynamic details can be obtained by an experienced echocardiographer that cardiac catheterization and angiography are usually unnecessary. Echocardiography allows an accurate evaluation of the tricuspid leaflets and subvalvar apparatus (displacement, tethering, dysplasia, absence), the size of the right atrium including the atrialized portion of the right ventricle, and the size and function of the right and left ventricles. Doppler echocardiography and color-flow imaging allow detection of an atrial septal defect and the direction of shunt flow. The principle echocardiographic characteristic that differentiates Ebstein's anomaly from other forms of congenital tricuspid regurgitation is the degree of apical displacement of the septal leaflet at the crux of the heart ($\geq$0.8 cm/m^2).[37] In addition, color-flow imaging allows assessment of the site and degree of tricuspid valve regurgitation.[32] Echocardiography provides the best method for assessing which patients are amenable to a valve repair and which will require tricuspid valve replacement[38] (Figure 127-2). Factors that are favorable for valve repair include a large, mobile anterior leaflet with a free leading edge. Significant leaflet tethering and the presence of tricuspid leaflet tissue in the right ventricular outflow tract make successful valve repair unlikely.

Cardiac Catheterization

The right atrial pressure is usually moderately elevated, and the pulse contour may show a dominant V wave with a steep Y descent. However, in patients with a greatly dilated right atrium, the atrial pressure pulse may be normal despite the presence of severe tricuspid regurgitation. Right ventricular pressure is most often normal, although the end-diastolic pressure may be elevated. Pulmonary arterial pressure is normal or decreased. In patients with an associated atrial septal defect and right-to-left shunt, oximetry shows systemic arterial desaturation, and intracardiac dye-dilution curves from the venae cavae confirm the shunt. A minority of cases has a left-to-right shunt through an atrial septal defect, which can be shown by oximetry and dye-dilution curves.

Angiography

Injection of contrast medium into the right atrium shows enlargement of this chamber and normal position of the tricuspid annulus. An indentation on the inferior wall of the right ventricle some distance to the left of the tricuspid annulus represents the site of origin of the displaced leaflets of the tricuspid valve. The leaflets sometimes appear as radiolucent lines laterally and superiorly within the body of the right ventricle. Contrast medium often moves back and forth between the right atrium and the right ventricle, and right-to-left shunting at the atrial level may be found in the presence of an atrial septal defect or a patent foramen ovale. Flow through the right side of the heart and lungs is slow.

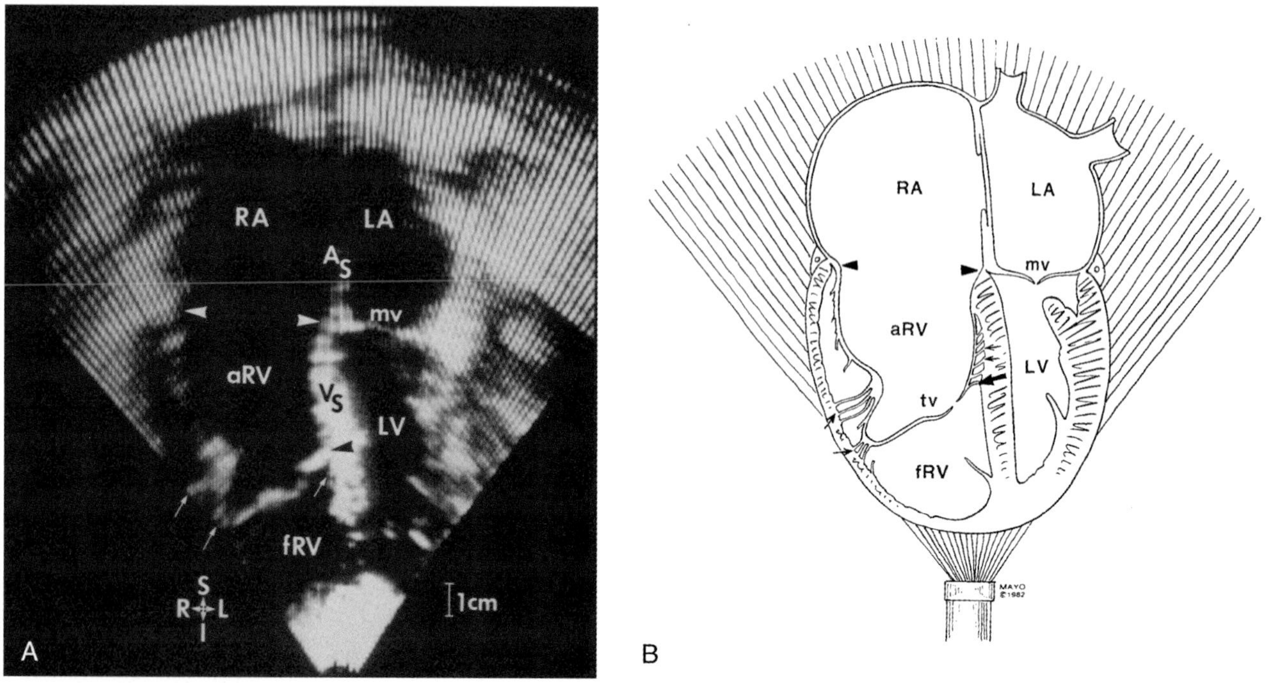

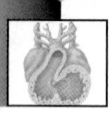

Figure 127–2 Two-dimensional echocardiogram (four-chamber view) (A) and interpretive diagram (B), showing features typical of Ebstein's anomaly. RA, Right atrium; LA, left atrium; mv, mitral valve; LV, left ventricle; fRV, functional right ventricle; tv, tricuspid valve; aRV, atrialized right ventricle; A_s, atrial septum; V_s, ventricular septum; arrows, tethering of leaflets. *(From Shiina A, Seward JB, Edwards WD, et al: Two-dimensional echocardiographic spectrum of Ebstein's anomaly: Detailed anatomic assessment. J Am Coll Cardiol 3:356–370, 1984.)*

Currently, cardiac catheterization is rarely done unless associated lesions are present or a previous shunt has been performed. In the latter case, angiography is desirable to define areas of pulmonary artery distortion, and angiography may also be helpful to assess patients with suspected pulmonary artery hypoplasia.

ELECTROPHYSIOLOGICAL EVALUATION

Atrial and ventricular arrhythmias are common in patients with Ebstein's anomaly; they often present therapeutic problems and may eventuate in sudden death, a common mode of mortality. Twenty-four hour ambulatory electrocardiographic monitoring is suggested for rhythm assessment in patients with palpitations or tachycardia. Invasive electrophysiological study is performed for all patients with Ebstein's anomaly who have preexcitation on their electrocardiogram or who have a history of recurrent supraventricular tachycardia, undefined wide-complex tachycardia, or syncope as aspects of their clinical presentation.[18]

TREATMENT

Medical management has little to offer patients with Ebstein's anomaly, except for management of fluid retention and some arrhythmias. The prognosis is poorest for NYHA classes III and IV patients and for those who have congestive heart failure, marked cyanosis, associated cardiac anomalies, significant cardiomegaly (cardiothoracic ratio greater than 0.65), and diagnosis of the condition in infancy.[16,24] Serious cardiac arrhythmias without congestive failure or hypoxemia may also be life-threatening.

Surgical attempts to treat Ebstein's anomaly began in the 1950s with the use of systemic-to-pulmonary artery shunts for relief of cyanosis. For the minority of patients with obstruction of blood flow through the right heart caused by pulmonary valvular or subvalvular stenosis or a stenotic or imperforate tricuspid valve, a shunt in infancy could be lifesaving. In the absence of obstructing lesions, systemic-pulmonary shunts have usually not benefited patients or have ended fatally.

A superior vena cava-right pulmonary artery (classic Glenn) shunt was proposed as a more physiological means of improving oxygenation; with this, approximately one third of the unoxygenated venous return would be diverted away from the right side of the heart and directly into the pulmonary circulation. In a collected series of 36 cases of vena cava-pulmonary artery shunts performed for this anomaly, 17 patients survived the operation and 14 were benefited by it.[17]

The first direct surgical approach to Ebstein's anomaly was made by Wright and his colleagues[44] in 1954. A single suture was taken in the atrial septum in an attempt to close a patent foramen ovale. The patient survived, but a residual shunt at the atrial level was demonstrated.

Reconstruction of the deformed tricuspid valve, directed toward total correction of the hemodynamic abnormality, began in 1958, when Hunter and Lillehei attempted to create a competent valve by repositioning the displaced posterior and septal leaflets.[21] Their method, employed in two patients, also entailed excluding the atrialized ventricular chamber. Both patients developed heart block and neither survived.[27] Later, Hardy and his colleagues[20] revived and modified the Hunter-Lillehei operation. They placed interrupted sutures close together on the spiral line of the displaced posterior and septal cusp bases and wider apart in the annulus. Tying of the sutures created multiple tucks in the leaflets, narrowing the tricuspid orifice somewhat, and pulled the displaced leaflets back to the tricuspid annulus. The technique was utilized in six patients, four of whom survived; one of the survivors had complete heart block.[19] Although some good early results have been reported with this procedure, it has not been generally effective in establishing a competent valve in the moderate and severe forms of Ebstein's anomaly. With suture placement in the septum as originally shown, heart block may occur. Moreover, it is not possible to transpose the septal leaflet and medial portions of the posterior leaflet to the tricuspid annulus because the ventricular septum cannot be plicated in the same way as the free wall of the right ventricle. Finally, direct approximation of the displaced leaflet to the tricuspid annulus along the free wall does not obliterate the atrialized ventricle, which protrudes below the heart as an aneurysmal sac and, despite efforts to the contrary, usually remains in communication with the right ventricle.

Replacement of the deformed tricuspid valve with a mechanical prosthetic valve was done successfully in two patients by Barnard and Schrire[5] in 1963. In their technique, the sutures anchoring the prosthesis were deviated cephalad to the coronary sinus and atrioventricular node to avoid injuring the conduction system. With the sutures thus placed, blood from the coronary sinus drained directly into the right ventricle. The atrialized portion of the ventricle was not obliterated.

In 1967, Lillehei replaced the tricuspid valve with a Starr-Edwards ball valve in five patients.[27] In two patients, the prosthetic valve was sutured to the true annulus, causing complete atrioventricular dissociation. One of the two died; in the remaining three patients, attachment of the prosthesis according to the Barnard and Schrire technique avoided heart block.

Other surgical techniques used for Ebstein's anomaly include atrioventricular plication combined with tricuspid valve replacement[42] and replacement of the tricuspid valve with a tissue valve together with obliteration of the atrialized portion of the right ventricle and closure of the atrial septal defect.[33] The severely symptomatic neonate has been successfully managed with tricuspid valve repair or replacement and atrial septal defect closure.[23] For selected neonates, closure of the tricuspid valve, atrial septectomy, and an aortopulmonary shunt have been advocated, and the patient is subsequently managed as a single ventricle.[39]

Prosthetic valve replacement, although remaining the most popular way to repair Ebstein's anomaly, has given less-than-ideal results for some patients. Mechanical valves in the tricuspid position are associated with a higher frequency of valve malfunction and thrombotic complications than they are in other cardiac positions.[34] Tissue valves do not have the thromboembolic complications of mechanical valves, but they do have a limited life expectancy, particularly in infants and children. In our experience, the overall failure-free rate of porcine heterograft valves in children is only 58.5% at 5 years,[43] although current results indicate the longevity of porcine valves is more favorable in the tricuspid position. Prosthetic valves are also undesirable in the small patient, because reoperation may be required for replacement of the valve because of somatic growth.

In 1972, we developed a repair that consists of plication of the free wall of the atrialized portion of the right ventricle, posterior tricuspid annuloplasty, and excision of redundant right atrial wall (right reduction atrioplasty)[8] (Figure 127-3). The repair is based on the construction of a monocuspid valve by the use of the anterior leaflet of the tricuspid valve, which is usually enlarged in this anomaly. The early and late (up to 25 years follow-up) results of our experience have been reported.[9,40] We believe repair is preferable to valve replacement whenever it is feasible because it avoids the problems of prosthetic valve dysfunction, anticoagulation, and, in children, outgrowth. More recently, other types of valve reconstruction have been proposed,[6,31,36] but late results of these procedures in significant numbers of patients have not yet been reported.

No two hearts with Ebstein's anomaly have exactly the same anatomy. While the basic principles of our original repair remain the same, we have frequently incorporated various modifications in the repair as numerous anatomical variants of the anomaly have been encountered and our experience has grown (more than 469 consecutive cases). The original posterior purse-string annuloplasty may be modified by bringing the tricuspid annulus at the appropriate point on the right ventricular free wall directly to the ventricular septum where it is anchored with a pledgeted suture; the remainder of the posterior tricuspid annulus is then obliterated with running sutures. The original ventricular plication technique results in maximal reduction of right ventricular size. Other, more limited, internal apex-to-base (transverse) or side-to-side (longitudinal) plications may be employed to elevate the papillary muscles, obliterate noncontractile portions of the atrialized right ventricle, or reduce annular size. Repairs may be done with or without internal plication of the atrialized right ventricle. If internal plication is not performed and thin areas of atrialized right ventricle are present between the coronary artery branches, especially posterolaterally, external plication may be added at the completion of the intraventricular repair. External plication has the advantage of preserving coronary arterial supply to all contracting portions of the right ventricle.

Other modifications we have employed more recently include bringing the anterior papillary muscle(s) toward the ventricular septum with one or more pledgeted sutures to facilitate closure of the anterior leaflet against the septum, and the addition of an anterior pursestring annuloplasty to the repair of those hearts that have extensive dilation of the right ventricular outflow tract and anterior portion of the tricuspid annulus (Figure 127-4). Occasionally, when leaflet tissue is adequate, a two leaflet repair is possible. Rarely, a three-leaflet repair can be performed; this is usually accomplished with an annuloplasty technique at the level of the displaced annulus.

Whether plication (or actual excision) of the atrialized right ventricle is necessary or desirable is still controversial. Potential advantages include (1) reduction in the size of the nonfunctional portion of the right ventricle which speeds transit of blood flow through the right heart; (2) reduction of compression of the left ventricle (pancake effect), thus improving left ventricular function; (3) elevating the papillary muscles, which facilitates closure of the anterior leaflet against the septum in systole; and (4) providing more space for the lungs (especially important in infants). All internal forms of right ventricular plication by necessity interrupt some coronary arterial supply to right ventricular musculature, and many have the potential risk of kinking the right

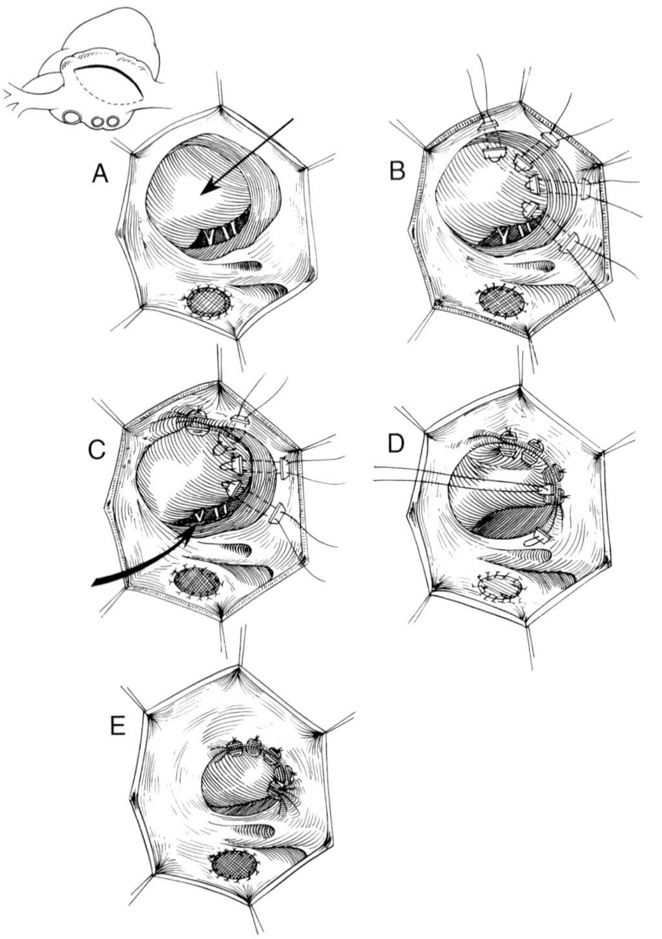

Figure 127–3 Diagram of original repair. A, *(Left)* The right atrium is incised from the atrial appendage to the inferior vena cava. The redundant portion of the right atrium is excised at the conclusion of the repair *(dotted line)* so that the final size of the right atrium is normal. *(Right)* The atrial septal defect is closed with a pericardial patch. The large anterior leaflet is indicated by the arrow. The posterior leaflet is displaced down from the annulus and the septal leaflet is hypoplastic and not visible in this view. **B,** Mattress sutures passed through pledgets of Teflon felt are used to pull the tricuspid annulus and tricuspid valve together. Sutures are placed in the atrialized portion of the right ventricle as shown so that when they are subsequently tied, the atrialized ventricle is plicated and the aneurysmal cavity is obliterated. **C,** The sutures are tied down sequentially. The hypoplastic, markedly displaced septal leaflet is now visible *(arrow)*. **D,** A posterior annuloplasty is performed to narrow the diameter of the tricuspid annulus. The coronary sinus marks the posterior and leftward extent of the annuloplasty, which is terminated there to avoid injury to the conduction bundle. One or more additional sutures may be required to obliterate the posterior aspect of the annuloplasty repair to render the valve totally competent. The tricuspid annulus at this time will admit two or more fingers in the adult. **E,** Completed repair that allows the anterior leaflet to function as a monocusp valve. **F,** Operative photograph of completed repair. The large anterior leaflet forms a competent monocusp valve *(arrows)*.
(Modified from Danielson GK, Maloney JD, Devloo RAE: Surgical repair of Ebstein's anomaly. Mayo Clin Proc 54:185–192, 1979.)

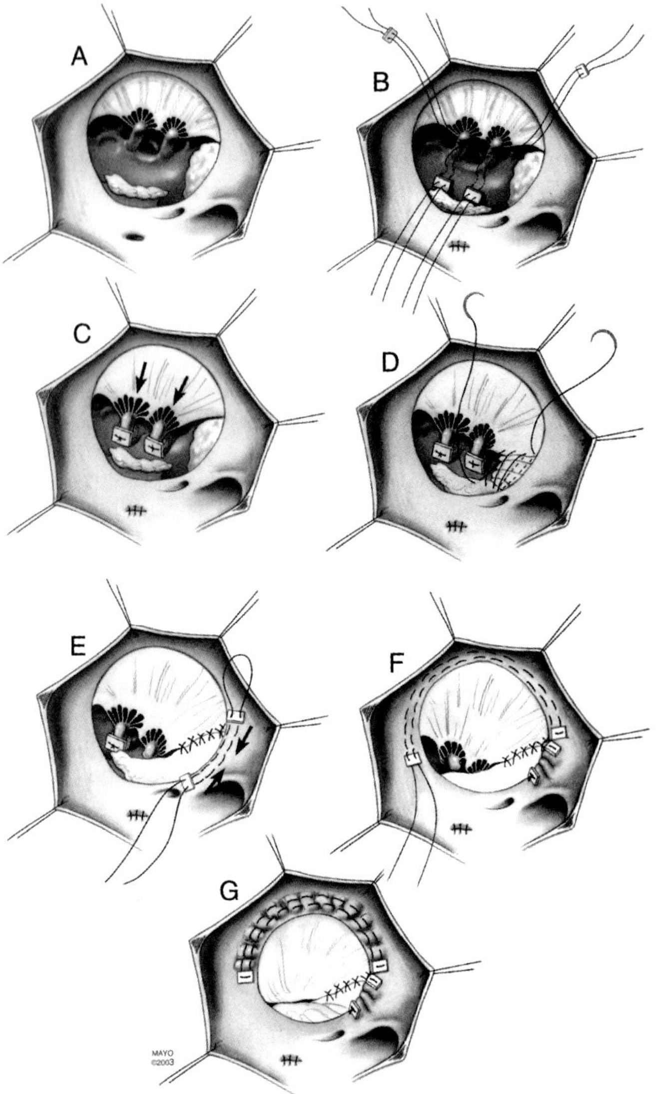

Figure 127–4 Diagram of current repair technique. A, Two papillary muscles arise from the free wall of the right ventricle with short chordal attachments to the leading edge of the anterior leaflet. The septal leaflet is diminutive and only a ridge of tissue. The posterior leaflet is not well formed and is adherent to the underlying endocardium. A small patent foramen ovale is present. **B** and **C,** The base of each papillary muscle is moved toward the ventricular septum at the appropriate level with horizontal mattress sutures backed with felt pledgets. The patent foramen ovale is closed by direct suture. **D,** The posterior angle of the tricuspid orifice is closed by bringing the right side of the anterior leaflet down to the septum and plicating the nonfunctional posterior leaflet in the process. **E,** A posterior annuloplasty is performed to narrow the diameter of the tricuspid annulus. The coronary sinus marks the posterior and leftward extent of the annuloplasty. **F,** An anterior pursestring annuloplasty is performed to further narrow the tricuspid annulus. This annuloplasty stitch is tied down over a 25-mm valve sizer in an adult to prevent tricuspid stenosis. **G,** Completed repair that allows the anterior leaflet to function as a monocusp valve.

coronary artery, problems that may generate ventricular arrhythmias and compromise ventricular function. The decisions regarding whether to plicate the atrialized right ventricle and how much to plicate are based on the anatomy encountered and the surgeon's personal philosophy.

In general, we believe repair is preferable to valve replacement whenever repair is feasible. However, if there is failure of delamination of more than 50% of the anterior leaflet or if the leading edge of the anterior leaflet has hyphenated or linear attachment to the right ventricle, a durable repair may not be obtainable with valvuloplasty techniques; valve replacement is then preferred. Valve replacement is performed when there is inadequate delaminated leaflet tissue for valve repair. Valve replacement must be performed in a manner that protects the conduction tissue and the right coronary artery.

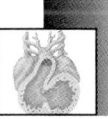

The late results of bioprosthetic tricuspid valve replacement in 158 patients with Ebstein's anomaly have been reviewed and reported.[22] The freedom from bioprosthesis replacement was 97.5% ± 1.9% at 5 years and 80.6% ± 7.6% at 10 and 15 years. Interestingly, freedom from reoperation at 10 and 15 years after tricuspid replacement (both bioprosthetic and mechanical) was not significantly different from tricuspid valve repair (81.9% versus 83.1%). In our early experience with surgery for Ebstein's anomaly, we made every effort to repair rather than replace the tricuspid valve because of the reported overall poor durability of bioprostheses in young patients in our experience[43] and that of others.[15] In many instances, we accepted a repair that only reduced the tricuspid regurgitation to moderate degrees to delay the time of valve replacement. In our experience, tricuspid bioprostheses in patients with Ebstein's anomaly have greater durability in both pediatric and adult populations compared to bioprostheses in other cardiac positions and even when compared with bioprosthetic tricuspid valve replacement for other cardiac diagnoses. We speculate that this favorable experience may be related to the large size of the bioprosthesis that can be implanted relative to patient somatic size and to the normal, low right ventricular systolic pressure after repair in patients with Ebstein's anomaly. Both of these factors would tend to reduce turbulence and stress on the bioprosthesis.

As our experience evolved and the improved longevity of bioprostheses in the tricuspid position in Ebstein's anomaly became apparent, we began to be more liberal with bioprosthetic valve replacement as opposed to leaving moderate tricuspid regurgitation after valve repair. Currently, we perform tricuspid valve repair whenever a good-to-excellent result can be obtained. If not, tricuspid replacement with a bioprosthesis is a reasonable alternative, particularly in older patients. For adult patients who are taking warfarin anticoagulation for other reasons and who want to minimize the need for a subsequent reoperation for bioprosthesis deterioration, a mechanical valve is a reasonable alternative.

INDICATIONS FOR OPERATION

Observation alone is usually advised for asymptomatic patients with no right-to-left shunting and only mild cardiomegaly. Most patients in functional Classes I and II can be managed medically, as was done for the majority of patients with the diagnosis of Ebstein's anomaly who were seen at this institution during the interval covered by this surgical experience. Operative correction is offered when symptoms progress, increasing cyanosis becomes evident, or if paradoxic embolism occurs. Operation should also be considered if there is objective evidence of deterioration such as decreasing exercise performance by exercise testing, progressive increase in heart size on chest X-ray, progressive right ventricular dilation or reduction of systolic function by echocardiography, or appearance of atrial or ventricular arrhythmias. In borderline situations, the ability to reconstruct the tricuspid valve, as determined by echocardiography, makes the decision to proceed with operation easier. Once symptoms develop and progress to Classes III and IV, medical management has little to offer; operation then becomes the only chance for improvement. A biventricular repair is usually possible, but in some circumstances when significant left ventricular dysfunction has occurred, cardiac transplantation may be the best option.

OPERATIVE MANAGEMENT

Our operative management of patients with Ebstein's anomaly consists of (1) electrophysiological mapping for localization of accessory conduction pathways in patients with ventricular preexcitation; (2) closure of any atrial septal communications; (3) correction of associated anomalies such as pulmonary stenosis, ventricular septal defect, and patent ductus arteriosus; (4) performance of any indicated antiarrhythmia procedures such as surgical division of accessory conduction pathways, cryoablation of AVNRT, or right-sided maze procedure[18]; (5) consideration of plication of the atrialized portion of the right ventricle; (6) reconstruction of the tricuspid valve when feasible, or valve replacement; and (7) right reduction atrioplasty. Intraoperative transesophageal echocardiography is used routinely.

After a median sternotomy, adhesions are freed and the external cardiac anatomy is confirmed. Electrophysiological mapping is performed if preexcitation has been diagnosed on preoperative electrophysiological study. Mapping of the ventricles is performed with a multi-electrode sock during sinus rhythm and atrial pacing; mapping of the atria is performed during ventricular pacing and reciprocating tachycardia. Immediate results are available through computer analysis of the recorded data (CR, Bard Inc., Murray Hill, NJ). When necessary, endocardial mapping on the atrial and/or ventricular side of the tricuspid valve annulus is accomplished on cardiopulmonary bypass at normothermia. The ascending aorta is temporarily cross-clamped as the right atrium is opened and all atrial and ventricular septal defects are rapidly closed. Any air on the left side is then aspirated, the cross-clamp is removed, and the heart is allowed to be perfused and beat. The atrioventricular junction is mapped with a rigid probe, and points of earliest activation are noted. Surgical ablation of accessory pathway(s) is performed by transmural incisions made in the right atrium 2 mm from the tricuspid annulus and carried 1 cm down over the right ventricle. The dissected areas are lightly electrocoagulated and repaired by suture. Alternatively, for pathways near the conduction system, cryoablation is often employed with the heart beating in order to avoid permanent heart block.

For patients with AVNRT, perinodal cryoablation is performed after institution of cardiopulmonary bypass, right atriotomy, and closure of intracardiac septal defects. Multiple applications of the cryoprobe (freezes) are made around and within the coronary sinus and then carried anteriorly toward the proximal atrioventricular node until temporary complete heart block is noted, at which time rewarming is begun immediately. Normal atrioventricular conduction returns shortly thereafter. When indicated, supplemental freezes are made superior and anterior to the atrioventricular node and His bundle.

For patients with atrial fibrillation or flutter, two techniques are employed. For most patients without previous cardiac surgery, a right-sided maze procedure is performed as previously described.[41] If there are dense adhesions as a result of previous cardiac surgery, a cryoablation procedure, which includes the right atrial isthmus, is performed. Multiple cryoprobe freezes are placed to produce blocking lines from the posterolateral tricuspid annulus to the coronary sinus to the inferior vena cava and the inferior atriotomy, from the anterolateral tricuspid annulus to the superior atriotomy, and from the fossa ovalis to the superior vena cava and superior atriotomy.

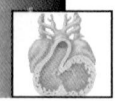

When cardiopulmonary bypass is instituted, techniques including aortic and bicaval cannulation with moderate hypothermia are used (28° to 34° C, depending upon anticipated complexity and length of procedure). The left side of the heart is vented with a catheter inserted through the right superior pulmonary vein, and an aortic tack vent is placed. The aorta is temporarily cross-clamped, and the myocardium is protected with multidose cold blood cardioplegia and topical hypothermia. The right atrium is opened from the appendage to the inferior vena cava. Repair is carried out as shown in Figure 127-3, or according to subsequent modifications as shown in Figure 127-4. When an atrial septal defect is present, the remaining atrial septum is usually thin and dilated; in this case, we prefer to excise the attenuated atrial septal tissue and close the resulting defect with an autologous pericardial patch. A patent foramen ovale often is repaired by direct suture. The valve anatomy is then carefully inspected. When a valve repair is performed, the heart is kept arrested and the field is kept bloodless to optimize exposure of the anatomy. For tricuspid valve replacement, the cross-clamp is removed after suture placement has been completed in the region cephalad to the conduction tissue, and the heart is allowed to be perfused and beating.

In the original repair, ventricular plication sutures are placed posterolaterally in the atrialized right ventricle to bring the hinge point of the displaced tricuspid valve toward the tricuspid annulus, thereby elevating the papillary muscles of the anterior leaflet and allowing the leaflet to close against the septum. Care is taken to avoid large branches of the right coronary artery and the posterior descending coronary artery. The epicardial arteries are inspected after each plication suture is placed; the suture is removed and relocated if an important coronary artery branch has been compromised. There has been a trend in our recent cases to replace internal plication with the technique of bringing the anterior papillary muscle toward the septum, as described previously. The posterior annuloplasty (see Figure 127-3D and E; Figure 127-4, E and F) is a critical part of the procedure. The posterior aspect of the annulus may first be narrowed with an annuloplasty suture and then obliterated by additional running sutures from the free-wall annulus to the septum, as originally described. Alternatively, the tricuspid annulus at the appropriate point on the right ventricular free wall may be approximated directly to the ventricular septum, where it is anchored with a pledgeted suture. The remainder of the posterior tricuspid annulus is then obliterated with running sutures, taking care to avoid the right coronary artery.

Because this repair is based on a satisfactory anterior leaflet, significant abnormalities of the leaflet may compromise the result. For most patients with fenestrations or perforations in the anterior leaflet, the defects can be repaired satisfactorily with fine running sutures. Small anterior leaflets may permit construction of a competent tricuspid valve but at the expense of creating some (usually acceptable) degree of tricuspid stenosis. The most important feature for a satisfactory repair is the presence of a mobile and free leading edge of the anterior leaflet. Leaflets with hyphenated attachments of the leading edge to the underlying endocardium or linear attachment currently are not considered appropriate for reconstruction. The presence of short papillary muscles and chordae does not preclude a satisfactory repair if the remaining leaflet tissue is well formed; however, direct insertions of the papillary muscle heads into the leading edge of the anterior leaflet severely restrict leaflet motion, making repair difficult. A few patients will have enough posterior leaflet tissue to permit a bileaflet repair and, rarely, all three leaflets will be moderately well formed but displaced, permitting a trileaflet repair. In the latter case, repair is usually accomplished with an annuloplasty technique at the level of the displaced annulus.

After the reconstruction is completed, the tricuspid valve is tested by temporarily clamping the pulmonary artery and injecting saline under pressure into the right ventricle with a bulb syringe and large catheter. The result is routinely reassessed by intraoperative transesophageal echocardiography after discontinuation of cardiopulmonary bypass.

When the tricuspid valve cannot be reconstructed, valve leaflet tissue toward the right ventricular outflow tract (which can cause right ventricular outflow tract obstruction) is excised and a prosthetic valve (bioprosthetic more often than mechanical) is inserted. The suture line is deviated to the atrial side of the atrioventricular node and membranous septum to avoid injury to the conduction mechanism (Figure 127-5). A small vein crossing the tricuspid annulus adjacent to the membranous septum typically marks the atrioventricular node. To avoid injury to the right coronary artery, the suture line may be deviated cephalad to the tricuspid valve annulus posterolaterally where the tissues are frequently very thin. The coronary sinus can be left to drain into the right atrium if there is sufficient room between it and the atrioventricular node; if the distance is short, the coronary sinus can be left to drain into the right ventricle. The struts of the bioprosthesis are oriented so that they straddle the area of the membranous septum and conduction tissue. The valve sutures are tied with the heart beating to detect any disturbances in atrioventricular conduction.

A right reduction atrioplasty is performed as the atriotomy is repaired. For patients not receiving a right-sided maze, care is taken not to incise or suture into the crista terminalis, which can produce the substrate for atrial flutter.[12,14] Temporary pacing wires are placed on the free wall of the right atrium and right ventricle for postoperative monitoring of rhythm, for pacing in selected cases, and for electrophysiological testing to confirm the absence of pathway function in those patients who underwent ablation of an accessory conduction pathway. Because pericardial effusions are common after repair of Ebstein's anomaly, particularly when there is gross cardiomegaly, a portion of the anterior pericardium on the right side is removed to allow free drainage of pericardial fluid into the right pleural space.

What the best treatment is for the neonate born with Ebstein's anomaly is still debated. Our philosophy is to try to bring the infant through the first few weeks of life by reducing pulmonary vascular resistance with nitric oxide or other pulmonary vasodilators. If this is not successful, we offer operation. Based on recent experience elsewhere of success-

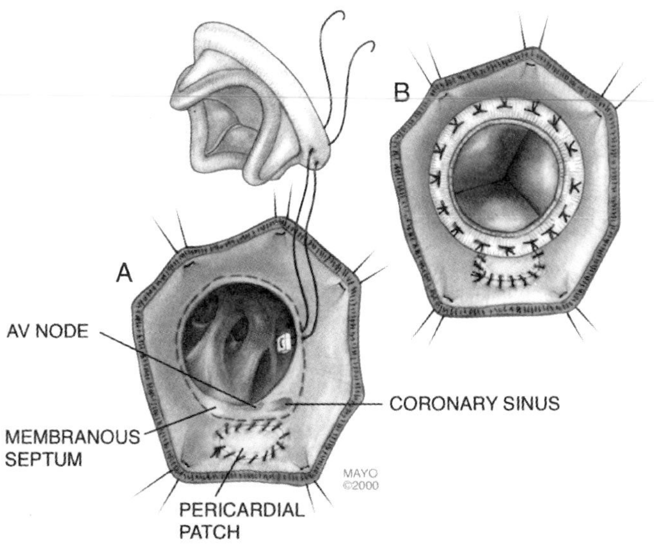

Figure 127–5 Diagram of technique for tricuspid valve replacement in Ebstein's anomaly. A, The valve suture line is placed on the atrial side of the membranous septum and atrioventricular node to avoid injury to the conduction system. The suture line is also deviated cephalad to the tricuspid annulus posterolaterally when the tissues are thin, to avoid injury to the right coronary artery. When there is sufficient distance between the coronary sinus and the AV node, the coronary sinus may be left on the atrial side of the suture line. **B,** The sutures are tied with the heart perfused and beating to ensure that a conducted rhythm is preserved. AV, Atrioventricular.

ful operations on neonates with Ebstein's anomaly,[23] and on our own recent success in infants, we prefer a biventricular repair to the single ventricle approach. Adjunctive use of atrial fenestration or a bidirectional cavopulmonary shunt is controversial; neither is used routinely in our practice. We occasionally use bidirectional cavopulmonary shunt selectively when the right ventricle is severely dilated and functioning poorly. Because concomitant left ventricular dysfunction may be present when the right ventricle fails, it is important to document by direct pressure measurements that the pulmonary arterial and left atrial pressures are low; otherwise, the bidirectional cavopulmonary shunt will not be feasible.

In patients with normal hearts, mechanical prostheses in the tricuspid position have a higher incidence of malfunction and thrombotic complications than they do in either the aortic or mitral position. However, tricuspid mechanical valves have functioned better in patients with Ebstein's anomaly, perhaps because the right ventricles are larger and there is less tendency for fibrous tissue ingrowth into the prostheses.

Table 127–1

Age Distribution

Ages	*Number of patients*
11–23 months	9
2–9 years	44
10–19 years	54
20–29 years	46
30–64 years	36
Total	189

CLINICAL DATA

Between April 1972 and January 2003, 469 consecutive patients with Ebstein's anomaly have undergone operation on our surgical service. The results of the first 189 patients have been analyzed.[9] Patients ranged in age from 11 months to 64 years (median 16 years, mean 19.1 years) (Table 127-1).

Table 127–2

Associated Cardiac Defects

Defects	*Number of patients*
Atrial septal defect	169
Accessory conduction pathway(s)	28
Pulmonary stenosis	16
Ventricular septal defect	7
AV nodal reentry tachycardia	4
Partial atrioventricular canal	4
Absent coronary sinus	3
Anomalous pulmonary venous connection	2
Bilateral superior venae cavae	2
Pericarditis	2
Patent ductus arteriosus	2
Other	10

AV, atrioventricular

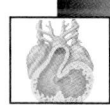

Hemoglobin values ranged between 10.8 and 23.4 g/dl, cardiothoracic ratios ranged between 0.49 and 0.96, and arterial oxygen saturations ranged between 65% and 98%.

Associated cardiac defects are shown in Table 127-2, and previous cardiovascular operations are shown in Table 127-3. These data show the wide age range of patients undergoing repair of Ebstein's anomaly and the large number and variety of associated cardiac defects and prior palliative operations they may have.

RESULTS

Early and late results of the first 323 patients with Ebstein's anomaly who underwent surgical treatment have been reviewed.[40] Ages at operation ranged from 9 months to 70.1 years (median, 17.3 years). In 42.7% a tricuspid valve reconstruction was possible; in 54.8% a prosthetic valve, usually a bioprosthesis, was required; and in 2.5% a modified Fontan or other procedure was performed. There were 21 early deaths (6.5%). Concomitant procedures included successful ablation of accessory conduction pathways (WPW syndrome) in 45 patients, a right-sided maze procedure for atrial flutter/fibrillation in 14 patients, and ablation of AVNRT in 8 patients, all without mortality. There were 23 late deaths (7.6%) in a follow-up extending up to 25 years (mean, 7.1 years). Late echocardiography showed the atrial septum was intact in all patients. Of the 138 patients who underwent valve repair, 23 (16.7%) subsequently required reoperation 1.5–17.7 years (mean, 9.4) later.

At late follow-up, atrial arrhythmias were reduced, and 92.1% of patients were in NYHA functional Class I or II. Postoperative reduction in heart size was usual and occasionally considerable (Figure 127-6). Nine female patients are known to have undergone a total of 12 successful pregnancies with delivery of normal children.

Table 127–3

Previous Cardiovascular Operations

Operations	*Number of patients*
Blalock-Taussig shunt	10
Closure of atrial septal defect	8
Glenn anastomosis	6
Pacemaker	6
Attempted repair elsewhere	5
Waterston shunt	5
Partial pericardiectomy	2
Other	7

Maximum exercise testing showed a significant increase in work performance, exercise duration, and maximum oxygen uptake after operation.[11] Maximal oxygen consumption increased from a mean of 47% of predicted value before operation to a mean of 72% at follow-up. Repair of Ebstein's anomaly also favorably affects cardiac output, particularly in

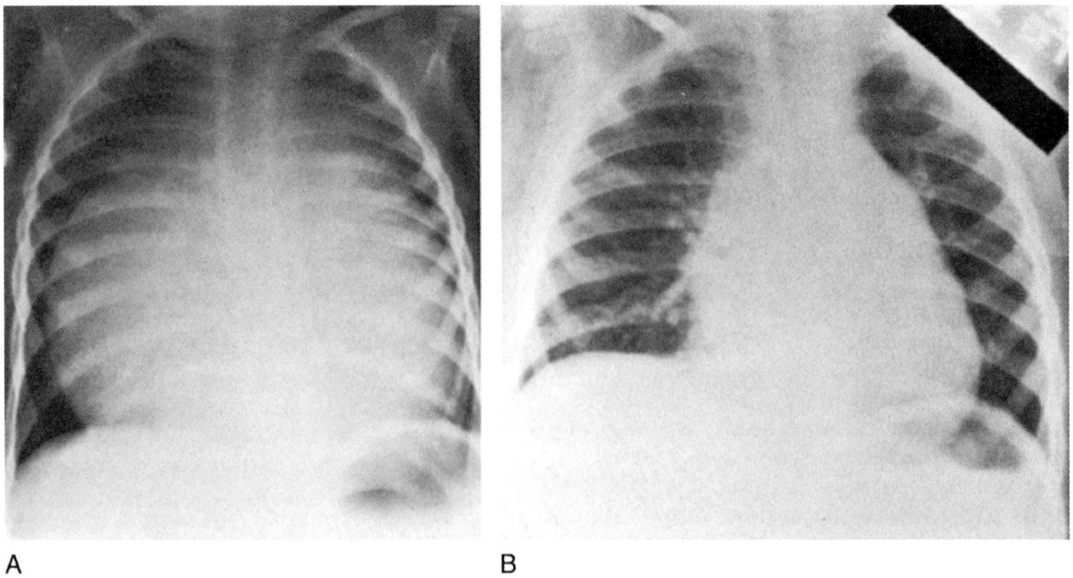

Figure 127–6 The patient was a 2-year-old girl with Ebstein's anomaly and a history of pneumonia, cardiorespiratory arrest, and failure to thrive. Chest films: **A,** Preoperative (cardiothoracic ratio—0.9). **B,** Thirteen days postoperatively (cardiothoracic ratio—0.55). Right ventricular angiogram, anteroposterior view.

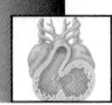

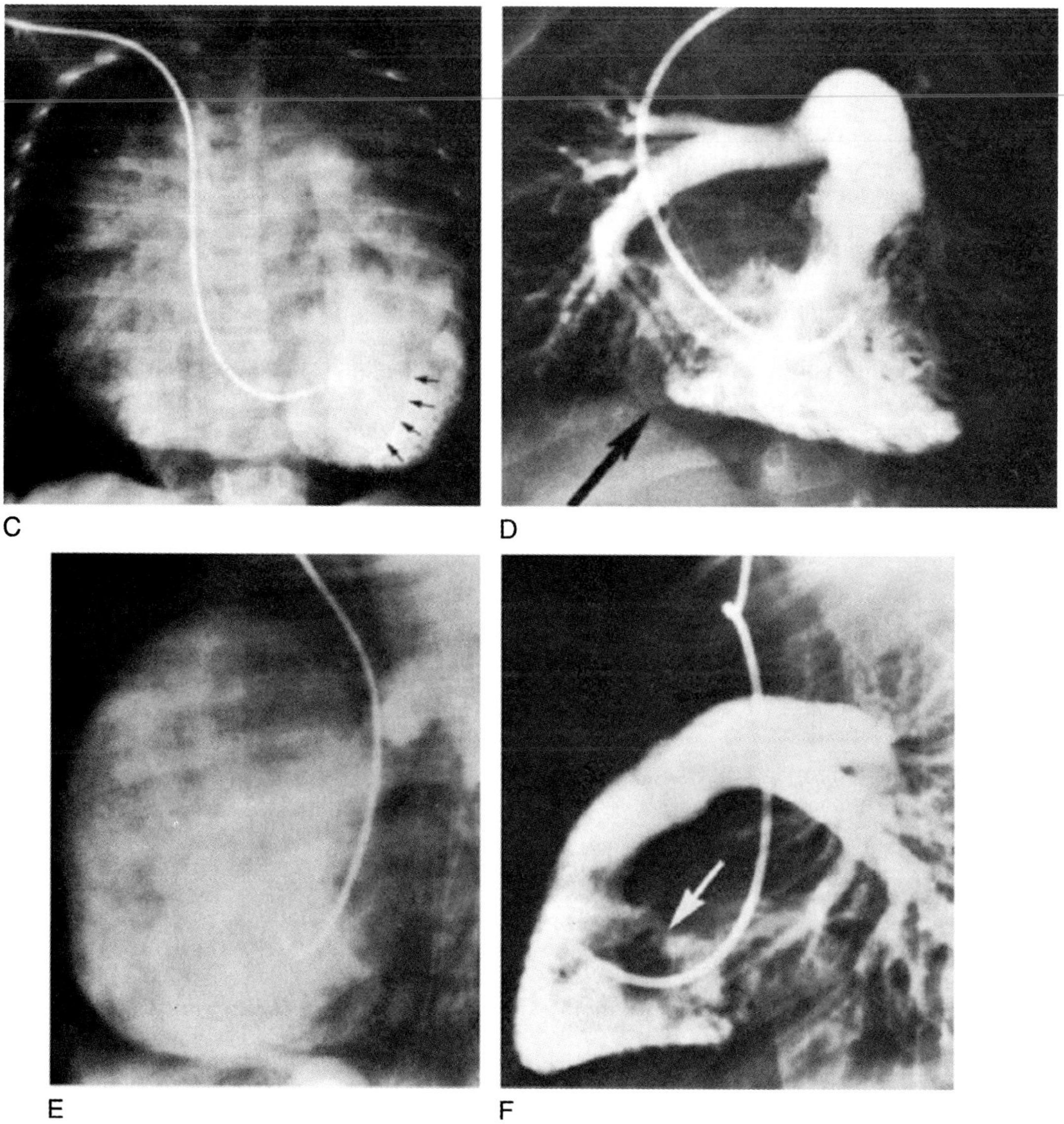

Figure 127–6 cont'd **C,** Preoperative. The contrast medium refluxes through the tricuspid valve to fill the entire cardiac silhouette. A radiolucent line within the cavity of the ventricle shows the location of the displaced tricuspid leaflets *(arrows)*. **D,** Postoperative. There is rapid transit of contrast medium from the right ventricle to the pulmonary arteries with only a trace of tricuspid insufficiency. The arrow indicates the new plane of the tricuspid valve. Right ventricular angiogram, lateral view: **E,** Preoperative. **F,** Postoperative. The tricuspid valve is competent. The arrow points to a filling defect created by the anterior leaflet. This patient is now 31 years old and is married. She is asymptomatic, is taking no cardiac medications, exercises regularly, and is employed full time.
*(**A-F,** from Danielson GK, Maloney JD, Devloo RAE: Surgical repair of Ebstein's anomaly. Mayo Clin Proc 54:185, 1979.)*

response to exercise, normalizes systemic arterial oxygen saturation, and reduces excess ventilation at rest and during exercise.

Results of the right-sided maze procedure for atrial arrhythmias in congenital heart disease have been reported.[18,41] Forty-four patients have undergone a concomitant right-sided maze procedure for paroxysmal (73%) or chronic (27%) atrial flutter/fibrillation during repair of cardiac lesions associated with right atrial dilation. The majority of patients had Ebstein's anomaly (70%). Early mortality occurred in one Ebstein patient (2.3%) who had giant cardiomegaly, ventricular arrhythmias, and inducible ventricular fibrillation on preoperative electrophysiological evaluation; death occurred from intractable ventricular fibrillation in spite of amiodarone administration. A permanent pacemaker was required in one patient for tachycardia/bradycardia syndrome. Mean follow-up was 17 months with a maximum follow-up of 66 months; cardiac rhythm was sinus in 85%, junctional in 8%, atrial flutter/fibrillation in 6%, and paced in 1%. There were no late deaths or reoperations.

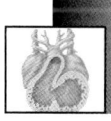

In summary, repair of Ebstein's anomaly eliminates right-to-left intracardiac shunting with its attendant risks, improves exercise tolerance and functional class, and reduces supraventricular arrhythmias. In addition, quality of life and longevity are improved.

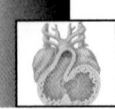

SELECTED BIBLIOGRAPHY

Special review of Ebstein's anomaly. Mayo Clin Proc 54:163, 1979.

This monograph describes the historical, clinical, and morphological aspects of Ebstein's anomaly. The clinical features and natural history of 67 consecutive patients with Ebstein's anomaly who were monitored for a mean of 12 years are described. This monograph gives a good overview of our knowledge of Ebstein's anomaly.

Danielson GK, Driscoll DJ, Mair DD, et al: Operative treatment of Ebstein's anomaly. J Thorac Cardiovasc Surg 104:1195–1202, 1992.

This article analyzes the largest surgical series of patients operated on for Ebstein's anomaly. Valve repair by plication of the atrialized right ventricle and valvuloplasty was accomplished in 58.2% of the 189 patients.

Ebstein's anomaly. Prog Pediatr Cardiol 2(1):1, 1993.

This monograph is an excellent current review of Ebstein's anomaly and includes a chapter on the neonatal expression of Ebstein's anomaly.

REFERENCES

1. Anderson KR, Lie JT: The right ventricular myocardium in Ebstein's anomaly. A morphometric histopathologic study. Mayo Clin Proc 54:181–184, 1979.
2. Anderson KR, Danielson GK, McGoon DC, Lie JT: Ebstein's anomaly of the left-sided tricuspid valve: Pathological anatomy of the valvular malformation. Circulation 58:87–91 (Suppl I), 1978.
3. Anderson KR, Zuberbuhler JR, Anderson RH, et al: Morphologic spectrum of Ebstein's anomaly of the heart: A review. Mayo Clin Proc 54:174–180, 1979.
4. Anderson RH, Becker AE, Arnold R, Wilkinson JL: The conducting tissues in congenitally corrected transposition. Circulation 50:911–923, 1974.
5. Barnard CN, Schrire V: Surgical correction of Ebstein's malformation with prosthetic tricuspid valve. Surgery 54:302–308, 1963.
6. Carpentier A, Chauvaud S, Mace L, et al: A new reconstructive operation for Ebstein's anomaly of the tricuspid valve. J Thorac Cardiovasc Surg 96:92–101, 1988.
7. Celermajer DS, Bull C, Till JA, et al: Ebstein's anomaly: presentation and outcome from fetus to adult. J Am Coll Cardiol 23:170, 1994.
8. Danielson GK, Maloney JD, Devloo REA. Surgical repair of Ebstein's anomaly. Mayo Clin Proc 54:185–192, 1979.
9. Danielson GK, Driscoll DJ, Mair DD, et al: Operative treatment of Ebstein's anomaly. J Thorac Cardiovasc Surg 104:1195–1202, 1992.
10. Dearani JA, Danielson GK: Congenital heart surgery nomenclature and database project: Ebstein's anomaly and tricuspid valve disease. Ann Thorac Surg 69:S106–117, 2000.
11. Driscoll DJ, Mottram CD, Danielson GK: Spectrum of exercise intolerance in 45 patients with Ebstein's anomaly and observations on exercise tolerance in 11 patients after surgical repair. J Am Coll Cardiol 11:831–836, 1988.
12. Durongpisitkul K, Porter CJ, Cetta F, et al: Predictors of early- and late-onset supraventricular tachyarrhythmias after Fontan operation. Circulation 98:1099, 1998.
13. Ebstein W. Ueber einen sehr seltenen Fall von Insufficienz der Valvula tricuspidalis, bedingt durch eine angeborene hochgradige Missbildung derselben. Arch Anat Physiol 238–254, 1866.
14. Gandhi SK, Bromberg BI, Rodefeld MD, et al: Spontaneous atrial flutter in a chronic canine model of the modified Fontan operation. J Am Coll Cardiol 30:1095, 1997.
15. Geha AS, Laks H, Stansel HC, et al: Late failure of porcine valve heterografts in children, J Thorac Cardiovasc Surg 78:351, 1979.
16. Giuliani ER, Fuster V, Brandenburg RO, Mair DD: The clinical features and natural history of Ebstein's anomaly of the tricuspid valve. Mayo Clin Proc 54:163–173, 1979.
17. Glenn WWL, Browne M, Whittemore R. Circulatory bypass of the right side of the heart: Cava-pulmonary artery shunt–indications and results (report of a collected series of 537 cases). In: Cassels DE (ed): The Heart and Circulation in the Newborn and Infant. New York: Grune & Stratton, 1966, pp. 345–357.
18. Greason KL, Dearani JA, Theodoro DA, et al: Surgical management of atrial tachyarrhythmias associated with congenital cardiac anomalies: Mayo Clinic experience. Semin Thorac Cardiovasc Surg 2003 (in press).
19. Hardy KL, Roe BB: Ebstein's anomaly: further experience with definitive repair. J Thorac Cardiovasc Surg 58:553–560, 1969.
20. Hardy KL, May IA, Webster CA, Kimball KG: Ebstein's anomaly: a functional concept and successful definitive repair. J Thorac Cardiovasc Surg 48:927–940, 1964.
21. Hunter SW, Lillehei CW: Ebstein's malformation of the tricuspid valve: study of a case together with suggestion of a new form of surgical therapy. Dis Chest 33:297–304, 1958.
22. Kiziltan HT, Theodoro DA, Warnes CA, et al: Late results of bioprosthetic tricuspid valve replacement in Ebstein's anomaly. Ann Thorac Surg 66:1539, 1998.
23. Knott-Craig CJ, Overholt ED, Ward KE, et al: Repair of Ebstein's anomaly in the symptomatic neonate: An evolution of technique with 7-year follow-up. Ann Thorac Surg 73:1786–1793, 2002.
24. Kumar AE, Fyler DC, Miettinen OS, Nadas AS: Ebstein's anomaly: Clinical profile and natural history. Am J Cardiol 28:84–95, 1971.
25. Lamers WH, Viragh S, Wessels A, et al: Formation of the tricuspid valve in the human heart, Circulation 91:111, 1995.
26. Leung MP, Baker EJ, Anderson RH, et al: Cineangiographic spectrum of Ebstein's malformation: its relevance to clinical presentation and outcome, J Am Coll Cardiol 11:154, 1988.
27. Lillehei CW, Kalke BR, Carlson RG: Evolution of corrective surgery for Ebstein's anomaly. Circulation 35, 36(Suppl I): 111–118, 1967.
28. Mann RJ, Lie JT: The life story of Wilhelm Ebstein (1836-1912) and his almost overlooked description of a congenital heart disease. Mayo Clin Proc 54:197–204, 1979.
29. Netter FH, Van Mierop LHS: Embryology. In: Yonkman FF (ed): The Ciba Collection of Medical Illustrations, Vol 5. Summit, NJ: Ciba Pharmaceutical, 1969, p. 125.
30. Oh JK, Holmes DR Jr, Hayes DL, et al: Cardiac arrhythmias in patients with surgical repair of Ebstein's anomaly. J Am Coll Cardiol 6:1351–1357; 1985.
31. Quaegebeur JM, Sreeram N, Fraser AG, et al: Surgery for Ebstein's anomaly: the clinical and echocardiographic evaluation of a new technique. J Am Coll Cardiol 17:722–728, 1991.
32. Reeder GS, Currie PJ, Hagler DJ, et al: Use of Doppler techniques (continuous-wave, pulsed-wave, and color-flow imaging) in the noninvasive hemodynamic assessment of congenital heart disease. Mayo Clin Proc 61:725–744, 1986.
33. Ross D, Somerville J: Surgical correction of Ebstein's anomaly. Lancet 2:280, 1970.

34. Sanfelippo PM, Giuliani ER, Danielson GK, et al: Tricuspid valve prosthetic replacement: Early and late results with the Starr-Edwards prosthesis. J Thorac Cardiovasc Surg 71:441–445, 1976.
35. Schiebler GL, Gravenstein JS, Van Mierop LHS: Ebstein's anomaly of the tricuspid valve: translation of original description with comments. Am J Cardiol 22:867–873, 1968.
36. Schmidt-Habelmann P, Meisner H, Struck E, Sebening F: Results of valvuloplasty for Ebstein's anomaly. Thorac Cardiovasc Surg 29:155–157, 1981.
37. Seward JB: Ebstein's anomaly: ultrasound imaging and hemodynamic evaluation. Echocardiography 10:641–664, 1993.
38. Shiina A, Seward JB, Tajik AJ, et al: Two-dimensional echocardiographic-surgical correlation in Ebstein's anomaly: Preoperative determination of patients requiring tricuspid valve plication vs. replacement. Circulation 68:534–544, 1983.
39. Starnes VA, Pitlick PT, Bernstein D, : Ebstein's anomaly appearing in the neonate. J Thorac Cardiovasc Surg 101:1082–1087, 1991.
40. Theodoro DA, Danielson GK, Kiziltan HT, et al: Surgical management Ebstein's anomaly: 25-year experience. Circulation 96(Suppl I):I–121, 1997.
41. Theodoro DA, Danielson GK, Porter CJ, et al: Right-sided maze procedure for right atrial arrhythmias in congenital heart disease. Ann Thorac Surg 65:149–154, 1998.
42. Timmis HH, Hardy JD, Watson DG: The surgical management of Ebstein's anomaly. The combined use of tricuspid valve replacement, atrioventricular plication, and atrioplasty. J Thorac Cardiovasc Surg 53:385–391, 1967.
43. Williams DB, Danielson GK, McGoon DC, et al: Porcine heterograft valve replacement in children. J Thorac Cardiovasc Surg 84:446–450, 1982.
44. Wright JL, Burchell HB, Kirklin JW, Wood EH: Symposium on physiologic, clinical and surgical interdependence in study and treatment of congenital heart disease; congenital displacement of tricuspid valve (Ebstein's malformation): report of a case with closure of an associated foramen ovale for correction of the right-to-left shunt. Proc Staff Meet Mayo Clin 29:278–284, 1954.

Table 128–1

Primary Cardiac Diagnosis in 1289 Adults Undergoing Surgery for Congenital Heart Disease Between 1973 and 2003 at the Toronto Congenital Cardiac Center for Adults, University of Toronto

Primary cardiac diagnosis	*N*	*% of Total*
Hypertrophic obstructive cardiomyopathy	322	25
Atrial septal defect[a]	291	23
Tetralogy of Fallot	140	11
Ventricular septal defect	99	8
Univentricular heart	65	5
Fibromuscular subaortic stenosis	45	4
Congenitally corrected transposition of great arteries	42	3
Ebstein anomaly	40	3
Coarctation of aorta	38	3
Pulmonary stenosis	29	2
Complete transposition of great arteries	25	2
Aortic valve stenosis or insufficiency	23	2
Double outlet right ventricle	22	2
Patent ductus arteriosus	15	1
Sinus of Valsalva aneurysm	13	1
Pulmonary atresia-ventricular septal defect	9	<1
Vascular ring	9	<1
Tricuspid insufficiency	8	<1
Coronary artery anomaly	8	<1
Arrhythmia	5	<1
Cor triatriatum	4	<1
Mitral stenosis	4	<1
Truncus arteriosus	4	<1
Other	31	2
Total	**1289**	**100**

[a]Including partial anomalous pulmonary venous drainage.

TRENDS IN ACHD SURGERY

Between 1973 and 2003 at the Toronto Congenital Cardiac Center for Adults (TCCCA), University of Toronto, we have performed 1342 operations (including reoperations during the same admission) in 1289 adults. Primary cardiac diagnoses are listed in Table 128-1. During this experience, we have observed several important trends in ACHD surgery.[4] Averaged over the 30-year experience, overall ACHD surgical volume increased at an annualized rate of 7%. The trend in ACHD volume closely parallels available American Heart Association data for adult acquired cardiac surgical volume (Figure 128-1A).[1] The proportion of adult congenital heart surgery compared to pediatric cardiac surgery at our institution is increasing and is between 10 and 20% (see Figure 128-1B). The demand for ACHD surgery continues to rise, and increasing levels of resources are required to meet this demand.

There is also a trend toward fewer primary repairs in ACHD. Most ACHD patients will have had previous surgery, and this will be increasingly the case because of earlier diagnosis (including intrauterine detection) and because of the more frequent primary repair in the neonate and infant. Conversely, re-operation is becoming progressively more common in ACHD surgery (see Figure 128-1C). The increasing prevalence of adults presenting for reoperation is because of residual lesions that cause late deterioration many years after previous, otherwise successful intracardiac repair (see Figure 128-1D). Whether the requirement for late reoperations will be lessened or simply delayed to a

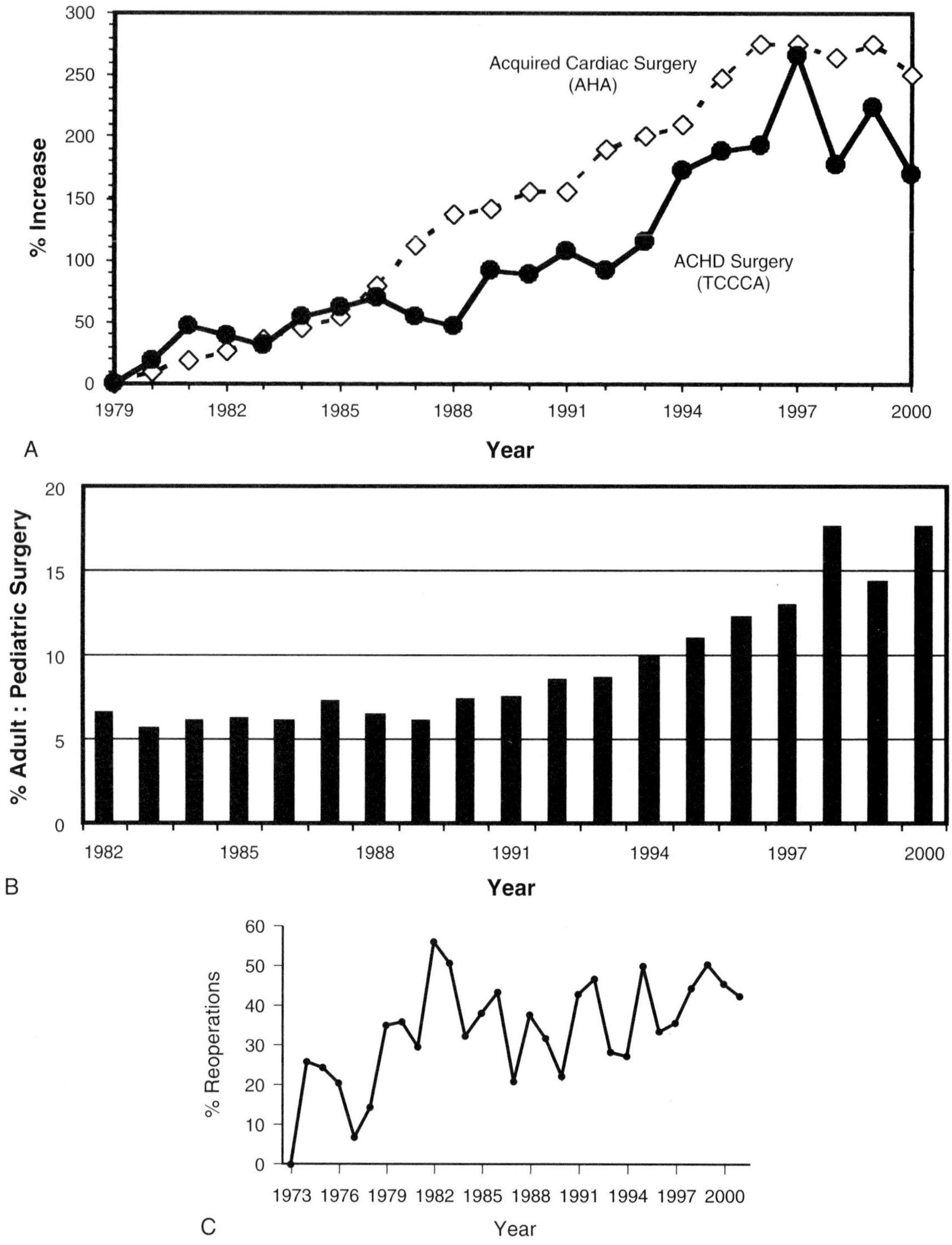

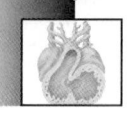

Figure 128–1 Trends in ACHD surgical volume at the Toronto Congenital Cardiac Center for Adults (TCCCA). A, Overall growth in volume compared to the growth in acquired cardiac surgical volume reported by the American Heart Association. The plateau in ACHD volume in recent years is not representative of decreasing demand but of limited resources allocable for ACHD surgery. **B,** Concomitant increasing proportion of ACHD surgery at TCCCA to pediatric cardiac surgery at the Hospital for Sick Children. **C,** Reoperation accounts for an increasing proportion of ACHD surgery.

later age by earlier definitive repair, refinements in operative techniques, and the use of intraoperative echocardiography is of great interest but is yet to be determined.

The number of previously palliated adults presenting for late definitive repair or repalliation has decreased (see Figure 128-1D) because in more recent years most of these patients have been repaired during childhood.

Overall mortality in our series is 4%, and there have been significant improvements in operative risk over time. Between the earlier and latter half of the experience, oper-

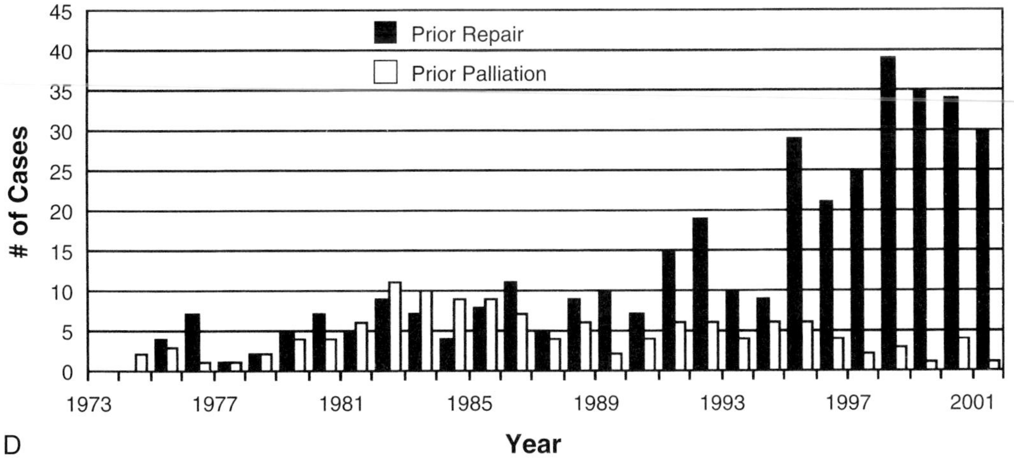

D

Figure 128–1 cont'd D, Most adults returning for reoperation have had prior intracardiac repairs *(black bars)*. Previously palliated adults returning for late definitive repair or repalliation are becoming less prevalent *(white bars)*.

ative mortality decreased from 4.2 to 1.2% for initial operations and from 11.3 to 3.3% for reoperations.[4]

ORGANIZATIONAL STRUCTURE TO SUPPORT AN ACHD PROGRAM

Medium- and high-risk ACHD patients should be seen in a supraregional referral center that has a multidisciplinary team committed to life-long care for these patients.[93,104,105] Surgery, diagnostic and interventional catheterization, full service EP management including ablation intervention, and magnetic resonance imaging (MRI) facilities must be available. In addition, related specialized anesthetic services, obstetrical care, psychology support, and vocational guidance counseling must be readily available. Service must be available 7 days per week. We estimate that a general population of 10 to 15 million people is required to support a supraregional centers.[105]

The principles of care are that patients with complex congenital heart disease require continuous and lifelong care, and that the adult patient with congenital heart disease has different needs than the child.[29] The organizational structure should be regionally coordinated so that regional centers looking after adults with less complex lesions can easily consult and refer to the supraregional centres.[58,105] A "critical mass" of patients is necessary to achieve and maintain expertise in every discipline required in the care of ACHD. Only surgeons that are experienced in all aspects of congenital heart surgery should perform adult congenital heart surgery.[88,89]

SURGICAL INDICATIONS IN ACHD

As in other areas of cardiac surgery, the decision to proceed with surgical repair of adult congenital heart disease is multifactorial. The need for surgery in congenital heart disease is primarily driven by an attempt to improve the natural history of the presenting lesion(s). Severe sequelae of uncorrected defects may include cyanosis (with its attendant complications), stroke, arrhythmia, heart failure, pulmonary vascular disease, and ventricular dysfunction (pulmonary or systemic). The absence of symptoms is less important than in acquired heart disease because symptoms occur late in the progression of some lesions and may indicate an irreversible state. A patient who has never been "normal" may not recognize symptoms. In other words, operation for an "asymptomatic" patient may be justified to modify, or improve upon, the natural history and to prevent or decrease the risk of late complications. As an example, an asymptomatic adult with aortic valve prolapse in association with a doubly-committed ventricular septal defect (VSD) in the outlet septum should have surgical repair of the VSD to prevent development of progressive aortic insufficiency. Unfortunately, available data on the natural history of ACHD is very limited compared to the well-known natural history in the neonate, infant, and child.

Other considerations in the decision to recommend surgery include the functional status of the patient confirmed by objective exercise testing, the requirements for and risk of long-term medications, and important medical comorbidities. Ultimately, the potential benefit of surgery must be tempered by operative risk of death and postoperative morbidity.

Because congenital heart disease encompasses many diverse lesions, each of which may have considerable morphologic variation, specific indications for surgical management must be individualized. Guidelines may be found in the 2001 update of the Canadian Cardiovascular Society Consensus Conference.[92,93,96]

PREOPERATIVE EVALUATION

Preoperative evaluation must establish a complete diagnosis of the cardiac condition and the identification of associated cardiac and noncardiac lesions, as well as an assessment of factors that may affect operative risk and long-term benefit. Baseline data are collected from a complete history and physical examination, electrocardiogram, chest X-ray, and echocardiogram. These data dictate further diagnostic studies that may be required.

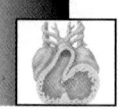

Coronary angiography is indicated for adults over 40 years of age or those with a history of angina, myocardial infarction, or prior coronary repair. Coronary angiography is also useful for assessing intramyocardial bridges associated with hypertrophic cardiomyopathy and in diagnosing congenital coronary artery anomalies. As many as 33% of ACHD may have an asymptomatic coronary arterial abnormality that is only detected at angiography and may provide vital information in interpreting symptoms or planning surgery.[56]

The prevalence of arrhythmia, both supraventricular and ventricular, increases with age in patients with congenital heart disease.[86] Adults with known arrhythmia or those with a history of palpitations, near-syncope, or syncope require further evaluation with 24-hour Holter monitoring if electrocardiography is not diagnostic. Complete preoperative characterization of the arrhythmia is essential for optimal planning and management, and may require catheter-based electrophysiological study.

Cardiac MRI is playing an increasingly important role in evaluation of ACHD.[43] MRI provides useful data on cardiac chamber size, volume, and function. MRI also gives anatomically detailed views of mediastinal vasculature including branch and peripheral pulmonary arteries as well as aortopulmonary collaterals. MRI is especially useful in the assessment of aortic arch anatomy after coarctation repair. It is also commonly used to evaluate postrepair TOF patients to quantify right ventricle dilation, evaluate branch pulmonary artery size and stenosis, and define aortic root morphology.

In patients requiring repeat sternotomy, MRI is probably the most helpful modality to assess the risk of inadvertent injury to the right heart structures or ascending aorta.

Preoperative duplex ultrasonography of the femoral and iliac arteries and veins provides important information in all patients having repeat sternotomy in whom peripheral cannulation for bypass may be necessary and lifesaving.

▸ PERIOPERATIVE MANAGEMENT

The cardiopulmonary physiology of patients with congenital heart disease is often complex and labile. Therefore a dedicated and experienced anesthetist should provide induction, intraoperative care, and postoperative support. The anesthetist must have first-hand experience in managing interrelated shifts in pulmonary and systemic vascular resistances, dynamics of intracardiac shunt, and blood gas and intravascular volume status. Control of postoperative hemostasis begins with induction of anesthesia. Prophylactic aprotinin infusion for all reoperations and for all cyanotic patients is critical.

The surgeon must be continuously mindful of the anatomy and physiology of ACHD. The surgeon must appreciate all anomalous morphology that may predispose to intraoperative injury—particularly for reoperative surgery where pericardial integrity is lost. Many congenital lesions are associated with enlarged, hypertensive right heart structures that predispose to injury during repeat sternotomy. For example, patients with prior atrial repair of complete transposition of the great arteries (D-TGA) have a morphological right ventricle generating systemic pressure which may be apposed to the posterior shelf of the sternum. Malposition of great vessels such as the aorta in transposition complexes, TOF, or double outlet right ventricle (DORV) must also be recognized preoperatively because they are at risk of injury during sternotomy. Knowledge of the extent of mediastinal and pulmonary collaterals is helpful in lesions naturally associated with reduced pulmonary blood flow. The surgeon should also be aware of and anticipate the presence of previously placed extracardiac conduits and/or shunts that may increase the risk of catastrophic injury. Location of anomalous coronary arterial branches such as LAD from the right coronary artery in TOF should be considered as these may impact aspects of the planned repair.

Sternal Reentry Protocol

Coordination of the operating room team in planning and completing successful sternal reentry is essential. Most ACHD will have had one or several previous median sternotomies.

Anticipation and Preparation

Every patient undergoing repeat sternotomy is at risk of injury to the heart and great vessels. Some are at greater risk such as those with enlarged or hypertensive right heart structures, aortic malposition or transposition where the ascending aorta may be close to the sternum, and previous conduit implants.

Although the lateral chest radiograph and MRI may be useful in predicting the potential for injury, one should assume injury could and will happen during any sternal reentry.

If injury occurs peripheral cannulation for bypass may be necessary, and the status of femoral and iliac vessels should be known preoperatively. Cannulae, pump tubing, and appropriate connectors for peripheral cannulation must be immediately available. The presence or absence of intracardiac shunting should be known to evaluate the risk of paradoxic air embolization from venous bleeding. If bypass is required to facilitate sternal reentry, venous filling pressure must be controlled above zero to avoid entraining air into the circulation.

Electrocautery, mechanical stimulation, or traction near the heart during sternal reentry may cause ventricular or supraventricular arrhythmia. Immediate defibrillation may be required. Internal paddles may be used if the heart has been exposed, and defibrillator pads positioned on the chest wall outside of the sterile field facilitate rapid defibrillation in the undissected mediastinum.

The patient should be heparinized for bypass prior to sternotomy.

The "Moving-V" Incision

Resternotomy begins with exposure and preservation of previous sternal wires. After untwisting the wires, traction on these by the assistant is useful for pulling the sternum away from the cardiac structures. The wire behind the sternum is also an important gauge for determining the appropriate depth of sawing. The linea alba is opened next, and a plane of dissection deep to the posterior wall of the rectus sheath is established from the midline to a lateral width of 10–15 cm on each side. This lateral plane of dissection is carried cephalad in a broad V-shape with the wide apex of the V in the midline behind the sternum. Electrocautery is used for much of the dissection, and the power should not be excessive nor should "spray" mode be used to lessen the chance of causing ventricular fibrillation. Dissection behind the sternum proceeds cephalad and after 2–4 cm of midline sternum is free of adhesions, the oscillating sternal saw with a narrow blade is used with light vertical pressure to divide the sternum over the clear area. After each vertical cut, the saw is lifted to the adjacent site and should not slide sideways to avoid tearing the tissue deep to the sternum. The saw is used to divide the outer table of sternal bone, the marrow, and the inner table of bone. The saw should not divide the inner table of periosteum. The surgeon should be able to feel the saw's progress and timing through each sternal layer.

The inner periosteum of the sternum should be divided with heavy straight scissors under direct vision. As each section of the sternum is divided, the newly exposed adhesions are dissected laterally from the midline and the V moves further cephalad to expose more of the deep surface of the sternum so that more can be safely divided.

With experience, most resternotomies are successful without resorting to peripheral cannulation. However, one should not be reluctant to support the circulation electively if adhesions are particularly difficult.

Management of Bleeding During Resternotomy

Inadvertent injury to cardiac and mediastinal structures may result in life-threatening venous and/or arterial hemorrhage. The source of bleeding, whether arterial or venous, is important.

Venous Bleeding

Sources of venous bleeding include right atrium, right ventricle, innominate vein, or pulmonary conduit. Lacerations causing venous bleeding can usually be repaired and may not require peripheral cannulation for bypass. Bypass suckers can be used to salvage blood loss, and unless massive venous bleeding is present, further dissection may provide sufficient exposure to control the laceration. Venous bleeding threatens the patient by blood loss. Less obvious, but more important, is the risk of venous bleeding allowing air into the circulation thereby leading to paradoxic air embolism. Therefore in the presence of intracardiac shunts, bypass with careful control to maintain a positive venous pressure is indicated for the control of massive venous bleeding. In addition, the patient should be placed in Trendelenburg's position and the table rotated to the patient's left side.

Arterial Bleeding

Bleeding from the mammary arteries is not infrequent and can be managed by further exposure and suture ligation. However, major arterial bleeding demands an immediate halt in dissection, compression of the bleeding site as well as possible, and immediate peripheral cannulation for institution of cardiopulmonary bypass. Once on bypass, systemic cooling is initiated and all further dissection in the mediastinum is avoided until the heart stops ejecting or fibrillates. Any attempt to repair a laceration to the aorta while the heart is ejecting will result in systemic air embolism.

With control of the circulation, low flow bypass is usually sufficient to complete the resternotomy and repair the aortic laceration. Total circulatory arrest is usually not required and the maintenance of some circulation decreases the risk of introducing air into the circulation. Once arterial bleeding is controlled, rewarming should be initiated so the heart can be defibrillated. Manual compression of the heart may decrease its distension until it is ejecting.

In summary, resternotomy requires a preplanned, coordinated effort from all members of the operating room team. Important injury to mediastinal structures will occur in some patients and initiation of the plan will be successful in salvaging an otherwise fatal situation.

POSTOPERATIVE CARE OF THE ACHD PATIENT

A multidisciplinary team of consultants, including specialized nursing care dedicated to adult congenital patients, provides postoperative management. The bedside critical care nurse is the front-line manager of patient care and adjusts medication and volume infusions to achieve stated objective endpoints. Arbitrary doses of drugs are avoided.

The physiology of the circulation in congenital heart defects will dictate the objectives in postoperative care. Monitoring of mixed venous saturations and lactate levels supplement direct measurement of cardiac output by thermodilution. Manipulation of peripheral and pulmonary resistances by control of ventilation parameters, (pCO_2 and pH) is as important as judicious infusions of vasodilators or vasopressors. Inotropic drugs are sometimes contraindicated (e.g., in dynamic subaortic stenosis) and selection of appropriate support drugs is based on the patient's underlying circulatory physiology and needs.

Arrhythmia control is vital. All ACHD patients should have atrial and ventricular temporary pacing wires for both diagnostic and therapeutic use. Suppression of SVT is frequently required, and an increasing proportion of these patients will have had a Maze procedure.

Postoperative bleeding remains an important source of morbidity, particularly after complex reoperative surgery. Anticipation of bleeding with early and adequate clotting factors is required. Aprotinin should be continued and fresh frozen plasma and platelets are almost always required in all but simple cases. Return to the operating room for postoperative bleeding is required if there is any evidence of tamponade. Bleeding should decrease after the first 4 h. Blood loss in excess of 6 cc/kg./h for the first 2 h and 3 cc/kg/h for the next 2 h will probably require reexploration.

SPECIFIC LESIONS

To provide continuing care to congenital heart patients in adulthood, adult congenital heart surgeons should be experienced in all aspects of congenital heart disease that are encountered in a pediatric surgical practice. Although a full review of specific lesions encountered in adults is beyond the scope of this chapter, the management of several common lesions are mentioned below. It must be noted that little data on surgical indications in adulthood are available to guide the surgeon. Despite this limitation, an excellent resource for managing this population is the synthesis of existing data and subsequent "recommendations" published from the Canadian Cardiovascular Society Consensus Conference (convened by an international team of experts and updated in 2001).[92,93,96] Although not individually referenced, many indications discussed in the subsequent sections reflect those recommendations.

Atrial Septal Defect

Physiology and Natural History

Clinical presentation of patients with ASD is dependent upon the type of defect, the magnitude of intracardiac shunt, and presence or absence of associated anomalies.[12,20] The volume overload from interatrial shunting is generally well tolerated for long periods of time. Asymptomatic patients with small intracardiac shunt (Q_P:Q_S < 1.5:1), no cardiomegaly on chest X-ray, and only minimal enlargement of the right ventricle have little to no risk of developing symptoms or pulmonary vascular complications and repair is unnecessary. For patients with larger shunts (Q_P:Q_S > 1.5:1), onset of symptoms may be expected beyond the second decade of life. The magnitude of intracardiac shunting may increase with age as left ventricular compliance decreases. The most common presenting symptom is reduced exercise tolerance with dyspnea and fatigue resulting from chronic volume overload of the right ventricular. Beyond 30 years of age, there is increasing risk of palpitations and arrhythmia resulting from atrial dilation. The onset of arrhythmia, either atrial flutter or fibrillation, usually causes a rapid deterioration in functional status because of loss of coordinated atrial contraction in the setting of right ventricular dysfunction. Patients who develop SVT will probably have persistent arrhythmia after successful ASD closure, especially if beyond 40 years of age.[37] These patients should be considered for arrhythmia ablation during ASD repair.

Older patients with an unrepaired hemodynamically important ASD may develop pulmonary vascular occlusive disease, although this is far less common and delayed in comparison to patients with VSD. Pulmonary vascular disease leads to a reversal of intracardiac shunting and systemic desaturation. Overall, patients with unrepaired ASD with Q_P:Q_S > 1.5:1 have a decreased life expectancy with an average life expectancy of 45 to 50 years.

Associated Lesions

Frequently older patients with an ASD develop tricuspid insufficiency and subsequent atrial arrhythmia. Other long-term complications of ASD such as mitral valve incompetence, pulmonary valve complications, and systemic arterial hypertension may be observed. Because of the potential for bidirectional shunting at the atrial level, patients with ASD are at increased risk of paradoxic embolization. Emboli within the systemic venous circulation that are normally cleared by the lungs may cross the ASD and enter the systemic arterial circulation. Cryptogenic stroke (i.e., a stroke with no source other than a paradoxic embolus) may occur in patients with patent foramen ovale (PFO).

Surgical Closure

The indications for ASD closure in the adult have been debated.[106] In the absence of firm guidelines, most centers advocate closure of hemodynamically important ASDs with the goal of averting the long-term complications noted previously.

In those few patients with pulmonary vascular disease, ASD closure is contraindicated unless the disease is reversible. Limits of reversibility are difficult to define. Measured pulmonary vascular resistance greater than 8 Woods units is unlikely to improve, and repair may actually shorten life expectancy. In patients with elevated pulmonary arterial pressure (i.e., greater than two thirds of systemic arterial pressure) and Q_P:Q_S < 1.5:1, ASD closure should be undertaken only after fixed pulmonary vascular resistance has been excluded. Pulmonary artery reactivity to oxygen or nitric oxide or, less commonly, lung biopsy evidence of reversible arterial changes, may be helpful in patient selection.[81] Documented cryptogenic cerebrovascular event may also warrant ASD or PFO closure.

Results of Closure

Surgical closure of ASD should be accomplished with operative mortality below 1%. Among 243 adults with ASD (secundum 62%; primum 19%; sinus venosus 11%) repaired at the TCCCA, there has been one death. Functional improvement occurs in a majority of patients. In 88 adults having surgical ASD closure, Jemielity and colleagues documented improvement in NYHA classification from 62% in NYHA class III or IV preoperatively to 82% in NYHA class I or II at a mean follow-up of 6.9 years.[52] Objective evidence of normalization of cardiopulmonary performance in adults with ASD was reported by Helber and associates, although they found that complete recovery may take up to 10 years.[45]

Although long-term outcomes after ASD closure are generally excellent, benefits of closure appear to depend upon the timing of closure. A survival benefit has been demonstrated for closure prior to 25 years of age compared to later closure, and closure prior to 40 years of age appears to confer protection from later onset atrial arrhythmias. In a classic study, Murphy and colleagues showed that patients repaired before age 25 had similar 27-year survival to a normal control population; however, 27-year survival for those repaired between 25 to 41 years and beyond 41 years was 84% and 40% respectively—both significantly less than the normal control population.[69] It is important to note that preoperative atrial arrhythmias persist after ASD closure in 60% of patients in whom a preoperative arrhythmia was present. Risk factors for persistent postclosure atrial arrhythmias include preoperative arrhythmia, older age (>40 years), and perioperative onset of arrhythmia.[37] Therefore arrhythmia ablation should be considered in adults during ASD repair if they have preoperative atrial arrhythmia, and perhaps in all adults over 40 years of age at the time surgery.

Ventricular Septal Defect

Physiology and Natural History

Although the clinical course of patients born with VSD is variable, presentation of an isolated VSD in adulthood

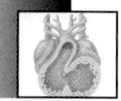

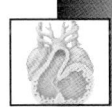

is uncommon. The natural history of a VSD is that 50% will close spontaneously by preschool years.[13] Defects remaining open beyond this time are unlikely to close spontaneously. The natural history of patients with an isolated VSD depends upon the size and location of the defect. The magnitude of left-to-right shunt is dictated by the size of the defect, the ratio of pulmonary-to-systemic vascular resistance, and the presence and severity of right ventricular outflow tract (RVOT) stenosis. The intracardiac shunt will remain left-to-right as long as there is absence of severe RVOT obstruction or advanced pulmonary vascular disease.

Surgical Closure

Most patients with clinically important VSDs are diagnosed and surgically repaired within the first year of life. Closure is indicated for signs and symptoms of congestive heart failure within the first 1 to 4 months of life and before age 9 to 12 months in the presence of pulmonary hypertension. For patients over 2 years of age, surgery is required only for the development of complications of the VSD or for the occasional patient with a persistently high left-to-right shunt. Lesions associated with a VSD include development of RVOT obstruction, aortic valve prolapse or aortic insufficiency, sinus of Valsalva aneurysm, and endocarditis.

The indications for surgical repair of VSD in adults are noted in Box 128-2. Most adults with a small VSD are asymptomatic and have normal pulmonary artery pressure and normal heart size if the $Q_P:Q_S$ is less than 1.5:1. These patients do not need closure in the absence of complicating features, have an excellent prognosis, and need only endocarditis prophylaxis over the long term.[61,103,108]

Adults with larger shunts ($Q_P:Q_S > 1.5:1$), increased pulmonary artery pressure, or cardiac chamber enlargement should be considered for VSD repair. Repair is safe and should restore normal ventricular size and function and prevent future deterioration and the risk of endocarditis.

Although pulmonary vascular disease is uncommon in patients with a VSD, the development of Eisenmenger's syndrome in the adult results in a very poor outlook and is a contraindication to VSD repair.[70,108] The limits of reversible pulmonary disease are difficult to define, but pulmonary artery pressure greater than 80 to 90% of systemic arterial pressure in the presence of a small shunt ($Q_P:Q_S < 1.5:1$) or a calculated pulmonary vascular resistance greater than 6 to 8 Wood units is unlikely to be reversible. Pulmonary artery reactivity to oxygen or nitric oxide may be useful in patient selection and in borderline cases, lung biopsy may be helpful.[81]

Box 128–2. Indications for Surgical Closure of Ventricular Septal Defects in Adulthood.

- **Presence of a hemodynamically important VSD**
  - Symptoms
  - $Q_P:Q_S \geq 2:1$
  - Pulmonary artery systolic pressure ≥50 mm Hg with a left-to-right shunt
  - Deteriorating ventricular function
    - Right ventricle due to pressure overload
    - Left ventricle due to volume overload
- **Important right ventricular outflow tract obstruction**
  - Peak-to-peak gradient ≥50 mm Hg
  - Echo peak instantaneous gradient ≥70 mm Hg
- **Aortic valve prolapse with a doubly committed subarterial defect**
- **Aortic insufficiency with an outlet muscular or perimembranous defect**
- **History of endocarditis**
- **Sinus of Valsalva aneurysm**

Associated Lesions

In the adult with a VSD, the most common associated lesion is RVOT obstruction (Figure 128-2). Some of these patients will also develop fibromuscular subaortic stenosis. The increase in right ventricular pressure may result in ventricular arrhythmia, tricuspid valve insufficiency, and atrial arrhythmia. Rarely, the obstruction may be so severe that right-to-left shunting occurs and causes desaturation or even peripheral cyanosis (so-called "acquired tetralogy of Fallot"). Repair of VSD with RVOT obstruction is indicated in patients with an RVOT pressure gradient greater than 50 mm Hg. Because the pulmonary vasculature has been protected and the pulmonary valve is nearly always normal, repair is safe and long-term outlook following repair is excellent. In some adults with RVOT obstruction, the VSD may have closed spontaneously, and they require only "isolated" RVOT resection.

The risk of endocarditis among patients with a VSD is very small and not an indication to recommend VSD repair. However, once endocarditis occurs, it is more likely to recur and is an indication for VSD repair. Endocarditis after successful VSD closure is very rare.

Associated Aortic Insufficiency

Patients with a VSD may develop aortic valve prolapse and subsequent aortic valve insufficiency (AI). The risk of developing AI is much higher in patients with a doubly committed subarterial outlet VSD than for other types of VSD (Figure 128-3A and B). Therefore we recommend closure of doubly committed subarterial defects if prolapse of the aortic valve is present. For patients with an outlet muscular VSD or perimembranous VSD, prolapse may not progress to AI, and we do not recommend VSD repair unless there is associated AI. In these cases, repair of both the VSD and of the aortic valve is recommended. Repair of the aortic valve in the adult may not be as durable as in the child.[82] The onset of aortic valve prolapse may restrict the size of the defect and the flow through it. The prolapsing leaflet itself may cause RVOT obstruction.[97]

Results of Closure

At the TCCCA, we have operated upon 103 adults with VSD. All had VSD closure, and 79 (77%) required 94 concomitant repairs (Table 128-2). The most common associated repairs include relief of RVOT obstruction (n = 36, 35%) and valvular repair or replacement (n = 32, 31%). Mortality was limited to one patient (1%) with a concomitant lung transplant.

Surgical closure of uncomplicated VSD should be accomplished with operative mortality of <2%.[103] Increased

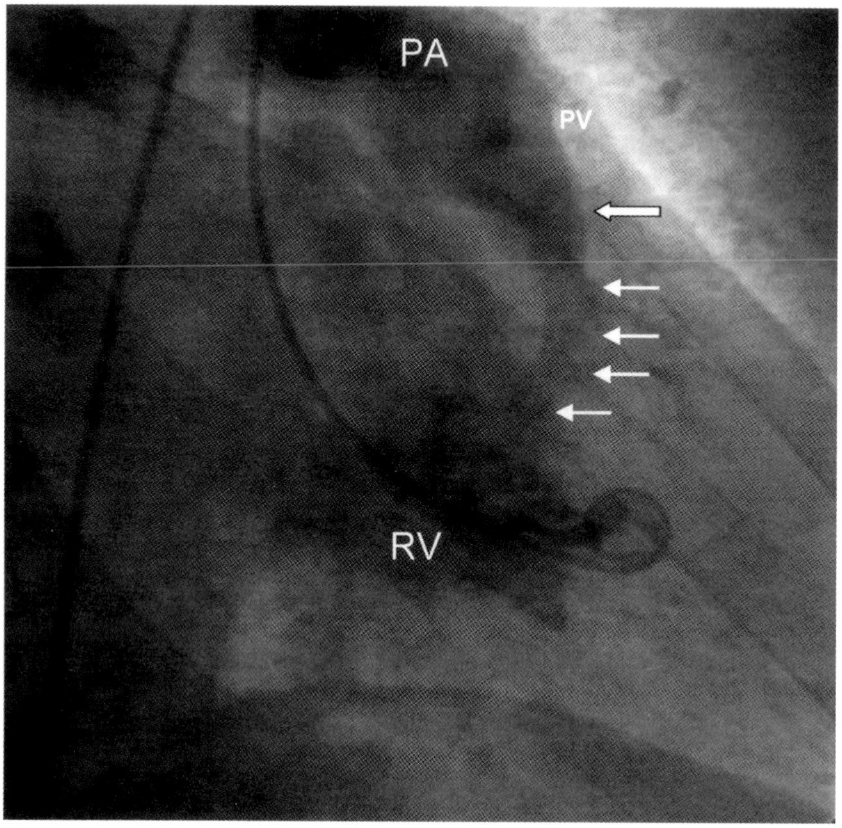

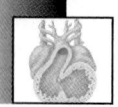

Figure 128–2 A right ventricular angiogram illustrates the severe RVOT stenosis below the well-expanded infundibular chamber supporting a normal pulmonary valve. The catheter is placed retrograde from the aorta and across the perimembranous VSD. The patient is a 35-year-old male with minimal symptoms but signs of right ventricular hypertrophy and strain on ECG. At repair he had a patch closure of the VSD, RVOT resection, and also required resection of LVOT fibromuscular stenosis.

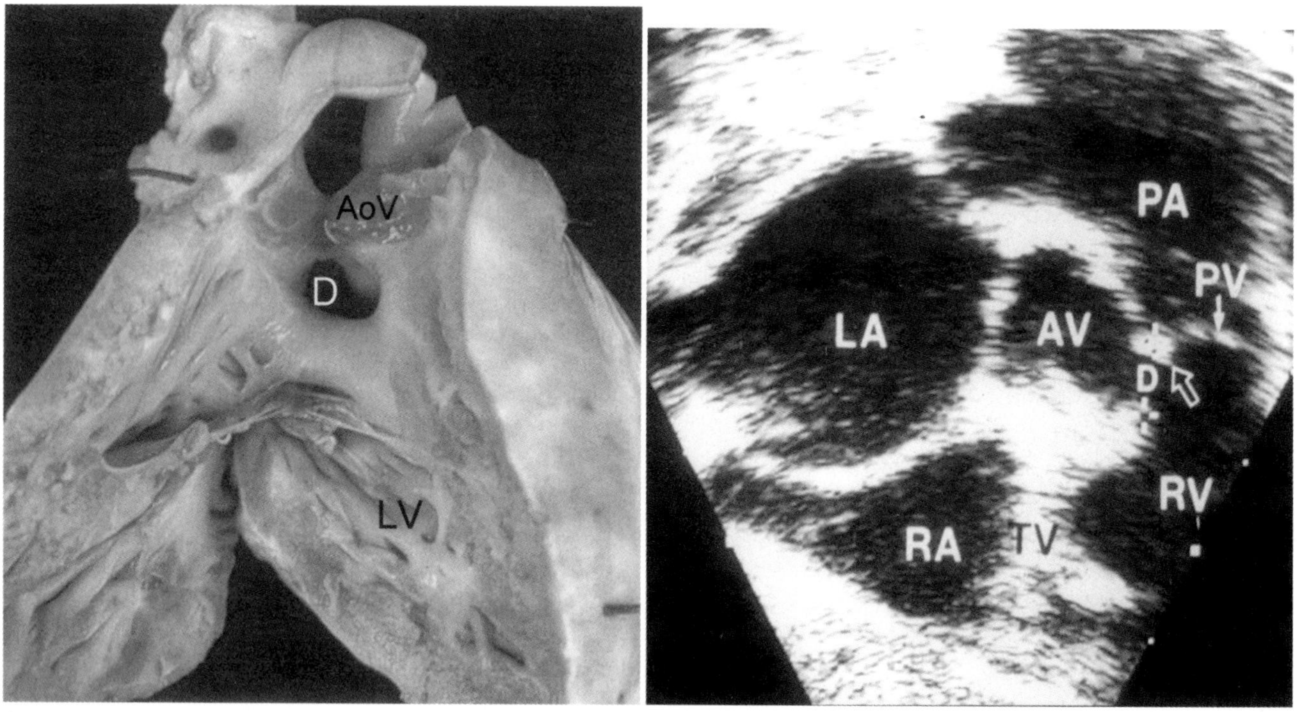

Figure 128–3 Aortic valve insufficiency in subarterial doubly committed ventricular septal defect (VSD). A, The anatomy specimen viewed through the right ventricle (RV) demonstrates the position of a doubly committed subarterial defect (D). There is fibrous continuity between the aortic (AoV) and pulmonary valve, and the VSD is adjacent to both great arteries. **B,** The echo illustrates the position of the VSD (D) relative to the pulmonary and aortic valves (PV and AV). The arrow marks the fibrous continuity between the valves. The close proximity of the aortic valve to the VSD usually results in aortic valve prolapse that progresses to aortic regurgitation. (See color plate.)

Table 128–2

Concomitant Repairs Performed During VSD Closure in 103 Adults[a]

Repair	*N*
Relief of RVOT obstruction	36
Aortic valve operation	16
Repair	10
Replacement	6
Tricuspid valve repair	9
Mitral valve operation	7
Repair	4
Replacement	3
ASD closure	6
Relief of LVOT obstruction	5
Sinus of Valsalva aneurysm repair	4
Partial anomalous pulmonary venous return	2
Coronary artery bypass graft	2
Lung biopsy	2
Lung transplant	2
Arrhythmia ablation	1
Other	2
Total concomitant repairs	**94 (in 79 adults)**

[a]24 adults (23%) had repair of an isolated VSD with no associated lesions.
ASD, Atrial septal defect; LVOT, left ventricular outflow tract; RVOT, right ventricular outflow tract.

risk is conferred by moderate or greater elevation of pulmonary artery pressure, multiple defects, and aortic regurgitation. Long-term outcomes after VSD closure are generally excellent. Survival to 25 years after closure has approached 90% in second natural history studies.[54] Otterstad and colleagues reported 5% long-term mortality as well as preservation of functional status and lower incidence of valvular complications and endocarditis compared to unrepaired VSDs in adolescents and adults followed an average of 15 years.[75] Potential late complications include residual shunt, conduction defects, and risk of tachyarrhythmia, and rarely subaortic obstruction. When present, residual shunt is often small and hemodynamically insignificant but requires continued prophylaxis for endocarditis. Reoperation should be considered for residual lesions with $Q_P:Q_S \geq 1.5:1$ and/or elevated pulmonary artery pressure.

Tetralogy of Fallot

Historical Perspective

Most adults with TOF will have been repaired during childhood. In most adults intracardiac repair would have been at a much older age than the current elective age of repair of 3 to 9 months. Repair of TOF in that early era was likely done through a generous right ventricular incision and, compared to current practices, was less likely to preserve the pulmonary valve. In recent years, adults in North America rarely present for initial repair of TOF. Surgical intervention in the adult with TOF will be predominantly for late deterioration many years after intracardiac repair.

Physiology and Natural History

TOF results from anterior and cephalad deviation of the infundibular septum. It is characterized by a malalignment subaortic VSD, RVOT obstruction, right ventricular hypertrophy, and an overriding aorta. The RVOT obstruction results in right-to-left intracardiac shunting and cyanosis. Rarely, TOF with mild RVOT obstruction results in desaturation without cyanosis (so-called "pink tetralogy"), and these patients may present later in life. Tetralogy-like physiology may be observed in adults with long-standing unoperated VSD in whom RVOT obstruction develops in later decades of life (see VSD section).

Late Primary Repair

Complete repair should be considered for adults who present with no prior surgery or with prior palliation. Indications for repair include worsening symptoms such as fatigue and dyspnea. Increasing level of cyanosis is less common than in childhood and is probably due to decreasing cardiac output from left ventricular dysfunction or increasing pulmonary vascular resistance, rather than outgrowth of pulmonary blood flow as is commonly seen in children. For patients with long-standing shunt palliation, evaluation of pulmonary artery anatomy and physiology is imperative because of the potential for pulmonary artery distortion, stenosis, aneurysm, or hypertension. Late palliative shunt complications such as pulmonary artery branch stenosis, left ventricular dysfunction, and aortic root dilation with aortic regurgitation may complicate late repair.

Late primary repair of TOF is associated with gratifying results if left ventricular function is not compromised and there is no major coexisting comorbidity.[72] Irreversible pulmonary hypertension and nonreparable anatomical lesions, such as severely hypoplastic or nonconfluent hypoplastic pulmonary arteries, must be excluded prior to late primary repair.

Late Repair of Residual Lesions

It is estimated that 10 to 15% of patients with repaired TOF require reoperation by 20 years after repair.[93] The second natural history of TOF demonstrates that the presence and magnitude of residual lesions affect late outcomes. Essentially all patients after TOF repair have some degree of residual RVOT stenosis and/or pulmonary valve insufficiency. Although residual lesions are usually well tolerated for many years, there appears to be an increasing prevalence of adults with repaired TOF who develop progressive cardiac symptoms after age 30 years. Symptoms result from deleterious effects of residual RVOT lesions (Figure 128-4), most commonly pulmonary valve insufficiency. The chronic volume load from pulmonary insufficiency results in right ventricular dilation, decreasing contractility, and eventually ventricular arrhythmia and tricuspid regurgitation followed by atrial tachyarrhythmia. In adults with RVOT stenosis, long-standing ventricular hypertrophy may lead to myocardial fibrosis, subendocardial ischemia, and ventricular tachycardia. The rate of right ventricular decompensation may be accelerated by branch pulmonary artery stenosis or residual atrial and/or VSDs. Reduced exercise tolerance and dyspnea may develop, and late sudden death is not uncommon. Gatzoulis et al have shown in a multiinstitutional study of postrepair TOF patients that a QRS width >180 ms and prolonged QT dispersion are risk factors for ventricular arrhythmia and late sudden death.[36] A subsequent report revealed that the combination of QRS width >180 ms and significant left ventricular systolic dysfunction are highly predictive of sudden cardiac death in TOF patients.[42]

Chronic right ventricular failure also produces dilation of the tricuspid annulus and distortion of the subvalvular apparatus with resultant tricuspid valve insufficiency. Worsening tricuspid regurgitation accelerates right ventricular failure as well as right atrial dilation—a risk factor for atrial arrhythmia.[36]

Left-sided cardiac lesions may also occur late after TOF repair. These lesions tend to occur in patients after age 40 years in whom the primary repair was at an older age. Approximately 15% of adults with repaired TOF develop progressive aortic root dilatation due to long-standing volume overload of the aortic root and to intrinsic histological abnormalities of the aortic wall. Aortic root dilation may lead to aortic valve insufficiency.[71]

Indications for reoperation in adults with previous intracardiac repair of TOF are noted in Box 128-3. Adults with repaired TOF are the most prevalent congenital cardiac group requiring late reoperation, accounting for 42% of reoperations in our series at the University of Toronto.[109] Residual lesions of the RVOT were the predominant indication for reoperation, and pulmonary valve replacement was performed during 87% of late reoperations in adults with repaired TOF. The primary technique for pulmonary valve implantation was orthotopic placement of the largest porcine valve, generally 29–33 mm. Patch enlargement of the pulmonary annulus and main pulmonary artery is usually required to accommodate a large pulmonary prosthesis. Most of these TOF adults (>75%) have multiple lesions requiring concomitant repair, on average 2.9 procedures per patient per reoperation.[73] The most common concomitant procedures include branch pulmonary arterioplasty (42%), arrhythmia ablation (31%) (see Arrhythmia section), tricuspid valve repair or replacement (22%), closure of residual VSD (9%), and aortic root repair (5%). Operative mortality is approximately 2% with two of three deaths occurring in patients requiring aortic root replacement. The number of prior cardiac operations, the number of concomitant procedures, tricuspid valve repair or replacement, and arrhythmia ablation do not appear to be important risk factors for death in our series.

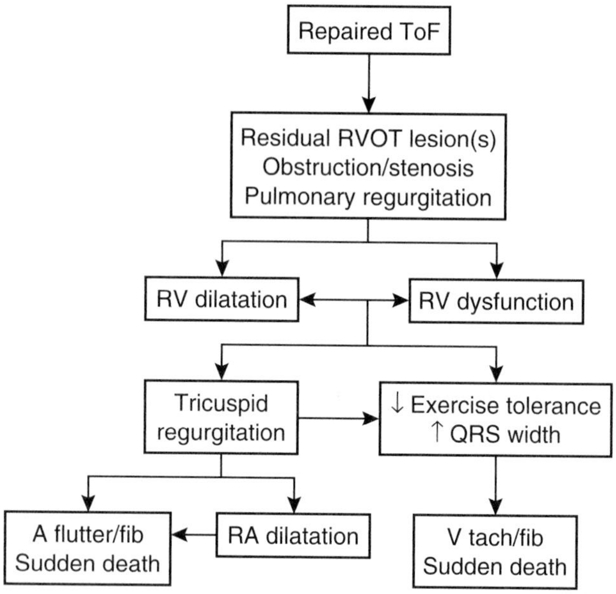

Figure 128–4 Schematic illustrating the chronic impact of residual hemodynamic lesions of the right ventricular outflow tract in patients with previously repaired tetralogy of Fallot. *(Modified and reprinted with permission from Ashburn DA, Harris L, Downar EH, et al: Electrophysiologic surgery in patients with congenital heart disease. Semin Thorac Cardiovasc Surg Ped Card Surg Annua 6:51–58, 2003.)*

Box 128–3. Indications for Reoperation in Adults with Previously Repaired Tetralogy of Fallot.

- **Pulmonary valve regurgitation accompanied by:**
  - Progressive symptoms
  - RV enlargement
  - Tricuspid valve regurgitation
  - Arrhythmia: VT or SVT
- **Residual pulmonary stenosis**
  - RV:LV pressure ratio ≥0.66
- **Residual VSD with Q_P:Q_S ≥ 1.5:1**
- **Aortic root dilatation ≥5.5 cm**
- **Aortic valve regurgitation**
  - Progressive symptoms
  - LV enlargement or dysfunction
- **RVOT aneurysm**
  - Rapid enlargement or pseudoaneurysm
  - Evidence of infection
- **Atrial or ventricular arrhythmia**
  - QRS duration >180 ms

LV, Left ventricle; RV, right ventricle; RVOT, right ventricular outflow tract; SVT, supraventricular tachycardia; VSD, ventricular septal defect; VT, ventricular tachycardia.

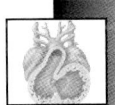

Although multiple aspects of outcomes after reoperation in patients with TOF have been reported, further late follow-up of this population is important.[6,49,73,110] Because pulmonary valve replacement has limited durability, repeat pulmonary valve replacement will be necessary. We have estimated that pulmonary valve survival in the adult population is 90% at 10 years after implant.[113] Patients report symptomatic improvement after pulmonary valve replacement, although objective evidence of functional improvement has been difficult to ascertain.[95]

Univentricular Heart and Fontan Surgery

Natural History

The adult survivor with univentricular heart (UVH) has defied the lesion's usually fatal natural history. Warnes and colleagues reported a small number of adults with UVH and perfectly balanced systemic and pulmonary circulations who survived into their sixth decade.[2] The rare patient with tricuspid atresia and, less commonly, other forms of UVH may be seen de novo during their adult years. However, the vast majority of adults with UVH will have undergone palliative operations, usually culminating in the Fontan/Kreutzer operation.

Surgical Palliation of Adults with UVH

Although surgical palliation in the adult with UVH may be indicated, the fact that some patients reach adulthood indicates that their pulmonary and systemic circulations must be ideally balanced or that they are surviving with pulmonary vascular disease. Clinical deterioration prompting reinvestigation of these patients usually confirms failing ventricular function in contrast to the common pediatric scenario of "outgrowing" pulmonary blood flow. Secondary effects of the failing ventricle may be the onset of atrioventricular valvular regurgitation and arrhythmia.

If the pulmonary artery pressure is low (<15 torr), the adult with UVH may be improved by a bidirectional cavopulmonary shunt (BCPS). BCPS may increase pulmonary blood flow and improve intracardiac mixing, thereby increasing systemic arterial oxygen saturation. Long-term palliation is sustained, and intermediate survival may be improved and is comparable to that for the Fontan operation.[39,100,112] The major advantage of BCPS is an increase in effective pulmonary blood flow without volume loading the systemic ventricle. Conversely, an aortopulmonary shunt increases ventricular volume loading and may accelerate ventricular failure. Arterial shunts in the adult are used rarely, and their size must be carefully controlled.

Fontan/Kreutzer Operations in Adults

The adult with UVH should be considered for the Fontan operation. Indications for performing a Fontan operation in the adult with UVH are a progression in symptoms, onset of complications, and/or deteriorating ventricular function. All criteria for success required in the younger candidate remain important in adulthood.[14] The effects of long-term volume loading including ventricular hypertrophy and diastolic dysfunction, which are risk factors for poor outcomes after Fontan completion, are especially relevant in the older patient. Even in the normal heart, left ventricular end diastolic pressure increases after the third decade at a rate of 2 mm Hg per decade. The relationship between diastolic dysfunction, ventricular hypertrophy, and ventricular compliance is complex and not easy to calculate, but is vital in determining the outcomes for ACHD patients.[33] Reported experience with the Fontan operation in adults is limited.[10,35,47,100] Early mortality does not appear to be different than in children (approximately 5% or less), and intermediate survival is between 70 and 80% at 10 years after Fontan, which is perhaps less satisfactory than in children. At 10 years post-Fontan, up to 90% of survivors are in NYHA functional class I or II. Late problems after Fontan operation in adulthood potentially include arrhythmia (in up to 60%) and deteriorating ventricular function (in up to 33%), although such complications are less common than among non-Fontan-palliated cohorts.[55]

As in other long-term studies, these are the outcomes achieved from an earlier era, and how these observations will change with better techniques applied at an earlier age remains unknown.

The Adult Late after Fontan Operation

Most adults with UVH will have had a Fontan operation during childhood. At the University of Toronto, 340 patients underwent Fontan operation between January 1977 and December 1991. From this population 228, or 67%, survived to adulthood (>age 18 years). The largest reported series of adults post-Fontan included 217 patients from 19 centers.[101] During a mean follow-up of 12 years, 9% died, 18% required Fontan revision, and 4% had a transplant. Functional class was 43% class I and 40% class II, and over 95% were meaningfully employed. There were 18 pregnancies with 15 live births.

Potential complications occurring late after Fontan operation are many.[31,32] Patients operated upon early in the Fontan experience who received a Fontan pathway via either a direct right atrium-pulmonary artery anastomosis or a right atrium-right ventricle conduit are at highest risk for late complications such as functional or mechanical pathway obstruction, thrombosis, and arrhythmia.[21] Complications in these technical modifications of the Fontan operation are attributed to incorporation of the native right atrium, which may severely dilate, into the Fontan pathway. Newer methods of constructing total cavopulmonary connection such as the lateral tunnel and extracardiac conduit provide improved flow characteristics and decreased atrial suture load aimed at reducing complications observed with previous technical modifications.[22,62] It is anticipated that lessons learned from earlier experience will substantially avoid or delay the risk of complications in future cohorts.

Adults with previous Fontan operation who present with hemodynamically important lesions of the Fontan pathway should be evaluated and considered for revision surgery. Complications such as exercise intolerance, arrhythmia, thrombosis, protein-losing enteropathy, and effusions may be harbingers of underlying hemodynamic lesions in the Fontan pathway. Once hemodynamic lesions are discovered, the decision to revise a failing Fontan connection should be made early in symptomatic patients before irreversible ventricular failure develops.

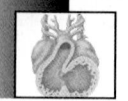

Fontan revision may include conversion of the Fontan circuit to a more hemodynamically favorable connection—usually an extracardiac connection between the inferior vena cava and pulmonary artery using an aortic homograft or polytetrafluoroethylene tube graft. Fontan revision may be performed safely and has been shown to improve hemodynamic performance and functional status.[63] Other important lesions such as moderate or greater atrioventricular valve regurgitation or pulmonary artery stenosis should be corrected at the time of Fontan conversion. However, in patients with failing Fontan circulation and atrial tachyarrhythmia, anatomic revision alone results in recurrent arrhythmia in as many as 75%. Mavroudis and colleagues have demonstrated that concomitant arrhythmia ablation at the time of Fontan revision is highly efficacious in managing coexisting pathway obstruction and arrhythmia.[65] As part of the Fontan conversion, they recommend a modified right-sided atrial Maze procedure in patients with atrial reentrant tachycardia and a Cox III Maze procedure for patients with atrial fibrillation.[18] Using this strategy in 40 patients followed up an average 2.5 years after surgery, they achieved 87% freedom from arrhythmia recurrence, 90% freedom from long-term antiarrhythmic medications, and significant improvement in exercise capability.

Irreversible ventricular systolic and/or diastolic dysfunction and elevated pulmonary vascular resistance post-Fontan represent an unsalvageable condition without cardiac transplantation.

Arrhythmia in Adult Congenital Heart Disease

Physiology and Clinical Importance

Arrhythmia is a very important late complication of congenital heart disease that negatively impacts the outcomes of affected patients. There is increasing risk of arrhythmia with aging, either with or without intracardiac repair.[86] Potential causes of arrhythmia in ACHD include residual lesions causing atrial or ventricular chamber dilation, ventricular hypertrophy, surgical scar, prosthetic material, intramyocardial fibrosis, and ischemia. Each of these factors may disrupt the natural equilibrium between conduction velocity, refractory period, and circuit length or circumference that predisposes to micro or macro reentry phenomena.[5,40,83,85] Arrhythmia almost always results in important, often sudden, deterioration in functional capacity and a risk of thromboembolism including stroke. Antiarrhythmic medication is expensive and fraught with important side effects. Arrhythmia is a common cause of premature death in ACHD and accounts for 26% of late deaths.[74,86]

The surgical management of arrhythmia is of increasing importance because of the growing prevalence of adults living with congenital heart disease. Many will have residual hemodynamic lesions and are candidates for cardiac reoperation. The type of residual lesion(s) determines whether they are at risk of atrial, ventricular, or both arrhythmias.

Atrial (Supraventricular) Tachyarrhythmia

Detection and management of supraventricular tachycardia (SVT) in ACHD presenting for repair or reoperation is important for three reasons: (1) SVT is an important cause of morbidity and mortality; (2) atrial arrhythmias have a propensity to persist or recur despite repair of the underlying defect; and (3) there are effective techniques for ablation of SVT.[37]

The arrhythmia must be accurately characterized to permit appropriate surgical planning and therapy. Adults presenting with a history of palpitations, presyncope, or syncope should undergo electrocardiogram and 24-hour Holter monitoring. Those with atrial fibrillation or typical atrial flutter do not require preoperative catheter-based electrophysiological study (EPS). However, those with an atypical atrial flutter need an EPS to define the mechanism and pathway of the flutter circuit.

Adults with less common arrhythmia such as accessory conduction pathways, dual atrioventricular nodes, and atrial ectopic tachycardia require preoperative EPS and may be candidates for preoperative catheter-based ablation.

The appropriate technique for surgical ablation of SVT depends upon the nature of the arrhythmia. Typical atrial flutter may be treated by cryoablation of the atrial isthmus. A 15-mm cryoprobe is used to apply overlapping cryolesions (−60° C for 2 minutes each) to the atrial myocardium between the inferior vena cava, tricuspid valve annulus, and the atrial septum to the right of the coronary sinus. For patients with atypical atrial flutter in whom the left side of the heart is normal, a right-sided atrial Maze operation as described by Theodoro and colleagues is performed.[91] Using this approach in 33 adults, combined with repair of concomitant cardiac defects, freedom from SVT recurrence at our institution has been 94% at 6 months, 89% at 1 year, and 84% at 3 years with no late deaths.[3]

Optimal surgical management of atrial fibrillation in ACHD is a debated subject. Some advocate a right-sided Maze operation for lesions predominantly located on the right side of the heart, while others advocate a bilateral Maze operation.[19,55,65,91] Our experience in managing atrial fibrillation in ACHD patients has been less satisfactory than for those with atrial flutter. In a group of 20 patients managed mostly by right-sided Maze operation (n = 14), our experience is less satisfactory than for atrial flutter. Freedom from SVT recurrence in patients with atrial fibrillation is 65% at 6 months, 57% at 1 year, and 46% at 3 years.[3] The experience includes isthmus cryoablation early in the series. Our current approach using a right-sided or complete Maze operation may improve late outcomes.

Accessory atrioventricular bypass tracts causing reentry tachycardia may be surgically interrupted using the techniques described by Sealy.[84] Such operations are rarely necessary in the modern era of catheter-based mapping and ablation.

Ventricular Arrhythmia

Intraoperative EPS mapping and ablation of ventricular arrhythmia in adults has primarily been applied to patients with previously repaired TOF. These patients are known to be at high risk of developing ventricular arrhythmia, usually in association with residual hemodynamic lesions.[94] Approximately one third of adults with prior repair of TOF presenting late for reoperation have a history of VT. In adults with repaired TOF requiring reoperation for hemodynamic residua, ventricular arrhythmia detected by intraoperative mapping permits cryoblation. Ablation may decrease postoperative morbidity and mortality.[26] An approach that combines repair of underlying hemodynamic lesions and arrhythmia ablation is optimal management.[44] However, in contrast to atrial arrhythmia, repair of the underlying hemodynamic lesion decreases the prevalence of ventricular arrhythmia even if operative ablation is not done.

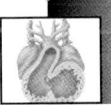

Preoperative screening for sustained ventricular tachycardia (VT) begins with a complete history and physical examination. Electrocardiogram and 24-hour Holter monitoring are indicated in adults with a history of palpitations, presyncope, or syncope. If these studies are diagnostic or a high index of suspicion remains, a preoperative EPS is performed. If monomorphic inducible VT is elicited, the patient is a candidate for intraoperative EPS and surgical ablation. In patients with known sustained VT the rate of preoperative inducibility averages only 70%. Therefore intraoperative EPS is performed even if VT could not be induced preoperatively. Intraoperative ablation is not indicated if VT is polymorphic (indicating multiple ectopic foci), and the patient is then managed with medication, with or without implant of an automatic implantable cardiac defibrillator (AICD).

Intraoperative management of ventricular arrhythmia begins with locating the site of origin of sustained VT. Prior to inducing VT, the patient is prepared for cardiopulmonary bypass so that circulatory support is immediately available. Electrophysiologic mapping is performed after induction of VT by programmed electrical stimulation. If induction of monomorphic VT is successful, epicardial and endocardial mapping are performed to define the site of origin.[27,76] The site of the reentry circuit in >90% of patients was in the infundibular septum adjacent to the VSD patch suture line and the tricuspid valve.[3] The site of VT origin is cryoablated (−60° C for 2 minutes) using three to six overlapping lesions. During cryoablation, the heart is arrested with cardioplegia to provide maximal depth and area of the cryolesion. Intraoperative ablation is not performed if intraoperative induction is unsuccessful, or if more than two sites of VT are identified.

Of 43 adults with CHD and sustained VT undergoing reoperation at the University of Toronto, intraoperative induction, mapping, and ablation of monomorphic VT was performed in 33 (77%). In the remaining 10 patients, failure to induce VT or identification of polymorphic VT precluded surgical ablation. Survival free of recurrent VT is 88%, 88%, and 80% at 6 months, 1 year, and 3 years, respectively, and to date is not significantly different for those who were not ablated.[3]

Complete Transposition of the Great Arteries

Historical Perspective

Most adults with complete transposition of the great arteries (TGA) have undergone either previous atrial repair (Mustard or Senning) or Rastelli operation. The transition to arterial switch operation occurred in the mid-1980s, so arterial switch patients are now just reaching adulthood. Surgical experience in the adult with TGA is limited (Table 128-3).

Table 128-3

Operations in Adults with Complete Transposition of the Great Arteries

Operation	*N*
Rastelli operation	9
Conduit replacement	6
Late conversion to arterial switch	3
Mitral valve replacement	3
Palliative Mustard operation	2
Tricuspid valve replacement	2
Fontan operation	2
Late arterial switch	1
VSD repair	1
Total	29

Atrial Repairs for TGA

Rarely, adults with TGA, VSD, and pulmonary vascular disease present with increasing cyanosis and are candidates for a palliative atrial switch operation.[11] An atrial switch changes the intracardiac mixing and transposes the higher preoperative oxygen saturation in the pulmonary artery to the systemic circulation, usually resulting in an increase of approximately 10%.

Adults with previous atrial repair (Mustard or Senning) have a very high prevalence of atrial arrhythmia that increases with age.[29,45,47] Many require both medication and atrial or antitachycardia pacing. Ablation of atrial arrhythmia has been performed in this setting, but the long-term success in this complex condition may be limited to providing better control rather than a cure.[87]

Baffle-related complications of atrial repair, particularly stenosis of the pulmonary or venous pathways, usually require reoperative management during infancy or early childhood. Some adults may have residual shunting through a baffle leak, although the shunt is usually incidental. The presence of a residual shunt precludes transvenous pacing because of the risk of paradoxical embolism.

Our oldest post-Mustard patient presented at age 52 years with sudden onset of morphological tricuspid regurgitation due to a ruptured chorda (Figure 128-5). He under-

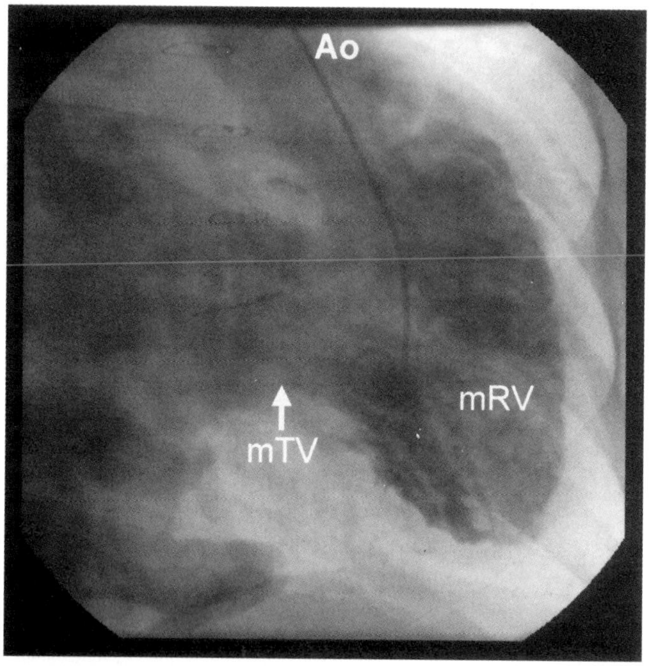

A

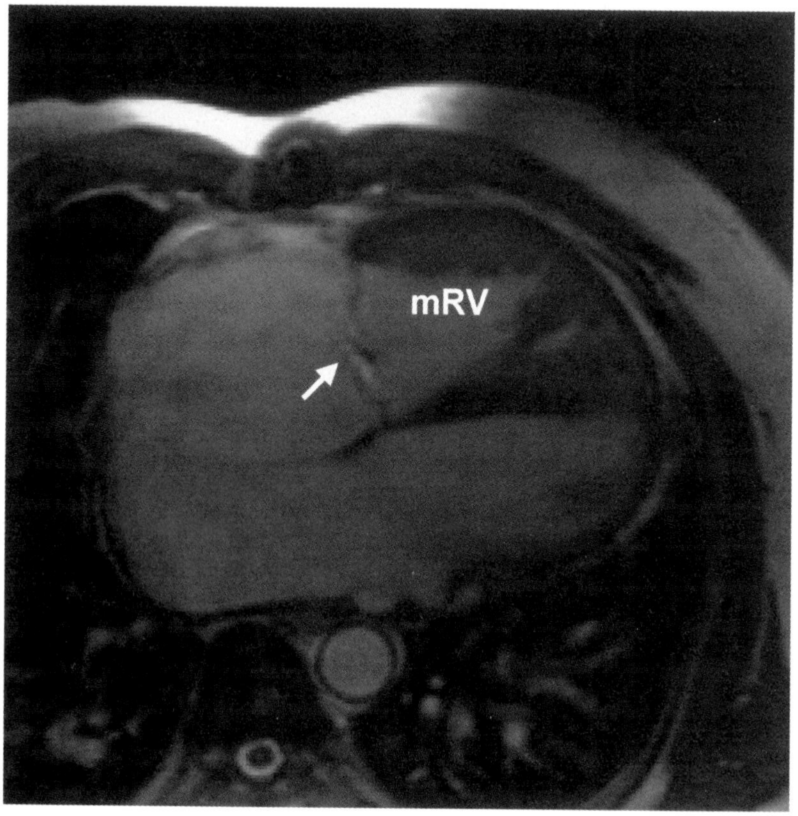

B

Figure 128–5 Images from evaluation of a 52-year-old man who presented with sudden onset of severe dyspnea 40 years after a Mustard operation for simple TGA. A, Retrograde angiogram shows a morphological RV (mRV), grade 2 function, supporting the aorta (Ao). There is severe morphological tricuspid valve (mTV) insufficiency with contrast seen within the pulmonary venous baffle. **B,** MRI demonstrates a ruptured chorda of the morphological tricuspid valve *(arrow)*. He underwent urgent tricuspid valve replacement and repair of a baffle leak.

went successful tricuspid valve replacement. Only one other adult with TGA had a tricuspid valve replacement—also for a torn chorda. Two adults required mitral valve replacement for endocarditis, one on two occasions for endocarditis.

The major concern for the adult with TGA after atrial repair is failure of the systemic morphological right ventricle and consequent atrial arrhythmia and right atrioventricular (morphological tricuspid) valve regurgitation.[44,60,78] These complications occur at an earlier age and are more prevalent in patients who required a VSD repair compared to patients with isolated TGA. Management options for these patients are cardiac transplantation or arterial switch conversion.

Conversion to Arterial Switch

Late arterial switch conversion requires preliminary preparation of the left ventricle (LV) by pulmonary artery banding.[15,66,79] Although the infant LV can be "prepared" to support the systemic circulation within 7 to 10 days, the time course for the older patients is much longer and is approximately 12 to 18 months in the adult.[25] Usually the pulmonary artery band must be tightened, and a remotely adjustable band would be preferable but is not yet commercially available.[16]

We have attempted pulmonary artery banding in only 5 of 556 Mustard patients. One was abandoned at operation because of cardiac arrest on induction of anesthesia, and she subsequently underwent cardiac transplant. One developed severe LV dysfunction after achieving systemic left ventricular pressure (two bandings in 18 months), and he was debanded and had a successful tricuspid valve replacement. Three other patients, ages 24 to 28 years, have had a successful late arterial switch conversion.

Overall experience with adult late switch conversions is limited although reported results are promising. Among 39 patients with failing systemic right ventricle after atrial repair of TGA, Poirier and Mee reported overall mortality of 33% (13 deaths: 8 early, 5 late) for a protocol of staged ventricular retraining.[79] Older age at staged conversion was a risk factor for death, suggesting that institution of such a protocol may be best performed early in the progression of systemic ventricular failure. Their data also suggest that biventricular function may be preserved in up to 90% of patients. Others have shown that tricuspid valve dysfunction is abated by arterial switch conversion.[99]

Rastelli Operation

Occasionally adults with TGA, VSD, and pulmonary stenosis (PS) will present for a Rastelli operation. An intraventricular baffle is constructed to direct blood from the left ventricle across the VSD and into the aorta, and right ventricle to pulmonary artery continuity is restored using a valved conduit. In our series there are 9 adults repaired at a mean age of 22 years (range, 19 to 37 years). Conduit replacement after a previous Rastelli was required in 6 other adults. The long-term outcomes for these older patients are not favorable.[23,57] Reoperating to replace the pulmonary conduit is inevitable.

Arterial Switch Operation

The late problems of the arterial switch population who are presently reaching adulthood are unknown. The fate of the neoaortic valve and of the surgically transferred coronary arteries is as yet unknown and requires ongoing follow-up of these young adults.

Congenitally Corrected Transposition of the Great Arteries

Physiology and Natural History

Congenitally corrected transposition of the great arteries (CC-TGA) consists of coexisting atrioventricular discordance and ventriculoarterial discordance. Despite the anatomical abnormalities of isolated CC-TGA, the circulation is physiologically correct (i.e., systemic venous blood is ejected into the pulmonary artery and pulmonary venous blood is ejected into the aorta). The systemic ventricle and atrioventricular valve are the morphologic right ventricle and tricuspid valve. Unlike complete TGA, CC-TGA may be undetected for decades; this is particularly true if there are no associated lesions.[80] Such adults may not present until the fourth or fifth decade of life when symptoms of rhythm disturbance, left atrioventricular valve regurgitation, and/or systemic ventricular dysfunction develop. Adults presenting with CC-TGA may not have had previous repair. Of 41 adults who have had intracardiac surgery at TCCCA for lesions associated with CC-TGA, 50% had no previous surgery and 32% had previous palliation only.

Associated Lesions

Patients with CC-TGA usually have associated VSD, tricuspid regurgitation, pulmonary stenosis, and atrioventricular conduction block, either alone or in combinations. We have previously reported the timing and results of surgery for lesions associated with CC-TGA.[111]

Surgery for CC-TGA

At the TCCCA, we have performed 46 operations in 41 adults (Table 128-4). Tricuspid regurgitation tends to increase in prevalence and severity as patients with CC-TGA age. We have performed tricuspid valve replacement in 17 adults. Mean age at surgery in our series is 36 years

Table 128–4

Operations Performed in 41 Adults with Congenitally Corrected Transposition of the Great Arteries

Operation	*N*
Conduit repair of VSD/PS[a]	17
Tricuspid valve replacement	17
VSD closure	7
LV-PA conduit replacement	3
Double switch operation	1
Fontan operation	1
Total operations	**46** (in 41 adults)

[a]Classic or physiological repair.

LV, left ventricle; PA, pulmonary artery; PS, pulmonary stenosis; VSD, ventricular septal defect.

(range, 20 to 63 years). Increasing symptoms of fatigue and dyspnea prompted operation. Failing systemic ventricular (morphological right) function is of particular concern in the adult with tricuspid valve dysfunction, and intervention should occur prior to deterioration of ejection fraction to 40% or less.[98] In spite of the systemic ventricle being a morphological right ventricle, long-term survival and functional results are reasonably good and approximately that for adults with normal AV connection.

Physiological Repair

Adults with CC-TGA, VSD, and pulmonary stenosis or atresia have traditionally been managed with VSD closure and bypass of the left ventricular outflow tract (pulmonary) obstruction by placement of a left ventricle-pulmonary artery valved conduit.[90,111] This type of operation is considered a physiological repair because it corrects circulatory physiology but does not correct the underlying atrioventricular and ventriculoarterial discordances. Our adult population of 17 patients undergoing physiological repair were operated upon at mean age 32 years (range, 22 to 45 years). Although this technique has been effective and is associated with an operative risk of <10%, long-term complications of conduit stenosis and progressive tricuspid valve regurgitation, as well as concern for the morphological right ventricle's ability to support the systemic circulation in the long term, have generated enthusiasm for the double switch operation.

Anatomical Repair

The double switch operation is an atrial switch operation (Mustard or Senning) combined with either an arterial switch operation (Figure 128-6) or, in the presence of pulmonary stenosis, a Rastelli operation.[7,24,48] The underlying anatomical defects, or atrioventricular and ventriculoarterial discordances, are corrected while preserving a physiologically normal circulation. The double switch operation circumvents the problems of the morphological right heart structures supporting the systemic circulation by transposing them to the pulmonary circuit; however, the problem of pulmonary conduit durability persists. Results with the double switch operation are encouraging, but its superiority to the classic approach will not be known until after 10 years of follow-up.[28,50,51,59,64]

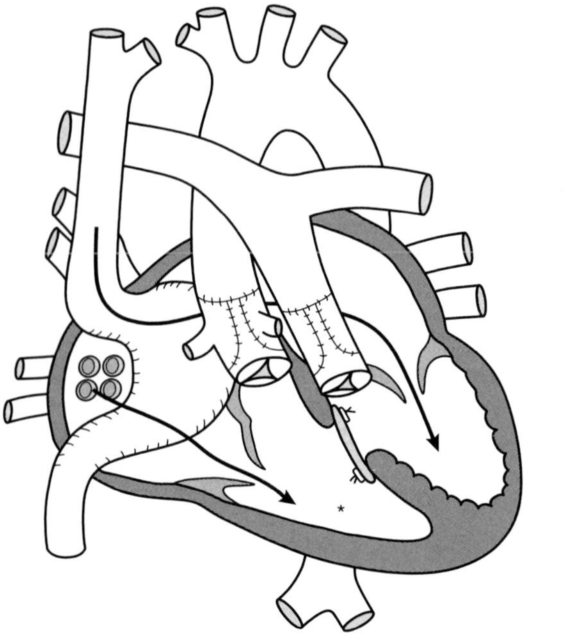

Figure 128–6 Double switch operation for anatomical correction of congenitally corrected transposition of the great arteries. After "retraining" the morphologic left ventricle using pulmonary artery banding to generate a pressure load, combined atrial switch operation (Mustard or Senning operation) and arterial switch operation place the morphological left ventricle (★) in the systemic circulation. The operation inverts both atrioventricular and ventriculoarterial discordance, and arrows denote the flow of blood through the repaired heart: systemic venous return—across tricuspid valve into morphological right ventricle (positionally left-sided) and pulmonary artery; pulmonary venous return—across mitral valve into morphological left ventricle (positionally right-sided) and aorta.
(Reprinted from Karl TR, Weintraub RG, Brizard CP, et al: Senning plus arterial switch operation for discordant [congenitally corrected] transposition. Ann Thorac Surg 64:495–502, 1997 with permission from the Society of Thoracic Surgeons.)

SUMMARY

Adult congenital cardiac surgery is a growing discipline with increasing clinical relevance. Many ACHD patients are at risk for poor outcomes because of natural progression of uncorrected defects and/or progression of hemodynamically important residual lesions. Once identified, surgical intervention in these patients can decrease the risk for, or delay, unfavorable outcomes. Further definition of the modified natural history of repaired congenital heart disease, operative indications, and long-term outcomes after operation in adulthood must occur if care for ACHD is to be optimized. Because this unique population is rapidly growing in the present era, ongoing requirements in health care delivery for ACHD such as resource allocation and development of specialized centers of care need to be met.

REFERENCES

1. American Heart Association: Heart Disease and Stroke Statistics—2003 Update. Dallas, TX: 2002.
2. Ammash NM, Warnes CA: Survival into adulthood of patients with unoperated single ventricle. Am J Cardiol 77:542–544, 1996.
3. Ashburn DA, Harris L, Downar EH, et al: Electrophysiologic surgery in patients with congenital heart disease. Semin Thorac Cardiovasc Surg Ped Card Surg Annua 6:51–58, 2003.
4. Ashburn DA, Webb GD, Van Arsdell GS, et al: Cardiac surgery in adults with congenital heart disease.
5. Bharati S, Lev M: Conduction system in cases of sudden death in congenital heart disease many years after surgical correction. Chest 90:861–868, 1986.
6. Bove EL, Kavey RE, Byrum CJ, et al: Improved right ventricular function following late pulmonary valve replacement

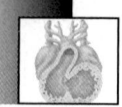

for residual pulmonary insufficiency or stenosis. J Thorac Cardiovasc Surg 90:50–55, 1985.
7. Brawn WJ, Barron DJ: Technical aspects of the Rastelli and atrial switch procedure for congenitally corrected transposition of the great arteries with ventricular septal defect and pulmonary stenosis or atresia: Results of therapy. Semin Thorac Cardiovasc Surg Ped Card Surg Annua 6:4–8, 2003.
8. Brickner ME, Hillis LD, Lange RA: Congenital heart disease in adults. N Engl J Med 342:256–263, 2000.
9. British Cardiac Society Working Party: Grown-up congenital heart (GUCH) disease: current needs and provision of service for adolescents and adults with congenital heart disease in the UK. Heart 88(Suppl I):I-1–I-14, 2002.
10. Burkhart HM, Dearani JA, Mair DD, et al: The modified Fontan procedure: early and late results in 132 adult patients. J Thorac Cardiovasc Surg 125:1252–1259, 2003.
11. Burkhart HM, Dearani JA, Williams WG, et al: Late results of palliative atrial switch for transposition, ventricular septal defect, and pulmonary vascular obstructive disease. Ann Thorac Surg 77:464–469, 2004.
12. Campbell M: Natural history of atrial septal defect. Br Heart J 32:820–826, 1970.
13. Campbell M: Natural history of ventricular septal defect. Br Heart J 33:246–257, 1971.
14. Choussat A, Fontan F, Besse P, et al: Selection criteria for Fontan's procedure. In: Anderson RH, Shinebourne EA (eds): Paediatric Cardiology. Edinburgh: Churchill Livingstone, 1977.
15. Cochrane AD, Karl TR, Mee RB: Staged conversion to arterial switch for late failure of the systemic right ventricle. Ann Thorac Surg 56:854–861, 1993.
16. Corno AF, Sekarski N, Bernath MA, et al: Pulmonary artery banding: long-term telemetric adjustment. Eur J Cardiothorac Surg 23:317–322, 2003.
17. Congenital heart disease after childhood: an expanding patient population: 22nd Bethesda Conference, Maryland, October 18–19, 1990. J Am Coll Cardiol 18:311–342, 1991.
18. Cox JL, Boineau JP, Schuessler RB, et al: Modification of the maze procedure for atrial flutter and atrial fibrillation. J Thorac Cardiovasc Surg 110:4473–4484, 1995.
19. Cox JL, Jaquiss RD, Shuesler RB, Boineau JP: Modification of the maze procedure for atrial flutter and atrial fibrillation. II. Surgical technique of the maze III procedure. J Thorac Cardiovasc Surg 110:485–495, 1995.
20. Craig RJ, Selzer A: Natural history and prognosis of atrial septal defect. Circulation 37:805–815, 1968.
21. de Leval MR: Right heart bypass operations. Semin Thorac Cardiovasc Surg 6:8–12, 1994.
22. de Leval MR, Kilner P, Gewillig M, Bull C: Total cavopulmonary connection: a logical alternative to atriopulmonary connection for complex Fontan operations. J Thorac Cardiovasc Surg 96:682–695, 1988.
23. Dearani JA, Danielson GK, Puga FJ, et al: Late results of the Rastelli operation for transposition of the great arteries. Semin Thorac Cardiovasc Surg Ped Card Surg Annua 4:3–15, 2001.
24. Devaney EJ, Ohye RG, Bove EL: Technical aspects of the combined arterial switch and Senning operation for congenitally corrected transposition of the great arteries. Semin Thorac Cardiovasc Surg Ped Card Surg Annua 6:9–15, 2003.
25. Di Donato RM, Fujii AM, Jonas RA, Castaneda AR: Age-dependent ventricular response to pressure overload. Considerations for the arterial switch operation. J Thorac Cardiovasc Surg 104:713–722, 1992.
26. Downar EH, Harris L, Kimber S, et al: Ventricular tachycardia after surgical repair of tetralogy of Fallot: Results of intraoperative mapping studies. J Am Coll Cardiol 20:648–655, 1992.
27. Downar EH, Parson ID, Mickleborough L, et al: On-line epicardial mapping of intraoperative arrhythmias: Initial clinical experience. J Am Coll Cardiol 4:703–714, 1984.
28. Duncan WB, Mee RB, Mesia CI, et al: Results of the double switch operation for congenitally corrected transposition of the great arteries. Eur J Cardiothorac Surg 24:11–19,90, 2003;
29. Flinn CJ, Wolff GS, Dick M, et al: Cardiac rhythm after the Mustard operation for complete transposition of the great arteries. N Engl J Med 310:1635–1638, 1984.
30. Foster E, Graham TP, Driscoll DJ, et al: Special health care needs of adults with congenital heart disease. J Am Coll Cardiol 37:1176–1183, 2001.
31. Freedom RM, Hamilton R, Yoo SJ, et al: The Fontan procedure: analysis of cohorts and late complications. Cardiol Young 10:307–331, 2000.
32. Freedom RM, Yoo SJ: Complications of the Fontan procedure. In: Freedom RM, Mikailian K, Yoo SJ, Williams WG (eds): The Natural and Modified History of Congenital Heart Disease. London: Blackwell Futura, 2003, pp. 460–470.
33. Freedom RM, Yoo SJ, Williams WG: The Fontan-Kreutzer procedure. In: Freedom RM, Mikailian K, Yoo SJ, Williams WG (eds): The Natural and Modified History of Congenital Heart Disease. London: Blackwell Futura; 2003, pp. 723–746.
34. Garson A, Allen HD, Gersony WM, et al: The cost of congenital heart disease in children and adults: a model for multicenter assessment of price and practice variation. Arch Ped Adol Med 148:1039–1045, 1994.
35. Gates RN, Laks H, Drinkwater DC, et al: The Fontan procedure in adults. Ann Thorac Surg 63:1085–1090, 1997.
36. Gatzoulis MA, Balaji S, Webber SA, et al: Risk factors for arrhythmia and sudden cardiac death late after repair of tetralogy of Fallot: a multicentre study. Lancet 356:975–981, 2000.
37. Gatzoulis M, Freeman MA, Siu SC: Atrial arrhythmia and surgical closure of atrial septal defects in adults. N Engl J Med 340:839–846, 1999.
38. Gatzoulis MA, Hechter S, Siu SC, Webb GD: Outpatient clinics for adults with congenital heart disease: increasing workload and evolving patterns of referral. Heart 81:57–61, 1999.
39. Gatzoulis MA, Munk MD, Williams WG, Webb GD: Definitive palliation with cavopulmonary or aortopulmonary shunts for adults with single ventricle physiology. Heart 83:51–57, 2000.
40. Gatzoulis MA, Till JA, Somerville J, Redington AN: Mechanoelectrical interaction in tetralogy of Fallot. QRS prolongation relates to right ventricular size and predicts malignant ventricular arrhythmias and sudden death. Circulation 92:231–237, 1995.
41. Gatzoulis MA, Walters J, McLaughlin PR, et al: Late arrhythmia in adults with the Mustard procedure for transposition of the great arteries: a surrogate marker for right ventricular dysfunction? Heart 84:409–415, 2000.
42. Ghai A, Silversides C, Harris L, et al: Left ventricular dysfunction is a risk factor for sudden cardiac death in adults late after repair of tetralogy of Fallot. J Am Coll Cardiol 40:1675–1680, 2002.
43. Haramati LB, Glickstein JS, Issenberg HJ, et al: MR imaging and CT of vascular anomalies and connections in patients with congenital heart disease: significance in surgical planning. Radiographics 22:337–347, 2002.
44. Harrison DA, Harris L, Siu SC, et al: Sustained ventricular tachycardia in adult patients late after repair of tetralogy of Fallot. J Am Coll Cardiol 30:1368–1373, 1997.
45. Helber U, Baumann R, Seboldt H: Atrial septal defects in adults: cardiorespiratory exercise capacity before and 4 months and 10 years after defect closure. J Am Coll Cardiol 29:1345–1350, 1997.
46. Helbing WA, Hansen B, Ottenkamp J, et al: Long-term results of atrial correction for transposition of the great arter-

ies. Comparison of Mustard and Senning operations. J Thorac Cardiovasc Surg 108:363–372, 1994.
47. Humes RA, Mair DD, Porter CP, et al: Results of the modified Fontan operation in adults. Am J Cardiol 61:602–604, 1988.
48. Ilbawi MN, DeLeon SY, Backer CL, et al: An alternative approach to the surgical management of physiologically corrected transposition with ventricular septal defect and pulmonary stenosis or atresia. J Thorac Cardiovasc Surg 100:410–415, 1990.
49. Ilbawi MN, Idriss FS, DeLeon SY, et al: Long-term results of porcine valve insertion for pulmonary regurgitation following repair of tetralogy of Fallot. Ann Thorac Surg 41:478–482, 1986.
50. Ilbawi MN, Ocampo CP, Allen BS, et al: Intermediate results of the anatomic repair for congenitally corrected transposition. Ann Thorac Surg 73:594–599, 2002.
51. Imai Y, Seo K, Aoki M, et al: Double-Switch operation for congenitally corrected transposition. Semin Thorac Cardiovasc Surg Ped Card Surg Annua 4:16–33, 2001.
52. Jemielity M, Kyszkiewicz W, Paluszkiewicz D: Do patients over 40 years of age benefit from surgical closure of atrial septal defects. Heart 85:300–303, 2001.
53. Karl TR, Weintraub RG, Brizard CP, et al: Senning plus arterial switch operation for discordant (congenitally corrected) transposition. Ann Thorac Surg 64:495–502, 1997.
54. Kidd L, Driscoll DJ, Gersony W, et al: Second natural history study of congenital heart defects. Results of treatment of patients with ventricular septal defects. Circulation 87:138–151, 1993.
55. Kobayashi J, Yamamoto F, Nakano K, et al: Maze procedure for atrial fibrillation associated with atrial septal defect. Circulation 98(Suppl II):II-399–II-402, 1998.
56. Koifman B, Edgell R, Somerville J: Prevalence of asymptomatic coronary arterial abnormalities detected by angiography in grown-up patients with congenital heart disease. Cardiol Young 11:614–618, 2001.
57. Kreutzer C, De Vive J, Oppido G, et al: Twenty-five-year experience with Rastelli repair for transposition of the great arteries. J Thorac Cardiovasc Surg 120:211–223, 2000.
58. Landzberg MJ, Murphy DJ, Davidson WR, et al: Organization of delivery system for adults with congenital heart disease. J Am Coll Cardiol 37:1187–1193, 2001.
59. Langley SM, Winlaw DS, Stumper O, et al: Midterm results after restoration of the morphologically left ventricle to the systemic circulation in patients with congenitally corrected transposition of the great arteries. J Thorac Cardiovasc Surg 125:1229–1241, 2003.
60. Lubiszewska B, Gosiewska E, Hoffman P, et al: Myocardial perfusion and function of the systemic right ventricle in patients after atrial switch procedure for complete transposition: long-term follow-up. J Am Coll Cardiol 36:1365–1370, 2000.
61. Magee AG, Fenn L, Vellekoop J, Godman MJ: Left ventricular function in adolescents and adults with restrictive ventricular septal defect and moderate left-to-right shunting. Cardiol Young 10:126–129, 2000.
62. Marcelletti C, Corno A, Giannico S, Marino B: Inferior vena cava-pulmonary artery extracardiac conduit. A new form of right heart bypass. J Thorac Cardiovasc Surg 100:313–314, 1990.
63. Marcelletti C, Hanley FL, Mavroudis C, et al: Revision of previous Fontan connections to total extracardiac cavopulmonary anastomosis: a multicenter experience. J Thorac Cardiovasc Surg 119:340–346, 2000.
64. Mavroudis C, Backer CL: Physiologic versus anatomic repair of congenitally corrected transposition of the great arteries. Semin Thorac Cardiovasc Surg Ped Card Surg Annua 6:16–26, 2003.
65. Mavroudis C, Backer CL, Deal BJ, et al: Total cavopulmonary conversion and maze procedure for patients with failure of the Fontan operation. J Thorac Cardiovasc Surg 122:863–871, 2001.
66. Mee RB. Severe right ventricular failure after Mustard or Senning operation. Two-stage repair: pulmonary artery banding and switch. J Thorac Cardiovasc Surg 92:385–390, 1986.
67. Moller JH, Taubert KA, Allen HD, Clark EB, Lauer RM, a Special Writing Group from the Task Force on Children and Youth AHA. Cardiovascular health and disease in children: current status. Circulation 89:923–930, 1994.
68. Moodie DS. Diagnosis and management of congenital heart disease in the adult. Cardiol Rev 9:276–281, 2001.
69. Murphy JG, Gersh BJ, McGoon MD, et al: Long-term outcome after surgical repair of isolated atrial septal defect. Follow up at 27 to 32 years. N Engl J Med 323:1645–1650, 1990.
70. Niwa K, Perloff JK, Kaplan S, et al: Eisenmenger syndrome in adults: ventricular septal defect, truncus arteriosus, univentricular heart. J Am Coll Cardiol 34:223–232, 1999.
71. Niwa K, Siu SC, Webb GD, Gatzoulis MA: Progressive aortic root dilatation in adults late after repair of tetralogy of Fallot. Circulation 106:1374–1378, 2002.
72. Nollert G, Fischlein T, Bouterwek S, et al: Long-term results of total repair of tetralogy of Fallot in adulthood: 35 years follow-up in 104 patients corrected at the age of 18 or older. Thorac Cardiovasc Surg 45:178–181, 1997.
73. Oechslin E, Harrison DA, Harris L, et al: Reoperation in adults with repair of tetralogy of Fallot: indications and outcomes. J Thorac Cardiovasc Surg 118:245–251, 1999.
74. Oechslin EN, Harrison DA, Connelly MS, et al: Mode of death in adults with congenital heart disease. Am J Cardiol 86:1111–1116, 2000.
75. Otterstad JE, Erikssen J, Froysaker TJ, Simonsen S. Long term results after operative treatment of isolated ventricular septal defect in adolescents and adults. Acta Med Scand Suppl 708:1–39, 1986.
76. Parson I, Downar E: Clinical instrumentation for the intraoperative mapping of ventricular arrhythmias. Pacing Clin Electrophysiol 7:683–692, 1984.
77. Perloff JK: Pediatric congenital cardiac becomes a postoperative adult: the changing population of congenital heart disease. Circulation 47:606–619, 1973.
78. Piran S, Veldtman G, Siu S, et al: Heart failure and ventricular dysfunction in patients with single or systemic right ventricles. Circulation 105:1189–1194, 2002.
79. Poirier NC, Mee RB: Left ventricular reconditioning and anatomical correction for systemic right ventricular dysfunction. Semin Thorac Cardiovasc Surg Ped Card Surg Annua 3:198–215, 2000.
80. Presbitero P, Somerville J, Rabajoli F, et al: Corrected transposition of the great arteries without associated defects in adult patients: clinical profile and follow up. Br Heart J 74:57–59, 1995.
81. Rabinovitch M, Castaneda AR, Reid L: Lung biopsy with frozen section as a diagnostic aid in patients with congenital heart defects. Am J Cardiol 47:77–84, 1981.
82. Rao V, Van Arsdell GS, David TE, et al: Aortic valve repair for adult congenital heart disease: a 22-year experience. Circulation 102(Suppl III):III-40–III-43, 2000.
83. Saoudi N, Cosio F, Waldo A, et al: Classification of atrial flutter and regular atrial tachycardia according to electrophysiologic mechanism and anatomic bases. J Cardiovasc Electrophysiol 12:852–866, 2001.
84. Sealy WC, Anderson RW, Gallagher JJ: Surgical treatment of supraventricular tachyarrhythmias. J Thorac Cardiovasc Surg 73:511–522, 1977.
85. Shen WK, Holmes DR Jr, Porter CJ, et al: Sudden death after repair of double-outlet right ventricle. Circulation 81:128–136, 1990.

86. Silka MJ, Hardy BG, Menashe VD, Morris CD: A population-based prospective evaluation of risk of sudden cardiac death after operation for common congenital heart defects. J Am Coll Cardiol 32:245–251, 1998.
87. Sokoloski MC, Pennington JC, Winton GJ, Marchlinski FE: Use of multisite electroanatomic mapping to facilitate ablation of intra-atrial reentry following the Mustard procedure. J Cardiovasc Electrophysiol 11:927–930, 2000.
88. Stark J: How to choose a cardiac surgeon. Circulation 94(Suppl II):II-1–II-4, 1996.
89. Stark J, Gallivan S, Davis K, et al: Assessment of mortality rates for congenital heart defects and surgeons' performance. Ann Thorac Surg 72:169–175, 2001.
90. Termignon JL, Leca F, Vouhe PR, et al: "Classic" repair of congenitally corrected transposition and ventricular septal defect. Ann Thorac Surg 62:199–206, 1996.
91. Theodoro DA, Danielson GK, Porter CJ, Warnes CA: Right-sided maze procedure for right atrial arrhythmias in congenital heart disease. Ann Thorac Surg 65:149–153, 1998.
92. Therrien J, Dore A, Gersony W, et al: Canadian Cardiovascular Society Consensus Conference 2001 update: Recommendations for the management of adults with congenital heart disease—Part I. Can J Cardiol 17:940–959, 2001.
93. Therrien J, Gatzoulis M, Graham T, et al: Canadian Cardiovascular Society Consensus Conference 2001 update: Recommendations for the management of adults with congenital heart disease—Part II. Can J Cardiol 17:1029–1050, 2001.
94. Therrien J, Marx GR, Gatzoulis MA: Late problems in tetralogy of Fallot—recognition, management, and prevention. Cardiol Clin 20:395–404, 2002.
95. Therrien J, Siu SC, McLaughlin PR, et al: Pulmonary valve replacement in adults late after repair of tetralogy of Fallot: are we operating too late? J Am Coll Cardiol 36:1670–1675, 2000.
96. Therrien J, Warnes C, Daliento L, et al: Canadian Cardiovascular Society Consensus Conference 2001 update: Recommendations for the management of adults with congenital heart disease—Part III. Can J Cardiol 17:1135–1158, 2001.
97. Van Praagh R, McNamara JJ: Anatomic types of ventricular septal defect with aortic insufficiency. Diagnostic and surgical considerations. Am Heart J 75:604–619, 1968.
98. van Son JA, Danielson GK, Huhta JC, et al: Late results of systemic atrioventricular valve replacement in corrected transposition. J Thorac Cardiovasc Surg 109:642–652, 1995.
99. van Son JA, Reddy VM, Silverman NH, Hanley FL: Regression of tricuspid regurgitation after two-stage arterial switch operation for failing systemic ventricle after atrial inversion operation. J Thorac Cardiovasc Surg 111:342–347, 1996.
100. Veldtman GR, Nishimoto A, Siu S, et al: The Fontan procedure in adults. Heart 86:330–335, 2001.
101. Wang S, Foster E, Graham TP, for the International Society for Adult Congenital Cardiovascular Disease: Clinical status of adults with prior Fontan operation. Presented at American College of Cardiology, 2000.
102. Warnes CA, Liberthson R, Danielson GK, et al: 32nd Bethesda Conference. Task Force 1: the changing profile of congenital heart disease in adult life. J Am Coll Cardiol 37:1170–1175, 2001.
103. Warnes CA, Fuster V, Driscoll DJ, McGoon DC: Congenital heart disease in adolescents and adults. C. Ventricular septal defect. In: Giuliani EF, Fuster V, Gersh BJ, et al. (eds): Cardiology: Fundamentals and Practice. St. Louis: Mosby, 1991, pp. 1639–1652.
104. Webb GD: Challenges in the care of adult patients with congenital heart defects. Heart 89:465–469, 2003.
105. Webb GD: Care of adults with congenital heart disease—A challenge in the new millennium. Thorac Cardiovasc Surg 49:30–34, 2001.
106. Webb GD: Do patients over 40 years of age benefit from closure of an atrial septal defect? Heart 85:249–250, 2001.
107. Webb GD, Williams RG: 32nd Bethesda Conference. Care of the adult with congenital heart disease: Introduction. J Am Coll Cardiol 37:1161–1169, 2001.
108. Weidman WH, DuShane JW, Ellison RC: Clinical course in adults with ventricular septal defect. Circulation 56(Suppl I):I-78–I-79, 1977.
109. Williams WG, Ashburn DA, Webb GD: Cardiac reoperations in adults with congenital heart disease. In: Franco KL, Verrier ED (eds): Advanced Therapy in Cardiac Surgery. London: BC Decker, 2003, pp. 263–268.
110. Williams WG, Harris L, Downar EH: Reoperation late after repair of tetralogy of Fallot; indications, timing, and outcome. In: Gatzoulis MA, Murphy DJ (eds): The adult with congenital heart disease. New York: Futura Publishing, 2001, pp. 81–91.
111. Yeh T, Connelly MS, Coles JG, et al: Atrioventricular discordance: results of repair in 127 patients. J Thorac Cardiovasc Surg 117:1190–1203, 1999.
112. Yeh T, Williams WG, McCrindle BW, et al: Equivalent survival following cavopulmonary shunt: with or without the Fontan procedure. Eur J Cardiothorac Surg 16:111–116, 1999.
113. Yemets IM, Williams WG, Webb GD, et al: Pulmonary valve replacement late after repair of tetralogy of Fallot. Ann Thorac Surg 64:526–530, 1997.

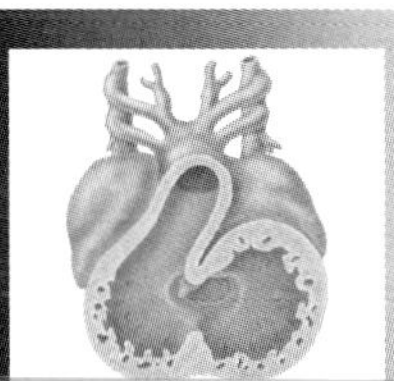

CHAPTER 129

Surgery for Arrhythmias and Pacemakers in Children

Constantine Mavroudis, Barbara J. Deal, and Carl Lewis Backer

INTRODUCTION

The advent of arrhythmia surgery and its evolution over the past 30 years expanded the options available for permanent arrhythmia management. Sealy and his associates from Duke University[12] are credited with the inauguration of arrhythmia surgery with ablation of the accessory connections that were responsible for the Wolff-Parkinson-White syndrome. Their anatomical studies in hearts free of structural heart disease resulted in 4 distinct ablation operations for manifest and concealed pathway dissection: (1) right anteroseptal dissection, (2) right free-wall dissection, (3) right posteroseptal dissection, and (4) left free-wall dissection. No accessory connections were found to traverse the shared annulus of the mitral and aortic valves, and therefore dissection between these structures was unnecessary. The outstanding success with the ablation of accessory connections[17,47] stimulated investigations into and the development of techniques for atrioventricular node modification for atrioventricular nodal reentry tachycardia,[93] atrial isolation techniques for automatic atrial tachycardia,[52] and ablative surgery in association with endocardial resection for ventricular tachycardia.[18,44]

The introduction of transcatheter radiofrequency (RF) ablation dramatically changed the therapeutic approach to arrhythmias. Transcatheter techniques mapped the offending arrhythmia and delivered RF energy to precise intracardiac locations to ablate accessory connections and foci of automatic atrial tachycardia and to create anatomical lines of block to treat atrial reentry tachycardia. For those patients with largely normal hearts and predictable anatomy, the results obtained with transcatheter RF ablation were—and remain—excellent.[41,53,54,61,70] During this period of transcatheter treatment of arrhythmias, research was ongoing in the field of surgical therapy of arrhythmias; Cox and associates[14,15,20] developed the Cox-maze operations for atrial fibrillation. Many patients with atrial fibrillation also had concomitant mitral valve disease that required surgery. Thus, a group of patients that could undergo concomitant reparative and arrhythmia surgery was identified. Added to this group were those patients who failed catheter ablation and/or had a wide arrhythmogenic focus not suitable for ablation. Integrating the knowledge gained from the catheter ablation technique into the surgical repair of congenital heart disease opened new pathways to the single-stage therapy of structural and rhythm abnormalities, particularly in patients with complex congenital heart disease.[23]

ANATOMICAL SUBSTRATES FOR ARRHYTHMIAS

Arrhythmia has been defined as "any cardiac rhythm other than the normal sinus rhythm. Such a rhythm may be either of sinus or ectopic origin, and either regular or irregular. An arrhythmia may be due to a disturbance in impulse formation or conduction, or both."[26]

Supraventricular Tachycardia

Supraventricular tachycardia (SVT) has replaced the term "paroxysmal atrial tachycardia" for describing tachycardia using the atrium or atrioventricular junction. Classification of the mechanisms underlying SVT requires understanding the cellular mechanisms of tachycardia: reentry, abnormal automaticity, and triggered reentry. Reentry, which accounts for approximately 80% of clinical arrhythmias, involves a circuit with limbs of functionally distinct conduction properties. Unidirectional block in one limb of the circuit allows an electrical impulse to traverse the second limb and reenter the blocked pathway from the other direction.[56] Reentrant rhythms can be initiated and terminated with pacing, thereby allowing for the electrophysiological study of the tachycardia circuit. Surgical treatment of SVT secondary to Wolff-Parkinson-White syndrome allowed for the elucidation of the reentrant circuit involving the atria, the atrioventricular node, the ventricles, and the accessory connection; surgical division of the accessory connection removed the second limb of tachycardia necessary for reentry to continue. Automatic rhythms involve enhanced firing of a relatively discrete focus and account for less than 10% of clinical SVT[56,63,116]; these rhythms are not amenable to pacing for termination or initiation.

Classification of SVT is important because of the distinctive clinical implications of the different arrhythmias and their specific therapies. Table 129-1 presents a classification system for SVT that combines cellular and anatomical considerations. Accessory connection-mediated tachycardia, which accounts for at least 80% of SVT in childhood (consistent with its congenital basis),[63] includes patients with manifest preexcitation (Wolff-Parkinson-White syndrome) and concealed accessory connections (not apparent on resting electrocardiogram but able to conduct retrogradely from ventricle to atrium). Atrioventricular (AV) nodal tachycardia is made up of reentry SVT using dual AV nodal physiology and automatic junctional tachycardia that can occur postoperatively or, rarely, in congenital form. AV nodal reentry tachycardia accounts for about half of paroxysmal SVT in adulthood, which correlates with the development of dual AV nodal physiology.[56,97,116] Primary atrial tachycardia, which accounts for 10–15% of SVT at all ages, is confined to atrial tissue and persists in the presence of AV block. Included in this group of rhythm disorders are reentrant rhythms such as atrial flutter or atrial reentry following atrial surgery and atrial fibrillation. Also included are automatic rhythms such as ectopic atrial tachycardia, which is often associated with cardiomyopathy. Junctional ectopic tachycardia is associated with congenital heart disease acutely postoperatively and with the later development of atrial reentry tachycardia.

Table 129–1

Classification of Supraventricular Tachycardia

Accessory connection-mediated tachycardia
Orthodromic reciprocating tachycardia
Permanent form of junctional reciprocating tachycardia
Antidromic reciprocating tachycardia
Preexcitation variants
Atrioventricular nodal tachycardia
Atrioventricular nodal reentry tachycardia
Typical: Slow—fast
Atypical: Fast—slow
Atrioventricular junctional: automatic
Junctional ectopic
Primary atrial tachycardia
Sinus
Automatic atrial
Atrial reentry
Atrial flutter
Atrial fibrillation
Multifocal atrial

From Deal BJ, Mavroudis C, Backer CL: Surgical therapy of cardiac arrhythmias. In Mavroudis C, Backer CL (editors): Pediatric Cardiac Surgery, ed 3. St. Louis: Mosby, 2003, pp.713–738.

Ventricular Tachycardia

The more complex classification of ventricular tachycardia is based on predisposing causes (e.g., post-repair tetralogy of Fallot), site of origin, cellular mechanism, and genetic ion-channel disorders (Table 129-2). In infancy, incessant life-threatening ventricular tachycardia is associated with ventricular hamartomas or histiocytosis.[32,33,117] Before the availability of intravenous amiodarone, such infants underwent surgical resection of the left ventricular endomyocardium, with some success.[32,33,117]

In older patients (usually adolescents with structurally normal hearts), idiopathic ventricular tachycardia generally arises from either the right ventricular outflow tract (left bundle branch block, normal- to rightward-QRS axis morphology) or the septal surface of the left ventricle (right bundle branch block, left axis morphology); both forms are amenable to catheter ablation techniques, with success rates of 70–80%.[8,61,88,102] Rarely, ventricular tachycardia may originate from the epicardial surface of either the left or right ventricle and thus limit use of the catheter ablation approach.

Patients who have undergone postintracardiac repair of tetralogy of Fallot or double outlet right ventricle are known to have late sustained ventricular tachycardia. The reported incidence is 5–8%,[34,36,50] with a risk of late sudden death of 2–6%.[55,85,87] Older age at initial repair, residual right ventricular hypertension, right ventricular outflow tract patch or aneurysm, significant pulmonary regurgitation, prolonged QRS duration of more than 180 msec on resting electrocardiogram, abnormal signal-averaged electrocardiogram, and longer duration of follow-up have been identified as risk factors for the development of ventricular tachycardia.* Rarely, patients with congenital heart disease may have sustained ventricular tachycardia before surgical repair.

Atrioventricular Conduction Disorders

AV conduction disorders are of 2 types: congenital and acquired (e.g., after repair of congenital heart disease).

*References 34, 36, 50, 55, 85, 87.

Table 129–2

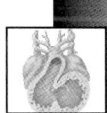

Classification of Ventricular Tachycardia

Scar-mediated
Postsurgical
Tetralogy of Fallot
Double outlet right ventricle
Postinfarction
Cardiomyopathy
Right ventricular dysplasia
Dilated
Bundle branch reentry
Hypertrophic
Electrical
Long QT syndrome
Idiopathic
Right ventricular outflow
Left ventricular outflow
Septal (Belhassen's)
Idiopathic ventricular fibrillation
Brugada's syndrome
Inflammatory
Secondary
Drug-induced
Electrolyte imbalance
Inflammatory
Ischemic
Traumatic

From Deal BJ, Mavroudis C, Backer CL: Surgical therapy of cardiac arrhythmias. In Mavroudis C, Backer CL (editors): Pediatric Cardiac Surgery, ed 3. St. Louis: Mosby, 2003, pp. 713–738.

Congenital complete atrioventricular block occurs in 1 out of every 15,000–22,000 live births and is associated with structural heart disease, particularly corrected transposition of the great arteries and heterotaxy syndromes, in up to 50% of cases.[81,86] Among infants with structurally normal hearts, the association with maternal antibodies SSA/Ro and SSB/La is well documented.[100] In older children with heart block, it is necessary to take a detailed history to elicit symptoms of bradycardia (e.g., prolonged naps, sleep disturbances), because children may modify their lifestyle to accommodate their limitations. Surgical AV block (complete or advanced second-degree block) persisting beyond 7–10 days postoperatively is a Class I indication for pacing. Without pacing, 53%–65% of patients will die suddenly.[51,72] Surgery involving ventricular septal defect closure (particularly in infants weighing less than 10 kg) or atrioventricular valve replacement accounts for most cases of surgically acquired heart block. Weindling and associates[114] have reported that 65% of patients with postoperative AV block will recover normal conduction, with the majority resolving by the eighth postoperative day.

INDICATIONS FOR SURGICAL INTERVENTION

Supraventricular Tachycardia

Surgical ablation of accessory connections achieved success rates of 95% or more before being supplanted by the widespread use of the RF catheter ablation technique.[16,17,45,46,74,75] At this time, surgical ablation of SVT is performed for patients failing both medical and catheter ablation techniques and for patients with complex congenital heart disease undergoing surgical repair. Certain accessory connections, especially in the posteroseptal region, may have an epicardial course[68] that limits the ability to successfully ablate using an endocardial catheter approach. Right-sided accessory connections in patients with Ebstein's anomaly tend to be multiple, with an increased likelihood of antidromic reciprocating tachycardia posing a therapeutic challenge. As compared with accessory connections in other locations, right-sided accessory connections are associated with significantly higher recurrence risks for preexcitation after ablation procedures,[9,96] and these often require multiple ablation procedures. Whether to persist with multiple ablation procedures or opt for surgical repair is an individualized decision.

Patients who have manifest accessory connections and who are to undergo surgical repair of associated congenital heart disease risk refractory tachycardia occurrence during the early postoperative period. Current recommendations are to assess the characteristics of the accessory connection and to perform ablation in those patients with inducible SVT and rapidly conducting accessory connections before surgical repair.[31,111] In the presence of associated complex congenital heart disease, more than 1 ablation procedure may be required, or the ablation procedure may pose technical difficulties that require prolonged fluoroscopy times.[11,71,109,110] Decisions must be made on an individual basis with regard to the optimal way to treat both the arrhythmia and the congenital heart defect, thus minimizing the number of procedures and the risk to the patient.

Patients with refractory atrial tachycardia failing catheter ablation procedures and patients with tachycardia requiring repair of associated intracardiac defects are considered to be candidates for surgical arrhythmia intervention. In rare cases of tachycardia in the neonate with structural heart disease (in which the ablation procedure poses significant risk to the infant), surgical ablation may be safely performed. In the structurally normal heart, atrial reentry tachycardia is uncommon, and it is usually amenable to RF catheter ablation procedures. If the area of reentry encompasses a wide area of atrial tissue, the catheter technique may not be successful, and resection with cryoablation may be effective.

Atrial reentry tachycardia occurs in 20–50% of postoperative Mustard or Senning patients,[37,94] 40–50% of Fontan patients,[38,91] and 34% of tetralogy of Fallot patients.[98] In the absence of hemodynamic problems, atrial reentry tachycardia is most often successfully treated using RF catheter ablation. However, if patients have residual hemodynamic abnormalities, consideration should be given to integrating catheter ablation into the surgical repair to minimize interventions for the patient. In contrast with nonsustained ventricular arrhythmias that may improve after the repair of residual hemodynamic problems, atrial arrhythmias tend to persist after surgery.

Catheter ablation of atrial reentry tachycardia after surgical repair of congenital heart disease has acute success rates of 30–80%,[3,108] with short-term recurrence rates of more than 50% for certain types of heart disease.[106] The catheter approach is more likely to fail in hearts with residual hemodynamic problems and markedly thickened atria. The Fontan population is particularly problematic as a result of significant atrial arrhythmias occurring in as many as 50% of patients with long-term follow-up[38,91] and limited success of the catheter approach, with high recurrence of tachycardia.[57,106] Factors contributing to the disappointing results of the catheter approach include chronic atrial hypertension and dilatation, distorted anatomy, multiple reentrant circuits, restricted catheter access (particularly after lateral tunnel-type repairs), and the inability to deliver RF lesions of sufficient depth to create a line of block. The ability to perform 3-dimensional mapping of the multiple reentrant circuits and to track the continuity of the ablation lines of block[29,99,107]—coupled with newer types of energy delivery enabling deeper lesions—may improve the results of catheter ablation in the future.[69]

The majority of Fontan patients with disabling atrial arrhythmias have significant hemodynamic abnormalities, including obstruction of the right atrial-to-pulmonary artery connection, pulmonary venous obstruction, and massively dilated right atria with sluggish venous flow, which predisposes them to atrial thrombosis.[91] In addition, in some patients, atrial reentry tachycardia may degenerate into atrial fibrillation, which is not currently amenable to catheter ablation in this population. The loss of atrial contractility is particularly debilitating in patients with single ventricle anatomy. Our center and others have attempted to treat the disabling arrhythmias with surgical revision of the Fontan anastomosis, without direct intervention for the arrhythmia substrate*; this approach resulted in improved hemodynamics but almost uniform recurrence of the atrial tachycardia.* The association of hemodynamic abnormalities and recurrent tachycardia after surgical repair has led our center to combine a surgical approach to arrhythmia therapy with revision of the Fontan hemodynamics in postoperative Fontan patients with refractory atrial tachycardia.[22,76,77] We have now performed 74 Fontan revisions in combination with arrhythmia surgery during the last 10 years.

In adults with unoperated atrial septal defects, atrial flutter/fibrillation occurs in 14–22% of patients.[5,7,35] Atrial fibrillation will persist in a high percentage of patients after surgery[5,7,35] if direct arrhythmia intervention is not performed.[6,64] Performance of right atrial arrhythmia surgery is ineffective for preventing the recurrence of atrial fibrillation. Therefore careful evaluation of older patients undergoing atrial surgery is necessary to determine the presence of atrial fibrillation and to assess the need for left atrial arrhythmia surgery.

Surgical treatment of tachycardia localized to the atria may involve resection or cryoablation of atrial tissue in addition to isolation procedures. Some authors had good results with simple cryoablation and excision of automatic foci, when found.[39,40,73] Multiple ectopic foci arrhythmia recurrence led surgeons to apply more extensive techniques[92] such as pulmonary vein isolation (Figure 129-1), left atrial isolation (Figure 129-2),[115] right atrial isolation (Figure 129-3),[48] and His bundle cryoablation, with pacemaker insertion in difficult cases. In general, refractory cases are rare and require an individualized treatment plan for accurate diagnosis and ablation.

*References 4, 13, 22, 59, 66, 79, 112, 113.

Ventricular Tachycardia

Patients with ventricular tachycardia refractory to medications and transvenous catheter ablation techniques and

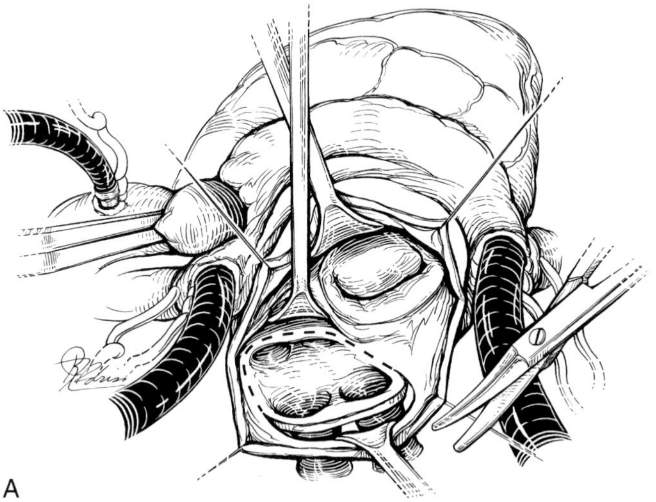

A

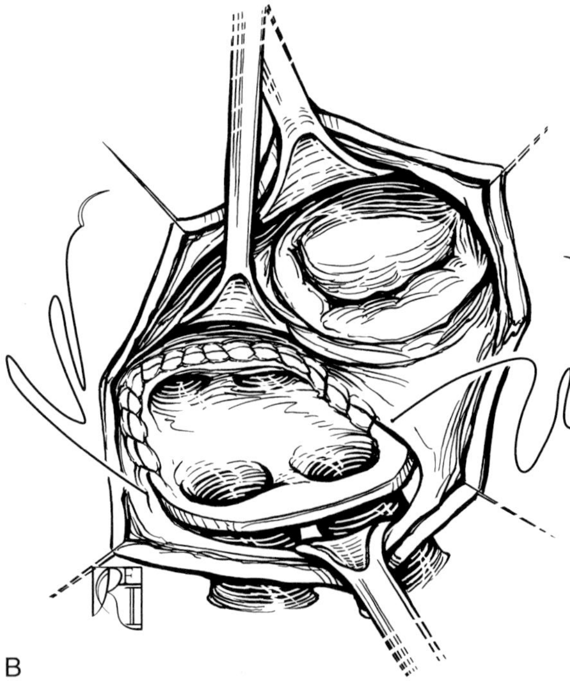

B

Figure 129–1 Isolation of an arrhythmogenic focus adjacent to the pulmonary veins.
(From Deal BJ, Mavroudis C, Backer CL: Surgical therapy of cardiac arrhythmias. In Mavroudis C, Backer CL, eds. Pediatric Cardiac Surgery, ed 3. St. Louis: Mosby, 2003, pp. 713–738.)

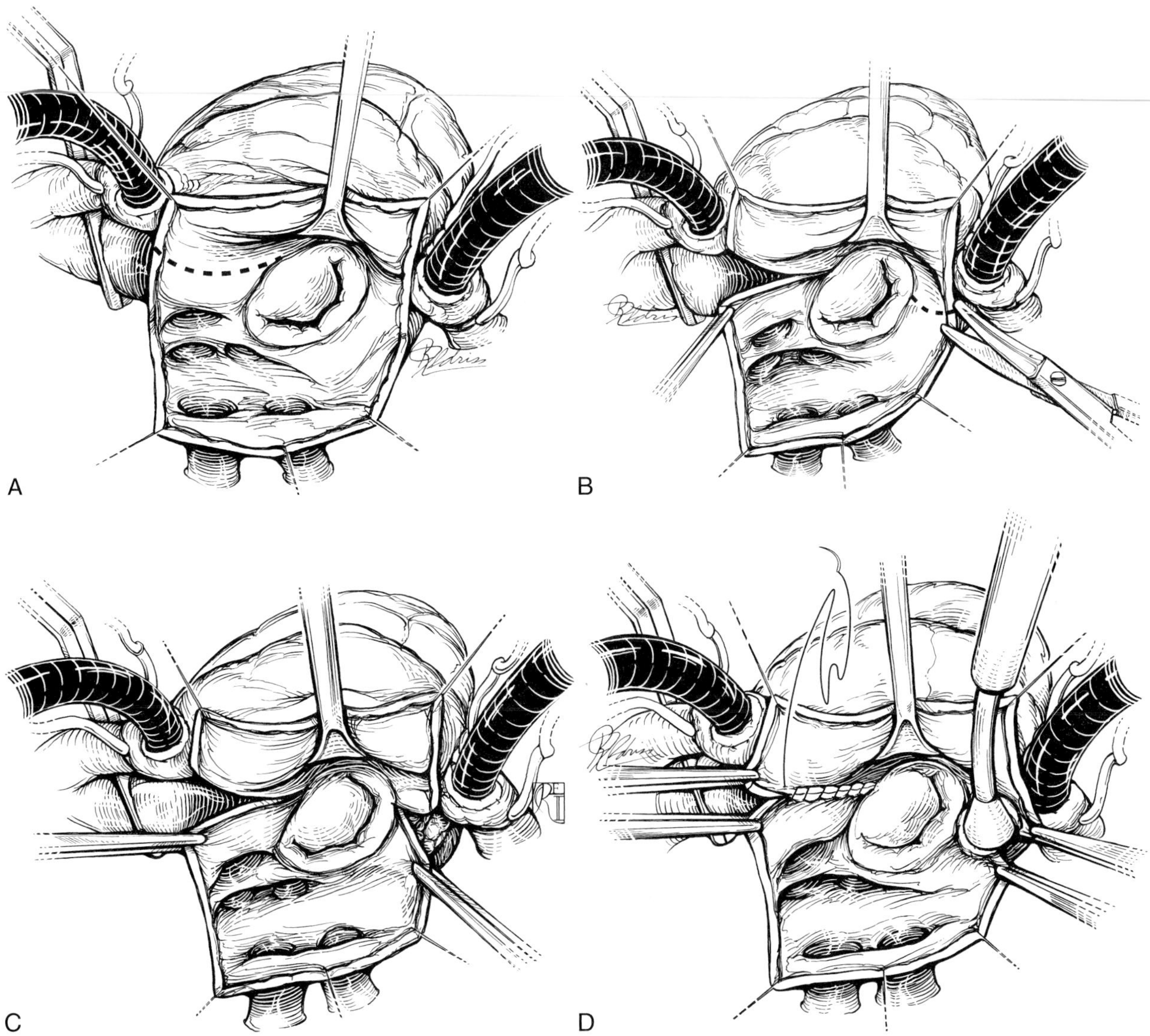

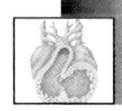

Figure 129–2 Left atrial isolation procedure. A, After standard left atriotomy incision, the interatrial septum is retracted gently and the atriotomy is extended anteriorly *(dotted line)* across Bachmann's bundle to the level of the mitral valve annulus just to the left of the right fibrous trigone. **B,** The anterior extension of the standard left atriotomy was completed. The base of the aorta and its juxtaposition with the anterior leaflet of the mitral valve are demonstrated. Note that the anterior atriotomy extends across the mitral valve annulus. The main body of the left atrium has been separated anteriorly from the remainder of the heart. **C,** The transmural left atriotomy is extended posteriorly to the level of the coronary sinus. The remaining portion of the incision is made through the endocardium and extends across the mitral valve annulus posteriorly just to the left of the interatrial septum. At this point, electrical activity continues to be propagated in a 1:1 fashion between the right and left atria because of the presence of interatrial muscular connections accompanying the coronary sinus. **D,** A cryoprobe is positioned over the endocardial aspect of the posterior atriotomy, and its temperature is decreased to –60° C for 2 minutes to ablate the endocardial interatrial fibers accompanying the coronary sinus. A similar cryolesion is created on the epicardial aspect of the atrioventricular groove on the opposite side of the coronary sinus to ablate all remaining interatrial epicardial connections. The left atriotomy is closed with a continuous 4-0 nonabsorbable suture.
(From Williams JM, Ungerleider RM, Loffler GK, et al: Left atrial isolation: new technique for the treatment of supraventricular arrhythmia. J Thorac Cardiovasc Surg 80:374–380, 1980.)

patients undergoing concomitant repair of structural heart disease are considered for the intraoperative ablation of ventricular tachycardia. Approximately 15% of repaired tetralogy of Fallot patients undergo reoperation for residual defects[62,89,118]; because these patients are at increased risk for sustained ventricular tachycardia, they should undergo preoperative assessment for significant ventricular (and atrial) arrhythmias, with a minimum of 24-hour continuous ambulatory monitoring and exercise testing. Electrophysiological studies are indicated for patients with symptoms due to arrhythmia, syncope, cardiac arrest, or sustained wide QRS tachycardia during evaluation. Sustained ventricular tachycardia may be ablated preoperatively; if catheter ablation fails, direct endocardial resection and cryoablation may be

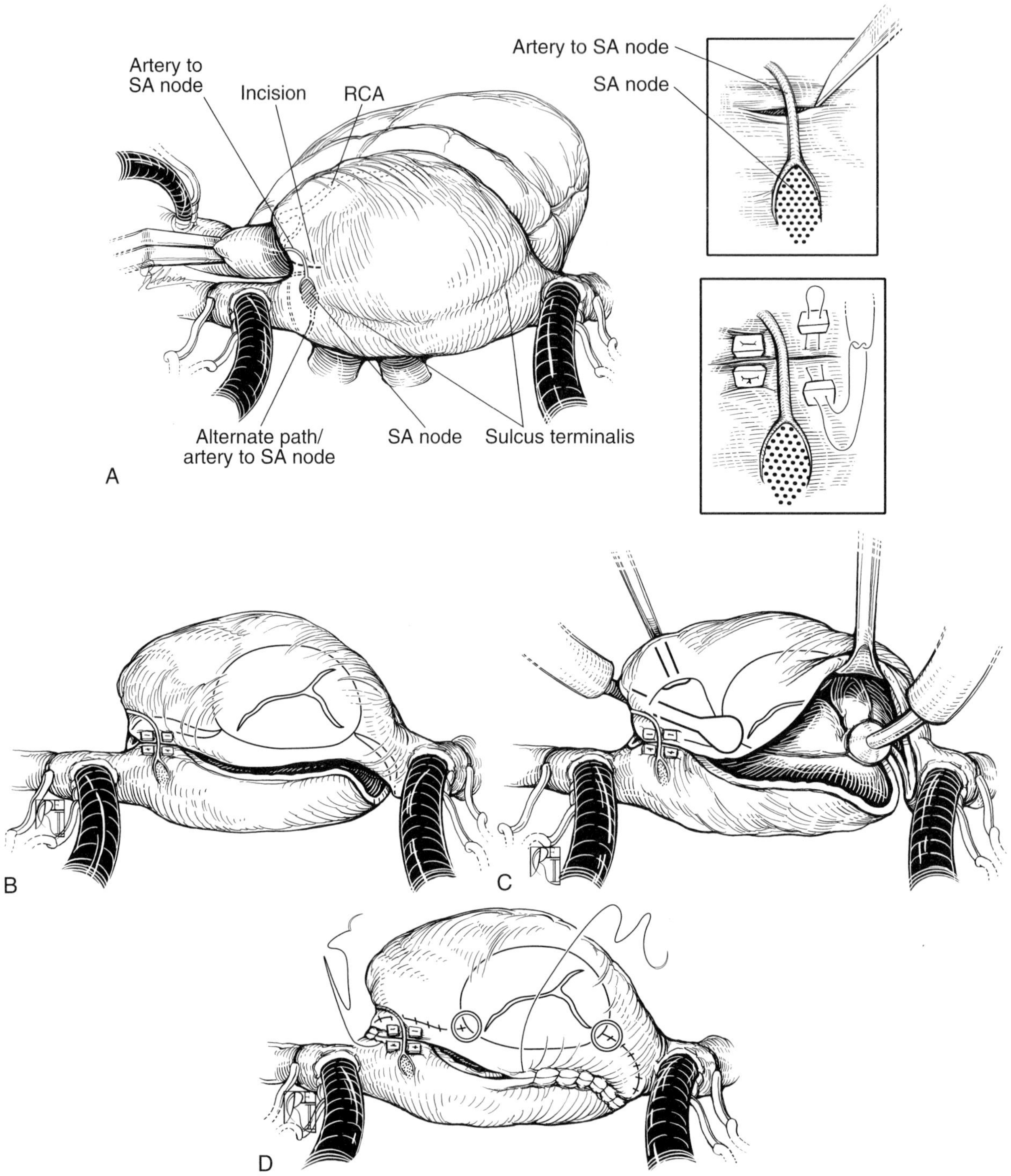

Figure 129–3 Right atrial isolation. A, The sinoatrial node artery is dissected free from the atrial tissue 5 mm anterior to the crista terminalis. A 2-cm incision parallel to the crista terminalis is placed beneath the artery (upper inset). **B,** The incision beneath the sinoatrial node artery is closed with a continuous nonabsorbable suture, and care is taken to not damage the artery. Small pledgets are used above and below the artery to reinforce the incision (bottom inset). The right atriotomy is then extended to a point anterior to the junction of the superior vena cava and the base of the right atrial appendage. **C,** The atriotomy is extended along the anterior limbus of the fossa ovalis to the anteromedial tricuspid valve annulus, just anterior to the membranous interatrial septum. Caudad extension of the right atriotomy around the posterior right atrial-inferior vena caval junction to the posterior-lateral tricuspid valve annulus is performed. A cryolesion (−60° C for 2 minutes) is placed at the end of the incision to ensure complete interruption of connecting atrial muscle fibers between the body of the right atrium and the remainder of the heart. **D,** The atriotomy is closed with a continuous 4-0 nonabsorbable suture. RCA, right coronary artery; SA, sinoatrial.
(From Harada A, D'Agostino HJ Jr, Schuessler RB, et al: Right atrial isolation: a new surgical treatment for SVT. I. Surgical technique and electrophysiologic effects. J Thorac Cardiovasc Surg 95:644–650, 1988.)

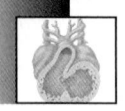

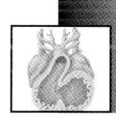

performed intraoperatively. Our center and others[25,30,49,83,118] have performed the surgical revision of residual hemodynamic abnormalities in the adult patient with tetralogy of Fallot at the same time as resection and cryoablation of the focus of ventricular tachycardia. Careful preoperative and intraoperative mapping of tachycardia is necessary; common sites of arrhythmia origin are related to the ventriculotomy, outflow tract patch, and perimeter of the ventricular septal defect. Postoperative ventricular stimulation is necessary to determine efficacy, with defibrillator implantation occurring if sustained ventricular tachycardia remains inducible.

Atrioventricular Conduction Disorders

The most frequent indication for pacing in childhood is for the prevention of bradycardia, either congenital or acquired advanced second- or third-degree AV block, usually as a result of cardiac surgery, infections (myocarditis), or autoimmune disorders. Indications for pacing in congenital complete heart block include a wide-QRS escape rhythm, ventricular dysfunction, a resting ventricular rate of less than 50–55 bpm in the infant with a normal heart or of less than 70 bpm in the infant with structural heart disease, and, in older children, an average heart rate of less than 50 bpm or abrupt pauses of 2–3 times the basic cycle length. A multicenter, long-term, follow-up study[82] has recommended pacemaker implantation in older adolescents to avoid ventricular dysfunction, syncope, or sudden death in adulthood. Determination of the timing of surgical intervention is based on periodical evaluations with exercise testing, ambulatory electrocardiographic monitoring, and echocardiogram. Currently pacing is most frequently performed for postoperative complete heart block followed by symptomatic sinus bradycardia or tachycardia-bradycardia syndrome occurring after atrial surgery, such as Senning, Mustard, or Fontan procedures.[95] Certain patients with long-QT syndrome and pause-dependent ventricular tachycardia or bradycardia as a result of beta-blocker therapy require pacemaker implantation that possibly includes defibrillator implantation.

SURGICAL MANAGEMENT

Multiple reports have introduced slight modifications to the extant surgical atrial ablative techniques[60,65,103]; these modifications have included alternative energy delivery systems for ablation and differing anatomical ablative sites. In patients with congenital heart disease, anomalies in embryological development can result in varying types of anatomical and physiological atrioventricular conduction systems. In addition to the congenital lesions are the acquired problems of cavitary dilatation and increased atrial wall thickness. In particular, atrial wall thickness, which is sometimes up to 1.5 cm, represents a significant challenge for achieving adequate transmural ablation, especially for alternative forms of energy delivery systems, such as RF ablation. It is for this reason that incision and cryoablative techniques are used to ensure transmural lesions. Large atria resulting from abnormal hemodynamics are surgically reduced, and previous atrial scars are resected, especially if the electrophysiological study shows corresponding areas of slow conduction. However, patients with heterotaxy syndrome (occasional absence of the coronary sinus), tricuspid atresia (absence of the tricuspid annulus), anomalous venous drainage (both systemic and pulmonary), gross anatomical thickening of the atrial wall, and endocardial fibrous anatomical jet lesions require alterations of standard techniques based on the preoperative and intraoperative electrophysiological study.

Specifically, patients with heterotaxy syndrome and absence of the coronary sinus are treated without the obligatory cryoablation lesions that connect the coronary sinus with the inferior vena cava and the tricuspid valve. These patients can be approached by way of the following: (1) isolation of the superior and inferior venae cavae, (2) linear lesions that connect the orifice of the inferior vena cava with the medial and proximate atrioventricular valve (often a common atrioventricular valve), (3) a linear lesion that connects the atrial septal area with the base of the resected right atrial appendage, and (4) a linear lesion that connects the atrial septal area with the posterior incised atrial wall across the crista terminalis.

Patients with tricuspid atresia have a "tricuspid dimple" in about a third of cases.[90,104] Some authors[60] have elected to treat this dimple as a diminutive valve and apply cryoablation lesions to connect the coronary sinus with the dimple. However, the anatomical dissections performed by Orie and associates[90] showed the atrioventricular node in very close proximity to the proposed cryoablation area. Our approach to patients with atrial reentry tachycardia and tricuspid atresia is to omit the cryoablation lesion that connects the coronary sinus with the presumed diminutive tricuspid annulus.

Anomalous systemic and pulmonary venous drainage to the atria are approached as additional anatomical barriers, in much the same way as the pulmonary vein orifices. They are therefore treated using isolation techniques (either by transection and reanastomosis or by orifice cryoablation) as the case dictates. The other therapeutic cryoablation lesions are added to these ablations, as indicated.

Gross anatomical thickening of the atrial wall, which was found in our patients with automatic atrial tachycardia, was successfully treated with resection.

The basic tenets of surgical atrial arrhythmia ablation in congenital heart patients are as follows: (1) a thorough understanding of the anatomical features referable to the specific congenital anomaly, (2) resection of excess atrial tissue, including previous atrial incisions, (3) establishing lines of block in areas that have been previously shown to be critical parts of a reentrant circuit, and (4) establishing atrial pacing, especially when sinus node dysfunction exists. Operative strategies to minimize cross-clamp times can be planned to apply right-sided lesions before cross-clamp placement (assuming that there exists no communication between the right and left sides of the heart), to apply lesions during exposure for other left-sided problems (e.g., mitral valve surgery), and to use newly adapted cryoablation probes that can deliver longer lines of block with each application.

Accessory Connections

The goal of surgical therapy for the Wolff-Parkinson-White syndrome/concealed bypass tract is to divide or cryoablate accessory connections that are responsible for the reentry phenomenon and clinical tachycardia using the *endocardial* or *epicardial* techniques (Figure 129-4). The endocardial technique requires cardiopulmonary bypass and, depending on the anatomical location of the bypass tract, it is performed within the right or left atrium.[16,17,74] The epicardial technique may or may not require cardiopulmonary bypass, depending on the location of the accessory connection, and it is performed on the epicardial surface of the heart at the atrioventricular junction by dividing the atrial end of the connection.[45,46,75] Excellent results can be achieved with both techniques; the choice is dependent on the surgeon and the institution.

Left Free-Wall Accessory Connections

Ablation of left free-wall accessory connections is usually performed by the endocardial technique from within the left atrium using cardiopulmonary bypass and cardioplegic arrest. The exposure is through a left atriotomy, usually performed at the interatrial (Sondergaard's) groove, and it is similar to that used for mitral valve repair/replacement. After proper exposure, a curvilinear incision parallel to and 2 mm away from the posterior mitral annulus is made, extending from the left fibrous trigone to the posterior septum (Figure 129-5, *A* and *B*). A dissection plane is developed between the fat pad of the atrioventricular groove and the superior portion of the left ventricle, extending to the epicardial reflection throughout the entire length of the initial incision (Figure 129-5, *C*). The dissection is completed by extending the ends of the incision and the dissection, "squaring off" to the mitral annulus to divide any accessory connection that might be located at the juxta-annular area.[16] This dissection exposes the entire left free-wall space to the respective boundaries, thus ensuring the division of any or all accessory connections. The endocardial incision is sutured to complete the procedure (Figure 129-5, *D*).

The epicardial approach (Figure 129-6) for left free-wall accessory connections requires upward and rightward cardiac retraction for proper exposure, which frequently results in severe hemodynamic instability. As a result, despite the fact that no intracavitary exposure is required for this technique, most surgeons prefer to use cardiopulmonary bypass. After exposure is achieved, the epicardial reflection of the atrium is entered, and a plane of dissection is established between the atrioventricular groove fat pad and the atrial wall. Coronary sinus tributaries often require ligation and division, and care must be taken to avoid coronary artery injury. The dissection plane is extended to the level of the posterior mitral valve annulus and carried slightly onto the top of the posterior left ventricle. This maneuver divides the atrial end of all accessory connections in this area, except for those that lie immediately adjacent to the mitral valve annulus. If present, these juxta-annular connections can be interrupted by a cryosurgical probe that is placed at the level of the mitral valve annulus. The atrial epicardial reflection is then reapproximated by suture technique.

Both techniques have their respective advantages and disadvantages,[16,45] and they can be applied selectively, depending on the anatomical circumstances governing the operation. Anatomical variation may be especially important in the case of the simultaneous repair of congenital heart disease and ablation of accessory connections. Under these circumstances, the atrioventricular anatomical connections may vary, especially in cases of a subaortic muscular conus,

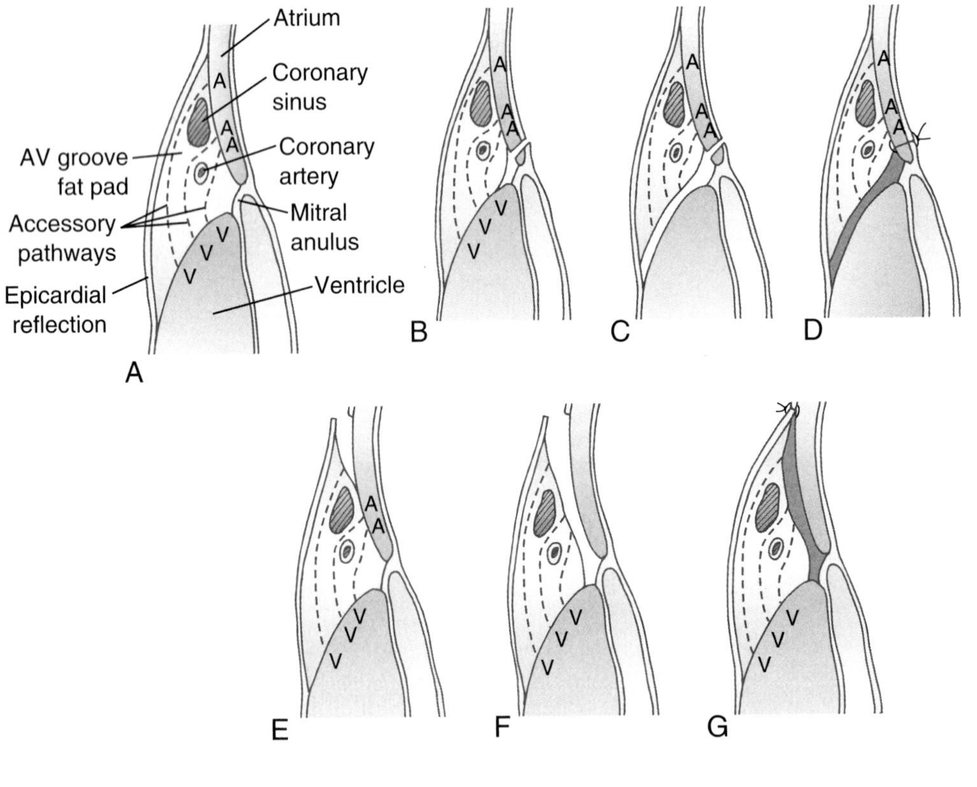

Figure 129–4 Diagrammatic representation of a cross-section of the posterior left heart. A, The different depths at which left free-wall connections can be located in relation to the mitral annulus and epicardial reflection are shown. **B, C,** and **D,** The endocardial surgical technique. **E, F,** and **G,** The epicardial technique.
(From Cox JL: The surgical management of cardiac arrhythmias. In Sabiston DC Jr, Spencer FC, eds.: Surgery of the Chest, ed 5. Philadelphia: WB Saunders, 1990, p. 1872.)

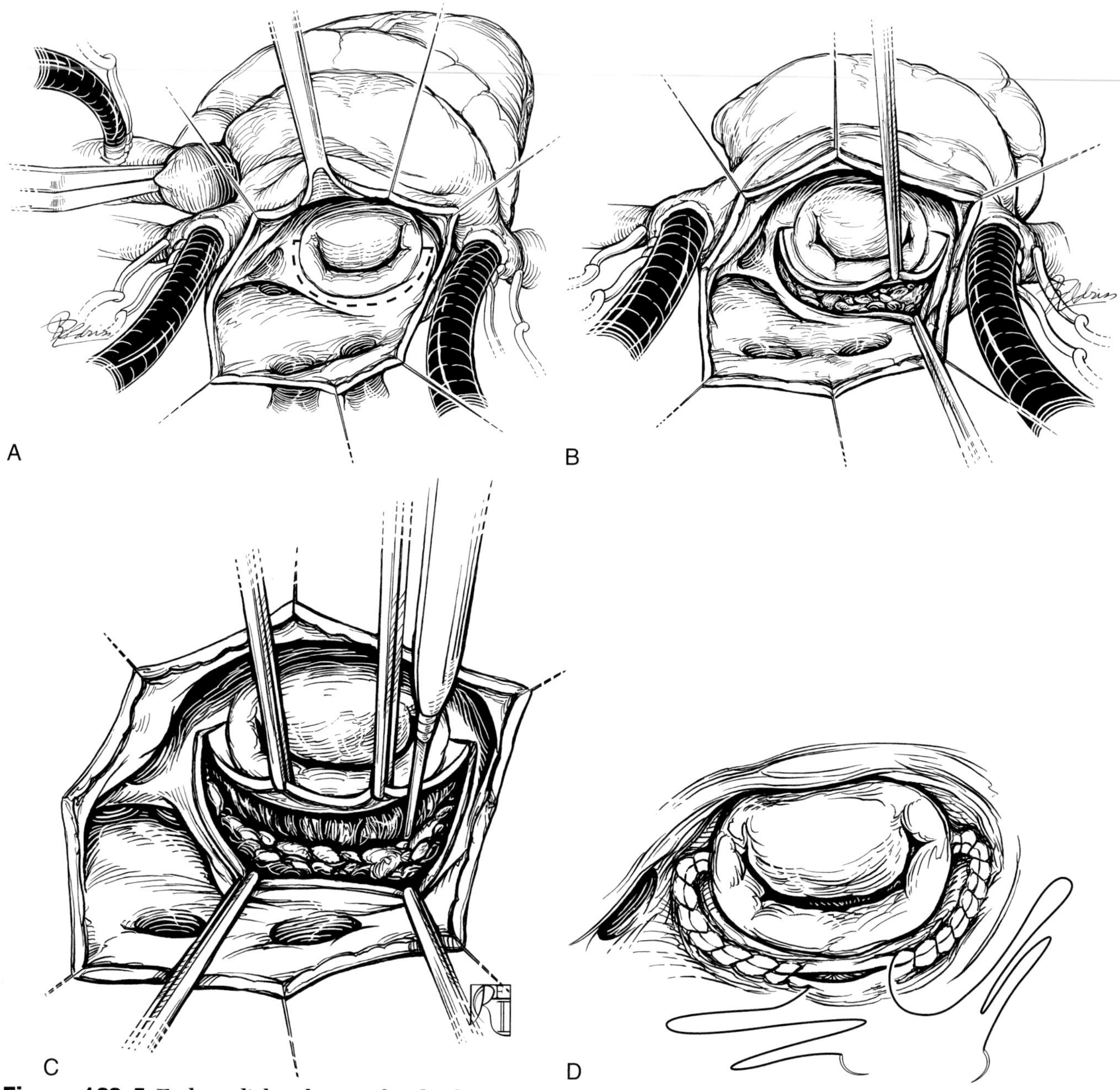

Figure 129–5 Endocardial technique for dividing left free-wall accessory connections in the Wolff-Parkinson-White syndrome.
(From Deal BJ, Mavroudis C, Backer CL: Surgical therapy of cardiac arrhythmias. In Mavroudis C, Backer CL, eds.: Pediatric Cardiac Surgery, ed 3. St. Louis: Mosby, 2003, pp. 713–738.)

atrioventricular discordance, and juxtaposition of the atrial appendages. The surgeon should be familiar with both techniques and be ready to alter the procedure, depending on the pathoanatomy.

Posterior Septal Accessory Connections

The endocardial approach to posterior septal connections is through the right atrium. Normothermic cardiopulmonary bypass is usually used, with certain precautions taken, including closure of any intracardiac shunts before proceeding with the operation. Preoperative evaluation—particularly transthoracic echocardiography—may not always detect the presence of a patent foramen ovale. Care is taken to fibrillate the heart shortly after cardiopulmonary bypass and before right atrial entry to check for and close a patent foramen ovale; this maneuver will ensure that no air is introduced to the left ventricle during a beating cardiac cycle. After complete patent foramen ovale closure, the heart can be defibrillated and the operation continued. After completion of the endocardial mapping, a supraannular incision is made 2 mm above the posterior medial tricuspid valve

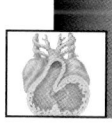

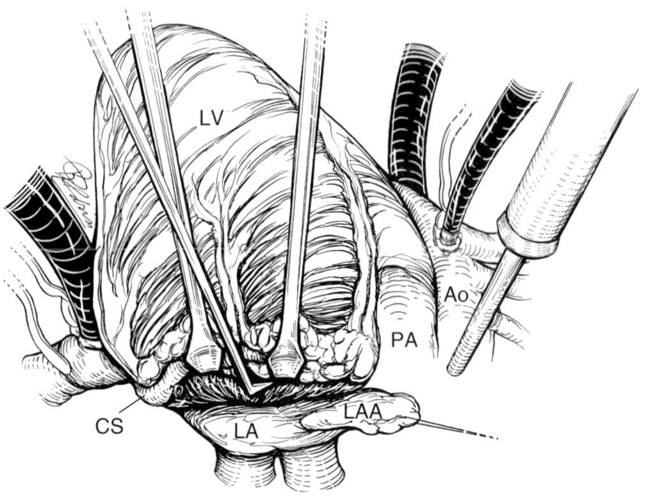

Figure 129–6 The epicardial approach to left free-wall accessory connections. A schematic of the left ventricle, viewed from an operative position. The fat pad is mobilized and the atrioventricular junction exposed. Ao, aorta; CS, coronary sinus; LA, left atrium; LAA, left atrial appendage; LV, left ventricle; PA, pulmonary artery.
(From Deal BJ, Mavroudis C, Backer CL: Surgical therapy of cardiac arrhythmias. In Mavroudis C, Backer CL, eds.: Pediatric Cardiac Surgery, ed 3. St. Louis: Mosby, 2003, pp. 713–738.)

annulus, beginning at least 1 cm posterior to the His bundle (Figure 129-7). The supraannular incision is extended counterclockwise onto the posterior right atrial free-wall. This incision provides exposure to the posterior septal space near the left ventricle and the epicardial reflection at the posterior right ventricle near the crux of the heart. The posterior septal space fat pad is dissected away from the top of the posterior ventricular septum while the heart is beating or during hypothermic cardioplegic arrest, depending on the vascularity of the dissection plane and the preference of the surgeon.

Except for the location, the epicardial approach to posterior septal accessory connections is very similar to that for the left free-wall connections. The posterior septal accessory connections are divided by developing a dissection plane between the fat pad and the top of the posterior ventricular septum, following the mitral annulus over to the posterior superior process of the left ventricle, and following the epicardial reflection from the posterior right ventricle across the crux and onto the posterior left ventricle. Cryolesions are placed at regular intervals around the annulus to ensure complete division of all accessory connections.

Right Free-Wall Accessory Connections

Epicardial dissection for right free-wall accessory connections can be performed without cardiopulmonary bypass in the majority of cases. An incision is made in the epicardium, thereby establishing a dissection plane between the right atrial wall and the atrioventricular groove fat pad to the tricuspid valve annulus (Figure 129-8) throughout the entire length of the right atrial free wall. Cryolesions at appropriate intervals can ensure complete accessory connection ablation.

The endocardial technique can be used if there is concern about epicardial bleeding or if a concomitant intracardiac repair is necessary. Under cardioplegic arrest, a supraannular incision is placed 2 mm above the tricuspid valve annulus and extending around the entire right free-wall. A dissection plane is then established between the underlying atrioventricular groove fat pad and the top of the right ventricle throughout the length of the supraannular incision. The dissection is extended to the epicardial reflection off the ventricle, thereby dividing all of the penetrating fibers in this area. The incision can then be closed.

Anterior Septal Accessory Connections

The epicardial approach to anterior septal accessory connections was less successful than the endocardial approach.[46] Except for location, the endocardial dissection is similar to that for the right free-wall lesions. A supraannular incision is made just anterior to the His bundle, 2 mm

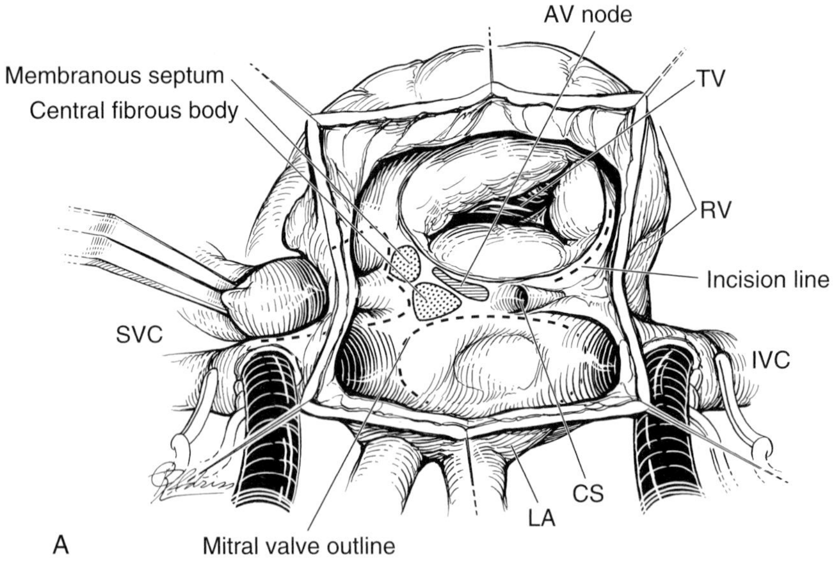

Figure 129–7 Endocardial technique for surgical division of posterior septal accessory connections in the Wolff-Parkinson-White syndrome. The junction of the posterior medial mitral and tricuspid valve annuli forms an inverted V at the posterior edge of the central fibrous body, and the fat pad comes to a point at the apex of that V. The apex of the V is always posterior to the His bundle, although the distance between the apex of the V and the His bundle may vary.

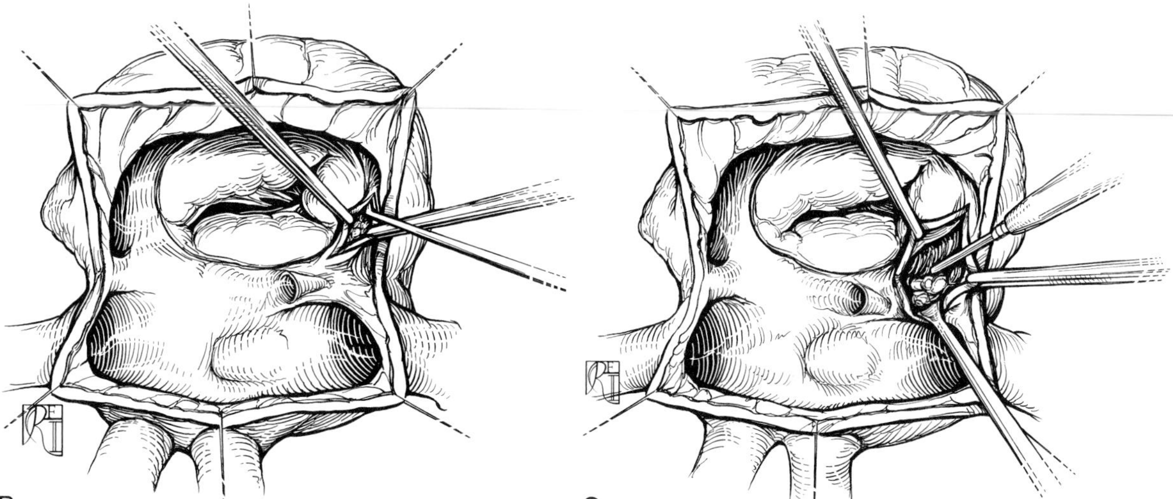

B C

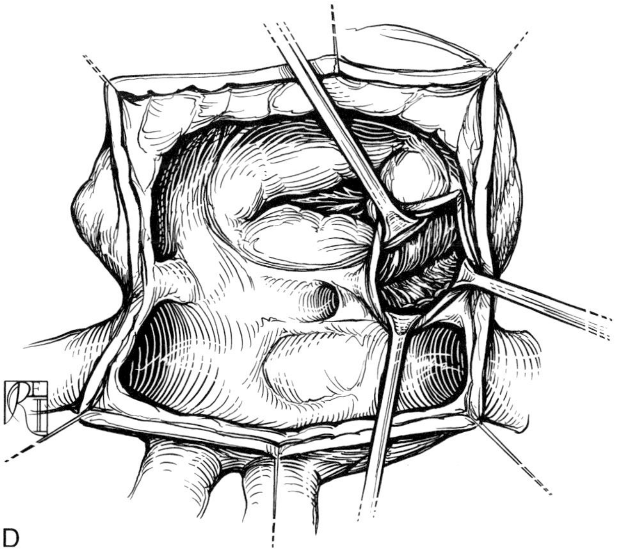

D

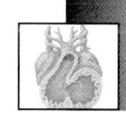

Figure 129–7 cont'd As long as the dissection in this region remains posterior to the central fibrous body, the His bundle will not be damaged. After the anterior point of the fat pad is gently dissected away from the apex of the V (i.e., away from the posterior edge of the central fibrous body), the mitral valve annulus comes into view at the point at which it joins the tricuspid valve to form the central fibrous body. AV, atrioventricular; CS, coronary sinus; IVC, inferior vena cava; LA, left atrium; RV, right ventricle; SVC, superior vena cava; TV, tricuspid valve.
(From Cox JL, Gallagher JJ, Cain ME: Experience with 118 consecutive patients undergoing operation for the Wolff-Parkinson-White syndrome. J Thorac Cardiovasc Surg 90:490–501, 1985.)

above the tricuspid annulus and extended in a clockwise direction onto the right anterior free-wall. The dissection plane is established between the fat pad occupying the anterior septal space and the top of the right ventricle and developed to the aorta medially and to the epicardial reflection off the ventricle anteriorly. Great care is required to avoid injury of the right coronary artery that courses through the fat pad in this area and the aortic wall at the right coronary sinus of Valsalva.

Atrioventricular Nodal Reentry Tachycardia

An anatomical approach to slow pathway modification effectively treats AV nodal reentry tachycardia: lesions are delivered inferior and anterior to the os of the coronary sinus, with slow pullback from the tricuspid annulus towards the inferior vena cava. Currently, the cryoablation technique for patients with AV nodal reentry tachycardia is used,[19] although intraoperative RF catheter ablation techniques may replace cryoablation in the future. The surgical approach uses normothermic aortobicaval cardiopulmonary bypass in a beating heart after patent foramen ovale closure, if present.[10,21] A series of discrete cryolesions (90 seconds at –60° C) are placed near the posterior inferior rim of the coronary sinus os (Figure 129-9). It is not desirable to attain prolongation of the PR interval; instead, an anatomical approach to modifying the posterior inputs to the node is used. The occurrence of 2:1 block during lesion application mandates immediate cessation of that particular cryolesion, because it may be too close to the fast pathway inputs to the atrioventricular node. After a short period of recovery, the cryoablation may continue until all of the lesions are placed and remapping confirms success. The surgical cryoablation modification of the atrioventricular node as described above requires less than 5 minutes. In patients with prior Mustard or Senning procedures undergoing reoperation, we have elected to perform ablation of AV nodal reentry tachycardia directly intraoperatively and to avoid the retrograde catheter approach to the pulmonary venous atrium.

Atrial Flutter

Direct intervention for atrial arrhythmias at the time of surgery is highly effective and relies on four techniques: (1) inferomedial right atrial ablation for typical atrial flutter,

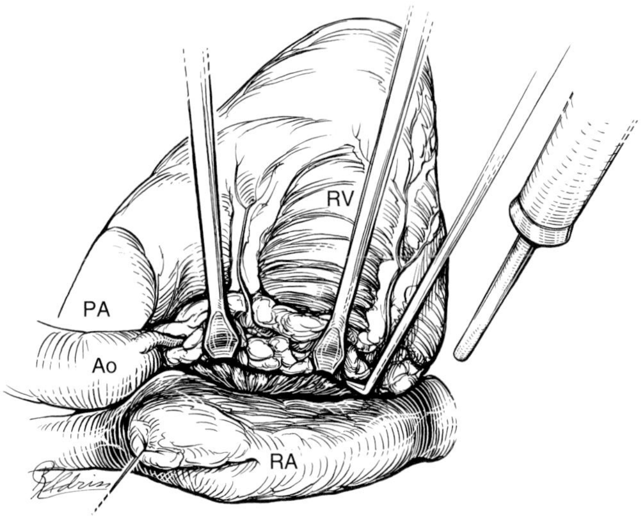

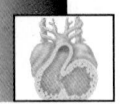

Figure 129–8 Epicardial approach for right free-wall accessory connections. A schematic view of the exposure of the right coronary fossa and anterior right ventricular atrioventricular sulcus. Ao, Aorta; PA, pulmonary artery; RA, right atrium; RV, right ventricle.
(From Deal BJ, Mavroudis C, Backer CL: Surgical therapy of cardiac arrhythmias. In Mavroudis C, Backer CL, eds.: Pediatric Cardiac Surgery, ed 3. St. Louis: Mosby, 2003, pp. 713–738.)

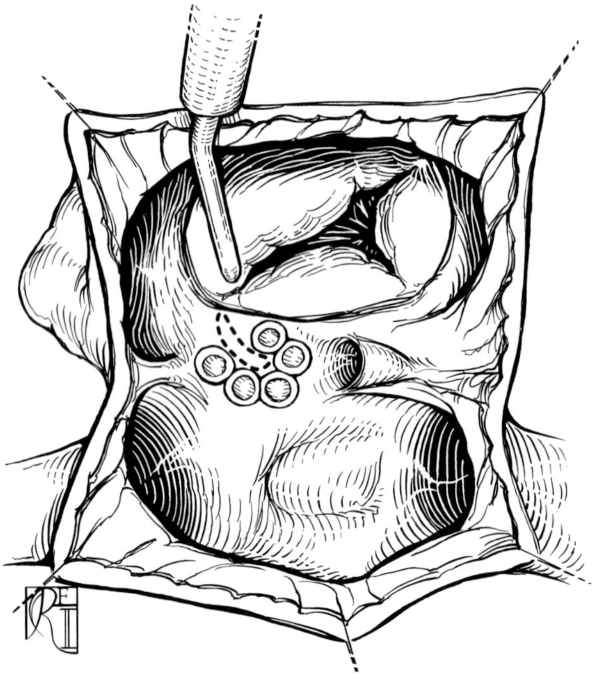

Figure 129–9 Cryolesions are placed around the coronary sinus and the area of the atrioventricular node. During application of cryothermia, prolongation of the atrioventricular intervals begins to occur, which should trigger cessation of the cryothermia to avoid complete heart block.
(From Deal BJ, Mavroudis C, Backer CL: Surgical therapy of cardiac arrhythmias. In Mavroudis C, Backer CL, eds.: Pediatric Cardiac Surgery, ed 3. St. Louis: Mosby, 2003, pp. 713-738.)

(2) a modified right atrial maze procedure for multiple atrial reentrant circuits, (3) a Cox-maze III procedure for atrial fibrillation, and (4) atrial pacemaker implantation, either to avoid bradycardia or as an antitachycardia device.

We have experience with a small number of patients with atrial reentry tachycardia originating near the rim of an unrepaired atrial primum or secundum septal defect. Because of the need for atrial surgery, we elected to ablate under direct vision intraoperatively. After mapping the tachycardia preoperatively, surgical repair includes excision of the rim of the atrial defect, with localized cryoablation of the involved perimeter of the defect. Cryoablation is performed using 3-, 5-, and 15-mm circular probes (Frigitronics, Cooper Surgical, Inc., Shelton, Conn) at –60° C for 90 second lesions. Anatomical ablation of the inferomedial right atrial isthmus between the os of the coronary sinus and the inferior vena cava may successfully treat atrial flutter. We have also performed right atrial cryoablation for an infant with recurrent atrial flutter at the time of initial repair of tetralogy of Fallot.

More commonly, atrial tachycardia occurs as a late sequela of intracardiac repair of congenital heart disease. Atrial reentry tachycardia after the Mustard or Senning procedure is amenable to catheter ablation, although a retrograde catheter approach via the aorta and across the tricuspid valve into the pulmonary venous atrium is often necessary,[58,109] with the attendant risk of creating aortic insufficiency. If the patient requires reoperation for hemodynamic problems (e.g., atrial baffle leak repair), direct surgical cryoablation between identified anatomical barriers can be successfully performed with minimal prolongation of the surgical repair; this is in contrast with lengthy fluoroscopy time.

Patients with atrial reentry tachycardia after the Fontan procedure undergo a modified right atrial maze procedure (Figure 129-10). The modified right atrial maze is intended to interrupt critical areas of reentry specific to the Fontan patient: the atriotomy scar, the rim of the atrial septal defect and the lateral right atrial wall, and the prior atriopulmonary connection. In addition, the area of "typical" atrial flutter is addressed with cryoablation lesions between the inferior vena cava and the os of the coronary sinus and between the inferior vena cava and the region of the tricuspid valve or atrioventricular groove.

Atrial Fibrillation

Atrial fibrillation typically occurs in the presence of markedly dilated left atria, usually in the setting of significant mitral regurgitation, and is due to either ventricular dysfunction or valve abnormalities. The Cox-maze III procedure is designed to eliminate atrial fibrillation while preserving intact AV nodal conduction and atrial contractility. Use of the cryoablation probe or RF catheter intraoperatively, instead of atrial incisions, considerably shortens surgical time. Patients with atrial fibrillation after the Fontan procedure undergo a complete Cox-maze III procedure (Figure 129-11) involving the right and left atria. The Cox-maze III procedure is designed to limit the ability of the microreentrant circuits of atrial fibrillation to propagate while allowing for the normal conduction of an atrial impulse to the atrioventricular node and preserving atrial

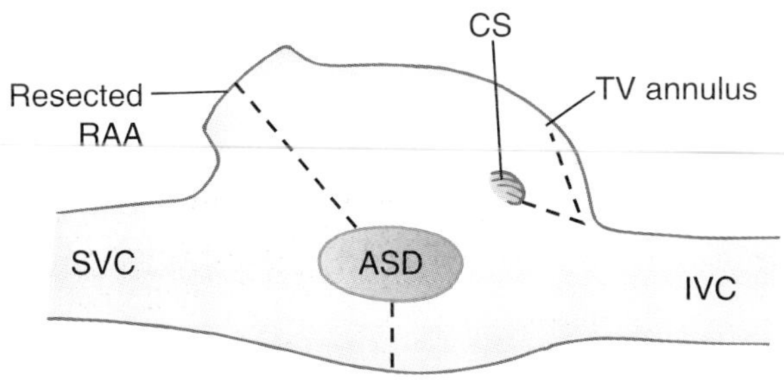

Figure 129–10 Modified right atrial maze procedure for atrial reentry tachycardia. Large section of anterior right atrial wall is resected, including the incision from the superior vena cava to the inferior vena cava. Cryoablation lesions are indicated by dotted lines. ASD, Atrial septal defect; CS, coronary sinus; IVC, inferior vena cava; RAA, right atrial appendage; SVC, superior vena cava; TV, tricuspid valve.
(From Deal BJ, Mavroudis C, Backer CL, et al: New directions in surgical therapy of arrhythmias. Pediatr Cardiol 21:576–583, 2000. Reprinted with permission.)

contractility.[14,15,20] The modified right atrial maze procedure can be completed in less than 10 minutes, whereas the Cox-maze III procedure has required an additional 35–55 minutes of surgery. The use of linear ablation probes or RF catheters can considerably shorten the procedure.[80,105]

Ventricular Tachycardia

Our experience in patients with ventricular tachycardia is confined to 5 individuals: 3 with repaired tetralogy of Fallot and severe pulmonary insufficiency resulting from a transannular patch, 1 with a ventricular jet lesion caused by an unoperated ventricular septal defect, and 1 with an oncogenic site near the course of the left anterior descending coronary artery. Endocardial resection and cryoablation techniques were employed for the tetralogy patients. Ventricular septal defect closure together with endocardial resection/cryoablation and epicardial resection with localized cryoablation techniques were used for the remaining 2 patients.

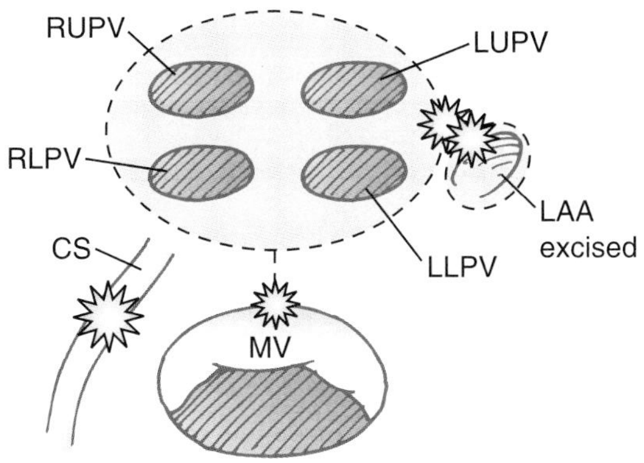

Figure 129–11 Left atrial incisions and cryoablation lesions of Cox-maze III procedure for atrial fibrillation. Incisions are indicated by dotted lines, cryoablation lesions by stars. CS, coronary sinus; LAA, Left atrial appendage; LLPV, left lower pulmonary vein; LUPV, left upper pulmonary vein; MV, mitral valve; RLPV, right lower pulmonary vein; RUPV, right upper pulmonary vein.
(From Deal BJ, Mavroudis C, Backer CL, et al: New directions in surgical therapy of arrhythmias. Pediatr Cardiol 21:576–583, 2000. Reprinted with permission.)

RESULTS

The 2003 *Pediatric Cardiac Surgery Annual* published reports from 3 centers[2,42,78] about their experience with arrhythmia surgery in patients with associated congenital heart defects. The Mayo Clinic[42] limited their report to a subset of patients with congenital cardiac anomalies who had right atrial dilatation and associated paroxysmal or atrial tachyarrhythmias who underwent repair of the congenital cardiac anomaly and an isolated right atrial maze procedure. They used an isolated right-sided maze in these patients because of the shorter cardiopulmonary bypass time, the limitation of the number of atrial suture lines, and the ability to avoid a possible noncontractile left atrium and to minimize dissection of adhesions and suture lines behind the heart, thus avoiding additional potential bleeding sources. At the Mayo Clinic, the biatrial maze procedure is considered for patients with congenital cardiac anomalies who have chronic atrial fibrillation with left atrial or biatrial enlargement.

Greason and colleauges[42] reported on 45 patients with atrial tachyarrhythmias who underwent a right-sided maze procedure at the time of cardiac repair of congenital cardiac anomalies: Ebstein's anomaly was seen in 37 patients (82%), non-Ebstein's tricuspid regurgitation in 5 patients (11%), and isolated atrial septal defect in 3 patients (7%). Associated cardiac defects included atrial septal defect in 27 patients, accessory conduction pathway(s) in 6 patients, pulmonary stenosis in 5 patients, pulmonary regurgitation in 5 patients, left superior vena cava in 2 patients, tetralogy of Fallot in 2 patients, ventricular septal defect in 2 patients, partial anomalous pulmonary venous return in 1 patient, and mitral regurgitation in 1 patient. Forty percent of patients (18 out of 45) had previous cardiovascular operations, and 9 patients had undergone previous catheter or surgical ablation of accessory conduction pathway(s). There were 2 early deaths (4%) from ventricular fibrillation as a result of coronary artery problems. Both of these patients had Ebstein's anomaly with giant cardiomegaly. There was 1 late death from disseminated intravascular coagulation 16 months after operation in a patient who had no atrial arrhythmias postoperatively. There was no surgical heart block; however, 1 patient who had undergone atrial septal defect closure had a preoperative history of syncope and had sick sinus syndrome after operation. He underwent pacemaker implantation on postoperative day 8. Another patient who underwent tricuspid valve repair for non-Ebstein's tricuspid regurgitation required pacemaker placement 22 months postoperatively for bradycardia. Electrocardiographic follow-up was available in 39 out of 42 late survivors (93%) at a median follow-up of 22 months, and this showed sinus rhythm in 33 patients (85%), paced rhythm in 2 patients (5%), junctional rhythm in 1 patient (3%) and atrial fibrillation in 1 patient (3%). Establishment of a rhythm other than atrial flutter or fibrillation was achieved in 36 out of the 39 survivors (92%), obviating the need for warfarin therapy in those patients.

In a broad review of the experience with arrhythmia surgery at the Hospital for Sick Children and the Toronto

General Hospital's Congenital Cardiac Center for Adults in Ontario from 1984 to 2001, Ashburn and others[2] discussed outcomes for the surgical ablation of accessory bypass tracts and the operative protocols and outcomes for the management of supraventricular and ventricular arrhythmias. Among 69 patients who underwent ablation of accessory bypass tracts, there was 1 early and 2 late deaths, all of which occurred in patients with structural heart lesions. The most commonly associated heart lesions were Ebstein's anomaly, congenitally corrected transposition, and ventricular septal defect. Reoperation for persistent or recurrent arrhythmia was required in 5 patients during the early postoperative period and in 4 patients late postoperatively. In survivors, the long-term freedom from arrhythmia approaches 90%. Of 32 patients with atrial flutter who underwent ablation, all had concomitant repair of associated congenital heart disease. The method of ablation was either isthmus cryoablation (25 patients) or right atrial maze (7 patients). There were 2 operative deaths, 1 in a patient with tetralogy of Fallot, atrial flutter, and ventricular tachycardia and 1 in a patient with congenitally corrected transposition, ventricular septal defect, and pulmonary stenosis. There were no late deaths. Freedom from arrhythmia recurrence was 94% at 6 months, 89% at 1 year, and 82% at 3 years. Twenty patients underwent ablation of atrial fibrillation and concomitant repair of associated congenital heart defects. Thirteen patients (65%) had undergone prior cardiac surgery. Right atrial maze was performed in 14 patients, isthmus cryoablation (early in the series) in 4, and bilateral maze in 2. Freedom from arrhythmia recurrence was 65% at 6 months, 57% at 1 year, and 46% at 3 years. Of note is that recurrence in the atrial fibrillation subset occurred earlier (median interval, 3 months after ablation) than it did in the atrial flutter subset. Forty-three patients with sustained ventricular tachycardia underwent surgery for congenital heart defects; 33 of these had monomorphic ventricular tachycardia induced and mapped intraoperatively. Ten patients had either failure to induce ventricular tachycardia or inducible polymorphic tachycardia and did not undergo ablation. In the patients with polymorphic ventricular tachycardia, ablation was not indicated; management options included medical therapy and/or automatic implantable cardioverter-defibrillator. Thirty-one patients (94%) who underwent ablation had the reentry circuit involving the myocardium adjacent to the ventricular septal defect patch and the infundibular septum. There was 1 operative death. Freedom from arrhythmia recurrence was 88% at 6 months, 88% at 1 year, and 80% at 3 years.

At the Children's Memorial Hospital (Chicago),[78] between July 1992 and August 2002, we performed arrhythmia surgery on 34 patients for refractory atrial (29 patients) or ventricular (5 patients) arrhythmias, excluding patients who underwent arrhythmia surgery with concomitant Fontan conversion. Thirty-two patients had various forms of complex congenital heart disease, whereas 2 had structurally normal hearts. Twenty-two patients (65%) had undergone previous cardiac procedures. Anatomical correction of congenital heart disease was performed concomitantly with arrhythmia surgery in 32 patients. Mortality was 5.9% (2 out of 34 patients); 1 patient died as a result of low cardiac output following Mustard takedown and arterial switch operation, and 1 neonate died the day of surgery after tricuspid valve isolation for Ebstein's anomaly. There was 1 late death 11 months postoperatively after an attempted Mustard-to-arterial switch conversion at another institution. No patient developed heart block. No patient was returned to the operating room for postoperative bleeding. Early postoperative tachycardia occurred in 4 patients (12%) while they were receiving inotropic therapy: 2 out of the 14 patients with atrial reentry tachycardia, 1 out of the 5 patients with atrial fibrillation, and 1 out of the 5 patients with an accessory connection. Supraventricular tachycardia was inducible at postoperative electrophysiology studies in 1 out of 20 patients (5%): a patient with a concealed accessory connection, atrial reentry tachycardia, dextrocardia, and heterotaxy syndrome who underwent a primary Fontan procedure at 9.3 years of age. Recurrence of tachycardia using the concealed accessory connection occurred early postoperatively and was inducible at pacing study; atrial reentry tachycardia was not inducible. Ventricular tachycardia was inducible in 2 out of 5 patients after tetralogy of Fallot repair. One patient had 3 morphologies of inducible ventricular tachycardia before surgical repair; only 1 morphology was adequately mapped to the right ventricular outflow tract. Both patients received implanted automatic defibrillators before discharge. During the median follow-up duration of 23 months, documented recurrence of the clinical supraventricular tachycardia occurred in 2 out of 27 patients (7%) and in none of the 4 ventricular tachycardia patients. However, new-onset atrial reentry tachycardia developed in 2 patients, 1 who had undergone arrhythmia surgery for ventricular tachycardia and the other for accessory connections (Table 129-3).[24] Two patients (5.9%; 2 out of 34) underwent pacemaker implantation for the late development of sinus bradycardia.

INDICATIONS FOR PACEMAKER INSERTION IN CHILDREN

The American College of Cardiology/American Heart Association Task Force on Practice Guidelines[43] has prepared guidelines for the implantation of cardiac pacemakers and antiarrhythmia devices; the pediatric indications are summarized in Table 129-4. Class I indications include conditions for which there is evidence and/or general agreement that the device will be useful. Class II indications include conditions for which there is conflicting evidence or divergence of opinion; in IIa the weight of evidence/opinion favors implantation, whereas, in IIb, the usefulness or efficacy is less well established. In Class III there is evidence or general agreement that implantation is not indicated.

In addition to antibradycardia pacing, certain pacemakers can be programmed to recognize tachycardia and to initiate a pacing protocol to interrupt the arrhythmias. Pacing at rates faster than the tachycardia cycle length is an effective means of terminating reentrant tachycardia, particularly atrial reentry/flutter. The success of the RF catheter ablation technique for treating these forms of tachycardia has limited the application of antitachycardia pacing. In addition, cardiac asystole is a more common cause of cardiac arrest in young patients than ventricular fibrillation, which is in contrast with adult patients. In pediatric patients,

Table 129–3

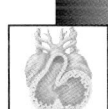

Incidence of Postoperative Arrhythmias by Preoperative Arrhythmia Site[a]

Arrhythmia (incidence per site)	*AF (n = 5)*	*ART (n = 11)*	*AAT (n = 3)*	*AVNRT (n = 2)*	*VT (n = 5)*	*AC (n = 6)*
Perioperative						
Transient; while on inotropes	1	2	–	–	–	–
Inducible at EPS						
No clinical arrhythmia	–	–	–	–	2[b]	–
Persistent recurrence; on amiodarone	–	–	–	–	–	1
Late						
Transient, 1 month postop; resolved with course of sotalol	–	1	–	–	–	–
Palpitations, no documented recurrent arrhythmia; on beta blockers	–	1	–	–	–	–
New-onset ART	–	–	–	–	1[b]	1[c]
Persistent recurrence 5 years postop; underwent RF ablation of AV node, pacemaker	–	1	–	–	–	–
Total persistent recurrent or new-onset arrhythmias	0 out of 5	1 out of 11	0 out of 3	0 out of 2	1 out of 5	2 out of 6

[a]In 29 patients operated on at the Children's Memorial Hospital between July 1992 and January 2002 for refractory atrial (n = 24) or ventricular (n = 5) arrhythmias.[24]
[b]One of the 2 patients with VT inducible at EPS developed new-onset ART late postoperatively.
[c]Patient was on digoxin.
AF, Atrial fibrillation; ART, atrial reentry tachycardia; AAT, automatic atrial tachycardia; AVNRT, atrioventricular nodal reentry tachycardia; VT, ventricular tachycardia; AC, accessory connections; EPS, electrophysiological study; RF, radiofrequency; AV, atrioventricular.
From: Deal BJ, Mavroudis C, Backer CL: Beyond Fontan conversion: surgical therapy of arrhythmias including patients with associated complex congenital heart disease. Ann Thorac Surg 76:542–553, 2003.

defibrillator implantation has centered on 3 types of heart disease: (1) cardiomyopathies, (2) primary electrical disease (long QT syndrome, Brugada syndrome, idiopathic ventricular fibrillation, resuscitated cardiac arrest, strong family history of sudden death), and (3) repaired congenital heart disease. Defibrillator implantation may be used as a bridge to cardiac transplantation in patients with severe ventricular dysfunction and ventricular arrhythmias or syncope at risk for sudden cardiac death.

However, in patients with atrial reentry tachycardia after surgical repair of congenital heart disease (e.g., Mustard, Senning, or Fontan procedures), antitachycardia atrial pacing may be the only effective therapy, short of surgical intervention. Since their introduction in 1980, the efficacy of implantable defibrillators for reducing the incidence of sudden cardiac death due to ventricular tachycardia/fibrillation is well established.[1] Electrophysiology study to determine the efficacy of atrial pacing to terminate tachycardia and optimal pacing sites is mandatory. A transvenous or epicardial atrial pacing lead is implanted. Tachycardia detection and termination algorithms are programmable, with efficacy verified at postimplantation study. A typical protocol recognizes atrial rates of more than 200 bpm and delivers a train of 6–8 atrial impulses at 80% of the tachycardia cycle length to terminate. The termination algorithm is automatically programmed to continue pacing at faster rates until termination is achieved or to a predetermined, minimum-paced cycle length. To avoid initiating inappropriate pacing therapy, tachycardia detection criteria need to account for sinus tachycardia at rates of up to 200 bpm in pediatric patients; beta-blocker therapy may be necessary to ensure that sinus rates do not exceed 160–180 bpm. Because of the small numbers of patients benefiting from this therapy, continued industry support for the technology is limited.

SURGICAL TECHNIQUE

Historically, pediatric pacing systems have been epicardial, with the generator implanted in the abdomen.[27] However,

Table 129–4

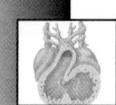

Indications for Permanent Pacing in Children and Adolescents

Class	Indication
Sinus node dysfunction	
I	Sinus node dysfunction with correlation of symptoms during age-inappropriate bradycardia. Definition of bradycardia varies with patient's age and expected heart rate.
IIa	Asymptomatic sinus bradycardia in child with complex congenital heart disease with resting heart rate of <35 bpm or pauses in ventricular rate of >3 seconds.
IIa	Bradycardia-tachycardia syndrome with need for long-term antiarrhythmic treatment other than digitalis.
IIb	Asymptomatic sinus bradycardia in adolescent with congenital heart disease with resting heart rate of <35 bpm or pauses in ventricular rate of >3 seconds.
III	Asymptomatic sinus bradycardia in adolescent with longest RR interval of <3 seconds and minimum heart rate of >40 bpm.
AV conduction disorders	
Congenital heart block	
I	Congenital third-degree atrioventricular (AV) block in infant with ventricular rate of <50–55 bpm or with congenital heart disease and a ventricular rate of <70 bpm.
I	Congenital third-degree AV block with a wide QRS escape rhythm or ventricular dysfunction.
IIa	Congenital third-degree AV block beyond the first year of life with an average heart rate of <50 bpm or abrupt pauses in ventricular rate that are 2 or 3 times the basic cycle length.
IIb	Congenital third-degree AV block in asymptomatic neonate, child, or adolescent with an acceptable rate, narrow QRS complex, and normal ventricular function.
Postoperative AV block	
I	Postoperative advanced second- or third-degree AV block that is not expected to resolve or that persists at least 7 days after cardiac surgery.
IIb	Transient postoperative third-degree AV block that reverts to sinus rhythm with residual bifascicular block.
III	Transient postoperative AV block with return of normal AV conduction within 7 days.
III	Asymptomatic postoperative bifascicular block with or without first-degree AV block.
Other conduction disorders	
I	Advanced second- or third-degree AV block associated with symptomatic bradycardia, congestive heart failure, or low cardiac output.
III	Asymptomatic type I second-degree AV block.
Long QT/ventricular tachycardia	
I	Sustained pause-dependent ventricular tachycardia, with or without prolonged QT, in which efficacy of pacing is thoroughly documented.
IIa	Long QT syndrome with 2:1 AV or third-degree AV block.

From Deal BJ, Mavroudis C, Backer CL: Surgical therapy of cardiac arrhythmias. In Mavroudis C, Backer CL (editors): Pediatric Cardiac Surgery, ed 3. St. Louis: Mosby, 2003, pp. 713–738.

epicardial leads required early and frequent replacement because of exit block. Transvenous lead longevity was favorable as compared with epicardial leads; this, in combination with the smaller generators that have been developed, resulted in increasing numbers of transvenous pacing systems implanted in the pediatric population. Disadvantages of the transvenous leads include the potential for caval obstruction or thrombosis, especially in smaller patients. As leads fail and replacement leads are placed, a young patient could expect to undergo lead extraction procedures, which carry some risk. In addition, small patient size, unfavorable venous anatomy, or previous surgery (e.g., Glenn or Fontan

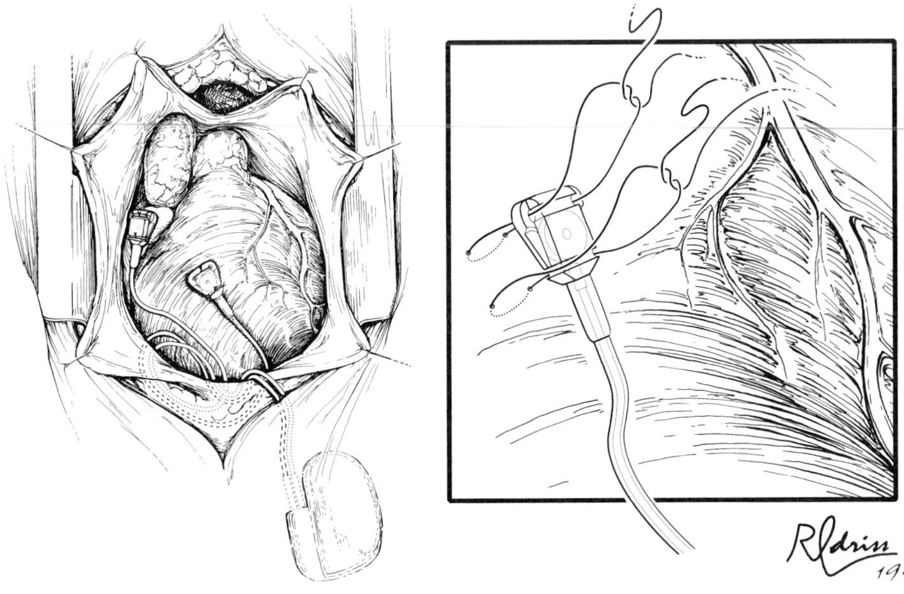

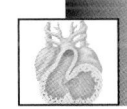

Figure 129-12 Dual-chamber pacemaker leads placed through a full sternotomy in a patient who also underwent intracardiac surgery. Steroid-eluting lead is affixed to the epicardium with two 5-0 polypropylene sutures.
(From Dodge-Khatami A, Johnsrude CL, Backer CL, et al: A comparison of steroid-eluting epicardial versus transvenous pacing leads in children. J Card Surg 15:323–329, 2000.)

operations) could preclude access to right-sided chambers, which is necessary for endocardial lead insertion. The introduction of steroid-eluting epicardial leads, with their potential for longer lead life, defers the need to use transvenous caval leads until later in life. A recent study recommended the use of steroid-eluting epicardial leads for as long as practically feasible before using the transvenous approach in children who will require a lifetime of pacing.[28]

Epicardial

Epicardial leads are placed through a limited lower median sternotomy incision, with placement of the generator occurring in a subrectus pocket. Steroid-eluting leads are sutured to the epicardial surface using a pair of 5-0 polypropylene sutures, 1 in the proximal groove and 1 through the 2 distal lateral holes (Figure 129-12).

Transvenous

Transvenous leads are placed surgically under fluoroscopic guidance (Seldinger technique) through the subclavian vein (right or left).

Implantation of Automatic Implantable Cardioverter Defibrillator

Initial devices were bulky (>230 g) and required a thoracotomy for the placement of epicardial patches, thus limiting their use in young patients. Improvements in technology have permitted a transvenous lead approach, smaller implantable generators (<130 g), and the incorporation of antibradycardia pacing capability, thereby resulting in the dramatic expansion of defibrillator use in pediatric patients over the last decade.[67,101] Initial devices required thoracotomy for the implantation of large epicardial ventricular patches and abdominal generator placement to deliver "shock-only" therapy for ventricular fibrillation. Current devices employ transvenous dual-chamber leads with pectoral generator placement, which are capable of delivering "tiered" therapy: antitachycardia pacing, low- and high-energy cardioversion (up to 30 j), antibradycardia pacing, and device diagnostic memory with telemetry. To avoid delivering shocks for nonsustained arrhythmias, devices are "noncommitted," and they perform a "second look" after device charging to confirm that the arrhythmia is ongoing before delivering a shock. Detection algorithms incorporate high rate, rate stability, sudden onset, and duration criteria; incorporating atrial lead information reduces inappropriate shocks for sinus tachycardia. Shock delivery using biphasic rather than monophasic waveform allows for lower defibrillation thresholds. Newer devices will incorporate atrial defibrillation therapy for atrial fibrillation, with the potential for application in late survivors of repaired congenital heart disease.[84]

SUMMARY

The introduction and development of transcatheter RF ablation to treat the various forms of supraventricular and ventricular arrhythmias have supplanted routine surgical ablative therapy and redefined its role. Presently, only a small population of arrhythmia patients will require surgical ablation; this includes patients for whom catheter ablation has failed, patients with concomitant congenital heart disease in association with arrhythmias, patients with atrial fibrillation, and very young patients for whom transcatheter techniques are prohibitive due to small size, cyanosis, and distorted anatomy. The general approach to these patients is to apply the principals of corrective surgery in concert with standard and adaptive surgical ablative techniques based on the type of arrhythmia and the diagnostic (preoperative and intraoperative) electrophysiological studies.

Because many of these patients require complex repairs (often with long cross-clamp times), the surgeon's dilemma is whether to add cryoablation and incisional lesions to the operation. However, variations in atrial and ventricular anatomy that may limit the catheter approach can be directly addressed surgically, thereby ensuring lesion depth and the continuity of anatomical lines of block. Patients who require surgical intervention for hemodynamic abnormalities can be spared a lengthy catheter ablation procedure by careful preoperative arrhythmia mapping and definitive surgical arrhythmia therapy, with results comparable with or superior to results achieved in the catheterization laboratory. Patient size or anatomical complexity should not be limiting factors when it comes to the combined surgical arrhythmia approach. Furthermore, because older patients undergoing surgical revision of prior surgical repairs of congenital heart disease are at increased risk for the later development of atrial arrhythmias, incorporation of arrhythmia therapy into planned surgical revision should be considered.

REFERENCES

1. The Antiarrhythmics versus Implantable Defibrillators (AVID) Investigators: A comparison of antiarrhythmic-drug therapy with implantable defibrillators in patients resuscitated from near-fatal ventricular arrhythmias. N Engl J Med 337:1576–1583, 1997.
2. Ashburn DA, Harris L, Downar EH, et al: Electrophysiologic surgery in patients with congenital heart disease. Semin Thorac Cardiovasc Surg Pediatr Card Surg Annu 6:51–58, 2003.
3. Baker BM, Lindsay BD, Bromberg BI, et al: Catheter ablation of clinical intraatrial reentrant tachycardias resulting from previous atrial surgery: localizing and transecting the critical isthmus. J Am Coll Cardiol 28:411–417, 1996.
4. Balaji S, Johnson TB, Sade RM, et al: Management of atrial flutter after the Fontan operation. J Am Coll Cardiol 23:1209–1215, 1994.
5. Berger F, Vogel M, Kramer A, et al: Incidence of atrial flutter/fibrillation in adults with atrial septal defect before and after surgery. Ann Thorac Surg 68:75–78, 1999.
6. Bonchek LI, Burlingame MW, Worley SJ, et al: Cox/maze procedure for atrial septal defect with atrial fibrillation: management strategies. Ann Thorac Surg 55:607–610, 1993.
7. Brandenburg RO Jr, Holmes DR, Brandenburg RO, et al: Clinical follow-up study of paroxysmal supraventricular tachyarrhythmias after operative repair of a secundum type atrial septal defect in adults. Am J Cardiol 51:273–276, 1983.
8. Calkins H, Kalbfleisch SJ, el-Atassi R, et al: Relation between efficacy of radiofrequency catheter ablation and site of origin of idiopathic ventricular tachycardia. Am J Cardiol 71:827–833, 1993.
9. Cappato R, Schlüter M, Weiss C, et al: Radiofrequency current catheter ablation of accessory atrioventricular pathways in Ebstein's anomaly. Circulation 94:376–383, 1996.
10. Case CL, Crawford FA, Gillette PC, et al: Successful surgery for atrioventricular reentrant tachycardia in a small child. Am Heart J 116:187–189, 1988.
11. Chiou CW, Chen SA, Chiang CE, et al: Radiofrequency catheter ablation of paroxysmal supraventricular tachycardia in patients with congenital heart disease. Int J Cardiol 50:143–151, 1995.
12. Cobb FR, Blumenschein SD, Sealy WC, et al: Successful surgical interruption of the bundle of Kent in a patient with Wolff-Parkinson-White syndrome. Circulation 38:1018–1029, 1968.
13. Conte S, Gewillig M, Eyskens B, et al: Management of late complications after classic Fontan procedure by conversion to total cavopulmonary connection. Cardiovasc Surg 7:651–655, 1999.
14. Cox JL, Boineau JP, Schuessler RB, et al: Electrophysiologic basis, surgical development, and clinical results of the maze procedure for atrial flutter and atrial fibrillation. Adv Card Surg 6:1–67, 1995.
15. Cox JL, Boineau JP, Schuessler RB, et al: Modification of the maze procedure for atrial flutter and atrial fibrillation. I. Rationale and surgical results. J Thorac Cardiovasc Surg 110:473–484, 1995.
16. Cox JL, Ferguson TB Jr: Surgery for the Wolff-Parkinson-White syndrome: the endocardial approach. Semin Thorac Cardiovasc Surg 1:34–46, 1989.
17. Cox JL, Gallagher JJ, Cain ME: Experience with 118 consecutive patients undergoing operation for the Wolff-Parkinson-White syndrome. J Thorac Cardiovasc Surg 90:490–501, 1985.
18. Cox JL, Gallagher JJ, Ungerleider RM: Encircling endocardial ventriculotomy for refractory ischemic ventricular tachycardia. IV. Clinical indication, surgical technique, mechanism of action, and results. J Thorac Cardiovasc Surg 83:865–872, 1982.
19. Cox JL, Holman WL, Cain ME: Cryosurgical treatment of atrioventricular node reentrant tachycardia. Circulation 76:1329–1336, 1987.
20. Cox JL, Jaquiss RD, Schuessler RB, et al: Modification of the maze procedure for atrial flutter and atrial fibrillation. II. Surgical technique of the maze III procedure. J Thorac Cardiovasc Surg 110:485–495, 1995.
21. Cox JL: Surgery for cardiac arrhythmias. In Braunwald E (editor): Heart Disease Update 13 to Heart Disease: A Textbook of Cardiovascular Medicine, ed 3. Philadelphia: WB Saunders, 1991, p. 295.
22. Deal BJ, Mavroudis C, Backer CL, et al: Impact of arrhythmia circuit cryoablation during Fontan conversion for refractory atrial tachycardia. Am J Cardiol 83:563–568, 1999.
23. Deal BJ, Mavroudis C, Backer CL, et al: New directions in surgical therapy of arrhythmias. Pediatr Cardiol 21:576–583, 2000.
24. Deal BJ, Mavroudis C, Backer CL: Beyond Fontan conversion: surgical therapy of arrhythmias including patients with associated complex congenital heart disease. Ann Thorac Surg 76:542–553, 2003.
25. Deal BJ, Scagliotti D, Miller SM, et al: Electrophysiologic drug testing in symptomatic ventricular arrhythmias after repair of tetralogy of Fallot. Am J Cardiol 59:1380–1385, 1987.
26. Definition of terms related to cardiac rhythm. WHO/ISFC Task Force. Am Heart J 95:796–806, 1978.
27. DeLeon SY, Ilbawi MN, Idriss FS: Pacemaker implantation in infants and children: a simplified approach. Ann Thorac Surg 30:599–601, 1980.
28. Dodge-Khamati A, Johnsrude CL, Backer CL, et al: A comparison of steroid-eluting epicardial versus transvenous pacing leads in children. J Card Surg 15:323–329, 2000.
29. Dorostkar PC, Cheng J, Scheinman MM: Electroanatomical mapping and ablation of the substrate supporting intraatrial reentrant tachycardia after palliation for complex congenital heart disease. Pacing Clin Electrophysiol 21:1810–1819, 1998.
30. Downar E, Harris L, Kimber S, et al: Ventricular tachycardia after surgical repair of tetralogy of Fallot: results of intraoperative mapping studies. J Am Coll Cardiol 20:648–655, 1992.
31. Dubin AM, Van Hare GF: Radiofrequency catheter ablation: indications and complications. Pediatr Cardiol 21:551–556, 2000.
32. Garson A Jr, Gillette PC, Titus JL, et al: Surgical treatment of ventricular tachycardia in infants. N Engl J Med 31:1443–1445, 1984.
33. Garson A Jr, Smith RT Jr, Moak JP, et al: Incessant ventricular tachycardia in infants: myocardial hamartomas and surgical cure. J Am Coll Cardiol 10:619–626, 1987.
34. Gatzoulis MA, Balaji S, Webber SA, et al: Risk factors for arrhythmia and sudden cardiac death late after repair of tetralogy of Fallot: a multicentre study. Lancet 356:975–981, 2000.

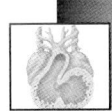

35. Gatzoulis MA, Freeman MA, Siu SC, et al: Atrial arrhythmia after surgical closure of atrial septal defects in adults. N Engl J Med 340:839–846, 1999.
36. Gatzoulis MA, Till JA, Somerville J, et al: Mechanoelectrical interaction in tetralogy of Fallot. QRS prolongation relates to right ventricular size and predicts malignant ventricular arrhythmias and sudden death. Circulation 92:231–237, 1995.
37. Gatzoulis MA, Walters J, McLaughlin PR, et al: Late arrhythmias in adults with the Mustard procedure for transposition of great arteries: a surrogate marker for right ventricular dysfunction? Heart 84:409–415, 2000.
38. Ghai A, Harris L, Harrison DA, et al: Outcomes of late atrial tachyarrhythmias in adults after the Fontan operation. J Am Coll Cardiol 37:585–592, 2001.
39. Gillette PC, Smith RT, Garson A Jr, et al: Chronic supraventricular tachycardia. A curable cause of congestive cardiomyopathy. JAMA 253:391–392, 1985.
40. Gillette PC, Wampler DG, Garson A Jr, et al: Treatment of atrial automatic tachycardia by ablation procedures. J Am Coll Cardiol 6:405–409, 1985.
41. Goldberger J, Kall J, Ehlert F, et al: Effectiveness of radiofrequency catheter ablation for treatment of atrial tachycardia. Am J Cardiol 72:787–793, 1993.
42. Greason KL, Dearani JA, Theodoro DA, et al: Surgical management of atrial tachyarrhythmias associated with congenital cardiac anomalies: Mayo Clinic experience. Semin Thorac Cardiovasc Surg Pediatr Card Surg Annu 6:59–71, 2003.
43. Gregoratas G, Abrams J, Epstein AE, et al: ACC/AHA/NASPE 2002 guideline update for implantation of cardiac pacemakers and antiarrhythmia devices: summary article: a report of the American College of Cardiology/American Heart Association Task Force on Practice Guidelines (ACC/AHA/NASPE Committee to Update the 1998 Guidelines). Circulation 106:2145–2161, 2002.
44. Guiraudon G, Fontaine G, Frank R, et al: Encircling endocardial ventriculotomy: a new surgical treatment for life-threatening ventricular tachycardias resistant to medical treatment following myocardial infarction. Ann Thorac Surg 26:438–444, 1978.
45. Guiraudon GM, Klein GJ, Sharma AD, et al: Closed-heart technique for Wolff-Parkinson-White syndrome. Further experience and potential limitations. Ann Thorac Surg 42:651–657, 1986.
46. Guiraudon GM, Klein GJ, Sharma AD, et al: Surgery for the Wolff-Parkinson-White syndrome: the epicardial approach. Semin Thorac Cardiovasc Surg 1:21–33, 1989.
47. Guiraudon GM: Surgical treatment of Wolff-Parkinson-White syndrome: a “retrospectroscopic” view. Ann Thorac Surg 58:1254–1261, 1994.
48. Harada A, D’Agostino HJ Jr, Schuessler RB, et al: Right atrial isolation: a new surgical treatment for supraventricular tachycardia. I. Surgical technique and electrophysiologic effects. J Thorac Cardiovasc Surg 95:643–650, 1988.
49. Harken AH, Horowitz LN, Josephson ME: Surgical correction of recurrent sustained ventricular tachycardia following complete repair of tetralogy of Fallot. J Thorac Cardiovasc Surg 80:779–781, 1980.
50. Harrison DA, Harris L, Siu SC, et al: Sustained ventricular tachycardia in adult patients late after repair of tetralogy of Fallot. J Am Coll Cardiol 30:1368–1373, 1997.
51. Hofschire PJ, Nicoloff DM, Moller JH: Postoperative complete heart block in 64 children treated with and without cardiac pacing. Am J Cardiol 39:559–562, 1977.
52. Holman WL, Ikeshita M, Lease JG, et al: Elective prolongation of atrioventricular conduction by multiple discrete cryolesions: a new technique for the treatment of paroxysmal supraventricular tachycardia. J Thorac Cardiovasc Surg 84:554–559, 1982.
53. Jackman WM, Beckman KJ, McClelland JH, et al: Treatment of supraventricular tachycardia due to atrioventricular nodal reentry, by radiofrequency catheter ablation of slow-pathway conduction. N Engl J Med 327:313–318, 1992.
54. Jackman WM, Wang XZ, Friday KJ, et al: Catheter ablation of accessory atrioventricular pathways (Wolff-Parkinson-White syndrome) by radiofrequency current. N Engl J Med 324:1605–1611, 1991.
55. Jonsson H, Ivert T: Survival and clinical results up to 26 years after repair of tetralogy of Fallot. Scand J Thorac Cardiovasc Surg 29:43–51, 1995.
56. Josephson ME, Wellens HJJ: Differential diagnosis of supraventricular tachycardia. Cardiol Clin 8:411–442, 1990.
57. Kanter RJ, Garson A Jr: Atrial arrhythmias during chronic follow-up of surgery for complex congenital heart disease. Pacing Clin Electrophysiol 20:502–511, 1997.
58. Kanter RJ, Papagiannis J, Carboni MP, et al: Radiofrequency catheter ablation of supraventricular tachycardia substrates after Mustard and Senning operations for d-transposition of the great arteries. J Am Coll Cardiol 35:428–441, 2000.
59. Kao JM, Alejos JC, Grant PW, et al: Conversion of atriopulmonary to cavopulmonary anastomosis in management of late arrhythmias and atrial thrombosis. Ann Thorac Surg 58:1510–1514, 1994.
60. Kawahira Y, Uemura H, Yagihara T, et al: Renewal of the Fontan circulation with concomitant surgical intervention for atrial arrhythmia. Ann Thorac Surg 71:919–921, 2001.
61. Klein LS, Shih HT, Hackett FK, et al: Radiofrequency catheter ablation of ventricular tachycardia in patients without structural heart disease. Circulation 85:1666–1674, 1992.
62. Knott-Craig CJ, Elkins RC, Lane MM, et al: A 26-year experience with surgical management of tetralogy of Fallot: risk analysis for mortality or late reintervention. Ann Thorac Surg 66:506–511, 1998.
63. Ko JK, Deal BJ, Strasburger JF, et al: Supraventricular tachycardia mechanisms and their age distribution in pediatric patients. Am J Cardiol 69:1028–1032, 1992.
64. Kobayashi J, Yamamoto F, Nakano K, et al: Maze procedure for atrial fibrillation associated with atrial septal defect. Circulation 98(19 Suppl):II-399–II-402, 1998.
65. Kopf GS, Mello DM, Kenney KM, et al: Intraoperative radiofrequency ablation of the atrium: effectiveness for treatment of supraventricular tachycardia in congenital heart surgery. Ann Thorac Surg 74:797–804, 2002.
66. Kreutzer J, Keane JF, Lock JE, et al: Conversion of modified Fontan procedure to lateral atrial tunnel cavopulmonary anastomosis. J Thorac Cardiovasc Surg 111:1169–1176, 1996.
67. Kron J, Oliver RP, Norsted S, et al: The automatic implantable cardioverter-defibrillator in young patients. J Am Coll Cardiol 16:896–902, 1990.
68. Langberg JJ, Man KC, Vorperian VR, et al: Recognition and catheter ablation of subepicardial accessory pathways. J Am Coll Cardiol 22:1100–1104, 1993.
69. Lesh MD, Kalman JM, Saxon LA, et al: Electrophysiology of “incisional” reentrant atrial tachycardia complicating surgery for congenital heart disease. Pacing Clin Electrophysiol 20:2107–2111, 1997.
70. Lesh MD, Van Hare GF, Epstein LM, et al: Radiofrequency catheter ablation of atrial arrhythmias. Results and mechanisms. Circulation 89:1074–1089, 1994.
71. Levine JC, Walsh EP, Saul JP: Radiofrequency ablation of accessory pathways associated with congenital heart disease including heterotaxy syndrome. Am J Cardiol 72:689–693, 1993.
72. Lillehei CW, Sellers RD, Bonnabeau RC, et al: Chronic postsurgical complete heart block. With particular reference to prognosis, management, and a new P-wave pacemaker. J Thorac Cardiovasc Surg 46:436–456, 1963.

73. Lowe JE, Hendry PJ, Packer DL, et al: Surgical management of chronic ectopic atrial tachycardia. Semin Thorac Cardiovasc Surg 1:58–66, 1989.
74. Lowe JE: Surgical treatment of the Wolff-Parkinson-White syndrome and other supraventricular tachyarrhythmias. J Card Surg 1:117–134, 1986.
75. Mahomed Y, King RD, Zipes DP, et al: Surgical division of Wolff-Parkinson-White pathways utilizing the closed-heart technique: a 2-year experience in 47 patients. Ann Thorac Surg 45:495–504, 1988.
76. Mavroudis C, Backer CL, Deal BJ, et al: Fontan conversion to cavopulmonary connection and arrhythmia circuit cryoablation. J Thorac Cardiovasc Surg 115:547–556, 1998.
77. Mavroudis C, Deal BJ, Backer CL, et al: The favorable impact of arrhythmia surgery on total cavopulmonary artery Fontan conversion. Semin Thorac Cardiovasc Surg Pediatr Card Surg Annu 2:143–156, 1999.
78. Mavroudis C, Deal BJ, Backer CL: Arrhythmia surgery in association with complex congenital heart repairs excluding patients with Fontan conversion. Semin Thorac Cardiovasc Surg Pediatr Card Surg Annu 6:33–50, 2003.
79. McElhinney DB, Reddy VM, Moore P, et al: Revision of previous Fontan connections to extracardiac or intraatrial conduit cavopulmonary anastomosis. Ann Thorac Surg 62:1276–1282, 1996.
80. Melo J, Adragao P, Neves J, et al: Surgery for atrial fibrillation using radiofrequency catheter ablation: assessment of results at one year. Eur J Cardiothorac Surg 15:851–854, 1999.
81. Michaëlsson M, Engle MA: Congenital complete heart block: an international study of the natural history. Cardiovasc Clin 4:85–101, 1972.
82. Michaëlsson M, Jonzon A, Riesenfeld T: Isolated congenital complete atrioventricular block in adult life. A prospective study. Circulation 92:442–449, 1995.
83. Misaki T, Tsubota M, Watanabe G, et al: Surgical treatment of ventricular tachycardia after surgical repair of tetralogy of Fallot. Relation between intraoperative mapping and histological findings. Circulation 90:264–271, 1994.
84. Morris MM, KenKnight BH, Warren JA, et al: A preview of implantable cardioverter defibrillator systems in the next millennium: an integrative cardiac rhythm management approach.Am J Cardiol 83:48D–54D, 1999.
85. Murphy JG, Gersh BJ, Mair DD, et al: Long-term outcome in patients undergoing surgical repair of tetralogy of Fallot. N Engl J Med 239:593–599, 1993.
86. Nakamura FF, Nadas AS: Complete heart block in infants and children. N Engl J Med 270:1261–1268, 1964.
87. Nollert G, Fischlein T, Bouterwek S, et al: Long-term survival in patients with repair of tetralogy of Fallot: 36-year follow-up of 490 survivors of the first year after surgical repair. J Am Coll Cardiol 30:1374–1383, 1997.
88. O'Connor BK, Case CL, Sokoloski MC, et al: Radiofrequency catheter ablation of right ventricular outflow tachycardia in children and adolescents. J Am Coll Cardiol 27:869–874, 1996.
89. Oechslin EN, Harrison DA, Harris L, et al: Reoperation in adults with repair of tetralogy of Fallot: indications and outcomes. J Thorac Cardiovasc Surg 118:245–251, 1999.
90. Orie JD, Anderson RH, Ettedgui JA, et al: Echocardiographic-morphologic correlations in tricuspid atresia. J Am Coll Cardiol 26:750–758, 1995.
91. Peters NS, Somerville J: Arrhythmias after the Fontan procedure. Br Heart J 68:199–204, 1992.
92. Prager NA, Cox JL, Lindsay BD, et al: Long-term effectiveness of surgical treatment of ectopic atrial tachycardia. J Am Coll Cardiol 22:85–92, 1993.
93. Pritchett ELC, Anderson RW, Benditt DG, et al: Reentry within the atrioventricular node: surgical cure with preservation of atrioventricular conduction. Circulation 60:440–446, 1979.
94. Puley G, Siu S, Connelly M, et al: Arrhythmia and survival in patients >18 years of age after the Mustard procedure for complete transposition of the great arteries. Am J Cardiol 83:1080–1084, 1999.
95. Rao V, Williams WG, Hamilton RH, et al: Trends in pediatric cardiac pacing. Can J Cardiol 11:993–999, 1995.
96. Reich JD, Auld D, Hulse E, et al: The Pediatric Radiofrequency Ablation Registry's experience with Ebstein's anomaly. J Cardiovasc Electrophysiol 9:1370–1377, 1998.
97. Rodriguez LM, de Chillou C, Schlapfer J, et al: Age at onset and gender of patients with different types of supraventricular tachycardia. Am J Cardiol 70:1213–1215, 1992.
98. Roos-Hesselink J, Perlroth MG, McGhie J, et al: Atrial arrhythmias in adults after repair of tetralogy of Fallot. Correlations with clinical, exercise, and echocardiographic findings. Circulation 91:2214–2219, 1995.
99. Schumacher B, Wolpert C, Lewalter T, et al: Predictors of success in radiofrequency catheter ablation of atrial flutter. J Interv Card Electrophysiol 4:121–125, 2000.
100. Scott JS, Maddison PJ, Taylor PV, et al: Connective-tissue disease, antibodies to ribonucleoprotein, and congenital heart block. N Engl J Med 309:209–212, 1983.
101. Silka MJ, Kron J, Dunnigan A, et al: Sudden cardiac death and the use of implantable cardioverter-defibrillators in pediatric patients. The Pediatric Electrophysiology Society. Circulation 87:800–807, 1993.
102. Smeets JL, Rodriguez LM, Timmermans C, et al: Radiofrequency catheter ablation of idiopathic ventricular tachycardias in children. Pacing Clin Electrophysiol 20:2068–2071, 1997.
103. Theodoro DA, Danielson GK, Porter CJ, et al: Right-sided maze procedure for right atrial arrhythmias in congenital heart disease. Ann Thorac Surg 65:149–153, 1998.
104. Thoele DG, Ursell PC, Ho SY, et al: Atrial morphologic features in tricuspid atresia. J Thorac Cardiovasc Surg 102:606–610, 1991.
105. Thomas SP, Nunn GR, Nicholson IA, et al: Mechanism, localization and cure of atrial arrhythmias occurring after a new intraoperative endocardial radiofrequency ablation procedure for atrial fibrillation. J Am Coll Cardiol 35:442–450, 2000.
106. Triedman JK, Bergau DM, Saul JP, et al: Efficacy of radiofrequency ablation for control of intraatrial reentrant tachycardia in patients with congenital heart disease. J Am Coll Cardiol 30:1032–1038, 1997.
107. Triedman JK, Jenkins KJ, Colan SD, et al: Intra-atrial reentrant tachycardia after palliation of congenital heart disease: characterization of multiple macroreentrant circuits using fluoroscopically based three-dimensional endocardial mapping. J Cardiovasc Electrophysiol 8:259–270, 1997.
108. Triedman JK, Saul JP, Weindling SN, et al: Radiofrequency ablation of intra-atrial reentrant tachycardia after surgical palliation of congenital heart disease. Circulation 91:707–714, 1995.
109. Van Hare GF, Lesh MD, Ross BA, et al: Mapping and radiofrequency ablation of intraatrial reentrant tachycardia after the Senning or Mustard procedure for transposition of the great arteries. Am J Cardiol 77:985–991, 1996.
110. Van Hare GF, Lesh MD, Stanger P: Radiofrequency catheter ablation of supraventricular arrhythmias in patients with congenital heart disease: results and technical considerations. J Am Coll Cardiol 22:883–890, 1993.
111. Van Hare GF: Indications for radiofrequency ablation in the pediatric population. J Cardiovasc Electrophysiol 8:952–962, 1997.
112. van Son JA, Mohr FW, Hambsch J, et al: Conversion of atriopulmonary or lateral atrial tunnel cavopulmonary anastomosis

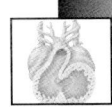

to extracardiac conduit Fontan modification. Eur J Cardiothorac Surg 15:150–157, 1999.
113. Vitullo DA, DeLeon SY, Berry TE, et al: Clinical improvement after revision in Fontan patients. Ann Thorac Surg 61:1797–1804, 1996.
114. Weindling SN, Saul JP, Gamble WJ, et al: Duration of complete atrioventricular block after congenital heart disease surgery. Am J Cardiol 82:525–527, 1998.
115. Williams JM, Ungerleider RM, Lofland GK, et al: Left atrial isolation: new technique for the treatment of supraventricular arrhythmias. J Thorac Cardiovasc Surg 80:373–380, 1980.
116. Wu D, Denes P, Amat-y-Leon F, et al: Clinical, electrocardiographic and electrophysiologic observations in patients with paroxysmal supraventricular tachycardia. Am J Cardiol 41:1045–1051, 1978.
117. Zeigler VL, Gillette PC, Crawford FA Jr, et al: New approaches to treatment of incessant ventricular tachycardia in the very young. J Am Coll Cardiol 16:681–685, 1990.
118. Zhao HX, Miller DC, Reitz BA, et al: Surgical repair of tetralogy of Fallot. Long-term follow-up with particular emphasis on late death and reoperation. J Thorac Cardiovasc Surg 89:204–220, 1985.

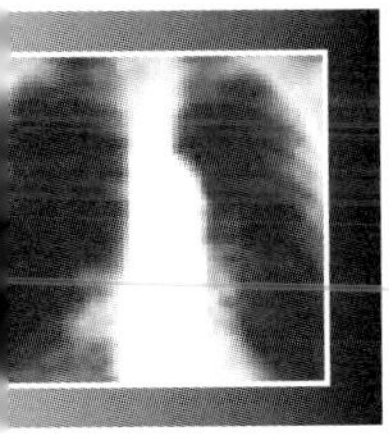

Index

Page numbers followed by "f" denote figures; "t" denote tables; and "b" denote boxes

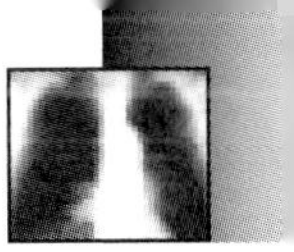

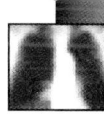

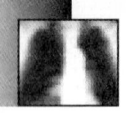

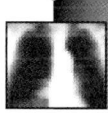

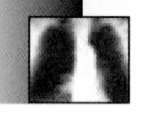

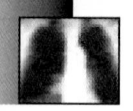

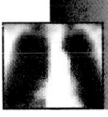

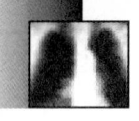

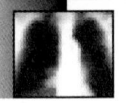

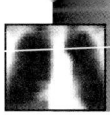

U

V

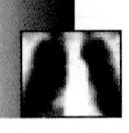